FAMILY-CENTERED CARE OF CHILDREN AND ADOLESCENTS
Nursing Concepts in Child Health

JO JOYCE MARIE TACKETT, B.S.N., M.P.H.N.
Associate Professor of Nursing
Blackhawk College
Kewanee, Illinois

Formerly, Assistant Professor of Nursing
University of Michigan
Ann Arbor, Michigan

MABEL HUNSBERGER, B.S.N., M.S.N.
Assistant Professor of Nursing
University of Michigan
Ann Arbor, Michigan

1981

W.B. SAUNDERS COMPANY   PHILADELPHIA LONDON TORONTO SYDNEY

W. B. Saunders Company: West Washington Square
Philadelphia, PA 19105

1 St. Anne's Road
Eastbourne, East Sussex BN21 3UN, England

1 Goldthorne Avenue
Toronto, Ontario M8Z 5T9, Canada

9 Waltham Street
Artarmon, N.S.W. 2064, Australia

Front and back cover illustration reprint from Psychology Today Magazine.
Copyright © 1978 Ziff-Davis Publishing Company.

Family-Centered Care of Children and Adolescents:
Nursing Concepts in Child Health

ISBN 0-7216-8740-7

© 1981 by W. B. Saunders Company. Copyright under the Uniform Copyright Convention. Simultaneously published in Canada. All rights reserved. This book is protected by copyright. No part of it may be reproduced, stored in a retrieval system, or transmitted in any form or by any means, electronic, mechanical, photocopying, recording, or otherwise, without written permission from the publisher. Made in the United States of America. Press of W. B. Saunders Company. Library of Congress catalog card number 80-51326.

Last digit is the print number: 9 8 7 6 5 4 3 2 1

To Jim, for being there and for his faith in me
To my sons, Bob and Ian, for their inspiration
 and love
To our unborn child

Jo Joyce

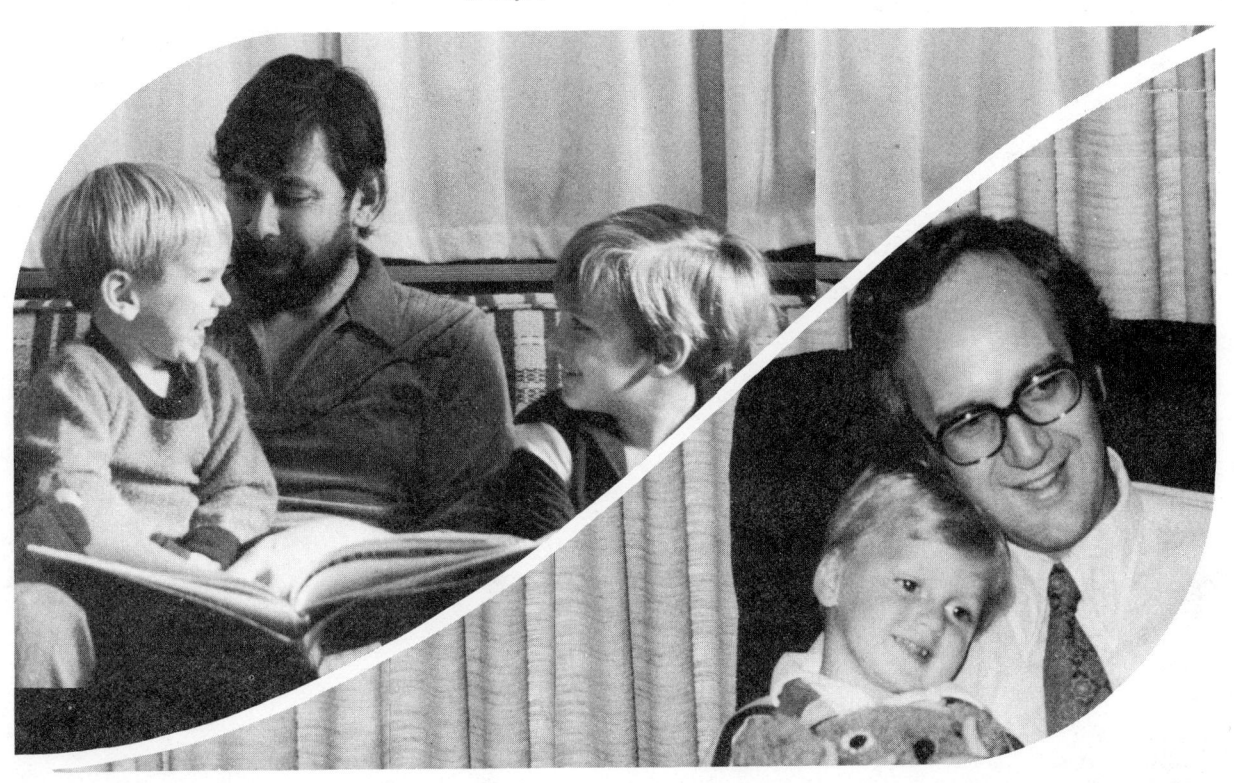

To Merrill, for his loving care of our son and for
 believing we could do it
To Jason, whose entry into our family has made
 this book come alive

Mabel

and
To our parents, who always care

CONTRIBUTORS

MARGARET ALDERMAN,
    Assistant Director of Nursing–Maternal-Child Health, University of California Hospital, San Francisco, CA

MARY ARBOUR, R.N., M.S.N.Ed.
    Associate Professor, Parent-Child Nursing, University of Michigan School of Nursing, Ann Arbor, MI

CLAUDELLA ARCHAMBEAULT-JONES, R.N.
    Director of Education, National Institute for Burn Medicine, Ann Arbor, MI

JANET ALLEN-LIA, R.N., B.S., M.S.
    Maternity Nurse Practitioner, Sterling Area Health Project, Sterling, MI

KATHLEEN UNDERMAN BOGGS, R.N., M.S.N.
    Assistant Professor, University of Michigan School of Nursing, Ann Arbor, MI

LINDA BOND, R.N., M.S.N.
    Assistant Professor, Parent-Child Nursing, University of Michigan School of Nursing, Ann Arbor, MI

DEBORAH L. BRAUNSTEIN, R.N., B.S.N.
    Staff Nurse–Pediatric Clinic, University Hospital, Ann Arbor, MI

MARY TAYLOR BURKHART, R.N., M.A., C.P.N.P.
    Formerly Nursing Co-Director, Pediatric Nurse Practitioner Program, University of Michigan School of Nursing, Ann Arbor, MI

ELLEN CHRISTIAN, R.N., M.S.
    Associate Professor, Southeastern Massachusetts University College of Nursing, North Dartmouth, MA

JUDITH CLARK, R.N., M.S.N.
    Associate Professor, Southeastern Massachusetts University College of Nursing, North Dartmouth, MA

ANITA CLAVIER, R.N., B.S.N.
    Head Nurse, Internal Medicine Clinic, University Hospital, Ann Arbor, MI

SARA CRISWELL, R.N., B.S.N.
    Assistant Professor, Department of Nursing, Black Hawk College, Moline, IL

CAROLYN PEDIGO DeLOACH, R.N., B.S.N., M.S.N.
    Associate Professor of Nursing, Eastern Michigan University, Ypsilanti, MI

CAROL M. EASLEY, R.N., A.M.
    Assistant Professor of Nursing, University of Michigan School of Nursing, Ann Arbor, MI

CHERYL E. EASLEY, R.N., A.M.
    Assistant Professor of Nursing, University of Michigan School of Nursing, Ann Arbor, MI

KATHLEEN TIGHE EDWARDS, R.N., B.S.N.
Masters Candidate, Nursing Care of Children and Adolescents, Wayne State University, Detroit, MI

THERESA ELDRIDGE, R.N., M.S., C.P.N.P.
Assistant Professor, Core Practitioner Program, University of Colorado School of Nursing, Denver, CO

IRVING FELLER, M.D.
Director, Michigan Burn Center; Clinical Professor of Surgery, University of Michigan, Ann Arbor, MI

MARY LOU FREY, B.S.N., M.S.
Formerly Assistant Professor, University of Michigan School of Nursing, Ann Arbor, MI

ELIZABETH B. GALL, R.N., B.S., M.A., P.N.P.
Nurse Preceptor, Liberty Pediatrics Pediatric Nurse Practitioner Program, University of Michigan School of Nursing, Ann Arbor, MI

MARIANNE R. GLASSANOS, R.N., M.S., C.P.N.P.
Clinical Nurse Specialist, Holden Newborn Intensive Care Unit, University Hospital, Ann Arbor, MI

FRANCES BONTRAGER GREASER, R.N., M.S.N.Ed.
Formerly Assistant Professor, Maternal-Child Health, Goshen College, Goshen, IN. Director of Nursing Services, Elkhart County Association for the Retarded, Elkhart, IN

LINDA NICHOLSON GRINSTEAD, R.N., B.S., M.N.
Assistant Professor, Grand Valley State College, Allendale, MI

ANNE E. HARTSON, R.N., M.A.
Associate Instructor, University of Iowa College of Nursing, Iowa City, IO

JUNE HAUGE, M.S.W., A.C.S.W.
Social Service Director, Moline Public Hospital, Moline, IL

ANNE KRABILL HERSHBERGER, R.N., M.S.N.
Associate Professor of Nursing, Goshen College, Goshen, IN

RUTH M. HEYN, M.D.
Professor of Pediatrics, University of Michigan Medical School; Head of Section of Pediatric Hematology/Oncology, Mott Children's Hospital, University of Michigan, Ann Arbor, MI

AMY L. HOFING, R.N., M.S.
Clinical Nurse Specialist, Pediatric Nursing Service, Mott Children's Hospital, University of Michigan, Ann Arbor, MI

GAIL K. INGERSOLL, R.N., M.S.
Assistant Professor of Nursing, School of Nursing, University of Michigan. Clinical Instructor, Young Adolescent Unit, Mott Children's Hospital, University of Michigan, Ann Arbor, MI

MARY SUE JACK, R.N., M.S.
Graduate Student and Teaching Assistant, University of Rochester, Rochester, NY. Formerly Assistant Professor, University of Michigan School of Nursing, Ann Arbor, MI

ANNE MURPHY KARR, R.N., M.S.
Diabetes Nurse Clinician, Diabetes Research and Teaching Unit, Mott Children's Hospital, University of Michigan, Ann Arbor, MI

EVAN J. KASS, M.D.
Assistant Professor of Urology and Child Health and Development, Children's Hospital, National Medical Center, Department of Child Health and Development, George Washington University, Washington, DC

KATHLEEN L. KING, R.N., M.S.N., P.N.P.
Formerly Instructor, Parent-Child Nursing, University of Michigan School of Nursing, Ann Arbor, MI

STEPHEN A. KOFF, M.D.
Assistant Professor of Surgery, Chief of Pediatric Urology Service, University of Michigan Medical Center, Ann Arbor, MI

EVELYN M. McELROY, R.N., Ph.D.
Associate Professor of Psychiatric Nursing, School of Nursing; Assistant Professor, School of Medicine, Department of Psychiatry, University of Maryland, Baltimore, MD

SANDRA I. MERKEL, R.N., M.S.N.
Clinical Nurse Specialist, Adolescent and Pediatric Nursing, University Hospital—Mott Children's Hospital, University of Michigan, Ann Arbor, MI

BARBARA MILLER, R.N., B.S.N., P.N.A., M.A.
Supervisor, Child Care, Visiting Nurses-Homemaker Association, Rock Island County, Rock Island-Moline-East Moline, IL

JANET S. MALINOWSKI, R.N., M.S.N.
Associate Professor of Nursing, Mercy College of Detroit, Detroit, MI

MARY LOU MOORE, B.S.N., M.A., F.A.A.N.
Nursing Coordinator and Instructor, North Carolina Perinatal-Neonatal Nursing Program, Bowman Gray School of Medicine, Winston-Salem, NC

LINDA MOWAD, R.N., B.S.N.
Masters Candidate, New York University, New York, NY. Independent Nurse Consultant.

JUDY COLTSON MOYER, B.S., M.S.
Instructor, University of Michigan School of Nursing, Ann Arbor, MI

FLORENCE NEZAMIS, R.N., B.S.P.A.
Assistant Head Nurse, Cardiac Toddler Unit, Mott Children's Hospital, University of Michigan, Ann Arbor, MI

LISA ROOT PARKER, R.N., B.S.N.
Pediatric Diabetes Clinician, Michigan Diabetes Research and Training Center, University of Michigan Medical Center, Ann Arbor, MI

CHESTER R. PEACHEY, R.N., M.S., B.S.N.
Doctoral Student, Western Michigan University. Associate Professor of Nursing, Goshen College School of Nursing, Goshen, IN

JOYCE PIAZZA, R.N., B.S.
Formerly Cardiac Surgery Nurse Clinician, Pediatrics Department, Mott Children's Hospital, University of Michigan, Ann Arbor, MI

JENNIFER PIERSMA, R.N., M.S., C.P.N.P.
Assistant Professor of Nursing, University of Colorado School of Nursing, Denver, CO

THERESA M. SARAHAN, B.S.N., P.N.P.
Nurse Clinician II, Pediatric Surgery, Mott Children's Hospital, University of Michigan, Ann Arbor, MI

MARCIA N. SHEETS, R.N., M.S.N.
Clinical Faculty, University of Washington School of Nursing. Staff Development Director, Outpatient Services, Children's Orthopedic Hospital and Medical Center, Seattle, WA

ELAINE C. SMITH, R.N., Ph.D.
Associate Professor, Department of Public Health Nursing and Assistant Dean for Regional Program, College of Nursing, University of Illinois, Urbana, IL

ANITA SPIETZ, R.N., M.S.N.
Research Assistant Professor, Newborn Nursing Models Project, Department of Maternal-Child Nursing, University of Washington, Seattle, WA

FRANCES WHITE THURBER, R.N., M.S.N.
Instructor, Parent-Child Nursing, University of Michigan School of Nursing, Ann Arbor, MI

MICHAEL DAVID TROUT, M.A.
Director, Center for the Study of Infants and Their Families, Alma, MI

LINDA L. UPTON, R.N., M.S.
Staff Development Coordinator, Department of Nursing, Children's Hospital of Michigan, Detroit, MI

MARY WASKERWITZ, B.S.N., P.N.P.
Pediatric Nurse Practitioner, Nurse Clinician II, University of Michigan Section of Pediatric Hematology/Oncology, Ann Arbor, MI

A. FRANCES WENGER, R.N., M.S.N.
Director, Division of Nursing, and Associate Professor of Nursing, Goshen College, Goshen, IN

DOROTHY WIERENGA, R.N.
Head Nurse, Maternity Unit, Illini Hospital, Silvis, IL

STEPHANIE WRIGHT, R.N., M.S.N.
Formerly Instructor, Parent-Patient Education, Magee-Women's Hospital, Pittsburgh, PA

MARY JEAN YABLONKY, B.S.N., C.R.N.A.
Associate Director, Program of Nurse Anesthesia, University of Michigan Medical Center. Clinical Instructor–Staff Anesthetist, Department of Anesthesiology, Mott Children's Hospital, University of Michigan, Ann Arbor, MI

FOREWORD

At a time of lively development in the field of child health nursing, when far-reaching changes are taking place in both practice and education, it is particularly important that we have a systematic up-to-date compilation of the basic knowledge in the field. In this text, Jo Joyce Tackett and Mabel Hunsberger, together with an outstanding group of contributors, have provided us with an authoritative, innovative and significant textbook that fully meets this need. It is long overdue.

The primary objectives of the book are to impart knowledge and skills central to parent-child nursing practice, to foster the development of meaningful and creative ideas and approaches to the care of children, and to cultivate an appreciation of the complexities and wide dimensions of this special area within nursing. From the following pages, the reader will come to appreciate both the art and science of child health nursing.

Following an initial section devoted to basic family, developmental and nursing concepts, each major phase in the development of children, from infancy to adolescence, is treated in depth. The authors have surveyed the full scope of knowledge and have dealt with every aspect of the nursing care of children from wellness to illness. The general approach they have taken will undoubtedly stimulate thoughtful analyses.

The unique and most penetrating efforts are in the area of family-centered care. In contrast to more traditional texts, this book integrates throughout its pages the critical role of the family in the adaptation, integration and development of the child. Fully explored is the concept that the family is society's primary agency in the provision of the growing child's biological, psychological and sociological needs and in the development of a child into an integrated person capable of living successfully and healthily in society.

This book also puts child health nursing in its proper perspective by offering a balanced approach, which includes the care of the well child and his family as well as the child with altered states of health. It represents a careful distillation of the variety of approaches that nurses, as members of today's health care team, employ. Use of the book will undoubtedly lead to a deeper awareness of the full scope of the pediatric nursing role.

Family-Centered Care of Children and Adolescents makes excellent use of the latest research. On the one hand it includes well-established findings and familiar concepts in child health nursing and related disciplines. Linkages have been established with numerous other fields, including sociology, anthropology and developmental psychology. In addition, extensive references to studies carried out within the last year or two, those less familiar to child health nurses, are included. These are of fundamental importance and serve to make the book valuable to both students of child health nursing and practicing child health nurses and educators.

The authors are ideally suited to writing this particular book. They have been engaged both in direct nursing care of children and their families and in the education of nursing students for many years. They have integrated the contributions of many knowledgeable practitioners with their own wide experience to build a highly relevant theoretical framework while incorporating practical guides for specific areas of practice.

In this book, students and practitioners have a tool for developing their professional knowledge and competencies. It points the way to many new directions in the nursing care of children and their families and is an important resource for today's and tomorrow's nurses.

BEATRICE J. KALISCH, R.N., ED.D., F.A.A.N.

Titus Professor of Nursing and
Chairperson, Parent-Child Nursing
University of Michigan
Ann Arbor

PREFACE

A family-centered approach to the study of children is essential to a well-prepared pediatric nurse. In this text we describe how families grow and develop and how their needs and the stresses on them change over time. We present the child in the context of the family to which he or she belongs, and we acknowledge the impact of that family's growth and development on the child's growth and development.

We portray the child and his or her family as a healthy unit that has the potential for adapting to any number of stresses, whether developmental or situational in nature. The specific developmental needs (physical, intellectual, emotional-social) of children are presented, including the nurse's role in nurturing each child's developmental potential. Guidelines are presented on which to base realistic anticipatory guidance for parents so that they can better understand their child's growth and development and can take action to prevent or best manage altered health states. Personal responsibility of the child for his or her own health, with encouragement of self-care activities appropriate to developmental stage, is also emphasized.

We believe health always exists but that altered health states can occur in response to developmental or situational stress. Emphasis is given to the nurse's understanding of those behaviors manifested during developmental crises. We describe illnesses as situational crises (temporary, reversible, irreversible; and life-threatening alterations). Specific illnesses, whether minor or critical, are not necessarily addressed at the age when they first appear, but rather at the stage when the altered state poses the greatest potential for impairment of the child's physical, intellectual, and emotional-social development. We believe that altered health states of children and adolescents are most appropriately studied within a growth and development framework, because understanding the development of the child is the foundation of understanding the rationale behind nursing actions.

Careful consideration has been given to using accurate, researched information as a basis for the practical nursing interventions recommended in this text. Our own background as students, practitioners and teachers has served to impress upon us the importance of research-based nursing practice. Our intent is to impart an appreciation for research to the readers of this text.

A teacher's guide prepared by Pamela Cross, M.S.N., Emory University School of Nursing, Atlanta, is available from the publisher for this book. In addition to containing chapter summaries and suggested learning activities, the guide presents behavioral objectives and a study guide for every chapter, directed at the student. The guide is designed so that the instructor can photocopy individual pages for distribution to students or can adapt the study guide questions to his or her own teaching methods.

We are especially grateful to the enduring efforts of the many people who helped make this book a reality. We first must thank our many colleagues in nursing, in medicine and in the other caring professions who have contributed, reviewed and shared their knowledge and experience with us. We thank the staffs of C. S. Mott Children's Hospital, Ann Arbor, and Emma L. Bixby Hospital, Adrian, Michigan, for their unfailing cooperation and assistance with photography. We especially thank the many families who allowed us to share their experiences, in health and illness, in photographs. Appreciation is extended to Joanne Dungey, Kathy Kohler, and Marilee Verstraete, who graciously tolerated the typing and re-typing of thousands of handwritten pages. We give our thanks to John Brady for his help in negative production, and to Robert Bensinger (Medical Photography of the University of Michigan) for hospital photography. Our gratitude is extended to the W. B. Saunders staff for the outstanding effort in the production of this text, especially to Larry Ward for his many fine illustrations and to Edna Dick for painstaking attention to manuscript detail. A very warm and special thanks to Ilze Rader, Associate Nursing Editor, for her persistent but understanding encouragement.

To our husbands, Jim and Merrill, we offer our love, admiration and appreciation for their enduring support of us and our book and for their many sacrifices in our behalf. Special gratitude is due for sharing their expertise in photography and to Jim for many long hours of darkroom work to produce most of the photographs. We acknowledge our continued indebtedness to each other for offering what was needed to bring this work to successful completion as a joint effort between two friends.

Jo Joyce Tackett
Mabel Hunsberger

CONTENTS

Part 1 FAMILIES GROW AND DEVELOP

1 Family Growth and Development 5

Family Theory 5
Historical View of Family Stages 6
Family Characteristics and
 Functions 8
Developmental Framework of
 Families 10
Roles in Families 10
Family Life Cycle 12
The Nurse and Families 20
 Jo Joyce Tackett

2 Influential Factors in Family Living 22

Space 23
Time 23
Communication Patterns 26
Family Environment 27
Finances 27
Work 29
Television 30
Religion 33
Public Policy 34
Culture 35
 Cheryl E. Easley
 Carol M. Easley

3 Parenting for the Socialization of Children 39

Roles of Parents 40
 Rules 41
 Punishment 43
 Reward 44
Functions of Parenting 45
Principles of Parenting 49
Parenting Styles 50
Assessing Parenting Capabilities 55
 Jo Joyce Tackett

4 Alternative Family Life Styles 60

Single Parent Families 61
 By Divorce 63
 By Death 65
Step-parents 67
Foster Parents 67
Migrant Children 68
Adoption 69
Communal Families 72
Homosexual Parents 73
 A. Frances Wenger

5 Families With Dysfunctional Life Patterns 76

Characteristics of Dysfunctional
 Life Patterns 77
The Nurse and Dysfunctional
 Families 79
Failure-to-Thrive Families 80
Child Abuse and Neglect 84
The Dance of Development 86
 Elizabeth B. Gall

Part 2 CHILDBEARING FAMILIES

6 Growth and Development Needs of the Childbearing Family: Maintaining Wellness 95

Adjusting to Pregnancy 95
 Labor Redistribution 95

xiii

Adapting Sexual Relations 96
Changing Relationships With
  Relatives and Friends 96
Preparing for the Parent Role 99
  Reallocating Resources 99
  Gaining Knowledge 100
  Changing Communication
    Patterns 100
  Planning for Future Children 102
Preparing Siblings 103
Janet S. Malinowski

7 Potential Family Stresses During Pregnancy 106

Unplanned Pregnancy 106
Difficult Pregnancy 107
Interrupted Pregnancy 108
Stillbirth 109
Teratogenic Agents 110
Janet S. Malinowski

8 Pregnancy in Adolescence 115

Incidence of Teen Pregnancy 116
Reasons for Teen Pregnancy 116
Interruption of Education 116
Effects on Family Relationships 117
Effects on Peer Relationships 117
Physical Risks to Pregnant
  Adolescent and Fetus 118
Challenge to Health
  Professionals 120
Sara Criswell
Dorothy Wierenga
June Hauge

Part 3 FAMILIES WITH CHILDREN: THE NURSE'S ROLE IN THEIR DEVELOPMENT AND HEALTH

9 Problem-Oriented Recording and Nursing Process 128

Nursing Process 128
  Assessment 128
  Problem Identification 128
  Developing a Plan 129
  Intervention 129
  Evaluation 129
Documentation of Health Care 130
  Source Oriented and Integrated
    Records 130
  Narrative Recording 130
  Problem Oriented Records 130
Amy L. Hofing

10 Growth and Development 135

Principles of Growth and
  Development 136
Factors Influencing Growth and
  Development 138
Natural Forces 139
Nurturing Forces 144
Developmental Theories of
  Physical Competency 144
  Intellectual Competency 145
  Language Development 149
  Emotional-Social Competency 151
Jo Joyce Tackett

11 Understanding the Play of Children 157

Theories of Play 157
Effect of Play on Physical,
  Cognitive and Emotional-Social
  Development 159
Social Character of Play 162
Content of Play 163
Role of Nurse in Promoting Play 164
Mabel Hunsberger

12 Communicating With Children and Parents 166

The Communication Process 166
Parent-Child-Nurse Relationship 166
Nonverbal and Verbal
  Communication 168
Communication Skills 169
  Observation 169
  Listening 170
  Silence 171
Principles of Communicating With
  Children 171
  Parents 175
Mabel Hunsberger

13 Health Appraisal 177

History-Taking 177
Physical Assessment 185
  Approaching the Child 188
  Measurements 188

Vital Signs 192
Physical Examination 193
Developmental Screening 238
Nutritional Assessment 242
Laboratory Screening 245
Theresa Eldridge
Jo Joyce Tackett
Mabel Hunsberger

14 Family Assessment 251

Approaches to Family
  Assessment 251
Guidelines for Family
  Assessment 253
The Family Apgar 253
Jennifer Piersma

15 Managing Health 258

Identifying Personal Health
  Needs 258
Developing Problem-Solving
  Skills 259
Nurse's Role in Promoting
  Health 262
Teaching 264
Counselling 268
Referrals 270
Jo Joyce Tackett

16 Managing Stress 273

Family Crisis Intervention 273
  Chester R. Peachey
When Behavior is a Problem 279
When a Child is Ill 283
  Jo Joyce Tackett
When a Child is Hospitalized 295
  Gail K. Ingersoll
When a Child is Dying 305
  Mabel Hunsberger
  Marcia Sheets
  Anita Spietz

17 Principles and Skills of Pediatric Nursing 315

Daily Care Considerations 315
  Mabel Hunsberger
  Judy Coltson Moyer
Fluid and Electrolyte Balance
  in Infants and Children 345
  Mabel Hunsberger
Total Parenteral Nutrition
  (Hyperalimentation) 365
  Anita Clavier

Nursing Care of Children
  Requiring Anesthesia 369
  Mary Jean Yablonky
Preoperative and Postoperative
  Nursing Care 373
  Mabel Hunsberger

Part 4 FAMILIES WITH INFANTS

18 Growth and Development Needs of the Family With an Infant: Maintaining Wellness 381

Accepting Responsibility for
  the Infant 383
Assuming New Roles 383
Forming an Attachment 386
Adjusting Family Life 388
  Anne Krabill Hershberger

19 Potential Stresses in Families With Infants 396

Lack of Support Structures 396
Fatigue 398
Division of Labor 399
Lack of Knowledge of Infant
  Care 399
Family Relationships 401
Finances 404
  Anne Krabill Hershberger

20 The Newborn Infant 406

The Normal Newborn 406
  Initial Assessment 407
  Apgar Score 407
  Later Assessment 411
  Neurological Examination 420
  Physical Care 424
    Carolyn Pedigo DeLoach
Variations in Gestational Weight
  and Age 429
  Preterm Infant 430
  Special Needs 435
  Post-Term Infant 442
  Variations in Gestational Age 443
  Intrauterine Growth
    Retardation 444
    Mary Lou Moore

21 Growth and Development of the Infant: Maintaining Wellness 447

Physical Competency 447
Intellectual Competency 457
Emotional-Social Competency 460
Helping Parents Promote
  Development 464
    Linda Upton

22 Potential Stresses During Infancy: Growth of Human Bonds 471

Normal Development of
  Social Relations 471
Breakdown in Attachment 475
Assessing Attachment 482
    Michael Trout

23 Potential Stresses During Infancy: Temporary Alterations in Health Status 493

Allergies 494
Dermatitides 499
Conjunctivitis 507
Common Infections 508
Gastrointestinal Problems 513
Neuromuscular Disorders 517
    Jo Joyce Tackett

24 Potential Stresses During Infancy: Reversible Alterations in Health Status 522

Nurse's Role with Family 522
    Mabel Hunsberger
Congenital Heart Anomalies 528
    Mary Burkhart
    Marianne Glassanos
Congenital Anomalies of the
  Respiratory Tract 558
    Mabel Hunsberger
Urinary Tract Anomalies 560
    Stephen Koff
    Mabel Hunsberger
Facial Anomalies 565
    Deborah Braunstein
Gastrointestinal Tract Anomalies 569
    Theresa M. Sarahan
    Mabel Hunsberger
Musculoskeletal Anomalies 599
    Stephanie Wright
Respiratory Infections 606
    Mabel Hunsberger
Neurological Infections 616
Gastrointestinal Infections 621
    Judy Coltson Moyer
Nutritional Alterations 624
    Mabel Hunsberger
Endocrine Alterations 630
    Kathleen U. Boggs

25 Potential Stresses During Infancy: Irreversible Alterations in Health Status 639

Impact of Diagnosis: Nurse's
  Role 639
Central Nervous System
  Alterations 648
Neurocutaneous Syndromes 653
Visual Impairment 657
Inborn Errors of Metabolism 662
Immune Deficiencies 664
Alterations in Reproductive
  Functioning 665
Maternal Infections 667
Gastrointestinal Alterations 668
    Ellen Christian
    Judith Clark

26 Potential Stresses During Infancy: Life-Threatening Alterations in Health Status 671

Infant's Response: Parent's
  Response 671
Genetic Disorders 672
Infectious Diseases 679
Sudden Infant Death Syndrome
  (SIDS) 682
    Marcia Sheets
    Anita Spietz

27 Hospitalized Infant 689
    Linda Nicholson Grinstead
Nursing Care Plan for Infant With
  Respiratory Alteration 698
    Kathy T. Edwards
    Amy L. Hofing

Part 5 FAMILIES WITH TODDLERS

28 Growth and Development of the Family With A Toddler: Maintaining Wellness 709

Adapting Resources 709
Reorganizing Relationships 714
Reworking Family Philosophy 717
    Jo Joyce Tackett

29 Potential Stresses in Families With Toddlers 722

Energy Depletion 722
Disagreements About Parenting 725
Dependence/Independence Balance 726
Unhealthy Toilet Training Patterns 728
Jo Joyce Tackett

30 Growth and Development of the Toddler: Maintaining Wellness 731

Physical Competency 731
Intellectual Competency 739
Emotional-Social Competency 743
Health Maintenance 754
Mabel Hunsberger

31 Potential Stresses During Toddlerhood: Managing of Toddler Behavior 764

Excessive Fears 764
Separation Anxiety 769
Sibling Rivalry 772
Temper Tantrums 776
Jo Joyce Tackett

32 Potential Stresses During Toddlerhood: Temporary Alterations in Health Status 780

Temporary Orthopedic Conditions 781
Iron Deficiency Anemia 785
Pica 788
Parasitic Infections 789
Jo Joyce Tackett

33 Potential Stresses During Toddler Years: Reversible Alterations in Health Status 797

Child With Burns 799
Claudella Archambeault-Jones
Irving Feller
Ingestions 818
Croup 823
Linda Mowad

34 Potential Stresses During Toddler Years: Irreversible Alterations 828

Impact of Diagnosis: Nurse's Role 828
Celiac Disease 832
Hemophilia 835
Nephrotic Syndrome 838
Frances White Thurber

35 Potential Stresses During Toddler Years: Life-Threatening Alterations in Health Status 843

Toddler's Response 844
Rhabdomyosarcoma 845
Retinoblastoma 845
Anita Spietz

36 The Hospitalized Toddler 849

Reducing Stress 849
Enhancing Normal Development 858
Keeping the Toddler Safe 859
Mabel Hunsberger
Nursing Care Plan For Toddler With Circulatory Alterations 868
Joyce Piazza

Part 6 FAMILIES WITH PRESCHOOLERS

37 Growth and Development Needs of the Family With a Preschooler: Maintaining Wellness 879

Resource Allocation 879
Communication 880
Realistic Expectations 882
The World Beyond the Family 884
Kathleen King

38 Potential Stresses in Families with Preschoolers 888

Dual-Career Families 888
Incest 891
The Aggressive Preschooler 892
Kathleen King

39 Growth and Development of the Preschooler: Maintaining Wellness 894

Physical Competency 895
Intellectual Competency 900
Emotional-Social Competency 903
Health Maintenance 908
Barbara Miller

40 Potential Stresses During Preschool Years: Managing Behavior 914

Respecting Ownership 914
Stuttering 916
Sleep Disorders 917
Excessive Masturbation 918
Jo Joyce Tackett

41 Potential Stresses During Preschool Years: Temporary Alterations in Health Status 921

Communicable Diseases 922
Rabies 931
Pediculosis Capitis 934
Hordeolum 936
Jo Joyce Tackett
Barbara Miller

42 Potential Stresses During Preschool Years: Reversible Alterations in Health Status 937

Reactions of Preschooler and Family 937
Respiratory Conditions 940
Mabel Hunsberger
Urogenital Problems 946
Evan J. Kass
Mabel Hunsberger

43 Potential Stresses During Preschool Years: Irreversible Alterations in Health Status 955

Family Reactions 955
Poliomyelitis 958
Visual Problems 961
Hearing Impairment 973
Sensory-Impaired Child in the Hospital 983

Bronchial Asthma 984
Rhinitis 995
Mary Lou Frey
Mabel Hunsberger
Jo Joyce Tackett

44 Potential Stresses During the Preschool Years: Life-Threatening Alterations in Health Status 999

Leukemia 999
Neuroblastoma 1006
Wilms' Tumor 1008
Support During Diagnosis and Treatment 1009
The Child Who Dies 1013
Mary Waskerwitz
Ruth M. Heyn

45 The Hospitalized Preschooler 1016

Impact of Hospitalization 1016
Minimizing Developmental Trauma 1020
Jo Joyce Tackett
Nursing Care Plan for the Preschooler with a Urinary Alteration 1028
Margaret Alderman

Part 7 FAMILIES WITH SCHOOL-AGE CHILDREN

46 Growth and Development Needs of the Family With School-Age Children: Maintaining Wellness 1041

Adapting to an Expanding World 1041
Nurse's Role in Facilitating Adjustment 1047
Letting Go 1048
Financial Solvency 1050
Evelyn McElroy
Jo Joyce Tackett

47 Potential Stresses in Families With School-Age Children 1052

Inappropriate Adjustment to School 1053
Prejudice 1055
The Latch-Key Child 1055
Sexual Assault 1056
Evelyn McElroy
Jo Joyce Tackett

48 Growth and Development of the School-Age Child: Maintaining Wellness 1060

Physical Development 1060
Intellectual and Language Development 1070
Emotional and Social Development 1076
Health Maintenance 1085
Elaine C. Smith

49 Potential Stresses During School-Age Years: Managing Behavior 1090

Enuresis 1091
Encopresis 1093
School Phobia 1095
Antisocial Behavior 1098
Mary Sue Jack

50 Potential Stresses During School-Age Years: Temporary Alterations in Health Status 1103

Cutaneous Problems 1103
Trauma 1107
Legg-Calvé-Perthes Disease 1112
Precocious Puberty 1113
Anne E. Hartson

51 Potential Stresses During School-Age Years: Reversible Alterations in Health Status 1116

Reversible Inflammatory Processes 1117
Fractures 1126
Childhood Obesity 1134
Dental Problems 1136
Anne E. Hartson

52 Potential Stresses During School-Age Years: Irreversible Alterations in Health Status 1140

Osteogenesis Imperfecta 1142
Minimal Brain Dysfunction: Learning Disabilities 1144
Developmental Disabilities 1149
Frances Bontrager Greaser
Diabetes 1166
Sandra Merkel
Lisa Parker
Anne Karr
Juvenile Rheumatoid Arthritis 1179
Anne E. Hartson

53 Potential Stresses During School-Age Years: Life-Threatening Alterations in Health Status 1184

How the School-Age Child Perceives Death 1184
Intracranial Tumors 1189
Tumors of Soft Tissues 1195
Reye's Syndrome 1196
Marcia Sheets
Anita Spietz

54 The Hospitalized School-Age Child 1201

Impact of Hospitalization 1201
Nursing Actions to Facilitate Adjustment 1204
How the School-Age Child Views His Body 1207
Jo Joyce Tackett
Nursing Care Plan for the School-Age Child with Neurological Alteration 1214
Florence Nezamis

Part 8 FAMILIES WITH ADOLESCENTS

55 Growth and Development Needs of the Family With Adolescents: Maintaining Wellness 1221

Reallocation of Resources 1221
Division of Labor and Responsibility 1223
Maintaining Communication 1224
Mary Arbour

56 Potential Stresses in Families With Adolescents 1226

Parent-Adolescent Differences 1227
Adolescent Sexuality 1227
Drugs 1228
Peer Relationships 1229
The Alienated Adolescent 1230
Mary Arbour

57 Adolescent Growth and Development: Maintaining Wellness 1232

Physical Growth and Development 1232
Cognitive Development 1236
Emotional Development 1238
Social Development 1240
Maintaining Health 1243
Janet Allen-Lia

58 Potential Stresses During Adolescence: Managing Behavior 1249

Delinquency 1250
Suicide 1252
Abuse 1253
Sexual Activity 1255
Runaways 1257
Drug Misuse 1259
Linda Bond

59 Potential Stresses During Adolescence: Temporary Alterations in Health Status 1263

Acne Vulgaris 1263
Infectious Diseases 1266
Menstrual Disturbances 1270
Jo Joyce Tackett

60 Potential Stresses During Adolescence: Reversible Alterations in Health Status 1273

Spinal Abnormalities 1274
  Kyphosis and Lordosis 1274
  Scoliosis 1276
Communicable Diseases 1288
  Hepatitis 1288
  Venereal Diseases 1292
Obesity 1293
Jo Joyce Tackett

61 Potential Stresses During Adolescence: Irreversible Alterations in Health Status 1298

Delayed Puberty 1299
Schizophrenia 1300
Depression 1303
Systemic Lupus Erythematosus 1304
Tuberculosis 1308
Kathleen U. Boggs

62 Potential Stresses During Adolescence: Life-Threatening Alterations in Health Status 1314

How Adolescent Perceives Death 1314
Bone Tumors 1316
Hodgkin's Disease 1319
Muscular Dystrophy 1321
Cystic Fibrosis 1324
Marcia Sheets
Anita Spietz

63 The Hospitalized Adolescent 1331

Adolescent Development 1331
Impact of Illness 1333
Impact of Hospitalization 1335
Nurse and Adolescent 1336
Sandra Merkel
Nursing Care Plan for Adolescent With Musculoskeletal Alteration 1340
Sandra Merkel

Appendices 1359

Index 1389

FAMILY-CENTERED CARE OF CHILDREN AND ADOLESCENTS
Nursing Concepts in Child Health

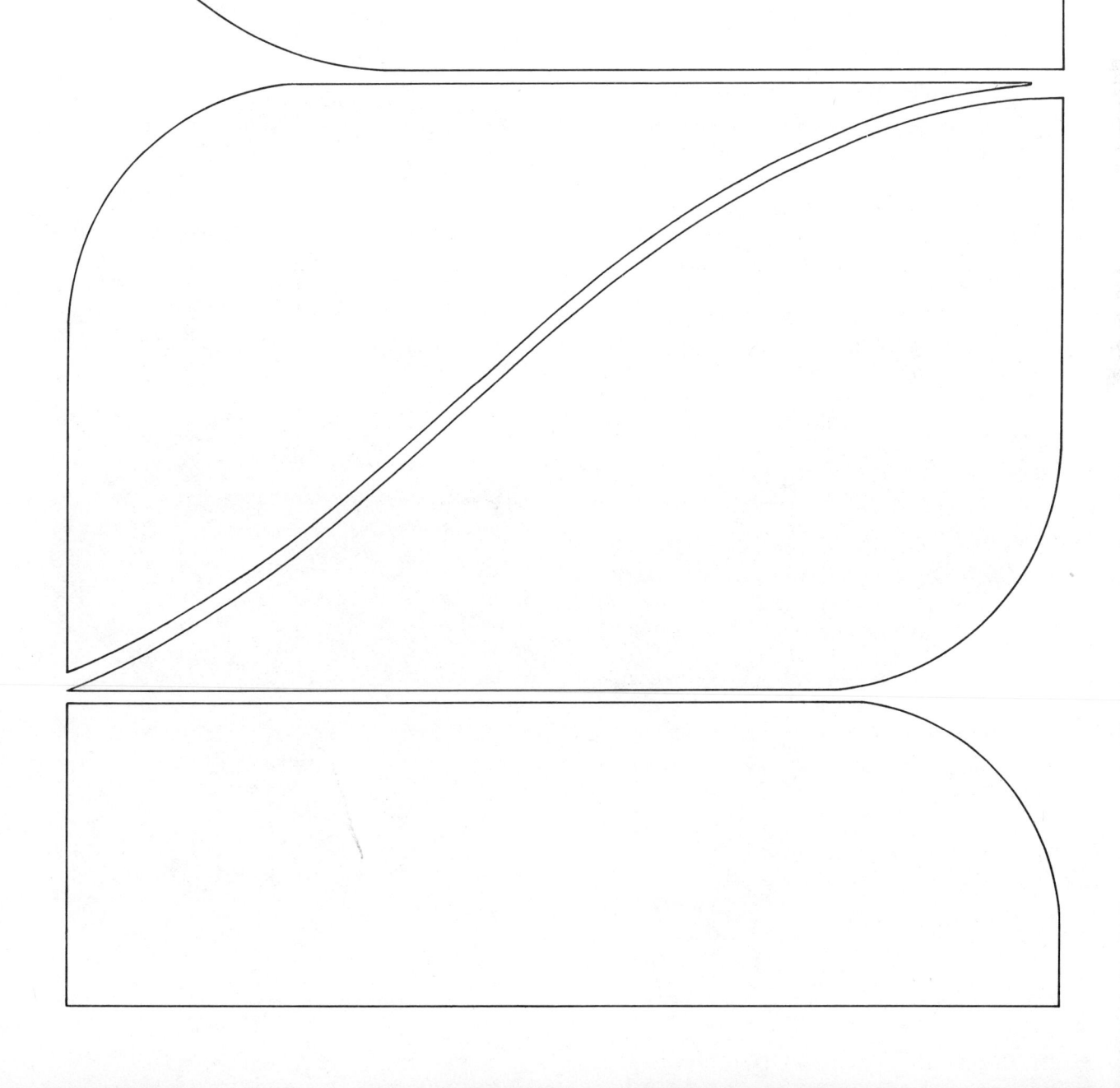

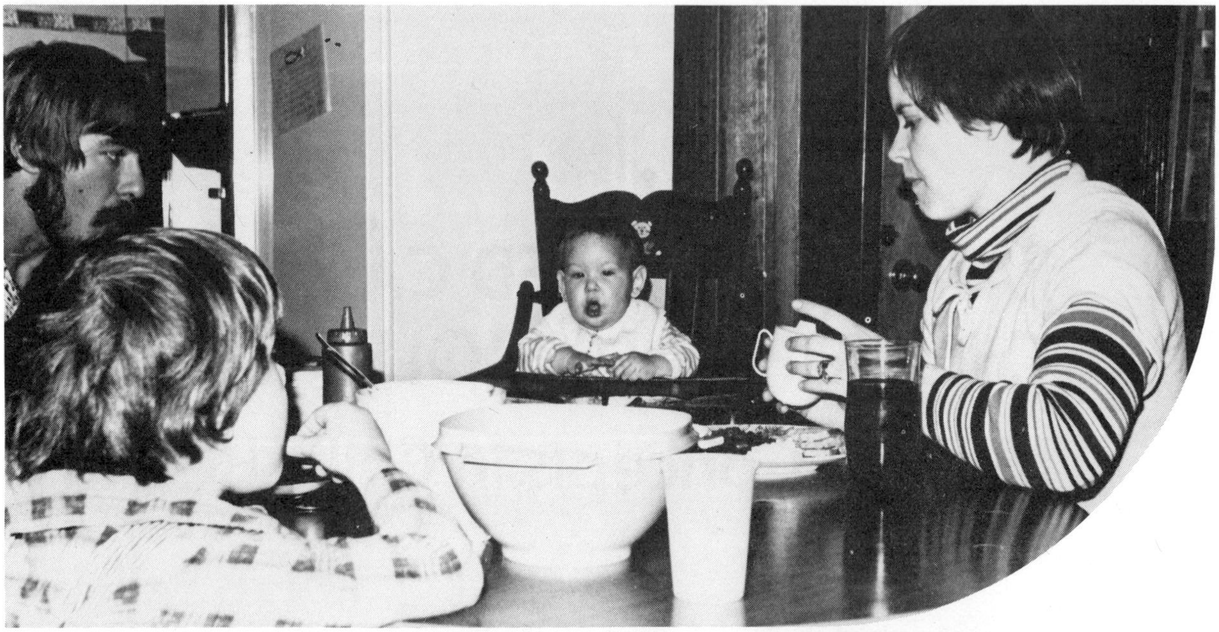

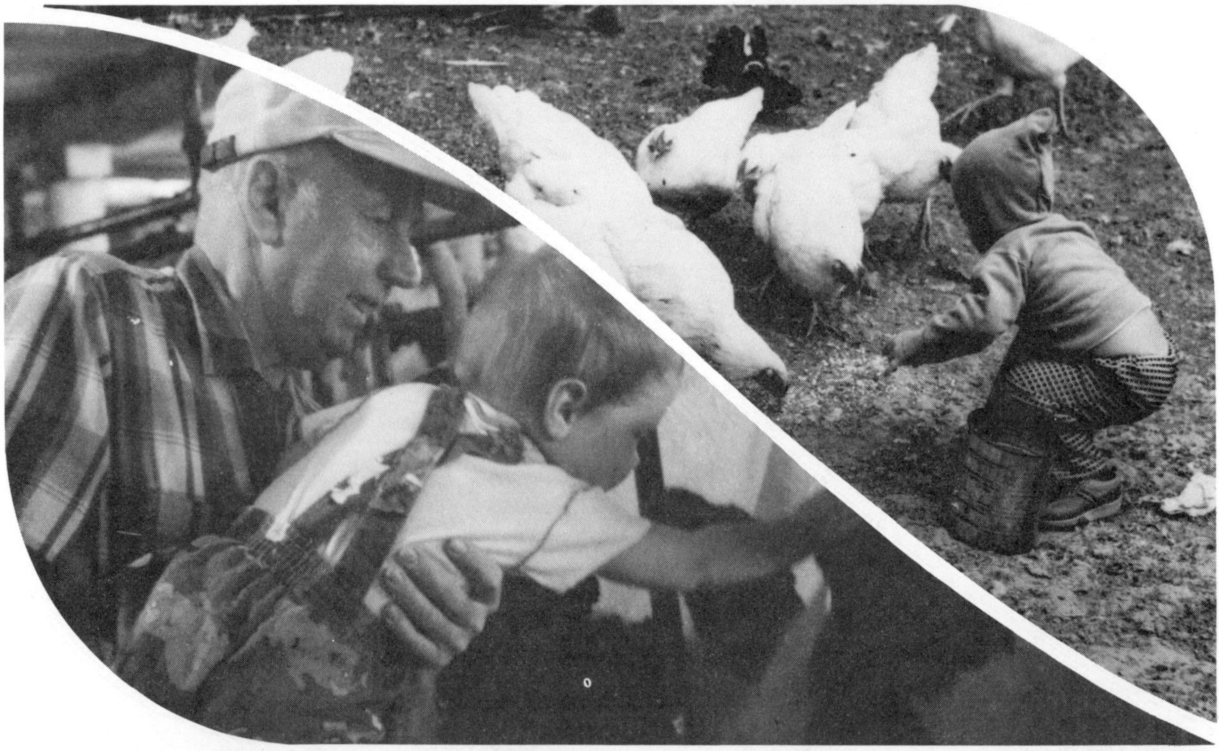

PART 1

SETTING THE EXAMPLE

I'd rather see a sermon than hear one—any day.
I'd rather you would walk with me, than merely show the way.
The eye's a better pupil and more willing than the ear,
Fine counsel is confusing, but example is always clear.
The best of all the teachers are parents who live their creeds,
For, to see good in action is what every child needs.
I can say, I'll learn how to do it if you'll let me see it done;
I can watch your hand in action though your
    tongue too fast may run.
Although the lectures you deliver may be very
    wise and true,
I'd rather learn my lesson by observing what
    you do;
For I may misunderstand you and the fine
    advice you give,
But there's no misunderstanding how you
    act and how you live.

— AUTHOR UNKNOWN —

FAMILIES GROW AND DEVELOP

FAMILY GROWTH AND DEVELOPMENT

by Jo Joyce Tackett, RN, MPHN

WHY STUDY FAMILY?

One of the fundamental goals of nursing is to provide family-centered nursing care. This is in part based on the premise that, since the family is a system, no one individual member can be effectively cared for if that care does not consider the other members who both affect and are affected by the member seeking nursing care. Practitioners who care for the children in families must necessarily acknowledge this relationship because it is the family that is largely responsible for that child, that most significantly enhances or hinders that child's development, and to which that child must ultimately be accountable.

The premise of this book is that the family unit, *whatever its form,* still thrives and is even growing in its significance to society and its own members and in the functions it bears in this modern world. We acknowledge that the family and its meaning are continually changing, as is true of any living, open system, but we believe that its demise, although often predicted, is unlikely. In fact, the multitude of rapidly occurring changes of recent years has proved the family to be a highly flexible, adaptable unit.[3]

Throughout history, the family has been the basic unit in society. Families shape the direction of society (through values, beliefs, customs) and are also shaped (alterations in role expectations, functions) by these same factors in society.[20] It is this symbiotic relationship between the family and society that makes it hard to decipher which exerts the greater influence.

> A child is a transient who comes into the lives of parents for a brief period. He stays only a few years before he must be on his way to his own fulfillment. Mothers and fathers should live with each child so that they are happy to greet that child when he comes to them and happy to see him go when the time comes for going.
> Marguerite and Willard Beecher

DEFINING FAMILY

In a world that places ever-increasing and changing demands on the family, a very fluid definition of that unit is paramount. The following definition adheres to that requirement.

The family unit is a living, open system of reacting and interacting persons who group themselves together with a central purpose to create and maintain a common culture which promotes progressive and holistic development of each of its members.

Regardless of how the members of family units group themselves together or whether they reside in the same household, their effect upon each other is significant and generically similar. In each family unit there are: (1) relationships that are distinctly purposeful and highly intimate, (2) shared values and goals, and (3) extensive communication systems to which each member makes a contribution.[13, 18]

This concept of the family as an open system with an intimate environment gives a view of the family as an interacting whole that encourages the nurse to work with the client in the context of his* family, (i.e., family-centered nursing). This focus will direct the nurse toward more comprehensive planning, yielding more effective interventions of longer-lasting impact. Furthermore, because families are highly individualistic in terms of structure, life style, interactions and so forth, viewing them in a developmental sequence helps the nurse make some predictions about a family's behaviors, needs and potential conflicts.

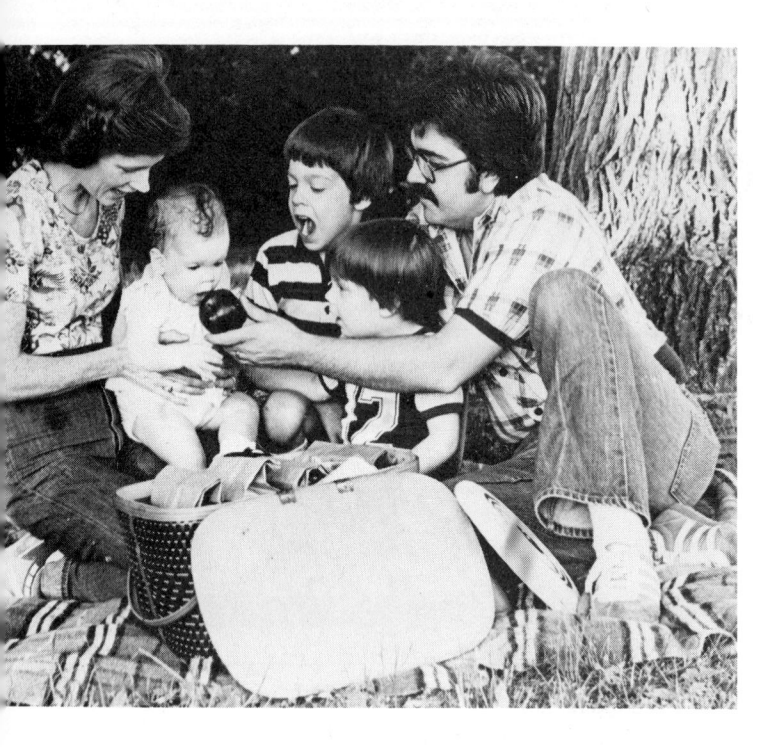

FAMILY: A HISTORICAL PERSPECTIVE

The family has always existed, and even though analysis of iconography concludes that its structure as a cohabitable unit with intimacy and emotional sharing did not occur until the fifteenth century, the family has never been successfully dissolved.[1] Historically the family has been a succession of extensions (extended family pattern in which parents, children and other related kin sustain themselves either under the same roof or on attached land homesteads with shared daily activities) and contractions (nuclear family pattern in which a couple and their children exist separate from other relatives and maintain their own separate routine of daily activities) whose rhythm follows the modification of the political order and economic conditions.[1, 18, 20] Throughout time, people have continually exercised imagination in the construction of various styles of family living and different ways of relating the family to the larger community, each experiment again reaffirming the family as the basic unit of human living, of social stability and of health.[4, 14]

Actually, in the United States most families have generally consisted only of parent(s) and child(ren). Even in colonial days only 6 per cent of colonial U.S. families had more than the nuclear unit and the latest census shows that extended families still compose about 6 per cent of U.S. families. Then, as now, most children moved out of their parents' homes to set up their own household.[8, 11] Nor is mobility new. Historically, statistics repeatedly indicate approximately 20 per cent of the population "on the move" and today, as a hundred years ago, most moves are over short distances (only about 4 per cent move to another state) and most moves are made by young people.[8, 12, 17]

Other aspects of family living have not remained unaltered through time. A growth process is continually in evidence, moving the family, in its hundred variations, toward a more symmetrical form of living. We have progressed from a preindustrial (agricultural) family, housed rurally, to an industrial (traditional) family in urban residence, and, further, to a postindustrial (modern) family with a suburban or small town abode. Table 1-1 illustrates some of the differences exhibited in each stage of this historical growth process.

These stages are presented here as a frame of reference to the nurse because, even though we are today in a postindustrial social era, the socioeconomic status of an individual family will often influence what particular stage a given family is in, with the accompanying characteristics of that stage. For example, a family of lower socioeconomic status in this postindustrial era still may closely resemble an early industrial (Stage II) family with some Stage I (preindustrial) elements; a "blue-collar" middle class family in this postindustrial era still often resembles the Stage II (industrial) family; the "white-collar" middle and upper

---

*This book acknowledges the potential roles of both sexes; however, for convenience and consistency, the nurse is identified by the feminine word form and the client or child by the masculine word form.

TABLE 1-1 A HISTORICAL PERSPECTIVE ON THE STAGES OF SYMMETRICAL GROWTH IN FAMILY LIVING

Family Stage	Purpose	Goal	Motivation	Structure/Roles	Orientation	Societal Expectations
I Pre-industrial (agricultural)	Economic unit of production	Self-sufficiency	Survival	Closed system; patriarchal structure; dictatorial governance; rigidly defined roles; childrearing = 54% of married life	Children were economic necessities, assets, viewed as possessions. Treated as miniature adults with early indoctrination into adult responsibilities and strong lines between right and wrong.	Economic security; protection; religious training; recreation; education; reproduction; health care
II Industrial (traditional)	Consumptive unit; work oriented	Success, domesticity	Quantity of living; accumulation of goods	Emerging open system; less patriarchal, but husband still head of household and final authority. Autocratic governance; clearly defined roles but not rigid	Children seen as an economic liability after enactment of child labor laws. Early assumption of adult role—contribute to the family income by 16 or 18.	Reproduction; religious training; class and status-conferring; privacy; identity-conferring
III Post-industrial (modern)	Consumptive unit; leisure oriented	Self actualization of members and independence; enhancing potentials of members	Quality of living	Open symmetrical system; shared equalitarian structure. Democratic governance, de-differentiation of roles—flexible and negotiable, depending on who is available and the situation; childrearing = 18% of married life	Children seen as an economic liability had by choice, viewed as persons in their own right. Late assumption of adult role, average at 21–22 years. Obligation to family is to develop own potentials.	Provision of physical needs; fulfillment of emotional and love needs. Nurturing—preparing child's personality for modern world; companionship

FAMILY GROWTH AND DEVELOPMENT

classes are most likely to reflect the Stage III (postindustrial) family in their life style. Familiarity with the characteristics that accompany these stages of family living will help the nurse to identify the life style patterns and attitudes that the family with whom she is interacting is likely to show. She can then relate to them in a way that accommodates their living patterns and considers their family attitudes.

Regardless of its life style, the family provides for some satisfactions that are hard to come by and sustain anywhere but in a family setting.[9] The healthy family unit provides "roots" for its members, offering them love, intimacy and companionship that is ongoing and noncontingent. A link between the past and future, one's family offers a foundation for the present and for one's continuity and stability through time. The family will continue to be the most economical and efficient agent for the raising of children, although child care responsibilities will change, owing to factors such as decreased family size, increased leisure hours and increased numbers of mothers in the work force.

What would happen to the childbearing role of families in an era of biological revolution remains to be seen. If a future society accepts as commonplace embryo transplants, genetic designing, cloning and "test tube" babies, babies might very well become a purchasable commodity, not requiring a couple for their conception and birth but only for their progressive development after birth. Certainly this is an ethical issue worth serious consideration by families, the helping professions and society at large.

SHARED CHARACTERISTICS OF FAMILIES

As the definition of family presented earlier in the chapter implies, families, regardless of their structural organization or life style, have in common three facets to their existence. These are intimacy, interaction-communication patterns and shared, or common, goals and values.

Intimacy

The rapidly changing expectations and demands on all segments of life today make this characteristic of families highly appealing. In an era when little else remains constant and most relationships outside the family are temporary and founded on numerous contingencies, which lends them a fragile nature, the real source of security is usually the noncontingent, love-based, enduring and close relationships at home. It is in the realm of a healthy intimate climate that spouses learn to live in harmony despite their differences, that children become social beings and that the foundation for happiness and health is derived. In this home each member can be himself, experience and express a diversity of feelings and know that he is still accepted. No other institution in modern society allows this degree of intimacy or unconditional caring.

Interaction-Communication Patterns

This is the process by which a family relates to life outside itself and through which one member's actions are stimulated by the behaviors of other members within the family. In simplest terms, family interaction is the sum total of all the roles performed within a given family.[5] The roles (goal-directed patterns of behaving that an individual carries out in his interactions with a given role partner) of family members are defined by the norms within the family and by those established in larger society.[13]

One's position in a given situation is the basis for the role(s) assumed, and thus both position and role prescription may fluctuate, depending on who the role partner is in an interaction. For example, a man might enact roles as follows with the accompanying role partners:

Position Role	*Role Partner*
Husband	Wife
Father	Child
Son	Father
Brother	Sibling
Employee	Employer

A broader discussion of role prescriptions within a family unit will be presented later in this chapter.

The roles either acquired (e.g., oldest child, female) or electively achieved or adopted (e.g., breadwinner;* parent; spouse) by family members largely determine the nature of the communication that occurs among family members and with whom it occurs. As a society

---
*A role open to either or both spouses in many homes today.

takes over more of the functions of a family or its members through agencies outside the family unit, fewer roles are required of each member. As the number of roles a family member has decreases, those roles left to him become increasingly significant and are performed more ardently. This societally imposed decrease in roles tends to produce within the family relationships that are more intense. Simultaneously, having fewer roles with their entailed responsibility allows for more freedom and time to experiment with the remaining roles (role flexibility) and for role fluidity (exchanges in role tasks among members as the family situation dictates).[4, 20]

Shared or Common Goals and Values

The goals of a family are derived to satisfy the affiliation needs of each member and to maintain family cohesiveness. They determine the way a family accomplishes its activities of daily living (life style) and the degree to which a family relies on other institutions for its socialization (e.g., family-created recreation as opposed to recreation obtained at the "Y" and the park recreation program). These goals reflect the family members' social status, their value systems and their orientation regarding their reason for being. Knowing a family's goals tells the nurse where the family places its priorities in life. For example, is present gratification most important or has the family a future orientation? Are children valued as important members of the family or are they seen primarily as expensive liabilities produced and tolerated out of social expectation? Are healthy life habits a purposeful part of family behavior or merely present by accident or circumstance?

Family goals also profoundly influence developmental tasks at every phase in the family life cycle.[5] In the emerging family, the way two individuals go about adjusting to living as a married couple (a developmental task) is greatly dependent on the family goals they have formed. An expanding family can be expected to care for and nurture its children to the extent that such activities are consistent with family goals and values. A contracting family will release its young adults from the family unit in a manner that does not compromise family goals.

UNIVERSAL FAMILY FUNCTIONS

All families are obligated to certain societally defined functions in order to assist their members to develop socially acceptable relationships. These functions are significant because they validate the necessity for and existence of families.[13, 19, 21] These functions of the family unit can be categorized into four major areas of responsibility.

Security and Survival Functions

The family unit is responsible for its own physical and biological maintenance. This involves providing for food, clothing, shelter; managing reproductive considerations of planning and controlling family size; recruiting and releasing family members; obtaining health care for members; apportioning of both tangible (goods, facilities, income) and intangible (space, affection, authority) resources; and maintaining reasonable division of labor (assigning responsibility for income, household tasks, child care and so forth).

Emotional and Social Development and Maintenance

Responsibilities of this function include support to family members during periods of stress (morale maintenance), enforcement of a system of social controls that involves rewards and punishment (motivation maintenance), support and acknowledgement of efforts to achieve (ego maintenance), channelling of sexual and affectional drives and establishing effective patterns of communication (maintenance of order), enculturation, and placement of members in the larger society by offering protection to them from undesirable outside influences and by establishing each member's ties and status within the family, the community and its institutions.

Sexual Differentiation and Teaching

This function involves the family's responsibility for nurturing of its members, especially child care and rearing. Teaching members their roles and responsibilities, fostering the development of conscience and supporting the learning of hobbies and skills that will produce healthy, capable adults are also part of this function.

Growth of Individual Members

Responsibility here is directed toward guiding the internalization of increasingly mature and acceptable patterns of physical, intellectual and emotional-social behavior in each member (socialization, personality development) by fostering gradually expanding independence, encouraging problem solving and supporting each member's efforts to adjust to his changing body.

The manner in which these four functions are performed and the degree to which they are accomplished varies with the family's socioeconomic status, cultural orientation and where it is within its life cycle; but these responsibilities do confront all families regardless of the integrative or destructive factors involved.

Division of family functions into these four categories facilitates the nurse's assessment of where the family is in its development of responsibility for itself and its members. How this assessment is used to implement the nursing process will be dealt with in the dicussion of family assessment in Chapter 14.

FAMILY LIFE CYCLE AND DEVELOPMENTAL TASKS

Families, like children, are born, develop, mature and age. At each stage families, like children, are faced with new developmental tasks requiring a reorganization of roles, communication patterns and goals. Families, like children, are affected by situational crises (illness, change or loss of income, change in family composition), maturational crises of individual members or altered social and environmental conditions (inflation, war, move to a new locale).[18]

Duvall's eight stages in the family life cycle are presented in Table 1–2, as they are reflective of the organization and philosophy of this book.[5] However, remember that clear-cut stages can be described only for families with one child. In families with more than one child there are overlaps in stages and in family developmental tasks. Still, the family life cycle approach emphasizes the dynamics of family interaction as shifting and changing from one period to another in a family's life span. The life cycle approach also helps to illustrate how family developmental tasks parallel those of individual family members, sometimes complementing each other. For example, in beginning families a developmental task of the unit is the establishment of satisfactory sexual relations, a task which complements or facilitates the individual spouses' developmental task of achieving intimacy. At other times tasks are in conflict: for example, in a childrearing family a family developmental task is to provide sufficient income to meet the increasing costs of family living, which usually requires that one or both spouses be away from home a great deal, yet the individual task of each spouse now is to become an effective parent (generativity), which requires time investments within the home.

The nurse's role is to act as facilitator or change agent to promote acceptance and successful accomplishment of tasks by the family and its members. Table 1–2 depicts the eight stages in a family's life cycle and the developmental tasks or crises — individual, positional and family group — that predominate at each stage.[5, 10, 16]

At whatever stage in the life cycle a family is when a nurse interacts with it, the family's developing relationships should be assessed and supported. Interventions should be planned in such a way that the family members can be kept together as much as possible, and actions should be initiated that will promote progressive mastery of individual member and family group tasks by the family unit. Ongoing *anticipatory guidance* at each stage facilitates the nurse's aim of helping the family members to help themselves and to accept assistance confidently when it is needed.

FAMILY ROLE PRESCRIPTIONS

Traditional roles, that is, roles clearly defined on the basis of sex and family position, are not functional in most families today. Clearly defined roles do not allow for individual uniqueness or particular family needs, both of which are major concerns in modern families. Research has documented that rigidly fixed roles suppress valuable aspects of the role-bearer's personality and foster guilt when the individual's feelings and desires do not jibe with the rigid role expectations.[9] Contrary to earlier beliefs, clearly differentiated roles do not seem necessary for development of a secure sexual identity. What is important is how fully one incorporates the notion of one's sex, how acceptable that gender is to one and how comfortable one is being that sex. These are factors which are primarily dependent on how one's original family accepted one and the sex one is and if the family allowed one to develop at

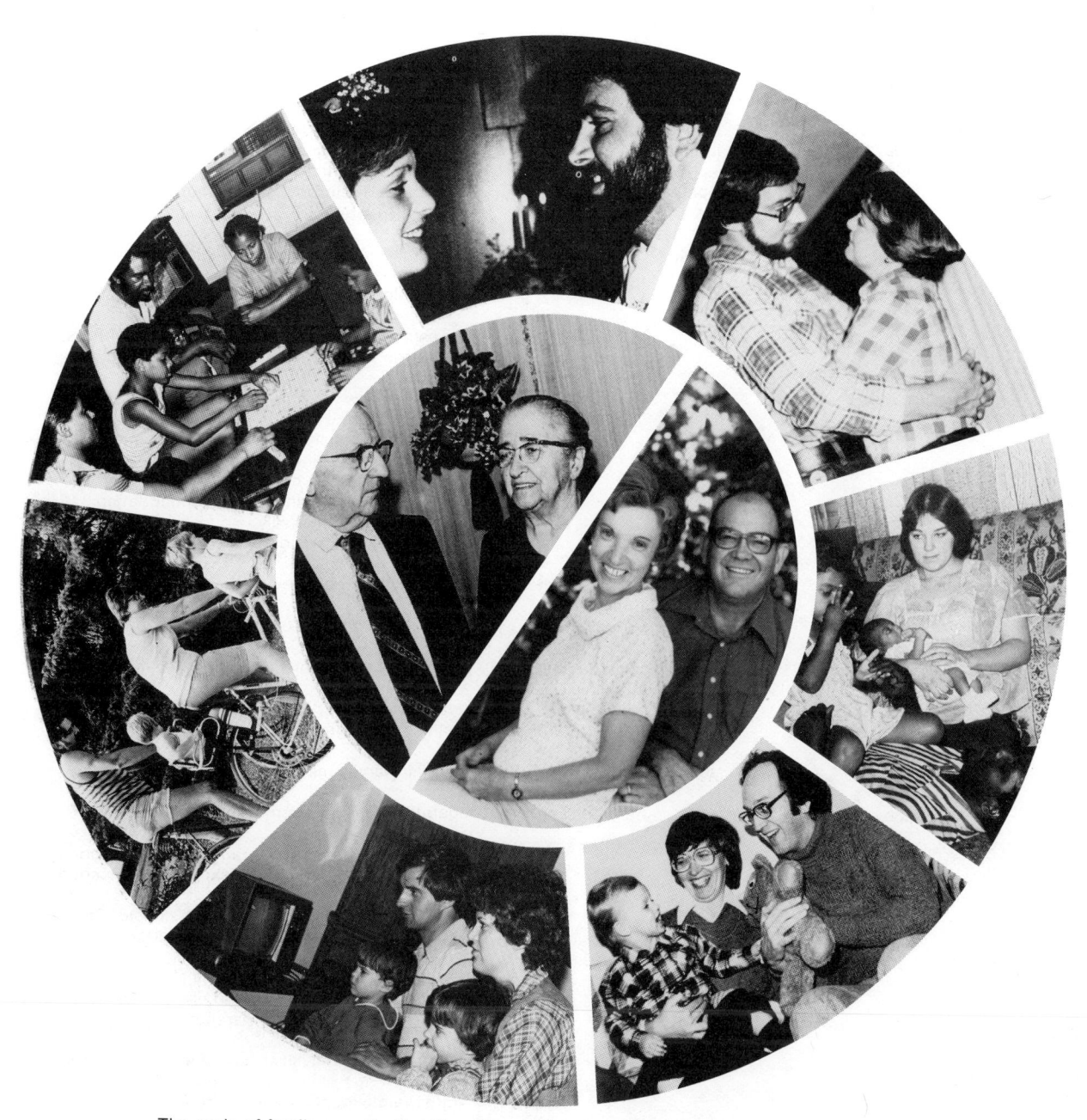

The cycle of family growth: Families, like children, are born, develop, mature and age.

FAMILY GROWTH AND DEVELOPMENT 11

TABLE 1-2 THE FAMILY LIFE CYCLE AND ASSOCIATED DEVELOPMENTAL TASKS[2, 5, 11, 16]

Stage	Time Span	Individual/Positional Developmental Tasks	Family Group Developmental Tasks
THE EMERGING FAMILY *Stage 1: Beginning Family* (Married couple without children)	2± years		

Establishment phase (Wedding day to confirmation of first pregnancy)		Individual adults: intimacy
		
		Spouses: adjustment to life as a couple without loss of individual identity
			Establishing the marriage
			  Making sexual adjustment
			  • relinquish childhood inhibitions, prohibitions
			  • achieve reciprocal gratification
			  • family planning
			
			  Reshaping relational and social relationships
			  • establish own home unit
			  • develop workable philosophy of life as a couple
			  • accept separation from parents
			  • establish mutual friends compatible with the marriage
			
			  Accepting new roles as husband and wife and as potential parents
			  • mutually satisfying, realistic economic arrangement (income and budget)
			  • system of open communication
			  • ways of expressing and accommodating differences creatively
			  • satisfactory division of labor, responsibility

Expectant phase (Confirmation of pregnancy to birth of baby)		Individual adults: continuing intimacy and emerging generativity
		
		Spouses: maintaining a basic relationship as a married couple while beginning integration of a perception of selves as parents
			Adjustment to pregnancy
			
			Re-evaluate division of labor and responsibility
			
			Adapt sexual relations to pregnant state
			
			Adapt relationship with relatives and friends to realities of pregnancy
			
			Maintain family members' morales
			
			Preparation for the parent role
			
			  Develop new economic arrangements to accommodate changes in income/expenses as needed
			
			  Expand communication system to consider present heightened emotional needs and addition of new child
			
			  Acquire knowledge about and plan for specifics of pregnancy, childbirth, parenthood
			
			  Arrange for the physical care of the expected baby
			
			  Adjust family goals to incorporate new roles

THE EXPANDING FAMILY *Stage 2: Childbearing Family* (From birth of first child until he is 30 months old)	2½± years		

TABLE 1-2 THE FAMILY LIFE CYCLE AND ASSOCIATED DEVELOPMENTAL TASKS (*Continued*)

Stage	Time Span	Individual/Positional Developmental Tasks	Family Group Developmental Tasks
Exaltation phase (From birth until parents take baby home)		Individual adults: accept parenthood (generativity) Spouses: accept each other as parents and companions Parents: learn basic infant care Infant: trust; develop physiological skills of survival (sleep, suck, swallow, primitive coordination)	Realizing the child really exists Accept new or added responsibility (Re)orient to parent role Begin bonding with child
Homecoming phase (From time child is taken home to third month)		Spouses: regain intimacy and develop marital relationship Parents: develop confidence and competence in parenting role and child care; learn baby's cues Infant: settling into a routine Siblings: trust → autonomy; begin separation from mother; make room for new baby in relationships with parents	Adjusting family life to incorporate new baby Support during members' mood swings (post-partum blues, baby's settling in, sibling jealousy) Realignment of division of labor and responsibility to compensate for member fatigue and 24-hour care Father accept provider role at least temporarily
Stabilization phase (Third through 30th month of baby's life)		Parents: learning to accept growth and development of child(ren), to accept his display of selfhood, to recognize "teachable moments" in child's development Child(ren): learn to handle self and own will	Establishing a stable family unit; making a home for all members Adapt resources to accommodate child(ren) • provide adequate housing—space for parents' privacy • childproof home environment • adjust budget • reshape division of labor and responsibility to include care of children without taxing any one member and provide opportunities for child to contribute as able • plan for future children Re-establishing relationships to include children but retain parental privacy • maintain working relationships with relatives that allow exposure to child(ren) • revitalize mutually satisfying sexual relations • allocate time and funds for spouses to get away occasionally and participate in social, community activities Rework family philosophy to: • see satisfaction in parenthood • value persons above things • establish healthy independence among members • resolve conflicts in developmental tasks of members and unit in constructive ways • accept help in a spirit of appreciation and growth

Table continued on following page.

TABLE 1-2 THE FAMILY LIFE CYCLE AND ASSOCIATED DEVELOPMENTAL TASKS (Continued)

Stage	Time Span	Individual/Positional Developmental Tasks	Family Group Developmental Tasks

Stage 3: *Family with Preschooler* (Oldest child 2½ to 5 years; usually one or two other children)	3½± years	Individual adults: expanding generativity (concern for children generally in the community, not just one's own)
		
		 Spouses: marital maintenance
		
		 Parents: nurturing children; learning to separate from children
		
		 Preschooler: initiative
		
		 Younger children: trust → autonomy
		
		 Siblings: adjustment to shared relationship with parents and to ordinal position roles
			Supplying adequate space, facilities, equipment for a larger and progressively more active family
			
			 Meeting predictable and unexpected costs of family life
			    more illness and health maintenance costs
			    home ownership costs
			
			 Maintaining satisfactory sexual relations, setting controls on family affectional behaviors (oedipal period), and planning for future children
			
			 Creating and maintaining effective communication that allows for the increasing expressive skills of the children and yet allows for individual privacy
			
			 Cultivating fuller relationships with relatives as resources to help impart cultural and familial values and enrichment between generations
			
			 Realistically apportioning responsibilities and home duties among members, including children but not overburdening any one member
			
			 Enjoying contacts outside home
			
			    Time away from each other
			
			    Time for developing individual friendships, interests

Stage 4: *Family with School Child* (Oldest child between 5 or 6 and 12; may have younger children in all developmental stages)	7± years	Individual adults: fostering a home atmosphere of love; continuing own development of skills; enlarging generativity to concern for all children in nation
		
		 Spouses: continue to satisfy each other as married persons
		
		 Parents: socialization and education of children; learning to accept rejection by school child without deserting him
		
		 School child: industry
		
		 Younger children trust → industry depending on age
		
		 Siblings: continued adjustment to shared relationships with parents and sibs and to occasional changes in ordinal position roles
			Reorganizing to adapt family living to expanding world of school-age child
			
			    Provide for children's activities and parents' privacy
			
			    "Let go" of school child so he can grow socially
			
			 Cooperation by all members to get things done
			
			 Participation in parent-child affairs/activities
			
			 Feeling close to relatives
			
			 Tying in with life outside the family (PTO, athletic groups, clubs)
			
			 Keeping financially solvent
			
			    Mother may go to work
			
			    Father may moonlight or hold two jobs
			
			 Effectively utilizing family communication
			
			    Time for each child to get individual attention
			
			    More verbal discussion of member differences
			
			    Try to see life through child's eyes
			
			    Increased effort for spouse companionship

TABLE 1-2 THE FAMILY LIFE CYCLE AND ASSOCIATED DEVELOPMENTAL TASKS (*Continued*)

Stage	Time Span	Individual/Positional Developmental Tasks	Family Group Developmental Tasks
THE MATURING FAMILY *Stage 5:* Family with Teenagers (Oldest child 13 until time he leaves home; may have children in all developmental stages)	7± years	Individual adults: keeping "up to date" while adjusting to realities of impending middle age; generativity evolved to concern for children throughout world Spouses: remaining compatible allies in the midst of developmental conflicts among family members Parents: balancing teen's freedom and responsibility; building a new life that allows release of young adults Teenager: identity; beginning emancipation from parents; establishing self with peers of both sexes Other children: trust → identity, depending on ages Siblings: adjusting to sharing of resources with sibs who have increased demands for them	Loosening family ties to allow readiness for releasing young adults in-the-making Provision of facilities for widely differing needs of members Assignment of greater responsibility and freedom to children in the division of labor and responsibility Keep communication systems open • allow nonjudgmental exchange of ideas among members • members keep themselves available to each other to listen and support • alter affectional guidelines among family members and with friends and dates • allow each member space for his private thoughts • maintain contact with extended family as a valuable support system Work out money conflicts during this period of escalated school and personal expenses • part-time jobs for children • reasonable allowances • democratically determined family budgeting Put marriage relationship into focus • spouses manage time alone and to get away together • get reaquainted, re-establishing common interests • reorganize social relations with peers
THE CONTRACTING FAMILY *Stage 6:* Family as Launching Center and Recruiter (Oldest child leaves home until last child leaves home)	6½± years	Individual adults: adjust to middle age; develop post-parental interests Spouses: rediscover each other as a couple and as friends Young adults: identity → intimacy Other children: trust →identity, depending on ages Siblings: adjusting to absence of other sibs from home and to changing availability of resources in the home once shared with sibs	Reorganize family to maintain unity while releasing matured and maturing children into lives of their own Rearranging physical facilities and resources in accordance with decreased need or use Managing income to meet costs during this peak expenditure period • determine how costs of college/marriage will be covered • plan for retirement expenses Reallocate responsibilities and household tasks among grown and growing children Widen family circle by recruiting new members through marriage of children Come to terms with selves as husband and wife • accept reality of gradual alterations in body appearance and function • adapt to menopausal changes • adjust to decreased vigor and health

Table continued on following page.

TABLE 1-2 THE FAMILY LIFE CYCLE AND ASSOCIATED DEVELOPMENTAL TASKS (Continued)

Stage	Time Span	Individual/Positional Developmental Tasks	Family Group Developmental Tasks
			Maintain open communication within family and the family members recruited • keep a secure home where children and their families are welcome • accept comfortably the way of life children choose • reconcile conflicting values and loyalties among members
Stage 7: *Family in the Middle Years* (Empty nest until retirement)	15± years	Individual adults: maintain activity that promotes self-fulfillment and moves one toward ego integrity Spouses: reignite conjugal relations; re-establish marital dyad Parents: accept separation and individuation of children as they establish their own families and colleagueships Grandparents: contribute to enrichment of grandchildren's concepts of life and to their historical roots	Re-emergence of the marital dyad Maintain a pleasant, comfortable home • share household responsibilities and decrease their number • reaffirm those values and routines that have meaning Assure security for later years while income is at its peak • provide for care of aging parent(s) • arrange for steady income after retirement • arrange for coverage of health costs that are predictable as aging occurs Keep a system of open communication within and outside of family unit • maintain links with older and younger generations • invest energy in new interests and peer relationships • participate in community life • keep in touch with siblings and aged parents • maintain periodic contact with grown children and their families • draw closer together as a couple
THE DECLINING FAMILY			
Stage 8: *Family in Later Years* (Retirement until death of one or both spouses)	16± years	Individual adults: ego integrity; learning ways to constructively deal with aging, loneliness, death Spouses: helping each other find life meaningful after retirement Grandparents/great grandparents: develop a feeling of kinship in warm, meaningful interactions that transmit the familial history and orientation	Adjust to and accept retirement Adjust to retirement income Establish comfortable household routines Find a satisfactory home for later years Face aging, loneliness, death and manage grief constructively Cope with final independence from own parents as they die Cope with final independence from spouse when he/she dies Accept own impending infirmity and death Maintain communication within and outside of family Nurture each other as spouses Maintain contact with children and their families Involve self with people and activities outside family (senior citizens groups, religious groups)

one's own rate, not on how precisely roles were defined in the family unit.[9]

The husband and wife roles that prevailed (and still do in homes that reflect a preindustrial or industrial character) before the 1970s described the wife's role as being expressive and integrative. She fulfilled that role if she kept the home in order and did most of the childrearing, healed the emotional wounds of family members and offered unconditional love. A husband's role was instrumental or task oriented. He complied with the description of his role if he maintained a position of final authority at home, resided as breadwinner and taskmaster and offered his love to members on a conditional basis that demanded respect for his contribution and authority in the family.

Postindustrial society added a role to the position of wife, primarily out of economic necessity, to allow her to hold at least a part-time job outside the home, but this role addition did not shift any of her other clearly defined tasks to the husband; it simply added one more task to those she already performed.

The shared role ideology that has emerged to accommodate the looser-knit "equalitarian" marriage of the late seventies involves sharing economic, household and childrearing tasks and responsibilities by both spouses. Although the loosely defined roles of this ideology produce tension (some strain exists in all roles, regardless of how well prescribed they are), they allow for much greater flexibility, creativity and general happiness among family members.[9, 19] There are many possible causes for role strain, and knowing the source of the conflict can aid the individual (with the nurse's help if she is involved) in abating the conflict. Common sources of role strain include:[15]

1. The role is acquired too quickly for the modification in self-concept to occur that is necessary for acceptance of the role. Many rituals have been developed to assist persons to adapt their self-concept more rapidly (bridal and baby showers, capping ceremonies).
2. The role demanded by a position is in conflict with a characteristic of the individual's personality, as when a man of mild temperament is placed in a position requiring assertiveness.
3. Conflicting pressures of the "middleman role" are present that make role fulfillment difficult (woman as arbitrator between her child's needs and her husband's demands).
4. A person has two antagonistic roles, making it difficult for adequate performance in either role (a woman who is both housewife and jobholder).
5. The role is incongruent with the person's emotional needs (an ill child who tries to continue carrying out his role as a child in his family).

How well a person resolves role conflicts or adjusts to a new role is largely determined by the quality and consistency of responses the role evokes, especially from the "significant others" in his life; how well his and his partner's roles complement each other; the extent to which the role either satiates his emotional needs or stimulates his creative tendencies and how much energy he invests in learning the role.

The following family role prescriptions are discussed here: spouse, mother, father, child, sibling and grandparent.

Being a Spouse

The condition of a marriage lays the foundation for the successes or failures in a family's development. Therefore, how well a man and a woman perform the role prescription of spouse is crucial to the family's well-being. Research related to measurement of marital success has illustrated that a spouse role prescription that bears the following features is most likely to produce happy, healthy interactions.[6, 7] Each spouse is able to accept affection from and express affection for the other, has confidence about the mate's fidelity and is committed to his own fidelity. Each spouse also displays a democratic or equalitarian attitude toward the other, performs sexually in a manner that satisfies both and exerts energy to maintain harmony with the spouse and to develop shared interests. The spouse's actions are judged with charity, attempt is made to remain attractive to the spouse through the years and each is committed to the permanence of the marriage. Communication is open and honest, offering outlet for both intellectual and emotional expression.

As most married couples will attest, achieving this role prescription requires hard work, and performance of the prescription must endure the ups and downs of daily living, obviously a task requiring maturity.

Being A Mother

The mother role is best performed when the mother combines those attitudes she learned from observation of and interaction with her own mother, the development of motherliness (a feeling of emotional bond with the child) and the acquisition of child care skills and some knowledge of child development. Enacting the mother role prescription effectively requires resolution of some basic conflicts inherent in being both a person and a mother.[15] Some of these basic conflicts include: (1) the idealized mother projected by mass media onto the woman's own fantasies about motherhood against her feelings of inadequacy as a mother; (2) vacillation between her own need to be dependent and the need to be independent and responsible; (3) love for versus resentment of the child; (4) demands made by the child for her love and energy versus those made by her husband and (5) self-actualization versus successful motherhood.

From the arbitration of these conflicts, the modern mother carries out a role prescription characterized by either *providing* or *obtaining* child care that satisfies the child's growing needs and enhances his development. She also allocates time with her child(ren) that emphasizes quality rather than quantity. Her role involves allowing her child(ren) enough freedom to develop autonomy, initiative and independence; supporting him when he succeeds and when he fails; permitting her child to experience life and the continuum of feelings associated with living fully and providing a role model of acceptable adult behaviors.

Margaret Mead summed up the mother role prescription when she said, "Every act of motherhood contains a dual intent, as the mother holds the child close and prepares it to move away from her, as she supports the child and stands it firmly on its own feet, as she guards it against danger and sends it out across the yard. Unless a mother can do both — gather her child close and turn her child out toward the world — she will fail in her purpose."[14]

Being A Father

To be more human, more responsive and more fully functional is a freedom being offered men by equality of the sexes that will surely add gratification to and complement the role of father. The new measures of a man's masculinity are no longer based on sexual exploits or stoic unemotionalism but on how he manages his life, whether his conduct with other people recognizes his and their humanness, his ability to make decisions and how perceptive he is as to the consequences of those decisions.[9] Measuring up to this yardstick of manliness supports rather than compromises his effectiveness as a father. In fact, it is my contention that, within the next generation, one will speak of being a parent rather than being a mother or a father, because of the blending of role prescriptions that will by then be desirable.

A man's role prescription as a father can, by today's emerging standards, reflect his manliness. That prescription involves his role as a beloved friend and teacher to his child and a stimulating source for awakening the emotional potential in his child. His father role requires that he be a model of mature social and vocational behavior, an ego ideal for masculine love, ethics and morality and a protector and counselor as his child develops. The father's role, like the mother's, is best performed when it

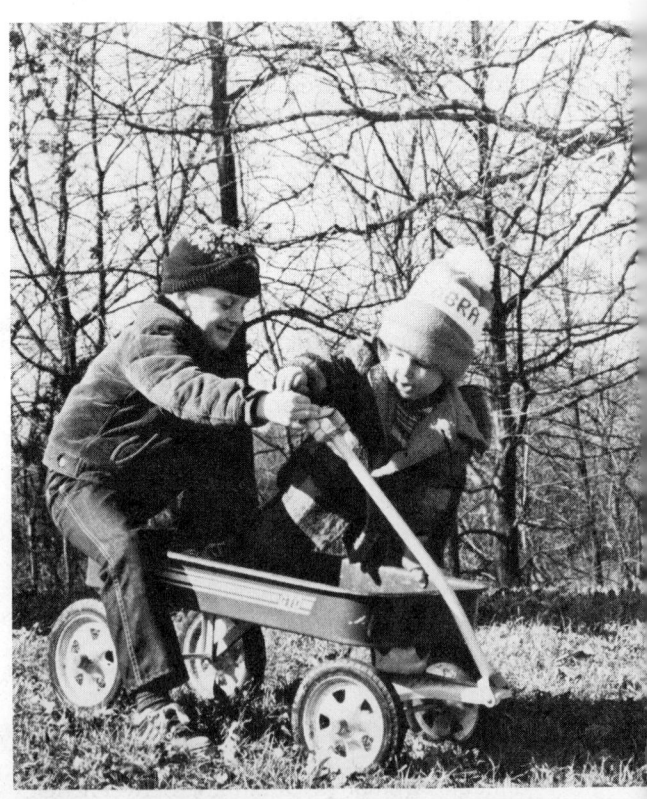

A feature all siblings have in common is that they must learn to share.

blends the attitudes he learned from observing and interacting with his own father, the development of fatherliness (a feeling of emotional bond with his child, more easily achieved when he has been actively involved at all stages of the pregnancy and birth) and the acquisition of child care skills and some knowledge of growth and development.

The shared role ideology permits a fluidity between the mother role and father role that allows the two people involved in parenting to exchange components of the two role prescriptions, without fear of personal or social reprisal, as family need or circumstance demands and on either a temporary or permanent basis. Since no society has yet devised a foolproof system within which all men and women become equally felicitous and satisfactory parents for all their children, this ideology is a contemporary solution in the individual's and family's best interests.

Being A Child

Although a child's role in the family is not static, there are some aspects of his role prescription that remain constant. The child role requires behaviors that will result in acquisition of (1) a psychic structure that produces a secure identity and constructive self-esteem, (2) skills for independent functioning, (3) an education and (4) experience in peer relationships.[2] Other components of the child role prescription fluctuate depending on the child's age and the techniques of parenting with which he must cope. The age-related role prescriptions of being a child are discussed in those chapters that correspond to each age.

Being A Sibling

Every child in a family learns different lessons about himself and about life depending on his ordinal position (eldest, middle, youngest child), his sex, the age span between him and his sibs, whether or not he was a planned or wanted child and the socioeconomic state of the family at his birth. But beyond all the prescription features unique to his sibling role, every sibling has a feature in common with his brothers and sisters: he must learn to share. He has to learn to share his parents, his toys, his space and what seems to him to be his entire world with his siblings. The younger he is, the more conflict this sharing involves. The wider the age span between him and his sibling(s), the less threat his sib prescription to share creates for him.

Being A Grandparent

Although the majority of families do not house the grandparents, the parents do, at intervals, either visit or bring to their home these special people in a child's life. The role prescription of grandparents — "to teach their grandchildren how the whole of life is lived to its conclusion . . . by a readiness to run each day, each week, each year a new and untried course" — provides the grandchild with one of the richest experiences of his childhood.[14]

Grandparenting tends to be characterized by two styles of interaction.[11] One style is the indulgent grandparent who seeks pleasure and enjoyment from grandchildren. The other style is portrayed in grandparents who remain aloof, preferring infrequent contact, usually during holidays or ritual occasions. Whichever the style, the grandparents should keep in mind the

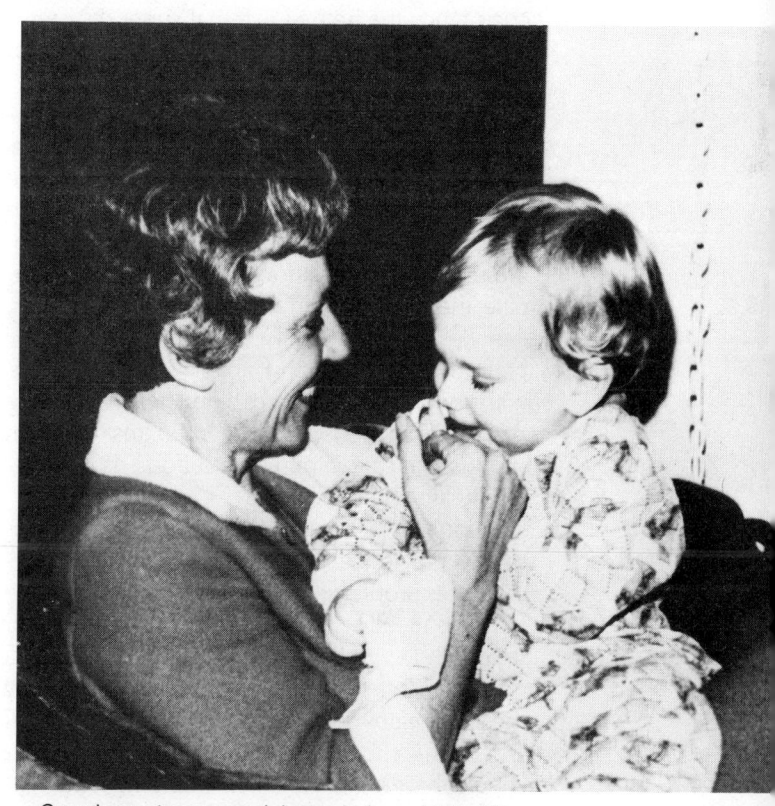

Grandparents are special people in a child's life.

FAMILY GROWTH AND DEVELOPMENT

parents' primary position with their children and be aware of those rules of childrearing that the parents do not want breached under any circumstances. Grandparents also may serve, at least temporarily, as parent surrogates during intervals when the parents seek further education or experience illness. The role may be more enduring in cases in which there is divorce or if the grandparents are providing child care for dual-career spouses' children.[11]

FAMILY LIVING: AN ADAPTIVE PROCESS

Family living is an adaptive process that involves establishing an equilibrium between the family's integrative features (strengths) and its disruptive aspects (limitations). When family members' strengths predominate in their daily living, they evidence capacity and motivation to successfully master their individual and family group developmental tasks. When the family's strengths waiver because of disruptive events (role conflict, loss of a support system, maturational changes, accidental interruptions such as illness), its members experience a period of crisis when the help of external support systems (extended family, community agencies, health professionals) may be needed.

The nurse who understands the roles, functions and tasks of families and the changes inherent in periods of transition from one life stage to another can be useful to families in times of crisis. During periods of equilibrium, the nurse with this knowledge base can anticipate the needs of families and their members, can help them identify ways to satisfactorily perform their roles and adapt to role changes with minimal stress, can help them recognize their present and potential strengths and can support their developmental efforts as a growing, healthy family unit.

During times of crisis the nurse can apply this same knowledge base to help the family surmount its problem(s). By assessing how well the family is meeting its own and society's goals for it and how well the family is achieving its developmental tasks, the nurse can identify those strengths in the family that can be organized to combat the problem. These strengths should be drawn on when planning interventions. Family members and their support systems should be included in the planning process and ways to involve other potential resources should be devised. The nurse's intervention measures should include support to family members as they apply their strengths and resources to the problem, and positive reinforcement for attempts to develop latent strengths should be offered. The evaluative process is an opportunity for the nurse to help the family accept the fact that sometimes help is needed and that seeking help at those times is itself a strength. It also affords the nurse the opportunity to help family members determine how this crisis has prepared them to handle future crises by sharpening or adding to their store of strengths.

Hopefully, this chapter has helped the reader to see that family life at its best fulfills a human need not fully met by any other arrangement or institution and that the family remains, despite all its limitations, the most powerful influence in the lives of most of us.

References

1. P. Aries. Centuries of Childhood. Alfred A. Knopf, Inc., 1962.
2. R. Blanch and G. Blanch. Marriage and Personal Development. Columbia University Press, 1968
3. P. Chinn. Child Health Maintenance: Concepts in Family-Centered Care, 2nd edition. C.V. Mosby Co., 1980
4. R. Coser. The Family: Its Structures and Functions. St. Martin's Press, 1974
5. E. Duvall. Marriage and Family Development. J. B. Lippincott Co., 1977
6. J. Fawcett. The family as a living open system: an emerging conceptual framework for nursing. International Nursing Review, October 1975, p. 113
7. D. Goldstine, et al. The three stages of marriage. Family Circle, 3 May 1977, p. 10
8. E. Gottschalk, Jr. Exploding the myths about the American family. Family Circle, 13 December 1977, p. 72
9. L. Howe, editor. The Future of the Family. Simon & Schuster, Inc., 1972
10. D. Hymovich and M. Barnard. Family Health Care: General Perspectives, Volume 1. McGraw-Hill Book Co., 1979
11. D. Hymovich and M. Barnard. Family Health Care: Developmental and Situational Crises, Volume 2. McGraw-Hill Book Co., 1979
12. K. Keniston and the Carnegie Council on Children. All Our Children: The American Family Under Pressure. Harcourt Brace Jovanovich, Inc., 1977
13. K. Leahy, M. Cobb and M. Jones. Community Health Nursing. McGraw-Hill Book Co., 1972
14. M. Mead and K. Heyman. Family. Macmillan, Inc., 1965
15. A. Reinhardt and M. Quinn. Family-Centered Community Nursing: A Sociocultural Framework. C.V. Mosby Co., 1973
16. D. Schulz. The Changing Family: Its Functions and Future. Prentice-Hall Inc., 1976

17. J. Simpson. The American Family: A History in Photographs. Viking Press, 1976
18. E. Sobol and P. Robischon. Family Nursing: A Study Guide. C.V. Mosby Co., 1975
19. J. Tapia. The Nursing process in family health. Nursing Outlook, April 1972
20. C. Tinkham and E. Voorhies. Community Health Nursing: Evolution and Process. Appleton-Century-Crofts, 1972
21. A. Toffler. Future Shock. Random House, Inc., 1970
22. M. Young and P. Willmott. The Symmetrical Family. Pantheon Books, 1973

Additional Recommended Reading

D. Hymovich and M. Barnard. Family Health Care. McGraw-Hill Book Co., 1973

C. Kirkpatrick. The Family as Process and Institution. Ronald Press, 1963

D. Papilia and S. Olds. Human Development. McGraw-Hill Book Co., 1978

D. Sutterley and G. Donnelly. Perspectives in Human Development: Nursing Throughout the Life Cycle. J. B. Lippincott Co., 1973

2 INFLUENTIAL FACTORS IN FAMILY LIVING

by Cheryl E. Easley, AM, RN
and Carol M. Easley, AM, RN

An examination of factors that are influential in family life requires that we first gain a perspective of the nature of the family, the nature of the environment and the nature of the interaction between the two. The family may be considered as a system. It is an open system, since it has the ability to exchange matter and energy with its environment. For instance, the family takes in food and clothing and gives off items produced through family enterprise, and refuse. The family also produces children who are eventually released into the larger society as workers. In addition, the family exchanges energy with its environment. Emotional energies such as patriotism, community pride and "feeling tones" such as the "Christmas spirit" are a few examples. The family contributes energy to the environment as it develops and enacts its particular life style. Compare the different feeling tone produced in a community by a family that makes a special effort to help other community residents to that of a family that is continually quarrelling with its neighbors. Since the family can be said to consist not only of a group of individual members but also of the interactions between these members, it is more than and different from the sum of its parts.

The family environment is anything external to the family unit. It includes other people, the material world, and nonmaterial factors such as social systems, institutions, political structures and value systems, to name a few. The family and the environment are constantly in a state of mutual interaction in which both are simultaneously shaping and being shaped. Each individual family has arrived at its present condition through a process of development and interaction with the environment through time. In addition, the family as a social institution has been shaped by a long historical process of interaction with other social institutions down through the ages.

As families interact with their particular environments, there exists a range of possible outcomes, or end results, for both the family and the environment. Some of these potential outcomes are positive and some are negative. If nursing is viewed as a science, the goal is to produce knowledge that will allow us to make predictions. Through a study of the family and the environment with which it interacts, we hope to increase our ability to predict the outcomes of this interaction. Knowledge of outcomes will aid us in making nursing judgments and planning and evaluating nursing interventions.

THE NATURE OF THE FAMILY

Family Structure

Much is heard today of the changing structure of the American family — the shift from extended to nuclear family as society has changed over time from agrarian to industrial and from an industrial to a postindustrial era. The increasing mobility of families, both geographically and socially, the trend toward urbanism and suburbanism, changes in the role of women and contraction of living space have all contributed to the prevalence and functionality of the nuclear family. More recently, statistics have seemed to challenge the primacy of the nuclear family. In addition, studies of diverse cultural groups have revealed the importance of other family forms. Even families that seemed to fit the nuclear pattern are found to have created social support systems among neighbors and friends that are strongly reminiscent of the extended family.

In assessing families, it is important to view them from a perspective of their strengths. No family should automatically be considered weak or fragmented simply because it does not fit the traditional nuclear mode. A much more useful approach is to view the family as it functions within its environment in terms of its internal interaction. The outcomes and process of family functions must be placed within the context of the family's values, goals and cultural milieu.

Space and Time

Each family, like each individual, exists in a four-dimensional matrix of space and time. How the family structures and is influenced by these factors is the subject of this section.

There are a number of vantage points from which to study family space. One might consider the amount of personal space required by each individual member, the availability, perceived adequacy and use of household space, and the extent to which the family or its members or both extend spatially into the neighborhood, the community and the world.

Each individual person has need for a certain amount of space over which he maintains territorial control. Invasion of this territory by others against his will can lead to feelings of anxiety, resentment or hostility. A common example of this is the fact that many family members occupy specific seats at the dinner table and experience distress if these places are usurped by others without their consent. The amount of space one perceives himself to require is probably related to many factors, including age, culture and family characteristics. Personal space needs determine the amount of physical distance the person needs to maintain in his interaction with others. Territorial dominance needs relate to the extent of space over which a person desires to maintain control, such as a bedroom or an office. Since a family is made up of interacting individuals with differing spatial requirements, these concerns may be potential sources of conflict. Many adolescents, for instance, pass through a developmental period when the need for privacy and control of their own bedroom is greatly valued and fiercely defended, a situation that may lead to clashes with siblings or parents.

The structuring of space in the family home is dependent on several factors. A major consideration is the amount of space available in relation to the number of persons who must occupy it. The trend of increasing urbanization and the evolution of the nuclear family have led to decreases in the number and size of the rooms in many family dwellings. The large rambling farm house with its spacious grounds has for many families given way to the compact urban apartment. Certainly, economic factors play a major part in the amount of living space the family occupies.

Among the very poor the number of persons in the household can exceed the number of rooms in the dwelling; members may be obliged to share bedrooms or beds or both with multiple roommates or may even sleep in the living room or kitchen. There may be no place in the house where a person can be entirely alone during much or all of the day. Limited opportunities for privacy in such instances may have an effect on the ability of family members to study or concentrate and may also have an impact on the sexual behavior of the parental pair. In some cases the family must share certain household facilities, such as the kitchen or the bathroom, with other families, a situation that may lead to inconvenience and stress.

On the other end of the spectrum are affluent families who may be able to provide multiple rooms per person. In some homes abundant space can be used as a barrier for isolation from interaction with other family members. Between these two extremes lie the vast majority of families in the United States, with varying degrees of available living space. The perception and use of this space is of more importance to the family than the absolute amount of space available. The structuring of space, which the family does by arrangement of furnishings and by designation of certain areas for certain purposes, is crucial.

Another important factor is the family members' feeling of ownership or personal responsibility for their dwelling and its environs. Apathetic or negative reactions to their housing can lead to family demoralization and inadequate upkeep of the home. The importance of the family domicile as it relates to family integrity cannot be overemphasized. It is against this background that the drama of collective family interaction is played out. The shape of that interaction is in part determined by the space that the family occupies.

The final aspect of family space involves the extension of the family into the larger society. Not only the size of the family's home but its location plays a part in influencing the nature and quality of family life. Moves by many families to different regions and from urban to rural settings or vice versa can lead to feelings of rootlessness and alienation, unless the families become adept at establishing support systems in their new communities. In both urban and rural settings there exist advantages and disadvantages with which the family must cope.

While some families seem to be quite adventurous and value travel and exploration of novel and fascinating regions, others tend to remain close to familiar locations. Finances influence the extent of family mobility, but this is not the sole consideration. It is possible that families in large cities such as New York have never seen neighborhoods that might be only a subway ride away. Travel to distant areas or outings to a park or recreational facility nearby are possibilities that the nurse can suggest to these families. Such activities offer opportunities for shared relaxation, learning and sheer fun that serve to strengthen family ties and provide memories to be cherished.

Consideration of family space characteristics should be included in the nursing assessment, plan and intervention. The following questions may be relevant: (1) What are the perceived spatial needs of individual family members and to what extent are these being met? (2) What is the relationship of the amount of living space to the size of the family group? (3) Does the family perceive this space as being adequate? (4) If there is a lack of space, does this represent a problem to the functioning of the family or its members? (5) Is space organized and used to promote or inhibit family interaction? (6) Is the allocation of space a source of conflict for the family? (7) Are there areas in the home for both privacy and family togetherness? (8) Do members tend to congregate in certain areas for common or individual pursuits? (9) What is the family's perception of and level of satisfaction with its home area and neighborhood? (10) How does the family interact with neighbors? (11) Does the family take advantage of opportunities to explore the community and utilize its resources? (12) Do its members extend themselves to whatever degree possible into the larger society?

The impact of time on family life can be studied from a number of perspectives. A historical consideration of the family can serve to document the evolution of family structure, function and interaction in a general sense through the varying epochs of human civilization. Historical changes have impinged upon the timing of family events by providing the institutional or social conditions under which such transitions can be implemented or impeded.[9] An example of this is the movement of children out of the home at approximately six years of age as a result of compulsory education. It may also be of interest in some contexts to trace the development of a particular family through time in the manner of the genealogist. This approach to family study has recently grown in popularity as a result of the well-known book and television series *Roots,* which sent many in search of the story of their family origins.

A more intimate view of the relationship of time to the family may be gained by placement of the family as a whole and its individual members on their respective life-cycle continua. The family has basic tasks to perform, some of which are always required, such as the provision of shelter and physical care for its members. In addition, it has developmental tasks (stage-critical tasks) which are crucial to its function and cohesion at specific stages of its growth. An example of such a stage-critical task is the need for the family with teenage children to achieve balance between dependence and independence as their adolescents mature and strive for autonomy.[5] One can also readily understand that the developmental tasks implied for a married couple with school-age children will differ markedly from those of a middle-aged family whose youngest child is about to marry. From a slightly different stance, an understanding of individual stage-critical tasks enables one to differentiate the needs of the teenage couple facing a first pregnancy from those of a couple at the same phase of family development who are in their mid-thirties. (See Chapter 1 for a review of family developmental tasks.)

It is also important to be aware of recent changes in the onset and length of various phases of the family life cycle, such as the increasing postponement of marriage by women and the lengthening of the empty nest phase.[7,8] These changes in family timing have a profound effect on the lives of individuals and families in general. For instance, the prolongation of postchildrearing years means that more middle-aged women may be free to enter the labor market for longer periods of time than was previously the case. It also means that couples have more years to spend alone together and are more likely to share in the lifetimes of their grandchildren.[9]

Other systems affect families in terms of time. Work or school, because they demand or purchase time, can determine the amount of time that family members control. This is a factor of major importance as the family attempts to structure the temporal aspects of its life.[19]

A major concern with regard to the increasing number of working mothers continues to be the demand on the quantity and quality of their time contribution to the family. Advocates of the needs and rights of women to pursue career goals with the same intensity as men emphasize the relatively greater importance of the quality of time spent with family and children than the quantity of such time. In some families the perceived obligation of the male parent to contribute time to child care and other home duties is being considered as more or less equal to that of the woman.

In circumstances in which the father works some distance from home, as is the case in many suburban families, a good portion of his time may be expended in travel, thus limiting available family time. Some more affluent parents may also restrict family contact during summer months by sending children to camp for extended stays or by obtaining summer residences for the mother and children, with the father taking the role of weekend visitor.

It is possible also for the family to have an effect on the time structuring of the larger society. The impact of the family on timing in the educational system can be seen, for example, in the nine-month school year, a schedule originated to accommodate farm families who required the labor of their children during the summer months. This pattern has been consistently retained in a nonagrarian context to provide a time for family vacations and recreational activities.

An interesting view of the relationship between family size and time economics has been proposed by Sawhill.[22] In underdeveloped agricultural societies children are seen as workers, future producers of income for parents. This valuation of children as workers leads to high fertility rates, since parents are willing to invest time in childrearing. In the more industrialized nations children are expected to supply future satisfactions in much the same manner as does a house or car. Children are not an economic asset in such societies; on the other hand, time has great personal and monetary value. The amount of time necessary for childrearing has led to a reduction in family size. Also, various alternatives to expenditure of parental time with children, such as day care centers and entertainment devices like television and records, have come into general use.

Families structure time for their members in three ways: they orient members to past, present and future; they develop regulatory patterns

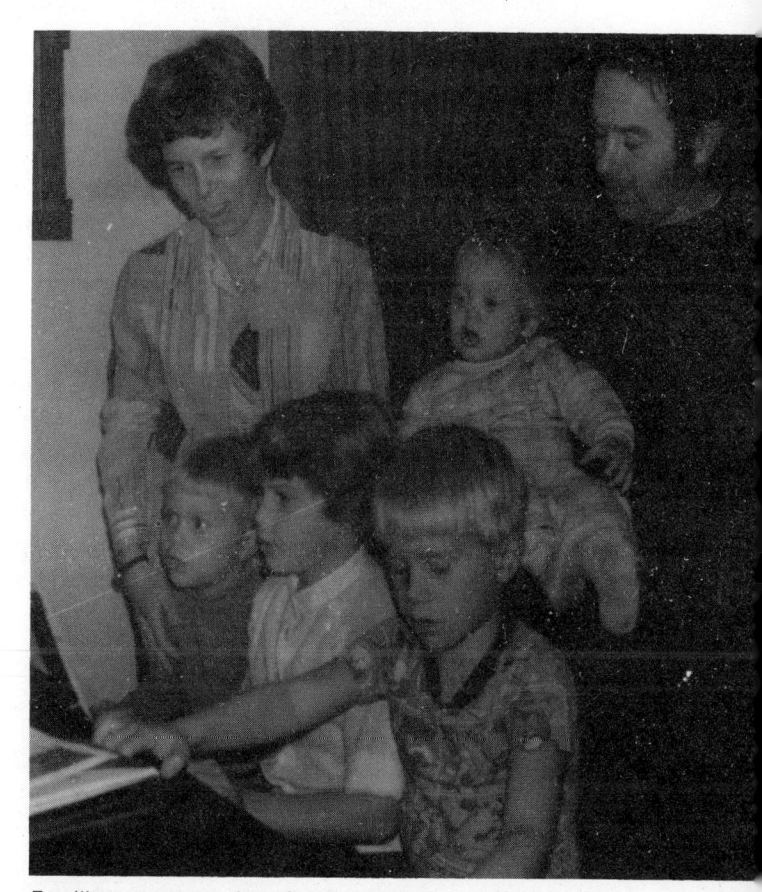

Families structure time for their members. Strong families plan frequent joint activities.

INFLUENTIAL FACTORS IN FAMILY LIVING

for the sequence, frequency, duration and pace of family activities and they establish guidelines for the evaluation of the use of time as either constructive or wasteful.[6] A study of the relationship characteristics of strong families found the allocation of time for family interaction to be a major factor. Such families were noted to actively plan for joint activities and to limit those that cut into time spent together. Meals and leisure pursuits were family events, and it was obvious that a high value was placed on family time.[25]

There are a number of important time-related assessments that the nurse can make in her work with a family. The nurse should obtain a comprehensive view of how family time is structured: (1) In what types of activities is the family together and how much time is used for them? (2) Are meals, recreation or religious occasions a time for family interaction? (3) Are there periods during the day for quiet or private communion between husband and wife, parent and child or for individual solitude? (4) What value do the family members seem to place on time and how are they oriented to its use? (5) Are they extremely relaxed or very compulsive in their modes of responding to time commitments? (6) How much freedom is accorded individual family members to schedule their own personal activities? (7) Is there satisfaction or dissatisfaction in the family concerning its overall use of time? The answers to these questions will aid the nurse in assessing the effect of time on family function. According to one view, areas of potential problems affecting families in modern society such as effects of urbanization and excessive time devoted to watching television and commuting are "basically problems of time rather than problems of interpersonal competence, and time structuring holds the solution to these problems.[27]"

Family Communication

Many who study communication begin with the assumption that when people interact communication is inevitable.[3,24] The need to be involved in communication characterizes most humans and is also seen in the animal and perhaps even the plant world. Since the family provides the primary orientation to and training for communication and since communication is critical to family functioning, it is necessary to include an assessment of communication patterns in the provision of nursing care.

Families communicate verbally and nonverbally. The characteristic patterns through which this takes place are in some ways unique to each individual family and bear the imprint of cultural, educational and interpersonal aspects of the family's experience. Appalachian families, for example, have been noted to use relatively little verbal communication because value is placed on actions rather than words.[17] For other families verbal messages may predominate and members may feel inhibited in the nonverbal expression of attitudes or emotions. When the nurse interacts with families and observes their communication patterns, she may tend to assess and understand these behaviors in the light of her own particular cultural and familial orientation. Thus it may be easy for her to misunderstand or misinterpret what is happening in a situation unless she is sensitive not only to the content but also to the meanings that are attached to the communication by the participants.

Stinnett's study of strong families revealed positive communication to be a major factor in their makeup. Parents in these families were noted to share time and activities with their children and to engage in active listening. Positive verbal messages and the expression of appreciation characterized their communication. Conflict was handled by discussion and mutual problem identification.[25] Families experiencing interactional problems often exhibit communication patterns that are negative in content, confusing, contradictory or restricted. The members may share comments that are mainly of a complaining or devaluing nature. They may confuse each other by giving incongruent messages on verbal and nonverbal levels: a mother may give her child a verbal command that her behavior implies he need not obey. The communication may be contradictory, leading to anxiety and uncertainty on the part of the person to whom it is directed. For example, children may be instructed not to resort to the use of falsehoods, whereas they observe the parents in the act of prevarication. Parents may limit their opportunities for communication through the employment of physical distancing maneuvers or by restricting the amount of time spent with the family.

Families can differ tremendously in the ways

they communicate nonverbally. For some the physical expression of affection is ongoing, spontaneous and unlimited with regard to age or family position. In these families, for example, it may be a commonly accepted practice for the father to embrace his teenage son. In other families any physical contact beyond a handshake may have been restricted between father and son after the son achieved school age. Families may also vary in the ways in which they express feelings symbolically through behaviors such as gift giving or locking doors.

Geographical mobility of families has meant that many may be isolated from extended family or kinship groups. This has necessitated the use of long-distance communication devices such as letters, telephone calls, and mailed tape recordings as families attempt to maintain contact. In addition to internal communication, families must also communicate effectively with the external environment if they are to survive and progress. It may be of interest to note which family member is designated to act as spokesman for the family in certain situations. Some families seem quite adept at dealing with various social institutions such as the school or the economic system and are able to realize their goals in relation to these structures. For other families these skills may be lacking.

Another problem in communication is often experienced by immigrant families who may not speak English or by United States families with regional or cultural speech patterns that differ from those of the community with which they interact.

A need may be indicated in these situations for the professional nurse to enact the advocate role to ensure that families and agencies or systems are communicating in such a way that family needs are recognized and met and that family rights and responsibilities are protected.

FAMILY ENVIRONMENT

Family Economics

Finances "One of the obvious and most basic facts about marriage in the United States is that for perhaps 98 per cent of families there will never be enough money."[23] It has been said that as a worldwide trend, most people feel that they could be financially secure if their income were increased by 25 per cent. As incomes rise for United States families, their perceived needs also rise, and with increased affluence, spending and indebtedness increase rapidly. Thus higher-income families tend to be more in debt than do middle- or lower-income families. Much of this debt results from attempts to meet the family's demands for more and better goods and services. The general affluence of society, the ready supply of luxury items and services and constant advertising pressure that creates artificial needs combine to generate an almost irresistible urge to acquire. The general lack of expertise in financial management means that for most families financial distress may be present to some degree all of the time. It has been estimated that during the husband's lifetime approximately half a million dollars will pass through the hands of the typical United States middle class family, and yet most of the time the family will be experiencing financial problems. Without skills in preparing and maintaining a budget, most families have limited knowledge of how their money flows or how they could improve their money management.[23]

Money is the most frequent subject of quarrelling among married couples, and economic instability is a major cause of marital failure. Effective handling of personal finances, along with sexual harmony and satisfactory food man-

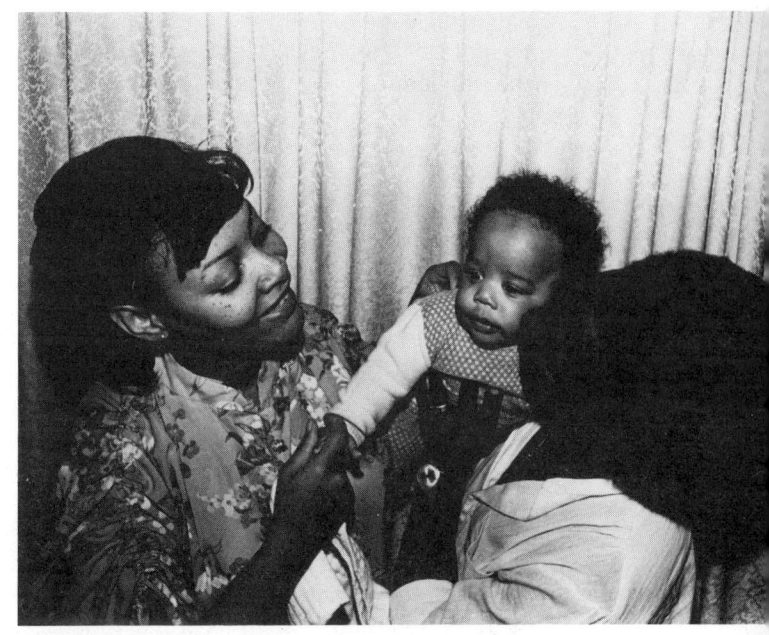

Families differ in the way they communicate affection nonverbally.

agement, is one of the three major areas that are critical to marital success. Another aspect of the problem is that approximately one in seven families in the United States is in such financial distress that its major concern is bare subsistence.[23]

Saxton sees three major areas of economic conflict arising in families after the birth of the first child. The couple is in conflict over bills, over the allocation of limited resources and over power. The arrival of a child means that there are basic expenditures that the family must make. Arguing and bitterness may occur as the family strives to pay its bills. Personal expenditure becomes a source of conflict as each partner vies to meet his or her individual needs within the limited available resources. If the wife gives up her job to care for the child, there is a realignment of power in the marriage with the control of cash as its primary focus. All of these factors produce strain in the marital relationship.[23]

The consequences of poor financial management are obvious: discord, lack of family cohesiveness and inability to provide high-quality health maintenance services for family members. Nurses have often been reluctant to involve themselves in the financial situations of the families they serve. With increasing acceptance of holistic ideas of health care, nurses must begin to view their role as one of involvement with the total family in all major aspects of its life process. The nurse must be aware of the interaction of family economics with other factors critical to family health and welfare. Family financial assessment is an important part of the nurse's data-gathering. As many community health nurses can attest, a frequent problem identified by the families they visit is that of financial distress. This distress is not limited to lower-income families, but is particularly felt among middle class families as well. Nurses must utilize their knowledge of available community resources to refer the family appropriately for help.

Poverty The Census Bureau has specified the poverty line so that family income should be sufficient to provide an adequate diet. The line is defined in relationship to the number of family members and is adjusted each year to the cost-of-living index. Twelve per cent of the total population is below the poverty line and 43 per cent of this low-income group is made up of racial and ethnic minorities. These poor families are more likely to live in urban or rural areas than are the nonpoor. They tend to be characterized by lack of education, high unemployment rates, families that are larger and headed by females, residential crowding and lack of adequate bathroom facilities. The poor are five times more likely than the nonpoor to perceive their health status as only fair or poor. Poverty and minority status are inversely related to life expectancy. Those residents in poverty areas show higher crude death rates for tuberculosis and homicide than residents in nonpoverty areas. Infant mortality rates among certain ethnic minorities, namely blacks and native Americans, remain significantly higher than the rates for whites and Asian Americans, despite an overall decrease in infant mortality rates in past years.[10]

As the nurse plans to provide services to families that are poor, she should be aware of the special health problems that may be implied. She must know the relationship between lack of adequate income and the family's inability to provide itself with resources to maintain and restore health. When subsistence is a problem, health is not a primary family goal. When the family is struggling to pay the rent and provide food, clothing and other basic necessities, the parents may not be vitally interested in keeping the children's immunizations up to date, especially when this involves long waits, paternalistic and condescending attitudes displayed by health care providers and transportation problems that a public clinic visit often entails. Nurses who are white, middle class females need to constantly remember that their values are different from those of the poor families they serve, to avoid the labelling and blaming that often result when the nurse evaluates the family's behavior in light of her value system.

Another facet of nursing care for poor families is *advocacy*. The nurse who assumes the advocate role represents the family's interests as it seeks to cope with the health and welfare systems. In this role the nurse perceives herself as primarily accountable to the family rather than to an institution or agency. Intervention by the nurse-advocate is often vital to the effective functioning of the poor family. Faced with a bewildering array of health and social welfare agencies, the family is often at a loss as to how to proceed. A nurse with the ability to coordinate the family's interaction with the health department, Big Brothers or Big Sisters, and the many offices of governmental social service departments such as Protective Services and Aid for Families with Dependent Children (AFDC), performs an invaluable service.

In a larger sense the nurse may act as advocate for poor families by her participation in the political process. Individually and collectively, nurses may actively support legislation to ameliorate the social and economic stresses affecting poor families while concomitantly affirming the dignity of each family and maintaining family integrity. Political action is necessary at local, state and federal levels by nurses who have knowledge of the legislative process and skill in the application of pressure to gain political ends.

Work The world of work and the world of the family are usually not in contact with each other. While those researchers working with families are very aware of the impact of work on the family, there has been very little recognition of this impact by organizations.[21] Employers are only recently beginning to notice the effect of the family on workers' effectiveness and to appreciate how the work situation affects the total family.

Although work and family situations may sometimes be mutually supportive, at other times they are in conflict.[21] The demands of the workplace may create severe strains on family relationships. In most traditional nuclear families, the father spends more time at work than with the family. In fact, if a man desires to reduce his interaction with the family, he may use work as an excuse to withdraw.[8]

Shift work can produce a variety of problems for the family, depending on the particular shift that is worked. Working the night shift can increase friction between the marital pair, while afternoon work can lead to conflict over family roles. Alternating work on afternoon and night shifts may lead to the inability to establish regular eating and sleeping patterns. Night work leads to a decreased social life but increases time available for housework and child care. For those who want isolation, shift work often provides relief from family and community responsibilities.[12]

The demands of the job often present problems for families. Transfers, promotions and work-related travel may all subject the family to stress.[12, 21] Transfers uproot the family and may cause life style alterations. Children must leave neighborhood and school friends and establish new social ties. This often involves a temporary loss of status for the child. While the father may have a slightly easier transition, since he fits into an organizationally structured niche, the nonworking mother will, like the children, be faced with making new friends and seeking a place in a new community network. Promotion also demands a change in life style. The entertaining demands on the couple are often increased, leaving less time for parent-child interaction. If the husband is promoted to a high position or elected to high political office, the wife often assumes the role of "corporate" or "political" wife. She is increasingly drawn into the husband's occupational sphere, a situation that places severe demands on her time and adds stress that relates to the projection of the correct wifely image. All of this detracts from time available for parenting. Even if the demands on the mother are not excessive, the occupational requirements for some fathers are so high that the mother often pursues a life style like that of a single parent.[12]

Extensive work-related travel leads to changes in family roles and functions. The responsibilities of the mother are markedly increased. Fathers experience guilt and travel fatigue. An important effect is that the father misses first-hand knowledge of significant family experiences. Prolonged absence may lead to marital infidelity, and the lack of experiences and information shared as a couple may cause strain in communication, even when both partners remain faithful. In some families the mother and children close ranks, leaving the father out, and his re-entry may pose problems.[12, 21]

The trend toward upward mobility is pressing more and more people into the middle class. The rise in status carries an associated increase in consumption, which locks the family into work. The more a family consumes materially, the more the parents are committed to the work setting. This means that there is less emotional energy available for family disposal. As a reaction, the family turns to material consumption to compensate for the emotional void. This leads to further dependence on work to procure the material goods that the family now demands.[8, 21] An important result of the increase in material consumption by the family and rising inflation in contemporary society is the trend for more and more mothers to enter the labor force. Once the children are in school, the majority of women living with their husbands take jobs. Since the early 1950s wives with children have been more likely to work than are those with none. The numbers of working mothers with children under 3 years of age is increasing rapidly. Two-thirds of working mothers work full time.[4]

Younger mothers (those under 25), often with young children, are frequently found in the workplace. Many of these women have husbands who earn low wages. Most of the working mothers tend to have at least a high school education. Of course, those without this minimal educational level also need employment, but they have poor success in the labor market and tend to secure extremely low-paying jobs that are often undesirable. As a result, it may not be financially worthwhile for these women to work in light of employment-related costs such as transportation, child care, lunches and appropriate clothing. In addition, increased income taxation may negate any earnings that the mother realizes. So, although these women are likely to be in families with incomes below the poverty line, the family does not benefit financially from their working.[4]

Middle- and high-income mothers are also showing an increasing pattern of employment. Many in this group are single parents who, as a result of death or divorce, must work to maintain the family's standard of living.[4] Women drawn into the labor market after years of household tasks and child care are often at an educational and psychological disadvantage and may need counselling and emotional support.

When mothers work, child care becomes a problem. Although ideally both parents are equally involved in child care, in reality the mother is usually the main caretaker. Substitute child care usually falls far short of the need, unfortunately. Millions of children under 6 come home to empty houses from kindergarten or day care. Millions in the school-age group are also "latch-key" children. Bronfenbrenner associates this with academic and behavioral problems in children, as well as reading difficulties, high drop-out rates, drug use and juvenile delinquency.[4]

How can the detrimental effects of work on family life be ameliorated? The 1970 White House Conference on Children and Youth recommended that employers recognize the impact of work on families and strive to change occupational demands in ways that will strengthen family ties.[21] Nurses may have an advocate role in interpreting family needs to employers when appropriate. Family and work interaction is a significant factor in family assessment. The nurse must investigate the work roles of both parents and seek to ascertain how such roles affect the parents as individuals, their marital functioning and their parenting experiences. Awareness of work-related stresses can aid the nurse in helping the family to identify potential problem areas and to plan preventive strategies. Referrals to social and educational agencies is a typical nursing intervention when the problem is economic, and referrals can be a valuable form of intervention. But these referrals, as with other nursing interventions, must be made in a manner that considers the family's motivation, the power structure within the family and the family's economic value system.

Television (A Mass Medium)

A powerful modern influence is television. The power of this medium is felt in both individual and family life. Despite the many studies that have been done to investigate the manner and extent of television's influence, we continue to have a very poor understanding of its effect. Such questions as what the relationship is between the sex and violence portrayed on television and violent crime in society, what effect child-oriented advertising has on the children's minds and how involvement with visual imagery affects desire and ability to relate to the written word are among the many queries to which we have no answers.

The vast financial investment in this medium and the powerful interests involved in its control create tremendous pressure that may, unfortunately, contaminate the objectivity of some investigations. The tension between the Federal Communications Commission (FCC), a regulatory body of the federal government charged with guarding the public interest, and the huge monied corporations and advertising interests concerned with amassing wealth and control often leads to conflict. In addition, various public interest organizations have entered the arena, seeking to promote or safeguard certain ideas or groups. For instance, the American Academy of Pediatrics is currently asking for a ban on television advertising directed to children, and this is being strongly opposed by those industries that are dependent on advertising appeals to the young, such as cereal and toy manufacturers.

Action for Children's Television (ACT) and other groups are also pressuring the Federal Trade Commission to regulate television advertising aimed at children, beginning with control of ads for heavily sugared candy and cereal. In response, some manufacturers have produced research findings which they say prove that sugar is not harmful to the general health of children and does not predispose to dental caries. Some religious groups are attempting to apply moral censorship in the areas of sexuality, violence and profanity. A basic dilemma revolves around the issue of safeguarding the public interest while maintaining First Amendment guarantees of free speech and freedom of the press.

Television is said to be the most pervasive force in United States society. There is at least one television set in 95 per cent of homes, and many homes have several sets. The average child in the United States spends more time in front of the television set than he does in school. A child from a home in which television is not available will often watch at the home of a friend. The financial importance of children's television is demonstrated by the fact that advertisers spend $600 million a year on children's shows. Broadcasters realize 25 per cent of their overall profits from the 7 per cent of their programming aimed specifically at children.[13]

The effect of television watching on family life is of increasing concern. Many parents and children argue over what to watch, and there is speculation that mass communication may be replacing interpersonal communication.[13] Rosenblatt and Cunningham see television contributing to troubled family relationships in two ways.[20] The operation of a television set creates frustrations rising from the noise and distraction it produces as well as the tension caused by differing preferences for programs or sound volume. There may be difficulties in carrying on other activities in close proximity to the television set, such as reading, conversing, telephoning or sleeping. If living quarters are cramped, this problem is intensified, since alternative space for other activities may not be available. The second problem area that television creates for the family lies in its use as a coping mechanism that allows one to escape from family problems. The family may use television watching to avoid tension-laden interactions and to provide an outlet for anger and aggression.

Rosenblatt and Cunningham found a strong positive correlation between the amount of time television sets were on in the home and scores on a scale measuring family tension.[20] Families with few members in relation to amount of available space tended to operate the set less than families with relatively high population density. The authors note: This is consistent with the hypothesis that, despite the frustration that may stem from TV set operation, television set operation is used to head off tense interaction.[20] They conclude that in families with a great deal of space in the dwelling to get away from each other, television set operation is frustrating, but in families with little space, operation of the set is an acceptable avoidance mechanism to escape unpleasant interaction.

There is an average of six times more violence during one hour of children's television than there is in one hour of adult television.[26] The "catharsis hypothesis," a well-known psychological theory on aggression reduction, suggests that people can make unconscious impulses less harmful by bringing them to the surface. According to this theory, children will becomes less likely to act out aggressive impulses if they view violence and aggression on television.[11] In reviewing the literature in this area, Heaps found only one study that supports this hypothesis.[11] By contrast, the majority of studies on the subject have shown that aggressive tendencies are stimulated rather than reduced by viewing television violence. In fact, it has been found that children actually learn aggressive behavior from "film-mediated models."[11] Two processes are involved in the child's response to the observation of television violence.[11] The first relates to the child's learning of new aggressive modes of behavior that were previously not part of his repertoire. He becomes an imitator of novel types of violence that he observes on the screen. The second process involves the release of inhibitions revolving around violent and aggressive patterns of behavior already in his repertoire. In other words, the child not only may learn new patterns of aggressive behavior but also is stimulated to act out those patterns he already knows.

Another consideration raised by viewing many of the cartoons that children watch is the unrealistic portrayal of the physical and moral consequences of violence and aggression. Cartoon characters are virtually indestructible. Humans and animals are beaten, shot, bombed, knifed, thrown from windows, pushed over cliffs, smashed with jackhammers, squashed by falling boulders and subjected to any number of other traumas, and yet, after a brief period of looking frazzled and a bit foolish, they are competely restored to their former condition. The character who perpetrates this mayhem is often the hero of the episode. What does this teach the child about the result of violent behavior? It certainly does not show him that it is harmful in an immediate or long-range sense. Nor does it teach him that there is anything morally wrong with the infliction of pain and harm on others. He is stimulated to perform actions without accurate information as to the results.

Kittrell compares television watching to drug-taking.[13] Both of these activities tend to withdraw the child from the environment and to obliterate the real world, and may be used as a means of escape. Both are basically passive states that require little thought or preparation. The desired effect is achieved with no exertion or commitment. Television, like a drug, can act as a stimulant or a sedative, depending on the child and the program he is watching. A parent may prescribe a dose of television to relax a child. Most parents are aware of the various effects of television on their children, but they do not know how to deal with them. Kittrell views this "narcotic" effect of television on children as the fundamental issue, not violence or advertising. He contends that television violence and advertising can be handled through laws and regulations, but "dealing with the effects of television, on the other hand, will require creative, individual responses from parents and children."[13]

Kittrell raises several questions regarding the effects of television viewing on children. What role does television play in the development of role models and value systems? Does television produce a passive attitude to life, blunt the imagination or inhibit the child's ability to engage in creative play? Do "flashy" educational programs such as "Sesame Street" or "The Electric Company" cause lack of interest in the more mundane, regimented and difficult world of classroom learning? Does television, by occupying the child's leisure time, discourage personal emotional discoveries that he could be making?[13] These are questions to which we have no answers at present, but certainly parents should be made aware of these issues as they make decisions about television for their children.

O'Bryant and Corder-Bolz report research findings which indicate that the most effective control of television's influence on children can be exerted from the home rather than by outside organizations.[18] A research project revealed that only about a third of parents studied tried to control the amount of television that their children watched. The study showed that children are most likely to adopt the television habits of their parents. Adolescents were the only group who did not display this behavior, probably as part of the rebellion against parents that characterizes this developmental stage.

Parents were found to be using television as reward and punishment. This practice was viewed as detrimental in several ways. A general rule of discipline is that reward and punishment should be specifically related to the behavior to which the parent is responding. Granting television viewing privileges as a reward may become a crutch to parents too lazy or unimaginative to think of other means of showing approval. Denial of viewing privileges as punishment may mean that the child misses a documentary or a show that has been assigned in school. A major consideration is that use of television viewing as reward and punishment places too much emphasis and value on television viewing.

O'Bryant and Corder-Bolz suggest that parents interrupt during television programs and interpret what is seen by the child to help him to understand and organize his visual perceptions, and to separate the real and the unreal. By becoming an active participant the parent can influence what the child learns and retains, and the attitudes that he develops.

Indirect mediation is recommended as a technique that parents can use to intervene in the television watching of teenagers. This is accomplished by a parent making a comment to the spouse or another family member in the teenager's hearing. The comment should express approval or disapproval of things seen on television in relationship to family values. This gives the teenager the opportunity to compare what he is watching with values the parent hopes to impart. Silence by the parent when television presents material that conflicts with family values and attitudes is misleading to the adolescent, since he is likely to interpret this silence as consent or agreement. O'Bryant and Corder-Bolz suggest that parents should view television purposefully, selecting and planning what is to be watched; that they critically evaluate what is seen and verbally express their criticism; and that they use television to lead to the discussion of topics that might otherwise be postponed or neglected, such as drugs, rape, teenage pregnancy and other controversial or sensitive issues.[18]

What are the nursing implications related to the effects of television on the family? If comprehensive family care is a nursing goal, the nurse must critically evaluate the often contradictory findings of research in the area and present accurate information to families. Here are a few recommendations that may help guide the nurse as she counsels:

1. Parents should be in control of the use of television. They have the responsibility to guide their children in wise choices.
2. Parents need to spend time with their children, both when they are watching television and when engaged in other activities.
3. Television watching must not be allowed to completely occupy the time individuals and families need for exercise, reading, talking together and pursuing other activities.
4. Television should not be used as reward and punishment.
5. Television should not be used as a babysitter.
6. Parents should be able to inculcate their own values and attitudes; if television interferes with this process, they must re-evaluate its use.
7. Children as they develop should be learning progressively to appreciate the difference between reality and unreality. Parents must be careful that use of television does not impede this process.

Nurses should include an investigation of the type and amount of television watching as a part of the history-taking phase of family assessment. This is especially important in families with communication problems or those in which behavioral problems with the children exist. Nurses must teach parents to use television selectively and creatively.

Religion

Religion has always played an enduring and important part in our idealized conception of family life in the United States. Religious belief and practice range from the traditional Judeo-Christian forms to numerous variants of Eastern mysticism, to religious agnosticism and atheism. Our national history reveals our fundamental position on the freedom of religious expression for all, in theory if not always in practice.

The impact of religion on family life in general and on behavior related to health and sickness in particular is readily evident. Often religious preference is also intermeshed with the ethnic or cultural background of families, making it an even more salient aspect of the life style. Among the family patterns affected by a family's religion are proper relationships between its members, family power configurations, responsibilities of parents and children, diet, use of leisure time and finances, attitudes toward family planning and divorce, beliefs regarding health and illness and use of health care resources.

In general, religion is seen as supportive of family strength by its tenets that place value on respect for others, mutual helping, commitment and other such interpersonal behaviors. Religion also provides activities in which all family members may participate, thus increasing the time that families can spend together. In some faiths divorce or extramarital sexual activity or both are strongly prohibited. On the other hand, recent years have seen conflicts between individual religious liberty and family power as numerous parents took forcible steps to retrieve their children from commitment to nontraditional religious groups that were negatively viewed by the families.

A number of religious groups place emphasis on the proper roles and power relationships within the family. For instance, some of the more fundamentalist groups advocate the father as family leader and primary decision maker and tend to emphasize the mother/homemaker roles as most desirable for women. Various groups provide rules regarding the use of family planning methods or stress values related to optimum family size or both. The duty of adult children to care for aging parents is enjoined on some religiously conscientious families in the light of the biblical fifth commandment.

Groups such as the Church of Jesus Christ of Latter-Day Saints (Mormons) or the Seventh-Day Adventists advocate such practices as proper dietary habits and abstinence from stimulants and depressants. These, along with other life style factors, seem to have had the effect of prolonging the life expectancy of the adherents of these faiths beyond national averages.

A number of religions affect family health care behavior through precepts determining which, if any, medical or health-related procedures are appropriate for their followers. This has often led to conflict between families and health care providers, especially when certain interventions were refused on behalf of dependent children. Such situations have sometimes been resolved by having the child declared temporarily a ward of the court.

In assessing the religious aspects of an individual family the nurse must be careful to maintain an open and nonjudgmental attitude. Often the family may value adherence to their religious convictions much more highly than a conflicting health goal that is valued by the nurse. It is also important to avoid the pitfall of religiously stereotyping the family: that is, failing to accurately assess the extent to which each individual family adheres to the tenets of their religious preference and the extent to which they may have made alternative decisions. The nurse should be alert to cues that the family or its individual members are experiencing guilt or conflict in relation to religious concerns. In these instances as well as others involving interpersonal or intrapersonal distress, the nurse should keep in mind the possibility of collaboration with or referral to a clergyman or other family-designated religious advisor in a team approach to family care implementation.

Public Policy and Programs

A factor that has the potential to impact profoundly on family life is public or governmental policy and programs. While the federal government has no policy explicitly addressing families, many public programs affect family functioning.[30] United States families are constrained by the legalities surrounding such issues as compulsory education, marriage, divorce and child custody, child support and protection and the provision of financial subsidies from governmental sources. Mandatory education has a marked effect on family life, since from approximately the age of 6 the child spends a large portion of the day in school and receives a large measure of socialization there. As a result the child is exposed to authority figures, information and values beyond what parents and family provide. Child support and child protection laws obligate parents to care for their offspring, and attempt to establish basic standards for that care. The statutes regarding divorce, which vary considerably from state to state, regulate the manner in which families become legally disconnected and control subsequent management of their interrelated finances and the care of dependent children. As the nurse considers individual families, she must assess the influence of factors such as these in more specific detail. It is important to note here that families are not merely passive in their relationship to governmental decisions. Changes in collective family behavior and values have led to alterations in laws or policies. An example of this is the changes in divorce and child custody laws that reflect the increasing value placed on more equitable privileges and responsibility for both partners in the divorce.

It is helpful to view public programs as they have affected changing trends in family characteristics. A study by Moore and Caldwell assessed the effect on out-of-wedlock sex and pregnancy of government programs such as Aid to Families with Dependent Children (AFDC), liberalized abortion, and subsidized family planning services. No support was found for the hypothesis that AFDC benefits were associated with greater incidence of pregnancy or the probability of carrying an out-of-wedlock pregnancy to term. In other words, public welfare was not found to act as an economic incentive to childbirth outside of marriage. The availability of subsidized family planning services was related to decreased out-of-wedlock pregnancy among black teenagers but had no effect on similar rates among whites. This was thought to be associated with the more frequent economic disadvantage among blacks. No clear support was noted for the idea that public policies affect the initiation of sexual activity by adolescents. This instead seemed to be related to the educational level of the adolescent's father, church attendance, race, location of residence and intactness of the family.[16]

Another study looked at the effect of the source of income on the degree to which female single parents felt in control of their lives. Besides the amount of dollars available, the manner in which the money was provided was found to affect the family's sense of autonomy and independence. The provision of money by methods that impair these perceptions, that are unreliable or unstable or that involve degrading or stigmatizing factors can negatively affect the self-esteem of the family. Income sources such as AFDC or child support, because they may be characterized by one or more of the aforementioned factors, can serve to weaken rather than strengthen the woman's feeling of control over her own future and that of her family. Income earned through work, on the other hand, allows the woman to fulfill the provider role in a way that enhances her feelings of personal fate control. Work-related income does not entail the demeaning or stigmatizing effects of public welfare. In addition, social security finances provide stability and reliability, which do not always characterize child support payments.[2]

In terms of this study and in the case of many other public programs, while the intent is to be helpful, little attention is paid to the possibility of negative side effects for families. In addition to this, the absence of a defined policy by the national government regarding positive family-related goals and the absence of an agency specifically designated to deal with family welfare means that often policies or programs are developed with inadequate consideration of the impact they might have on family health collectively. A familiar example is the relationship between AFDC regulations and family disruption. In some regions AFDC benefits are available only if there is no adult male present in the home. For many families in which unemployment is a problem or in which the man's wage earning capacity is low, he feels encouraged to abandon the family in order for them to be eligible for public assistance.

One facet of the advocate role of the nurse is to assist the family in coping with governmental policies that might tend to impair its integrity or functioning. A related professional responsibility involves providing knowledgeable and active input, either individually or through organizations that aid in the development of public policies and programs which are sensitive to and supportive of family well-being.

Culture

The impact of culture on the individual and the family and implications of culture for nursing practice are topics about which there is much current concern. They are also topics that are rather hard to define, owing to the diversity and complexity of cultural modes that characterize the pluralistic society of the United States.

Culture has been defined many times and in varying ways. One of the most comprehensive definitions is given by Ashley Montagu:

> Culture represents man's response to his basic needs. Culture is man's way of making himself comfortable in the world. It is the behavior he has learned as a member of society. We may define culture as the way of life of a people, the environment which a group of human beings occupying a common territory have created in the form of ideas, institutions, pots and pans, language, tools, services and sentiments.[15]

Some authors also differentiate readily observable or overt cultural products (e.g., dress, religion, childrearing practices) from those that are covert or not as obvious (e.g., ideals and values).[14, 29]

It is important to bear in mind that the production of culture is a human enterprise. In a very real sense man creates his culture and is created by it. Culture is invented and transmitted by humans who are themselves shaped by the culture in which they participate. Culture is probably the most important part of the human environment, as it defines the way of life for a group of people.[29]

When viewed over a short span of time, cultures seem stable, so that one might mistakenly conclude that they are static or unchanging. On the contrary, cultures are dynamic, although some seem to change more slowly than others. The direction and shape of future alterations grow out of present cultural forms. In other words, the seeds of a given cultural epoch can be identified in earlier periods of the group's history. Since culture is not a completely harmonious system, change can result from internal conflict, strains or maladjustments.[29] In the words of Benedict, "It is, so far as we can see, an ultimate fact of human nature that man builds up his culture out of disparate elements, combining and recombining."[1]

Culture can be viewed as a pervasive, dynamic aspect of social interaction. It forms the material and nonmaterial matrix of life for the individual and the family. It includes all facets of the man-made environment that are learned and transmitted from generation to generation.

As the nurse attempts to individualize care based on cultural understanding, it may be helpful for her to focus on a few areas in which cultural differences are important. The discussion that follows does not cover all of the possible cultural differences but will suggest some areas that have particular relevance for health care.

First of all, the nurse should understand the typical family constellation and power structure of a given cultural group. It is important to know who the family members are. Although the nuclear pattern is becoming more common in non-Western cultures, many families still reside in extended groups. On the basis of how authority is allocated in the family, any member may hold the reins of power. For instance, among some American Indian tribes the grandmother, not the parents, has authority over the grandchildren. Should consent for surgery be required, for example, the grandmother must be consulted. In other cultural groups the maternal uncles or some other nonparental relative may hold power. If the nurse does not know whom to approach for health care decisions, she may feel that the family is being evasive or uncooperative as nonauthority members hesitate to make crucial decisions.

The sex roles ascribed to males and females by the culture present another area of health concern. Family planning practices, the nature of the marriage relationship, division of labor within the family and variations in training and discipline of male and female children are only a few of the areas affected by what are considered proper roles for males and females. As all societies become more industrialized, there is a tendency toward increased symmetry in sex roles (i.e., the expected behaviors for men and women are becoming more and more alike).[24] Despite this trend, even in the most industrialized nations differences persist in male and female roles. The nurse must be aware of these differences as she plans family-centered care. If an overworked mother with several children is encountered in the well-child clinic, the nurse may think it appropriate to discuss family planning methods with her. However, if the mother is Latino, her husband may have control over decision-making in this area and well may be affronted when he is not consulted as the decision maker.

Nutritional practice is an obvious focus of cultural difference, yet many nurses tend to forget this as they care for or counsel clients. The selection, preparation and consumption of food has deep social and psychological meaning for the individual and the family. The hospitalized client from a particular culture may be served food that is to him unfamiliar, unpalatable, forbidden or even repulsive. For example, the typical client in the United States would be shocked at the practice of eating dog meat that is common in some Asian cultures; and yet mayonnaise, used in most diets, is so disgusting to many Vietnamese that they will try to avoid the sight of it. Other cultural differences revolve around the timing of meals, the manner of food service and the correct use of eating utensils. The nurse has an obligation to see that these cultural values of the client are not violated.

As the nurse seeks to counsel families, she must be aware that much of what she has learned and has available in printed form about nutrition is culturally biased toward food preferences of white middle class individuals. Nutritional counselling must begin with the identification of the typical diet and food consumption patterns of the family. Then the nurse is able to assess the nutritional value of what family members are eating and plan with them to enhance or correct their diet, on the basis of recognition and support of their cultural patterns. The use of culturally appropriate literature or consultation with a nutritionist or both may be necessary.

Communication barriers are obvious when caring for a non-English-speaking client, but nurses often fail to realize that caring for English-speaking clients from diverse cultural backgrounds presents similar communication problems. Black and Appalachian Americans, for example, have patterns of speech and word usage that are unique and illogical to the typical white American nurse. If the nurse makes no effort to "learn the language," she will miss important information that the client is seeking to convey. This inability to communicate becomes critical when the client is seeking to discuss his health status. If the nurse fails to realize that for the Appalachian client "high blood" is related to blood volume, not blood pressure, with the approved remedy being ingestion of brine (salt water), she may be surprised at the client's behavior following a diagnosis of hypertension.[28]

Finally, the nurse must be prepared to encounter cultural differences in beliefs and behavior related to health and illness. Not only are illness states culturally defined, but who will be consulted and which kinds of treatment are appropriate are culturally determined. Health professionals are slowly beginning to realize that traditional practitioners such as shamans, witch doctors and medicine men are often sought in preference to physicians and nurses. In the past the typical reaction has been to discourage and ridicule the use of the traditional practitioner. As more is learned about the relationship between belief and healing, progressive health professionals are learning to work cooperatively with traditional practitioners for the benefit of the client. Even if families are willing to accept Western health care providers, they often wish to use folk remedies or have treatment applied in ways that do not violate cultural beliefs. For example, the southern black woman may come to the hospital for delivery but continue to hold the belief that a knife placed under the bed will "cut the pain."

Many of the herbs and healing compounds in traditional systems of healing have beneficial physiological effects, while other remedies seem to be successful because the client has faith that they will work. The nurse should include in her assessment the identification of health practices and practitioners that the family or client believes to be appropriate for care. She should be sensitive to the religious basis for family beliefs related to health. When family values have been explored the nurse is able to add an important dimension to her care planning by incorporating the family's cultural health beliefs.

In the effort to interact with and provide health care to clients from cultures other than our own, the failure to consider the import of cultural differences can prove disastrous. The preceding discussion has pointed out a number of critical areas that must be considered in the provision of transcultural nursing care. It is the responsibility of the professional nurse to identify the various cultural groups in the population which she serves and to educate herself about their beliefs and practices.

An error which often occurs in working with culturally diverse clients is the assumption that all members of a given culture fit very strictly into a textbook description of the culture's typical behavior. This kind of stereotyping can inhibit the nurse-family relationship. Behaving as if all black families, regardless of socioeconomic or regional variation, share consistent value systems, patterns of speech and dietary practices or expecting all Spanish-speaking families to adhere to traditional folk beliefs regarding illness are examples of such cultural stereotyping. According to Montagu, "No single individual ever gains a knowledge of the whole of his culture. As a member of his culture, the individual is equipped to participate in it, not to become a mere repository of it."[15] This concept can be applied to families also. Each family modifies the culture of the larger social group in ways that are uniquely its own. Some practices, beliefs and materials are maintained, while others are altered or relinquished. While it is helpful for the nurse to have a basic understanding of the culture of a given family, this should not blind her to what actually characterizes that family in a cultural sense. Assumptions or biased expectations must not replace accurate assessment of each individual client and family.

References

1. R. F. Benedict. An Anthropologist at Work: Writings of Ruth Benedict (edited by Margaret Mead). J. B. Lippincott Co., 1959
2. S. Bould. Female-headed families: personal fate control and the provider role. Journal of Marriage and the Family, May 1977, p. 339
3. N. I. Brill. Working with People: The Helping Process, 2nd ed. J. B. Lippincott Co., 1978
4. U. Bronfenbrenner. The changing American family. In E. M. Hetherington and R. D. Park, eds. Contemporary Readings in Child Psychology. McGraw-Hill Book Co., 1977, p. 315
5. E. M. Duvall. Marriage and Family Development, 5th ed. J. B. Lippincott Co., 1977
6. D. Finkelhor. Book review of Inside the Family: Toward a Theory of Family Process by D. Kantor and W. Lehr. Harper and Row, 1975. In Journal of Marriage and the Family, May 1977, p. 423
7. P. Glick. Updating the life cycle of the family. Journal of Marriage and the Family, February 1977, p. 5
8. S. H. G. Golden. Pre-school families and work. Doctoral dissertation, University of Michigan, 1975
9. T. K. Hareven. Family time and historical time. Daedalus, Spring 1977, p. 57
10. Health of the Disadvantaged: Chartbook. U.S.D.H.E.W., (HRA)77-628, 1977
11. L. K. Heaps. Effect of exposure to television violence on

aggressive behavior. Family Perspective, Winter 1977, p. 35
12. R. M. Kanter. Jobs and families: impact of working roles on family life. Children Today, Mar/Apr, 1978, p. 11
13. E. Kittrell. Children and television: the electronic fix. Children Today, May/June 1978, p. 20
14. M. Leininger. Transcultural Nursing: Concepts, Theories, and Practices. John Wiley & Sons, 1978
15. A. Montagu. Man, His First Two Million Years: A Brief Introduction to Anthropology. Columbia University Press, 1977
16. K. A. Moore and S. B. Caldwell. The effect of government policies on out-of-wedlock sex and pregnancy. Family Planning Perspectives, Jul/Aug, 1977, p. 164
17. R. L. Nolan and J. L. Schwartz, eds. Rural and Appalachian Health. Charles C Thomas Publisher, 1973
18. S. L. O'Bryant and C. R. Corder-Bolz. Tackling "the tube" with family teamwork. Children Today, May/June, 1978, p. 21
19. C. S. Piotrowski. Jobs, families and everyday life. Doctoral dissertation. University of Michigan, 1977
20. P. C. Rosenblatt and M. R. Cunningham. Television watching and family tensions. Journal of Marriage and the Family, February 1976, p. 105
21. J. R. Renshaw. An exploration of the dynamics of the overlapping worlds of work and family. Family Process, March 1976, p. 143
22. I. V. Sawhill. Economic perspectives on the family. Daedalus, Spring 1977, p. 115
23. L. Saxton. The Individual, Marriage, and the Family, 3rd ed. Wadsworth Publishing Co., Inc., 1977
24. A. Skolnick. The Intimate Environment: Exploring Marriage and the Family, 2nd ed. Little, Brown and Company, 1978
25. N. Stinnett and K. H. Sauer. Relationship characteristics of strong families. Family Perspective, Winter 1977, p. 3
26. Television and the family. Family Perspective, Winter 1977, p. 1
27. Time and family life. Family Perspective, Spring 1975, p. 1
28. T. Tripp-Reimer and M. C. Fridel. Appalachians: A neglected minority. Nursing Clinics of North America, March 1977, p. 41
29. R. S. Zais. Curriculum: Principles and Foundations. Thomas Y. Crowell Co., 1976
30. S. L. Zimmerman. Reassessing the effect of public policy on family functioning. Social Casework, October 1978, p. 451

Additional Recommended Reading

K. W. Bartz and W. C. Witcher. When father gets custody. Children Today, Sept/Oct, 1978, p. 2

P. J. Hiebert. Cultural Anthropology. J. B. Lippincott Co., 1976

D. Kantor and W. Lehr. Inside the Family: Toward a Theory of Family Process. Harper and Row, 1975

R. E. Spector. Cultural Diversity in Health and Illness. Apple-Century-Crofts, 1979

PARENTING FOR THE SOCIALIZATION OF CHILDREN

3

by Jo Joyce Tackett, RN, MPHN

THE COMMITMENT TO PARENT

To become a parent is probably the biggest commitment in any adult's life. Raising children is one of the most complicated, intricate and challenging tasks to be performed by family and society and compares with no other in terms of consequence. The task encompasses a gradual shaping of the neonate into a person capable of living in our society and the generational perpetuation of the values, skills, knowledge, beliefs and activities deemed useful for happy, healthy living.

A child's socialization begins in a family, is sustained by that family but ultimately moves outside the family as his life cycle propels him beyond family care. The child's unique temperamental traits, coupled with his family and social climate, determine in large measure how much he will be influenced by previous generations and what he ultimately will pass on to the generation he creates. Thus the unfolding social nature of man rests upon the character and quality of parenting, making parenting responsibility an awesome proposition.

In the past, society exerted great pressure on couples to become parents — often before they were ready to take on the responsibility. Many people did not think about what parenting involved until a child was on the way. Today, alternate life styles and scientific advances make options available to young people. They may choose to delay parenting until they feel ready and then parent only as many children as they feel they can skillfully socialize, or choose not to become parents.

Many couples now talk about having a child before they make the decision. A realization of the awesomeness of the parenting responsibility has surfaced, which is motivating more couples to seek self-knowledge and some understanding of the parenting task (minimally, knowledge of human growth and development) to make them more capable of successfully meeting the demands of parenthood. The option of choice and the acquisition of preparatory skills promise to make life better for children and more rewarding for parents.

The stresses of modern living and children's earlier exposure to the conflicts of our world make the demanding work of childrearing more difficult. However, arousal of societal awareness of parents' needs for assistance is resulting in many supportive actions. Increasing education for parenting is being done in high schools (kindergarten through 12 curricula exist in some regions) and by organizations devoted to the preservation and health of the family in changing society. Professionals in the health, psychology and sociology fields are helping people to become better parents by providing anticipatory guidance education, seminars and literature. The women's liberation movement and the changing attitudes it has created are freeing fathers to become more active parents and mothers to be happier persons and, consequently, more effective parents. Business leaders are becoming more aware of the life style changes that will make it necessary for them to do their part to support family life and healthy parenting. A few large corporations are already providing quality day care centers and accommodating part-time and split-shift schedules, especially for parents of young children. Supportive changes such as these should, over time, make being a good parent less difficult and more rewarding.

Whatever the support society gives, however, the quality of parenting still depends largely upon individuals. Nurses have a responsibility to assist individuals to be successful parents and to reinforce those attitudes and behaviors in parents and children that will promote healthy socialization within the context of a happy family. This chapter is an attempt to give the nurse who deals with children and parents some insight into the special roles parents play in the development of a human being and the methods available to parents to carry out those roles, and to suggest interventions the nurse and parents can employ to redirect unhealthy parenting practices into healthier awareness.

SOCIALIZATION AND PARENTAL ROLES

A Working Definition of Parenting*

Parenting "includes the broadest ideas on training . . . and educating the child during his early, formative years. It is (the consistent daily) love and affection which develop one's own self-esteem and self-image. It includes the pangs of guilt and punishment and the heady feelings of praise and success."[20] Parenting is shaped out of the experience of living and interacting with people of various ages in play, activities of daily living and family and sociocultural rituals. This definition implicates four essential elements of the parenting process, regardless of parenting style, which interact to socialize children. Table 3–1 defines these elements and describes the major function of each in socializing the child.

The nurse's assessment of parenting skills requires an evaluation of each of these four elements. Therefore, each of these is

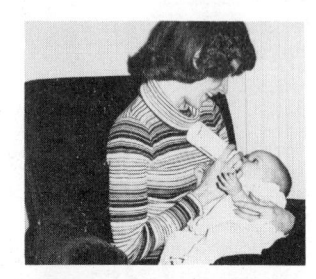

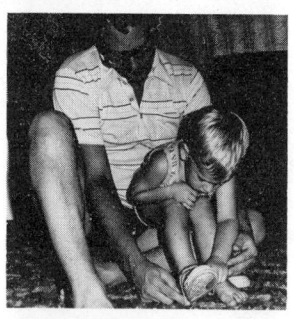

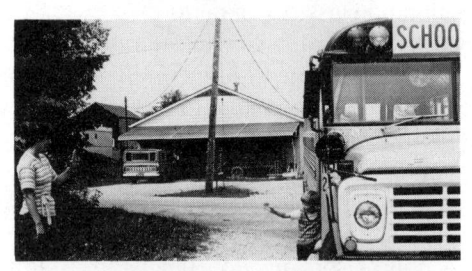

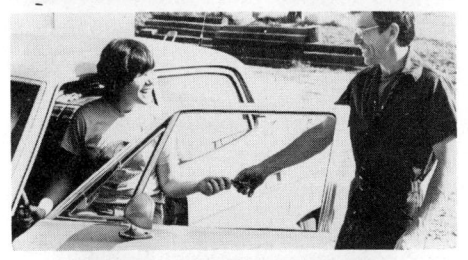

---
*Parenting has many synonymous terms, including child-rearing, discipline, socialization.

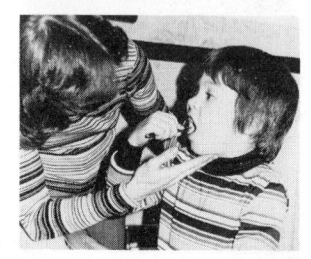

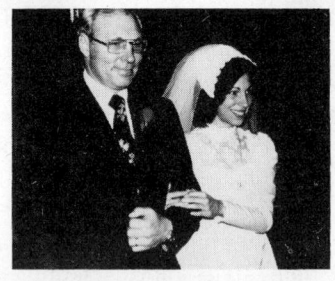

A child's socialization begins in and is sustained by his family but ultimately propels him beyond the family. This series portrays the changing parent-child relationship in that socialization life cycle.

TABLE 3-1 ESSENTIAL ELEMENTS OF PARENTING AND THEIR FUNCTION IN SOCIALIZATION

Element	Definition	Functions in Socialization
Rules	Guidelines for behavior. May differ depending on setting and situation. Establishes what is and is not permitted.	*Educates* child by identifying behaviors acceptable to cultural and social milieu. *Restrains* misbehavior by placing limits or boundaries on behavior. Develops *moral conscience*.
Consistency: • in rules • in required compliance • between parents in parenting methods	Maintaining uniformity or persisting in expectations for child; enforcing rules; retaining authority by using parenting methods congruent with rules, child's unique character and situation.	Speeds *learning* process by regular reinforcement and repetition. Provides *security* since child knows what is expected of him and what he can expect from person in authority. Fosters *respect* for rules and authority (essential to social survival).
Punishment	Negative consequences, natural or artificial, of breaking rule (misbehavior).	*Educates* by emphasizing which behaviors are not acceptable following the misbehavior. *Restricts* repetition of unacceptable behavior, at least temporarily. *Motivates* appropriate behavior following misconduct, at least temporarily.
Reward	Reinforcement of behavior by physical, emotional, social or material means that the child finds pleasurable or satisfying.	Powerful *motivation* of acceptable behavior; *stimulates repetition* of desirable behavior after such behavior has occurred.

discussed in some detail, with direction given to what the nurse should look for and evaluate within each element of the parenting process.

Rules Rules are essential to the child's mental development. Similarity in use of rules — the more frequently the same rule can be applied in a variety of circumstances — makes them easier for the child to integrate into his general moral code.[13] When the number of rules or the character of a rule differs from one situation to another, it is harder for the child to conceptualize and incorporate the principle into his developing moral code. For example, "Be kind to others" is a rule that can be applied in the majority of situations and is therefore internalized at a fairly early age — a toddler can learn to share, not to bite or hit, to offer a friendly smile. However, "Tell the truth" varies in character depending on the situation, and the child requires many years to gain the intuition that tells him which degree of truth is appropriate for any given situation. Before adolescence, children have not learned when to use the absolute truth and when to avoid and modify absolute truth. One does not tell the lady at the grocery store that she is fat.

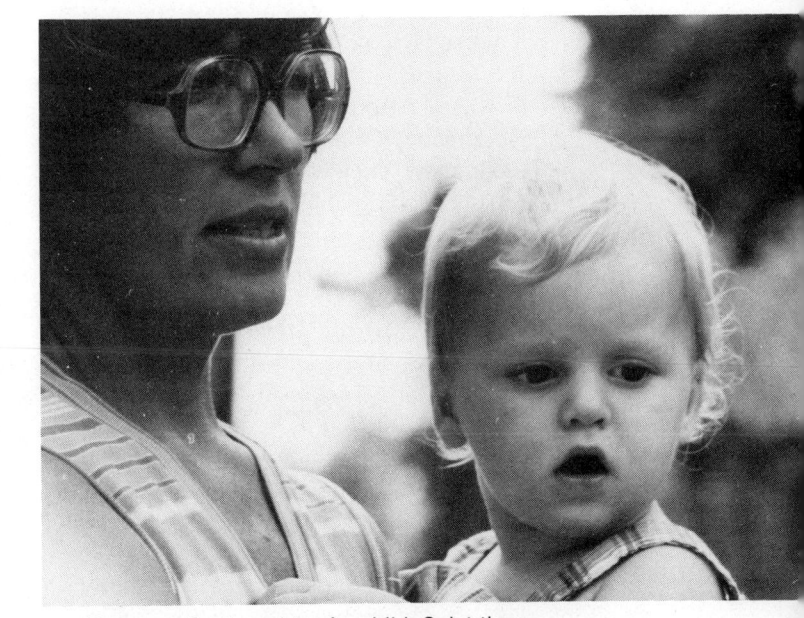

> Bitter are the tears of a child:
>   Sweeten them.
> Deep are the thoughts of a child:
>   Quiet them.
> Sharp is the grief of a child:
>   Take it from him.
> Soft is the heart of a child:
>   Do not harden it.
>   From "A Child"
> by Lady Pamela Wyndham Glenconner

Deep are the thoughts of a child. Quiet them.

Learning rules advances the child toward greater freedom and more mastery of his environment. Although frustration is created in the process of learning rules, it is unavoidable and is not a harmful side effect. The rules the child masters will ultimately make it easier for him to get along in the world, because each rule he masters allows him more responsibility for his own behavior, readying him for greater independence from external (parents and other adults) guidance and control.

Clearly established rules (i.e., limit setting) give the child guidelines as to what is acceptable and not acceptable.[11] He learns that some actions are never acceptable because they are endangering, illegal, unethical or antisocial. Conversely, he learns that some behaviors are always acceptable. He also gradually learns that a gray area exists in which some behaviors are acceptable at certain ages or in some circumstances and are unacceptable at other times.

Rules can be conveyed in a number of ways. The method most frequently used with infants and young toddlers is environmental control. Confinements in space, restrictions on play materials and childproofing are measures taken to convey rules by environmental control. Direct verbal communication is used increasingly as a child masters language. Even though this is the most common method of teaching rules, it is the least effective. Younger children respond to a tone of voice when reprimands and explanations are given; however, direct verbal methods do not take on much clout until the child reaches an age (usually school age) when he can comprehend simple explanations that accompany verbal commands.

An extremely effective but seldom utilized method of teaching rules is the "overheard" technique,[12] whereby a limit or rule is discussed in front of the child but is not directed specifically at him. The most efficient method of teaching rules is by role modelling, since children emulate their parents through imitation from infancy on. This method also has the advantage that illustrative examples occur 24 hours a day, so the child receives regular reminders as he watches his parents' behavior. Imitated rules are also more readily internalized.

The nurse's evaluation of parents' childrearing skills should include observation and discussion of the rules being communicated by the parents. The nurse can use the following guidelines to evaluate this:

1. Are the parents aware of the rules they are currently teaching their child? Are they able to establish rules? To say "no" when appropriate?
2. Are the rules they verbalize consistent with their own behaviors?
3. Are the number and type of rules they are currently working on realistic in terms of the child's age, temperament and mental capacity?
4. Are the parents using age-appropriate methods to communicate the rules? Are rules being clearly communicated?
5. Are the rules logical and enforceable?
6. Is the child showing evidence of rule mastery? If so, is he being given the opportunity for self-regulation in that area of living?

Parents should be given positive reinforcement for those aspects of the guidelines in which they evidence parenting skill (a "yes" answer). In those areas in which their skills are lacking (a "no" answer), the nurse should institute interventions to help them develop skills.

Consistency in Rules Rules are learned much faster when they are consistently upheld by and applicable to all family members. Some breaches of limits may be tolerated by children when rules are first being learned or in certain circumstances, and relapses can be anticipated during illness or fatigue. It is easier to be consistent when there are not too many rules to be maintained.

Of particular importance is the consistency of messages between parents and between parents and other caretakers. Parents need to agree on rules. They should seek help if they cannot agree, or the child will likely end up needing help. Rules should be consistently endorsed until the child learns and accepts the rules as his own. Parental or family rules should be conveyed to other caretakers along with the expectation that they will enforce and model the rules while caring for the children.

Consistency in Enforcement Children usually respond more favorably to situations when they can predict the outcome. Rules or limits should be consistently enforced and with the same degree of force each time. Demands should not be made that parents cannot or do not intend to enforce. However, consistency in enforcement does not mean that consideration should not be given to the circumstances involved — that would be rigidity, not consistency. Breaches of limits or rules should be dealt with immediately, first with a warning and, if the behavior does not stop, then by applying either natural or artificial negative consequences. Warnings ideally state what should be done rather than what should not. The enforcement of rules should occur without obvious anger by the reinforcer and with a minimum of words. Explanations of "why" should follow the consequence, provided the child is old enough to understand. Even then, explanations should be simple and brief. Through consistently employed enforcement of rules, the child slowly learns to connect the act with the consequence and changes his behavior to avoid discomfort.

Consistency in Parenting Methods The methods used to enforce rules should be consistent with the seriousness or value placed on the rules. Fair parenting methods foster respect in the child for rules and for authority. Methods should also recognize children's individual temperaments, since some temperaments thrive better on more firmness and consistency while other temperaments are relatively adaptable and less dependent on consistency of method.

The following checklist is helpful in assessing parents' ability to be consistent.
1. Do parents display a code of conduct that is congruent with what they are enforcing for their children?
2. Are rules realistically enforced with consideration for age, newness of rule, circumstances?
3. Do parents follow through by enforcing rules?
4. Have parents communicated rules to other caretakers?
5. Do parents agree on the rules to be enforced and share their enforcement?
6. Is enforcement promptly enacted?
7. Is rationale shared with the child age-appropriate? Simple? Concise?
8. Are enforcement methods congruent with the rules involved? The child's temperament?
9. Does the child display evidence of developing respect for rules? Authority?

Punishment The first ground rules of punishment, if it is to be effective in encouraging desirable behavior, are that the child be informed of what his punishment will be if misconduct occurs and that he know why he is being punished once the punishment has been enacted.

Punishment is the "fine," or price paid for deviating from established rules. It may be in the form of artificial consequence such as disapproval, withdrawal of privileges, isolation, substitution or physical punishment. *Disapproval* may be verbal or nonverbal. Often tone of voice alone conveys that the parent "means business." Numerous facial expressions and gestures can be used; their meanings are learned quickly even by young children.

Older children are more likely to respond to *privilege withdrawal*. Something they would like to do or have is withheld. The privilege withheld should be reasonable, not something critical such as a birthday party or long-anticipated special event such as a prom, and the punishment should occur fairly soon after the misdeed. When possible, the withheld privilege should be something associated with the misconduct.

Isolation works with some children. As a general rule isolation periods of longer than an hour breed contempt for the parent rather than redirecting the offender's behavior. This method is not usually easily carried out before preschool age.

Substitution is a form of environmental control generally used with infants and young toddlers. The parent bodily removes the child from the situation prompting inappropriate behavior or diverts him with another activity or toy. It is often coupled with a disapproval action.

A discussion of whether *physical punishment* — spanking, specifically — is an acceptable punishment measure would be irrelevant. It can be safely assumed that almost every parent has hit their child at some time or another. What is relevant is that spanking, as well as any other form of punishment, should not be used excessively or carried to extremes. Some believe spanking cancels the crime, freeing the child to repeat the act.

Natural consequence may also be used as a form of punishment and is probably most effective in helping the child see self-regulation as his own responsibility. For example, if a child refuses to eat at mealtime, he gets extremely

THE FAMILY CIRCUS By Bil Keane

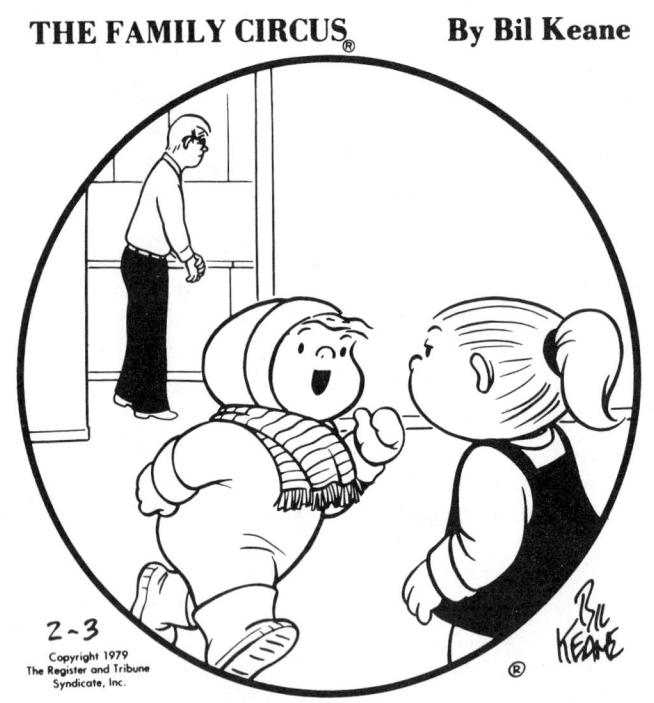

"I just got a spanking. Daddy hurt his hand and I didn't feel a thing."

hungry before the next meal when he can again have food. This approach does require restraint on the parents' part to not intervene but allow the natural consequence to occur. This approach is usually most successful with preschool and early school-age children.

Having the child use *positive practices* (apologizing, repairing the results of the misdeed, correcting inappropriate behavior, practicing correct behavior several times) as a part of punishment is often realistic and has the double advantage of also reinforcing desirable behavior.[21]

When possible, punishment should be presented unemotionally. However, parents are only human and circumstances sometimes make unemotional intervention extremely difficult to achieve. Fairness (i.e., punishment that fits the crime) is an important factor in determining how severe the punishment should be. This does not mean all children in a family need the same form or degree of punishment; what is right for one child is not necessarily right for another.

A misdeed should be punished promptly, then the act should be forgotten. Children do not need reminders of their wrongdoings on a long-term basis.

The following checklist can assist the nurse's evaluation of parents' use of punishment in the parenting process.
1. What forms of punishment are usually employed?
2. Is the punishment used age- and developmentally appropriate?
3. Is the parents' goal in punishing to educate or motivate desirable behavior or to impart revenge?
4. Is the reason for punishment explained to the child?
5. Are the parents usually able to apply punishment without emotional display?
6. Is the punishment realistic to the misdeed?
7. Are misdeeds immediately followed by punishment measures?
8. Do the parents attempt to employ positive practices as punishment whenever possible?
9. Does the child express through words or behaviors that he understands the consequence if he breaks a rule of conduct?

Reward *Rewarding* is really another means of enforcing rules or setting limits. All of us, but especially children, need praise, encouragement and rewards for behaving properly. Rewards should be differentiated from *bribes*. A bribe occurs when a child is either told before the act that he will be rewarded or is actually rewarded ahead of time for a promise to avoid misbehavior. A reward means the child is or has conducted himself properly and now receives the reward. The reward is given spontaneously during or after the act.[20]

The use of rewards creates an increased likelihood that a child will repeat desired behavior. It also communicates to the child what the desired behavior is without a lot of confusing verbal exchange.

Rewards fall into five general categories. Table 3–2 describes the advantages and disadvantages of each type of reward.

To be effective, a reward must meet certain criteria: (1) it must be something the child finds satisfying and desirable, (2) it must be readily available and (3) it must be accessible to the child only when the desired behavior occurs.[21] When and how frequently the reward is offered also determines the effectiveness of rewards as a reinforcement. Whatever its form, the reward should be given the child while he is still

TABLE 3-2 ADVANTAGES AND DISADVANTAGES OF REWARDS

Reward Category	Advantages	Disadvantages
Objects (Food, toys, trinkets, clothing)	Since object is visible, reinforcement continues each time object seen or used. Stimulates several sense modalities.	Can be costly. If food is used, calories involved. Cannot always be given immediately after the desired behavior.
Activities (TV, theatre, roller skating, whatever activity the child finds rewarding and parents approve)	Usually inexpensive. Perceived as desirable by most children. May be contingent upon earning so many tokens or points.	What appeals can change rapidly; avoid problem somewhat by giving child choices or by letting child suggest activities.
Social (Hugs, kisses, pats, smiles, praise)	Can use lavishly without any cost.	Must be sure to give only when earned. Needs to be combined with tangible rewards occasionally to retain effectiveness.
Personal (Self-satisfaction, feeling good)	Most desirable; fosters self-regulation.	Must be learned, cannot be given by another. Seldom effective in child with poor self-concept.
Token (Stars, check marks, points)	Good for all ages, can be promptly given.	Final reward to be earned by accumulated tokens can be expensive.

engaged in the desired action or immediately after he completes it. In the beginning the behavior must be reinforced regularly, preferably each time it occurs. Gradually the reward can be given only occasionally (intermittent reinforcement). Eventually the desired behavior will become a habit, requiring no external reward.

Accentuating the positive aspects of a child's behavior (i.e., catching him in the act of being good) can eliminate a lot of parent-child conflicts. A child who perceives his parent as one who supports his growing self is more apt to imitate that parent's values and beliefs. However, the psychology laboratory has produced evidence that both rewards and punishment have strong motivational effects on socializing behavior.[8] Unfortunately, scientific investigation has revealed no simple formula for when to use each — that is still left to parents' intuition and judgment.

The following checklist may assist the nurse to evaluate parents' use of rewards in their parenting.
1. Do parents offer rewards or bribes? Do they know the difference?
2. What type of rewards do the parents employ? Are they appropriate to the child's developmental level?
3. Does the child communicate verbally or through his behaviors that he perceives the rewards as worthwhile?
4. Are the rewards realistic and given only when merited?
5. Do the parents know how and when to wean the child from external rewards?

Goals and Functions of Parenting

The parenting process is guided by some basic goals or purposes. The goals most directly motivating parenting activities are: (1) to keep the child safe, (2) to instill familial beliefs and standards (includes those social and cultural aspects the family has internalized), (3) to teach social behaviors and roles[5] and (4) to help the child become self-regulating and independent.[7]

Which of these goals is the strongest motivator varies with the child's age, the parents' intellectual and social levels, the parents' interests and individual personalities, the child's temperament and familial attitudes about parenting. These same factors determine which parenting methods are selected and influence how effective those methods are (see discussion of methods later in this chapter).

Discipline functions to organize the child's world. Rules consistently established and enforced make his world predictable and give him boundaries within which to grow and develop.

The predictability and boundaries increase the child's security and reinforce his developing trust of others and himself. The feelings of security and trust that result from repetition of these experiences (outer controls with parent as policeman) help him learn to cope and solve problems independently out of a sense of self-control (inner controls with parent as counselor) and self-confidence. As the child progressively masters the rules and roles of living, he experiences a sense of accomplishment and acceptance that builds his self-esteem. Positive self-esteem encourages a child to make his own decisions on the basis of his own good judgment and inner convictions rather than peer suggestion or impulse, readying him for healthy adult independence.

Parental Roles

A child is a unique individual with his own special potential; that factor makes parenthood

---

HELPING A CHILD PROBLEM-SOLVE TO ELICIT APPROPRIATE BEHAVIOR

Unsolvable Problems

1. Accept the child's problem as real to him.
2. Express empathy.
3. Try to help the child understand the situation, why it cannot be resolved.

Solvable Problems

1. Have the child describe the situation from his own perspective; get perspectives of others involved if helpful.
2. Help the child identify his options.
3. Help the child determine the likely consequences of each option.
4. Use simulation—parent and child role-play ways the child may respond to his problem if it occurs again. This helps the child gain experience in handling and realizing that options exist in resolving problems and that each has its own consequences. The child can then select the option he feels comfortable with the next time the problem arises.
5. Sometimes talking and simulation are not enough guidance for the child and the parent needs to structure a program of change to help the child improve his response to the problem.

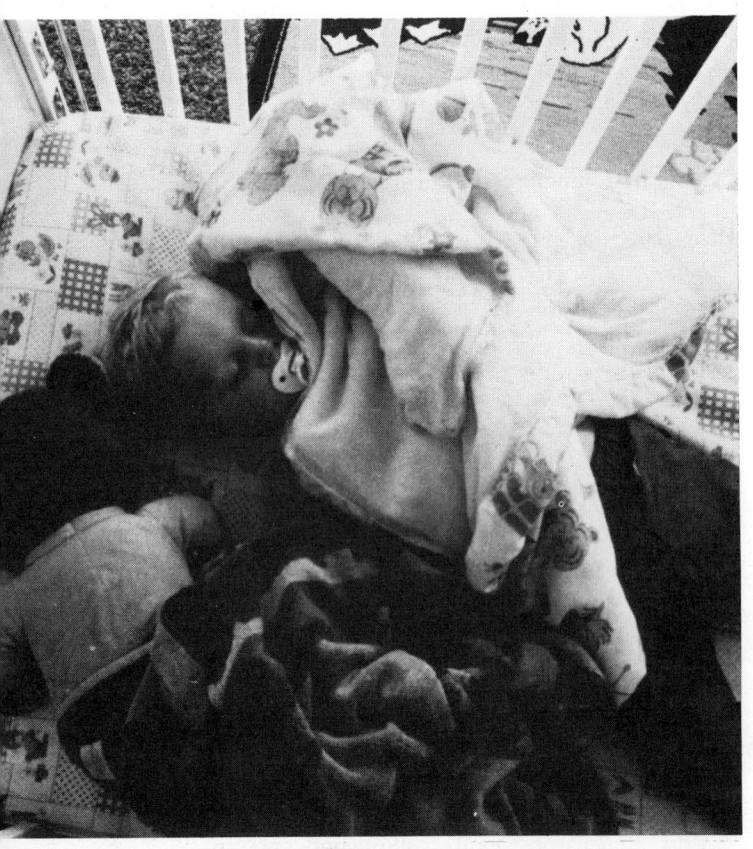

Rules consistently established and enforced make the child's world predictable, reinforcing his developing sense of security and trust.

an exciting endeavor for those who choose to make the commitment to parent. However, successful parents keep in mind that they are persons first and parents second.

The skills of parenting are not sex-specified. Male and female parents should combine their individual capabilities, each contributing those parenting behaviors with which they feel most comfortable and competent. As stated by Perdue et al., "Women are no more understanding, patient, secure or loving than men. Men are no more competent to make decisions, earn wages, negotiate family status within the community and set limits than women."[23] A couple must balance these qualities between them and contribute these behaviors to their parenting according to each parent's strengths, not on the basis of sex — these qualities do not "belong" to one or the other sex.

Providing a home and food is only the beginning of being a parent. The most important role of parenting is the *nurturing* of personality and development in a climate of *love* and *security* that starts a child on the road to healthy adult-

TABLE 3-3 CRUCIAL PARENTAL ROLES AT EACH STAGE OF CHILDHOOD

Stage	Parental Roles
Infancy	Physical caretaker — affirm love and acceptance. Stimulator of motor development; builder of trust by being predictable and consistent.
Toddlerhood	Physical helper — affirm developing selfhood. Stimulator of self-regulatory body functioning; facilitator of exploration within set limits.
Preschool	Physical ↔ psychological helper — affirm creative efforts. Facilitator of emotional self-control, moral and sexual development; stimulator of self-care skills with limits.
School age and preadolescence	Psychological helper — affirm capacity to be productive. Stimulator of mental, social, on-going moral development; facilitator to acceptance of changing skills and body image; progressive freedom-giving with reasoned limit-setting.
Adolescence and young adulthood	Psychological supporter — affirm developing adult image. Facilitator of open communication; freedom-giver; reinforcer of moral limits.

hood. The paradox of parenting is that we live with our children so we can teach them to live without us. This nurturing begins before the child's birth as the parent(s) prepares emotionally and intellectually for the parenting role.

We are all products of our own childhood. For a parent raised in a loving home, repeating that atmosphere with his own child is usually easier. If one has experienced an unloving or insecure childhood, successful parenting may be more difficult, but it is not an impossibility. None of us chose our backgrounds, but by understanding the importance of giving love in a way children can perceive and receiving education for parenthood, one can compensate for one's own childhood deprivations.

Parents are their children's first teachers. They teach the most important lesson of living: how to interact with other humans. They also teach children to be happy and loving by providing them with happiness and love. Expressions of love can be woven into all the things parents do for or with their child.

An effective parent cannot be passive but must participate in the child's learning process. How a parent participates (parental role) in the learning process will change as the child grows and develops. Table 3-3 describes the primary parental roles at each developmental stage of childhood. Encouragement, approval and positive interaction are needed by children at all ages from their parents.

Parental roles have traditionally been differentiated into mothering roles and fathering roles. In modern society this is steadily changing so that the relative impact of each parent on a child's development is also undergoing change. However, this modern concept of

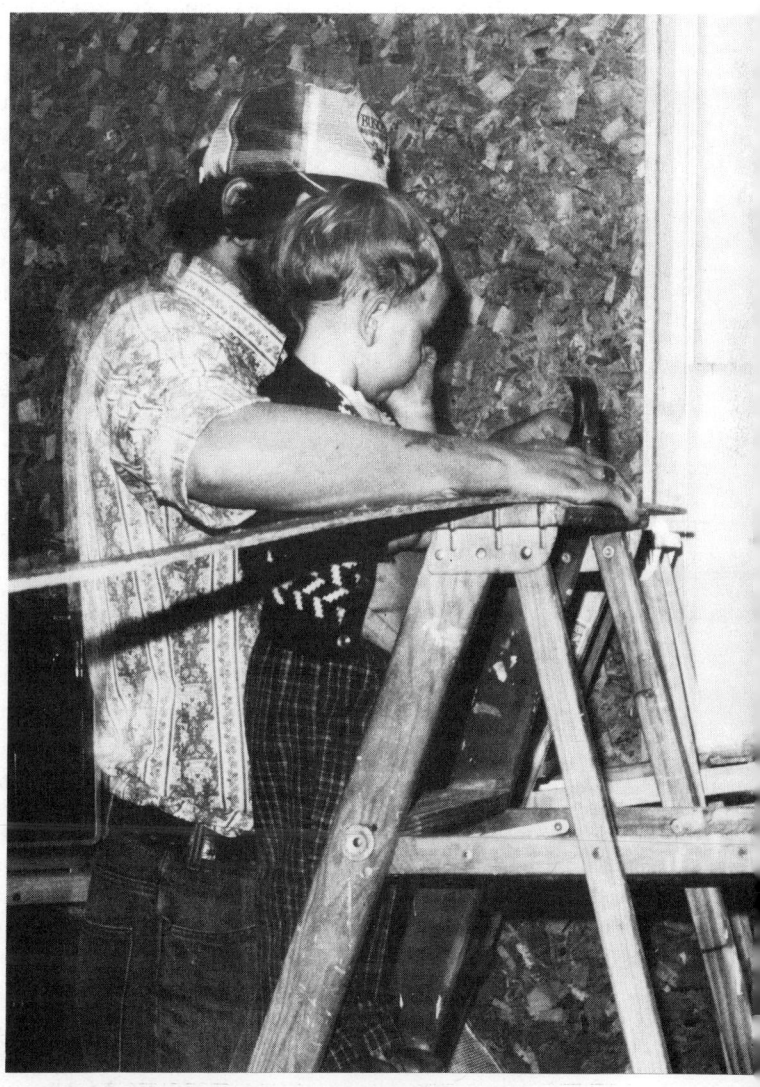

Parents are their children's first teachers.

parenting has not existed long enough for adequate researched documentation of what the changes it produces actually are. Many families, particularly at lower-middle and lower class levels, are still functioning by basically traditional parenting standards. Therefore, a discussion follows on the traditional mothering and fathering roles and the impact each has had on children's development.

Traditional Mothering Role A mother's functions have been labelled as *expressive*, involving keeping the family functioning smoothly as a unit.[19] Her traditional role requires that she maintain family relationships, referee conflicts among family members, offer emotional support based on unconditional love and keep home strains and stresses under control. She is unquestionably the primary caregiver and manages most of the parenting tasks. Research suggests that, in the traditional mothering role, she has the greatest impact on the development of sexuality in her children, regardless of their sex, probably because she is more consistently available to model and reinforce related behaviors. She also strongly influences the father-child relationship by how she feels about the father. In father-absent or -present homes in which the mother reinforces a negative image of the father, children display more antisocial behavior and poorer self-concepts.[19]

Traditional Fathering Role The traditional father's role is an *instrumental* one, involving binding the family as a unit and its individual members into society.[17, 19] He is the parent who incites his children to incorporate the rules and values of society and who symbolizes the authority of society. He is responsible for earning the family income, making major family decisions, and inflicting disciplinary measures. His love is conditional, requiring adequacy of performance by family members before it is given. Even though his impact on his children's sexuality development is less than the mother's, he has the greatest concern that his daughters be feminine and his sons masculine.[19] Although they see themselves as important to their children's development, traditional fathers often take insufficient advantage of the time available to them to spend with their children.[17, 19] Fathers are also twice as likely to be abusive toward their children.[19] Research indicates that the traditional father's influence is predominantly in the area of the child's moral development, in the child's tendency to express or inhibit aggression and in whether or not the child becomes delinquent.[19]

Shared Parenting Many couples today, as a result of the human liberation movements that have precipitated identity changes for both sexes, are rejecting the role models their parents gave them because these models no longer seem adequate in today's rapidly changing world. Some major changes that directly affect parenting are the increasing numbers of working mothers, the increased amount of leisure time available to family units, the increasing numbers of divorces involving paternal custody, the smaller size of family units. Current society exerts relentless and often contradictory pressures on parents to "get ahead" on the one hand and to become more involved in family life and child-nurturing on the other.

Statistics from basic research and criminal justice data confirm that children of either sex who receive warm affection and nurturing from their fathers as well as their mothers are most likely to become generous, morally sensitive and creative persons.[17, 19, 26]

Of course there have always been warm fathers, free of the machismo mystique, who enjoyed both a closeness to and a responsibility for the full care of their children, but traditional

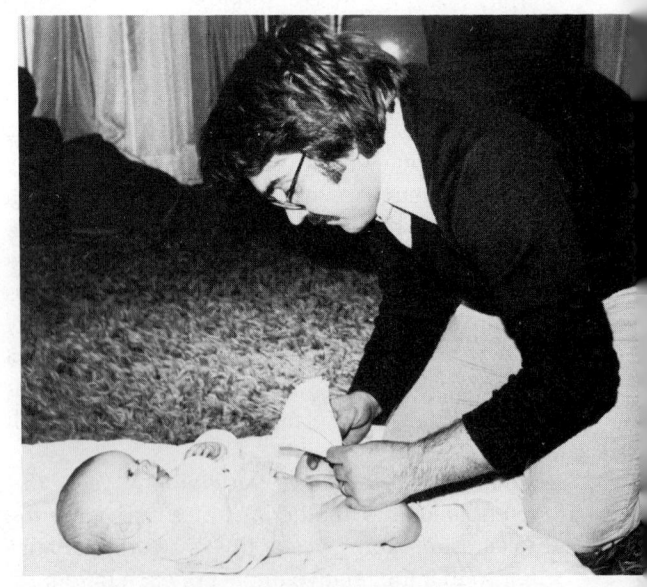

Many fathers, even in traditional homes, enjoy the closeness that helping care for their children allows them.

FAMILIES GROW AND DEVELOP

institutions and attitudes have made involvement in shared parenting difficult for such fathers.

Today men are increasingly demanding to have their full share of parenting, while more women are insisting on taking more responsibility in the world outside the home (fortunately for children, these changing images are congruent to parenting).[14, 15, 26] Early indications are that both the boys and the girls in shared parenting situations value tenderness, nurturing and compassion.[26, 29] Since fathers can affect all aspects of their children's development, those who want to have an impact in the lives of their children need to involve themselves in all aspects of their children's needs and pleasures.[17, 19] The result of shared parenting is a balanced, firmly founded relationship with the child by both parents.

PRINCIPLES OF PARENTING

Any set of principles to help parents select parenting techniques can only be a guide and not a blueprint. Nor can the most timely child-rearing manual be adopted for all children or in all homes. Any effort to do so will soon find parents filled with resentment, guilt, lowered confidence or all three because most manuals offer guidelines that are too vague to be useful or that do not take into account differences in parents or uniquenesses of children.[9, 27]

Some guidelines have been offered to parents, however, that come from children themselves and that have applicability regardless of the child involved or the parenting methods preferred by parents.[9]

1. *"Don't blow your class,"* or keep the dignity of your parenthood. The first rule to maintain parental dignity is for parents to present a united front regarding rules and the disciplinary measures taken to enforce them. Although differences are likely to exist in a couple's attitudes and parenting methods, they should be resolved by compromise outside the child's hearing and, ideally, before he is even born.

A second rule to retain parental dignity is to avoid arguing with the child. Confrontations force someone into submission, which is deflating to self-esteem. If a parent firmly believes in the stance he has taken on an issue, it should simply be enforced. If the issue cannot be enforced, it should be dropped and forgotten. And if the parent has no definite stance on the issue, the child's opinion should be heard to arrive at a joint decision.

Parents should also avoid threats, promises, bribes and sarcasm. Threats only invite misbehavior. The use of promises invalidates the parent-child relationship. Bribes communicate doubt to the child of his ability to behave on his own initiative and insure only short-term cooperation. Sarcasm blocks communication and encourages revenge fantasies. All of these diminish parenting as a teaching-learning process.[11]

A final rule for maintenance of parental authority is to talk less and listen more. Authority calls for brevity in the administration and enforcement of rules. Brevity requires conciseness that facilitates the child's comprehension of what is expected of him or why the reinforcement occurred. When words are used to socialize children the emphasis should be on what must be done. Words should be kept to a minimum and accompanied by action; they should be descriptive, not general.[7]

2. *"Bug me a little,"* or use firm but fair, loving discipline. Such discipline remembers that everyone needs successes and that positive attitudes and expectations are contagious, especially to children. Loving discipline does not see everything that happens but rather ignores some things and laughs at still others. Fair discipline respects each child as a unique person and allows him room within which to learn the rules of happy living. Firm, fair discipline allows the experience of feelings but sets limits on the actions taken to express them, channelling expression into acceptable forms (symbolic release, talking it out, or play). Fair discipline also respects the child's ability to absorb only a few rules at a time. Four or five rules are manageable by the average child, although those children with mental or intellectual handicaps may be able to handle only one to three rules at a time and may require a longer period for mastery. Above all else, fair and loving discipline does not involve comparisons between children.

3. *"Call my bluff,"* or let the child see that you mean what you say. Children need limits set on their behavior until they have learned to be self-regulatory; they expect to bear the consequences of misbehavior despite the temporary anger, frustration or disappointment it

causes them. Once a rule is established and conveyed to the child, it should be promptly and consistently enforced. Rules that cannot be enforced should not be made. Parents should also allow children to own and solve their own problems to the extent that they are ready and able.

4. "Light me a candle," or show the child the way to maturity and faith. The vast majority of a child's learning occurs as a result of imitation of the significant others in his life. Thus, if parents wish to effectively socialize their children, they need to model behaviors consistent with what they are attempting to teach. Children also behave in a manner consistent with the injunctions and permissions their parents project upon them, usually unconsciously.[12] These injunctions and permissions are conveyed to the child indirectly through the conversation he overhears about himself that the parent is addressing to someone else.

Research findings and observations of children's instinctual behavior support the validity of two other principles of parenting.[8, 12] First, parents need not waste time teaching those things that the child will teach himself when he is developmentally ready (toilet training, weaning). Instead, parents should consider what attributes society will judge once the child is an adult (dependability, honesty, creativity, ambition) and teach those. Second, parents are wise to avoid extremes — overpermissiveness or strict authoritarianism, bribery or revenge, pampering or being overly strict — as these invariably produce unhealthy responses in children.

PARENTING STYLES

No one method for instructing in the rules of living and conveying right or wrong has proved more effective than another, as long as the method used was not carried to extremes, and none will work until a child holds respect for his parent(s) and the authority a parent represents.

Three parenting themes can be derived out of the parenting behaviors within families. Any one of them, if extreme, can result in incomplete or unhealthy socialization of children. Conversely, any of them, if conducted in an atmosphere of love that positively reinforces desired behavior, can effect the healthy socialization of children.[12, 21] Table 3–4 summarizes these three styles.

FACTORS IMPORTANT TO SELECTION OF PARENTING STYLE

Children are very different and have their own unique responses to all of life's experiences and challenges, including the parenting with which they must cope on a daily basis. Parents also differ with regard to the parenting styles they can effectively and comfortably employ and in how they respond to each individual child. Thus there can be no one right or wrong parenting style, nor can a given parenting style be used with all children.

A child's temperament and developmental stage as well as parental interests and sociocultural values are factors that influence the effectiveness of the various parenting styles. The discussion that follows is intended to offer some guidelines that the nurse can utilize as she offers guidance and counsel to parents in their efforts to socialize their children. To use the guidelines appropriately, the nurse must assess the child and parents in terms of each of the these factors. (See Chapter 10 for guidance in assessment.)

Temperament or Basic Personality Parenting methods have impact on whether children's traits develop into assets or problems. Table 3–5 describes management of the three temperaments to derive the most positive functioning of the child. The following temperament-related considerations are also useful to parents as they construct a parenting plan for each child:

1. Make demands and expectations consistent with the child's temperament, i.e., realistic for him.
2. Encourage children to function at their potential; do not foster complacency or underachievement.
3. Accept that some temperaments are more demanding of tolerance than others, that some are more at risk for behavior problems and that it is all right to seek professional help and important to identify and correct problems as soon as they appear.
4. Try to accept the nature of each child and to channel negative features in a desirable direction. Occasional frustration is normal, but seek help if it is prolonged or chronic.

Age and Developmental Stage Parents will need to adapt their basic parenting plan for

TABLE 3-4 THREE PARENTING STYLES[7, 13, 21]

Parenting Styles	Main Theme	Predominant Approach to Teach Socialization	Primary Teaching Methods	Comments
Autocratic or authoritarian	Obedience; respect	Favors punitive measures to curb self-will when child does not comply with code of conduct	State rules. Declare expectations. Assert parental values. Apply negative reinforcement for noncompliance, usually physically. Occasionally grant privileges or increased responsibility for compliance.	Behavior evaluated in accord with a set standard of conduct, often theologically based. Tends to employ primarily negative reinforcement.
Democratic or authoritative	Autonomous problem solving based on self-regulation and disciplined conformity	Shares rationale for desired behavior with child; affirms child's efforts to comply but sets limits or boundaries for acceptable behavior	Describe problem or explain rules. Help child find his own solutions to problem or way to comply with rule based on his uniqueness. Reinforce positively for compliance, negatively for noncompliance: verbally (declare pleasure or indignation), physically (actions that communicate satisfaction or dissatisfaction with behavior), in writing (notes of praise or recommended change in behavior).	Least likely to be carried to extremes. Encourages development of child's own inner controls over behavior, self-reliance. More verbal exchanges; employs both positive and negative reinforcement.
Permissive		Uses reason; punitive measures seldom (if ever) used to teach socialization	Suggest rules, giving reasons for them. Give child choice of complying or not complying. Sometimes positively reinforce compliance, usually ignore or tolerate noncompliance.	Does not foster development of inner controls. Few demands made for responsibility unless child chooses to have it. Tends to leave child on own, reinforcing neither positively or negatively.

each child as the child grows and matures. The need for external (parent-initiated) reinforcements diminishes as a child gets older, and the external reinforcements that are provided can become gradually less action-oriented and more reason-oriented as the child develops intellectually. Keeping a child's developmental tasks in mind at each age helps parents determine what adaptations to the basic parenting approach are needed. Table 3-6 clarifies realistic parental expectations at each age and stage of development.

Sociocultural Values and Interest of Parents Values and roles become less rigidly defined with increasing socioeconomic status and when parents perform at higher intellectual levels. This seems particularly evident in the areas of parenting related to parenting style, developmental competency emphasis and parental protectiveness.

Parenting Style Lower class parents tend to use more power-oriented reinforcements, especially with their sons.[4] Although a good mix in preferred parenting styles exists with the middle class, the tendency is to use a democratic approach, especially with daughters.[8] The middle class parent uses more body contact in nurturing activities. Upper class parents show a preference for the permissive parenting style, although they are also strictest about sexual training.

Developmental Competency Emphasis Lower class parents tend to value early self-control (physical competency), while middle and upper class families value earlier mastery of problem-solving skills (emotional, intellectual competence) by their children.

TABLE 3-5 TEMPERAMENT OR BASIC PERSONALITY AS A FACTOR IN PARENTING[3, 12, 28]

Easy Child	Slow-to-Warm Child	Difficult Child	Mixed Child
1. Adapts to almost any parenting approach and is easy to manage as long as expectations are clearly defined and consistently endorsed; this avoids confusion for child.	1. A patient, relaxed, persevering approach is most effective. New situations or rules should be presented gradually, but repeatedly, without much pressure. (One reassuring feature of this child is that he gradually adapts and his noncooperation or nonparticipation until he does is usually nonbelligerent and silent.) Because of some common elements in the traits of difficult and slow-to-warm personality types, some management guidelines apply to both. Nos. 2–8 in this column apply to both.	1. A firm, consistent approach that emphasizes the positive works best. Those aspects of child's temperament that may have undesirable consequences if allowed unrestricted expression should be controlled and limited in a calm but firm and consistent manner.	Respond to whichever of the other three personality types seems to predominate in this child.
2. Learns rules quickly unless intellectually impaired.	2. Refuse to compete with the child or force adherence to every rule of the home to its more rigid interpretation. Such action only increases negative display of behavior.	2. Patience is essential. (This child is two times more likely to receive parental criticism.) Active effort is necessary to avert negative parent-child relationships from arising out of child's constant stressful behaviors. (Nurturing a child of this temperament places special demands on parents and interactions are usually perceived as stressful between parent and child.)	
3. Realistic parenting that will not be incongruent with what child finds in the world outside his home is an important consideration. These children seldom develop behavior problems, but when they do it is most often due to a conflict between home-taught values and those of the outside world.	3. Try not to explode at the child, as such fury only exaggerates his inappropriate behavior.	3. Parents of this "testy" child cope best if they take turns coping with child's behavior and give each other a daily chance to get away from child.	
4. Because this child adapts so readily, it is important not to initiate any practice or ritual that is undesirable to continue over time as this child will quickly incorporate that practice into his living pattern.	4. Clearly identify on a regular basis what behaviors will be accepted and what behaviors are unacceptable. (A picture chart or checklist posted in rooms the child spends much time in are creative ways to regularly reinforce expectations.) This child also needs help identifying what behaviors are contingent on the situation at hand; do this clarifying at times when the child is not misbehaving so that he is not so tense that he cannot hear the rules. Then carry through consistently in enforcing established limits. (A democratic approach is least overwhelming to this child. However, an autocratic approach also suits difficult child as long as autocratic approach is not extreme.)	4. In those activities that predictably cause negative behavior, parents are wise to take turns handling the child; it is important to persist in introducing the child to this situation or expectation, however, so that he can eventually learn control.	
	5. Since this child learns slowly much repetition is needed.	5. This child needs gradual and repeated reinforcement (positive and negative) of expected behaviors before he can internalize them. (Problems in behavior usually arise from conflict between the child and almost any aspect of his environment, whether it be parents, new situations or the world outside.)	
	6. Build in success experiences for this child daily.	6. This child can manage only a minimum number of rules at a time (1–3). The rules need to be straightforward, unencumbered by explanations or choices.	
	7. Maintain established routines while child is mastering a rule or behavioral expectation.	7. Provide constructive avenues for excess emotions and energy.	
	8. Key words to management: • Firmness • Repeated exposure • Consistent reinforcement • Patience		

TABLE 3-6 AGE AND DEVELOPMENTAL STAGE AS A FACTOR IN PARENTING[6]

Parenting Goals	Infant (0–1 yr)	Toddlers (1–3 yr)	Preschooler (3–5 yr)	School-age Child (6–12 yr)	Adolescent/Young Adult (13–21 yr)
Safety	Protect from falls, injuries, etc., as motor skills increase	Place limits on investigations and mobility; child-proof home.	Assist in protecting self. Teach safety rules.	Allow unassisted activities but with safe levels of limits, as riding bike on road but not on heavily traveled streets.	Self-responsibility for safety.
Family beliefs and values	Child can adapt to routine ADL	Child can begin integrating religious and cultural values through practice and participation in rituals.	Child can conform to home routines, take responsibility for helping with some. Able to learn manners, feel guilt. Increased participation in family practices and rituals.	Ready to comprehend reasons, explanations behind values, beliefs, practices. Ready for involvement in group activities and practices.	Ready to decide or choose for self what beliefs and values to accept–time to let go and allow that choice. Enforce morality rules of family until he learns to trust his own moral judgment.
Social behavior and role	Enforce cooperation in ADL and care procedures. Child can learn some patience	Expect obedience most of the time. Child is able to learn respect for other's belongings, and to accept substitute caretakers.	Able to cooperate, learning to share. Can increasingly control anger and aggression. Tries many roles during play. Needs sexual questions answered; will investigate.	Can have regular responsibility for some home chores. Needs some limits set on friend selections. Expect acceptable school behaviors, peer tolerance.	Needs limits on sexual expressions; don't expect mature judgments. Avoid overreacting to typical teen crises. Expect acceptable social behavior.
Self-regulation and independence	Dependent on others to meet his needs; no self-control	Can take increasing responsibility for regulation of body functions; needs to learn proper language for body and its functions. Learns to accept, respect limits. "Do it myself" really means "let me do what I can, then help me."	Can accomplish most self-care in ADL. Will need help in more complex tasks.	Able to increasingly accomplish ADL without aid; anticipate occasional regression. Increasingly socialized (internal enforcement) in behaviors, but still heavily guided by imitating significant others.	Has internalized most rules of living. Able to maintain own ADL and many of home chores if given opportunity. Needs faith in his abilities reinforced and support during failures; otherwise, independent, self-regulating.

PARENTING FOR THE SOCIALIZATION OF CHILDREN

Democratic parenting predominates:
more paternal involvement likely

```
Parenting yielded almost                                          Parenting either over-
full time to substitute                                           permissive (indulging)
caretakers or no care-                                            or overcontrolling
takers                                                            (extreme autocratic,
                                                                  dominating)

              Parenting incidental;    May be any of three styles,
              laissez faire or over-   although permissive style
              permissive               is less likely

              Primarily self-centered;  Primarily child-centered;
              most involvement is with  most involvement is with
              own activities and        child care activities and
              interests                 children's interests
                                                                  Completely child-
                                                                  centered; total involve-
                                                                  ment in children; no
                                                                  interests or activities
Completely self-centered;                                         not involving children
total involvement in own
activities and interests
                        Balance between own activities
                        and interests and those
                        involving children
```

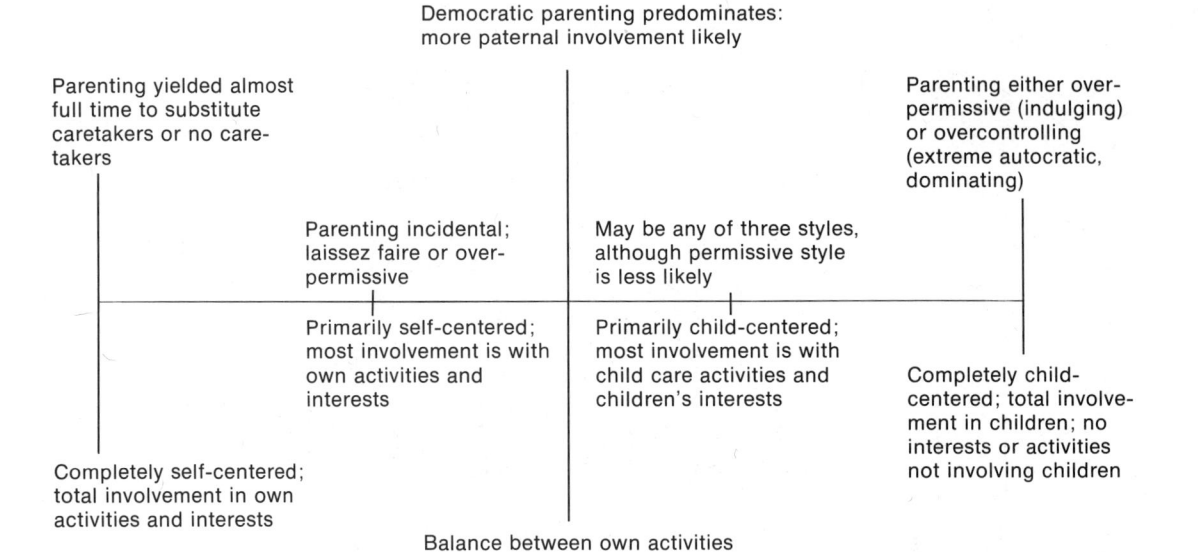

Figure 3-1 Relationship between parent interest level and parenting style.

Parental Protectiveness Lower class parents tend to underprotect their males and overprotect their females.[16] Middle class parents are the ones most frequently involved in motivating social agencies to promote a safe environment for children. Upper class families tend to be overprotective of their children.[16]

Specific cultural practices influencing parenting are dependent on the family's cultural background. Whether cultural or societal values are given precedence in parenting depends on how strong the family's bond is with their cultural heritage. A parent's personality structure influences parenting preferences. The more rigid a parent's personality is (difficult or slow-to-warm temperament), the more likely that person is to employ strict or autocratic parenting methods.

Whether a parent's interests are primarily child-centered or self-centered also affects parenting style. Figure 3-1 illustrates the relationship that usually exists between parental interest level and parenting style.

RESPECTING RIGHTS

Parents and children who acknowledge and accept each others' rights are healthier, happier parents and children. The "child's bill of rights" and "parent's bill of rights" are useful guidelines to parenting activities.

Child's Bill of Rights Children need love, discipline and gradual independence from their parents. Parents who attempt to adhere to the following bill of rights for their children will most likely meet those needs regardless of the parenting style they employ. A child should be able to expect that his parents will:[13, 21]

1. Be consistent in their interactions with him so that he can feel secure,
2. Show affection to him in a manner that communicates he is accepted and valued as an individual,
3. Accentuate the positive in the child rather than criticize or humiliate; respect his efforts,
4. Understand and tolerate his childish behaviors yet provide direction and limits as necessary so he can learn to behave in ways that earn him acceptance, develop his conscience and prepare him for independence,
5. Model healthy, competent adult behavior.

Parent's Bill of Rights Parents need to feel respected as authorities and as persons by their children. Parents can help their children develop that respect by adhering to the following bill of rights for themselves regardless of their parenting approach.

A parent should be able to expect that his child will behave within the guidelines his

parents establish, and respect his parents' efforts to raise him to healthy adulthood.[1, 7, 21] Further, parents should model respect by themselves respecting their right to:[1, 7]
1. Be an authority with their children,
2. Hold their rights to be equally as important as their child's rights,
3. Be a person of worth who has strengths and limitations,
4. Have some daily private times away from children,
5. Seek ambitions and accomplishments outside of parenthood,
6. Make it unprofitable for their child not to mind his own business with regard to the spouse relationship,
7. Be authentic in expressions of feelings, including constructive venting of anger.[7, 11]

ASSESSING PARENTING CAPABILITIES

Raising a family should not be approached as an exercise in perfection. Parenting will be affected not only by parents' strengths and flaws but also by their children's strengths and weaknesses. No family is perfect and yet the great majority of parents do a more than adequate job of raising their children to be successful adults — sometimes against tremendous odds. Health professionals have a responsibility (1) to help parents free themselves from unjustified guilt when their child does not always measure up; (2) to help parents develop self-confidence and trust in their parenting instincts, enhanced by accurate information and professional guidance and (3) to help parents find a compromise between what they expect of themselves and their children and what is realistic.

Reassurances That Parents Need

Research and surveys of parents indicate that parents need information in four areas in order to relax and enjoy realistic, guilt-free parenting enacted with self-confidence.[5, 8, 9, 18, 22, 29] They need to know (and the health professional is in an ideal position to inform them):
1. It's ok not to be perfect.
2. It's ok to exert authority.
3. It's ok not to be rich.
4. It's ok to work or not to work.

It's OK Not To Be Perfect Parents need reassurance that it is all right to be themselves with their children. No one is perfect; all parents make mistakes with their children. If parents are able to admit to their human failings and imperfections, they are modelling genuineness — a useful adult concept that the child will imitate and incorporate into his own moral code. Being genuine frees a parent to admit that a situation was handled badly, to be released from brooding or guilt and to apologize to the child. (Such action builds rather than diminishes a child's respect.)

Genuine parents can continue being "husband and wife" as well as "mother and father" without feeling guilty that they may be inadequate parents by doing so. After all, parenting has built-in time limits; marriage does not.[22] The modelling of a healthy male-female relationship that this action provides to the child is also a valuable learning experience, preparing him for successful adulthood.

Real parents need real children. Parents who accept self-imperfections are more able to accept the imperfections of their child and the stimulation their "real" child provides in his inventiveness, unpredictability and mischievousness. Knowledge of child growth and development facilitates parents' adaptation to their real child's changing self, allowing them to relax their anxieties about those behaviors they know are a part of their child's stage of growth and guiding them in the establishment of realistic rules and limits. Parents should also realize that this knowledge of development, although it makes them more self-confident, flexible, resilient and resourceful, cannot produce the perfect child. Setting aside in a personal "memory bank" or "emotional savings account" the wonderful things their child does gives parents a reservoir to draw from to retain their optimism on the days when their child is not so wonderful.[20]

Parents who are able to accept that neither they nor their children are perfect can feel comfortable accepting that their parenting actions will not always be perfect either and that this is all right. Although there are certain minimum elements that parents must provide for satisfactory parenting — rules, consistency, positive and negative reinforcements, all based on love — there is no single recipe for providing those ingredients. Parents should periodically evaluate the impact their approach is having on their child; whether unpleasant feelings, increased misconduct, an atmosphere of family tension are building up. If they are prepared to modify their approach if it seems to be damaging, regardless of what manuals, relatives or psycholgists say, they can trust that their own recipe is a good one. That trust will help their child grow to trust himself.

When parents are genuine enough to teach their child all they honestly know and believe, they have no need to feel guilty when the child chooses a different path from their own.

It's OK To Exert Authority To raise children takes lots of energy and ingenuity and is rarely a peaceful endeavor, but parents who feel comfortable setting limits for themselves and their children make the tasks of learning and growing easier. (A sense of humor kept handy is also helpful. A smile or laugh can lighten serious moments, ease tension, reduce anger, restore perspective.) To successfully raise their children parents sometimes need to exert authority. Relationships that are loving and caring readily withstand acts of authority with the end result being respect and cooperation: two desirable characteristics to be developed as children grow into adults. An important aspect of parental authority is the recognition by parents and children that parents can use different parenting styles with each child and react differently to each and still be loving. Effective parenting does not require equal or identical parenting behaviors for each child in a family.[5]

Expert advice from professionals can be helpful and even lifesaving, but children are not all alike, and the expert does not know a child as his parents do. Parents should not be condemned if their approach does not match the latest manual recommendations or the professional's beliefs. The professional's obligation is to objectively ascertain that the parental approach is not having a negative impact on the child or family. If it is not, the parents' approach should be reinforced. If a negative affect exists, parents need to be provided insight into the conflict, offered information that will give them broader parenting options to choose from and supported in their efforts to change.

It's OK Not To Be Rich The conflict between children's desires and the realities of the budget is a common frustration to most families today. It is important for parents to recognize the influence of finances on their parenting decisions. Parents need to realize and be reassured that children do not need everything they desire; in fact, they are often better off without the majority of things the glamorous ads make them believe they need. Every family's budget has a limit. Parents who recognize that fact are able to set priorities, ignore the cajoling media and retain some genuine experiences rather than substituting artificial or inanimate ones for them. These positive actions establish values that will be important to the children's ability to handle money as adults.

Parents should not protect their children from the budget; it is an important skill to be learned along with the other skills of successful adult living.[18, 29]

It's OK To Work Or To Not Work The following discussion addresses the mother; however, the statements made are equally applicable to whichever parent chooses to stay home or to work.

Parenthood is itself a profession (human development specialist). It does not have to be a parent's (usually the mother's) only career, but it is certainly worthy of recognition as a chosen profession. Full-time mothers should be encouraged to keep growing through some investment in personal interests or activities and not to sacrifice their dreams for the sake of their children. Children need to learn that mother has personal worth aside from her parent role, that she is capable of other interests and has other talents.

Society also needs to relax judgments on the mother who chooses to stay home, even if she does have advanced education or training that makes her well qualified for the work world. Mothers who choose to work need to be assured that, except for the extreme situation when the parent(s) is almost never available to the children, no research exists that shows a positive correlation between the amount of time spent with a child and his security, or that the fact that a mother works injures her child's development.[8, 24]

Children do not measure whether they are accepted or rejected, cared for or neglected by how much time their parent(s) spend with them but rather in terms of (1) the amout of love they are shown, (2) how well their parents listen to them with interest, (3) how proud their parents are of their achievements, (4) what their parents do during the time they are with them, and (5) the willingness of their parents to discuss their problems or worries with them.[8]

Whether a mother chooses to stay home or to work is not the real issue. What does matter is whether she feels comfortable and useful in whichever decision she makes. Her satisfaction with her decision and the roles it demands of her influence her self-image and how she interacts with family members, particularly children. What is the best arrangement in one family may not be in another. Society has an obligation to leave this a family matter without advocating or discouraging one life style or the other.

Using their natural strengths as parents, coupled with all the information and support available to them from the helping professions, parents can help their children become what they were meant to be with a minimum of frustration and turmoil and a maximum of pleasure and joy, whether they work away from home or not.

Parenting Problems

As with any aspect of living, problems in parenting can and do arise. Statistics of basic research and criminal justice allow classification of parenting problems that produce disturbances in socialization into four general categories. Table 3–7 lists those categories and describes the kind of parenting activities that are symptomatic of these problems. Nurses and other professionals who work with children and families should be watchful for any of these symptomatic behaviors each time they observe and interact with their clients.

TABLE 3–7 PARENTING PROBLEMS AND SYMPTOMATIC PARENTAL BEHAVIOR

Unrealistic Expectations

- Parent requires more self-control from child than age, development or circumstances make reasonable.
- Parent expects immediate obedience.
- Parent enforces too many rules at once or provides no rules. (Children need rules for behavior and will seek them elsewhere, often in gangs.)
- Parents request social skills of the child that they do not model owing to lack of knowledge or experiences.

Inconsistency

- Family disharmony.
- Parents lack a united front in goals, values, parenting philosophy or moral stance about right and wrong.
- Parents model behaviors and values incongruent with what they teach verbally and in rules established.
- Enforcement is not consistently carried out.
- Distortions in communication—too vague, too long, contradictory or void.

Extremes in Style, Methods

- No limits established or no guidance and reinforcements to help child comply with limits; overpermissive.
- Lack of firmness; parent not respected as authority.
- Limits too rigid; power replaces authority and fear or anger replaces respect.
- Reinforcements (positive or negative) do not match deed; too excessive, too long, teach wrong lesson.
- Primary disciplinary methods employed are bribes, promises, threats, sarcasm.

Disturbed Relationships

- Parent is too close to child to permit growth—intrusive control, dominance—exemplified by parent who always (1) wants to change child, (2) demands to know child's activities and conversation, (3) interferes in child's problem-solving or decision making, (4) reminds child of his misdeeds.
- Basically unfriendly or ambivalent interaction.
- Interaction inappropriate for child's age, stage or temperament.
- Parent is too distant for child to develop respect (1) parent preoccupied with self and own activities or wishes, (2) child feels isolated or unwanted.

The child's overt behavior can also be a direct barometer of the state of health of the parenting he is experiencing. The nurse, through her knowledge of normal development and temperament, can learn to differentiate temporary deviant behavior that is equivalent to growing pains or temperamental character and that deviant behavior which indicates problems. The nurse should offer guidance or help parents and child to obtain guidance from appropriate sources whenever she observes and/or receives parental reports of the following persisting behaviors:[5]

1. A child who continually behaves outside the stereotyped norms for children his age and temperament. Even if the behavior is later established to be normal, parents are usually grateful for guidance in how to accept and constructively interact with their perceived "atypical" child.
2. Bizarre behavior or speech that persists or receives frequent negative social response, or both.
3. Unexpected, atypical reactions to situations for age and temperament.
4. Prolonged adverse reactions to common situations or experiences (ADL* disturbances).
5. An accumulation of several related or unrelated troubling behaviors — unhappy, confused, rebellious, "ornery" without regard for others' responses, stubborn beyond reason, lazy, oversensitive, aggressive, delinquent activities — that seem to be lingering, getting worse or involving steadily more of the child's time.

Seeking professional help should be a first-aid measure rather than a last resort; this often requires alertness and initiative on the professional's part to help the family acknowledge that the problem potentially exists or is developing.

Intervening in Parenting

Parenting is not a topic to be evaluated and discussed at the third yearly visit, or when punishment is not working or after deviant behavior is observable. The nurse should approach the topic with the parent(s) early in the parenting relationship. Ideally, parents would have sought information before deciding to

*Activities of daily living.

have children. However, very few parents discuss such things before their infant arrives. The parenting process begins when the infant is born, so parents need information by this time, at least, and additional information can be added as the nurse and parents together anticipate the child's changing needs throughout his developing years.

As the nurse counsels parents through their child's developing years, she should bear in mind that, within a loving, secure home (ensured through adequate bonding and attachment) with routines, parents can try any style of parenting with which they feel confident and comfortable and most children will respond favorably as long as extremes are avoided. Occasional "mistakes" do not destroy a child for life.

In her early counselling the nurse should listen sensitively, observe the parent-child relationship and the individual temperaments involved and then help the parents find the style thay can live with and feel comfortable with on a daily basis.[20] Ongoing assessment of the parenting process and its impact on the child should occur at each contact, with particular attention given to symptoms in the four areas mentioned earlier in which problems frequently occur.

If symptoms are suggested either by the nurse's own observations, parental report or the child's deviant behavior, the nurse should intervene early to reverse unhealthy parenting patterns. Her intervention may involve helping the family see the problem area and referring its members to a competent resource for assistance. Problems that are minor, identified early or that she is competent to intervene directly in should be promptly managed. Intervention should begin with a general physical (special attention should be given to the child's hematocrit, height and weight progression) and developmental (DDST)* assessment of the child and of the physical and emotional status of the parents. (She should watch for any debilitating factors that deplete the parents of the stamina needed for parenting activities.)[2]

The support systems available to the parents — moral, direct, personal and professional — and whether these are having a positive or negative effect on the parenting efforts should be ascertained. If support systems exist that appear detrimental, the parents should be aided to reshape or get rid of them. If support systems

*Denver Developmental Screening Test (see Chapter 13).

appear inadequate, resources available to the family should be evaluated to strengthen those already existing or create additional ones.

The current level of parenting needs to be assessed for deficits in the categories listed in Table 3–7. If symptoms document that unrealistic expectations exist, education should be provided so that the parents can alter the parenting techniques to consider the age and development of their child(ren). If parents lack social skills, they should be assisted to develop a program to strengthen these skills.

If the conflict revolves around the problem of parents' inconsistency in treatment of the child, they need to be informed of the effect the inconsistency has, and they should be provided with guidance to develop uniformity and consistency, wherever their weakness lies. Often marital or family counselling is required to resolve these conflicts.

When evidence exists that parenting style or method is extreme, having a negative impact on the child, parents need help in realizing that their actions are motivating their child's misconduct. A multidisciplinary approach is often required to help these parents modify their parenting behaviors and to reverse the child's response pattern. Behavior modification programs designed for both parents and child are often successful, particularly when the problem is identified and the behavior pattern interrupted early.

Disturbances in parent-child relationships also usually require multidisciplinary intervention on a long-term basis. If disturbances are identified in the early weeks and months of the infant's life, corrective success is easier and faster.

When teaching or correcting parenting skills, the nurse should always work with and emphasize the strengths of the parents and child. In addition, she is responsible for locating appropriate resources capable of offsetting their deficiencies. It is impossible to predict and teach all the skills germane to parenting. But if the nurse can help parents develop an ability to sort out problems, look at options and negotiate suitable interventions, she has brought them a long way toward effective preparation for the challenges of parenthood.

References

1. M. Beecher and W. Beecher. Parents On The Run. Grosset and Dunlap, 1967
2. B. Bishop. A guide to assessing parenting capabilities, American Journal of Nursing, November 1976, p. 1784
3. J. B. Brown. Infant temperament: A clue to childbearing for parents and nurses, American Journal of Maternal Child Nursing, July/August 1977, p. 228
4. M. S. Brown. Childrearing in cross-cultural perspective. Health Values: Achieving High Level Wellness, March/April 1977, p. 77
5. S. Chess, T. Alexander and H. Chess. Your Child Is A Person. Penguin Books, 1976
6. E. Erikson. Childhood and Society. W. W. Norton & Co., Inc., 1963
7. A. Faber and E. Mazlish. Liberated Parents Liberated Children. Avon Books, 1975
8. S. Fisher and R. Fisher. What We Really Know About Childrearing. Basic Books, 1976
9. G. Fletcher. What's Right With Us Parents. William Morrow & Co., Inc., 1972
10. S. Fraiberg. The Magic Years. Charles Scribners' Sons, 1968
11. H. Ginott. Between Parent and Child. Avon Books, 1972
12. W. Homan. Child Sense. Basic Books, 1977
13. E. Hurlock. Child Development. McGraw-Hill Book Co., 1978
14. H. Keshet and K. Rosenthal. Fathers: a new study. Children Today, May/June 1978, p. 13
15. B. Kierman and M. Scaloveno. Fathering. Nursing Clinics of North America, September 1977, p. 481
16. M. Koller. Families: A Multigenerational Approach. McGraw-Hill Book Co., 1974
17. M. Lamb. The Role of the Father in Child Development. John Wiley & Sons, Inc., 1976
18. E. LeShan. How To Survive Parenthood. Random House, Inc., 1965
19. D. Lynn. The Father: His Role in Child Development. Wadsworth Publishing Co. Inc., 1974
20. M. A. Murphy. When parents ask about discipline. Pediatric Nursing, December 1976, p. 28
21. G. Norton. Parenting. Prentice-Hall Inc., 1977
22. E. Peck. The Parent Test: How To Measure Your Talent For Parenthood. Putnam Books, 1978
23. B. Perdue, J. Horowitz and F. Herz. Mothering. Nursing Clinics of North America, September 1977, p. 491
24. L. Salk. What Every Child Would Like His Parents To Know. Warner Paperback Library, 1973
25. J. Segal and H. Yahroes. A Child's Journey: Forces That Shape the Lives of Our Young. McGraw-Hill Book Co., 1978
26. E. Stein, editor. Fathering: Fact or Fable. Abingdon Press, 1977
27. G. Strozier. A critical look at childraising books. Detroit Free Press, 19 November 1976, p. 1-C
28. A. Thomas and S. Chess. Temperament and Development. Brunner/Mazel Inc., 1977
29. L. Yarrow. Trust yourself! You're a better parent than you think. Parents, April 1979, p. 52

Additional Recommended Reading

H. Biller and D. Meredith. Father Power. Doubleday Books, 1975
F. Dodson, How To Parent With Love. Rawson, Wade, Publishers, Inc., 1978
T. Gordon. P.E.T. In Action. Wyden Books, 1976
M. LeBow. Behavior Modification: A Significant Method in Nursing Practice. Prentice-Hall Inc., 1973
E. LeShan. Raising Your Child Without a Script: Natural Parenthood. New American Library, Inc., 1970
P. Smith et al. Childrearing attitudes of single teenage mothers. American Journal of Nursing, December 1979, p. 2115

4
ALTERNATIVE FAMILY LIFE STYLES

by Frances Wenger, RN, MSN

Will the traditional nuclear family be supplanted in its importance by some alternative family style? How many variant styles will society tolerate and support? What is the relationship between family life style and child development? Is one life style more conducive to effective childrearing than another? These and many more questions are being asked by various segments of society.[2, 34] The topic appears frequently in the news media as documentaries on television and feature articles in newspapers and magazines. Professional journals and textbooks are increasingly reporting on research in what is referred to as alternate family styles, variant family styles or emergent family styles. These include single parent (male or female), single parent by divorce, single parent by death, single parent by choice, communal families, adoptive parents, single parent adoption, biracial adoption, transcultural adoption, migrant families, gay marriages, foster parents, and stepparents.

In this chapter we define the more prevalent alternative family life styles in contemporary Western society, giving particular attention to childrearing practices and child-adult relationships. Some of the unique aspects of the variant styles will be compared to the traditional nuclear family, which was discussed in Chapter 1. The goal of these descriptions is to provide a basis for nurse interaction with many differing family systems. Therefore, whenever applicable, suggestions for nurse interaction patterns are included. Most of the suggestions are general and could be used by any health care provider. However, the educational preparation of the professional nurse and the unique contribution of nursing practice to health care have been considered in formulating the specific suggestions.

CHANGING PATTERNS

Change in family patterns is increasing in most societies. At a time when Western societies seem concerned about the demise of the nuclear family, Safilios-Rothschild[29] reports that the nuclear family is becoming the predominant family structure in societies that are entering industrialization. This should not be confused with the contemporary Western nuclear family. The traditional extended family has been replaced by a "modified" extended family rather than a strictly nuclear one. The "modified" extended family involves residential separation of the nuclear family from kin, while at the same time a close relationship is maintained between the couples and their parents through patterns of frequent visiting and communication, mutual financial assistance, babysitting and household services and a variety of other exchanges and obligations.[29]

In the United States and other Western societies, emerging styles seem to reach in two directions, with some persons searching for more extended family-like relationships and responsibilities (communes, group living arrangements) and others actualizing self-fulfillment needs and mobility (some single-parent, gay marriages). Families are systems with at least two and usually more persons, each with his own needs and aspirations, thereby making them complex. The dichotomy of extended and nuclear is only a generalization to permit some analysis. Likewise, the classification of the family styles discussed in this chapter serves only to identify some unique aspects of the particular family system. The nurse should always attempt to interact with the family holistically as a unique group of people.

SINGLE PARENT FAMILIES

Parents Without Partners,* an organization with chapters in most communities, defines the single parent family as consisting of one parent who is caring for his or her children, in his or her home, and who is a single parent due to widowhood, divorce or separation, or who is unmarried.[31] The current concern about the increasing incidence of single parent families — 16 per cent of all households in the United States today — ignores the fact that there have always been single parents in this country. High death rates and mobility of the bread winner who sought an improved livelihood by westward migration meant that more children in early America had fewer parental surrogates than today.[34] Single parenting because of death is not increasing, but as society embraces more values for individual fulfillment, the incidence of divorce and remaining single by choice has increased. The number of children reared in single parent families increased by 100 per cent between 1960 and 1970.[25]

Male Single Parent Families

The general assumption that children should live with mothers is being challenged daily in families working through the process of separation. The feminist movement has given impetus for women and men to discard traditional roles. New laws on custody provide indication that single male parenting will likely increase.

Mendes[25] reports on a research study that was conducted in Southern California from 1974 to 1975. The most important factor in the health of the family was whether the situation was chosen by the father or was accidental. The father's initial reaction to the child is based on that factor. The assenters (acceded but did not seek

---

*Parents without Partners, Inc., is an international nonprofit, nonsectarian educational organization devoted to the welfare and interests of single parents and their children. A journal, *The Single Parent*, is published bimonthly. The headquarters is at 80 Fifth Avenue, New York, New York 10011.

the role) needed assistance most but were least likely to seek out supportive services. These fathers wanted to prove their abilities as single parents. The seekers (chose the role) more readily expressed their needs and concerns about parenting, such as concern about normal childhood, adolescent behavior, disciplinary problems and daughters' sexual development.[25]

In recent research studies of motherless families, it was shown that the fathers take on homemaking, child guidance and nurturing responsibilities as well as the more traditional father roles of financial support and house maintenance.[21, 22, 25, 32] The most difficult area of responsibility for single male parents is nurturing of the children. Many expressed insecurity in responding to their children's feelings. The men usually report that they feel closer to their children as a result of increased nurturing responsibilities.

A growing number of single male parents are voicing the need for supportive care, which can take many forms. For some, it may be commu-

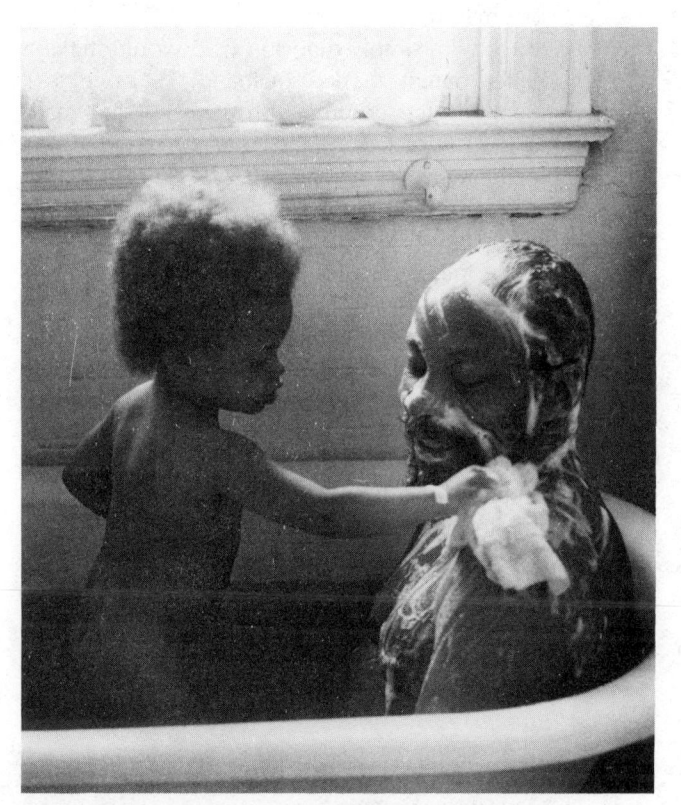

Today more single fathers are taking on homemaking, child guidance and nurturing responsibilities. (Anna Kaufman Moon/Stock, Boston, Inc.)

ALTERNATIVE FAMILY LIFE STYLES 61

nity support groups such as Parents Without Partners or Parent Effectiveness Training.* It is important that these support groups have masculine role models. In the past, many of the support groups were dominated by women whose needs, although similar, are distinctly different because of socialization factors.

Others may benefit from group living arrangements with dual parent families or with other single parent families. One father reported the he actually has "the best of two worlds." He lives in a small house with his son. Five other families, one single, live nearby in similar houses. Two of the women in these families care for six children while the others work outside the homes. They are paid by the group for this function. The other adults help with special projects with children that require more time and specialized supervision. Evenings and weekends, each family is on its own. This particular father states, "I spend a lot of time with Billy as just the two of us and have the security as he does of having many other people to trust and care for him." He adds, "If my own family had worked, I wouldn't have chosen this for myself, or more importantly, for Billy. Maybe I'm simply a person who would make a better parent than a husband."[22] Table 4-1 identifies the common problems of the male single parent family and nursing roles that can facilitate resolution of those concerns.

The roles of father and husband have usually been viewed as inseparable and compatible. Some fathers are finding it necessary to challenge this assumption. Some are successfully demonstrating that they can and want to care for and nurture their children without the support of a wife. As society includes emotional responsiveness as a male trait as well as a female trait, single male parents will be better prepared for the nurturing responsibilities and privileges of parenthood.

Female Single Parent Families

Families headed by a single woman are more common than those headed by a single man.

---
*In hundreds of communities, Parent Effectiveness Training classes are being taught Dr. Thomas Gordon's system of specific skills in solving family conflicts and encouraging healthy parent-child relationships.

TABLE 4-1 THE NURSE'S ROLE IN MAXIMIZING THE MALE SINGLE PARENT FAMILY EXPERIENCE

Situational Factors	Nurse Role Factors
Father's need for support in child nurturing.	Identify community support groups.
Support groups need masculine role models.	Influence community agencies to include males in organizing and conducting groups for single parent fathers.
Assistance needed in learning physical care of children and homemaking tasks.	Assess family needs for child care. Teach physical care of children and/or mobilize community resources.
Children's need for mother role models.	Assist in identifying surrogate mothers and adult women role models within father's support group of relatives, friends, schools.

Since homemaking, child care and nurturing have traditionally been female family responsibilities, mothers who have become heads of household by accident or by choice continue to assume these important family functions. In addition, they are confronted with the burden of economic provision and other traditional male family tasks (automotive repair, house maintenance and some child discipline).

In divorce situations, courts have generally granted custody of children to mothers rather than to fathers. This practice is changing, but the majority of single parent families are still headed by women.

Mothers who become single parents by accident (not by choice) often find it necessary to work outside the home, sometimes for the first time. Home and child care tasks that formerly consumed all their time now are relegated to marginal time, often when they are tired. The children's view of the change in their mother's priorities can be interpreted as rejection, making the emotional climate even more unstable. Nurses relating to these families can be helpful in encouraging the mothers and the children to verbalize their views of the home responsibilities and relationships. The mothers and children may need assistance in setting priorities and in securing help from friends and relatives or other community resources.

The purported negative impact on male children in female-headed families has been a focus of research and discussion.[17, 22] Hill cites research ambiguities which demonstrate that the data are far from conclusive. Studies on father absence have focused on sanctioned and honorable absences and temporary absences rather than on morally disapproved and permanent absences, such as divorce and desertion. Hill reports on a study in which extensive interviews were conducted with groups of young married and unwed mothers, consisting largely of Appalachian whites and blacks from the Bluegrass region of Kentucky.[17] A high degree of normal psychosocial development was found in the female-headed single parent families that had the support of other family members and relatives. In fact, such families functioned better than many two-parent families. The key seems to be support from relatives and friends, who serve to strengthen the mother's parental role and who serve as male and female role models.

Research into the sexual attitudes of one-parent children concludes that "inappropriate" attitudes result less from having been raised by only one parent than from the attitudes of that parent.[22] Children may experience a variety of problems that relate to poor sexual identification if single parents have conflicting feelings toward the opposite sex. This conflict may focus on one member of the opposite sex, such as the absent father. A mother may react to her son negatively because of her unresolved feelings toward her absent spouse. Some mothers react with overprotection of the son, while others may reject the son. The nurse's responsibility is to assess the family interaction patterns, to assist the family members in finding professional counselling and to encourage widening the circle of their relationships. The foregoing discussion on sexual identification and attitudes pertains to both sexes but was presented in this section because of the popular concerns about single parent mother-son relationships. Table 4–2 identifies the major concerns in the female single parent family and appropriate nursing roles that help such families manage those problems.

TABLE 4–2 THE NURSE'S ROLE IN MAXIMIZING THE FEMALE SINGLE PARENT FAMILY EXPERIENCE

Situational Factors	Nurse Role Factors
Mothers may need assistance with financial matters and home repair.	Assess need areas. Identify resources such as financial counselling, home repair courses or community groups who assist in home repair.
Children's need for father role models.	Assist in identifying surrogate fathers and adult male role models within the mother's group of relatives, friends, schools.

Single Parent Families by Divorce

In 1976 the number of children under the age of 18 whose parents were not in an intact marriage had soared to 20 million in the United States.[16, 18] Only 50 years ago divorce was scandalous. Now it is commonplace in every classroom to find some children who have experienced marital separation of their parents, often ending in divorce. In fact, these children are referred to as a distinct category, "Children of Divorce," in professional literature.[18, 20]

The attitudinal and economic barriers against divorce have weakened in the last decade partly because of the women's rights movement. Women and men are increasingly concerned about self-fulfillment; it is almost an obligation to realize one's potential for growth. Weiss refers to this sense of obligation as the ethic of self-realization.[38] For some persons who are struggling with disenchantment with their marriage, professional marriage counselling and support from friends and family do not seem to be enough to stabilize the marriage. For some, economic factors, too-early marriage commitments, the demands of parenting and the lack of support systems seem to make dissolution of the marriage the only viable option.

Children of these families are caught in the matrix of the parents' frustration and changing life styles. The responses of the children depend on several variables such as the developmental stages of the children, elapsed time since event of separation, predivorce family interaction and postdivorce family structures. The adjustment of children of divorced parents tends to be measured against the norm of children from intact, presumably well-functioning families rather than against children in homes in which there is considerable parental dissension, the predivorce norm.[18] In addition, there has been little follow-up study of children after the initial crisis.

A longitudinal study following 131 children from 60 divorced families over a four-year period has been done in California by Wallerstein and Kelly.[20, 35, 36, 37] This study is age related and involves children's responses in four developmental periods: preschool, early latency, later latency and adolescence. (For discussion of developmental periods see Chapter 10, "Emotional-Social Competency.") The sample is composed of 92 per cent white families, 3 per cent black and 5 per cent interracial, including Oriental and Hispanic parents. Although replication in samples with a broader class and ethnic base is needed, some salient factors can be noted from this significant piece of research.

The latency period was divided into two distinct groups because of the evidence from the interviews. The latency period is usually viewed as one developmental stage, but the children's responses to divorce were significantly different in the early latency (7 to 8 years) and later latency (9 to 10 years) periods. The children and their parents were seen by an interdisciplinary team during four to six individual clinical sessions conducted over a six-week span of time. Independent information was obtained with parental consent at the time of the initial counselling and one year later. Most subjects were interviewed a second year later as well.[30] Table 4–3 is my compilation of some of the common responses noted in the interviews with the children and their parents.

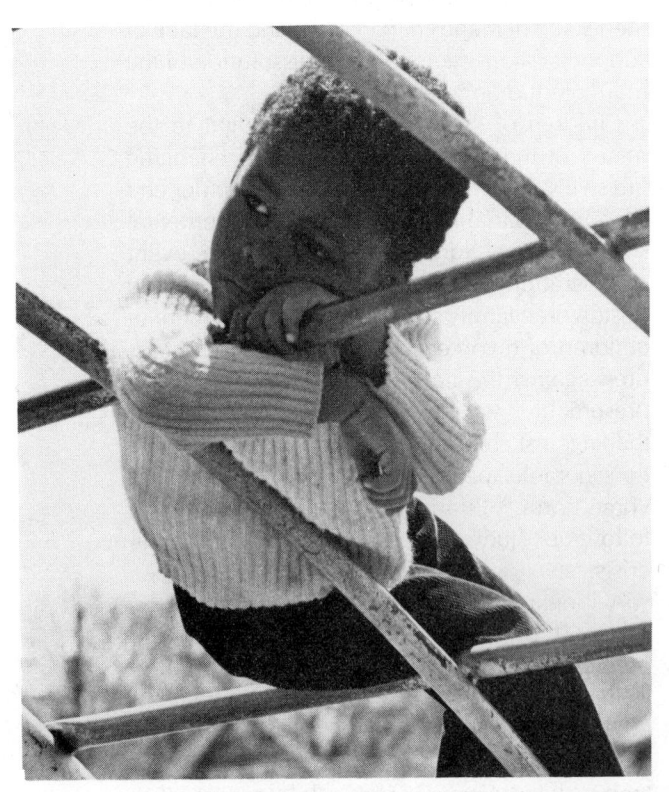

Pervasive sadness tends to be the characteristic response of children when divorce occurs during the child's early latency period. (Jim Ritscher, Stock, Boston.)

The fact that more than 50 per cent of the 7- and 8-year-old boys acutely missed their fathers is of particular interest. The researchers postulate that it may be because of the closeness in time to their "oedipal resolution."* Developmentally considered, the boy in early latency has only recently renounced the gratification of his mother, but in divorce he may lose his father as well.[19] It may also threaten to disrupt the process of identification with his father that has been evolving since birth.

As was mentioned before, these responses of a middle class, largely white sample cannot be used as generalizations for other social classes and ethnic or racial groups. However, they do serve as a model for raising questions about other groups of families enmeshed in the complexities of divorce. Professional nurses can be cognizant of the probable differences between the early and later latency responses and the resulting needs of the children. In this study no consistent parallels between behavior at home and in school could be noted. The effect of divorce on school performance also showed wide variation. Sometimes there was increased success in school and in other cases a decline in school achievement was noted. This is of importance because too frequently expectations for children's behavior in school are formed according to what is known about their home situation.

The nurse's role in the dilemma of divorce will depend on the period of time elapsed since the parental separation, the child care arrangements and the ages and sexes of the children. When the nurse is the primary care provider, she may be the key person who can assist the family members to obtain professional counselling. In the community she may be instrumental in the development of support groups for divorced parents or children of divorce or both. She may often serve as the liaison between the home and the school when the reasons for a child's behavior are being sought. The effects of divorce on the well-being of the client should always be a concern for the nurse.

Divorce remains a topic for continued concern and careful research. Predictions are that marital separation will continue to increase. The parents and the children affected need various levels of support not only during the initial crisis, but until some measure of equilibrium is

---

*The psychological stage in a boy's development in which he has a sexual and emotional fixation on his mother, normally resolved when the child is between 8 and 12.

TABLE 4-3 CHILDREN'S RESPONSES TO DIVORCE AT THE TIME OF INITIAL COUNSELLING AND ONE YEAR LATER

Developmental Period	Initial Responses	One Year Later
Preschool	Use of denial through fantasy. Assumed responsibility for precipitating the divorce. Rise in aggression and irritability.	5-6-year-olds cling to hope of reconciliation.
Early Latency (7-8-year-olds)	Pervasive sadness. Awareness of their own suffering with difficulty gaining relief. Family dissolution perceived as threat to their whole life; fantasies of deprivation. Absent father missed acutely, especially by young boys. Anger toward custodial mother (most lived with mother). Fear of antagonizing mother. Conflicts with loyalty, need to hold on to both parents.	Modified responses. Sad, resigned attitude. Reluctantly accept finality of divorce. View life as more difficult; less gratification. Cling to absent fathers, even when fathers are disinterested.
Later Latency (9-10-year-olds)	Initial poise, presence and courage. Age-available coping noted: denial, courage, bravado keeping in motion, conscious avoidance, seeking support. Layering of psychological functioning, use of coping mechanisms and simultaneously succumbing to anguish or pain. Conscious, intense anger; organized and object-directed moral stance in judgment against parents. Feelings of vulnerability and lack of security. Variety of somatic complaints.	Muted responses; accepting situation. Align with custodial parent. Precocious thrust into adolescent preoccupation with sexuality and assertiveness. Reject absent fathers if they do not receive gratification from them.
Adolescence	Conflicts in feelings toward parents. Some psychological independence. More freedom to challenge custodial parent's position, if they disagree.	Use both parental homes to their advantages. Reject absent fathers if they do not receive gratification.

found in which all family members feel a sense of identity, security and encouragement for growth.

Single Parent Families by Death

The possibility of losing a parent by death is seldom discussed in families and yet it is a reality for many children. The reactions and adjustments of children to the death of a parent are dependent on their developmental stages, the openness with which their dual-parent family discussed death and the support that they have to discuss their feelings after the death of the parent.

Published resource material on the topic of death and dying is rapidly increasing. In the last decade professional literature and popular magazines have contained many articles encouraging people to deal openly with fears of death and to consider death as a part of life. Probably the researcher who has had the greatest impact, especially among professionals, is Elisabeth Kübler-Ross. Kübler-Ross is a psychiatrist who has conducted a series of research projects in which she has learned about the experience of imminent death from children and adults who are dying. She and her fellow researchers carefully record and analyze the responses of dying persons and their families. She says that we routinely shelter children from death and dying, thinking we are protecting them from harm. But it is clear that we do them a disservice by depriving them of the experience. By making dying a taboo subject and keeping children away from people who are dying, we create unnecessary fear.[28]

Grieving is necessary for all children who are separated from a parent by death. Preschool children faced with death of a parent cannot comprehend the finality of death. For them, it is reversible. If encouraged, these young children will verbalize and, in their play, act out their fantasies of the return of the parent. Children in the latency period who understand the finality of death may react with sadness, withdrawal, regression and anger. They may be very reluctant to verbalize their feelings but often become adept at drawing pictures depicting their emotions. Adolescents are more sophisticated in their range of coping mechanisms and may feel the need to mask their intense feelings of loss. They respond according to what they think is an appropriate adult response (that is, denial of death). They too need supportive persons around them who will listen but not insist on verbalization.

The remaining parent may be so involved in his own grief that it is difficult to respond to the developmental level of the children's needs. Nurses involved in the situation should assess this burden for the remaining spouse and assist each family member to find resource persons who can be available to them.

The children's later responses to living in a single parent family will largely depend on their ability to work through the grief process. This is essentially the same as for children who must deal with parental separation because of divorce. There is some difference in that children of divorce often continue a relationship with the parent who no longer lives with the child. The finality of death, even though painful and difficult, needs to be psychologically dealt with by children of all ages. It is essential that the children receive sustained and open support as they incorporate this painful experience into their lives.

Never-Married Single Parent Families

In considering persons who are parents but have never been married, the factor of choice and nonchoice is also relevant. Although questions have often been raised about the covert psychological need of the unwed mother to bear a child, the fact remains that it is the woman who bears the child. Therefore, unless she chooses to have the child adopted, she becomes a single parent. In the past, the majority of unwed mothers did not consciously choose that role and society at large did not accord single unwed mothers respect. In fact, children born out of wedlock have been referred to as illegitimate children or bastards, a stigma that adversely affected their lives. It is interesting to note that under the principle of legitimacy the focus is on the function of the economic provider, a role assigned to the father.[30] Changing female roles are having an effect on the principle of legitimacy. As women establish themselves socially and in the work place, the single woman who opts to have children is more able to provide them with an acceptable access to the social world and the resources once considered solely a father's contribution. Although the term illegitimate is still used in the courts and in federal statistics, the social stigma is decreasing.

Second only to divorced persons, the most rapidly growing category of single parenthood, especially since 1970, has been the never-married mother.[6] In part, this has been due to the changing values in American society, such as increasing acceptance of extramarital intercourse, single mothers keeping their babies in lieu of adoption or abortion and single parent adoption of children. Single parent adoptions are discussed later in this chapter in the section on adoption.

The most important factor in discussing parenthood outside of marriage is the preparation and desire of the parent to provide for and nurture children. When parenthood is voluntarily chosen by a single person who is equipped to provide the child with the necessary resources, the experience can be beneficial and satisfying to both parent and child.[30] Some women choose to bear children without the sanction of marriage. These women consider parenting a role that will give them satisfaction and believe that they, personally, have a contribution to give their children in nurturing them without the support of a spouse. Other women do not consciously choose to become parents, but when they find themselves pregnant do not consider adoption or abortion viable options.

Eiduson reports distinct categories of single mothers:

Three groups could be identified: nest builders — women who consciously chose and planned to have a baby and start a new household; post-hoc adaptors — women who had not planned to become pregnant but adjusted happily to this circumstance; and a small group of unwed mothers, women who were more like the unwed mothers of yesteryear in attitudes and circumstance. The levels of education and of professional development, income status and general life style were distinctive for each group, with the nest-builders being the women who were most self-sufficient and whose goals were most closely tied to those of the women's movement. Roles and responsibilities toward the child also differed among the groups, depending on the availability of economic, psychological and social support.[10]

The social support system for never-married single parents is a key factor in the care and nurturing of the children. Sometimes these mothers have extended family who share in the care of the children. But for those unmarried mothers whose family has rejected them or who choose to leave familiar settings in order to begin a new life with their children, the social supports are often few or nonexistent. Many of these young mothers are teenagers who have difficulty meshing their adolescent needs with the parenting role thrust upon them. Nurses relating to these families can assist the mothers in evaluating their needs for supportive assistance and in locating adequate help.

STEP-PARENTS

The process of assimilation should be a major concern for families in which there are various combinations of birth-parent and step-parent relationships with children. Two one-parent families may be brought together into a single household, or a single parent may marry a spouse without children. The family system becomes even more involved if there are birth-parents of the children living elsewhere with whom the children continue a viable relationship. Some children live regularly in homes with a birth-parent and a step-parent and spend weekends or other designated time periods with the other birth-parent and a step-parent. A step-parent is defined as a parent married to the birth-parent of the child.

When a parent dies and the remaining parent remarries, the step-parent may have to deal with the overidealization of the dead parent by some of the children.[8] Some children make comparisons between the idealized parent who is gone and the step-parent as a way to hold onto the memory of the dead parent. The best way to cope with the situation is to discuss the good points of the deceased parent and yet not agree to the comparison. This is often very difficult unless the step-parent feels secure in the relationship with the spouse and children.

The responses and needs of the children depend to a great extent on the relationships established in the previous family system. If there was unresolved hostility and anger, with little parental support for the children, they may respond with eagerness to a new avenue of love. Or they may have difficulty trusting the step-parent, afraid to invest in another failure. Some of the child's anger at the absent birth-parent may be displaced onto the step-parent, since the child may feel safer in doing this. The nurse should encourage the step-parent not to take this anger personally, because he is obviously not responsible for it. To react angrily in retaliation may only verify the child's feelings that he was correct in the first place, and this may interfere with his full acceptance of his good feelings about the step-parent.[8]

The ages of the children also determine their responses to the step-parent. Developmental tasks may be interrupted by the change in family relationships. At some ages the bonding between parent and child seems to be more crucial. For instance, the 10-month-old infant who has been cared for primarily by the mother and enters a relationship with a step-father may be able to adjust rather quickly because of the sustained relationship with the birth-mother. However, the 5-year-old son who is sorting through oedipal relationships and begins a new relationship with a step-father may have more difficulties in the assimilation process. Adolescents who are in the process of self-identity and are fluctuating between the need for parental guidance and self-reliance sometimes find the relationship with the step-parent most difficult.

Recognition of the problems and potentials in the step-relationship is necessary for the parents as well as the children. Sussman[34] summarizes the strengths and limitations as follows:

Strengths:
1. Previous marital experiences may result in an increased number (actual incidence unknown) of stable marriages.
2. Parenting, which may formerly have been the function of a single adult, may be shared with the new partner and his or her older children.
3. For some, there is improved economic status as a consequence of shared income.

Weaknesses:
1. The difficulties in blending two formerly independent households into one functioning unit may result in extreme psychic stress for some members.
2. Formations consisting of two large families may require substantial economic help, counselling and other supports in order to survive.
3. Economic and social commitments to individuals of previous marriages may restrict the development of adequate, stable relationships in the new marriage.

FOSTER PARENTS

Foster care of children refers to parenting by persons who are not the biological or adoptive parents of the children involved. The foster child is not an orphan; he has one or both birth-parents living.[13] For various reasons the care of the child by the birth-parents or parent has been interrupted temporarily or permanently. This has necessitated placement of the child in another family.

Placement in families can be a formal or informal process. If a social agency assumes jurisdiction for the child's welfare, the placement process is a carefully detailed procedure whereby the foster parents must meet criteria before becoming approved as a foster care home. Payment, usually minimal, is involved. Some persons or families assume foster parenting responsibilities through friendship or familial ties or both with the birth-parent who is unable to care for the child. This arrangement is more often temporary; for instance the child stays with the foster family until the birth-parent again gets a job or remarries or recovers from some other family crisis.

Permanence is increasingly becoming a major issue in foster care.[12, 15, 19, 39] In the recent past and even today, many foster children are moved from foster home to foster home, sometimes with intermittent periods of time with their birth-parent. Anyone with even limited knowledge of the developmental tasks and needs for nurturing of children can speculate about the problems of these children. There is an important difference between protecting children from the extremes of neglect or abuse and providing care that ensures permanency in living arrangements and continuity of relationships.[39]

Fanshel and Shinn[14] report in their longitudinal study of children in foster care that:

It is no longer considered sufficient that a child be afforded a placement situation in which his basic needs are being cared for in terms of shelter, food and clothing, and a benign environment in which positive emotional growth can be enhanced. A newly emphasized criterion is being used to assess the adequacy of an agency's performance, namely whether a child can be assured permanency in his living arrangements and continuity of relationship. It is not enough that he might be placed in a foster family home that offers him family-like care. If he cannot regard the people he is living with as *his* family, on a permanent basis, his situation is increasingly regarded as reflecting something less than an adequate resolution to his life situation.

Permanency planning must begin early in foster care. This means intensive work with the birth-parents to achieve a decision on their child's future. Care must be given to balancing the rights and wishes of the parents and the rights and needs of the children, especially when the child's need for continuity is added to his rights. The concept of continuity encompasses the issue of time with consideration given to the child's sense of time if the meaning of continuity is fulfilled from the child's perspective.[39]

The pediatric nurse who cares for foster children should be aware of the physical and psychological impact of foster care.[14] If permanency in foster care has not been realized, the nurse must be aware of the psychological effects of transience. Large segments of the past may not be known or may be incomplete. The child may be beset with chronic feelings of inadequacy, unworthiness and low self-esteem. He may have difficulty relating emotionally, often developing shallow relationships, afraid to get attached to any person because of fear of loss or separation.

The efforts of the nurse must be directed toward potentiating a nonthreatening environment. The foster parents need support in understanding that the anger which the child may display toward them is rarely a direct attack against them as caretakers. These children have often been hurt, disappointed and deserted. They need an environment where they can express themselves and receive loving care and guidance. The nurse and foster parents need to watch for clues of past trauma. The present situation may awaken emotional reactions of the past. The child needs safe and acceptable avenues to express his feelings from the past without being rejected. This attitude requires investment of time and effort. In many nonverbal and verbal ways the child forces the issue, asking, "You really care about me, don't you?" The foster parents' and the nurse's gratification comes with the glimmer of hope in the eyes of the child and the increasing times when the child can be free to trust others in his world.

MIGRANT CHILDREN

Children of migrant laborers know transience as a way of life. The transience in their lives usually comes about through changes in the geographical location of their home, since the family moves with the job. The jobs are frequently farm labor and, therefore, are seasonal. The change in location may mean moving to another state or from one section of a state to another, such as do the fruit harvesters in Florida, or it may mean travelling from Mexico to the northern midwestern states. In this case, the change means contact with a different culture and language.

These children are sometimes referred to as "children who follow the sun" or "children of the road."[28] They are born into one of the grimmest poverty situations in the country.[28] The living accommodations are often makeshift, minimal and crowded. Illnesses such as rickets, scurvy, pinworms, anemia and malnutrition abound. At an early age these children join their parents in the fields and many spend the rest of their lives working in similar situations. Their school life is interrupted frequently — in fact, every few weeks at the peak harvest season. School records seldom move with the children, increasing the problems of continuity. Lack of health records poses the same problem, sometimes necessitating repeated immunizations; at other times tests and immunizations are missed.

Since 1966 the federal government has taken special interest in the welfare of migrant children. Title I of the Elementary Education Act was amended to give the U.S. Office of Education authority and funds to improve educational programs and to offer supplemental services for these children.[28] Continuity of instruction, health care, nutrition and psychological services have high priority.

In 1974, Public Law 93–380 authorized the use of the Migrant Student Record Transfer System, a computer data bank located in Little Rock, Arkansas, which can trace the whereabouts of each child as he migrates.[28] This service makes student placement easier, indicates where special help is needed and eliminates repetition of tests and physical examinations. In one instance it was used to find more than 200 children who were potential victims or carriers of typhoid fever.

There has been improvement in educational, health and social services for migrant children; however, the greatest barrier remaining is the manner in which these services are delivered. Ida Brownlee Bragdon, herself once a migrant child and now an oral language specialist working with migrants, identifies the masks these children wear and suggests ways to lift the masks.[5] She identifies the masks of nonverbal behavior, periodic tuning-out, blank stares, ignorance and hostility. Environmental economic and social factors as well as lack of communication between the migrant children and providers of education and health services help to produce these defense mechanisms. The most effective way to reach these children is to recognize their strengths.[5] Health care strategies should be built on the positive attributes of these families. In Table 4–4 Bragdon lists strengths and sources of those attributes.

TABLE 4–4 POTENTIAL STRENGTHS OF MIGRANT CHILDREN

Strength	Source
Eager to please	Families emphasize respect for authority.
Responsible	Care for younger children, contribute to family income.
Loved	Families welcome children with enthusiasm.
Adaptable	Move frequently, adjust quickly.
Perceptive and sensitive	Language barriers increase need to read visual cues.
Express themselves vividly with family	Little contact outside migrant group.
Want education	Encouraged to continue to enroll in school.
Curious	Have had many and diverse living situations.
Possess a culture	Beliefs, values and behavior based on survival in life they know.

These strengths may not apply to all migrant children. Other positive attributes will then need to be identified to serve as a basis for health care strategies.

ADOPTION

Adoption refers to the process of surrogate parents assuming legal custody of children who were not born to them. There are many types of adoptive situations, including dual parents, single parents, transracial adoptions, transcultural adoptions, intercountry adoptions and stepchild adoptions. The adoption process is also varied, involving adoptions through public and private adoption agencies, adoptions arranged through physicians and lawyers and some adoptions arranged by other intermediaries functioning between the birth-parents and the adoptive parents. The laws governing adoption are state laws and, although generally similar, they vary in specific details that should be known to all involved in the adoption process. Intercountry adoptions sometimes involve a prolonged process during which each country's adoption laws are being satisfied.

The overt and covert reasons for the formation of adoptive families are also many and varied. Some persons adopt children for social conscience motives: population control or assisting handicapped children, breaking race barriers and poverty cycles. Others adopt because of needs for personal fulfillment through parenting when bearing children is not possible or feasible: infertility problems, personal choice to circumvent pregnancy and labor, single parenthood. Still others respond to extended family or god-parent commitments when children are separated from birth-parents by death or desertion.

Each adoptive family is the result of a unique combination of factors, all of which have a bearing on the relationships. The nurse may not know these factors, but she should be sensitive to the complex and unique qualities of each adoptive situation. These will not be discussed here in detail. The following discussion describes some aspects of adoption that can help the nurse to interact positively with these families.

Development of Entitlement

The purpose of adoption is the creation of a continuing relationship not formed by birth.[11] This relationship needs to be viewed as being as real as the biological one. The length of time it takes for entitlement (the right of adopted children and adults to fully belong) to develop varies according to the age of the child at the time of adoption and the psychological reaction of the parents to the adoption. If the parents feel that conception and pregnancy are necessary for complete parent-child bonding, they may never view the adopted child as really "theirs." The child will always be "their adopted child," rather than simply "their child." If the sense of belongingness is not developed, the adults can never be successful parents. If it is partially developed, the adults can parent some of the time but may have problems with discipline, with allowing the child to separate from them or with telling him about his adoption.[11]

Persons outside the family sometimes verbalize their awe or disbelief or both that the parents and sibling actually do not differentiate their feelings of belonging between children born into the family and those adopted. Families with only adopted children do not know how they might feel with children born to them, but families with children both born to them and adopted by them can attest to their bonding with each child in the family. If there are other children in the family, they need to be included in the development of entitlement.

It is best for the family members to openly acknowledge their feelings of belongingness with each other. This may be difficult for some, but if adoption is an acceptable topic of discussion and related to the developmental age of the children, it can be a rewarding process, a growth experience for all members of the family. All persons need to acknowledge their self-identity at various stages in life. The family with adopted members is forced by circumstances to deal with this issue and can be healthier for it. Some may need assistance in discussing their relationships and feelings about adoption. Nurses can encourage and guide this process or assist the family to find professional counselling services in the community.

Adoption does not have a negative effect on self-concept. Studies have shown no significant difference in self-concept of adolescent adoptees and nonadoptees.[27] The initial motives of the parents to adopt is the most important factor in successful adjustment. Therefore, nurses should carefully assess the parents' views of bonding with their adopted children and assist parents in developing realistic and healthy attitudes in their parenting roles.

Telling or not telling children about their adoption has been an ongoing topic of discussion among professionals and lay persons. In most communities stories are still circulated with variations on the theme of tragic results when persons learned of their adoptive state at inopportune times in their lives. Many of these accounts are partially, if not totally, true. Some families and communities have not fully dealt with entitlement.

To tell or not to tell is no longer the focus of the question, but rather how and when. No one can tell a parent when or how to tell the child of his adoption. It must be done in a manner in which the parent and child are comfortable with their relationship. Recently, the idea that all children should be told at an early age is being questioned.[4, 16] Children under 5 have an active fantasy life and are not verbal enough to discuss feelings. After 6 the developmental tasks of children seem to be more quiescent. However, the longer one waits to tell children of their adoption the greater the possibility that they will be told by someone else in the community. Braff[4] questions the practice of giving adoption information to children under 7 or 8 if they have not asked.[4]

Probably the best counsel is to inform parents of the advantages and disadvantages of telling at different ages, and to discuss the child's developmental status and the likelihood of community interference.[16] Parents can then make their own decision about when and how to tell their children.

Transracial Adoption

Some families adopt children whose race is different from their own. These families cannot as easily choose when to tell their adopted child about adoption. The family and the community are always aware of the adoption status because the child's skin color or other physical features are unlike those of the parents. Strangers will often assume that they are not a family.

One family tells of an incident in which their 4-year-old child (he was mulatto and they were white) wandered about a restaurant until the waiter brought the family's food, whereupon he again joined his parents to eat. The proprietor came to the table and said, "Friendly little fellow, just comes and eats with you." "But he is our son," the mother replied. "No, he is not," the proprietor insisted, "he belongs to that other family." There had also been a Mexican-American family in the restaurant. After some further discussion, the proprietor was convinced that the child and parents indeed belonged together.

Such parents and children must in their own way establish their relationship when others question their identity as a family unit. One child who was becoming aware of his appearance with the family would often look at himself in the mirror, sometimes calling himself derogatory names. His mother once asked, "If you could have anything in the world you wanted, what would it be?" He laid his brown arm alongside her pale one and said, "To look like you, Mommy." With love and with constancy, yet not without sadness and hurts, this family supported each other in recognizing the child's identity as he continued to work through who he was. At age 12, the same child responded in a classroom situation when the teacher asked the class which skin color is the best. "The color you are," he volunteered.

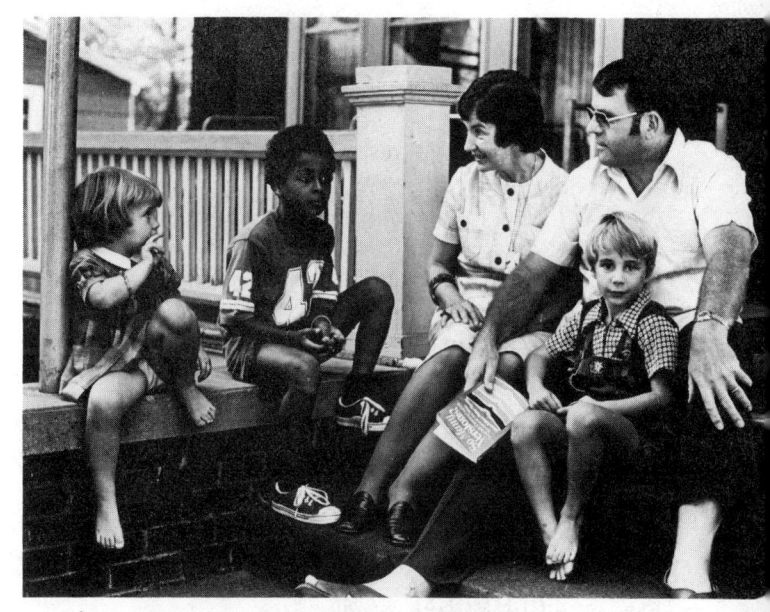

In adoptive families parents and children must in their own way establish their identity as a family unit. Parents are able to bond with each of their children, whether the child is born to them or adopted, of the same race or different. (Photograph by Alice Roth.)

Some professionals, as well as some racial groups, are very critical of transracial adoptions. There is little question that it is preferable for children to be adopted into families who are as similar to the child as possible, if these families are capable of providing loving support and encouragement. If such parents are not available, the child's present need for food, shelter and a home of his own is considered by some to be more important than future psychological and pyschosocial needs.[7] When the parents are comfortable in the parenting role and recognize the problems in transracial adoption, they can support the child as he develops his identity in the transracial setting. In fact, the home can become a microcosm of what the world community is really like. Multiracial appreciation is not only discussed but acted upon.

Single Parent Adoption

What makes single women or single men choose a role that many divorcees and widowed persons find depressing? Dougherty sought the answer to this question and reports on the increasing incidence of single parent adoptions.[9] The majority of mothers were willing to accept responsibility for the child and all were highly educated. Other single parents, friends and family provided the needed support. Moral support was a recognized need, but few wanted institutional help. Adjustments focused on scheduling, new financial arrangements and change in friends. Some of these persons experienced a broadening of their circle of friends to include couples with children, but they also lost some of their previous friends who did not care to adjust to the needs of children in the single parent's home.

COMMUNAL FAMILIES

Communes are intentional communities that are formed of biologically unrelated people who live together in order to build a kind of large chosen family.[30] Commune members have interdependence and expect a commitment from one another. Communal living is not a new phenomenon; the practice stretches far back into history, even to Biblical times (Acts 2:44–45). The best known modern communal society is the kibbutz movement in Israel. In the United States, communal experiments have flourished in the past 15 years.

Communes are organized for a variety of reasons. Many have been organized to avoid, challenge or replace the highly competitive materialistic atmosphere spawned in the urban-industrial society. Others have sought family systems that foster individual growth. Whatever the goals, communes tend to be formed by groups of people who are actively searching for a better way of life.[26] Their motivation may be religious, political, economic, psychosocial or a combination of these.

Childrearing

Communal childrearing is a convenient way of caring for children, since the responsibility is shared by the group.[26] It is often the means by which the commune's ideals are taught. This is exemplified by the Oneida community,* in which a basic tenet was for all people to love each other equally. A special relationship between parent and child was considered out of keeping with universal love. This view is different from that of the kibbutz, in which childrearing is shared but parents can visit young children in the Children's House at any time and have special times when the children can join them in their private quarters.[33]

Spiro contends that the kibbutz is a child-oriented society par excellence.[33] Children are prized above all else and no sacrifice is too great to make for them. Collective education may be strict and formal but the amount of energy, money and services provided for the children is noteworthy. The functions of the parent and the "nurse" (nurse in the sense of caretaker for children) can be divided into four categories: caretaking, nurturing, training and values. The "nurse" is responsible for nurturing and caretaking only. After the child is 2 years old, the sole responsibility of the kibbutz parent is "to love" his child.

The identity formation of the child is a result of continuity in the kibbutz educational-childbearing process and the ideals upon which the kibbutz is founded. There is consistency between the child's world and the community and from this follows consistency between childhood and adulthood. Adolescents are involved in the social and work ideals of the community. By contrast, many Western adolescents are isolated in their own world of peers during adolescence. Kibbutz children learn by doing — how to work, think, relate to others and take responsibility. Kibbutz youth criticize the adult society, but their criticism is thoughtful and specific, usually including their views on solutions to problems.[3]

Children in "hippie" communes tend to be viewed as autonomous, independent persons, largely capable of caring for themselves.[26] Young children's needs are responded to by any member of the group. This corresponds to adult values concerning freedom, independence and

---

*The Oneida Community was a mid-nineteenth century commune located in New York State along the Oneida Creek. It survived for more than a generation, disbanding in 1879 because of lack of an adequate leader and increasing external pressures. Some of the features of the community included group marriage, scientific breeding and sexual equality. It succeeded in a business sense, as well as socially. Oneida, Ltd. was formed in 1880 and continues today to manufacture Oneida Community Silverware.

nonorganization. The "hippie" theory of children is in some respects distinctive.[1] It does not fit preindustrial, agricultural (lower class) or industrial (middle class) attitudes. Young people are seen as separate from the biological parents, but not as members of an autonomous category of children. Their status is that of a person, a member of the commune equal to other members.

Age makes an important difference. In Berger's research study,[1] infants and early toddlers were almost universally in the charge of their mothers. Children from 2 to 4 years of age belonged to the commune to greater extent. They received a lot of fathering. There were strong norms that required fathers to be involved in child-nurturing. After age 4 or 5, the child was the responsibility of any adult in the group. All children were viewed as intrinsically worthy of love and respect, but not necessarily of attention.

In these communes, the extent to which the child belongs to the extended family or to parents is due to the sequential developmental stages of the child rather than to the type of commune. The role of parents is to facilitate child development, which is essentially exemplary rather than paternalistic or didactic. Every attempt is made to allow children to grow naturally, to be as autonomous as possible.

An important comparison is made by Berger and his co-workers in their studies of parent-child relationships in communal families and traditional nuclear families.

The single most important belief governing the relation between children and adults is that the experiences had by children not be fateful or self-implicating for adults, that adults cannot be legitimately characterized in terms of what they do with or to their children — in rather clear contrast to both preindustrial and middle class views in which the behavior of children reflects upon their parents who are in some sense responsible for it.[1]

Communards generally say communes are good for children. There may be important continuity between generations. Most studies of contemporary communes, except for the kibbutzim, have involved only preadolescent children. Longitudinal studies may provide data for distinctive child development practices. Professional nurses who have contact with communal families should make every effort to understand the basic values of the specific commune as they respond to the families' health care needs.

HOMOSEXUAL PARENTS

Bisexuality and homosexuality have been discussed most often in terms of abnormal behavior. Because professionals and lay persons are discussing their views on the subject more openly, some believe that bisexuality and homosexuality are increasing. There is no evidence that the number of homosexuals has grown proportionately to the general population. What has happened is that homosexuality as an alternate life style is receiving a higher degree of acceptance from the general public.[22] Normality versus abnormality is not the topic of this discussion. Rather, it is the recognition that homosexual marriages exist and that children are being reared by homosexual parents.

The greatest concern most researchers have about sexual preference of the parents is its influence on the children. In response to the query about whether a homosexual parent could raise a heterosexual child, a young lesbian answered, "What kind of homes do homosexuals come from now?"[22] The obvious answer is that many children develop homophile sexual preferences even though they grow up in heterosexual homes. Because of a deep concern for their children's freedom to develop their own sexual identity, many homosexual parents carefully keep their relationship secret even when living with a partner. Others openly discuss their situation with their children. Some professionals suggest waiting until after the children have worked through their own sexual identity between ages 3 and 8.[24] The parent has then to consider the risk of the children learning of his homosexuality from other persons. When and how the parent discusses the situation with the children is dependent on the parent's comfort with his own homosexuality and his maturity in response to the demands of the children, the lover and society.

Martin and Lyon,[24] themselves lesbians, discuss the prejudices, the community responses and the fears of lesbian mothers in many case studies reported in their candid book, *Lesbian Woman*. Martin's daughter learned of her mother's sexual preference when she was a late adolescent. The daugher said she had often thought that if she never married, she hoped she would find as warm and loving a relationship with another woman as her mother had, not knowing that the relationship had a sexual dimension. The daughter's fiance had more difficulty accepting his future mother-in-law's life style. In the end, he stated that he actually had two mothers-in-law!

When the children of homosexuals first learn of their parents' life style, the response is often shock and wonder. If the parent-child relationship has been one of mutual love and the parent is comfortable in his sexual orientation, the first reaction is short-lived. As one child stated, "As time went on, I realized how unimportant that fact was. She didn't suddenly become something twisted and evil. She is still the same wonderful person, and I love her."[24]

Despite the fact that gay marriages are not recognized as legal, many lesbians and male homosexuals do form lasting same-sex unions that they think of as marriages. Many have permanence, faithfulness and a shared life. Some courts refuse lesbian mothers custody of their children, while other courts allow it. Some lesbian women have combined families of two mothers, and others who want children have gotten pregnant by a willing male.[30] There are greater problems for male homosexuals who want children, because adoption agencies give preference to heterosexual parents, and courts are more likely to grant custody to the mother rather than to the homosexual father. Much research is needed on the parent-child relationships and needs of these families.

References

1. B. Berger et al. The communal family. The Family Coordinator, 19 October 1972, p. 419
2. J. Bernard. The Future of Marriage. World Publications, 1972
3. J. Blasi and D. Murrell. Adolescence and community structure. Adolescence, Summer 1977, p. 165
4. A. Braff. Telling children about their adoption: new alternatives for parents. American Journal of Maternal Child Nursing, Jul/Aug 1977, p. 254
5. I. Bragdon. How to help migrant children. Today's Education, Jan/Feb 1976
6. U. Bronfenbrenner. The Changing American Family. In Contemporary Readings in Child Psychology by Hetherington and Parke. McGraw-Hill, 1977, p. 317
7. A Chimezie. Transracial adoption of black children. Social Work, July 1975, p. 296. Discussion September 1975, May 1976
8. Committee on Public Education Groups for the Advancement of Psychiatry. Charles Scribner's Sons, 1973
9. S. A. Dougherty. Single adoptive mothers and their children. Social Work, July 1978, p. 311
10. B. Eiduson. Child development in emergent family styles. Children Today, Mar/Apr 1978, p. 24
11. C. Eldred et al. Some aspects of adoption in selected samples of adult adoptees. American Journal of Orthopsychiatry, April 1976, p. 279
12. D. Fanshel and E. Shinn. Children in Foster Care: A Longitudinal Investigation. Columbia University Press, 1978
13. J. Fuentes. The need for effective and comprehensive planning for migrant workers. American Journal of Public Health, January 1974, p. 2
14. R. Geiser and M. N. Malinowski. Realities of foster care. American Journal of Nursing, March 1978, p. 430
15. J. Goldstein et al. Beyond the Best Interest of the Child. New York Free Press, 1973
16. C. Hammons. The adoptive family. American Journal of Nursing, February 1976, p. 251
17. R. C. Hill. The Strength of Black Families. Emerson Hall Publishers, 1972
18. S. Jenkins. Children of divorce. Children Today, Mar/Apr 1978, p. 16
19. M. Jones. Finding permanent homes for children in foster care. Children Today, Mar/Apr 1979, p. 8
20. J. Kelly and J. S. Wallerstein. The effects of parental divorce: experiences of the child in early latency. American Journal of Orthopsychiatry, January 1976, p. 20
21. H. Keshet and K. Rosenthal. Fathering after marital separation. Social Work, January 1978, p. 11
22. C. Klein. The Single Parent Experience. Walker & Co., 1973
23. E. Kübler-Ross. Death: The Final Stage of Growth. Prentice-Hall Inc., 1975
24. D. Martin and P. Lyon. Lesbian Woman. Bantam Books, 1972
25. H. A. Mendes. Single fatherhood. Social Work, July 1976, p. 308
26. G. Nass. Marriage and Family. Addison-Wesley Publishing Co., Inc., 1978

> When one is confronted with so many family life styles and childrearing practices, it is difficult to remain objective. One's own values influence how one perceives and reacts to situations. The nurse must attempt to understand her own values about the single parent's ability to parent, the decisions of families to become divorced, the mobility of migrant families, foster parents' attachment to the children, adoptive parents' ability to love their children unconditionally, communal sharing of childrearing responsibilities and children being reared by homosexual parents. To examine one's values does not mean one agrees with the choices other persons have made regarding life styles. It does mean that one attempts to understand the grid through which one views another's life style. In doing so, the nurse will be able to focus on the assessment of the family system and respond to the basic needs of the children for nurturing, caretaking, education and development of values.

27. M. Norwell and R. Grey. Comparison of self-concept in adopted and nonadopted adolescents. Adolescence, Fall 1977, p. 443
28. J. Park. Children who follow the sun. Today's Education, Jan/Feb 1976, p. 53
29. C. Safilios-Rothschild. Trends in the family: A cross cultural perspective. Children Today, Mar/Apr 1978, p. 38
30. L. Scanzoni and J. Scanzoni. Men, Women and Change: A Sociology of Marriage and Family. McGraw-Hill Book Co., 1976
31. B. Schlesinger. One Parent Family. University of Toronto Press, 1970
32. B. Schlesinger. Single parent fathers. Children Today, May/June 1978, p. 12
33. M. Spiro. Children of the Kibbutz. Schocken Books, Inc., 1967
34. M. B. Sussman. The family today. Children Today, Mar/Apr 1978, p. 32
35. J. Wallerstein and J. Kelly. The effects of parental divorce: the adolescent experience. In The Child and His Family: Children at Psychiatric Risk. John Wiley and Sons, Inc., 1974
36. J. Wallerstein and J. Kelly. The effect of parental divorce: experiences of the preschool child. Journal of American Academy of Child Psychiatry, April 1975
37. J. Wallerstein and J. Kelly. The effects of parental divorce: experiences of the child in later latency. American Journal of Orthopsychiatry, April 1976, p. 256
38. R. S. Weiss. Marital Separation. Basic Books, Inc., 1975
39. K. Wiltse. Foster care in the 1970's: a decade of change. Children Today, May/June 1979, p. 10

Additional Recommended Reading

L. Afek and J. Hickey. Health classes for migrant workers' families. American Journal of Nursing, July 1972, p. 1296

B. Eiduson. Child development in emergent family styles. Children Today, Mar/Apr 1978, p. 24

An interim report of a longitudinal study of 200 children who are growing up in a variety of life styles that illustrate the pluralistic development of the family in the United States today. A significant study that should be followed by professional nurses.

W. Feigleman and A. Silverman. Single parent adoptions. Social Casework, July 1977, p. 418

H. Finklestein Keshet and K. M. Rosenthal. Single parent fathers. Children Today, May/June 1978, p. 13

M. Gill. Adoption of older children: the problems faced. Social Casework, May 1978, p. 272

K. Lewis. Children of lesbians: their point of view. Social World, May 1980, p. 198

M. McRae. An approach to the single parent dilemma. American Journal of Maternal Child Nursing, May/June 1977, p. 164

Presents an approach based on Piaget's theory of child development that the nurse can apply in the clinical setting for the assessment of normal and abnormal emotional development in children, and in educating parents.

H. Mendes. Single-parent families: a typology of life styles. Social Work, May 1979, p. 193

Presents a beginning conceptualization of five distinct life styles of single parent families. Describes the psychosocial risks and the unique opportunities of each life style.

S. Moss and M. Moss. Surrogate mother-child relationships. American Journal of Orthopsychiatry, April 1975, p. 382

M. Ward. Large adoptive families — a special resource. Social Casework, July 1978, p. 411

R. Youngblood. Children of the road. The Education Digest, March 1979, p. 20

B. M. Zimmerman. The exceptional stresses of adoptive parenthood. American Journal of Maternal Child Nursing, May/June 1977, p. 191

5 FAMILIES WITH DYSFUNCTIONAL LIFE PATTERNS

by Elizabeth B. Gall, RN, BS, MA, PNP

DEFINING DYSFUNCTION

Defining dysfunction precisely is not always possible, because family interactions are complex and the professional nurse's contact with families is relatively brief. All families have phases when they function well and other periods when they function poorly, even to the extent of disintegration. So nurses need to distinguish whether a dysfunctional pattern is temporary, situational or chronic, and foresee whether the ultimate outcome of a particular family's interaction is likely to have reversible or irreversible effects on its members.[5]

This chapter discusses family units that are not carrying out the universally accepted tasks of families and their members. Such families display behaviors that place their children in jeopardy — physically, emotionally, socially and intellectually. Parents in these families are unable or unwilling to assume the responsibility for their own actions and life outcomes that is expected of families in our social structure today.

An emphasis in this chapter is on the *interactional patterns* in such families, because *disturbed relationship* is the common denominator of altered health states of families in dysfunction.

Common disturbances in relationships frequently affiliated with family dysfunction are (1) inflexibility in parenting style, (2) parental misperception regarding the child, (3) inappropriate expectations of parents, and (4) parent-child mismatch.

An inflexibility in parenting style invites dysfunctional interaction within a family. The nurse may see parenting practices that are functional for one of the children and quite dysfunctional for another child. One basis for these differences lies in the children's temperaments, or their basic individual approaches to life.

Disturbed functioning may be stimulated by parental misconception regarding the child. We know that a child affects his parents by his unique responses to them and by the way that the parents perceive the child. Their perception may be related, not objectively to the child's looks or behavior, but to a projected attribution.[7] "He looks like Uncle John. I don't like him!" or, "She's so cute! She acts just like I did at this age," are common expressions of parents. The parents begin to prescribe injunctions (prohibitions) and permissions that the child either accepts or rejects to develop his own life plan, or script.*

The Gouldings[14] have described recognizable life injunctions that influence people's behavior:

Don't be (exist or live); Don't be you (the sex you are); Don't be a child (be a parent instead, take care of me); Don't grow (stay little); Don't make it (out in the world); Don't (fearful); Don't be important; Don't be close (to others, or be sexually responsive); Don't belong (here or anywhere); Don't be well (or sane); Don't think (don't think about "X" — forbidden subject — don't think what *you* think, think what *I* think); and Don't feel (don't feel "X" — mad, sad, glad — don't feel what *you* feel, feel what *I* feel).

The author gratefully acknowledges unique contributions to this chapter from Della Cowing, M.S.W.; Sara Gibb, B.S.: Deborah Thornton, M.S.W.; Madelyn Haynes, M.S.N., P.N.P.; Steve Bhaerman, M.A.; and John Gall, M.D.

*A "script" is a life plan people develop out of their responses to injunctions and permissions.

The positive opposites of these injunctions are *permissions* for living, for uniqueness, and for thinking, feeling and doing. The *injunctions* and *permissions* are either verbalized by the parents so the child hears them as messages or the child infers them from sensory cues and behavior. The child then makes decisions and develops his changeable script. This script dictates how he will think, feel and act.

Dysfunction can result when parents relate to their child(ren) in a manner that reflects inappropriate expectations for the child in relation to his age or capabilities. Often they lack the knowledge they need to be able to anticipate what their child can be expected to do or comprehend. During periods of stress, even informed parents sometimes relate inappropriately to their child.

A mismatch in family members' personalities may prompt conflict. One particular child may not "fit" his parents, but he could be loved and nurtured by another set of parents for the very qualities that set off stressful interactions within his biological family.[29]

Cultural and ethnic differences cannot be overlooked in defining family dysfunction. A well-functioning family may be unable to adapt successfully when it is transplanted into another cultural setting. Subcultures exist in every society, and their members may suffer deprivation and loss as a result of subtle and systematic discrimination against their efforts to "make it" in the mainstream society.[28]

CHARACTERISTICS OF FAMILIES WITH DYSFUNCTIONAL LIFE PATTERNS

Crisis and Stress Response

A striking feature of families in dysfunction is crisis: either a series of crises or multiple crises.[20] The family members' coping mechanisms are inadequate to meet the challenges posed by their environment in ways that foster life and health. In fact, stress response in the form of either altered health states or psychosomatic disease may be one indicator of dysfunction.[31] When confronted with what they perceive to be painful and stressful events, family members may respond with panic, anger or apathy. They may say, "This is just the way life is!" They may see no other way to look at their situation or feel that they have no other choice of action. They often operate in rigid, prescribed patterns learned in their family of origin. Their learned patterns limit the child's ability to think, solve problems or leave the scene of action.

Some families seek out the stimulation of stressful activities for excitement. However, they may overextend their energy resources and become fatigued so that their children are neglected. The nurse may be able to help them plan alternate periods of rest and recreation with stressful activities so that they experience pleasure. Their children, in turn, will experience more pleasant responses from their parents.

At times, dysfunctional families present a dizzying merry-go-round of activity to health professionals, making it difficult to see where intervention is possible. The sheer destructive energy and momentum of dysfunctional family systems, like centrifugal force, repel the best efforts of helping professionals to exert a counterforce.

The nurse involved with dysfunctional family systems may experience the contagion of stress, discovering in herself symptoms of the stress response. She may find her pulse racing with anger at the mother of twins who are failing to thrive. The nurse feels the urge to lash out with angry words, to blame the mother for getting herself into a helpless position with an alcoholic husband who does not care for her or provide for their babies. However, the nurse can use the energy generated by her anger constructively to help the mother plan better care for the twins and get help through community agencies. A person who succeeds in coping with a crisis builds up self-esteem and adds options in responding to different situations. The nurse can teach families how to draw upon resources within their environment of which they were previously unaware.[24]

Disturbed Communication Patterns

Families in dysfunction experience miscommunication, verbal and nonverbal. People who have not learned how to say what they think, believe, see, hear and feel seem to have difficulty exchanging valid information with others. The nurse may experience a sense of frustration when she talks with them. She cannot get a clear picture of what they are describing and she may feel confused. She may hear incomplete sentences, distorted ideas, grandiose or degrading epithets as she talks with family members. The nurse may check with several members to get information and may consult with other health professionals in order to get a realistic view of the family to plan its care.

Members of families with disturbed communication patterns tend to respond inappropriately to others and to situations. One woman laughed and giggled as she talked about the loss of her first expected baby and the severe illness of her newborn son. As a child, she had not been allowed to express her feelings or needs, especially sadness. Her parents expected her to cope on her own and not bother adults. Laughter at inappropriate moments often covers fear. Anger may also be used to cover fear or sadness and vice versa.

Some parents respond to their children in irritation and anger much of the time, an inappropriate mode that tends to destroy creativity and problem-solving. Other families have hidden "rules" that inhibit expression of feelings. Relationships between children and their parents in these families tend to be apathetic, revealing little affection or feelings. Children from such environments often seek inappropriate affectional exchanges (usually in excess) from casual acquaintances or strangers and do not portray the "stranger anxiety" that usually is characteristic of the child's developmental age.

Perpetuation of Dysfunction to Next Generation

Characteristically, families with dysfunction perpetuate their disruptive and destructive parenting practices to the next generation.[1] Thomas Gordon,[13] the originator of Parent Effectiveness Training, says:

Most parents, confronted with a situation where a child is experiencing a problem, respond the same way their own parents did. And because they have not had a chance to learn a better way, parents keep making the same mistakes *their* parents made.

Although the extended family can be supportive when a young family undertakes its parenting tasks, sometimes the family members are locked into dysfunctional interaction patterns. For example, well-meaning grandparents may take over care of a newborn baby and not allow the parents to establish bonding and attachment with their own child or re-establish their marital relationship in a new way following the birth of the baby. Relatives and friends are often unaware of how they may be compounding distress in the family by their efforts to be helpful.

Unhealthful parenting practices may be the parents' own unsuccessful solution to a developmental hurdle. The young parents may have gone through a difficult period at a particular age. When their own child comes to that age or stage, the parents have a difficult time nurturing the child. Instead, they react more as a sibling to their offspring. Unwed teenage mothers are often caught in this situation with their own mothers.

A woman who had a turbulent adolescence may discover that her parent had a similar upset at the same age. One mother expressed terror as her children approached their teen years, not because she herself had a hard time but because her sister did. Her sister acted out and caused much disruption in the family. This mother had been extra "good" as a teenager in order to compensate for her sister's "badness" in behavior. Reliving her compensatory behavior re-created pain for herself as her children began adolescence.

Parental guilt may lead to perpetuation of dysfunctional behaviors in the next generation. When parents feel guilty, they may overnurture their children, also a disruptive parenting practice. Parents, especially in the "middle class," work hard to give their children advantages they themselves may have missed. They are overinvested in their child's achievements. The children in these families may feel overwhelmed with expectations, or "swallowed up."

Lack of a Beneficial Support Group

Another characteristic of families in dysfunction is lack of a constructive support group, or enmeshment in a group having destructive effects on the family or its members. Leech-like relatives or friends may cling to a family that is already barely holding together. Two apparent opposites — isolation and overinvolvement in destructive relationships — are common. One woman in Parents Anonymous* belonged to a roller skating group of about 30 people. Social workers, noting that these friends were con-

---

*A group that, like Alcoholics Anonymous, reinforces healthy behavior patterns through mutual support. Its members seek to channel impulses to abuse their children into constructive action.

stantly in and out of the woman's house, at first thought she was not isolated. But as the caseworker got to know the woman's situation better, she discovered that this group was playing into the mother's system of neglect and abuse of her children by reinforcing it. If she could not find a baby sitter when it was time to go roller skating (she had four children under 7 years of age) her friends would urge her to go anyway and leave the children at home. Members of the group yelled at, spanked and generally "scapegoated" her children. As the caseworker discovered later, the mother was angry because she felt the children tied her down. The group responded to the anger the mother felt, and, by supporting her behavior in this way, joined her abuse system.

Disorganization of Family Living Pattern

Families in dysfunction and crisis experience disorganized daily living patterns. Often food is not provided for family members, meals are not prepared and sleeping arrangements are erratic or crowded or the children's sleep needs are disregarded in favor of adult social desires. Noise may disturb rest and sleep schedules of parents and children alike. General environmental disorder is visible. Children may have disturbed behavior such as nightmares, somnambulism, compulsive solitary rocking or head-banging and despairing crying, whining or wailing. These children may be ignored and their needs discounted by the parents.

These families are often disoriented as to time, space and sequence or social obligation, evident to the nurse by their missed appointments or their coming on the wrong day, wrong time or both. They move frequently; they may give relatives' addresses and phone numbers and cannot be located, or reached by telephone. They are often trying to avoid creditors and bill collectors; they may view health professionals with suspicion.

Children in Jeopardy

The most extreme characteristic we see in dysfunctional families is children in jeopardy. The underlying cause of jeopardy varies. Often dysfunctional families neglect or cannot manage the fulfillment of basic human needs for food, shelter, body protection from the elements; for security and protection from harm; for rest and for stimulation; and for recognition and self-identity. The nurse may be the crucial person in the health care field who advocates understanding of children. She can help break the chains of miscommunication that bind generations together with missed signals, anguish and despair.

PRIMARY NURSING ROLES IN WORKING WITH FAMILIES IN DYSFUNCTION

People who are taught dyfunctional life patterns fail to achieve developmental tasks within their complex family network. The outcome of their failures is often psychic pain and physical symptomatology, ranging from psychosomatic disease to physical trauma. By the time children in dysfunctional relationships receive medical or legal intervention, much damage may have been done to their bodies and minds.

The nursing profession has a unique advantage in helping families in dysfunction. Nurses can be eclectic and select from other disciplines interventions that will be helpful to clients. Nurses can continually enlarge their repertoire of interventions by drawing from various psychotherapeutic theories and methods.[26]

Casefinder

The nurse is often the first professional helper with which the family shares its dysfunction. Their request for help is often not direct; it may be a report of some symptom to a nurse that leads her to suspect dysfunction. The nurse must therefore be observant of family interactions* and alert in her history-taking for those patterns that characterize the dysfunctional family. She can then either employ her own skills to intervene or refer the family to resources that can help them.[23]

Role Model

The first intervention is the nurse herself — all her humanness, wholeness or incompleteness,

---

*Research on operational definitions of mother-infant interaction and a scale for scoring have been developed by Massie and Campbell at Children's Hospital and Medical Center, San Francisco. Called the Attachment Indicators During Stress (AIDS) Scale, it is designed for infants from birth to 18 months. Its purpose is to detect aberrant mother-infant responsiveness in stressful situations, particularly physical examinations. See Chapter 22 for the scale.

her experiences in her own family of origin and her particular stage of personal development. All are resources the nurse can use to intervene by modelling how to relate to others in an autonomous and caring manner. She can teach people how to look at things, hear things, feel, touch and respond in ways that bring them pleasure instead of the pain of dysfunction. She can model how to serve others best by serving her own needs for expression of what she really thinks, feels, needs and wants in a given situation.

Teacher and Counselor

The nurse's functions as teacher or counselor require that she intervene to help reverse the family's dysfunction. She can provide information to help parents correct knowledge deficits or misconceptions regarding parenting options or developmental expectations. (See Chapter 3 on parenting.)

Her counselling efforts can reinforce the fact that each child is unique. To these families, their child's uniquenesses can be emphasized. Parents should be assured that temperaments do clash, but ways to cope with those aspects of their child's personality that conflict with their own can be learned. Parents may also need guidance to develop realistic ways of interacting with their child during periods of stress.

Parenting the Parent

Nurses can lend themselves to families as parent-surrogates for a time. When a nurse intervenes to assist a mother or father with parenting tasks, she nurtures them in the present and also may be caring for parts of their personalities that suffered deprivations and unresolved hurts during their own childhood.[2, 3, 17, 20] Specifically, the nurse's interventions are aimed at giving parents permission to enjoy their children and instruction in how to relate to them. Together, nurse and parents can plan how to initiate actions whereby parents can meet their own needs so they can, in turn, give to their children. These experiences can stimulate the parent to take charge of his own life and decide how he will behave.

Team Member

Most family dysfunction requires lengthy treatment because of persisting patterns of interaction, and multiple interventions are required to effect change in them.[17] The nurse can increase her therapeutic effectiveness by participating in an interdisciplinary team. The team offers the advantage of combating the multiple problems of the dysfunctional family with the energies and expertise of those in several disciplines. The involvement of representatives of several disciplines also brings to bear on the family the implied pressure of society to achieve relief of their stress and to get on with being human in a humane setting. The team offers each individual professional the emotional reinforcement needed to withstand the exacerbations that typify this family unit. The nurse's specific role within the team and interaction with the family depend on several factors, including the team's composition and her particular expertise.

Child Advocate

The nurse keeps in mind the needs of the vulnerable child and acts in his behalf. She is responsible to act in the child's behalf during parental absence or whenever the child's development or survival is jeopardized, but within a context that attempts to preserve the family.

FAILURE-TO-THRIVE FAMILIES

The failure of a child to thrive without organic cause is one evidence of family disorganization and occurs in all socioeconomic and educational circumstances. The family's first mute plea for help may be to seek medical care for their child. Or they may be reported by a neighbor or professional person for suspected child abuse and neglect and thereby come to the attention of nurses through referral from social services.

All members of families in dysfunction fail to thrive in various ways. However, the home environment of newborns and young children may be so limited or threatening that they fail to grow and develop "without organic reason." Most children who fail to thrive are studied and treated by their primary physician. One to five per cent of all hospital admissions of children are for this condition, but figures on its occurrence in the population cannot be found, perhaps because it is not a medical diagnosis but an entity that is concurrent with other conditions. Unless adverse psychosocial factors are recognized and prompt treatment is begun, these children may suffer permanent physical, mental and emotional limitations that handicap them for the rest of their lives.[9, 22]

Establishing Diagnosis

The child with somatic symptoms usually comes to the attention of a nurse or is brought to a physician for medical diagnosis. Careful history-taking and hospital-based laboratory studies and observation will rule out organic disease. Simultaneously, the child should be treated as a suspected "failure to thrive" as the nurse pays special attention to the parent's feeding techniques and nurturing care. If the child responds with gain in weight and laboratory studies are within normal range, the diagnosis can be confirmed.[4]

Clinical Manifestations

Symptoms of "failure to thrive" in the infant are: weight below the third percentile; sudden or rapid deceleration in the growth rate; delay in developmental milestones, especially gross motor skills and vocalization; somatic symptoms such as muscular hypotonia, decreased muscle mass, generalized weakness and abdominal distention. The parents may give a history of feeding problems with the baby, including vomiting, ruminating and diarrhea.

Older babies, toddlers and preschool children who are failing to thrive may show unusual social behaviors such as avoiding eye contact or intense watchfulness; avoidance of physical contact with other people; repetitive self-stimulating behaviors like rocking, head-banging, head-rolling and intense sucking. The child's affect may be disturbed, demonstrating excessive irritability, apathy or extreme compliance. The parents may report sleep disturbances in the child. The nurse may observe disturbances of human attachment, such as lack of stranger anxiety or lack of preference for parents inappropriate for the child's age.[17]

Etiology

Even though failure to thrive may be due to a nutritional deficiency or organic disease, it most often is the result of a disturbance in the relationship between the primary caretaker (usually the mother) and the child.

The precipitating factors underlying the disturbance are varied. The infant may be the product of an unwanted, unplanned or stressful pregnancy. The child's birth may have been a difficult natural one, or by cesarean section. He may have been premature or he may have some birth-associated illness or congenital defect. His appearance or temperament may be displeasing to his parents, or they may attribute some defect to him when none is apparent. The mother and infant may have been separated after delivery for a time complicated by anxiety and uncertainty about life outcomes. Parents may have difficulty establishing affectional ties with their children when they have unresolved grief over separation from significant people, familiar places and important objects. They may lack information about infant care and development, and expect responses from their child that conflict with his needs, development and abilities. For example, some young parents are disappointed to discover their baby does not "love" them as they expected but demands a lot instead.

Nursing Interventions

History Taking The information the nurse gathers is based on etiological factors and signs and symptoms. The history should be comprehensive so that the psychosocial origin of the child's problem is not overlooked. This process, carefully done, can eliminate unnecessary laboratory testing for an organic cause. Care is taken not to order laboratory tests that would deprive the child of food for a period of time. However, environmental failure to thrive should not be assumed without sufficient data or in the absence of data. Table 5-1 describes tests commonly performed in an effort to identify organic cause.

The manner of questioning and the nature of the questions necessary to elicit the history may seem threatening to parents. The nurse must develop tact, and pace the parents adequately in her manner of questioning. A helpful attitude in which the nurse is concerned about the child and also about the parents' feelings will likely gain the most information. The nurse needs to know about the prenatal history and the perina-

TABLE 5–1 DIAGNOSTIC APPROACHES TO RULE OUT ORGANIC DISEASE IN FAILURE-TO-THRIVE CHILDREN

Diagnostic	Purpose/Rule Out
Initial Screening	
Physical examination	R/O congenital defects; data base and measurements on admission
Denver Developmental Screening Test (DDST)	Establish relation to developmental milestones
Tuberculin test	R/O tuberculosis
Bone survey x-rays; of long bones, joints, skull	R/O old or recent fractures; establish bone age; check epiphyseal development
Anterior/posterior and lateral chest x-ray	R/O pulmonary disease
Urinalysis	R/O urinary tract infection (UTI); diabetes
CBC and differential	R/O anemia, chronic or systemic infection
Sweat test	R/O cystic fibrosis
Stool testing:	
Reducing substance and pH	R/O mono- and disaccharide deficiency
Occult blood	R/O milk intolerance
Ova and parasites	R/O internal bleeding
	R/O parasitic infestation
Further Studies (When indicated, based on history or failure to gain in hospital)	
Repeat DDST; Bayley or psychometrics	R/O mental retardation; prescribe activities for development
Detailed urinalysis: culture, 24-hour catecholamines	R/O UTI; metabolic defects
Stool testing:	
72-hour fecal fat	Malabsorption
D-xylose test	
culture	Infection
PBI and T4	Hypothyroidism
Electrocardiogram; cardiac catheterization	R/O cardiac anomalies; circulatory defects
Upper and/or lower GI x-ray	R/O dysphagia; anatomical abnormalities; internal injuries
Intravenous pyelogram	R/O urinary tract abnormalities; internal injuries
Biopsy:	
Bowel	R/O Hirschsprung's disease; congenital muscular dystrophy; celiac disease
Muscle	

tal course, family history of the child and parents, the infant's feeding history and the child's health history. The nurse will construct an accurate growth chart and maintain it during hospitalization. The nurse will observe and also ask questions about parent-child interactions, the parents' relationship with their child and the child's developmental attainment at home.[15]

Care of the Child in the Hospital The nurses in charge should limit the number of caregivers to a primary nurse each shift with an assigned nurse to relieve them on their days off.

The basic care is the same as for any child of similar age, but it may take more time, especially for feeding, with extra attention to holding the child, cuddling him and eliciting eye contact. Special skin care is sometimes required because of general altered nutritional state, bulky, frequent acid stools or frequent vomiting.

During hospitalization, nursing care includes ongoing testing and monitoring of the patient. The nurse will record the number, character, color and consistency of the stools; she may test the stools for occult blood and for reducing substances. (If the infant is malabsorbing, sugar will be present in the stool.) She should check the pH of the stool. (If it is less than 5.5 this means that acid is present, which results when sugar breaks down into acids.) The weight of the child is documented at the same time each day, under similar conditions. An accurate record of intake and output, including weighing the diapers, is made. The nurse is responsible for monitoring the intake, keeping a calorie count of the food actually ingested and estimating the child's retention of calories when vomiting occurs. She may need to have a consultation and some help from the dietary department in regard to planning the diet so that the child will have an optimum intake for "catch-up growth" while at the same time overfeeding is being avoided.

In addition to physical examination, within 24 hours of admission a Denver Developmental Screening Test should be done to determine the child's level of attainment, and if more stimulation is indicated, a program initiated to foster the child's progression in development. A foster grandparent or a person responsible for a play program may also be brought in to stimulate positive interaction with the infant and to model interactions for the child's primary caregivers, the parents.[4]

Nursing Care of the Child's Primary Caregiver (Mother/Father) The child's caregiver(s) should be welcomed and included in the hospital program. However, parents should not be coerced into participating until they are ready. (On occasion a treatment program is instituted that requires parents to be absent temporarily. Feeding and nurturing is done by the nurses, and the weight gain is evaluated while the child has been separated from the parents.)

The caregiver may need "re-parenting" in those areas in which she is dysfunctional. The nurse "mothers the mother" by providing emotional nurturing. This is often done most effectively through role modelling, demonstration and positive reinforcement of the caregiver's mothering efforts by the infant's primary nurse.[6] This re-parenting can sometimes be done even better by a foster grandmother, who may be less threatening than the nurse and nearer to the age of the mother's own mother.

In spite of all the nurse's anticipatory guidance and tact, parents may feel threatened, particularly if the child improves during hospitalization when no treatment other than feeding, nurturing and stimulation has been provided. They need to have their insecurity alleviated and their self-esteem built up as they succeed in caring for the child. The nurse can specifically point out their healthy fostering behaviors and responses by the child. The parents can learn playfulness, joy and laughter responses to their child.

The nurse can listen to the mother and help her work through her negative feelings that have disrupted healthy interactions with the child. The nurse can help allay her feeling of guilt regarding the diagnosis and reinforce healthful changes for the present and future. The mother's life partner or spouse and relatives may also need guidance in relating to the child in ways that support the mother's self-esteem as an individual and as a parent.

Documentation of Observations During Treatment Nurses who care for the child must build upon each other's findings and findings of others in the care team. In the case of an infant, they should:
1. Document the ways in which the child is held and fed and how eye contact is initiated by the primary caregiver(s), and the

facial expressions of the child and of the caregiver during interactions.
2. Note what the caregiver does with the child — play, talk, hold, stroke — and the child's response.
3. Note how the caregiver refers to the baby and whether she talks of the baby at all. This is an indicator to others of how the caregiver perceives the child.
4. Record the responses of the caregiver to the baby's cues. For example, what is the mother's response when the baby looks at her, when he cries, when he reaches toward her, during motor activity?
5. Note the response of the infant to the mother's overtures, the baby's reaction to the mother's feeding rate and the way he is being held. What the nurse should be looking for is synchrony or disharmony, and, specifically, how this occurs.[23]

Prevention In the broadest sense, nurses can have an impact on the prevention of failure to thrive as community members and health care providers. Nurses can initiate prenatal classes for parents in obstetrical clinics and physicians' offices and in adult education departments of public schools. In these classes they can discuss not only physical effects but also psychological and social effects the infant may have on family life.

Nurses can intervene with counselling to parents in situations of high-risk pregnancy, premature birth and cesarean section and in instances of other early parent-child stress such as birth of a defective child.[8] Postnatally, nurses can help parents learn and interpret their child's cues and gain a sense of self-esteem from their interactions.[21] Nurses can praise parents for healthful, fostering interactions with their children. Well-child examinations by nurses provide excellent opportunities to model and teach positive parenting techniques.[2]

CHARACTERISTICS OF FAMILIES WHO NEGLECT AND ABUSE THEIR CHILDREN

A global definition of problems with parent-child interaction that result in abuse and neglect has been proposed by Helfer:[16] Any interaction or lack of interaction between a caregiver and child which results in nonaccidental harm to

---

NURSING INTERVENTIONS FOR FAMILIES IN DYSFUNCTION

For Parents

1. Listen to the parents.
2. Nurture parents by caring.
3. Model positive parenting techniques.
4. Teach normal development and child management and plan with parents for goal attainment.
5. Foster normal bonding and attachment of parents with their children.
6. Praise parents for desirable parenting efforts and behaviors that foster their own self-esteem.
7. Help parents to discover that they have options and allow them to decide.*

For Parents and Child

1. Consult and refer to other professions when appropriate.*
2. Community involvement with volunteer groups, lay therapy groups and Parents Anonymous, Alcoholics Anonymous and other appropriate, specific groups and agencies (child protective services).*

For Child

1. Age-appropriate, ongoing nursing assessment, diagnosis, prognosis, treatment.*
2. Positive nurturing and stroking for all life permissions: to exist and thrive, to feel, to think, to act.
3. Prevention of negative parental scripts enables child to make life-enhancing decisions about self and world. Assist child to independence at appropriate age.*

*NOTE: Many of these interventions for parents and children need to be carried out in a team approach, group teaching and group therapy.[17] In their book "The Abusing Family" the Justices point out that different therapists or nurses should care for the parents and for the child, especially in abusing families.[20]

the child's physical and/or developmental state.

In the United States alone, a total of more than one million cases of child abuse and neglect are reported annually: 800,000 children neglected, 200,000 physically abused, 60,000 to 100,000 sexually abused, and 4000 killed by neglect and abuse.[12]

Etiology

Three elements commonly are present in families in which abuse occurs: (1) abuse of the parent(s) themselves as children, (2) perception by the parent(s) that the child is different and (3) occurrence of family crisis that alters living conditions. First, the potential for child abuse often results from the parents themselves having been abused as children. They are isolated individuals who cannot trust or use other people beneficially. The parents have a poor self-image, are impatient and often in conflict with each other about many things: sexual difficulties, discipline of their children, in-laws and decision-making. Their family systems perpetuated discipline that utilized physical punishment. The spouse of the abusing parent may be so passive that he or she does not intervene to spare the child from abuse.

Second, these parents have unrealistic expectations of their children; the child who is abused may be perceived as different by the parent or parents. He often was an unwanted child, and his parents may have experienced stress at his birth. He may have special problems such as retardation, prematurity or a congenital defect that triggers the abusive pattern in the parent. A clash between the child's temperament and that of the abusive parent often exists, making the child seem unacceptable or undesirable to this parent. Sometimes the precipitating factor is simply a developmental task the child is attempting to master under unrealistic parental demand.

Third, the family often endures a crisis or a series of crises, such as drastic changes in its living conditions or financial status. The parents may have limited food, money, light or heat. They may have experienced separation or loss.[17]

Identifying and Diagnosing the Abuse or Neglect

The abused or neglected child's behavior depends on many factors, including his age, his developmental level, the specific pattern of relationships in the family, whether abuse has been an ongoing situation or a single event and what injuries he has received. Abused children may be irritable or apathetic. They usually show indiscriminate and superficial affection to strangers.

The index of suspicion for the nurse should be triggered by certain factors in the history and signs and symptoms. History indications include unexplained or evasive-contradictory accounts of how trauma occurred, especially pattern injuries caused by belt loops or electric cords and burns, or hand imprints; reluctance to give information; delay in seeking medical care; previous history of similar episodes or multiple visits to various hospitals; multiple poison ingestions or "accidents"; inappropriate reaction to severity of child's injury and abusive verbal exchanges between parent and child.*

Physical signs and symptoms include evidence of general neglect*; failure to thrive*; poor skin hygiene*; irritability; delayed motor, social, language and cognitive development; bruises, abrasions, burns, soft-tissue swelling, human bites, eye damage; lesions or injuries in various stages of healing; fracture or dislocation of extremities; unexplained genital or severe abdominal injuries; coma; convulsions, symptoms of drug withdrawal or intoxication; death.[12]

In order for sexual abuse to be identified, the child must be carefully inspected for evidence of oral, anal or genital penetration. Laboratory tests can be done to determine the presence of semen or venereal disease. State and federal statutes require immediate reporting to child protective services by anyone who observes children with such symptoms.[12, 17, 25]

Management and Nursing Interventions

Prevention Prevention is of primary importance. Nurses are in strategic positions to identify potential abusers and to employ supportive intervention.[25]

Prenatal Observation The nurse should assess the parents' attitude toward the pregnancy. She should determine if the pregnancy was wanted

---
*These are present in neglect and emotional abuse as well as in physical abuse.

TABLE 5-2 THE DANCE OF DEVELOPMENT

Child's Age	Psychological Stage[10]	What the Child Needs[20] Child's Developmental Tasks	Parent's Developmental Tasks[18]
0–6 months (or crawling)	Early oral (Existential)	To establish symbiosis Positive physical and verbal reinforcement To find that he has impact on environment Talk	Learn cues baby uses to express needs
6 months– 1½ or 2 years	Late oral (Exploratory)	Move around Get into things Drop things Self-feed	Anticipate baby's needs for safety and protection
1½ or 2–3 years	Anal (Separation)	Test and oppose Be negative Break symbiosis Learn to consider needs and feelings of others	Accept child's growth and development
3–6 years (can be 2½–5)	Genital (Imaginative)	Identify differences in self and others: sex; color hair, eyes Ask questions Move away more from parents physically Invent monsters	Learn to separate from child
6–12 years	Latency (Creative)	Argue, compete, achieve Do things, have companions Joint community activity	Learn to accept child's rejection (of parent) without deserting child
12–18 years (Puberty through teens)	Adolescence (Recycling)	Be contradictory Be part child, part adult Say in effect: "Go away—come closer" and "Tell me what to do—I dare you" Recycle previous stages	Learn to build new life with mate (independent of child)
18 years on through life	Adulthood and maturity		

FAMILIES GROW AND DEVELOP

TABLE 5-2 THE DANCE OF DEVELOPMENT *(Continued)*

What Parent Should Do[20] *Helpful Parenting Behaviors*	What Parent Shouldn't Do[20] *(Parenting Behaviors to Avoid)*	*Tasks of Parents of Adults*
Feed, fondle, talk to baby When baby cries, check to see what is wrong Try out different things to soothe child	Don't withhold strokes Don't feed on schedule Don't spank Don't hover over baby when there is no discomfort	Learn to relate to grown children as peers and accept their autonomy as parents Expand and/or contract own interests Resolve own developmental issues Learn to relate to grandchildren, maintain and grant autonomy to children and grandchildren Learn to pace self according to physical and emotional capacities Relearn dependency on others without establishing shifting symbiotic (unhealthy) relationships
Continue giving unconditional positive strokes "Baby-proof" the house Provide protection	Don't restrict mobility Don't force toilet training Don't spoon- or force-feed Don't spank	
Expect child to start considering others Expect child to use cause-and-effect thinking and problem-solving Institute discipline Begin toilet training	Don't fail to discipline (not punish) and give reason to convey expectations Don't make expectations so high that they are too demanding Don't be inconsistent with child	
Answer all questions with reasons Encourage problem-solving Teach how to get strokes	Don't answer questions with "Because I say so" Don't get upset over masturbation Don't tease	
Discuss values and state rules Listen to child's reasons Encourage task completion and setting priorities	Don't make rules and values too rigid Don't fail to discuss rules and values	
Stick by rules and values Encourage independence but still offer "protection" and guidance	Don't give up Don't be overprotective or underprotective	

or not, signs of depression in the parents and whether the pregnancy is publicly acknowledged or denied, with attempts to keep it hidden until this is no longer possible. Parents' overemphasized expectations for the baby as to its sex, development and appearance should alert the nurse to potential problems in the parent-child relationship that emerges.

Inquiries should be made about social supports for the pregnancy: Is a spouse present? Is he involved in pregnancy care for the expectant mother? What relatives or friends offer positive support and practical help? Nursing care includes recognition of family situations of excessive stress such as job loss by either or both expectant parents; inadequate income or housing; several children to care for or children born very close together that cause strain on the mother's energy; marital difficulties. Over time, the nurse will elicit a picture of the pregnant couple's own experiences with their parents as they grew up, their exposure to parenting role models and their opportunities to acquire parenting knowledge and skills. The nurse collaborates with the physician, social services agencies or other appropriate team members to help the couple resolve as many problems as possible during the pregnancy and counsels the parents to help them cope with those situations that cannot be changed.

Postnatal Observation The nurse needs to observe and participate with the parents in their initial responses to the baby. Do they talk to their baby, recognizes his cues, establish eye-to-eye contact, play with him? The nurse can help the parents see likeable characteristics in their infant and can point out the baby's capabilities. The nurse should note parents' reactions to caregiving: whether they recognize the baby's needs and the way they offer care. She will note verbal references they make to the baby; their talk of the baby; the baby's name, its meaning to them and their process and timing in agreeing on it; and their descriptions of the baby to others. The nurse will be alert for signs of anxiety related to the baby's presence: overconcern about the baby's condition, lack of confidence in their parenting tasks, spouse jealousy or sibling rivalry.[8]

Intervening in High-Risk Families The nurse may need to teach childrearing practices, beginning prenatally or in the newborn period. She can promote harmony among parents and children by praising positive interactions and parenting behaviors. She can help parents to identify the child's attributes and unique qualities. She can make the infant available to the parents for development of the bonds of attachment after delivery and in the postnatal period in the hospital. Anticipatory guidance that teaches developmental expectations and child care skills appropriate to the child's age are offered on an ongoing basis.

Those who display unhealthy parenting styles, who are dependent or have a diagnosed psychosis or mental deficiency or who seem to have a disorganized and ill-structured life style require multidisciplinary intervention and supervision to help them establish healthy relationships with their children.

An innovative and workable approach to the treatment and teaching of abusing parents has been developed by Rita and Blair Justice (Table 5–2).[10, 18, 20] Child abuse is a system involving the entire family; therefore, a systems approach is needed by professionals to break up the family's interlocking symbiosis and to change their dysfunction.

The Documentation of Abuse and Neglect The federal Child Abuse Prevention and Treatment Act of 1974 requires that all professionals report instances of child abuse. There are statutes in all the states that require lay persons as well as professionals to report child abuse to some designated agency such as child protection services. These agencies have legal authority to investigate and to protect children. Some states have penalties, including fine or imprisonment, for violations. The person who reports a suspected case in good faith is immune from legal reprisals by the persons he names.[17]

Whether abuse is found or not, the nurse needs to keep objective, factual, descriptive records of her observations. Photographs are almost essential to document bruising and injuries of the child. The nurse should record conversations with parents in suspected cases (preferably tape recorded) so that the records will be clear for scrutiny in the future.

Care of the Abused Child The child needs to have consistent behavior toward him by caregivers who are responsible for his treatment and restoration. Efforts at attachment must come

88 FAMILIES GROW AND DEVELOP

from an adult source, since this child will not usually risk initiating a relationship on his own. These caregivers can reinforce the child's appropriate behavior through a behavior modification program. For example, pleasant and positive stroking* of various kinds is offered consistently for constructive and healthful behaviors. The caregivers need to provide age-appropriate and developmentally appropriate stimulation.

Play is most effective in interacting with the child. The nurse should encourage positive interactions between the child and parents and pleasant feelings of the child toward the parents while this child is being cared for in the hospital setting.

Care of the Parent The nurse has a dual responsibility to model the role of caregiver and to demonstrate healthy interactions and expectations for the child. The nurse can reinforce any positive parenting efforts by actively involving the parents in the planning of care. On the other hand, the nurse should avoid forcing participation when the parents are not ready for caregiving. The nurse can praise the parents' interest in and concern for their child, and reinforce competent child care behaviors. As a team member the nurse provides mothering of the abusive parent to help fulfill that parent's unmet needs and models healthy mothering behaviors for the parent. The nurse can teach realistic growth and development expectations and childrearing options to the parents, mostly through demonstration and role modelling and discussions on management of the child's developmental tasks, such as toilet training.

The nurse may help the family members reduce crisis in the home by referring them to social agencies, employment agencies, housing assistance or other appropriate resources. The nurse can help the family to identify and get in touch with support groups such as Parents Anonymous, friends or religious groups. Often just helping the family identify their own actual and potential strengths is a useful nursing action. The nurse can help the parents to identify situational factors that have contributed to the abuse and to learn ways to control and constructively release their anger. The parents may need permission to express their anger in constructive ways; they may never have learned how to do that.[20]

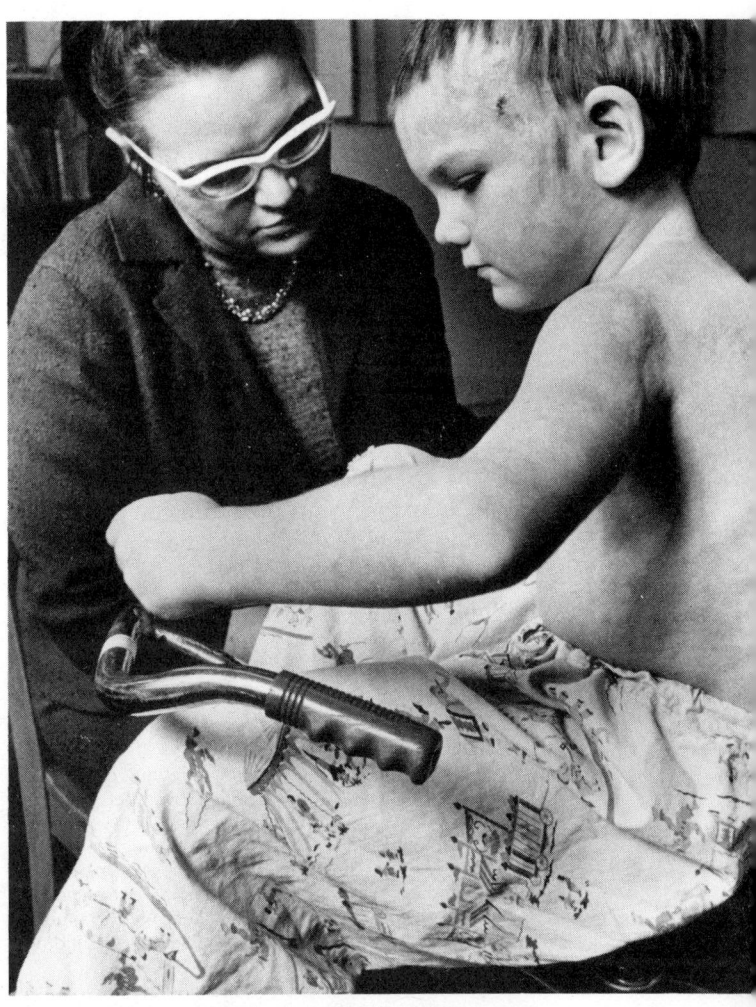

The abused child needs consistent behavior in the adults around him. A foster grandparent can initiate a positive relationship with such a child. (Photograph from Photo Researchers, Inc.)

Discharge Planning The nurse needs to begin to prepare the children and the parents as soon as a legal decision is made to release the child from the hospital. Even though one child usually is the victim in the family, when that child is removed another child can take his place as abuse victim because the real problem is dysfunctional parenting and not the specific child. Thus the nurse should be aware of the need for protection of all the children in a family until the adults have made changes in their parenting style. If foster home placement is the legal decision, the nurse can encourage continuing contact of the parents and siblings with the child. The nurse can help the family to understand the child's need to regress to earlier

---

*Words and gestures motivated by kindness that increase an individual's self-esteem and sense of well-being.

developmental stages to finish missed tasks. The parent's progress in forming healthier parenting behaviors must continue to be evaluated while the child is in the foster home.

When the child is to be returned to his own home, the nurse will participate with the team in continuing close supervision. She will help to monitor the family for signs of continued abuse of this child or transfer of abuse to another child. The nurse may need to make home visits, and the parents should be encouraged to visit her or to seek nursing assistance at any time, especially if they feel they are losing control of themselves.

In the case of a child having been removed legally from the home, the nurse can participate in counselling with all family members to help each of them to grieve and finish the process of mourning losses they may experience.[17]

References

1. E. Berne. What Do You Say After You Say Hello? Bantam Books, Inc., 1973
2. B. Bishop. A guide to assessing parenting capabilities. American Journal of Nursing, November 1976, p. 1784
3. M. S. Brown and J. T. Hurlock. Mothering the mother. American Journal of Nursing, March 1977, p. 439
4. G. Chipault et al. Guidelines for pediatric management of hospitalized infants and toddlers with "failure to thrive." University of Michigan, C. S. Mott Childrens' Hospital, Ann Arbor, Michigan 48109, 1979
5. K. E. Christiansen. Family epidemiology: an approach to assessment and intervention. In Family Health Care, Vol. I, D. H. Hymovich and M. U. Barnard, eds., McGraw-Hill Book Co., 1979
6. A. L. Clark. Recognizing discord between mother and child and changing it to harmony. American Journal of Maternal Child Nursing, March/Apr 1976, p. 100
7. C. Cropley, F. Lester and S. Pennington. Assessment tool for measuring maternal attachment behaviors. In Current Practice in Obstetric and Gynecologic Nursing, Vol. I, L. K. McNall and J. T. Galeener, eds., C. V. Mosby Co., 1976
8. M. A. Curry. Significance of early physical contact between mother and infant. In Current Practice in Obstetric and Gynecologic Nursing, Vol. I, L. K. McNall and J. T. Greener, eds., C. V. Mosby Co., 1976.
9. P. C. English. Failure to thrive without organic reason. Pediatric Annals, November 1978, p. 83
10. E. Erickson. Childhood and Society. W. W. Norton & Co., 1963
11. Failure to thrive. Pediatric Annals, November 1978 (Entire issue)
12. V. J. Fontana. Child abuse: an attack every two minutes. Pediatric Consult, January 1979, p. 2
13. T. Gordon. P.E.T. in Action. Bantam Books, Inc., 1976
14. M. M. Goulding and R. L. Goulding. Injunctions and counter-injunctions. In Changing Lives through Redecision Therapy, M.M. Goulding and R.L. Goulding, eds., Bruner/Mazel, Inc., 1979
15. L. L. Harrison. Nursing intervention with the failure to thrive family. American Journal of Maternal Child Nursing, Mar/Apr 1976, p. 111
16. R. E. Helfer. Putting abuse and neglect into perspective. Workshop outline prepared for the National Committee for the Prevention of Child Abuse, 1978
17. R. E. Helfer. The diagnostic process and treatment programs. USDHEW, Office of Child Development/Children's Bureau: National Center for Child Abuse and Neglect. DHEW Publ. No. (OHD) 76-30069, 1976
18. D. P. Hymovich. The family with a young child. In Family Health Care, Vol. II. D. Hymovich and M. Barnard, eds., McGraw-Hill Book Co., 1979
19. S. H. Johnson. The contemporary néonatal nurse. In Current practice in Obstetrics and Gynecologic Nursing, Vol. I. L. McNall and J. Galeener, eds. C. V. Mosby Co., 1976
20. B. Justice and R. Justice. The Abusing Family. Human Sciences Press, Inc., 1976
21. M. H. Klaus and J. H. Kennell. Maternal-Infant Bonding: The Impact of Early Separation or Loss on Family Development. C. V. Mosby Co., 1976
22. M. Levine. Failure to thrive. Pediatric Annals, November 1978, p. 8
23. H. N. Massie and B. K. Campbell. The Massie-Campbell scale of mother-infant attachment indicators during stress. Children's Hospital and Medical Center of San Francisco, P. O. Box 3805, San Francisco, CA 94119
24. S. McCabe. Anticipatory guidance of families with infants. In Family Health Care, Vol. I. D. Hymovich and M. Barnard, eds., McGraw-Hill Book Co., 1973
25. N. McKeel. Child abuse can be prevented, American Journal of Nursing, September 1978, p. 1478
26. R. J. McKeighen. Principles of family counseling. In Family Health Care, Vol. I. D. Hymovich and M. Barnard, eds., McGraw-Hill Book Co., 1979
27. R. Olson. Index of suspicion: screens for child abusers. American Journal of Nursing, January 1976, p. 108
28. C. Taylor. Cultural barriers: an anthropological perspective. In Family Health Care, Vol. I. D. Hymovich and M. Barnard, eds., McGraw-Hill Book Co., 1979
29. A. Thomas and S. Chess. Temperament and Development. Bruner/Mazel Inc., 1977
30. A. Ware. Using nursing prognosis to set priorities, American Journal of Nursing, May 1979, p. 921
31. R. L. Woolfolk and F. C. Richardson. Stress, Sanity, and Survival. Monarch (Simon and Schuster), 1978

Additional Recommended Reading

D. E. Babcock and T. D. Keepers. Raising Kids O.K.: Transactional Analysis in Human Growth and Development. Grove Press, Inc., 1976

R. Bandler, J. Grinder and V. Satir. Changing with Families, Vol. 1: A Book about Further Education for Being Human. Science & Behavior Books, 1976

M. U. Barnard. Supportive nursing care for the mother and newborn who are separated from each other. American Journal of Maternal Child Nursing, Mar/Apr 1976, p. 107

C. Blosser. Avoiding potential behavior problems in children. Pediatric Nursing, May/June 1979, p. 11

T. G. R. Bower. A Primer of Infant Development. W. H. Freeman & Co., 1977

G. Chipault. A better beginning: Helping the failure-to-thrive infant and family.

A color video cassette with accompanying booklet which includes a profile of the failure-to-thrive infant and of the family, a discussion of interaction between and intervention for parents and infant, guidelines for assessing the failure-to-thrive infant and a bibliography. Booklet available separately. Write to: Media Library-Peds., University of Michigan Medical Center, Towsley Center Box 57, Ann Arbor, MI 48109.

D. Dinkmeyer and G. D. McKay. Systematic Training for Effective Parenting: Parents' Handbook. American Guidance Service, Inc., 1976

N. B. Ebeling and D. A. Hill, eds. Child Abuse: Intervention and Treatment. Publishing Sciences Group, Inc., 1975

N. Edwards. The New Parent Class. The Pennypress, 1978.

Available from ICEA P. O. Box 20048, Minneapolis MI 55420

H. M. Halpern. Cutting Loose: An Adult Guide to Coming to Terms with Your Parents. Bantam Books, Inc., 1978

G. Handel. Sociological aspects of parenthood. In Family Health Care, Vol. I. D. Hymovich and M. Barnard, eds., McGraw-Hill Book Co., 1979

R. E. Helfer and C. H. Kempe, eds. The Battered Child. University of Chicago Press, 1974

S. J. Holt and T. M. Robinson. The school nurse's family assessment tool. American Journal of Nursing, May 1979, p. 950

A. Hurwitz. Child abuse: a program for intervention. Nursing Outlook, September 1977, p. 575

C. H. Kempe and R. E. Helfer, eds. Child Abuse and Neglect: The Family and the Community. Ballinger Publishing Co., 1976

C. H. Kempe and R. E. Helfer, eds. Helping the Battered Child and His Family. J. B. Lippincott Co., 1972

S. J. Mackenzie. A mother care class. Transactional Analysis Journal, January 1977, p. 68

B. Mitchell. Working with abusive parents: a caseworker's view, American Journal of Nursing, March 1973, p. 480

A. C. Mullins and R. E. Barstow. Care for the caretakers. American Journal of Nursing, August 1979, p. 1425

K. Neill and C. Kauffman. Care of the hospitalized abused child and his family. American Journal of Maternal Child Nursing, Mar/Apr 1976, p. 117

N. A. Polansky, D. Hally and N. F. Polansky. Profile of neglect: A survey of the state of knowledge of child neglect. USDHEW, Social and Rehabilitation Service, PSA Publ. No. (SRS) 76-23-37

C. P. Porter. Maladaptive mothering patterns: nursing intervention. From AJN Clinical Sessions, Detroit 1972. Appleton-Century-Crofts, 1973

N. Rothenberg. Opportunities for psychological prophylaxis in the neonatal period. Clinical Pediatrics, January 1976, p. 53

A. B. Savino and R. W. Sanders. Working with abusive parents: group therapy and home visits. American Journal of Nursing, March 1973, p. 1483

K. Scharer. Rescue fantasies: professional impediments in working with child abusers. American Journal of Nursing, September 1978, p. 1483

J. Schiff, et al. Cathexis Reader: Transactional Analysis Treatment of Psychosis. Harper and Row, 1975

T. Schleiker. Teaching parents to cope with behavior problems. American Journal of Nursing, May 1978, p. 838

C. M. Steiner. Scripts People Live: Transactional Analysis of Life Scripts. Grove Press, Inc., 1974

R. F. Stewart. The family that fails to thrive. In Family Health Care, Vol. I. D. Hymovich and M. Barnard, eds., McGraw-Hill Book Co., 1973

S. Streshinsky. Help me before I hurt my child. Redbook, June 1974, p. 85

A. Thomas, S. Chess and H. G. Birch. Temperament and Behavior Disorders in Children. New York University Press and University of London Press, Ltd., 1968

S. Woollams and M. Brown. Transactional Analysis (College edition). Prentice-Hall, Inc., 1978

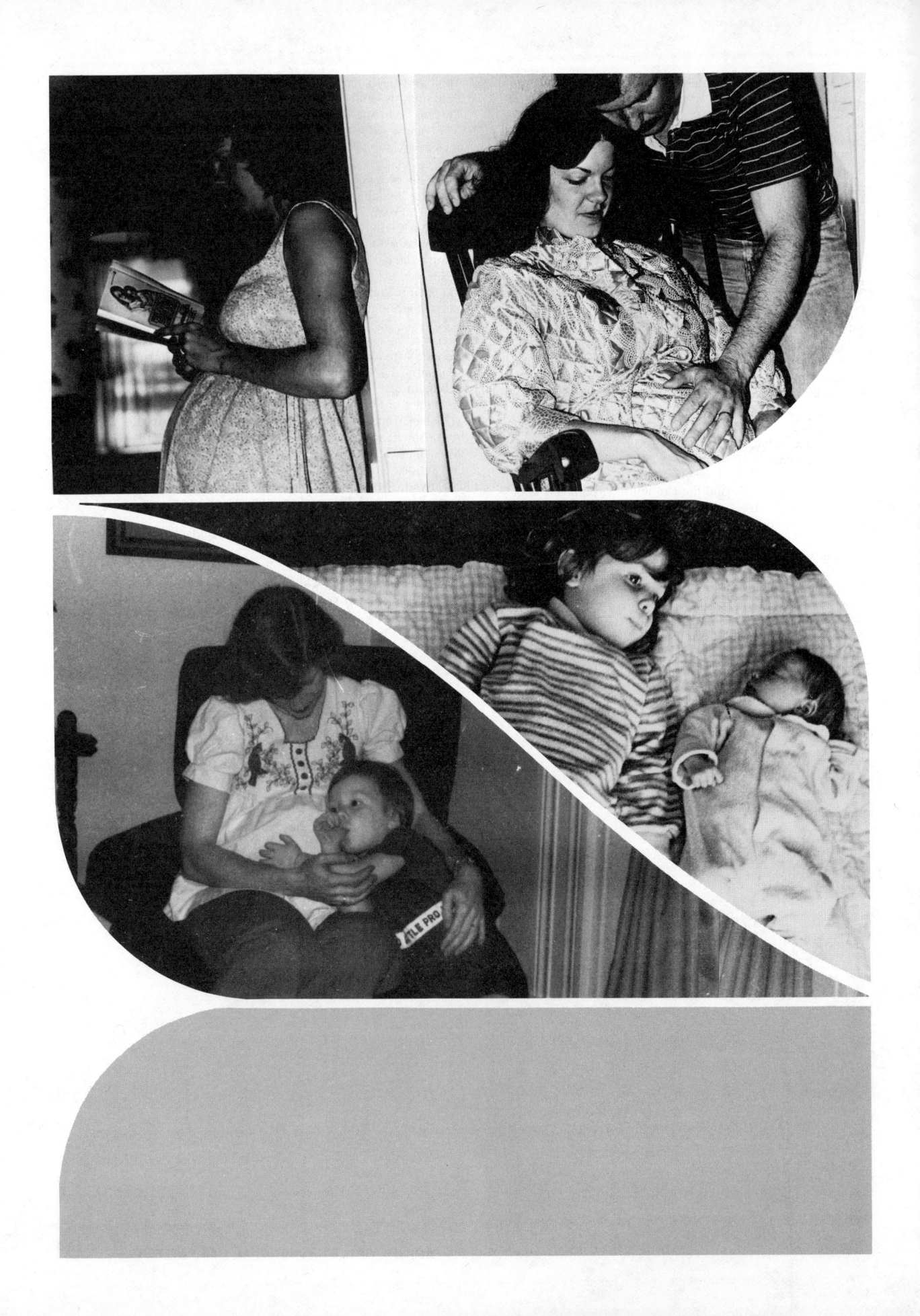

PART 2

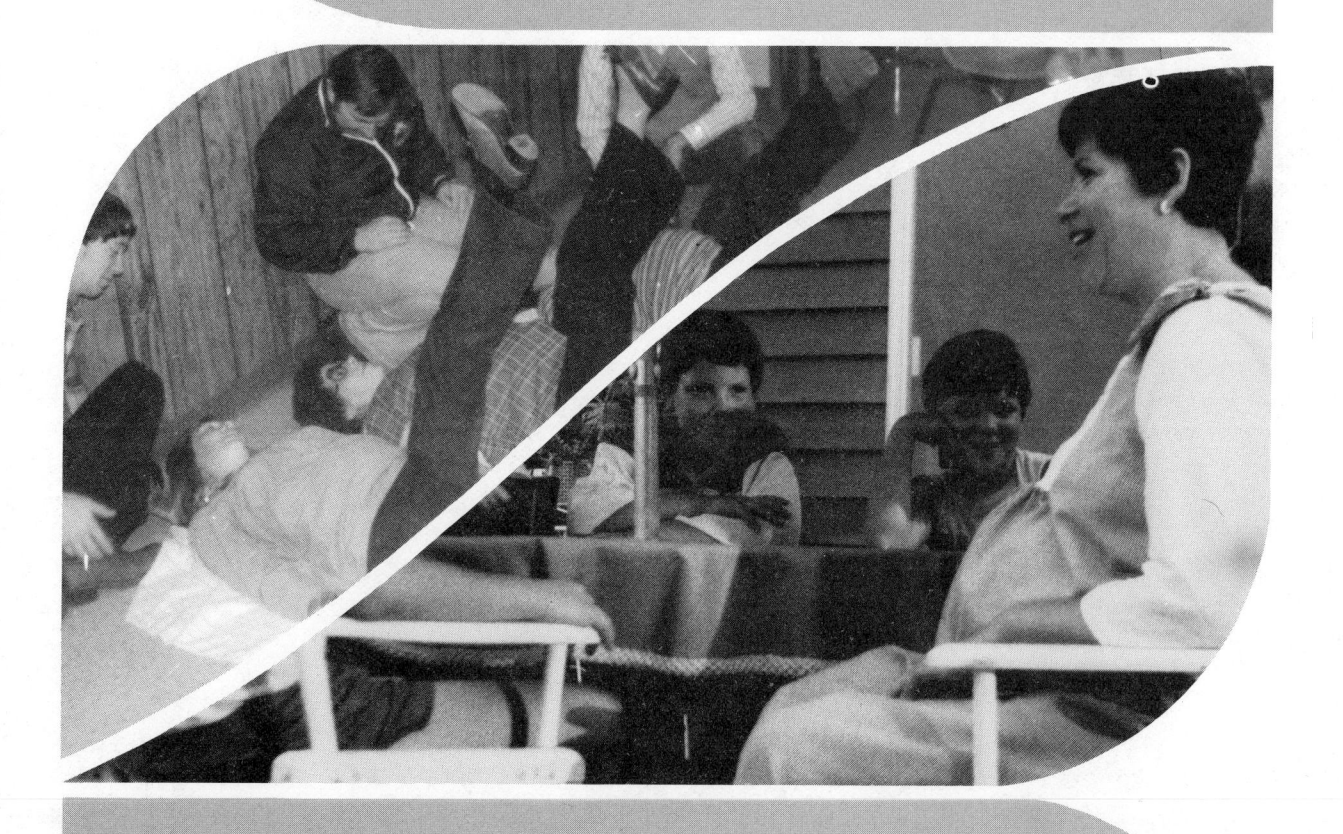

CHILDBEARING FAMILIES

GROWTH AND DEVELOPMENT NEEDS OF THE CHILDBEARING FAMILY: MAINTAINING WELLNESS

by Janet S. Malinowski, RN, MSN

INTRODUCTION

Throughout this chapter emphasis is placed on the adjustments the family must make during pregnancy. Successfully adapting to pregnancy and actively preparing for the parenting role will help a family have a healthy, happy childbearing experience and will facilitate integration of the baby into the family unit. Nurses can play an important role in maintaining wellness in the family by providing anticipatory guidance, along with closely observing the family unit for signs and symptoms of stress.

The nurse meets the family at various stages of pregnancy. For example, a nurse caring for a child in the hospital, in the clinic or in the community should focus on the entire family. When an ill child's mother is pregnant, the nurse must give special attention to the impact of the child's illness on the mother's health. The additional stresses of a sick child further complicate the adjustment to pregnancy with regard to managing household tasks, coping with economic stresses and fatigue and maintaining morale. The nurse requires an understanding of the needs of the family during the normal pregnancy cycle to enable her to intervene at a time when these additional stresses are encountered. Also, the nurse's understanding of the adjustments required before the birth of a child gives her a greater sensitivity to the meaning that the coming of a child has to his parents.

ADJUSTMENT TO PREGNANCY

The first attempt at anything is usually the most difficult. Parenthood for the first time is no exception. The couple has many adjustments to make, many developmental tasks to accomplish. The tasks of each parent are somewhat different, and the more harmoniously the two people work together, the more likely it is that their transition to parenthood will be a fulfilling one.

This does not negate the significance of adjustments to succeeding pregnancies. Similar physical and emotional adaptations are involved, but the ability to make these transitions is usually greater owing to knowledge gained during past pregnancies. There is one significant difference about succeeding pregnancies — they involve the children already born into the family.

Redistribution of Labor

Completion of household tasks is a joint effort in most families today. Who does what is determined somewhat by the family members' interest, competency and compatibility. Just the same, regardless of whether the mother works outside the home or not, in most family units she bears most of the responsibility for household tasks.

Pregnancy necessitates a redistribution of labor among family members. In a few cultures, pregnancy is viewed as a time of increased stress, vulnerability and debility for the woman. Women in these cultures therefore curtail their physical activities early in pregnancy. But more typically the woman with an uncomplicated pregnancy continues her usual tasks until one to two months before the expected delivery date.

Primary factors that determine the alteration of her tasks are her level of fatigue and physical mobility. Her routine long hours and physical activity eventually become more than she can tolerate. The heavy housework is then usually assumed by her spouse and, when appropriate, by their children. There is another reason why the father assumes additional responsibility within the household. He realizes that with the woman's increased dependency and passivity caused by the pregnancy there is a need for him to provide more nurturing. Ideally, he becomes more accommodating and tender, ministering to her needs and those of the children — a task which is usually that of the mother.

For the working mother pregnancy necessitates that she at least temporarily withdraw from the labor market and, as a result, be financially dependent upon her spouse. Usually she sees her job as being important to her, and often, if she quits too early, she becomes bored and feels apart from the mainstream of life. When she is not working the father becomes the main supporter of the family — a role which he takes pride in. Yet he realizes that with this role comes added responsibility for him.

The nurse can help families to learn what is safe for the mother to do at various stages in her pregnancy. This may involve setting specific limitations for the mother (no more scrubbing while on her knees) and instructions for the father (relieve her of strenuous tasks such as lifting). It may also include discussions about which activities should be continued (exercise in moderation, social and job functions that are not overly taxing) and assistance in making realistic alterations when necessary. Children in the family should be encouraged to assume responsibility within their capability; this will not only lighten the mother's workload but will promote their self-esteem. The nurse should encourage open discussion of the family's concerns about the physical maintenance of the household.

Adapting Sexual Relations to the Pregnant State

It is important that nurses realize that all cultures do not have the same views about sexual activity during pregnancy. At one end of the spectrum are those societies that prohibit sexual relations and enforce this by having the couple sleep in separate rooms or houses.[2] At the other end are those that encourage sexual activity because they believe it lubricates the birth canal[1] and provides strength to the fetus.[2]

But more typically the pregnant couple experiences comparatively minor alterations in their sexual feelings and activities. The father undoubtedly has feelings about his mate's changing physical appearance. At some stages of the pregnancy it might seem attractive; at others, unappealing. The nurse can help him to understand why his mate may experience nausea, increased frequency of urination and a decreased interest in sexual activity in the early stage of pregnancy. Knowledge that these factors will change by three to four months of pregnancy, when the mother's emotional outlook and physical comfort will usually improve considerably, often helps him cope more easily. During the third through seventh months of the pregnancy their sexual activity may be the most satisfying it has ever been. The constraint of fear of pregnancy has gone, and the increased vaginal lubrication caused by the pregnancy may result in pleasurable stimuli. Modification in coital positions will undoubtedly be necessary due to the enlarging abdomen and tender breasts, but as long as there is no bleeding, pain or rupture of membranes, usually coitus can be continued throughout the pregnancy without danger to the baby or mother.[5] The nurse should encourage open verbal expression between the couple because this will help them to accept their changing feelings about and physical approaches to sexual relations during pregnancy.

Adapting Relationships With Relatives and Friends to Realities of Pregnancy

Although parents of the couple may jovially talk about the pleasures of grandparenthood when they learn of pregnancy in their offspring, mixed feelings do exist in both the pregnant couple and their parents. One's daughter or son has obviously reached reproductive maturity once pregnancy has occurred. Although this is often a reason for joy, it carries with it numerous responsibilities for the younger couple, such as instilling values and norms, fostering self-esteem, providing adult role models.

Sharing the news with the prospective grandparents is obviously most difficult with the first pregnancy, as this is the time of most change in the couple's life style. The couple carefully considers the timing and wording of this news because they sense the need for acceptance. Regardless of what the couple's relationship has been with their parents before, there is now a heightened awareness of the parental role model that was portrayed throughout their lifetime, and the value of experience. One's appreciation of his own parents is invariably increased during pregnancy.

The response of the grandparents to the pregnancy varies. Some will enthusiastically share their time, material items and emotional support with the pregnant couple. This is especially helpful to the couple who already has young children. Some grandparents become overly indulgent — pushing their opinions and services on their children. Other grandparents view their child's pregnancy as a sign of their aging, an increased financial burden or a poorly managed act of sex. "Let the young people handle their problems on their own" seems to be their attitude.

It is important that pregnant couples receive positive support from their parents, other relatives and friends. There is an increased need for approval and the helpful advice that these significant others can provide. If a couple does not already have friends that have or are interested in children, this is the time that such friendships are usually established. There is a need to be able to discuss the feelings and physical changes that occur during pregnancy with people who have significant meaning to them and who understand the changes that pregnancy brings about.

Maintaining Each Other's Morale

Pregnancy imposes a testing of a family's ability to adapt psychologically to change. There is a potential for general family disequilibrium if efforts are not made to maintain each family member's morale.

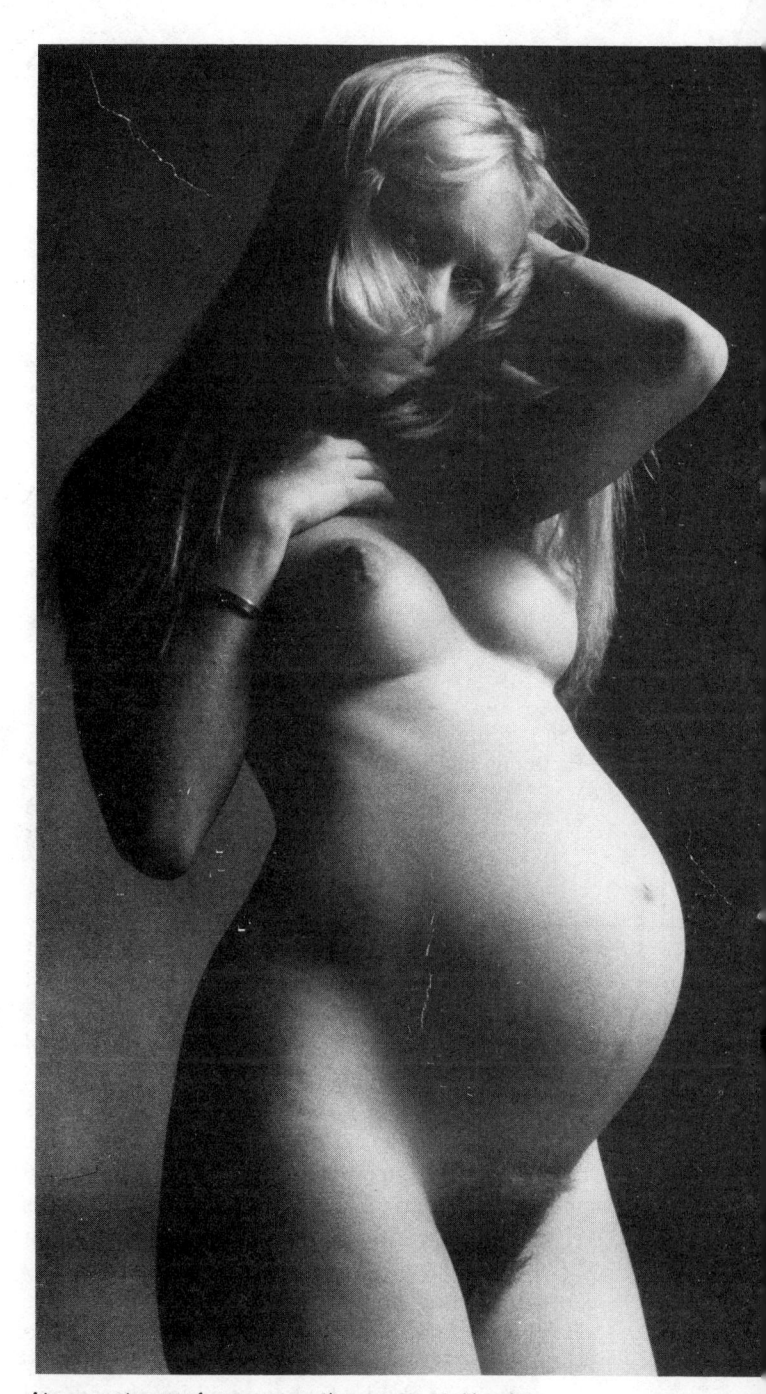

At some stages of pregnancy, the woman and her husband find her appearance attractive; at other times, unattractive. However, the pregnant woman continues to be a sexual being and needs to be accepted as such. (Photograph by Tony Kent.)

Both expectant mother and father commonly experience ambivalent feelings during the early pregnancy period. A woman's feelings are influenced by the alterations in her hormonal status. Moodiness or periods of happiness sud-

NEEDS OF CHILDBEARING FAMILY

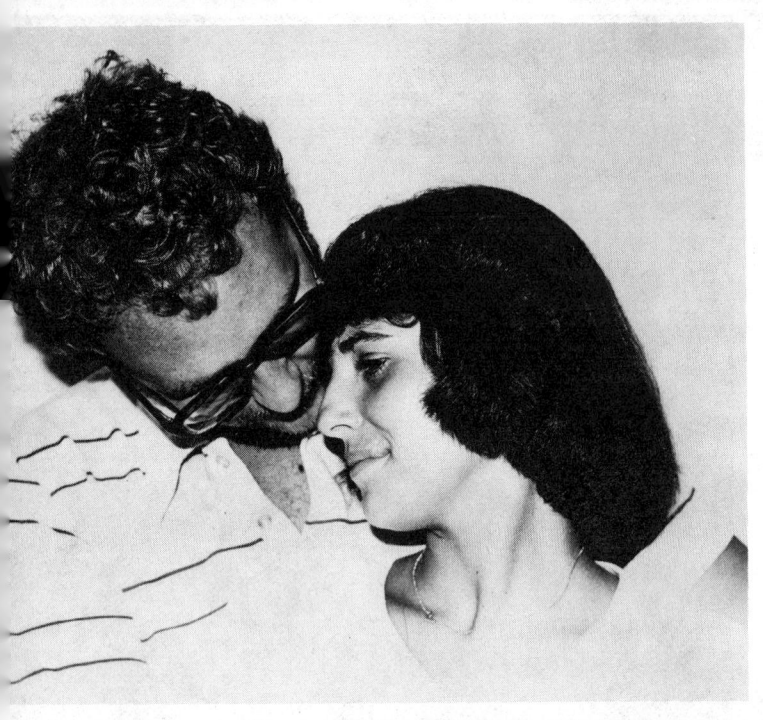

During the "binding into pregnancy" phase, the pregnant woman focuses her thoughts on herself. Her mate needs to understand this inward focus and the moodiness of this phase and quietly sustain her through it.

denly followed by depression may unexplainably occur. Factors such as an unwanted pregnancy, or the death or illness of another child may exaggerate the mother's negative feelings and actually interfere with the development of her mothering traits.

It is important that her mate as well as significant others understand the phases she is going through while pregnant. During the "binding into pregnancy" phase, she focuses her thoughts on herself. She realizes that when the baby comes she will not have time for many of the things that she is currently doing. If she already has children, she will once again have to face the confinement of having a totally dependent child. Her body will be altered and her energy will need to be reallocated. She realizes that there are both advantages and disadvantages to the pregnancy.

As she learns to accept the pregnancy and begins to feel better, she begins to incorporate the unborn baby into her thoughts and actions. This occurs around the fourth month of pregnancy and is referred to as "binding into the baby." She notices a necessity for maternity clothes. She begins to look for movement by the baby. Especially if this is her first pregnancy, she begins to think about what mothering will be like and begins to mimic the actions of other mothers — she drinks more milk, eats more liver, takes naps. She becomes increasingly receptive to information her mother and friends with children have to offer. She is also becoming protective of the unborn baby; only those things that would not harm "him" should be done.

Pregnant women become very attached to their pregnancies but need to accept that what is growing inside them is an individual who will have his or her own personality and appearance. Through fantasy women picture what their child will be like. Much thought is given to how the child will be raised; many ideals are established.

The final phase of development for a pregnant woman is to prepare for the unborn baby's separation from her. This "binding out of pregnancy" becomes increasingly acceptable to her as she experiences urinary frequency, shortness of breath, insomnia, and clumsiness. She begins to dislike her large appearance and has trapped-in feelings. These discomforts occur between the seventh and ninth months of pregnancy and cause her to await the onset of labor, although few pregnant women actually look forward to going through labor and delivery to have the baby.

The expectant father may also have alternating feelings about the pregnancy. He is undoubtedly pleased that his virile act has demonstrated his ability to procreate. Yet he probably has some doubts about his ability to fill his newly acquired role. The expectant father has a unique relationship with the unborn baby. He imagines what it will be like to have this child in his life. At times he may consciously or unconsciously prefer to be independent and carefree again. Yet, as he gets involved in the naming game, he considers the merits of continuing his own name and following family traditions; he imagines the personality of the child. What the baby will look like and what kind of a father he will be are things the expectant father often thinks about. Usually he does not share these ideas unless he is encouraged to do so.

Expectant fathers frequently sympathize or identify with their pregnant mates. They may exhibit psychosomatic symptoms such as nausea, vomiting, backache or headaches. In Liebenberg's study[4] 65 per cent of first-time expectant fathers experienced such symptoms. They

> **NURSING ACTIONS: FACILITATING ADJUSTMENT TO PREGNANCY**
>
> Redistribution of labor
>   Help family realize what is safe for mother to do at various stages of pregnancy
>   Discuss which activities should be continued and which alternatives could be adopted
>   Encourage father and children to assume responsibility within their capabilities
>   Encourage family members to discuss their concerns about their household tasks
> Adapting sexual relations to the pregnant state
>   Accept cultural variances
>   Help father to understand the physical and emotional changes that occur in the pregnant woman
>   Encourage sexual relations utilizing necessary modifications and inform the couple of contraindications.
>   Encourage communication of changing feelings about sexuality
> Adapting relationships with relatives and friends
>   Realize the need for a tactful sharing of the news of the pregnancy
>   Help the couple to understand their parents' response to the pregnancy
>   Encourage the couple to seek support (emotional and other) from significant others who are familiar with children
> Maintaining each other's morale
>   Accept ambivalent feelings in early pregnancy
>   Prepare family members for changing emotional phases of pregnant women
>   Realize that fathers have fantasies about the unborn child
>   Anticipate psychosomatic symptoms in fathers, especially the first-time father
>   Encourage a sharing of feelings among family members
>   Provide appropriate counselling when signs of maladjustment are noted

may also develop an intolerance for certain foods and gain weight, especially in the abdomen. These symptoms may occur without his mate even having them, and they may recur in succeeding pregnancies. These responses appear to be nature's way of bringing a pregnant couple closer together, helping especially the father to be more receptive of the woman's need for support during pregnancy.

In order for a couple to successfully adjust to pregnancy, they need to maintain high morale in each other. A secure marriage with harmonious goals and values is an immeasurable asset. A relationship in which there is a sharing of concerns, of happiness and sadness and of workloads helps them to make this adjustment. A positive relationship with their children and their parents further enhances the situation.

During the pregnancy it is possible for the nurse to identify signs of potentially poor parenting ability. Those parents who must have a child of a specific sex, who strongly reject certain physical characteristics and who indicate uneasiness about their ability to discipline a child need professional counselling.

PREPARING FOR THE PARENT ROLE

To prepare for the new baby, numerous tasks must be undertaken by the expectant family. The budgeting of finances and the use of household facilities must undergo change. Communication modes must be expanded and knowledge deficits regarding childbearing and childrearing erased by timely input from a variety of sources. The children already in the family need to be helped to adjust to their new roles, and consideration should be given to future family planning. The needs of the family as a whole, as well as those of each individual, need to be considered.

Reallocation of Resources

In previous generations the father assumed the role of primary financial provider, spending most of his time outside the home. Today which person works outside the home and how much varies from couple to couple. Many couples purposely delay pregnancy until a time that seems most advantageous to their life situation.

With the occurrence of pregnancy, many alterations in the family budget become necessary. Additional money must be available for medical expenses and baby supplies. Child care fees for existing children may increase. A move to another house may be desirable in order to provide adequate space and a more suitable neighborhood. Adjustments need to be made for at least a temporary curtailment in the mother's contribution to the monetary income. Expenditures for parental entertainment outside of the home may need to be decreased.

Although a pregnant woman may continue to work as long as she is physically able, a major concern of the expectant father centers on his ability to provide for his developing family. His financial well-being influences his feelings of self-esteem. In an effort to assume the added responsibility of expectant fatherhood with greater ease, he may assume a second job, put in more overtime on his primary job or take action to improve his job security by being more conscientious (punctual, thorough) or by obtaining additional education. His financial concerns extend into the future also; he may take out his first life insurance policy or get extra insurance coverage — a tendency anticipated by insurance salespeople!

Most couples are able to rearrange their budget on their own but nurses should be instrumental in providing realistic information about the mother's ability to work outside the home and in referring the family to a source of financial aid if necessary.

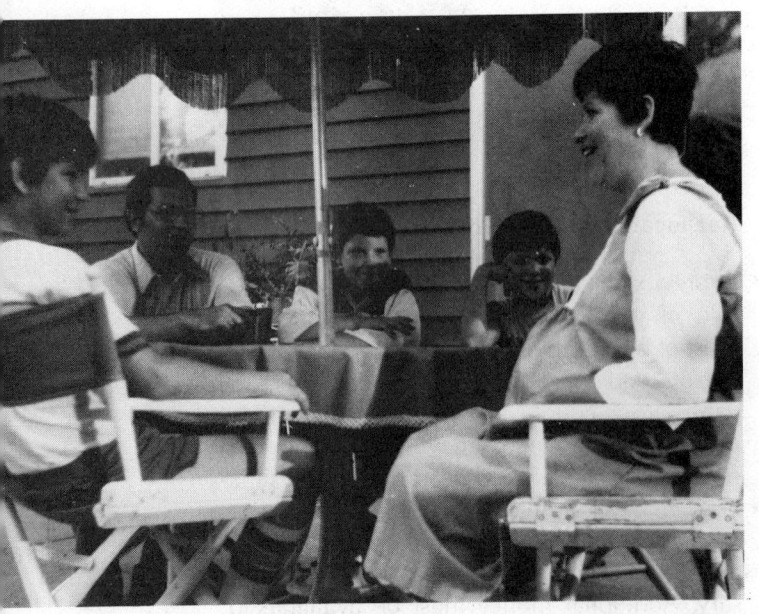

Open communication within the household is important — the pregnancy adds new dimensions and a new topic — the baby. (Photograph by Mike Malinowski.)

Arrangements for Physical Care of Baby

A new budgetary item is the physical preparation for the baby. Baby showers are commonly given for the first baby. They most often provide the extras, but essentials such as diapers, shirts and receiving blankets are often omitted. The future children usually manage to get along adequately with many hand-me-downs.

A frequent area of disagreement among pregnant couples is the amount of money that should be spent for the baby's things. The mother usually envisions more elaborate and expensive preparation than the father deems necessary. Nurses who provide guidelines about essential supplies for a newborn are helpful. The couple can then obtain the extras as their resources permit.

Nurses should be aware that there are instances when preparation for the baby is postponed until after the baby is born. In those of the Orthodox Jewish faith this is the case. For the couple who has experienced repeated failure to deliver a live or healthy child this is also likely true.

Expansion of Communication Patterns

Pregnancy adds many dimensions to communication within the family. There is a new topic to talk about — a baby. A need occurs for increased sensitivity to the needs of others — the pregnant woman whose personality is fluctuating, the father who may feel the stress of added responsibility, the children who will experience some alteration in their positions in the family constellation. There is also another significant person involved, the obstetrician. The high regard the pregnant woman has for this authority figure might make the father feel uneasy.

Open communication within the household is important. Family members should feel free to share their concerns and ideas. It is common for a father to accompany his mate to prenatal office visits and classes. Some health facilities also provide special sessions for the children.[7]

Acquisition of Knowledge

The primary source of information regarding the pregnancy should be the health care team — the nurse, the physician and others. At the time of her first prenatal visit and throughout pregnancy, a woman should be encouraged to discuss the discomforts she is experiencing, as they often can be alleviated or at least explained. Many of them (e.g., morning sickness, urinary frequency) are temporary. Often what appear to be major problems can be resolved with a little help from her mate and significant others. Throughout the pregnancy, the nurse should anticipate the concerns of the mother and her family. Questions should be answered and guidance appropriate to the phase of pregnancy should be given. In order to prepare for labor and delivery, most women eagerly accept childbirth preparation classes, literature, hospital tours and conversation with anyone who seems knowledgeable about what she and her baby are about to go through.

Most women vicariously try out the mother role during their pregnancy. If they already have children in the family, they may want to expose the children to the realities of having a baby in the household. The pregnant mother may get involved in changing diapers and giving baths to other young children. The family may even take in young children as weekend guests. It is likely that father will be included in this role-playing, since he too has some learning (or re-learning) to do.

Fathers, too, need to be prepared for the approaching labor and delivery. In some primitive societies, it is common for an expectant father to go through a ritual of moaning and groaning, as if having labor pains, near the time the baby is due. This practice of couvade (ko͞o väd′) is an acceptable way for him to be actively involved in the birth process and to gain recognition for his role in reproduction. In our society, many expectant fathers attend prenatal classes with their mates during the last two to three months of pregnancy. Many of these classes emphasize the father's presence during the birth process and include ways the father can be supportive during labor and delivery. But these classes are valuable in other ways. They provide factual information that helps to decrease the father's anxiety. If he understands the labor process, he experiences less apprehension. He also benefits from sharing his feelings with other expectant fathers in the class. He finds that he is not the only one who is very concerned about getting his mate to the right place in the hospital in time, but not too early!

Although many health personnel are enthusiastic about including fathers in every aspect of pregnancy, a word of caution must be given. Some men prefer to stay out of the sequence of events during pregnancy. Their cultural orienta-

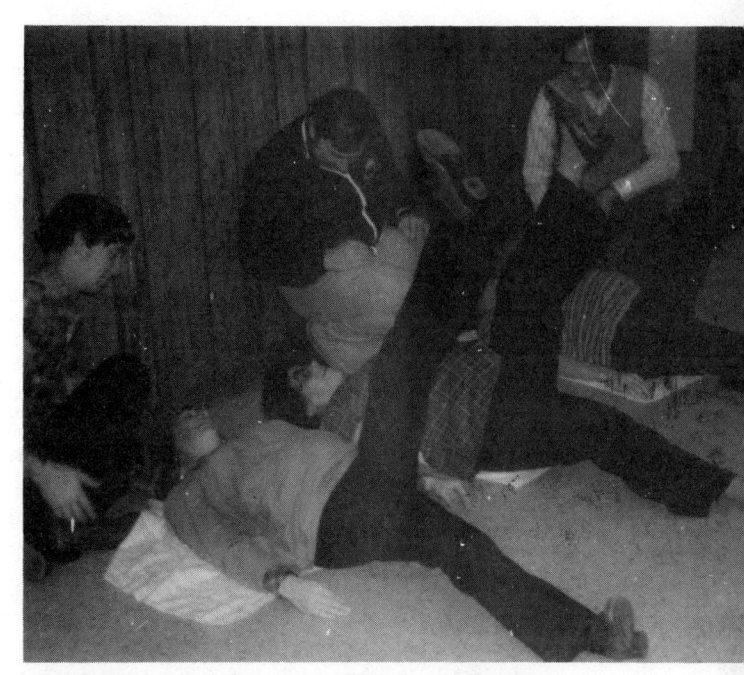

Expectant parents' classes help both spouses ready themselves for labor and delivery and gives them the opportunity to share their concerns with other couples.

tion may be that childbearing is the woman's concern. These fathers are sometimes pushed into a situation that they do not want to be in. This is not beneficial to the development of the family unit and may even be harmful. It is important that the individual needs of the expectant father be recognized. He should not be required to meet everybody else's expectations!

Even in a comparatively static period of history, parenting practices change from generation to generation. Not all couples have the advantage of nearby relatives, especially parents, who might serve as a significant support system. Instead there are numerous "parenting experts" available to the public. Unfortunately, many times their viewpoints conflict, and this creates confusion rather than clarity for prospective parents. The nurse can help the couple to recognize that no one practice is right and that they can select methods with which they can be comfortable and that they find appropriate for each unique child.

When the Child Is Adopted

A family who adopts a child prepares for the parent role by making adjustments similar to those of the childbearing couple. The timing of these adjustments, however, is considerably different and varies markedly with each family situation. Usually there is a lengthy period of waiting after the initial decision to adopt has been made. During this period the family prepares for adoption by talking and thinking about how it would be to have a child. Because there is an uncertainty about ever receiving a child for adoption, thoughts about becoming parents are merely vague fantasies. The tendency is to avoid any premature actual preparations for a child in the home.

While living under the conflict of wanting a child but not allowing themselves to become consumed by anticipatory thoughts, an adoptive family often receives an abrupt telephone call about a child for possible adoption. This results in a surge of emotions that leaves the family feeling excited, elated but also overwhelmed. At a time when family members are enthralled with the excitement of receiving a child, they must also use their rational powers to process information about the child and the child's family. When an older child is adopted, the child's physical, intellectual and emotional-social competencies become a concern to prospective parents. Whereas a childbearing family is concerned about having a healthy baby, an adoptive family may be concerned about the genetic and early environmental factors that have influenced and will continue to affect the child's growth and development. The adoptive family may experience some ambivalence about accepting a child because of factors in the child's history and general health status. The family, however, does have the option not to accept the child for adoption, whereas the childbearing family does not have that choice. This is an important difference between the adjustment of childbearing and adoptive families. The fact that the adoptive family *has* a choice increases the stress at the time of adoption, and the decision must be made at a time when its members' emotional states are labile.

The time between the initial phone call and the placement of the child is often a week or less. Important plans may need to be altered to make immediate preparations for the child. Regardless of the child's age, generally some physical preparation or rearranging within the home is required. There is an element of panic as the family plans to get the necessary furniture, equipment and clothing. Within a matter of a week there is a tremendous drain on money, time and emotional energy.

The adjustment to becoming parents when a child is adopted is complicated by the additional stresses as described during the preparatory phase of adoption. Adoptive families have the ongoing stresses unique to adoption. (See Chapter 4 for further discussion of adoptive families.)

PLANNING FOR FUTURE CHILDREN

Many couples set goals early in their relationship regarding the number and spacing of children, and the ages at which they wish to complete their family. However, events can occur that cause alteration of these goals.

Most people have unrealistic ideas about what parenthood will be like. Until becoming parents, they do not realize how much time, energy and money is required by one child alone. The fact that a 24-hour-per-day commitment for 18 or more years is begun again with each child makes a couple with a child seriously consider if, and when, they wish to have another.

Parenthood also involves responsibility for rearing an individual who has his own personality and physical characteristics. Some children are harder to raise than others. Some have major health problems. There is no guarantee that a future child will be similar to one born already, or will be easier to raise.

Although there always seems to be enough love in a family for another wanted child, as the number of children increases, so does the need to share resources. Some families find that this can easily be done; others find it stressful.

Usually children born three years apart are considered to be ideally spaced.[3] Yet some families prefer closer spacing, assuming greater companionship among the children or advantages to getting through the childbearing cycle more rapidly or both. Others prefer longer spacing so they can enjoy the early developmental years of each child and get them through college one at a time.

Among the 88 per cent of young married couples who use some form of contraception, only 20 per cent have only planned pregnancies at planned intervals.[2] The reasons given for this low percentage include lack of available birth control clinics, physicians' attitudes, uncon-

> **NURSING ACTIONS: FACILITATING ADJUSTMENT TO THE PARENT ROLE**
>
> Reallocation of resources
>   Provide information to the family about the mother's ability to work outside the home
>   Refer the family to a source of financial aid if necessary
> Arrangements for physical care of baby
>   Be aware that mothers tend to want more elaborate and expensive items for the baby than do fathers
>   Be prepared to provide guidelines for *essential* baby supplies
>   Accept that some families prefer to postpone preparation for the baby until after its birth
> Expansion of communication patterns
>   Encourage increased sensitivity to the needs of each family member
>   Provide for situations in which family members can share their feelings and ideas
> Acquisition of knowledge
>   Allow for the asking of questions and provide guidance on problems that may occur during pregnancy
>   Provide for participation in childbirth education classes, hospital tour
>   Encourage families to gain vicarious experiences with young children
>   Recognize the individual father's wishes regarding involvement in the pregnancy cycle
> Planning for future children
>   Provide families with information so they can make realistic family planning decisions
>   Encourage family members to share their viewpoints with each other

scious motivations, method failure, patient failure, cultural bias and religious dogma.[2]

Following delivery, ovulation may occur as early as day 36 in the bottle-feeding mother and on day 39 in the breast-feeding mother.[2] It is important that nurses warn couples that, without contraceptive precautions, a woman might be discovered to be pregnant at the time of her six-week postpartal examination. Abstinence from sexual activity is the most reliable method but, more realistically, a condom with spermicidal foam or cream is usually recommended for this interval. Common misconceptions are that breast feeding provides protection against conception and that the old diaphragm can be effectively used again following the pregnancy.

Although couples usually think about which contraceptive method they might use following a pregnancy, final decisions are usually made several days following birth or even later. The birth experience and the status of the newborn can be influential in determining when or if another child is desired.

An example of a situation that might alter plans for future pregnancies is the birth of a child with a genetic defect. All parents of such a child need help to recognize and accept their feelings about the implications of the condition. (See Chapter 25 for a discussion of how nurses can help families in their adjustment to this difficult situation.) The couple will need to consult a reliable authority on genetic counselling. Rarely is this one person; it usually is a team consisting of geneticists, pediatricians, the family physician, nurses and community service representatives. The nurse or physician may have the important role of recognizing the need for referral for the genetic counselling that can provide a correct diagnosis of the causes of the condition. Accuracy is imperative. The nurse can help family members prepare for the first visit to the geneticist by emphasizing the need for them to provide an extensive family history. It is beneficial for the nurse to be present during the counselling session. She is then better prepared later to reiterate, explain and elaborate on the information given. Interpreting the geneticist's findings and helping the family to develop a logical plan of action is the role of the whole team. Its members must be consistent in the information they provide in order not to confuse the couple. Depending on the prognosis, the couple may wish to bear other children or to utilize a very effective form of contraception (maybe even permanent sterilization).

PREPARATION OF SIBLINGS

Children already in the family have adjustments to make during pregnancy. The mother's physical and emotional status will likely alter the roles of the children. The children may be expected to assume added responsibility for some

> **NURSING ACTIONS: PREPARATION OF SIBLINGS FOR THE EXPECTED BABY**
>
> Role changes
>   Discuss ways that children's roles will be altered
>   Encourage normal responses from the children
> Feelings of jealousy
>   Discuss normal feelings of displacement
>   Encourage discussion of children's feelings
>   Suggest specific children's books that deal with the subject
> Children's curiosity about human sexuality
>   Encourage expression of the parents' feelings about discussing sex with their children
>   Help parents provide correct information at the appropriate level of development
>   Provide references if necessary
>
> Preparation for the mother's absence from home
>   Encourage parents to inform children of the planned sequence of events
>   Encourage keeping of the children in a familiar place by a caretaker who knows them and will maintain their routines
>   Discuss ways the mother can keep in touch with the children
> Expectations of what baby will be like
>   Encourage the parents to discuss with, and preferably show, the children what very young infants are like
>   Assist the children to understand what is appropriate behavior with a baby
>   Help the parents to anticipate the children's needs to express their hostile feelings

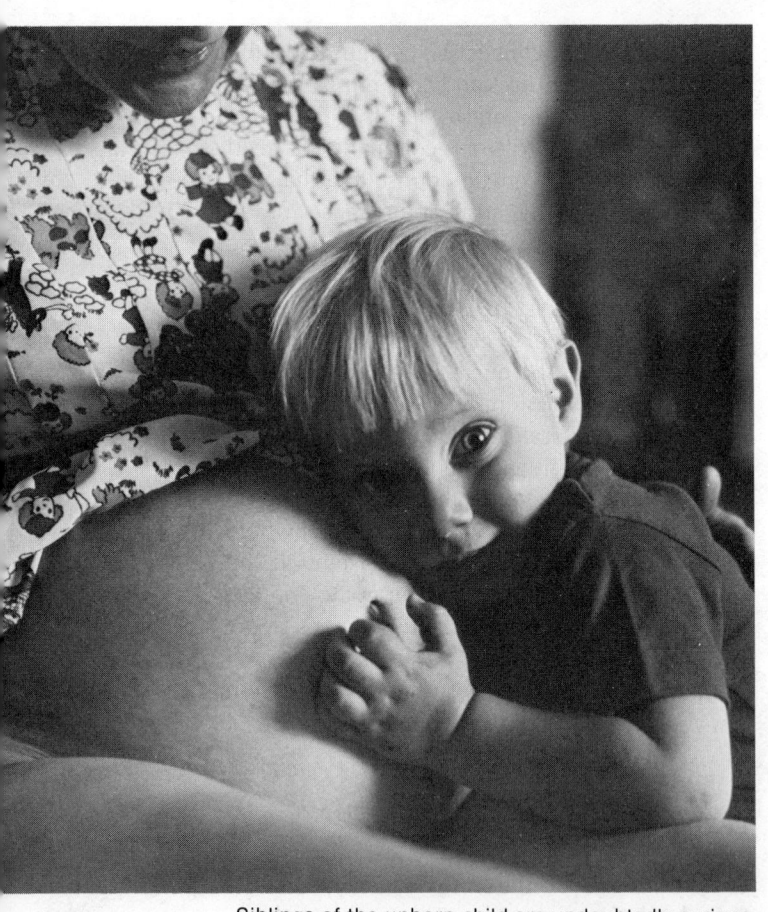

Siblings of the unborn child are undoubtedly curious. Their questions should be answered in as simple and natural a way as possible. (From A. Clark and D. Affonso; Childbearing—A Nursing Perspective, 2nd ed. F. A. Davis Co., 1979, p. 112.)

household chores and to adjust to the mother's mood changes. They will wonder what effect the baby will have on their relationship with their parents. Will the baby take their place? Is the baby coming because they are not good enough or not loved? There will probably be feelings of jealousy for this baby even before it is born.

The children are undoubtedly curious, at least to some extent, if they are 2½ years old or older, about what babies are like, how babies grow, how they get started, how they are born. When providing such information, the approach to use depends on their level of development. The nurse should advise the parents that these questions be answered with accurate information and correct terminology, and in the depth necessary to satisfy the child. Parents should use a natural tone of voice, considering what the child is asking as well as why it is being asked. Numerous children's books can be used to supplement the parents' verbal explanation. Although the child may be temporarily satisfied with the information provided, the parents should anticipate that the same questions may be asked many times.

The children also have a right to be prepared for the absence of the mother at the time of the baby's birth. Plans should be made ahead of time for their care, preferably by people familiar to the children and in their own home. Efforts should be made to continue with the children's usual routine. How long their mother will be gone and the possibility of telephone calls or hospital visits or both should be discussed.

The children's adjustment to the baby can be enhanced by familiarizing them with realistic explanations of what babies are like: they cry, wet diapers, feed by breast or bottle, depend on others for all their care. If the children are helped to realize that they were once babies themselves and that they have developed beyond that stage, they will probably see that there are many advantages to being a big sister or brother.

References

1. A. Clark, ed. Culture, Childbearing, Health Professionals. F. A. Davis Co., 1978
2. A. Clark and D. Affonso. Childbearing — A Nursing Perspective. F. A. Davis Co., 1979
3. E. Duvall. Marriage and Family Development. J. B. Lippincott Co., 1977
4. B. Liebenberg. Expectant fathers. Child and Family, Summer 1969, p. 264
5. J. Malinowski. Sex during pregnancy: what can you say? RN Magazine, November 1978, p. 48
6. R. Rubin. Cognitive style of pregnancy. American Journal of Nursing, March 1970, p. 502
7. P. Sweet. Prenatal classes especially for children. American Journal of Maternal Child Nursing. Mar/Apr 1979, p. 82
8. J. Wapner. The attitudes, feelings, and behaviors of expectant fathers attending Lamaze classes. Birth and the Family Journal, Spring 1976, p. 5

Additional Recommended Reading

J. Aldous. Family Careers: Developmental Change in Families. John Wiley & Sons, 1978

M. Barnard, B. Clancy and K. Krantz. Human Sexuality for Health Professionals. W. B. Saunders Co., 1978

J. Clausen, M. Flook and B. Ford. Maternity Nursing Today. McGraw-Hill Book Co., 1977

L. McNall and J. Galeener. Current Practice in Obstetric and Gynecologic Nursing, Vol. 2. C. V. Mosby Co., 1978

M. Moore. Realities in Childbearing. W. B. Saunders Co., 1978

C. Phillips and J. Anzalone. Fathering: Participation in Labor and Birth. C.V. Mosby Co., 1978

R. Rubin. Maternal tasks in pregnancy. Maternal and Child Nursing Journal, Mar/Apr 1975, p. 143

J. Stichler, M. Bowden and E. Reimer. Pregnancy: a shared emotional experience. American Journal of Maternal Child Nursing, May/June 1978, p. 153

7 POTENTIAL FAMILY STRESSES DURING PREGNANCY

by Janet S. Malinowski, RN, MSN

The pregnant family invariably undergoes stress when the pregnancy is unplanned, physically difficult for the mother, or terminated voluntarily, spontaneously, or for medical indications. Before or at the time of birth, the baby also may undergo stress from certain factors (some known, some unknown) in his environment. This chapter deals with some of the major causes of stress in pregnancy and the impact stress may have on the family. It is believed that a strong family unit will usually be able to cope with, and at times avoid, unexpected stressful events if the stated nursing interventions are adhered to. More complex intervention may be warranted when sufficient support systems do not exist. This is likely to be the case in the single parent family — a topic addressed in a later chapter.

UNPLANNED PREGNANCY

Despite wide dissemination of birth control information and devices, pregnancy continues to occur at unplanned times and intervals. Although intrauterine devices and spermicidal foams or creams used with a diaphragm or condom have high protection rates, their use is not a guarantee against pregnancy. Theoretically, "the Pill" is nearly 100 per cent effective, but the human factor (involving reliability in taking as prescribed) decreases its effectiveness. Miscalculation, inaccurate information, acts of impulse and conscious or unconscious motivation for pregnancy of one sex partner affect the incidence of unplanned pregnancies.

An unplanned pregnancy lacks the advantage of preparation — the development of a plan that considers anticipated advantages and disadvantages. Whereas planning often unites a family in a common endeavor, an unplanned event has the increased potential for generating stress.

The terms unplanned pregnancy and unwanted pregnancy are not synonymous. Some pregnancies are truly unwanted; however, initial ambivalent feelings toward an unplanned pregnancy are common and normal. The pregnant woman is likely to be upset and visibly moody in the early phase of this pregnancy. Family members may find her difficult to get along with because of unpredictable behavior. Members of the family who realize what effect this pregnancy has on the mother (and possibly the father) often can help other family members to accept, and adjust to, the family's temporarily unstable emotional climate. The pregnancy may interfere with the social, educational and recreational (athletic) calendars of events, especially of the mother, but possibly of each family member. Some rearrangements will undoubtedly need to be made.

A nurse may be of assistance to the family by discussing what effects this pregnancy is likely to have on each involved family member. Assuming the pregnancy will be continued, each member's role in the family will undergo some changes. The youngest child will no longer be the baby. In order for him to better understand what is occurring, he (and his siblings) may be encouraged to accompany their mother on her prenatal visits and be included in certain portions of the examination (e.g., listening to the baby's heart rate, discussing the hospitalization for the birth). Each sibling should be prepared to take on added responsibility, including that of sharing with one or more persons. The children should be helped to understand that their father's and mother's thoughts and actions will center on preparations to be made for the coming baby, and therefore they will have less time for them. By extending the family communication system, a workable plan of action can often be formulated. The major goal should be acceptance of the pregnancy and the resulting baby by the family as a whole.

Some families will elect to abort the conceptus of an unwanted pregnancy. Today this can legally be done. Most early abortions are done in a hospital outpatient department or during a short hospital stay. The procedures available for abortion are usually complication-free, although they are more hazardous than any acceptable contraceptive method! There are undoubtedly more psychological than physical sequelae to abortion.

It is important that the pregnant woman, preferably with her mate, be counseled by health personnel (frequently nurses) prior to the abortion. Not only should she understand what abortion is, but she should be sure that it is what she wants. It should not be a decision forced upon her. Her conscience and her values must be considered, since she must live with this decision for the rest of her life. Abortion is not the only solution; there are other alternatives, such as giving the child for adoption following birth. It is my opinion that this woman needs to be helped to reach the decision that is best for her, regardless of her family's opinions. If she decides to have the abortion, she will need help to carry it out. This may mean locating a place to go and a way to finance the abortion. It also means informing her of the procedure to be performed. Without adequate counselling, feelings of anger, guilt, fear and sadness are likely to result for the woman. These psychological sequelae may persist for many years if they are not properly managed around the time of abortion.

For the family with children, communication about the abortion may be difficult. It is likely that even the 2- to 3-year-old will sense that something unusual is occurring in the family. It is important that the child's feelings of security not be threatened. During the mother's visits to the health facility, the child should be with comforting caretakers. How much is said to the child about the abortion is dependent on his knowledge of the existing pregnancy, his comprehension level and the parents' preference and ability to share the information with him. Nurses should be prepared to discuss with such parents if and how they plan to share this information with their children.

DIFFICULT PREGNANCY

Even the accepted, uncomplicated pregnancy has certain physiological stresses. The possible nausea and vomiting of early pregnancy and the heartburn, backache, leg cramps and shortness of breath that come and go are discomforts that, unless understood and given proper attention, could be stressful to the pregnant woman as well as her family.

Normally, nausea and vomiting cease following the first three months of pregnancy, but some women continue to experience a gradual increase in their frequency and intensity. This condition is called *hyperemesis gravidarum,* or *pernicious vomiting of pregnancy.* This can lead to a drastic decrease in the mother's food intake, dehydration, acidosis and eventually fetal and maternal death. The cause of hyperemesis gravidarum is thought to be both physical and psychological. Effective management usually involves providing reassurance to the mother and increased rest, often facilitated by tranquilizers. If treatment at home is not successful, hospitalization is necessary so that intravenous fluids can be given and the restful (often lonely) atmosphere of a private room provided.

Another possible stressful occurrence during pregnancy is *threatened abortion.* Spotting or bleeding from the undilated cervix might cause the woman to fear for her own life but more realistically for that of the fetus. Management consists of strict confinement to bed, treatment with progesterone (a female hormone) and abstinence from coitus, although these measures have not been proved effective. The bleeding may stop and the remaining five or more months of the pregnancy progress with no further complications.

Such conditions as planned abortion, pernicious vomiting and threatened abortion cause a

> **NURSING ACTIONS: FACILITATING ADAPTATION TO AN UNPLANNED, DIFFICULT OR INTERRUPTED PREGNANCY**
>
> Recognize that each family member undergoes some degree of stress.
>
> Consider the strengths of each individual in the family unit.
>
> Encourage open communication within the family unit and with potentially helpful others (i.e., its own support system, professionals).
>
> Provide factual information as necessary, promoting a realistic outlook on the situation.
>
> Provide needed emotional support.
>
> Allow the family to make their own decisions if the situation permits.

temporary alteration in the family life style. The woman is no longer able to fulfill her usual role, and therefore other family members, and maybe people outside the family, are involved in meeting the family's daily needs. The perceptive pediatric nurse may not be told directly about these family occurrences but might recognize clues as she interviews or cares for a sad, lonely child or a frustrated parent. Leading statements such as: "You seem on edge today. I'd be interested in knowing if there is some way I might help you," might result in a sharing of feelings, the involvement of a helping professional (e.g., a public health nurse) or the suggestion of ways to handle the situation effectively.

INTERRUPTED PREGNANCY

Interrupting a pregnancy by electing to have an abortion is a voluntary decision. There are also conditions that bring about involuntary termination of a pregnancy.

What started out as a threatened abortion many times ends in *spontaneous abortion*, or miscarriage (a lay term). At least one in every five to seven conceptions aborts with no apparent external stimulus. Although the cause of spontaneous abortion is usually unknown, a fact that often helps families accept the loss of the pregnancy is that more than 50 per cent of the aborted fetuses are found to be abnormal. (There is a high incidence of chromosomal abnormalities in these fetuses.) Other potential causative factors are acute maternal infection, umbilical cord abnormalities, incompetent cervix (a condition that can be surgically treated) and inadequate progesterone levels to support implantation and development.

Once any part of the conceptual product has been expelled or excessive bleeding has occurred, the uterus must be evacuated. At times this is completed spontaneously; if incomplete, a dilatation and curettage (D and C) is done in the first three months of pregnancy and manual removal with instrumental evacuation is done following the sixteenth week of pregnancy.

For the woman who has aborted for the first time, the likelihood that she will abort a second time is no greater than that for anyone else in the general population. But once a woman has aborted three consecutive times, she is considered to be a *habitual aborter*. This is emotionally stressful to a family who wants to have more children, and it warrants further evaluation.

Another condition classified as interruption to pregnancy involves conception and what is thought to be a pregnancy because of the symptoms it presents but in fact does not result in a fetus. The woman's uterus grows larger than would be expected for the period of time elapsing since her last menstruation but no fetal heart tones are present. Instead of developing into a fetus, the product of conception has developed into a cluster of cysts, which resembles bunches of grapes, called a *hydatidiform mole*. This must be evacuated from the uterus either spontaneously or medically. A fear that exists even after the mole's removal is that this condition may predispose to carcinoma.

Ectopic pregnancy is another condition classified as interruption to pregnancy. In this case the fertilized ovum has not been implanted in the normal place — the uterus — but in a fallopian tube (the most common extrauterine site), an ovary, the abdomen or the cervix. Around two to three months into the pregnancy, the woman experiences cramping on one side of the lower abdomen and sudden excruciating

> **NURSING ACTIONS: FACILITATING SIBLINGS' ADAPTATION TO THE EVENT OF STILLBIRTH**
>
> Assess the parents' ability to cope with the death.
>
> Consider the ages of the children, what they know about their mother's pregnancy and the birth, how they have reacted to them.
>
> Help the parents to provide appropriate information to their children.
>
> Prepare the parents for the children's expression of mourning and need for increased assurance of safety and love.
>
> Prepare the parents for the children's repeated questions.
>
> Assist the parents to see the value of a trusting relationship and open communication.

pelvic pain, dizziness or shock or all three. The placental site bleeds and when the blood reaches the level of the diaphragm, shoulder pain may occur. Family members who observe the mother in this extreme pain become frightened. Medical care is immediately sought and, because of the often vague early symptoms, the condition may be confused with appendicitis. Surgery is necessary to remove the impregnated site. This may have implications for future pregnancies since the one affected tube or ovary may be the only functioning one the woman has. As a result, this woman would be unable to conceive future children by natural means.

All of these conditions that represent interruptions to pregnancy — spontaneous abortion, hydatidiform mole removal and ectopic pregnancy removal — have an impact on all members in a family. In most instances the children are not fully aware of these interruptions, which take place in the early part of pregnancy, but they sense the emotional stress the parents are experiencing and are caught up in a household that is temporarily not functioning according to its routine. Nurses should discuss with the parents the impact of the interrupted pregnancy on the children. Some parents need little more than encouragement to share their feelings and basic factual information with their children. Other parents initially need help to cope with their own feelings and then help with presenting the situation in a way that their children can comprehend realistically and nontraumatically. In such situations the nurse may be directly involved in the family discussions. She might act as the facilitator, thereby decreasing the emotional impact of the event and presenting accurate information, using terminology that is appropriate for the children's level of understanding while enhancing their knowledge related to health.

STILLBIRTH

Another stressful outcome of pregnancy is fetal death, or *stillbirth* (baby born dead). Some mothers are cognizant of the death shortly after it occurs; others learn about it from the examining physician.

The parents of a dead fetus normally experience grief. Initially they are shocked and do not believe the death is possible. A supportive nurse shows she cares by merely being present. Little verbal communication may be necessary. The couple needs to know the planned sequence of management (e.g., induction of labor or wait for the onset of spontaneous labor). Until the actual birth, however, few parents will fully accept that their baby is dead. The reason for the death is likely to remain unknown.

At the time of birth, the parents need to be helped to move into the next phase of the grief process: gaining awareness of the loss. Not only should they be told immediately that the baby is stillborn, but, if they are willing, they should be allowed to see, touch and even hold their baby. I vividly recall sharing with his parents an infant who had died three days before birth as a result of three tight knots in his umbilical cord. I wrapped him neatly in a clean blanket, held him as I would a live infant and showed him to his parents. They already had been told that he looked perfectly normal and had been shown the knots. My actions were taken to decrease their formation of undesirable mental images of their baby.

After the parents have been told of their loss, they begin to move through restitution and acceptance, the final phases of grieving. Tears and periods of depression — expressions of anger and guilt — typically occur. They must also confront the need to share the sad news with the other children in the family. Some of the children may be satisfied to hear that there will not be a baby joining the family at this time, but more likely there will be the repeated question of "Why?" Both the parents and the children need to be frequently assured that the baby's death was not due to anything they did or thought and that the baby's death was not an act of punishment.

As the family is ready, the baby's things should be removed from his place in the house. Friends who mean to be helpful should be discouraged from doing this immediately for the family. The family should not be led to believe that anything can totally replace this baby they have lost, not even another pregnancy. Ideally, a nurse will be able to continue to interact with this family unless they have successfully worked through the grieving process. Depending upon how the situation is handled, the children can learn to accept death or to fear it. As the subject is discussed, the children need to feel secure in their parents' presence so that future communication with and confidence in their parents will continue. Their feelings of well-being need to be re-established.

TERATOGENIC AGENTS

History has dramatically shown that certain factors in the environment can cause birth defects and fetal deaths:
1. Radiation in the population exposed to atomic irradiation at Hiroshima caused defects in the fetal central nervous system.
2. Rubella epidemics in 1941 in Australia and 1964 in the United States caused multiple defects, both structural and functional.
3. The thalidomide tragedy in West Germany, England and Scandinavia in the early 1960s caused phocomelia (children born without limbs or with limbs in embryonic stage of development. Thalidomide is a tranquilizer and sedative that was used to relieve morning sickness common in early pregnancy. The drug was not sold in the United States because the Food and Drug Administration would not authorize its approval due to insufficient evidence of its safety for human consumption.)

Any factor that adversely affects the fertilized ovum, the embryo or the fetus, whether it be chemical or physical, is called a *teratogen*. There is no complete list of teratogenic agents. A few agents have been definitely identified as teratogens (e.g., thalidomide and certain antifolic acid compounds),[6] and others, such as lysergic acid diethylamide (LSD), are highly suspected.

Sometimes potentially harmful drugs or other agents are used or encountered without the woman's knowledge of their potentially harmful effect. The nurse can provide valuable information to the expectant mother. She can also be instrumental in referring the woman for diagnostic studies (e.g., amniotic fluid studies) if they are so indicated. It is not the nurse's function to instill fear in the pregnant woman and her family, but measures that can be taken to decrease harm to the fetus should be observed. A nurse should not be judgmental; she should avoid condemning an act already done. At the time of birth, the baby should be thoroughly examined and the parents should be told what the findings are. If special care is required by the baby, professional guidance should be given.

There are certain factors that determine the effect of teratogens. *Exposure to the teratogen early in pregnancy is usually more hazardous than later in pregnancy.* The most hazardous time is between implantation in the uterine wall and complete development of vital organs. The brain, heart, eyes and kidneys develop between two and eleven weeks of pregnancy. This is so early in pregnancy that, unfortunately, most women do not even know they are pregnant. Detrimental teratogenic effects are less likely to occur as the pregnancy progresses beyond the third month.

The amount or strength of the teratogen may influence the amount of damage. For example, there is some radiation in our everyday environment and it causes no damage.

Specific teratogens sometimes attack specific tissues. Thalidomide concentrates on the limbs. Rubella has less specificity, having affinity for several organs.

Some agents enhance the teratogenic effects of each other (e.g., foods containing tryamine, such as aged cheese, red wine and chicken liver, potentiate monoamine oxidase inhibitors). Others (e.g., juices high in acid that slow the speed of absorption into the bloodstream) may decrease the teratogenic effect.

Teratogens can be direct in their influence

TABLE 7–1   DRUGS THAT ARE HARMFUL TO THE HUMAN FETUS*

Drug	Consequence
Alcohol	Fetal changes associated with chronic alcoholism
Aminopterin Amethopterin	Gross deformity or death
Chloramphenicol	Used near term may result in gray-baby syndrome; i.e., sudden collapse and death
Cyclizine Diphenidol Thiethylperazine	Anticonvulsants whose use is not recommended in pregnancy
Ethacrynic acid	Fetal and neonatal jaundice; thrombocytopenia
LSD	Evidence for teratogenicity not conclusive but grounds for caution
Mineral oil	Regular use may lead to reduced absorption of fat-soluble vitamins A, D, E and K; reduced absorption of vitamin K may cause hypoprothrombinemia
Morphine	Addiction in utero; withdrawal symptoms following birth; severe respiratory depression
Nicotine	May affect fetal growth
Novobiocin	Near delivery associated with thrombocytopenia and hyperbilirubinemia
Potassium iodide Radioactive iodine Propylthiouracil	Congenital goiter, with possible respiratory distress from pressure of enlarged thyroid on trachea
Reserpine	Nasal discharge, respiratory distress, lethargy, anorexia in newborn
Salicylates	Neonatal bleeding in high doses; possible salicylate intoxication in high doses
Streptomycin Dihydrostreptomycin Chloroquine	May affect inner ear of fetus
Sulfonamides	Avoid during last trimester; possible hyperbilirubinemia, thrombocytopenia, kernicterus if given near term
Testosterone Synthetic progestins (e.g., ethisterone, norethisterone)	Masculinization of the female fetus
Tetracycline and derivatives	Inhibition of bone growth; discoloration of teeth
Thalidomide	Phocomelia (seal-like limbs), amelia (absence of limbs), and other deformities
Thiazides	Long-term use may lead to hyponatremia; diabetogenic effect on mother may have an effect on infant
Trimethadione (Tridione) Paramethadione (Paradione)	A variety of defects may occur, including facial defects, cardiac defects, cleft palate, and intrauterine growth retardation

*From Moore, M.: Realities in Childbearing. W. B. Saunders Co., 1978.

(e.g., German measles acts on the fetus) or indirect (e.g., in maternal thyroid deficiency the fetus receives an inadequate amount of iodine).

Drugs   Numerous drugs have been assumed to be teratogenic to the fetus. A partial list is given in Table 7–1. Because the effect of most drugs on the fetus has not been ascertained, the pregnant woman should take certain precautions. She, as well as any female physically capable of pregnancy, should take drugs only when and in the amount recommended by a health professional who is aware of her (potential) pregnancy. This is true of both prescription and nonprescription drugs. Furthermore, the advantages of taking any drug must outweigh the disadvantages. Even if a woman is not immune to rubella, she should not take the live virus while pregnant; the fetus would contract the disease. Assurance that she is not pregnant and that she is not likely to become pregnant during the next two months should be obtained before rubella vaccine is given to any female of childbearing age. It would be wise to postpone the taking of even iron, folic acid and vitamin supplements until fetal organogenesis has been completed.

The term drug should be interpreted in its broadest sense. It includes medicated nose drops, topical medications containing hormones that are absorbed through the skin, vaginal and rectal suppositories, alcohol and nicotine.

Table 7-1 includes alcohol and nicotine (cigarettes). Heavy indulgence in these "social drugs" is known to be detrimental to the fetus. Chronic alcoholic mothers have been found to give birth to offspring with "fetal alcohol syndrome," which is characterized by growth deficiency affecting the head, heart and joints, as well as by retarded postnatal development.[4, 8, 9] Recent studies[7, 9] indicate that even moderate drinking (more than two ounces of 100 proof whiskey a day) during early pregnancy may cause harm to the fetus. Cigarette smoking by a pregnant woman decreases the infant's head circumference (which is related to intellectual function), causes low birth weight and small infant size, and increases fetal and perinatal death rates.[3, 5, 12, 18] If the mother decreases the average number of cigarettes smoked regularly following the fourth month of pregnancy, the risk to the baby can be decreased.[2, 17] The effects of alcohol and cigarette smoking on the fetus are discussed further in Chapter 8.

Radiation Radiation in the form of x-rays may cause a number of malformations in the fetus. Therefore, except in emergencies, all females of childbearing age should have abdominal x-ray films taken only during the first 10 days of their menstrual cycle, since this is the time they are least likely to be pregnant. For those pregnant women who are exposed to x-rays regularly at work or who need to have their teeth or limbs x-rayed, a lead apron should be used to shield the pelvis. Pelvic x-rays should not be done except at term and then only for diagnostic purposes.

Infections During the first three months of pregnancy, certain maternal infections are known to cause abortion and fetal abnormalities. The most common infections are termed the TORCHS*:

T = Toxoplasmosis
O = Others (measles, mumps, chickenpox, infectious hepatitis)
R = Rubella (German measles)
C = Cytomegalovirus (CMV)
H = Herpes simplex
S = Syphilis

Toxoplasmosis is discussed in detail in Chapter 27. It is a parasitic disease acquired from two primary sources: (1) the handling or ingestion of raw or undercooked fresh meat that contains a specific cyst and (2) direct contact with the feces of an "infected" common house cat (in cat litter box or vegetable garden). The disease causes swollen lymph nodes behind the ears. Once infected, a woman has a lasting immunity, which means that her future offspring will not be affected by it. But if she is infected while pregnant, the fetal effects are eventual blindness and deterioration of the brain.

Simple preventive measures include (1) proper cooking of meat and cleaning of raw vegetables, (2) handwashing following handling of raw meats and vegetables coupled with avoidance of contact with mucous membranes while handling these items, (3) daily discarding of cat litter box contents, avoiding of litter box contact by pregnant women or handling only with disposable gloves and (4) covers placed on sand boxes to prevent their use by cats to deposit feces as a part of public education and prenatal and child health maintenance counselling. If a rise in the titer occurs during the first trimester, a decision must be made regarding termination of the pregnancy.

When a pregnant woman has *measles (rubeola), mumps, chickenpox* or *infectious hepatitis*, there is no increase in fetal defects, although an increase in the number of early deliveries and fetal deaths is thought to occur. Therapeutic abortions are not considered to be necessary.

Rubella is a threat to the fetus during the first three months of pregnancy. According to one study,[16] there is a 50 per cent chance of fetal defects during the first four weeks following conception and no chance of defects occurring if the disease is contracted after the third or fourth month of pregnancy (although these fetuses will be born with a rash that warrants

---

*I have chosen to use the term as presented by Ramamurthy.[15] Syphilis is usually included in "Others" and thus the term TORCH results.

> **NURSING ACTIONS: PREVENTING TERATOGENIC EFFECTS ON THE DEVELOPING FETUS**
>
> Encourage limiting drug use to only those drugs that are prescribed and necessary for maternal and fetal health.
>
> Discourage use of cigarettes and alcohol, especially excessive use.
>
> Warn against x-rays, especially to abdomen, except when this is adequately shielded or when the x-rays are required for diagnosis at term.
>
> Suggest avoidance of contact with cat feces.
>
> Advise about the value of informing health personnel of any infectious diseases occurring during pregnancy.
>
> Assess for and encourage a satisfactory diet during pregnancy.

isolation within the nursery). Rubella syndrome consists of congenital cataracts, deafness, heart disease, microcephaly and stunted growth. A fetus will not be harmed if the children in the household are immunized for rubella during their mother's pregnancy, but the pregnant woman should wait to be immunized until after the pregnancy is completed.

Cytomegalovirus infection is discussed in detail in Chapter 27. The virus causes a small number (less than 2 per cent) of intrauterine infections but more commonly infects the infant during the birth process. Although the sequelae of the infection are usually thought to be few, a severe case can cause brain damage, perceptual organ damage or death.

A mother infected with *herpes simplex virus* will pass this infection to the infant at the time of delivery as the baby passes through the mother's infected genital tract. The mortality rate (for infants infected with herpes simplex) is 60 per cent; at least half of the babies who survive develop significant neurological and/or ocular sequelae.[19] Currently there is only one solution for those women who have, are suspected of having or have had the infection within three weeks of the onset of labor — namely, cesarean delivery.

Syphilis can be treated during pregnancy with the drug of choice, penicillin, just as in the nonpregnant state. The drug crosses the placental barrier but does not injure the baby. If serology tests determine the presence of the disease by 16 weeks' gestation, fetal infection can be prevented by treating the mother. It is at this time that the organisms begin to be transferred through the placenta to the fetus. After 18 weeks' gestation, there is an 80 per cent chance the fetus will have the disease. This means an increased likelihood of spontaneous abortion and stillbirth. If the fetus survives, the child is likely to be born deaf, blind, deformed or mentally retarded.

Maternal Malnutrition A final teratogen that warrants mentioning is maternal malnutrition. Severe restrictions in calories, protein, vitamins and iron intake may result in early abortion, intrauterine growth retardation (IUGR), malformation, perinatal mortality and abnormal development during infancy. A satisfactory diet during pregnancy includes moderate amounts of carbohydrates and fats and high intake of protein, vitamins and minerals.

References

1. L. Annis. The Child Before Birth. Cornell University Press, 1978
2. N. Butler, H. Goldstein and E. M. Ross. Cigarette smoking in pregnancy: its influence on birth weight and perinatal mortality. British Medical Journal, 15 April 1972, p. 127
3. Dunn. Maternal cigarette smoking during pregnancy and the child's subsequent development. Canadian Journal of Public Health, Jan/Feb 1977, p. 43
4. J. Hanson, K. Jones and D. Smith. Fetal alcohol syndrome: experience with 41 patients. Journal of the American Medical Association, 5 April 1976, p. 1458
5. J. Hardy and E. Mellits. Does maternal smoking during pregnancy have a long-term effect on the child? Lancet, April 1972, p. 1332
6. L. Hellman and J. Pritchard. Williams' Obstetrics. Appleton-Century-Crofts, 1971
7. J. Henahan. Mom's couple of drinks per day may produce an abnormal child. Medical Tribune, 16 March 1977, p. 1
8. K. Jones and D. Smith. Recognition of the fetal alcohol syndrome in early infancy. Lancet, February 1973, p. 999
9. K. Jones, D. Smith, A. Streissguth and N. Myrianthopoulos. Outcome in offspring of chronic alcoholic women. Lancet, January 1974, p. 1076
10. L. McNall and J. Galeener, eds. Current Practice in Obstetric and Gynecologic Nursing, Vol. 2. C.V. Mosby Co., 1978

11. M. McRae. An approach to the single parent dilemma. American Journal of Maternal and Child Nursing, May/June 1977, p. 164
12. M. Meyer. Maternal smoking, pregnancy, complications and perinatal mortality. American Journal of Obstetrics and Gynecology, 1 July 1977, p. 494
13. M. Moore. Realities in Childbearing. W. B. Saunders Co., 1978
14. A. Nahmias. The TORCH syndrome of perinatal infections. Hospital Practice, September 1974, p. 65
15. R. Ramamurthy. Infections in the neonate: perinatology — past, present, and future. Lecture presented at Third March of Dimes Perinatal Nursing Conference in Chicago, February 1978
16. A. Rhodes. Virus infections and congenital malformations. Presented at the First International Conference on Congenital Malformations, Philadelphia, J. B. Lippincott Co., 1961
17. D. Silverman. Maternal smoking and birth weight. American Journal of Epidemiology, June 1977, p. 513
18. Smoking threatens unborn children. University of Michigan Medical Center Report, Fall 1977, p. 5
19. A. Visintine, A. Nahmias and W. Jose. Genital herpes. Perinatal Care, Oct/Nov 1978, p. 32

Additional Recommended Reading

S. Babson and R. Benson. Management of High-Risk Pregnancy and Intensive Care of the Neonate. C. V. Mosby Co., 1975

J. Bahr. Herpes virus hominis type 2 in women and newborns. American Journal of Maternal and Child Nursing, Jan/Feb 1978, p. 16

A. Clark and D. Affonso. Childbearing: A Nursing Perspective. F. A. Davis Co., 1979

J. Dwyer. Human Reproduction: The Female System and the Neonate. F. A. Davis Co., 1976

J. Goerzen and P. Chinn. Review of Maternal and Child Nursing. C. V. Mosby Co., 1975

C. Hardgrove and L. Warrick. How shall we tell the children? American Journal of Nursing, March 1974, p. 448

K. Hope and N. Young, eds. Momma: The Sourcebook for Single Mothers. Plume Books — New American Library, 1976

C. Klein. The Single Parent Experience. Avon Books, 1973

K. Kowalski and M. Ross Osborn. Helping mothers of stillborn infants to grieve. American Journal of Maternal and Child Nursing, Jan/Feb 1977, p. 29

L. Martin. Health Care of Women. J. B. Lippincott Co., 1978

C. S. McGovern. Recognizing a tubal pregnancy. American Journal of Maternal and Child Nursing, Sept/Oct 1978, p. 303

S. Romney, M. Gray, A. Little, J. Merril, E. Quilligan and R. Stander. Gynecology and Obstetrics: The Heatlh Care of Women. McGraw-Hill Book Company, 1975

D. Schanche. Toxoplasmosis. McCall's, November 1971, p. 56

A. Scupholme. Who helps? Coping with the unexpected outcome of pregnancy. Journal of Obstetric, Gynecologic and Neonatal Nursing, Jul/Aug 1978, p. 36

S. Stagno. Toxoplasmosis. American Journal of Nursing, April 1980, p. 720

PREGNANCY IN ADOLESCENCE

8

by Sara Criswell, BSN, RN,
Dorothy Wierenga, RN and
June Hauge, MSW, ACSW

Evidence gathered during the last 10 years indicates that females today have more control over themselves and their lives, including their reproductive lives. In spite of this, there has been a significant increase in the number of pregnancies in the adolescent population, particularly among the 15 and under age group. In this teen population the birth rate is increasing rather than decreasing, as it is in all other age groups in the United States. Many health professionals feel that teen pregnancies in the United States have reached epidemic proportions. Latest statistics show that about 10 per cent of American teenage girls become pregnant yearly and approximately two-thirds of these pregnancies are unplanned. More than one in four teenage girls who have premarital intercourse get pregnant, reveals the Alan Guttmacher Institute, a division of the Planned Parenthood Federation of America.

For health professionals, especially the nurse, the pregnant teenage client represents an all-too-familiar and distressing situation. It is imperative that the nurse understand the teenage client. Before she deals with these clients, she should review basic human growth and development and understand developmental tasks of adolescence. Only with a thorough understanding of both physical and pyschological development in adolescents will the nurse be able to understand the motivations for pregnancy and the coping behavior patterns of the teen mother and father.

Adolescence encompasses a period of extensive accelerated physical and psychological growth, beginning at about the age of 10 in girls and 12 in boys. Modifications of the psychological structure take place at approximately the same time physical changes occur. Sexual interests become conscious and are discussed and explored according to the mores of the peer group.

The teenage years are a period in which all the earlier needs and phases of life are relived in some degree and in which conflicts, those of authority and dependency and those pertaining to sex, are reactivated and lived through, resulting in a general reorganization of the personality. If there has been a difficult childhood life experience that resulted in the adolescent's not being emotionally free to develop his self-dependence to the utmost, there will be a difficult teenage period.

In the early part of adolescence, pressures of physical, psychological and social changes are very intense, and the adaptive capacity of the individual is strained to the point of relative inadequacy. Once the physical aspects become somewhat stabilized, the person can become familiar with these changes; with this comes progressive mastery. In like manner, familiarity with social and emotional demands clarifies these issues and mastery is facilitated.

Competition exists between childish interests and childish need for dependency and adult interests and desire for independence. Parents are at a loss as to whether to treat the young person as a child or as an adult. Rebellion against too-firm control, floundering without guidance, and regression when the youth is faced too soon with adult responsibilities may be results of this conflict. Youth at a White House conference a number of years ago stressed that they seek neither control by nor independence from adults. They stated that they want the kind of support that backs them up and yet gives them freedom to move ahead independently to the extent that they can.

Adolescent parenthood may come as a result of unhealthy identification with role models (pregnant mother, sister, friend), vengefulness toward the family, or self-punishment. Often a feeling of isolation, increased by lack of warmth in her environment, can cause a girl to "seek something," which results in pregnancy.

During these years, establishment of a sense of identity is a primary problem: "Who am I? What will my role be in life?" These young people may search for examples of courage and high ideals on which to model themselves, or they may identify with criminal personalities and become delinquent. The peer group of the same sex has great importance for the adolescent, since he puts great value on what his peer group finds acceptable in behavior and philosophy in their mutual strivings toward adulthood. Because the values of the peer group are often at variance with the standards of the parents, conflicts frequently result. Interest in the opposite sex brings about rivalry and jealousy that threatens friendships. These conflicts are difficult to resolve because of the teen's feelings of general inadequacy and because of his questionable status as a sexual individual. However, the surer he becomes of himself, the more he seeks intimacy in the form of friendship and love, and inspiration.

At this age, life becomes particularly difficult for those teenagers of minority groups. When they begin to move out of the close family circle, they are exposed to the fact that they are often not considered equal to other people, and this is very disrupting to personality development.

Approximately 600,000 teenagers give birth each year. Often the "causes" of early pregnancies, whether outside of or within a marriage, are related to some of the struggles for identity, reactions to attitudes toward them by parents and other adults, peer pressures and many other factors that probably contribute to the occurrence of a pregnancy. The fact that many more sexually active teenagers do not become pregnant causes speculation that pregnancy in itself may have meaning. It has been speculated that this is true for older, married couples. Some women have said such things as, "The only time I feel like a worthwhile human being is when I am pregnant." Further discussion with such women might indicate that they have very poor self-esteem and the feeling that they increase in worth as they are able to "produce" something.

Pregnancies of teens often seem to occur when their parents are having marital or financial problems or problems related to the pressures of moving, changing jobs or coping with a death in the family.

Peer pressures — "everyone is doing it" — and the need to try to fit in and be accepted and not be seen as a person who is different contributes to some young people sexually "acting out." It must be realized that the young adolescent's capacity for impulse control is poorly developed. Improper sex education or no sex and family life education, lack of or inaccurate contraception information, and reluctance on the part of society to provide pregnancy testing and abortion information all contribute to particular problems in this age group.

THE SOCIAL EFFECTS OF ADOLESCENT PREGNANCY

Who is affected by a teenage pregnancy? The pregnant girl, the teenage father, the families of both, other family members on both sides, peers and society as a whole are all affected.

Those adolescents who continue pregnancy often do not complete their education or obtain vocational training. Often school dropouts are associated with pregnancy. Some schools are changing in their attitudes about pregnant students continuing in school; however, there are still schools in which a pregnant girl cannot continue with her education. Some girls choose to drop out of school, even if the school permits their remaining.

What about marriage? It is estimated that half of pregnant teenagers marry before the baby is born. The outlook for a stable marriage and family life is bleak. Divorce rates are two to three times higher for these couples than for any other age goup.

Family relationships, which may already be strained, may be further complicated and weakened by the pregnancy of the teenage girl or the responsibility for impregnation by a teenage boy. Goals for education, training or work may be interrupted or completely changed. This will affect the feelings of all concerned. A young man who has to quit school to go to work and support a child at the age of 17 may, at the age of 20, be taking out negative feelings about this on his wife and small child. The individual dreams and expectations of the young parents may be different, but they find themselves giving up or changing their goals and usually feel that they have failed their parents, families and themselves. The teenage boy's parents may be seeing the end of lifelong dreams when a son for whom education was planned must take an unskilled, dead-end job. Frustration and unhappiness may follow young and old for years to come. For another family, their daughter, who has been on the honor roll every year, is now a mother at 17, and instead of being a teacher is living in a small apartment alone with her child, with few friends and very little to give her satisfaction.

The teenage mother no longer has the same interests as her own peer group, but neither does early motherhood qualify her for peer attachment in an older age group. A critical part of adolescent development is the formation of peer relationships. Since her status in either peer group is questionable, it enforces a sense of alienation and isolation. In this isolated state the girl receives little if any positive feedback about herself or her mothering, leading to a lowered self-image. It is important for the nurse to intercede and help the girl see herself as her mother's peer. The girl should be encouraged to make her own decisions in the childrearing situation. To allow the girl's mother to actively intervene in the childrearing process is depriving the girl of developing her own mothering skills. This can cause inconsistencies in expected behavior for the infant that can be detrimental to his normal psychological development.

Nurses commonly do not recognize the needs of the extended family. A teenager's mother may need much support and understanding, because often this new grandmother feels guilty and imagines that she has failed

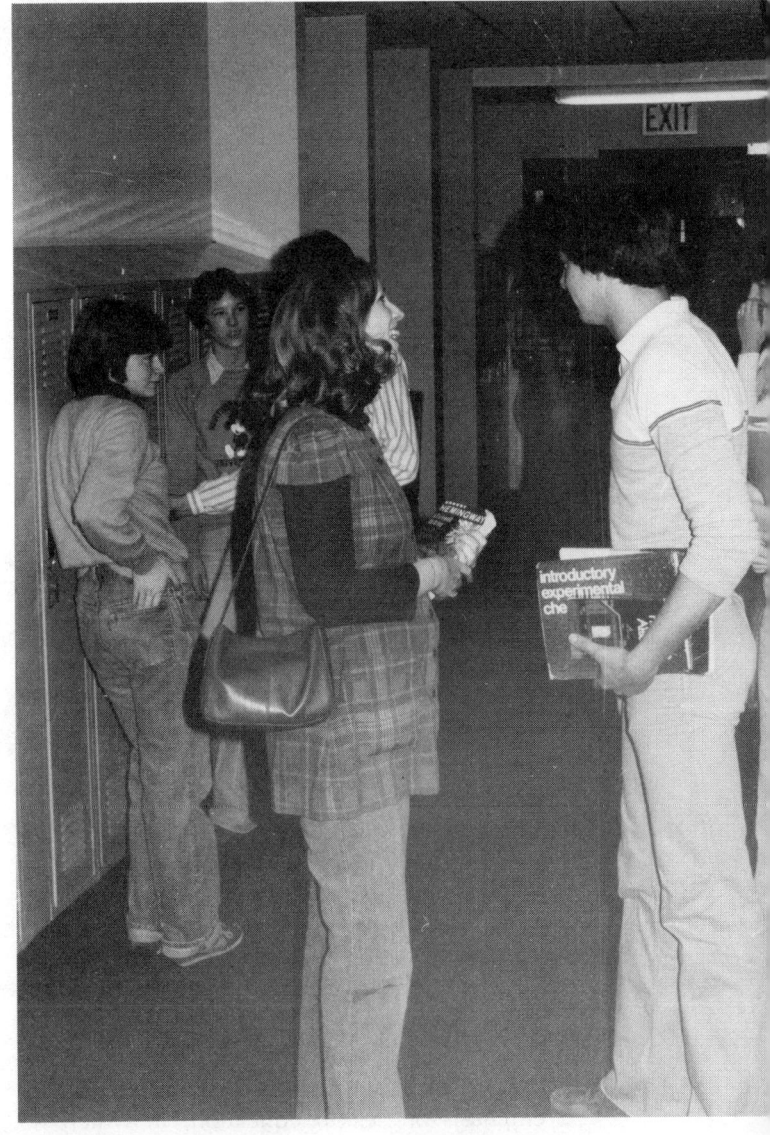

"I want to finish school" is the wish of many pregnant teens. Many high schools are providing opportunities for these girls to do so.

her daughter, and she questions her own parenting skills. On the other hand, she may feel a sense of pride in her new status. Many times the grandmother is feeling some sexual inadequacies as she approaches middle age and by becoming a grandmother, her feminine identity and ability to mother is reinforced. In this case, it is often difficult for the grandmother to allow the new mother to participate in the infant's care. The nurse, by teaching infant care and encouraging rooming-in, can strengthen the new mother's confidence. Only when the teenage mother feels confident in her ability to mother will she actively care for her newborn.

Grandparents of the young couple are affected, too. They have been watching their grandchildren with pride and hope and now may find themselves trying to respond with understanding and encouragement to their children and their children's children, or perhaps they find themselves over-reacting to what is happening. They often feel they have failed in some way.

Schools are affected by the problems of these young people who are coming to them for education. They must decide who can stay in school and who must drop out. They must re-evaluate their sex education programs and their counselling services, trying to determine if they have given too much sex education to their young people, or too little such education and guidance.

What about the community? Some interested and concerned segments of society find themselves trying to encourage schools to educate better in the area of sex and "relationship" factors. They encourage teachers with understanding and conviction that there is a need for help in these areas as young people grow into adulthood. The need for teachers who are concerned and caring and nonjudgmental in their approach, and who have the ability to teach young people without preaching, is recognized in some areas of the nation. There are other areas in which citizens continue to question the emphasis on sex in education, in which no consideration is being given to the attitudes of teachers and those responsible for our young people's lives, and very judgmental and restricted direction is allowed. The question becomes: How can sex be accepted as a normal and meaningful part of life without being exploited?

Some communities offer classes to young pregnant couples who remain in school so that they can be prepared as well as possible for what is to come, so that they can begin to understand what has happened and some aspects of why it has happened. Through these classes suggestions can be given to help prevent further pregnancies for which the young people are not prepared.

Regardless of how the community views teenage pregnancy, it must first recognize that the problem exists. The stresses that a teenage pregnancy places on a community are numerous and varied. Lack of education of young people, regardless of whether forced by school policy or by personal choice, leads to high unemployment. This, in turn, provides a low financial base for the teen family, which dictates the need for public support (welfare). The increased divorce rate and incidence of child abuse among teenage parents raises the need for social services.

If the community recognizes the problem and takes a positive attitude in trying to prevent and deal with teenage pregnancies, it will probably accept some financial responsibility for job placement, day care centers, maternal-child clinics and public education in family living.

PHYSICAL RISKS TO ADOLESCENT MOTHER AND FETUS

Increased rates of teenage pregnancy are of concern to medical and social agencies, since pregnancy is associated with a high rate of complications in the very young. The incidence of toxemia, prolonged labor and iron deficiency anemia in teenage mothers has been established. These mothers have a disproportionate number of infants of low birth weight, with associated mental retardation. The relationship of infant mortality to young maternal age has also been noted. There are also apparent linkages between young mothers and infants with epilepsy, cerebral palsy and an increased incidence of deafness and blindness. The fact that these pregnant girls are of an age of susceptibility to communicable diseases also places added risk to the fetus.

A pregnancy that occurs within the first two years of menarche may present definite medical problems, such as infants who are small for gestational age. Gynecological age is defined as the number of years between menarche and the first pregnancy: the teen mother of 14 who began menarche at age 12 would have a gynecological age of 2 years. Higher risks are associated with lower gynecological age. Due to the physical immaturity of the very young mother, cephalopelvic disproportionment may be a problem, necessitating a cesarean section or resulting in prolonged labor, increasing the risk of neurological handicaps in the neonate.

However, studies are still inconclusive in regard to the relationship of the age of the mother to the intelligence or physical and mental handicaps of the child. Physical and emotional immaturity of the mother coupled with inadequate prenatal care, poor diet and irregular eating habits are factors in the incidence of high-risk and low birth weight infants. There is evidence that indicates that with adequate prenatal care and proper diet this risk factor may be greatly reduced.

Many teenagers do not seek prenatal care until late in pregnancy, and their visits to their doctor or clinic may be erratic. The reasons for this are numerous. The girl does not want to admit that she is pregnant or accept this fact, and so refuses medical attention. She may be unable to receive care without parental consent or she may fear that the doctor will tell her parents of her condition. She may also lack the necessary funds for care and may not know about the availability of public funds or want this help. Transportation, either public or private, may not be available. Because she is immature and lacks knowledge about pregnancy, she may not understand the need for early and regular medical supervision. Another prime factor is the embarrassment encountered during the pelvic examination.

The young girl of today matures physically earlier than did the previous generation. After menarche, she is potentially capable of becoming a mother. The age for establishing menarche has become lower in the United States and Europe and the level of sexual activity has increased in the past several years. The major contributing factors for early menarche are adequate nutrition and improved health during the adolescent years. The ability to conceive (fecundity) and the capacity to avoid spontaneous abortion also contribute to a rise in the incidence of teenage motherhood.

The younger the girl, the greater the risk to her and her infant. The additional nutrient demands of pregnancy may compromise her growth potential and that of her fetus. A significant relationship has been found between protein intake of the mother and the condition of the infant. Mental deficiency in the fetus and low birth weight may be due to an inadequate protein intake during pregnancy. Thus, an appropriately balanced diet provides building material for the growth and development of a healthy child. There is increased need for calories for thermal balance in the mother and to provide energy necessary for building fetal and placental tissue and to maintain the mother's body and tissue processes. An additional 200 calories above the mother's usual caloric intake is recommended. This is consistent with the 20- to 25-pound weight gain recommended by the Committee on Maternal Nutrition, Food and Nutrition Board, National Council of National Research, Academy of Sciences (Washington, D.C.).

The National Institute of Health suggests that there is a correlation between the level of amino acids in the blood of the pregnant woman and the subsequent intelligence of her offspring.[5] It is recognized that good nutrition is important in any pregnant woman. Increased attention to nutrition in the pregnant adolescent is imperative because of her own growth spurts and because of her typically poor dietary habits. For example, teenagers tend to eat snack foods and to eat sporadically, and females particularly may practice fad diets for weight control.

Undernutrition in the young pregnant woman has been shown to interact with genetic factors during prenatal development, with irreversible results to the infant.[1] Long-term, large-scale studies seeking the causes of birth defects have discovered links between complicated multigenerational tangles of social, economic and biological factors that make some mothers "poor producers."[1, 2] These factors do not cause easily identifiable birth defects, but a combination of them probably accounts for many young mothers from disadvantaged homes lacking adequate prenatal care, adequate diet and ideal living conditions. Adverse living conditions interact with prematurity to increase retardation, behavior disorders, lower IQs and learning problems.

The adverse effects of cigarette smoking and alcohol consumption were mentioned in Chapter 7. Unfortunately, smoking and drinking often add to the physical problems of the pregnant adolescent. The Surgeon General's Report on Smoking and Health indicated that interactions between macro- and micronutrients and tobacco for pregnant patients are significant because of fetal malnutrition. Studies in the United States and Great Britain indicate that babies born to mothers who smoke are smaller and have greater risk of perinatal mortality. Partially responsible for low birth weight may

PREGNANCY IN ADOLESCENCE 119

be impairment of the mother's protein metabolism, as well as lower levels in maternal blood of amino acids, vitamins B_{12} and C, glucose, and fatty acids. In addition, it is postulated that the smoking mother's higher levels of carboxyhemoglobin and nicotine may decrease oxygenation of the fetus. The effects of cigarette smoking, unlike those of maternal rubella and certain drugs or medications, are most dangerous in the last six months of pregnancy, when the central nervous system of the fetus is developing.

Recent years have seen a significant rise in the occurrence of fetal alcohol syndrome. The pregnant adolescent often is unaware that alcohol affects her unborn child. Alcohol is readily available to teenagers, and peer pressures for drinking in this age bracket are strong. Fetal alcohol syndrome is a combination of physical and emotional anomalies found to consistently occur among children of moderate- and heavy-drinking mothers. Moderate to heavy drinking in this case is defined as consumption of more than 3 ounces of alcohol per day. Also, studies have indicated that binge drinking can have the same unfortunate results.[3] Severe manifestations of the disease are marked growth deficiencies, multiple birth defects and mental retardation. These children may be markedly shorter in stature, exhibit hyperactive behavior and learning or behavioral problems, and have short attention spans. The children often exhibit abnormalities of the eyes and face, with small eyes or drooping lids.

It has been determined that alcohol passes directly to the fetus through the placenta soon after being consumed by the mother. The concentration of alcohol passing to the fetus is the same as that which the mother drinks. However, because of the immaturity of the organs of the fetus, its metabolism of alcohol is much slower than in the adult. Consequently, the alcohol acts as a toxic agent that interferes with development of the fetus, or damages it.

The pregnant drug addict, in recent years, has tended to be the younger teenager and the young adult. The true prevalence of drug addiction in mothers is unknown, but there are indications there has been an increase in the number of these women in the past 15 years. Most drug-addicted patients delay perinatal care until near delivery to avoid being without their drugs during a long labor period. They often deliver in ambulances or at home and make considerable effort to nourish their addiction by hiding drugs or obtaining them from others outside the hospital during their hospital confinement. The physicians of some of these patients may prescribe tranquilizers or barbiturates to help control symptoms of withdrawal from drugs.

Greatest medical difficulties in these circumstances tend to occur after delivery, when withdrawal in the mother and infant puts them at risk. Narcotic use by the mother may lead to intrauterine growth retardation and the typical pregnancy outcome in those women nutritionally deprived and receiving inadequate prenatal care, with one important addition — congenital addiction of the baby. Even after withdrawal, detoxification and rehabilitation, the addicted individual remains at risk years later, because subsequent drug intake may result in the desire and immediate urge for more drugs. Detoxification of the newborn infant seems to be initially successful. The detoxified infant with supportive measures, including hydration and diminishing doses of sedatives, recovers, and a permanent cure may be assured because the infant has not developed a psychological dependence on drugs. Although methadone may be used to manage the pregnant addict, it only magnifies the effects on the fetus, who will have to experience withdrawal from the other drugs and from the methadone.

IMPACT ON HEALTH PROFESSIONALS

The pregnant adolescent provides challenges to health professionals. Health professionals find that they are providing services to adolescents who have suddenly been saddled with adult responsibilities. In helping all clients, it is important to consider their age when planning their care. One must take into account the developmental tasks of the specific age group to understand its behavior. I recall a student nurse who became quite upset because her patient, a teen mother, did not wish to keep her baby the full time allowed during the 9 o'clock feeding. The new mother was more involved in making phone calls to her friends. This close association with peers as exhibited through phone calls is behavior to be expected for teens. After looking at normal adolescent behavior, the student

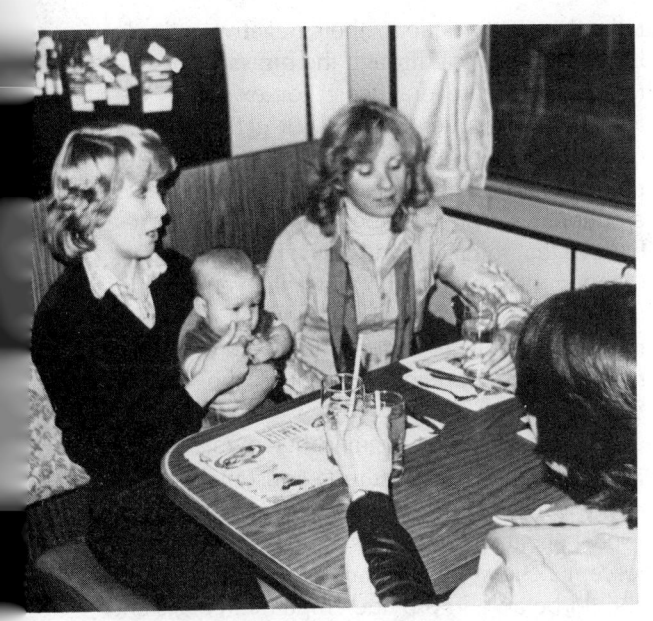

The teenager with a baby still needs close association with her peers. She needs to successfully master adolescence and its tasks to become a mature, responsible adult.

nurse became less judgmental and was better prepared to approach the teen mother with a positive attitude. Frequently, nurses, as well as other health professionals, assume that since the teen client is pregnant or has delivered a child, she has automatically reached adulthood. One should look at where the client is developmentally rather than at the client's age alone. Age, as we know, is no guide to level of maturity.

The nurse, in dealing with the pregnant teen, should not only teach routine prenatal care but must also help her meet the special problems she faces. This client will need special instruction in diet and exercise. She may have little, if any, knowledge of reproduction, and therefore anatomical terminology may be foreign to her. As most teens are fairly healthy, the pregnant teen may find this her first hospitalization. She may be frightened and feel intimidated by the nursing staff.

Of all the types of education necessary for this client, teaching family planning can be the most frustrating for the nurse. Of all childbearing females, adolescents probably have the greatest need for contraceptive counselling. They find themselves in a no-man's land. Physically they are developing and finding that they have sexual desires, but at the same time they are pressured by society to keep these sexual impulses under control. In many ways, the adolescent is expected to act as an adult and assume adult responsibility. Frequently, the adolescent sees her emerging adult role in conflict with her physically maturing body. Sexual privilege and freedom do not come with physical maturity. According to Woods, "The social conflicts over sexual morality only serve to intensify the confusion experienced by the adolescent as he or she attempts to cope with intense sexual feelings. The dilemma the adolescent faces is strong repression of sexuality versus rebellion against sexual mores."[6]

Since a number of psychological changes occur, such as alteration in body image and establishment of identity, that have a bearing on the adolescent's sexuality, it is imperative that health professionals be conversant with these changes. Many nurses find it difficult to talk to adolescents about contraceptive methods or other sexually related topics. The nature of contraceptive counselling implies that the nurse should be discussing such matters as frequency of sexual activity and sexual habits. This can be embarrassing, especially if the nurse has not had much experience in teaching contraception to adolescents. One must first be understanding of one's own sexuality and its implications on one's behavior before offering any help to someone else about sexual concerns. The nurse may feel some confusion over her role in teaching about contraceptives. She must recognize that she is giving information, and the decisions about the use of such information are strictly left up to the client. Some nurses hesitate to offer contraceptive information to unwed girls because they feel in doing so they have given their approval to sexual promiscuity and perhaps even encouraged it.

Since society in the main does not approve of premarital sexual activity, it is exceedingly difficult for adolescents to obtain adequate health services in the area of family planning and treatment of venereal disease. In most facilities, parental consent is needed before counselling or treatment or both are begun. It is our opinion that the requirement for parental consent is deterring many adolescents from seeking necessary health care. We also believe this is true in the case of a young girl who finds herself pregnant. Because she fears that the physician will report to her parents, she postpones prenatal care until late in her pregnancy and, in so doing, places herself and her infant in jeopardy. Approximately one-third of states now permit unmarried girls under 18 years of age and living at home to give consent for their own contraceptive care.[4]

Another reason adolescents, both male and female, do not seek contraceptive counselling is the fear of facing judgmental attitudes of health personnel. The attitudes of health professionals may discourage the girl or boy or both from contacting those agencies that are available to them. Also, facilities may not be geared toward adolescents, who may feel uncomfortable being with older married clients. Lack of financial resources may also hinder the teen from seeking and using contraceptives. Progress has been made in some areas of the country by the establishment of clinics especially for teens. These clinics are equipped to meet the health needs of adolescents, but only after they are more widely available will we see a change in teenage contraceptive practice.

Even if the adolescent receives contraceptive information, there is often a reluctance to utilize the contraceptive. Adolescents often idealize or romanticize love, and preparing for sexual activity seems to them to decrease the spontaneity of the moment. Teens frequently label the users of contraceptives as promiscuous.

Sometimes those teens who are having difficulty understanding changes in body image do not believe they are sexually mature enough to reproduce; hence, no precautions are taken. Naivety about her own physiology may cause the young teen to have a false sense of security. A frequent comment by these girls is, "I never thought it (pregnancy) would happen to me." Reality testing is common among adolescents. Being sexually active without benefit of contraceptives may be one way for the adolescent to test her sexual maturity.

Nurses can do much to help make the childbearing experience pleasant and satisfying for the teen mother and father. Nurses should be aware of prevailing attitudes toward teenage pregnancy in their home area and should also examine their own feelings toward the subject. Many nurses do not readily empathize with the young mother. Even though nurses with this attitude are not physically abusive to the hospitalized teenage patient, their negative attitude becomes apparent through the omission of certain nursing care practices. For example, the teen patient frequently does not get back rubs but will receive only absolutely essential nursing care. These patients infrequently receive emotional support. Some doctors and nurses believe that the labor and delivery and postpartum periods should be unpleasant, even painful, for the teen mother. This thinking certainly reflects a punitive attitude and is probably a result of the puritan heritage of the United States.

The nurse must recognize her own feelings and, regardless of her attitude, must make every effort to be nonjudgmental. Nurses should be especially accepting and supportive of the adolescent's choice in the matter of her baby. One should be able to provide empathic, consistent care regardless of the adolescent's decision about her future and that of her baby. Frequently these patients ask the nurse for her opinion as to what they should do with their future. The girl is really asking the nurse to make her decision, and the nurse should be careful not to do this. The nurse should help her identify the advantages and disadvantages of each possible choice and then *allow her time to make her own decision* without the influence of the nurse's attitudes. Frequently encountered by the pregnant adolescent patient is the stigma that she probably will "be on welfare." Nurses should not be critical of the patient's mode of support but rather should be supportive and, if appropriate, explain to the patient ways of saving money. For example, these girls often do not seek prenatal care because of limited funds, so it is important to explain that most physicians charge a flat fee regardless of the number of visits. Nurses should help contain patient costs regardless of how the patient is paying her hospital bill.

In dealing with pregnant adolescents, it is important to remember that they are individuals, each with a unique set of problems. The nurse should not generalize about these patients or categorize them. She should treat them with respect and convey a nonjudgmental attitude, and provide an atmosphere of confidentiality. Every effort should be made to supply the girl with all the information regarding diagnosis of the pregnancy, prenatal care, labor and delivery and future family planning. The nurse should ascertain the girl's level of knowledge concerning the birth process so that when she is teaching she will not be talking down to the girl. All procedures should be explained in advance and the girl allowed time to ask questions. This childbearing experience will affect the girl's subsequent pregnancies and, in order to minimize any adverse effects, every effort should be made now to reassure the girl that childbearing can be a pleasant and fulfilling experience.

Since the pregnant girl is the one undergoing the physical changes, she is the one most frequently seen by the various health professionals. However, this does not mean that the young father should be ignored. As a rule, the teenage parents are curious and anxious to learn about reproduction and infant care. Ideally, the father should be included in as much of the teaching and counselling as the mother, starting with the diagnosis and prenatal care. During hospitalization the father should be encouraged to support the mother.

This is a time when the nurse can begin having an influence on the couple. She has the opportunity to teach and reinforce positive attitudes toward parenting. One of the best ways of teaching parenting skills is through a rooming-in situation. This physical setting, whereby mother and baby are together for extended periods of time, affords an excellent opportunity for teaching infant care to both the new mother and new father. Many nurses feel that if the young couple is not married, the father should be excused from any teaching or active participation in infant care. If the father shows interest and the girl wants him included, then the nurse should not make judgments but include him as much as possible. If the couple is married and both will be assuming care of the infant, it is imperative that the husband receive the same teaching as the mother. Since in most situations rooming-in has extended or unlimited visiting hours for the father, it allows him more time for the necessary teaching and exposure to the infant so that he can begin the bonding process. The teaching is done with the couple only rather than in a large group situation. This frequently relieves some inhibitions and the couple feels more comfortable asking questions.

An important aspect of postpartum care is to foster confidence in the mother and father about their childrearing abilities. They must be given emotional support and praise when caring for the infant. Because of the stressful situation of pregnancy and birth the couple may lack the necessary self-esteem for parenting. Frequently when the mother has low self-esteem and the baby cries, she panics and feels she has done something wrong. She questions her ability to mother. On the other hand, when a mother has high self-esteem and the baby cries she responds to the infant, finding out what she can do for the baby, and she feels confident that she has something to offer.

The adolescent not only is forming her own new family unit, but still is an active part of another family unit. Therefore, the parents of the adolescent should not be ignored. The new grandparents should be included in teaching and counselling; this helps them in forming a positive attitude toward the new family unit. It is helpful for all concerned if they can be involved in long-range planning for the new family. All too often the grandparents are only involved when they are paying the bills. Probably one of the best ways to include the extended family is with a team approach. When the team approach is not available, the nurse should be aware of community agencies offering services to adolescents who are pregnant or who are parents or both. The nurse should not forget the availability of community nurses. The new adolescent family is a prime candidate for home agency referral. The follow-up on these adolescents is extremely important, especially with regard to information about family planning and counselling on parenting. Unfortunately, the follow-up period is probably not long enough. The teen parents can usually handle the baby's needs the first few months. However, when the infant becomes a toddler, the young parents may have extreme difficulty coping. Frequently this is the time when child abuse occurs. Fortunately we are beginning to see more emphasis on parenting and some agencies are offering classes or individual counselling or both.

One area frequently ignored by nurses is the law as it pertains to adolescent parents. Nurses should be familiar with the legal implications of childbirth involving adolescents. The young mother generally is given 72 hours after delivery before she can sign adoption papers. This ensures that she is not forced into signing the papers while under the influence of any delivery medication and allows her more time to make the best decision for her future. Nursing personnel should become familiar with the specific laws within the state in which they practice. Also, new fathers have certain legal rights that must be respected. Often nurses refuse the teen mother permission to see her infant if she is contemplating adoption. Legally, however, the mother has all rights to that infant until the adoption papers are signed. So when a young mother asks to see her infant, she should be allowed to do so regardless of the thoughts of the nurse. For example, some nurses feel that if the girl sees her infant she will not be able to give it up for adoption. This refusal, then, clearly implies that the nurse feels it would be best for the girl to give up her infant. This is not a decision the nurse should make.

It is generally accepted that parenthood is a period of crisis — crisis being any time when old patterns of behavior are no longer acceptable or usable. Parenthood calls forth a change demanding new behaviors, and unfortunately most individuals have had very little, if any, formal preparation for the change. Although research continues concerning family development and the need for preparedness in the parental role, most individuals face parenthood with only their experience with their own parents as their guide. In order to adapt to changes, the parents must rely on their maturity and support from spouse, family, friends and health professionals.

Little research has been done on the characteristics of teenage parents. Certainly the young adolescent parents' relationships with the child are influenced by the unique developmental tasks of adolescence.

Adolescent maturity is a development stage of life. The development of self-recognition is determined by the behavior of others toward the teenager. Maturation is a threefold process — physical, emotional and intellectual — and each one unfolds separately and independently Yet they are interwoven with each other.

Changes in glandular secretions bring about changes in height, weight, body contour and voice. Body development may seem strange to adolescents and may sometimes be embarrassing to them. Not all are pleased with these physical changes, but their concerns seem to be with their physical appearance, which is directly correlated with personal esteem. Experience helps to mold the young woman's perception of her physical self. The young girl of today may look older and more sophisticated; this may lead one to expect greater maturity of her than she is capable of having. The boy, her counterpart, is often so young that it is incongruous to picture him as a father. Nonetheless, he is her potential mate.

Early marriage and mating in the early part of this century was culturally acceptable by society when the young people involved were physiologically ready for sexual experience. This sanctioned behavior was adequate to assist the young couple to establish a home and a family. Readiness to assume responsibility to support a family today takes many more years to achieve. In the meantime, young people have all the usual sexual drives and desires. This may result in unwanted or unplanned pregnancy. Pregnancy is always accompanied by emotional changes produced by hormonal and metabolic changes. Emotional upsets may be evidenced by hostility, rebellion, anger and frequent psychosomatic complaints. The experience of an unwed pregnancy and the reaction of society to her situation may leave potent impressions on the adolescent's self-concept and may be responsible for even more psychological problems later in her life.

The adolescent girl has a definite need to develop her personal goals first. This is vital to her performance as a mother. The very young girl is indeed totally unready to mother a child. Every attempt should be made to educate and support the young girl or couple when keeping the infant is their choice. The nurse has not only a responsibility to provide a safe labor and delivery for the infant, she must also take some responsibility in providing a sound framework within which the family can develop.

References

1. V. Apgar. Is My Baby All Right? Simon and Schuster, 1972
2. A. Clark and D. Alfonso. Childbearing: A Nursing Perspective. F. A. Davis, Co., 1979
3. Fetal Alcohol Syndrome. Governor's Planning Council on Developmental Disabilities (Springfield) and Governor's Citizens Advisory Counsel on Alcoholism (Chicago), Illinois, 1978
4. E. House. Medical services for sexually active teenagers. American Journal of Public Health, April 1973, p. 285
5. United States Department of Health, Education and Welfare. FDA Drug Bulletin. U.S. Public Health Service, Feb/Mar 1979
6. N. F. Woods. Human Sexuality in Health and Illness. C. V. Mosby Co., 1975

Recommended Additional Reading

C. Anderson. The lengthening shadow: a case study in adolescent out-of-wedlock pregnancy. Journal of Obstetric, Gynecologic and Neonatal Nursing, Jul/Aug 1976

M. Barnard, B. J. Clancy, and K. E. Krantz. Human Sexuality for Health Professionals. W. B. Saunders Co., 1978

F. Barnes, ed. Ambulatory Maternal Health Care and Family Planning Services. American Public Health Association, 1978

F. Curtis. Observation of unwed pregnant adolescents. American Journal of Nursing, January 1974, p. 100

S. Dresen. Adjusting to single parenting. American Journal of Nursing, August 1976, p. 1286

C. Houde. Adolescent contraceptive counseling. Journal of Obstetric, Gynecologic and Neonatal Nursing, Jan/Feb 1976

N. Kandell. The unwed adolescent pregnancy: an accident. American Journal of Nursing, December 1976, p. 2112

S. Marinoff. Contraceptives in adolescents. Pediatric Clinics of North America, August 1972, p. 811

R. Mercer. Becoming a mother at sixteen. Journal of Maternal and Child Nursing, January 1976, p. 44

J. Parker and C. Cooke. The interdependent team approach in caring for the pregnant adolescent. Journal of Obstetric, Gynecologic and Neonatal Nursing, Jul/Aug 1976

J. Petrilla. Health care for adolescents. Journal of Obstetric, Gynecologic and Neonatal Nursing, Jul/Aug 1978

S. Reeder, et al. Maternity Nursing. J. B. Lippincott, 1980

E. Tankson. The adolescent parent: one approach to teaching child care and giving support. Journal of Obstetric, Gynecologic and Neonatal Nursing, May/June 1976

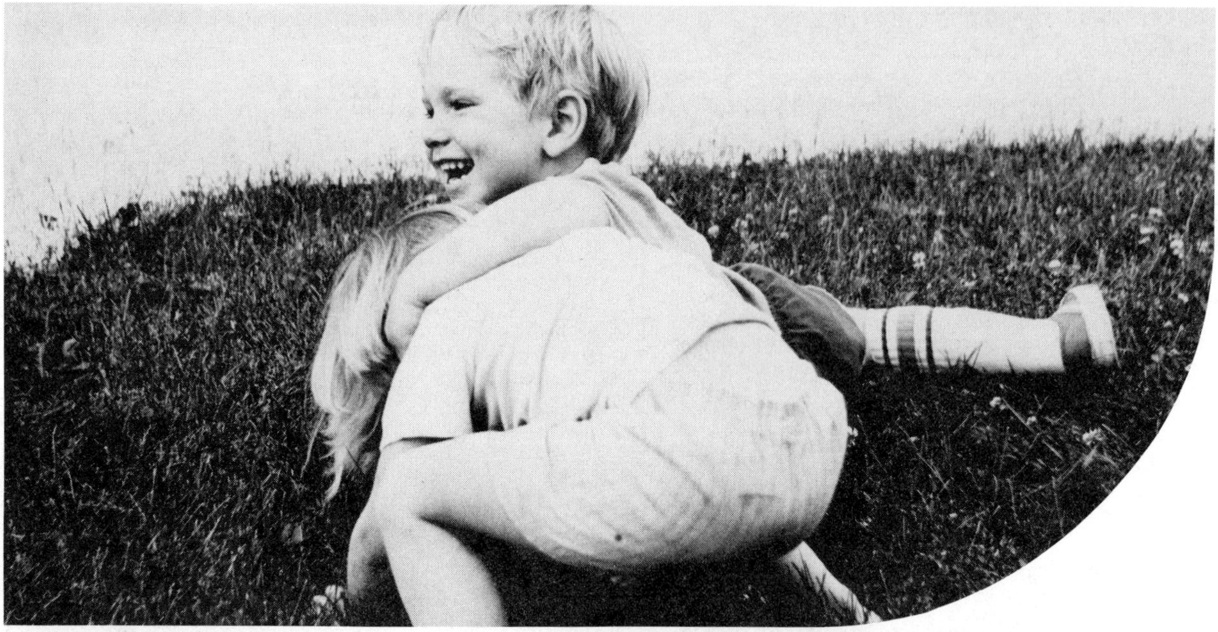

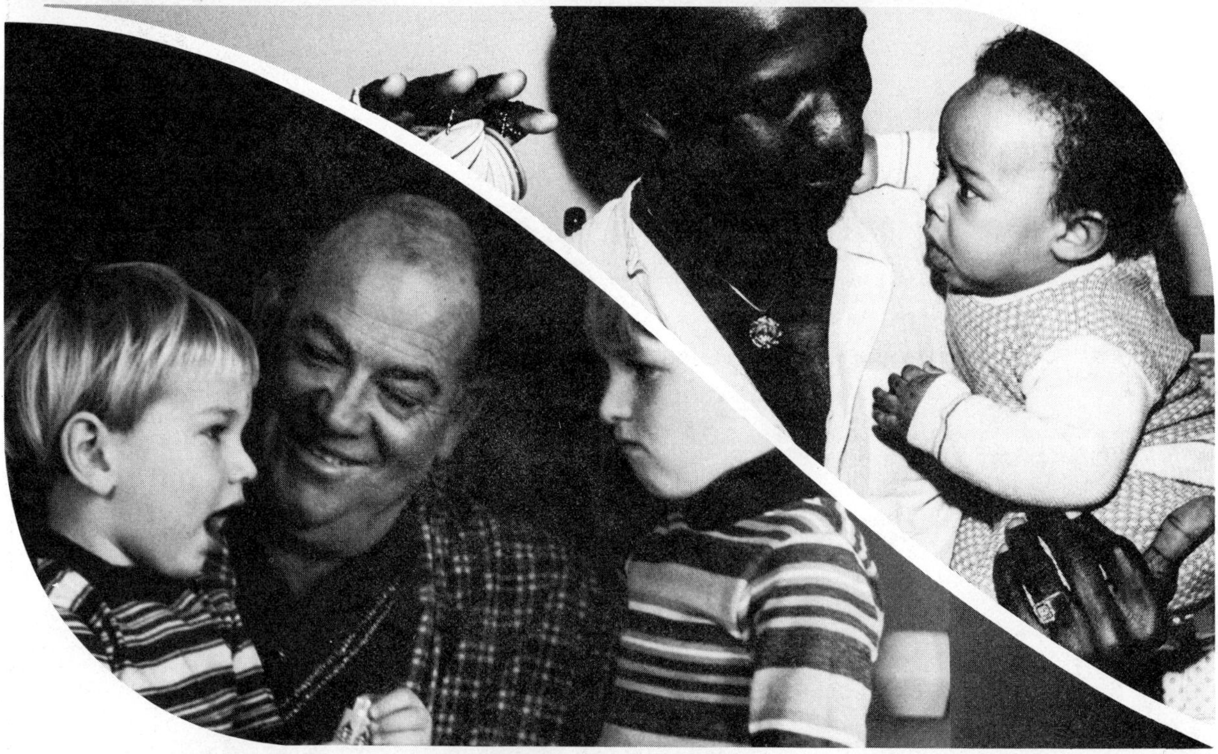

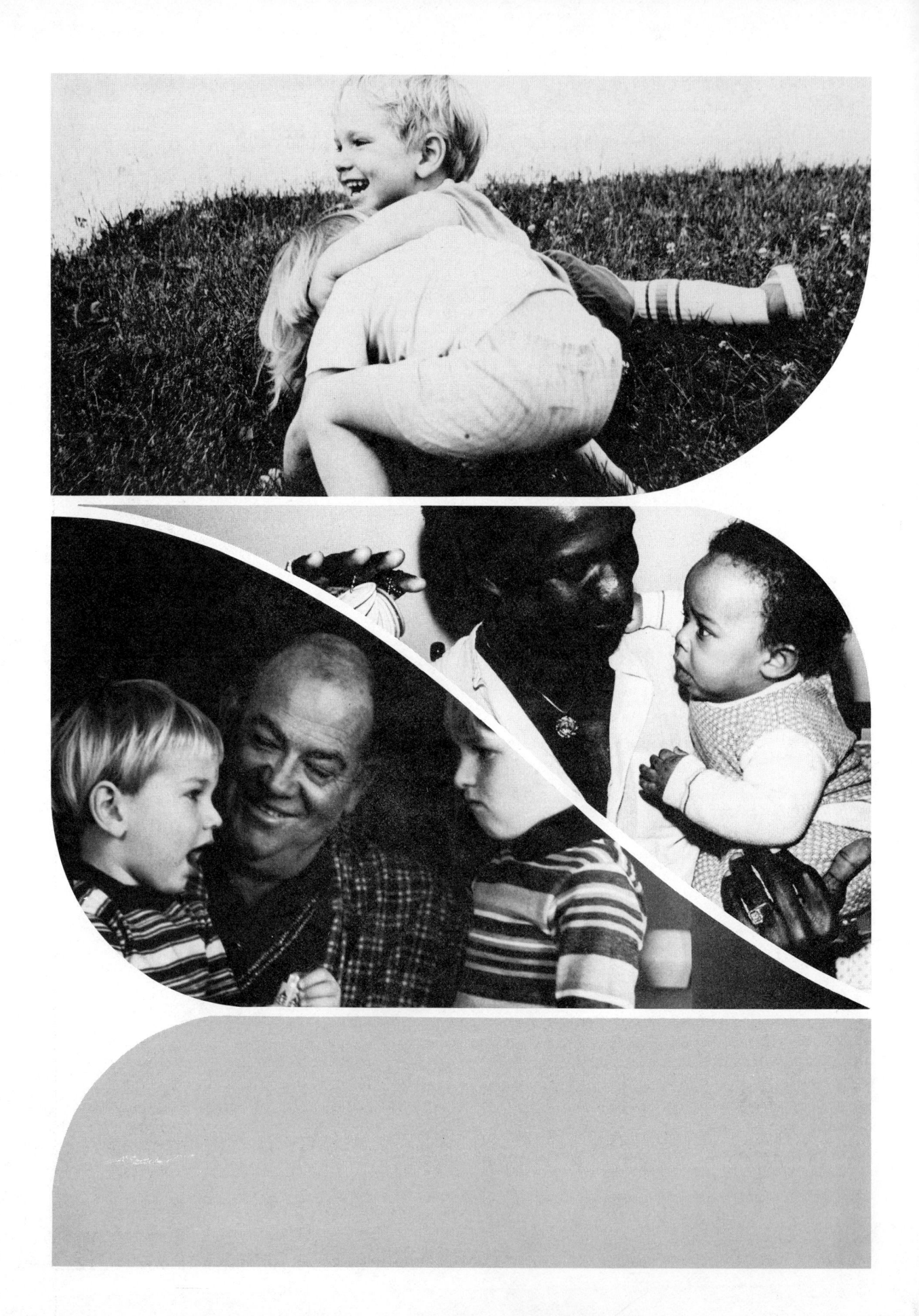

PART 3

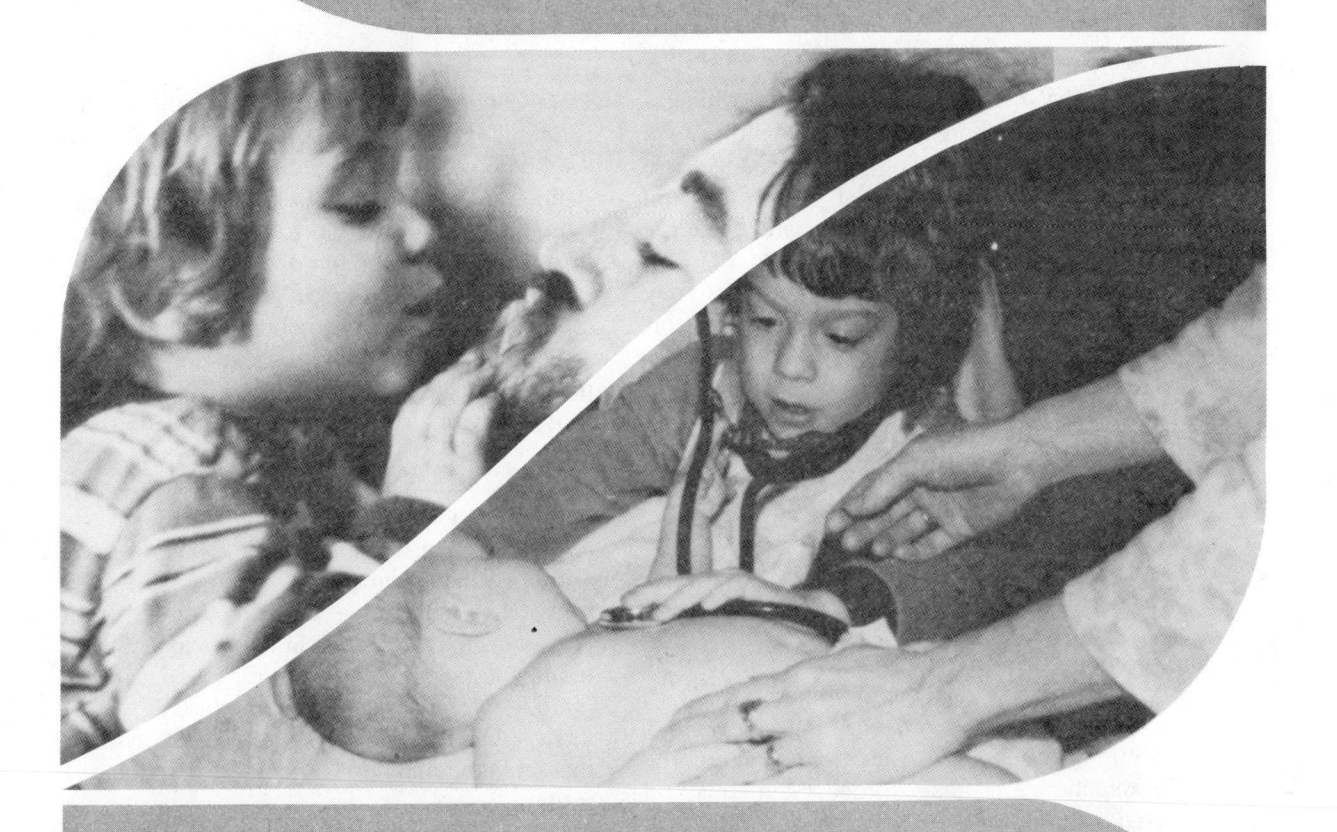

FAMILIES WITH CHILDREN
The Nurse's Role in Their Development and Health

9 PROBLEM-ORIENTED RECORDING AND NURSING PROCESS

by Amy L. Hofing, RN, MS

Planning and documentation are two vital aspects of nursing care. Both are sometimes seen as busywork or paperwork that takes the nurse away from the bedside. Yet if they are not components of the care of every patient, patient care becomes routinized and based only on physician's orders, or it changes from day to day or shift to shift, depending upon the person caring for the patient at any particular time. If the care given is not documented, there is no reliable means for reviewing or evaluating it — no mechanism for identifying the progress of the patient toward the goals of care or even knowing what these goals are.

NURSING PROCESS

An important point to remember about nursing process is that it really is a problem-solving or scientific method. In order for it to be effective, it must be thought about and used in an orderly, systematic way. Nursing process is the method used by nurses to identify, implement and evaluate the care required by a patient. The parts of the process may be known by various titles. Common terms used to classify the categories are assessment, planning, implementation and evaluation.

Assessment

Sometimes assessment is viewed in two parts: data collection and problem identification.

Data Collection Data collection must be purposeful if it is to be effective. The information to be obtained, called the *data base*, must be defined so that all problems that the nurse cannot afford to overlook will be identified through the information collected.

The data base collection may be an interdisciplinary effort, with members of various disciplines helping to define the data base and gather specific parts of it. More commonly, those individuals in each discipline define and collect their own data base. There is some overlap with this method, but each data base is defined so that information will be collected which will assist in identifying problems dealt with by that particular discipline. Thus, the physician's data base contains questions or categories that will assist in the diagnosing and treatment of disease. The nurse's data base includes physical signs and symptoms as well as the coping mechanisms and support systems that an individual has available in adapting to a disease.

Problem Identification (Nursing Diagnosis) The problems are developed by grouping items or cues from the data base. The groups of items are synthesized by formulating a term or statement that describes the group. The problem may be described at the level of a single symptom — for example, lethargy — or as a complex of signs and symptoms referred to as a *nursing diagnosis,* such as altered level of consciousness.

It is useful to think of the problem component as the *patient's* problems. Some authors refer to this category as "needs." This leads to identification of *nursing care* needs as well as the patient's needs. For example, "Inadequate fluid intake" might be listed in a category titled "Problems," while one might find "Encourage fluids" if the category were titled "Needs." The problem statement leads to thoughts about a variety of interventions; if the phrase "related to . . ." is added, the interventions can be even more specific. Such a problem statement might be "Inadequate fluid intake related to nausea." The need statement does not help one to identify any further interventions; planning is not facilitated by such a statement.

Nursing diagnoses may be used as problem statements. Nursing diagnoses are currently being identified and classified by the National Group on Classification of Nursing Diagnoses. This group (composed of nurses) was formed in 1972 and, at this writing, has accepted 37 classifications with more than 100 diagnoses. "Alterations in Parenting" and "Impairment of Mobility" are two examples of the categories.

Roy defines nursing diagnosis as a summary statement or judgment made by the nurse about the data she has gathered in her nursing assessment.[5] A nursing diagnosis is made up of three components. The first two parts are generally included in the written or identified diagnosis. The first part is the problem, or the term or terms, describing the patient's state or behavioral response. The second element describes the etiology or cause of the problem. A nursing diagnosis made up of these two parts is "Noncompliance related to knowledge deficit." The third component is the defining characteristics that are the observable signs and symptoms of the problem. The nurse must have, as part of her knowledge base, information about the signs and symptoms that must be present in order for a particular diagnosis to be represented. If a diagnosis is to be used accurately, it must be based on a valid assessment or data base and the defining signs and symptoms must be present.[4] For example, some of the defining characteristics or signs and symptoms that must be present in order to make the subdiagnosis "altered body image" are: the patient's negative verbalization about his body, expressions of grief over the loss of a body part or function, general reactions of poor comprehension of facts and explanations and use of nonpersonal pronouns.[3] Identification of nursing diagnoses and selecting and testing the defining characteristics are continuous.

Development of a Plan

The planning phase of the nursing process consists of identifying expected outcomes and the interventions that will help the patient to achieve those outcomes. The outcome must be measurable and achievable. In order for the outcome to meet this standard, it may sometimes represent maintenance of the current condition without further deterioration rather than resolution of the problem. An outcome that predicts restoration of health is meaningless for a patient with a terminal illness. A useful outcome in that instance might be one referring to maintenance of comfort. For example, "The patient will receive medication for pain at intervals that will permit participation in activities of daily living."

Nursing Intervention

The intervention part of planning may sometimes be identified as "Nursing Actions" or "Nursing Orders." Interventions that are written as specifically as possible are the most likely to be followed, since they convey the intent of the writer. For example, "Turn side to side every two hours" is a clearer order than "Turn side to side." The second order leaves the frequency completely to the discretion of the person caring for the patient. The caregiver is free to select any time interval and has no way of knowing the intention of the person who identified the need.

When writing orders for each problem, three things should be considered: which data must be obtained through observations or measurements, which activities must be carried out that will have a beneficial or therapeutic effect for the patient, and education or information that the patient or family or both will require. Consideration of these three dimensions for each problem will ensure a comprehensive approach.

Evaluation

Evaluation is the final step in the nursing process. For an individual patient, evaluation is a comparison of the actual outcome with the expected outcome for each problem. The result of evaluation determines whether the problem is resolved or the interventions are continued for a longer period of time. Evaluation may lead to a revision of any or all parts of the plan for that problem; perhaps the problem is incorrectly defined, the outcome is not achievable or measurable or the actions or orders will not result in the expected outcome.

Evaluation may be accomplished by a variety of means. It may be carried out concurrently while the patient is receiving care or it may be retrospective, after the patient has been discharged from care. The patient's chart may be monitored, and the results achieved are compared with the expected outcomes. Observation of the patient or an interview with him may also be useful evaluation tools. Whatever method or combination of methods is used, the results must be measured against the anticipated results. On the basis of this comparison, an individual patient's care plan may be modified if the evaluation is concurrent. If it is retrospective, the care of a number of patients can be reviewed, specific trends identified and general patterns of care changed.

The patient's health care record must contain documentation of the use of nursing process. Regulatory bodies and accrediting agencies examine the record for such evidence. The written record is the evidence of care given that is accepted by courts of law. If care is not documented, it is generally considered not to have been done.

DOCUMENTATION OF HEALTH CARE

There are two major methods of organizing the patient's health care record. They are known as source-oriented and integrated record systems. *Source-oriented* means that the record is divided into sections with each discipline having its own section. It is difficult to comprehensively follow a patient's progress when each health care specialist charts in a separate section of the chart. The care provided and the patient's response to the care on any given day may be found in two or more parts of the chart. Members of each discipline tend to concentrate on their own notes, paying little attention to information in other sections. Such a system tends to fragment the patient's care, since members of each discipline remain relatively unaware of the plans and activities of other professionals caring for a patient.

An *integrated record* is one in which members of all disciplines enter the care they give in one section of the patient's chart. The record can thus be read in chronological order.

Narrative Recording

Notes in either of these types of records may be written in a narrative style, including that information which the writer feels is pertinent. One note may include information related to several of the patient's problems. Patient responses, plans, care given, as well as miscellaneous information, may appear in the note.

The narrative style does not lend itself to documentation of the nurse's plans for patient care or patient education. Nurses' notes in such a system tend to provide a record of the nurse's activities rather than the patient's response to care.

Problem-Oriented Recording

Problem-oriented recording is another way of documenting patient care. This method may also be used with either a source-oriented or an integrated record. It is most effective when used in the integrated record, because it then provides a chronological account of the patient's problems, care planned and provided and the patient's response to care.

The problem-oriented record has components that correspond to the nursing process. It is a method of recording that follows a logical problem-solving sequence. It provides documentation of the recorder's thought process and allows the reader to evaluate both the data and the conclusions reached. Problem-oriented recording permits permanent documentation of nursing process.

The components of problem-oriented recording are the data base, problem list, initial plans and progress notes.

Data Base The data base corresponds to the data collection component of nursing process. Specific information to be collected from each patient is identified.

Some examples of general categories for data collection might be: Functional Abilities/

Surface Appraisal; Feeding Practices/Nutrition; Health Practices, Care and Understanding; Developmental Abilities; and Parent/Child Relationship. Under the category "Feeding Practices/Nutrition," the nurse would collect specific information related to birth weight, current diet and sleep pattern, feeding arrangements and aids, oral abnormalities, and feeding problems.[2] Collection of these data would be appropriate for an infant or young child on a general care unit. The major categories and the specific information will vary with the age of the patient and the reason for collecting the data. In any case, the data base must be defined and the same information must be collected about all patients who belong to the particular group.

Problem List The problem list is prepared using the data base. The problem component sometimes causes objection to problem-oriented recording. This is because "problem" is usually defined as a pathological condition. A more comprehensive and useful definition has been given by Dorothy Smith: "(A problem is) any condition or situation in which a patient requires help to maintain or regain a state of health or to achieve a peaceful death. It may concern the patient, family, and/or health team member and may be physiologic, psychologic, sociologic, or economic."[1] Such a definition allows one to list problems having to do with health maintenance and situations that may influence health.

Problems are listed at the level the data will support. This means that a symptom may be listed as a problem or, if the data will support it, a nursing diagnosis may be made. The level at which problems are identified is also dependent upon the practitioner's knowledge base. The beginning practitioner may more often list symptoms as problems, while the person with more experience may be able to identify several symptoms as being parts of a single entity.

Initial Plan After a beginning problem list has been made, an initial plan is developed for each problem. An example is seen in Figure 9–1. Each person contributing to the problem list writes an expected outcome and plan for the problems or aspects of the problems that he will deal with. Thus, a nurse writes an expected outcome and plans for nursing problems and also those aspects of medical problems with which nurses will be involved.

INITIAL PLAN

March 1, 1981 1500 (3:00 pm)
#3 Developmental delay
Expected Outcome: Current developmental achievements will be maintained and opportunities provided for further development within baby's capabilities.

dx: 1. Denver Developmental Screening Test to identify current abilities (done 3/1/81)
    2. Talk with parents about types of developmental activities they provide at home. Document these so they can be continued during hospitalization.

rx: 1. Explore possible Physical Therapy referral with physician.
    2. Provide cradle gym and other suspended small toys to encourage reaching.
    3. Up in infant seat at least four times on day and evening shifts.
    4. Place both of baby's hands on bottle during feedings to reinforce midline behaviors.
    5. Provide rattles and small toys that can be easily grasped.

pt. ed.: Share above activities with parents as well as additional activities and results of assessment.

_____ RN

Figure 9–1 Sample initial plan.

The expected outcome in the initial plan must be measurable and achievable. The outcome may be short-term or long-term, depending on the data available at the time of the assessment and what can be realistically predicted.

The second part of the initial plan is the *interventions*. These are divided into three categories in order to ensure a comprehensive plan just as they are in the planning aspect of nursing process. The diagnostic (dx) category refers to any order that specifies the collection of additional data. Vital signs, weight and calorie count are examples of diagnostic items, as well as are items such as "Observe parent-infant interaction." Therapeutic (tx or rx) items are those that provide some direct benefit or change for the patient. "Turn every two hours," "Use cross-cut nipple for feedings," and "Give pain medication one-half hour before physical therapy ap-

Treatments and Clinical Parameters	2400–0800 (12M–8A) 3/1/81	0800–1600 (8A–4P) 3/1/81	1600–2400 (4P–12M) 3/1/81	2400–0800 (12M–8A) 3/2/81
Observation and care of abdominal incision	dressing dry	dressing changed— wound clean and dry	dressing dry	dressing changed— small amount yellow drainage
Activity	turned every 2 hrs.	to bathroom X2 with assistance	ambulated X2 without help	slept until 7A
Cough and deep breathe	X4—nonproductive	X4—nonproductive	X2—nonproductive	X1—nonproductive
Temperature	99^2 (o)	98^6 (o)	99 (o)	98^4 (o)
Signature	_____RN	_____RN	_____RN	_____LPN

Figure 9–2 Sample flow sheet.

pointment" are therapeutic items. The patient education (pt. ed.) category contains any item related to informing or educating the patient, family or significant others.

Progress Notes and Flow Sheets The patient's ongoing care is documented using progress notes and flow sheets. Flow sheets can be found in a variety of formats. They vary from a simple graphic sheet on which vital signs are recorded to a sheet on which are listed numerous items such as blood sugar, insulin dose, diet and activity with spaces to record results and observations about the items. The flow sheet facilitates comparison of findings in regard to one item over a period of time or observation of the relationship among several items. Certain routines of care such as hygiene may also be documented on flow sheets. A detailed plan for patient education may also be written on a flow sheet, and the patient's progress with the plan may be monitored and recorded on this sheet. (Figure 9–2 is a sample flow sheet.)

Progress notes, often entitled S-O-A-P notes, are used to document the patient's progress in relation to each problem. Progress notes are not necessarily written daily or according to any routine. They must be written when there has been a change in the patient's condition or new data have been identified. They are also written when there is lack of progress; in this case the plan must be reviewed and changed as needed. For the long-term patient, progress notes should be periodically written, even if there has been no change, to document that this is the expected course of events and to review the existing data to be sure nothing has been overlooked. Progress notes are written for individual problems, comparing the patient's progress with the expected outcome of the initial plan and making modifications in the interventions of the initial plan. If new findings are recorded they may indicate a new problem, which must be added to the problem list.

The acronym SOAP stands for Subjective Objective Analysis Plan. The note is organized so that one first arranges the data about the problem according to what the patient or significant others report (Subjective) and what the professional observes or measures (Objective). One then analyzes the recorded data (Analysis) to arrive at an understanding of the data. The data are reviewed to identify a possible etiology of the problem. Sometimes it is more appropriate to indicate whether the data represent a positive or negative change for the patient, if progress is occurring and, if there is no progress, whether this is expected or not. The analysis is always based on the recorded data. Each professional makes an analysis using the knowledge base of his profession. It is inaccurate for one to make an analysis that goes beyond the recorded data or is not within the boundaries and responsibilities of one's own profession. The plan is formulated on the basis of the analysis and is composed of three components: further data-gathering (dx), nursing interventions (rx) and patient or family education (pt. ed.). Figure 9–3 is an example of a progress note.

> March 1, 1981 1900 (7:00 pm)
>
> #1 Parent-Infant Separation
>
> S   Mother remarked on some of baby's characteristics, e.g., long legs. Expressed delight when baby opened eyes. Both parents talked about baby, expressed realistic concerns, recognized changes in her appearance since they had last seen her at birth. Father able to restate accurately what he had been told by physicians about baby's cardiac defect and surgery. Mother considering rooming-in although she has not yet recovered completely from difficult delivery. Both expressed pleasure when told by physician they could anticipate taking baby home in about a week.
>
> O   Both parents held baby. Mother stroked baby's arms and legs and spoke softly to her.
> Mother was just discharged from hospital today. Father fed baby.
>
> A   Parents, especially mother, showing many signs of bonding with baby.
>
> P-dx: 1. Record parental visits and phone calls.
>
> rx: 1. Identify primary nurse who can be available to parents if further questions or concerns arise.
>   2. Encourage parents' continuing involvement in baby's care.
>
> pt. ed: 1. Develop education plan with primary nurse for parents to learn general infant care.
>
> _____ RN

Figure 9-3 Sample progress note.

Continuity of care is provided by summarizing the patient's care when he is transferred to another unit or when he is discharged. The components of both these summaries are the same. In the summary, each unresolved problem is reviewed individually in SOAP format. Subjective and objective data are reviewed, placing emphasis on the patient's condition or progress in relation to that problem. Members of each discipline summarize the problems that they have treated or aspects of a problem in which they have participated in treating. The analysis is an assessment of the discharge status of the patient in relationship to that problem. The plan outlines ongoing care such as physician's or clinic appointments, care to be given by a community health nurse, medications or self-care activities. Resolved problems are generally not summarized but are listed by their titles with the notation that they are resolved. The patient's record will not only facilitate coordination of care during hospitalization, but it will provide continuity for care needed after discharge.

The problem-oriented record facilitates use of nursing process. Its various components correspond closely to the components of nursing process. This makes it possible to provide permanent documentation of nursing process. The patient's health care record is a chronological record of his progress in relation to specific problems, accounting for data collected, the analysis of that data and evaluation of the patient's progress, and planning to facilitate further progress.

References

1. E. Becknell and D. Smith. System of Nursing Practice. F. A. Davis Co., 1975, p. 4
2. Data base for infants. C. S. Mott Children's Hospital, Pediatric Nursing Service, University of Michigan, Ann Arbor, 1979
3. K. Gebbie and M. A. Lavin. Classifying nursing diagnoses. American Journal of Nursing, Feb 1974, p. 252
4. M. Gordon. The concept of nursing diagnosis. Nursing Clinics of North America, Sept 1979, p. 490
5. C. Roy. A diagnostic classification system for nursing. Nursing Outlook, Feb 1975, p. 91

Additional Recommended Reading

K. S. Abrams, R. Neville and M. C. Becker. Problem-oriented recording of psychosocial problems. Archives of Physical Medicine and Rehabilitation, July 1973, p. 316

J. Atwood and S. R. Yarnall, eds. The problem-oriented record. Nursing Clinics of North America, June 1973, p. 213

M. Bertucci, M. Huston and E. Perloff. Comparative study of progress notes using problem-oriented and traditional methods of charting. Nursing Research, Jul/Aug 1974, p. 351

J. T. Bloom, et al. Problem-oriented charting. American Journal of Nursing, November 1971, p. 2144

L. S. Bootoy, et al. Documenting Patient Care Responsibly. Intermed Communications, Inc., 1978

M. K. Crabtree. The problem-oriented system. The Michigan Nurse, January 1974, p. 8

M. Durand and R. Prince. Nursing diagnosis: process and decision. Nursing Forum, Vol. V, no. 4, 1966, p. 50

B. W. Gallant and A. M. McLane. Outcome criteria: a process for validation at the unit level. Journal of Nursing Administration, January 1979, p. 14

M. Gordon, ed. Implementation of nursing diagnosis. Nursing Clinics of North America, September 1979, p. 483

B. Henderson. Nursing diagnosis: theory and practice. Advances in Nursing Science, October 1978, p. 75

F. Howard and P. I. Jessop. Problem-oriented charting — a nursing viewpoint. The Canadian Nurse, August 1973, p. 34

J. W. Hurst and H. K. Walker, eds. The Problem-Oriented System. Medcom Press, 1972

M. A. Lavin and K. M. Gebbie. Reflections on nursing diagnosis. The Missouri Nurse, June 1973, p. 10

J. C. McCloskey. The problem-oriented record vs. the nursing care plan: a proposal. Nursing Outlook, August 1975, p. 492

M. McGugin et al. POR and you: how to make POR work for your Pediatric Nursing Service, C. S. Mott Children's Hospital, University of Michigan, 1976

P. Mitchell and J. Atwood. Problem-oriented recording as a teaching-learning tool. Nursing Research, Mar/Apr 1975, p. 99

M. E. Nicholls and V. G. Wessells, eds. Nursing Standards and Nursing Process. Contemporary Publishing, Inc., 1977

J. S. Rothberg. Why nursing diagnosis? American Journal of Nursing, May 1967, p. 1040

J. B. Walter, G. P. Pardee, and D. M. Molbo, eds. Dynamics of Problem-Oriented Approaches: Patient Care and Documentation. J. B. Lippincott Co., 1976

GROWTH AND DEVELOPMENT

10

by Jo Joyce Tackett, BSN, MPHN

> . . . I look upon your creation in amazement
> For we are indeed fearfully and wonderfully made.
> All its secret, silent machinery —
> The meshing and churning —
> What a miracle of design!
>
> Alton Ochsner[12]

WHY STUDY GROWTH AND DEVELOPMENT? NURSING IMPLICATIONS

Anyone who has watched a sleeping infant, studied closely the determined way a toddler forces his whole body into mobility, listened attentively to the conversation of two preschoolers at play, tolerated the teasing and chiding of an active, alert school-age child, or cried in his heart over the tense struggle of an identity-seeking adolescent cannot deny the miraculousness of the fascinating beings called Homo sapiens. Researchers and professionals in the helping arts attest to the intricacies and complexities that interplay to create a whole being who is totally unique and yet exists because of his commonalities in living and dying with others of his species.

By studying these commonalities in our existence, we can better understand how we grow, develop and mature into unique individuals who seek to achieve our full potential. But the reward of knowledge alone is not adequate reason for studying human development. As health professionals, nurses must sometimes intervene in this growth and development relationship in order to deal with disease, abnormality or other factors threatening health, and we ought to know with what we are interfering. Nurses and other health professionals are not only expected to understand human developmental processes, but are also expected to capably treat and prevent those conditions that might adversely affect these processes. Therefore, studying human development helps the nurse to know what to expect of individuals at any given age. Such knowledge is needed for the nurse to develop and deliver a plan of care that is age-appropriate and relevant to the needs of the client. Understanding human developmental processes also helps us see the reasons why many conditions or illnesses are more prominent in certain age groups. Nurses working with childbearing and childrearing families require developmental knowledge to accurately teach parents, so that parents can contribute positively to their children's attainment of optimal growth and development.

The primary concern of the nurse working with children and their families involves the individual needs of that child-family unit in the development of life competencies (i.e., successful achievement of individual and family group tasks). Any factors enhancing or altering development of those competencies become essential aspects of the nursing assessment and contribute to the nursing diagnosis and plan of care. The foremost question to be considered by the nurse is, "How does this factor (health state, physical trait, temperament, parental disharmony, social condition) affect this child's ability to (1) perform physically and biologically, (2) learn and think, (3) perceive and accept himself in a way that allows him to relate socially to others,[1] and how does this factor affect his family's ability to support him in these tasks?" This approach maintains the focus on the whole child, including the family that is a part of his wholeness.

THEORIES ABOUT MAN AND HIS ENVIRONMENT

Research on growth and development has primarily arisen out of three basic theories about man and his environment, commonly referred to as developmental models.

The model reflected in the works of theorists such as Skinner and Pavlov is the *mechanical mirror model* or *mechanistic world view*.[9] This model compares people to machines, reacting to events in their environment rather than initiating them. This view perceives man as being shaped entirely by his environment. Cause and effect can be predicted. It is the quantity of stimuli that produces change in man, and his development is continuous. In other words, a family or an individual repeats a given behavior or practice because some factor in the external environment prompts or reinforces that action, or both.

The *organic lamp model* or *organismic world view* defines people as active organisms who, by their own actions, set in motion their unique development; they both initiate events and react to them.[9] Change is both quantitative and qualitative, is a fact of living and is experienced internally. This model defies the possibility of predicting cause-and-effect relationships. The theories of Piaget and Kohlberg (discussed later in this chapter) are based on this view that the environment does not cause development but that it can affect how easily developmental progress is achieved. Development is perceived in this model as discontinuous, involving a set sequence of phases or stages (also referred to as *stage theory*).

The *psychoanalytic world view* is a third model, which is reflected in the theories of Freud and Erikson.[9] This model sees the individual as being continually torn between activity and passivity and between natural instincts and social constraints. The way in which this conflict is resolved determines the person's personality development. Simply stated, this view reports man as a reactive organism who passes through stages of development. In reality the whole person is probably reflected in all these models, depending upon his behavior in a given situation and at a given point in time.

DEFINING GROWTH, DEVELOPMENT AND MATURATION

Growth and development are not synonymous terms, but in the healthy child these two processes do parallel each other and are interdependent in function. The ways the whole child changes over time are both *quantitative* and *qualitative* in nature.

Growth comprises quantitative change, involving an increase in size of the whole child or in size and number of any of his parts. The change is measurable — usually either in centimeters or inches (height), kilograms or pounds (increased organ mass, weight), or by an increase in numbers present (increased vocabulary, increased number of relationships with others, increased number of physical skills able to perform) — and is easily observed or studied.

Qualitative changes are the "leaps" (increased skill or capacity) in function that result from mastering a series of smaller steps.* The qualitative component, called *development*, is more complex and less easily measured or studied.

The timing of these quantitative and qualitative changes is to some extent controlled by a maturational process that involves the child's biological ability and environmental opportunity to relinquish previous functions and learning or to integrate new functions and learning into his existing structure for more mature performance, or to perform both these actions. For example, the child relinquishes the palmar grasp in favor of the more manipulative pincer grasp that will allow better investigation of his environment, but not until he has developed the biological structures — increased muscle cells and nerve cell specialization — necessary to perform this action.

PRINCIPLES EVIDENT IN GROWTH AND DEVELOPMENT

Primary to a discussion of the principles or commonalities in human development is the concept of the child as an open system who receives from and gives to his environment and who has adaptive potential (ability for both qualitative and quantitative changes) within the limits of his inheritance. A second relevant concept is that an interactive heredity and environment shape that open system into a unique human being. Another important concept is that self-realization or self-actualization (i.e., achieving one's potential) is the ultimate goal of human development.

---

*Piaget's steps of progressive intelligence, Erikson's stages of progressive sociability, Kohlberg's steps to adult morality, Freud's steps of sexuality formation illustrate qualitative change.

Derived from these concepts are some commonalities of development, typically referred to as *principles of growth and development*.

Development Is Complex

Human development is a continuous, irreversible and complex process that is lifelong. Inherent in this developmental process is aging, which, interestingly enough, is most rapid during the fetal stage, and is also lifelong.

Development Has Direction

Human development is progressive and orderly (i.e., follows a sequence). It proceeds:
1. From simple to complex
   This is exemplified in the child's ability to make basic "cooing" sounds before he learns to refine those sounds into speech.
2. From general to specific
   Illustrative of this principle is the infant's acquisition of palmar grasp before he learns the finer control of pincer grasp.
3. From head to toe (cephalocaudally)
   An example is the fact that an infant gains neck and head control before he can control the movements of his trunk and limbs (Fig. 10-1).
4. From inner to outer (proximodistally)
   This principle is similar to the cephalocaudal principle in that the child learns control of the near structures before the structures farther away from his center. He is able to coordinate his arms to reach for an object before he has learned the hand and finger coordination necessary to grasp it (Fig. 10-1).

Development Is Predictable

The orderly sequence of development is invariable and although the precise age for the sequential steps to occur varies for each child, there is a general chronology that involves wide norm ranges to allow for these individual differences. For example, the age range for learning to walk is usually given as 9 to 15 months, with the average age being 12 months.

A child will usually follow a consistent pattern with respect to either an early or late rate of development. Therefore, deviation from his own pattern may be more indicative of a problem than his conformance to the norm or lack thereof.

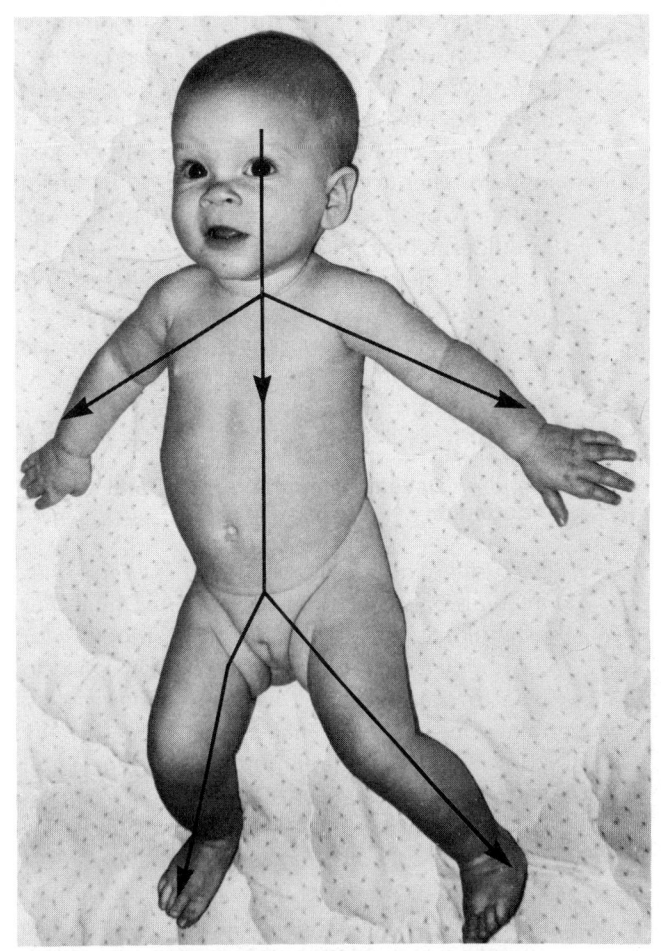

Figure 10-1 The development of muscular control proceeds from head to tail (cephalocaudal), from the center of the body to its periphery.

However, the characteristics of growth and behavior at each age, and the maturational changes that occur with increasing age, bear obvious resemblances among children. The child cannot walk until he has mastered creeping, regardless of whether he follows an early or late pattern for achieving these characteristic behaviors or changes.

Children Develop Uniquely

Each child has his own genetic potential for growth and development that cannot be exceeded but may be deterred or modified at any stage in the sequence. For example, although intellect is primarily set by genetic inheritance, a child's experiences during the critical periods will either stimulate or discourage his intellectual achievement. If he is beset by poor nutrition, confined to his crib or playpen and offered few interactions with the people in his environment, he may not achieve intellectually, regardless of his genetic potential. Conversely, offered opportunities to experience his world from a number of positions (crib, playpen, floor, shoulder, tabletop), sustained on a nutritionally balanced diet and provided with regular opportunities to interact (be spoken to, played with, cuddled) with the important people and objects in his environment, the child is on his way to achieving his intellectual potential.

Children Develop Through Conflict and Adaptation

Each stage in the developmental sequence has intervals of equilibrium and disequilibrium. For example, at 2 years life is running smoothly for the toddler. He has a calm willingness to do what he can but does not try too hard to do things he cannot manage. But at 2½ his life poses marked disequilibrium. He becomes rigid and inflexible, demanding rituals and routines that must not be altered. He shuttles endlessly between any two extremes of a situation.

Conflict arises out of the child's motivation to master his environment and his lack of the competency needed for that mastery. Equilibrium exists before the new environmental or maturational stimulus occurs that demands adaptation by the child, and after the child has developed the necessary competence to adapt to the stimulus. Disequilibrium exists in the interval from recognition of and desire to master (adapt to) the new stimulus until mastery is accomplished. Growing children repeatedly evidence their strength and competence to adapt and achieve if their environment gives them at least some support.

Development Involves Challenges

Social expectations for each developmental stage exist, called *developmental tasks*. The task of each stage is to overcome the problem or challenge that confronts a child because of his age. Delay or failure in task achievement makes further development more difficult. Examples of developmental tasks are: (1) Erikson defines the infant's emotional-social task as learning to trust; (2) Piaget defines the school-age child's intellectual task as learning to use symbols and the concepts they represent; (3) a physical task of the toddler is learning to walk without aid.

Development Requires Practice and Energy Investment

Developmental energy flow is invested most heavily in certain competency areas at any given time, so that different aspects of development progress at different rates. Earlier achievements in one competency area may even regress temporarily while some other aspect of that competency area or another competency area is being stimulated, because a strong preoccupation exists to practice and perfect the skill required for mastery of the newly confronted stimulus. For example, during infancy the central focus of energy is on sensorimotor and physical growth. The toddler's energy concentration is invested in his developing selfhood and body control, while the preschooler's investment is in language development. Cognitive development and sociability require the bulk of the school-age child's energy and the teenager exerts massive energy into development of his sexual and social identity and capacity for intimacy.

In summary, human development, although complex, is continuous, follows an orderly sequence and general chronological pattern, involves task mastery, and requires concentrations of energy upon the task confronting the child at that particular time. However, task achievement in one competency area is not accomplished in isolation but interacts upon skills in other competency areas simultaneously to result in characteristic ways of behaving.

FACTORS INFLUENCING GROWTH AND DEVELOPMENT

Anyone who has in some way been involved with the study of children has had exposure to the nature versus nurture controversy that has been a key developmental issue of the nineteenth and twentieth centuries. No one really knows the total effect of each of these forces upon developmental process and, considering the complex, open system of the human organism, perhaps the more crucial question is how these two forces interact with one another to affect development. One thing studies have revealed is that these forces are interactive with the individual organism to influence development.

It is generally accepted that nature sets the limits on potential development, while nurturing forces present the realm of opportunities or possibilities for attaining that potential. Research has demonstrated that physical development is primarily influenced by natural forces and that long-term deprivation in nurturing is required to interfere with physical development.[9] However, research to date also has shown that intellectual and emotional-social development, although controlled by nature with regard to ultimate capacity for development, is much more influenced by nurturing forces (i.e., environmental stimuli), allowing the individual either to maximize his genetic (natural) potential or allow it to depreciate.[12]

Natural Forces

The primary natural force in human development is one's inherited genetic endowment. One's genetic makeup, established at conception, determines one's sex and racial characteristics and many physical attributes such as eye color, hair color and stature. Behavioral geneticists have conducted research that strongly supports the argument for the existence of some biologically inherited behaviors, particularly ones related to temperament.[11, 13] Fairly well documented examples are the individual's personality traits related to degree of neuroticism (general nervousness or fearfulness), whether one tends to be introverted or extroverted, one's aggressiveness or shyness, one's tendency for moodiness and even one's smiling response.[5] Heredity also determines glandular action, and it is known that hormonal activity is necessary to stimulate growth at various stages in development.

Because of the virtually infinite number of gene combinations possible in the creation of a human being, this means that in organisms as complex as man, heredity represents not only the passing on of certain characteristics but also the transmission of individual uniqueness.

The genetic history of several generations goes into the genetic makeup of a given child, so the nurse who is evaluating the genetic forces at play in a child's development should include in the child's health history an assessment of inheritable factors present two, three or more generations before him. Her interpretation of those inheritable factors requires that the nurse have a basic understanding of the principles of inheritance.

Genetics Genes are small particles in the nuclei of the male and female reproductive cells which carry the information that establishes each characteristic of an organism and transmit that characteristic across the generations. Genes occur in pairs, one each obtained from the mother and the father during the reproductive process. Each pair of the thousands of genes received controls some specific cellular function. Each pair of genes is located along rod-shaped chromosomes, like a string of beads, within the reproductive cell. The location of each gene set on the chromosome is called its *locus*. The interaction that occurs between each pair of genes collectively produces the unique person.

Human beings have 46 chromosomes (23 sets), 44 of which are autosomes and two of which are sex chromosomes. The genes from each parent that share the same locus on the chromosome are said to be homologous because they possess codes for the same trait. However, since each gene of the pair comes from a separate parent, the genetic information carried by each is often for a different effect. For example, a pair of genes are homologous (at the same locus on the chromosome) for eye color. But one gene of the pair may carry genetic information for blue eyes, while the other gene carries information for brown eyes. Whenever the gene pair carry genetic material for different effects, the two genes compete for expression. Which of the two genes will express itself (become the visible characteristic) depends on which is dominant over the other. The gene that expresses itself is therefore referred to as the *dominant gene* of the pair, while the one that remains hidden or unexpressed is referred to as a *recessive gene*. Dominance is relative, however, since a gene may be dominant in combination with one gene but recessive in combination with another.

When a set of homologous chromosomes have a gene pair that carry information for the same trait effect (e.g., both are for blue eyes), the genes are *homozygous*. When the information carried by each gene of the pair is different (e.g., one for blue eyes and one for brown eyes), they are *heterozygous*. Characteristics that are manifested only when the gene pair is homozygous are considered recessive traits. In pairs that are heterozygous, the dominant gene is expressed so that the characteristic manifested is considered a dominant trait.

Genetic traits have variable expressivity. In other words, several family members may have the same trait but the trait is more obvious or, in the case of inherited disease, more severe in some members than in others. For example, several family members may have brown eyes, but some have *dark* brown eyes while others have *very light* brown eyes, or some gradation of brown in between these two shades. Several family members may have the same disease, but some are severely affected while others are only mildly affected. The reasons for this phenomenon are not clearly understood at this time.

Genetic traits may also be *pleiotropic*. This means that the genes for a certain characteristic set a series of secondary characteristics into action that are different from the primary effect of that specific gene. For example, a child with genetic information for phenylketonuria (PKU) will produce a secondary characteristic of very light blond hair regardless of the genetic traits for hair color inherited from his parents.

Genetic diseases can be categorized by the hereditary factors that cause them. *Chromosomal aberrations* occur in which there is an abnormality in the structure or number of chromosomes inherited. In a structural aberration there is a loss, increase, rearrangement or exchange of genes within a chromosome. Aberrations in chromosomal number result in the gain or loss of a chromosome. Deviations in chromosome number are identified by the suffix "-somy." Trisomies are the most frequently occurring and involve the addition of one chromosome to a pair. Usually these aberrations are apparent in the physical characteristics of the child, as in Down's syndrome (trisomy 21), although chromosomal analysis is sometimes required when the aberration is not physically manifested. The aberration is thought to occur during germ cell formation in the female, since the female is born with all the ova that ripen through the reproductive cycle, while the male produces fresh sperm continually. Numeric or structural aberrations may occur in either autosomes (e.g., Down's syndrome) or sex chromosomes (e.g., Turner's syndrome). When a characteristic that has never before existed appears in a family, the etiology is often a *mutation*. A mutation involves a change in the genetic material of a gene, usually for no identifiable reason. Once the mutation occurs, it persists and is transmitted through the generations. Hemophilia is the classic example of a disorder that originates from a gene mutation.

Still other genetic diseases are *multifactorial* — they are caused by a complex interaction between genetic and environmental factors, as in diabetes mellitus. Most structurally manifested defects are associated with a dominant gene and are manifested when the child inherits this gene from a heterozygous parent. Conversely, most metabolically manifested defects are caused by recessive genes, in which case the defect is manifested when the child inherits a homozygous gene from each parent. Structural defects occur more often than metabolic defects, but metabolic defects are usually more severely manifested.

Mendelian genetics explains four modes of inheritance from gene activity: (1) autosomal dominant, (2) autosomal recessive, (3) X-linked dominant, and (4) X-linked recessive.

Autosomal dominant inheritance involves the presence of a deviant gene on an autosome that dominates over a normal gene. The trait that this dominant gene defines is manifested by any person who possesses that gene in his genetic makeup, regardless of whether it is homozygous or heterozygous. It can be traced vertically through past generations (positive family history). Males and females are affected with equal frequency and, unless the condition is caused by a fresh mutation, persons who inherit this condition have a parent affected by that condition. Unaffected children of the affected parent(s) will not have the abnormal gene and will produce unaffected offspring. Half of the children of a heterozygous affected parent will receive the gene and be affected. (See Appendix I for a diagrammatic presentation of autosomal dominant inheritance with various mate combinations.) Some autosomal dominant disorders are so severe that affected persons are infertile or die young so that the condition soon becomes extinct in the family.

Autosomal recessive inheritance is manifested only when a person receives the recessive deviant gene from both parents (i.e., is homozygous for the trait) or is a carrier (i.e., is heterozygous for the trait) who can transmit the deviant gene but does not display evidence of the disorder because a normal gene dominates. The probability of homozygous mating is increased in mating between blood relatives, which explains the greater incidence of diseases such as PKU in societies that permit consanguineous marriages, such as in the Amish group. Males and females are affected with equal frequency. There is seldom any evidence of the trait in previous generations (negative family history). (See Appendix I for a diagrammatic presentation of autosomal recessive inheritance with various mate combinations.)

In *intermediate* inheritance the heterozygous recessive carrier has equal expression by both the normal and the recessive gene. In this situation, some symptoms or characteristics of the disorder are manifested but at a level that is relatively harmless and does not alter life expectancy as occurs when the person is homozygous (affected by the disease). An example of intermediate inheritance is the individual who possesses one gene for sickle cell anemia (is heterozygous for the anemia — a carrier). Because there are minor manifestations similar to those expressed in persons affected with the disease, as in someone who is homozygous for the anemia because he has two recessive genes, this individual is described as having the "sickle cell trait," while homozygous persons who manifest the full consequences of the disease have sickle cell anemia.

In sex-linked inheritance patterns, transmission of a deviant trait will depend on the sex of the individual who possesses the gene, because genes in the X chromosome differ from those in the Y chromosome. Females have two X chromosomes with similar gene constitutions. Males, however, have one X and one Y chromosome. The genes in the X chromosome have no counterpart in the Y chromosome so that a characteristic carried on the X chromosome is *always* expressed in the male.

X-linked dominant inheritance is not currently associated with very many diseases. Vitamin D–resistant rickets is the most frequently identified disease of this type of inheritance. All affected children have an affected parent, thus a positive family history occurs. An affected male transmits the gene to all his daughters but none of his sons. An affected mother transmits the disease to half of her daughters and sons. Normal children of an affected parent will have normal children. Because the affected males have no corresponding normal gene to modify the effect of the dominant gene, they usually experience more severe manifestation of the disease than females. So far no inheritable features have been attributed to the Y chromosome except that of maleness. (See Appendix II for a diagrammatic presentation of X-linked dominant inheritance with various mate combinations.)

A number of serious conditions are associated with *X-linked recessive* inheritance, which is determined by the recessive gene on an X chromosome. Since males have no counterpart for the recessive gene on their single X chromosome, if the X-linked recessive gene is received, they will be affected. The affected male cannot transmit the disease to his sons, since they receive a Y chromosome from him, but he transmits the recessive trait on his X chromosome to all his daughters, making them carriers. Males are most often affected, because they require only one recessive X chromosome to manifest the disease. When X-linked recessive inheritance does occur in a female, it is usually much less severe due to X inactivation.* (See Appendix II for a diagrammatic presentation of X-linked recessive inheritance with various mate combinations.)

The nurse plays a major role in detecting hereditary forces that are detrimental to the health and development of children. Situations indicating a need for genetic counselling should be identified and appropriate intervention or referral initiated. The nurse's role in detecting and counselling in genetic disorders is addressed elsewhere in this book.

As more is discovered about the natural forces affecting development, the implications for practice in the health professions will expand, and an understanding of how these forces interact with nurturing will become increasingly important.

Nurturing Forces

Research is yielding increasing support to the idea that the external environment has a very significant effect upon one's overall development. In the fetal stage of development intra-

---

*In all cells only one X chromosome is active. The other(s) is somehow inactivated very early in the cell division process.

ALTERED PHYSICAL COMPETENCY
A toddler experiences immobility that interferes with walking achievement

ALTERS EMOTIONAL-SOCIAL COMPETENCY
Interference with walking decreases his autonomy to investigate a larger world

CONTINUED ALTERATION OF EMOTIONAL-SOCIAL COMPETENCY
Diminished self-esteem as skills for establishing selfhood continue underdeveloped or underutilized

ALTERS EMOTIONAL-SOCIAL COMPETENCY
Delay in intellectual development places the child progressively behind his peers in the development of social and independence skills

ALTERS INTELLECTUAL COMPETENCY
Limited opportunity for exploration slows cognitive development; a child this age learns by doing

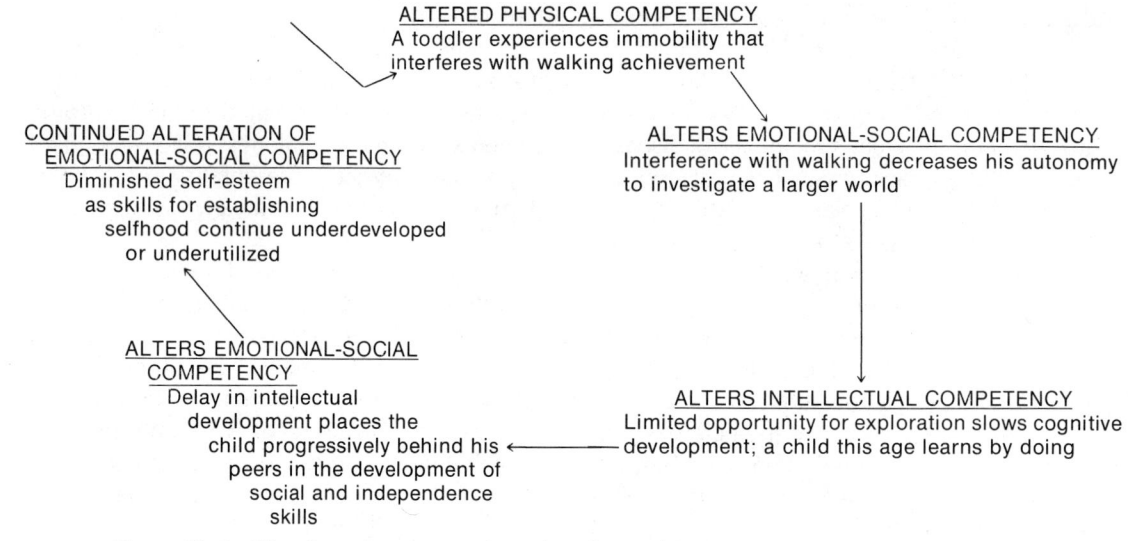

Figure 10-2 Alteration of one competency interferes with development of other competencies.

uterine conditions may exist that place development in jeopardy. Some obvious examples are nutritional deficits; malposition; maternal metabolic or endocrine imbalances; the impact of teratogenic agents such as maternal exposure to radiation, smoking or drug use during pregnancy and Rh incompatibility, to name a few.

Ordinal position in one's family has also been shown to have impact upon one's development. Exposure to older siblings fosters earlier and easier learning, particularly of motor, social and language skills. An only child usually has earlier intellectual development because of his constant exposure to adults but slower motor development because adults are doing things for him and he has no sibling to encourage his motor performance through active play. Youngest children are often slower in some areas of development (language, motor skills) because they have had less encouragement or opportunity to express themselves.

Exercise is influential because it stimulates muscular growth and reinforces emotional health.

Climate and season of the year also affect development. Climatic influences are secondarily related to sanitary problems posed by warm or temperate climates. Growth spurts are seasonally correlated; for example, height gains correlate positively with the coming of spring.

One's state of general health also has an impact upon developmental progression. Illness or injury with associated disability, nutritional impairment, immobility and energy diversion for recovery rather than learning all hamper progress in some facets of development.

Current research findings substantiate the very significant role of the social environment in developmental achievement.[7] Social input comes from a variety of sources. Parenting, including the quality of the parent-child relationship and management style, has been described as having the strongest impact upon development as a nurturing force. As the child grows older his siblings and, later, his peers have an increasingly greater impact. The school milieu contributes to his development in the form of skill training, cultural transmission and self-actualization. And of increasing concern today is the impact of mass media on development. A widely accepted belief is that parental guidance is required for the child to gain positive developmental benefits from mass media sources, particularly television. Cultural input* also contributes either constructively or deleteriously to development.

All of these components of the social environment are, however, redefined by the family itself, so that it is the "home culture" that ultimately influences a child's development, particularly during his early years.

---

*Cultural input refers to ethnicity, demographic setting, socioeconomic class, parental occupation, family structure.

CRITICAL PERIODS IN DEVELOPMENT

A third issue related to development is the *critical period hypothesis*. A critical period is a specific time frame during which certain environmental events or stimuli have their greatest impact upon a child's development. The time frame involved is that point when maximum capacity for a particular aspect of development is either first present or when the structures to be developed are undergoing their most rapid growth.

During these critical periods some form of minimal sensory stimulation is necessary for normal progression in development. If the stimuli are not introduced during this critical period, the task in question cannot be mastered, at least without much difficulty.[3] After this critical period the child can be totally unaffected by certain stimuli or resistant to them. For example, a fetus is not affected by maternally contracted rubella virus after the third month of fetal development. Deficits of appropriate sensory stimulation during the critical periods are cumulative and can progressively interfere with future development of other competencies besides the one competency involved during the critical period.[2] Figure 10–2 illustrates this relationship.

Conversely, sensory stimuli necessary to development of a particular skill or task that are exerted upon a child before the critical period will have negligible, if any, effect.[3] For example, an infant cannot learn to read regardless of how often he is exposed to the media that would produce reading skills, whereas a child at the right age and stage in his development has a "readiness" to read; that is, in his critical period he acquires reading skills fairly rapidly.

USING CHRONOLOGICAL AND COMPETENCY APPROACHES TO STUDY GROWTH AND DEVELOPMENT

As the discussion in this chapter has already implied, a child's development is a very complicated, intertwined process to study. To facilitate discussion and learning, this book is organized along chronological lines. Its content is presented in relation to the general chronological pattern with which researchers have found that growth and development tend to be associated.

The chronological division is somewhat arbitrary, but it is based upon the performance or competency criteria that signal change or progress from one developmental stage to another. It must be remembered that these chronological divisions and associated developmental stages are not so obviously divided in the real child's life. It is done here purely for convenience and ease of learning and discussion.

The chronological structure upon which this book is organized is defined as follows:

1. *Prenatal life* – period of life from conception to birth.
2. *Newborn* or *neonatal life* – period extending from birth through the first month of life.
3. *Infancy* – period beginning at the end of the first month of life and ending at one year of age.
4. *Toddlerhood* – period extending from one year through the thirty-sixth month of life.
5. *Preschool years* – period extending from the beginning of the third year to the end of the fifth year of life.
6. *School-age years* or *middle childhood* – period from the start of the sixth to the end of the eleventh year.
7. *Teenage* and *young adult years* – period from the beginning of the twelfth to the end of the twenty-first year of life.

Furthermore, the whole person is more easily understood if described in terms of broad categories. This book dissects the child's development into three facets of the self called *competencies*: physical, intellectual and emotional-social. Again, the division is arbitrary and rarely clear cut, since change in each developmental competency affects development in the other spheres as well.

The three competency areas described in this book are defined as follows:

1. *Physical competency* – This competency involves the child's ability to apply various motor, neurological and biological capacities to achieve steadily more mature self-care abilities requiring mobility and manipulative skills. Aspects of this competency include physical health, body build and configuration, size, strength, rate of motor, neurological and biological maturation and motor skill performance.
2. *Intellectual competency* – Development of language and reasoning to the point of mature abstract thought, perceptions and communication skills is the task in this competency area. Some aspects of intellectual competency are perceptual level, memory, problem solving

and reasoning ability, language skills, academic achievement and IQ.

3. *Emotional-social competency* – Development of an inner sense of security that is supported by self-awareness and acceptance, evidenced by the capacity to form productive interpersonal relationships with individuals and groups, is the goal in this competency area. Temperament, interpersonal relations skills, emotional adjustment, development of sexuality and morality are measures of this competency.

DEVELOPMENTAL THEORIES

It is the child's growing capacity to take in his world, rework experiences and give it out again in speech or song, craft or art, in all the activities in which men engage, that is the source of individuality.

Margaret Mead, From Family by M. Mead and K. Heyman, The Macmillan Co., 1965

Physical Competency

Intellectual and emotional-social competencies are both deeply rooted in and influenced by the capacities and needs of one's physical competency. Behind each developmental advance is a physical maturational or functional change. Likewise, a child's feelings and behavior are directly affected by his physical state and his current physical needs. An example of this is the peak period of misbehavior typical just prior to a child's usual mealtimes, when he has a physical need for food.

Because physical development is mostly quantitative, it is easily measured. Physical development also displays some conspicuous age uniformities, so it is a useful means of evaluating the relative health status of a child.* The level of physical competency achieved by a given child is compared with established norms or averages. These norms are defined from the mathematical average obtained by measuring many children of similar age on a given trait. The norm is more truly representative when the children measured are drawn from varying social and cultural groups. However, if a group of children digress significantly from the norm for a given trait, many of them should be measured for that trait to establish an average appropriate for them.

Growth charts for height and weight represent an example of norms established to determine physical competency. These grids are especially helpful when a pattern is obtained over a period of time for the child and compared for consistency in height and weight gains. Body weight has proved to be a useful index of nutritional status and correlates positively with height increases. For example, a child at 4 to 6 months is considered to have adequate caloric intake if his weight has doubled from what it was at birth. Beyond that age weight increases usually correspond closely to height increases.*

Head and chest circumferences are also measurements used to monitor physical development. Head circumference is usually a part of the physical appraisal until about age 4 or 5. This is because a composite of these measurements provides an estimate of the rate of brain growth for which the normal range is narrow for each age group. Brain and nerve cell growth and cell specialization are most rapid from birth to approximately 4 years of age, at which point there should be a significant slowing. Thus, this age span is considered a critical period for protein and caloric intake and for intellectual development.

Another measurement of physical development is skeletal or bone age. Skeletal growth is most rapid during infancy and adolescence. Norms have also been established for dental development and vital signs (temperature, pulse, respirations and blood pressure) for children at various ages, which are also measures of physical competency. Likewise, laboratory determinations important to routine health appraisal have established normative values for children at different ages. Normative ranges for vision and hearing performance at different ages also exist.

Nutritional patterns and intake needs at different ages also have been determined through averages. An estimation of the child's nutritional adequacy is an important aspect of the evaluation of physical competency.

Physical activity patterns associated with sleep, rest, exercise and elimination are also

---

*See Chapter 13, Physical Assessment, for examples of methods to evaluate physical competency.

significant features of physical competency for which normative ranges exist. However, these must be evaluated in context with the typical patterns of the family unit also.

In evaluating physical competency in those areas for which norms are not measurable, such as motor skills, screening tools are useful. The Denver Developmental Screening Test, which evaluates fine and gross motor development, is an example of such tools.

Specific norms of physical competency are presented in Chapter 13, in the age-related chapters on growth and development, and in the appendices.

Keen observation is required by the nurse assessing a child's physical development and physical needs. Children, especially those under 5 or 6,* have difficulty identifying and describing their physical discomforts or needs in ways adults can understand. Also, physical changes in children often occur quite suddenly and without any accompanying warning signs.

Obtaining accurate physical measurements from a crying, squirming infant or from actively protesting toddlers and preschoolers can be quite a challenge to even the most skilled nurse. However, knowledge of age-effective approaches to children, coupled with keen observational skills, usually yields successful evaluations.

The nurse caring for children should always keep in mind that the physical care she offers is not only supportive to the child's physical needs and development but is also a means of communicating support to his emotional-social and intellectual needs. The nurse's understanding of physical development and recognition of the alterations to physical development caused by stress — whether accidental (illness) or maturational (change in structure or function) or environmental (inadequate diet related to poor socioeconomic status of family unit) — will give direction for nursing interventions to prevent, minimize or remedy those stresses and for interventions to enhance the child's environment in ways that support healthy physical development.

Intellectual Competency

Intellect is a composite of skills, behaviors and adaptive abilities that makes it possible for an individual to adjust to new situations, to think abstractly and to profit from his experiences.[10] Although only ambiguous measures of intellect exist, it is demonstrable in the way a person solves problems and in how appropriate his response is in any given situation. By 1 year of age a child shows increasingly overt evidence of his developing mind. He is able to make some of his own decisions and can accept the decisions of others with whom he feels secure. He has achieved the ability to wait, because he can intellectually recognize the cues and sounds in his environment that assure him his needs will momentarily be met. His intellectual advances by 1 year have also taught him that he can anticipate certain routines from his environment. Evidence of a young infant's developing mind is seen when he registers the sounds of bottle preparation. He has learned that these sounds mean he will soon be fed, so he awaits the bottle in alertness rather than expressing his need by crying. He evidences here the rudimentary notion of cause and effect.

Intelligence, once believed to be genetically fixed, has been found, in recently reported longitudinal studies, to be fluctuating.[10] These findings illustrate the effect of environment on intellectual development and function. Neither can the maturational factor be ignored. Intellectual development cannot advance until the structures for thought exist to assimilate the experience. However, a variety of sensory and motor stimuli are needed before learning will occur. Learning cannot be accomplished for a child. He must do his own learning from his experiences with movement, touch, sounds, visual images and taste. It is from these manipulations that thoughts arise which are necessary for the formation of mental images. A child cannot intellectually categorize the mental image of a cow simply by being offered a verbal description of one. The image will not occur until he has at least seen a picture of a cow, or felt one or watched one in real life.

These findings on the effect of environment on intellect have resulted in a rising concern for the provision of primary or early learning opportunities. Evidence of this concern has been exemplified in the movements for development of Head Start or Get Set programs, preschool or kindergarten education, nursery schools, play programs for children during confinement and

---

*Language and intellectual development has not progressed enough before this age to allow clarity in verbalization of mental processes.

similar social structures whose aim is to counteract any sensory deprivations that a child might experience because of any sociocultural or physical limitations in his early life. Other programs that have arisen out of a recognition of the importance of motor and sensory stimulation early on are the stimulation programs for immature babies and infant-stimulation programs for any infant with signs of developmental lag.

Knowledge of intellectual development and intellectual needs of children at various ages is extremely valuable to the nurse who interacts with children. Understanding the child's level of intellectual thought and function helps the nurse to more meaningfully decipher a child's communications, to more accurately interpret his behaviors and the processes that motivate them and to realize more empathetically the meaning various experiences have for the child. This understanding should be demonstrated in the nursing interventions planned, the approach with which those interventions are offered and the age appropriateness of nurse-child communication. Because the nurse often deals with the child under circumstances that have placed limits on him and his environmental exposure, it is of utmost importance that the necessity for stimulating and interactional experiences be recognized and provided for as an essential aspect of nursing care.

Although most tests available for the measurement of predictive intellectual capacity or estimation of level of intellectual function are done by personnel in other health-related professions, the nurse should be familiar with existing tests and the cautiousness with which they must be interpreted.* She should also be aware of the variability of test results in young children and of the limited correlation that exists between results of these early tests and tests conducted later in the child's life, although more consistency usually exists after age 5.

The construct of the test will vary, depending upon the age of the child being evaluated. Performance type tests are usually used with infants and toddlers; the Denver Developmental Screening Test (DDST) is an example. Preschool and early school-age children who have not yet mastered reading cannot respond to the written tests offered literate school-age children. Young adults are usually given verbal tests. Any of these tests, however, are more fair measures of predictive capacity when interpreted in conjunction with achievement and school readiness tests.

The one individual who has perhaps contributed most toward our understanding of intellectual or cognitive development is the Swiss psychologist Jean Piaget. He and his Geneva colleagues, through a variety of ingenious studies, have derived the stage theory about children's intellectual activity and how it undergoes qualitative changes over the span of childhood. He stresses that throughout the hierarchy of gradual development, a variety of experiences must be available and active experiences must exist for learning to occur. Piaget's position is that the adaptation that occurs as a result of these two factors is the essence (i.e., the stimulus for development) of both intellectual and biological functioning. He further asserts that adaptation involves continuous twin processes, *assimilation* and *accommodation*. Assimilation is the process of incorporating new experiences or stimuli into one's current activity or way of thinking (making the unfamiliar seem familiar). Accommodation is the process of reaching out, responding to the requirements of the environment and allowing new ways of thinking to occur. Assimilation may occur without accommodation, but accommodation must always be preceded by assimilation. A child who sees a fire burning for the first time attaches meaning to that observation according to what he has perceived or what has impressed him, such as its brightness or redness — this is assimilation. He has now incorporated a visual image of fire and the properties of it that attracted his attention. This perception will tend to cause him to perceive other fires he sees in the same manner as he perceived the first, regardless of the actual characteristics of those fires. Then one time he reaches out to touch the fire and discovers it is hot. Through assimilation he now adds another perception and through accommodation his mental image of fire changes drastically. Both of these processes are ways the child goes about organizing his world by ordering and classifying his experiences. The end product of these processes, once organized in the child's mind, allows the child to alter old ways of thinking in order to solve new problems. Figure 10–3 illustrates the flow of the intellectual process for adaptation.

The following is an outline of the sequence

---

*See Chapter 13 for examples of intellectual measurement tools.

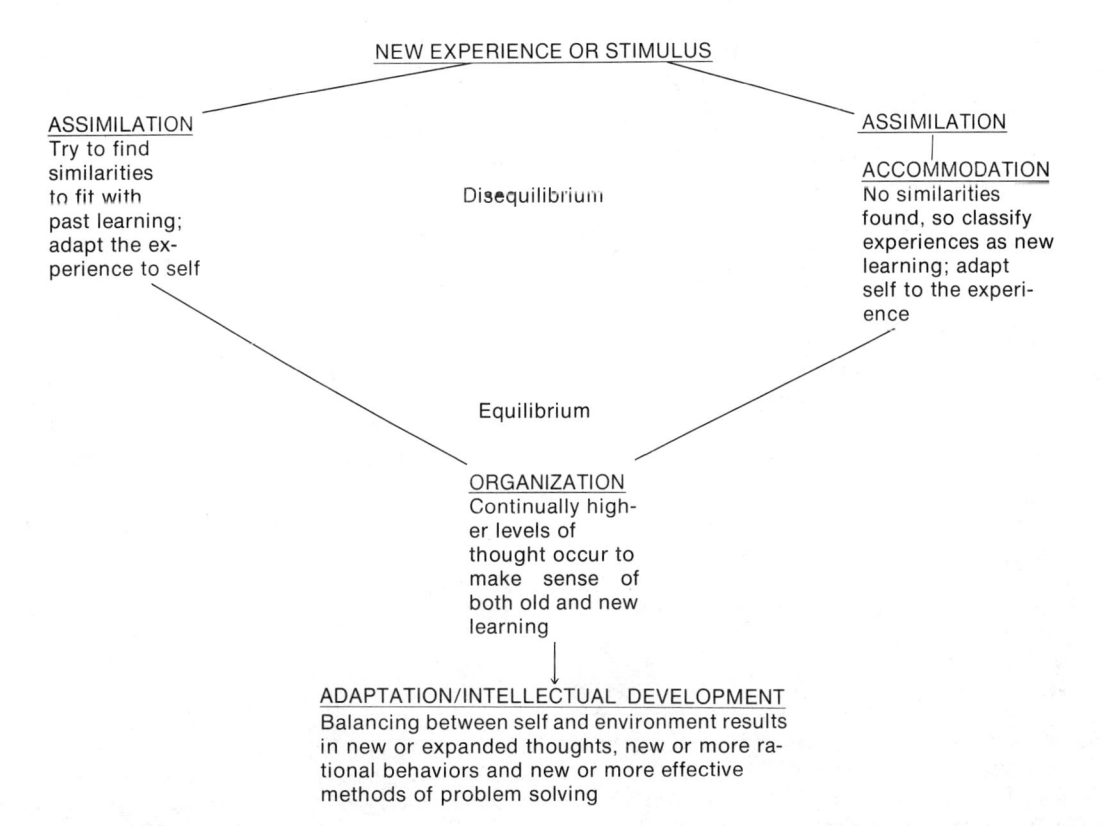

```
                    NEW EXPERIENCE OR STIMULUS
                   ╱                          ╲
    ASSIMILATION                                ASSIMILATION
    Try to find                                 ACCOMMODATION
    similarities        Disequilibrium          No similarities
    to fit with                                 found, so classify
    past learning;                              experiences as new
    adapt the ex-                               learning; adapt
    perience to self                            self to the experi-
                                                ence


                        Equilibrium
                   ╲                          ╱
                        ORGANIZATION
                        Continually high-
                        er levels of
                        thought occur to
                        make sense of
                        both old and new
                        learning
                              ↓
                    ADAPTATION/INTELLECTUAL DEVELOPMENT
                    Balancing between self and environment results
                    in new or expanded thoughts, new or more ra-
                    tional behaviors and new or more effective
                    methods of problem solving
```

Figure 10-3 Intellectual process in adaptation. (A diagrammatic presentation of Piaget's theory of intellectual development as an adaptive process.)

theorized by Piaget as the development of intellect.

Sensorimotor period – first 2 years of life

The child moves from neonatal birth reflexes to the construct of symbolic images. The task involved is mastery of coordinating simple sensorimotor activity. During this stage the child is dependent upon his body for self-expression and communication. He works to create an organized world that links his desires for physical satisfaction to his sensory experiences.

Stage 1 – Birth to 1 month
This stage is characterized by use of primitive reflexes and random body movements. Completely autistic, the child displays no awareness of self or of a world outside himself. The continual practice of these reflexes leads to their maturation and a sense of order for the neonate.

Stage 2 – 1 to 4½ months
Repetitive use of the primitive reflexes, coupled with neurological and physical maturation, tends to produce habits. These new behaviors, or habits, are learned by chance combinations of primitive reflexes and are repeated* purely for the pleasure they pro-

Primitive reflexes, accidentally produced (stage 1), are repeated for pleasure (stage 2) during the sensorimotor period.

*This initially reflexive behavior gradually becomes behavior that is consciously motivated, by about 2 months of age.

duce. For example, random arm movement places the infant's fist at his mouth at a moment he happens to be making sucking movements; he repeats this movement combination because he has discovered that sucking his fist is satisfying, thus the accidentally acquired behavior becomes a new sensorimotor habit.

Stage 3 – 4½ to 9 months

Eye-hand coordination is achieved during this stage. New behavior is repeated as a means of reproducing an interesting alteration in his environment that was initially discovered by accident. An example of this is when a rattle is placed in the infant's fist and random movement of his arm makes it rattle. He will repeat the arm movement over and over to recreate the noise that occurs — he has discovered he is a part of the action that produces a given result. He has also discovered play. The infant is beginning to associate events that occur close together, too. He recognizes that the position of cradling him at the breast means it is time to eat and he roots and makes sucking movements. In fact, his first notion of causality derives from recognizing that certain actions have certain results. He also gains a dim awareness of before-and-after in the sequence of events (i.e., a rudimentary notion of time). And recognizing the breast as a part of the sequence is evidence of a dawning recognition of symbols.

Stage 4 – 9 to 12 months

Coordinating of more complex behaviors occurs with development of perceptions. The baby will push aside obstacles or use sources close at hand to get what he wants. For example, he learns that by pulling toward him his mother's hand that has a bottle in it, he can bring the bottle into his reach. The beginning of object permanency is evident in the baby's search for vanished objects.

Stage 5 – 12 to 18 months

Rudimentary trial-and-error behavior occurs through active experimentation to discover different ways of getting results or solving simple problems. For example, he discovers that pulling at a blanket corner brings a toy into reach. These activities are evidence of beginning reasoning. Serious interest in the construction of objects fosters various manipulations of them — he pulls at a toy and pokes, pats and bites it. The concept of space is evident in the fact that the child now seeks an object in the place he saw it moved to, not in its original location. The fact that he continues to seek the nonvisible object indicates memory and retention.

Stage 6 – 18 to 24 months

The child can now form mental images that allow him to attach symbols to various experiences, usually involving only one or a few of its properties. He can think about a situation before acting and he can anticipate the possible movements of objects. He begins to see himself as separate from others in his environment, motivating emotional attitudes of competition and rivalry. Play becomes a purposeful means for discovery and not merely pleasure. Object permanency is now well developed. Intellectual function now allows him to imitate; usually the imitation is of actions. Imitation allows the child to begin to identify with his significant others by the end of this stage.

Preoperational period – 2 to 7 years

This period is characterized by egocentric* thought that is expressed in animism,† artificialism,‡ realism,§ and magic omnipotence.‖ The child at this state continues to seem illogical to adults. His task is to use language and memory to begin to understand the past, present and immediate future. He displays progressively more socialized behavior in this period as he moves steadily away from egocentric thought. The irreversibility of this stage evolves into a conception of reversibility in the concrete state. If a preschooler is asked if he has a brother, he will say "yes." If asked whether his brother has a brother, he will say "no."

Stage 1 (preconceptual stage) – 2 to 4 years

The child now forms mental images to stand for things he cannot see (symbolic thought), including their various properties. These concepts are reinforced through drawings, language, dreams and "make believe" and "imitative" play. Play involving language, action and symbolic imitation is this child's primary tool for adaptation and consumes most of his waking hours. Most play at this stage is

---

*The child sees things only from his own point of view.
†The child gives lifelike qualities to inanimate objects.
‡The child perceives that all things are designed by man.
§Everything is considered real by a child in this stage, even his dreams.
‖The child believes he can make things happen just by thinking them and that the world exists for him alone.

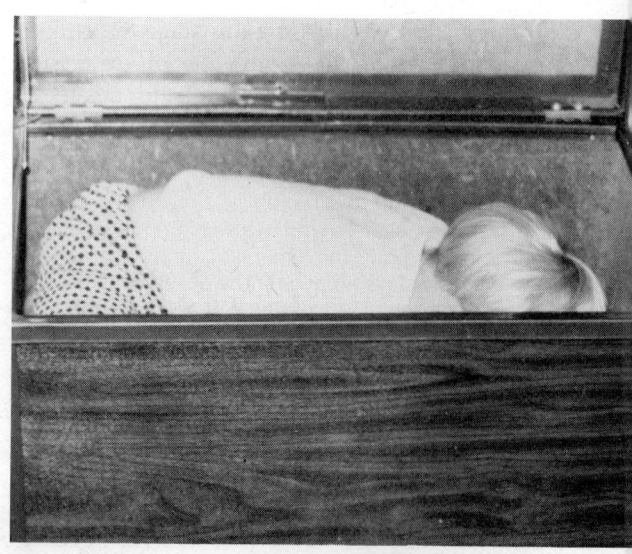

During the preoperational stage the child sees things only from his point of view. This child of 2½ thinks that because he cannot see anyone he cannot be seen.

parallel. Because of his egocentrism, he is engrossed in his own thoughts, feelings and experiences, so is not able to give attention to what someone else is doing or may want. His egocentrism is also operational in his perception of objects and events. For example, this child cannot visualize the other side of a box or the other side of a profile of a face. He wonders if the waves stop at night when he is asleep (i.e., all else in the world sleeps when he sleeps). He comprehends "doing what he is told" and relates it causally to pleasing his parents. He takes his instructions literally, so needs specific instruction in behaviors to be carried out; "be good" is not specific enough for him to enact.

Stage 2 (perceptual or intuitive stage) – 4 to 7 years

Prelogical reasoning appears, based on perceptions that do not acknowledge intrinsic aspects. Experiences and objects are judged by outside appearances and results. For example, given an equal number each of toothpicks and pencils, he will insist he has more pencils because they are bigger or because they take up more space. Nor can he accept that two 4 ounce glasses will both retain the same amount of water, because one is short and wide and the other is tall and narrow. Selective attention is also present in that the child can concentrate only upon one characteristic of an object at a time. For example, red balls cannot at the same time be rubber balls, even though his image of the object attributes to it multiple properties. This child begins to use words to express his thoughts, but during the first couple of years in this stage some of his thoughts are still acted out. During the first half of this stage the child still perceives anything that moves or is active as being alive. Play becomes gradually more social, demanding collective rules, organized games and fantasy enactments of the rules and values of his elders.

Concrete operational period – 7 to 11 years

The child at the beginning of this stage thinks and reasons with inductive logic; but by the end of this stage his thinking is deductive and his world shifts from "one of mythology to one of science," in which objects and events have explanations.[7] He can mentally perform tasks that previously had to be actually carried out. He learns to comprehend constancy,* reversibility,† and number conservation. He understands the value of rules and bases judgments on reason. The future and the abstract are still beyond his comprehension. He invests much energy into efforts to order and classify‡ the objects and experiences in his life, which is

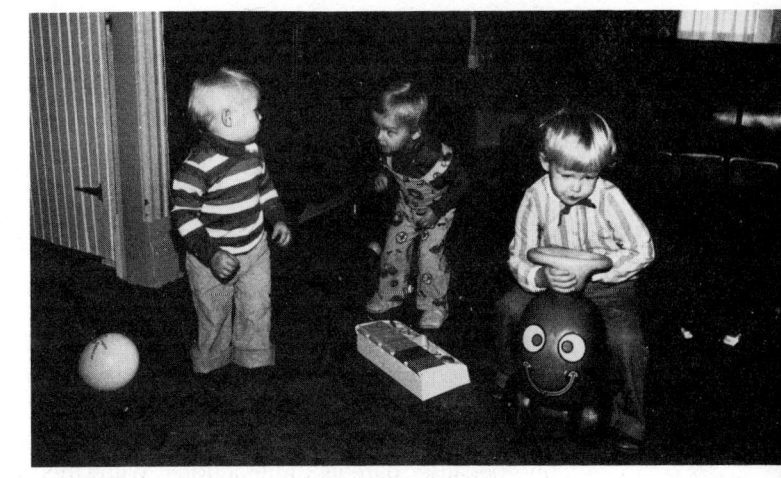

---

*This means that substances retain their properties regardless of change in shape or arrangements — also referred to as *conservation*.
†He realizes that the whole can be divided into its various parts and returned to a whole again or that if A equals B, B must also equal A.
‡He is able to sort objects into categories according to characteristics such as color or shape — also referred to as *seriation*.

Egocentric thought in the young child makes him frequently oblivious to other events and activities in his environment.

evidenced by his endless collections and scrapbooks. By the end of this stage he can comprehend that he belongs to a family, a city and a country simultaneously. Play and conversation now serve to establish progressive mutuality and equality in his relationships. Notions of animism and artificialism continue during this period.

Formal operational period – 11 years on

This stage is characterized by logical reasoning and the ability to think about the hypothetical and abstract. He can systematically analyze problems and arrive at their possible solutions. Relative realism exists by which he can separate what is thought from what is of the real world. Thought patterns incorporate the past, present and future.

Piaget's theories suggest ways that nurses should consider to better understand children's concepts about their bodies and their world and about health care experiences.

Development of Language Language is an important aspect of intellectual development that has only recently gained much attention by researchers and health professionals. Language development involves an increasingly complex expansion of receptive (comprehension of language) and expressive (speaking of language) skills over time. Social reinforcement of language efforts is extremely important, a fact that nurses should apply both in their own verbal interactions with children and in their child guidance instruction to parents.

GROWTH AND DEVELOPMENT

It is also known that receptive language skills are achieved earlier than expressive language skills, as is evidenced in the early toddler's ability to follow an instruction before he has learned the vocabulary skills to acknowledge that instruction. Nurses can apply this fact in their nursing care, too. Even an infant has a less stressful response to nursing procedures if he is spoken to before, during and for a brief interval after the procedure.

As with all other realms of development, language development is influenced by both nurturing and natural forces. Females evidence earlier language acquisition than males, probably because parents' interactions with their daughters tend to be more verbal, whereas their interactions with their sons more often are physical in nature.[6] Children in lower socioeconomic classes tend to acquire speech more slowly. Investigation has revealed this to be associated with the fact that their parents use less speech with these children, and when they do use speech, sentences are simple and offer little information.

Twins usually are slower in language achievement than are children born singly. This may be because there is less conversation between each of them and their mothers, most likely due to the fact that they are so close with each other that the mother addresses them as one.

Children's interaction with adults stimulates their language development, so when that interaction is diminished, language skills take longer to develop. Socioeconomic influences also exist, with language mastery occurring earlier in children from middle and upper class homes. Children from bilingual backgrounds may have difficulty with mastery of one or both languages. When children are expected to learn two languages at once with differing rules and letter pronunciation, they become confused. Learning a second language is usually easier once one language has been mastered well enough for the child to be comfortable with it. However, the single most influential factor is whether the child is receiving reprimand for his attempted usage of one of the languages.[6] Dialects (language variations) are structured by professional association (incorporation of professional jargon-terminology into language), age (adolescent slang is usually unique to that generation alone), geographic location (usually different inflections or pronunciations of the same words, called colloquialisms, from one locale to another), and socioeconomic class (more complex word forms are used in upper classes).

Three theories of language development seem equally viable to our current knowledge of language development.[3,5] Noam Chomsky's research supports an *innate theory* in which he depicts language development as genetically determined. Through this innate capacity of brain cells to act upon linguistic input, triggered by a system known as a *language acquisition device* (LAD), native language learning occurs. LAD enables the child to select and fit together properties of language and concrete experiences, eventually synthesizing them into language competency.

B. F. Skinner has applied *reinforcement theory,* also called behavior modification theory and stimulus-response theory, to language development. He supports the concept that language, as with all behavior, is acquired or learned as a result of one's environmental interactions through which behaviors that produce language are reinforced.

Social learning theory describes the development of language as a modelling process, resulting from the child's imitation of adult remarks and from his caretakers' expansion of his utterances. All three theories are most likely functioning in language development, each being a description of one facet of yet another complex component of human development.

All three theories are in consensus as to the approximate age range during which various stages of language acquisition occur. The progression of language development is seen in Table 10-1.

TABLE 10-1 AGE RANGES OF LANGUAGE DEVELOPMENTAL STAGES

Cooing stage	0-2 months
Babbling stage	2-6 months
First word, usually imitated	12-18 months
Rapid vocabulary acquisition	18 months-3 years
Open and pivot words	
Telegraphic sentences	
Steady word acquisition	3-5 years
Multiword sentences	
Basic mastery of language by end	
Progressively complex sentences	6-11+ years
Use of pronouns, proper nouns, prepositions	
Basic grammatical mastery by end	

TABLE 10-2 AN EXPANSION CHART OF THE EIGHT STAGES IN THE LIFE CYCLE OF MAN*

Stage	Approximate Age	Task and Subtasks	Task's Negative Counterpart	Significant Persons	Significant Supporting Experiences
Infancy (Oral)	0–1 yr	Sense of trust: realization of hope. Getting; tolerating frustration in small doses; recognizing mother as distinct from others and self	Mistrust	Maternal person	Consistency and quality in the care received
Toddler (Anal)	1–3 yrs	Sense of autonomy: realization of will. Child will try out new powers of speech; beginning acceptance of reality vs. pleasure principle	Shame and doubt	Paternal persons	Opportunity to attain some self-control based on a feeling of self-esteem rather than fear
Preschool (Oedipal)	3–6 yrs	Sense of initiative: realization of purpose. Questioning; exploring own body and environment; differentiation of sexes	Guilt	Basic family	Opportunity to do for himself with a balance between imaginative exploration and set limits
School age (Latent)	6–12 yrs	Sense of industry: realization of competence. Learning to win recognition by producing things; exploring, collecting; learning to relate to own sex	Inferiority	Neighborhood; School; same-sex peers; adult, nonparent idols	Opportunity to achieve success and recognition by engaging in manageable tasks in his social world so he can learn responsibility, social and work skills, cooperation and fair play
Adolescence (Mature)	12–? yrs	Sense of identity: realization of fidelity. Moving toward heterosexuality; selecting vocation; beginning separation from family; integrating personality (altruism, etc.)	Identity diffusion	Peer groups and out groups; models of leadership	Opportunity to establish who he is and what his purpose in society is to be through both private and social experiences that build self-esteem, foster increased need for independence and cushion his periods of feeling he does not belong
Late Adolescence and Young Adult	—	Sense of intimacy and solidarity: realization of love. Becoming capable of establishing a lasting relationship with a member of the opposite sex; learning to be creative and productive	Isolation	Partner in friendship, sex, competition, cooperation	Opportunity to experience close, shared relationships with individuals of own and opposite sex in which his own identity is verified and accepted and he accepts the identity of others
Adulthood	—	Sense of generativity: realization of care. Learning effective skills in communicating with and managing children; developing active interest in the next generation	Self-absorption and stagnation	Spouse; children; friends and work associates	Opportunity for involvement in activities that aroused concern for and advocacy for the next generation
Late Adulthood	—	Sense of integrity: realization of wisdom. Reconciling life accomplishments; learning to accept death; putting life in order; accepting retirement without quitting life	Despair	Spouse; children and grandchildren; friends	Opportunity to be acknowledged for life accomplishments by self, children, peers in a manner that looks at what was achieved rather than what was not so that end of life can be dealt with gracefully and peaceably

*Based on Erikson: Childhood and Society,[2] and Maier: Three Theories of Child Development.[5]

Emotional-Social Competency

A child's personality is the integration of feelings, attitudes and relationships as expressed by his behavior patterns. The adult measure of a healthy personality (i.e., the goal of emotional-social development) is one's capacity to love, to achieve and to become interdependent in function. And yet emotional-social development is not something that has been mastered by adulthood. It is, rather, a process that unfolds throughout the individual's lifetime, with each stage of life having its own tasks to be mastered and the leftover tasks of other life stages to be re-resolved.

Erikson's theory on the psychological development of man illustrates this lifelong struggle for emotional-social equilibrium. Table 10–2 illustrates his eight stages, the approximate age at which each task or crisis is experienced, the negative counterpart of unsuccessful task mastery and the significant interpersonal relationships and experiences in the environment of the person needed to support him in his task accomplishment. Erikson's theories descend from Freud's teachings on personality and sexual development. To show the relationship, Freud's stages are listed in parentheses with Erikson's stages.

Erikson stresses that the negative counterparts to each stage's task are never completely conquered but must be re-tackled at various times throughout life; however, it is healthy if favorable mastery exists most of the time and if compensations are healthy that are used when mastery totters.

Illness or accident can compound the problems confronting a child who is already at the peak of a psychological crisis. When the nurse is a part of the child's environment she can support his development if she knows the task he is facing. Regression to a previous task level, or reversion in the direction of the negative counterpart of a task level currently confronting the child, is common in children (and parents) during extreme or continued stress. The nurse should respect the individual's need to regress, help the child and his parents to accept that fact and the accompanying increased dependency, support them as they rework those tasks and provide an environment that fosters a return to their age-appropriate tasks.

As Erikson's model illustrates, parents too are in the process of developing and may require assistance from nurses in (1) building constructive relationships with each other and with their children, (2) feeling satisfaction and confidence in parenting skills, (3) learning to cope with the stresses confronting their children and in knowing their responsibility in helping the child manage those stresses.

Another component of a child's emotional-social development is his sexuality development. Although a child's sex is determined genetically at conception, his total sexuality is influenced by his developmental progress in all three competency areas (physical, intellectual, emotional-social). His sexuality also affects development of those competencies. Sexuality is a part of a person's everyday living behavior, taught to him more by the attitudes of those around him than by any specific information given. Sexuality development entails both the social and sexual aspects of one's biological gender. It is the attitudes and values learned from the significant role models in one's environment, the sexual orientation that results from the behavioral reinforcements one receives as one grows, and the sex role preference one acquires that eventually determine masculinity or femininity and whether one is heterosexual, homosexual, or bisexual.[3, 8] During infancy and early childhood biological changes in the genital and hormonal systems are few. However, significant differences in behavior do appear between male and female children as early as the first year of life, primarily as the result of sex typing* and parenting influences.

According to Freudian theory† the child experiences oral, anal, phallic and latency periods in psychosexual development. The first year of life, Freud proclaimed, is *orally* dominated, with all feelings and activities being focused on and expressed by the mouth. The toddler years are focused on control and expression via the child's anal region, with toilet training being a primary issue during the *anal stage*. The preschool years find the child's libido expression focused on the genital region and his general intrusive behavior toward his environment depicts this *phallic stage*. The sexual feelings and drives arising from his genital interests place him at conflict in his relations with his parents.* *Latency* describes the period of sexual development experienced by the school-age child. He has discovered that a sexual relationship with his parent is not plausible and turns his interests away from sexual concerns, investing his energy instead into the tasks of socialization. By the end of early childhood core gender identity has solidified and, if any problems exist in this realm of development, they are usually attributable to socioculturally perpetuated sex myths, misconceptions or gender identity disturbances evolving from home settings that give the child negative feedback about his gender.[14] Adolescence represents the period for development of *sexual maturity*, established biologically by means of widespread anatomical, hormonal and physiological changes. However, the adolescent usually finds himself "in a bind" in which he has a new set of sexual functions but is told he must wait for adulthood to enjoy them; conflicts in sexuality during this period usually arise out of that bind.

A third component of emotional-social development is moral development. Morality is composed of developmental tasks in two areas. The child must achieve a realistic acceptance of his social responsibility. He must also integrate personal principles of justice and reciprocity that are based on empathy, mutual respect and regard for the integrity and rights of others.

One of the leading theorists in the area of moral development is Lawrence Kohlberg.† He states that moral development is prefaced by the child's ability to reason, thus moral development follows a sequence that corresponds with the development of intellect. Kohlberg's model

---

*Sex typing means treating a child in certain ways because of the sex he is.
†Although the validity of Sigmund Freud's theory on personality and sexual development is currently being questioned, it is included in this text since it is the most complete theory presently available on the topic.

---

*This conflict is depicted in the Oedipus complex in the male, in which he loves his mother and his father is his competition, and by the female Electra complex in which she loves her father and her mother is the competitor.
†Because Kohlberg and Piaget have very similar theories about moral development, only one is discussed.

describes three phases of moral development. In the first phase, *preconventional* or *premoral morality* (4 to 7 years), children perceive rules as absolute and unalterable. This perception is congruent with the intellectual egocentrism and realism of children this age. A punishment and obedience orientation prompts acceptable moral behavior at this phase. This "do what's right or be punished" attitude, coupled with a naive instrumental hedonism (doing right earns one favor or rewards), makes the child in this phase fairly compliant to adult-set rules.

The *conventional morality* phase (7 to 11 years) is based on the child's perception of rules as existing for the good of all, to preserve order and to protect people. The child in this phase complies with rules because of his desire to please or help others and to maintain approval as a "good" child, which helps him to avoid the feelings of guilt he experiences by not "being good."

Principled morality (12 years on), the last phase in Kohlberg's schema, is the period when the individual accepts rules on the basis of his own judgments of what is universally ethical and on the basis of his personal conscience. His moral conduct is prompted by (1) a sense of obligation to social contract and democratic law and (2) a desire to avoid loss of respect among his peers and in the wider community.

Temperament is yet another facet of emotional-social development that needs to be discussed. A behavioral style that makes unique one's approach to people and situations, temperament is bound in those genetic or constitutional traits that cause individuality.[13] The characteristics of one's temperament are evidenced from birth and are predictive of one's adult personality. Although the traits that make up one's temperament may become less prominent over time, the chances of actually averting them is slim, and the fact that they continue to exist will be evident as they reappear during new or stressful situations.[13] Whether the behaviors typical of a given temperamental characteristic will present in acceptable or aberrant ways is dependent in large measure on how the significant others in one's life respond to those characteristics. Additionally, any situation* or demand that strongly conflicts with one's temperament produces severe stress, during which time signs and symptoms of behavior problems may arise.

Although temperament has been found to have a genetic origin,* it has been shown that one's environment can heighten, diminish or otherwise modify temperamental characteristics but not abolish them. In fact, some research even suggests that these apparent changes are in actuality only fronts enacted to gain social acceptance.[6, 13] This tendency of temperament to remain basically unchanged despite environmental pressures is called *persistence in personality and self-concept*. What modifications, if any, are possible in these genetically transmitted traits and the associated self-concept are more likely to occur in early childhood than at any other time in one's life — thus the importance of an environment that fosters these traits as assets and that positively reinforces self-concept from the beginning of life.

Extensive research conducted by Thomas, Chess and Birch[13] indicated nine clearly recognizable characteristics, or traits, of temperament. They are categorized according to reactivity. They include:

1. Motor activity – the intensity and frequency of activity or motility;
2. Rhythmicity – regularity of repetitive biological functions such as sleep and wakefulness, eating patterns, bowel and bladder patterns;
3. Approach to the new or withdrawal from or acceptance of it – the child's initial reaction to a new stimulus;
4. Adaptability – the ease or difficulty with which initial responses to new stimuli can be modified;
5. Intensity of response – degree or amount of energy invested in reactions to stimuli;
6. Threshold of responsiveness – level of external stimulation necessary to evoke an overt response;
7. Quality of mood – general cheerfulness or unhappiness, amount of pleasant and friend-

---

*Such situations might include inconsistent care, inappropriate performance expectations, a series of traumatic events, imitations of aberrant behavior in other member(s) at home.

*Similar research studies carried out in Norway by Ann Torgurson and in America by Thomas and others resulted in remarkably similar findings. The same distribution of temperament types was found, despite marked differences in culture, parenting style, socioeconomic status and racial factors.

GROWTH AND DEVELOPMENT

TABLE 10-3 INCIDENCE AND CHARACTERISTICS OF THE THREE PERSONALITY TYPES*

Personality Type	Incidence	Characteristics
Easy child (sanguine, endomorph)	40% of all children; 18% develop maladjustments	Well adjusted psychologically and physically; adapts rapidly Friendly, likes company Seeks people during stress May need urging to complete ambitions Sleeps and eats well; highly regular biological rhythm, good candidate for demand feeding as infant; easily toilet trained Displays low to mild intensity of response Positive mood predominates; smiles and laughs much more than he cries; caregiver can usually be sure something is amiss when he does cry; tends to find good in any situation, even disappointing ones
Difficult child (choleric, mesomorph)	10% of all children;† 70% develop maladjustments	Slow to adapt to any new situation, but can function well once he "learns the rules" of situation Likes people but is not dependent upon them and sometimes functions better alone—a natural leader Seeks activity during stress; needs acceptable outlets for his vigor and aggressive motor drive; competitive Seems to be constantly moving and highly destructive; intense in reactions; needs unbreakable, well-constructed toys and clothing Displays mostly negative withdrawal responses to new situations; frustration expressed in tantrums or destruction; pleasure expressed loudly and boisterously, but these outbursts do not necessarily reflect the value of the situation to him—his responses simply have an "all or nothing" quality Has irregular biological functioning; sleeps poorly and lightly and requires less sleep; erratic in appetite and frequency of hunger; not a good candidate for demand feeding as an infant and much patience and time is required for toilet training, with more frequent accidents Negative mood predominates; seems to fuss or cry constantly; finds reasons to be unhappy; tends to be an "I can't" person; seldom a good scholar
Slow-to-warm-up child (phlegmatic, ectomorph)	15% of all children; 40% develop maladjustments	Slow adaptive capacity; usually quietly withdraws but is watchful and contemplative all the while Primarily a loner; usually prefers only one or two close friends; socially shy Seeks to be alone during stress; avid reader Often matures late; oversensitive and immature compared with most peers Poor relaxer; frequently experiences disturbed sleep and eating patterns Displays low intensity of reaction Fairly high frequency of negative mood, although it sometimes is not immediately noticeable because of low intensity with which it is expressed

*Information for this table was gathered from Gesell et al.: Infant and Child In the Culture of Today;[4] Segal and Yahroes: A Child's Journey;[11] and Thomas et al.: Temperament and Behavior Disorders in Children.[13]
†Research by Someroff and Zax at the University of Rochester showed that women who were highly anxious or who had a psychological disorder during the prenatal period have a higher incidence of difficult children.

ly behavior as opposed to unpleasant and unfriendly behavior;
8. Distractibility – effectiveness of extraneous environmental stimuli in altering the direction of ongoing behavior;
9. Attention span and persistence – length of time an activity is pursued whether self-initiated or planned or structured, and the amount of frustration tolerated in activity despite obstacles.[13]

These traits tend to combine to form three clearly different personality structures.* Table 10-3 describes the incidence and traits of these three personalities.

The nurse who is able to recognize these three personality structures or temperaments is able to make a more reasoned judgment about the child's behavior and about the approach to him that will be most effective. Knowledge of temperament is especially helpful to parents. Knowing that some aspects of their child's behavior are due to his nature helps to relieve many parents of guilt feelings and of undue pressure caused by their belief that their parenting methods are creating the behavior. Understanding the parenting methods most effective with the various personality types can aid parents in adopting the method most appropriate for each of their children. (See Chapter 3 for further discussion of temperament and parenting style.)

A child's feelings may appear irrational at times; nonetheless they are very real. The most loving thing adults can do is to let a child experience the full range of all these feelings — the sad as well as the happy. This deepens his sense of himself and helps him to discover that feelings change. Acknowledging and respecting the feelings a child is experiencing allows him to do the same. This acknowledgement and respect also comforts the child, because he then knows he is not alone in this experience. In the long run this freedom to express his feelings allows him to use his own inner resources to manage the challenge at hand; he feels less burdened by the feelings themselves and can focus more of his energy on dealing with the problem.

Because the child's feelings are an expression of who he is, they are an important description of his emotional-social health status. Nurses

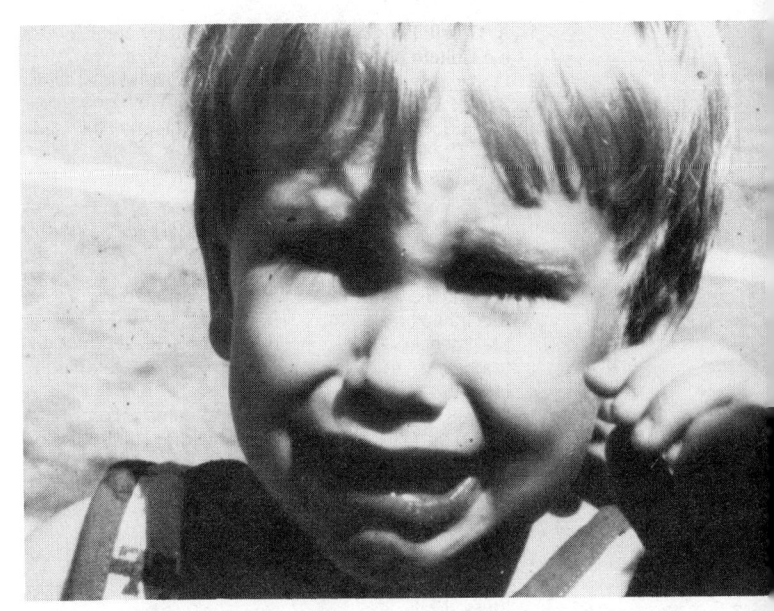

---
*Approximately one-third of the population does not fit into these three categories clearly but are instead blends not clearly separable.

Children need to experience the full range of emotions—the sad as well as the happy.

and parents who keep attuned to the child's feelings are given insight into where he is developmentally, which tasks are presently confronting him and in which areas he needs their support. The feelings and behaviors that the child uses to express himself are his cues to his significant others of where he is headed next. With her knowledge of human development, the nurse who heeds those cues can recognize signs of the child's readiness for new experiences that she or his parents can help to provide. The nurse's awareness of the child's cues, along with her understanding of every child's need for satisfying achievements and relationships, and her recognition of the importance of maintaining and protecting the child's relationships with his family, will bring the nurse a long way toward the construction of a holistic plan of care, effectively delivered.

References

1. P. Chinn. Child Health Maintenance: Concepts in Family-Centered Care, 2nd ed. C. V. Mosby Co., 1979
2. E. Erikson. Childhood and Society. Norton Publishers, 1963
3. E. Evans and B. McCandless. Children and Youth: Psychosocial Development. Holt, Rinehart & Winston, 1978

4. A. Gesell, F. Ilg and L. Bates Ames. Infant and Child in the Culture of Today. Harper & Row, 1974
5. D. Helms and J. Turner. Exploring Child Behavior: Basic Principles. W. B. Saunders Co., 1978
6. E. Hurlock. Child Development. McGraw-Hill Book Co., 1978
7. H. Maier. Three Theories of Child Development. Harper & Row, 1969
8. W. L. McNab. Sexual attitude development in children and the parent's role. Journal of School Health, November 1976, p. 537
9. D. Papilia and S. Olds. Human Development. McGraw-Hill Book Co., 1978
10. M. Spencer Pulaski. Understanding Piaget: An Introduction to Children's Cognitive Development. Harper & Row, 1971
11. J. Segal and H. Yahroes. A Child's Journey: Forces that Shape the Lives of Our Young. McGraw-Hill Book Co., 1978
12. D. Sutterly and G. Donnelly. Perspectives in Human Development: Nursing Throughout the Life Cycle. J. B. Lippincott Co., 1978
13. A. Thomas, S. Chess and H. Birch. Temperament and Behavior Disorders in Children. New York University Press, 1968
14. D. Winnicott. The Child, the Family and the Outside World. Penguin Books, 1964

Additional Recommended Reading

S. Ambron. Child Development. Holt, Rinehart & Winston, 1977

L. Bourne, Jr. and B. Ekstrand. Psychology: Its Principles and Meanings. Holt, Rinehart & Winston, 1976

L. Kayes. Developing Your Child's Temperament. Dell Books, 1979

E. LeShan. A child needs tears as well as laughter. Woman's Day, May 1974

S. Sahin. The multifaceted role of the nurse as genetic counselor. American Journal of Maternal Child Nursing, Jul/Aug 1976, p. 211

A. Scheinfeld. Heredity in Humans. J. B. Lippincott Co., 1972

A. Thomas and S. Chess. Temperament and Development. Brunner/Mazel, Inc., 1977

L. Whaley. Understanding Inherited Disorders. C. V. Mosby Co., 1974

D. Winnicott. The Family and Individual Development. Harper & Row, 1969

UNDERSTANDING THE PLAY OF CHILDREN

by Mabel Hunsberger, BSN, MSN

. . . you can be sure that you foster your child's development when you free yourself to sing a song, make up funny words, and scuff through falling leaves.

Bernice Weissbourd, in *Parents,* September 1979.

Watching children play is an encounter with the content of their lives. Play is a reflection of a child's developing physical, intellectual and emotional-social competencies. Through play children are in a continuous state of telling about themselves — what they can do, how they think and how they feel. Careful attention to the language of play gives an adult entrance into a child's world.

We are beginning to understand that, through the medium of play, a child "learns what no one can teach him."[6] One needs only to watch an inquisitive child examine the texture of each item on his plate at mealtime to appreciate his preoccupation with learning while he plays. Through play children orient themselves to their expanding world of people and objects and gradually learn how to relate to them effectively. Much of this learning is accomplished by the creation of a make-believe world in which children can assume roles that offer safe expression of their fears and re-enactment of the conflicts felt in the real world. In this way a child can adapt to the expectations of those in his environment. The beauty of childhood is that the "work" of growing and developing is done in the name of play.

THEORIES OF PLAY

Numerous theories have been offered to explain why and how children play. An examination of the various theories that have been developed over time gives one an appreciation for the complexity of an activity as seemingly simple as play.

Surplus-Energy Theory

Herbert Spencer, an English philosopher of the mid-nineteenth century, hypothesized that children play because of excess energy accumulation, necessitating energy release through play. The exuberant activities of children were recognized to be a normal part of their development, but play was not thought to accomplish any immediate goal.[5] The notion of surplus energy is identifiable in the high premium that schools and families pay to provide yards and gymnasiums for the physical activity of children.

Instinctive-Practice Theory

Karl Groos, a German philosopher and writer of the late nineteenth century, viewed play as instinctual and as a preparation for adult life.[2] To him the function of play was to exercise skills necessary for adult life. He was particularly cognizant of the imagination of children and interpreted such play as "pre-exercise" for adult living. The value of Groos's theory is that he recognized the functional value of play: practicing and perfecting the skills needed in adult life.

Psychoanalytic Theory

Psychoanalytic theorists, particularly Freud and Erikson, stress the cathartic benefit children gain through play. Freud stated that "in their play children repeat everything that has made a great impression on them in real life."[4] To illustrate, a child who has been punished for running onto a busy street may be later seen acting out the scene in doll play, in which the child first scolds the doll, then comforts it. The repetition of the experience affords an opportunity to express hostile feelings and provide assurance that the act of running onto the street does not warrant rejection. According to this theory, the playing out of such anxieties is thought to help a child gain mastery over fears, feelings, people and things. The use of play therapy to treat emotionally disturbed children is an outgrowth of the psychoanalytic view of play.

Cognitive Theory

According to cognitive theorists, a child's play is the way in which reality can be explored and assimilated into his mental structure. The Swiss psychologist Piaget distinguishes between play and imitation.[9] The process of assimilation predominates when a child is playing. Conversely, when accommodation predominates, the result is imitation. When assimilation and accommodation are in equilibrium, intellectual adaptation occurs. (See Chapter 10 for further discussion of assimilation and accommodation.) To illustrate, intelligent adaptation occurs when a child uses his mental processes to discover that he can get raisins out of a bottle by dumping them out. Once he has mastered this skill and repeats it for the pleasure and fun of doing it, Piaget describes that as play. If on the other hand a child has observed another person dumping raisins out of the bottle and then mimics the activity, that is imitation. Whether a single activity is play, imitation or intellectual adaptation is not easily discerned on random observation.

Piaget's theory of play correlates with his theory of intellectual development (see Chapter 10). The way a child plays and the nature of imitation vary throughout the stages of development. The games that characterize certain periods of development reflect one's intellectual processes. Practice games, which predominate in the sensorimotor period of development (0 to 2 years), are repetitive actions done for the pleasure they bring. Those activities that are to gain mastery or increase understanding are not considered by authorities to be practice games. It is when mastery has been achieved that play occurs. The period of symbolic games or make-believe play (2 to 7 years) is the stage when children are egotistical in thought and, through fantasy, transform reality to be consistent with their immediate need (assimilation). At a given time a child can pretend that an object is an animal and moments later transform that object into a person, whichever is consistent with the needs of the moment. In addition to meeting the conscious needs of a child, symbolic play functions in the realm of the unconscious. Emotional experiences are reproduced in play in an effort to diffuse the anxieties that are produced by the real world. These enactments of real-life impressions are often distorted owing to the egocentricity of thought that prevails during this stage. Gradually a child's increasing participation in the natural and social world eliminates the need for symbolic games, which are replaced by games with rules. Games with rules (7 to 11 years) are representative of a child's increased social interaction and developing reasoning abilities. These games have sensorimotor components (races, ball games) and intellectual ones (cards, chess) and are guided by rules, within which competition and cooperation can take place.

Enjoyment or Hedonic Theory

Hurlock[7] and the Sutton-Smiths[11] believe that play should be enjoyable and that its end result is of little consequence. According to this theory, an activity is not play unless the player is engaged merely for the enjoyment it gives. When actions are carried out with the end result as a primary goal, then the activity is more rightly called work. The differences between mastery activities and play activities are not easily identified, because one cannot be sure of the intent of the player. What this view brings to mind is that not all that children do is necessarily play. Whether a child's activity is for the purpose of mastery or play, a great deal of it does appear to provide enjoyment.

The foregoing theories provide a framework from which to formulate an understanding of play. Play is viewed from different perspectives but each theory contributes important ideas about play. The central recurring theme is that play should be pleasurable and enjoyable. If a child enjoys what he does, he is likely to do it again and experiment with variations of the activity. This is how play leads to discovery and subsequent advancement in growth and development. If, on the other hand, an activity is not pleasurable, it is not likely to be continued and the potential benefits of play are diminished. If play is not enjoyable, it follows that growth and developmental benefits will not be realized. The idea that play is practice for adult living is a plausible interpretation because of the contributions of play to the total child. As long as the end goal of developmental advancement does not take precedence over the value of the pleasure derived from play, then the activity is play. This is not to say that play does not contribute to growth and development. The important point is that a child should be allowed to play for enjoyment without the confines of adult standards of what he has to accomplish.

The question of how play contributes to what is not play (creativity, problem-solving, language learning) continues to motivate research. Although the exact dynamics of how play contributes to all aspects of normal growth and development is not clear, some observations can be made. The following discussion identifies major contributions of play to the physical, intellectual and emotional-social development of children.

CONTRIBUTIONS OF PLAY TO THE DEVELOPING CHILD

The varied theories of play conjure up the notion that play has something to do with every aspect of the developing child. Some theorists address one aspect of development more than another; however, combination of these theories acknowledges that play contributes to the physical, intellectual and emotional-social development of children. Although a single play activity is likely to contribute to all aspects of development simultaneously, each is discussed separately here to facilitate a clearer understanding of play.

Physical Development

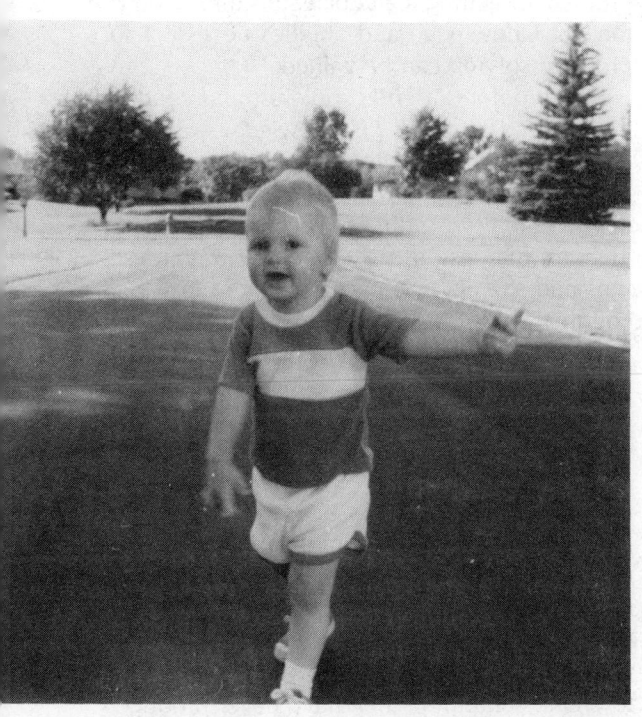

The physical activity of play contributes to the development and coordination of the body throughout the life span. Children's play varies from one developmental stage to the next due in part to the physical maturation of their bodies. During infancy play is dominated by sensorimotor activities such as looking, tasting, touching and manipulating the environment. Through reaching, grasping and mouthing objects repetitively, the *senses are developed* and *muscles are coordinated*. Hand-eye coordination is a competency that requires practice through play and maturation through growth. Through play children develop control of their bodies as they practice creeping, crawling and walking. The skillful movements and coordination required to take them to new territories for exploration are practiced incessantly. As children grow older they continue to increase their physical competency by engaging in activities that demand more precision, such as athletics, bicycle riding, swimming, dancing and skating. Thus through play a person progresses from a randomly reflexive repertoire of behavior in infancy to skillfully coordinated movement in adulthood.

Cognitive Development

Through play a child *discovers the real world*. He learns about the composition of his world and relationships within that world. His earliest encounters with sound, movement, touch and visual experiences are the beginning phases of

The physical activity of play contributes to the development and coordination of the body throughout life.

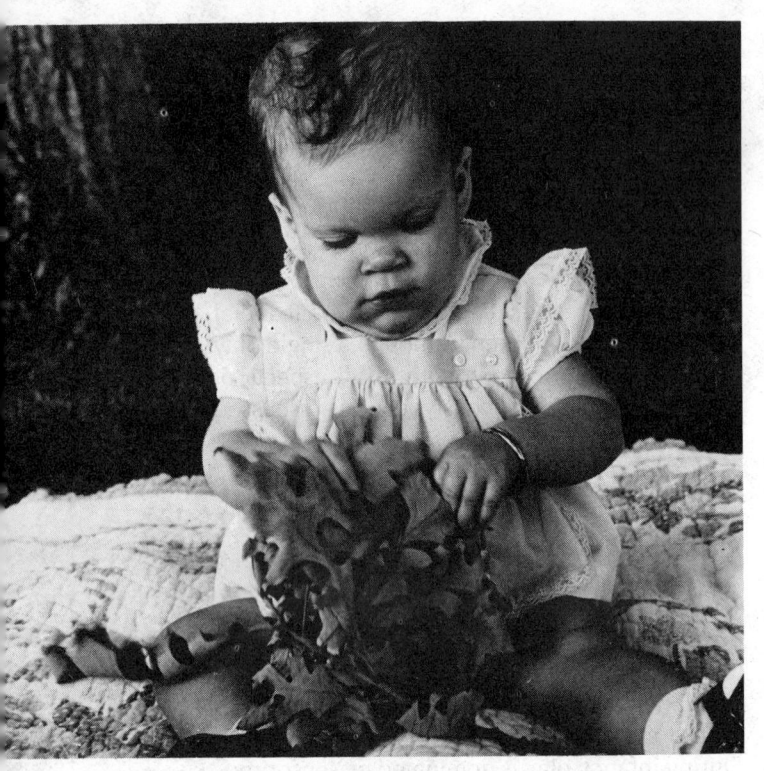

Through play the child discovers his world.

learning through play. It is through manipulation of objects and achievement of pleasurable sensations that a child learns about himself and the objects in his environment. The repetitive pastime of putting objects into a receptacle and then dumping them out is a pleasurable exercise of seeing how objects respond and how he can affect their response. There are strong indications that early sensory experiences contribute to a child's later skills of perception and abstraction necessary for reading.[3]

Play provides an arena for the *development of language.* Even before a child is able to use words to describe what he sees, his experiences with space, sound, color and relationships help him to form impressions about the environment. His experimentation with some objects gives him an opportunity to discover how soft and smooth they feel before he has the words to describe his perceptions. It is these early experiences and formation of multiple images that help him put words into use.[3] Play situations promote the use of words and phrases as children express their thoughts and wishes regarding the objects and events that comprise their play world. As children become more social in their play, they need to increase their word usage to make their ideas known to their playmates. As peer relations develop, language is an important tool in the expression of the innermost thoughts and secrets of their lives. Thus the world that children encounter through play from infancy provides a stimulus for the development of perceptions and progressive use of language.

Problem-solving has its beginnings in play. To understand how play contributes to problem-solving it is useful to define what constitutes a problem. It is feasible that a given set of circumstances is a problem for one child but not for another, because of differences within the child. A problem can be defined as a situation in which a child has no ready response to deal with a presenting set of stimuli.[2] Play contributes to problem-solving because experiences with objects, people and ideas give the child a familiarity with how things work and to what degree his own capacities can affect his environment. For example, if a child wishes to get a cookie out of a jar on a counter, he can solve the problem by drawing on previous play experiences even though this particular problem has never been solved by him. Based on his experience he knows (1) I can move the chair, (2) I can crawl onto the chair, (3) I can open a jar. Each of these experiences has been practiced in play, but now they can be combined to solve the new problem of getting the cookie. It is through play that the knowledge and abilities necessary for problem-solving can be gained.

Play *promotes a child's interest and concentration,* and *expands his knowledge.* Children have a natural tendency to explore and learn about their environment. It is easy to capture a child's attention with novel objects and new ideas for play. Exposure to books, trips to museums and strategy games are activities in which children happily participate. These activities increase their ability to concentrate and enlarge their mental capacity.

If a child is given the opportunity to be creative, play can be a natural avenue for *creative expression.* Creativity is so loosely defined that it is difficult to be assured of a mutual understanding without some clarification of its meaning. Creativity is the process of combining old ideas into forms that are new for the individual.[12] Through play children can experiment with new combinations of materials and ideas to create something they have never produced before. Children can be creative with very simple materials if left to their own imagination. Play opportunities provide many possibilities for creativity, some of which are object manipulation, dramatic play, drawing and painting, and daydreaming. Piaget suggests that it is advisable to supply appropriate materials for children's play but let them do their own experimenting in that "every time we teach a child something, we keep him from inventing it himself."[10]

Emotional-Social Development

Play allows a child to experiment with his thoughts, feelings and actions until he learns to adapt his emotions in a socially acceptable manner.

Self-awareness is developed through exploration of himself and of others in relationship to himself. The interpersonal experiences of smiling, crying, cooing and touching are the beginning behaviors that lead to an awareness of the various responses he can evoke within his environment. Through this exchange and experimentation a child learns a great deal about the specific effects of his own actions and thereby develops an increasing sense of who he is relative to his environment. As a child's territory widens and his relationships increase, so does his sense of self. Through play a child develops an increasing sense of who he is, what he can do and how others perceive him. These perceptions combine and contribute to his development of self-esteem.

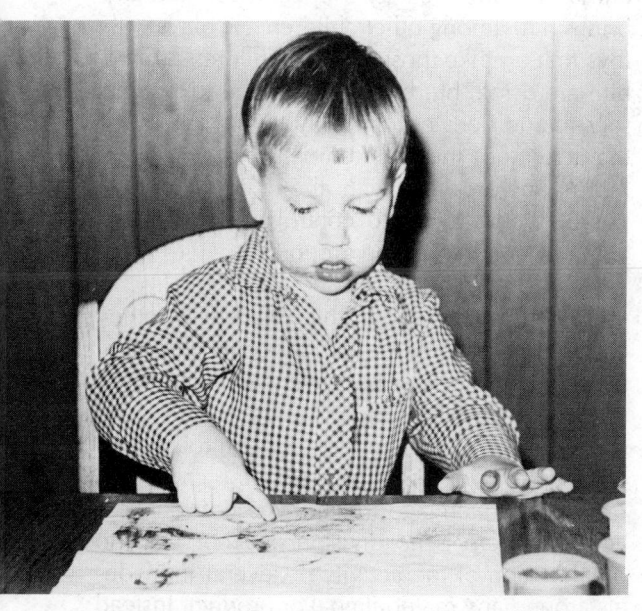

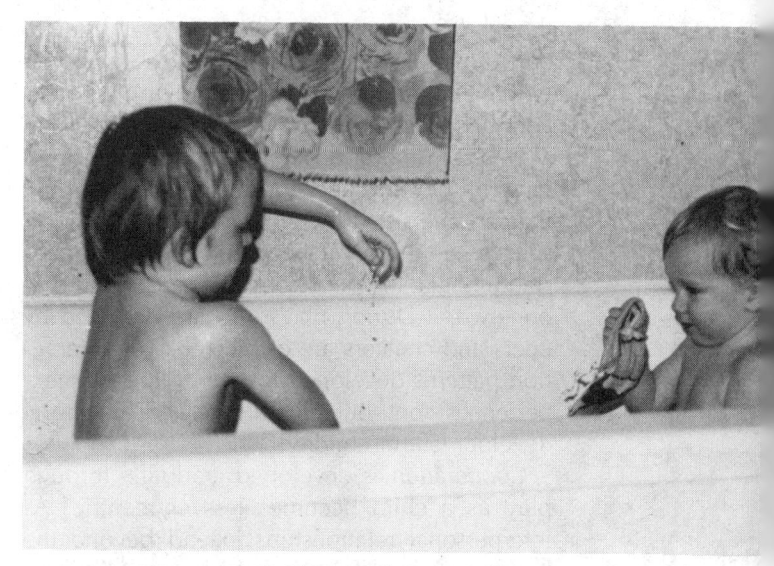

To Mother a wash cloth is for getting clean. To me it's a fuzzy that splashes and tickles and scrubs. And I can do it all by myself.

Expression of emotions is a life-long learning process. During the developmental process children engage in fantasy play to explore feelings, lessen fears and work through conflicts. In games of pretending, imaginary playmates are safe recipients of aggressive impulses. Experiences that have frightened or excited a child may be re-enacted in play with imaginary participants. Through such play activities a child can express those intense feelings that may not be perceived as acceptable forms of behavior in the real world.

Independence and self-care skills are learned and practiced in a child's play. The delight a child experiences in seeing his own accomplishments during play gives him the confidence to begin doing things for himself in other aspects of living. As a child realizes that he can stack his own blocks, he also demands that he be given control over his own body. In everyday activities of living such as eating, dressing, bathing and preparation for sleep, play continues as he experiments with his own skills and becomes increasingly more independent.

The *moral development* of a child is dependent on his intellectual development and on the social interactions he experiences. Children learn right from wrong in play because of the positive and negative reinforcement they receive from their family, peers and society. Some play is rewarded and some is punished. Al-

Play opportunities provide many possibilities for creativity.

though learning right from wrong is an integral part of moral or ethical behavior, moral development consists of more than obeying the rules and behaving properly. The significance that play has in moral development is that it helps children develop an understanding of the feelings of others and the ability to share. Ambron suggests that ethical behavior entails "understanding that the needs of others are as valid as our own."[1] During play rules are enforced by peers and cheaters are ostracized. The interaction patterns developed through these play experiences contribute significantly to the moral development of children.

Cooperation is developed gradually through play as a child becomes less egocentric. As interpersonal relationships extend beyond the home to peers, children quickly learn the give and take of life during play. They learn to share playthings, agree to make a sandcastle by another's specifications, and wait until later for their turn to fly a plane. Play gives children the opportunity to show regard for the ideas of another.

DEVELOPMENTAL CHARACTERISTICS OF PLAY

The kind of play in which children engage is largely determined by their developmental stage. Children progress through stages of play reflecting a range of thoughts and abilities. As a child grows and develops, his environment changes and so do his needs. The social character and the content of play provide two developmental classifications of play to use in examining these changes.

Social Character

In the 1920s Parten[8] observed a group of 2- to 5-year-old children during play and identified different types of play. These behaviors were observed in normal preschoolers and are considered typical for that age. It is common that the younger child spends more time in solitary and parallel play, whereas by 5 years of age a child is mostly cooperative in his play. As reported in Parten's 1932 article in the Journal of Abnormal and Social Psychology, the following descriptions of play behavior reflect a progression of sociability ranging from playing alone to playing alongside another child and finally to cooperative play.

"**Unoccupied Behavior** The child apparently is not playing but occupies himself with watching anything that happens to be of momentary interest. When there is nothing exciting taking place, he plays with his own body, gets on and off chairs, just stands around, follows the teacher, or sits in one spot glancing around the room."

"**Onlooker** The child spends most of his time watching the other children play. He often talks to the children whom he is observing, asks questions or gives suggestions but does not overtly enter into the play himself. This type differs from the unoccupied in that the onlooker is definitely observing particular groups of children rather than anything that happens to be exciting. The child stands or sits within speaking distance of the group so that he can see and hear everything that takes place."

"**Solitary Independent Play** The child plays alone and independently with toys that are different from those used by the children within speaking distance and makes no effort to get close to other children. He pursues his own activity without reference to what others are doing."

"**Parallel Activity** The child plays independently, but the activity he chooses naturally brings him among other children. He plays with toys that are like those that the children around him are using, but he plays with the toys as he sees fit and does not try to influence or modify the activity of the children near him. He plays *beside* rather than *with* the other children. There is no attempt to control the coming or going of children in the group."

"**Associative Play** The child plays with other children. The conversation concerns the common activity; there is borrowing and lending of play material, following one another with trains or wagons; mild attempts to control which children may or may not play in the group. All the members engage in similar if not identical activity. There is no division of labor, and no organization of the activity of several individuals around any material goal or product. Instead of subordinating his individual interest to that of the group, each child acts as he wishes. By his conversation with the other children one can tell that his interest is primarily in his associations, not in his activity. Occasionally, two or three children are engaged in no activity of any duration but are merely doing whatever happens to draw the attention of any of them."

"**Cooperative or Organized Supplementary Play** The child plays in a group that is organized for the purpose of making some material product, or of striving to attain some competitive goal, or of dramatizing situations of adult and group life or of playing formal games. There is a marked sense of belonging to the group or of not belonging to it. The control of the group situation is in the hands of one or two of the members who direct the activity of the others. The goal as well as the method of attaining it necessitates a division of labor, the taking of different roles by the various group members and the organization of activity so that the efforts of one child are supplemented by those of another."[8]

Content of Play

Stone and Church have provided a useful approach to play by categorizing it according to content. The six categories of play they identified are: (1) social-affective, (2) sense-pleasure, (3) skill, (4) dramatic, (5) formal, (6) competitive.[12]

They propose that play begins as *social-affective play*. Parents stimulate their infants by cooing, fondling and other playful gestures. The infant's responses of pleasure are a reward to the parent and a cyclic pattern of play develops.

Sense-pleasure play has been defined as nonsocial play that originates outside the infant. It is nonsocial in that it is stimulated by environmental variations in color, movement, sound, taste and texture. The experience of sensing these variations is pleasurable, thus the term sense-pleasure. For the infant, pleasurable experiences are expanded when he develops the manipulative and locomotor ability to experiment with the sensations derived from play with water, sand and food. Activities of movement such as swinging, bouncing and rocking are examples of sense-pleasure play, as is exploration of one's own body.

Skill play occurs when infants have developed the ability to reach out, grasp and manipulate. It consists of the repetitive practice of newly discovered abilities. There can be an element of sense-pleasure in skill play depending on the type of activity, but it is the practicing and accomplishment of a task that intrigues a child rather than the pleasure derived during the activity. For example, it is the challenge of learning to ride a bike rather than the sensation of riding it that motivates the child in skill play. The fascination that motivates skill play is the challenge of taking on a task which one is hardly capable of accomplishing. People of all ages are subject to this intrigue.

Various combinations of social-affective, sense-pleasure and skill play continue during the toddler and preschool years. It is also at this time that a new motif emerges: *dramatic play*. In dramatic play a child tries out roles and

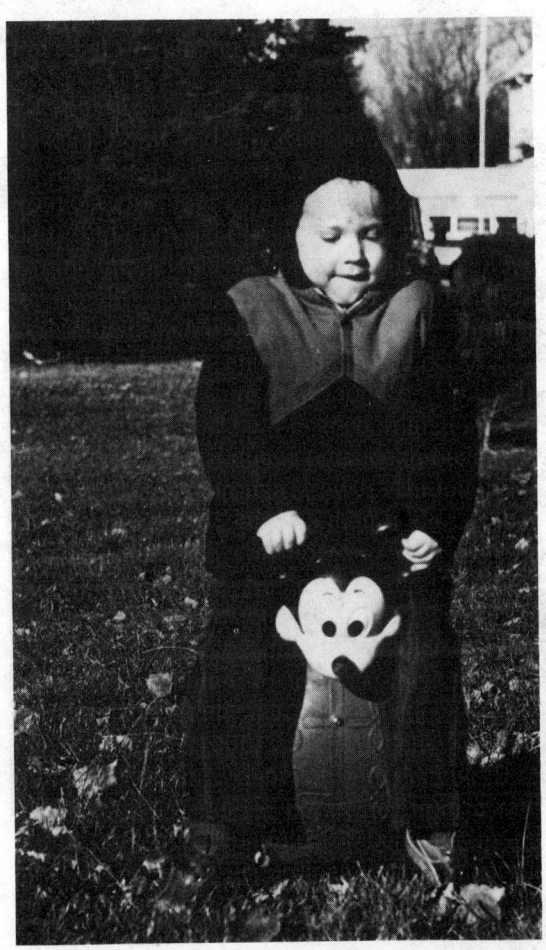

Pleasurable experiences are expanded when the child develops manipulative and locomotor ability to experiment in play.

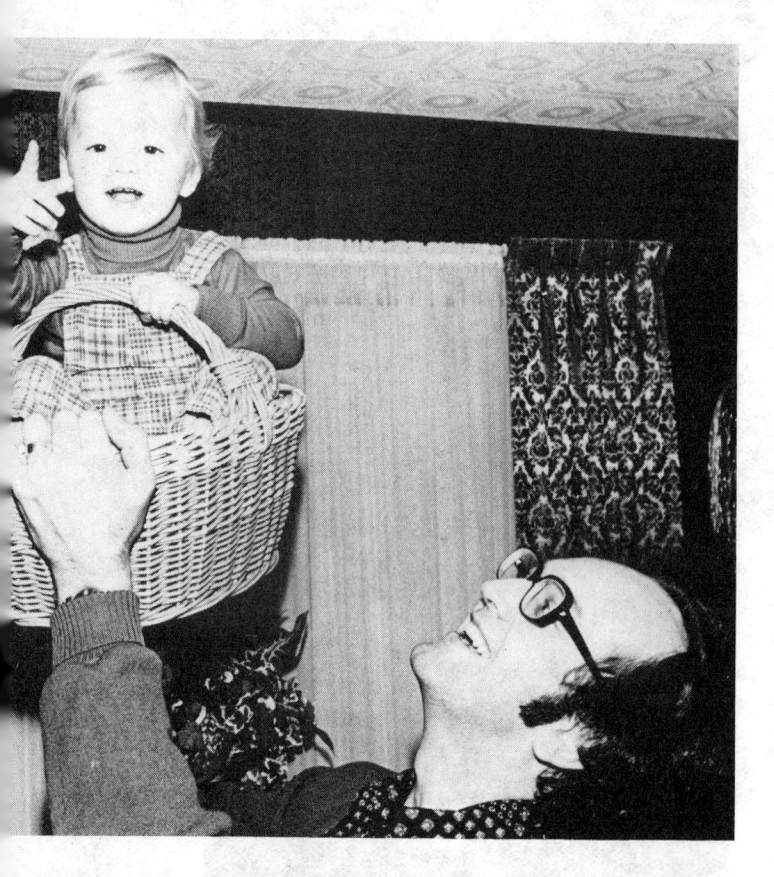

identities drawn first from domestic life and later from the world at large. The imitative quality of this play is obvious when a child mimics adults by talking on the telephone, pretending to be shaving and dressing up in adult clothing. Through imitation a child is identifying with those prominent persons in his environment.

When a child re-enacts scenes and events of everyday life, it may take the form of reproductive dramatic play or productive dramatic play. In reproductive dramatic play children try to re-create in their play a situation they have observed in real life or in the mass media. By contrast, in productive dramatic play children create characters and themes that may be taken either from real life experiences or from their imagination.[7]

Formal games are simple, noncompetitive exercise such as ring-around-a-rosy and London Bridge. As children get older, their play becomes competitive and ranges from table games to sports.

The progression from social-affective play to formal games and from solitary play to cooperative play reflects the child's developing physical, intellectual and social skills. This developmental process is influenced by the opportunities and nurturing provided by the family within which the child develops. Family relationships provide the basis for a child's social relationships with others and contribute to his developing sense of self-esteem. If parents play with their children, the excitement of discovery and creativity is shared and children feel accepted and encouraged in their play. If children feel that parents are interested in what they can do, they are also stimulated to try new things in play. The characteristics of play (social character and content) are determined by the stage of development of a child but are subject to the quality of relationships within the family.

HELPING PARENTS TO PROMOTE PLAY

The nurse's understanding of what constitutes normal, healthy play is fundamental to her role in the care of children and their families. She can prepare parents to expect the normal changes in the social character and content of play at various stages of development. The importance of providing opportunities for play appropriate for the age of the child cannot be overemphasized. It should be stressed that it is not necessary to buy expensive toys to promote the development of children. Use of common household equipment and the sounds and textures of the outdoors provide excellent opportunities. Parents should be encouraged to play with their children but also should be helped to realize that there are times when they should not play (when irritable and tired). There are times when a child's greatest desire is to have a parent watch him play. Whether parents encourage the play of children by playing with them or watching them, it should be pleasurable for parents and children.

Helping a parent to choose safe, durable toys suitable to the developmental level of the child is another important function of the nurse. Also, the proper use of toys is an area in which many families need assistance. Too many toys can be confusing and overstimulating to children. Excessive use of toys can also thwart the child's own resourcefulness to create play situations out of natural stimuli in the environment. Self-expression and the freedom to play according to their own needs is what is most beneficial to children.

The nurse's role is to encourage parents to provide opportunities for play, play with their children when appropriate, and participate in the thoughts and feelings of their children by watching them play.

References

1. S. Ambron. Child Development, 2nd ed. Holt, Rinehart & Winston, 1977
2. S. Bijou. Child Development: The Basic Stage of Early Childhood. Century Psychology Series. Prentice-Hall Inc., 1976
3. F. Caplan and T. Caplan. The Power of Play. Anchor Press, 1973
4. S. Freud. Beyond the Pleasure Principle. Translated by James Strachy, Liveright Publishing, 1961
5. C. Garvey. Play. In The Developing Child Series, J. Bruner et al., eds. Harvard, 1977.
6. R. Hartley and R. Goldenson. A Complete Book of Play. Thomas Y. Crowell Co., 1963
7. E. Hurlock. Child Development, 6th ed. McGraw-Hill Book Co., 1978
8. M. Parten. Social participation among preschool children. Journal of Abnormal and Social Psychology, March 1932, p. 243
9. J. Piaget. Play, Dreams and Imitation in Childhood. Translated by C. Gattegno and F. M. Hodgson. Routledge and Kegan Paul Limited, 1951
10. M. Piers. Play and Development. W. W. Norton & Co., Inc., 1972
11. L. J. Stone and J. Church. Childhood and Adolescence, 3rd ed. Random House Inc., 1973
12. B. Sutton-Smith and S. Sutton-Smith. How to Play With Your Children (And When Not To). Hawthorn Books, 1974

Additional Recommended Reading

E. Cass. Helping Children Grow Through Play. Schocken Books, Inc., 1973
B. Campbell. Child's play is serious business. American Baby, August 1978, p. 48
M. Gibbons. When parents ask about play. Pediatric Nursing, Nov/Dec 1977, p. 19
J. Gordon. Baby Learning Through Baby Play. St. Martin's Press, 1970
E. Hartley et. al. Understanding Children's Play. Columbia University Press, 1952
R. E. Herron and B. Sutton-Smith. Child's Play. John Wiley & Sons, Inc., 1971
S. Millar. The Psychology of Play. Penguin Books, 1968
C. Robeck. Infants and Children: Their Development and Learning. McGraw-Hill Book Co., 1978
J. Sparling and I. Lewis. Six learning games to play with your infant. Parents, October 1979, p. 35
M. A. Tauber. Parental socialization techniques and sex differences in children's play. Child Development, March 1979, p. 225
B. Weissbourd. As they grow/2 year olds: Playfulness spurs development. Parents, September 1979, p. 70

12 COMMUNICATING WITH CHILDREN AND PARENTS

by Mabel Hunsberger, BSN, MSN

Communication is the sharing of information between individuals. Thoughts, feelings and opinions are exchanged, whether consciously or unconsciously, through verbal and nonverbal means. Relationships are formed through a continuous process of learning about what others think and feel. We are always communicating something, whether we are aware of it or not. The way messages are interpreted in the process of communication is dependent on the relationship that exists between the communicants.

THE PROCESS OF COMMUNICATION

The process of communication with children and parents is affected by the relationships that exist between family members as well as the relationship that the nurse has with each member. The nurse's understanding of herself and her awareness of the effect of her own communication is a key to her relationship with children and their parents. The way messages are formed (coded) and interpreted (decoded) is subject to the acceptance one feels in the presence of another. It is the goal of the nurse to facilitate communication by creating an atmosphere of acceptance to potentiate the accuracy of communication.

In the communication process a stimulus causes an individual to form a message that he transmits to another person, the receiver. If a parent sends a message to the nurse in the presence of children, the nurse must decode that message with the realization that parents have an image to protect. Also, when the children talk in the presence of their parents, the nurse must recognize that communication is not only influenced by the nurse-child relationship but also by the acceptance the child senses from his parents. Thus the context within which the message is sent has an essential bearing on the way the message is decoded. Communication has not been accomplished until the message is received in the context within which it is sent. The receiving of a message involves decoding of both the verbal and the nonverbal content of the communication. Aside from the relationship that exist between communicants, each person's biases and life experiences always affect communication. In the case of children and parents it is the family within which they live that largely influences their communication with each other and with those outside the family unit.

THE PARENT-CHILD-NURSE RELATIONSHIP

Because communication is the heart of human relationships, it is one of the most important skills a nurse uses when dealing with children and their families. Much of what a nurse can accomplish depends on her ability to make parents and children feel accepted and comfortable in the relationship. Parents are unlikely to reveal true feelings about their children if there is even a slight possibility that they will feel judged as incompetent parents. Children also are sensitive to lack of recognition of their true feelings and response to these and become less communicative with persons who fail to respect their concerns. The nurse's communication ability prescribes the boundaries within which the relationship develops and therefore affects all that a nurse does with children and their families.

Respect for the individuality of each person within the relationship has particular relevance when dealing with parents and children. The way an individual thinks and feels, and therefore responds to a message, is a reflection of his total life experiences, including values of family, friends, community and society. Communicating respect involves recognizing that the views that parents hold regarding childrearing, health maintenance and children's roles may be in opposition to those of the nurse. To respect parents as individuals is to recognize that longstanding family and cultural patterns are an integral part of their way of life and affect their view of parenting. Children also need to be respected as individuals. It is easy to fall prey to the stereotype that because a child is a certain age he will behave in a prescribed manner. Each child is exposed to his own unique set of experiences that affects how he talks and feels and how he interprets what is communicated to him. It is when nurses can respond to the individuality of each family member as well as to their needs as a child or parent that communication contributes to an effective parent-child-nurse relationship.

Implicit in respect is the idea of *acceptance of the total person*. To be accepting of a parent, a nurse must be able to understand that the temper tantrums of a child produce intolerable frustration in the parent and lead to corporal punishment by the parent. The nurse does not have to agree with corporal punishment to be accepting of the parent but should not make the parent feel less worthy. What she does is accept the need that motivated the behavior and not condemn the parent for the behavior. The nurse can show acceptance by encouraging expression of the feelings that led to the incident and thereby help a parent to identify alternate ways of expression. Communicating with children involves a similar approach. The behavior of the child does not have to be condoned even

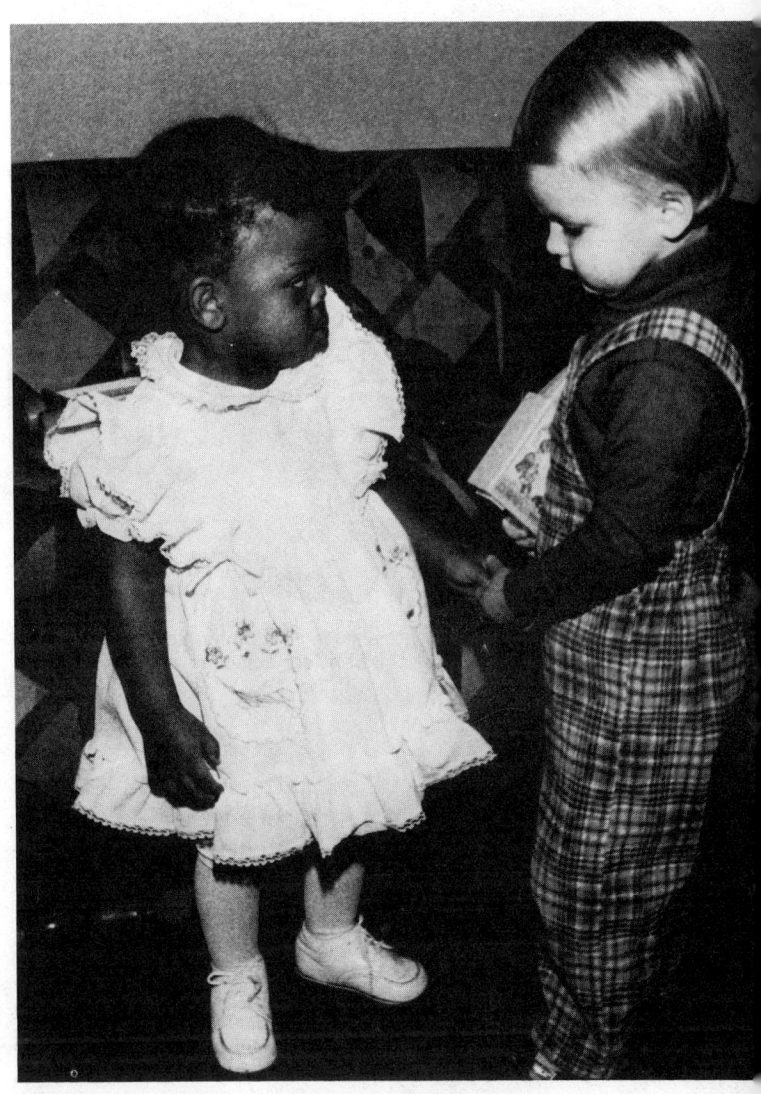

Relationships are formed as thoughts and feelings are communicated.

though the need of the child is accepted. When the nurse communicates acceptance of the individual, parents and children feel secure in the relationship and are likely to describe feelings and events more accurately.

Empathy is another essential element of the parent-child-nurse relationship. Empathy is communicated by the nurse when she can make parents and children feel that the meanings of their life experiences are being understood. The important feature of empathy is that the recipient feels it. Empathy involves being able to accurately perceive how it is for another person from that person's point of view. When dealing with children it means that one has to

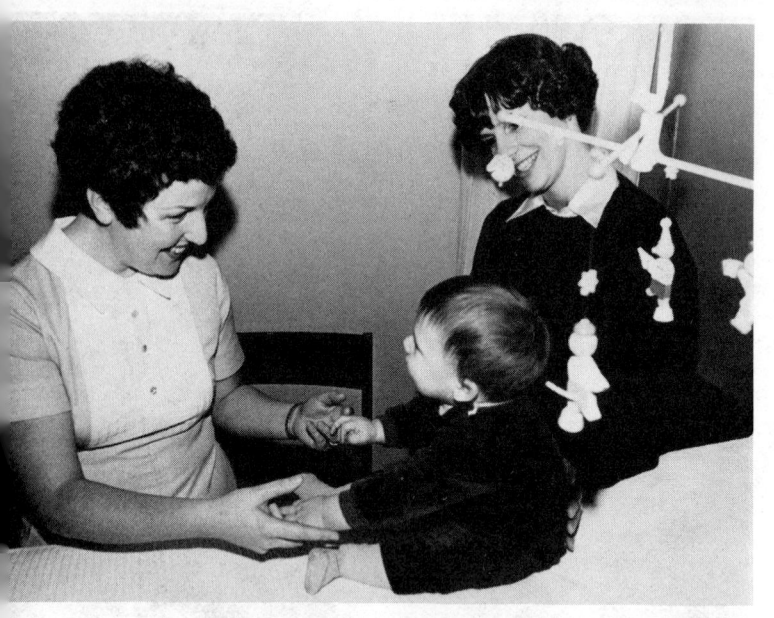

The nurse who is skilled in communication can make parents and children feel accepted and comfortable in a relationship with her.

be able to see the world through the child's eyes to grasp what an experience means to him. Children express how they feel when they are quiet, when they talk and especially when they play. To grasp how a child feels, attention must be given to all aspects of his behavior, not only his speech. It is only when the nurse spends sufficient time with a child that she has the opportunity to see and hear how the child feels and to gain enough understanding of the child's feelings to communicate empathy. Sensitivity to a child's nonverbal communication gives the nurse the most accurate sense of the child's true feelings, because children are often unable to verbalize how they feel. If a nurse is able to "tune in" and "be with" the child as his private thoughts and feelings are explored, he feels less lonely and alienated.[3] Providing this comfort is one of the most important things a nurse can do for a child.

Parents also feel a sense of relief from loneliness if they feel understood. When dealing with parents empathically a nurse does not offer advise or try to change a parent's way of thinking. Attempting to alter another person's thinking in accordance with one's own biases and beliefs is an evaluative gesture and is not empathic. To establish a relationship in which communication can ensue, a nurse does not wish to make the parent into what the nurse feels is a good parent but to create a secure environment within which parents can realize their own potential and chart their own course. It is through empathic understanding that people can be helped to become less dependent on the opinions of others and to be able to clarify their own thinking and course of action.[3, 6]

The attitudes that the nurse holds regarding parents and children determines the quality of the relationship she can expect to develop. Her respect for the individual and acceptance of each family member in his own right are necessary before empathic understanding can be communicated. It is the nurse's use of self and individuality that determines how the attitudes of respect, acceptance and empathy will be communicated. The parent-child-nurse relationship is shaped by the nurse's ability to use her own personal attributes in combination with her skills of communication.

TYPES OF COMMUNICATION

Nonverbal Communication

For a nurse to communicate effectively she must learn how to use and be responsive to verbal and nonverbal communication. Invariably it is gestures, facial expressions and tone of voice that add important dimensions to what is said. Nonverbal communication is less easily governed by conscious control than is verbal communication and is therefore more reliable. Children particularly show by their actions how they feel even before they have the language to verbally express such feelings. Communication through nonverbal means is a child's most natural mode of expression. Adults exercise more control over their nonverbal messages than do children but tone of voice, facial expressions and body language are hard to control even for an adult. Thus, even though parents do not necessarily verbalize their true feelings, their nonverbal communication remains an important dimension of communication with their children and with the nurse. The nurse who works with children and their families needs to become adept in identifying incongruities between verbal and nonverbal messages. Parents do not necessarily verbalize their true feelings because they often feel compelled to respond in prescribed ways owing to their role as parents or to respond in a way that they believe will please the nurse. An incongruity between ver-

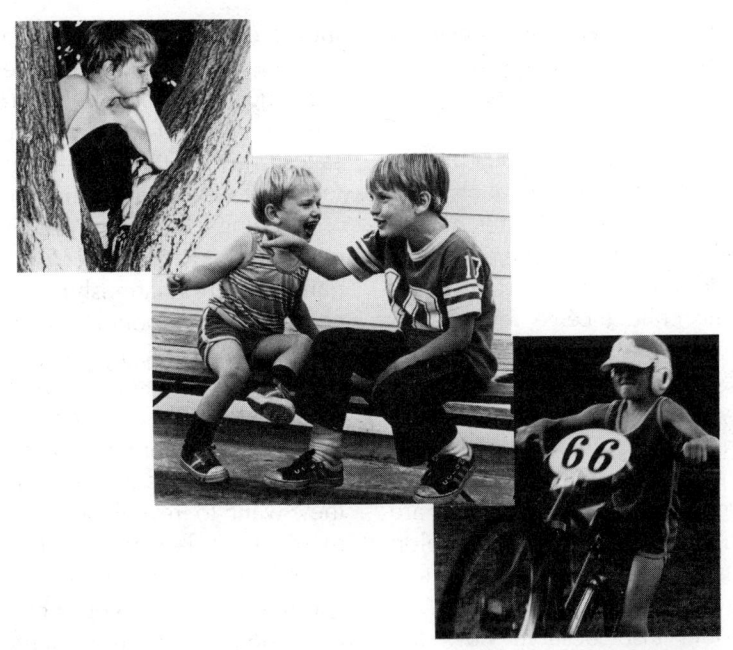

Children express how they feel when they are quiet, when they talk, and especially when they play.

bal and nonverbal communication may be the nurse's only indication that parents hold feelings they hesitate to verbalize.

Verbal Communication

Communication through the spoken word is the most obvious expression of thoughts and feelings, but it is not necessarily the most accurate. Individuals vary in their ability to use language as a way to communicate, so that the person who is reluctant to talk may be telling his listener something about his limitation in self-expression rather than about his mood. The nurse must also recognize that minimal verbal expression has cultural significance. In some cultures, such as certain parts of Appalachia, communication with few words is the accepted mode of behavior. When verbal communication is hampered by language barriers, the nurse must be sensitive enough to recognize when a nod of the head and lack of verbal communication really means that the client does not understand. When caregivers communicated with refugees from Southeast Asia, it was found that patients comprehended health instructions best when the nurse gave them in the family's home, where they felt comfortable.[7] When a language barrier is the reason for reduced verbal expression, the nurse should search for interpreters. She also should make an effort to communicate within the given limitations by speaking slowly and softly, using gestures and having bilingual dictionaries available for herself and the family.

Persons from different cultures or value systems may use the same words to communicate, but the meaning of the words varies. The parent, the child and the nurse each have their own life experiences and values that affect the use and meaning of words. To use words effectively in communication, it is therefore important for the nurse to recognize when her own words have not been understood and to clarify the intent when others have used language in a way that is not clear to her.

SKILLS OF COMMUNICATION

Observation

Observation of nonverbal communication provides meaningful clues to what children and parents are saying to each other and to the nurse. Children communicate with us by the *way* they do things as well as by *what* they do: observing their eyes, quality of voice, facial expressions and body posture and movements tells us how they feel about situations and people. Does a child say "I feel disappointed," or does he show us this by his saddened eyes, quiet mood or sobbing cry? We cannot wait for him to reach the maturity to identify his emotions and tell us about them before we respond to his feelings.[1]

The interaction between parents and children is an integral part of communication at all times and should be the focal point of the nurse's observations. The nurse should observe how the parents respond to their child's requests for attention. Does the child receive rewards for good behavior or is attention granted only when unacceptable behavior ensues? The way a parent physically handles a child, the way questions are answered or whether they are answered at all, and the manner in which the parent elicits cooperation from the child are clues that the nurse should observe to develop an understanding of how these parents feel about their children.

The nurse should also observe how the parents react to her; for instance, how they respond when the nurse demonstrates affection and care for their child. Is there a response of pride and joy, or is there some indication that the nurse's attention to their child is causing some conflict because they do not feel equally affectionate to the child? Does a parent resent attention given by the nurse because it is viewed as competition with the parent's relationship with the child? The nurse's sensitivity to the parents' nonverbal expression of how they feel when she shows affection and attachment to their children is an often-neglected link to effective communication with parents and children. Observation of the multidirectional flow of nonverbal clues provides the nurse with important information to which she should respond in her communication with children and their parents.

Listening

To listen carefully, attention must be given to the words, the tone of voice and the predominant theme of a conversation. Listening to communication between parents and children makes apparent whether the child is encouraged to speak for himself or whether the parent completes sentences, corrects the child and shows little regard for the ideas of the child. The nurse should listen for the kind of discipline employed. Does the parent threaten the child into good behavior or does an explanation of why the good behavior is necessary accompany the request? The verbal interchanges between the parents and children are important messages to which the nurse should respond in her feedback when communicating with them.

Listening to concerns requires special skills of openness and acceptance by the nurse, because parent-child relationships are often highly charged with emotion and frequently parents have difficulty acknowledging problems. The concerns that parents express verbally about themselves, their children and each other may therefore be distorted because they do not wish to be regarded as incompetent parents, nor do they want to reveal personal difficulties in a marriage. It is only by the nurse's sensitive assessment of what she hears and sees that she can develop a true perspective of how parents feel. The messages from parents should always be received with the realization that they are under a great deal of stress trying to conform to the abstract model of "good parenting."

When listening to children, an understanding of their level of language development and cognition is fundamental. Listening to the cry of an infant and trying to interpret it are the beginnings of sensitive communication with children. When children begin to talk, it is important to take the time to listen to what they say to adults and other children.

Perhaps the thing that causes the most problem for adults is not so much when children cannot use language, but rather when they *can* speak. Children speak early in life and it is easy to assume that the thinking that underlies the speech is the same as that of an adult.[1] The child's way of thinking changes as he develops, and it is important to respond to children on the basis of how they think and not how adults think. For example, a child may ask the nurse for a drink of water or ask to see her stethoscope or to listen to her watch. To hear what the child is asking may involve more than to meet only the obvious request. The child may be thirsty when he asks for a drink and he may be curious when he asks to see the stethoscope and hear the watch; on the other hand, he may be trying to delay the nurse because he is afraid of what is coming next, or he may be asking her to stay awhile because he is scared or lonely.

The greatest disservice we can do a child is not to listen at all. Ignoring a request without any explanation will not only cut off communication but will interfere with the basic trust relationship that is so important when dealing with children. If one does not have time to listen to the child, it is important to tell him why and when there will be time. Rules and limits can be set to regulate when it is appropriate to talk, but they should be clear to both parties. Just as a child can accept that others have the right to speak, adults must accept a child's right to be heard.

Silence

Silence is a common medium of communication when dealing with parents and children. Children may be quiet because they are afraid, angry or shy or because they are busy. Therefore silence cannot be understood without taking into account the individuality of the child and the surrounding stimuli. The age of the child, the usual behavior of the child and the nature of the situation are important elements of the meaning of silence. Perhaps the parent or the child does not wish to speak about a certain topic in front of the other, or it may be that the topic is a point of conflict within the family. When silence is used to block communication it is important for the nurse to be sensitive to the unreadiness of the child or the parent to discuss the problem. Her role is to resume conversation at a level that is more comfortable, thereby allowing the regaining of composure.[2]

Silence can be used positively by the nurse to facilitate communication. Silence is needed for the processing of thoughts and feelings; during silence people seek to understand the content of what has been said. For a child, thoughtful silence may be primarily filled with fear of the unknown and the inability to express that fear. Often words do not dispel fear in a child, but it is the nurse's presence that brings comfort. The nurse's silent presence can be one of the most effective ways for her to share the difficulties and fears of another's thoughtful silence. The nurse's use of silence allows the child or the parent to feel accepted in the presence of a caring person. To use silence most effectively the nurse must evaluate its meaning with regard to the age of the child, the relationships between family members and the nature of the situation at hand.

COMMUNICATING WITH CHILDREN

In communicating with a child it is important to recognize that he is an individual. Each child reacts to a unique set of stimuli, which combine to form his personality. What has happened to a child within his family creates the most important force in his development and it is within his family that a child develops his style of communication. According to Satir, all communication is learned. It is from his family that a child develops ideas about himself (self-concept), has experiences of interacting with others, and learns how to deal with the world around him.[10] Families develop patterns of communication that have a large impact on how children relate; therefore for a nurse to have a realistic expectation of a child's style of communication it is important for her to begin with an assessment of the family.

The attitude of parents toward their children within the home is the fabric from which patterns of communication evolve. Children who come from homes in which they have been deprived of attention and affection may be overwilling to please and to comply with the wishes of others.[5] When dealing with a child who interacts in this way the nurse should respond to the need that the behavior indicates.

Communication patterns are further affected by the relationships between siblings. When sibling rivalry persists, the internal family relationships deteriorate. Friction develops between husband and wife as well as between parent and child as blame is attributed to various family members. A child who comes from a family in which relationships are strained often has difficulty developing relationships outside the home.[5]

The child who is encouraged to participate in decision-making in the home is likely to take an active role in decisions outside the home. A more dependent role is to be expected when the child comes from an adult-centered home in which children are expected to be submissive and are allowed little opportunity for input into family matters.

Principles of Communication with Children

The principles used in dealing with children derive from the premise that communication with a child is affected by the facts that (1) he is an individual, (2) he comes from a certain family and (3) he is at a particular developmental level. The following principles of communication can be applied when relating to children.

The most basic principle is that adults need to *take time to listen and talk with children*. It is most distressing for a child to be in the presence of adults and to be shown no recognition. Children are people, have ideas, and need to feel important. Young[12] asserts that children's resentment is not due to the fact that adults "disagree and deny" but that they "disregard and ignore." When decisions are being made that affect children, they should be consulted. Children have ideas and should be made to feel that their thoughts are important enough to be heard and considered. Not all wishes need to be granted to give a child a sense of well-being, but he does need to be given the opportunity to talk and be heard.

A child's view about health needs to be heard and considered when health care is being planned. Natapoff found that children as young as 6 years of age have ideas about health and can talk about health matters. The children in this study defined health in a positive way with "feeling good and being able to participate in desired activities" as the most important components of health.[8] A child's concept was noted to change with maturation. Six-year-old children saw health as things you do pertaining to eating, exercise and cleanliness. Nine-year-olds were more concerned with an overall health state in which they felt good and were in good shape. Twelve-year-olds saw health to include feeling good and being able to participate in desired activities but also showed evidence of abstract thinking in their concern for mental health.[8] Taking time to listen and talk to children about their views of health is an important step toward having children participate in their own plan of care.

For a nurse to develop a relationship with a child in which she is trusted, she must *be honest*. It is not likely that one willfully chooses to be dishonest with a child, but rather adults tend not to tell children the truth because they wish to protect them from hurt. A fair approach to a child's question is an honest, straightforward answer. For example, if a child asks whether a shot will hurt the honest answer is "Yes," but coupled with a reassuring statement such as "Yes, a shot hurts, but it is over quickly and I am going to be right here with you." It is the touch, the facial expression and the few words of simple explanation and encouragement that can make that "yes" seem tolerable. A child can accept the truth even if it means discomfort as long as the nurse communicates a sense of caring and stays with the child.

An adult must *be reliable* in his relationship with a child so that an environment of trust is created in which the child feels secure. Promises that cannot be kept are a great disappointment to children and make them feel deceived. If you tell a child you will be back to play a game it does not matter so much when, but you must return to fulfill the promise. Should it be absolutely impossible to do so, a broken promise must be explained. Another area of potential deception is offering a choice when there is no choice. Small choices can be offered to a child and can give him a sense of importance and some control. For example, asking a child whether he wishes to take the pink medicine or the orange medicine first is significant and should not be overlooked by the nurse.

To *set limits* is to demonstrate respect and care to a child, while setting no limits produces feelings of insecurity. A child feels in isolation and out of communication when those responsible for his care do not know about his activities. The "testing" of adults by children should be recognized as a normal part of how children receive feedback. Trying to crawl up on a forbidden table one more time and being prevented from doing so may be a test of whether or not that child can feel confidence in adults. It is consistency and fairness in limit-setting that provide security in child-adult relationships and are beneficial to the child.

Communication by touch is a sensitive dimension. Treating children as objects to be indiscriminately patted, kissed and picked up without giving them a choice can communicate disrespect for them as persons.[12] Adults are often unaware of the inappropriateness of their well-intended actions. A child may be engaged in planning an important course of action just when an adult comes by and abruptly picks him up. When adults meet their own needs of holding and cuddling with little regard for where the child was going or was about to do, touch has been used indiscriminately. A sensitive adult will keep in mind the child as a person, observe what a child is doing and then use touch as a response to the needs of the child and as a way to communicate affection. This method shows respect for the child and simultaneously teaches a child self-respect and self-importance.

Recognition of a child's *need for privacy* must not be overlooked. While recognizing that a child needs stimulation and communication from adults, the important right for privacy must also be preserved. Even at a young age a child's private thoughts should not be interrupted. According to Young, children need a private world for many reasons. They need safe retreats in which fantasies can ensue or quiet can be used to sort out the stormy emotions. When the big world outside gets too confusing, they may need a psychological refuge. When a typical child is asked the question "What were you talking to your sister about?" he expresses his need for privacy with a retort such as "Oh, we were just talking." To have privacy is a child's right. It is his right to open or close a door. To communicate sensitively with children is to realize that the door cannot be commanded to be opened. The respect and confidence that children develop in their relationships with adults cannot be forced — it must be won.[12]

In relating to children effectively it is important to *respect their emotions*. Children gradually become socialized and learn to control their emotions and translate their feelings into actions as well as words. To communicate with children it is important to realize that emotions change rapidly, with the hate existing one moment and love the next. Respecting his emotions means that a child is allowed to cry when hurt and to become angry when thwarted. It does not mean that he is allowed to be destructive or cause injury. If aggressive acting out becomes a pattern of behavior, attempts need to be made to channel the aggression into constructive play and exercise or positive verbal communication and problem-solving.

The fears of a child make it imperative to *avoid rushing a child into a relationship*. Children need time to become acquainted and check out a new environment. An infant or a toddler may be frightened if approached and spoken to directly. When a child fears strangers it is more effective to first speak to the parent in the presence of the child and to gradually become acquainted with the child through the parent. The approach can be made by first glancing at the child while speaking to the parent and gradually moving closer to the child while making reference to him. It is important not to block the child's view of the parent so

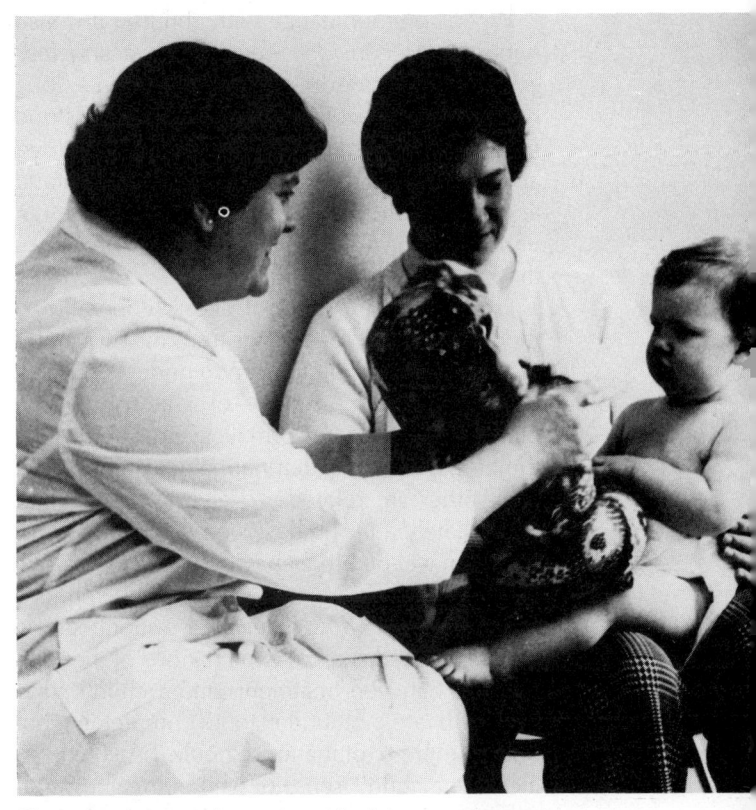

The nurse interacts by gestures, facial expression and tone of voice to develop a relationship prior to examination as the mother provides security for her infant. (Photograph by Cynthia Stewart.)

that he will not fear the parent has disappeared.

A preschool child can often be approached through the medium of play, while a school-age child and an adolescent need different approaches. School-age children and adolescents feel a sense of importance and respect when one addresses them directly, speaking secondly to the parent.

Meeting a child at his level physically facilitates communication. A child's height is a disadvantage to feeling any sense of power. Consequently, to make a child feel that he has something to say about the discussion at hand, every attempt should be made to meet him at eye level. Because children are highly sensitive to nonverbal communication it is important for them to be able to see the person's face for additional clues. Meeting a child on his level gives him a greater sense of equality and facilitates the exchange from child to adult and from adult to child.

When communicating with children it is also important to *consider their cognitive and language abilities.* Adults speak to infants long before they expect their words to be understood because it is a means of communicating love and attention. As children begin to understand and use words, it is important to have an understanding of the child's thought processes that affect his communication.

From 2 until 7 years of age (preoperational thought), a child sees things from his own point of view. It is difficult for him to understand why he cannot have a drink of water before a diagnostic test. He also makes causal errors by thinking that events that happen in proximity to each other are related. To give a child a shot immediately after he has been reprimanded for some unacceptable behavior is an insensitive and destructive thing to do, because the child is likely to think that he received the shot because he misbehaved. Verbal explanations of the relationship between treatments and a child's state of health are not understood completely, but brief, simple explanations should be given. To increase a child's sense of well-being and security it is paramount that acceptance and affection are communicated both verbally and nonverbally before, during and after any hurtful event. Although a child does not understand the full implication of the words spoken to him, he understands (receptive language) more than is indicated by his speech (expressive language).

During the preoperational stage a child engages in pretending; this is a form of communication often difficult for adults to understand. A child's natural tendency to act out his feelings and experiences helps him to cope with the real world and can provide important information to others. Allowing a child to act out that which is about to happen to him is frequently more beneficial than verbal explanation. If he can see and imagine the events that will occur by producing them with dolls or puppets or conversations, he has an acceptable and bearable perception, and he has been able to diffuse some of his emotions pertaining to the event.

One of the most challenging aspects of communication with children at this stage of development is that of answering the "why" question. The difficulty of answering why questions comes in the difference between the ways a child and an adult interpret the meaning of why.

According to Piaget, an adult perceives why to have two distinct meanings: the goal ("Why are you going?") and the cause ("Why is the car moving?"). When a child asks why he is implying both meanings at the same time but does not appear to differentiate between the goal and cause.[9] Children often ask questions pertaining to phenomena even when there is no "because." Children are also thought to use why questions to learn the meaning of why. Concrete objects are easily labeled with words but children of this age have difficulty understanding the abstract concept of such words as why and how.[11]

When answering why and how questions, it is important not to read too much into the questions and to avoid explanations that require abstract thinking. For example, "Why is that truck stopping?" is most simply answered with "Because there is a stop sign." A child of this age often responds with "But why?" Additional information such as "Because the truck will hit the car on the other road," may be sufficient to satisfy the child, but sometimes the answers stimulate further questions. Providing simple, concrete answers helps the child to understand relationships and satisfies his curiosity. To answer the question is of greatest importance. It must not be ignored.

Children may ask questions to satisfy curiosity or for other reasons. Children sometimes practice language and make social contacts by asking questions without expecting an answer. For example, a young child who sees his mother returning from the grocery store with obvious purchases of food may ask "Why did you go to the store?" This may be an effort to make his presence known rather than to discuss the activity of shopping. On some occasions it is apparent that children ask questions to gain attention or that they ask them as a request for help with a problem. Persistent questioning may be done out of curiosity, to practice language or to make social contact, but it may also be an indication of fear, insecurity or unresolved concern. It is only through an attempt to answer a child's questions that we gain insight into what is motivating the question.

Explanations that are given to a child need to be given in concrete terms with reference to familiar happenings in his life experience. For example, time is understood when it is explained in relation to after you wake up, have your breakfast and brush your teeth. Explanations such as "There will be bright lights, the room will be cool, and they will take your picture with a large camera," give the child concrete facts to think about and do not leave his thoughts to an imagination that is capable of visualizing an event as being far more injurious than it is in reality. Because of a child's difficulty in separating fact from fantasy, it is important to explain a painful procedure just prior to its occurrence and to follow it with physical comfort.

During the state of concrete operations (7 to 11 years) important cognitive advancements are made that affect communication. At around age 7 a child is better able to cooperate because he begins to comprehend a viewpoint other than his own. He is now able to engage in a discussion about an event because he is able to focus on more than one aspect of an experience. He can also comprehend explanations that describe an event, but he is still bound to concrete thought. For example, he can understand that it is not painful to have a chest x-ray but he cannot comprehend how repeated x-rays may be harmful to his body.

His cognitive ability enables him to explore and consider many alternatives to a problem. A school-age child needs to be given the opportunity to question and explore what is being said and what will happen to him. An increased understanding of his body and environment requires that details be painstakingly explained when describing an event that pertains to his body. It is especially important to encourage expression of fears when his body integrity is threatened by invasive procedures. His increased use of word symbols makes it possible for him to use language to express his concerns and understand more complex explanations. All such communication, however, must be confined to concrete phenomena, because he cannot solve problems or understand ideas that involve abstract thinking.

The period of formal operations (11 to 15 years) is when abstract thinking begins so that hypothetical situations can be created. It is important to remember that there is an increased need to express feelings verbally during this stage. The adolescent, no longer bound to concrete phenomena, wishes to discuss his values and ideals. He now can hypothesize about how things should be done and especially does so when it involves his own destiny. He does not wish to be told what to do but will be much more cooperative if he is included in the decisions that are made regarding him.

One of the major difficulties that arise during adolescence is the confusion between ideals of how things should be and how they actually are. It is this preoccupation with what "could be" that characterizes the thinking during the stage of formal operation and sometimes produce conflict with other people. An adolescent needs to have the opportunity to express his thoughts of how things should be to help him evaluate his own ideas. Putting his ideas into words is how he formulates what they actually are and eventually resolves the confusion between the real and ideal.

An adolescent's thinking is again characterized by egocentricity, as it was early in life. He often imagines other people to have thoughts and feelings that they do not have but that are in reality his own.[5] He has the need to engage in egocentric thinking and needs the privacy to do so. A special respect for his private thoughts should be communicated by avoidance of prying into personal matters. Because of his egocentricity he often misinterprets the meaning of someone else's communication by not differentiating his own thinking from the thoughts of others. He is highly sensitive to nonverbal communcation and needs an environment of acceptance within which he will feel the freedom to express personal views if he so desires.

COMMUNICATING WITH PARENTS

The nurse who hopes to relate to parents in a way that is beneficial must begin from the premise that parents are individuals. The way a parent thinks and feels about his role as a parent differs with each individual. This role is a manifestation of each person's total life experiences, including cultural, moral and ethical dimensions. This accounts for phenomena that nurses may find troublesome; parents are individuals and therefore may disagree with each other on parenting issues. The nurse should promote the individuality of parents by encouraging individual expression and giving feedback that gives equal recognition to each parent. The nurse's acceptance and respect for individual opinions can serve as a role model for parents to also respect each other's individuality.

When in communication with parents, the nurse must recognize that the way parents perceive their role will affect the communication process. Parents may think that they are expected to have certain feelings and respond in prescribed ways because they are parents. The nurse can dispel some of these erroneous ideas by acknowledging that their frustrations with parenting are normal reactions.

Positive feedback from the nurse that reflects acknowledgment of effective parenting serves to give the parents needed assurance. Most parents need to hear that their children are growing and developing normally, but it is equally important for the nurse to attribute the health of children to the care and nurturing of parents. Small recognitions of positive parent-child relationships provide a significant source of encouragement to parents.

Frequently nurses do not grant such assurances because they fail to realize the regard that parents have for the professional opinion of a nurse. Comments such as "You handle your baby very confidently," "You seem very calm when Mark insists on his own way," and "I notice you are careful to pay attention to your children's questions," are incidental observations that give parents added confidence in their parenting skills. This kind of feedback provides a feeling of basic acceptance that can encourage parents to express the less admirable feelings they hold regarding their children.

The nurse whose goal it is to establish an atmosphere that encourages communication will be careful to avoid an attitude of "talking to" but rather will use an approach that facilitates "talking with" parents. To minimize "talking to" parents, the nurse should use the skills of silence, listening and observation in conjunction with her own personal characteristics of acceptance of others, respect for them and empathy with them. A nondirective approach (using open-ended questions) often creates an environment within which a parent feels accepted and is able to think through a problem and consider new ways of approaching it. The nurse's role then is to reflect the parent's thinking so that the issues can be more easily clarified and decision-making by the parent can be facilitated. The goals parents can set for themselves are more likely to be reached and to bring beneficial results to the family than are those the nurse can establish for the parents.

References

1. D. H. Cohen, and V. Stern. Observing and Recording the Behavior of Young Children. Teachers College Press, 1958
2. M. Collins. Communication in Health Care. C. V. Mosby Co., 1977
3. K. M. Dimick, and V. E. Huff. Child Counseling. William C. Brown Company, Publishers, 1970
4. K. S. Farr. Communication pitfalls in routine counseling. Pediatric Nursing, Jan/Feb 1979, p. 55
5. E. B. Hurlock. Child Development. McGraw-Hill Book Co., 1978
6. B. J. Kalisch. What is empathy? American Journal of Nursing, September 1973, p. 1548
7. R. B. Leyn. The challenge of caring for child refugees from Southeast Asia. American Journal of Maternal Child Nursing, May/June 1978, p. 178
8. J. N. Natapoff. Children's views of health: A developmental study. American Journal of Public Health, October 1978, p. 995
9. J. Piaget. Six Psychological Studies. Translated by Anita Tenzer. Edited by David Elkin. Random House Inc., 1967
10. V. Satir. Peoplemaking. Science and Behavior Publishers, 1975
11. M. S. Smart and R. G. Smart. Children: Development and Relationships. Macmillan Inc., 1977
12. L. R. Young. Life Among the Giants. McGraw-Hill Book Co., 1965

Additional Recommended Reading

M. N. Blondis and B. E. Jackson. Nonverbal Communication with Patients: Back to the Human Touch. John Wiley & Sons, 1977

G. Burton. Interpersonal Relations: A Guide for Nurses, 4th ed. Springer Publishing Co., 1977

P. L. Chinn and C. J. Leitch. Child Health Maintenance: A Guide to Clinical Assessment, 2nd ed. C. V. Mosby Co., 1979

T. Chopoorian. Communication beyond the assessment process. In P. A. Brandt, ed., Current Practice in Pediatric Nursing. C. V. Mosby Co. 1978

D. E. Costello. Communication patterns in family systems. Nursing Clinics of North America, December 1969, p. 721

T. J. Kenny and R. L. Clemmens. Behavioral Pediatrics and Child Development. Williams & Wilkins Co., 1975

D. R. Klinzing and D. G. Klinzing. The Hospitalized Child: Communication Techniques for Health Personnel. Prentice-Hall Inc., 1977

A. C. Mitchell. Barriers to therapeutic communication with black clients. Nursing Outlook, February 1978, p. 109

P. C. Pothier. Mental Health Counseling with Children: A Guide for Beginning Counselors. Little, Brown and Co., 1976

J. Rich. Interviewing Children and Adolescents. Macmillan Inc., 1968

L. F. Smith. Communicating with young children: An experiment with play therapy, Part 3. American Journal of Nursing, December 1977, p. 1963

E. Wiedenbach and C. E. Falls. Communication: Key to Effective Nursing. Tiresias Press, 1978

HEALTH APPRAISAL

by Jo Joyce Tackett, BSN, MPHN,
Mabel Hunsberger, BSN, MSN,
Theresa Eldridge, RN, MS, CPNP

Nursing assessment is fundamental to the nursing process. The phrases assessment and appraisal of health are often used interchangeably; both mean the act of evaluating the quality or status of health. The health appraisal allows the nurse to gather data about the child's past and current health status and present problems and plan for actions that may prevent future problems or identify conditions that may need follow-up assessment. The appraisal focuses primarily on the child but also explores family dynamics and cultural, environmental, socio-ecologic and religious variables that may affect the child's development.

The major goal of a comprehensive assessment is to evaluate the competencies of the child. These competencies — physical, intellectual and emotional–social — provide a framework from which the nurse can approach the assessment process.

The information gathered by the nurse is the data base. This data base must be recorded in a systematic way so that it could be used by another health team member. A modification of the Problem-Oriented Medical Record (POMR) facilitates a well-organized format. The data base and clinical summary are recorded as follows: (1) subjective data (history), (2) objective data (physical examination, family and developmental assessment and other screening tests), (3) assessment (a problem list is developed and recorded; sometimes this is called nursing diagnosis or impression). Then a plan for each problem is developed and recorded. (See Chapter 9 for further discussion of POMR.) Other formats are equally functional for recording assessment findings. The nurse is responsible for learning the format used in her work setting.

TAKING A HISTORY

Interviewing

Interviewing the child or adolescent presents a special challenge because information must be gathered from both the child or adolescent and his caretakers. Equal value should be placed on the information received from the child and from the adult. If inconsistencies between information offered by the child and parent arise, the nurse must gather more data to determine the reliability of each informant. Inconsistencies should be explored further, as they may direct the nurse to underlying problems of inadequate communication within the family.

The interview is not only a time to gather information but also a time to establish trust between the nurse, the child and the parents. The nurse should be warm and friendly and provide a relaxed accepting atmosphere. Privacy must also be ensured. It may be necessary to seek the assistance of an interpreter if the child and family speak another language.

There are several kinds of interviews, each devised to meet different needs and situations. The well-child interview is most frequently conducted by nurses and pediatricians working in ambulatory care settings. It initially includes a complete history, which is modified at subsequent visits to obtain updated information. Following this interview anticipatory guidance is often provided to the child and his family.

The problem interview, or interim health history, focuses on an immediate physical or emotional problem that has been identified by the child, his family or a health care provider. Information obtained pertains primarily to a specific problem but should not be restricted to the problem. Sufficient data should be collected for the nurse to determine the general health status of the child and the family. The length of time of such an interview varies with the particular circumstances. If the child is seen for regular well-child visits the interview may be relatively brief, but if the family generally seeks health care only when problems arise, the nurse is responsible for obtaining a total health history.

Once a problem has been identified and is being managed, a therapeutic interview may be needed. This is generally used to obtain information about how a problem, especially one that is persistent or long term, is responding to treatment.

Communicating by health caregivers with a child and his family requires active listening. The nurse must listen to what the child or parent says and tell them her perceptions of what has been said or implied. This allows the child or parent to verify the nurse's interpretation and provides the opportunity for clarification of any misinterpreted statement.

The interview approach should also be based on the developmental levels of the child and the adult. Questions should be asked in a clear and concise manner, avoiding use of jargon and medical terminology. They should also be asked in a way that is nonthreatening and nonjudgmental. For example, instead of asking the child, "Are you having any problems in school?" the nurse might ask, "What is school like for you?" This approach does not judge or threaten the child by presupposing a problem or making the child feel inferior.

How questions are asked is very important. The type of question may either facilitate the interview process or make it difficult and tedious. One example is the use of open as opposed to closed questions. Open questions allow the child or parent the opportunity to express views, opinions, thoughts and feelings. The closed question does just the opposite: instead of developing rapport, it has a tendency to make the interview too clinical and concise if used excessively. An example of an open-ended question is: "How do you like school?" A closed question would be: "Do you like school?" This allows for only a yes or no answer.

There are also direct and indirect questions. Direct questions are stated in a manner that generally requires a yes or no answer or specific information, such as: "How old are you?" and "When did Johnny first sit alone?" Indirect questions are questions that do not seem to be questions. They permit the client to select or elaborate on information. For example, "You must have some thoughts about discipline," or "It must be difficult to have twins," are indirect questions that do not end with question marks but obviously invite a response. Such questions express the interviewer's interest in what the child or parent has to say and permit the client or parent to express information in his own way. Double questions provide for a choice of one of two alternatives (e.g., "Do you want me to examine your ears or your nose first?"). Such questions enable the child to control part of the interview or the examination, thus providing him with a sense of security and lessening his anxiety.

In an interview, a variety of these techniques and types of questions can be used, depending on the situation and the style of the interviewer. Certain kinds of data lend themselves to a particular technique. For example, direct questions may be used when collecting the data in the review of systems, whereas an open-ended question may be better when collecting data about family or social relationships. When an indirect, open-ended approach is not obtaining the information desired, it may be obtained by asking more direct or closed questions. The nurse should not overuse either technique.

Although every child is approached on the basis of his unique character, some general principles exist regarding the child's ability to contribute to the interview that are determined by his age and stage of development.[7] The infant and early toddler are not interviewed verbally because they have not adequately mastered language; however, they do contribute a volume of information through their behavior and other forms of nonverbal communication that the observant nurse can note and document. The preschooler is verbal enough to tell the nurse about his daily routines if questions are put in terms he can understand. He may also be able to relate some characteristics of symptoms if they produce sensations he is currently experiencing (e.g., a stomachache); however, recall of past sensations is vague at this age. The preschool child relates best to the nurse if his parent remains present throughout the interview.

School-age children can provide the majority of the current information about themselves and their family, school and daily life. The older school-age child can also accurately report past events, making him a significant informant about his own health history and systems review. Involving him in the interview conveys to the school-age child that the nurse thinks him competent and responsible regarding his own health care. Parents can remain present during most of the interview; however, the school-age child should have some time alone with the nurse so that he can share things he feels unable to express in his parent's presence. Whether the parent is present during the physical examination should be decided during the child's time alone with the nurse, so that the child is not pressured by the parent's presence when he makes this decision.

Generally, the adolescent can be independent in contributing the necessary information to the interview. Once the interview is complete, the examination done and a clinical summary has been shared with the youth, he and the nurse together can discuss the problem and any management with the parent. A parent should remain nearby to provide any information the youth is unsure about or does not know. Some teens prefer a friend to be present during the interview or physical or both and may not be accompanied by a parent. How much independence and responsibility the teen can assume for the prescribed care will depend on his maturity. (See Chapters 12 and 15 for further discussion of age-appropriate communication.)

The interview incorporates not only verbal communication but also nonverbal communication. Body posture and facial expressions may influence the flow of the interview. Distancing (how far apart the interviewer and interviewer are from each other) also contributes to the effectiveness of communication. Most interviewers select a distance of approximately two to three feet from the parent and child. It is difficult to establish rapport or listen when the child and parent are sitting at some distance across the room. In summary, a successful interview is based on appropriate verbal and nonverbal communication skills, establishing appropriate environmental conditions, using a variety of direct and indirect interviewing techniques, and establishing rapport with the parent and the child.

The Health History

The following discussion focuses on the type of information obtained in each category of a pediatric history. (See Table 13-1 for one example of a history format.) It is one approach for gathering data in an organized manner. Titles of categories may vary in different settings, but the content usually remains unchanged.

Demographic Data or Identifying Data Prior to beginning the interview the nurse introduces herself, ensures the child's and parents' comfort, explains the purpose of the interview, and then begins to collect basic demographic data. Much of this data may already be found in the child's chart and may only need verification as being correct. The informant(s) should be identified and the reliability of that informant(s) indicated. In many instances, the informants may be both parent and child. An example of the type of statement used for informant is: "Mother and Todd, reliability questionable; mother answers hesitantly, speaks primarily Spanish. Todd speaks no English. Interpreter present for history."

Reason for Contact The reason for contact is the specific reason for the visit to the office, clinic or hospital. It is a brief statement recorded in the child's or the parent's own words. The reason for contact is often referred to as the chief complaint. It should be elicited by asking open-ended neutral questions such as "How may I help you?" or "Why have you come here today?" If there are multiple problems or complaints, it may be necessary to have the informants identify the one problem or reason that caused them to seek health care.

TABLE 13-1 PEDIATRIC HISTORY-TAKING OUTLINE

Demographic Data
1. Name (nickname or preferred name)
2. Address
3. Date and place of birth
4. Sex
5. Age
6. Race/Nationality
7. Religion
8. Date of interview
9. Primary language spoken
10. First names of parents
11. Source and reliability of informant(s)

Reason for Contact (Chief Complaint)
1. Statement in child's or informant's own words of the reason health care is presently being sought— problem or symptom.

Present Illness (Analysis of Chief Complaint)
1. Onset – events coincident with onset, sudden or gradual, previous episodes, when began.
2. Characteristics of chief complaint (analysis)
    a. Type, or *character,* of complaint (pain: dull, sharp, aching, burning, radiating, itching, tickling).
    b. *Location* (if applicable). Should be anatomically precise (ask child to point to affected area).
    c. *Severity* (annoying, uncomfortable, incapacitating) and effect on normal daily activities (eating, sleeping, elimination, playing, mood).
    d. *Duration* (intermittent, persistent or continuous, interval between if intermittent).
    e. *Influencing factors* (precipitating, aggravating, relieving, ameliorating, recent illness exposure).
    f. *Past treatment* or evaluation of complaint. (When, where, and by whom, what studies were performed in the past and what were the results (blood studies, x-ray, etc.), results of past treatment, past diagnosis).
    g. *Current treatment* or evaluation of the complaint (treatment, medications, tests) and response of condition to these measures.
3. Present status of complaint (getting worse, better, unchanged).
4. Reason for seeking care now.

Past Health History

Birth History (prenatal)
1. Mother's state of health during pregnancy
    a. Illnesses (fever, rash, vomiting, infection); month in pregnancy when occurred; treatment prescribed.
    b. Hospitalizations; month in pregnancy when hospitalized; treatment prescribed.
    c. X-rays; month in pregnancy when taken.
    d. Medications taken (over-the-counter or prescribed); month in pregnancy when taken; reason(s) taken.
    e. Diet during pregnancy; amount of weight gained.
2. Previous obstetrical history
    a. Gravida including this pregnancy
    b. Para including this pregnancy
    c. How long before this pregnancy were there any still births, abortions or miscarriages and their causes, if known?
    d. Have any live-born children died? How long before this pregnancy and cause if known?
    e. Length of this pregnancy
3. Prenatal care received
    a. Mother's age with this pregnancy
    b. When was prenatal care initiated and for how much of pregnancy was it maintained?
    c. Bleeding or complications (toxemia) during this pregnancy and blood type of both parents
4. Attitude toward this pregnancy
    a. Mother describes as easy or difficult pregnancy
    b. Planned or unplanned pregnancy
    c. Child wanted by either or both parents

Birth History (natal)
1. Circumstances of birth
    a. Where was baby born (e.g. home, birthing room, hospital)?
    b. Natural or induced labor; length of labor; any problems during labor
    c. Was fetal monitoring used? Why?
    d. Any drugs given during labor?
2. Characteristics of delivery
    a. Natural, assisted (forceps used) or C section delivery
    b. Was the father present?
    c. Mother concious during delivery? Unconscious?
    d. Was baby in normal position? Breech?
3. Condition of baby at birth
    a. Birth weight
    b. APGAR score
    c. Did baby cry immediately?
    d. Was mechanical suctioning or oxygen required?
    e. Was the baby put in an incubator?
    f. Any abnormalities noted at birth?

Table 13-1 PEDIATRIC HISTORY-TAKING OUTLINE *(Continued)*

Birth History (*postnatal*)
1. Weight loss or gains and amount during hospital stay
2. Any difficulties during stay in nursery   (Feeding or sucking problems; cyanosis, jaundice, rashes)?
3. Length of baby's hospital stay? Nursery or rooming in? Baby and Mother went home together?
4. Bottle-fed? Breast-fed?

Past Illnesses
Accidents
1. Age at each accident.
2. Circumstances surrounding accident (cause, where occurred).
3. Facts regarding accident
    Extent of injury
    Treatment received
    Complications or residual problems
    Child's reaction
4. Any current problems associated with accident(s)?

Illnesses
1. Names of illnesses or infections
    Age when occurred
    Treatment received
    Complications or sequelae
2. Names of childhood diseases
    Age
    Severity
    Treatment
    Residual problems

Operations
1. Date and age at each operation.
2. Why was surgery done?
3. Outcome of surgery
4. Child's reaction to each surgery
5. Any follow up or complications?

Hospitalizations
1. Reason for each hospitalization.
2. Dates and child's age at each.
3. Length of each.
4. Child's reaction to hospitalization(s).
5. Outcome.
6. Complications.

Allergies
1. Untoward response to medications, foods, animals, insect bites.
2. Type of reaction (Hives, rash, swelling, rhinitis, nausea).
3. Do symptoms occur seasonally?
4. Do symptoms occur immediately or a few to several hours after exposure?

Immunizations
1. Type received (see Table 13-2)
2. Dates received
3. Untoward reactions

Developmental History
1. Motor development milestones
2. Language development milestones
3. Social development milestones
4. Current developmental status with regard to activities of daily living
    a. Diet
       How is child's appetite?
       Bottle-fed? Breast-fed?
       If breast-fed, mother's diet and fluid intake? If bottle, what kind, how much, how formula mixed?
       Amount in 24 hours? Number of feedings in 24 hours, length of each feeding, how progressing?
       If taking solids, what kind, portion size, how often?
       What kinds of foods in diet—meats, vegetables, fruits, cereals, juices, eggs, milk, snacks?
       How often? What portion size? How does child eat (spoon, fork, fingers, knife)? How well does
       child feed himself? Is he messy, neat? Does he use a cup?
       When does child eat (alone, with family)?
       Does child take vitamins (kind, how often, with or without iron)?
       Food dislikes, food likes, food jags?
    b. Elimination
       What are child's bowel patterns? Frequency? Consistency? Discomfort?
       Is child toilet trained? (At what age? Accidents? Day or night trained?) How was child toilet trained?
       Any associated stresses with elimination habits? Enuresis? (A more detailed history is found
       in the review of systems.)

Table continued on following page

TABLE 13-1 PEDIATRIC HISTORY-TAKING OUTLINE *(Continued)*

    c. Sleep
        When does child go to bed? Does he sleep through night?
        Nightmares, night terrors?
        Difficulties with putting the child to bed?
        How many hours does child sleep in 24 hours? Naps (when, how long)? Difficulty falling asleep?
        Insomnia? Where does child sleep? Does he have his own bed?
        How does the child awaken (alert, fussy)?
        Any change in sleep patterns?
    d. Development
        How does child compare to siblings, peers?
        What can child do now? (This should be age appropriate: 15-month-old walks, 3-year-old rides a tricycle, and so on.)
        What new tasks has child accomplished since the last visit?
        What does child like to do? The developmental patterns should cover fine and gross motor activities, intellect and speech, and personal-social.
        What kind of games does child like to play? How does he play with peers?
    e. Personality/school performance
        Unusual behaviors (thumbsucking, nail biting, masturbation)?
        How does child describe himself? How does parent describe child's personality?
        What are child's school interests? Grades? School performance?
        How does child interact with teachers, classmates?
        How does child get along with family members?
        What chores does child do?
        Does he get an allowance?
        What does child do when he's mad, sad, glad, scared?
    f. Discipline
        How is the child disciplined (verbal, physical)? When is he disciplined? How often?
    g. Sexuality
        What questions is child asking?
        What are parent's responses?
        What is family's attitude toward masturbation, nudity?
        What does child or adolescent know about secondary sexual development, sexuality, menstruation, sexual exploration?
        Is adolescent sexually active? Using birth control (type, frequency of use, problems)?
        Does the adolescent female know how to examine her breasts?

Child Review of Systems (see Table 13-3)
1. General appearance
2. Skin and lymphatics
3. Eyes, ears, nose and throat
4. Cardiopulmonary system
5. Gastrointestinal system
6. Genitourinary system
7. Musculoskeletal system
8. Neurologic status

Family Profile
1. Family members
2. Familial and hereditary diseases
    a. Glaucoma, cataracts, other eye disorders
    b. Tuberculosis, asthma, heart disease, hypertension
    c. Ulcers, colitis
    d. Kidney disease
    e. Arthritis, muscular dystrophy
    f. Mental disorder, epilepsy, learning disorders
    g. Allergies, diabetes, sickle cell disease, cancer, congenital anomalies
3. Family social history (see Table 13-4)
    a. Finances
    b. Resources
    c. Family relationships
    d. Residence
    e. Health attitudes and practices

Present Illness This portion of the history is obtained if the child presents with a specific physical, intellectual or language, emotional, or social problem. It is not always included in a health maintenance visit unless the child is also ill or has a specific complaint. The present illness history should include four components: (1) a description of the onset and progression of the problem or symptom, (2) an analysis of the problem or symptom, (3) the present status of the problem or symptom (better, worse, the

TABLE 13-2 RECOMMENDED IMMUNIZATION SCHEDULE FOR INFANTS AND CHILDREN*

Condition	2 Mo.	4 Mo.	6 Mo.	1 Yr.	15 Mo.	1½ Yr.	4–6 Yr.	14–16 Yr.
DTP	✔	✔	✔			✔	✔	
Polio	✔	✔				✔	✔	
Measles					✔			
TB test				✔				
Rubella					✔			
Mumps					✔			
Tetanus-Diphtheria								✔

*Recommended by the American Academy of Pediatrics, October 1980.

same) and (4) the reason for seeking care now.[2] If more than one problem or symptom exists, the nurse must investigate their order of occurrence. Table 13–1 summarizes the type of information to be gathered for these four components of the present illness.

Past Health History *Birth History.* The birth history should include data concerning the mother's health during pregnancy, labor and delivery, and the infant's condition immediately following birth. Whenever asking questions it is helpful to explain the relevance of the questions and the importance of having this information. An explanation should be given to the parent that prenatal influences and the child's early life experiences may have significant effects on the child's physical, intellectual and emotional development. Table 13–1 lists questions that should be covered in a comprehensive birth history.

Past Illnesses The past health history includes a summary of any diseases, accidents, operations or hospitalizations the child has experienced before the present health history. Table 13–1 summarizes crucial questions to be documented in these areas.

Immunizations The type of immunizations the child has received as well as the dates of the initial series and last booster dosage (if appropriate) should be noted. Any reactions and the treatment that followed should also be documented. A record of tuberculin skin testing is included with the immunizations. Table 13–2 summarizes the recommended schedule of immunizations for infants and children.

Developmental History Documentation of the age at which the child mastered developmental milestones in all three competencies is also included in the health history. Although parental recall may be hazy, such information may give insight into a current abnormality. Milestones usually recorded include three categories: motor development, language development and social development. Motor development milestones are: held head up, rolled front to back and back to front, sat alone, crawled, pulled to stand, walked holding on and alone. For the older child motor documentation should include the age at which he rode a tricycle, hopped, skipped, ran, jumped, and climbed stairs.

Language development milestones are: babbled, used first word, used two-word sentence, major method of communication (e.g., sounds, words, actions), present vocabulary.

Social development milestones are: child's/parent's description of child's basic personality (usual mood, strong features, difficult or weak features); present or persisting fears, nervous behaviors; how feelings are expressed (verbally, behaviorally, aggressively); how child gets along with parents, siblings, peers, at school; what type of discipline is effective with child, how often punishment is employed; type and quality of play, who child plays with; school performance and adjustment; age of onset and resolution of separation anxiety; typical response to new situations; moral attitudes; degree of independence demanded and achieved.

A review of the child's current developmental status is also summarized, particularly with regard to skills relevant to daily living (Table 13–1). Specific questions asked will depend on the child's age and development.

HEALTH APPRAISAL 183

TABLE 13-3 OUTLINE OF CHILD REVIEW OF SYSTEMS

General
Overall state of health? Fatigue? Growth patterns? Recent or unexplained weight loss or weight gain? Contributing factors (illness, dieting change in appetite)? Fevers? Chills? Exercise tolerance? General ability to perform normal daily functions?

Skin and Lymph
Skin problem such as excessive dryness, pruritus, skin sensitivity? Rashes? Acne? Skin color changes? Tendency for bruising? Petechiae? Abnormalities of nail color, nail growth? Hair loss? Hair color change? Use of hair dyes, chemicals for hair straightening? Swollen lymph glands?

Eyes
Known visual problems? Behaviors that may indicate visual problems: turning head to one side, sitting close to the television set,* squinting, rubbing the eyes, bumping into objects? Crossed eyes (strabismus)? Lazy eye (amblyopia)? Wears glasses or contact lenses? Eye infections? Excessive tearing or absence of tears? Burning? Edema of eyelids? Redness?

Ears
Earaches, ear infections, ear discharge? Hearing loss? Behaviors that may indicate this: turning radio or television very loud, requests to repeat in conversation, loud speech, inattentive behavior, decreased or no response to loud noises?

Nose
Nosebleeds (episodic, recurrent, severe)? Frequent nasal congestion or runny nose? Nasal obstruction or difficulty with breathing? Frequent sneezing, sinus pain, sinus infections?

Throat
Mouth breathing? Bleeding gums? Toothaches? Teething? Sore throats, infections, strep throats? Hoarseness? Difficulty swallowing?

Cardiorespiratory
Trouble breathing, choking, turning blue? Difficulty feeding, tires easily, difficulty running or playing? Cough (where, when, position, wet, dry)? Wheezing? Keeps up with other children? Number of colds per year? Heart murmur? Anemia? Date and result of last blood count? Blood type? Blood transfusion? Rheumatic fever?

Gastrointestinal
Bowel patterns, frequency, color, discomfort? Abdominal pain, diarrhea, constipation? Flatulence, bloody stools, bleeding, fissures, nausea, vomiting?

Genitourinary
Urinary stream, frequency, pain on urination, urgency, periods of dryness (as opposed to dribbling or constant wetness), bleeding, enuresis? Menstruation (when started, how often, amount, length of each menses, discomfort, problems)? Vaginal discharge, pruritus? Pain or discharge from penis? Swelling or pain of testicles? Change in testicular and penile size? Pubic hair?

Musculoskeletal
Weakness, history of fractures, strains, sprains? Painful joints, swelling, redness of joints? Clumsiness, lack of coordination, tremors, abnormal gait, restricted or painful movement?

Neurological
Convulsions, febrile seizures? Fainting, tremors, twitches, blackouts, dizziness, frequent headaches? Learning problems, clumsiness, coordination problems? Numbness, memory loss, speech problems, unusual habits? Taste, tactile sense? Sees, hears, smells?

*Young children tend to sit close to TV even though no visual problem exists. In school-age or older children it may indicate a visual problem.

Child Review of Systems   The child review of systems is specific for the child for whom the history is being obtained. It is important that this be differentiated from the family review of systems. The review of systems is done for a complete data base in a well child as well as for a child who presents with an illness or specific complaint. It focuses attention on any deviations from health, thus allowing the nurse a more comprehensive picture of the child's health status and potential problems. The information received in this part of the history is invaluable even when it may appear unrelated to the problem at hand.

Table 13-3 is an outline of suggested areas for review of each body system. The nurse should use terms that are easily understood by the parent and child, even though information is recorded in medical terminology. The questions will vary depending on the age and developmental level of the child.

Family Profile   The primary purpose for obtaining a family health history is to discover potential hereditary or familial diseases that could affect the health of the child.

A second purpose for a family health history is to identify possible stress factors that could affect the child and his family. A recent death or chronic illness of one of the family members may interfere with the normal function of the child and his normal developmental progress. Because of the impact of family stress on the child's development, this information should also be obtained even if the child is adopted. A

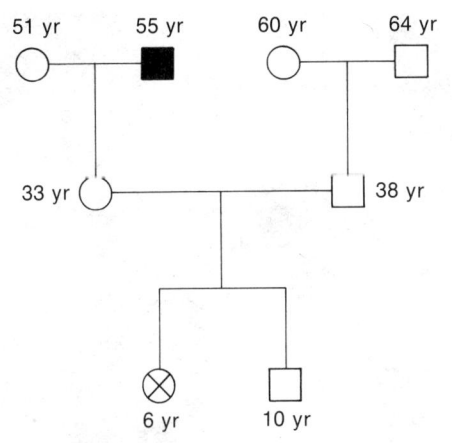

Figure 13-1 A family genogram.

family health history may be represented in written form or pictorially by a genogram or both.

Family Members A list or diagram of family members, including their ages, sex, and state of health is made. If a genogram is used, a circle represents a female and a square represents a male. Marriage is represented by a horizontal line and a vertical line indicates a descendant. A blacked circle or square indicates that an individual is deceased. An "X" indicates the child or client with whom this particular history is concerned. (See Figure 13-1 for an example of a basic family genogram.)

Familial or Hereditary Diseases Information on existing or past conditions that are of a familial or hereditary nature in parents, maternal and paternal grandparents, first aunts and uncles, and siblings should be obtained. A review of systems is often a helpful and organized approach to gathering this data (Table 13-1).

Family Social History This portion of the history includes information on environmental, economic, personal and social factors that influence the child's and family's overall development and health. Table 13-4 summarizes the pertinent data in this area.

The nurse should ignore no information offered during the social history. If it is said, it is probably important and should be recorded. While it is crucial that the nurse gather complete information, she should be aware that there is often as much important information contained in the inaccuracies of a child's or parents' stories as there is in the accurate factual data. These inaccuracies may reflect areas of conflict for a family. It is also important to recognize that the giving of information and the sharing of stories and recollections is therapeutic for many families. As a result a bond is often formed with a good interviewer. It should be understood that the interviewer is someone who will be available to the family later and not a clerk from a separate department.

PHYSICAL ASSESSMENT

Approaching the Child

When doing an examination on a child it is important to provide a comfortable atmosphere

TABLE 13-4 FAMILY SOCIAL HISTORY

Finances
1. Who is employed? Where? Occupation?
2. Does the family have enough money to do the things that are important to its members?
3. Are they receiving financial assistance (welfare, food stamps)?
4. Do they have health insurance?

External Resources
1. What schools, day care or preschool facilities are being used?
2. Are there babysitters? How often used?

Family Relationships
1. Who lives at home (parents, grandparents, significant others)?
2. What are the family interrelationships?
3. What is the marital status?
4. What is the home atmosphere like (happy, sad, cooperative, antagonistic, chaotic)?
5. Who shares in household chores?
6. Who within the family shares in caring for the children?
7. What is the level of education?
8. What are some of the family activities?
9. How were the parents disciplined as children?

Residence
1. Type of housing (house, apartment, room)?
2. Is there a yard and is it fenced?
3. Are there stairs?
4. Is a busy street nearby?
5. What is the proximity to transportation, shopping, playground, schools, health care facilities?
6. Is it a safe neighborhood?
7. Is there city or well water? Is it fluoridated?

Health Attitudes and Practices
1. How does the family regard health services and personnel?
2. How is the family's role as health consumer perceived?
3. Who makes decisions about health issues, management of illness, when to seek health care?
4. What cultural or religious traditions exist that affect health care or childrearing practices?
5. What is the family's attitudes and participation in preventive health practices?
6. How is safety stressed in home and family living?

HEALTH APPRAISAL

and to conduct the examination as quickly, efficiently and with as little anxiety as possible. To do this the nurse must determine what approach is developmentally appropriate for the child being assessed.

It is helpful to take full advantage of opportunities as they arise. For example, it may behoove the nurse to listen to a small child's heart and lungs when the child is lying quietly in his mother's arms because the child may begin to cry later during the examination. Another example would be to observe the neurological, growth and developmental status of the child while he is playing with toys in the room. The nurse may also listen to the child's speech and articulation when he talks to a parent or siblings in the room or when he answers questions during the history.

Children at any age may exhibit modesty that should be respected. Gowns should be offered to children beyond infancy. Infants generally are not aware of being unclothed and often like being without clothing. As much of the examination as possible should be done without touching the child who is extremely anxious or uncooperative.

It is essential that the nurse explain each step of the physical examination and, if possible, make a game out of it. A young child may enjoy playing "This little piggy went to market" with his toes while the nurse is examining the feet and lower extremities. Initially doing part of the neurological exam or a Denver Developmental Screening Test that allows active play may make the examination go smoothly. Allowing the child to participate actively in the examination process also promotes rapport and cooperation. It allows the nurse to make observations about the child's coordination and other neurological skills at the same time.

Whenever an examination is done it is important to take a systematic approach. This may vary depending upon the age of the child and the amount of cooperation received. The child should be kept dressed until the time of the physical examination. It is very uncomfortable for a child to have to sit in a gown or unclothed while the nurse is taking a comprehensive health history. Also, it is much less threatening for a toddler or a preschooler to remove just his socks and shoes and then continue to remove additional pieces of clothing as the examination

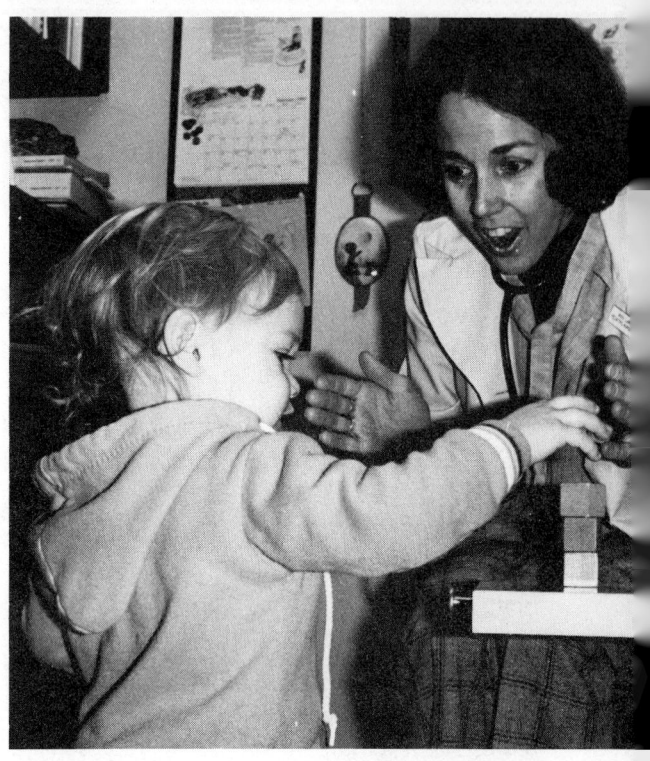

Initially doing part of the Denver Development Screening Test that allows active play may encourage rapport between the child and the nurse before the physical examination. (Photograph by Jennifer Piersma.)

progresses. The nurse should never ask, "Jane, will you take off your clothes?" but rather, she should say, "It's time to take off your clothes." Giving the child an opportunity to say no will only frustrate the nurse and the child when there is actually no choice in the situation. However, the nurse can provide the child with choices in other areas, such as "Shall I look at your ears or your nose first?" or "Shall I listen to your heart first or look at your feet?" In this way the child feels that he has some control in the examination process. A child who feels in control is much more likely to be cooperative.

Some techniques may be very helpful in examining the younger child or the anxious child. When the examiner examines the child while he is on the lap of the parent or another adult, the laps of the examiner and the parent can become the examination table. The adults generally will sit facing each other with knees touching to form a flat surface upon which the child may be placed for examination of the abdomen and musculoskeletal system. Even if restraint is needed, it is also possible to examine the child in the parent's arms. With the child's head on the parent's shoulder, the parent can firmly but gently restrain his head and body while the examiner examines his ears. For the ear examination the child may be held on the mother's lap with both legs between her knees. One of the mother's arms then restrains the child's chest and arms while her other arm restrains the child's head against her chest. The child may feel more secure or less threatened being restrained in the parent's arm than being restrained on the table. However restraint is accomplished, it is important to be sure that the uncooperative child is adequately restrained during the physical examination so that injury does not occur.

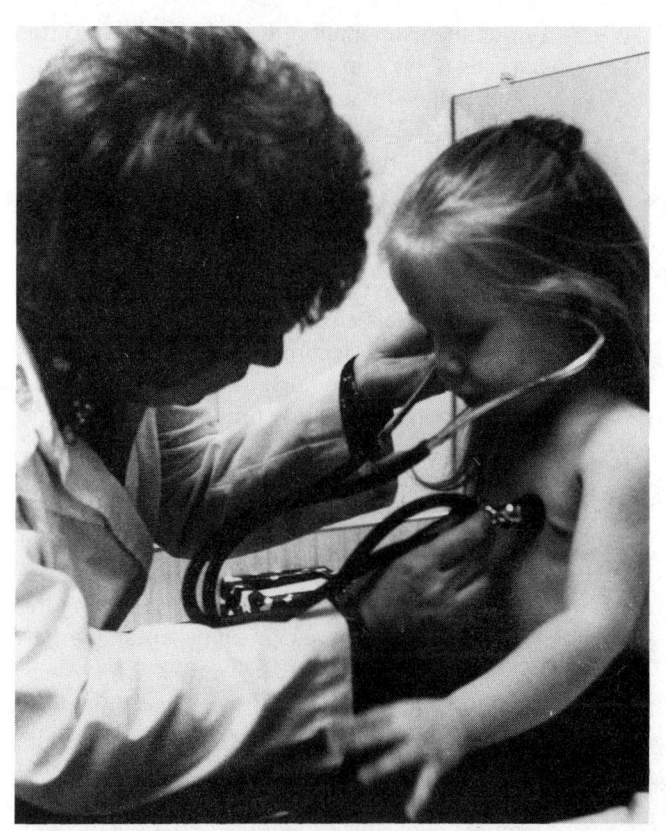

It may be helpful to let the child examine and handle the equipment to be used — otoscope, stethoscope and reflex hammer — so that he is less anxious about these instruments. The nurse can also play several games with the child, such as having the child pretend to blow out the light of the otoscope. This is not only a good way to set the child at ease but the nurse may also use this information to determine the child's lung capacity and also his ability to follow directions. When examining the abdomen, the nurse may play games with the child by pretending to guess what the child had for breakfast or for lunch. When palpating the abdomen the nurse may say, "See if I can figure out what you had for breakfast," and may guess several foods. If she guesses the right one, the child is delighted and generally is enthralled with the process of the nurse trying to figure out what is in his tummy.

The young child may also respond to the game of pretending that something is caught in his ear, such as a bird, a monkey or a puppy. The nurse may be able to make noises of animals or birds that distract the child and allow for a more cooperative examination.

Many children like to be involved in the health examination and like to listen to their own heart. Such involvement provides an excellent opportunity to do health teaching. (Photograph by Jennifer Piersma.)

Many children also like to be involved in the health examination and may wish to listen to their heart or their parent's heart or lungs. This is also an excellent time to do health teaching, especially for the older child. This may be a good time to explain what is located in the abdomen and what the nurse is palpating. The school-age child and the adolescent are very interested in knowing why the abdomen is being palpated and what the nurse is looking for.

The examiner may wish to employ a variety of tools to assist her in the physical examination. These may be items such as a doll with a heart embroidered on the chest. Many children will respond to doll play to lessen their anxiety

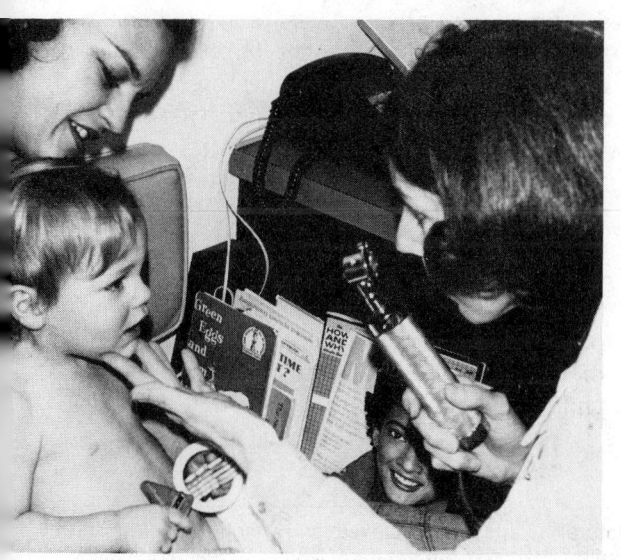

A parent's lap is preferred by the young child to an examination table. (Photograph by Jennifer Piersma.)

HEALTH APPRAISAL 187

during the examination. It is also helpful to use puppets to explain procedures and let the puppet hold the stethoscope or the tongue depressor during the examination. The child may wish to examine the puppet by using the tongue depressor to look down the puppet's throat or listen to the puppet's heart or examine its ear. Ordinary sock puppets made at home or some of the commercial puppets such as Sesame Street characters can be used.

Whatever the techniques used to complement the style of the nurse, a variety of toys and examination techniques should be used for the different age groups so that the examination progresses smoothly, with as much of the child's cooperation as possible. The nurse should always be firm and confident and not allow the child to control the progress of the examination. This is best done by allowing the child to participate and become an active part of the interaction process.

Following are specific physical examination suggestions for each age group. These are some general guidelines that may vary with the exact age of the child, his developmental level and temperament, his previous experiences with nurses and examinations, and his parent's attitude toward the examination.

Newborn or Infant: Generally does not object to having clothes removed. Can be distracted by moving objects, noises or games such as peek-a-boo during listening to the heart and lungs and palpating the abdomen. The quiet child may be examined head to toe or toe to head. The older infant (6 to 8 months and older) may be developing stranger anxiety and might best be examined on the parent's lap. Observe the child playing for objective data — for example, pincer grasp, transfer of one object hand to hand. Observe the parent-child interaction.

Toddlers: May or may not object to removing clothing. May wish to undress himself, which is another opportunity to observe for developmental, musculoskeletal and neurological capabilities. The examiner may wish to establish rapport first by playing games or performing a developmental test. Toddlers generally do not like being touched by strangers and are often frightened or anxious. The examiner cannot reason with or generally comfort a child this age. If the child cries or is uncooperative, it is best to proceed as quickly as possible. The child should be told that it is all right to cry but he cannot bite, pinch or kick. Toddlers resist being supine, so do as much of the examination as possible with them upright. It is helpful to distract the child and if possible demonstrate parts of the examination on the parents, a sibling, or a toy animal or doll. If a cooperative older or younger child is present, the examiner may examine that child first to lessen the toddler's fears. The ear and throat examination should be done last, since it causes increased stress and fear. The toe-to-head approach is frequently better.

Preschoolers: Most preschoolers are cooperative about removing their clothing but may be sensitive about examination of the genitalia. The underpants should be left on until this examination, which is best saved until last. This child may wish to use a gown. The preschooler will generally sit on the examination table if the parent is nearby. There is usually no complaint about sitting or lying down. These children like to be talked to, like to participate in the examination and may demonstrate interest in listening to their hearts, looking in eyes with penlights, and so on. The toe-to-head approach is often best used here because of the ear and throat examination, or the throat examination can be postponed until near the end.

School Age and Adolescent: These children are often sensitive about the genitalia examination, so this may be postponed until last. Girls are often sensitive about exposing their chest. Adolescents need constant reassurance that they are all right; they are intensely interested in body concerns. Both boys and girls should be robed. Either the head-to-toe or the toe-to-head method can be used without difficulty. Children in this age group are generally very cooperative and interested in the examination. Adolescents may wish to be examined without parents in the room.

Measurements

Height and Weight For the child, the measurements of height and weight should be obtained and plotted on a standardized anthropometric chart at each physical examination (at least five times during the first year of life and one to two times a year thereafter through adolescence). Height and weight measurements reflect overall growth of the child. (See Figure 13-2 for height and weight charts.)

The method of assessing the child's height varies with age. The infant and young child is stretched out and his knees are extended. Using a sliding tool is a preferred method to obtain height measurement. The child's head is firmly placed at the headboard while the movable end of the measuring stick is stretched until the child's heel touches the footboard. It is impor-

Figure 13-2 Charts for boys and girls of length (or stature) by age (upper curves) and weight by age (lower curves), each curve corresponding to the indicated percentile. (Adapted from National Center for Health Statistics: NCHS Growth Charts 1976. Monthly vital statistics Report. Vol. 25, No. 3, Supp 76-1120. Health Resources Administration, Rockville, MD, June 1976.)

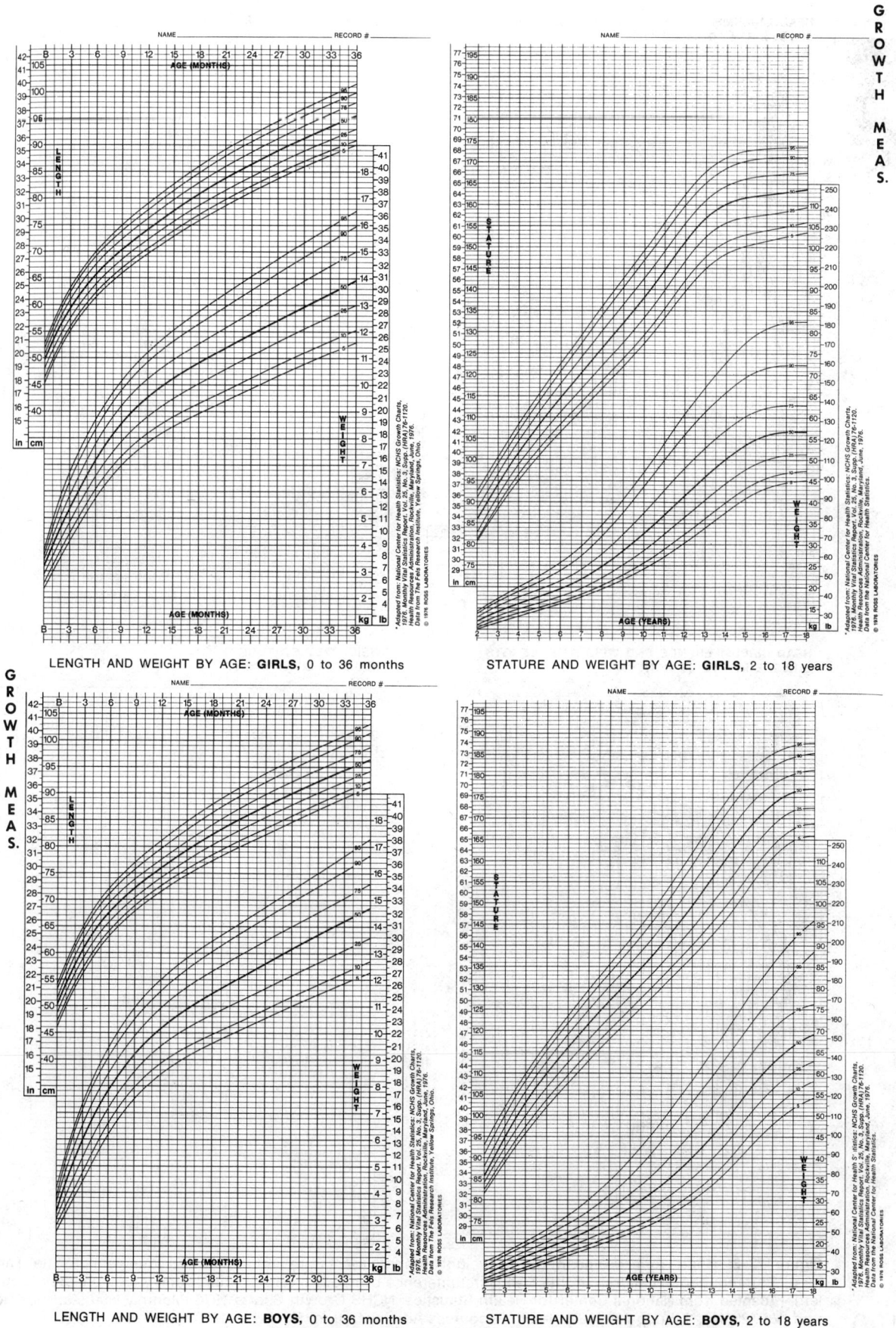

LENGTH AND WEIGHT BY AGE: **GIRLS**, 0 to 36 months

STATURE AND WEIGHT BY AGE: **GIRLS**, 2 to 18 years

LENGTH AND WEIGHT BY AGE: **BOYS**, 0 to 36 months

STATURE AND WEIGHT BY AGE: **BOYS**, 2 to 18 years

Figure 13–2 *See legend on opposite page*

189

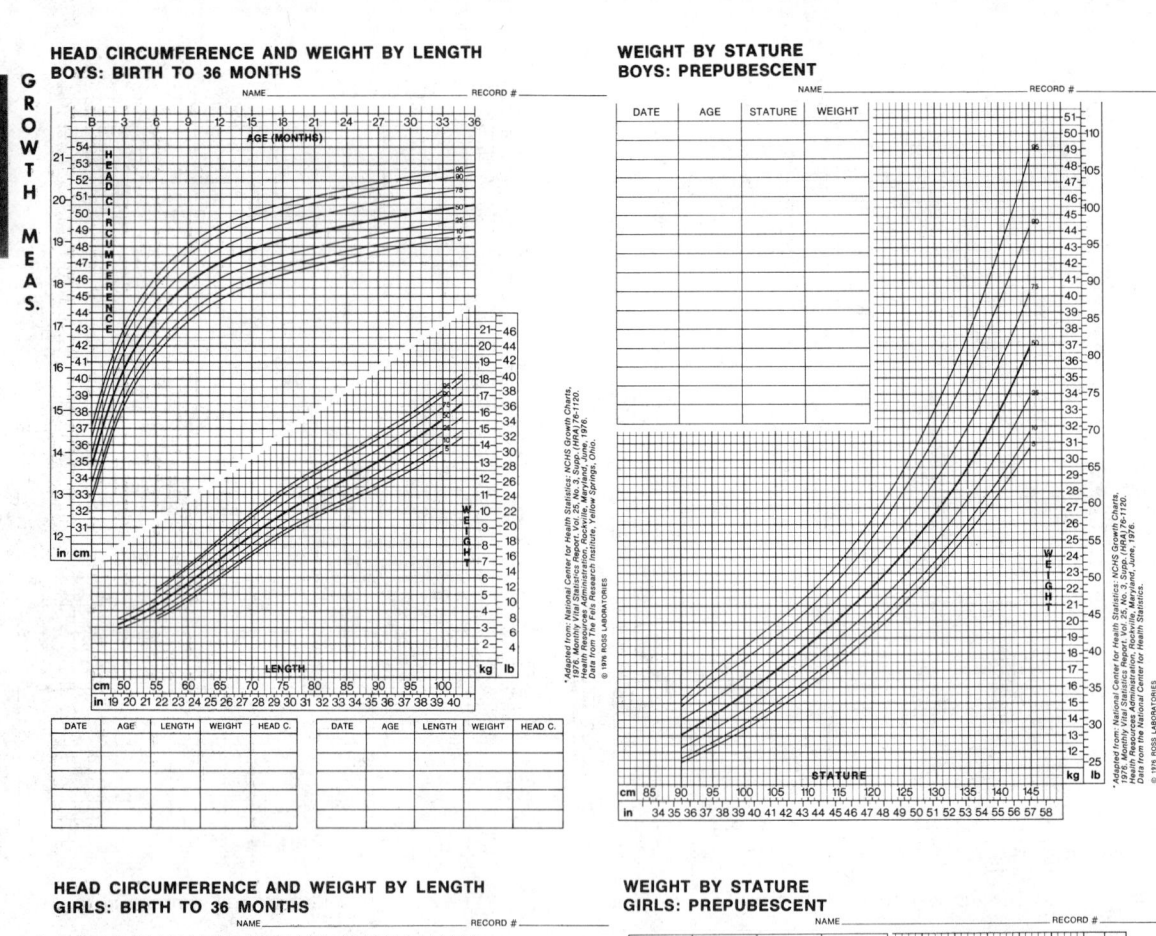

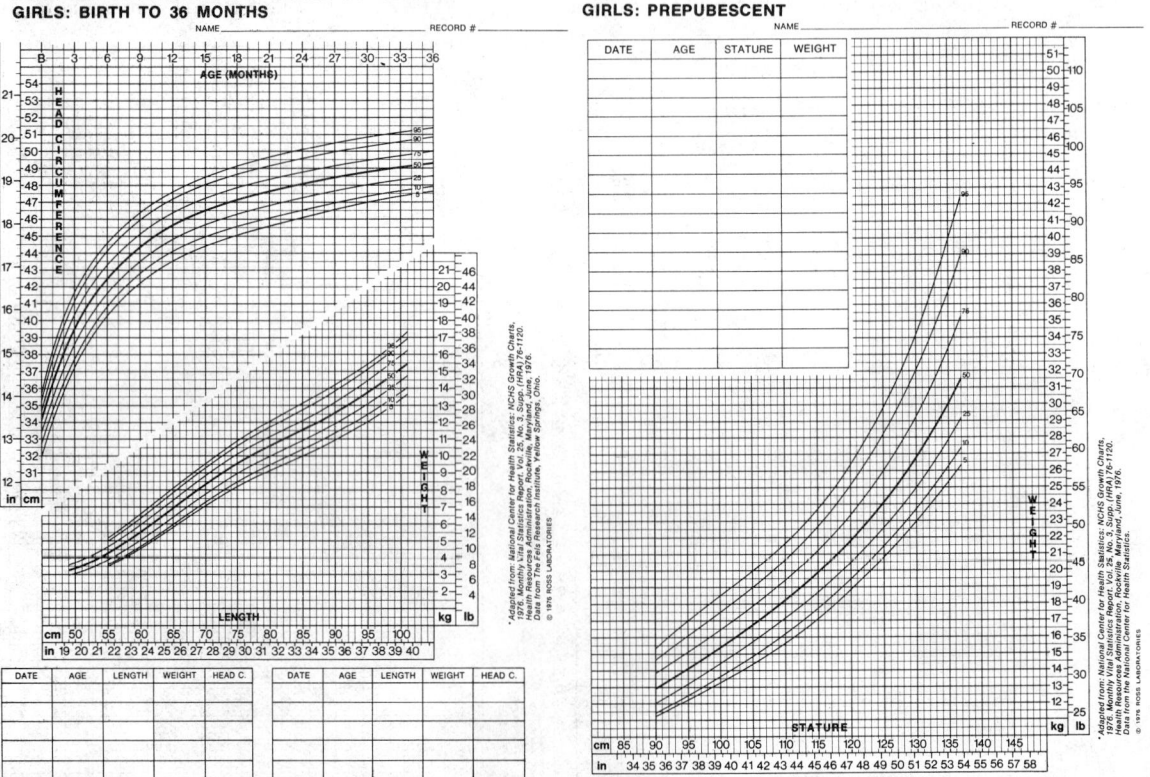

Figure 13–2 Charts for boys and for girls of weight by length (or stature), for infants and young children (left) and for older (prepubertal) children (right). Head circumference by age is given for infants and young children (upper left). (Adapted from National Center for Health Statistics: NCHS Growth Charts 1976. Monthly vital statistics Report. Vol. 25, No. 3, Supp 76–1120. Health Resources Administration, Rockville, MD, June 1976.)

tant during this measurement that the child's head be at a right angle, with the parietal areas touching the top of the headboard and not the occipital area. Another method is that the small infant is placed on his back with one person at his head and another at his feet. A mark is made at the infant's head and heel. The distance between these two marks is measured with a tape measure. The older child can stand on a standard balanced adult scale with a movable rod. If a standard scale is not available a tape measure can be taped to the wall for the child to stand against and a flat object can be placed on the child's head at the level of the tape measure to identify the appropriate height.

After the height is measured, it is recorded and plotted on a growth grid. Percentile charts with height, weight, and head circumferences are frequently used by health care facilities. The percentile charts use percentiles to show the distribution of height, weight and head circumference for a typical series of 100 children. For example, the 25th percentile indicates that 75 children are taller and 25 children shorter than the child being measured. In general a child in the 25th percentile will continue at about this percentile throughout his life. A child who suddenly has an increase to the 90th percentile or a drop to the 3rd percentile requires further investigation. If a measurement differs greatly from previous visits, the nurse should check the technique and re-evaluate the measurement. Often the measurement has been taken incorrectly or plotted on the graph wrong.

Heredity is a major factor influencing a child's stature. Tall parents usually have taller children than shorter parents; however, abnormal shortness may also be due to chronic illness, heart disease, liver or kidney disease, allergies, malnutrition or growth hormone deficiencies.

Weight is also an important index of the child's growth and should be measured with every examination whether the child is well or sick. It is a more easily obtainable measurement and usually is more accurate than height. The same general considerations of growth and development that applied to height also apply to weight.

Infants are weighed without any clothing on a balanced infant scale. Older children can remain clothed without shoes and be weighed on an adult balanced scale. Depending on the child's age and the amount of privacy available, the child can undress down to the underpants.

Once a measurement has been taken, it is plotted on the growth chart. The weight generally follows the same percentile from one time to the next; any sudden decrease or increase should be evaluated. Percentile decrease may indicate malnutrition, acute illness, dehydration, emotional problems or chronic illness. Percentile increase may be related to overnutrition, edema or endocrine disorders.

Some general rules exist regarding height and weight:

1. Average weight from 1 year to puberty is derived by multiplying the age in years by 5 plus 18; this answer is the child's desirable weight in pounds.
2. Average height in inches from 2 to 14 years is figured by multiplying 2 times the age in years plus 32.
3. Height and weight measurements provide important information, but a single measurement is of less importance than a series of measurements.
4. The relationship between height and weight is significant. A child who falls at the 90th percentile for height and at the 3rd percentile for weight requires a more detailed assessment.

Head Circumference The brain achieves 75 per cent of its adult size by 3 years of age. One-half of total head growth occurs during the first year of life. Therefore, the head circumference should be taken at each well-child visit during the first 3 years. It is usually not taken after 3 years of age unless some abnormality exists.

A reliable reading of head circumference is obtained by using a metal or paper tape measure around the broadest part of the head. The tape is placed over the occipital protuberance and the frontal bones. An accurate measurement is often difficult to obtain, so it is best to take three measurements and use the largest. A newborn's head circumference is equal to or slightly larger than the chest circumference until the child is about 3 years of age, when the chest circumference becomes larger than the head size. Head circumference increases 4 inches in the first year and only 2 inches between the ages of 1 and 7.

The head circumference is plotted on a growth chart (Fig. 13-2) like the height and weight. Head circumference is usually plotted in centi-

TABLE 13-5 NORMAL PULSE AND RESPIRATORY RATES FOR SPECIFIC AGES*

Age	Pulse (Beats per Minute)	Average Pulse	Respirations (Breaths per Minute)
Newborn	70–170	120	30–40
2 years	80–130	110	25–32
4 years	80–120	100	23–30
6 years	75–115	100	21–26
8 years	70–110	90	20–26
10 years	70–110	90	20–26
12 years	70–110	85	18–22
14 years	65–105	85	18–22
16 years	60–100	85	16–20
18 years	50–90	80	12–24

*These are averages and vary with the sex of the child.

meters because this is more accurate. As with the height and weight, serial measurements provide more information than a single measurement, and marked differences should be investigated.

Other Measurements Occasionally, special measurements are needed to evaluate unusual characteristics of the child. One such measurement is the sitting height. In older infants and children this is easily obtained by having the child sit against a wall and measuring the distance between the vertex of the head and the sitting surface. This is used when children are suspected of having an abnormality in their growth rate. It can help distinguish true dwarfism from small stature. Sitting height normally accounts for approximately 70 per cent of total body length at birth, 60 per cent at 2 years of age, and about 52 per cent at 10 years of age and through adulthood.

Another special measurement is the chest circumference. The chest circumference is measured only at birth unless growth problems are evident. The tape measure is placed around the chest and across the nipple line. This measurement is not significant unless compared with head circumference. At birth the chest circumference is approximately 2 cm less than the head circumference until about 2 years of age. The chest circumference then continues to grow rapidly while the head circumference increases minimally.

Assessment of Vital Signs

As in other areas of the physical examination of children, there are special approaches that reduce anxiety and gain cooperation when vital signs are being obtained. Older children and adolescents are usually treated much the same as adults. They will, however, need to be reassured of the results and will need adequate explanation of what is being done. Younger school-age children may wish to participate. For example, they may participate in taking their blood pressure by helping to press the cuff down, holding the gauge or squeezing the bulb. Smaller children, particularly preschoolers, demonstrate fear of body mutilation with any intrusive procedure. The rectal temperature, for example, often arouses anxiety and stress in this child. In young children it is usually advisable to check respirations and pulse first, next blood pressure, and temperature last. Following this order will produce greater accuracy, since temperature-taking can produce sufficient anxiety and crying to alter the respiratory and pulse rate.

The normal oral temperature is between 35.5 to 38° C (96 to 100.4° F). Rectal temperatures are one degree higher and axillary temperatures are one degree lower than oral temperatures. When the temperature is recorded, the method for obtaining it must be recorded. (No notation after the temperature denotes an oral temperature; (R) denotes rectal; and (A) an axillary temperature).

The length of time allowed for accurately measuring temperature depends in part on custom in various settings. The advantage of the electronic thermometers is that they require only seconds to register accurate temperatures, regardless of the route, and thus are especially helpful with young children.

Children commonly demonstrate elevated temperatures after vigorous playing or after eating. They may also have an increased temperature on very warm days. Fever may also be

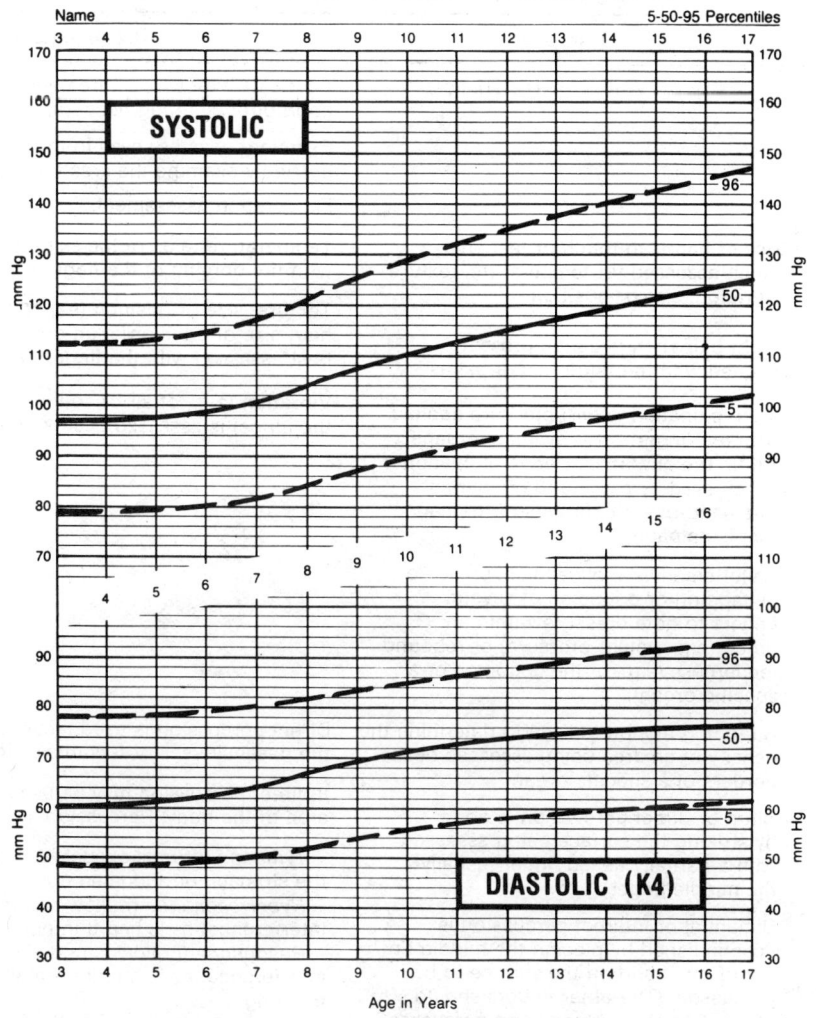

Figure 13-3 Children's blood pressure chart. (From A. Jaworski. New boy-girl blood pressure chart for pediatric office use: a single sheet graph for all children. Clinical Pediatrics, September 1978, p. 699.)

produced by viral or bacterial infections, dehydration, tumors, poisoning or chronic infections. Hypothermia is seen in children who are in shock or chilled or it may be seen in infants with infections. If fever or hypothermia exists, it should be evaluated and followed closely.

Table 13-5 and Figure 13-3 describe average pulse rates, respiratory rates and blood pressure readings at various ages. Chapter 17 describes in more detail some of the special techniques used in assessing vital signs in children.

THE PHYSICAL EXAMINATION

Physical examination utilizes five basic assessment techniques (1) inspection, (2) palpation, (3) percussion, (4) auscultation and (5) measuration. Table 13-6 describes these techniques.

General Appearance

The examination should begin with an overall impression of the child. Observation of the child is done to formulate an impression that can be verified or disproved following a more extensive examination. The following are examples of some areas used to develop a general appearance statement: physical appearance (ill or well), nutritional status, behavior and degree of activity, facial expression, interactions with parents or nurse, developmental status, consciousness level, speech or nature of cry, gait and coordination and posture. The general appearance focuses on physical characteristics or behaviors of the child and should be a brief

TABLE 13-6 TECHNIQUES UTILIZED IN PHYSICAL ASSESSMENT

Technique	Purpose	Comments
Inspection	Evaluation of visible characteristics.	Adequate exposure of area being visualized and good direct lighting necessary.
		Examiner uses her eyes to thoroughly and unhurriedly examine the area being inspected.
		First step in assessment.
Palpation	Use of hands to touch or feel area being assessed for temperature, texture, vibration, size or position.	Temperature (e.g., of the skin) is assessed best with the dorsum of the fingers.
	Light palpation is gentle pressure applied with the fingertips or palms	Texture, size or position (e.g., texture of the hair, size or position of an organ or mass) are best assessed with the fingertips.
	Deep palpation is firm pressure applied with the fingertips to evaluate organs within the abdomen. Deeper palpation is achieved by placing the fingers of one hand over the fingers of the hand that is palpating.	Vibration (e.g., of air or sound moving through the lungs) is assessed best with the palms.
	Ballottement is application of pressure by tapping or bouncing of several fingers to note pressure within an organ (e.g., ocular pressure) or rebound tenderness (e.g., of the abdomen or a specific organ).	
Percussion	A rapping motion utilized to determine the density of an area being assessed or the borders of a specific organ.	Direct percussion is used most often to percuss the nasal sinuses or tendons or inflamed organs.
	Blunt or direct percussion is done by striking the surface being assessed with a partially flexed finger (usually the middle finger).	Indirect percussion may be used to percuss any area of the body. Percussion sounds include:
	Bimanual or indirect percussion is accomplished by placing the middle finger of one hand on the surface to be percussed. (The other fingers should not rest on the surface to be percussed as this will diminish the sound created by percussion.) The middle finger or index and middle fingers of the other hand strike the middle finger resting on the body surface on the upper phalange. Only the very tip(s) of the striking finger(s) is used.	*Tympany* (drumlike) such as is heard over the stomach or abdomen normally. *Hyperresonance* (hollow sound with air interference) as is heard in pneumothorax. *Resonance* (hollow sound without air interference) as is heard normally over the lung. *Impaired resonance* (diminished hollow sound) as is heard when fluid has accumulated in a hollow cavity such as the lung. *Dullness* is heard normally over muscle or a thick or solid tissue organ such as the liver. *Flatness* is heard normally over bone.
Auscultation	Listening to or studying the sounds arising from organs via the direct contact of the ear on the body surface over the organ or, more commonly, with the aid of a stethoscope.	Auscultation is done over the lungs, heart and abdomen to determine the functional status of these organs. The skull, thyroid gland and carotid arteries are auscultated for bruits (swishing sounds).
	The diaphragm (flat side) of the stethoscope picks up high frequency sounds and is used for auscultation of most organs.	
	The bell (curved or cupped side) of the stethoscope picks up low frequency sounds such as heart murmurs.	
Measuration	Clinical measurement of body surfaces to determine size, amount of asymmetry or amount of swelling. Clinical measurement of vital signs or lab values.	Measurements of height and weight and of blood pressure, temperature, pulse and respiration should be a part of every physical examination.

summary statement. An example of a general appearance statement is as follows: *Alert, smiling, well-developed, well-nourished toddler playing on mother's lap and in no acute distress.*

Skin (Integumentary System)

The skin is examined as a whole to determine its overall condition and then more specifically as each body part is assessed. For example, when the head is assessed, the skin of the head and the face is examined. When the lower extremities are examined, the skin of the lower extremities is checked and so on. All skin findings, however, are recorded under one heading. When a body part is inspected, it is examined generally, then more specifically. For example, the skin of the head and face are examined, followed by a more detailed and specific survey of an area of the face, for instance the nose. The skin is inspected and palpated for color and pigmentation, moisture, turgor, texture, sensitivity, lesions, temperature and edema.

Color Normal skin color varies from whitish pink to brown depending on the race. Dark-skinned children such as those of American black, American Indian, Mexican, Oriental, Mediterranean or Latin descent have varying pigmentations from brown, red, olive green to bluish skin tones. Accurate skin assessment must take into consideration the variations in skin of each race. For example, children who are of Oriental descent have a yellow skin tone that may appear to be jaundiced. Black children may often have a bluish pigmentation around the gum lines or palate. Often the sclera of a black child has a brown or blue-brown pigmentation that may resemble petechiae or hemorrhages.

The skin should be inspected for signs of hyperpigmentation or hypopigmentation; if present, the pigment abnormality should be evaluated as to whether it is diffuse or localized. Hyperpigmentation is often seen in Addison's disease, hyperthyroidism or pregnancy, or it may be the result of exposure to the sun or an ultraviolet lamp. Hypopigmentation is seen in children with vitiligo, which is a patchy lack of melanin, or in children with albinism, which is a diffuse lack of melanin.

Erythema is an increased amount of oxygenated blood in the vasculature of the dermis. It is found in children who are febrile, have a sunburn or localized infection, or who have been exposed to the cold. Body parts exposed to the cold become a bright pink or red.

When examining the skin the nurse should note any sign of cyanosis or erythema. Cyanosis is a bluish tint of the skin due to a large amount of reduced hemoglobin in the capillaries. It is most evident in the mucous membranes, conjunctivae of the lower eyelids and the nail beds. Children with congestive heart failure or congenital heart disorders frequently are cyanotic. Cyanosis may also be found in children with pneumonia or other respiratory disturbances. Acrocyanosis, the bluish discoloration of the hands and feet frequently seen in newborns, is normal for the first few days of life; it is caused by inadequate peripheral vasculature.

Skin that is very pale demonstrates a decrease in hemoglobin content, often seen secondary to anemia or shock. In white-skinned persons pallor is noted by a loss of pink skin coloring; in black-skinned persons the skin becomes an ashen gray. Jaundice is seen as a yellow-green hue; this usually means an increased bilirubin. It occurs in children with liver disease or hemolytic blood disease. Jaundice is best discerned by blanching the skin and observing the blanched area for a yellow or yellow-green appearance. Examination of the skin for jaundice should be done in natural sunlight as opposed to fluorescent light, which gives some normal skin tones a yellow color. Areas in which jaundice is easily observed are the sclera and the hard palate and the gums, particularly in dark-skinned races. Skin that appears like yellow squash may also be the result of carotenemia.

Another skin discoloration seen by the nurse is a grayish color that may be the result of an increased concentration of metal salts such as silver, gold, and bismuth. If these metal salts are given as medication it may result in deposits of the salt in the skin. Tattoos will also change the skin color. These are seen more frequently in adolescents than in younger children.

Moisture The skin is inspected and palpated for the presence or absence of moisture and the degree of moisture present. Often the nurse will see an increase in moisture in combination with temperature findings such as cool wet hands, which usually indicate a vasoconstriction often found during anxiety. Dry parchment-like skin is often associated with rising fever, whereas hot, moist skin typifies the diaphoretic process of a resolving fever.

Texture Inspection and palpation of the quality and character of the skin surface is necessary for the evaluation of skin texture. Normal skin is smooth, soft and flexible. Skin that is rough and dry often indicates an endocrine problem or is also seen in children who bathe very frequently or who are exposed to cold weather. Rough, dry skin is also seen with vitamin A deficiencies. If scaling is found it should be described as to the extent and location. Scaling only present between fingers and toes could be a sign of a fungal infection. Scaling of the palms and soles might be associated with scarlet fever. Eczema often causes scaling of the cheeks and behind the ears, knees and elbows. Thick yellow oily scales on the scalp may indicate seborrhea, which can spread into a red maculopapular rash on the face and trunk.

Children with a velvety smooth skin may have hyperthyroidism. Palpation of the skin may also produce a crackling sensation if the child has subcutaneous emphysema caused by a lung disorder. The crackling sensation may also indicate a bone fracture of an underlying structure. The nurse may find striae when examining for texture. Striae are pale white stripes often seen in children who are obese or in adolescents who have heavy breasts or who are pregnant.

Turgor One of the best indicators of nutrition and hydration is skin turgor. Normal skin turgor is elastic and taut. Turgor is evaluated by pinching the skin between thumb and forefinger, usually of the lower abdomen or calf, and noting the reaction of the pinched skin. If the skin returns promptly to the normal position it is assessed as elastic. Skin that does not promptly return may indicate a loss of turgor due to dehydration or excessive exposure to ultraviolet rays. Skin that stays pinched or tented for a few seconds after the skin is released is considered flabby or decreased in turgor and may indicate chronic disease and muscle disorders.

Edema Excess water that is stored in the skin in the form of edema is evaluated according to whether it is pitting or nonpitting. The nurse's thumb is firmly pressed over the medial aspect of the child's malleoli (ankle protuberance) for at least five seconds. After releasing the skin, any sign of indentation that lasts several seconds indicates pitting edema. Puffiness or edema that does not remain indented is termed nonpitting edema. Any body surface area can be edematous and should be evaluated using the technique just described. Generalized edema, however, is often evaluated by examining the lower extremities. Edema is seen in children who have allergies, kidney or heart anomalies, and malnutrition.

Temperature Palpation of the skin to determine its temperature is best completed by comparing body parts. Skin temperature is not an accurate reflection of the internal temperature of the body but may reflect a maladjustment in the thermoregulating mechanism of the body. Localized hyperthermia, an indication of increased blood flow, may be secondary to a burn or a cellulitis. Generalized hyperthermia may be the result of generalized sunburn, fever or hyperthyroidism. Localized hypothermia is seen in peripheral arterial sclerosis and is an indication of decreased blood flow. Children in shock may exhibit generalized hypothermia.

Lesions Examination of the skin is not complete unless it has been inspected and palpated for skin lesions. Any lesions or markings on the skin should be noted and described in detail as follows: size, color, shape, location, surface characteristics, anatomical distribution, configuration and morphology. Lesions are classified as primary, secondary, and special lesions (Table 13-7). Primary lesions are the initial lesions evident in a disease process, whereas secondary lesions are altered primary lesions that result from scratching or in response to medication or the normal healing process. Primary lesions include macules, papules, wheals, vesicles, petechiae, pustules and bullae. Examples of secondary lesions are scales, crusts, striae, excoriation, erosion, ulcers, fissures, lichenification, and scars. Plaques may be either primary or secondary lesions. Comedones (blackheads) and milia (whitish nodules) are examples of special lesions.

Many skin lesions can be normal, such as capillary hemangiomas (birthmarks), mongolian spots, freckles, and nevi (moles). Other skin lesions such as cysts, port wine stains or large hairy moles require further evaluation and possible referral. Lesions in the form of a skin rash are seen frequently in children of all ages. Heat rash and diaper rash are common in infants and young children. Another common condition is acne. It generally begins during adolescence and can range from mild to severe. There is also a skin rash that newborns have that is frequently labeled *neonatal acne.*

Hair Hair is examined for color, length, distribution, cleanliness, amount and for texture. Scalp hair should be examined to determine if it is clean and shiny and if it covers the entire head. Hair texture is noted as being thick or thin, fine or coarse, soft or brittle. Nutritional and endocrine disturbances may affect hair texture. The scalp and body hair is also closely inspected for alopecia (bald areas), which may indicate systemic pathology or a skin infection.

Body hair is also evaluated. Hair on the eyebrows and eyelashes and any hair associated with a lesion such as a mole should be examined. Any hair on the face, axillae, pubic area and chest should also be examined carefully at all ages. Pubic hair usually appears when the child is between 8 and 12 years of age. Axillary hair appears shortly after the onset of pubic hair. Adolescent males begin to develop facial hair approximately six months after the appearance of axillary hair. Hair that has appeared earlier than normal or excessive hair may be an indication of precocious puberty or could signify an endocrine problem. The spine is inspected and palpated for hair tufts of the sacral area, which are seen in children with spina bifida.

Nails Nails are examined as part of the integumentary system. Nails are inspected and palpated for their size, shape (convex or concave) and color (pink, cyanotic, pale). Characteristics such as smoothness, pitting, ridging and clubbing are carefully noted. Clubbing is generally a sign of chronic lack of oxygen often seen in children with congenital heart disease or chronic pulmonary disease (see Fig. 24–3). It can also be a normal familial trait. Any change in color should be noted. Adolescents and children who smoke heavily may have yellow nail tips. The cuticles should be assessed for intactness, smoothness and any splitting or hangnails.

Lymphatic System

The lymphatic system provides important information about the child's health status. A large lymph node or generalized lymphadenopathy may be the first sign of disease. Lymph nodes are inspected and palpated during the examination of the part of the body in which they are located. They are examined for size, mobility, tenderness, warmth, redness, distribution and consistency. Palpable lymph nodes on children may be normal but should be evaluated carefully. It should be noted whether lymphadenopathy is localized or generalized. The physical examination should include evaluation of five major lymph node areas: head, neck, axillae, inguinal, and arms and legs (Fig. 13–4).

Lymph nodes are palpated by using the distal portion of the fingers (finger pads) and gently but firmly pressing in a circular motion along the regions in which the nodes are normally present. When the nodes of the neck are palpated, the child's head should be straight with slight upward tilting without tension in the sternocleidomastoid or trapezius muscles. The examiner may find it helpful to turn the child's head 10 or 20 degrees toward the side being examined to relax the skin and muscles. The head is tilted downward slightly to allow easier palpation of the occipital chain. In order to inspect and palpate the lymph nodes located in the submental and submaxillary areas, the head may need to be tilted backward slightly.

Another examination technique used to evaluate the lymph system is to have the child shrug his shoulders slightly so the nurse may palpate the fossa when examining for supraclavicular nodes. Axillary nodes are palpated with the arms relaxed and slightly adducted, with the child's forearm resting on the examiner's forearm to eliminate pull and tension on the axillae. Often this area is very ticklish and the child may need to be distracted. Epitrochlear nodes are best examined with the arms slightly flexed. Inguinal nodes are palpated when the child is supine. Finally, the less frequently palpated popliteal nodes are located slightly medially in the popliteal fossas. These are best palpated with the knees bent at a 45-degree angle so that the muscles and tendon are relaxed. The examiner places her thumbs on the patella and reaches with the fingertips of both hands behind to the fossa, palpating deeply toward the medial aspect.

Shotty, moveable, cool, nontender discrete nodes up to 3 mm in diameter are normal in all of these areas; however, cervical and inguinal nodes may normally be as large as 1 cm. Lymph

TABLE 13-7 BASIC TYPES OF SKIN LESIONS

PRIMARY LESIONS (May arise from previously normal skin)

CIRCUMSCRIBED, FLAT, NON-PALPABLE CHANGES IN SKIN COLOR

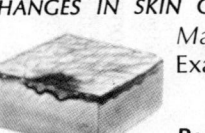

Macule—Small, up to 1 cm. Example: freckle, petechia

Patch—Larger than 1 cm. Example: vitiligo

PALPABLE ELEVATED SOLID MASSES

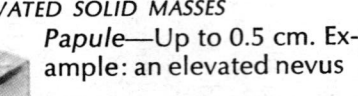

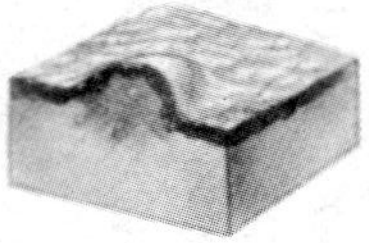

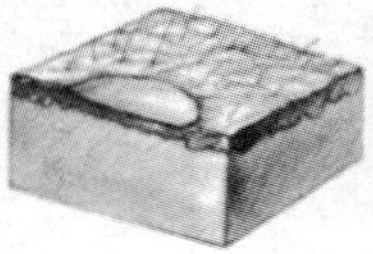

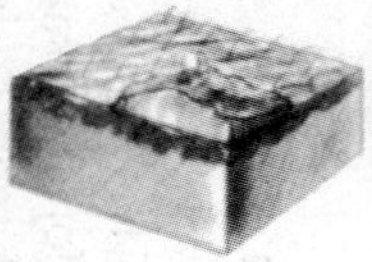

Papule—Up to 0.5 cm. Example: an elevated nevus

Plaque—A flat, elevated surface larger than 0.5 cm, often formed by the coalescence of papules

Nodule—0.5 to 1–2 cm; often deeper and firmer than a papule

Tumor—Larger than 1–2 cm.

Wheal—A slightly irregular, relatively transient, superficial area of localized skin edema. Example: mosquito bite, hive

CIRCUMSCRIBED SUPERFICIAL ELEVATIONS OF THE SKIN FORMED BY FREE FLUID IN A CAVITY WITHIN THE SKIN LAYERS

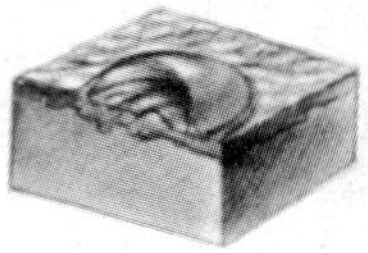

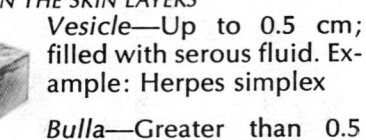

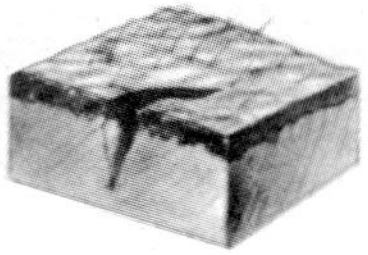

Vesicle—Up to 0.5 cm; filled with serous fluid. Example: Herpes simplex

Bulla—Greater than 0.5 cm; filled with serous fluid. Example: 2nd degree burn

Pustule—filled with pus. Examples: acne, impetigo

SECONDARY LESIONS (Result from changes in primary lesions)

LOSS OF SKIN SURFACE

Erosion—Loss of the superficial epidermis; surface is moist but does not bleed. Example: moist area after the rupture of a vesicle, as in chicken pox

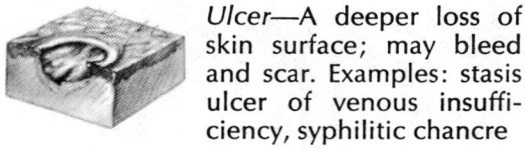

Ulcer—A deeper loss of skin surface; may bleed and scar. Examples: stasis ulcer of venous insufficiency, syphilitic chancre

Fissure—A linear crack in the skin. Example: athlete's foot

MATERIAL ON THE SKIN SURFACE

Crust—The dried residue of serum, pus or blood. Example: impetigo

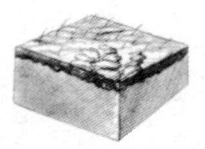

Scale—A thin flake of exfoliated epidermis. Examples: dandruff, dry skin, psoriasis

SECONDARY LESIONS (Result from changes in primary lesions)

MISCELLANEOUS

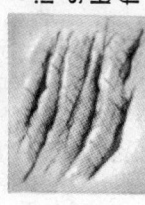

Lichenification—Thickening and roughening of the skin with increased visibility of the normal skin furrows. Example: atopic dermatitis

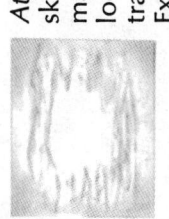

Atrophy—Thinning of the skin with loss of the normal skin furrows; the skin looks shinier and more translucent than normal. Example: arterial insufficiency

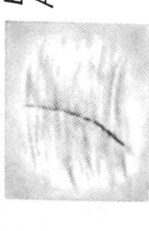

Excoriation—A scratch mark

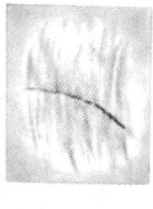

Scar—Replacement of destroyed tissue by fibrous tissue

Keloid—A hypertrophied scar

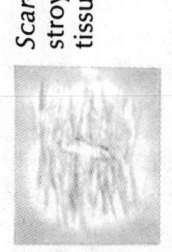

From B. Bates. A Guide to Physical Examination. J. B. Lippincott Co., 1974, pp 14–15.

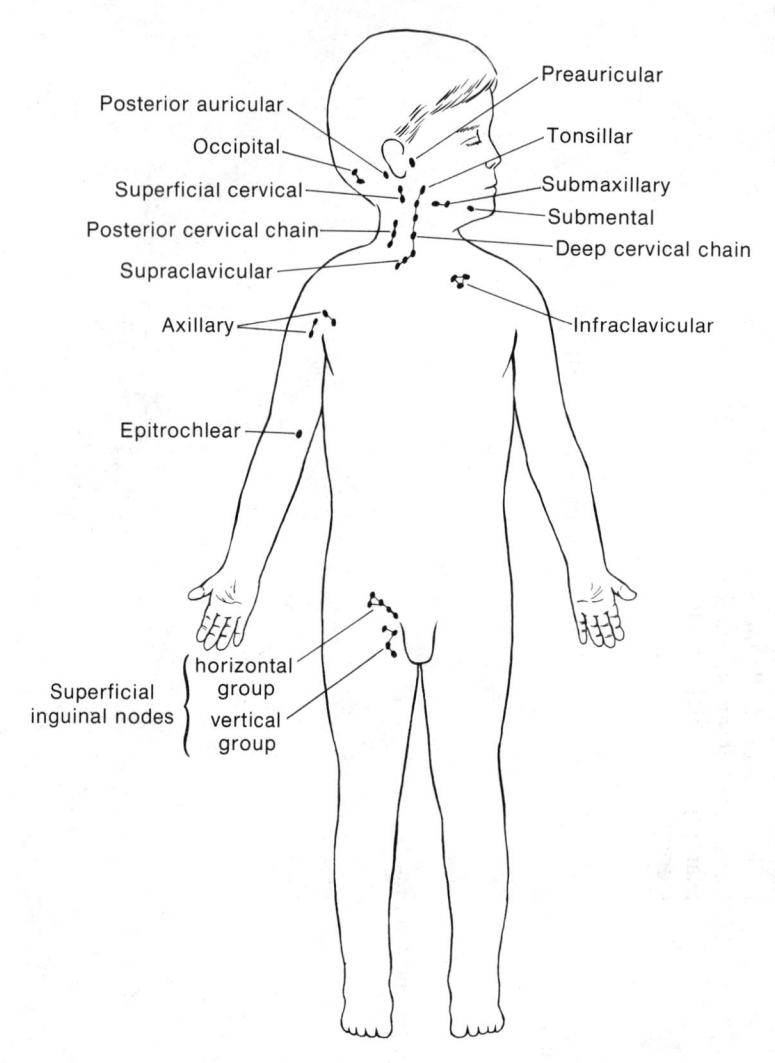

Figure 13-4 Lymph nodes of the body.

nodes that are large, tender, warm or red are usually an indication of infection and the source should be determined. Lymphadenopathy distribution can be characteristic of certain infections (Table 13-8). The occipital, posterior cervical and auricular lymph nodes become inflamed and enlarged when a rubella infection is present. Cervical adenitis is found in children with scarlet fever. Generalized lymphadenopathy can be seen in systemic illnesses such as leukemia, salmonellosis, syphilis, mononucleosis and measles.

Head, Face and Neck

Head Inspection from all angles is necessary to determine the size, shape and symmetry of the head. The shape of the skull is generally round but may be long or broad. Newborns frequently have asymmetrical heads due to intrauterine positioning and to molding, which may occur during the birth process. Size is best determined by obtaining a measurement of head circumference.

Suture lines and fontanels are inspected and palpated during examination of the infant's and young child's head. (See Fig. 20-6.) The head should be carefully palpated to determine if the suture lines are closed, over-riding or separated. They are frequently over-riding or separated at birth. Premature closure of suture lines can vary the shape of the head depending on which sutures are closed. The first two years of a child's life are important for brain growth; any sign of premature closure of sutures should be thoroughly investigated.

There are six fontanels but generally only

two, the anterior and the posterior, are of clinical significance. Fontanels are inspected and palpated for size, shape, number and location. They are also palpated and inspected for bulging, tenseness, pulsation or depression.

Occasionally a third fontanel is also found. It should be evaluated in the same way as the anterior and posterior fontanels. A fontanel that is depressed may be indicative of malnutrition and dehydration. Children who have a bulging fontanel may have hydrocephaly, meningitis, lead poisoning, vitamin A poisoning or a subdural hematoma.

Children under 6 months of age may normally have a fontanel over 4 to 5 cm in diameter, but it may also be diagnostic of increased intracranial pressure, subdural hematoma, rickets, hypothyroidism, or osteogenesis imperfecta. Small anterior fontanels should be checked closely for premature closure.

Fontanels are generally diamond-shaped and should be measured in two dimensions, anterior-posterior and horizontal. The examiner uses a tape measure to measure the two dimensions.

The average anterior fontanel may be very small or absent at birth but generally enlarges to an average size of 2.5 cm by 2.5 cm. It should remain open for at least 9 to 10 months to allow for adequate head growth. Approximately 97 per cent of all anterior fontanels close between 9 and 19 months of age. Very large fontanels may not close until 2 years of age. The posterior fontanel is often not palpable at birth. If present, it averages 1 cm by 1 cm in size. It generally is not palpable after 1 to 2 months of life.

The child's scalp is inspected and palpated for scaliness, infections and hair. The scalp should be inspected closely for signs of cradle cap by scraping the scalp lightly with a fingertip. Hair is examined as discussed in the section on examination of the skin. Scalp hair should be examined closely for signs of alopecia, nits and lice, and for excessive hair and low-set hairlines which may be indicative of congenital anomalies. The head should be inspected and palpated for any bulges or swellings. Cephalohematomas and caput succedaneum may be seen in the newborn period (see Chapter 20).

Control, movement and position of the head is also observed. An infant may be observed for head lag when pulled from a supine to a sitting position. Little or no head lag should be evident after 3 months of age. The position in which the child holds his head may also indicate abnormalities. Persistent positioning at an angle may indicate torticollis (stiff neck with head drawn to one side) or visual problems. The head should also be evaluated for full range of motion. The examiner must rotate the head of the newborn for passive range of motion, but for the older child the nurse can elicit active range of motion by having the child follow a toy or a bright light. The head should move smoothly from an extended or flexed position and from side to side. Jerky or limited movement warrants further investigation.

After fontanel closure a "cracked pot" sound on percussion of the skull at the junction of the frontal and temporal and parietal bones may indicate increased intracranial pressure. Percussion is accomplished by using the direct method, in which the middle finger directly percusses the child's skull.

The skull may also need transillumination if there is concern about head growth or shape or fontanel size. A flashlight is fitted with a sponge-rubber collar so that there is a tight fit when it is placed against the skull. The procedure must be done in a very dark room, preferably with the child in the parent's lap for comfort. The flashlight is then placed snugly on the skull and moved; both sides and the front and back are covered. The expected transillumination in the occipital area is 1 cm and 2 cm in the fronto-parietal area. Any increased area of light denotes an abnormality.

Face The face should be inspected for shape, symmetry, paralysis, placement of features, distribution of hair and skin color and texture.

Symmetry and placement of features should be evaluated from the front and each side. The eyes should be set at the same level and not set wide apart or close together.

The nose should be midline with symmetrical nares; the mouth should be symmetrical and the ears set at the same level on both sides of the head. The top of the pinna (external ear) should meet or cross an imaginary line that extends from the lateral corner of the eye to the most protuberant part of the occiput. This is the eye-occiput line — ears that do not cross this line are low set and may indicate mental retardation or kidney anomalies.

Facial paralysis and asymmetry of facial movement should be closely observed. This is

TABLE 13-8 LYMPHATIC SYSTEM

Chain	Location	Areas Drained	Clinical Significance of Enlargement
1. Occipital	At nape of neck (lower occipital bone)	Occipital region of scalp	Pediculosis, seborrhea, tick bites, chickenpox, rubella, external otitis, scalp lesions
2. Posterior auricular	Mastoid, posterior to pinna	Posterior part of temporoparietal region, pinna, posterior part of external acoustic meatus, scalp, facial skin	Rubella, skin lesions in area drained, external otitis, chickenpox, pediculosis
3. Preauricular	Directly in front of ear (anterior to tragus), temporal	Face, eye, lateral surface of curicula	Lesions of the eyelids (chalazions), conjunctivitis, infectious skin disorders of the face
4. Superficial cervical	Chain over sternocleidomastoid muscle at upper section of neck superficially	Tongue, tonsils, pinna, parotid scalp, neck, thorax	Scalp infections, pediculosis, lesions in areas drained, scarlet fever
5. Deep cervical (jugular)	Begins with *tonsillar* node at the angle of jaw and continues under sternocleidomastoid muscle, ending posterior to this muscle in supraclavicular chain	Most of tongue, tonsils, pinna, parotid, oropharynx, nose, paranasal sinuses, palate, larynx, trachea, esophagus, middle ear	Tonsillitis, pharyngitis, thyroid disease, inflammatory process of areas drained, scarlet fever
6. Submaxillary (submandibular)	Beneath body of mandible midway between chin and ear	Medial conjunctiva, cheek, side of nose, upper lip, lateral part of lower lip, gums, submaxillary gland, anterior margin of tongue	Stomatitis, conjunctivitis
7. Submental	Beneath chin	Central portions of lower lip, floor of mouth, apex of tongue	
8. Tonsillar	The first of the deep cervical chain at angle between ear and jaw	Mouth, pharynx, principal node for tonsil	Tonsillitis, pharyngitis
9. Parotid	Parotid gland; lateral wall of pharynx at junction of mandible and maxilla; occasionally in subcutaneous tissue over parotid gland	Parotid gland, tissues of face, root of nose, tympanic cavity, eyelids, frontotemporal region, external auditory canal	Parotitis, mumps, tumors
10. Supraclavicular	Directly over medial area of clavicle	Head, abdomen, breast, thorax, arm, lung	Dental infections

202

11.	Sentinel node	Left clavicle	May be first node enlarged with Hodgkin's disease
12.	Posterior cervical	Along anterior border of trapezium muscle	Pediculosis, scalp infections
13.	Infraclavicular	Below clavicle	Cancer, infection
14.	Lateral axillary	Along head of humerus	Infection or disease of hand, arm
15.	Central axillary	Adipose tissue of central axilla at base	Infection or disease of arm, chest, breast
16.	Subscapular (posterior axillary)	Posterior wall of axilla fossa and lateral edge of scapulae	Infections or disease of skin of neck and thorax
17.	Pectoral (anterior axillary)	Lateral border of pectoralis minor	Infection or disease of thorax or breast
18.	Subclavicular (medial)	Superior to and posterior to pectoralis minor	Disease or infection of breast or other areas drained by axillary nodes
19.	Epitrochlear	Medial aspect of inner elbow just above medial epicondyle of the humerus	Arm, hand, finger infection, congenital syphilis, cat scratch disease
20.	Horizontal inguinal	Parallels inguinal ligament, runs diagonally towards perineum	Infections of perineum or genitalia, VD, lice, diaper rash
21.	Vertical inguinal	Runs vertically at upper, inner aspect of the thigh	Infections of legs, feet, genitalia, anus, VD, lice, diaper rash
22.	Popliteal	Popliteal fossa	Infections of knee joint and heel and lateral aspect of posterior half of foot
	Generalized lymphadenopathy		Use of Dilantin; infectious mononucleosis, cancer/leukemia/Hodgkin's, cat-scratch fever, salmonella, eczema, histoplasmosis, syphilis, viral hepatitis, measles, bacteremia, sarcoidosis, lupus erythematosus, rheumatic fever, sickle cell anemia, hemolytic anemia, Cooley's anemia, cystinosis, Gaucher's disease, juvenile rheumatoid arthritis

Absence → Condition: Agammaglobulinemia

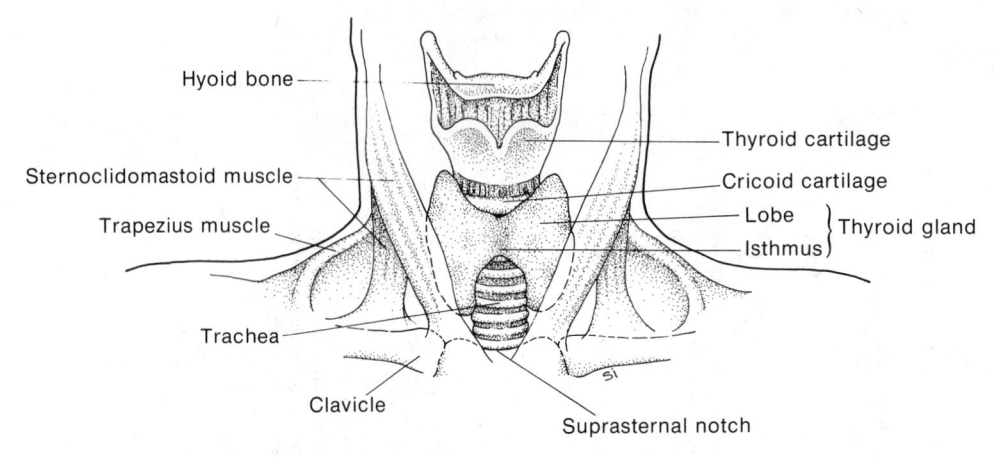

Figure 13-5 Structures of the neck.

easily done when an infant cries or yawns. An older child can smile and wrinkle his forehead so that the examiner can check for paralysis. Edema, twitchings and tics should also be observed for and palpated. Facial coloring is observed and any evidence of pallor, jaundice or cyanosis or any unusual marking is noted.

Neck Following examination of the head and face, the neck is inspected for control, mobility, pulsations, symmetry, size and shape. Palpation of the neck is used to determine strength, pulsations and position of structures such as the thyroid and trachea. The sternocleidomastoids and trapezius muscles are palpated for tone and presence of any masses or hematomas. Strength of these muscles is evaluated by having the child move them against the resistance of the nurse's hands. Range of motion should also be determined. A child with any nuchal (back of neck) rigidity or opisthotonos (spasm in which head and heels are bent backward and body bowed forward) should be referred. Enlarged veins or excessive pulsations can indicate cardiac problems.

The trachea is inspected and palpated to determine if it is midline. The examiner inspects the neck hyperextended and then palpates the trachea beginning at the suprasternal notch and moving upward. The thumb is placed on one side of the tracheal rings and the index and middle fingers on the other side to evaluate the tracheal rings and determine if the trachea is midline or deviated.

The thyroid is inspected and palpated. Inspection takes place in the hyperextended position. The examiner looks for bulges, asymmetry or enlargement. With the neck tilted slightly forward the examiner palpates for the hyoid bone, cricoid and thyroid cartilages; the thyroid isthmus; and finally the lobes of the thyroid gland (Fig. 13-5). The thyroid is palpated with the child in a supine or sitting position. The thumb is placed on one side of the thyroid and the index and middle finger on the opposite side. In the older child the examiner may stand behind the seated child and place the index and middle fingers of each hand on the sides of the thyroid. Having the child swallow some water moves the thyroid upward and allows for better palpation. Any nodules, enlargement or tenderness of the thyroid gland should be considered abnormal; these signs warrant further evaluation.

Examination of the lymph nodes is done during the examination of the neck. The examiner generally begins with palpation of the occipital nodes and progresses to the posterior auricular and preauricular lymph nodes. The examiner then continues to the anterior and posterior cervical triangles. (See Figure 13-4 for locations of these nodes.)

Auscultation of the neck is done to determine the presence of bruits or murmurs. The bell of the

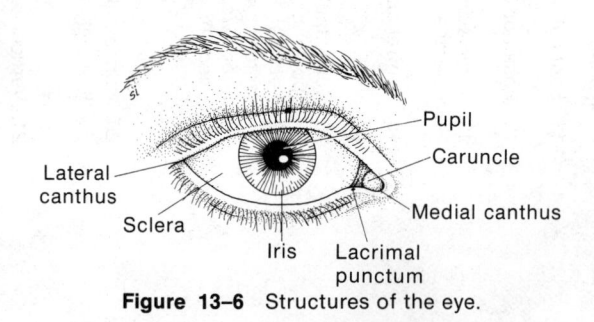

Figure 13-6 Structures of the eye.

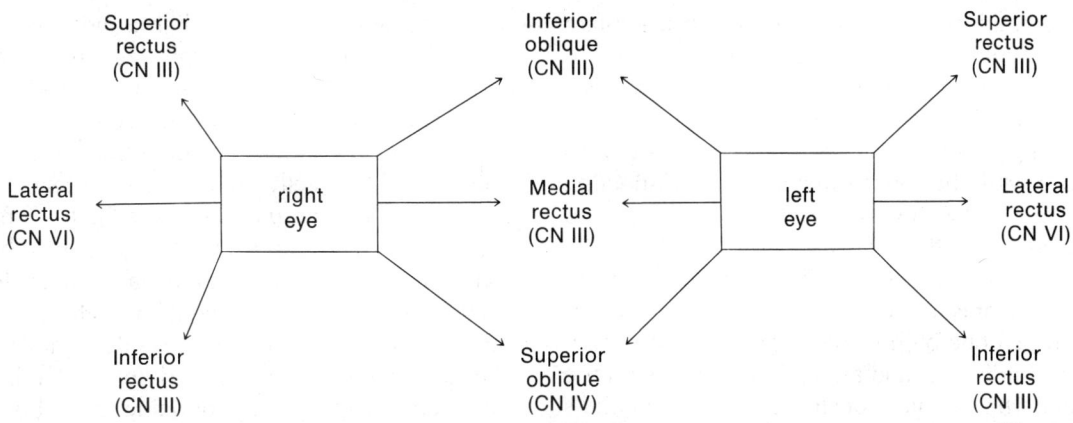

Figure 13-7 The visual fields of extraocular movement. If the child's eye is unable to move to any one of the positions, it indicates dysfunction of either that muscle or cranial nerve. (A young child may not be able to follow instructions to move only his eyes; the nurse then should hold the child's head still.)

stethoscope is placed over the carotids for this part of the examination. Finally, any hoarseness or stridor of the voice is noted. An infant's cry is evaluated for its quality. A high-pitched cry, a cat-like cry or a low, hoarse cry are indications of abnormalities. The older child is evaluated for voice quality and speech.

Eye Examination of the eyes (see Fig. 13-6) is accomplished through observation with the naked eye and an ophthalmoscope. A flashlight is needed to observe the pupillary light reflex and an ophthalmoscope to check the fundus and the lens.

Examination begins with the eyelids, which are inspected for ptosis (drooping), retraction, slanting, epicanthal folds,* edema or redness. They should also be inspected for styes (inflamed swellings of the eyelid), chalazions (eyelid masses), boils and blepharitis (eyelid infection). Edema of the lids may indicate serious problems such as renal failure or may be caused by allergies, injuries, drugs or infection.

Presence or absence of eyelashes is determined, as is their color and texture. The nasolacrimal duct should be inspected for patency, position, redness and swelling. Eyes that tear excessively or have any discharge should be investigated further. Excessive tearing before the age of 3 months may be due to a blocked nasolacrimal duct (dacryostenosis). It may also result from infections, a foreign body, allergies or exophthalmos (abnormal protrusion of the eyeball).

The palpebral (inner surface of the eyelid) and bulbar (covering the eye) conjunctivae are examined next for color, moisture and integrity. Chemosis (swelling of the conjunctiva) is seen with infections and allergies. The conjunctivae are also examined for pallor, inflammation, injection (dilated blood vessels), growths, enlarged follicles ("cobblestone" appearance) and drainage.

The orbit of the eye is also assessed. Children with sunken, blank eyes may be severely ill or malnourished. Small orbits (microphthalmia) usually indicate underlying pathology. Inspection of the eye orbits also determines hypertelorism (wide apart), hypotelorism (close together) and prominent supraorbital ridges. The globe of the eye and the ridges are palpated for tenderness, turgor and swelling. Exophthalmos (abnormal protrusion of eyeballs) and endophthalmos (abnormally deep-set eyeballs) are significant findings and should be referred for evaluation.

Full range of motion of the extraocular muscles is evaluated by having the child follow an object to each of the six visual fields (Fig. 13-7). The eyes are observed closely for smooth, symmetrical tracking and any sign of *nystagmus* (constant involuntary movement of eyeball). The direction of the nystagmus should be recorded.* A paralyzed extraocular muscle causes *paralytic strabismus*. The eye cannot follow to one or more visual fields. In *concomitant strabismus* the eyes do not move simultaneously but each eye can move to all quadrants during the range of motion exercises. Concomi-

---

*The epicanthus is a vertical fold of skin on either side of the nose, sometimes covering the inner canthus. Its presence is normal in certain races and sometimes indicates a congenital anomaly in others.

*Nystagmus may be induced during movement or may be spontaneous.

tant strabismus is frequently seen in the infant but should be minimal after 6 months of age.

Two screening tests are used to detect strabismus. The corneal light reflex is determined by shining a penlight at the bridge of the child's nose while he looks straight ahead. Inspection of the child's eyes should then be done to determine if the reflection of light falls at the same point on each pupil. Any deviation indicates strabismus or trophia. A cover test can also be done by holding a light 12 inches from the child's eyes and asking him to focus on the light. The examiner occludes one of the child's eyes (using a paper cup works well), making sure that both eyes remain open, and observes the uncovered eye for movement inward or outward. The occluder is then moved quickly over the other eye and the eye that had been covered is inspected for any inward or outward deviation. The test is repeated on the opposite eye. Normally no deviation occurs in either eye. The cover test is repeated having the child focus on a distant object. A cover test can be done on even the youngest child by having a bright, flashing object to attract his attention. Older children can focus on the examiner's finger or on a picture placed on the wall. Children having a wide nasal bridge or epicanthal folds may have the appearance of having strabismus. This is referred to as *pseudostrabismus*. A negative cover test and an equal corneal light reflex rule out this condition.

The cornea, sclera, iris and pupil are considered to comprise the eye proper and are examined next. The cornea (transparent eye covering) is inspected for clouding, enlargement, abrasions, lesions or change in color. Abrasions or lesions are best observed by shining a light from the side across the eye. The sclera (white part of eye) is observed for color, hemorrhage or discoloration. The sclera of newborns is often a light blue because of its thinness, but a dark blue sclera can indicate osteogenesis imperfecta or glaucoma. A yellow sclera is often the first clinical sign of jaundice.

The iris and pupil are examined together. The size, shape and color of the irises are noted. Any freckles, Brushfield's spots* or other irregularity should be noted. Pupils are examined for size, shape, equality, reaction to light, and accommodation. A difference in pupil size (anescaria) may be normal but can also be caused by central nervous system damage. The pupillary reaction to light should be done both directly (shining light directly in eye and noting response) and consensually (shining light in one eye and noting if other eye also responds by constricting). Accommodation (a change in dilation and medial movements of both pupils) can be tested even in the young child by having him focus on a brightly colored object at a distance and then quickly bringing the object toward the eye. The pupils constrict as the object is brought close to the eyes and are dilated when the child is focusing on an object at a distance. The eyes are accommodating from far to near vision. An older child can be asked to look far off into the distance (at an object out the window), then to focus on an object within 12 to 14 inches from the eyes.

The lens is examined by shining a light on the eyes and inspecting the lens for opacities. Finally, with the aid of the ophthalmoscope, the retina can be examined. The examiner holds the ophthalmoscope in her right hand and looks with her right eye into the right eye of the child. Examination of the left eye is accomplished by reversing the process. The examination is done in a semidark room. The child should be instructed to focus on a fixation object such as a fluorescent sticker.

The ophthalmoscope is dialed to 0. The examination begins by focusing the light into the child's eyes at a distance of about 12 inches from a position that is about 15 degrees to the side of his line of vision. A red reflex is obtained at this time. An absence of a complete, circular red reflex or the appearance of an opaque density surrounded by a red reflex indicates a cataract or other pathological condition requiring referral to a physician. In non-white races the red reflex (a reddish-orange color reflected from the fundus through the pupil) is normally paler and may have a pink or salmon-colored appearance. The ophthalmoscope generally has from 15 to 20 diopters in the black (positive lens) and in the red (negative lens). (A diopter is the refractive power of the lens with a focal distance of one meter.) The negative lens (red numbers) compensates for myopia (nearsightedness). The positive lens (black numbers) compensates for hyperopia (farsightedness). The refractive ability of the child's eyes plus the refraction of the examiner's eyes will determine

---

*Small white spots on the iris's periphery often seen in Down's syndrome.

which diopters of the ophthalmoscope will be be used during the examination.

Examination of the fundus (Fig. 13–8) of the eye requires an older child (most preschoolers can do this) who is cooperative and able to hold his eyes still and focused on an object for a short period of time. If the child can cooperate, the examiner approaches from the 12 inches used to obtain a red reflex to within 3 inches of the child. As the examiner approaches the child (progresses inward) each layer of the eye is inspected, beginning with the cornea, progressing to the lens and then the vitreous. As the examiner moves in, the dial of the ophthalmoscope is turned to smaller numbers until red minus numbers are reached. The exact number will depend on the refractive ability of the examiner's and the child's eyes.

During the internal examination of the fundus, the optic disc is located and observed for size, shape, color, margins and physiologic depression. The disc is usually round but occasionally may be vertically oval. It is a creamy pink or pale yellow color and has a depression slightly temporal (toward the temple) of the center that is the physiologic cup. The margins should be smooth and slightly darker than the rest of the disc.

The macula is a small circular area located 2 disc diameters temporal to the optic disc with the fovea centralis seen as a gleaming light in its center. The fundus is normally an orange-red color and should be uniform throughout. Lightness and darkness in color varies from one race to another. The fundus should be inspected for signs of hemorrhage or papilledema.

The arteries and veins should also be examined. The arteries are narrower than the veins and exhibit a light reflex from their center. Veins do not normally have a light reflex and are wider than arteries with a 3:2 ratio. As the vessels cross, the veins are under the arteries. Abnormalities such as tortuous vessels, hemorrhages, hypertrophied vessels or excessive dilatation should be referred for further evaluation.

Finally, visual acuity is tested. Vision screening should begin early in life and continue at regular intervals. The infant's vision can be evaluated by watching the child's ability to focus and follow brightly colored objects or a light. The infant should be followed closely for any sign of developmental delay or an obvious lack of response to his environment, which could indicate visual problems.

Vision testing consists of assessing light perception, visual acuity and color perception. Light perception is tested generally in the newborn by shining a light into the eyes and noting responses such as blinking, following the light and increased alertness. A rotating striped drum placed in front of the newborn's face should cause nystagmus if vision is present. The nurse should be aware of signs that may indicate visual loss, such as fixed pupils, marked strabismus, constant nystagmus and "setting-sun" sign.

Visual acuity is defined as the ability to see near and far objects clearly. The Snellen Alphabet Chart (Fig. 13–9) consists of nine lines of letters in decreasing size. The child must be familiar with the alphabet in order to perform this test. The child stands 20 feet from the chart and reads each line, which is given a value. Line 8 for example is "20" so that if the child can read this line from a distance of 20 feet, his vision is 20/20. This is accepted normal vision for children after age 6.

The Snellen E (Fig. 13–9) is another version of the Snellen Chart that is used with older toddlers, preschoolers, first graders and children for whom English is not the first language. The limbs or legs of the letter E point in four different directions and are of sizes corresponding with the size of the alphabetic Snellen letters. The child indicates the direction the E (table legs)

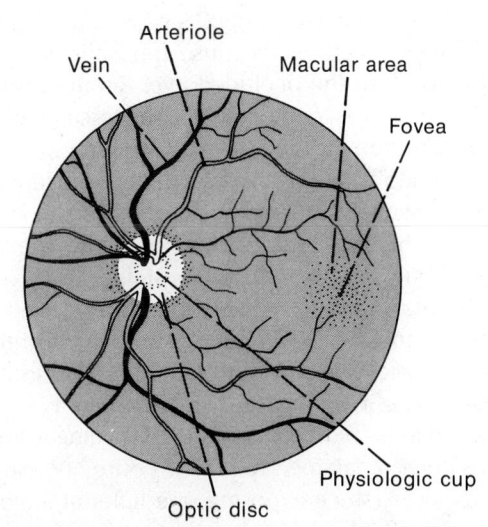

Figure 13-8 Landmarks of the ocular fundus. (From J. Luckmann and K. Sorensen. Medical-Surgical Nursing: A Psychophysiologic Approach. W. B. Saunders, 1980, p. 327.)

LETTER CHART FOR 20 FEET
Snellen Scale

SYMBOL CHART FOR 20 FEET
Snellen Scale

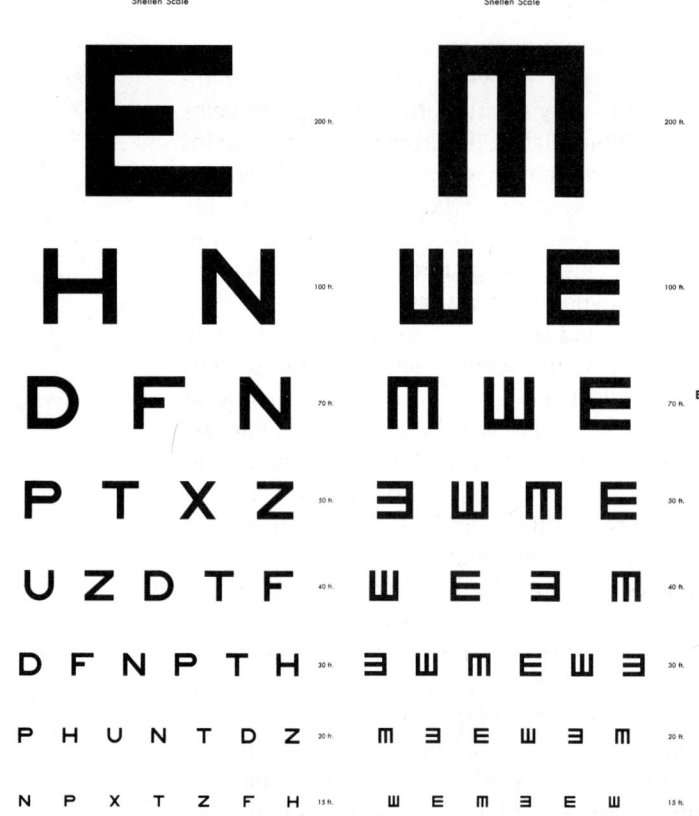

Figure 13-9 Two types of visual acuity charts. The standard Snellen alphabet chart (left) can be used as early as the child's ability to name letters allows. The Snellen "E" chart can be used with younger children. The child is asked to point with his hand or fingers in the direction the E points. (Courtesy National Society to Prevent Blindness, 79 Madison Avenue, New York.)

is pointing. This may be difficult for toddlers and preschoolers owing to their confusion in identifying the direction and inability to read the chart should not be misinterpreted as an inability to see. The child is often helped to identify direction if given concrete items to refer to (the table legs are pointing toward the door, the ceiling, the floor or the window). The child should practice pointing in the various directions with a practice E card before testing. The testing procedure is the same as with alphabetic letters. The Titmus Vision Tester also has both the alphabetic and the preschool E chart, so it can be used if available. The advantage of a machine like the Titmus is that the child is less distracted during its use because it is a closed machine, and it can be used in a much smaller area.

The Stycar Chart is much easier to use in the preschool period, with very little preparation of the child. The letters (HOUTX) are on a card held in front of the child. The chart with these same letters is placed 10 feet away. The examiner points to a letter on the chart and the child is asked to find the corresponding letter on the card. It has been determined that these letters are among the most easily recognized.[14]

Allen Cards are probably the best of the available picture tests. The test consists of a series of black and white pictures (a birthday cake, telephone, Christmas tree) that are shown to the child by the examiner as she slowly moves toward the child. The distance at which the child is first able to recognize three of the pictures determines the numerator over the denominator of 30. A 3-year-old is expected to achieve a score of 15/30; a 4-year-old, 20/30. A child who cannot identify the pictures or has a 5 feet difference between eyes should be referred.

Whatever test is employed, appropriate test technique should always be used. Adequate illumination is essential. The light should fall evenly on the chart without glare. The chart is placed at the child's eye level. Each child should be tested individually so that memorization of the chart while waiting will not be a problem. For children under 6 two examiners are usually required. One sits in a chair beside the child. (The child may stand on a set of footprints on the floor or with the tips of his toes behind a marked-off line, or be seated in a child-sized chair beside the examiner.) This examiner occludes one eye at a time while the child keeps both eyes open. A paper cup works well as an occluder because the child is less likely to close the occluded eye. Reminders to keep both eyes open may be necessary with some children.

The child is then instructed to read the letters slowly, without guessing, as the line is uncovered by the second examiner. The examiner should begin with at least the 20/40 or 20/50 line and move either up or down depending on how well the child does. The child should be tested as far down on the chart as he is capable of reading. Reading the majority (one more than half) of letters in the line being tested constitutes a passing score. The entire line must be exposed, since exposing one letter at a time may not effectively test a child for amblyopia. Visual acuity becomes increasingly organized as the child develops. Most infants are able to see objects clearly at close range, usually 12 to 14 inches. Binocular vision is clearly established between 4 to 7 months of age and mature function of the eye muscles is generally developed by 1 year of age.

Table 13-9 outlines the development of visual acuity during childhood. These standards differ from those used in the past. Children have better vision than was previously believed. Any child who does not have the visual acuity expected for his age should be referred. Also, any child who has a two-line difference between eyes should have further evaluation. This may indicate poorer vision in the one eye, which may be compensated for and the vision eventually lost completely without correction.

Screening for heterotropia is another important vision test. In heterotropia the child's eyes do not focus together to provide binocular vision. Heterophoria is the latent tendency for heterotropia. The corneal light reflex is one of the most important screening tests to determine a tropia. The cover test is another screening test to help rule out a tropia or a phoria. These screening tests are discussed in detail in the examination of the eye and should always be part of every well-child examination.

The Denver Eye Screening Test (Fig. 13-10) may be used to summarize findings from vision acuity screening and heterotropia testings to determine the need for referral. The form is especially useful in evaluating children before they are literate or developmentally ready to cooperate fully with visual testing methods.

Finally, color vision is assessed in every child, usually at preschool age. Although color blindness is rare in females, it is important to determine the child's ability to determine colors. The child who has color blindness will need counselling for safety purposes such as interpreting traffic signals and also later regarding occupational choices. This child will also need assistance in developing the ability to coordinate colors of wearing apparel so that he is not ridiculed by peers. The Ishihara Plates are plates with figures composed of dots hidden in a background of similar dots. The figure is a different color so that the only way to distinguish the figure is by color. These plates are useful in children who have the skills to discriminate figure ground, letters, numbers and geometric figures. The younger child may not be able to do this. Other tests such as matching colored yarns or putting colored tennis balls in similarly colored muffin tin compartments can be used; however the Ishihara is the only standardized color vision test at this time.

Ears Examination of the ears begins with inspection for shape, position and placement of the external ears. The pinna (external ear lobe) should cross the eye-occiput line and should be no more than 10 degrees posterior to a perpendicular line drawn from the eye-occiput line to the lobe. (Fig. 13-11). The pinna is also inspected for color and structural anomalies. Mumps, mastoiditis, cellulitis or congenital anomalies may cause the auricle to stand out. The pinna is palpated for cartilage formation, masses, tenderness and cysts.

The bony prominence located immediately posterior to the ear lobe is the mastoid process. This area is inspected and palpated for erythema, swelling and tenderness. The outer canal of the ear is then inspected for discharge. Bloody discharge is seen with a perforated tympanic membrane, foreign body in the canal, irritation or scratching of the canal or basilar skull fracture. Purulent drainage commonly denotes a fungal or bacterial infection.

Internal structures are examined with the aid of an otoscope. The procedure is usually painless unless an infection or furuncle exists in the ear canal, or the otoscope touches the bony part of the ear canal. Children may become anxious during this part of the examination, but adequate explanation and allowing time for the child to become familiar with the instrument often alleviates anxiety.

A child who is not able to be cooperative should be adequately restrained. The young infant can be placed on his abdomen with his head to one side. The examiner can retract the pinna with her left hand and also keep the head still while holding the otoscope in her right

TABLE 13-9 VISUAL ACUITY AT VARIOUS AGES

Age	Vision
Birth	Differentiates light and dark; fixates on objects 8–10 inches away
16 weeks	20/200
20 weeks	20/200
1 year	20/100
2 years	20/40
3 years	20/30
4–6 years	20/20

DENVER EYE SCREENING TEST

Name
Hospital No.
Ward
Address

Lit. 217	1ST SCREENING:DATE						RESCREENING:DATE					
	Right Eye			Left Eye			Right Eye			Left Eye		
Vision Tests	Normal	Abnormal	Untestable	Normal	Abnormal	Untestable	Normal	Abnormal	Untestable	Normal	Abnormal	Untestable
1. "E" (3 years and above-3 to 5 trials)	3P	3F	U	3P	3F	U	3P	3F	U	3P	3F	U
2. Picture Card (2 1/2 - 2 11/12 yrs.-3 to 5 trials)	3P	3F	U	3P	3F	U	3P	3F	U	3P	3F	U
3. Fixation (6 months - 2 5/12 years)	P	F	U	P	F	U	P	F	U	P	F	U
4. Squinting		yes			yes			yes			yes	
Tests for Non-Straight Eyes	Normal		Abnormal			Untestable	Normal		Abnormal			Untestable
1. Do your child's eyes turn in or out, or are they ever not straight?	NO		YES			U	NO		YES			U
2. Cover Test	P		F			U	P		F			U
3. Pupillary Light Reflex	P		F			U	P		F			U
Total Test Rating (Both Eyes)												
Normal (passed vision test plus no squint, plus passed 2/3 tests for non-straight eyes)	Normal						Normal					
Abnormal (abnormal on any vision test, squinting or 2 of 3 procedures for non-straight eyes)	Abnormal						Abnormal					
Untestable (untestable on any vision test or untestable on 2/3 tests for non-straight eyes)	Untestable						Untestable					
Future Rescreening Appointment for Total Test Rating (Abnormal or Untestable)	Date:						Date:					

Figure 13–10 Denver Eye Screening Test. (Courtesy of William K. Frankenberg, M.D., and Josiah B. Dodds, Ph.D., University of Colorado Medical Center.)

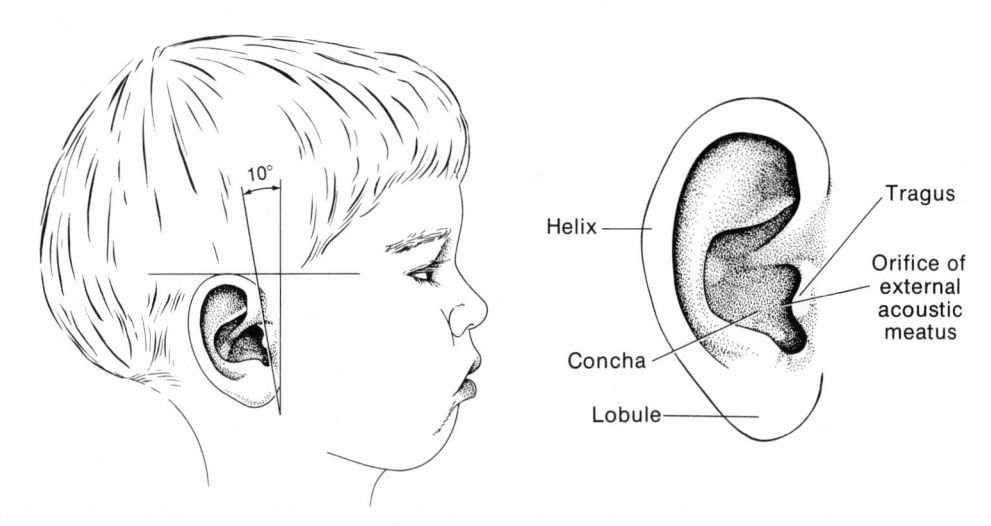

Figure 13-11 Line indicating normal placement of the external ear.

hand. The otoscope is held like a pencil with the right side of the hand and fifth finger resting on the child's head to cushion the otoscope if the child should move his head. The toddler or preschool child can sit on the parent's lap with his legs held firmly between the parent's legs. The parent places an arm firmly across the child's trunk and arms; and the other arm is used to hold the child's head firmly against the parent's chest. This age child can also be restrained while lying supine on an examination table with this arms extended above his head and held firmly by the parent. The examiner then leans over the child's trunk and restrains the head to one side. The examiner should be careful not to put weight on the child's chest; this could frighten the child and cause respiratory distress. The child who will sit on the examination table needs only to tilt his head to one side to allow for better visualization.

Once the child has been appropriately restrained, the ear canal be examined. The ear canal is normally curved and must be straightened before the nurse can visualize the canal and tympanic membrane. In infants and toddlers the auricle is pulled down and in the child over 3 the auricle is pulled up and back to straighten the ear canal (Fig. 13-12). The canal is then examined internally for erythema, lesions, furuncles or discharge. The amount and consistency of cerumen (wax) is also noted and described.

Once the canal has been inspected, the examiner proceeds to the tympanic membrane. The tympanic membrane is assessed for color, the landmarks, and mobility.

A normal tympanic membrane is a light, pearly gray color. An erythematous membrane may be seen in the child who has been crying or the child with otitis media. A dull gray or yellowish color is often seen with serous otitis and a vivid red in suppurative otitis. The landmarks are the umbo, light reflex, long process, short process, pars flaccida, annulus and the anterior and posterior malleolar folds (Fig. 13-13).

The light reflex is a small, triangular cone of light that is seen at the anterior inferior quadrant. It is located directly below the umbo. A diffuse, spotty or absent cone of light may indicate infection or fluid in the middle ear. The

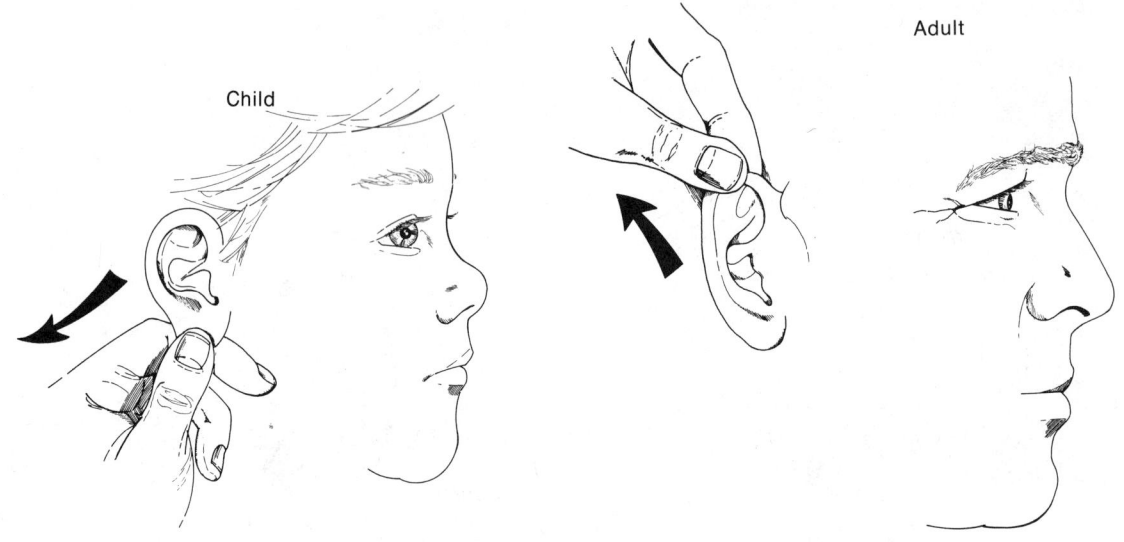

Figure 13-12 Examination of the external ear in the child under 3 and the older child or adult.

umbo, found at the top of the cone of light, appears as a round white fibrous area. The long process (handle of the malleus) can be seen above and nasally of the umbo. The short process of the malleus looks like a sharp white protuberant bone through the membrane. When the membrane is retracted the landmarks appear more pronounced; bulging makes them more obscure. A bulging or retracted tympanic membrane requires referral.

The annulus is a white fibrous ring surrounding the periphery of the drum. The three small bones, or ossicles (malleus, incus and stapes), lie directly behind the membrane. The incus and stapes may be seen only if the drum is very translucent or if it is retracted.

Evaluating the mobility of the eardrum is useful in determining the presence or absence of fluid in the middle ear. Fluid will cause the membrane to move in a restricted fashion or not at all. Mobility of the eardrum is assessed by using a pneumatic headpiece on the otoscope. This device is a piece of rubber tubing that is attached to the head of the otoscope. It must be used with a tight-fitting speculum so that the ear canal is sealed off. Air is puffed through the tubing while the examiner observes the movement of the tympanic membrane. Absent or decreased mobility indicates fluid (negative middle ear pressure).

Hearing is an essential part of the well-child examination. Since learning and language are so closely related, it is important for the nurse to be alert to clues indicating a possible hearing disorder. Children who evidence characteristics summarized in Table 13-10 should be tested for possible hearing problems. Hearing testing should be done at all ages to evaluate hearing accuracy.

For young infants and toddlers, testing is often accomplished by using a noisemaker. The child is seated on the parent's lap and distracted visually from the front. A noisemaker is then used to one side. The child should be distracted visually by one examiner while another examiner produces the sound to one side at 18 to 24 inches from the child. The first examiner observes for the response. (Table 13-11 summarizes the characteristic responses of infants who can hear.)

The sounds produced should be of high, medium and low frequency and should be repeated on each side. The examiner should reproduce the sound approximately 8 to 12

Figure 13-13 Normal tympanic membrane.

TABLE 13-10 CHARACTERISTICS OF CHILDREN WHO MAY HAVE HEARING OR LANGUAGE DEFICITS

Response to Auditory Stimuli
(See Table 13-15 for normal development of hearing responses)
Inattentive to speech.
Does not react with a startle to loud noises during first year.
Does not react to name or commands by 6-9 months.
Does not turn to source of sound by 4 months.
Does not understand commands or instructions by 18 months.
Inconsistent responses to environmental sounds during first 2 years of life.
Turns up volume on radio or TV.

Voice Characteristics
Voice quality is poor.
Voice is loud or monotone.

Speech Characteristics
Babbles normally until 6 months then gradually decreases sound production.
Not talking at all by age 2 years.
Speech highly unintelligible after age 3 years.
Uses mostly vowel sounds after 1 year of age.
Speech that is difficult for others to understand.
Consistently drops word endings.
Constantly misses high-pitched consonants and fricatives such as *th, ch, s, sh, b,* and *k*.
Omits initial consonants after age 3.

Medical Characteristics
History of prenatal infections, birth anomalies, prematurity, birth trauma, birth anoxia, kernicterus.
History of treatment with ototoxic drugs during infancy.
Familial history of congenital hearing impairment.
History of frequent upper respiratory or ear infections.

TABLE 13-11 DEVELOPMENT OF HEARING RESPONSES[5, 10]

Age	Hearing Response
Birth	Startle reflex; blinking of eyes; attends to voice.
12 weeks	Eye movement toward sound when prone.
12-18 weeks	Eye movement toward sound when upright.
4 months	Widening of eyes; quieting; listening posture; slight head turning; looks in same direction as sound.
6 months	Turns head to source of sound; may have beginning localization; downward localization occurs before upward localization.
8-12 months	Turns head 45° or more in direction of sound; localizes sound source above and below; rapid automatic response to sound by one year.
12-36 months	Rapid speech development and language patterns based on hearing input.

inches above and below the level of the ear to determine if the child can localize the sound.

Toddlers and preschoolers are difficult to examine for hearing, but it is important that adequate hearing testing is done because hearing is critical to appropriate speech development. Play audiometry is used for children over 15 months of age. The child can be tested with or without earphones; however, more specific information about each ear is gathered if the child will allow earphone testing. The child is conditioned through a play technique to respond to sound stimuli. Once the child has been conditioned to respond to the sound (by dropping the block in a box or putting a ring on a peg), the examiner can test the child with the earphones in place. Often the examiner places several toys in front of the child, places the earphones on him, and then requests that the child pick up a certain toy. This is done at different frequencies and decibels. The child's responses are then recorded. By 3 to 4 years of age the child can frequently have routine audiometric pure tone testing with a minimum of preparation. Hearing and hearing loss are further discussed in Chapter 43.

Tuning forks can also be used to identify conductive or neurosensory hearing loss. This can be done only on an older child (at least 5 years of age) who can follow directions and give appropriate responses. The Weber test is performed by placing an activated tuning fork (struck on the hand to set it in vibration) on the midline of the skull. The child should indicate if he can hear it equally in both ears (the normal response) or if the sound is localized to one ear. If the sound is lateralized to one ear, that ear may have a conductive hearing loss. Lateralization to the affected ear occurs because room noise, which is blocked out in that ear, does not interfere with bone vibration. Lateralization to one ear may also indicate a sensorineural loss in the opposite ear. The inner ear or nerve is affected; therefore vibrations are not as well detected from the bone. The sound is heard better in the unaffected ear.

The Rinne test is performed by striking the tuning fork and placing the stem on the child's mastoid process until he indicates he can no longer hear it. The tuning fork, still vibrating, is then placed one to two inches from the concha (ear opening). The child is asked if he can still hear it. He should be able to hear the vibrations

HEALTH APPRAISAL 213

in the air longer than he can the vibration on bone because air conduction is normally two times longer than bone conduction. This is repeated on the opposite mastoid and ear. Any child who cannot hear the sound via air conduction longer than bone conduction should be referred.

Although the information received from using tuning forks is very helpful, it is not a precise assessment of the child's hearing. Audiometric hearing testing is the most reliable method to evaluate hearing. Pure-tone audiometry is done by presenting electronically generated pure tones of various frequencies (measured in Hertz) and intensities (measured in decibels) to a child through earphones. The child is instructed to raise his hand as soon as he hears the sound. For children younger than 5 years, a play activity should be substituted for raising the hand. The child should not be able to see the audiometer controls. The usual procedure is to present the various frequencies at an intensity of 20–25 dB; however, a 15–20 dB tone is required to identify minor hearing loss caused by otitis media. Testing at 15 dB is often not done because it requires a more sound-proof room. Various methods of testing are used. Downs (Early identification of hearing loss. In *Speech Language and Hearing*. N. Lass et al., eds., W. B. Saunders Co., 1981) recommends the following procedure:

1. Present a pure tone of 50 dB at 1000 Hz; this acquaints the child with the procedure. Praise the child for raising his hand.
2. Set the dial to 15 dB and present tones at 1000, 2000, and 4000 to one ear.
3. Switch ears; present tones in reverse sequence: 4000, 2000, and 1000 Hz.

Test results are marked on a graph (audiogram) for each frequency. A child who fails to respond to any of the tones at 15 dB in either ear fails the test. The child should be retested later the same day; if he fails again, referral is necessary.

Nose Determining whether the child is breathing through his nose or mouth is the first step in the examination of the nose. Patency of the nares of the newborn is assessed by placing the diaphragm of the stethoscope against one naris while blocking the other naris and listening for breath sounds. An infant who does not have patent nasal passages may experience respiratory distress. Flaring of the nares also indicates respiratory distress and can be caused by obstruction, pneumonia, fever, anoxia and acidosis. A child who mouth breathes may have nasal polyps, allergies, enlarged adenoids or a deviated septum.

The shape of the nose is inspected. A flat or saddle-shaped nose is indicative of congenital anomalies, congenital syphilis, cleft palate and other conditions. A crease across the nose may be a result of the allergic salute, in which a child frequently pushes against the tip of his nose because of rhinitis or itching. The nose is also palpated for crepitus, tenderness and stability.

Internal examination of the nose requires a penlight or an otoscope with a nasal speculum. The otoscope provides a better visualization of the internal structures. The examiner gently pushes the tip of the nose up and places the speculum at the opening of the naris to inspect the nasal mucosa. Normal mucosa are pink and moist. Inflamed mucosa indicate irritation or infection. Pale, boggy mucosa are seen in children with allergies, and swollen gray mucosa indicate chronic rhinitis.

The examiner also determines the type and amount of nasal secretions. Thin watery secretions are seen in children with allergies, colds, or foreign bodies high in the nose. Purulent discharge is commonly seen with nasal and sinus infections or foreign bodies that have been lodged for a period of time. Nasal bleeding occurs at Kesselbach's plexus, which is located at the anterior tip of the septum. Trauma, allergies, dry climate or blood dyscrasias will cause epistaxis from this point. The septum should be inspected for deviations or perforations. Septal deviations are seen rarely in children unless perforation has been caused by injury of the nasal septum, a foreign body, syphilis or tuberculosis. The examiner should also inspect the turbinates and meatal openings. Any swelling, color change, or discharge should be noted.

Finally, palpation and percussion of the sinuses is performed. The maxillary and ethmoid sinuses are developed in infancy. The frontal sinuses develop around 7 to 8 years of age, while the sphenoid sinuses do not develop until after puberty. Firm pressure is applied along the supraorbital ridge, maxillary area and on the infraorbital ridge nasally (Fig. 13–14). Any indication of tenderness with percussion or palpation may indicate a sinus infection.

Mouth Examination of the mouth and throat

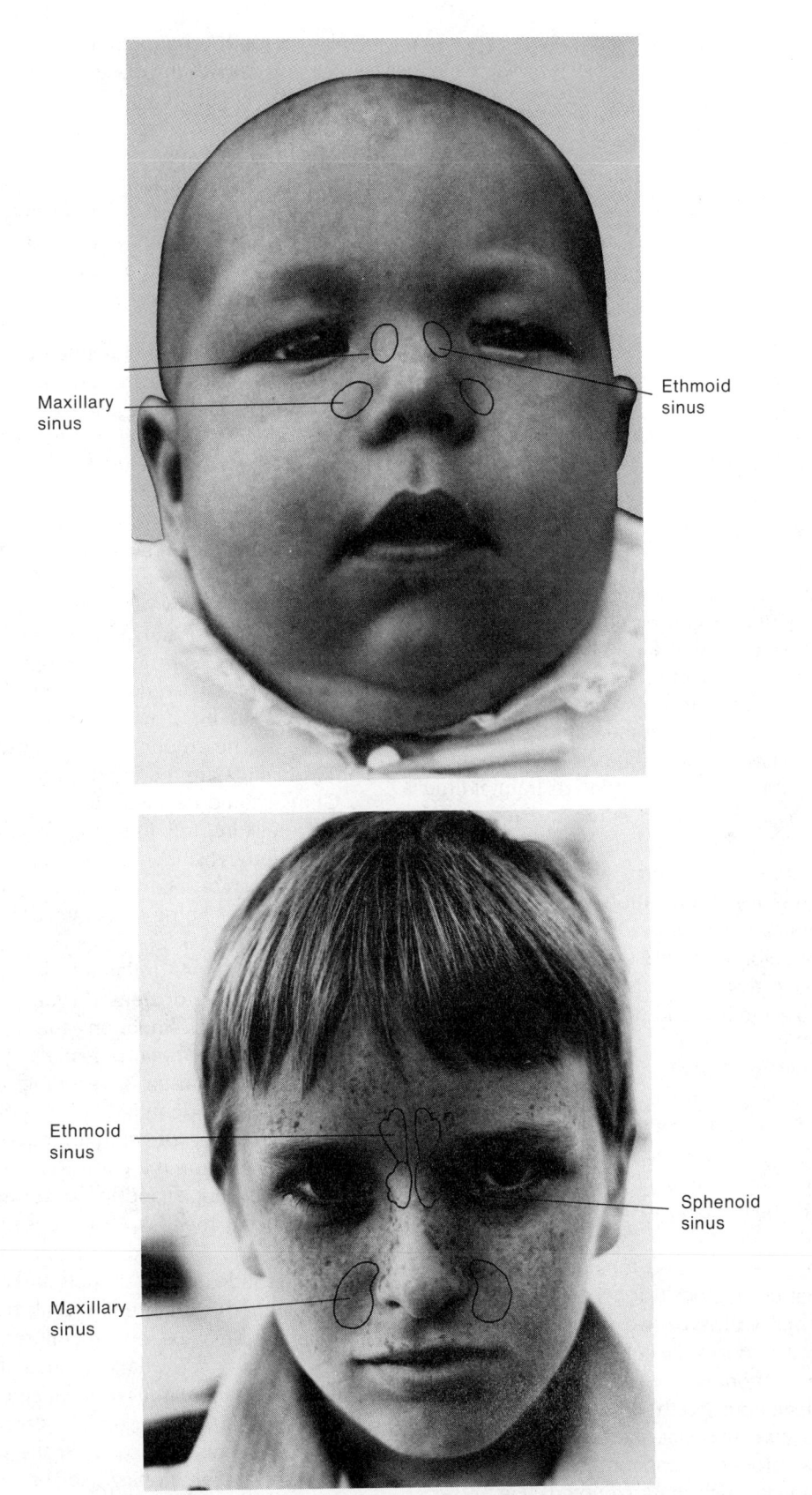

Figure 13–14 Facial sinuses indicated on an infant and a child.

HEALTH APPRAISAL 215

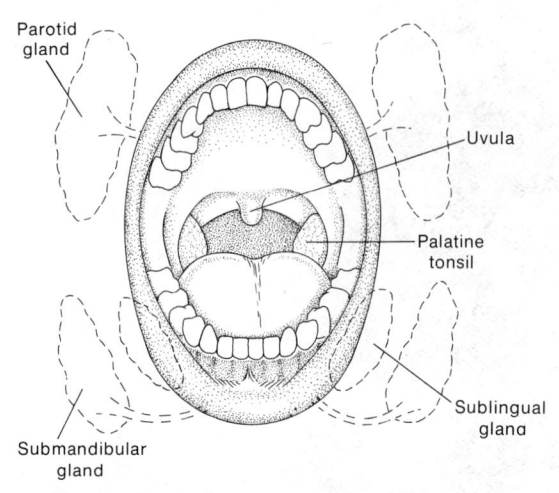

Figure 13-15 Structures of the child's mouth.

(Fig. 13-15) is often difficult and traumatic for the child. This part of the examination, along with the otoscopic examination, may be done last. An uncooperative child should be adequately restrained to allow for a safe examination. The infant can be examined while in the supine position, arms held above the head. The young child can sit on the parent's lap and be restrained as was described for the ear tests. The older child generally needs no restraint if time is taken to explain the procedure and acquaint the child with the equipment. A tongue depressor and a good light source are essential for this portion of the examination.

Examination begins with inspection of the lips for color, moisture, size, shape, asymmetry, drooping, fissures, clefts, edema or lesions. In addition, the lips and the surrounding area are inspected for pallor or cyanosis. Cherry-red lips are seen in children with acidosis or carbon monoxide poisoning. Unusual mouth odors should be noted as they can be clinically significant. Unusual odors are present in children with poor oral hygiene, dental caries, sinusitis, allergies, diabetic acidosis, malnutrition and diphtheria.

Teeth are inspected for number, type, position, caries, malocclusions, color and hygiene. The child will have two sets of teeth; the first teeth, or deciduous teeth, begin eruption around 6 months of age (Fig. 13-16). All 20 of the deciduous teeth usually are erupted by 2½ to 3 years of age. Permanent dentition begins at around 6 and progresses until all 32 permanent teeth have erupted (Fig. 13-16).

Delay in tooth eruption can be genetic or significant of underlying disease processes.

Teeth with flattened edges are usually seen in children who grind their teeth. Malocclusion is often caused by persistent thumbsucking. To determine malocclusion, the examiner inspects the alignment of the teeth. In normal occlusion the top posterior molars meet and rest snugly on the opposing bottom molars and then the upper central incisors just overlap and touch the lower incisors.

Teeth that are mottled (white flecks) or pitted are seen in children who have ingested excessive fluoride. Iron ingestion, antibiotic ingestion, or severe jaundice at birth can cause a green or black discoloration of teeth. The teeth should be percussed for tenderness. A tongue depressor is tapped on the crown and sides of teeth to elicit tenderness. Salivation is noted. Salivary secretion is limited until 3 months of age when the salivary glands become more active. Absence of salivation may be caused by fever, dehydration or atropine ingestion. Excessive salivation is frequently seen in children who are teething or who have caries or mouth infections. The amount, color, consistency and odor of saliva are recorded if abnormal.

Gums should be inspected and palpated for color, moisture, inflammation, swelling, bleeding, tenderness and ulcerations. Inflammation and swelling are secondary to infection or poor oral hygiene. A herpesvirus infection or improperly fitting dental corrective appliances may cause ulcerations. Inflamed, bleeding gums may be a result of decreased vitamin C intake or pyorrhea. A black line along the margin of the gum may signify metal poisoning such as lead poisoning. Any raised or receding areas of the gums should be identified. It is important to use the tongue depressor gently to move the buccal mucosa away from the gums to allow adequate inspection of upper and lower gums.

The buccal mucosa (inner cheek region) is inspected and palpated for color, moisture, lesions, parotid (Stensen's) ducts and masses. The buccal mucosa is normally pink but black or brown areas may be seen in children with Addison's disease and in dark-skinned children. An enlarged, erythematous or swollen parotid duct is seen with parotitis. Koplik's spots (a group of gray-white spots) are seen on the buccal mucosa opposite the molars in the prodromal stage of measles. White patches on the oral mucosa, especially the tongue and hard palate, that cannot be scraped off indicate a yeast (monilial)

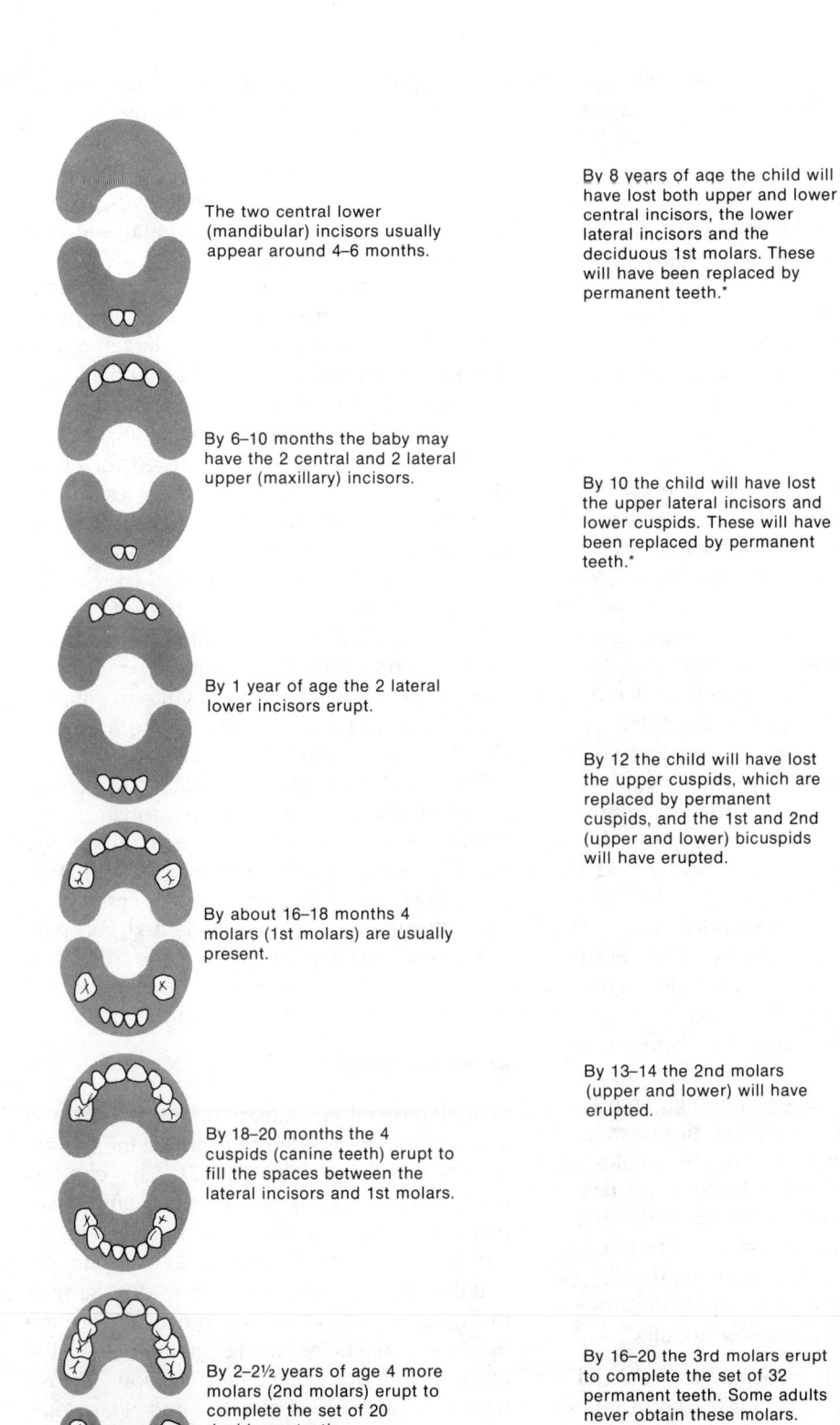

The two central lower (mandibular) incisors usually appear around 4–6 months.

By 6–10 months the baby may have the 2 central and 2 lateral upper (maxillary) incisors.

By 1 year of age the 2 lateral lower incisors erupt.

By about 16–18 months 4 molars (1st molars) are usually present.

By 18–20 months the 4 cuspids (canine teeth) erupt to fill the spaces between the lateral incisors and 1st molars.

By 2–2½ years of age 4 more molars (2nd molars) erupt to complete the set of 20 deciduous teeth.

By 8 years of age the child will have lost both upper and lower central incisors, the lower lateral incisors and the deciduous 1st molars. These will have been replaced by permanent teeth.*

By 10 the child will have lost the upper lateral incisors and lower cuspids. These will have been replaced by permanent teeth.*

By 12 the child will have lost the upper cuspids, which are replaced by permanent cuspids, and the 1st and 2nd (upper and lower) bicuspids will have erupted.

By 13–14 the 2nd molars (upper and lower) will have erupted.

By 16–20 the 3rd molars erupt to complete the set of 32 permanent teeth. Some adults never obtain these molars.

*Although the diagram represents only the erupted permanent teeth, the reader should recognize that the mouth also contains the remaining deciduous teeth.

Figure 13-16

infection called thrush. The floor of the mouth is inspected and palpated for cysts, masses or calculi of the submaxillary glands. (This is the major location of oral cancer.)

Inspection of the tongue is done to determine color, moisture, size, tremors, coating, size of papillae, and the presence of lesions. The normal tongue is pink and should fit in the mouth. A large protruding tongue is seen in children with Down's syndrome. Normally the tongue has conical filliform papillae; large red papillae resembling a strawberry are seen with scarlet fever. The tongue becomes tender and red with riboflavin deficiency, niacin deficiency or severe anemia. A geographic tongue has gray, irregular borders and can be considered normal or caused by allergies, fever or drug ingestion. The tongue should also be examined for furrows and scars. Deep furrows are seen in children with Down's syndrome. Scars could be the result of trauma or previous convulsions. Gross tongue tremors when the tongue is stuck out are seen in children with cerebral palsy; fine tremors are seen with chorea or hypothyroidism. The examiner should observe the tongue closely to determine mobility. The frenulum is checked for tongue-tie and is considered abnormal if the tongue cannot extend beyond the lower alveolar ridge. The ventral surface of the tongue is inspected for distended veins. The older child is instructed to push against the tongue depressor laterally on each side to determine the tongue's strength.

The hard and soft palates are inspected and palpated for color, shape, clefts, and the presence of lesions. An abnormally high arch may be associated with congenital disorders and may result in speech problems. The palates are usually a striated pink color. Epstein's pearls are seen as firm white nodules in the midline and are of no significance. Examination of the palates is not complete until both hard and soft palates have been completely palpated (use a disposable glove) for masses or nodules.

Throat The uvula is inspected as the child is gagged or is told to say "ahh." The examiner should not attempt to gag the child until the very end of the examination. A gag reflex should also not be obtained if there is a suspicion of epiglottitis, since this may cause increased swelling and occlude the airway. The soft palate and uvula should rise when the patient gags or says "ahh." Paralysis of the soft palate or uvula, which is indicated by no movement or movement that is not midline, may signify diphtheria, poliomyelitis or abnormality of the glossopharyngeal or vagus nerves. An exceptionally long uvula is congenital and may cause gagging or coughing.

If present, tonsils are inspected for color, size, symmetry, inflammation or exudate, and possible lesions. Tonsils are much larger during childhood and begin to shrink between the ages of 8 and 12 years. Tonsillar crypts (small sac or cavity) usually indicate past infection.

The posterior pharynx is checked for color, drainage, edema and abnormal lesions or growths. Lymphoid hyperplasia and inflammation are seen in infection. A pale, puffy mucosa usually denotes edema. Ulcers and vesicles are seen in children with viral infections. Postnasal drainage may indicate either allergy or infection of the nasopharynx or sinuses, depending on the type of discharge seen. A white membrane over the pharynx or tonsils may be a sign of diphtheria or bacterial infection.

The child is gagged by placing a tongue depressor over the root of the tongue. This allows for visualization of the epiglottis. If the child has symptoms or epiglottitis, examination is not done; the child is referred if necessary. An epiglottis that is swollen, inflamed, or pale requires referral to a physician. If the soft palate and uvula have not previously been inspected for movement, it can be done at this time.

Chest and Lungs

Skillful inspection, palpation, percussion and auscultation are needed to examine the thorax, breasts and lungs (Fig. 13–17). The chest is inspected for size, shape, symmetry and movement. The shape of the chest is round in the newborn with the anterior-posterior diameter equaling the transverse diameter. With growth the chest shape becomes more oval with the transverse diameter being greater than the anterior-posterior diameter. Pigeon breast, barrel chest, funnel breast and Harrison's groove are examples of abnormal chest structure (Fig. 13–18). Asymmetry such as precordial bulging may indicate chronic localized chest disease, enlargement of the heart or pneumothorax. Other causes of asymmetry include tumors, scoliosis, and congenital absence of the chest muscle. The posterior chest wall is inspected and palpated to determine equality of the scapulae, and any deformity is noted. The

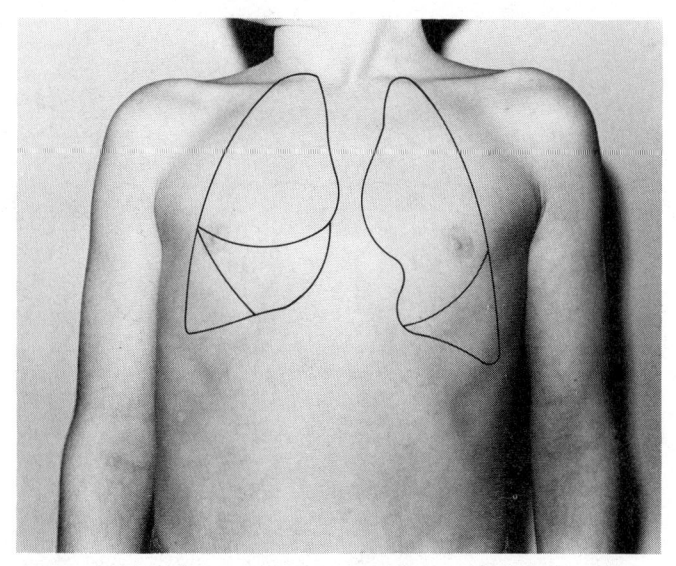

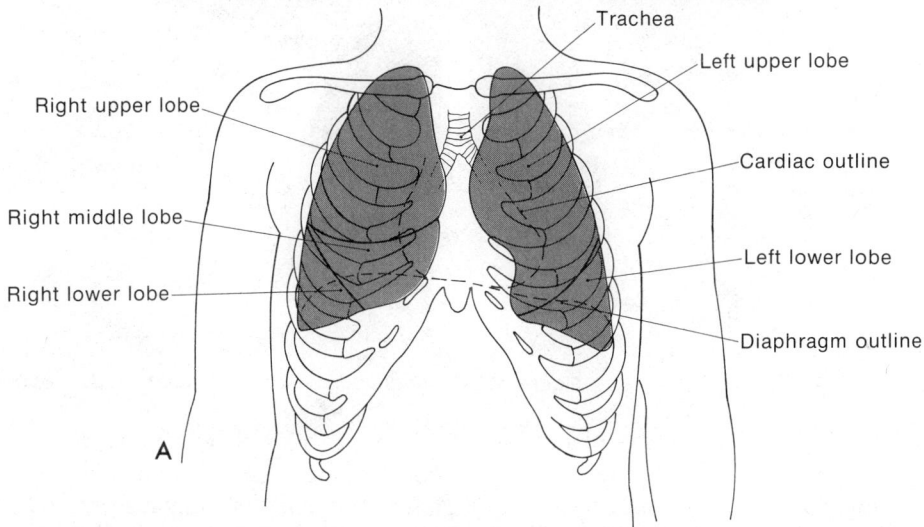

Figure 13–17 The four parts of the lung within the chest. *A*, Anterior thorax, *B*, Posterior thorax; *C*, left lateral thorax, *D*, right lateral thorax.

Illustration continued on following pages

chest should be inspected during inspiration and expiration. Normal inspirations occur as the chest expands, the sternal angle increases and the diaphragm descends. With expiration, the process is reversed. Paradoxical respirations (diaphragm rises on inspiration and descends on expiration), or any signs of respiratory distress, should be noted. Normal respirations are generally abdominal in the infant and young child and become thoracic around 7 years of age, although both are normal. Thoracic breathing is seen predominantly in females and when in the prone position.

Respiratory motion is also observed both during quiet respirations and during deep respirations. It is important to note the type, rate, rhythm and depth of respiration as well as the use of any accessory respiratory muscles in the neck. Retractions, if present, should be described as to their location and depth. Retractions are usually suprasternal and severe in the presence of a high obstruction. They are usually less intense and infrasternal when there is low obstruction.

The chest is palpated to determine if any cysts, tenderness, tumors or abnormal growths exist. Sharp angular bumps at the junction of the rib and its cartilage (costochondral junction) are seen in children with vitamin D deficiency. The clavicles are palpated for crepitus and tenderness to rule out a fracture. Palpation of the ribs will indicate the number of ribs and the presence of tenderness. Lung expansion is

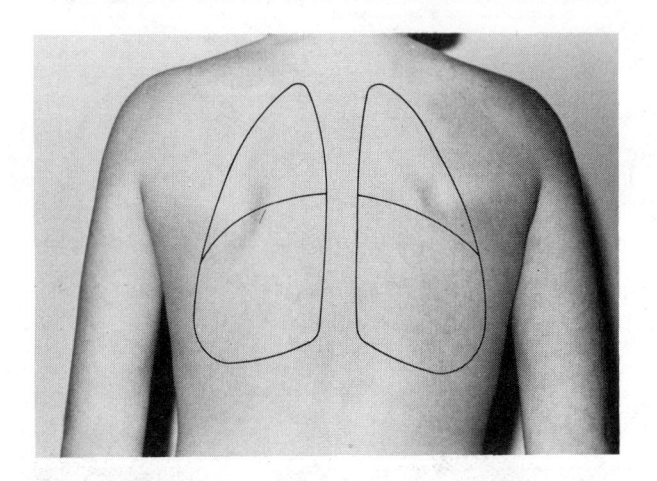

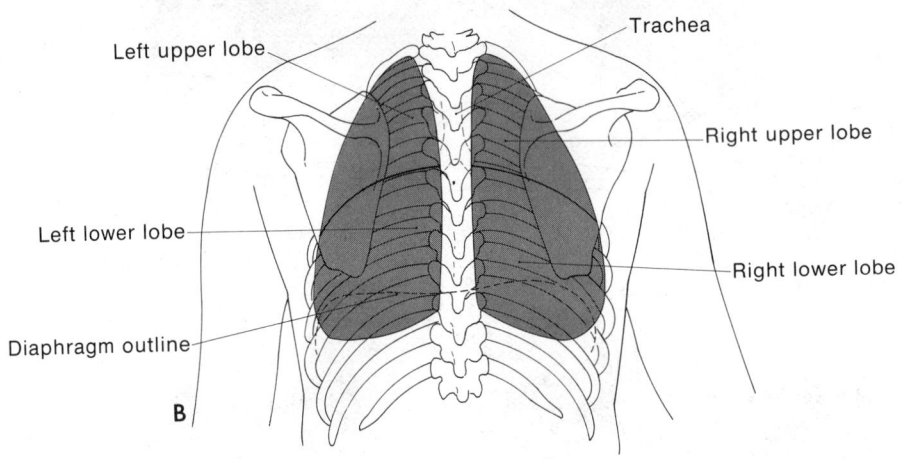

Left upper lobe
Trachea
Right upper lobe
Left lower lobe
Right lower lobe
Diaphragm outline
B

Figure 13-17 Continued   Illustration continued on opposite page

evaluated by the examiner as she places her hands, palms down, on the child's chest, thumbs resting on the costal margin (for the anterior chest) or midspinally at the tenth rib (for the posterior chest). The fingers are spread and placed on symmetrical areas of the chest. As the chest expands with deep inspiration, the examiner observes her thumbs to see if their movement is equal. Thumb movements should be equidistant in an upward, outward direction.

The conduction of vocal sounds through the chest wall (tactile fremitus) is palpable by placing a hand palm down on the child's chest. Vibrations are felt best with the joints of the hands. Fremitus is felt as a tingling sensation as the child cries or when the words "99" or "blue moon" are said. The examiner's hands are placed in symmetrical bilateral positions as the chest is palpated from top to bottom both anteriorly and posteriorly. Absent or decreased tactile fremitus is seen with bronchial blockages, asthma, pleural effusion and pneumothorax. Increased vibrations are seen with consolidation, such as pneumonia or atelectasis. The chest should also be palpated for pleural crepitus, which is felt as a coarse, crackling sensation when pressure is applied.

The indirect method of percussion is used to percuss the chest. Percussion proceeds symmetrically from side to side and downward to determine the presence, size and density of underlying structures. Percussion should be done in the intercostal space, not on the rib, and should be just lateral to the sternum anteriorly and the spine posteriorly. Percussion starts in the supraclavicular area on the anterior chest. Dullness is percussed over the diaphragm, liver and heart, and tympany over the stomach. The liver is percussed beginning at the right fifth or sixth intercostal space in the midclavicular line. Percussion from this point downward to a point where the sound changes indicates the size of the liver. Beginning as resonant sounds, percussion sounds change to dullness over the liver, then return to resonance beyond the liver border.

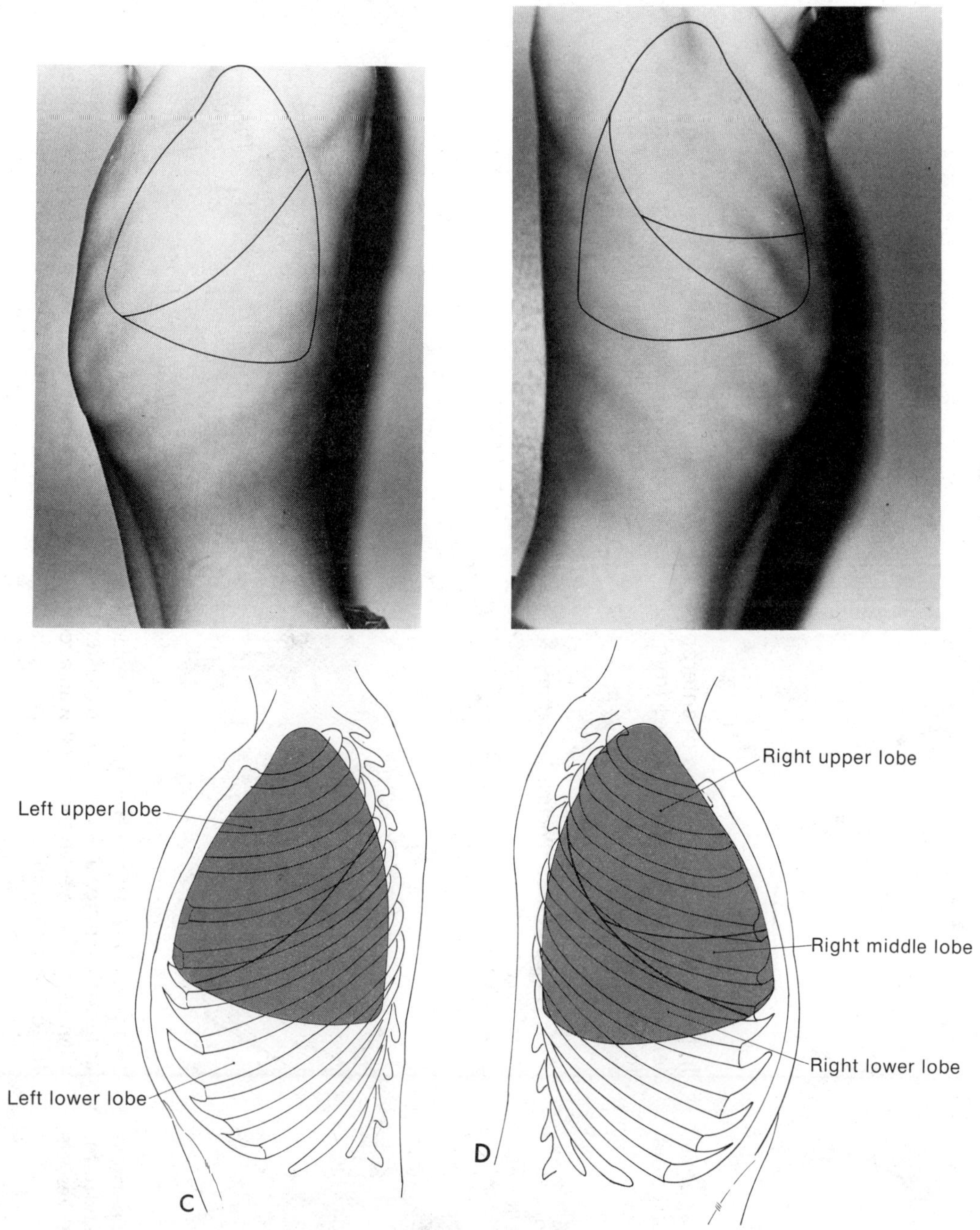
Left upper lobe
Left lower lobe
C
D
Right upper lobe
Right middle lobe
Right lower lobe

Figure 13–17 *Continued*

Posterior percussion begins at the shoulder level. The diaphragm is percussed posteriorly at the level of the eighth to tenth rib. The lateral chest is percussed in symmetrical areas, moving from the top of the axillae downward. Percussion of the lung fields should be heard as resonant. Hyperresonance or dullness in unexpected areas should be considered abnormal. Hyperresonant lung sounds are normal in the newborn, however, due to the thin chest wall. The examiner should listen for obvious respiratory sounds, such as grunting or wheezing, before auscultating the chest.

Auscultation is done using the diaphragm of the stethoscope. The chest is auscultated in a systematic fashion from side to side moving from top to bottom, including anterior, posterior and the lateral aspects. Respiratory rate and depth are recorded. Table 13–5 summarizes average respiratory rates by age. These can be obtained by observing thoracic or abdominal movement, placing a hand on the thorax or abdomen and observing the movement of the

Normal Infant

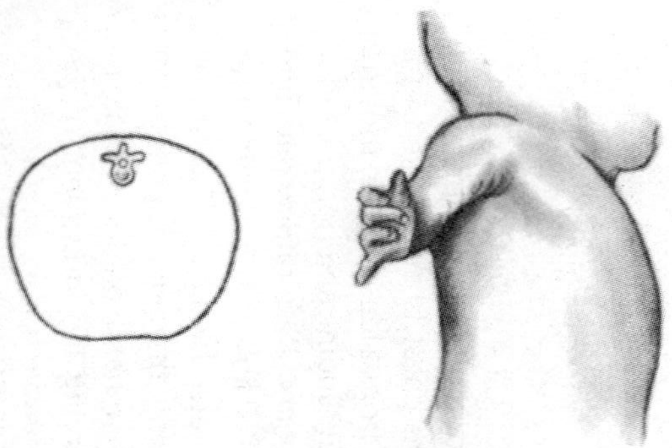

CROSS SECTION OF THORAX

CLINICAL APPEARANCE

The chest of the normal infant is approximately round or barrel-shaped in cross section.

Normal Adult

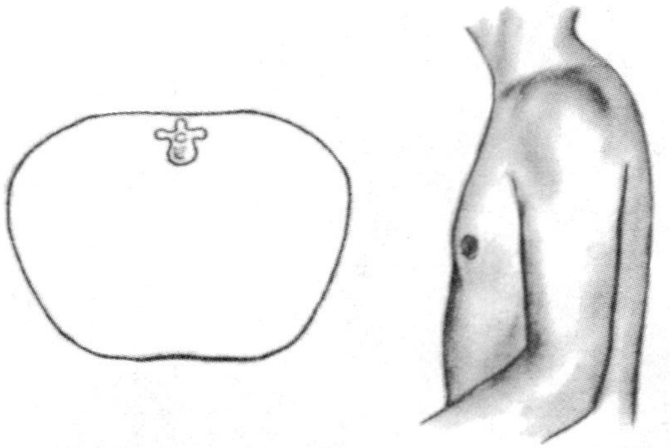

CROSS SECTION OF THORAX

CLINICAL APPEARANCE

In the normal adult the ratio of anteroposterior to lateral diameter ranges from 1:2 to 5:7.

Barrel Chest

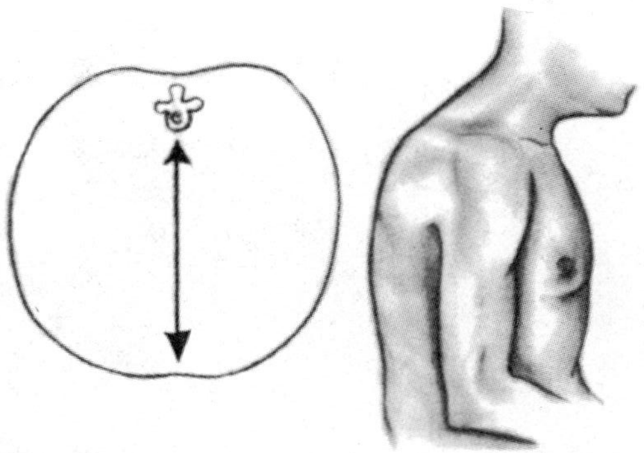

CROSS SECTION OF THORAX

CLINICAL APPEARANCE

A barrel chest is associated with pulmonary emphysema or normal aging. The ratio of anteroposterior to lateral diameter approximates 1:1.

Funnel Chest (Pectus Excavatum)

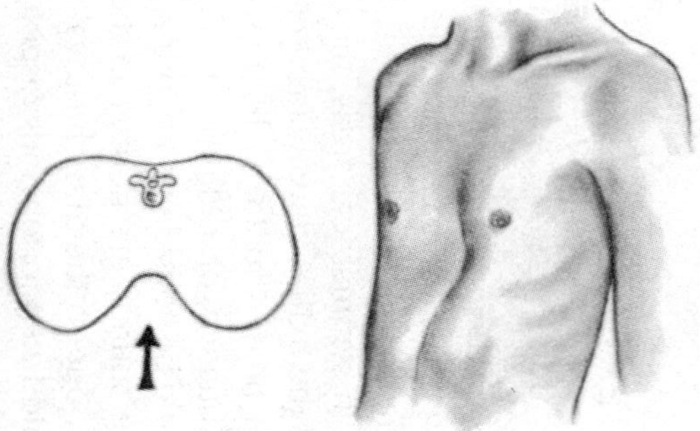

CROSS SECTION OF THORAX

CLINICAL APPEARANCE

A funnel chest is characterized by a depression in the lower portion of the sternum. Compression of the heart and great vessels may cause murmurs.

Pigeon Chest (Pectus Carinatum)

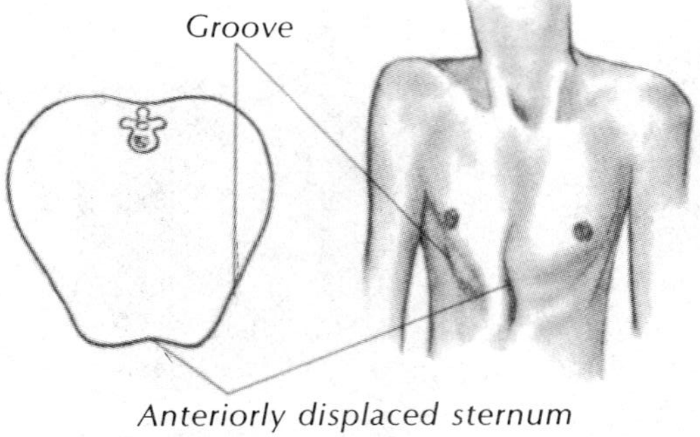

CROSS SECTION OF THORAX

CLINICAL APPEARANCE

Groove

Anteriorly displaced sternum

In a pigeon chest the sternum is displaced anteriorly, increasing the anteroposterior diameter. Grooves in the chest wall accentuate the deformity.

Thoracic Kyphoscoliosis

CROSS SECTION OF THORAX

CLINICAL APPEARANCE

High shoulder
High scapula
Thoracic convexity to right
Interspaces flared

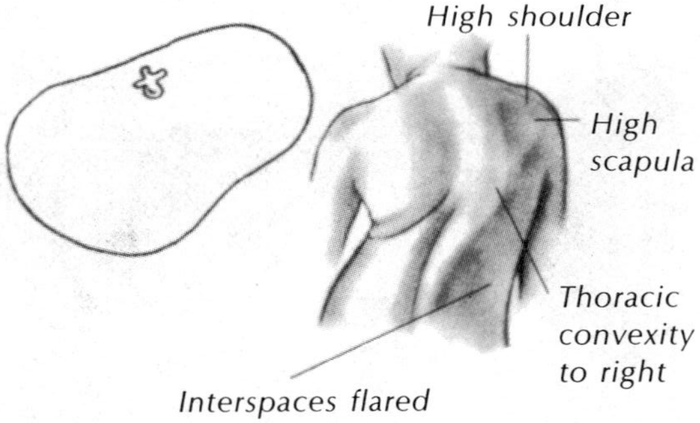

In thoracic kyphoscoliosis the spine is curved and the thorax shows corresponding deformities. Distortion of the underlying lungs may make interpretation of lung findings very difficult.

Figure 13-18 Deformities of the thorax. (From B. Bates. A Guide to Physical Examination. J. B. Lippincott Co., 1974, p. 93.)

TABLE 13-12 CHARACTERISTICS OF BREATH SOUNDS

Type	Length of Inspiration and Expiration	Quality and Intensity	Normal Location
Vesicular	loud ╲ soft	Softest; swishing sound	Throughout lung fields except over sternum and scapulae
Bronchial	soft ╱ loud	Loudest; blowing, hollow sound	Trachea
Bronchovesicular	same	Louder and higher pitched sound than vesicular; tubular quality	Sternum, upper intrascapular area

examiner's hand, or auscultating the breath sounds for rate, rhythm and depth.

Breath sounds are evaluated as to type, quality, pitch, duration and intensity. Breath sounds are normally louder in children under 6 years of age due to the thin chest wall. There are three types of breath sounds: vesicular, bronchial and bronchovesicular. Table 13-12 summarizes the characteristics of each. Vesicular breath sounds are louder, longer and higher-pitched in inspiration and are shorter, softer and lower-pitched in expiration. This type of breath sound is normally found all over the chest except in the areas of the sternum anteriorly and scapulae posteriorly. The ratio of the length of inspiration to the length of expirations is about 5:2. Vesicular sounds are exaggerated in the late stages of pneumonia, emphysema, and in tuberculosis. In the early stages of pneumonia vesicular breath sounds are diminished.

Bronchial breath sounds are shorter on inspiration than on expiration. They are usually louder than the other types of breath sounds. This type of breath sound is normally heard over the trachea. If heard in other areas, it may indicate atelectasis or consolidation. Bronchovesicular breath sounds are a combination of the bronchial and the vesicular breath sounds. Bronchovesicular sounds are equal on inspiration and expiration and are louder and higher pitched than vesicular sounds. They are heard over the sternum and upper intrascapular area.

Additional respiratory sounds not normally heard are adventitious sounds. These sounds are superimposed on normal breath sounds when air being exchanged passes through secretions (rales), through a narrowed lumen (rhonchi), or when the pleura loses its normal lubrication (friction rub). See Table 13-13 for a description of these sounds. Rales and rhonchi

TABLE 13-13 ADVENTITIOUS LUNG SOUNDS

Type	Cause	Description
Rales (Crackling or bubbling sound produced by air flow through secretions.)		
Fine	Watery secretions in the alveoli.	Fine, minute crackling. It is a sound similar to that of several strands of hair being held up to your ear and rubbed together through your fingers. Heard at end of inspiration.
Medium	Watery secretions extending from the alveoli pathway up the tracheobronchial tree.	A loose, crackling sound heard in mid and late inspiration.
Coarse	Secretions in the trachea and bronchi.	Low, rumbling bubbling sound on early inspiration and part of expiration.
Rhonchi (Sounds heard as air passes through the trachea, the bronchi, or bronchioles in which the lumen has been narrowed, irrespective of cause.)		
Sibilant	(1) Anatomical narrowing of trachea, bronchi, or bronchioles or (2) bronchospasm	High-pitched wheezing or musical sound primarily in mid or late expiration but may be present throughout respiratory cycle.
Sonorous	Originates in larger bronchi and the trachea. The flow of air continuously vibrates thick secretions along the airway.	Loud low-pitched gurgling sound throughout the respiratory cycle that can be cleared by coughing or suctioning.
Friction rub	Inflamed pleural surface with diminished lubricating fluid.	A grating sound, as if leather is being bent or rubbed together. It is heard near the end of inspiration at the lower anterolateral chest wall.

can be heard while auscultating the chest anteriorly and posteriorly as described. A pleural friction rub is best heard by placing the stethoscope at the base of the lungs on each lateral chest wall. A description of the sound and whether it occurs during inspiration, expiration or both should be noted. Children having adventitious breath sounds should have further evaluation.

Decreased or absent breath sounds are abnormal. Breath sounds are absent or decreased when the flow of air is obstructed and the sound of air exchange is not transmitted. Obstruction of air flow can be caused by a foreign object or mucus, air in the lung cavity (pneumothorax) or fluid (pleural effusion). To avoid overlooking these conditions, the chest should be symmetrically auscultated from side to side with careful comparison of breath sounds from one side to the other.

Breasts

Breasts should be examined in both males and females. During inspection of the anterior chest, the nipples should be checked for color, spacing, placement, symmetry, fissures, inversions, secretions, scaling and lumps. Breast bud formation usually begins around 10 to 14 years of age (see Table 57–2). One breast may begin to develop before the other and is often tender. Precocious breast development may be normal but can also indicate diethyl stilbesterol ingestion or ovarian tumors. The breasts are inspected and palpated for redness, heat, tenderness and masses. For palpation the child or adolescent lies in a supine position with the right arm extended above the head. The examiner lightly palpates the right breast with her fingertips in a rolling circular motion. Examination is begun at the center of the nipple and progresses in a counterclockwise manner in concentric rings until the entire breast and area surrounding the breast has been examined. (Alternate methods of examination may be used as long as the method is systematic to ensure complete assessment of breast tissue.) The axilla is also palpated for swelling, tenderness and lymphadenopathy. The procedure is repeated on the left breast.

Breasts should be examined with the child in various positions: (1) in a sitting position with hands raised above the head, (2) leaning forward, and (3) with the hands resting on the hips pressing the elbows back and toward the midline. Inspection for dimpling, asymmetry, masses, discharge and color takes place in each of these positions.

The male breast should also be inspected and palpated for abnormalities. Any increased size should be noted, since it may be indicative of endocrine problems. The adolescent male also normally has some breast development during puberty.

Heart

Inspection and palpation of the precordium is done to detect precordial bulging, thrills, lifts or heaves, precordial friction rubs, and the apical impulse known as the point of maximal impulse (PMI). The PMI is palpable in the fourth or fifth intercostal space at or just medial to the midclavicular line and may be visible in thin children.

A lift or heave is seen and felt when the cardiac action is abnormally forceful, actually lifting the ribs and sternum with each heart beat. A thrill is a palpable heart murmur. It is a vibration and is often described as similar to the feel of a cat purring. Other observations related to the examination of the heart include respiratory distress, finger clubbing, edema and cyanosis.

Percussion of the heart may be done using the direct or indirect percussion technique. Percussion of the heart outlines its size and shape. The heart normally is in the shape of an inverted triangle with the right border extending along the right side of the sternum from the second to the fifth ribs and from the right sternum (fifth rib) to the left midclavicular line at the fifth rib. The hypotenuse of the triangle is extended from the right sternum at the second rib to the left midclavicular line at the fifth rib (see Fig. 13–19). The heart in an infant lies slightly more horizontally with the apex to the left of the nipple line. Percussion dullness that is located other than in the expected area could mean cardiac enlargement or heart displacement.

Auscultation is the most informative method of assessing cardiac function. It is used to evaluate the quality, rate and rhythm of the heart and to detect abnormal heart sounds. There are five areas of the heart to examine when evaluating function (Fig. 13–19): (1) aortic, (2) pulmonic, (3) Erb's point, (4) apical (mitral), and (5) tricuspid (epigastric). First, the apical pulse

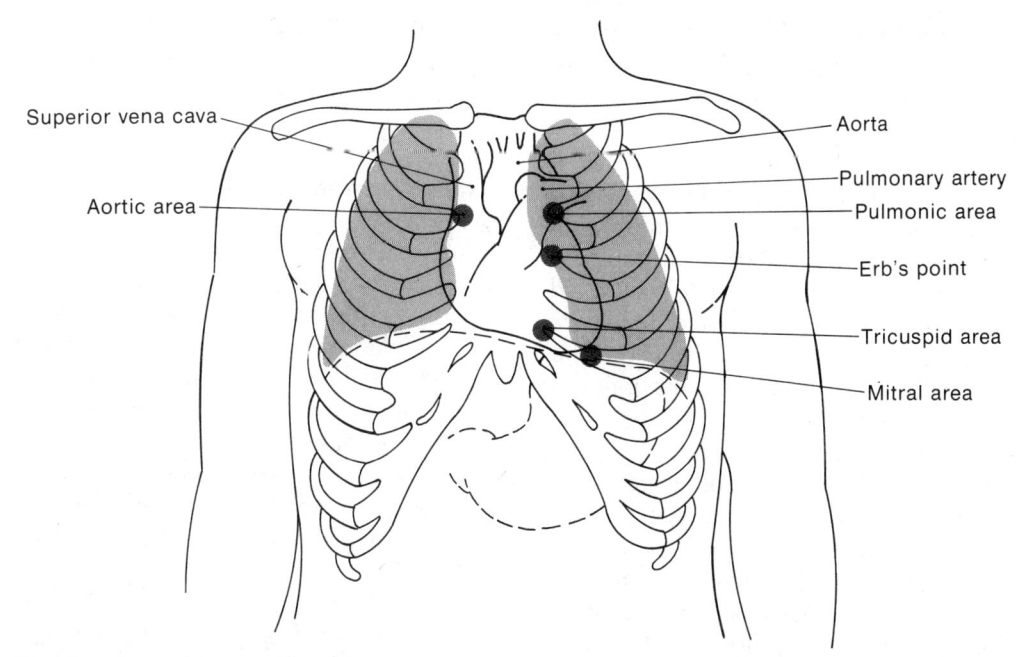

Figure 13-19 Position of heart in chest. The five areas of heart sounds are marked with black dots.

rate, intensity and rhythm are noted. Rapid or decreased pulse rates may be normal or may indicate pathology. The heart is auscultated with both the bell and the diaphragm of the stethoscope. The bell picks up low frequencies and the diaphragm picks up high frequencies. The heart may be examined with the child in several positions: standing, sitting, leaning forward, supine and left-lateral lying position. The heart should also be auscultated after exercise. For routine examination the child may be examined supine or on a parent's lap. The examiner begins by evaluating heart sounds for quality, intensity, rhythm, and unusual sounds.

The first heart sound, S_1, indicates the systolic portion of the cardiac cycle; it is the "lub" of the "lub-dub." This sound is normally louder at the apex and is long and low-pitched. The first heart sound is synchronous with the carotid pulse. It is caused by a closing of the mitral and tricuspid valves. The second heart sound, S_2, is louder than S_1 at the base (aortic and pulmonic areas). This second sound reflects the diastole of the cardiac cycle and is the "dub" of the "lub-dub." It is shorter and higher in pitch than S_1 and is caused by closure of the semilunar valves (aortic and pulmonic valves). A third heart sound, S_3, is occasionally heard due to blood rushing through the mitral valve and rapidly filling ventricle. The third heart sound is low-pitched and occurs early in diastole. It is heard best at the apex. It can be normal in a child but is almost always abnormal in an adult.

A fourth heart sound, S_4, may exist but is seldom normal. It is caused by an audible atrial contraction at the end of diastole and is heard best at the apex. The heart sounds are evaluated for quality, intensity and splitting. The first and second sounds should be clear and distinct. Any muffling or indistinctness may indicate pathology. Intensity refers to where each heart sound is heard best. S_1 should be heard best at the apex and S_2 heard best at the base of the heart. If this is not the case the heart should be evaluated in more depth for a possible abnormality.

The rhythm of the heart is evaluated by listening carefully to determine if any irregularity exists. If an irregular rhythm is present, the examiner should attempt to determine a specific pattern. Sinus arrhythmia is a common irregularity in which the heart speeds up with inspiration and slows down with expiration. It should disappear when the child holds his breath and is considered normal in children.

One classification of unusual or abnormal heart sounds is heart murmurs. Review the six heart murmur classifications in Chapter 24 in the section on heart anomalies. A heart murmur originates within the heart or its great vessels. The flow of blood is altered, causing an abnormal sound that is audible on auscultation. Murmurs are usually caused by (1) flow across a partial obstruction, (2) flow across an irregularity within the heart or vessel, (3) an increased amount of blood flow through a normal passageway, (4) flow from a normal passageway into a dilated area, (5) regurgitation (backward) flow through a valve or defect and (6) flow of blood from a high pressure area through an abnormal passageway. The relationship of murmurs to other events should be noted. Murmurs may disappear or be accentuated by activity or crying or may vary with respirations. There are two types of murmurs: innocent and organic. Differentiation of the two types requires evaluation by a physician.

Finally, the cardiovascular pulses are palpated for presence or absence, and regularity and intensity. (See Table 13-5 for normal pulse rates.) The carotid, radial, femoral, popliteal, and pedal pulses are palpated and compared. The femoral and radial pulses are frequently palpated simultaneously to determine if a lag exists between the two. A femoral-radial lag or absent or diminished femoral pulses are characteristic of coarctation (stricture or contraction) of the aorta. Temperature and color of the extremities should also be assessed. Cold, pale or cyanotic extremities suggests cardiac disease or peripheral vascular disease.

A thorough examination of the heart should include blood pressure (see Figure 13-3 for normal values) and observation of the child before and after exercise or eating. Any color changes or fatigue should be noted.

Abdomen

Examination of the abdomen requires inspection, auscultation, palpation and percussion of its four major divisions: right upper quadrant, right lower quadrant, left upper quadrant and left lower quadrant. It is essential that the child be quiet and cooperative if the examiner is to evaluate this system thoroughly. The abdominal muscles are relaxed by flexing the child's knees slightly. The infant can be distracted or be given a bottle to quiet him and relax the abdominal wall for examination. Before beginning the examination the examiner should warm her hands.

Inspection allows the examiner to determine shape and contour, movement and peristalsis, distention, bulges and diastasis rectus (splitting of the rectus muscle). Children normally have a pot belly that should begin to disappear by 4 or 5 years of age. The abdominal wall moves with respiration until 6 or 7 years of age; failure to do so may indicate appendicitis, peritonitis, paralytic ileus, diaphragmatic paralysis or a large amount of air in the abdominal cavity.

Peristalsis is not generally visible in children. Visible peristaltic waves usually indicate an obstruction in the gastrointestinal tract. Pyloric stenosis is suspected if peristaltic waves occur from left to right.

Abdominal distention may be a sign of pregnancy, feces, organomegaly (enlargement of an organ), ovarian cysts, ascites, or air in the abdominal cavity. The abdomen should be inspected from the front and the sides to determine the extent of the distention; it is then palpated and percussed. Diastasis (splitting) of the rectus muscle is a protrusion in the midline from the xyphoid to the umbilicus and can be inspected and palpated. The split can be part way or the entire length between these two points. The width of the bulging can be one-half to two inches and still be considered normal. However, it may also be caused by a congenital weakness of the muscle or a chronically distended abdomen. Close follow-up with measurement of the length and width should be done.

The umbilicus is inspected closely for bulging, color and discharge. A bluish umbilicus can be caused by intra-abdominal hemorrhage. In the newborn the umbilical cord should be inspected for bleeding or signs of infection and for the presence of one vein and two arteries. Protrusion of the umbilicus usually indicates a hernia. Palpation of the hernia should be done to confirm a hernia after auscultation of the abdomen has been completed. Hernias are seen normally in children up to the age of 2 or 3 years. They persist longer in black children, being seen until 7 or 8 years of age. Drainage from the umbilicus should be checked for color, odor, amount and consistency. If infection is suspected the fluid may be cultured. In addition to infection, a patent urachus* or a urachal cyst may be the cause of umbilical drainage.

Finally, the abdomen is inspected for distended veins and obvious pulsations. The skin is examined thoroughly as discussed earlier in this chapter.

Auscultation follows inspection of the abdomen so that peristaltic sounds are not disturbed

---

*A canal in the fetus connecting the bladder apex and the umbilicus.

by palpation or percussion. The diaphragm of the stethoscope is placed firmly over the abdomen and the examiner listens in all four quadrants for peristaltic sounds. These are metallic, short, tinkling sounds. Normally an average of 15 to 34 bowel sounds are audible per minute. High-pitched, frequent or hyperactive sounds are heard in children with diarrhea, gastroenteritis and intestinal obstruction. Absence of peristaltic sounds may indicate a paralytic ileus or early peritonitis. Peristaltic sounds are very irregular and before concluding that they are absent, the examiner must listen for at least 5 to 10 minutes.

Vascular sounds are also auscultated for in the abdominal examination. A venous hum may indicate abnormality of the umbilical vein or portal obstruction. Murmurs may indicate coarctation of the aorta or a renal artery defect. Friction rubs and bruits heard in the abdomen are also abnormal and should be referred.

Percussion follows auscultation and is done with the child supine, either on his parent's lap or on the examination table. The examiner begins with the child's thorax at the left midaxillary line and percusses downward. The spleen is generally percussed as well, between the ninth and eleventh interspaces in the left midaxillary line. The diaphragm is percussed above the spleen. Occasionally tympany under the left diaphragm is percussed if a stomach bubble is present.

This procedure is then repeated in the right side where liver dullness is expected at the sixth interspace anteriorly and ninth rib posteriorly. The lower edge of the liver should be percussed at the right costal margin or occasionally 2 to 3 cm lower. With respiration the liver moves about two finger breadths. Asking the child to take a deep breath and hold it facilitates percussion. The remainder of the abdomen is then percussed. Dullness encountered anywhere other than where it can be expected may indicate feces or a mass. Percussion should be used to outline the border and size of underlying structures. Tympany usually indicates air in the stomach and may be more pronounced in children who swallow air excessively or who have a gastrointestinal obstruction.

The final method of examination is palpation. Light palpation begins the examination and should proceed in a systematic fashion. The examiner uses her fingertips, gently and superficially examining the lower left quandrant, then the left upper, right upper and right lower quandrants in that order. Initially, the examiner notes if the abdomen is soft or hard, tender or distended.

After completing light palpation, the examiner proceeds in the same systematic way using deep palpation. Deep palpation is accomplished best during deep inspiration and deep expiration. The examiner may wish to place one hand on top of the other to provide firmer pressure for this examination technique. Deep palpation is useful in discovering masses, tenderness, deep vessels and palpable organs. A pyloric tumor would be palpable at the right costal margin just to the right of the midline of the abdomen. Wilms' tumor may be palpated adjacent to the vertebral column in the kidney area.

The liver, if palpable, is felt for size, consistency and tenderness. Any liver palpable below the costal margin should be percussed for size and evaluated for possible pathology.

The spleen can be palpated more easily if the child lies on his right side and takes a deep breath. The examiner lightly places her fingers just below the left costal margin at the midaxillary line and palpates the tip of the spleen. If more than the tip of the spleen is palpable it is considered abnormal. In some children, the tip is not normally palpated.

To palpate the kidneys, the examiner must use very deep palpation. They are adjacent to the vertebral column and will descend slightly with inspiration. The lower pole may be felt particularly on the right, since this kidney is lower than the left. The child's flank should be firmly supported with the examiner's left hand while the right hand palpates the abdomen deeply. Normal kidneys are rarely palpable except in the newborn immediately following birth. However, palpation of the kidneys should always be attempted, since enlargement indicates significant pathology.

It is also possible to palpate the bladder in early childhood for possible distention. The intestines may also be palpable and, in intussusception, a sausage-shaped tumor may be found. Palpation is not complete until the child is checked closely for hernias. Umbilical hernias may be located and inspected with palpation. The examiner places a finger into the umbilicus and palpates for protrusion of intestines. Hernias vary in size and should be measured at each visit to see if they are resolving. Occasionally epigastric hernias are palpated as

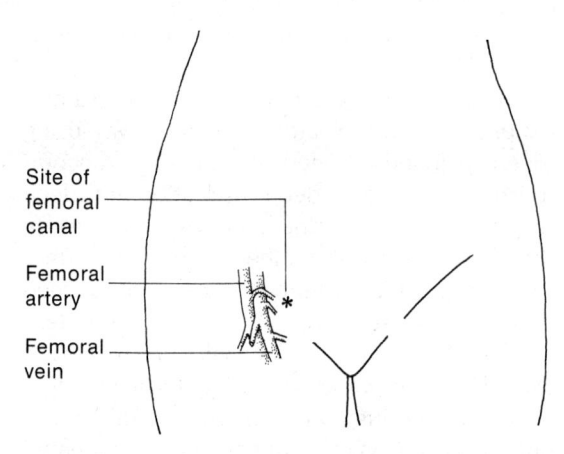

Figure 13-20 The femoral area in the female. A femoral hernia, more common in females, is felt or seen as a small bulge at the site of the femoral canal.

a small nodule protruding between the fibers of the linea alba and are often felt best when the child is standing. Examination for a femoral hernia is done by placing the right index finger on the child's femoral artery. The next finger then lies atop of the femoral vein and the ring finger is directly over the femoral canal. The standing child is then asked to strain as if having a bowel movement or to cough in order to elicit the hernia if one exists. The femoral hernia is felt or seen as a small bulge that results from a weakness in the musculature at the femoral canal. The child should be standing for this procedure (see Fig. 13-20). A femoral hernia is more common in females. Technique for palpating inguinal hernias is described with assessment of male genitalia.

Female Genitalia

Every child should have a thorough examination of the genitalia. The examiner can complete this portion of the examination last if the child or adolescent is shy or embarrassed. This should be accomplished in a matter-of-fact manner that will put the child at ease. The female genitalia are inspected and palpated with gloved hands for presence or absence and symmetry of the external structures (Fig. 13-21). Evidence of edema, color changes, moisture, lesions and masses should be identified and recorded. The examiner begins by inspecting the mons pubis for any masses or abnormality. The presence or absence of pubic hair should be noted. Hair should be described according to color, quantity, texture and distribution. It should also be inspected for lice.

The vulva is inspected for erythema, swelling, masses and varicosities. The labia minora are normally quite large in the infant and may protrude from behind the labia majora. Swelling of the vulva could be a sign of sexual molestation, infection, a foreign body, trauma or lymphedema.

Next Bartholin's and Skein's glands are inspected and palpated. They are not normally seen or felt. If visible or palpable, enlargement exists and is due to infection, usually gonorrhea.

The clitoris is inspected carefully to determine if its size is abnormal. It may normally be large in the newborn, while a hypertrophied clitoris in an older child may indicate labioscrotal fusion or pseudohermaphroditism. Because of its sensitivity the clitoris should not be palpated unless there is a specific reason for doing so.

The vestibule is inspected and palpated for lesions and masses. There will be few abnormal findings here until the child is older, when the examiner may find ulcerated venereal lesions. Important also is the examination of the urethral meatal opening for inflammation, erythema and discharge. Location of the meatus should be noted for possible epispadias. Finally, the vaginal opening and hymen are checked for congenital absence of the vagina or for imperforate hymen. Newborns may have a small amount of bloody vaginal discharge until one month of age. Foul-smelling discharge may be due to infection, the presence of a foreign body or pinworms.

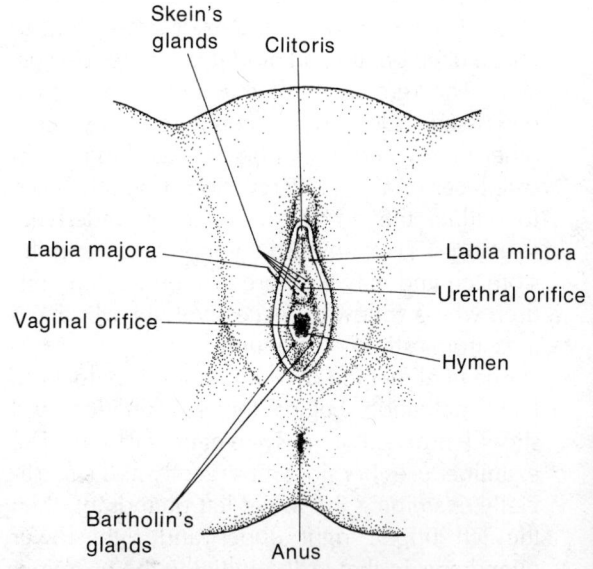

Figure 13-21 The female genitalia.

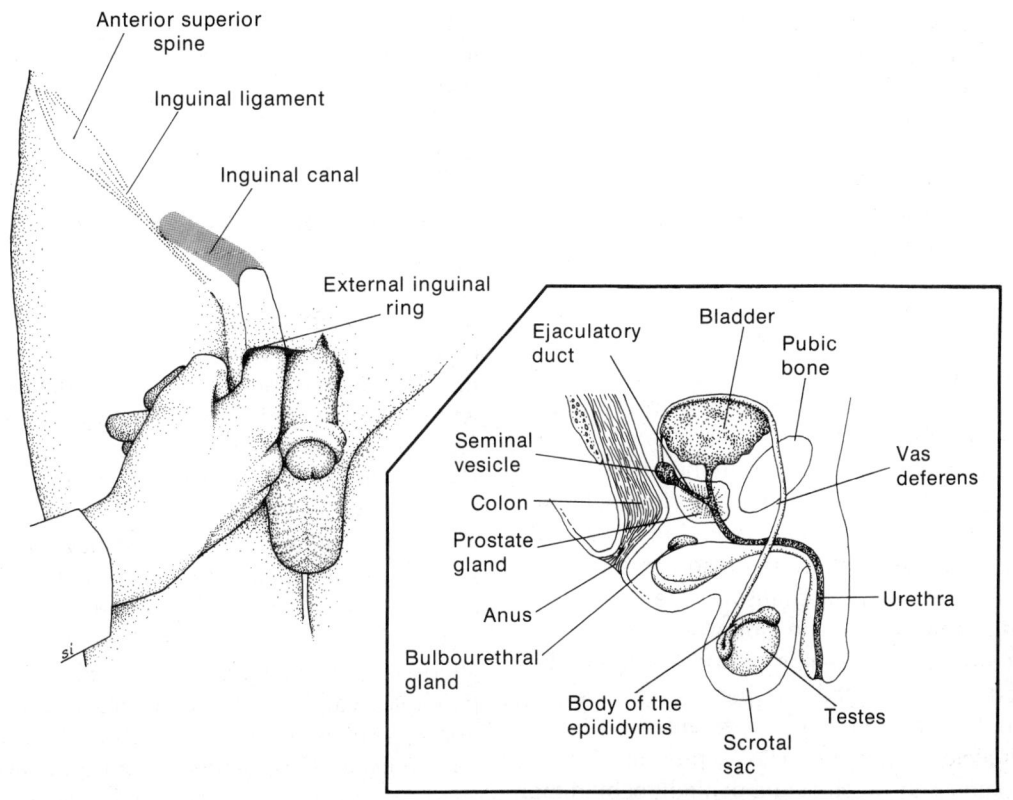

Figure 13-22 The male genitalia. The inguinal canal is palpated to check for a possible hernia. In a younger child, the little (fifth) finger would be used.

Digital and speculum examination is seldom done until puberty unless suggestion of pathology exists. The adolescent girl seeking oral or intrauterine contraception, and the girl whose mother received diethylstilbestrol (DES) during pregnancy may also need periodic internal and bimanual examination. This examination can be very traumatic for a young girl and should be carried out by a skilled practitioner who has explained the procedure in detail. Regional lymph nodes and femoral pulses may be examined after the genitalia examination.

Male Genitalia

The male genitalia (Fig. 13-22) are also examined thoroughly in a matter-of-fact and efficient manner. The examiner should begin by first inspecting and palpating the penis for size and consistency. An enlarged penis may be due to precocious puberty, central nervous system lesions or testicular tumors. It should be noted if the child has been circumcised and if not whether the foreskin is retractable or if adhesions are present. Even circumcised males may develop adhesions due to the adherence of part of the foreskin to the glans. In the uncircumcised newborn, the foreskin remains tight for the first three to four months and gradually becomes freely retractable by the age of 2 years.

The meatal opening is inspected for its size, position and any discharge. Hypospadias or epispadias is present if the opening is either on the ventral or dorsal surface of the glans penis. These conditions require medical evaluation. A pinpoint meatal opening may cause urinary obstruction. If possible, the child's urinary stream should be observed or information obtained from the child or parent during the history. A urinary stream that dribbles or is not a steady, strong stream may be seen with meatal stenosis or other anomalies. The glans is also inspected for lesions, swelling or venereal warts.

The shaft of the penis is examined for size, varicosities and masses. The infantile penis is approximately 2 to 3 cm long when nonerect. Any penis smaller than this should be examined for the possibility of hermaphroditism. During puberty, the penile shaft lengthens and widens. Pubic hair, if present, should be described in the

HEALTH APPRAISAL

same way as the female pubic hair. Assessment of pubertal changes is very important in both the male and the female child. See Chapter 57 for illustrations and discussion of staging in secondary sex characteristic development.

The scrotum is inspected and palpated for edema, inflammation, masses and color. The rugae are inspected also. A smooth, shiny scrotum without rugae may indicate undescended testes (cryptorchidism), which requires referral. The scrotal sac should be palpated for the presence or absence of testes and for their size and any masses or tenderness. To keep the testes from becoming stimulated and retracting into the inguinal canal, the examiner places her fingers on the inguinal canals, occluding them. Retractile testes may not be found in the scrotal sac during examination; this disorder is referred to as pseudocryptorchidism. The spermatic cord can be palpated and followed to the testes. Any swelling, thickening or nodules should be noted. An enlarged or pendulous scrotum should be transilluminated to determine if a hydrocele, hernia or mass is present. This is accomplished by placing a penlight behind the scrotal sac. Illumination occurs in hydrocele but not in hernia or masses. Swelling and discoloration of the scrotum that has developed suddenly may be a sign of spermatic cord torsion, which requires immediate attention by a physician.

The inguinal canal is palpated to rule out a possible hernia (see Fig. 13–22). A hernia of this type is indirect and may be congenital. It is seen in males nine times more frequently than in females and occurs more commonly on the right side. The examiner should place her finger (in a young child, the fifth [little] finger should be used) in the scrotal sac and gently approach the inguinal canal, following the spermatic cord. The finger tip should not be able to enter the canal through the external inguinal ring unless the ring is abnormally dilated. Weakness of the ring may signal a potential hernia. This weakness is tested by having the child cough or strain. The external ring is palpated for tone. The examiner also palpates the inguinal canal, noting by pressing through the side of the abdominal wall if any abdominal contents can be felt pressing down into the inguinal canal or if a bulge is palpable. These findings would indicate a hernia. Regional lymph nodes and the femoral canal and pulses should also be examined at this time if they were not during the abdominal survey.

Rectum and Anus

The rectum is inspected for fissures, prolapse, hemorrhoids, polyps, inflammation, rashes and lesions. Patency should also be determined, both with data from the history and rectal examination. Signs of scratching or irritation may be due to pinworms. A rectal examination will determine sphincter tone and existence of an imperforate anus. This is accomplished by inserting the little finger (gloved and lubricated) slowly into the rectum. Sphincter tone and the character, amount and consistency of feces should be identified. Presence of masses, tenderness or a lack of sensation should be investigated further. Fecal masses are present in children with mental deficiency, anal stenosis, psychological difficulties and chronic constipation. Complete absence of feces in the rectum may indicate ileus, peritonitis or obstruction.

Musculoskeletal System

Extremities A general inspection of the skeletal system begins with observation of the child as he walks into the examination room. The child is also observed during his play activities and while performing tasks such as undressing. Symmetry of movement, position, general alignment, deformities, gait, extra digits and unusual posture are observable while the child is unaware of the examiner's scrutiny.

During the actual examination soft tissues and muscles are inspected and palpated for symmetry, contractures, erythema, swelling and tenderness. Muscles are inspected and palpated for symmetry, mass, tone, strength and paralysis. The bones are palpated for shape, outline, thickening, abnormal prominence or indentation. The examiner should determine if the temperature of one extremity seems higher than the others. All joints should be inspected and palpated for swelling, redness or tenderness and should be actively and passively placed through full range of motion. The upper extremities are compared for equality of strength, length, and symmetry of movement.

Having the child (simultaneously with the right and left hands) squeeze the examiner's fingers allows the examiner to evaluate strength and symmetry.

The examiner palpates the clavicles for crepitus or tenderness that would indicate a fracture. The arms are examined carefully for subluxation and for an increased carrying angle; the child is instructed to hold his arms straight out at his sides at a right angle with his palms facing forward. The arms should form a smooth, continuous line of approximately 180 degrees. If the lower arm is bent upward forming an angle of less than 180 degrees, the child has an increased carrying angle. This may be normal but is also associated with gonadal dysgenesis.

The hands are checked closely for extra digits (polydactyly), webbing, missing digits (syndactyly) or abnormally short or long digits. Creases of the hands are inspected closely. Evidence of a simian crease may indicate Down's syndrome but is also normal in some individuals. The knuckles should be inspected for their presence and any anomalies. Examination of the upper extremities should incorporate examination of the regional lymph nodes, skin, nails, hair and pulses.

The examiner also applies pressure to the arms of the child while they are raised above his head, out to his sides and out in front of him. The child should be able to maintain his arms in these positions while the examiner tries to force the arms in the opposite direction. The child can also flex his arms close to his trunk while the examiner tries to straighten them. This process is reversed and the child extends his arms in front of him at a 180 degree angle while the examiner exerts pressure to prevent the child from flexing his arms.

The lower extremities are observed for shape. Genu varum (bowleggedness) is present when the medial malleoli (bony protuberances on either side of the ankle) are touching and the knees are more than 1 inch apart. A child has genu valgum (knock-knees) if the knees are together and the medial malleoli are more than 1 inch apart. Genu valgum is normally seen in the child between 2½ to 3½ years of age, while genu varum is often seen in a child until after he has been walking for a year. The tibia should be inspected and palpated for torsion. See Chapter 32 for torsional assessment technique.

The lower extremities are also checked for equality in length. The child should lie supine and then extend his legs. The four malleoli should be in the same plane. The child may also be requested to stand while the examiner inspects the patellae and the crease in the popliteal fossas for symmetry. This should be done with the child standing straight with the knees and feet together. The examiner can place her hands on each side of the pelvic rim and, while at eye level with the pelvis, examine for equality.

Strength of the legs is checked in much the same way as in the upper extremities. The legs are flexed and the examiner tries to straighten them. This process is reversed by having the legs extended while the examiner exerts pressure in trying to prevent the child from flexing his legs.

Range of motion of the hips, knees, ankles and toes should also be checked. It is particularly important to evaluate hip rotation in the infant to rule out congenital hip dislocation. See Chapter 24 for detailed assessment for congenitally dislocated hip.

The feet are inspected for equality of size and shape and for position. If possible the feet should be examined with the child standing. The arch is examined for unusual height or a flat arch. Children have a fat pad under their medial arch until they have been walking one to two years, which gives them the appearance of having flat feet. The examiner should be able to fit at least one finger under the medial arch. An arch that allows more than one finger is high. An arch that does not allow at least one finger is considered flat. The child can also wet his feet and stand on a piece of newspaper; this will outline his arches.

The position of the feet should be noted. Pes valgus (toeing out) and pes varus (toeing in) refer to the entire foot turning either in or out and are caused by structural anomalies. Metatarsus varus, and valgus on the other hand, is turning in or out of the forefoot only. The heel is straight and midline, while the forefoot turns inward or outward. These conditions should be referred for further consideration. The heels of the child's feet should be closely observed from the posterior angle. The child should stand while the examiner inspects the heel cords for deviation. Slight medial slanting before the age of 5 or 6 is normal, but after this age may be an indication of pronation. A child who has pronated feet looks as if he is standing on the inner aspects of his heel and arch. The medial malleoli are frequently lower than the lateral malleoli.

Finally, the child is observed for gait, balance and stance. Children should walk, run and skip while the examiner observes. The beginning walker (between 12 to 18 months) generally demonstrates a broad-based gait with poor balance. By 3 or 4 years, the gait is narrow-based and the child should be able to maintain his balance on one foot for several seconds. Most children are able to skip fairly well by 5 or 6 years of age.

The child's gait and stance should be inspected from all points of view, particularly side view. The phases of the gait should be inspected for symmetry, coordination, and position of arms and legs. Any deviation should be identified in relation to the appropriate phase and stage.

Spine

At birth the spinal curve is in the shape of a C rather than the double S seen in later life. The curves present in the neonate are the thoracic and pelvic curves. Around 3 to 4 months of age the cervical curve develops. This is the time when the child begins to hold his head upright. The lumbar curve appears between 12 to 18 months when the child begins to walk. The four curves then are the cervical, which is a convex line, the thoracic, which is concave, the lumbar, which is ventrally convex, and finally the pelvic curve, which is a concave curve directed caudally and ventrally. The cervical and lumbar curves are secondary or compensatory curves because they do not develop until after birth. It is important to remember this evolution of spinal curvatures when examining the spine in a young child.

Inspection and palpation of the spine should be done with the child standing if possible. The examiner checks for symmetry of bony landmarks, alignment and for other skin manifestations such as dimples, cysts and tufts of hair. The spine is inspected and palpated for the presence or absence of each spinous process and for masses and tenderness. The child's posture is examined from the front, back, side and when the child is in a flexed position. A child with an exaggerated concave curve in the thoracic region has kyphosis. On the other hand, an exaggerated convex curve on the lumbar region indicates lordosis, which may be normal in some children. Poor posture, commonly seen in adolescence, may appear as kyphosis but is usually not a permanent skeletal deformity. Scoliosis is a lateral curvature of the spine that requires medical follow-up. Positional evaluation of scoliosis is described in Chapter 60.

Neurological

A complete neurological examination involves all body parts. The examiner should be familiar with the total assessment of the neurological system in order to integrate it into the physical examination as well as to perform a more extensive evaluation when indicated. The neurological examination involves testing of function within six major areas: the cerebrum, the cranial nerves, the cerebellum, the motor system, the sensory system and reflex action.

The basic neurological examination begins with assessment of general cerebral functions. Developmental tests and interviews with the child are important aids in evaluating this area. The child's state of consciousness, intellectual performance and mood give the examiner a general impression of his cerebral function. The examiner should note closely the child's posture, state of cleanliness, facial expressions, gestures, movements, hypo or hyperactivity, speech and distractibility. The older child can be examined for orientation to time, place and person. Memory is also a part of general cerebral function; immediate, recent and remote memory should be evaluated. Immediate recall refers to the retention of an idea or thought for a brief time; this is tested by having a child repeat numbers or sounds. A child of 4 years can usually repeat 3 numbers (4, 3, 1), while a child of 5 years can repeat 4 numbers and a child of 6 can usually repeat 5 numbers correctly. Memory of an idea that lasts slightly longer is recent memory. The child can be shown an object and told that he will be asked later to tell what the object was. The examiner can also tell the child a "secret word" that he can be asked to repeat later. The examiner usually waits 5 minutes before asking the child to recall the object or secret word. Remote memory refers to memory for longer periods of time. The child can be asked what he had for dinner last night or an older child can be asked his birthday or his address.

Evaluation of specific cerebral function includes testing three functional areas: cortical sensory interpretation, cortical motor integration and language. Cortical sensory interpretation is the ability to recognize objects through the rise of senses. Visual sensory interpretation can be accomplished by playing the "find it" game. The examiner places several objects on a table and then instructs the child to hand her the objects as they are named. The child should not name the object himself since this would involve expressive language skills as well. Tactile sensory integration (stereognosis) is done by placing one of several objects in the child's hands and having him identify the object. This should be done with the child's eyes closed. Familiar objects such as coins, bottle caps and buttons should be used. Graphesthesia is the ability to identify shapes traced in the palm or on the back of the hand. School-age children can usually identify the numbers 0, 1, 3, 7 and 8. Younger children usually identify geometric forms, parallel lines or crossing lines. If the child cannot identify the shape, the examiner does the tracing twice and asks the child if the two are the same or are different.

Evaluation of the auditory sense is done by having the child listen with his eyes closed and identify different common sounds such as a whistle or a hand clap.

Body part perception, or somatic sensory perception, can be accomplished by observing the child's response to tactile stimuli. The child's eyes are occluded and his hands placed in front of him. The examiner touches one or two fingers and the child is asked to show which finger(s) were touched. By the age of 6 children may still occasionally confuse the third and fourth fingers, especially if two fingers were touched.

Kinesthesia (the ability to perceive direction of movement or weight) is evaluated in children over 5 by manipulating the child's finger to either an up or down position. The child's eyes should be closed for this test and the examiner should be careful to handle only the sides of the child's fingers so that the weight of her fingers does not give the child a clue to the direction. Texture discrimination can be done by having the child feel different textured items with his eyes closed and tell whether they are smooth or rough. Visual motor integration and cortical motor integration (ability to perform purposeful acts) can be tested by having the child copy various designs which are first drawn or shown to him. The child 3 years of age can usually draw a circle. By the age of 4 years he can draw a square, and by 5 years the child can draw a triangle. Children 6 years of age can draw a diamond and 7-year-olds can usually draw a British flag design.

The last specific cerebral function to be tested is the child's ability to communicate and understand both spoken and written language (receptive and expressive). Screening tests for articulation and speech may be used and are described later in this chapter. Having the child repeat numbers or nonsense syllables, testing his ability to follow directions, and testing his language discrimination are other ways of evaluating language ability. An inability to repeat may indicate that the child has poor ability to perceive what he hears. Discrimination is evaluated by saying two similar words such as fright and flight. The child is then asked if they are the same or different words.

The infant's cry may also be neurologically significant. A high-pitched shrill cry may indicate intracranial damage, while a high-pitched screeching cry may indicate cri-du-chat syndrome (a syndrome of genetic congenital defects), especially if associated with microcephaly, low-set ears or micrognathia (abnormally small jaw).

Evaluation of the 12 pairs of cranial nerves is easily integrated into the nurse's physical examination. Children and adolescents enjoy the active participation required for testing cranial nerve functions. Difficulty is encountered in the assessment of cranial nerves in infants and young children owing to the child's developmental level; however, cranial nerves are tested if feasible. Specific nerves and procedures for testing are indicated in Table 13–14.

Tests for cerebellar function involve primarily assessment of balance and coordination. Developmental screening tools provide an accessible, standardized method of assessing fine and gross motor balance and coordination skills. General cerebellar examination begins with observing the child's gait, watching him walk heel to toe, and checking his ability to dress and undress, button, stack blocks, throw and kick and so forth. Balance is specifically evaluated by observation of gait and having the child stand with his eyes open and then closed. This test of sensory equilibrium (Romberg test) is positive if the child begins to fall.

Examples of coordination tests are finger-to-nose, heel-to-shin, and alternating motion. For

TABLE 13-14 ASSESSMENT OF CRANIAL NERVES

Nerve	Distribution	Test for Function
I Olfactory (S)*	Olfactory nerve, mucous membrane of nasal and turbinates	With eyes closed child is asked to identify familiar odors such as peanut butter, orange, peppermint. Test each nostril separately.
II Optic (S)	Optic nerve, retinal rods and cones	Check visual acuity, peripheral vision, color vision, perception of light in infants, fundoscopic examination for normal optic disc.
III Oculomotor (M)*	Muscles of the eye (superior rectus, inferior rectus, medial rectus, inferior oblique)	Have child follow an object or light with his eyes (EOM)* while head remains stationary. Check symmetry of corneal light reflex. Check for nystagmus (direction elicited vertical, horizontal, rotary). Check cover-uncover test.
	Muscles of iris and ciliary body	Reaction of pupils to light, both direct and consensual, accommodation.
	Levator palpebral muscle	Check for symmetrical movement of upper eyelids. Note ptosis.
IV Trochlear (M)	Muscles of eye (superior oblique)	Check the range of motion of the eyes downward (EOM). Check for nystagmus.
V Trigeminal (M, S)	Muscles of mastication (M)	Have child clamp his jaws and palpate jaw muscles and temporal muscles for strength and symmetry. Ask child to move lower jaw from side to side against resistance of the examiner's hand.
	Sensory innervation of face (S)	Test child for sensation using a wisp of cotton; warm and cold water in test tubes; a sharp object on the forehead, cheeks, jaw. Check corneal reflex by touching a wisp of cotton to each cornea. The normal response is blink.
VI Abducens (M)	Muscles of eye (lateral rectus)	Have child look to each side (EOM).
VII Facial (M, S)	Muscles for facial expression (M)	Have child make faces: look at the ceiling, frown, wrinkle forehead, blow out cheeks, smile. Check for strength, asymmetry, paralysis.
	Sense of taste on anterior 2/3 of tongue. Sensation of external ear canal, lacrimal, submaxillary and sublingual glands	Have child identify salt, sugar, bitter (flavoring extract) and sour substances by placing substance on anterior sides of tongue. Keep tongue out until substance is identified. Rinse mouth between substances.
VIII Acoustic (S)	Equilibrium (vestibular nerve)	Note equilibrium or presence of vertigo (Romberg sign).
	Auditory acuity (cochlear nerve)	Test hearing. Use a tuning fork for the Weber and Rinne tests. Test by whispering and use of a watch.

Table continued on opposite page

TABLE 13-14 ASSESSMENT OF CRANIAL NERVES (*Continued*)

Nerve	Distribution	Test for Function
IX Glossopharyngeal (M, S)	Pharynx, tongue (M)	Check elevation of palate with "ah" or crying. Check for movement and symmetry. Stimulate posterior pharynx for gag reflex.
	Sense of taste posterior third of the tongue (S)	Test sense of taste on posterior portion of tongue.
X Vagus (M, S)	Mucous membrane of pharynx, larynx, bronchi, lungs, heart, esophagus, stomach, kidneys	Note same as for glossopharyngeal. Note any hoarseness, stridor. Check uvula for midline position, movement with phonation. Stimulate each side of uvula on each side with tongue depressor — should rise and deviate to stimulated side. Check gag reflex. Observe ability to swallow.
	Posterior surface of external ear, external auditory meatus	
XI Accessory (M)	Sternocleidomastoid and upper trapezius muscles	Have child shrug shoulders against mild resistance. Have child turn his head to one side against resistance of examiner's hand. Repeat on the other side. Inspect and palpate muscle strength, symmetry for both maneuvers.
XII Hypoglossal (M)	Muscles of tongue	Have child move his tongue in all directions. Have him stick out tongue as far as possible; check for tremors or deviations. Test strength by having child push tongue against inside cheek against resistance on outer cheek. Note strength, movement, symmetry.

*S = sensory, M = motor, EOM = extraocular movement.

the finger-to-nose test the child stands erect with arms extended at the sides and touches his index finger to his nose. He uses one index finger and then the other. This test is repeated with the eyes closed. An abnormal response would be "past pointing," in which the child completely misses touching his nose. In the heel-to-shin test the child lies supine on the examination table and places one heel rapidly down the shin from the knee to the ankle. This is repeated using the other heel. Uncoordinated or inaccurate movements suggest a cerebellar dysfunction.

Rapid alternating motion is tested by having the child rapidly alternate pronation and supernation of the hands on the knees. One hand should be tested and the other observed for mirroring movements. Slow and inaccurate movements are considered abnormal. Additional information can be obtained by having the child stand erect and balance on one foot. By the age of 4 years a child should be able to balance for about 5 seconds. By the age of 6 he should be able to balance on one foot with arms folded across his chest. The child should balance on the right and then the left leg to evaluate symmetry. Another test would be to have the child touch each finger to the thumb of the same hand in rapid succession. This should be done with each hand to check for symmetry. The hand not performing the task should also be observed for mirroring. The cerebellar function of the infant may be grossly assessed by observing coordination in sucking, swallowing, reaching and grasping.

Examination of the motor system includes evaluation of muscle size, muscle tone, muscle strength and abnormal muscle movements. Most of the motor system evaluation is accomplished through the examination of the extremities and spine and developmental screening tools. Muscles should be checked for hypertrophy, atrophy and asymmetry. Any abnormality or asymmetry should be referred.

Muscle strength is discussed in examination

of the extremities. Any abnormality would be recorded in this section as well. Involuntary movements are done by observing a child in a stationary state with hands resting on the knees or stretched out in front. Occasionally involuntary movements can be better elicited by involving the child in a stressful conversation. Any choreic, twitching or convulsive movements should be referred. Tremors or tics are also abnormal.

Primary sensation and discriminatory sensation must be tested when evaluating the sensory system. When doing a thorough neurological examination, the face, trunk, arms and legs must be tested for primary sensation. Five types of sensation are tested: superficial tactile sensation, superficial pain, temperature, vibration, deep pressure pain, motion and position (cerebellar function). A wisp of cotton is brushed on the skin of symmetrical areas of the body to evaluate superficial sensation. Superficial pain is evaluated by lightly pressing a sharp and a blunt point of a safety pin and asking the child to identify sharp or dull. Since this may cause anxiety in the young child, a tongue depressor may be broken and the rough and smooth ends used to simulate sharp and dull. This may be less frightening to the child. Temperature can be evaluated by filling test tubes with warm and cold water and having the child identify each. The temperature should be rechecked frequently to be sure the test is valid. Vibration is evaluated by placing a large tuning fork on the sternum, elbows, iliac crests, knees and toes. The child is asked to tell when the vibration stops. The examiner then places the tuning fork on a similar body part of her own to see if she can still feel it.

Deep pain can be evaluated by strong pressure on bone and tendons, testicular pressure, or pressure on the eyeballs or on calf and forearm muscles. This should never be done unless indicated by clinical symptoms such as decreased level of consciousness.

A test for discriminatory sensation is one-point discrimination. One part of the body is touched and the child is asked to point to the area where he felt something touch him. This should be done with the child's eyes closed. This can be easily integrated into the primary sensation testing when the wisp of cotton or test tubes are used.

Finally reflex action is evaluated. For the older child and adult, reflexes fall into two categories: superficial and deep. Examples of superficial reflexes include abdominal reflexes, the cremasteric reflex, the plantar grasp reflex and the gluteal reflex. The abdominal reflex, usually active after the first two days of life, is elicited by stroking the four quadrants of the abdomen around the umbilicus. This is done with a sharp point, and the strokes should form a diamond or a square. A normal response is for the umbilicus to move toward the stimulus in the quadrant that is currently being stroked. Absent or asymmetrical movement may not necessarily be significant but should be noted.

The cremasteric reflex is obtained by stroking the inner aspect of the thigh with a sharp object (broken tongue depressor or fingernail). The testis on the stimulated side moves out of the scrotal sack into the inguinal canal. Both sides should be tested; any abnormality could indicate pathology. This reflex is often stimulated by cold or anxiety.

The plantar reflex is elicited by stimulating the balls of the feet, usually by pressing the thumb firmly against this area. Plantar flexum, or a "grasping" response, is normal in the infant up to 3 months of age.

To obtain a gluteal reflex (anal wink) the examiner separates the buttocks and strokes the perianal area. Normally, there is a brisk contraction of the anal sphincter.

Deep tendon reflex responses are usually graded using the following scoring system: $0 =$ absent, $+1 =$ sluggish, $+2 =$ active, $+3 =$ hyperactive, $+4 =$ transient clonus, and $+5 =$ permanent clonus. Deep reflexes are evaluated for strength and symmetry from side to side and from upper to lower extremities. The tendon should be slightly stretched and briefly tapped with a reflex hammer. The expected response is contraction of the muscle. Only five of the most common deep tendon reflexes are discussed here: triceps, biceps, brachioradialis, patellar and achilles. The triceps is elicited by flexing the child's arm at the elbow and striking the tendon just above the olecranon process (Fig. 13–23). Usually the muscles of the forearm contract. The biceps reflex is done with the child's arm semiflexed at the elbow and slightly pronated with the elbow resting in the examiner's palm (Fig. 13–23). The examiner places a thumb over the tendon and strikes her thumb for contraction of the biceps and forearm. Striking the semipronated arm just above the styloid

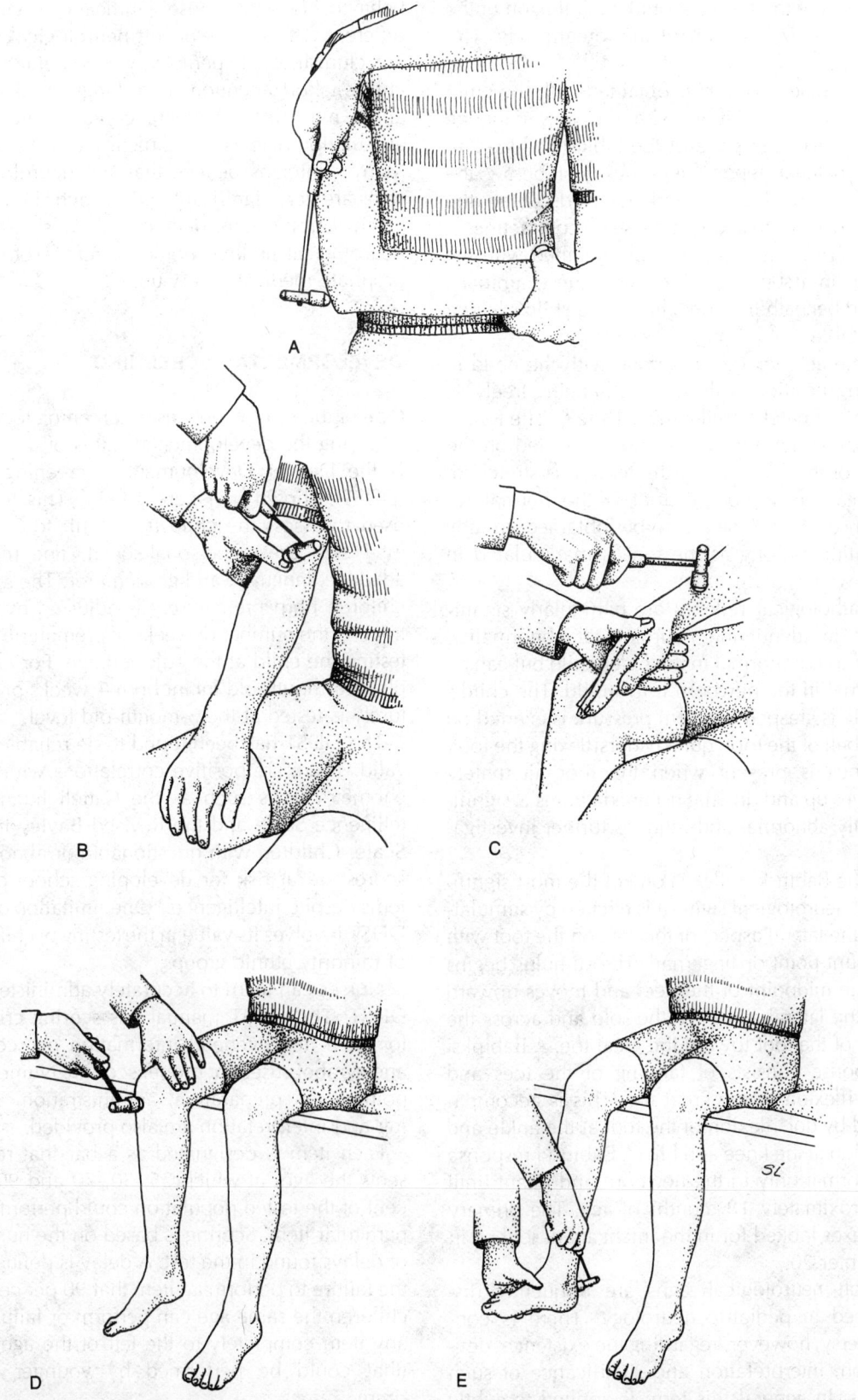

Figure 13-23 The deep tendon reflexes: *A.* triceps; *B.* biceps; *C.* brachioradialis; *D.* patellar; *E.* achilles.

process of the radius should elicit flexion of the elbow and pronation of the forearm (Fig. 13-23).

The patellar reflex is obtained with the child in a sitting position with the legs dangling freely over the edge of the table (Fig. 13-23). The patellar tendon is struck just below the patella; the leg will jerk forward. Often the quadriceps muscle can be seen contracting as well. This reflex can also be obtained with the child in a supine position with the examiner's hand beneath the knee, lifting the child's leg off the table.

The achilles reflex is done with the child in sitting position with the legs hanging freely as with the patellar reflex (Fig. 13-23). The foot is grasped and upward pressure is exerted on the ball of the foot so that the tendon is stretched. Plantar flexion of the foot is the normal response. This reflex can be obtained in any position as long as the foot is manipulated in this way.

Pathological reflexes are particularly significant in identifying neurological abnormality. Clonus is abnormal in the older child but can be normal in the newborn if it is mild. The child's ankle is grasped and firm pressure is exerted on the ball of the foot, quickly dorsiflexing the foot. Clonus is present when the foot alternately moves up and down. Sustained clonus is significantly abnormal and requires further investigation.

The Babinski reflex is one of the most significant neurological signs. It is elicited by stimulating the lateral aspect of the sole on the foot with a blunt point or fingernail. The stimulus begins at the midpoint of the heel and moves upward on the lateral aspect of the sole and across the ball of the foot toward the great toe. A Babinksi response consists of fanning of the toes and dorsiflexion of the great toe. This is accompanied by dorsiflexion of the foot at the ankle and flexion at the knee and hip. A Babinski response is normal only in the newborn and infant until approximately 18 months of age. The primary reflexes looked for in the infant are described in Chapter 20.

Soft neurological signs are frequently discussed in pediatric neurology. There is controversy, however, regarding the existence, definition, interpretation and significance of such signs. In general this term is applied to subtle behaviors or signs whose significance is viewed differently. Examples of soft neurological signs are clumsiness, hyperactivity, perceptual difficulties, short attention span, language disturbances, mirroring movement, confused laterality, articulation defects and difficulty with balance. Many clinicians believe that soft neurological signs are very significant and as such should be given careful consideration. Any significant neurological finding should be referred for appropriate medical follow-up.

DEVELOPMENTAL SCREENING

One of the most widely used screening tools for assessing the developmental status of the child is the Denver Developmental Screening Test (DDST), shown in Figure 13-24. This tool is used to assess the child from birth to 6 years in 4 skill areas: personal-social, fine motor-adaptive, language and gross-motor. The age of children born prematurely is adjusted by subtracting the number of weeks of prematurity and testing the child at the adjusted age. For example, a 6-month-old infant born 4 weeks prematurely is tested at the 5-month-old level.

The DDST has been found to be reliable and valid. There are positive correlations with psychometric tests such as the Cattell Infant Intelligence Scale and the Revised Bayley Infant Scale. Children with questionable or abnormal scores are at risk for developing school problems despite intelligence.[4] One limitation of the DDST involves its value in the testing of children of minority ethnic groups.

Nurses can learn to accurately administer the DDST. The DDST manual has scoring criteria for each item, general information on scoring and symbols used for proper scoring. Numerous pointers on preparation, administration, scoring and interpretation are also provided.

Each item is designated as a bar that represents the ages at which 25, 50, 70 and 90 per cent of the tested population could perform the particular item. Scoring is based on the number of delays found in the test. A delay is defined as the failure to perform an item that 90 per cent of children the same age can perform or failure in any item completely to the left of the age line (that could be performed by younger children).

Before beginning the test, the nurse must be sure to adequately explain to parents the purpose of the test and how it is performed. The

DDST is not an intelligence test and this should be clearly stated to the parent. The parent should also understand that the child will be asked to perform tasks below and above his expected performance so that the best possible performance is obtained. DDST results should be completely explained to the parent, reinforcing the child's satisfactory performance. Children with abnormal or questionable results should be rescreened before referral for diagnostic testing (Fig. 13-24).

The child's performance is affected by factors such as fatigue, anxiety, illness, shyness or separation from the parent. Also, undetected visual or hearing problems or neurological or familial developmental problems may influence the child's performance and should be considered.

Another screening tool frequently used is the Denver Prescreening Developmental Questionnaire (PDQ). It is an easy questionnaire of 97 questions that can be answered rapidly. The questionnaire is divided according to the child's age and is given to the parent to fill out. The parent answers 10 questions from the appropriate age category. The nurse then reviews the answers and provides time for the parent to express concerns or ask questions. This inexpensive tool is a modification of the DDST and assesses the same four categories but can be done with minimal professional time. Indications that a child has a developmental delay require follow-up with a complete DDST.

The Developmental Profile is a developmental screening tool consisting of 217 items arranged in five scales: physical developmental age, self-help developmental age, social developmental age, academic developmental age and communication developmental age. This test was standardized by Alpern and Ball[1] for children from the newborn period through 12 years of age. It relies largely on verbal responses from the parent, teachers, older sibling, or other individuals acquainted with the child. It provides an individual profile that can be compared to data on what is normal for specific ages at which children in the standardized population perform developmental skills.

Although much attention has been focused on assessing the child's development, concern is also directed at assessing his environment, which may foster or impede his developmental processes. Using both clinical and home visit observations, Dr. Bettye Caldwell developed an assessment tool designed to identify characteristics of the environment of children from birth to 3 years and 3 to 6 years. The instrument is the Home Observation for Measurement of the Environment (HOME) (see Appendix III for these forms). The birth to 3 years inventory measures six subscales: emotional and verbal responsiveness of the mother, avoidance of restriction and punishment, organization of physical and temporal environment, provision of appropriate play materials, maternal involvement with the child and opportunities for variety in daily stimulation.

The inventory for 3 to 6-year-olds measures seven subscales: provision of stimulation through equipment, toys and experience; stimulation of mature behavior; provision of stimulating physical and language environment; avoidance of restriction and punishment; pride, affection and thoughtfulness; masculine stimulation; and independence from parental control. The purpose for both scales is to identify certain aspects of the quantity and quality of the social, emotional and cognitive environmental supports available to the young child in his home.

This tool must be administered by a person who goes into the home and observes the child when awake during his normal daily routine. It takes approximately an hour to obtain the data. The parent should be notified of the forthcoming visit. The HOME can be used in combination with other screening tools to assist parents to solve current problems and prevent development of other problems by providing anticipating guidance for appropriate parenting.

Obtaining a profile of the infant's temperament can also be useful in planning his care. The Carey Infant Temperament Questionnaire* (developed by Dr. W. B. Carey) is a clinical screening instrument used to study the temperament of the infant between 4 and 8 months of age. Carey identifies temperament as an important variable in infant development that influences the relationship between parents and infant and other caregivers. The child's feeding, sleep, elimination and play patterns are some of the areas identified in the questionnaire completed by the parent. The items also look at the infant's responses to different situations.

The Washington Guide to Promoting Devel-

---

*This questionnaire can be obtained from Dr. W. B. Carey, 319 W. Front St., Media, PA 19063.

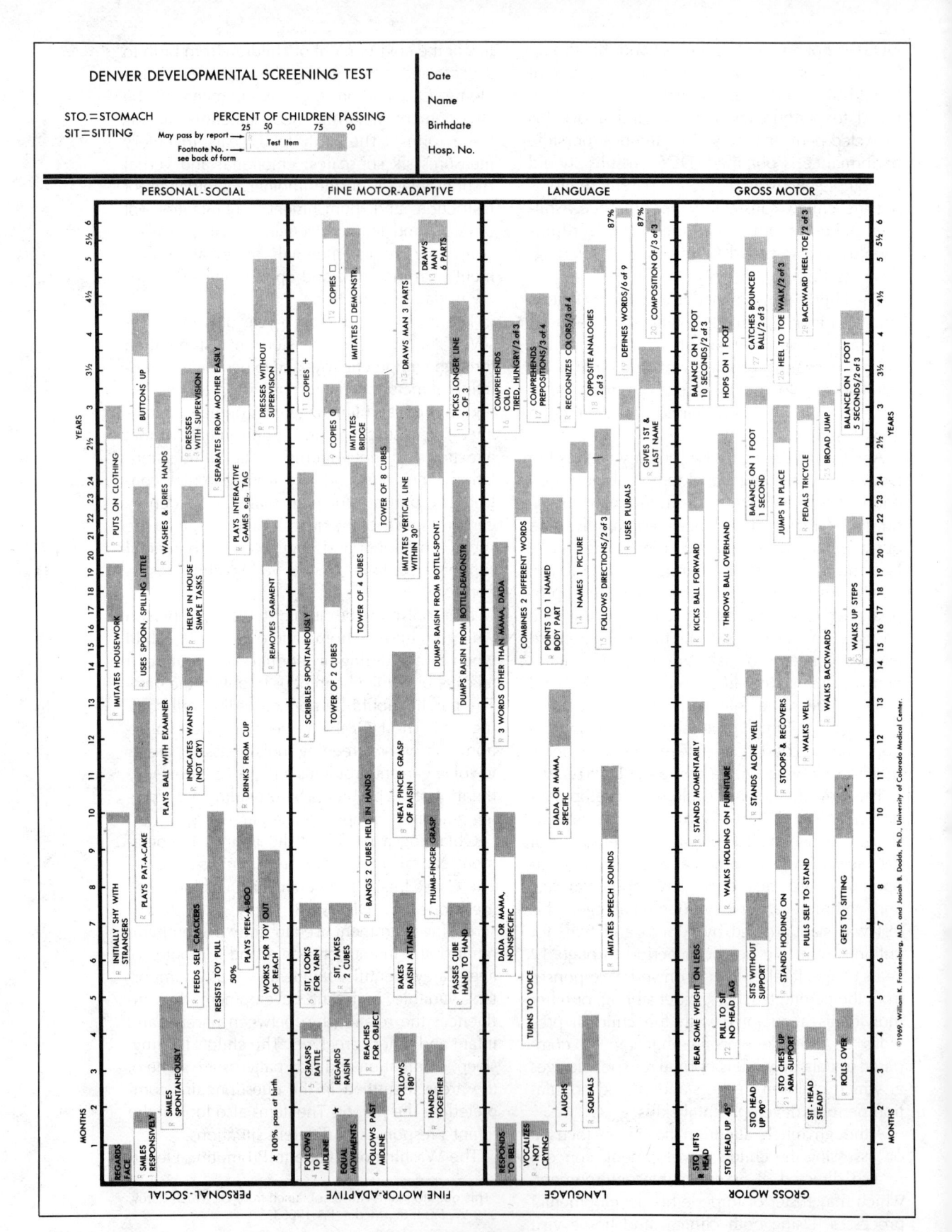

Figure 13-24

FAMILIES WITH CHILDREN

Illustration continued on opposite page

1. Try to get child to smile by smiling, talking or waving to him. Do not touch him.
2. When child is playing with toy, pull it away from him. Pass if he resists.
3. Child does not have to be able to tie shoes or button in the back.
4. Move yarn slowly in an arc from one side to the other, about 6" above child's face. Pass if eyes follow 90° to midline. (Past midline; 180°)
5. Pass if child grasps rattle when it is touched to the backs or tips of fingers.
6. Pass if child continues to look where yarn disappeared or tries to see where it went. Yarn should be dropped quickly from sight from tester's hand without arm movement.
7. Pass if child picks up raisin with any part of thumb and a finger.
8. Pass if child picks up raisin with the ends of thumb and index finger using an over hand approach.

9. Pass any enclosed form. Fail continuous round motions.
10. Which line is longer? (Not bigger.) Turn paper upside down and repeat. (3/3 or 5/6)
11. Pass any crossing lines.
12. Have child copy first. If failed, demonstrate

When giving items 9, 11 and 12, do not name the forms. Do not demonstrate 9 and 11.

13. When scoring, each pair (2 arms, 2 legs, etc.) counts as one part.
14. Point to picture and have child name it. (No credit is given for sounds only.)

15. Tell child to: Give block to Mommie; put block on table; put block on floor. Pass 2 of 3. (Do not help child by pointing, moving head or eyes.)
16. Ask child: What do you do when you are cold? ..hungry? ..tired? Pass 2 of 3.
17. Tell child to: Put block <u>on</u> table; <u>under</u> table; <u>in front</u> of chair, <u>behind</u> chair. Pass 3 of 4. (Do not help child by pointing, moving head or eyes.)
18. Ask child: If fire is hot, ice is ?; Mother is a woman, Dad is a ?; a horse is big, a mouse is ?. Pass 2 of 3.
19. Ask child: What is a ball? ..lake? ..desk? ..house? ..banana? ..curtain? ..ceiling? ..hedge? ..pavement? Pass if defined in terms of use, shape, what it is made of or general category (such as banana is fruit, not just yellow). Pass 6 of 9.
20. Ask child: What is a spoon made of? ..a shoe made of? ..a door made of? (No other objects may be substituted.) Pass 3 of 3.
21. When placed on stomach, child lifts chest off table with support of forearms and/or hands.
22. When child is on back, grasp his hands and pull him to sitting. Pass if head does not hang back.
23. Child may use wall or rail only, not person. May not crawl.
24. Child must throw ball overhand 3 feet to within arm's reach of tester.
25. Child must perform standing broad jump over width of test sheet. (8-1/2 inches)
26. Tell child to walk forward, heel within 1 inch of toe. Tester may demonstrate. Child must walk 4 consecutive steps, 2 out of 3 trials.
27. Bounce ball to child who should stand 3 feet away from tester. Child must catch ball with hands, not arms, 2 out of 3 trials.
28. Tell child to walk backward, toe within 1 inch of heel. Tester may demonstrate. Child must walk 4 consecutive steps, 2 out of 3 trials.

<u>DATE AND BEHAVIORAL OBSERVATIONS</u> (how child feels at time of test, relation to tester, attention span, verbal behavior, self-confidence, etc,):

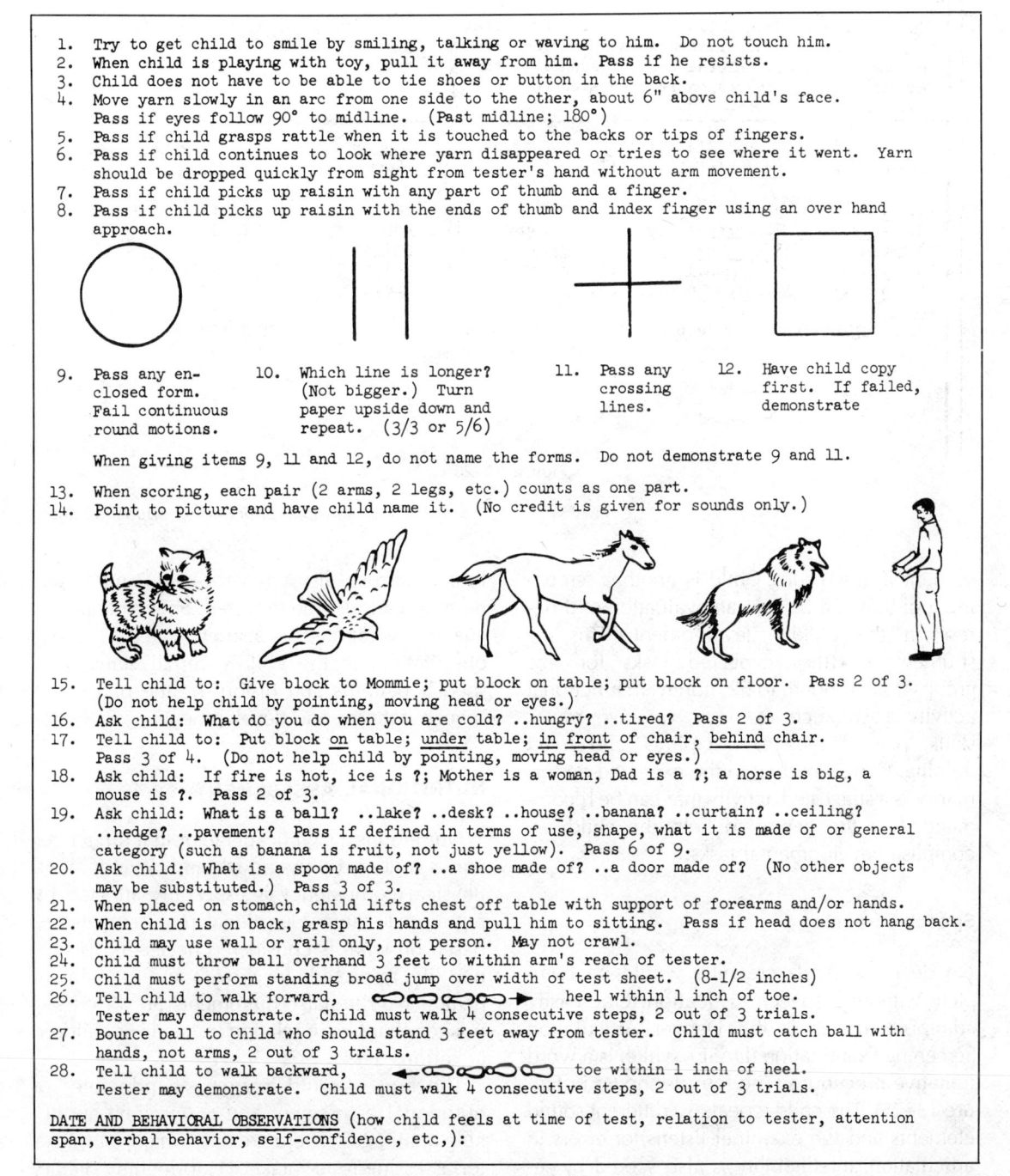

Figure 13-24 The Denver Developmental Screening Test. (Courtesy of William K. Frankenberg, M.D., and Josiah B. Dodds, Ph.D., University of Colorado Medical Center.) A summary of scoring instructions is presented in Appendix IV.

```
DENVER ARTICULATION SCREENING EXAM          NAME
    for children 2 1/2 to 6 years of age
                                            HOSP. NO.
Instructions: Have child repeat each word after
you. Circle the underlined sounds that he pro-  ADDRESS
nounces correctly. Total correct sounds is the
Raw Score. Use charts on reverse side to score
results.
```

Date: _____ Child's Age: _____ Examiner: _____ Raw Score: _____
Percentile: _____   Intelligibility: _____ Result: _____

1. table   6. zipper   11. sock   16. wagon   21. leaf
2. shirt   7. grapes   12. vacuum   17. gum   22. carrot
3. door   8. flag   13. yarn   18. house
4. trunk   9. thumb   14. mother   19. pencil
5. jumping   10. toothbrush 15. twinkle   20. fish

Intelligibility: (circle one)   1. Easy to understand   3. Not understandable
                                2. Understandable 1/2   4. Can't evaluate
                                   the time.

Comments:

Figure 13–25

Illustration continued on opposite page

opment in the Young Child is another screening tool that can help in an evaluation of progress in the child's development. This instrument identifies expected tasks for age groups from 1 month to 52 months in functional activity areas such as sleep, feeding, motor skills, play, language, discipline, and toilet training. Corresponding to the expected performance is a suggested activity that can be recommended to the parent to help the child accomplish developmental tasks.

Speech Screening

No developmental screening would be complete without a speech evaluation. One easily administered test is the Denver Articulation Screening Examination (DASE), which is a word imitative procedure (The form is shown in Figure 13–25). The child repeats 30 different sound elements and the examiner listens for errors in articulation. Intelligibility is also scored by selection of one of four categories ranging from easy to understand to cannot evaluate. The DASE is designed to pinpoint significant speech delays and normal variations in the acquisition of speech sounds. Abnormal conditions such as tongue thrust, lisp, hypernasality and hyponasality can also be detected. Speech and language development is also evaluated by direct observation of the child's verbal skills, and speech patterns and history by the parents of speech patterns and development.

NUTRITIONAL ASSESSMENT

Nutrition is a significant factor that influences and is influenced by growth and development. Physical competency is especially affected by nutritional status. Nutritional requirements are based on what is considered necessary to support life, to provide for growth and to maintain health. Nutritional requirements are discussed in later chapters in relation to needs of children at various ages.

The nurse should learn basic principles of nutritional assessment and counselling applicable at all ages. There are three major purposes for assessing food intake: (1) to identify dietary practices of the family, (2) to obtain baseline data on the caloric and nutrient intake of a specific child from which a plan of therapy can be developed and progress measured and (3) to provide parents with the opportunity to ask questions about nutrition and feeding behaviors.

A nutritional history is obtained for a

To score DASE words: Note Raw Score for child's performance. Match raw score line (extreme left of chart) with column representing child's age (to the closest previous age group). Where raw score line and age column meet number in that square denotes percentile rank of child's performance when compared to other children that age. Percentiles above heavy line are ABNORMAL percentiles, below heavy line are NORMAL.

PERCENTILE RANK

Raw Score	2.5 yr.	3.0	3.5	4.0	4.5	5.0	5.5	6 years
2	1							
3	2							
4	5							
5	9							
6	16							
7	23							
8	31	2						
9	37	4	1					
10	42	6	2					
11	48	7	4					
12	54	9	6	1	1			
13	58	12	9	2	3	1	1	
14	62	17	11	5	4	2	2	
15	68	23	15	9	5	3	2	
16	75	31	19	12	5	4	3	
17	79	38	25	15	6	6	4	
18	83	46	31	19	8	7	4	
19	86	51	38	24	10	9	5	1
20	89	58	45	30	12	11	7	3
21	92	65	52	36	15	15	9	4
22	94	72	58	43	18	19	12	5
23	96	77	63	50	22	24	15	7
24	97	82	70	58	29	29	20	15
25	99	87	78	66	36	34	26	17
26	99	91	84	75	46	43	34	24
27		94	89	82	57	54	44	34
28		96	94	88	70	68	59	47
29		98	98	94	84	84	77	68
30		100	100	100	100	100	100	100

To Score intelligibility:

	NORMAL	ABNORMAL
2 1/2 years	Understandable 1/2 the time, or, "easy"	Not Understandable
3 years and older	Easy to understand	Understandable 1/2 time Not understandable

Test Result: 1. NORMAL on Dase and Intelligibility = NORMAL

2. ABNORMAL on Dase and/or Intelligibility = ABNORMAL

* If abnormal on initial screening rescreen within 2 weeks. If abnormal again child should be referred for complete speech evaluation.

Figure 13–25 Denver Articulation Screening Examination for Children 2½ to 6 years of age; percentile rank. (Courtesy of William Frankenberg, M. D., and Josiah Dodds, Ph.D., University of Colorado Medical Center.)

24-hour period of intake. For recall, questions about when the child got up and activities that took place at different times during the day can be asked. If more specific information is needed, a 3-day or 7-day food diary is kept and submitted for evaluation. A food diary is helpful in establishing food intake and the time of day and type of food consumed. Methods of preparation and household measures (cup, teaspoon) of amounts of food consumed are recorded. Mixed dishes should have the recipe or in-

TABLE 13-15 FORMAT OF A NUTRITIONAL HISTORY*

I. Age
II. Concerns of parents or child about current nutrition or feeding behaviors
III. Infant history (used when client is an infant)
   A. Type of feeding method (bottle, breast)
   B. Formula feeding
      1. Type used
      2. How prepared
      3. When formula was started
      4. Other formulas used
      5. Number of bottles and ounces consumed in 24 hours
      6. Frequency of feedings and number of ounces at each feeding
      7. Amount of time required for feeding
      8. Approach to feeding (propped bottle, held in arms, etc.)
   C. Breast feeding
      1. Number of times nursed in 24-hour period
      2. Length of time nursed at each breast, at each feeding
      3. Problems with breasts (cracked nipples, swollen breasts)
      4. Diet, medications and fluid intake history of mother
      5. Notice of milk letdown reflex by mother
      6. History of stress, fatigue in mother
   D. Additional intake
      1. Vitamins, iron, fluoride supplements
      2. Solid foods
         a. Type
         b. Frequency
         c. Amounts
         d. When started and how introduced
         e. How fed (feeds crackers, solids in bottle)
      3. Other fluids (juices, water, sugar water)
   E. Feeding behaviors/habits
      1. Satisfaction of child following feeding
      2. Use of pacifier or thumbsucking
      3. Nighttime nutrition
      4. Sleeping through night
      5. Elimination patterns
      6. Vomiting, spitting up
      7. Response to foods (spitting, colic, diarrhea, rash)
      8. Activity and personality (crying, irritable, sleeping) after feeding
   F. Family involvement with feeding
      1. Family attitudes/beliefs of food, feeding practices (how food is used)
      2. Participation in feeding (father, siblings)
      3. Response of family to feeding
         a. Breast feeding
         b. Self-feeding by infant and inevitable mess
         c. Response of parent/child to new foods when introduced
IV. Toddler, preschooler, adolescent history
   A. Number of meals eaten per day
   B. Where meals are eaten (school, fast-food chain, home)
   C. Method of feeding (fingers, utensils used)
   D. Amount of milk intake in 24 hours
   E. Snacking
      1. Type of foods
      2. Amounts
      3. Where snacks eaten
      4. Frequency and nearness to mealtimes
   F. Food preferences and dislikes
   G. Who plans, buys and cooks food
   H. Finances
      1. Amount of money available for food
      2. Food programs (food stamps, Head Start Breakfast, school lunch)
   I. Dietary recall for past 24 hours
   J. Developmental behavior of eating (utensils, chewing)
   K. Habits (same as infant)
   L. Response of family to eating behavior of child
   M. Last dental visit
V. Past medical history
   A. Prenatal nutrition of mother
   B. Birthweight
   C. PKU results
   D. Developmental history
      1. Feeding behaviors (use of cup, spoon, finger-feeding)
      2. Age of weaning
      3. Pica
   E. Allergies
   F. Chronic problems
VI. Family history
   A. Hypertension
   B. Obesity
   C. Stroke
   D. Diabetes
   E. Heart problems
   F. Allergies
   G. Hyperlipidemias
   H. Anorexia nervosa

*Adapted from J. Fox and C. Elsberry. Primary Health Care of the Young, McGraw-Hill Book Co., 1980.

gredients included. Additional supplements such as vitamins or minerals should also be recorded. Although this method provides more comprehensive information, its disadvantage is that it is time consuming and requires much cooperation and motivation on the part of the child and parents. It is especially helpful, however, in working with obese children to help them see exactly how much they consume. Another interview method is to ask about the frequency with which specific foods are eaten. The specific foods are grouped in the major categories and the person is asked to respond to whether they are rarely eaten (less than once a week), sometimes eaten (once a week) or eaten every day.

A total assessment of the child's nutritional status includes a record of dietary intake, clinical evaluation including anthropometrical measurements, and biochemical evaluation of nutrients within the body. Table 13-15 identifies information that a nutrition history would include. It is essential that this information be obtained in a nonjudgmental manner. It is also important to remember that parents have been exposed to many ideas about nutrition and may be confused by the diverse and often conflicting information available. Direct questions should be avoided if possible; open questions should be asked instead, such as, "What do you add to the cereal?" This approach avoids suggestion, criticism or judgmental statements. The interviewer's attitude and nonverbal cues are frequently helpful in alleviating parental anxiety. A calm, accepting attitude helps parents provide accurate data without feeling defensive.

Additional information can be obtained by observing the parent-child interaction during feeding. Observing a mother breast-feeding or bottle-feeding may provide useful information from which an assessment may be made and counselling provided. Feeding behaviors frequently reflect the child's development; delays in feeding behaviors may also indicate delays in other areas. Also, children may not be provided the opportunity to develop certain skills such as using a cup or spoon and the parent may need counselling in this area.

The nurse also determines nutritional status through objective examination. A thorough physical examination should identify areas of concern if undernourishment or overnourishment exists. The measurements of height, weight, head circumference and the measurement of skin folds using a caliper provide essential information for evaluation of nutritional status. (See Figure 13-26 for instruction and evaluation of skinfold measurements.) Plotting these measurements and following them serially is an important aspect of nutritional assessment. Physical indications of nutritional status are shown in Table 13-16. One or more of these signs indicates the need for a careful interview about food intake and eating habits. Additional helpful information about nutritional status may be obtained from hematocrit or hemoglobin tests to detect anemia; routine analysis for albumin and sugar; and, in children at risk, cholesterol levels.

Once data have been gathered, the nurse evaluates the diet to see if the recommended dietary allowances (RDA) are being met (see Appendix V). Also any feeding behaviors that are of concern should be dealt with. Parents are the decision makers for the young child, but the older child has practical decision-making powers regarding nutrition. The parent and child should be counseled regarding modification of the child's diet if necessary. It is important to include both the parent and the child in the plans for change. It is also important that they know the reasons why change is needed and how their beliefs, attitudes and actions are affecting the nutrition of the child. The parents and the child may need support and help in dealing not only with their feelings and behaviors but also those of friends and relatives.

LABORATORY SCREENING

Laboratory tests are used as diagnostic or screening aids; when combined with subjective and objective findings, they provide a complete data base. Many of the laboratory specimens needed for diagnostic examination of children are obtained the same as they are for adults. The older child is often able to cooperate and follow directions adequately to assist in obtaining the laboratory specimens. Infants and small children, however, are usually unable to help the nurse obtain some specimens. Appendix VI gives normal laboratory values for children.

Blood Specimens

Most blood samples are obtained by the laboratory staff or physicians. The nurse is often responsible for making certain the parent and child understand the procedure, assisting in restraint, and making certain that the correct equipment is available. In some areas, however, such as the intensive care and outpatient clinics, the nurse is responsible for collecting specimens needed.

Venous blood samples are obtained by venipuncture or by aspiration from an intravenous infusion site. If the sample is obtained from an intravenous infusion site, the nurse must be sure the specimen collected is not inaccurate due to the type of fluid being infused in the catheter. For example, a catheter that contains a glucose solution would invalidate a blood specimen withdrawn for a glucose determination.

Microtechnique capillary blood specimens are excellent for many blood tests because they require less blood and are less difficult to ob-

MEASUREMENT OF TRICEPS SKINFOLD THICKNESS

General Considerations
The use of skinfold thickness in the assessment of nutritional status of children is based on the assumption that increased subcutaneous fat, resulting from either high calorie intake or low energy expenditure, reflects a greater calorie reserve.* Measurements of skinfold thickness can provide an indirect estimate of the amount of body fat, and they can be used as an index of nutritional status. To be most useful, skinfold measurements should be taken regularly during routine health supervision visits.

Instructions
With practice and patience, accurate skinfold measurements of infants and children can be obtained. The following instructions should help to obtain reliable, accurate figures.

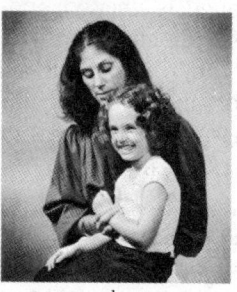

1 For a child, have an attendant hold the child's left hand or forearm with the elbow flexed to approximately 90 degrees and pressed gently against his or her abdomen. The child can be either standing or sitting.
For an infant, have an attendant (preferably the mother) hold the infant in a semi-upright position, with infant's right side next to but not touching mother's body, and with infant's head facing forward. Gently restrain the infant's left hand or forearm with the elbow flexed to approximately 90 degrees and pressed gently against his or her abdomen.

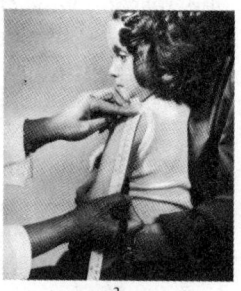

2 Marks are placed at the left acromion (shoulder) and olecranon (elbow). The distance between these marks is measured and the midpoint marked.

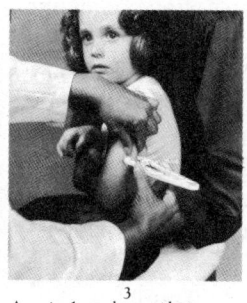

3 At a site 1 cm above midpoint, grasp a layer of skin and subcutaneous tissue with the first finger and thumb of one hand, gently pulling it away from the underlying muscle, and continue to hold until measurement is completed.
Place caliper jaws over the skinfold at the midpoint mark and apply pressure with the thumb to align the lines on the caliper. Do not apply excessive pressure.

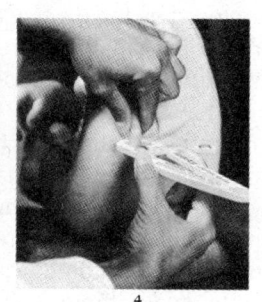

4 Estimate reading to nearest 1.0 mm, 2 to 3 seconds after aligning lines. Three readings should be taken, averaged, and recorded. Compare present measurement with previous triceps skinfold measurement(s) to determine possible change.
Reference data below is presented to assist in interpretation of reading.

TRICEPS SKINFOLD PERCENTILES*

(Triceps skinfold measurements based on data obtained using Lange skinfold calipers on white subjects included in the Ten-State Nutrition Survey, 1968-1970.)

Interpretation
Skinfold measurements between the 15th and 85th percentiles are probably within normal limits for age and sex. Those greater than the 95th percentile may be considered representative of obesity, particularly when weight for length or stature also exceeds the 95th percentile.

* Frisancho AR: Triceps skinfold and upper arm muscle size norms for assessment of nutritional status. Am J Clin Nutr 27:1052-1058, 1974.

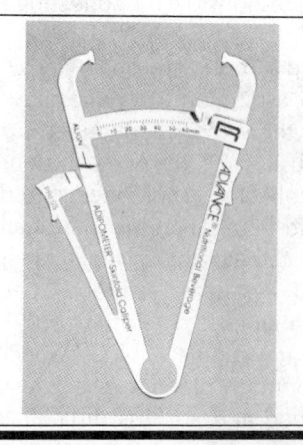

AGE (years)	MALES PERCENTILES(mm)					FEMALES PERCENTILES(mm)				
	5th	15th	50th	85th	95th	5th	15th	50th	85th	95th
Birth-	4	5	8	12	15	4	5	8	12	13
0.5-	5	7	9	13	15	6	7	9	12	15
1.5-	5	7	10	13	14	6	7	10	13	15
2.5-	6	7	9	12	14	6	7	10	12	14
3.5-	5	6	9	12	14	5	7	10	12	14
4.5-	5	6	8	12	16	6	7	10	13	16
5.5-	5	6	8	11	15	6	7	10	12	15
6.5-	4	6	8	11	14	6	7	10	13	17
7.5-	5	6	8	12	17	6	7	10	15	19
8.5-	5	6	9	14	19	6	7	11	17	24
9.5-	5	6	10	16	22	6	8	12	19	24
10.5-	6	7	10	17	25	7	8	12	20	29
11.5-	5	7	11	19	26	6	9	13	20	25
12.5-	5	6	10	18	25	7	9	14	23	30
13.5-	5	6	10	17	22	8	10	15	22	28
14.5-	4	6	9	19	26	8	11	16	24	30
15.5-	4	5	9	20	27	8	10	15	23	27
16.5-	4	5	8	14	20	9	12	16	26	31
17.5-24.4	4	5	10	18	25	9	12	17	25	31

Figure 13–26 Measurement of skinfolds. (Reproduced by permission of Ross Laboratories, Columbus, Ohio.)

TABLE 13-16 PHYSICAL INDICATIONS OF NUTRITIONAL STATUS OF THE CHILD

Physical Aspect	Well-Nourished Child	Malnourished Child	Deficiency
Height and Weight	Within growth norms — steady gain and increase from year to year	Above or below growth norms — failure to gain or excessive weight gain each year	Protein, calorie, other essential nutrients
Skin	Clear, smooth, elastic and firm	Rough, dry, scaly, xerosis	Vitamin A
	Reddish-pink mucous membranes	Petechiae, ecchymoses, poor wound healing	Vitamin C
		Depigmentation of skin	Protein, calorie
		Lesions	Riboflavin
		Dermatitis, sensitivity of skin to sunlight	Niacin
		Pallor	Vitamin B_{12}, iron, folacin
Musculoskeletal	Well-developed, erect posture	Head sags, winged scapula, bowed legs, costochondral beading, cranial bossing	Calcium, Vitamin D
	Shoulder blades flat		
	Arms and legs straight		
	Skull and jaw well developed	Epiphyseal enlargement of wrists	Vitamins D, C
	Firm muscles with good tonus	Small flabby muscles, muscle weakness	Phosphorus, protein
	Moderate amount of fat	Faulty epiphyseal bone formation	Vitamin A
		Pretibial edema bilateral	Protein, calorie, thiamine
Head	Hair — smooth, good amount, lustrous	Dull, dry, depigmented, abnormal texture, easily pluckable, thin	Protein, calorie
	Eyes — clear and bright	Dull with dark circles and hollows. Bitot's spots, conjunctivitis, xerosis, night blindness (nyctalopia), light sensitivity (photophobia)	Vitamin A, riboflavin
	Mouth — pink, moist lips; pink, firm gums; full set of teeth	Cracking and scaling lips, cheilosis, fissuring of mouth corners	Riboflavin
		Spongy, swollen gums, bleed easily (gingiva)	Vitamin C
		Irregular or missing teeth with cavities; defective tooth enamel	Vitamins D, A
		Glossitis	Folacin, B_{12}, niacin, iron
		Tongue fissuring	Niacin
Neck	Normal size	Enlarged thyroid	Iodine
		Enlarged parotids	Protein, calorie
Neurological		Listless	Protein, calorie
		Loss of ankle- and knee-jerk reflexes, motor weakness, sensory loss	Thiamine
		Headache	Niacin, thiamine
		Polyneuritis, motor weakness	Thiamine
Abdomen	Flat	Distended, protrudes, hepatomegaly	Protein, calorie
Cardiac	Normal heart size and sounds	Cardiac enlargement and tachycardia	Thiamine, potassium
		Murmur	Iron

Source: Pearson, Gayle A. Nutrition in the middle years of childhood. *The American Journal of Maternal Child Nursing,* 2(6):383 (1977). (12)

tain. The toe or lateral heel is used for infants, while the older child may have capillary blood drawn from the lateral side of the third or fourth finger or the tip of the earlobe. Whatever method is used, it is essential that the parent and child be adequately prepared for the procedure and adequate restraint of the child be provided if he is unable to cooperate.

Once the site is selected, the nurse may wish to warm the toe or finger by placing it in warm water or wrapping it with a warm washcloth to increase blood flow. The older child can open and close his hand several times to increase blood flow. The finger, if used, is placed lower than the elbow and the toe is placed at a lower level than the knee. It is best if the examiner's hand is supported on the table or resting on her own knee.

The area is washed with the alcohol sponge and left to air dry or is wiped with a dry cotton ball or gauze. The finger (or other site) is firmly grasped by the examiner and swiftly and firmly jabbed with the lancet. The finger, toe or heel pads should never be used as use of these may cause increased pain or scar if repeated testing is done. It is better to plunge firmly through the skin the first time so that adequate blood flow is achieved. The first few drops of blood are wiped free and the capillary tube held to the site for drawing the blood sample. Two tubes are usually obtained for comparison or in case one breaks. The finger or toe should not be "milked" because this damages the red blood cells and may alter the test results. Upon completion of the procedure a dry cotton ball is held firmly over the site for a few minutes. A Band-Aid is then offered to the child. The young child should be carefully checked to be sure the Band-Aid is not removed and swallowed.

Hematocrit One of the most frequently used laboratory screening tests is the hematocrit. The hematocrit is a comparison of packed red blood cell volume and the volume of whole blood. This is generally a screening test used for anemia. Using the procedure described previously for obtaining capillary blood, the nurse draws two capillary tubes of blood to be centrifuged. Normal hematocrit values are expressed in percents. Normal values are usually 33 per cent and above and abnormal values are any numbers below 33 per cent or above 50 per cent.

Hemoglobin A hemoglobin refers to the measurement of hemaglobin, a protein, within each blood cell. Since the hematocrit measures the number of red blood cells and the hemoglobin measures the hemoglobin within each cell, it is frequently important to measure both to determine if anemia is present. Depending on the type of method used to determine the hemoglobin, either capillary or venous blood is obtained. Hemoglobin values are expressed in grams per dl of blood.

The hemoglobin and hematocrit are always done if there is a suggestion of possible anemia by history or physical findings. The child should be screened at 6 to 9 months of age, between 12 and 18 months, and again during adolescence. These are the ages that the child is most frequently at risk for developing iron deficiency anemia.

Sickledex A simple screening procedure for sickle cell anemia is the Sickledex. This disease is a defect in the structure of the red blood cell, which loses its rounded shape and becomes sickled by stress or lack of oxygen. Approximately 10 per cent of the black American population has this condition. The test is done only on black children over 6 months of age due to the amount of fetal hemoglobin present before that age. The Sickledex is a screening test and any positive test should be referred for more specific diagnostic testing.

Testing for Venereal Disease One of the most common screening tests for syphilis is the flocculation test developed by the Venereal Disease Research Laboratory (VDRL) of the United States Public Health Service. A venous blood sample of 5 ml of blood is necessary for most VDRL testing. The tests are then processed by specially trained laboratory technicians. Results are recorded and returned to the health care provider.

Bilirubin The destruction of red blood cells within the liver results in a byproduct called bilirubin. Bilirubin that has not been processed by the liver is unconjugated or indirect. In the liver, bilirubin is conjugated (direct) and excreted through the biliary ducts to the gut. When the level of bilirubin in the blood exceeds 5 mg/100 cc, the child becomes jaundiced. This occurs most frequently in the newborn and is the result of an increased destruction of red blood cells (from which bilirubin is formed), by immaturity of the liver (which processes bilirubin), or by obstruction of the biliary system (which allows excretion of bilirubin into the small intestine). High levels of serum indirect bilirubin (over 20 mg per cent) are associated with kernicterus and permanent brain damage. Elevated direct bilirubin levels (bilirubin processed by the liver) are found in infants with congenital anomalies of the biliary tract that prevent excretion of bilirubin into the gastrointestinal tract.

Total bilirubin measures the concentration of bound and unbound bilirubin in the serum. Specimens to measure bilirubin levels are now obtained by laboratory technicians with small hematocrit-sized pipettes and require only a lancet stick of the infant's heel or toe. A normal direct bilirubin level would be 0 to 0.3/dl, an indirect level would normally be 0.1 to 1.0 mg/dl, and the total bilirubin level 0.1 to 1.2 mg/dl.

Phenylketonuria Phenylketonuria (PKU), a disorder of amino acid metabolism, causes an abnormal accumulation of the amino acid phenylalanine in the blood, resulting in brain damage. Testing for PKU has become mandatory on all newborns in most states. Blood levels of phenylalanine are measured by the Guthrie test between the second and sixth day of life after the child has ingested any protein substance (usually milk formula) for 24 to 48 hours. The infant's heel is pricked with a lancet and three drops of blood are pressed to a special absorbent filter paper. PKU testing may be repeated at 3 to 6 weeks of age in newborns with a negative Guthrie test using ferric-chloride-treated paper strips that, if absorbed by urine with phenylalanine content above 15 mg/100 ml, turns green.[9] (Chapter 25 describes the details of this test.) Newborns with a positive Guthrie test must be retested with the blood test to show evidence of persistently elevated blood levels of phenylalanine.

Lead Screening for lead toxicity is done by both blood and urine testing. Blood testing requires venous blood; evaluation is done by a trained laboratory clinician. A normal lead value is 10 to 20 mg/100 ml of whole blood. Levels above 40 mg/100 ml represent excessive exposure and absorption of lead and may produce symptoms of lead poisoning. Levels exceeding 80 mg/100 ml represent clinical lead poisoning.[13] Tests such as that measuring free erythrocyte porphyrin (FEP) have been devised that need only a capillary blood sample. In general a value 10 times greater than the normal FEP value is indicative of lead poisoning. Values 5 to 10 times greater may be the result of lead poisoning, iron deficiency anemia or both. All children with an elevated FEP level must have a more specific blood level study done to accurately rule out the possibility of lead poisoning.

Urine Specimens

One of the most painless and effective ways to evaluate the functioning of the entire body is examination of the urine. The various techniques for collecting urine specimens are described in Chapter 17. Older children and adolescents can readily provide a specimen with correct instructions but may be embarrassed by carrying specimens through hallways. If this is the case, a paper bag should be provided or the nurse should retrieve the specimen as discreetly as possible. Adolescent females who are menstruating should delay providing a specimen or a notation should be made on the laboratory slip to explain the presence of red blood cells.

School-age children are cooperative but, like adolescents, are very curious and concerned regarding the reasons for obtaining the specimen. Explanations of the method and reasons for obtaining a urine sample will greatly expedite the procedure.

Preschoolers and toddlers are less cooperative and often have difficulty following directions and so need more assistance. Before trying to obtain a specimen, the nurse should offer liquids and wait 20 to 30 minutes. The parent should be questioned as to the child's terminology for this bodily function, and these words should be used, such as "pee-pee" or "tinkle." Children who have difficulty voiding in an unfamiliar receptable may be provided with a clean or sterilized potty chair or bed pan placed on the toilet. Toddlers may have difficulty voiding in an unfamiliar receptable since they have undoubtedly been admonished for voiding in places not approved by parents during the toilet training phase. The parents may need to reassure the child it is all right to void in the bed pan.

A standard urinalysis includes an examination for the color, pH and specific gravity; testing for glucose, ketones and protein; and a microscopic determination for cells, bacteria and crystalline content. Simple qualitative screening tests can be done for pH, glucose, protein, blood and other substances by using reagent-covered test strips that are dipped directly into the urine or pressed between two urine-saturated surfaces of a diaper. The presence of the test substance causes a color change on the strip, which is then compared to the colors identified on a chart or on the test strip bottle. The odor should also be noted, as it can indicate an abnormality. Microscopic examination of the urine is done by an experienced laboratory clinician.

Cultures Urine cultures are done on children who are suspected of having a urinary tract infection and on children with routine urinalysis results indicating abnormal microscopic findings. Techniques for obtaining urine specimens for culture are described in Chapter 17.

Many specific laboratory tests are used today. The nurse should acquaint herself with the proper collection methods and normal values specific to her clinical setting, as these may vary. Normal values for some of the most common laboratory tests can be found in Appendix VI.

References

1. G. Alpern and I. Ball. Developmental Profile. Psychological Developmental Publications, 1972
2. American Academy of Pediatrics, Standards of Child Health Care. American Academy of Pediatrics, 1977
3. B. Bates. A Guide to Physical Examination. J. B. Lippincott Co., 1979
4. B. Camp et al. Preschool developmental testing in prediction of school problems. Clinical Pediatrics, March 1977, p. 257
5. M. Downs and H. Silver. The A,B,C,D's of H.E.A.R. Clinical Pediatrics, October 1972, p. 563
6. S. M. Erickson. Assessment and Management of Developmental Changes in Children. C. V. Mosby Co., 1976
7. J. Fox, ed. Primary Health Care of the Young. McGraw-Hill Book Co., 1980
8. W. Frankenburg et al. Reliability and stability of the DDST. Child Development, April 1971, p. 1315
9. J. Hughes. Synopsis of Pediatrics, 4th ed. C. V. Mosby Co., 1979
10. R. S. Illingsworth. The Development of the Infant and Young Child — Normal and Abnormal. Williams and Wilkins Co., 1972
11. G. Nichols and D. Kucha. Oral measurements. American Journal of Nursing, June 1972, p 1091
12. G. Pearson. Nutrition in the middle years of childhood. American Journal of Maternal Child Nursing, Nov/Dec 1977, p. 383
13. R. Ravel. Clinical Laboratory Medicine - Clinical Application of Laboratory Data. Year-book Medical Publishers, Inc., 1978
14. M. Sheridan. Vision screening of very young or handicapped children. British Medical Journal, 6 August 1960, p. 453
15. J. Wasson et al. Common Symptoms Guide. McGraw-Hill Book Co., 1975

Additional Recommended Reading

M. Alexander and M. Brown. Pediatric History and Physical Diagnosis for Nurses. McGraw-Hill Book Co., 1979

J. Brown. Child health maintenance. Nurse Practitioner, Jan./Feb. 1980, p. 33

M. S. Brown and M. A. Murphy. Ambulatory Pediatrics for Nurses. McGraw-Hill Book Co., 1975

B. Bates, A Guide to Physical Examination. J. B. Lippincott Co., 1979

S. Blumental et al. Report of the task force on blood pressure control in children. Pediatrics (Supplement), May 1977, part 2

P. Chinn. Child Health Maintenance. C. V. Mosby Co., 1979

C. Kempe et al. Current Pediatric Diagnosis and Treatment. Lange Medical Publications, 1980

M. O'Pray. Developmental screening tools: using them effectively. American Journal Maternal Child Nursing, Mar/apr 1980, p. 126

P. Pipes. Nutrition in Infancy and Childhood. C. V. Mosby Co., 1977

S. Tilkian et al. Clinical Implications of Laboratory Tests. C. V. Mosby Co., 1979

V. Vaughn et al. Textbook of Pediatrics. W. B. Saunders Co., 1979

Free Films (Loaned)

To Nourish a Child: Nutrition from newborn through teens. (16 mm; 20 min; color and sound)

Be Foodwise and Follow the Basic Four (16 mm; 20 min; color and sound)

Both available from Tupperware Educational Services; Tupperware Home Parties, Dept. HT, Orlando, Fl 32802.

FAMILY ASSESSMENT

14

by Jennifer Piersma, RN, CPNP, MS

The family may be reviewed from several different perspectives, or frameworks. The majority of these frameworks focus on the family as a group or on the subgroups of the family system (e.g., sister-brother subgroup, parent-child subgroups). Hill and Hansen[5] identified five frameworks used in studying the family: interactional, structure-functional, institutional, situational and developmental. Nye and Berardo[7] identified six additional perspectives from which to view the family: economic, religious, legal, social psychological, anthropological and psychoanalytic. Whereas none of these frameworks offer a holistic view of the family, they do offer alternative ways to describe its many different facets.

A comprehensive family assessment includes data pertaining to all these frameworks. Family data must be obtained in a thorough and systematic manner. Before beginning actual data collection with a specific family or family members, the nurse must first learn as much as she can about the family in general. Keeping abreast of current literature and research on the family will assist the nurse in designing her own systematic approach to family assessment. The reader is referred to Chapters 1, 2 and 4 for a review of family development, function and life styles.

The discussion that follows is a summary of several possible approaches to family assessment. A format for use by the beginning practitioner is then described, along with guidelines in how to obtain the assessment data.

APPROACHES TO FAMILY ASSESSMENT

A Family Developmental Framework

The family developmental framework is a useful one for the nurse to employ when describing families and family members. This approach allows the nurse to analyze the family system at different periods in its development as well as to anticipate changes in the family group over time. Aldous[1] discusses four systematic characteristics of the family: (1) family interdependency, (2) selective boundary maintenance, (3) adaptability to and initiation of change and (4) family task performance.

Family interdependency varies according to the stage of family development. For example, parent-child interdependency will be greatest during the child's younger years and will lessen as the child prepares for launching from the family group. The degree of interdependency will also vary according to the individual's and family's stage in the life cycle. Power in family decisions may indicate the dependence of certain family members on each other as well as the stage of family life. *Selective boundary maintenance* refers to the identity of the family system. Aldous describes several characteristics of the family that contribute to its boundary maintenance: a separate residence, kinship terminology (e.g., dad, mother, kid brother), shared experiences, shared rituals. Family boundaries may be impinged upon by external agencies; however, external interactions do contribute resources to the family unit to retain its identity.

Adaptability to change depends on the interdependencies of family members and its boundary-setting characteristics. The family must set goals for itself that do not conflict with goals of individual members and the expectations of external agents. If there is conflict between any of these, the family must utilize feedback processes to adapt to or initiate change. Such events as the birth of a baby, marriage of a child, or a mother taking a job outside the home will require the family unit to change such things as communication patterns or decision-making processes.

Family task performance refers to the tasks, or functions, the family system must perform to meet family goals (see Chapter 1). Family tasks or functions vary in difficulty and in importance throughout the family life cycle. For example, physical maintenance is a major task in early infancy and childhood and in retirement, whereas social control is important in early childhood and later in adolescence. Also, external influences (see Chapter 2) on family boundaries may complicate or facilitate the family's ability to adapt to or initiate change when meeting its tasks.

Duvall's[3] theory of family development can be used to assist the nurse in assessing the family's stage of development and in planning with the family for tasks currently being dealt with or to be anticipated. Evaluation of the family is assisted by determining whether a family is achieving these developmental tasks. (An adapted summary of the tasks is described in Table 1–2, Chapter 1.) The nurse should also evaluate the extent or quality to which those tasks are being achieved. If family composition differs from the nuclear makeup, the developmental tasks must be adapted to the family group represented. It is important to examine the functions within each family and to gain insight into the family members' understanding of their responsibility and role development in respect to identified functions.

A Family Systems Framework

A systems approach views the family as the system and individual family members as subsystems. Lego[6] identifies four basic issues for the nurse to investigate utilizing the systems approach. The first issue is termed *individual boundaries*. This involves determining if the family unit allows the individual family member to develop an individual identity while sustaining a desire within that family member to contribute to the family identity. A continuum with "the family" focus on one end and "the individual" focus on the other is one way to picture this concept. A second concept is the *multi-generational transmission process*. This concept refers to identifiable family patterns that have recurred or are recurring in different generations of the family. The third issue, *triangling*, assists the nurse in identifying family interrelationships. Triangles assist the nurse in assessing areas of fusion versus differentiation in the family. A family genogram may be adapted to identify perpetuating family behaviors or interaction patterns throughout generations. For example, Lego's fourth concept is the *level of family differentiation*. This involves identifying the individual family member's sense of worth or separateness. This concept refers to people being attracted to people like themselves, that is, people with similar family backgrounds and systems, similar ways of thinking and feeling. Bowen[2] discusses the differentiation in the individual as ranging from little sense of self or lowest level to a high sense of self. The level of differentiation a family member has will infleunce his proneness to physical versus mental illness. A low level of differentiation will complicate a parent's ability to meet the basic functions of the family.

Crisis as a Framework

Crisis theory also represents a valuable resource for the nurse. It assists in anticipating normal maturational developmental and situational crises. It also assists in identifying and anticipating the individual's or family's ability to cope effectively with any identified crisis.

Family Strengths Framework

Otto[8] presents a framework for the assessment of family strengths and resources. Thirteen assessment criteria are identified that contribute to family unity and the development of family potential:

1. The ability to meet physical, emotional, spiritual needs.
2. Joint responsibility for childrearing.
3. Effective communication.
4. Ability to provide support, security and encouragement.
5. Ability to initiate and maintain growth-producing relationships within and outside the family.
6. Formation of responsible community relationships.
7. Use of home as a growth matrix for adults and children.
8. Ability to help themselves and to accept help when needed.
9. Flexibility in performing functions and roles.

TABLE 14-1 WHAT IS MEASURED BY THE FAMILY APGAR?

Component	
Adaptation	How resources are shared, or the member's satisfaction with the assistance received when family resources are needed.
Partnership	How decisions are shared, or the member's satisfaction with mutuality in family communication and problem solving.
Growth	How nurturing is shared, or the member's satisfaction with the freedom available within the family to change roles and attain physical and emotional growth or maturation.
Affection	How emotional experiences are shared, or the member's satisfaction with the intimacy and emotional interaction within the family.
Resolve	How time* is shared, or the member's satisfaction with the time commitment that has been made to the family by its members.

*Besides sharing time, family members usually have a commitment to share space and money. Because of its primacy, time was the only item included in the Family APGAR; however, the nurse who is concerned with family function will enlarge her understanding of the family's resolve if she inquires about family member's satisfaction with shared space and money.

Modified from G. Smilkstein. Assessment of family function. In G. Rosen et al, eds., Behavioral Science in Family Practice. Appleton-Century-Crofts, 1980.

10. Mutual respect for individuality of each member.
11. Use of crisis as a means of growth.
12. Concern for family unity, loyalty, cooperation.
13. Flexibility of family strengths.

Family Function Framework

Another tool, Family APGAR[9], is a brief screening questionnaire designed to give an overview of five areas of family function: Adaptability, Partnership, Growth, Affection and Resolve (Table 14-1). It is designed to assist physicians in the clinical setting with general assessment of the child's perception of his family's functional state. The Family APGAR consists of five close-ended questions that may be used with members of any type of family group. The individual family member's responses are scored and indicate that member's satisfaction with the five areas of family function (Table 14-2). It is important to emphasize that this is a screening tool that alerts the health professional to do further evaluation of the family and is not diagnostic of family dysfunction.

GUIDELINES FOR FAMILY ASSESSMENT

The following guidelines are presented to identify significant areas to be assessed when inter-

TABLE 14-2 FAMILY APGAR QUESTIONNAIRE

	Almost Always	Some of the Time	Hardly Ever
I am satisfied with the help that I receive from my family* when something is troubling me.	_____	_____	_____
I am satisfied with the way my family discusses items of common interest and shares problem solving with me.	_____	_____	_____
I find that my family accepts my wishes to take on new activities or make changes in my life-style.	_____	_____	_____
I am satisfied with the way my family expresses affection and responds to my feelings such as anger, sorrow, and love.	_____	_____	_____
I am satisfied with the way my family and I spend time together.	_____	_____	_____

Scoring: The patient checks one of three choices which are scored as follows: "Almost always" (2 points), "Some of the time" (1 point) or "Hardly ever" (0). The scores for each of the five questions are then totaled. A score of 7 to 10 suggests a highly functional family. A score of 4 to 6 suggests a moderately dysfunctional family. A score of 0 to 3 suggests a severely dysfunctional family.

*According to which member of the family is being interviewed the nurse may substitute for the word "family" either spouse, significant other, parents, or children.

From G. Smilkstein. Assessment of family function. In G. Rosen et al., eds., Behavioral Science in Family Practice. Appleton-Century-Crofts, 1980.

viewing the family. They serve as a beginning baseline for the nurse to expand upon. As her knowledge base and clinical expertise increase, she becomes more adept at identifying the unique needs of families.

Assessment information may be gained through interview and questioning, through observation of parent-child interactions and by careful listening to family members' comments. A clear picture of some aspects will require a visit to the home if this is feasible in the nurse-family relationship (community health nurse, family nurse practitioner, school nurse, hospital nurse visiting a patient before admission to or discharge from the hospital), or through feedback from other professionals who have visited the home (social worker, mental health worker).

Ideally, a family assessment should be obtained from all members within the family group. It is best completed entirely within the family's home environment. Within the home setting, the nurse can gather a more complete observational data base in regard to such things as environment, sociocultural variables and interaction patterns of family members. These observations must be documented and assessed, as must all other components in the data base. In Chapter 13 (see History Guidelines), significant content areas in the family and social histories are outlined. It is anticipated that basic demographic data have been collected before a family assessment.

The Family Unit Age (chronological and developmental), sex, and the relationship of each family member to the other is recorded. The family unit is comprised of all individuals who reside in the home itself as well as significant others who interact regularly with the family unit. Significant others may include babysitters or close friends who spend a significant amount of time with the child. This information assists the nurse in determining the type of family unit the child is part of — nuclear, extended, single-parent, blended, and so on. Ordinal (birth order) position of the child is also valuable information to be obtained.

Residence A description of the dwelling (house, apartment, room) and its environment is included. There should be a description of the home and its condition, developmental stimuli apparent in the home (books, games, toys) and number of rooms in the dwelling. The neighborhood (location, community resources located in or near the neighborhood, general level of upkeep) should be described. Any environmental hazards present in the home and neighborhood environs (stairs without railings, busy intersection only 20 feet from house, no fenced-in play area) should be identified. The nurse may ask the family members to list hazards they are aware of to get an idea of their recognition of health hazards. (See Chapter 13 under Family Social History for further description of data appropriate to this section.)

Significant Family Events Separations, divorce, marriage, a new child, a move, a death — major life events may all significantly influence the family's and child's behavior patterns. These events may also influence the family's socioeconomic resources, coping mechanisms and decision-making process in respect to health care. Identification by the family of these significant events will assist the nurse in assessing the family's perceptions of its own strengths, weaknesses and potential problems. Questions to ascertain what the family members have done or think they could do to resolve any problems or crises also gives the nurse information about the family's level of problem-solving skills. The nurse may also evaluate the family's readiness for and interest in information or education that would help with problem resolution.

The nurse should remember that shared family experiences, rituals and even crises may contribute to family solidarity and identity.

Health History This information includes past and present illnesses in any family member significantly influential to family unit functioning. It provides information in regard to stressors the family and child are exposed to as well as illnesses or problems that are hereditary or familial. The nurse also should gain information about the family's past experiences with and understanding of health and health care, compliance with therapy, and decision-making in respect to health issues.

Interrelationships It may be difficult to obtain an accurate picture of family interrelationships during a single home visit. A continuing professional relationship with the family will increase the level of trust that facilitates collection and verification of data. As mentioned earlier, a family pedigree or genogram can give the health care professional a visual representation of family relationships and of behaviors that are recurring patterns through generations. The following are significant aspects of interrelationships to be observed or discussed with the family unit:

1. What bonds keep this family together (family identity)?
2. How closely bonded is each member to the family unit?
3. How are decisions made within the family? Who contributes?
4. Who or what represents power in this family unit? How is this power displayed? Is this power an indicator of appropriate dependency of the family member on other members? Is this dependency appropriate to the family stage?
5. Are family roles or interdependencies clearly defined or overlapping? Are they appropriate for the chronological and developmental age of each member?
6. Are family roles assigned or are they developed out of circumstance?
7. Are there role conflicts?
8. What are the functional requirements (developmental tasks) of this family? Are they being satisfied?
9. Do family members communicate? How? Is it effective communication? What triangles exist?
10. How are resources shared in this family?
11. How are affection, anger, sadness, fear shared between family members? (Is any member used as a scapegoat during stressful times?) Who does each family member approach with problems or during crisis? During times of elation?

Resources Each family unit requires external and internal support to adapt to and initiate change. In general it is important to identify the resources that are known to the family and that are given priority by it. Decision-making regarding their use is also explored.

Economic support (can the family "make ends meet?") is a significant external resource. Size of income is not a good indicator of a family's ability to maintain itself. Today, economic stress is common and may be due to inability of an income to meet rising costs rather than to the amount of the income. Economic stress may undermine other family strengths.

It is important to identify who the wage earners are in the family. Does the family rent or own its own home? Do members desire to budget? Have they sought assistance with budgeting? What financial resources are used by the family (food stamps, Medicaid, infant supplement programs, and so on)?

Education may provide greater flexibility and mobility in the occupations of family members. The educational level of the parents or other family members may also negatively or positively affect the child's educational motivation and experience. It is important to assess how education is viewed by the family. Is it viewed as personal growth or a way of "moving up?" Did the parents do well in school? Do they promote achievement in all areas or primarily academic achievements? Educational level and cognitive ability of the family will influence how and where the nurse begins health education and counselling as well as to what degree the family can participate actively in problem-solving.

The family's relationship with the health care system may provide them with yet another resource. However, factors such as language barriers, inadequate income, lack of transportation, low priority in the family for health needs, and dissatisfaction with past health care may all cause health care to be an ineffective resource for that particular family. It is important to make sure the family is aware of health resources that they may be able to use.

Another resource area for the family includes social interaction. This area includes well-balanced communication with friends, relatives, community organizations, clubs, and so on outside of the family group itself. Does the family know where to go to get help or assistance when needed? Does this increase the family's selective boundary maintenance and strengthen its identity?

Cultural or ethnic background may also be a valuable resource for the family during stress. It is also important for the nurse to determine how culture or ethnic background may influence family relationships, childrearing practices, health beliefs, and so on.

Values and goals represent another area to be assessed by the nurse. Is the family "present-oriented" or "future-oriented?" What is important to this family — what goals do they have? What are family plans to meet these goals? Are these goals appropriate to the family's stage? What is the commitment of each individual family member to identified goals? How is this commitment demonstrated? How do these values positively or negatively affect the family's health status and the status of the child's health?

Religion, or the family's religious preference, may successfully provide spiritual and social strength to the family. It is also necessary to observe for evidence of religion in the home and to determine if the family's view of the importance of religion in life influences its values and functions and the interactions between individual members. The problem-solving ability of the family may be limited by certain doctrinal beliefs. Overcommittment or undercommittment to religious activities may alienate individual family members and decrease their value as a resource to the family. In regard to health care, such issues as birth control, abortion and blood transfusions may be affected by religious belief.

Childrearing Practices It is important to assess how discipline is exercised and who is responsible for discipline in the family. Does the family use verbal or physical discipline or a combination? How were the parents disciplined as children? How is acceptable behavior rewarded? Another area is how the child is expected to learn in life (by example or role-modeling, experimentation, through error and so on). This may also include what the parents think a child must learn in life (to be strong, to be sensitive, to be successful). Do parents disagree about any areas of childrearing? How have they resolved these areas of disagreement? It is also vital to assess the parent's description of each child. What do parents cite as the best aspect of their child's personality? Is there any aspect that they would change? How well do they understand their own and their child's developmental stage? How has this affected their interactions with the child? What changes are they anticipating in the next year for the child? For themselves?

Activities of Daily Living Daily activities give insight into the family's identity and task development. Sleeping, eating and recreational activities are important areas to consider. What are the sleeping patterns of family members? Where do members sleep? Do family members receive enough rest for their individual and developmental needs? On the subject of food, does culture influence food practices? Does the family eat together? Who is responsible for preparation of meals? Are individual nutritional demands met? Are meals served at regular times? What group and individual recreational activities are enjoyed? How often? How many hours of television does the family watch per week?

These guidelines are a basic assessment outline for the nurse. If data collection has been done systematically with an appropriate factual and conceptual knowledge base, the nurse will be able to interpret and assess the unique family unit. The family and nurse will then be able to identify family strengths, weaknesses and problem areas. This is most readily accomplished by using information from the assessment to determine how well the family is accomplishing both family developmental tasks (see Table 1–2 in Chapter 1) and family member developmental tasks (see Table 10–2, Chapter 10). Family members who are not fulfilling their responsibilities in a given task may be identified from the data in those areas in which family or individual member functioning is inadequate.

Planning intervention necessarily involves family members, since they will be the ones required to take action to change. Developing interventions drawn from family strengths and positive support systems is important to success. Mobilization of potential strengths and support systems may also be necessary. The nurse can help family members identify ways they can work to correct existing weaknesses or limitations. If resources outside the family are required, the nurse can inform the family of the use of these resources and help them make contact if necessary.

Implementing the plan is primarily up to the family. However, the nurse can motivate the family by increasing their knowledge base, backing them in the solutions they choose to try, and reinforcing them with praise and encouragement throughout the course of the intervening activities. If several resources are being utilized, the nurse can help the family coordinate those contributions.

As the nurse grows in knowledge, she will develop more precise, well-organized concepts in regard to the family and develop greater expertise in applying them to "fit" the unique family unit, both in terms of family assessment and intervention.

References

1. J. Aldous. Family Careers. John Wiley & Sons, 1978
2. M. Bowen. Use of family theory in clinical practice, In Changing Families, J. Haley, ed., Grune and Stratton, 1971
3. E. Duvall. Marriage and Family Development, 5th ed. J. B. Lippincott, 1977
4. M. Good et al. The family APGAR Index: a study of construct validity. Journal of Family Practice, June 1978
5. R. Hill and D. Hansen. The identification of conceptual frameworks utilized in family study. Marriage and Family Living, 1960 p. 299
6. S. Lego. Family theory and application. In Comprehensive Psychiatric Nursing. J. Haber, et al., McGraw-Hill, 1978
7. I. Nye and F. Berardo. Emerging Conceptual Frameworks in Family Analysis. Macmillan, 1966
8. H. Otto. Criteria for assessing family strength. Family Process, September 1963, p. 329
9. G. Smilkstein. The family APGAR: a proposal for a family function test and its use by physicians. Journal of Family Practice, Nov/Dec, 1978, p. 1231

Additional Recommended Reading

N. Ackerman. Psychodynamics of Family Life. Basic Books, 1958

E. Eichel. Assessment with a family focus. JPN and Mental Health Services, January 1978, p. 11

J. Eshleman. The Family: An Introduction. Allyn and Bacon, 1978

G. Francis and B. Munjas. Manual of Sociopsychologic Assessment. Appleton-Century-Crofts, 1976

S. Holt and T. Robinson. The schools nurse's family assessment tool. American Journal of Nursing, May 1979, p. 950

D. Hymovich, and M. Barnard. Family Health Care, 2nd ed. McGraw-Hill Book Co., 1979

R. Moos et al. Preliminary Manual for Family Environment Scale. Consulting Psychologists Press Inc., 1974

W. Ogburn. The changing family. The Family, July 1938, p. 139

H. Otto. A framework for assessing family strengths. In Family Centered Community Nursing by A. Reinhardt and P. Quinn. C. V. Mosby Co., 1973

15 MANAGING HEALTH

by Jo Joyce Tackett, BSN, MPHN

Health, or wellness, is something each of us experiences and is an accepted fact of life for most. It is manifested in our behaviors. However, health is not guaranteed or automatic, regardless of how we behave or the quality of our living style. To be healthy, a person must be able to display behavior that helps him adapt in a healthy manner to life situations (i.e., health-promoting behavior). Health-promoting behavior is manifested when the individual (1) identifies and accepts reality, (2) actively adjusts when his environment (internal or external) changes, (3) holds a wholesome outlook or attitude toward himself and life in general, and (4) takes on developmentally appropriate responsibility for managing his own health.[2, 11]

HEALTH PROMOTION AS A NURSING GOAL

There are several factors that justify and in fact necessitate a health promotion orientation in the nursing care of children. Our children are the future of our world, and its positive progress requires not just their survival but their development as persons who are healthy physically, psychosocially and intellectually.

Most of the diseases that cause morbidity or mortality in children are preventable when health-promoting practices are employed, and their reduction alone significantly decreases the economic and social burdens on the nation. Since young children are unable to articulate or identify their own health needs, parents and other caretakers must learn and adopt behaviors that promote their own health. They are then more likely to be sure that the health needs of their young children are met. Likewise, the use of rational health practices early in life (mostly achieved through emulation of caretaker role models) significantly increases the likelihood that these practices will be retained throughout the child's life. Because of these factors, the goals of nursing practice with children and their families should be to promote individual motivation for health and facilitate the use by family members of their own resources to identify their health needs, and to effectively cope and take responsiblity for maintaining their own health (self-care).

Identifying Personal Health Needs (Decision to Act)

Identifying what one considers healthy and what one needs or is required to do to preserve health is determined by subjective reality. What a child or his caretakers believe to be good or right for him influences whether or not he will engage in health-promoting activities. The health needs a child or his family recognizes vary with their age, sex, educational level, cultural orientation, and the parents' financial status and occupations. The more susceptible the child is believed to be to a health problem and the more serious the perceived consequence if health promotional behavior is not performed, the more readily will parents or the child himself adopt the behavior.

The nurse's task then is to help the child or his parents or both recognize the child's susceptibility and the potential consequences if health behaviors are not enacted. Deciding whether a problem exists that merits their attention is ultimately the family's responsibility. The nurse must work within the framework of their values and beliefs to help them see health as being a salient need. The nurse's efforts will be more successful if the action required to maintain health is made feasible in relation to the family's life style and economic status.

Developing Problem-Solving Skills (Direction Action Will Take)

Recognizing a health need does not guarantee that the child or his parents will take any action to meet that need. A prerequisite to action is knowing the possible action(s) to be taken to resolve the need. The process necessary to arrive at action alternatives is called problem-solving. The family derives its problem-solving options from a variety of sources, each of which the nurse must consider in order to understand and support the decision made by the child or family. Common sources include:

1. Family or cultural tradition. The option a family has used in the past to deal with a health need persists as long as it seems to work. The family is most familiar with and best able to employ this option. Repetition of that option is encouraged by the endorsement received from the extended family or cultural group.
2. Social or peer incentives. The group with which the child or family identifies presents a recommended option. The more a child or parent feels the need for that group's approval, the more likely this option is to be selected. The role the individual holds within that group also influences to what extent he is expected to adopt the recommended option.
3. Information from mass media, including health media to the extent that the child or family is exposed to it. The degree to which mass media information influences the option chosen depends upon how much personal meaning the message has to the child or parent. Studies have shown that mass media appeals that stress personal and social consequences are more effective in influencing behavior than those stressing bodily damage.[12] For example, an advertisement that discourages smoking because it decreases the person's ability to maintain endurance during active sports or because it causes bad breath will have more impact than an ad that discourages smoking because it leads to cancer or heart disease. The exception to this is the case of an individual who knows someone who has experienced the bodily damage or for whom the recommended healthy behavior has worked.
4. Information from a source whom the child or parent respects as knowledgeable and whom he believes cares sincerely about him as an individual. For the infant and young child his primary caretaker(s) is that significant source. To the extent that the child's basic needs are met consistently and adequately, he is informed that those needs and the practices employed to meet them are important (valued, given priority). Figure 15–1 shows the relationship of these early experiences to the development of behavior promoting or not promoting health.

The task of the nurse becomes one of assisting the family or child to evaluate the various options in terms of the probable consequences of each and then to nonjudgmentally support efforts to carry out the option. The nurse can aid the child and the family to evaluate consequences. This is done by asking them to enumerate the things they can expect to do or can continue to do that they enjoy if the option is carried out. They are then asked to identify the things they could not expect to do or could no longer do that they enjoy if that option is not carried out. This approach, rather than a focus on potential pathology, to which they cannot relate because they have not experienced it, allows them a personal identification with each option evaluated, since they can relate the option to experiences with which they are familiar (things they enjoy).

The nurse must be ready to handle her feelings when the option the child or family chooses is not the one she considers most desirable. Recognition that there is no one right way to maintain health, that many possible actions may achieve that goal, is essential. The nurse must also realize that her "ideal" option is often not the most *feasible* option for a family or for an individual child. There are levels or

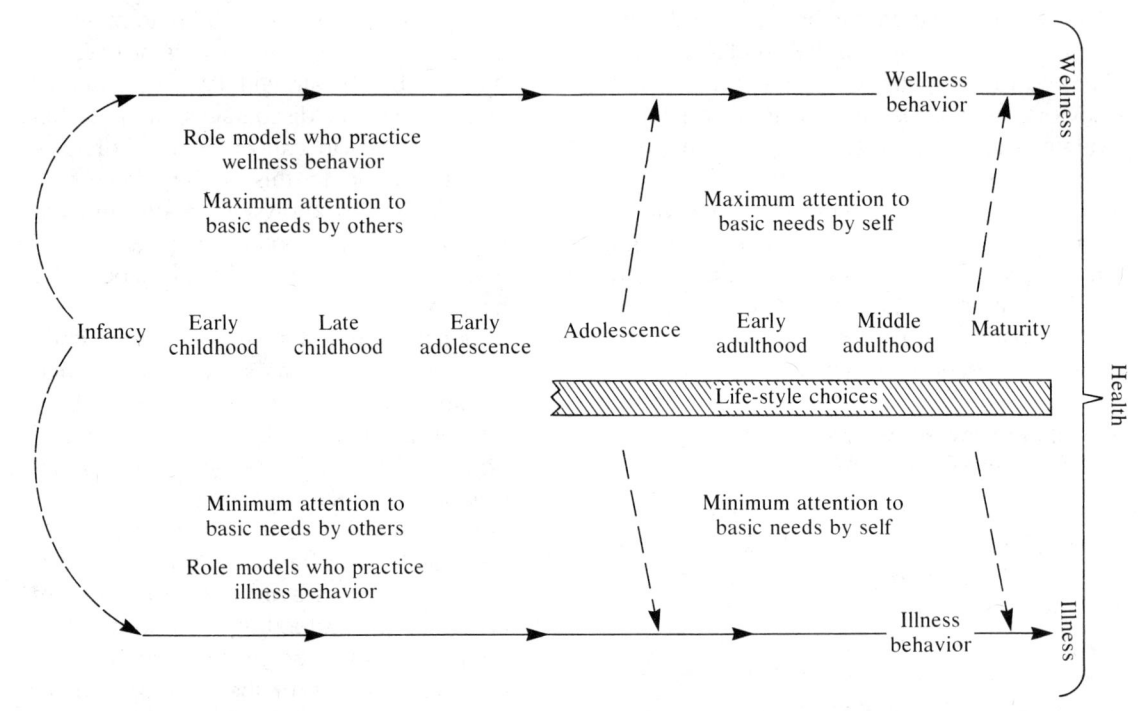

Figure 15-1 Development of wellness or illness-seeking behavior. (Reprinted with permission of Charles B. Slack publishers and the authors John J. Bruhn and F. David Cordova.)

degrees of ideal, and action taken at each level is healthier than no action taken to promote health. If the nurse helps the child and the family to carry out the option they choose, even though it does not measure up to her ideal, she has helped them move toward health. Success in that option readies them to try next a higher-level option (closer to the ideal established by the health profession). When optimal courses of action are not chosen, the nurse can evaluate with the individuals why they chose the course they did and offer additional information to clarify misconceptions, convey that the option chosen may not be the best one, and augment more informed decision making. Reasonable choices should be reinforced and encouraged.

The extent to which the nurse actively participates in the child's and the family's problem solving decreases as their skill in that process increases. Temporary dependence on the health professional can sometimes be healthy and necessary; we should expect parents and children to be dependent in some situations, especially during crises, and in other situations they should be expected to be independent and self-reliant. Allowing some dependence on health care personnel while the child and the family is learning greater skill in problem solving or decision making is important to their health care and health education.

Responsibility for Self-Care (Taking Action)

Once behaviors have been identified that aim to promote health, action must be taken to carry out those behaviors. To carry out a behavior requires knowledge of how it is performed and the ability to resolve any barriers that interfere with enacting it. Table 15–1 summarizes major factors (potential barriers) influencing behavior enactment.

In the early months of life, the child is totally dependent on his caretakers to carry out the behaviors that will ensure his health, but as the child develops and acquires skills of daily living himself, he becomes increasingly able to assume more responsibility in maintaining his own health. Thus, by the time a child reaches young adulthood he is also capable of being fully responsible for his own health maintenance.

Achieving this level of responsibility requires that caretakers and health personnel allow the growing child progressively more opportunity to (1) be involved in his own health care (identify his own health needs, determine how to meet those needs, and acquire knowledge, skills and attitudes essential to meet those needs), (2) assume responsibility for his own

TABLE 15-1   FACTORS INFLUENCING PREVENTIVE HEALTH ACTION

Personal Readiness	Social Factors (Influence of the Environment)	Situation Factors (Attributes of the Action)
1. Recognize consequences of not adopting behavior and consider them personally important	1. Family/cultural pressure to carry out behavior	1. How likely the behavior is to maintain health
2. Accept personal vulnerability to unhealthy state	2. Social or peer group pressure to carry out behavior	2. Pleasure gained in performing the behavior
3. Adopt positive attitude about doing something to decrease that vulnerability	3. Are congruent with perceived role expectations	3. Effort required to perform it
4. Believe that behaviors do exist that can decrease vulnerability or satisfy health need	4. Are not in conflict with personal values and beliefs, lifestyle	4. Environmental conditions (middle column) make carrying out the behavior possible (feasibility)
5. Prove to be intellectually, emotionally and physically able to carry out behavior	5. Economic resources to carry out behavior exist	5. How appealing the behavior is to the individual
6. Know behavior(s) that will satisfy health need or decrease personal vulnerability		6. How promptly behavior can be carried out once the decision has been made to act; how often behavior must occur

Adapted from R. Wu. Behavior and Illness. Prentice-Hall, Inc., 1973.

MANAGING HEALTH   261

healthy and unhealthy habits and their consequences and (3) assume responsibility for contacting and relating effectively to health care providers.

NURSING PROCESSES IN HEALTH PROMOTION

Promoting personal responsibility for health by children and their families may occur in a variety of settings, including the clinic, hospital, home, doctor's office, school, or any other setting where the nurse interacts with children and families.

The processes by which the nurse motivates this responsibility for self-care are also the same regardless of the setting. They include establishing rapport and providing support, teaching, counselling and therapeutic referral.

Establishing a Working Relationship

The essentials for a working (cooperative) relationship are trust, empathy and genuineness shared mutually by each person involved in the interaction. Each participant comes with his own values, needs and perceptions of what the relationship will accomplish. Trust is most quickly established when the nurse responds in a consistent, nonjudgmental manner that conveys acceptance of and alliance with the child and parent. Empathy is communicated to the child or parent when the nurse takes seriously the concerns expressed, whether they are expressed verbally or nonverbally. The nurse's questions, asked to help her discover the child's and parent's perceptions of their needs, show that she cares, that she considers them worthwhile and that she wants to understand how they are feeling. Being genuine is extremely important when dealing with children, as they are particularly alert to insincerity. The nurse should be honest with the child and the parent at all times and make no promises that cannot be carried out. If possible, the nurse should position herself at the child's level during any interaction with him and avoid artificial barriers between herself and her clients, such as desks or counters. A working relationship is seldom established immediately, and the child will frequently test the nurse to assure himself that the relationship with her is still stable. Often, the best approach to the child is through the medium of shared play. Parents respond more quickly when the nurse's approach considers their needs first (even small ones such as making sure they are comfortable or that they have a cup of coffee).

When the nurse models the behaviors necessary to a good working relationship, her client, whether a child or adult, is given guidelines for his behavior in the relationship. Once he becomes comfortable in this behavior, cooperative interaction is possible.

SUPPORTIVE NURSING ACTIONS

The modern family not infrequently feels isolated from the resources that might help them make decisions regarding health, especially from the wisdom of the older generation extended family. The health profession has recognized this fact and accepted greater responsibility for providing information and support services that were formerly readily available within the family itself.[4] Parents now expect the health professional to understand and reinforce their own strategies of parenthood and childrearing. Becoming well acquainted with the

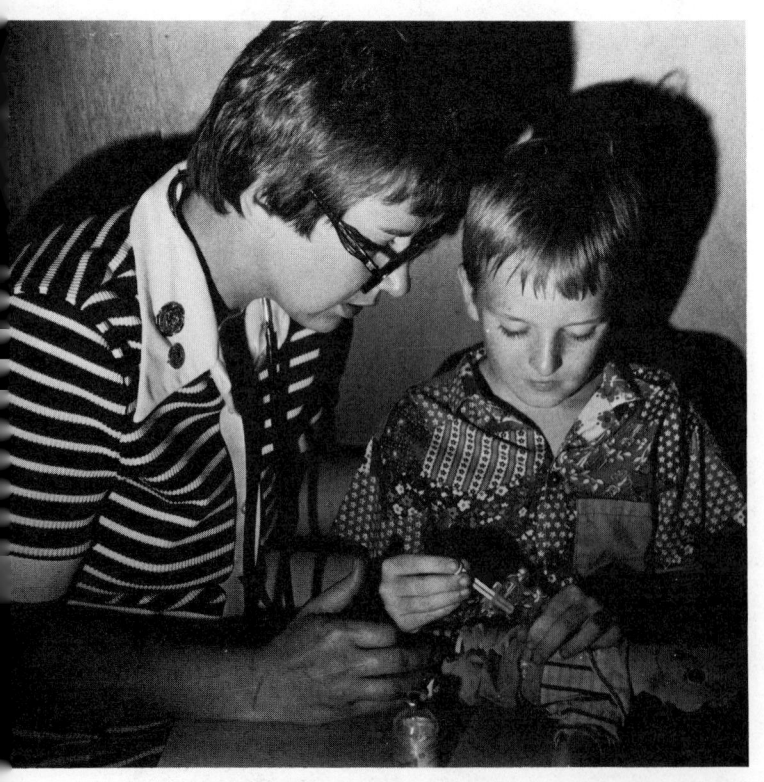

Whenever possible, the nurse should position herself at the child's level during any interaction with him.

characteristics of the family that so strongly influence a child's health is economical of both the nurse's time and resources. Unless caretakers have their dependent needs met, we cannot expect that they will do well in meeting their children's developmental needs.

The support that parents or caretakers request from the nurse involves building up their confidence and self-esteem as persons and parents, providing information on successfully meeting their child's needs and encouraging him to steadily assume responsibility for his own health, and giving reinforcement of their own credibility as parents.

Building Parental Self-Esteem

Very simple actions by the nurse, if genuinely employed, will build parents' self-esteem. These actions can be carried out during even brief contacts with them. The most gratifying experience for any of us is to be addressed by our name. When the nurse addresses the parent (or child) by name, she communicates that she acknowledges him to be a recognizable, unique person rather than "just another parent." Casual statements by the nurse such as "Mrs. Jones, you are feeding Bobby properly. He is gaining just the amount in weight and height that he should be for his age" reassure the caretaker that positive changes are occurring in the child because of her care. It takes five seconds to say, but it adds immeasurably to the caretaker's confidence. Equally supportive are comments that help the family see their child's positive responses to them: for example, "See how Tommy follows you with his eyes? You are important to him. He seeks you out," or "Beth talks of you frequently and pretends she is you in her play at the day care center. You are obviously very special to her." Not only do such statements support the caretaker's confidence as a parent, they also stimulate positive feelings in the parent toward the child.

An approach that acknowledges the feelings, needs and well-being of the family and not just the child is also a supportive action. A statement such as "How is the rest of the family reacting to Susie's temper tantrums?" or "How are you managing your need for rest while David is ill?" communicates the nurse's understanding that the child's needs and behaviors affect all family members.

Phone calls or home visits that are initiated by the nurse also build parents' self-esteem. These convey her personal interest in the family and their child and her willingness to take their needs seriously. An additional benefit to the nurse is that her assessment and diagnostic capacities are increased by this exposure to the family.

Information to Increase Parenting Success

The specific kinds of information parents (and children) need to promote the child's health are discussed later in this chapter. In addition to the specific skills the nurse can teach parents, supportive actions can be taken to enhance the parent-child relationship within which successful parenting occurs.

The nurse should use every possible opportunity to develop parents' awareness of their child's assets as well as his deficits. Establishing the child's assets (physical, mental or social) helps to personify him to his parents in a positive manner. Stressing the developmental normalcy of their child's behaviors as well as those behaviors that convey his own individual personality reassures parents that their child is progressing and that any developmentally associated negative behavior is only temporary and not caused by faulty parenting techniques.

Allowing parents (especially first-time parents) telephone access to a health professional on a 24-hour basis during stressful times is also a supportive action. Such action is seldom abused by parents; each call a parent makes to a health professional resource is a cry for support at some level.

Reinforcing Parental Credibility

The nurse has an obligation to support families within the context of their cultural beliefs, parenting practices and selected life style. Associated with that support is a responsibility to gently and tactfully introduce those scientific practices and facts essential to health in such a way that they do not conflict with the family's beliefs and values. This task admittedly challenges the nurse's most creative abilities, but it is essential if the goal of self-initiated healthy living is to become a reality. The nurse can begin by favorably accepting the caretaker's (or child's) intentions as well as abilities. For example, during an examination of an infant with an umbilical hernia the nurse may note that the mother has taped a coin over the hernia (a culturally motivated behavior). She compliments the mother on her good intention by saying, "I see you're taking measures to attempt to correct your baby's hernia. You are right to be concerned." She then gently introduces scientific facts that complement rather than conflict with the mother's belief that measures must be taken to reduce the hernia by saying, "It has been discovered that placing the baby on his tummy frequently each day will help reduce the hernia by strengthening his tummy muscles. Most babies like to be on their tummies anyway so this measure is easy for the mother and the baby is comfortable since he does not have to contend with itching or pulling from tape or a binder. This position also helps him learn the head control he needs before he can sit." Thus the nurse has praised the mother's intention to care for her baby, she has given her an easier way to do so, and she has done this without being in conflict with the cultural attitude that measures should be taken to reduce umbilical hernias.

Another example of complimenting intent is demonstrated in the following situation. A mother brings her child to the clinic with an ear infection. When the nurse enters to get a history and examine the child, the mother states that she was going to bring the child in two days ago but she could not get transportation until today. An appropriate statement from the nurse might be "It was good that you tried to bring her in two days ago. The earlier we begin treating infections, the quicker they are brought under control and the less likely the child is to have serious consequences." This statement compliments the mother on her intentions and gives her factual information to utilize the next time she must make a similar decision regarding her child's health. The statement also avoids judgment or blaming by the nurse.

The nurse should make use of every opportunity to convey confidence in the parents' ability to make health judgments and to trust their own feelings and their ability to act to promote the child's health. The feeling of success the nurse helps to engender in the child's caretakers in one situation encourages them to act successfully in others.

The supportive actions identified here to promote healthy parenting are equally functional in supporting children as they attempt to assume self-initiated care.

THE NURSE'S TEACHING ROLE

A large amount of nursing care in any setting is teaching. Through teaching the nurse fosters an atmosphere of personalized caring and attempts to help families gain information to competently initiate their own problem solving and overcome the barriers to healthy change in their lives. There is a wealth of information that parents and children can use to their advantage, and the nurse is pressed to communicate it all in the brief contacts she has with family members. Because of the brevity of contact, the nurse should recognize that all moments while a parent waits are precious teaching opportunities, and each procedure or treatment offered lends itself to simultaneous teaching.

Teaching may be done formally in a planned situation such as a parent education or school health class. Teaching more often is informal or incidental, occurring at any opportune moment and prompted by immediately identified need. The three most prominent forms of incidental learning are imitation of role models, task repetition and positive environmental feedback. In any situation, active teaching is usually more effective. Active teaching utilizes actions more than words to convey the necessary information.

A technique the nurse may use to teach actively is role modelling. At any age, individuals learn more from the teacher's actions than from her words. This is especially true of children and adults who feel insecure in the parent role, since they tend to capitalize on imitation to learn skills. A second technique is demonstration to clarify verbal instruction. A third is role playing, puppet play, games using role reversal, and psychodrama. These take more time but are extremely effective in increasing the learner's sensitivity to others' feelings or circumstances. A fourth technique is learner participation in tasks, reinforced by visible or tangible rewards for effort as well as accomplishment. One learns best when one performs or practices under supervision those skills one must eventually manage on one's own. Rewards can be used to motivate repetition to master the task. As a general rule of thumb, the more educated the learner is the more likely he is to be able to learn through verbal or written instruction and logical explanation, with or without the use of active teaching techniques.

Teaching Caretakers

Wellness behavior is learned. The overall concept of health and the value it is given indirectly influence health behavior and how readily it is learned. The values parents hold toward health, the level of knowledge they have about health, and the extent to which they practice wellness behaviors greatly influence their child's development of healthy attitudes and behavior. These facts indicate the relevance of teaching parents the facts of healthy living if the goal of developing self-initiated responsibility for health in their children is to be reached.

Parents expect health professionals to be sources of information and education. Hansen and Aradine have identified several critical areas in which parents expect assistance.[4] They want information about:

1. Child development and the parents' role in fostering positive development;
2. Childrearing issues and the rationale for approaches that the health profession recommends;
3. Child behavior, including school, social and learning behavior and how to manage it;
4. The steps to take when caring for an ill child at home and the rationale for this management;
5. Family issues and balancing the needs, care and problems of all family members;
6. How best to utilize and relate to health professionals and other community resources;
7. Identifying and managing problems and needs that parents themselves experience;
8. Family relationships related to issues such as personal and interpersonal crises, illness, divorce or separation, single parenting and extended family issues.

These issues are addressed throughout this book, including nursing actions to help meet the family's informational needs.

Underlying these many expectations brought to the health professional is the parents' desire to succeed in the care of their child and to receive encouragement from the professional that their parenting strategies can succeed. Health-related topics are abundant in consumer media. The nurse should stay abreast of these sources, since parents are likely to apply that information. Then the nurse should answer questions that parents have about such information, validate accurate sources and supply facts when the family has been misled. The nurse can also utilize a variety of techniques in assisting parents to gain knowledge and skills in parenting, applying teaching-learning theory to her approach. But the teaching she does as a role model, demonstrating to parents how to respond to their child through cuddling, talking, listening, touching and praise, is probably the most pertinent knowledge she can impart.

Teaching Children

Too often health teaching about children is directed mostly toward their parents. As Pigeon notes, "Like sponges they (children) silently absorb and ruminate over what they hear.... health teachings should be aimed at children as well as their parents."[9] The child's thoughts should be explored and his concerns, questions and opinions elicited.

If we expect children to steadily assume more responsibility for their own health as they grow, we need to teach them how to manage stress. They must learn ways to reduce stress in their environment, acquire effective coping skills and develop an attitude that is oriented toward health rather than illness. Children need information about what to expect (what they will hear, feel, smell and see) during health care experiences. And, if they are to initiate their own health care, they must learn how to approach health care providers and be assertive with them.

Acquisition of healthy behavior by the child involves four processes. He must develop an *awareness* of health from his role models. He must be exposed to developmentally appropriate *information* about wellness and health practices. If he is to learn responsibility, he must be included as an *active participant* (as early in life as possible) in making health choices so that he can master the problem-solving required to make healthy decisions about his life. And, finally, he must be *reinforced* for his attempts and his successes in practicing wellness behaviors.

Health teaching aimed at children must consider the child's thinking ability at various ages, the concept of health that is characteristic of his

TABLE 15-2 CHARACTERISTIC HEALTH CONCEPT AND COGNITIVE SKILL ON THE BASIS OF AGES, AND EXPECTATIONS FOR TAKING RESPONSIBILITY AND APPROACH TO TEACHING

Age (Years)	Health Concept (8)	Cognitive Level (9)	Age-Related Teaching Approach (9)	Realistic Expectations of Responsibility for Self-Initiated Care (2)
Infancy (0-1)	No concept; learns to value needs on basis of how well and how consistently they are met.	Egocentric.	Consistently and fully meet basic needs.	None—totally dependent on caretakers.
Early childhood (1-4)	No concept; merely imitates behavior of role models that are satisfying and/or earn reward.	Egocentric; preconceptual; does not question own perceptions.	Continue meeting basic needs but steadily demand that child master skills of daily living; role model wellness behaviors; reward his imitation. Play with child to learn his perceptions since he cannot verbalize them adequately.	Some capacity to carry out tasks to promote own health if taught skills and allowed opportunity to take responsibility; likes to practice wellness behaviors.
Middle childhood (5-8)	Concept is that health involves a series of health practices (eat right, brush teeth, stay clean) and health is apparent when the person is able to perform his usual activities.	Egocentric; transductive reasoning; centration: concrete reality predominates.	Encourage his account of what his health needs, what caused it, what he might do to resolve that need—correct misperceptions; use teaching techniques that provide him with tactile, visual, auditory and motor experiences.	Can carry out many tasks to promote own health, seeks responsibility; practice important. Can take independent action to identify many health needs and can identify some realistic solutions.
Late childhood and preadolescent (9-13)	Concept of health as sense of physical well-being as evidenced by "feeling good" or being in shape.	Objective, systematic thought; questions and seeks validation and correction of own perceptions; gradual increase in causal reasoning; decentration but still favors concrete reality.	Share assessment and/or findings; this allows him to perceive changes in health status. Allow time for him to validate his perceptions of his needs and what actions should be taken; respect his views and opinions. Give simple rationale for health practices/procedures. Make invisible processes of health real with diagrams, models. Teach the skill/procedure (tangible, concrete) then give the rationale (abstract) for the skill/procedure in simple terms.	Can plan for and take initiative to carry out most health needs if has learned trust and autonomy. Can actively participate in managing his own health needs. Acute interest in health education. Can consider possible risks and benefits of health behaviors if allowed to participate in problem solving.
Adolescent and young adult (14-21)	Concept of health as physical, emotional, social stability that is long term though superimposed brief illness may cause temporary instability. Evidenced by "feeling good," being in control of self, being able to participate in desired activities.	Realizes realm of possible and hypothetical as well as the real. Develops theories. Craves details for egocentric purposes primarily.	Significant other role models of wellness behavior crucial to overcoming peer pressures. Inform of realities of health problems and the possible outcomes; honesty imperative to his cooperation. Present all details; relate them to him personally. Especially likes theoretical explanations and discussions. Allow discussion of the effects of health problems and health behaviors on him and his future. Let him determine the possible resolutions to his health needs and collaborate with him to determine management. Begin by presenting rationale for a skill/procedure then give details of performing it.	Can assume full responsibility to identify his health needs, determine possible resolutions and carry them out. Can experientially apply wellness to life choices.

266 FAMILIES WITH CHILDREN

age, and the degree of independent action that he is realistically capable of for his stage in development. Table 15-2 describes these various characteristics for children in the various age groups and their relevance in selecting an appropriate teaching approach.

Whatever and wherever the teaching opportunity with a child is, the nurse can take the same basic steps to assist the child to develop problem-solving and coping abilities in health promotion. The only alteration required is in the teaching approach taken, which must be adjusted to the child's age and cognitive capabilities. These steps are:[7]

1. Ask the child what he thinks his problem or need is (he learns problem identification) and whether the problem is important to him (he learns to make health a priority).* This information gives the nurse an understanding of the child's perception of his situation and the priority that health currently is given in his family. This tells the nurse how much health information the child needs before he is likely to cooperate.

2. The nurse then gets an additional history, preferably from the child and then augmented by his caretaker, and does whatever assessment is indicated. Teaching occurs throughout this process as the nurse gives truthful explanations of what the child will see, hear, feel, smell, taste during assessment procedures. Age-appropriate rationale is also given for each procedure. Because young children acquaint themselves with the world through their physical senses, teaching should focus on this aspect of procedures. These children also require visual examples (for example, a procedure done on a doll) and sample sensations (e.g., what a pinch of the skin feels like) to comprehend what to expect. Older school-age children still need explanations regarding expected physical sensations, but they can usually comprehend from verbal explanations alone. Adolescents, although they want to know what physical sensations to expect, are much more interested in the rationale and consequences of each procedure.

3. The child is presented with the important findings uncovered in the nursing assessment. This is a good opportunity to teach names of body organs or explain body processes or both, and what it means when they are altered. How simple and concrete or complex and abstract this teaching must be will depend on the child's age.

4. The nurse interprets the findings to the child in terms of probable cause. For the young child who still perceives people as the cause of all events, the explanation should be prefaced by reassurance that the cause was not himself, his wishes or the wishes of others upon him. The child in late childhood or preadolescence has usually mastered casual relationships enough to grasp a simply presented scientific explanation. The adolescent or young adult will want a detailed scientific explanation. The provision of health information is critical at this time because it now has maximal relevance to the child personally.

5. The nurse elicits the child's opinions of what he thinks ought to be done. Usually the best approach is to have the child list the alternatives he can think of and why he thinks each would help (he learns problem-solving). This task should be the child's responsibility, with the nurse assisting only if the child cannot think of any alternatives on his own. Table 15-3 gives examples of some alternatives children have selected that reflect age-appropriate understanding of their problem or need. Health education is then offered to correct any misconceptions, to increase the child's knowledge of the situation so he can identify more realistic or additional alternatives, or to reinforce accurate perceptions of what will work and why.

6. The child selects the alternative(s) he will carry out, alone or with assistance (he learns decision-making). Before he makes his selection, he should be informed if any of his alternatives are not acceptable because of rules of the setting in which they must be carried out. The child's selection should be written down for him (and/or for those who will assist him to carry it out) and documented in the nurse's records. This becomes a contract between the child, nurse and others involved as to what must by done by each. (See the box on page 269 for a discussion of contracts).

7. The child is asked to identify the resources (personal or in his external environment) that he will need to utilize to carry out his alternative(s). Health teaching that helps the child to become knowledgeable about personal, family or community resources available and how to use them is appropriate.

---

*The question can be stated as "important to his health" once the child is old enough to have a concept of health (see Table 15-2).

TABLE 15–3 EXAMPLES OF REALISTIC HEALTH BEHAVIORS CHILDREN HAVE IDENTIFIED AT VARIOUS AGES

Early Childhood
1. I will brush my teeth after breakfast and at bedtime.
2. I will cover my coughs and sneezes with my hand or a Kleenex.
3. I will drink a glass of milk at breakfast, lunch and supper.

Middle Childhood
1. I will try to remember to wash my hands after using the toilet and before eating.
2. Whenever possible I will change wet shoes and socks or stockings for dry ones.
3. I know what a good breakfast is, and I will try to eat one every day.
4. I will go to bed willingly when I am told to do so.

Late Childhood and Preadolescence
1. I will try to learn to eat some foods that are new to me or that have been prepared in a way which is new to me.
2. I will listen to the morning weather report and dress accordingly.
3. I will try to cooperate with my parents and other adults who help to keep me well.
4. I will keep my hands clean and will also keep them away from my face, especially from my eyes, nose, and mouth, and away from any sores.

Adolescence and Young Adulthood
1. I will study my own posture and try to do the things that will improve it.
2. I know about the four food groups (meats, vegetables, fruits and milk) and I will try to eat foods from each every day.
3. I will take frequent baths and wash my hair at least once each week.
4. I will listen to my parents' point of view in areas in which we disagree and seriously evaluate their points.

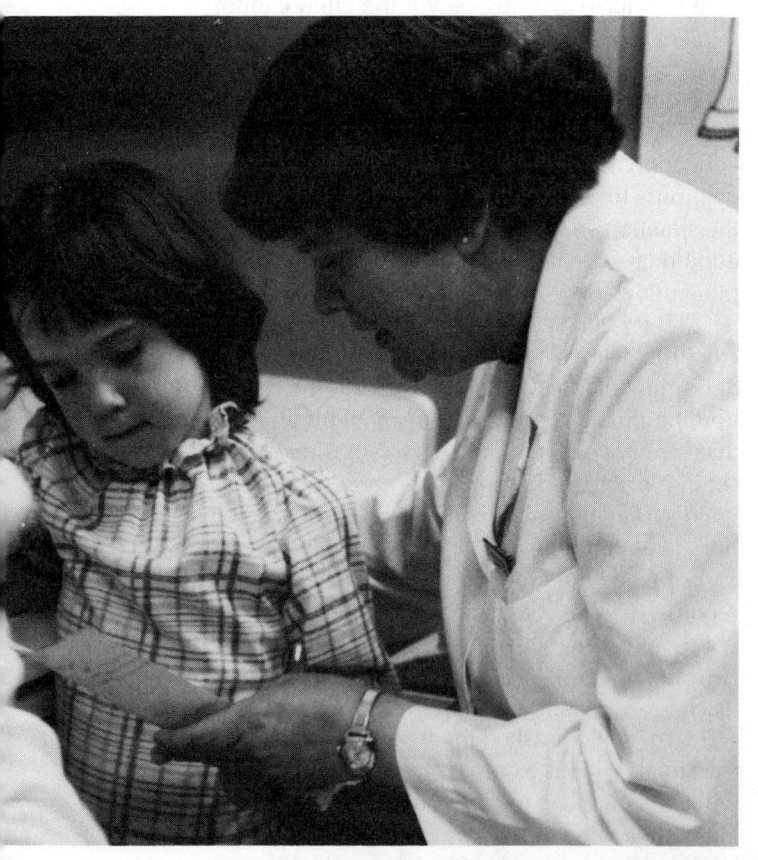

The child selects the alternative(s) she will carry out. This is written down and becomes a contract between the child, nurse and others involved as to what must be done by each.

8. The nurse asks the child what he will do if the same problem or need recurs (reinforces child's ability to be responsible to initiate his own health care).

When the child selects optimal alternatives, this should be reinforced. Inappropriate decisions are not reinforced, and the nurse provides additional information to further clarify the problem and its cause and to help the child see the inappropriateness of his decision.

This approach involves the child actively in identifying his health needs, finding viable solutions and carrying them out. The nurse applies learning, reinforcement and decision-making theories to assist the child to become responsible for his own wellness behaviors.

THE COUNSELLING ROLE

A counselling relationship, whether with a child or his parent, is a two-way interaction involving both verbal and nonverbal communication. Its purposes are (1) to come to a realistic definition or resolution of a problem or both, (2) to increase the client's awareness of himself and his needs, or (3) to get a broader understanding of a situation causing conflict for the client. Many times counselling is the intervention initiated during developmental or situational crises. (Table 15–4 describes common developmental conflicts in families for which the nurse

USING A CONTRACT TO MOTIVATE HEALTHY BEHAVIOR

A contract is a partnership between two parties (nurse and child, parent and child, teacher and child, nurse and family) that specifies mutually agreed upon goals or behaviors and each person's roles in fulfilling the contract. The contract may be informal and verbal (*mutual agreement*) or formal, written and signed by both parties (*contract*).* If positive or negative reinforcers or both are included in the contract, it is called a *contingency contract.* The intent of the contingency contract is to sustain the child's motivation to specific self-care or self-control activities by providing planned consequences for attaining or not attaining the desired goal or behavior.

The contents of the contract depend upon whether it is a mutual agreement, contract or contingency contract. A mutual agreement usually includes a statement of the goal to be reached, the date by which it is to be reached, and each person's responsibilities in achieving the goal. A contract has these same features with the addition of each person's signature to the written document. A contingency contract has all the features of the contract but specifies in addition what the child will gain (reward) for fulfilling his part of the contract and what he will forfeit if he does not fulfill his obligation. The second party to the contract (nurse, parent, teacher) dispenses the rewards or forfeitures as designated in the contract.

Stuart and Homme and co-workers from their research on the effectiveness of behavioral contracts formulated several rules that increase the likelihood of successful behavior change in contingency contracting.[5, 11] These rules can guide the nurse in making contracts with children and their families.

---

*A nursing care plan is a *mutual agreement* if jointly developed with the client and a *contract* if it is jointly developed, written and signed by the nurse and client.

Rule 1. The reward should be immediate.
Rule 2. Initial contracts for a behavior should reward small approximations of the behavior.
Rule 3. The contract should be devised so that rewards are frequent and small amounts.
Rule 4. Performance should be rewarded after it occurs. There is a tendency for the reinforcing party to become lenient or ease up on contract specifics. Such action usually dooms any success in changing behaviors.
Rule 5. The contract should be mutually devised and genuinely agreed on by both parties. Neither should comply out of fear.
Rule 6. Each party must clearly understand what is expected of him and what he can expect in return.
Rule 7. The contact must be followed consistently; otherwise the child interprets forgotten or missed reinforcements as condoning undesirable behavior. (Neglect of contract reinforces and perpetuates the undesired behavior.)
Rule 8. The goal or behavior contracted for as well as the reinforcers must be realistic and achievable.

The contract approach to obtain healthy behaviors in children has several benefits. It clearly identifies the requirements necessary to achieve the goal or solve the problem. The clarification of responsibility a contract affords minimizes confusion, contributes to a trust relationship and provides a vehicle to help the child make a transition from behavioral management by others to self-regulation.[3, 10] The contingency contract is especially successful because human beings, like animals, tend to behave in ways that pay off for them.

---

is most often consulted. Table 15–5 describes situational crises requiring counselling.)

The nurse counselor, to be successful, must develop skills of astute observation, tactful questioning, objective listening, and foremost, allowing the client to choose his own alternatives and solutions. (Refer to Chapters 11 and 12 for a review of play and communication theory, both of which are useful in counselling.) In determining the family members who should be included in a particular counselling situation, a general rule is that all who will be affected by the situation or its resolution should participate in the decision-making. This mutual participation is most successful because it allows each involved family member to gain perspective on the problem and his particular role in its management. An indirect effect is that this approach motivates a cooperative partnership among all members of the counselling relationship, including the nurse counselor.

TABLE 15–4 POTENTIAL DEVELOPMENTAL AREAS OF CHILD-PARENT CONFLICT*

Newborn and Young Infant
Feeding
Crying
Sleeping
Bathing and dressing
Schedules

Older Infant
Feeding
Weaning
Separation
Toilet needs
Sleeping
Crying
Safety measures

Toddler
Self-feeding
Decreasing appetite
Toilet training
Separation
Tantrums
Negativism
Breath-holding
Aggressive behavior
Discipline
Childproofing

Preschooler
Speech
Independence
Sibling rivalry
Sexual curiosity
Bad dreams
Phobias
Discipline
Safety rules

School-age
School adjustment
Conduct disturbances
    Lying
    Cheating
    Stealing
    Bad language
Aggressive behavior
School achievement
Discipline

Adolescent
Independence (adolescent rebellion)
Sexual activity
Drug experimentation
Peer group choices
Delinquent behaviors
    Truancy
    Shoplifting
Nutrition

*Adapted from J. Browden. Needs and Technics for Counseling Parents of Young Children. Clinical Pediatrics, October 1970, p. 601.

TABLE 15–5 SOME SITUATIONAL PROBLEMS REQUIRING COUNSELLING*

Birth of a sibling
Death in the family
Adoption
Divorce or separation
Rape, incest, promiscuity
Child with handicaps
Entry into school and school readiness
Preparation for hospitalization

*Adapted from J. Browder. Needs and Technics for Counseling Parents of Young Children. Clinical Pediatrics, October 1970, p. 601.

The environment can be a valuable adjunct in promoting the counselling relationship and the desired problem-solving. The decor, furniture arrangement, and opportunity the environment allows for the client to initiate contact with the nurse all have significant impact.[6] Colors used, style and texture of furniture and play equipment, and lighting help to convey that the client is welcomed, that his comfort and privacy (not isolation) are the nurse's concern, and that his needs as well as those of the staff have been considered. The decor should emphasize living and health rather than illness and morbidity. Decor and furnishings can also be effective in reminding staff of the needs of the children and families they serve. Any room arrangements or approaches to clients should encourage eye-to-eye contact and conversation; an "assembly line" approach must be avoided. When choices are feasible (which nurse to confer with, which room to have the meeting in) they should be offered, since choices permit the client some sense of control.

The nurse's responsibility as a counselor lies in helping the family attain the counselling goals by evoking their sense of security and self-confidence in handling problems, by offering health information that will help them solve problems, and by guiding them in the decision-making process. However, she is not to be a decision maker for them.

THE NURSE'S ROLE IN REFERRALS

Health promotion is a multi-profession, interdisciplinary responsibility that requires a sharing of skills and cooperative division of labor. The nurse alone cannot possibly manage the complexity of needs that can exist in a family. When it becomes necessary or advantageous to solicit assistance that goes beyond what the nurse has directly available, the appropriate action is to refer family members to resources that can help them.

Such action by the nurse does not absolve her of responsibility for the family but rather adds to her role. To refer appropriately, the nurse must acquaint herself with the many potential health team members on a local, regional and statewide basis. She must know what each resource offers, what its capabilities are (its record of success in handling the problems it professes to be able to manage) and how the family can obtain those services. When a family is to be referred to the resource, the nurse is responsible for informing the family. To attain or maintain the needed services, the nurse may be called upon to act as an advocate for the client or as a liaison (negotiator, mediator) between the client and the resource provider.

If several resources are needed by the family, the nurse is often the team member selected to coordinate the various services in a manner that does not overwhelm the family. (Table 15-6 lists several types of resources.) Collaboration with those in other disciplines is not always easy; it demands that the nurse apply diplomacy and creativity if the family is to obtain the help it needs.

TABLE 15-6 SOME COMMON RESOURCES AVAILABLE TO FAMILIES*

Parenting Education
College and school academic and nonacademic courses
Hospital and clinic classes
Red Cross classes
Mental Health Center classes
Planned Parenthood
Cooperative Extension Services
State and local health departments

Parent Support
Voluntary self-help organizations
Parents Without Partners
Psychologists, social workers, physicians, nurses in private or group practice
Health department nursing services

Children's Self-Initiated Care
School health programs
Children's clinics
Teenage clinics
Walk-in clinics
Alanon
Youth Services Bureau
Project Grow
Head Start, Get Set

Crisis Assistance
Hot lines
Crisis centers
Family and children's services
Clergy
Mental health centers
Project Now
Social services departments of hospitals, government
Runaway and youth counselling services
Legal Aid Society

Financial Assistance/Reduced Fee Health Care
City or County Health Department
　WIC Program
　Well-Child Clinics
　Immunization clinics
　Communicable disease clinics
Crippled Children's Services
　(government program usually located in health department or family and children's services)
Health collectives
Local civic clubs

*To find what is available in a specific area, begin with the yellow pages of a phone book (social services organizations, psychologists, city or county listings, Health Services headings).

SUMMARY

One of the goals of nursing is promoting the health of children and their families wherever and whenever the opportunity exists. Development of wellness behavior is achieved by helping the child and his family learn to identify their health needs, to do realistic problem-solving, and to be responsible for their own health. The nurse's supportive role, as well as her roles as teacher, counselor, and advocate, liaison, and coordinator in referrals, facilitates healthy family living.

References

1. J. Browder. Needs and technics for counseling parents of young children. Clinical Pediatrics, October 1970, p. 599
2. J. Bruhn and F. Cordova. A developmental approach to learning wellness behavior. Part 1: Infancy to early adolescence. Health Values: Achieving High Level Wellness, Nov/Dec 1977, p. 246
3. D. Gelfand and D. Hartmann. Child Behavior. Pergamon Press, 1975
4. M. Hansen and C. Aradine. The changing face of primary pediatrics. Pediatric Clinics of North America, February 1974, p. 245
5. L. Homme et al. How to Use Contingency Contracting in the Classroom. Research Press, 1970
6. M. Johnston. Toward a culture of caring: children, their environment, and change. American Journal of Maternal and Child Nursing, Jul/Aug 1979, p. 210
7. M. Lewis. Child-initiated care. American Journal of Nursing, April 1974, p. 652

8. J. Natapoff. Children's views of health; a developmental study. American Journal of Public Health, October 1978, p. 995
9. V. Pidgeon. Characteristics of children's thinking and implications for health teaching. Maternal-Child Nursing Journal, Spring 1977, p. 1
10. A. Sheridan and R. Smith. Student-family contracts. Nursing Outlook, February 1975, p. 114
11. R. Stuart. Behavioral contracting within the families of delinquents. Journal of Behavior Therapy and Experimental Psychiatry, February 1971, p. 1
12. R. Wu. Behavior and Illness. Prentice-Hall, Inc., 1973

Additional Recommended Reading

M. Birchfield. Headstart health: a process for health education. American Journal Maternal and Child Nursing, Sept/Oct 1977, p. 307

J. Cowley et al. Teenagers today: health education at school — the present, the future. Nursing Times, 10 May 1979, p. 138

J. Johnson et al. Easing children's fright during health care procedures. American Journal Maternal and Child Nursing, Jul/Aug 1976, p. 206

H. Kitzman. The nature of well child care. American Journal of Nursing, October 1975, p. 1705

J. Krumboltz and C. Thoresen. Counseling Methods. Holt, Rinehart & Winston, 1977

H. Mauksch. A socio-scientific basis for conceptualizing family health. Social Science and Medicine, August 1974, p. 521

K. O'Leary and G. Wilson. Behavior Therapy. Prentice-Hall, Inc., 1975

M. Komalker. Communication block revisited. Nursing 79, June 1979, p. 1077

R. Skinner. Lifetime health monitoring, preventive care: age one through adolescence. Patient Care, 30 April 1979, p. 201

E. Stone et al. Children's concepts of illness, internal body parts. Maternal-Child Nursing Journal, Summer 1979, p. 115

M. Zangari and P. Duffy. Contracting with patients in day-to-day practice. American Journal of Nursing, March 1980, p. 451

MANAGING STRESS

FAMILY CRISIS INTERVENTION

by Chester R. Peachey, RN, BSN, MS

WHAT IS STRESS?

Stress is a phenomenon that is universally experienced by all persons and groups of persons. There is no anticipated or common response to stress, since all persons respond in a highly individualistic manner. What is stress for one person may not be for another. So it is with the family group: what generates stress for one family may not for another.*

Hans Selye has defined stress as "the daily wear and tear on the body, the effects of the rate at which you live at any moment, positive or negative, physical, emotional or mental."[6] Selye elaborates by stating that stress is the nonspecific response of the body to any demand that is made on it.[8] The demand made is specific but the stress response is nonspecific. Stress is not to be avoided; rather, it is part of life and living. When stress is experienced as negative it is more correct to call it *distress*. Selye's work has dealt with biological stress. The *general adaptation syndrome* (GAS) is created by the release of certain adaptative hormones. The GAS is viewed in three stages: (1) alarm, (2) resistance and (3) exhaustion.[7] Body organs are affected by this response. Changes are evidenced in gastrointestinal functioning and in the adrenals and thymus. Specific physiological signs and symptoms of stress are dilated pupils, diaphoresis, increased heart rate, increased rate and depth of respirations, dry mouth, decreased peristalsis and muscular tension. Stress can also be demonstrated in a local reaction or, as Selye calls it, *local adaptation syndrome* (LAS).

The factor that produces stress is called a *stressor*. Stressor function is what disturbs the body's equilibrium; it is immaterial whether the agent or situation faced is pleasant or unpleasant. All that counts is the intensity experienced that demands readjustment or adaptation. Adaptation does mean adjustment.[8]

Stress also demands psychological adaptation and adjustment. Not only are physiological functions affected by stress, but psychological and behavioral responses occur. There is a demonstrated decrease in intellectual functioning. Signs of this decreased ability are seen in the lack of clear thinking, inability to remember information and difficulty in making decisions.

THE FAMILY AS A SYSTEM

It is important for the nurse to view the family, in whatever form, as a system. Systems theory has contributed much to nursing in terms of understanding the behavior and functioning of a variety of groups. The family is only one of these groups. Miller states that the family is considered an open system as opposed to a closed system.[5] An open system is defined as one that continually interacts and exchanges information with the environment. A closed system is

---

*Understanding stress theory is basic to understanding nursing interventions to facilitate adaptation. Only a brief review of theory is given here; it is assumed that the reader has studied stress theories in earlier nursing courses. If an introduction to stress theory is needed, see the referencs and suggested readings at the end of this section.

isolated, cut off from its environment. Sedgewick states that if the family is approached as a system, then organizational theory and principles of psychosocial learning can be applied.[7] Within the system there is an order established that contributes to the effective and efficient functioning of the persons involved. The family as a system is made up of persons who are interdependent. Each member has a role to fulfill. The clarity of this role for each member is necessary and useful so that the family system can function as a group of healthy individuals. The clarity of roles contributes to the family maintaining a steady state as a system.

The family, as a social unit, consists of persons who have interdependent relationships. Through the acceptance of this interdependence, policies are determined, feelings are honored, skills are respected and comfort is given. These four activities contribute to the success and strength of the family unit.

Communication is an important determinate in the successful functioning of the family system. The established channels for communication within the family must be respected and utilized by each member. Valuable information can only be processed if the communication network is functioning adequately. For the nurse, it is imperative that assessment of the communication network within the family system take place. It is important to utilize the strengths of the communication system. When roles, functions and communication network operate effectively, the family system is in equilibrium. The nurse must understand the intricacies of interpersonal relationships in the family. The strengths and limitations of each member must be assessed.

THE FAMILY AND STRESS

When stress is introduced into the family system, significant changes and reactions occur. Within the communication network, stress affects the transfer of information.[5] Inadequate message transmission and reception occur as stress is increased. Ineffective transmission of messages results in communication network breakdown.

Sedgewick states that other types of stress situations which bring about dysfunction in the family system are lack of role clarity, vagueness of expectation, unresolved conflict and conflict between the family system and other systems, such as church, school, police.[7] The lack of role clarity results in family members being unable to identify their positions within the family structure. For younger family members, if there is a vagueness of what is expected from them, individual stress levels can increase and result in dysfunctional interpersonal relationships. Conflicts that are unresolved add to the dysfunctional quality of interaction. The continued elevation of stress level in unresolved conflicts draws enormous amounts of energy from the family system that could otherwise be used in problem solving. Within the family system, when one member experiences stress all members experience stress. It must be remembered that stress does not automatically lead to crisis. It is only when the family coping mechanisms are inadequate that crisis occurs. The adaptive response of the family as a system, so that it can deal successfully with stress and crisis, is what makes for individual member growth. As families allow themselves the freedom to engage in problem solving, which results in growth, they will also allow and encourage individual members to engage in problem solving and resultant growth. Although stress is extremely uncomfortable, it is rarely fatal, nor does it continue at an intolerable level forever. The nurse should keep this in mind when working with families who are experiencing stress.

As the nurse assesses families to determine the level of stress within the system, it must be remembered that not all stress will lead to a crisis situation. However, within all crisis there is stress. Stress does not involve merely damage but also the adaptation to damage and change, and it can be positive and life promoting. It is recognized that most crises occur in a family (group) context and seldom occur in isolation. It is important for the nurse to remember that a distinction between stress and crisis must be made for effective intervention to occur.

WHAT IS CRISIS?

Crisis is defined as a turning point in the life of a person or group, when a conflict is perceived as threatening and its solution is not possible by the usual coping mechanisms.[4] Gerald Caplan, one of the original formulators of crisis theory, has defined crisis as a period of disequilibrium in which a person feels overwhelmed by a problem that is not solved by available coping mechanisms.[2] Crisis can be chronic or acute in nature. It may be internal, interpersonal or in any combination. Caplan also has stated that crisis is self-limiting and tends to last four to six weeks, during which time adequate resolutions should take place.[1]

PHASES OF CRISIS

Crisis can be separated into four phases.[3, 5] The first is the initial impact or *shock* phase. It is during this phase that there is difficulty comprehending what has occurred. *Defensive retreat* follows as the next phase. The emotional response is one of denial and emotional moving away from the event that has occurred. The third phase is *acknowledgment* — an acceptance that a disruptive event has occurred. The fourth and final stage is called *resolution*, adaptation or change. It is during this phase that an acceptance of what has happened occurs and life goes on. These phases may not be sharply demarcated for each person, yet each is predictable. The family undergoes the same phases of crisis as an individual, although the intensity of timing may be different.[6]

What precipitates a crisis in one family may not do so in another. Families who are successful in dealing with crisis have found ways to use the process as a growth-promoting experience. Successful families do this by exercising control in order to regulate their subsystems. Members in the family are highly committed to the family group and its goals. Also, the family who successfully deals with crisis retains a functional family coalition. The members work together and support each other and thus provide a safe environment in which to function and grow. Parents assume parenting functions and do not abdicate this responsibility.

The communication process is the third aspect that aids in growth from a family crisis event. For the members to be open and speak directly to the issues at hand leaves no double message or hidden agenda in the communication process. All nurses should understand how families can successfully negotiate a crisis period in their growth together. The nurse can help negotiate a family crisis by (1) raising the level of family awareness of the crisis, (2) supplying helpful facts about the crisis so the family will see it in clearer perspective, (3) aiding family members to support each other and (4) presenting alternatives so the members can choose a course of action that will induce growth while helping them cope with the crisis.

In order for the nurse to give assistance to a family in crisis, there must be an understanding of the dynamics that are at work. Failing to understand the dynamics is a severe handicap to the nurse who is attempting to aid the family. In addition to knowing the dynamics, the nurse must be aware of personal limitations. Coming to terms with one's limitations assists in realistic appraisal of the skills possessed as a professional.

Crisis intervention, in order to be most effective, should be based on a wide range of theories. There is no single theory that will serve the nurse in dealing with all family crises. It becomes a responsibility of each nurse to have a broad appreciation and understanding of the most current theories of crisis intervention so as to best meet individual family needs.

Aquilera and Messick state that the minimum goal of crisis intervention should be the resolution of the immediate crisis and a restoration of functioning to the level that existed before the crisis period.[1] The maximum goal would be an improvement in functioning that exceeds the precrisis level.

TYPES OF CRISES

There are two major types of crisis events that occur within the family. They are *maturational* and *situational*. Maturational crisis is also called developmental or normative; the situational crisis is also known as accidental.

Maturational Crisis and Intervention

Murray and Zentner have defined maturational crisis as the "transient points, the periods that every person experiences in the process of biopsychosocial growth and development and that are accompanied by changes in thoughts, feelings, and abilities."[6] It can most simply be said that maturational crisis periods occur as a part of normal life. The onset of crises is gradual, as the person or family moves from one stage to another. Examples of maturational crises include the following: entry of the child into school, puberty, start of a career, marriage, pregnancy, parenthood, children leaving home, community involvement, involutional period in life, retirement and facing the death of others and self. Inherent in each of these situations is a role change and shift.

When a family or person is moving to another developmental stage, a maturational crisis may occur when the person or family is unable to assume a role change that is appropriate for the new maturational level. As the nurse works with families, the family and its members must be adequately assessed so that it can be determined *what* the crisis is and *who* is in crisis.

In determining who is in crisis, it is important to examine factors that may contribute to the inability of the family or family member to make a role change.

First is the *person's inability to picture himself in a new role*. Because the person has learned appropriate role behavior and is now asked to learn a new role, stress is experienced. Roles that persons have learned are comfortable and contribute to intrapersonal equilibrium. To change roles generates disequilibrium. *Lack of interpersonal resources* is a second reason that a person is unable to make a role change. The greatest interpersonal resource that individuals and groups need is communication skill. A lack of skill in communication limits, if not totally negates, change. The nurse must bear in mind that assisting others in developing effective communication is a basic nursing responsibility and skill. Thirdly, role changes may be thwarted *by the refusal of significant others to see the person in a different role*. Stereotyping by society of role and function continues to be a deterrent to nonstressful role change. It becomes clear to the nurse that for individuals and families to change roles, there must be support from those involved in or affected by that change.

The process of growth and development and the accompanying maturational stresses are a normal part of life. The changes that occur *may* produce a crisis in the life of a family. Whether the stress that maturation generates becomes a crisis for a family depends on the resources available to the family as a group and as individuals.

Situational Crisis and Intervention

A situational crisis occurs when an unexpected or sudden event presents an overwhelming threat to the individual or family.[9] The stressful event has nothing to do with growth, development and the maturational process. Stress on an individual generates stress in those persons intimately involved with him. For example, an infant born with a congenital deformity precipitates a situational crisis for the new parents. Another example is hospitalization, which generates a situational crisis for the patient, since there is a threat to self-identity and self-esteem. For the family, hospitalization is equally a threat. Questions related to who is caring for the family member and what type of care is being given are raised.

Other situations that precipitate a crisis include: experiences of physical and emotional illness, congenital or acquired handicaps, relocation, chronic illness, death of a family member, divorce, suicide, losing a job, rape, adoption and child abuse. In addition, situations related to natural disasters such as wars, floods and hurricanes increase stress, since these experiences increase feelings of insecurity and loss of personal control over life events.

To further understand a situational crisis, a nurse needs to understand the operational steps of this experience.[7] The first operational step is the *threat* or damage posed *to life goals*. Events that constitute a threat are unexpected; they are not anticipated as being part of life experience.

The evoked *tension* and *anxiety* from the threat is the second step that needs to be recognized. Tension and anxiety are unique experiences to individuals and families. What generates tension and anxiety for one family may not for another. This points out the need for careful assessment and not anticipating what the "usual response should be." There is no typical response to anxiety. The nurse must appreciate the significance of the threat to the individual and family in order to understand the degree of anxiety evoked. The last step is that *unresolved problems and crises* from the past *are brought into awareness*. Since the past is reawakened, present situations are viewed in terms of what has occurred earlier. Individuals and families have unique methods in moving through operational steps of situational crisis. The nurse who understands the operational steps will have a basis to begin effective intervention.

When the nurse has determined that a family is in crisis and assessed how each member is affected by the crisis, the basis for planning intervention is established. It should be remembered that the nursing process — assessment, planning, implementation, and evaluation — serves as a framework for dealing with family crisis. (The nursing process is reviewed in Chapter 9.)

Aquilera and Messick state that there are four steps in the crisis intervention process: assessment, planning intervention, intervention, and resolution of the crisis.[1] These steps can be applied to both maturational and situational crises. The first step, thorough and adequate assessment, determines what the crisis is and how it affects each member of the family.

Second, planning must be done for therapeutic intervention. In planning for intervention, the nurse must accurately evaluate the resources that are available to the family. Resources can generally be viewed as personal, interpersonal and institutional.[9] Personal resources involve the use of cognitive skills in thinking through issues and solving problems. Problem solving is a basic skill that the individuals and the family as a group must develop. Interpersonal resources involve persons who are significant to others and who can provide support during times of stress. Health agencies, community support groups and religious organizations can be institutional resources.

Carrying out the intervention is the third step. For the planned intervention to be effective, it must be based on sound principles. One of the basic principles is that the nurse must show unconditional acceptance (a deep respect not limited by "shoulds" or "oughts") of the family and establish a positive, helping relationship. In receiving unconditional acceptance, the family experiences a decreased level of stress and anxiety. The family's crisis must be viewed as unique, and the nurse should not try to minimize what is presently happening. The nurse can assist the family by engaging the members in talking about the situation. The nurse conveys the belief that talking about the crises can reduce stress. So can sharing the disruptive life event with someone who cares.

The nurse must assist the family to face the crisis situation, but only as much as the family can manage. Two common errors are made in assisting a person or family in crisis. First, often the situation is forced into confrontation, which serves to increase defense behavior — basically, denial. Forcing a confrontation may seriously interfere in the establishment of a healthy working relationship between family and nurse. Second, underplaying the significance of the crisis event in family life may encourage the family in the unhealthy use of denial. Neither defensive retreat by the family nor oversimplification help solve the problem.

For the nurse working with the family in crisis, it is important not to fall into the trap of personalizing the behavior and feelings that may be exhibited. Denial is to be recognized as a normal reaction to confronting a crisis and should not be interpreted by the nurse as a personal issue with the family. It is equally important to not become involved in giving false reassurance to the family or allowing the family to blame others and see themselves as the victim of a situation. The family group must realize that they are responsible for their own behavior and for the decisions they make. A healthy intervention principle for the nurse is not to fall into the trap of "laying blame" on certain family members or outside factors. When the crisis specifically involves a maturation event, intervention must be directed toward the increase of support for the new role that the individual family or member is to assume.

The last step in the crisis intervention process is the resolution of the crisis. Upon reaching resolution, the family and individual members will have confronted the feelings they experienced and explored new ways of coping, and will have grown as a result of the crisis event.

LEVELS OF PREVENTION

It is imperative that the nurse examine the levels of prevention and understand that services are involved in each area. The *primary level* is concerned with the reduction of conditions that lead to unsatisfactory and ineffective growth experiences for the family. Examples are the use of premarital counselling groups in which couples can realistically deal with the issues of marriage, and prenatal classes in which expectant parents are better prepared for maturational crisis. The nurse must carefully assess families during interaction with them to identify those that are vulnerable to developmental crises. The timing of intervention is critical, as anticipatory guidance (teaching and counselling) is most likely to be received and acted upon by the family during the time they are working on establishing coping patterns. For example, anticipatory guidance relative to toddlerhood is best timed and most usefully received by the parents when an infant becomes a toddler, not before that. This does not mean parents of infants cannot be prepared for what to expect once their infant is a toddler. What it does mean is that the parents will not relate to or deal with that information until their infant is in fact a toddler. Therefore, any information given earlier will need repeating at this time because now is when the parents feel, and can therefore acknowledge, the stress and learn how to minimize it.

Secondary level of prevention involves early diagnosis so that effective intervention can begin for a recognized crisis. The most useful way the nurse can intervene is to help the family realize that there are problem-solving options to choose from. Knowing this can put the stress in perspective for the family members and may allow them to transfer their energy from worrying about the problem to solving it. By giving emotional support, the nurse helps the family to mobilize its own resources to implement its chosen option and to secure aid from personal or professional support systems without losing self-respect or pride. Postpartum clinics and community professionals that assist parents to deal with specific problems that the family encounters are examples of secondary level prevention resources.

Maintaining the family in the community as a functioning unit and preventing decompensation is the goal of *tertiary prevention*.

The nurse's purpose at this level is to intervene to alleviate any further family disturbance created by a crisis. Intervention at this point usually necessitates a team approach with other helping professions (physicians, social workers, legal professionals). The team approach offers the family with a complex problem several ego-strengthening support systems to help find and act upon options. Child abuser groups and support groups for families who are experiencing chronic illness are examples of services available to families at this level.

At all three levels of prevention the kind of help the family gets significantly influences the outcome, regardless of extenuating factors. Ideally, help should be directed toward turning the stressful situation and the problem-solving activities into growth-producing experiences for the family, in which it builds its strength, confidence and coping capacity to handle future stresses or crises succcessfully and independently. Nurses dealing with families during stress must realize that the right answer to each crisis lies within that unique situation. The family, with the nurse's support and assistance, needs to appraise the situation confronting them and then decide on the most constructive move they can make to improve or prevent it, without interfering with the rights of others. The goal of professional helping is for the family and its members to learn to think and act for themselves, not to maintain dependence on the professional helper.

This text is divided into parts according to stages of growth of the family and child: infant, toddler, preschooler, school-age child, and adolescent. In each part, a chapter is devoted to considering the potential stresses the family may encounter. As you study those chapters, try to apply the principles of stress and maturational crisis and how they affect the family system.

References

1. D. Aguilera and J. Messick. Crisis Intervention: Theory and Methodology. C.V. Mosby Co., 1978
2. S. DiFabio. Crisis: a complex process. The Nursing Clinics of North America, March 1974, p. 47
3. S. Fink. Crisis motivation: A theoretical model. Archives of Physical Medicine and Rehabilitation, November 1967, p. 592
4. J Haber et al. Comprehensive Psychiatric Nursing. McGraw-Hill Book Co., 1978
5. J. Miller. Systems theory and family psychotherapy. In Psychiatric/Mental Health Nursing: Contemporary Readings. D. Van Nostrand Co., Inc., 1978
6. R. Murray and J. Zentner. Nursing Concepts for Health Promotion. Prentice-Hall Inc., 1979
7. R. Sedgewick. The family as a system: a newtwork of relationships. In Psychiatric/Mental Health Nursing: Contemporary Readings. D. Van Nostrand Co., Inc., 1978
8. H. Selye. Stress Without Distress. The New American Library Inc., 1974
9. F. Williams. Intervention in situational crisis. In Nursing of Families in Crisis, G. Hall and B. Weaver, eds. J. B. Lippincott Co., 1974

Additional Recommended Reading

F. Bower and E. Bevis. Fundamentals of Nursing Practice. C.V. Mosby Co., 1979

G. Burton. Families in crisis - knowing when and how to help. Nursing 75, December 1975, p. 36

J. Hall and B. Weaver. Nursing of Families in Crisis. J. B. Lippincott Co. 1974

M. Hazzard and M. Scheverman. Family system therapy. Nursing 76, July 1976, p. 22

J. Luckman and K. Sorensen. Medical-Surgical Nursing: A Psychophysiologic Approach. W. B. Saunders Co., 1980, Chapters 3 through 6

K. Sorensen and J. Luckmann. Basic Nursing, A Psychophysiologic Approach. W.B. Saunders Co., 1979. Chapters 5 through 15.

F. Williams. The crisis of hospitalization. The Nursing Clinics of North America, March 1974, p. 37

F. Williams. Intervention in maturational crisis. In Nursing of Families in Crisis, G. Hall and B. Weaver, eds. J. B. Lippincott Co., 1974

WHEN BEHAVIOR IS A PROBLEM

by Jo Joyce Tackett, BSN, MPHN

SOMETHING IS WRONG WITH THIS CHILD

"Problem child" is a label adults attach to the child whose behavior they cannot understand. But children are frequently troublesome from an adult perspective, so what differentiates some children as "problem children?"

There is no rigid distinction between problem children and other children. The difference is that some children behave in ways adults judge as unacceptable or inappropriate. The behaviors that represent a child's emotional distress are essentially exaggerations of, deficiencies in, or a maladaptive combination of behavior patterns common to all children. The difference is in the degree.

The emotional upsets and behavioral disturbances this child displays are byproducts of the unsuccessful strategies he had chosen to cope with the difficulties of life. The problem arises out of the fact that the behaviors he uses to cope are ineffective, inappropriate or self-defeating, resulting in unfavorable consequences for the child (and frequently for others). Societal expectation is that behaviors be understandable, consistent and controlled. The emotionally distressed child chooses instead behaviors the motivation of which is at least illogical, if not unintelligible, and he acts unpredictably and inconsistently. His behavior is frequently uncontrollable, usually in any setting.

The behavior choices the child makes are very much bound by what he thinks of himself and how he perceives his relationships with others. If he does not see himself realistically, the social interactions that are difficult for all children to cope with become distressful, distorting the child's judgments as to what behaviors are appropriate.

Criteria have been identified by our society that distinguish maladaptive behavior from that of the norm. These criteria must be considered relative, however, since "maladaptive" is differently defined by various cultures and socioeconomic groups, by each sex, and according to the age of the person displaying the behavior.

The criteria used to diagnose emotional disorder are:[1, 3-5]

1. The behavior is to be condemmed and is unacceptable regardless of how rarely it occurs (incest, intentional damage to person or property).
2. The behavior is not inappropriate in and of itself but is inappropriate because of its frequency, because it is exaggerated, or because of when or where it occurs.
3. The behavior is absent or deficient in that the person rarely or never displays a behavior society deems necessary and normal (never smiles, never or rarely talks, seldom pays attention).
4. The behavior is a regular source of tension to the child or family members or both.
5. The behavior is inappropriate for the person's age and stage of development, intelligence or social situation.
6. The behavior is compulsively enacted, appearing to "come out of the blue" without any precipitating circumstances (obscure or bizarre motivation). The child seems unable to avoid or stop the behavior even though he knows it is futile or that it will inevitably bring disapproval or punishment.
7. The behavior is one of several others that together affect several areas of the child's life. The behavior(s) brings suffering to the child and others and interferes with his socialization and development.

ETIOLOGY AND IMPACT OF PROBLEM BEHAVIOR

Once a child is described as having problem (deviant) behavior, the inevitable question is "Why does this child display problem behavior?" Herbert has used the "loaded gun" concept to illustrate the vulnerable child.[3] What happens is that the child perceives a crisis

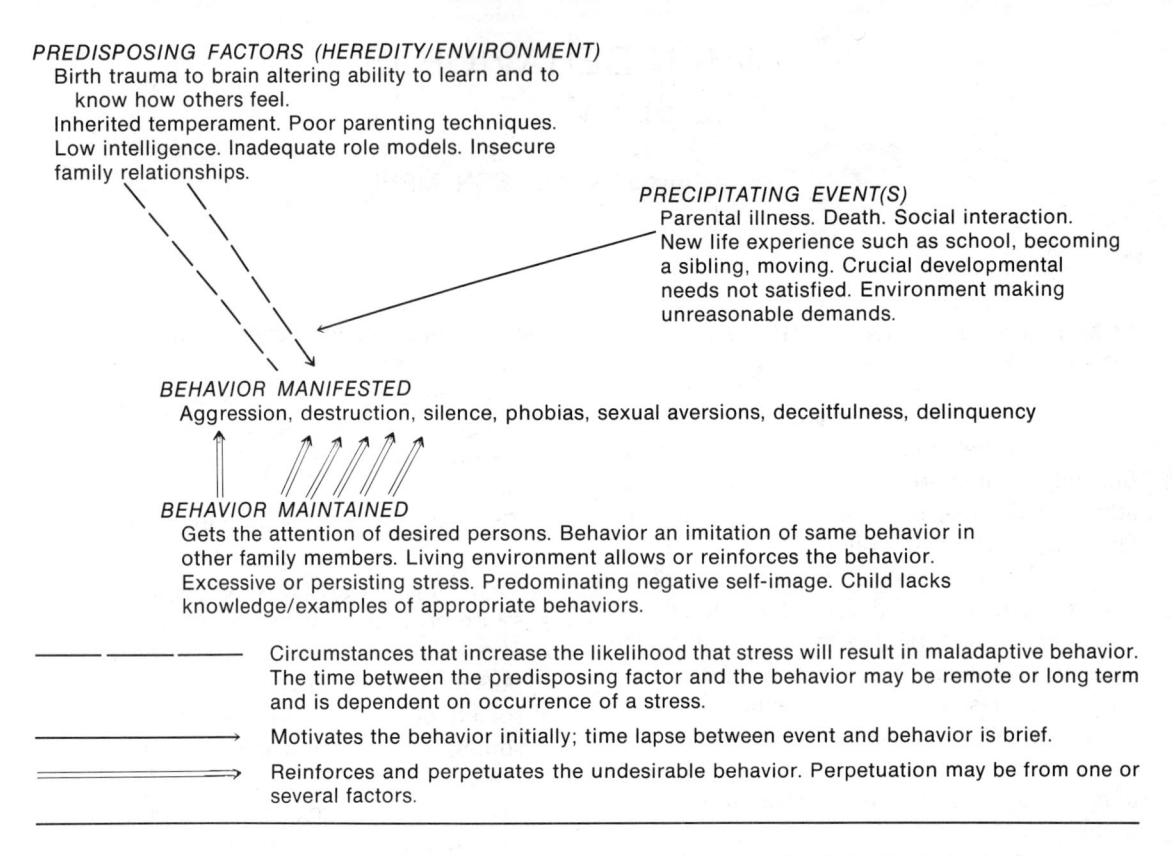

PREDISPOSING FACTORS (HEREDITY/ENVIRONMENT)
Birth trauma to brain altering ability to learn and to know how others feel.
Inherited temperament. Poor parenting techniques. Low intelligence. Inadequate role models. Insecure family relationships.

PRECIPITATING EVENT(S)
Parental illness. Death. Social interaction. New life experience such as school, becoming a sibling, moving. Crucial developmental needs not satisfied. Environment making unreasonable demands.

BEHAVIOR MANIFESTED
Aggression, destruction, silence, phobias, sexual aversions, deceitfulness, delinquency

BEHAVIOR MAINTAINED
Gets the attention of desired persons. Behavior an imitation of same behavior in other family members. Living environment allows or reinforces the behavior. Excessive or persisting stress. Predominating negative self-image. Child lacks knowledge/examples of appropriate behaviors.

— — — — Circumstances that increase the likelihood that stress will result in maladaptive behavior. The time between the predisposing factor and the behavior may be remote or long term and is dependent on occurrence of a stress.

⟶ Motivates the behavior initially; time lapse between event and behavior is brief.

⟹ Reinforces and perpetuates the undesirable behavior. Perpetuation may be from one or several factors.

Figure 16–1 Dynamics in the development and perpetuation of maladaptive behavior.[6]

(precipitating event). The trigger (precipitating event) only fires the already loaded (predisposing factors) gun, releasing the bullet (deviant behavior). Predisposing factors may exist long before their effects are seen, but they set the stage for the trigger to snap when a crisis comes along. Once the crisis occurs, the behavior promptly follows. If circumstances exist to perpetuate the behavior, it will be repeated again as a coping behavior, regardless of its effectiveness. Figure 16–1 diagrams the relationship of all these elements.

The child who is emotionally dependent uses his problem behavior as a crutch because he discovers that the behavior gains him consideration or attention (even if it is negative) that he is unable to get in any other way or that he perceives would otherwise be given to his siblings instead. The child will "shop around" to find those behaviors that get the most response from those in his environment whose attention he seeks. Also, the behavior is a way to dominate or manipulate people or situations toward which he otherwise feels powerless or it reinforces the perception he has of himself (self-fullfilling prophesy — "I think I'm bad... I act bad... I'm told I'm bad... I must be bad.")

The impact of the child's behavior on other family members depends on how maladaptive they perceive the behavior to be, how much the behavior disrupts family living, and how much negative feedback about it that the family receives from society (friends, school, legal institutions, organizations concerned with children's health). Many other factors unique to the particular family may also have impact on the family's reactions. At the very least the family must contend with an unhappy child who has not been socialized into the norm of society. Attempts to deal with their "problem child" fosters improved communication and better understanding of each member's developmental needs in some families; however in many families the effect is further disruption of family functioning or even disbanding of the family unit. With assistance the family may learn healthier coping patterns and develop constructive and supportive relationships with the child that help him overcome or adapt to the predisposing factors that led to his maladaptive behavior.

THE NURSE'S ROLE IN ASSISTING THE FAMILY

The nurse often has more contact with the child and family than do other health providers. Therefore she frequently can be the major identifier of problem behavior and the team member who directly intervenes with the family. Intervention is usually at two levels. One aspect is directed toward teaching family members, especially parents, how to help the child. The second aspect is aimed at directly influencing the child to help him learn healthier coping behaviors.

Assisting Parents

It takes tremendous patience and understanding for parents to work out differences with their child, especially when his behavior is unpredictable and obscurely motivated. It is even more difficult for parents to acknowledge that a problem exists in their child's adjustments to life experiences. The most difficult feature with which the nurse and other members of the health team must contend is in motivating the family to seek and utilize professional help. Ideally families can receive help preventively when the nurse identifies the vulnerable child or family or both. The nurse should astutely observe for attachment difficulties during the child's infancy, for communication breakdown among family members, and for personality conflicts between parent and child or in the way they interact. If she finds problems, she can intervene by: (1) reinforcing and pointing out the child's positive features and the strengths of the parenting efforts, (2) providing anticipatory guidance that helps parents maintain realistic expectations of the child and reassures the child that he can handle the tasks of living and growing, and (3) counselling parents to take care of their needs as well as to learn to interpret their child's needs.

Observations that indicate there is a problem that needs prompt diagnosis and intervention include evidence that parents do not know basic parenting techniques or do not apply their knowledge (how to role model desired behavior, how to be consistent and realistic in treatment of child); the lack or scantiness of affection, smiles and praise between parent and child; and a deficit in reinforcement or rewards for healthy behavior. (7) The nurse then must apply her own skills or those of referral resources (parent education classes and support groups) to assist the couple to learn appropriate parenting skills. (See chapter 3 for discussion of parenting.)

Assisting the Child

Once the child demonstrates behavior that fits the criteria described earlier in this chapter, intervention must be directed toward the child himself. Two intervention approaches are popular.[5] The traditional or *evocative approach* (psychoanalysis) attempts to alter the child's maladaptive behavior indirectly by first changing the child's intrapsychic organization (the way he thinks or feels about himself and therefore perceives social situations). The *behaviorist approach* (behavior modification) is based on the premise that behavior is learned and can therefore be unlearned or replaced by healthier behaviors through planned changes in the child's present external environment. This approach of altering the behavior directly is called *behavior modification*. Treatment may also use a combination of the psychoanalytic and the behavior modification approaches. Psychoanalysis is conducted by professional psychiatric personnel, although the nurse certainly can teach parents and teachers how to recognize and reinforce the positive attitudes and behaviors the child does display.

Behavior modification techniques can be mastered by most parents. The nurse is often responsible for using these techniques and teaching them to parents, teachers and other significant persons in the child's environment. The first step in behavior modification is to identify the problem behavior, the elements in the child's environment that provoke and reinforce it, and the behavior that is needed to replace it so the child gains social satisfaction and self-satisfaction. Consistently reinforcing the desired behavior and ignoring or negatively reinforcing the problem behavior is required over time to extinguish the problem behavior. This approach has had documented success[2,5,6,8] in changing behavior; however, it demands energy and patience on the part of the reinforcer(s) and is successful only if the program is consistently employed over time.

Parents should be forewarned that the undesirable behavior often escalates initially before it begins receding. If warning is not given, parents (or other reinforcers) often discard the program at this point. (Chapter 3 discusses the types of reinforcement possible and the advantages or disadvantages of various rewards.) The child's problem behavior was initiated because he knew no other behavior to satisfy the need he felt. Behavior modification fills the gap in the child's knowledge by teaching him other more socially and personally satisfying behaviors that may be used to meet his coping needs.

The nurse may be involved in designing the behavior modification program, implementing the program, or teaching and supervising other reinforcer agents (parents, teachers, significant members of child's environment). Teaching parents these techniques is a valuable component of the program, with long-term benefits.[3-5]

References

1. M. Beecher and W. Beecher. Parents on the Run. Grosset and Dunlap, 1967
2. R. Hawkins et al. Behavior therapy in the home: amelioration of problem parent-child relations with the parent in the therapeutic role. Journal of Experimental Child Psychology, April 1966, p.99
3. M. Herbert. Problems of Childhood. Pan Books, Ltd., 1975
4. L. Hersoo. Emotional disorders in childhood. Nursing Times, 9 June 1977, p. 864
5. M. LeBow. Behavior Modification: A Significant Method In Nursing Practice. Prentice-Hall Inc., 1973
6. G. Patterson et al. Reprogramming the social environment. Journal of Child Psychology and Psychiatry, August 1967, p. 181
7. I. Schleicher. Teaching parents to cope with behavior problems. American Journal of Nursing, May 1978, p. 838
8. L. P. Ullman and L. Krasner, eds. Case Studies in Behavior Modification. Holt, Rinehart & Winston, Inc., 1965

Additional Recommended Reading

S. Ambron. Child Development. Holt, Rinehart & Winston, 1977
C. Blosser. Avoiding potential behavior problems in Children. Pediatric Nurse, May/June 1979, p. 11
M. Krajicek and A. Tearney, eds. Detection of Developmental Problems in Children. University Park Press, 1977
D. Shulz. The Changing Family. Its Functions and Future. Prentice-Hall, Inc. 1976
D. Sutterly and G. Donnelly. Perspectives in Human Development. Nursing Throughout the Life Cycle. J. B. Lippincott Co., 1977
A. Thomas et al. Temperament and Behavior Disorders in Children. New York University Press, 1968
R. Turner. A method of working with disturbed children. Am. Journal of Nursing, October 1970, p. 2146

WHEN A CHILD IS ILL

by Jo Joyce Tackett, BSN, MPHN

Illness is an event experienced by people of all ages and cultures. It is characterized by changes in the body that cause impaired ability to meet minimal physical, physiological, emotional-social and intellectual requirements for functioning at the level appropriate for one's age, sex, development and physiological state.[16] Illness may be temporary, reversible, irreversible or life-threatening. Table 16–1 identifies the general categories of nursing responsibility for each type of illness.

The child's and family's behavioral response to illness in a child depends on (1) the nature of the illness (curable or not, brief or long-term, amount and location of discomfort, extent to which activities of daily living are interrupted); (2) age and sex of the child; (3) previous experiences with illness, personally or in others; (4) sociocultural frame of reference held regarding illness; (5) perception of what the illness means and what is happening to the child; (6) preconceived ideas about health care providers; (7) how much they know and understand about the illness; and (8) how the significant others in their environment respond to the illness.[1, 16]

Illness always poses a threat to a child's emotional well-being because of the many unfamiliar and often frightening sensations and experiences to which he is subjected and the unfamiliar people involved. Parents will inevitably experience guilt and helplessness when their child is ill. The extent to which these are experienced depends on the age of the child, the nature of the illness, and how others, especially health professionals, respond to them and their needs.

Siblings of the ill child experience guilt; they feel they had something to do with the sibling becoming ill. They also fear getting the illness themselves. The degree to which these feelings are experienced depends on age and the quality of the sibling relationship. Jealousy is commonly experienced while the ill child is receiv-

TABLE 16-1 NURSING RESPONSIBILITIES ACCORDING TO TYPE OF ILLNESS

Type of Illness	Major Nursing Responsibilities
Temporary	Support family unity. Implement preventive course of action. Help family develop a treatment plan; teach home care skills.
Reversible	Support family unity. Facilitate normal growth and development. Implement preventive course of action. Participate in developing and administering treatment plan.
Irreversible	Support family unity. Facilitate optimal growth and development. Implement prevention course of action. Participate in developing and administering treatment plan in collaboration with other disciplines.
Life-threatening	Support family unity. Facilitate comfort and progressive development. Implement preventive course of action. Participate, in collaboration with other disciplines, in developing and administering a plan of care that insures comfort, preserves dignity, and allows open confrontation with this last stage of living.

ing extra attention. A study by Brodie[4] revealed that well children perceive illness differently from their ill counterparts. She found that when children are ill, they usually see the illness as punishment or, at the very least, that they themselves are personally responsible for their plight. The sick child sees illness as a disruptive force in his life. Healthy children, however, frankly denied the possibility of misbehavior or self-causation as the source of illness or that illness was disruptive to their lives. Brodie suggests that the distortion in perception during illness is caused by the anxiety the illness creates, especially since these findings were consistent regardless of age, cognitive ability or past experience with illness. Table 16-2 describes the typical fears, responses and coping abilities of children during illness according to developmental stage.

Specific nursing interventions that facilitate the child's coping and diminish fears are also included in Table 16-2. Interventions, with the emphasis or focus altered depending on the child's developmental level, fall primarily into four categories: (1) informing the child of what to expect and how he can help; (2) encouraging caretaker availability; (3) providing emotional and physical assistance to help the child maintain control; and (4) allowing expression of the child's feelings.

Nursing interventions should also be directed toward reducing parental guilt and anxiety. Again, although the specific needs of parents are individual, four types of intervention can successfully reduce their guilt and anxiety and helplessness and give them confidence in their ability to support the child. These are (1) use a friendly approach that is nonjudgmental and positively reinforces the intended as well as actual measures they have taken to improve their child's health state; (2) keep the parents objectively informed of their child's situation, teach about the illness and its management, discuss with the parents the responses that their

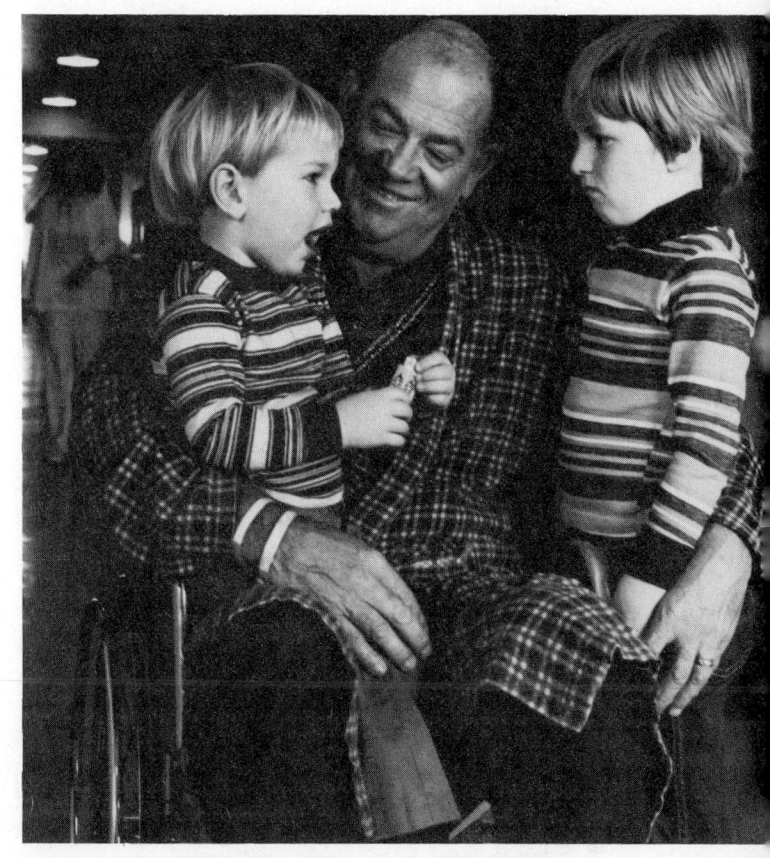

Children react differently to illness according to their past experience. As the expressions on these children's faces reveal, children also perceive illness differently as they get older.

MANAGING STRESS

TABLE 16-2 DEVELOPMENTAL DESCRIPTION OF CHILDREN'S RESPONSES AND COPING ABILITIES DURING ILLNESS EXPERIENCES AND SUPPORTIVE NURSING ACTIONS

Age	Main Fears	Verbal Response[1]	Nonverbal Response[1]	Ability to Cope	Nursing Actions To Facilitate Coping During Stressful Situations[2]
Infant and toddler (0–2)	Sudden movements Loud noises Separation from caretaker* Strangers*	Cries, yells, "No!" protests	Clings to caretaker. Tries to return to and visually searches for caretaker if separated. Tries to get away.	Limited ability to cope, especially with pain. Cannot hold still on own during stress.	Simple explanations of what is to be done and what sensations will occur; actively involve child if old enough. Keep caretaker present to calm child with touch and voice and preferably by holding child. Gentle restraint introduced as "Let me help you hold still." Perform what must be done as promptly, painlessly and quickly as possible. Allow presence of special object or toy during experiences. Explain source of any loud noise and reassure while noise exists. Keep number of strangers in room minimal.
Preschooler (3–5)	Dark Body harm* Being alone* Moving appliances	Cries, whimpers, screams. Verbalizes pain, fear, anger. Groaning, whining protests. Uses postponement tactics.	Seeks caretaker verbally and with eyes. Holds rigidly still. Turns away, shuts eyes. Kicks, bites, scratches, frowns, flinches, pulls away. Preoccupied with where he hurts and nurse's actions.	Believes he is being punished for wrongdoing. Will try to cooperate if he senses care given is trustworthy. Needs some assistance to hold still.	Give alternative outlet for pain (cry, yell, squeeze hand). Keep caretaker present. "Let me help you hold still" approach to restraint. Permit special object, toy or invisible friend during experience. Allow him to see and handle equipment before procedures or to see facility before he goes there for care. Brief verbal preparation before and during stressful experience; stress what he will experience with his senses; involve him actively. Be honest, friendly, reassuring. During stressful experience continually reassure and praise child's efforts to cooperate. Avoid reprimands or after-the-fact statements that reinforce child's concept of experience as punishment. Allow child to take home clean, disposable supplies for therapeutic play. Tangible rewards after stressful situation at least occasionally; not based on his being cooperative but because makes him feel good.
School-age (6–10)	Large machines Body injury Loss of self-control*	Verbalizes pain, anger, fear. Protests and trys to postpone. Whines, cries, screams.	Passively seeks support and body contact from caretaker by facial expression, not verbally. Sits or lies quietly, concentrating on maintaining control. Holds rigidly still. Turns away, closes eyes; kicks, pulls away.	Will try to cooperate if he knows what to expect. Progressively more able to hold still on own. Tries to control anxiety.	Give alternative outlet for pain (squeeze hand, count, talk about topic of interest). Describe or allow him to see equipment before procedure and the health facility before he receives treatment there. Verbal explanations before a stressful situation; stress sensations to be expected and what child can do to help. Keep caretaker present. Encourage verbalization of fears, questions. Ascertain child's perception of what will happen. Correct erroneous thinking. During stressful situation periodically reassure, remind child how he can help, and praise cooperation efforts. Allow him to take home clean disposable supplies for therapeutic play and to display before friends.
Preadolescent and adolescent (11+)	Loss of self control* Disturbance to body appearance* Death Drugs	Verbalizes pain and fear in adult manner. Tries to postpone until gains control. Groans.	Sits or lies quietly in attempt to maintain control, be brave. Turns away, winces.	Able to recognize and control anxiety. Tolerates pain poorly.	Prepare with explanations as would an adult. Encourage verbalization of questions. Describe procedures and instruments, stressing effect they will have on body's appearance and for how long. Tell youth how he may assist (gives sense of self-control) Caretaker's presence or absence the child's choice.

*Those particularly significant during illness.

child is likely to exhibit toward his illness because of his age, and help them identify how they can reduce their child's fears and anxiety; (3) prepare them for and encourage active participation in meeting their child's needs and providing treatment during his illness (this should never be forced on parents, however); and (4) provide opportunity for and encourage parents to verbalize their needs, fears and questions.

Siblings of the ill child are too often overlooked, which places them in double jeopardy if their parents must spend extra time away from them or provide extra attention to the ill child. The nurse should regularly inquire as to the siblings' adjustment to their sibling's illness and to the disruptions in home interactions and routines. Specific interventions are required to help the siblings deal with their guilt, fear and jealousy, even if these conflicts are not expressed.[15] The well child's guilt is managed by providing age-appropriate explanations of what is causing the sibling's symptoms of sickness and reassurances that nothing he himself did, said, thought or wished caused the sibling's illness. Allowing the sibling to help provide treatment (under whatever supervision his age and development make necessary) also helps to reduce his guilt.

The sibling's fear of contracting the illness must also be dealt with by reassurances that he is not likely to get the illness, if this is the case. If his contracting the illness is a real possibility, he should be honestly told (by his parents, with or without the nurse's assistance as they prefer) that the possibility exists. He should be informed of the symptoms that are important to tell his parents about if he experiences them and instructed on what, if anything, he can do to prevent getting the illness.

Involvement in his sick sibling's illness not only helps to reduce guilt, it also allows him to have a better understanding of what his ill sibling is going through and why the sibling needs his parents' attention, thereby minimizing jealous feelings. His involvement also allows the siblings to maintain contact with each other, increases the helping sibling's self-esteem and the sick sibling's morale, and permits all the family members to share in the crisis. Involvement includes keeping siblings informed of their sick sibling's progress or lack thereof, including them in teaching about the disease and its management, permitting them to interact with the sibling on a regular basis, and allowing them to assist in direct care to the extent it is feasible. When it is not possible for siblings to have direct contact with the sibling because of the contagious nature of the illness, hospital policies (many hospitals do not allow children under 12 to visit), or distance factors, indirect methods of maintaining involvement should be instituted. Examples include daily phone calls, tape recordings, written notes or pictures, snapshots and other creative approaches developed by the nurse, parents or siblings.

Siblings who have direct contact with the sick child should be prepared beforehand for what to expect (what they may see, hear or do while visiting the child at the hospital) and for their sibling's physical appearance.

If the sick child is old enough for peers to be significant, the same techniques can be used to help him maintain contact with them. The nurse or parent can also keep the school nurse informed so that she can help the teacher or peers or both understand any changes in the well siblings' behavior and help them plan ways to assist the ill sibling to adjust. The school nurse can also help plan the ill child's eventual return to school.

The nurse has an opportunity at the time of the history taking or after diagnosis to prepare parents to anticipate their well children's needs during the sibling's illness and guide them toward maintaining an adequate relationship with their well children while their ill child demands more of their time. The nurse can encourage the parents' own problem-solving to identify ways to maintain those relationships. If they need assistance, the nurse might suggest any or all the following measures: (1) demonstrate a continued interest and support for the well children's usual activities and feelings through acknowledging comments, asking questions and attendance at some of the children's activities; (2) celebrate in the usual manner any special events such as birthdays and holidays that occur during the sick child's illness; (4) encourage well siblings to continue their social activities; (5) spend 15 to 20 minutes each day with each child in some mutually enjoyable activity if possible; (6) recognize and express appreciation for the things each child does to help out during the sibling's illness; (7) generously praise the well siblings' flexibility during the crisis; (8) bring home occasional small gifts to the well children — sick children are frequent recipients of gifts, which can breed envy or jealousy in well siblings who receive none; or (9) if a parent must be absent from home because of one child's illness, maintain contact with well siblings at home every day or two. (The same measures used to keep siblings in communication can be utilized.)[14]

Parents should also be cautioned by the nurse that well children express their feelngs regarding the sibling's sickness and the family disruption in many nonverbal ways. Characteristic nonverbal expressions of their distress include: (1) somatic distress (sighing, weakness, fatigue, gastrointestinal complaints); (2) preoccupation with the image or memories of the sick sibling when he was well (especially if treatment must be conducted away from home); (3) self-blaming evidenced by irritability, impatience, social withdrawal, frequent crying; or (4) inability to maintain normal patterns of conduct and function (overactivity, restlessness, lack of initiative, regression, escalation of usual misbehaviors).[13]

The nurse's objective in meeting the needs of the sick child, his parents and his siblings, regardless of the duration of the illness or the setting for care, is to promote or regain family unity, or both, during the course of the child's illness. When each family member's needs are considered and met, more energy is available for each not only to adjust to the crisis but also to work together to help the sick child adapt to the stress of being ill.

TEMPORARY ILLNESS

Temporary illnesses are generally manifestations of the growth and development process and are minor and self-limiting. Examples of developmentally related ailments would be the dermatitide disorders associated with the infant's immature immune system, the parasitic infections of the toddler caused by his investigations of objects by mouth, the childhood communicable diseases of preschool and early school-age years brought about by broadened social exposure, the musculoskeletal injuries of the active school child, and the acne and menstrual disorders associated with the hormonal changes of adolescence. These ailments are self-limiting in that the body resolves the illness itself (although symptomatic interventions are desirable) or the condition is "outgrown" once the child progresses to a new developmental stage. Symptomatic treatment is usually carried out at home by the child himself or by the child's caretakers.

Most temporary illness causes a brief disruption to the child's usual activities and routines. Caretakers may experience interruption of sleep when called upon to soothe their irritable, uncomfortable or sleepless child or to administer the necessary symptomatic treatments. Particularly while symptoms are most acute, parental anxiety exists regarding whether or not to seek help from a health professional, whether or not their judgment is adequate to determine if the child is improving or getting worse, and concerning measures they should take to relieve their child's discomfort. Since care is usually administered at home, the caretaker who works away from home must either miss work or secure an adequate substitute caretaker for the sick child at home during work hours. The sick child tolerates his confinement during the acute stage of his illness but finds the confinement aggravating and monotonous during the recuperative stage. The sick child or his siblings may have difficulty understanding why the child must be confined or isolated.

Anticipatory guidance early in parenthood should cover some basic information that will be useful to parents when their child becomes ill. This information should include: (1) when to seek nurse or physician assistance, (2) facts to gather before calling for assistance, (3) what to do during the office or clinic visit and (4) instruction and practice in basic treatment of common symptoms (measures to reduce fever, evaluating respirations) and symptom assessment (temperature taking, throat inspection). The nurse also plays an active part in offering education and health services that can prevent many of the temporary illnesses.

When to Seek Assistance Parents need to know the early signs of illness if they are to make judgments about intervention. Illness is usually preceded by a change in the child's normal behavior, especially behaviors related to play and eating. Sudden or dramatic decrease in appetite and unusual irritability and lassitude are sure signs that all is not well. Fever and pain are also common precursors to illness. Pediatricians recommend that the parent call a health professional if:[6, 8]

1. The child is under 6 months of age and has any fever (37.8° C, 100° F).

2. The child is over 6 months and has a persistent fever over 39.2° C (102.5° F) rectally or 38.6° C (101.5° F) orally.
3. The child is persistently irritable or lethargic without obvious cause.
4. The child receives any serious injury or a hard crack on the head.
5. The child is developing signs of dehydration after prolonged vomiting or diarrhea.
6. The child is having respiratory difficulty: seek help immediately.
7. The child is obviously in pain: call for assistance even if it is midnight.
8. The parent is worried or does not know what to do.

Facts to Gather Before parents seek assistance they should look their child over for symptoms, take his temperature, and take note of his behavior so that they can answer the nurse's or doctor's questions. Table 16-3 outlines the observations caretakers should be taught to note and write down just prior to seeking assistance, whether by phone or by clinic visit. According to Tripp, from this information "the nurse can decide within minutes whether the child needs

TABLE 16-3 INFORMATION PARENTS SHOULD BE PREPARED TO PROVIDE BEFORE SEEKING ASSISTANCE[15]

CHILD'S AGE	(Symptoms may change suddenly in children under 6 months; age may affect treatment prescribed.)*
WHEN CHILD LAST WELL	(If symptoms are mild and recent, physician or nurse will probably follow by phone. If symptoms worsen or have lasted several days, child should be seen.)
BEHAVIOR	Is the child irritable? Lost interest in play? Decreased appetite? For how long has this been the case? (Child acting sick more than 24 hours should be seen by doctor or nurse even if symptoms are minor.)
FEVER	What is child's temperature? Rectally or orally? How long has the fever existed? What has been done for it—results? (Consult physician if fever is high, longer than 3 days, if infant under 6 months, if accompanied by a stiff neck and if child is dehydrated).
PAIN	Difficulty swallowing? Stiff neck? Pulling or holding ear—which one? Headache? Stomach ache—where? Pain when extremities moved? Hurt to breathe? (Consult physician immediately for acute, persistent pain; physician or nurse if child presents with no other symptoms or if trauma is associated.)
BREATHING	Slow or fast? Any noise? Coughing? Stuffy or runny nose? Unable to eat or drink? Any extra effort made to breathe? Any blueness around mouth? (See physician immediately if any distress or noise! See physician or nurse if interferes with feeding, cough interrupts sleep, persists more than 3 days without improvement.)
SKIN	Cool or hot? Dry or moist? Blotchy? Any rash—flat or raised, color, location, single or several together, itchy? (See physician or nurse if stiff neck too, swollen glands; if child looks very sick.)
ANY VOMITING/DIARRHEA	How many times today? How long has it been occurring? Any mucus? What does it look like? (See physician or nurse if frequent or constant, blood present, dehydration exists, possible poison or drug ingestion.)
EYES	Dull? Tearing? Discharge—amount and color? Partly closed? (See physician or nurse if discharge present or if, coupled with other symptoms, dehydration suggested.)
OTHER	Any other family members ill presently or recently (past 2 weeks)? Any similar illness in neighborhood or school? Any major changes in routines? Any recent family crises? Child have any chronic conditions? (A chronically ill child should be seen by physician even if symptoms are mild.)
WHAT HAS BEEN TRIED	Any medicines given? Have any of the things tried helped? (Gives some clue to caretaker's judgment re interventions. If questionable child should be seen, as other observations may be inaccurate.)
WHAT IS CARETAKER MOST WORRIED ABOUT	(If other family situations are being affected by the illness (party, trip, work) it may be important to the family for the child to be seen even if symptoms are mild.)

*The material in parentheses is a guide to the nurse in determining whether the child should be seen and by whom.

to be seen by a doctor immediately, needs to be seen by a nurse or doctor for further assessment but not necessarily immediately, or that the child may be observed and cared for at home."[15] Table 16-3 can also be used as a guide as to what to ask when parents seek assistance regarding temporary illness.

During an Office or Clinic Visit If the child is to be seen by a nurse or doctor, parents should bring along the observations they had written down as well as a list of any questions they have. The nurse who establishes the appointment can make this suggestion and encourage promptness in meeting the appointment time so the child has to wait as little time as possible. The nurse should assure the caretaker that she will call to adjust the appointment time if any unforeseeable delays come up before the appointment that would cause a long wait and then make sure she does this if necessary. Waiting is hard for any child, but especially for the ill child. The nurse might also suggest the child be allowed to bring along a couple of toys, books or other time-occupying security items. If the child is suspected of having a contagious disease, he should be kept away from other children in the waiting room. In fact, since the caretaker does not know what the other waiting children have, keeping the child occupied during the clinic visit is a wise action anytime, not just when he is ill. Some offices or clinics have the waiting area arranged to keep ill chidren in one area and children on wellness visits in another area.

The caretaker should be discouraged from threatening the child with doctor or nurse visits. Such threats disrupt the positive interaction desired between the child and the health care provider.

Teaching Parents Symptomatic Care The ultimate success of the family's involvement in home treatment is largely determined by their ability and preparation to participate in it.[10] All instructions in home care of symptoms or in procedures to assess symptoms should be written out, demonstrated (preferably with return demonstration by the caretaker) and opportunity given for the caretaker to seek clarification of any points not perfectly clear. In addition to teaching evaluation of a child for signs of illness, including rectal and oral temperature, the nurse may teach treatment of common symptoms. (Specific treatment is included throughout this book.) Included among these are fever control; dietary measures for mild vomiting or diarrhea; emergency first aid procedures (including those for bleeding and choking, and artificial respiration and circulation); aseptic measures, including the management of contagions; and how to measure and administer medicines according to the child's age. Obviously caretakers cannot absorb all this information at one time, but the nurse should try to instruct in all these areas in the early weeks of parenthood, then review them with the caretaker as the need arises or at periodic intervals. Many school health curricula are now including such information so that perhaps eventually adults will enter parenthood already knowledgeable about home management measures during minor illness.

Caretakers may also need assistance in developing convalescent activities for their recuperating youngster. The key elements of successful convalescent activities is that they encourage age-appropriate motor development, keep the child's fingers busy and keep his mind active. Many household items lend themselves to creative play and help him pass the time. Macaroni, paper plates, paper bags, old magazines or catalogues or fabric scraps (the possibilities are almost endless) coupled with scissors, paste, water paints and crayons can occupy many hours. Have the child make up stories based on a name, a character, a situation or write his own life story. If he is too young to write, he can dictate the story into a tape recorder or draw pictures.

Most children enjoy games. The parent can use words, birds, flowers, cities, or states, then give the child the challenge of learning a new word an hour or a bird a day to draw. Books can also hasten the passage of time; the young child who cannot read still enjoys pictures. One parent this author knows periodically tape-recorded the stories read to her children when they were well so that they had a stock supply of stories to listen to during illness. Use of these was, of course, interspersed with ones actually read to the child while he was sick.

The child is also helped through his convalescence if he is allowed to get at least partly dressed every day and to be occasionally on the living-room couch, if possible. If the child cannot join the family at mealtimes, each member (with the exception of those susceptible to the disease if it is contagious) can take turns having dinner with him. Perhaps everyone can join him for a bedside meal at special times.

A bedfast child should still have family responsibilities: sorting socks, snapping beans, sewing buttons, licking stamps. Even very small children should be given a chance at some tasks, and if achievement expectations are not too great, they will succeed. Older children can take charge of answering the phone on an extension during their waking hours and taking messages or calling members to the phone with a small bell. Some time to watch favorite television shows can be allowed, but bedfast children soon tire of the TV as their only source of entertainment. Human contact at regular intervals is imperative to their recovery and emotional needs. Usually parents need only a few examples of ways to occupy their child before their own imaginations take over.

REVERSIBLE ILLNESS

Reversible illness, usually brief, may require hospitalization but does not cause long-term (over a period of years) stress to the child and his family. Many of the reversible illnesses during infancy relate to the repair of anomalies, while those during toddlerhood are predominately accident-related. Preschoolers with reversible illness tend to have a predominance of infections, particularly of the genitourinary system. The major reversible illnesses of school-age children have musculoskeletal involvement, while the adolescent experiences more reversible illnesses contracted from other people. Reversible diseases are usually not self-limiting and require direct medical and nursing interventions for recovery to occur. Intervention may be on an outpatient basis, but often hospitalization, at least for a short time, is necessary. Typically acute or corrective care is conducted in the hospital, with recuperative care carried out on an outpatient basis or at home.

Most reversible illness causes a disruption to the child's routine that may last a few weeks to several months. Family life is interrupted long enough that family plans and role responsibilities must be at least temporarily revised. For the older child reversible illness may mean prolonged separation from peers (rheumatic fever) or damage to the self-image because of the social stigma attached to the illness (venereal disease) or the visibility of the treatment (scoliosis brace). Reversible illness usually lasts long enough for the young child to become cranky and "tired of being sick;" regression is almost inevitable, although the degree varies. Each family member must deal with the stresses that a hospitalization causes (discussed under hospitalization later in this chapter). Parents usually fail to get enough rest, either because of the juggling of usual family routine necessary with being at the child's hospital bedside, or if the child is treated at home, the interruptions of sleep that come with "around-the-clock" treatments and listening at night to be sure the child is all right. Parental anxiety is often worsened by the fear that the child's illness will not improve or that complications will arise.

Certainly families of children with reversible illness need to know how to evaluate and report symptoms and entertain the convalescent just as the family with a temporarily ill child does. In addition, they need support to maintain family unity for the duration of the illness (see Chapter 15 for a discussion of the nurse's supportive role) and during hospitalization (see section on hospitalization later in this chapter). The family may also need financial assistance to meet hospital expenses, and the informed nurse can direct them to appropriate resources. Most reversible illnesses require medical and nursing cooperation to develop and administer the treatment plan; involvement of other health disciplines may or may not be required.

IRREVERSIBLE ILLNESS

Irreversible illness is enduring or chronic illness which, while not life threatening, affects the lifelong adjustment process of the child and his family. Irreversible disease is not self-limiting or curable—the child must contend with it throughout life. The illness causes long-term stress, requires periodic hospitalization, and involves life-long medical and nursing management. During intervals of nonhospitalization, the child's condition (and later the adult) is managed on an outpatient basis and at home. An interdisciplinary approach that utilizes a variety of health, school and social service personnel is needed to adequately plan and administer the treatment regimen. The nurse is often given a coordination role on the team. Because many of the irreversible illnesses

TABLE 16-4 SCALE FOR DETECTING FAMILIES AT RISK FOR ADAPTING POORLY TO CHRONIC ILLNESS*

Factors	Rating	4	3	2	1	0
1	Age	<20	20–25	26–30	31–35	>35
2	Income	<5000	5000–7500	7501–10,000	10,001–15,000	>15,000
3	Race	Black		Other		White
4	Years married	<2	2–4	5–7	8–10	>10
5	Strength of marriage	Weak		Average		Strong
6	Number of children	1	2	3	4	>4
7	Education level	<High school	High school	1–2 yrs college	3–4 yrs college	>4 yrs college
8	Religious conviction	None		Average		Strong
9	Community involvement	None	One group	Two groups	Three groups	>Three groups
10	Support from maternal grandmother	None		Average		Strong
11	Husband/wife experiences with and feelings about chronic illness	Negative		Neutral		Positive

*From Chronic Illness in the School-Aged Child: Effects on the Total Family by B. Lawson. Copyright © 1977, American Journal of Nursing Company. Reproduced with permission from MCN; The American Journal of Maternal Child Nursing, January/February 1977, Vol. 2, No. 1.

are hereditary, genetic counselling and substantial family support is essential to the safeguarding of family relationships. Frequent hospitalizations, extensive treatment regimens and the illness itself present a terrific challenge for the health team and the family to help the child attain his optimal growth and development. Genetic counselling and close health supervision from conception help to prevent or minimize the effects of a majority of the irreversible illnesses of childhood.

The Family This type of illness demands frequent medical visits, expensive medication or other treatment, and periodic hospitalization, creating psychosocial fatigue and economic hardship. The family is always affected: some are strengthened, many face some degree of breakdown, a few are destroyed and all are strained. Litman found that the more chronic and complicated the illness, the more likely it is that the illness and its associated problems will have an appreciable affect on family functioning and role allocation. Most significantly affected is the primary caretaker.[10]

The greatest stress comes from the fact that the illness and its consequences must be dealt with on a daily basis. The drain on the ill child and on each family member over such an infinite amount of time can stretch their human resiliency almost beyond endurance, especially if the illness offers no periodic improvement or causes deterioration of the child's health over time. Lawson states that when one family member becomes chronically ill, the entire family to some degree becomes ill and requires attention and comfort from professional sources.[9] Table 16-4 is a scale that Lawson has developed to use in detecting those families at risk for adapting poorly to chronic illness. The higher the score on the scale, the greater is the family's risk for poor adjustment. When families at risk for poor adaptation are identified early after the diagnosis of irreversible illness, the health team can act promptly to make available to this family the resources needed to maintain its integrity.

The Child The most critical factor that determines how a child experiences and adapts to his chronic illness is the degree to which his parents accept his chronic condition and its consequences and still see him as a child who needs what any other child needs — love, discipline and independence. Mattsson has identified three behavior patterns that appear in children with irreversible illness whose parents have not resolved their resentment, guilt feelings and fears and accepted the normalcy of their child's needs. Those patterns are:[11]

1. The child is fearful, inactive and markedly dependent on his family, especially his primary caretaker. He neither participates in nor has any interest in outside activities. A vicious cycle builds that makes the child increasingly dependent, which in turn elicits resentment in family members involved in his care. The resentment is repressed much of the time but periodically is released in outbursts of disproportionate anger toward the child. The angry outburst instills greater guilt that prompts more overindulging, overprotective actions toward the child, which in turn heighten his dependency.[17]
2. The child rebels against his oversolicitous, guilt-ridden caretakers by becoming overly independent and daring, engaging in prohibited or risk-taking activities. The child strongly denies the real dangers of his activities or the true limitations placed on him by his illness.
3. Less commonly, the child behaves in a shy manner, seems lonely and resentfully directs his hostilities toward normal people because his family persistently places undue emphasis and attention on his handicaps and hides or isolates him from extended family, friends and the community. The child develops, then, a concept of himself as a defective outsider.

Successfully adjusted parents enforce necessary and realistic restrictions and expectations, encourage self-care, enforce school attendance, and facilitate the child's socialization with healthy peers as well as with peers who also are experiencing irreversible illness. Their successful adjustment supports similar adjustment in other family members and especially in the ill child. This environment allows the child to feel accepted and loved, to learn rules and adjust to his world in a socially approved manner, to build internal controls that acknowledge his limitations without destruction to his self-concept, and to feel secure in progressively caring for himself and venturing into the larger community. This child experiences a world that sees him for more than just his handicap, that will not stifle his development with overindulgence, and that acknowledges the reality of his illness so his energy can be spent not in hiding it but in overcoming it.

The Parents Parents of a child with an irreversible illness experience sorrow throughout their lives. This is a natural response to irreversible illness in their child. The intensity of that sorrow will vary over time, but it can dissolve only if the child dies. The intensity is directly influenced by the degree to which the child can accomplish the activities of daily living and how much he deviates from being a typical well child.[9]

The parents' first task is to come to terms with the painful truth and the grief that does not end. During the process of coming to grips with the truth, parents commonly evidence denial, forgetfulness and intellectualization of the disease. The health team can recommend or provide a consultation to get a second opinion on the diagnosis. Team members' openness and willingness to get a second opinion helps them gain the parents' trust and cooperation and helps the parents overcome their denial.

Because of the forgetfulness that accompanies parents' acute distress over the diagnosis, the health team must offer frequent reminders and repetition of information shared with the parents during the first days or weeks after diagnosis, when the parents are ready and able to hear it. Parents who intellectualize the illness, talking about it without emotion, are merely hiding the anguish they feel until they are ready to openly deal with the facts. Health personnel should be careful not to judge the parents as cold or uncaring during this period of intellectualization — they care so much and hurt so badly that this is the way they must cope until they have gained control over some of their anguish. The grief and sorrow is reciprocal between the child and his parents. They fear not only the potential loss of the child (not necessarily from his illness but from the complications the illness subjects him to), but also the loss of hopes and dreams for their own and the child's future. The anger, fear, hurt and despair that comes from their grieving must be shared in words and tears. They desperately need human closeness during the ups and downs of this lifetime illness.

Guilt also predominates in the parents' emotions. The guilt stems at various times from a sense of personal responsibility for their child becoming ill, from the negative feelings they periodically experience toward the child, or from the resentment because the child demands so much of their time. The nurse should provide regular opportunities for the parents to verbalize these feelings, should reassure them often that all relationships contain some negative feelings, and should repeat to them the real causes of the child's illness as frequently as seems necessary.

Throughout the animal world it is natural to be aggressive when one's young are in jeopardy, so that the anger expressed by human parents should be expected and accepted as a natural phenomenon by health personnel. Anger may be vented in any one or a combination of directions. Often the anger is taken out on those with whom the parent feels most secure — the spouse or other family members. The anger may be expressed through criticism, hostile interactions, aloofness or abuse. The anger may be vented at God or, in bitterness, at their religious community. Frequently the anger is directed at health personnel. Parents may attack the health team's slowness at deriving a diagnosis, insist that they are doing nothing that relieves the child's misery, search continuously for any signs of incompetency or noncompassionate actions, or insist that medical costs are unduly high.

The first approach to managing the anger is to allow the parents to talk it out, first with an objective listener and then with the recipient of the anger. If verbal expression is difficult for the parents, they can be encouraged to find release by writing down their feelings. Preventively or palliatively, parents can be encouraged to productively channel their anger. Vigorous body activity in the form of hard labor, physical exercise or aggressive sports (tennis, racket ball, volleyball) is an excellent release for angry feelings. Another approach is to fight for the child by mastering home treatment skills and planning actively for the child's future needs. Associating with others to educate the public about irreversible disease and to push for related research, or becoming involved in sociopolitical activities to influence school and hospital policies and to accommodate the physical environment of public places to the needs of children and adults with irreversible disease are also constructive approaches through which parents can release their anger.

Extreme apprehension also characterizes parents whose child is diagnosed with irreversible disease, especially during the early stages of coping.[12] Early in their adjustment many parents describe a sense of utter confusion, an inability to make even simple decisions, disorganization and forgetfulness (putting eggs in the pantry and flour in the refrigerator). There is acute fear that they will fall to pieces, be unable to handle all that the illness will demand of them. Many express that they too feel sick (more predominant in mothers, perhaps a residual element from the symbiotic relationship during pregnancy), or that they are "going crazy."[12] Another source of apprehension is the overwhelming sense of total helplessness and yet total responsibility they feel for their child's predicament.

During this time the nurse should be ready to provide comfort, reminding the parents often through word ("I'm here if you need me ... can I do anything to help you?") and deed (providing a cup of coffee, a pillow, a more comfortable chair) that they are not alone. Anticipating the parents' sense of sickness, the nurse can incorporate in her teaching the fact that our bodies express emotional stress through physiological changes (flushing, heart palpitations, dizziness), thus reassuring the mother that physical changes she might experience are probably a consequence of her emotional stress and not physical illness. To ease parents sense of helplessness and responsibility, the nurse should bolster their confidence by involving them in the planning and giving of care, teaching them as much as is known about the disease and its management, and in techniques of care.

One of the most prevalent negative patterns of parental response to a child's irreversible illness is overprotection.[3] Holaday describes several features that characterize the overprotective parent.[7] Table 16–5 summarizes those features.

A certain degree of dependency of the child and protection by the parents is sometimes necessary in caring for the child with irreversible illness. However, persistent or exaggerated encouragement of dependency by parents is an overreaction that demolishes the child's drives for self-esteem, self-control and independence.

The nurse must be alert to early signs of overprotective parenting, providing support and education that will assist the parents to achieve a healthy balance between dependence and independence for the child. From the time of diagnosis the nurse should take preventive measures to discourage overprotection by em-

TABLE 16-5 CHARACTERISTICS OF OVERPROTECTIVE PARENTING

Centered on Affected Child
1. Parents set unrealistic goals for this child because they do not or will not accept his limitations and capabilities.
2. Sacrifice selves and family for this child.
3. Protect child from every imaginable hurt or difficulty.
4. Use different (often inconsistent) types and patterns of discipline for this child than for normal siblings.

Overcontrolling
1. Monopolize the child's life, in constant attendance.
2. Hover over the child's activities, interceding in situations the child could handle himself.
3. Speak for the child, answer all questions directed to him.
4. Make decisions for child without considering his wishes.
5. Discourage child from personal or social activities that will help him grow up. They feed, bathe or dress him when he can master those skills himself. They may sleep with him, choose his friends, keep him home from peer gatherings.
6. Play is restricted either from fear for the child's safety (love-prompted overprotection) or to frustrate or punish the child (rejection-prompted overprotection).

---

phasizing the child's normal features, helping the parents identify the child's capabilities realistically and evaluate his progress in overcoming his limitations on a regular basis. Introducing the parents to a parents support group and exposing them to children with a similar disability who are achieving self-sufficiency may help the family set realistic goals and allow opportunities for their child to gain increased responsibility for himself. If overprotection has progressed to a pathological level, referral for psychological counselling becomes a nursing responsibility.

Marital strain, divorce and suicide are more prominent in families in which irreversible illness exists than with any other type of illness.[9] Several factors can contribute to this strain. As a way of coping, each spouse may blame the other (inheritance, neglect of the child, delay in seeking health care) for their child's illness. Spouses often have different coping styles that tend to conflict. For example, one spouse may cope best by experiencing closeness, sharing emotions, and talking about their plight, while the other spouse may cope best by staying aloof and working through the stress internally.

The illness causes a need for long-term changes in role expectations for each spouse, a fact one or both spouses may resent or be unwilling to accept. The extra attention and care required by the child, the disruption to home routines during hospitalization, the extra costs incurred that may mean a second job or longer work hours for one spouse all serve to decrease the frequency of or impair spouse communication at a time when it is so badly needed. Spouses may disagree over what to expect of their child or how the responsibility of his care should be divided. The nurse should regularly assess the family for signs of marital breakdown and refer those couples at risk for professional counselling. The nurse can also help the spouses become involved in a parents support group or organization early in the course of the disease as one means of helping to prevent or minimize marital and family discord. Exposure to parents in a similar situation helps reduce their sense of isolation and strengthen their sense of self-worth. It offers reassurance that their concerns are valid and shared by others. The sharing these parents do provides them with insights into handling daily situations and reinforces their parenting skills, in addition to affording each parent a source of caring support. Affiliation with parents in similar circumstances gives them opportunities to learn how to deal with their fears when treatment is not working, how to know when their child can handle more independence, and how to overcome their fear of leaving their child with a babysitter. (It also provides a source of knowledgeable babysitters.) They also learn from other couples how to cope with the regimented life style the illness imposes, how to handle people's negative reactions to their child and how to overcome many fears.

The Siblings Like the siblings of children with temporary or reversible illness, siblings of a child with irreversible illness experience guilt, fear for their own health, and are jealous because of the parental attention and time the ill child receives. However, the siblings of a child with irreversible illness must contend with and re-resolve these feelings for a lifetime because their sick sibling does not get well, and the chances are that he may even get worse. The sorrow they share with their parents after diagnosis is real but short-lived. Children simply have a short sadness span. The nurse should prepare parents for this fact and encourage them to let the siblings know that it is all right that their grief does not linger. Siblings of an irreversibly ill child must come to terms with the fact that there will be many times when their wants and wishes will have to take second place to the more immediate needs of their sick brother or sister. Parents should be guided to accept this fact, too, and to encourage their children to openly discuss their feelings about this with them. The siblings' acceptance is facilitated when parents state that they understand their feelings and appreciate the sacrifices that are made for their sick sibling.

Siblings should be expected and encouraged to help with the ill child's care, praised for their involvement, and reassured that sometimes he will have poorer health despite treatment and that it is not because of the care they gave. Such participation helps the well sibling to understand how long treatments do take, how fatiguing they can be and what their sick sibling's needs really are. This experience helps the siblings understand the realities of their sibling's care and makes the occasional taking of second place easier to tolerate. Siblings should be given age-appropriate information about their sibling's disease and treatment; many children's books are available that help to explain how the sick sibling feels, that teach more about the disease, and that urge the development of a positive, accepting attitude about handicapped people.* (A partial listing of some well-written children's books on irreversible diseases is included at the end of this section.)

The Grandparents Grandparents are an important resource to families who have an irreversibly ill child. Grandparents may initially be an additional emotional burden to the family when irreversible illness is diagnosed in their grandchild because they too go through denial, lack understanding of the disease (many of the reversible and irreversible diseases today were fatal during the grandparents' childrearing years), or need comforting themselves instead of being a source of comfort. They may experience guilt similar to the child's parents if the disease is hereditary. They may find it difficult to offer compassion because the child's illness forces them to face their own mortality. Many grandparents find it difficult to permit their adult children dependence during this crisis once they have finally accepted their child's independence from them. The grandparent's reaction may be either to overindulge or avoid the ill grandchild. In such a case, the parents must confront them to alter this behavior for the child's sake, although such directness toward their own parents may not be easy for them.

Many grandparents, however, are an invaluable source of emotional and tangible support to their children and grandchildren when irreversible illness occurs. They often serve as a sounding board for the sick child's distraught parents. They may provide transport or accompany the child and parent during outpatient care or hospitalization. Help with house routines is usually greatly appreciated. They may babysit or provide special attention to the siblings to help fill the void when their parents are occupied with the ill child. Grandparents often model the strength, patience and faith that the family needs to learn as they adjust to living with irreversible illness.

Recommended Children's Literature Pertaining to Children's Special Needs and Disabilities

Fiction

"Deenie" by Judy Blume, Bradbury Press, 1973, ages 10 to 14. (Scoliosis)

"Why Me?" by John Branfield, Harper and Row, 1973, ages 10 to 14. (Diabetes)

"Rachel," by Michael Charlton, Bradbury Press, 1975, ages 5 to 8. (Adjustment to wheelchair)

"A Dance to Still Music," by Barbara Corcoran, Atheneum Publishers, 1974, ages 10 to 14. (Deafness)

"Burnish Me Bright," by Julia Cunningham, Pantheon Books, 1970, ages 9 to 12. (Muteness)

"The Stronghold," by Mollie Hunter, Harper and Row, 1974, ages 10 to 14. (Crippling disease)

"The Treasure of Green Knowe," by L. M. Boston, Harcourt Brace Jovanovich, 1958, ages 9 to 11. (Blindness)

"Father's Arcane Daughter," by E. L. Konigsburg, Atheneum Publishers, 1976, ages 10 up. (Cerebral palsy)

"From Anna," by Jean Little, Harper and Row, 1973, ages 9 to 12. (Partial sight)

"The Top Step," By Gunilla Norris, Atheneum Publishers, 1970, ages 8 to 11. (Asthma)

"Sing Down The Moon," by Scott O'Dell, Houghton Mifflin Co., 1970, ages 10 to 14. (Crippled arm)

"David in Silence," by Veronica Robinson, J. B. Lippincott Co., 1965, ages 10 to 13. (Deafness)

"Let the Balloon Go," By Ivan Southall, St. Martin's Press, 1968, ages 9 to 14. (Cerebral palsy)

"Heidi," by Johanna Spyri, Charles Scribner's Sons, 1958, pages 9 to 12. (Crippling disease)

"A Little Demonstration of Affection," by Elizabeth Winthrop, Harper and Row, 1975, ages 11 to 14. (Asthma)

"A Single Light," By Maia Wojciechowska, Harper and Row, 1968, ages 11 to 14. (Deafness and muteness)

"Goldengrove," by Jill Paton Walsh, G. K. Hall and Co., 1973, ages 12 up. (Blindness)

---

*Much of the traditional children's literature depicts the handicapped person as the bad guy, evil, possessed and ugly.

Non-Fiction

"Handtalk: An ABC of Finger Spelling and Sign Language," by Remy Charlip, Parents' Magazine Press, 1974, ages 6 and up. (Deafness, muteness, blindness)

"What If You Couldn't. . . ? A Book About Special Needs," by Janet Kamien, Charles Scribner's Sons, 1978, ages 10 up. (Physical, mental and emotional handicaps)

"Lisa and Her Soundless World," by Edna S. Levine, Human Sciences Press, 1974, ages 4 to 8. (Impaired hearing)

"A Button in Her Ear," by Ada Litchfield, Albert Whitman and Co., 1976, ages 6 to 9. (Hearing loss)

"Wheelchair Champions: A History of Wheelchair Sports," by Harriet May Savitz, John Day Co., 1978, ages 10 up. (Wheelchair)

"About Handicaps: An Open Family Book for Parents and Children Together," by Sara Bonnett Stein, Walker and Co., 1974, ages 4 to 7. (Cerebral palsy and other handicaps)

"Connie's New Eyes," by Bernard Wolf, J. B. Lippincott Co., 1976, ages 9 to 12. (Blindness)

"Don't Feel Sorry for Paul," by Bernard Wolf, J. B. Lippincott Co., 1974, ages 8 to 12. (Artificial limbs)

References

1. J. Bellack. Helping a child cope with the stress of injury. American Journal of Nursing, August 1974, p. 1491
2. T. Brazelton. Anticipatory guidance. Pediatric Clinics of North America, August 1975, p. 533
3. D. Boone and B. Hartman. The benevolent over-reaction. Clinical Pediatrics, November 1972, p. 268
4. B. Brodie. Views of healthy children toward illness. American Journal of Public Health, December 1974, p. 1156
5. B. Burtoff. Are only bad guys disabled? Kids disabilities in print. Fort Wayne News Sentinel, 17 March 1980, p. 2C
6. V. Fontana. When your child doesn't feel well. Parents, July 1979, p. 80
7. B. Holaday. Parenting the chronically ill child. In Current Practice in Pediatric Nursing. Vol. II. P. Brandt et al, C. V. Mosby Co., 1978
8. M. Kelly. Answers to the 20 questions all parents ask. Parents, November 1978
9. B. Larson. Chronic illness in the school-age child, effects on the total family. American Journal of Maternal and Child Nursing, Jan/Feb 1977, p. 49
10. T. Litman. The family as a basic unit in health and medical care: a social-behavioral overview. Social Science and Medicine, August 1974, p. 495
11. I. Mattsson. Long-term illness in childhood: a challenge to psychosocial adaptation. Pediatrics, November 1972, p. 801.
12. A. McCollum. Coping With Prolonged Health Impairment In Your Child. Little, Brown and Co., 1975
13. B. Schoenberg et al., eds. Loss and Grief: Psychological Management in Medical Practice. Columbia University Press, 1973
14. J. Shulman. Coping With Tragedy: Successfully Facing the Problem of a Seriously Ill Child. Fallett Publ. Co., 1976
15. S. Tripp. What to ask and what to do when parents call about children's illnesses. Nursing 74, June 1974, p. 73
16. R. Wu. Behavior and illness. Prentice-Hall, Inc., 1973
17. W. Yancy. Approaches to emotional management of the child with a chronic illness. Clinical Pediatrics, February 1972, p. 64

Additional Recommended Reading

M. Avery. Primary care for handicapped children. American Journal of Nursing, April 1973, p. 658

V. Buchan. Don't sit on Randy. Home Life, October 1976, p. 34

M. Craft. Help for the family's neglected "other" child. American Journal of Maternal-Child Nursing, Sept/Oct 1979, p. 297

B. Dominguez and J. Perrin. Advocate for the crippled child. American Journal of Nursing, October 1973, p. 1750

S. Dube and S. Pierog. Immediate Care of the Sick and Injured Child. C. V. Mosby Co., 1978

M. Hartman. Folk health and illness beliefs. Nurse Practitioner, Jul/Aug 1979, p. 250

P. Keapovich. Immunosuppression in the child who has cancer. American Journal Maternal and Child Nursing, Sept/Oct 1979, p. 288

J. Miller. Cognitive dissonance in modifying families' perceptions. American Journal of Nursing, August 1974, p. 1468

E. Perrin et al. Telephone management of acute pediatric illness. New England Journal of Medicine, January 1978, p. 130

O. Simpson and M. Smith. Lightening the load for parents of children with diabetes, American Journal of Maternal and Child Nursing, Sept/Oct 1979, p. 293

H. Sultz et al. Long-Term Childhood Illness. University of Pittsburgh Press, 1972

WHEN A CHILD IS HOSPITALIZED

by Gail K. Ingersoll, RN, MS

Hospitalization is always a stressful experience for children and adolescents and their families. Normal routines are altered, strangers interrupt the parent-child relationship to provide care, unfamiliar equipment and surroundings are introduced, mobility is often hampered, and frightening or painful procedures must be endured. Improperly managed, the hospitalization experience can be emotionally and developmentally damaging to the hospitalized child and to his family.

Hospitalization of children should be avoided whenever other feasible alternatives exist.

Unavoidable hospital stays should be minimal in duration and should be managed in a way that is *responsive to the child's uniquenesses, to his developmental needs and to his cultural background.* If the hospital care providers are responsive to these factors and understand the needs of children and their families during illness and stress, the hospital experience can afford the child and his family an opportunity to grow, as new and better ways of dealing with problems are learned.

The goal of the nurse is to assist the child and family to adapt positively to the hospital experience and to facilitate their growth. This goal is accomplished by encouraging the child and family to draw upon their strengths and healthy support systems to develop positive coping mechanisms. They can also be assisted to utilize the problem-solving process to convert limitations into strengths as they attempt to adapt to the new and stressful situations hospitalization poses.

Understanding the child's or adolescent's developmental stage is, of course, central to providing appropriate care and support. This section discusses the general principles of coping with the stress of hospitalization. Chapters 27, 36, 45, 54 and 63 discuss in detail the specific needs of hospitalized children at various stages of development. Each of these chapters also includes a nursing care plan tailored to the particular needs of children of various ages.

THE STRESS OF HOSPITAL ADMISSION

The admission process has three aspects to which the child and his caretakers will react. These are: (1) the social environment of the admission setting, (2) the physical environment of the hospital unit to which the child is assigned and (3) the nature of the admitting procedures to which the child is subjected. The nurse plays a critical role in influencing the child's and family's experience with each of these factors.

The Social Environment

When the child is admitted to the hospital, it is important that the experience be made as pleasant as possible. First impressions often linger, and a rushed, depersonalized approach is likely to have a lasting negative effect. An appropriately handled admission interview fosters the child's and family's confidence in the ability of the staff to provide adequate care. Throughout the interview, the nurse should be sensitive to body language and convey an atmosphere of acceptance. Approach by a warm, caring person helps the child and family to cope with the admission in a positive way, and encourages their cooperation.

Time should be allowed for the child and family to ask questions so they do not feel rushed or pressured by the nurse's busy schedule. The child, especially the school-age child and adolescent, should also be given an opportunity to ask questions privately, without the parents' presence. The child should be introduced as early as possible to his primary nurse and/or some other hospital personnel with whom he can count on regular and frequent contact during his hospital experience (director of hospital play program, volunteer grandparent, hospital teacher). He should be introduced to his roommate and to other children of similar age who are likely to be present during his hospital stay.

The Physical Environment

The actual hospital environment is another factor that may be stressful for the child and family; there are many unfamiliar sights, sounds and smells. In addition, the child is admitted to a strange room, either alone or with children he does not know, and to an unfamiliar bed. He is removed from the objects and people he is used to at home that make him feel secure.

The nurse should encourage the child's parents to stay with him at least until he has investigated his new environment, claimed a few of the hospital's play items as temporarily his own, and arranged his bed area to make him feel he has established his own little "place to live."

Feelings of security are often threatened by the stress that accompanies hospitalization. Parents should be encouraged to bring a favorite toy or blanket for younger children. School-age children may enjoy bringing a favorite item such as a pocket radio or a game. Teenagers may enjoy having a poster of a favorite sports or movie star on a wall near their bed. These kinds of items represent the security of home and have special meaning to the child. Allowing the child to have some of his belongings, and permitting decoration of his space, helps to personalize it and makes him feel more secure.

Because the hospital must be concerned with preventing injury or preventing the spread of communicable diseases to children who are admitted for treatment, certain protocols may be required. These regulations, while they exist for the child's safety, may increase the child's and family's stress. For example, a child who has outgrown a crib or side rails on his bed at home may need them in the hospital because of the nature of his illness or injury. Nevertheless, the child might feel that he is being treated like a baby, especially if he is not provided with a reasonable explanation. Belts or ties may be used for a child in a wheelchair to prevent a fall; the child may perceive this action to mean that he is not trusted. Sometimes these restraining devices are used even when the child is alert and in little danger of injuring himself, simply because it is hospital policy. The nurse as the child's advocate has an obligation to motivate revision of policies that are outdated, unrealistic or serve no useful purpose.

If the child's or adolescent's health permits, he should be given a tour of the unit and introduced to the use of his call bell, bed controls, bathroom facilities and the play area. Any rules about unit routines or restrictions should be explained to the child on admission and repeated as necessary during his hospital stay.

Parents will be concerned that the child's home routines and limits are continued during his hospitalization. The information should be solicited during the admission interview and incorporated into the child's plan of care.

The child should be given opportunity to play out his admission fears with age-appropriate play materials as a part of his adaptation process. Whether he is allowed to act out his fears through active or quiet play will depend on his illness and the play facilities available.

Isolation alters the physical environment either to protect a child with an impaired immune system from contracting disease or to prevent a child with an infectious disease from spreading pathogenic organisms to other children. Nevertheless, isolation does increase stress for the child and family, particularly for the young child who has not yet developed the cognitive ability to understand its purpose. He may wonder why his mother's face is hidden behind a mask, why her hair is covered with a cap, and why her familiar clothes are under a long gown. The monotony of everyone dressing alike and of being confined to his room are additional stresses to which the child must adapt. Therapeutic play becomes an extremely valuable intervention that helps to entertain the isolated child while simultaneously providing an outlet for fears and frustration.

ADMISSION PROCEDURES

Admission x-rays, blood work and collection of urine specimens, as well as removing the child's clothing and taking blood pressure and temperature, especially rectally, are examples of procedures that may be unpleasant or frightening to the newly admitted child. Admission procedures should be preceded by an age-appropriate explanation to the child and completed as quickly as possible. The parents should also receive an explanation of the procedure and how they may assist. If it is not possible for a parent to be with the child during the procedure, a nurse to whom the child has already been introduced should stay with him during the procedure and offer comfort afterward.

Preadmission Preparation

One method of reducing the stress of hospitalization is a preadmission tour. It is beneficial for children to visit and tour the hospital, even if there is not a planned admission in the near future. Major areas such as the emergency room, the x-ray department, the laboratory, operating and recovery rooms, as well as patient rooms, can be visited. Staff in these areas can be introduced and simple explanations of their roles given. With an opportunity to see procedures (application of a cast to a doll and its removal) and to handle equipment (IV tubing or an oxygen mask), the child can begin to work through some of his fears regarding illness and hospitalization.

At the end of the tour, refreshments can be served in the play room area, and staff can be present to interact with the children, answer questions or clarify information. Various child-sized articles of nurse's or doctor's clothing and

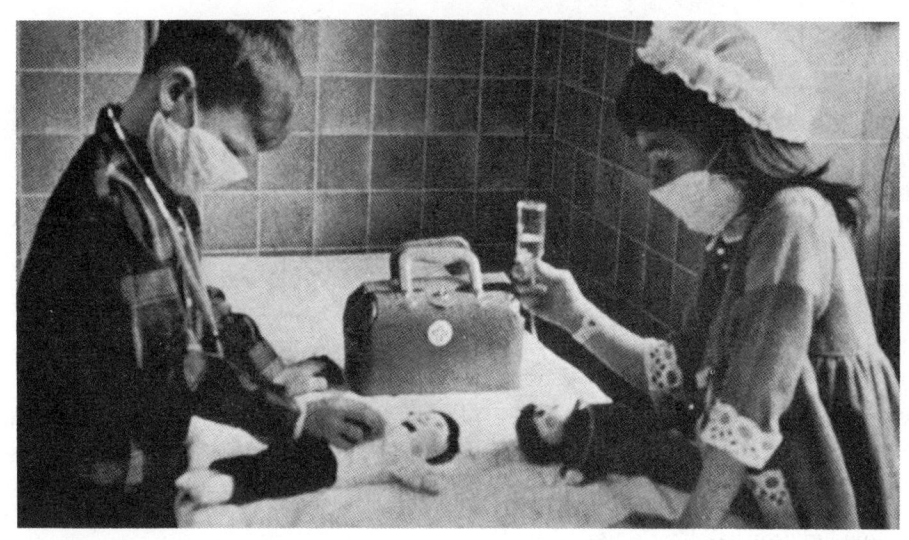

Treatment procedures are less frightening to children when they can act them out. (From M. Petrillo. Preventing Hospital Trauma. American Journal of Nursing, July 1968, p. 1472.)

a variety of equipment can be made available to the children at this time for examining and dramatic play. Since many children have contact with the hospital on an emergency basis due to acute illness or an accident, the general hospital team can be helpful in preparing the child for any experience with the hospital.

When admission to the hospital is planned for diagnostic work or surgery, the tour and parent-child teaching can be developed around that theme.

Books also provide a useful means of teaching and preparing the child for hospitalization. Lists of age-appropriate books are available through the hospital's play or library resource person or through the local children's library. (A recommended list is included at the end of this section with which the nurse may wish to become acquainted). These books could be utilized at home before admission, during hospitalization and again when the child and family return home.

Parental Needs During Admission

Parents need an introduction to the people who will be caring for their child, to the facilities available for their use, and to at least one other family who has a child hospitalized on the unit. They also need information about the policies of the hospital or unit or both that affect them.

A warm, caring approach to parents that makes them feel welcome will considerably lessen the stress they feel at admission. Nursing staff should convey from the beginning their recognition of the unique caretaking role of parents and provide ongoing understandable information and support that will enable the parents to utilize their strengths in supporting their child. Nursing attitudes and unit policies and facilities should provide for and encourage the presence and participation of parents and other persons most significant to the child. Most hospitals have tried in recent years to increase visiting hours for parents; many provide 24-hour open visiting for parents, and some include grandparents and siblings.

Facilities for parents should include a lounge separate from but close to their child's room, where they can relax. Health care booklets, magazines or light reading material, television or games provide a diversion for parents. A kitchen in which parents can make a cup of coffee, toast, or a cup of soup may also help them to feel welcome. Some hospitals are also able to provide a shower and dressing area for parents. In addition, some hospitals provide sleeper-lounge chairs, cots or sleeping bags for parents, as space permits. Although comfortable facilities for parents are particularly helpful in reducing their stress, most parents respond favorably to even small attempts and gestures to make them comfortable while they stay close to their child. Referrals to appropriate resources such as the hospital's social service department can also help parents work through the day-to-day problems of transportation, lodging, finances and home management.

THE STRESS OF HOSPITAL EXPERIENCES

The Child's Response to the Hospital Environment

There are a wide range of possible responses of the child to hospitalization. Factors influencing that response are the child's age, his personality, the preparation he received before hospitalization and his previous experiences with health professionals and the hospital environment. The severity of his illness and length of his hospital stay also affect his response. The greatest influences, however, tend to be how his parents respond to his hospitalization and how health professionals approach him.

Babies under 6 months of age tend to show less anxiety than in later months. They are less likely to cry when a parent leaves and are more easily comforted by a stranger. These babies do respond with fear to loud noises or sudden movement. When they get home they tend to be subdued, quiet, and have an extreme preoccupation with their surroundings. They are not easily distracted by their mother's voice or with a toy. Babies over 6 months fret and cry when their mother leaves. Children from around 6 months to 4 years show the maximum adverse effects of separation and the stress of hospitalization.

Robertson has coined the term *settling-in* to describe how young children react to the stress of hospitalization.[20] The first stage is *protest*. The child has a strong conscious need for his caretaker, and cries intensely when the caretaker leaves, does not accept the attempts of nurses or staff to comfort him, and will go to the farthest corner of his bed or crib to avoid their contact. The second stage is *despair*. The child still has a conscious need for his caretaker, but when that person does not come the child cries monotonously. The child becomes less active, withdraws and becomes apathetic. He may sob intermittently, rock back and forth, or engage in other repetitive behaviors. His grief for his caretaker is intense, but because he is now quieter than before, it may falsely be assumed that he is adjusting.

The third stage is *denial*. The child shows more interest in his surroundings, relates to the nurses and staff as well as to other children, and is perceived by others as happy. This behavior may be interpreted to mean that the child is settling in and adjusting well to the hospital. It is a danger signal, however, because the child is repressing his intense feeling for his caretaker. When his caretaker comes to visit, he will tend to ignore or reject her because she has failed to meet his needs. Relationships with nurses, staff and other children tend to be only superficial. When the young child is allowed to progress through all three steps of "settling in" behavior, he is in danger of experiencing long-term negative effects.

If possible, hospitalization for elective procedures should be avoided until after the child is 5 years of age. Other alternatives would include day hospitals or surgeries in which the child is admitted and treated, usually in one day, and goes home with his parents at night. Parents are usually allowed and encouraged to stay with their child as much as possible. The other alternative is for the parents to stay with the child (room-in) during his hospitalization. A grandparent, other relatives or a close neighbor could substitute for the parent during short periods of time. When it is not possible for parents to stay near, the nurse should substitute for them to meet the child's emotional needs, provide support to the parents when they can visit, and spend extra time with the child to hopefully prevent the second and third stages of "settling in." Therapeutic play may be useful in helping the child express some of his intense feelings.

Older children and teens tend to adapt more easily to separation from parents, fearing instead the possibility of bodily injury or deformity. These children also have a more realistic understanding of death, but they fear that they may die, being permanently separated from friends and family. Older children may also experience anxiety about treatment involving drugs, fearing that they may become addicted.

Wolff found that certain children are more vulnerable to the stress of hospitalization than others.[25] These vulnerable children are: (1) only children, (2) youngest children, (3) children living with extended families, (4) those with a history of responding poorly to strangers, (5) those who are exposed to other people only rarely and (6) those who have experienced recent trauma, such as death of a parent or divorce. Children with a history of poor adjustment tend to respond most adversely to hospitalization. The nurse should be alert for these relationships as the data base is obtained in the admission interview so that intervention can be initiated early to prevent long-term trauma associated with the hospitalization.

Children who have major physiologic stresses such as burns, malignancies requiring mutilating surgery, or chronic illness requiring frequent hospitalizations are also more vulnerable to the traumatic effects of hospitalization.[25] These children develop fears based on a combination of factual information and fantasy. The perceptive nurse will be alert for the child's expression of fear and will provide play opportunities or a time for talking to help the child work through his fears. The child may perceive alterations in body image that may or may not be real. The child must be helped to positively accept any necessary changes in body image after treatment. The nurse can provide the means for and observe play, listen, accept negative feelings, clarify misinformation and help the child explore ways to maximize his abilities.

Regardless of their age, most children will react to hospitalization with regression. The nurse should respect the child's need to regress and help him and his parents to accept the regressive behavior. Support and encouragement should be offered the child to help him recover from his regressive behavior and continue progressing developmentally during the course of his hospitalization. Parents are extremely important resources to the child during this time; the nurse should avoid interrupting parent-child interactions whenever possible.

The Child's Response to Procedures and Pain

Fears about procedures and pain result in stress for both the child and his parent. Often misconceptions exist about the purpose of the procedure and what is to be done. To a young child whose treatment involves daily blood work, it may seem that so much blood is withdrawn each time that he will not have any left. Showing the child that 5 millimeters is only about a teaspoonful and explaining how his body replenishes its blood supply will help to reduce his fears. Assuring the child that pain from a needle will only last for a moment, as well as providing him an opportunity to play with the syringe, will help him to cope with this fear. The child should be assured that for more painful procedures such as surgery he will be given medicine to make him sleep so that he will not feel pain, and assured that special medicine will be given to him to relieve discomfort after the treatment.

Other procedures, such as taking vital signs or collecting urine or stool specimens, will be fairly easy for most children to accept if they are given simple explanations. Telling a young child who needs frequent vital signs taken that the nurse has to watch him closely is usually sufficient explanation. An infant or very young toddler however might not understand why he needs to be restrained for such procedures and adapts best when a parent stays to provide comfort during and after the procedure. Older children and teens will need more thorough explanations of why various procedures are done if their cooperation is to be obtained.

The Nurse's Role in Relieving the Child's Stress

Turning passive experiences into active ones that facilitate the child's healthy adjustment to hospitalization is a major responsibility of the nurse. Through play, group activities and actual participation in his own care and some of the decisions regarding it, the child becomes a "doer" and a person with some control rather than a frightened, helpless victim.

Play Play provides a natural medium for the child to explore his feelings, express himself, and to work through the stress of hospitalization. According to Erikson, to work through problems utilizing play is one of the most self-healing measures found in childhood. When the opportunity for play is not available, destructive and unmanageable behavior, with potentially serious psychological effects, is frequently the outcome. Therapeutic play is any play activity that helps the child deal with the stress of hospitalization in a way that yields growth. Many aspects of hospital life can be made more familiar and less fear-provoking, and the child can be helped to understand some of the mysteries or distortions of his illness and treatment. It is therapeutic when a child can explore his feelings at his own pace, and when he begins to become desensitized to an object or procedure that formerly was frightening or painful. Sometimes just handling the equipment, as in play with a syringe, can help reduce stress. The child's natural desire for physical play can be used in the hospital to help him regain use of a body part after surgery or removal of a cast or to vent some of his anger. Dramatic play offers a good resource for the hospitalized child. He decides whose role he wishes to play, manipulates equipment that may be associated with painful or frightening treatment and re-enacts procedures.

Creative art play with individual or groups of children could include traditional free painting, cut-and-paste activities or work with crayons, as well as creative writing and poetry or interpretive dance. A pediatric mental health nurse, a play therapist or an art therapist can interpret the deeper feelings conveyed in these activities. This becomes especially helpful for understanding the needs of children with serious long-term and life-threatening illness.

Play can also be a useful diagnostic instrument for the nurse. By observing the child's play the nurse gains insight into the meaning of the hospital setting and hospital events for the child. The child's play also reveals to the observing nurse any distortions or misinterpretations he has regarding his illness, the procedures of treatment, or hospital personnel. Using these observations, the nurse can identify problems needing intervention and gain feedback about the effectiveness of preprocedural teaching or therapeutic play activities previously offered the child.

Group Activities Group activities help to reduce the stress of hospitalization for many children. The child sees how other children with problems adapt and cope, and this provides him with ideas for adapting. Children can encourage and offer support to each other, especially when the nurse reinforces these supportive behaviors.

Age-appropriate group activities also provide opportunities for socialization with a number of children and help the child learn to relate to children of the opposite sex. The children learn to share responsibilities and carry out tasks, and to respond to peer pressure in setting limits on behavior. Young children enjoy movies and arts and crafts, and older childen might enjoy working on a hospital unit newspaper. Since most children enjoy eating together, regular meals can be served in the play room or classroom. Children enjoy planning and preparing food and decorations for special events or parties. This activity also helps children begin to utilize organizational skills. Younger children might enjoy a clown's visit or a presentation by a magician, whereas older children might enjoy a concert by a rock band.

Group activities are especially meaningful to a child who must remain hospitalized during holidays or his birthday. Whenever possible, parties at these times should be arranged or at least allowed. Perhaps more visitors can be permitted on that day or visiting policies extended to allow visits by family members or friends who are usually not permitted to visit.

Active Participation The child who is forced to comply with treatment and hospitalization without any involvement in his own care suffers a loss of control and lowered self-esteem that thwarts his development and reinforces his regressive behaviors. Children should be given age-appropriate explanations of their illness. Instruction and demonstrations should be provided that will help them understand treatments and procedures and master at least some degree of self-care. Children are naturally curious about their bodies, and they enjoy explanations about what the nurse or doctor sees during an examination or procedure. A child enjoys listening to his own heart with a stethoscope, or seeing another child's eardrum as the nurse holds the otoscope. Since the seriously ill or injured child may be able to hear and understand a great deal more than his response indicates, he too should receive explanation. As the child's condition improves, he will be able to more actively participate in his own care.

Self-care helps to maintain and improve coordination, muscle tone and circulation, and it fosters positive self-esteem and a sense of self-control. The child may have a residual chronic health problem that will require continued treatment at home. Active participation in his own hospital care gives the child a sense of adequacy to cope positively after hospitalization.

Parental Response to a Child's Hospitalization

The parents of a hospitalized child also experience an increase in stress as a result of a number of factors. Freiberg's research revealed that parental anxieties were increased when they lacked information about or feared the procedures and treatments their child experienced and when they lacked information about the diagnosis and its impact on his future.[2] In addition, parents often feel guilty about their child's illness or injury, even when they could have done nothing to prevent it. The child may cry when they approach or leave, resulting in the feeling that their presence only adds to their child's discomfort, thereby reinforcing their guilt feelings. Stress is further increased if the admission is an emergency rather than a planned event. The pressure to hurry and the confusion that usually accompanies emergencies add to the parent's anxiety.

Initially, parents are concerned primarily about their child's physical condition. The prolonged waiting for diagnostic procedures or surgery to be completed or for the results of tests adds to the parents' stress by perpetuating their sense of helplessness. Parents have a right to know about the current condition of their child, the findings from diagnostic studies, the possible and actual effects of treatments, and their child's progress. This information should be offered as soon as possible after it is available so that the parents have concrete facts with which to deal rather than the fears and fantasies that arise from not knowing. During the waiting period a nurse should be available to the family to discuss concerns, answer questions and clarify misconceptions. This increases the family's confidence in and cooperation with the health care staff.

Parents may be concerned about whether or not a particular treatment, especially if it involves much pain, is helping their child or merely increasing his suffering. Treatment may also involve controversial or experimental procedures, necessitate restriction of movement or temporarily make the child's condition worse. In addition, parents may have unrealistic fears about the risk of a procedure, or have unrealistic expectations with regard to its results. For example, surgery may merely reduce pain or stop progression of a deformity, whereas the parent may expect it to provide a cure. The nurse can listen, accept parent's feelings and offer additional or clarifying information.

The Nurse's Role in Relieving Parental Anxiety

The nurse is a primary source of information and support to parents during their child's hospitalization. The explanations of care and the role modeling she provides help to involve the family in their child's care. She helps them understand their child's illness and prepares them to assume his care after discharge. Active participation by parents in providing some of the child's care during his hospitalization helps them develop confidence in their ability to provide even complex care. When the child is discharged, the parents feel comfortable because they have performed care procedures. Parents' feelings of frustration and helplessness can be prevented because they are actively contributing to their child's recovery.

Parents experience stress when their child is hospitalized and their roles of primary caretakers are assumed by the hospital staff. For this reason, too, parents should be encouraged to assist with the child's care to the extent they are willing and able. They must not feel, however, that unless they provide some care their child will receive less than optimal care from the staff. The nurse should remember that parents may feel inadequate or too frightened to physically care for their child, especially if his condition is serious. In these circumstances it may be advisable to allow the parent to observe the nurse caring for the child. The nurse can utilize the observation time to explain the purpose of various procedures and demonstrate how they are done. As parents feel more comfortable they may wish to increase their participation. When the parent begins to participate more actively, the nurse should assist and offer encouragement, as the parent will continue to need support and positive reinforcement. The parent also need the opportunity to ask questions and clarify information. As the parent becomes more comfortable in the role of care provider, the nurse should allow more independence, but she still assumes responsibility for all care given.

Parents often have useful suggestions about special approaches that may work well with their child. Some hospitals are providing care by parent units. Nurses are available if needed, but parents provide most of the care. These can be especially helpful when the child does not require complex care or when he has a chronic problem requiring complex care that parents have learned to provide.

Parent support groups composed of parents of children suffering from the same or different problems can be extremely helpful in reducing stress. These groups may be planned and supervised by professionals or develop spontaneously as parents with similar needs begin to share

> ### NURSING ACTIONS: FACILITATING COPING WITH THE STRESS OF HOSPITALIZATION
>
> Throughout the hospitalization experience, assess the child's developmental stage, and plan care according to these needs.
>
> **Admission**
>
> Allow adequate time to conduct an unhurried admission interview, if not an emergency. Allow time for and encourage the child and the parents to ask questions.
>
> Provide orientation to facilities. Be specific and use age-appropriate language. (Terms such as "lavatory," "bowel movement," or "vomit" may be completely unknown to the child.)
>
> Remember that people under stress may not remember everything said to them. Be ready to repeat information, without embarrassing the child or parent.
>
> **The child's hospital experience**
>
> Provide age-appropriate explanations of diagnostic tests, treatment and rules and restrictions. Assess each child's level of understanding individually, considering age and maturity, language ability, cultural background and family relationships.
>
> Observe the child's play to gain insight into the meaning of the experience for the child and to identify problems needing intervention.
>
> Provide opportunities for play, including handling equipment, dramatic play, and creative expression.
>
> Provide opportunities for age-appropriate group activities, including group play, eating meals with others, or special entertainment activities.
>
> Encourage and teach as much self-care as the child's age and condition allows.
>
> **The parent's experience**
>
> Recognize and acknowledge the stress parents are experiencing. Let the parents know that it's ok to be worried, to be afraid.
>
> Respect and reinforce the unique caretaking role of the parents. Provide for and encourage the presence and participation of parents.
>
> Identify the relationships within the family group. Respect the individual family's cultural, religious, and social values in regard to the child's care.
>
> Provide timely, *accurate* information about all aspects of the child's illness and care. Coordinate your information with other members of the health care team (dieticians, therapists, radiology technicians, physicians), so that the parents are not given conflicting instructions or information.

concerns and mutually experience a relief of tension. They discuss their feelings about a treatment or test and hear how another person has coped successfully. Some of these groups continue to meet even after the child is discharged from the hospital to provide information and support.

Keeping the Family Intact

When a child is hospitalized the family's routine, as well as the child's, is altered. Family life tends to revolve around the needs of the hospitalized child. This can be particularly stressful for the family when the hospital is a long distance from the home and visiting requires that some members be absent from home for several days at a time.

Although the family worries about the hospitalized child and initially all work together on their extra responsibilities, they soon become weary of the extra tasks and the siblings may begin to resent the extra attention given to the hospitalized child. Parents may feel overwhelmed trying to keep up with the demands of work, home responsibilities, and being with their sick child. Siblings may begin to feel that they are being ignored. They should be kept informed of their sibling's illness and his progress. Allowing siblings to visit the hospitalized brother or sister can be helpful in reducing stress. Seeing that their brother or sister is really ill helps them understand the reason for their parents' absence. They are often a source of cheer to the sick sibling as they tell the child he is missed and relate school, home and neighborhood events. Older siblings may become actively involved in providing care to their sick sibling under adult supervision. Sibling visiting also provides an opportunity for the children to share in a family crisis and provides a time that parents and children can be mutually supportive.

Allowing the hospitalized child to keep photographs of his siblings at his bedside also helps to keep them in his thoughts. Likewise, photographs taken of the sick child and sent home to siblings keeps him present in their thoughts. Notes, tape recordings and phone calls can also help siblings and peers keep in touch with and be supportive to the hospitalized child.

Recommended Reading to Prepare Children for Hospitalization

Madeline by Ludwig Bemelmans. Viking Press, 1939 and Penguin Books, 1977 (ages 3 to 9)
Michael's Heart Test by Children's Hospital of Philadelphia. Children's Hospital, 1967 (ages 3 to 12)
Margaret's Heart Operation by Children's Hospital of Philadelphia. Children's Hospital, 1969 (ages 3 to 12)
Pop-Up Going To The Hospital by Bettina Clark. Random House, 1971 (grades K to 3)
A Hospital: Life In a Medical Center by Paul Deegan. Amecus Street, Inc., 1971 (grades 4 to 7)
Linda Goes To The Hospital by Nancy Dudley. Coward-McCann and Goezhegan, Inc., 1953 (grades K to 4)
The Ambulance by Ann Falk. Burke Publishing Co., Ltd., 1966
Lets' Find Out About The Clinic by Robert Froman. Franklin-Watts, Inc., 1968 (grades K to 3)
Doctors and Nurses: What Do They Do? by Carla Greene. Harper and Row, 1963 (grades K to 3)
The Hospital Book by Barbara Hoar. The John Street Press, 1970 (ages 4 to 10)
Bittena's Secret by Britt Hollquist. Harcourt, Brace and World, Inc., 1967 (grades 3 to 7)
The Clinic by Eleanor Kay. Franklin Watts, Inc., 1971 (grades 4 to 6)
The Emergency Room by Eleanor Kay. Franklin Watts, Inc., 1970 (grades 5 to 7)
The Operating Room by Eleanor Kay. Franklin Watts, Inc., 1970 (grades 4 to 7)
Jimmy and Susie At The Hospital (A Child's First Hospital Stay) by Marguerite Lerner. Media Medica, 1969 (ages 3 to 7)
Your Children's Hospital Book by Rebecca Ludwick and Donna Rogers. The Children's Hospital of Vanderbilt University, 1976 (ages 6 to 12)
Brian's Trip to the Hospital by Ruth Odor. Standard Publishing Co., 1977 (ages 3 to 6)
Curious George Goes to The Hospital by H. A. Rey. Houghton Mifflin Co., 1966 (ages 3 to 8)
My Doctor by Harlow Rockwell. Macmillan Inc., 1973 (ages 3 to 7)
Richard Scarry's Nicky Goes to the Doctor by Richard Scarry. Western Publishing Company, Inc. 1971 (ages 3 to 6)
I Know a Nurse by Marilyn Schima. G. P. Putnam's Sons, 1969 (grades 1 to 3)
Johnny Goes To The Hospital by Josephine Sever. Houghton Mifflin Co., 1953 (ages 4 to 10)
I Want Mama by Marjorie Sharmat. Harper and Row, 1974 (ages 3 to 8)
It Can't Hurt Forever by Marilyn Singer. Harper and Row, 1978 (ages 10 to 14)
What Happens When You Go To The Hospital by Authur Thay. Reilly and Lee, 1969 (ages 3 to 10)
Pablito's New Feet by Dawn Thomas. J. B. Lippincott Co., 1973 (ages 5 to 8)
I Went To The Hospital by Ellie Simmons. Thompkins County Hospital Auxiliary, 1958 (ages 2 to 5)
Jeff's Hospital Book by Harriet Sobol. Henry Walch, Inc. 1975 (ages 4 to 10)
Emergency Room by Julie Steedman. EPM Publications, Inc., 1974 (ages 4 to 10)
A Hospital Story by Sara Stein. Walker and Company, 1974 (ages 3 to 10)
I Think I Will Go To The Hospital by Joan Tamburine. Abingdon Press, 1965 (ages 3 to 10)
It's No Fun To Be Sick by Phyllis Tickle. St. Lukes Press, 1975.
My Friend the Doctor by Jane Watson, Robert Hirschberg, J. Cotter. Golden Press, 1972 (ages 2 to 5)
Crocodile Medicine by Marjorie-Ann Watts. Frederick Warne, 1977 (ages 3 to 6)
Elizabeth Gets Well by Alfons Weber. Thomas Y. Crowell Co., 1970 (ages 5 to 9)
Wendy Well and Billy Better Say 'Hello Hospital!''; Wendy Well and Billy Better Visit the Hospital See-Through Machine; Wendy Well and Billy Better Meet the Hospital Sandman; Wendy Well and Billy Better Ask a ''Mill-Yun'' Hospital Questions by John Welzenbach and Nancy Cline. Med-Educator, Inc., 1970 (ages 3 to 12)
Mom! I Broke My Arm! by Angelika Wolff. The Lion Press, Inc. 1969 (grades K to 4)
At the Hospital: A Surprise for Krissy by Sandra Ziegler. The Child's World, 1976 (ages 3 to 7)

References

1. E. H. Erikson. Studies in the interpretation of play. Genetic Psychology Monographs, October 1940
2. K. Freiberg. How parents react when their child is hospitalized. American Journal of Nursing, July 1972, p. 1270
3. J. Robertson. Young Children in Hospital. Basic Books, Inc. 1958
4. S. Wolff. Children Under Stress. Pelican Books, 1973

Additional Recommended Reading

A. Altshuler and A. H. Seidl. Teen meetings: a way to help adolescents cope with hospitalization. American Journal of Maternal and Child Nursing, Nov/Dec, 1977
M. S. Andette. The significance of regressive behavior for the hospitalized child. American Journal of Maternal and Child Nursing, March 1974
P. Azarnoff. Mediating the trauma of serious illness and hospitalization in childhood. Children Today, Jul/Aug 1974, p. 12
T. Bowlby. Separation: Anxiety and Anger. Basic Books Inc., 1973
E. Branstetter. Separation anxiety in hospitalized children: comparison of three conditions of separation from mothering. Doctoral dissertation, University of Chicago, 1969
B. J. Chadivich et al. Maintaining the hospitalized child's home ties. American Journal of Nursing, August, 1978
J. Coffman Piche. Tell me a story. American Journal of Nursing, July, 1978
A. Costello Gallergan. Books for the hospitalized child. American Journal of Nursing, December, 1975
C. Crawford and M. Palm. Can I take my teddy bear? American Journal of Nursing, February, 1973, p. 286
F. H. Erikson. Play Interviews for Four-year-old Hospitalized Children. Child Development Publishing, 1978
L. Fischer Smith. An experiment with play therapy. American Journal of Nursing, December, 1977
H. Geist. A child Goes to the Hospital: The Psychological Aspects of a Child Going to the Hospital. Charles C Thomas, 1965

D. D. Gerbing. Putting play to work in pediatrics. American Journal of Maternal and Child Nursing, Nov/Dec, 1977

J. A. Haller. The Hospitalized Child and His Family. The Johns Hopkins Press

C. C. Hames and M. Ingham. The colorful creatures of continuous child care. American Journal of Maternal and Child Nursing, Nov/Dec, 1977

C. B. Hardgrove and R. B. Dawson. Ideas A to Z for personalizing pediatric units. Nursing 76, April, 1976

C. B. Hardgrove and R. B. Dawson. Parents and children in the hospital: the Family's role in Pediatrics. Little, Brown & Co., 1972

J. Johnson et al. Easing children's fright during health care procedures. American Journal of Maternal and Child Nursing, Jul/Aug 1976, p. 206

D. R. Klingzing and D. G. Klingzing. The Hospitalized Child; Communication Techniques for Health Personnel. Prentice-Hall, 1977

I. Koss and M. Teter. Welcoming a family when a child is hospitalized. American Journal Maternal and Child Nursing. Jan/Feb 1980, p. 51

R. Linheim et al. Changing Hospital Environments for Children. Harvard University Press, 1972

M. Caruso-McGillicuddy. A study of the relationship between mother's rooming-in during their children's hospitalization and changes in selected areas of childrens behavior. New York University Press

K. Oremland and J. Oremland, eds. The Effects of Hospitalization on Children. Charles C. Thomas, 1973

E. Payne, Art Therapy Intern, Mott Childrens Hospital, University of Michigan. Interview on Art Therapy, December, 1980

M. Petrillo. Preventing hospital trauma in pediatric patients. American Journal of Nursing, July 1968, p. 1469

M. Petrillo and S. Sanger. Emotional Care of Hospitalized Children, 2nd ed., J. B. Lippincott Co., 1980

H. Selye. Stress Without Distress. Signet Publishing, 1975

S. Shufer. Communicating with children: teaching via the play-discussion group. American Journal of Nursing, December 1977

P. Stelzer. Reminders for personalizing pediatric care. American Journal of Maternal and Child Nursing, Jul/Aug 1979, p. 252

I. Sweig. A new way to get acquainted with the hospital-pediatric open house for well children. American Journal of Maternal Child Nursing, Jul/Aug 1976, p. 217

WHEN A CHILD IS DYING

by Mabel Hunsberger, BSN, MSN
Marcia Sheets, RN, MSN
Anita Spietz, RN, MSN

Death is a subject that people try to avoid or repress until they are faced with their own death or that of a loved one. When the loved one happens to be their child, the emotional upheaval created by the threat of loss or actual loss of the child is immense. Because the child's death also affects his family and his caregivers, it is important for the nurse to have a working knowledge of the meaning of life-threatening illness and death and what the loss of the child means to his family.

The process by which a family copes with a child's life-threatening illness and impending death is influenced by many factors. To fully understand the reactions of various family members it is often necessary to explore the child's uniqueness to the family unit. The way a child is perceived and appreciated by the family may indirectly affect the attention and care he receives from them during the course of illness. Factors that influence a child's status within a family include the events surrounding his birth and delivery, his birth order, ages of other children, parents' relationship, economic situation at home, and how easy the child is to nurture and love. The child's role in the family and the circumstances surrounding his birth provide insights into the dynamics of the parent-child relationship that will help in understanding the meaning the child's death has for his parents and siblings.[2]

The family members' reactions and responses to life-threatening illness vary according to their unique life experience and the type and length of illness involved. Elisabeth Kübler-Ross has identified five stages of coping that are usually experienced by people facing a life-threatening illness.[6]

The child (depending on his age), parents and siblings, and anyone experiencing the child's death (grandparents, nurses, doctors, significant others) go through these five stages in preparation for death: denial, anger, bargaining, depression and acceptance. The important point about these stages is that they do not necessarily take place in sequence but may be repeated again and again. Each episode of acute illness, relapse or regression is capable of triggering the mechanism for repeating the stages.

STAGES OF COPING WITH LIFE-THREATENING ILLNESS

Denial Shock and disbelief overwhelms an individual when life is threatened by illness.

Denial of the diagnosis and prognosis is the usual initial method of coping when confronted with the findings that confirm a life-threatening illness. If possible, the nurse to be involved in the child's care should be present when these findings are related to the family. Since it is not unusual for the child and family to hear only the diagnosis and block out the course of treatment and prognosis, the nurse can provide the consistent, supportive environment needed and interpret, restate, refocus or clarify any information related by the physician.

The nurse's response to denial is crucial to the child and family's ability to eventually relinquish the denial. If the nurse continues to need denial to cope during this stage, so will the family. It is the nurse's acceptance of the family's need to use denial without reinforcing it that brings the child and family to a gradual awareness and eventual psychological adaptation to the fact that the threat to life by illness is a reality.

Anger When a gradual awareness of the reality of the diagnosis and prognosis penetrates, the angry reaction "Why me?" or "Why my child?" prevails. In contrast to the period of impact characterized by indecisiveness, searching and immobilization, this stage is associated with feelings of sadness, depression, guilt, anger and somatic complaints. Guilt and anger are probably the most universal or typical reactions of parents when their child is dying. Parents need to be assured and reassured by the nurse that the child's illness is not their fault. Feelings of guilt may lead to many reactions that can cause problems for their child, one of which is the tendency for parents to become overly permissive or overly protective of their dying child.

Anger is closely associated with guilt and may be directed toward spouses, caregivers, relatives or toward the dying child. The most common displacement of parental anger is on the nurse, mainly because she is available and involved in the child's day-to-day care. The most appropriate reaction to this is to recognize that the parents may need to criticize in order to feel less guilty themselves. Listening to parents ventilate their angry feelings in an accepting manner helps them maintain confidence in those providing their child's care and gives release to their feelings of guilt.

The dying child as well as those experiencing his death express anger and guilt in various ways. His anger may be expressed through open verbal hostilities, by withdrawal, rejection, or a variety of complaints. The nurse must intervene by respecting and allowing expression of these angry feelings without compounding the guilt that the child or family member is feeling.

Bargaining During this stage the dying person and his family are attempting to make a bargain (with God, the health team or significant others) that will postpone the threat to life. There is a plea for additional time to right some wrong or change that which is viewed as a possible reason for the illness. Bargaining can be associated with a feeling of guilt about a past deed by the parent or the child and is typically expressed by "if, . . . , then I will . . . ."

Depression There are two phases of depression, namely, *reactive depression* (thinking of past losses) and *preparatory depression* (thinking of impending losses). During the phase of reactive depression there is a concern for loss of the happiness and joy experienced before illness (physical activity, body image, general sense of well-being). The preparatory depression phase is characterized by the impending loss and separation from loved ones. It is during this phase that those experiencing death become quiet and sorrowful. Attempts to cheer and brighten their day are inappropriate — it is a time to be present and quiet so that their sorrow can be felt.

Acceptance This is the time when there is little interest in present or future activities. It is a time when children wish only for their parents to be present and parents want each other or a significant other. The child and family are not happy but not terribly sad. This stage is a time for tender loving care when touch, quietness, attention to comfort and gentle handling become the avenue of communication.

DECISIONS AFFECTING CARE OF THE DYING CHILD

Decision to Discontinue Treatment At some point the physicians caring for a child with a life-threatening illness may make a decision to discontinue treatment based upon the lack of response to medical therapy. This decision is usually made in conjunction with the family. There may also come a time when the family reaches this decision before the physician mentions it. At this time the family may request that no further treatment be undertaken so as to avoid further pain, frustration or unnecessary stress for their child. This decision is actually a statement that the family is giving up hope for survival — an acceptance of death as an inevitable end. It is also based on the realization that the child is not responding to treatment. This is always a difficult decision for the family and for the health team to deal with. It is an area which preprofessional students must deal with throughout their education and also well into their professional practices. Respect for the quality of the child's remaining life must be the basis of the decision. Ultimately, the choice must be the family's. The nurse can be supportive to the family during this difficult decision by helping them clarify their own thoughts and feel comfortable in their decision.

Decision on Alternative Environments for Terminal Care The option of receiving supportive care and symptom management care in a hospitalized situation or in the home should be discussed with the family. Some communities have or are developing community-based programs or hospice* groups to provide home care for dying children and adults. The hospice concept promotes the idea that when the goal of curing cannot be realized, more appropriate circumstances than the traditional hospital settings can provide the care that is vital during this critical time. Some cities provide hospice care to families of dying children by providing space within their hospitals, while others have special places set aside, such as an extended care facility. Other cities have developed a hospice program that is essentially a home care program. Many public health nurses are currently involved in providing support to parents who are caring for their dying children in their own homes.

Allowing a child to die in his home provides an opportunity for the family to design and control the environment. According to Ida M. Martinson, "the home is often the more natural place for a person, especially a child, to die. At home children can have their parents at hand; be surrounded by a familiar environment, have the company of brothers and sisters, pets, friends and relatives; eat what and when they want or are able to and participate in the normal family activities as much or as little as desired."[8]

Regardless of the environment that is chosen for terminal care for the dying child (if that choice is actually made), the needs of the whole child must be considered: his physical needs, his cognitive needs and his emotional and social needs. At the same time, the resources and needs of other family members must also be considered. The nurse must work with family members to gain an understanding of the resources within the family unit as well as their anxieties, concerns and fears. It is important for the health of the family that guilt is not assigned for choices that may be different from the usual choices and that may not include hospital care.

At the University of Minnesota, Dr. Martinson has developed a home care project in conjunction with many other health professionals. Criteria for the choice of home care are as follows:[9]

1. Cure-oriented treatment has been discontinued.
2. The child wants to be at home.
3. The parents desire to have the child at home.
4. The parents recognize their own ability to care for their ill child; the fact that they can care for the child until death is frequently not recognized until later.
5. The nurse is willing to be available 24 hours a day to facilitate care.
6. The child's physician is willing to be an on-call consultant.

Making the decision to care for the dying child at home is an extremely difficult one. During the dying process the parents may sometimes feel inept at providing the best care possible; they may wonder about their decision and may feel guilty that their child is not in the hospital. Inability to relieve pain is often a major reason why parents feel they cannot care for their child in the home, but with proper instruction and support, pain management can be achieved without much difficulty. Medications for the relief of pain, either in oral, rectal or parenteral form, can be provided to the family.

---

* A hospice was a way station for travelers during medieval times. In regard to care of the dying, it refers to programs and approaches (especially home care) as alternatives to care within a hospital.

The nurse can teach the family how to administer the drugs. If the child can be kept free from pain, the family and the child usually feel that the right decision has been made.

Home visits are made whenever the family or the nurse deems them necessary. The nurse may be asked by the family to assist in making plans prior to the death for funeral arrangements or whatever method of memorial the family prefers. Often the nurse or hospice team is on call for the family providing home care. Twenty-four hour service seven days a week provides the kind of support that parents need. They may never use the service, but they need the reassurance that someone is always there to help at any time of the day or night.[8]

If the family members indicate that they are absolutely unable to manage the care at home, then hospitalization should certainly be provided as an option. Hospitals have round-the-clock staff coverage to care for the child. Many hospitals are able to assign a private room with cots or hide-a-beds for parents. Unlimited visitation by siblings and friends also assists the family unit to deal with the stresses of the final days and hours. If the decision is made to hospitalize a child, the nurse should clarify with the family what expectations they have of the hospital and hospitalization. Many times family members assume that hospital care will be of higher quality and will make the child more comfortable than care provided at home. Each family must make the final decision and the nurse should assist the family by providing information and supporting them in their decision.

AFTER DEATH: THE GRIEVING PROCESS

The normal grieving process, as described by Lindemann, includes five types of symptoms: (1) somatic distress* experienced for periods of 20 minutes to an hour; (2) preoccupation with the image of the deceased; (3) feelings of guilt that develop from self-accusatory thoughts of having failed the deceased in some way; (4) hostile reactions, including feelings of irritability, anger, and loss of warmth toward others; and (5) displacement of usual patterns of conduct with aimless, restless behavior that cannot find significance.[7]

Morbid grief reactions of two types were also identified by Lindemann.[7] One is a *delay in reaction* and the other is a *distorted reaction*. Delayed reactions were found to be the most common and most dramatic. Distorted reactions comprise a variety of reactions including physical symptoms, altered psychological states (agitated depression, extreme hostility) and altered social interactions with progressive social isolation.

Engel has described grief and mourning responses to real object loss (persons, jobs, valued possessions, home, membership in a group, country and ideals).[3] The unexpected death of a loved one causes severe stress to a family, especially when the loss of a child is experienced. The responses (shock and disbelief, developing awareness and restitution) as described by Engel follow a fairly consistent sequence, although pre-existing conditions influence the course of successful grieving and sometimes can prevent it altogether.[3]

The first response of *shock and disbelief* is expressed according to each person's style of behavior, including numerous cultural variations. Grief-stricken individuals may sit motionless and dazed, engage in verbal denial, or display physical expressions such as throwing themselves on the body of the deceased. The engrossment in the appropriate activities that surround a death (funeral arrangements, comforting friends and relatives) often serves to foster the disbelief or denial that operates to protect the grievers against overwhelming stress at this time.

The second phase of a *developing awareness* is characterized by an acute sadness expressed in various ways. Crying is typical of this phase, but the anguish and despair that is felt is expressed within cultural restraints so that some families may respond with a public display of lamentation, whereas others may choose to cry when alone. Anger is another emotion experienced and may be directed to persons who are viewed as being responsible for the death of the loved one. When a mourner holds himself responsible in some way, he carries a sense of guilt during this phase of mourning.

The third phase, *restitution*, completes the resolution of grief. The reality of the death is accepted and the mourner is able to carry on with life and develop new relationships. The restitution phase involves the mourner in sever-

---

*Frequent sighing, loss of appetite, loss of strength, choking sensation and shortness of breath.

al experiences. With an increased awareness of the object loss, a painful void is felt. He may now experience various bodily sensations compared to his previous state of numbness. The mourner may develop symptoms similar to those experienced by his loved one; thereby he maintains a tie with the loved one. By experiencing some of the dead person's suffering the mourner also rids himself of guilt that may be present as a result of any aggressive feelings held toward the deceased. These symptoms are usually brief, if they occur.

During the phase of restitution there is also a predominance of thinking and talking about the deceased loved one. The memory of the lost object is idealized and only positive and desirable attributes are remembered. The mourner may take on certain mannerisms of the lost person, or carry on his ideals and good deeds. The lost object is now more of an intellectual memory and more detached from the self of the mourner. Many months are required to arrive at a state in which the mourner is less preoccupied with the loved one so that he can begin to get on with his own life. When mourning is successfully completed (this may take 6 to 12 months), both the pleasures and disappointments of the lost relationship are remembered realistically.

THE NURSE'S ROLE DURING LIFE-THREATENING ILLNESS

Helping the Family Cope with the Prognosis When parents first learn that their child has a life-threatening illness they often feel a need to protect him and make him feel that nothing is amiss. They approach the child with a forced cheerfulness and evade discussions of any serious nature. They may demonstrate behavior that is inconsistent with their usual pattern. For example, a permissive approach is adopted pertaining to sleep routine and a gift that was thought to be too expensive now appears. Parents may omit a procedure because they think it may disturb the child to have it done.[1] The nurse must understand that parents are convinced that they are doing what is best for the child.

The nurse is in a crucial position to help parents understand that their child perceives their anxiety and probably knows that his condition is worsening. The nurse should strive to provide an environment in which the child can express his awareness and anxiety of his impending death. She should be prepared to help parents deal with their own anxiety so that the parents and nurse can together identify and meet the child's needs.

Not all families are able to openly discuss death or dying, nor should they be forced to if they choose not to or if they feel it is inappropriate. The nurse should respect the wishes of the parents in this regard and remain available as the family moves toward the child's death. Even at the terminal moment, many families are still not at the point of being able to discuss death with the child or with each other.

Another phenomenon that exists is the parents' search for additional medical opinions. Parents are often reluctant to ask for another opinion, but they can be helped to express their concern and made to feel comfortable in their request.[10] They often are satisfied to seek one other opinion, and they should be helped to do so. They should, however, be counselled that going from doctor to doctor in a frantic search for a more favorable prognosis may be exhausting, especially for the child, and end in disappointment for them.

During the course of illness parents ask the same questions over and over again. Much of the information relayed at the time of diagnosis is not heard and needs to be reviewed frequently. Sometimes parents tend to blame themselves for their child's illness; therefore a nurse must be alert for questions in which information is asked for to confirm their sense of blame. Information should be presented in a clear, factual, understandable manner so that parents will not need to seek answers elsewhere. Often the nurse is the one who plays the important role of getting a family into contact with their physician, especially in large institutions, and she must not take lightly a parent's request to speak to the physician.

The nurse must understand how a family deals with stress during the course of a life-threatening illness, recognizing that each crisis and each family's ability to cope with stress is unique. Some families wish to remain extremely private about their feelings and find solace only in each other's support. In other situations the pattern of handling stress may necessitate outside sources to help the family cope during these darkest hours.

The nurse should be sensitive to the particular

wishes of a family regarding support from a religious source. Some families need such support and appreciate when a nurse offers to help them contact their own clergyman or the hospital chaplain. Respecting the family's wishes in this regard is a professional responsibility of every nurse who cares for the family of a dying child.

Although clergymen are viewed as experts in helping families during such times of crisis, the nurse should be aware that sometimes a clergyman is not trained to or is personally unable to help a family. Cliches can be meaningless and even disturbing to a family. If a family is told repeatedly that "It is God's will," they may feel guilty about expressing feelings that may be viewed as wrong or unacceptable.[4] The nurse should remain in touch with the family and cannot assume that once the clergyman is on the scene her responsibilities have ended. The team approach is essential to provide the comprehensive caring and support that families deserve during the stress of life-threatening illness.

Helping Siblings Cope With Life-Threatening Illness Siblings' reactions to the dying brother or sister will vary depending on their age, level of development and relationship to the dying child. The reaction of the parents and the severity and length of the child's illness influence a sibling's coping ability. More important, however, is the child's awareness of the seriousness of the sibling's illness. If parents choose not to tell the siblings and do not involve them in visits to the hospital nor in discussions about the dying child's condition, the siblings may become resentful and jealous because the brother or sister in the hospital receives special treatment and undivided attention from the parents. Unless the parents provide reasonable explanations for their absence and altered relations within the family, the sick child is often looked upon as responsible for the disruption of home life. The nurse working with dying children needs to assess and discuss with parents their responsibilities to their other children so there are healthy relationships for them to return to once the child has died. Stressing that the quality of time spent with their children is more significant than quantity may alleviate guilt parents experience in trying to divide their attention and time equally among the children. The nurse needs to encourage parents to be honest and open with their children, reassuring them of their love. Parents should be made aware that the siblings may be fearful of having wished the sibling ill or dead, or of becoming sick like their sibling. Some parents may need assistance in discussing the death with their children.

Helping the Family Cope With the Length of the Illness The parents' grief reaction and pattern of adaptation will depend a great deal on the course of illness. If the death of their child is sudden and unexpected, a variety of shock responses can be anticipated from those involved. These responses may range from immobilization or hysteria to complete control of the situation. Although their reactions vary, it is clear that family members do not fully comprehend what is communicated during this shock stage. Once the shock begins to diminish they have a dire need to communicate their feelings regarding what has happened. The nurse in emergency care may be the only person available to help the grievers work out their feelings and thoughts about what has occurred. Because they have not had time to prepare for the death, they are deprived of the advantages of anticipatory grief.* They also may feel great remorse or guilt for not having done things differently for their child. The nurse may be able to physically and psychologically comfort them through touch, active listening, or by providing a comfortable, private place for the family to grieve.

If the death of the child is not immediate but extends into days or weeks, family members have the advantage of beginning their anticipatory grief work, if they have accepted the diagnosis and are encouraged to mourn. On the other hand, a long-term life-threatening illness brings additional stresses. Parents of these children not only have to live with the uncertainty of the future but also provide care for the child while they are actively mourning his expected death.

Several interventions are effective with these parents and can direct their grief into constructive actions. The first of these is encouraging parents to meet in groups. Such groups consist of parents whose children have the same medical problems or prognosis. Within the group,

---

*Grieving that begins before the actual death of a loved one and may even be completed before death.

reactions, fears and feelings are shared with others who have experienced or are experiencing them. The second constructive action is to involve parents in the care and planning of their child's treatment. Mothers may be more willing to enter into these activities, but it seems to be healthiest for all concerned when both parents are involved in the care. When parents are a part of the plan, their anxiety, guilt or anger subsides and they usually become more cooperative, outgoing and accepting of the treatment. Parents' wishes and desires regarding the care of their child should be respected; they should be allowed to take part in determining whether certain treatments should be continued if there is little hope for improvement. Parents need to be given the option to take the child home to die if they feel he cannot be cured. In such cases, parents should be provided with information regarding possible problems or complications they may experience at home and be assured that someone will be available if help is needed. (See previous discussion on alternative environments for terminal care.)

Helping Families Cope During the Final Stages of Illness During final stages of death parents may withdraw from their children; their fears of death and pain are overwhelming. Perhaps the greatest fear at this time is a fear that their child is experiencing pain. Although the child may appear comfortable, it is important to understand that the parents' anxiety may center on their child's pain, but that it may also reflect the parents' sense of inevitable loss. Providing the child maximal comfort and relief of pain during this period is critical.

The parents' physical involvement in their child's care may lead to difficulties within the family structure. The stress placed on families with life-threatening illnesses requires altered patterns of living and a shift in expectations. Many changes are caused by illness, ranging from financial problems to changes in social status due to increased social isolation. Because these illnesses often require much time and energy on the part of those providing care (usually the mother), marital and parent-child relationships may suffer. Problems with siblings generally arise because of the time factor associated with the illness. The well child's perception of the mother having limited time leads to feelings of hostility and rejection, especially when he has a poor understanding of the illness of his sibling.

Helping the Family Cope After the Child's Death Following death there may be feelings of relief as well as defeat, particularly if the child has suffered for a long period of time. Common reactions are anger and periods of intense sorrow. Mourning takes on a finality that was not evident in anticipatory grief. It is during this time that hospital staff members have a tendency to withdraw from the family. It is crucial that the family not be abandoned. This is a period during which many decisions need to be made and a time to refocus on the family, parents and siblings alike. Parents need to vent emotions and talk about their dead child with those who were involved in caring for him. A nurse's presence and willingness to listen are important interventions with these families. When the responsibility of providing day-to-day care for their dying child is ended, parents may feel relieved and sense a genuine lessening of their pain. The nurse can help to clarify the normalcy of these feelings so that additional guilt is not experienced by the parents.

The help of other parents can be particularly appropriate after the death of a child. Parents have shared their thought that there is no one who understands what they are going through except another parent who has gone through it. There are parent groups and individual parents who can help the family during this phase of their growth. Other parents can assist by saying to the parents by their very presence that they have survived the loss and have coped. Not much more than that needs to be shared at this time except that they have coped and that they will continue to cope.

The nurse should pay special attention to assisting the family in their coping with the needs of their other children. The family may or may not have chosen to have siblings remain with the dying child. This will depend upon the environment in which the death occurs, the time of day, and the siblings' wishes to do so. Siblings must be helped to realize that if the death occurred in their absence they do not need to feel guilty because they were involved in their own daily activities. Depending upon the age and the developmental level of the siblings, they may think that since the energies of their parents were directed toward the dying child, their own energies should also have been expended in this way. Siblings may also need help with the ongoing hostility they feel toward the dead sibling who took so much time from their parents, leaving them so little time. To dissipate this hostility, siblings may need to talk to parents or the nurse or both about it. They need to be reassured that this hostility and these feelings are normal and that they are not bad for feeling them.

Siblings may or may not want to attend the funeral of the dead child. The choice should be theirs. Even very young children (preschoolers) may benefit from attending the funeral, but this choice must be made by the family and the sibling.

The deceased child's toys, books and clothing may be shared with surviving siblings. Young children (those with the concept of reversibility of death) may be afraid that the deceased child will return to reclaim the toys. Parents may need help understanding why a sibling may be so concerned about this happening.

Siblings may need time to think about what has happened within the family. They may need reassurance that they will not also die of the disease that has claimed brother or sister (unless, of course, the child also has a genetically caused disease). If this is the case, special follow-up help will be needed as the child prepares for his own life and death.

The interactions of parents with siblings may change after the death of one child. They may become overprotective of the surviving children. The sadness that they feel is of a different nature than the sadness of the siblings. Parents may mourn well beyond the time that siblings are actively mourning, and unconscious anger may result toward the siblings.

The severe stress placed upon the entire family continues to have a profound impact after the death of a child. The period after death is critical for continued support and involvement of hospital staff, if possible. Parents often complain that once their child has died they are forgotten by the staff. This period is characterized by intense grief and mourning that calls for a renewal of socialization, reorganization and decision-making on the part of the family. The nurse may wish to share in the funeral services or public memorial services. Following the death, subsequent phone calls, letters or visits to the family may be appropriate and therapeutic.

Receiving of phone calls, letters or visits from family members must be met with supportive encouragement to assist them in the separation from their child. Continued support can be coordinated through community services such as parent special interest groups, public health nurse referral, or other appropriate community resources.

THE NURSE'S RESPONSE DURING LIFE-THREATENING ILLNESS

Recognizing Her Own Needs The greatest disservice that a nurse can do herself and a dying child and family is to disregard her own personal needs. Denying one's own feelings makes one less than human and takes away the child's and family's right to experience the support of a truly human relationship. Each nurse has stresses and experiences in day-to-day living that shape her unique way of relating to those in stress. It is inhuman to expect nurses to somehow be unaffected by those minor mood changes and "bad days" that we afford the rest of society the right to experience. When a nurse can acknowledge that some days she feels limited or unable to cope with a dying child and family, she can then seek support from other professions to help her through the day or week. It is important to recognize that "We can give to others only from our abundance, and some days the cupboard is bare."[5]

Feelings of the Nurse Aside from a nurse's vulnerability to the usual vicissitudes of life, she will also experience a myriad of feelings associated with caring for a dying child and his family. A particular child may remind the nurse of her own child or a relative's or close friend's child. The particular illness causing the suffering may remind a nurse of an experience within her own family. Thus the dynamics of each parent-child-nurse relationship are unique, and when death is imminent the feelings that emerge are intense and stressful.

Nurses cope with stress in a manner similar to that of the child and family. Denial is used for protection from the reality of impending death. Real feelings are suppressed and a facade of "all is well" pervades in dealings with the child, family and health team members.

Anger and guilt are commonly felt by nurses who care for a dying child. In our culture these are results of the sentiment that it is a tremen-

A NURSE'S FEELINGS ABOUT CARING FOR A DYING CHILD: STATEMENTS FOR NURSES TO RESPOND TO IN A GROUP SESSION

1. I expect to feel uncomfortable when I have to talk to a dying child and to his family.
2. I feel at a loss to know what to say, especially when the child and family are aware that death is imminent.
3. I cannot imagine that anyone is ever free of the fear of dying.
4. I think I can help a child and family cope with the reality of death.
5. I am frightened at the thought of caring for a dying child.
6. I am afraid the child will ask me whether he is dying.
7. I feel terrible about causing tiny discomforts during a treatment when I know a child is dying anyway.
8. I feel I have to hide my own feelings of sadness so as not to make the child and family feel upset.
9. If I cry with a child or family member it disturbs me for the rest of the day.
10. I don't really have anyone to tell how I feel about (child's name) suffering.

dous injustice when a child suffers or dies. The nurse may direct anger toward a supernatural being, or she may blame parents for not seeking treatment earlier. While the nurse is struggling with the complexity of accepting the death of a child she may become intolerant of the many questions and demands from parents. Anger may also be directed toward the physician or to herself for not being able to cure the child. The nurse may feel guilty because painful procedures need to be done, the child is hurting, and yet there is no hope. These feelings of anger and guilt emerge out of a sensitive, caring nurse who is groping to right the wrong.

When given the needed support from other nurses and team members, the nurse can feel free to acknowledge her own struggle in dealing with death. When a nurse can share her feelings of anger and guilt and can break out of the shield of denial, the work of grief ensues.

The Nurse's Expression of Grief Each person expresses grief according to his own style of coping. Grief expression by nurses also varies according to the degree of involvement with a particular child and family, a variation that must be respected from one nurse to another. Grief is always a complex emotion but, when people have overextended themselves, behaviors of one nurse may appear inappropriate to another; each must recognize that the other needs to resolve grief in her own way.[5]

Grief needs an outlet such as the health care team, in which support is ready-made if "stuffy professionalism" does not thwart the process of grieving.[5] The pretense of successful coping can seriously hamper the grieving process among professionals.

Nurses need to become increasingly aware of the toll of what Kavanaugh describes as *institutional grief*.[5] An entire staff can become depressed and lose sight of their goals if grief remains unresolved. Opportunities must be provided for nurses to share their feelings and anxieties about working with special families in stress. Support systems cannot be left to each individual's personal contacts such as family and friends. These are usually not prepared to hear out the feelings and expressions regarding a child who is dying. Professional support groups must be deliberately planned — institutional grief cannot be left to resolve itself. These periods of professional sharing should be ongoing, so that feelings during the process of death as well as after the death can be shared.

If a nurse can ventilate her feelings in an atmosphere of openness, the child and family will gain. The sensitive exchange of feelings may bring to light that a nurse needs a period away from a particular child and family. It is the nurse who cares enough about the child and family who is willing to take the professional risk of reaching out for help to face a new day; it may mean a temporary change of assignment to a unit away from dying children.

Nurses can help each other to take these important steps toward dealing effectively with personal feelings about working with a dying child. Nurses must take an active role in planning group sessions. Group members can be asked to privately respond to a group of statements and then provide an opportunity for the sharing of feelings. Statements with reference to a particular situation could easily be developed by the primary nurse to facilitate sharing of personal needs and feelings about experiences with other families.

It is the sharing of feelings and personal difficulties in regard to care of the dying that brings human experiences into focus. The nurse who respects her own humaneness recognizes that she is vulnerable to the same feelings of denial, anger, fear, depression and grief that the family experiences. If nurses can support each other during these experiences, the pain of caring for a dying child and his family can be experienced rather than repressed. When the nurse feels the pain of loss she can provide what the child and family need — the presence of a human being.

Helpful Literature For Parents of Dying Children

L. Buscaglia. Love. Charles B. Slack Inc., 1972
M. Colgrove et al. How to Survive the Loss of a Love. Lion Press, 1976
W. Easson. The Dying Child: The Management of the Child or Adolescent Who is Dying. Charles C Thomas, 1970
E. Grollman. Talking About Death: A Dialogue Between Parent and Child. Beacon Press, 1970
G. Hunt. Don't Be Afraid to Die. Zondervan Publishing, 1971
E. Jackson. Telling a Child about Death. Hawthorn Books, 1965
N. Klien. Sunshine. Avon Books, 1974
E Kübler-Ross. On Death and Dying. MacMillan, Inc, 1969
E. Kübler-Ross. Questions and Answers on Death and Dying. MacMillan, Inc., 1974
R. Levit. Ellen: A Short Life Long Remembered. Bantam Books, 1974
D. Lund. Eric. Dell Books, 1974
J. Morris. Brian Piccolo: A Short Season. Dell Books, 1971
D. Evans Rogers. Angel Unaware. Fleming H. Revell Publishing, 1953
E. Valens. The Other Side of the Mountain. Warner Publishing, 1966

References

1. R. Caughill. The Dying Patient. Little, Brown & Co., 1976
2. P. Codden. The meaning of death for the parent and child. Maternal and Child Nursing Journal, Spring 1977, p. 9
3. G. Engel. Psychological Development in Health and Disease. W. B. Saunders Co., 1962
4. J. Gyulay. The forgotten grievers. American Journal of Nursing, September 1975, p. 1476
5. R. Kavanaugh. Dealing naturally with the dying. Nursing '76, October 1976, p. 23
6. E. Kübler-Ross. On Death and Dying. Macmillan Inc., 1969
7. E. Lindemann. Symptomatology and management of acute grief. American Journal of Psychiatry, September 1944, p. 141
8. I. Martinson et al. Home Care for Dying Children: A manual for Parents. University of Minnesota, 1979
9. I. Martinson et al. When the patient is dying; home care for the child. American Journal of Nursing, November 1977, p. 1815
10. V. Vaughn. The care of the child with a fatal illness. In Nelson Textbook of Pediatrics, 11th ed. by V. Vaughn et al. W. B. Saunders Co., 1979

Additional Recommended Reading

J. Bernstein. Loss and How To Cope With It. The Seabury Press, 1977
M. Bluebond-Langer. The Private Worlds of Dying Children. Princeton University Press, 1978
M. Buchanan. Pediatric hospital and home care. Easing parent's problems. Part 2. Nursing Times, 17 March 1977, p. 39
W. Easson. The family of the dying child. Pediatric Clinics of North America, November 1972
F. Erickson. Stress in the pediatric ward. Maternal-Child Nursing Journal, 1: 113–116, Summer, 1972, p. 113
S. Everson. Sibling counseling. American Journal of Nursing, April 1976, p. 644
H. Feifel, (ed.) The New Meanings of Death. McGraw-Hill Book Co., 1977
J. Fryer. The International Work Group in Death, Dying and Bereavement. Assumptions and principles underlying standards for terminal care. American Journal of Nursing, February 1979, p. 296
E. Furman. A Child's Parent Dies: Studies in Childhood Bereavement. Yale University Press, 1974
E. Furman. Helping children cope with death. Young Children, May 1978, p. 25
E. Kübler-Ross. Questions and Answers on Death and Dying. Macmillan, Inc., 1974
E. Kübler-Ross. Death: The Final Stage of Growth. Prentice-Hall/Spectrum Press, 1975
E. Kübler-Ross. To Live Until We Say Goodbye. Prentice-Hall Inc., 1978
E. Patterson. The Experiences of Dying. Prentice-Hall Inc., 1977
L. Pincus. Death and the Family. Vintage Books, 1974
H. Schiff. The Bereaved Parent. Crown Publishers, 1977
E. Schneidman. Death: Current Perspectives. Jason Aronson, 1976
B. Schoenberg et al. Bereavement. Columbia University Press, 1975
D. Wetzel and I. Martinson. Meri. University of Minnesota, 1975

PRINCIPLES AND SKILLS OF PEDIATRIC NURSING

DAILY CARE CONSIDERATIONS

by Mabel Hunsberger, BSN, MSN,
and Judy Coltson Moyer, RN, BS, MS

Nursing care of children requires that the caregiver take into account the unique needs of children. A child's response to nursing intervention is influenced by his or her physical, intellectual, and emotional and social developmental level. Nursing care must be adapted to maintain the safety of the child, support normal growth and development of the child and family, foster healthy family functioning, and gain the desired therapeutic effect of the intervention. In other words, the goal of nursing intervention is to attain the maximum therapeutic benefit with the least amount of disruption to the life of the child and the family.

The unique developmental needs of children dictate precautions that must be taken and serve as a guide for determining how to approach the child. Many procedures need to be altered in terms of size of equipment, amount of solution or medication, and speed of administration. There are also numerous procedures that are specific to the care of children (e.g., application of urinary collection bag, scalp vein insertion for an intravenous line). The manner of approaching a child for a procedure must be a central focus for the nurse who cares for children. See age-specific chapters (Chapters 27, 36, 45, 54, 63) on the hospitalized child for discussion of age-appropriate approaches.

BATHING AND HYGIENE

Bath time for the hospitalized child can provide a number of useful opportunities. For the child it meets hygiene needs and often provides an enjoyable playtime. For parents the bath is an opportunity to participate in the child's care, and for the nurse it is a time to observe the child's physical and emotional status and provide appropriate stimulation.

The child's bath should be as similar to the home routine as possible. Adhering to the home rituals of bath, sleep and mealtime as closely as possible may help minimize the trauma of hospitalization. Unless the child's physical condition contraindicates a tub bath or shower, either may be given.

The parents of the patient should be allowed to provide as much of the child's care as possible. Parents frequently are unsure of their role in the hospital or reluctant to participate because of the child's physical condition. It is important for the nurse to provide the parents with the opportunity to care for the child and to demonstrate any modifications necessary due to the child's condition.

As with all procedures, the initial task is to gather all the necessary equipment before beginning, both for efficiency and to ensure that the child is not left unattended. The bath temperature should be about 37.8° to 40.6°C (100° to 105°F) although checking the water with a thermometer is usually not necessary. The water can be checked for comfort with the wrist, or an older child can check the water himself.

During the bath, certain areas need attention; the nurse should either give the care herself or supervise the child in taking his own bath. The eyes should be wiped with a clean wash cloth, without soap, working from the inner canthus out. The auricle and external canal of the ears are washed with soapy water and a cloth. Do not use cotton swabs as this may impact the cerumen and could possibly damage the tympanic membrane or canal. To clean the female genitalia, separate the labia and gently wipe from front to back. To wash the genitalia of an uncircumsized male, gently retract the foreskin and wash with soap and water. After washing the penis the foreskin is gently drawn forward to its original position. This is done daily to prevent adhesions and is taught as a necessary part of daily hygiene.

Bubble bath products and other additives are frequently requested by children. These are contraindicated for use by children with frequent urinary tract or vaginal infections. At the first sign of skin irritation the use of these products should be discontinued. There is routinely no need for creams or powders after a bath. Occasionally a lotion is applied to dry skin, or a medicated lotion is ordered for specific dermatologic conditions.

For any child who is hospitalized or confined to bed for a period longer than several days, hair care is important. Black children with thick, coarse or very curly hair need particular attention because this hair type mats and tangles easily, which may cause breakage. Before matted hair is shampooed, the tangles should be removed as much as possible. To do this use a wide tooth comb and work in small sections. Beginning at the ends of the hair, gently fluff and lift the hair. Repeat this step each time, inserting the comb farther into the hair. Pulling on the scalp is painful; *be gentle*. Application of a lubricant (Dermassage, mineral oil or commercial hair preparations) to the hair may help disentangle it. This process may have to be done in several sittings, as it is uncomfortable and difficult for a child to remain still long enough for the entire head of hair to be finished. If the child's hair is dry, breakage can be prevented by using a lubricant. Braiding the child's hair may prevent further tangles, but care must be taken to prevent breakage from braiding the hair too tightly.

ASSESSMENT OF VITAL SIGNS

Temperature The child's temperature may be taken orally, rectally or in the axillae. A rectal temperature is the method of choice in infants and toddlers, with several exceptions. These exceptions are children with diarrhea or recent rectal surgery, low birthweight infants, and toddlers who are unable to remain still long enough to avoid damage to the rectal mucosa. An oral temperature most closely reflects the arterial temperature and so is the method of choice if it can be safely used. The oral route is used in children old enough to hold the standard glass thermometer in the correct position and not bite it. An oral reading may be inaccurate if taken immediately after the child drinks or eats. Wait 15 minutes after anything is taken by mouth before measuring temperature orally. Furthermore, any condition that causes the child to mouth breathe is a contraindication to taking a temperature orally. Oxygen therapy by tent or nasal cannula has been reported not to cause a significant change in oral temperature.[8] Mask-administered oxygen may cause an oral reading that does not reflect the true body temperature. The axillary method is used for preschoolers (rectal temperatures are generally avoided in the oedipal stage). The axillary method is probably least accurate in determining true body temperature because of errors in technique.

To take a rectal temperature, the child is positioned prone or supine with the hips flexed. The supine position is preferable as it allows the individual to talk to the child and to maintain eye contact, but the most important consideration is that the child is held securely to prevent squirming. The thermometer is shaken down to below 96°F (35.6°C) and then lubricated with a water-soluble jelly. The thermometer is then inserted about one-half inch into the rectum. Frequently this stimulates the child to defecate. If the child passes stool, remove the thermometer, allow the child to complete the bowel movement and begin again. Hold the thermometer in place for at least three minutes. Gently withdraw the thermometer and re-dress the child. The rectal temperature is recorded, indicating the route, e.g., 99.2 (R).

When taking an oral temperature the thermometer is left in place at least five minutes. In most institutions, no notation following the temperature indicates that the temperature was taken by mouth.

The axillary route is used with less resistance from the child, yet because it requires a longer period of time it frequently results in a falsely low reading. The thermometer is placed in the axillae against the skin. Care must be taken to assure that the thermometer remains in contact with the skin during the entire procedure. The thermometer is left in place for 7 to 10 minutes. This reading is recorded as, for example, 99.4 (Ax).

The development of electronic temperature recording devices has made it possible to obtain an accurate temperature reading on a child in a short time. One commonly used device is the IVAC Electronic Clinical Thermometer. This is a hand-held rechargeable unit that is taken to the bedside to be used. The unit has a probe with disposable covers. Positioning and indication of selection of route are similar to the use of a glass thermometer. The major advantage is that it takes only several seconds to obtain the temperature reading and this is indicated by an audible signal. After use, it is necessary to return the device to the storage unit, where it is recharged.

Pulse When assessing a child's pulse, not only is the rate considered, but also the rhythm and quality. The pulse should be assessed when the child is quiet, as activity or crying increases the rate. For this reason it is best to take it before beginning any procedures to be done at the same time. Common descriptive terms for quality of the pulse are "thready," "bounding" or "faint."

The apical pulse rather than peripheral pulse is usually assessed in young children. To do this, palpate the point of maximum impulse (PMI) and place the diaphragm of the stethoscope on this point. (Palpation of PMI is discussed in Chapter 13.) Listen closely, noting the rate, rhythm and quality of the pulsation. If the pulse is of regular rhythm, it is acceptable to listen for 30 seconds and multiply by two to find the beats per minute. An exception to this procedure is when the child has a cardiac problem, in which case auscultation for a full minute is recommended.

Respiration Respiratory rate is assessed by noting the number of inspirations per minute. Activity or excitement may cause an increase in the respiratory rate, so this assessment should be done when the child is quiet. In addition to rate, it is important to observe for increased respiratory effort. Indicators of this are retractions (e.g., substernal, intercostal and supraclavicular), nasal flaring and use of abdominal muscles to breathe. Respiratory difficulty may cause grunting or wheezing and apprehension. These signs should be noted as signals of distress that may indicate the child is in need of prompt attention.

An accurate respiratory rate for a newborn is obtained during sleep or quiet rest, usually through auscultation (placing a stethoscope on the infant's thorax and counting respirations) or palpation (placing the hand on the abdomen to count respirations). It is also possible to observe the abdominal respiratory rate in some infants. (Infants have primarily diaphragmatic respirations, which are observed by abdominal movement.) An infant's respirations are frequently irregular and must be counted for a full minute. After infancy the respiratory rate of a child is obtained by observing chest movement for 30 seconds and multiplying by two unless the child has a respiratory illness; in this case auscultation for a full minute is recommended. Rapid respirations may be an indication of respiratory distress from severe infection.

Blood Pressure Blood pressure measurement is a reading often neglected in children unless the child presents with a diagnosis such as renal disease, cardiac disease or head trauma. The American Academy of Pediatrics recommends that all children 3 years of age and older have their blood pressure measured annually as part of their routine health assessment. This is a necessary step in identifying individuals at risk for developing hypertension as adults and to prevent the long-term complications for hypertensive individuals.

The most important factor in taking an accurate blood pressure is the size of the cuff. The cuff refers to the inflatable bladder and not the cloth cover. It must be wide enough to cover one-half to two-thirds of the upper arm and long enough to completely encircle the arm. A cuff that is too narrow or too short may result in a falsely high reading and a too-large cuff may cause a falsely low reading.

The first step in taking a blood pressure reading for a child is to explain the procedure to the child and to allow him to handle the equipment. Apprehension can cause the blood pressure reading to be higher than is normal for the child; therefore, every effort should be made to help the child relax. As with adults, the child is seated with the right arm resting at heart level. The right arm is used whenever possible, as this is the arm used in the development of standardized charts. The procedure from this point is identical to that used with adults.

Occasionally blood pressure cannot be auscultated. Blood pressure measurement by palpation is an alternative method. The steps in this method are:

1. Place the proper size cuff on the arm.
2. Palpate the brachial pulse and keep fingertips placed over pulse site with sufficient pressure to feel the pulse but not obliterate it.
3. Inflate the cuff until the pulse is no longer felt.
4. Deflate the cuff until the pulse is again felt. This point is the systolic pressure and is recorded 98/P indicating the palpation method has been used.

Obtaining blood pressure measurement on an infant is a more difficult procedure and is not routinely done during well-child examinations. When it is necessary electronic units are most accurate. If this equipment is not available and attempts to auscultate the blood pressure are not successful, a "flush" blood pressure can be obtained. This method is less accurate and reveals only the mean pressure. The steps in this procedure are:

1. Proper size cuff is placed on the arm.
2. The arm is raised and an elastic bandage snugly wrapped, starting from the fingers and proceeding up to the cuff.
3. The cuff is inflated and the elastic bandage removed. The arm should be blanched (paler than its normal coloring.)
4. The cuff is slowly deflated.
5. The point at which the arm flushes is noted. This is the mean pressure.

It is possible to obtain a blood pressure reading by placing a cuff on the thigh of a child. This is done if there is no access to the arms or if a cardiac abnormality is suspected. The proper size cuff is placed around the thigh and the femoral artery in the popliteal space is palpated. The procedure then is the same as that used to obtain a reading with the arm. In infants under 1 year the reading is normally the same as in the arm. After age 1, the systolic reading is normally higher in the thigh than in the arm. If the thigh reading is lower it is suggestive of coarctation of the aorta.

SAFETY MEASURES APPLIED TO CHILDREN

Measures that must be taken to keep a child safe vary according to the developmental level of the child. Age-related safety measures have been included in those chapters that address normal growth and development. When a child is hospitalized the nurse and parents must recognize potential dangers. Needles, glass bottles, medications and various types of machinery basic to any hospital environment are common dangers to children. Safety measures to be taken that are specific to each age group are discussed in each age-related chapter on hospitalization (27, 36, 45, 54, 63) Included in this section are general safety practices that apply to any child in any health care setting. The discussion that follows includes safety measures pertaining to environment, transportation of children within the health care setting and restraining and positioning a child for a procedure.

Environmental Safety The hospital environment is unfamiliar to the child and family; thus it is more difficult for them to predict what might happen and where dangers lie. Furthermore, because a child is ill, parents and health team members alike may assume that he will be less active and less inquisitive. Consequently, when fewer precautions are taken accidents are more likely to happen. Regardless of the degree of illness, safety measures should be taken that are consistent with the child's development and usual level of activity (as described by parents).

For example, one cannot necessarily assume that an ill child will lie quietly in his crib while the nurse briefly turns or walks a short distance away from the crib.

To achieve environmental safety for children special attention must be given to (1) floors, sockets and cords; (2) furniture (especially cribs), supplies and equipment; (3) toys and recreational supplies; (4) faucets and bath tubs; (5) eating arrangements and utensils; and (6) stairways, elevators and doors. Precautions in these areas affect safety regarding the child's mobility, play and recreational activities and activities of daily living.

The mobility of children in hospitals is to be encouraged and should not introduce unnecessary dangers. Floors should be free of clutter; they should be clean but not slippery. A highly polished, waxed floor is inappropriate for a children's unit. Children should not be allowed to walk around in bare feet or socks. Properly fitting disposable slippers or skid-free shoes from home should be worn. Slick-soled shoes can be made safe by placing a wide strip of tape along the sole. Children should be instructed to walk, not run, in corridors and they should never be allowed to be mobile with objects on a stick (e.g., lollipops and Popsicles) in their mouths.

Numerous cords and sockets are necessary in most hospitals. Young children in cribs are sufficiently mobile to reach sockets — cribs need to be placed so that children cannot reach them (Fig. 17-1). Young children out of bed must be supervised to protect them from falling over cords.

In most hospitals children may leave the unit for short periods to go to the gift shop or snack bar if attended by a family member or hospital personnel. On the unit children must be protected from wandering into dangerous areas such as treatment rooms, stairwells, and elevators.

Safe toys and recreational equipment are basic to the care of all children. The potential problem in hospitals is that toys and equipment are in poor repair and not cleaned properly because no one in particular is assigned this responsibility. Thus each nurse must take individual responsibility to ensure that play equipment is maintained and properly cleaned and that activities are safe for the age of the child. (See chapters on growth and development for age-appropriate toys and activities.) Common sources of danger are removable parts that can be swallowed (especially the metal insert on squeak toys), rough and sharp edges, movable parts that readily pinch fingers, and toys and

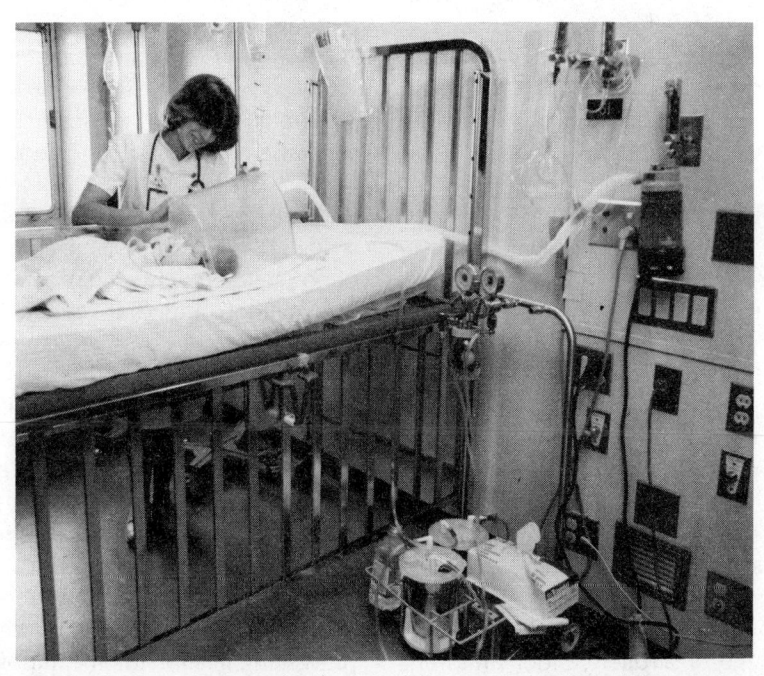

Figure 17-1 The wheels of cribs must be locked and the crib placed a sufficient distance from electrical outlets to prevent young children from poking objects into sockets. (Note: the crib side is in the down position for the photograph only.)

PRINCIPLES AND SKILLS OF PEDIATRIC NURSING

equipment that are too advanced for the child's age.

Daily care needs of the child in the hospital are the same as at home, but the unfamiliar environment may introduce additional dangers. Even a young child often knows which faucet is hot and which is cold at home but in the hospital he may inadvertently turn on hot water. Older children who are relatively independent at home may need more supervision in the hospital because of differences in the height and contour of the tub and the placement of faucets.

Mealtime requires supervision to protect children from unfamiliar dangers. For example, some hospital kitchens use metal covers that are hot and must be removed before the meal is served. Also, a child may not be accustomed to the size of fork or cup that is used in the hospital, or he may inadvertently be served food that is not age-appropriate, resulting in a choking episode.

One of the greatest dangers to a child anywhere involves use of supplies, equipment or furniture that is hazardous. Cribs must be in good repair and need to be used appropriately. For example, depending on the age and size of a child, an enclosed crib (see Chapter 36) or pads around the edge of the crib may be necessary to prevent falls and injuries. *These decisions are made by the nurse and require immediate attention on admission of a child to the unit.* Any crib with a broken latch must immediately be sent for repair; taping the side rail in place, regardless of how firmly, is an unsafe practice. Furniture should be sturdy, and child-sized tables and chairs should be available for playing and eating. Dangerous supplies such as electrical equipment, medications, soaps and shampoos, needles, razors and scissors must be appropriately stored to keep children of all ages safe.

Transportation of Children The hospitalized child must frequently be transported to another unit within the hospital for diagnostic or therapeutic procedures. An infant should not be carried to another part of the hospital because the person carrying him could slip and fall. Appropriate ways to transport infants are by crib, baby carriage or stroller. Older children can be transported in their bed or by stretcher, wheel chairs, wagons, or specially made carts that provide for a semi-Fowler's position. Regardless of the type of transporting device used, the child must be securely belted for safety.

The usual precautions of safety used in transporting adults should be applied for children. Of particular importance is being certain that the child is adequately identified, that the IV chamber will not run dry while the child is off the unit, and that the child will be attended while waiting in another department. Children will be less resistive to procedures if they are forewarned when and where they are going. Thus an indirect form of maintaining the child's physical safety is to prepare him psychologically before transporting him.

Caring for Children Who Require Restraints
Restraints are necessarily applied to children but should not be used without careful evaluation of alternatives. They are used to immobilize the child for diagnostic and therapeutic procedures of varying types and duration. The nurse generally makes the decision as to whether restraint is needed and which type of restraint is most appropriate.

Type of Restraint Commonly used restraints in the care of children are (1) mummy restraint, (2) elbow restraint, (3) jacket restraint and (4) arm and leg restraints.

A mummy restraint is used to immobilize an infant or small child for a short time as is required for examination or treatment of the head, neck or chest. The purpose of this technique is to secure the arms and legs within a blanket in a way that prevents the child from wriggling free. The nurse is thus free to hold the child securely to prevent movement of his entire body without attending to flailing arms and legs. This technique is particularly useful for jugular punctures, insertion of nasogastric tubes, scalp vein needle insertion, and detailed examination of the eye, ear, nose and throat (Fig. 17–2).

The modified mummy restraint is used for procedures that require an exposed chest. Figure 17–3 details steps in securing the infant in a modified mummy restraint.

The purpose of an elbow restraint is to keep the child from reaching his face or head by preventing flexion of the elbow. This type of restraint may be needed to preserve plastic surgery of the face, a scalp vein needle, eye patches, or to prevent scratching of the face in various skin disorders. The restraint usually

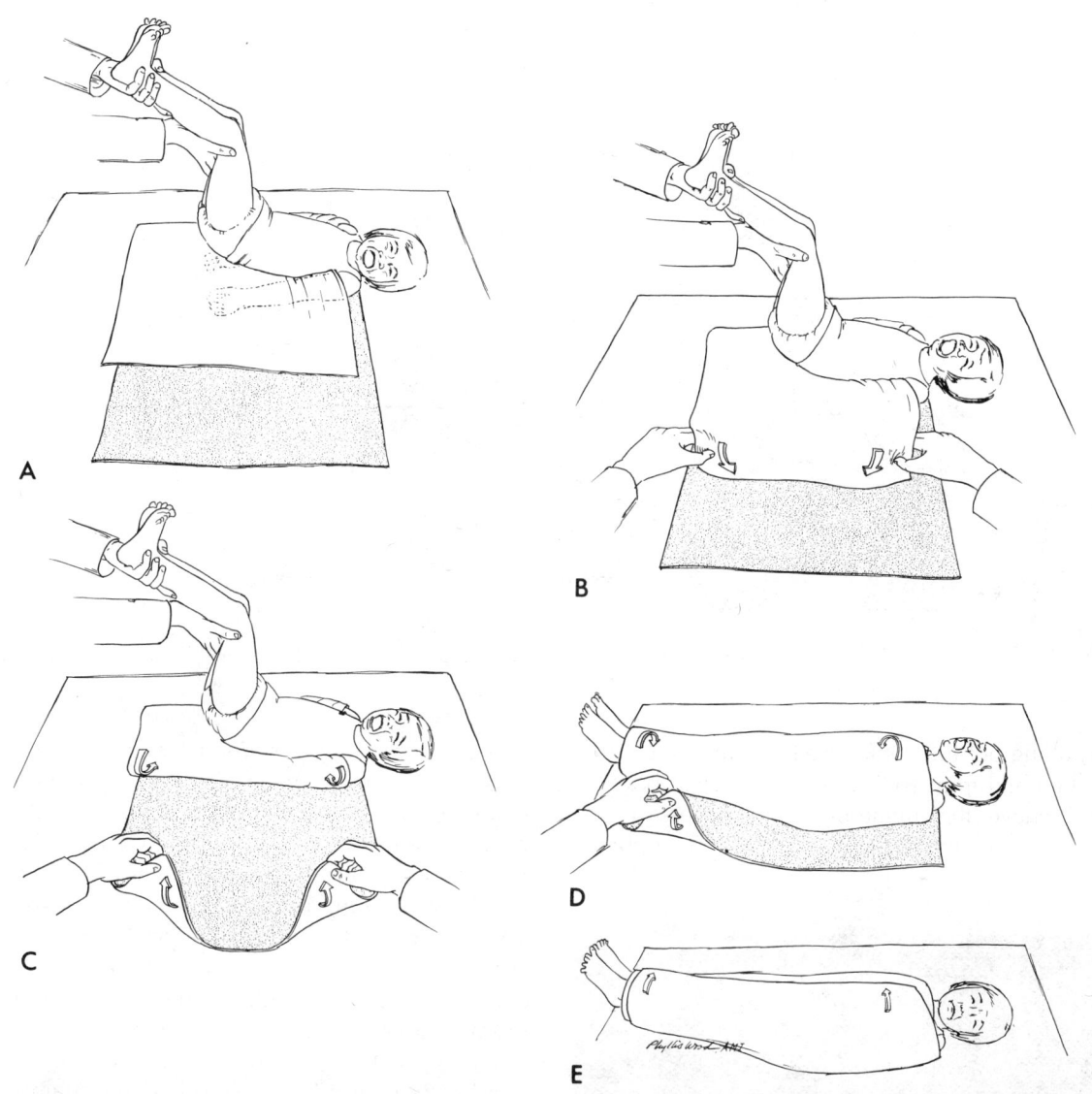

Figure 17-2 Mummy restraint. The restraining sheet is placed under the child and folded back, pinning the arms down (*A*). Next the sheet is tucked back under the child's left arm (*B*). The sheet is then wrapped around the child's entire body (*C, D, E*) and fastened with a safety pin. (From D. W. Smith, 2nd ed. Introduction to Clinical Pediatrics, W. B. Saunders Co., 1977.)

covers most of the arm, but it should not push into the child's axilla nor should it rub the wrist. A cloth (usually muslin) restraint with pockets for tongue depressors is commonly used (Fig. 17-4). A tongue blade must be placed into each pocket. Large blades made especially for these restraints should be used, or two tongue blades should be taped together. The tongue blade *must* extend the entire length of the pocket to prevent them from slipping to a position above or below the child's elbow. Care must also be taken to avoid using a tongue blade that is too long, which would result in pressure in the axillae. Similar types of restraints can be improvised. A padded cylinder can be made out of cardboard or a plastic container. Such a restraint must be placed over the child's shirt and secured with pins, ties or tape to prevent it from slipping off.

A jacket restraint is used to keep the child flat in bed or safe in a highchair or wheelchair. It is preferable not to use a jacket restraint to keep a child from climbing out of a crib. An enclosed crib should be used instead.

A jacket restraint is tied at the back to keep the child from untying it and the long tapes should be tied to the crib frames and not to the side rails. Jacket restraints are used for IV infusions to keep the child from sitting up and

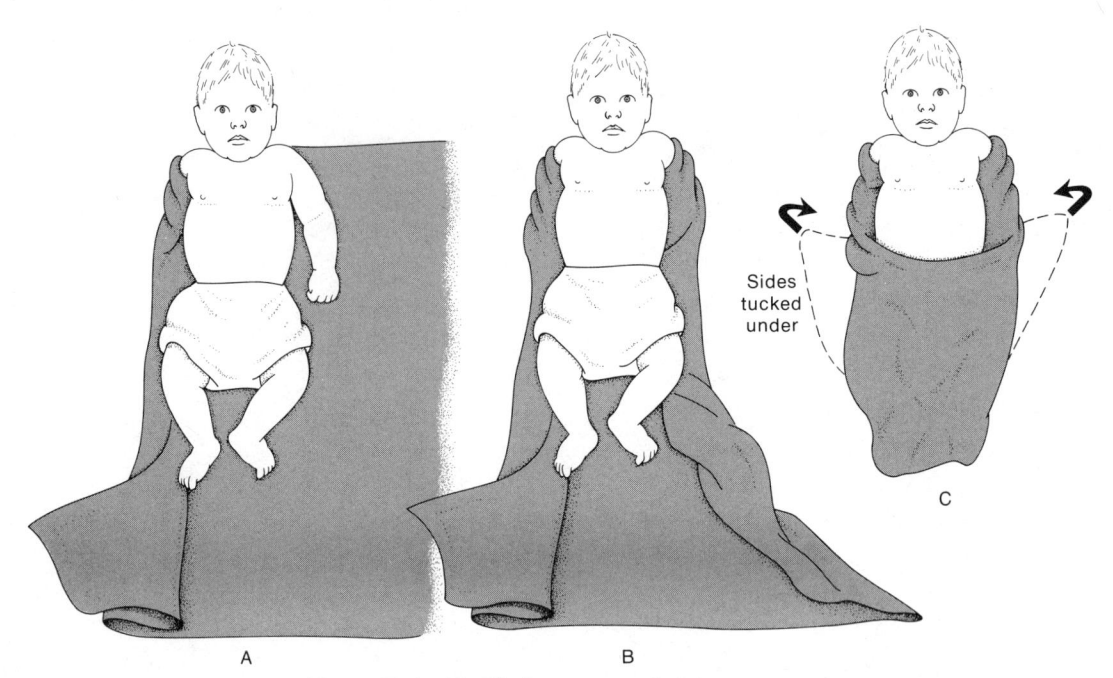

Figure 17-3 Modified mummy restraint.

pulling out the IV, for cleft lip surgery to keep the child from rolling onto the Logan bow, or whenever the supine position is necessary.

Arm and leg restraints are used to immobilize one or more extremities. The restraint can be a muslin strip, roller gauze, Kerlix, or similar material. First the wrist or ankle is padded with gauze (one or two 4 by 4's opened and folded lengthwise) a cut abdominal (ABD) pad, or a small wash cloth. The restraint is applied by using a clove hitch technique (Fig. 17-5). The clove hitch is not a slip knot and if applied correctly does not tighten. The ends of the restraint are tied to the crib frame.

Nursing Responsibilities The child in restraints must be continually re-evaluated to see whether restraint is still needed. The minimum amount of restraint necessary to meet the therapeutic goal should be used.

The nurse should work closely with the family to help them understand the need for restraints. Depending on the reason for the restraint, parents can be permitted to release the child from restraints for varying lengths of time.

Circulatory checks of the restrained limb must be done frequently by the nurse. If restraints are applied properly the potential for complications is minimized. If the child is not restless, each extremity should be checked at least every hour, but for a restless child extremities should be checked every 15 minutes. The nurse should also periodically remove restraints to exercise the involved extremity and give the child freedom of movement. It has been sug-

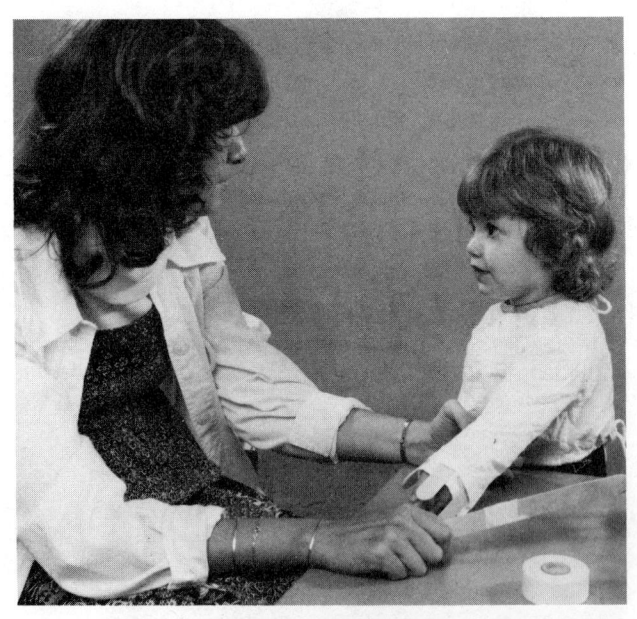

Figure 17-4 Applying an elbow restraint. Note the individual pockets in the sleeve for each tongue blade. This child requires two tongue blades taped together to provide sufficient length to keep her from bending her elbow.

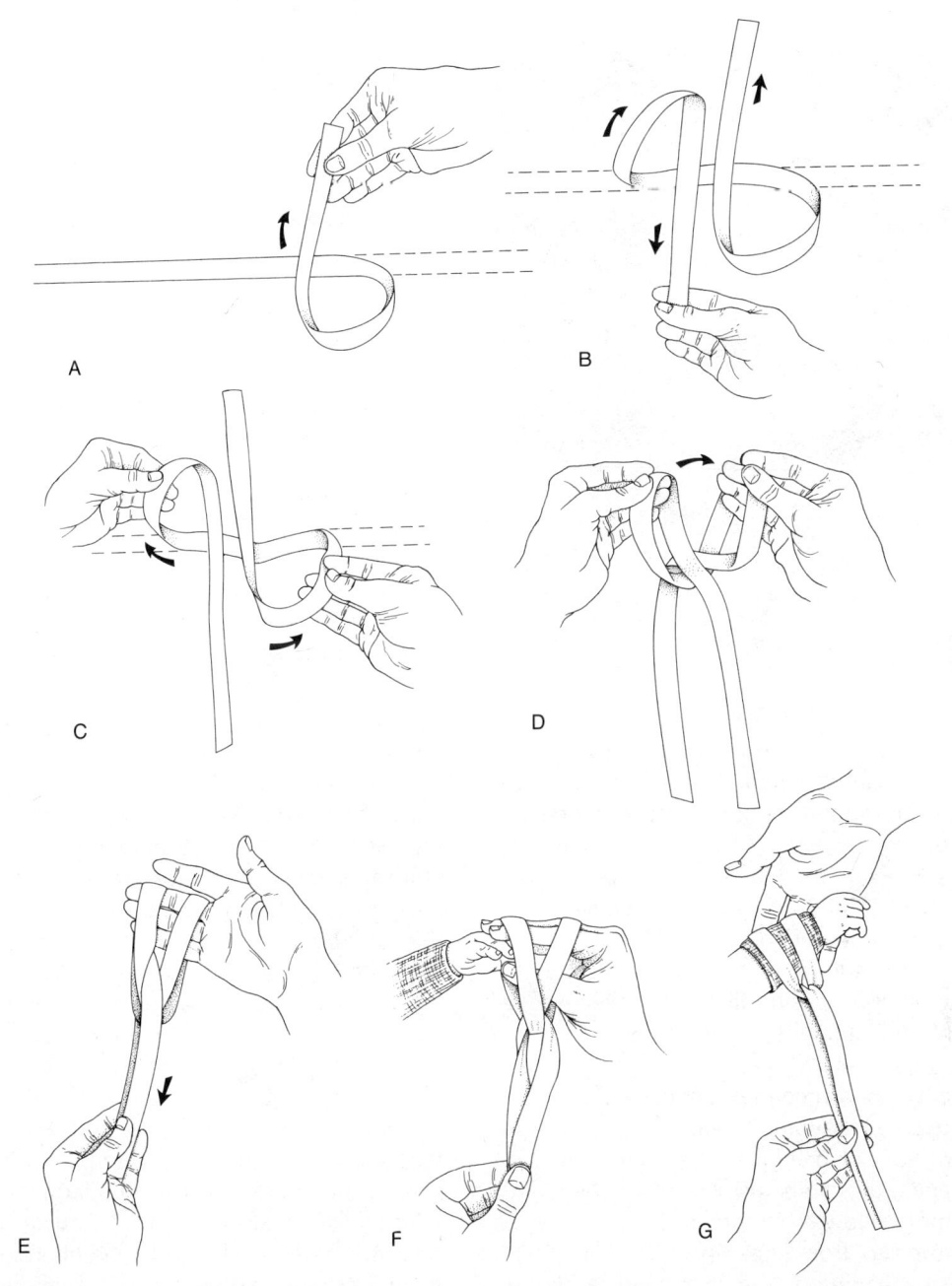

Figure 17-5 Clove hitch restraint. **A,** lay or hold restraint in a straight line. Make a loop by bringing one end across straight line. **B,** bring other end across straight line, making loop on opposite side of straight line. **C,** pick up both loops at once. **D,** bring hands together and let ends drop down. **E,** place fingers through both loops and pull ends firmly. **F,** slip clove hitch over padded wrist or ankle. **G,** tighten restraint by pulling alternately on the ends of the restraint. The knot is firmly secured against the padded extremity but should not impair circulation.

gested that this should be done under supervision every 2 hours for a 10-minute period.[7]

Nursing interventions for a child in restraints should be directed toward reducing the negative effects of immobility. Development of physical, intellectual and emotional and social competencies are all affected by the child's inability to be mobile. When restrained a child loses his major form of expression. He cannot defend himself by running away or by physically striking out; often he cannot even suck his thumb for comfort.[7] He feels helpless, frustrated and anxious. Immobility at a young age has also been identified as a factor in language delay and problems of articulation.[18] Limitation of activity reduces muscle strength and increases excretion of calcium, potassium and sodium.[7] The nurse has a responsibility to ensure that children are released for short periods, that parents are

PRINCIPLES AND SKILLS OF PEDIATRIC NURSING

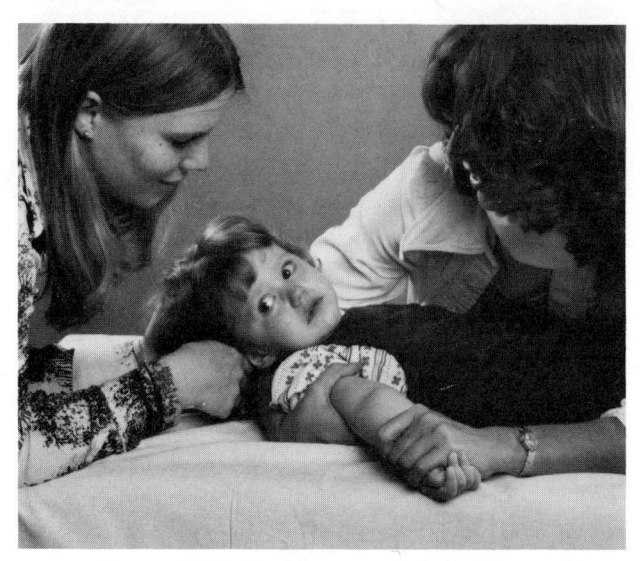

Figure 17-6 Venipuncture. If the child is properly restrained, both the child and the nurse can be comfortable, while the arm is securely held to permit a safe venipuncture.

taught how to release restraints and protect their child while unrestrained, and that children are not kept in restraints of unnecessary degree and duration.

Positioning Children for Procedures The nurse plays a major role in making it possible for procedures to be performed safely and efficiently. Proper positioning and effective restraint to maintain the position avoids injury to the child and shortens the procedure. One can generally not assume that a child will hold still without some assistance. The nurse's grip must be firm but not painful to the child. Her own torso and arms can be used to block the child's movement. However, care must be taken to avoid pressure from fingertips, injury to internal organs by leaning on the child, and respiratory embarrassment from occluding the airway.

Before beginning a procedure the nurse must assess the child for level of cooperation and potential strength with which he is likely to resist. In many instances one nurse can position and restrain a child effectively; however, for some children additional help may be needed. It is the young child who does not understand an explanation but has sufficient physical strength to resist with his whole body who particularly needs careful restraint. The nurse should summon additional help before beginning a procedure for these children.

Before a procedure the child and the parent is given an explanation of the procedure. Whenever possible and appropriate, parents should be encouraged to support the child by their presence. The appropriateness of a parent's presence varies with the type of procedure and wishes of the child and the parent.

Procedures should be done in the treatment room whenever possible rather than at the child's bedside. The child's bed should be, in his mind, a place that is safe and comfortable. Although children cannot be taken to a treatment room for each intramuscular injection, the nurse should ensure that the more lengthy traumatic procedures are done in the treatment room. This practice keeps the unit more comfortable and safer for all children in that trauma is not observed by other children and needles and equipment are not inadvertently left at a child's bedside.

Venipuncture With the child in a supine position the nurse can extend the child's arm and stabilize the wrist. The other hand is used to grasp the child's shoulder by placing it around the back of the child's neck (Fig. 17-6). The child's unused arm is secured behind the nurse's back. The nurse's torso can lean across the child but her weight is on her elbow, not on the child. This position is effective to restrain for the venipuncture and also allows the nurse to talk to the child and maintain eye contact because her face is in direct alignment with the child's face.

Procedures Involving the Perineal and Rectal Area The child is placed in a supine position with the nurse at his head. The nurse stretches her arms along each side of the child, grasping the thighs. The legs are flexed and abducted for exposure of the anus and perineum. A folded diaper is laid across the perineum and another diaper placed under the child. The upper diaper can thus be removed or positioned to allow access to the particular area required in that procedure.

Lumbar Puncture The technique of performing a lumbar puncture (spinal tap) does not vary from that in an adult. The puncture is made into the subarachnoid space at the level of the fourth or fifth lumbar vertebra. A lumbar puncture is contraindicated when elevation of cerebrospinal fluid (CSF) pressure is suspected. The abrupt release of the pressure by removal of spinal fluid may cause the brain stem to be drawn into the spinal column, compressing the medulla or cardiorespiratory center.

A correct position can be attained by placing the child on the side with his face toward the nurse and as close to the far edge of the table as possible (Fig. 17-7). The child's neck is gently flexed forward and the knees should be drawn up toward his chest. This results in a slight rounding of the back, which is the desired position. The child should be positioned so that his body is in alignment with the edge of the table. The nurse may appear to be placing her weight on the child as she leans forward across the child's body; however, her weight is actually placed on her elbows. His respirations and color should be observed during the procedure to ensure that the restraint does not compromise chest expansion. The nurse's position makes it difficult for her to see the child's face. If checking the child necessitates slight alteration of the nurse's position, it is better for her to inform the physician that she must move slightly rather than not to check the child.

For some children, especially premature infants, an alternate position may be used. The child is placed in a sitting position with the neck flexed forward. The child's buttocks are placed at the edge of the table. The nurse stands on the opposite side of the table facing the child and stabilizes his body and legs to maintain the position.

Children who can comprehend explanations should be forewarned of the position that is required. They should also be told about the cold sensation that occurs when the skin is cleansed, and the importance of keeping as still as possible. They should be told to squeeze the nurse's hand, but not to wriggle their bodies nor move their extremities. It may not always be appropriate for parents to be present during this procedure. In those circumstances in which the procedure is done frequently, as may occur in a long-term illness, parents become very familiar with the procedure and their presence may be of therapeutic benefit for the child.

Following the procedure, vital signs should be taken as ordered by the physician. If there are no specific orders or a standard routine to follow, the nurse should take vital signs and do a neurological check every 15 minutes for an hour, then every half hour for another hour. If the signs are stable the usual routine can then be resumed. Vital signs should include blood pressure, pulse and respirations. A neurological check should include evaluation of pupils, of

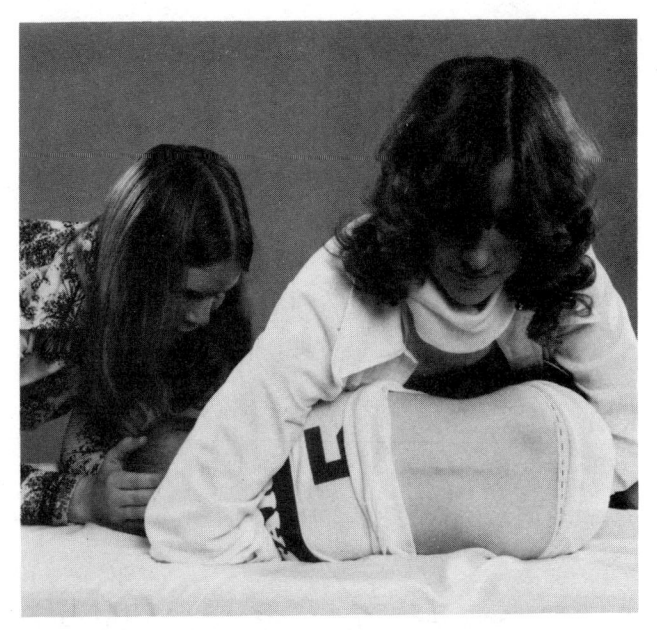

Figure 17-7 Lumbar puncture. If parents are present for this procedure, they can support the child by focusing on him rather than the procedure.

level of consciousness, and of motor abilities. Children are usually allowed to assume a position of comfort after the lumbar puncture.

COMMON PEDIATRIC PROCEDURES

Many of the procedures used to care for children are similar to those for adults. Procedures discussed in this section are those that are most commonly performed or those that require special adaptation when performed on children or both. For basic step-by-step instructions on how to perform various procedures, the reader is referred to texts on basic skills (fundamentals) of nursing.

Nursing Skills to Facilitate Respiration and Oxygenation*

Maintaining adequate pulmonary function in some children requires constant vigilance and specialized nursing skills. The nurse must focus on providing maximum pulmonary benefits with the least possible energy depletion and trauma to the child. Chest physical therapy can be adapted so that good pulmonary hygiene is integrated into the infant's total nursing plan

---

*Acknowledgement is given to Peggy Clough, MS, RPT Supervisor, Chest Service, Physical Therapy Division, University Hospital of Michigan, for her assistance in the preparation of this section.

A
UPPER LOBE
Apical segment
(Anterior)

45°

B
UPPER LOBE
Apical segment
(Posterior)

45°

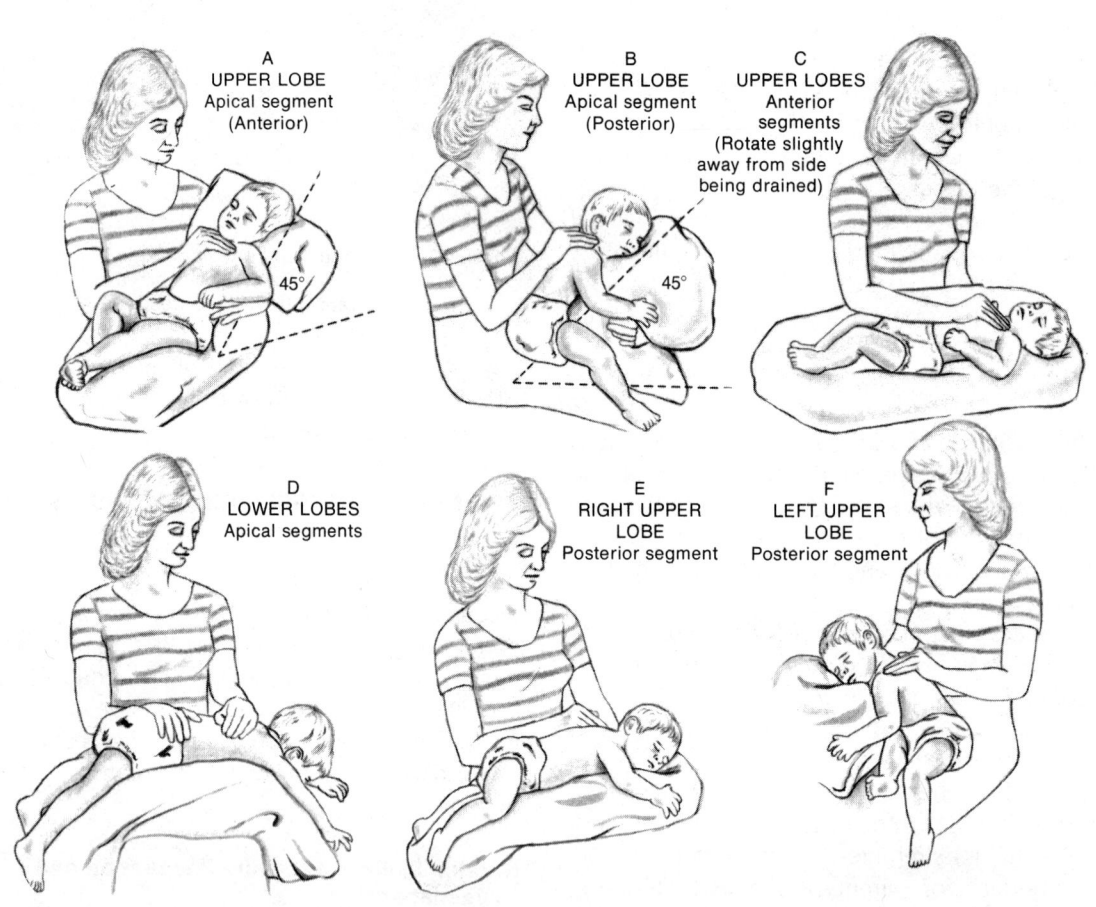

C
UPPER LOBES
Anterior segments
(Rotate slightly away from side being drained)

D
LOWER LOBES
Apical segments

E
RIGHT UPPER LOBE
Posterior segment

F
LEFT UPPER LOBE
Posterior segment

Illustration continued on the opposite page

326   FAMILIES WITH CHILDREN

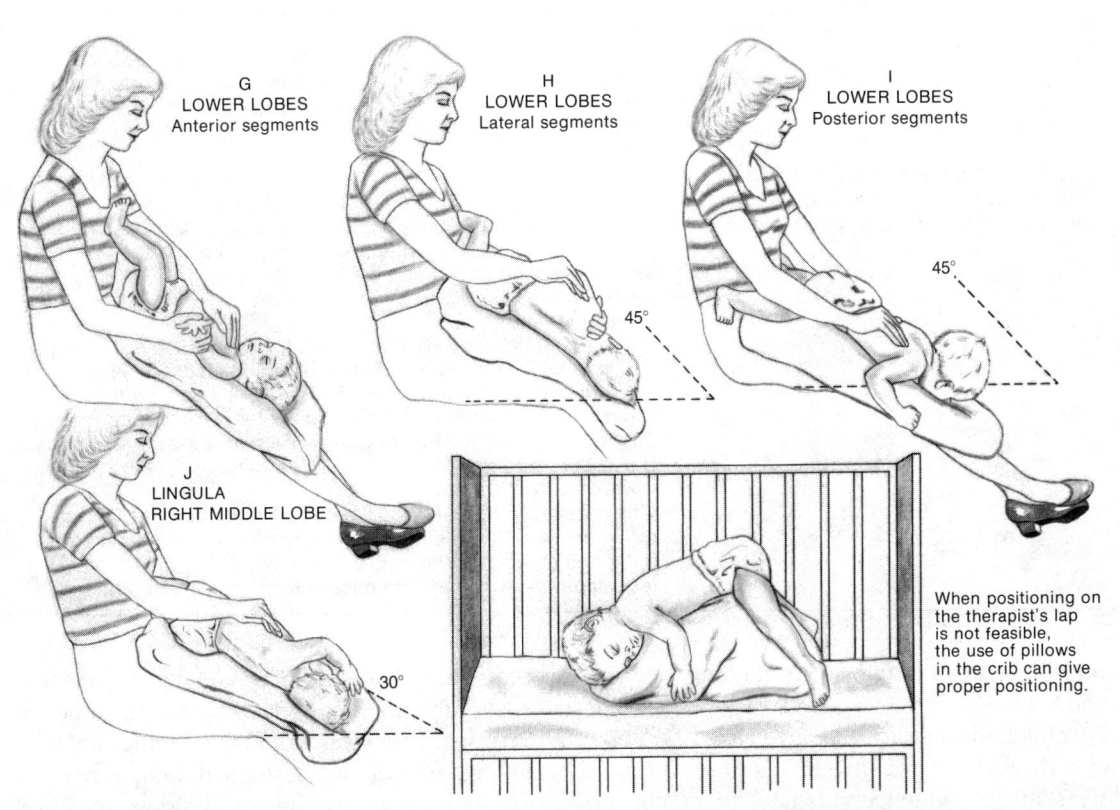

Figure 17-8 Postural drainage. The positions for postural drainage are correlated with the segment being drained. See Figure 17-9. In positions H and J the child is shown on his right side; however, he must also be turned to his left side to drain both lobes. (Adapted from materials used by the Chest Physical Therapy Department, Physical Therapy Division, Department of Physical Medicine and Rehabilitation, Hospital of the University of Michigan, Ann Arbor, MI.)

TABLE 17-1 NURSING ACTIONS RELATED TO DEEP BREATHING, COUGHING AND SUCTIONING

Developmental Considerations	Related Nursing Actions
1. Infants and young children do not cognitively understand the directions take a deep breath or cough.	A cough can be stimulated by slowly passing a sterile catheter through child's nose until it reaches the pharynx or trachea. A natural cough reflex can be stimulated by exerting firm pressure over trachea at sternal notch during expiration.
2. Even when child does understand the direction to take a deep breath and to cough, he often needs to be encouraged to do so by being engaged in developmentally appropriate activities.	To facilitate deep breathing, the nurse can provide: • Balloons • Soap bubbles • Spirometer • Pinwheels • Variety of blowing games. To facilitate an effective cough, the nurse should: (a) Place child in an upright sitting position to provide for maximum expansion of chest and mechanical advantage for abdominal muscles. (b) Prepare child with appropriate pain medication and, in postoperative cases, splint the operative area with a pillow. (c) Demonstrate the desired cough and ask the child to imitate.
3. Mucous membranes are thin and easily traumatized; special precautions must be taken in technique of suctioning.	• Oral suctioning: Insert catheter at each side of the mouth and advance to the back of the mouth. Gently rotate catheter; do not poke in and out of back of mouth. Suction each area once and then reassess the child and allow him to rest. Repeat procedure only if secretions are abundant. • Nasopharyngeal suctioning: Catheter is measured by spanning it from tip of child's nose to his earlobe. The measured distance on catheter is inserted through one nostril, then the other, smoothly and gently. On withdrawal suction is applied and catheter is rotated between the fingers. Avoid a jerky in-and-out motion. Assess respiratory status and repeat procedure only if indicated. • Nasotracheal suctioning: This potentially traumatizing procedure must be done with extreme caution (can result in laryngospasm and/or bradycardia). It is not a routine pediatric procedure but rather a specialized technique usually used for children in intensive care units.

and does not interfere with feeding or nap schedules.

A child's developmental level must be considered when intervening to maintain respiratory status. A young child may be unable to verbalize his difficulty in breathing and may be unable to produce a cough or to cooperate during these specialized procedures. Respiratory procedures involving catheters for aspiration are particularly resisted with squirming, kicking and body thrashing because of the irritating and choking sensation produced. The more proficient and skilled the nurse, the more effective the treatment and the less likelihood that the child will be traumatized.

Deep Breathing, Coughing and Suctioning These are discussed in Table 17-1.

Chest Physical Therapy Chest physical therapy (CPT) is a frequently used intervention in the pulmonary care of children and can include any or all of the following: deep breathing games or exercises, coughing, huffing, splinting, tracheal tickling, suctioning, postural drainage, percussion and vibration. These techniques are used singly or in combination in an effort to assist the infant or child in clearing excess or abnormal secretions from the lungs. The techniques involved in chest physical therapy often need to be modified for children both because of their size and their inability to follow verbal instructions.

Chest Physical Therapy Techniques Chest physical therapy includes a combination of techniques. Positioning, along with mechanical stimulation of the chest is necessary to attain the desired results.

Postural drainage is the placement of the child in a series of positions so that gravity will assist in moving secretions from the periphery of the lung centrally toward the trachea. There are 18 lung segments and 12 classical postural drainage positions. In each classical drainage position one or more segmental bronchi are perpendicular to the floor so that the force of gravity is optimal. Figures 17–8 and 17–9 show correlation of the segment being drained and the position of the child. The recommended positions used for a particular child will vary according to the lung segments most involved. Children are generally not able to tolerate more than four to six positions at one session; therefore, it may be necessary to rotate positions from one session to the next. For a young child, a comfortable position can be attained by placing him on a pillow while in bed or on the therapist's or parent's lap. A neonate in an isolette can be positioned by using a rolled blanket and by raising and lowering the isolette tray. With older children and adolescents, use of the knee gatch and pillows facilitates effective positioning for postural drainage. At home,

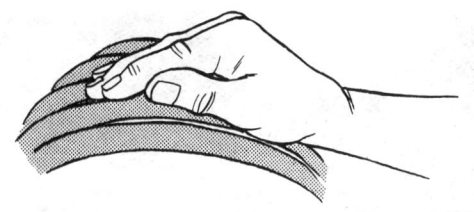

Figure 17–10 Position of hand cupped for percussion. The wrist movement involves a brisk relaxed flexion and extension. The examiner should be careful not to use only the fingers or only the heel of the hand. (From G. Leifer. Principles and techniques in Pediatric Nursing, 3rd ed. W. B. Saunders Co., 1977.)

an inverted chair, a home-made padded board, or a stack of newspapers with couch cushions over them may be used.

Percussion is performed intermittently during postural drainage to speed movement of the mucus. Percussion must always be comfortable for the child so that deep breathing can continue throughout the postural drainage treatment. To protect the skin from irritation, the child's chest should be covered with a light cotton shirt and no jewelry should be worn by the therapist or the nurse. To percuss, the hand is tightly "cupped" (Fig. 17–10) and is "clapped" against the chest over the area being drained. (Percussion is also called "cupping" and "clapping.") This procedure should produce a hollow sound (not a slapping sound), indicating that air is being compressed between the therapist's hand and the child's chest wall. The compression wave is presumably transmitted to the bronchi, stimulating turbulence in the air the child is moving in and out with each breath. The turbulent air flow catches the secretions adherent to bronchial walls and moves the secretions in the direction of gravitational pull. Care should be taken to percuss only over lung tissue. In an infant the lower ribs cover liver and kidneys; therefore percussion even for the lower lobes should be performed two to three finger breadths above the lowest rib. When the size of the infant's chest does not accommodate the therapist's hand, other means of percussion are used. To percuss an infant's chest, two or three fingers are tented together (Fig. 17–11) or a small cup-shaped object can be used. Objects that have been suggested in the literature for percussion are an anesthesia mask, a small padded medicine cup, a padded nipple, or the padded bell of a stethoscope.

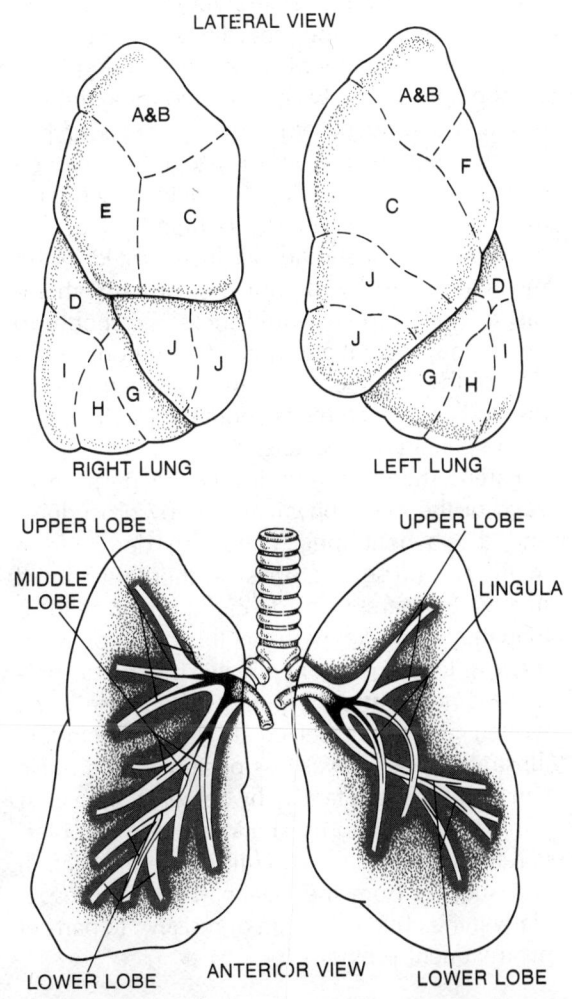

Figure 17–9 Lung segments. The upper diagram is labeled by letters to correlate the segment being drained with the position of the child in Figure 17–8. The bottom diagram shows the position and main segments of the lower airways of the tracheobronchial tree.

PRINCIPLES AND SKILLS OF PEDIATRIC NURSING

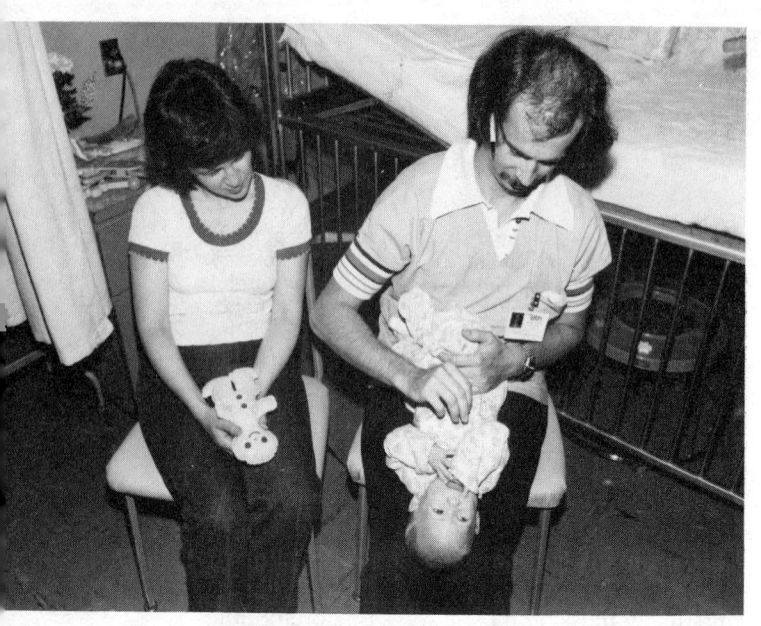

Figure 17-11 Chest percussion of an infant. To percuss, two or three fingers are tented together. Parents can learn to perform the procedure at home by observing and practicing the technique.

Vibration is a rapid quivering movement of the therapist's arms and hands applied to the chest wall during the exhalation phase of respiration. Hand positions for vibration are variable; hands can be placed over each other, side by side, or on either side of the chest. To initiate the vibration the therapist contracts all the flexor and extensor muscles of the arm and shoulder. Because the infant's respiratory rate is so fast and the chest wall small, various types of mechanical vibrators have been substituted for manual vibration. An electric toothbrush with the bristle portion padded has been suggested for vibration of neonates.[6] Vibration is a more difficult procedure than percussion and is not always taught to parents unless bronchial drainage will be required for months or years. Bronchial drainage with percussion and vibration is often fatiguing to the child; therefore, the areas of greatest involvement should be treated first.

Removal of secretions completes the process of chest physical therapy. This is accomplished by coughing or suctioning or both. Tracheal tickling is an effective way to stimulate a natural cough reflex in infants and small children. Tracheal tickling is performed by exerting firm pressure over the trachea at the sternal notch during expiration.

Nurse's Role in Chest Physical Therapy The nurse participates in chest physical therapy in a variety of ways, depending on the patient's needs and the setting. She may be in complete charge of carrying out the procedures; however, in many centers a physical therapist will perform the procedures and play a major role in teaching the family. Regardless of the type of setting, the nurse retains responsibility for the total care of the child. This means that the nurse should listen to chest sounds to identify any child who could benefit from chest physical therapy. According to Waring, "Persistent crackles in a given segment or lobe constitute sufficient indication in themselves for drainage of the involved bronchi."[21] The nurse should also evaluate the effectiveness of chest physical therapy and assist the physical therapist in teaching the family the necessary home program. Furthermore, the nurse should be sure that the chest physical therapy is being done and that it is being coordinated with other treatments the patient is receiving. Chest physical therapy is usually done two to three times a day and should be done before meals or just before bedtime or both. The child should be encouraged to drink fluids to help liquefy pulmonary secretions, unless contraindicated.

The treatment should be documented in the medical record by the nurse or physical therapist or both. Notes should include response to treatment, amount and type of secretions, duration of the treatment, the lung segments being drained and a statement about the participation of the patient and parents.

Parents need to understand the purpose of each of the chest physical therapy procedures and the benefit their child can derive from them. The nurse and physical therapist should involve the parents in the care of their child so that they learn to perform the chest physical therapy techniques effectively. If a home program is necessary, the parents should be given written guidelines before discharge, including illustrations of the various positions. The nurse can also assist the family by demonstrating with puppets, dolls, horns, balloons and bubbles. Parents of a critically ill child need information and support from the health care team, especially if the child is in pain or resistive to parts of his treatment program.

Caring for a Child with a Tracheostomy The nurse caring for a child with a tracheostomy must be skilled to provide the care associated

RESEARCH ON CHEST PHYSICAL THERAPY IN NEONATES

Chest physical therapy (CPT) for neonates is a special problem that requires ongoing nursing research. Below is a synopsis of one study that was done to evaluate chest physical therapy:

Study Synopsis

Purpose: To evaluate the difference between two methods of chest physical therapy in the neonate with respiratory distress syndrome.

Basic design: Experimental

Population: Infants in a neonatal unit with a verified diagnosis of respiratory distress syndrome who were in fluid balance and had no other major problems or congenital anomalies.

Sample size: 6

Method: Selection of subjects was based on physician diagnosis. Infants were randomly assigned to one of two groups — the first received vibration of the chest wall using an electric toothbrush, the second vibration using a padded nipple. If no vibration was ordered, infants were placed in a third, control group. Infants receiving vibration therapy did so every two hours for one minute, followed by suction both immediately and prn (as needed). Infants in the control were suctioned every two hours and prn. Staff nurses did both the vibrating/suctioning and collection of data, which included color, respiration and heart rates, level of activity, amount of secretion, weight, urinary output, and blood gas values. Blood gas values were obtained at least three times in a 24-hour period. Color, respiration and heart rates, and level of activity were noted before the vibration/suctioning procedure and 15 minutes after suctioning. Each infant was followed for a total of 18 testing sessions.

Data analysis: Analysis of variance.

Conclusions:
1. pO_2 and pCO_2 — levels highest in the toothbrush group.
2. Apical pulse — all groups had a significant increase in apical pulse rate 15 minutes after suctioning.
3. Respiratory rate — significantly higher in all groups 15 minutes after suctioning.
4. Breath sounds — significantly clearer in toothbrush group immediately after suctioning.
5. Color — toothbrush group had best color.

C. L. Curran and M. K. Kachoyeanos. The effects on neonates of two methods of chest physical therapy. Copyright © 1979, American Journal of Nursing Company. Reprinted with permission from MCN, The American Journal of Maternal Child Nursing, Sept/Oct, Vol. 4, No. 5, p. 313.

---

with the period of hospitalization, and in many instances she may need to assist families to provide home care. Whether a child needs a tracheostomy temporarily or for a long time, the nurse should involve the parents from the beginning. It is a frightening experience for the child and parents when they have little understanding of the purpose of the tracheostomy and the care that is required. Parents readily adapt to identifying their child's need for suctioning and perform the procedure effectively with assistance.

Tracheal tubes are made of soft, pliable materials that comfortably conform to the contour of the trachea. Most tubes used for children today do not have an inner cannula. The inner cannula is unnecessary because the smooth plastic surface reduces collection of secretions and crust formation. Generally it is not beneficial to place a gauze pad between the skin and the tube. If secretions are heavy, patting the area dry with gauze is preferred; a gauze placed under the tube quickly becomes saturated and contributes to skin excoriation. The skin around the tracheostomy must be kept clean and inspected for excoriation.

Infants and young children may need to be restrained (elbow restraints are preferable to wrist restraints) to prevent pulling at the tracheal tube. Special precaution is taken to have the child avoid small toys or those that have removable parts that could be inserted into the tracheal tube. The tube must be protected from food spillage during mealtime by using a bib that fits the contour of the neck and has short ties. For infants with particularly chubby necks a small towel rolled to support the neck prevents occlusion of the opening by skin folds.

Emergency equipment including an extra tracheotomy tube and equipment, a suction machine and suction catheters and obdurator are standard supplies kept at the bedside. A hemostat is placed in a location in which it is clearly seen. It is used to keep the trachea open in an emergency.

The normal process of filtering, warming and humidification of air by the upper airway is bypassed when a tracheostomy is necessary. Air can be humidified in a variety of ways depending on the age and mobility of the child. A mist tent, a collar (special mask) placed over the tracheostomy opening or a mechanical ventilator may be used. Humidification prevents drying of the tissues and aids in loosening secretions.

The nurse must check a child with a tracheotomy frequently to detect the need for suctioning. An increased pulse, restlessness, bubbling of secretions from the tracheotomy, changes in color (cyanosis or pallor), dyspnea, retractions, and noisy respirations are indications that the child's airway is being occluded with secretions. Infants and children require constant surveillance to identify these signs. Adults and older children have various means of summoning help. An infant or young child has only his cry to alert his caretaker of discomfort; with a tracheotomy he has a silent cry. Consequently these children must be placed where the nurse can easily see their movements.

A silent cry is particularly anxiety-producing to parents who care for their child at home. Some parents have been reported to become less anxious about not hearing their child's cry when they discovered that even during the night they could hear their child breathing and moving.[2] Two of the families in an investigation by Aradine installed intercom systems to facilitate hearing their child.[2]

Suctioning Suctioning for infants is done in a similar manner as for adults. A child's vulnerability to infection is great; therefore, sterile technique must be carefully observed and trauma to the tissues must be minimized. Although the exact procedure may vary, the following guidelines can be used for suctioning infants and children:
1. Sterile technique is used to prevent secondary infection.
2. Normal saline 0.5 to 2 cc is instilled into the trachea just before suctioning to loosen secretions. (This may produce coughing and gagging.)
3. After saline is instilled the child should be suctioned with a sterile catheter moistened by saline.
4. The child's head is turned to the right side to suction the left bronchus and vice versa.
5. The suction catheter is inserted (without applying suction) and then withdrawn in a continuous rotating motion while suction is applied intermittently. Withdrawing of the catheter should take no more than approximately 15 seconds.
6. The child is allowed to rest, air exchange is listened for and the child's general condition is evaluated before repeating procedure.
7. It may also be necessary occasionally to suction the oropharynx to remove accumulated secretions.

Closing a Tracheostomy The tracheostomy tube is generally removed after daily insertion of a tube that is smaller than the previous one. Eventually the tube is plugged, after which it is left in place for 24 hours. If there are no apparent difficulties and the plug is well tolerated, the tube can be removed. Air leakage through the wound is not uncommon but generally ceases within 72 hours after removal of the plugged tube.[21]

Parents who care for these children at home require a great deal of assistance to adapt to the additional stresses. Two major themes identified by Aradine that underlie the frustrations expressed by parents were the extremely time-consuming care required and the severe isolation that they experienced.[2] These parents benefit from speaking to parents of other children with tracheostomies and may require the assistance of a public health nurse. The nurse can maintain the continuity of care that these families need. She can contact other community resources and maintain contact with the hospital or clinic personnel. The nurse should emphasize the child's need to attain normal developmental milestones and can help parents prepare for and cope with various developmental changes in their child.

Nursing Care of a Child with a Gastric Tube

Nasogastric tubes are used with pediatric patients to provide a route for gavage feedings

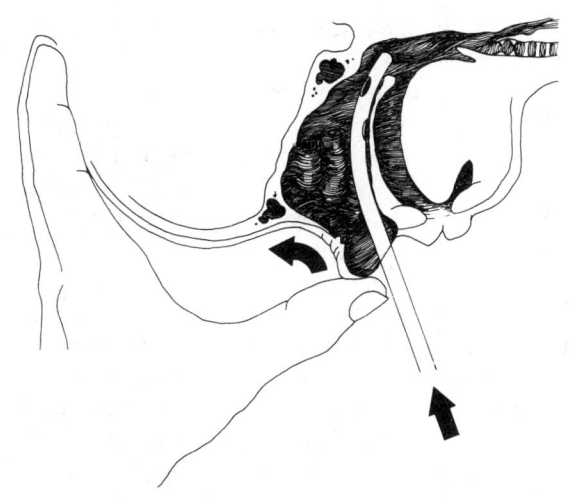

Figure 17-12 Nasal passage of tube. The tip of the nose is pressed slightly upward to enlarge the nasal opening. The tube is directed to slide along the base of the nose. If resistance is encountered, the tube must be withdrawn and redirected. (From W. T. Hughes and E. S. Buescher. Pediatric Procedures. W. B. Saunders Co., 1980, p. 246.)

(given when a child is unable to take nourishment by mouth), for abdominal decompression or for lavage (washing out of the stomach). Regardless of the intended use, the principles for insertion are the same. Insertion of this tube is a frightening experience and should be explained to the child and the parents. The explanation to parents should include information on how they may assist. The child should be told of the sensations he will experience during and following the insertion. It is often helpful if parents remain during the insertion to comfort the child. The child should be helped by his parents or a nurse to sit quietly during the insertion. He may feel like he is choking as the tube stimulates the gag reflex, but this will subside as the tube passes beyond the pharynx.

To determine the length of tubing required to reach beyond the cardiac sphincter of the stomach, use the tube to measure from the tip of the nose to the child's earlobe and down to the xiphoid process or from the earlobe to the tip of the nose and down to the xiphoid process. Mark this point on the tube with tape.

To insert the nasogastric tube, position the child in a high Fowler's position. An infant may be positioned with his neck hyperextended. Inspect the nares for patency, obstruction or deviated septum. The tube may be slightly lubricated with water. Nasal secretions usually make further lubrication unnecessary. As the tubing is advanced the child should be instructed to take small sips of water, as swallowing will help advance the tube. The tube is inserted to the point marked with the tape. At any time during the procedure, if resistance is encountered the nurse should withdraw the tube and after a brief rest period for the child, try again.

After insertion it is necessary to verify the placement of the tube. This can be done in three ways. With a syringe, attempt to aspirate stomach contents. If there is no return, advance the tube and aspirate again. Aspirate is obtained when the tube is properly placed. The second method is to place a stethoscope over the stomach and, using a syringe, introduce a small amount of air into the tube. The amount of air inserted varies with the size of the child. Approximate amounts of air used are 0.5 cc for prematures, 1 to 2 cc's for infants, and 3 to 5 cc's for older children. If the tube is positioned in the stomach, insertion of air will result in a "whoosh" sound. Placement can be further tested by placing the distal portion of the tube in a glass of water. If the tube is in the lungs, bubbles will result when the child breathes. Lack of bubbles verifies only that the tube is not in the lungs and not that it is correctly positioned in the stomach. A tube in the lungs will cause the child to cough and choke; therefore, this situation is usually recognized immediately. Aspiration of stomach contents or a "whoosh" sound of air adequately ensures correct tube placement.

After the tube is correctly positioned, it is taped to either the nose or the cheek. The tube is secured in this way to ensure that it remains in the same position. Tape is wrapped around the tube and secured just below the nose. (See Figure 17-12 for pathway). The tube is then looped to the cheek or the bridge of the nose. In either case it is important that the tube does not create pressure on the nares, as this may cause necrosis.

An older child may complain of a sore throat and earache or dry mouth and lips. Providing frequent mouth care and lubrication for the lips will lessen the discomfort. With the permission of the physician, a child can be allowed to suck on hard candy or ice chips to soothe the sore throat.

Nasogastric Tube Feeding Nasogastric feeding may be a continuous drip feeding or an intermittent feeding. The formula and amount are prescribed by the physician. The continuous drip formula should be infused slowly to avoid distention or discomfort. If the patient complains of nausea, the feeding should be slowed or discontinued temporarily. The amount of formula that is hung should not exceed that which will be used in four hours because the milk-based formula is an excellent medium for bacterial growth.

When administering feeding to an infant it is important to provide the same stimulation he would receive if he were able to take the feeding orally. The infant should be held and talked to during the feeding. If it is not contraindicated, the infant may suck on a pacifier during the feeding. With intermittent feeding of infants, the tube may be inserted before each feeding and taken out after the feeding is completed. In this instance, the tube is usually inserted through the mouth rather than the nose.

If a tube is to stay in place between feedings it should be cleared with several cc's of water after the feeding is completed. To remove the tube from an older child the procedure is explained to the child, then the tube is clamped and gently withdrawn. Mouth care is provided to the child as soon as possible following removal of the tube.

Decompression by a Nasogastric Tube A nasogastric tube may be inserted to remove air and secretions from the stomach and intestines (decompression) preoperatively or postoperatively or both to prevent vomiting and bowel distention. Following abdominal surgery peristalsis is inhibited owing to handling of the abdominal organs, necessitating decompression by a nasogastric tube. Drainage is achieved by intermittent suction or by gravity drainage. Continuous suction is not used because it irritates the mucosal wall of the stomach.

When a child has a nasogastric tube for decompression, the amount, consistency and color of drainage are observed and recorded. The drainage contains important electrolytes; therefore, it must be measured accurately to allow replacement. Drainage is replaced by giving an amount of intravenous fluids as ordered by the physician equal to the amount of drainage. (This is in addition to the daily 24-hour IV fluids.) Ensuring patency of the tube is accomplished by irrigating the tube with normal saline according to the physician's order.

The usual order is for irrigation with a specified amount of normal saline every two hours and as necessary. The saline is gently instilled with a syringe (without a needle) and then gently drawn back. The same amount that is instilled is withdrawn to ensure accurate calculation of the drainage. An alternate method is to reconnect the tube to suction after instilling saline, noting that the fluid is freely drawn back by suction. The amount of saline instilled each shift or each 24 hours must then be calculated and subtracted from the total amount of drainage to calculate the actual drainage. In either method force is never used while instilling nor while drawing back because the stomach mucosa is easily damaged. The ease with which the tube irrigates and the consistency, color and amount of the fluid returned at the time of irrigation are recorded. Bowel sounds should be checked whenever a child has a nasogastric tube for abdominal decompression.

Lavage by Nasogastric Tube When a nasogastric tube is inserted as a consequence of poison ingestion, the child is positioned with his head to one side and slightly lowered to avoid aspiration in the event of vomiting. Suction should also be available for immediate removal of vomitus whenever stomach contents are removed by lavage.

Feeding a Child with a Gastrostomy Tube A gastrostomy tube is a catheter that enters the stomach through a surgical incision in the abdominal wall. The gastrostomy tube is used for long-term management of children who are unable to receive adequate nutrition through oral feedings.

The catheter is secured in place. It may be taped into place by using one-half inch tape. The tape is wrapped around the tube and secured to the skin. The tube may also be secured by using a nipple. A slit is cut into a 4 by 4 gauze pad and placed around the tube. A hole is cut in the top of a nipple and small holes into the side. (The holes at the side are to provide for air circulation.) The tube is put through the hole in the top of the nipple. The nipple is then moved along the tube until it is firmly positioned on the gauze placed around the tube. Using one inch paper tape, the nipple and gauze are secured to the skin.

The tube may come out regardless of the method used to secure it. If this happens with a child on tube feedings at home, the family should be instructed as follows:
1. Stomach contents may leak out; do not be alarmed.
2. Cover the opening with a diaper or other absorbent cloth.
3. Go to the emergency room of the local hospital or to the clinic of the hospital at which the tube was inserted. Do this before the next feeding time or within two hours.
4. Take the old tube with you; this will help the staff know the size of tube the child needs. You may have been given an extra sterile tube when the child was discharged. If you were, take this tube to the clinic or emergency room.

A reddened area about the size of a quarter around the tube is normal. There may be a small amount of drainage around the tube, but if it has a bad odor or if it changes in any way it should be checked for possible infection. A fever may also indicate an infection. To keep the area clean, wash around the tube with a 1:1 solution of hydrogen peroxide and water. The child can be bathed as usual.

During feedings, an infant should be held and cuddled; an older child can sit in a highchair. Type and amount of formula will be prescribed by the physician. The position of the tube can be checked by gently pulling until resistance is felt. To complete the feeding:
1. Wash your hands.
2. Check the temperature of the formula. It should be room temperature.
3. Attach the end of the tube to a syringe (10 to 50 cc's varying with size of the infant).
4. Clamp the tube.
5. Fill the syringe with formula.
6. Holding the tube above the height of the opening, unclamp the tube.
7. Add more formula to the syringe before it empties to prevent air from getting into the stomach.
8. Follow the formula with one-half ounce of water to clear the tube.
9. Clamp the tube, fold it over, wrap it with a 4 by 4 gauze pad and secure it with a rubber band.
10. Wash the materials in hot soapy water, rinse well and store in a clean place.
11. The feeding should take approximately as long as a feeding by mouth.
12. Infants should be allowed to suck on a pacifier to satisfy normal developmental needs.

Medication may be given through the tube. Using the same syringe, give one-half ounce of water after the medicine to assure that the medication is not in the tube.

The tube can be pinned to the child's undershirt or covered with a soft stretchy band of fabric. With a gastrostomy tube the child can resume his regular play activities.

Nursing Skills to Facilitate Elimination

Enema Administration An enema is used for the same purpose in children as it is in adults: (1) to facilitate defecation when normal physiological processes of elimination are ineffective and (2) to cleanse the bowel in preparation for surgery or diagnostic procedures. Specific differences between children and adults and related nursing actions to consider are discussed in Table 17–2.

There are three special considerations in the giving of an enema. First, comparing the sensation of the catheter tip insertion to the taking of rectal temperature is useful for some children, but the child should not be led to believe that an enema is "just like having your temperature taken." Second, a potty-trained child should be encouraged to expel the enema while sitting on a potty chair. Also, a potty-trained child needs special reassurance that it is OK if he does not make it to the potty chair to expel the enema. Third, preschoolers require special explanations and understanding because they do not clearly mentally separate rectal and genital regions of the body. Administration of an enema thus has the potential to arouse fears related to the genitalia.

*Colostomy Care** A colostomy is the surgical creation of an opening between the colon and the surface of the body. In many instances, a colostomy is a temporary procedure done during infancy, with the definitive procedure being performed at a later time (often when the child

---
*This section on colostomy care was contributed by Terry Sarahan.

TABLE 17-2 NURSING ACTIONS IN PROVIDING AN ENEMA

Developmental Considerations	Related Nursing Actions
1. The child's bowel capacity and anal opening varies according to his size. A young child's rectal mucosa is thin and easily traumatized.	Approximate solution amounts according to age of child: • Infant 150–250 • Toddler and preschooler 250–350 • School age 300–500 • Adolescent 500–750 Enema tips should be soft, well lubricated, and appropriate in size for age of child (French catheter No. 10–12 for young children). For older school-agers and adolescents, the standard enema tip can be used. The enema tip is inserted 1½ to 4 inches (3.7 to 10 cm), varying according to size of child.
2. Young children are particularly vulnerable to fluid and electrolyte imbalances.	An isotonic (normal saline) solution is used to prevent rapid fluid shift from bowel. Plain water is hypotonic and with repeated enemas water intoxication and fluid overload can result.
3. A child's bowel is more easily perforated under pressure.	The enema reservoir is elevated gradually until the solution begins to slowly flow by gravity. For young children, greater control of administration is achieved by using a 50 ml syringe attached to a catheter.
4. Young children do not have the cognitive nor physiological ability to "hold" the enema.	With child in supine position, head and back can be supported with pillow. The bedpan must be in position during administration because there is immediate return of the solution. After the solution has been administered, the buttocks can be gently pinched together to facilitate "holding" of the enema. A child who is old enough (school age and adolescent) to understand the explanation "hold the enema" is positioned on the left side with right leg flexed.

reaches 1 year of age). A colostomy may also be necessary for various reasons later in childhood. Parents and children, including siblings, benefit from explanations and demonstrations, using a doll or special models designed for teaching about a colostomy and colostomy care.

After surgery, the child and parents are encouraged to look at the stoma and gradually increase their involvement in its care. Extra care is taken to provide an atmosphere that encourages them to discuss their concerns, fears and feelings about caring for a colostomy. Adjustment by the child and parents is affected by the reason the colostomy is required and whether it is to be temporary or permanent. A child's adjustment also is determined by his particular developmental level and by how well his parents can accept his need for a colostomy.

As much as possible, nursing care should be provided by the same individuals to ease the adjustment of the family and facilitate learning. Table 17–3 provides specific directions for care of an ostomy.

Colostomy irrigation is performed before surgery to completely cleanse fecal material from the bowel. The equipment necessary for this procedure includes enema bag, warmed irrigation solution, a soft pliable catheter, a nipple, lubricant and an IV pole. The irrigation solution is placed in the enema bag and the tubing is filled with fluid. The pliable catheter is attached to the enema tubing. The tip of the enema tubing is cut off so that the irrigation solution will run continuously through both the tubing and the catheter. The catheter is inserted through the nipple. The catheter is then inserted into the stoma and the nipple is placed into the stoma. The nipple is used to prevent leakage around the catheter as the enema is administered. The enema bag is placed 18 inches above the stoma and the enema is administered gradually. This procedure should be done slowly. If the child complains of crampy abdominal pain, the enema should be stopped for several minutes and then restarted.

Clean Intermittent Catheterization*   Clean intermittent catheterization (CIC) has gained general acceptance as a safe and effective method of managing bladder-emptying problems in children.† It is most frequently used in children with neurogenic bladder dysfunction and permits most of these children to remain dry while

---

*Consultation given by Evan Kass, MD, for the preparation of this section.
†J. Lapides et al. Clean intermittent self-catheterization in the treatment of urinary tract disease. Journal of Urology, March 1972, p. 458.

TABLE 17-3 DIRECTIONS TO PATIENTS OR PARENTS FOR CARE OF AN OSTOMY*

Putting on the Bag
1. Wash your hands.
2. Have Karaya ring or Stomahesive (protective seal) ready to use. With clean scissors, cut openings in Stomahesive and bag. Guides are provided in the colostomy bag box. Cut hole in the Stomahesive slightly smaller than opening in bag so that Stomahesive fits closely around stoma. Cutting several at a time to have ready for future bag changes is easiest.
3. Remove the old Stomahesive or Karaya ring and bag, pulling gently. This is a good time to check to see that stoma is pink.
4. Wash skin with warm water. A tub bath may be taken at this time. Pat skin around stoma dry. Cover the stoma with Kleenex to prevent stool from leaking onto the skin.
5. Apply "Skin Prep" to skin around stoma and fan it dry.
6. Remove the white paper backing from the Stomahesive. Remove Kleenex from the stoma and place the Stomahesive or Karaya rings on the skin, centered around stoma. Push on one area at a time so it sticks to skin and has no wrinkles.
7. Remove white paper backing from bag. Put sticky side of bag onto the Stomahesive or Karaya ring; smooth it down to remove all wrinkles.
8. Roll bag up (turning edges to the outside) until you can see stoma, then sprinkle Karaya powder directly on the stoma. Then unroll bag.
9. If bottom of bag is open, fold bottom up twice horizontally, then fold it like a fan vertically. Use a rubber band to hold bag closed.
10. To dispose of old bag, rinse out in the toilet and then throw in the trash. Do not flush it down the toilet.
11. Wash your hands.

Emptying the Bag
1. Remove rubber band from end.
2. Empty the stool into a container or right into the toilet if you can stand next to it.
3. Pour warm water into bag, gently washing water around in bag. For an infant or young child, bag can be rinsed by using a 50 cc syringe. Empty the water into the container or toilet.
4. Special deodorants are available to use if you wish.
5. Dry end of bag and close it again.

Skin Maintenance
1. Always use a protective seal over the skin (Stomahesive), placing it right up to stoma with bag placed on top 1/8 inch away from stoma.
2. Change bag promptly if any leakage occurs.
3. Avoid use of ointments or lotions around stoma.
4. Clean and dry skin area around stoma before applying bag.
5. If excoriation occurs, apply Mycostatin powder or Kenalog spray and dry the area with cool setting on hair or blow dryer.

*Extracted from Ostomy Care for Infants and Children. T. Sarahan et al. University of Michigan Printing Department, 1979, p. 9. Additional sources for information on colostomy care: B. Bolinger, A teenager's Ostomy Guide, Hollister Inc., 1978. Guide for the Colostonate. Coloplast Brand Ostomy Products, 1977. Managing Your Colostomy, Hollister Inc., 1971. Ostomy Related Skin Problems, Hollister Inc., 1977.

their kidneys are protected from damage, thereby eliminating the need for surgical urinary diversion in most cases. The technique is based on the concept that the urinary bladder is normally resistant to bacterial invasion as long as overdistention and high pressures within it are avoided. Certainly bacteria are introduced into the bladder with each catheterization; however, as long as the bladder is emptied frequently and overdistention is avoided, these bacteria are not harmful.‡

Any child is a potential candidate for intermittent catheterization; age, sex and status of the urinary tract have not proved to be absolute contraindications to a successful program.§ The only absolute requirement is the complete willingness of the patient or the patient's family to perform the catheterizations as directed. Although catheterizations are usually performed every three to four hours, it is important to remember that the program is individualized, depending on the type of neurogenic bladder dysfunctions, bladder capacity, sphincter dysfunction, fluid intake and status of the upper urinary tract.

The nurse who works with patients on intermittent catheterization should be prepared to deal with the parents' and child's initial fear of the procedure. (Often other families who have experienced similar problems can be very helpful in this regard.) This technique requires frequent catheterizations. Even though the catheter is not sterile, CIC is effective only because with it bladder overdistention can be avoided. If bladder distention occurs because a catheterization is missed or too much fluid is consumed, septic urinary tract infection may result. The nurse should keep in mind one cardinal rule: avoid bladder overdistention. Emphasis should not be placed on cleanliness if it proves to be a barrier to catheterizing at the appropriate intervals.

The nurse who works with children on a self-catheterization program or one in which parents perform the procedure should adapt her nursing care as shown in Table 17-4.

Specific directions for clean catheterization are outlined in Table 17-5.

‡E. Kass et al. The significance of bacilluria in children on long-term intermittent catheterization. Journal of Urology, in press.
§E. Kass et al. Intermittent catheterization in children less than 6 years old. Journal of Urology, June 1979, p. 792.

TABLE 17-4 NURSING ACTIONS RELATED TO A SELF-CATHETERIZATION PROGRAM

Developmental Considerations	Related Nursing Actions
1. Urethral size varies with age.	A rubber catheter is used, size nos. ranging from 8–14 French. For infants and young children, No. 8 clear plastic feeding tube is more appropriate for size of urethra. A clear tube allows for immediate visualization of urine.
2. Developmental level must be appropriate to accomplish task of self-catheterization successfully.	The nurse should assess child's ability in telling time, fine motor skills, and level of independence in self-care. By 8 some children can be independent in self-catheterization.[3]
3. Informed, understanding school personnel are central to child's successful self-catheterization program.	A referral to school nurse with instructions of needed facilities: • Privacy in a room with a sink. • Place to store equipment, including a change of clothing.
4. It is difficult to control a young child's fluid intake.	Parents should be taught to encourage fluid intake early in day and limit fluids after 7 P.M.

Collection of Specimens

Children are frequently unable to cooperate to produce the needed specimen. Usually they do not have the cognitive ability to understand instructions and in many instances lack the physiological capability to produce the specimen requested. Thus specimen collection for the child is often an intrusive, frightening experience requiring some degree of body manipulation and restraint. Special adaptations are necessary to collect specimens from children in a way that is technically accurate yet produces minimal disruption and frustration to the child.

Specimens, once collected, must be clearly labeled and immediately processed. The nurse should be sure that the correct laboratory slip accompanies the specimen when it is sent to the laboratory.

Collection of Urine Specimens * Urine specimens are collected in various ways, depending on the age of the child and the purpose of the specimen. The major difficulty is the collection of specimens from children who are not toilet trained. Routine urine specimens are collected by using a clean plastic urine bag. Twenty-four–hour urine specimens require a special collecting bag with tubing. Specimens for culture are collected by using a sterile urine bag. In some instances either catheterization or a suprapubic needle aspiration of urine from the bladder is indicated.

If contamination by skin does not alter the results of the required test (e.g., specific gravity), urine can be squeezed from a diaper or drawn out of a diaper with a syringe from which the needle has been removed. One drop of urine squeezed from a diaper is sufficient to test specific gravity with a fractometer.

Routine Urine Specimen A specimen for routine urinalysis is collected from an infant or young child by using the following guidelines:

1. Wash hands well, then cleanse the perineum or penis with soap and water; rinse and dry. This should be done before collection of any urine specimen from a child who is not toilet trained.
2. The bag can be applied with various techniques. If applied from side to side, the paper backing from one side is peeled off and folded back. That side of the bag is then attached to the skin starting at the bottom and moving upward.

TABLE 17-5 DIRECTIONS FOR CLEAN CATHETERIZATION

1. Wash hands with soap and water or with a towelette, if possible.
2. Lubricate catheter.
3. Wash genital area (optional).
4. Insert catheter.
   A. Male: Grasp penis, holding on sides, and hold it erect, then insert catheter slowly.
   B. Female: Separate labia and insert catheter. A mirror may be helpful while learning but child can usually learn to locate meatus by palpation.
5. Insert one to two inches farther than point at which urine begins to flow.
6. Allow urine to flow into a cup or other container until flow stops.
7. Remove catheter slowly and immediately hold catheter tip up to avoid spilling of urine.
8. Wash catheter with soap and water; rinse and dry. Store in a dry clean bottle or plastic bag (optional).
9. Catheters are changed approximately monthly.
10. *Cardinal rule:* Avoid bladder overdistention. Always catheterize at appropriate intervals even if unable to wash.

---
*Acknowledgement is given to Evan J. Kass, M.D. for consultation and review of this section.

The paper backing is then peeled off completely and the other side of the bag is attached similarly. If applied from bottom to top, the paper backing from the lower half of the bag is removed and the lower portion is secured. Once the lower part is carefully secured the paper backing from the upper portion is removed and the top half of the bag is secured. In either method the single most important factor is that the bag securely adheres to the skin, especially along the lower edge where leakage and contamination are most likely to occur. For females the perineum is pulled slightly taut during application of the lower portion of the bag. In young male infants, placing the penis and scrotum inside the bag facilitates a better seal at the lower edge. For older male infants and toddlers, the bag can be applied on top of the scrotum with only the penis inside.

3. Secure a diaper over the bag to prevent loosening of the bag by pulling or kicking.

4. Place the infant or child into a semi-Fowler's position to facilitate flow of urine by gravity into the urine bag.

5. Give the usual amount of fluids. Overhydration may give inaccurate results.

6. Check urine bag frequently (every 20 to 30 minutes) because the weight of the urine in the bag may cause it to loosen. Also, urine should be collected as soon after the child has voided as possible for the most accurate laboratory analysis.

7. After the child voids, remove the bag gently to avoid skin irritation; then cleanse the area and re-diaper the child.

8. When the desired specimen has been obtained, transfer it to a clean specimen container. Either refrigerate it or deliver it to the laboratory promptly. The maximum time that should elapse between voiding and testing of urine kept at room temperature is 4 hours. A urine specimen that is stored in the refrigerator is preferably not stored longer than 8 hours; the maximum length of time is 24 hours.

Clean-Catch Specimen for Culture With older children the collection of a clean-catch or midstream urine specimen is done in a similar manner as in adults. The major differences are that more supervision is required and that the required supervision may embarrass the child.

Careful explanation is given as to why the specimen is needed and what the procedure entails. A forewarning should be given regarding the coldness of the cleansing solution. Parents should be invited to accompany the child to collect the specimen if the child so desires; however, it is preferable that the nurse take responsibility for supervision to ensure that the urine is collected properly. Proper collection of a clean voided specimen may obviate the need for catheterization of a child.

Girls are asked to sit in the usual position on the toilet. The nurse wears a sterile glove to spread the labia for cleansing of the meatus. The perineum is cleansed with an antiseptic by wiping from front to back along each side of the meatus and directly across the meatus using a clean sponge for each wipe. The perineum is then rinsed with sterile water or saline and patted dry with a sterile gauze sponge. It is important to dry the area well because the presence of an antiseptic in the urine specimen may prevent bacterial growth, giving a false-negative report. The girl is then asked to void while the labia are spread apart. After the stream is started a sample (midstream) of urine is collected in a sterile container, after which the child finishes voiding.

Boys are asked to stand in the usual position to void. The meatus and glans penis are cleansed with an antiseptic. If the boy is uncircumcised the foreskin is retracted sufficiently to cleanse the meatus and glans penis. The area is then rinsed, patted dry, and midstream urine sample is collected. For an uncircumcised boy care is taken to slide the foreskin to its original position to prevent constriction of the penis.

During specimen collection for urine culture the open edge of the container used to collect the voided specimen is not permitted to touch the child's skin. The nurse immediately closes the container with a sterile lid and care is taken not to touch the open edge or the inside of the container. The specimen should be delivered to the laboratory as soon as possible.

For infants and young children urine for culture is collected by using a sterile urine bag. The perineum or penis is cleansed in the same way as just described for a clean-catch urine specimen using an antiseptic. After the area is thoroughly dry a sterile urine bag is applied in the same manner as for a routine urine specimen. A sterile urine bag has a small hole on the lower edge to one side of the bag that is covered with a blue tab (Fig. 17–13). To empty the bag it is held in such a way that the area with the tab is free of urine. The tab is pulled off, the bag is

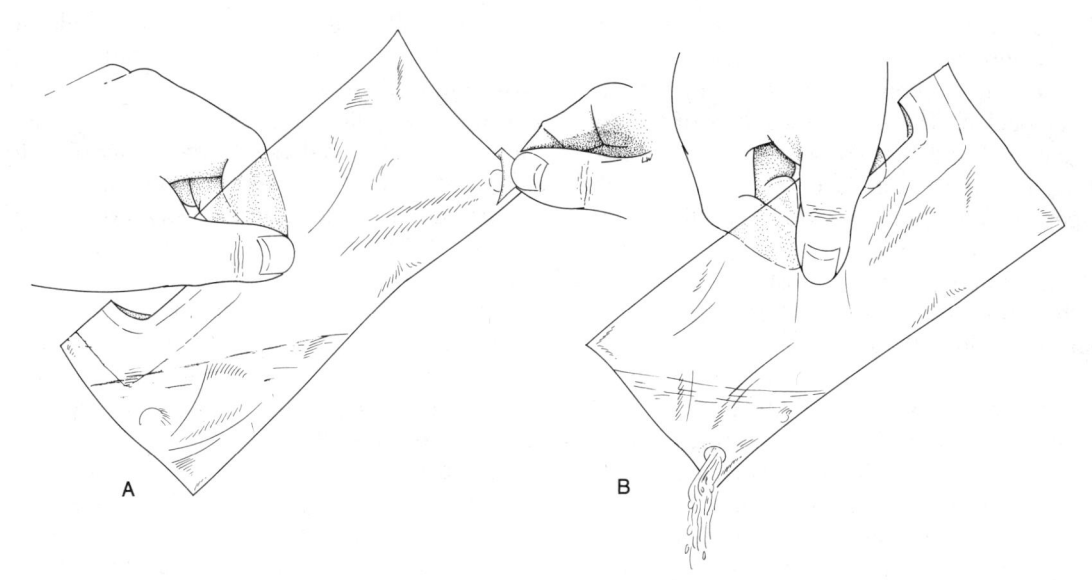

Figure 17-13 Emptying urine for culture from a sterile urine bag. (*A*) To drain urine into a specimen bottle, tip the bag to one side with blue tab at upper edge. Remove blue tab. Care is taken to avoid spilling or contaminating urine at large opening of bag. (*B*) Turn bag with exposed small hole at lower edge and pour into sterile container. Apply lid, label and send to laboratory.

then tipped into a position that permits drainage of the urine through the small hole that has been uncovered by pulling the tab. At least 1 to 2 ml of urine is needed for a urine culture.

Urethral Catheterization Catheterization may be necessary if bacteria are present on a clean-catch specimen. Catheterization of a child is done the same as for an adult. The major differences are in the way the child is psychologically prepared, in the type of restraint necessary and in the size of catheter used. The smaller meatus makes catheterization in children somewhat more difficult than in adults. Rarely is catheterization necessary to obtain an adequate urine specimen in a male.

Toddlers and preschoolers may be resistive when procedures involving the genitalia are done. They are fearful that they will be injured and they abhor restraint. Consequently their physical strength is used in an attempt to flee. Before trying to catheterize a child of this age the nurse must explain in simple terms to the child what is to be done. It is beneficial for the parents to reinforce this by repeating the explanation. The catheter, sponges and containers can be shown to the child just before the procedure. Whether parents stay or not is an individual matter, but they make that choice. At least one other person must be present to help restrain the child.

School-age children and adolescents generally cooperate, but the nurse should recognize that they may also be fearful and will likely be embarrassed. Explaining the procedure and getting it done quickly is what is most appreciated at this age. Older school-agers and adolescents may need specific technical questions answered to feel comfortable about the procedure; therefore, the nurse should expect to spend extra time to provide the necessary information that they request.

The size of the catheter varies with the size of the child. Approximate-sized catheters to use are a size No. 8 clear plastic feeding tube for an infant and a size No. 8 to 14 Foley for an older child.

Collection of a 24-hour Urinary Output A special collecting device is used to collect urine output for a 24-hour period. The plastic urine bag is similar to those used for routine urine collection except that a long drainage tube is connected to one corner of the lower edge of the bag (Fig. 17–14). As the child voids the urine can be drained via this tube without removing the bag.

The urine bag is applied using the same technique as for a routine urine, except that an adhesive skin preparation such as tincture of benzoin is routinely used to form a sticky surface before applying the bag. Tincture of benzoin (or a similar material) is applied to the area that comes in contact with the sealing edge of the urine bag. The benzoin is painted onto the skin with a cotton-tipped applicator and within a few minutes the area is sticky, providing an adhesive surface for attachment of the urine bag.

It is of prime importance that the bag be securely attached to prevent leakage, contamination or loss of the entire voiding. Once the bag is applied nursing care is directed toward preventing loss or contamination of urine. Numerous methods are employed in practice to maintain the bag in position, many of which require some form of restraint. When the long tube is uncoiled and attached to a drainage bottle, arm and wrist restraints are generally necessary to prevent the child from grasping the tube with his hands or creating a pull on it with his feet and legs.

Contamination by stool is one of the most frequently occurring problems that necessitates restarting the 24-hour urine collection. Various forms of restraint on a sling or frame are used to avoid contamination with stool. In this method a bedpan is placed beneath the frame and the child is placed on the frame without a diaper, allowing the stool to fall away from the urine bag. This method is frustrating to the child and parents and is usually unnecessary. An alternate method not involving restraint is to leave the tube coiled within the diaper. The tube has a removable cap that is opened periodically to drain the urine from the bag. With this method the bag must be checked and emptied frequently because the weight of the urine creates a pull on the bag. Frequent checking of the urine bag also decreases the likelihood of losing the specimen due to contamination by stool. Parents can help the nurse decide how frequently the urine bag must be checked because they are generally aware of how frequently their child's diaper needs to be changed. This method is usually effective, presenting a problem primarily when a child has diarrhea.

The nurse is responsible for managing the collection of a 24-hour urine specimen. It is started just after the child has voided. Urine from this first voiding is discarded, but the time of the voiding is recorded as the starting time. For infants and children it is more difficult to know the exact time of voiding. A dry diaper is checked frequently until the child voids. The bag is applied immediately after the wet diaper is noted.

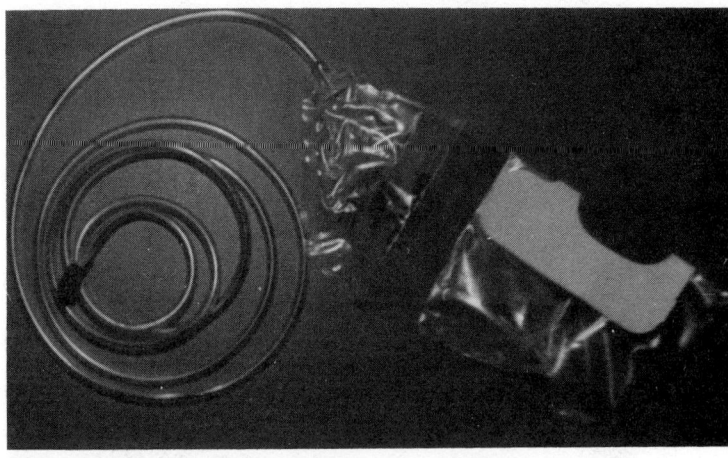

Figure 17-14 Urine collector for 24-hour specimen. The tube can remain coiled inside the child's diaper. The end of the tube has a cap that is removed frequently to empty urine. After the paper backing is removed the designated edge must form a tight seal against the skin by use of an adhesive dressing. The lower edge of bag is applied first, using either side-to-side or bottom-to-top method.

During the collection period the nurse must ensure that the urine is being stored according to specification from the laboratory. If the nurse is not certain how to store the urine she should call the hospital laboratory. The bag is removed 24 hours after the time of the discarded specimen or wet diaper and the specimen is delivered promptly to the laboratory. Improperly managing the collection of a 24-hour urine specimen may cause delay in the discharge of a child; thus every attempt must be made to apply the bag securely, check the bag frequently, store the urine properly and deliver it to the laboratory promptly.

Throat, Nasopharyngeal and Sputum Specimens Specimen collection from the nose and throat is unpleasant. It should be done as efficiently and accurately as possible to avoid the necessity of repeating the procedure. A brief explanation just before performing the procedure is appropriate for all ages. To obtain a throat culture a sterile Culturette swab is used (Fig. 17-15). This swab contains transport medium to prevent the throat material from drying before reaching the laboratory. To culture the throat, the swab should touch the most inflamed and purulent area. The swab should be passed with a rolling motion deep into the throat and across the tonsils without touching the tongue on entry or exit of the mouth. This procedure

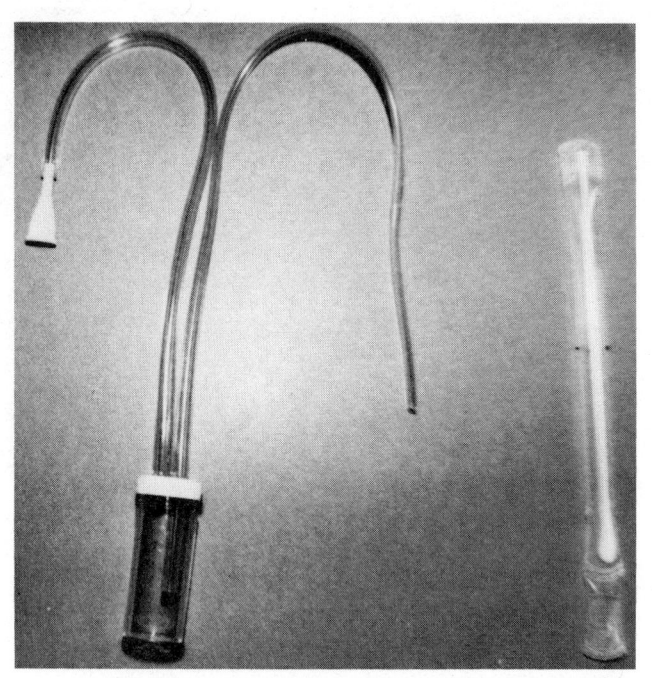

Figure 17–15 Devices used to collect throat and sputum specimens. Left, a mucus trap for sputum collection. Suction is applied via the tube curved to the left; the tube on the right side is the catheter tip that is inserted to the trachea. Right, sterile culture swab with transport media used for culture.

should result in stimulation of the gag reflex if done properly. If the child cannot cooperate by opening his mouth wide, a tongue depressor should be used to hold the tongue down while the throat is entered with the swab. The swab is returned to the holder and pushed into the lower chamber, which holds the transport media. Various types of tubes are available whose operation is similar in principle.

To culture the nasopharynx a swab on a flexible wire is used. Entry can be made through the nasal passages, flexing the wire downward to the nasopharynx or through the mouth and bending the wire upward to pass under the uvula.

To collect a sputum specimen from children who are too young to cooperate in coughing and expectorating, a device called a mucus trap can be used (Fig. 17–15). The catheter is inserted to the trachea, stimulating a cough reflex. Suction is applied to the other tube by placing the mouth over it and sucking as on a straw. A sputum specimen is drawn through the catheter into the mucus chamber. (It is not drawn up the tube to which suction is applied.) When a child can cough up a specimen, the nurse should be present while the specimen is being collected to avoid getting a specimen that has been merely cleared from the back of the throat. Sputum is located within the bronchi and lungs and can be removed only by a deep cough.[13] The best time to collect a sputum specimen is when the patient awakens in the morning. Specimens from the respiratory tract are collected in sterile containers. The edges and inside of the container should be kept free of contamination. The outside of the container should also be free of contamination from secretions to protect personnel handling the specimen. Collection time should be marked on the container, and the container should be delivered to the laboratory immediately.

Stool Specimens To obtain a sample of stool the tip of a tongue blade is used to transfer stool into a clean cup (a sterile container is not necessary for stool specimens). Frequently, a stool specimen is needed when a child in diapers has diarrhea—a sample of stool can be obtained by scraping a tongue blade across the diaper. If a minute amount of stool remains on the blade, this can be broken off into the cup. When it is not possible to obtain a stool specimen a rectal swab is done; however, only in shigellosis, gonorrhea and a few other infections do the organisms live on the rectal walls rather than exclusively in the feces.[13] A rectal swab is done by gently inserting a swab into the rectum and slightly twisting it as it is removed. The swab is inserted approximately as far as when a rectal temperature is taken. Stool specimens and rectal swabs should be sent to the laboratory immediately; this is especially important when the stool specimen is for ova and parasites.

NURSING CARE OF A CHILD WITH A FEVER

Fever is one of the most apparent indicators to parents that their child is sick. It is the symptom that prompts families to seek medical care in 30 per cent of visits.[20] A fever is an abnormal elevation of the central body temperature caused by (1) metabolic heat production that exceeds the heat loss capabilities of the body or (2) impairment of the body's heat loss capabilities.

Fever from infection rarely poses a threat to the child. It has been hypothesized that a fever may be beneficial by providing poor environment for pyrogen growth, although this has not been supported by research.[20] Although some physicians believe that because of the possible benefits of fever a child should not be given symptomatic treatment, the usual practice is to treat the fever along with the cause.

Nonpharmacologic measures to reduce a fever begin with removing the child's clothing down to diapers or light pajamas and cooling the child's environment. This allows for radiation of heat away from the body. A second step in reducing fever is to sponge the child with tepid water. The child is placed in a tub of plain tepid water and sponged completely, including the head, for approximately 15 minutes. The evaporation of water from the skin surface has a cooling effect. In the past sponge baths to reduce a fever included the use of alcohol in the water. This was believed to speed cooling by more rapid evaporation. This practice is now discouraged because of the danger of absorption of alcohol and too-rapid heat loss. It is important to use tepid water and not cold, as cold water may cause shivering. Shivering is a natural mechanism that occurs with rapid cooling and causes the body temperature to increase. Thus whenever a child begins to shiver, cooling treatments should be discontinued.

Hospitalized children with persistent high fevers are frequently placed on hypothermia mattresses. These are pads with internal coils to circulate cool water. The pads should be covered with a bath blanket; the child is never placed directly on the pad because this can cause burns. It is important to watch for shivering and to discontinue the treatment if this occurs.

During a febrile episode the body needs more fluid because of its increased metabolic rate and increased respiratory rate. The child should be offered oral fluid frequently. Parents who are treating their child's fever at home should be told to offer fluids and not to be concerned about a child's refusal to eat solids. The nurse should review the signs of dehydration with parents and encourage them to call if they have any further questions.

Antipyretic medications are frequently used to control fever. The most common are acetylsalicylic acid (ASA or aspirin) and acetaminophen (ACM or Tylenol). These medications are available in a variety of forms and dosages (Table 17–6). A rule of thumb is to give one grain of ASA or ACM per year of age every 4 hours. The maximum single dose for a 10-year-old or older child is 10 grains.[15] Recently it has been proposed that using a combination of ASA and ACM is more effective in sustaining a temperature reduction than either drug alone.[15] Used in combination the drugs can be given in one of two ways. The first is to alternate doses of ASA and ACM at two-hour intervals. For example, a 1-year-old child would receive 1 grain of ASA at 2 P.M. and 1 grain of ACM at 4 P.M. In the second way the child simultaneously receives 1 grain of ACM and 1 grain of ASA every 6 hours. The second method has the advantage of requiring administration of medication less frequently, which may mean longer periods of sleep for the child.

The use of these medications is common but not without dangers. Parents treating a febrile episode at home must be given clear and precise instructions regarding the dosage and use of medication. "Baby aspirin" is the leading cause of accidental poisoning in children. Any teaching regarding the use of such drugs must include instructions on safe storage and the use of childproof containers.

TABLE 17–6 ACETAMINOPHEN (TYLENOL) AND ACETYLSALICYLIC ACID (ASPIRIN) PREPARATIONS

Acetaminophen Preparations (Tylenol)

Tempra drops	0.6 cc = 60 mg (1 grain)
Tempra syrup	5 cc = 120 mg (2 grains)
Liquiprin	2.5 cc = 120 mg (2 grains)
Tylenol chewable tablets	1 tab = 80 mg (1¼ grain)
Tylenol Tablets or Datril	1 tab = 325 mg (5 grains)
Tylenol Extrastrength	1 tab = 500 mg (8⅓ grain)

Acetylsalicylic Acid (Aspirin) Preparations

Chewable tablets (Baby Aspirin)	1 tab = 80 mg (1¼ grains)
Adult tablets	1 tab = 325 mg (5 grains)

CARDIOPULMONARY RESUSCITATION OF INFANTS AND SMALL CHILDREN

Cardiopulmonary resuscitation of infants and small children is similar to that for adults. Resuscitation of an older child or adolescent is the same as that for adults.

Breathing To give mouth-to-mouth resuscitation to an infant or small child, the neck is tilted backward and both the nose and mouth are covered with the rescuer's mouth. An infant's neck is particularly pliable. Care must be taken to avoid excessive backward tilting, which can block the respiratory passages rather than opening them. Small breaths (puffs) are given at the rate of approximately 20 per minute.

Circulation In infants and small children the left nipple area is palpated to determine the presence or absence of a pulse. The child's back can be supported with one hand while the other hand is used for compression. An alternate method is to place the child on a firm surface. Using a ratio of five cardiac compressions to one ventilation, the chest is gently compressed at the rate of 80 to 100 compressions per minute.

For infants the tips of the index and middle fingers of one hand are placed at midsternum and sufficient pressure is applied to depress the sternum one-half to three-fourths inch. For small children the heel of only one hand is used, making sure to keep the fingers off the chest. The sternum is depressed three-fourths to one and one-half inches depending on the size of the child.

One lung inflation is interjected after every fifth chest compression for infants and young children, whether there are one or two rescuers. This procedure is continued until the infant responds or until mechanical resuscitation can be initiated.

References

1. American Heart Association. Cardiopulmonary Resuscitation, 1977
2. C. Aradine. Home care for young children with long-term tracheostomies. American Journal of Maternal Child Nursing, Mar/Apr 1980, p. 121
3. A. Altshuler et al. Even children can learn to do clean self-catheterization. American Journal of Nursing, January 1977, p. 97
4. G. G. Blainey. Site selection in taking body temperature. American Journal of Nursing, October 1974, p. 1859
5. C. L. Curran and M. K. Kachoyeanos. The effects on neonates of two methods of chest physical therapy. American Journal of Maternal Child Nursing, Sept/Oct 1979, p. 309
6. M. Davis. Getting to the root of the problem. Nursing '77, April 1977, p. 60–66
7. E. L. Dowd et al. Releasing the hospitalized child from restraints. American Journal of Maternal Child Nursing, Nov/Dec 1977, p. 370
8. S. Graas. Thermometer Sites and Oxygen. American Journal of Nursing, October 1974, p. 1867
9. M. Grier. Hair care for the black patient. American Journal of Nursing, November 1976, p. 1781
10. M. Hartman. Intermittent self-catheterization. Nursing '78, November 1978, p. 72
11. C. Katz and N. McIntosh. Care of the gastrostomy tube and incision. Gastrostomy Feeding Guide. Mott, Women's, and Holden Standardized Care Plan Committee. University of Michigan, 1978
12. J. Lapides et al. Clean intermittent self-catheterization in the treatment of urinary tract disease. Journal of Urology, March 1972, p. 458
13. K. Marchiondo. The very fine art of collecting culture specimens. Nursing '79, April 1979, p. 34
14. Report of the Task Force on Blood Pressure Control in Children. Pediatrics (Supplement) May 1977.
15. L. A. Robinson et al. Nursing considerations in the use of nonprescription analgesic-antipyretics: Aspirin and acetaminophen. Pediatric Nursing Jul/Aug 1977, p. 18
16. E. J. Ruley. Diseases of the urinary system. In Principles of Pediatrics, R. A. Hoekelman et al., (eds). McGraw Hill Book Co., 1978, p. 1569
17. T. Sarahan et al. Ostomy Care for Infants and Children. University of Michigan Printing Department, 1979
18. M. S. Sibinga and C. J. Freedman. Restraint and Speech. Pediatrics, July 1971, p. 116
19. M. Shannon. The gastrointestinal system. In Comprehensive Pediatric Nursing, G. Scipien et al., McGraw-Hill Book Co., 1975, p. 757
20. R. C. Stern. Pathophysiologic basis for symptomatic treatment of fever. Pediatrics, January 1977, p. 92
21. W. W. Waring. Diagnostic and therapeutic procedures. In Disorders of the Respiratory Tract in Children, E. Kendig and V. Chernick, eds. W.B. Saunders Co., 1977
22. B. J. Whitson, and J. M. McFarlane, The Pediatric Nursing Skills Manual. John Wiley & Sons, 1980

FLUID AND ELECTROLYTE BALANCE IN INFANTS AND CHILDREN

by Mabel Hunsberger, BSN, MSN

The nurse who cares for infants and children requires an understanding of the body's regulatory mechanisms to enhance her assessment skills and decision-making ability. The reader is referred to basic science texts of biology, chemistry and physiology for in-depth discussions of fluid and electrolytes. Included here is a discussion of fluid and electrolyte balance and intravenous therapy as it applies to infants and children. Those processes that have particular significance in children and the unique characteristics of children that affect fluid and electrolyte balance will be addressed.

BODY WATER COMPARTMENTS AND INTERNAL DISTRIBUTION

Total body water (TBW) at birth comprises 75 to 80 per cent of body weight. During the immediate postnatal period there is a weight loss of approximately 19 per cent of body weight. The infant's proportionate rapid weight gain during the first year of life is primarily due to an increase in adipose tissue. Since there is an inverse relationship between total body water and total body fat, the infant's weight gain is accompanied by a proportionate reduction in fluid volume. In the child of around 2 years of age both the percentage of total body water and its internal distribution approximates that of an adult. See Table 17–7 for a comparison of fluid volume and its distribution at birth, at 1 year of age, and after 2 years of age.

The internal distribution of fluids in an infant makes him vulnerable to high losses of fluid. It is an increase in extracellular (primarily interstitial) fluid that accounts for the vast difference in TBW before 1 year of age. Extracellular fluid is easily lost and in the event of illness, trauma or stressful environmental conditions the infant is extremely vulnerable to fluid and electrolyte imbalances.

REGULATION OF FLUIDS AND ELECTROLYTES

Infants and young children are more vulnerable to rapid fluid and electrolyte imbalances than adults for various reasons; a major difference is their higher basal metabolic rate. The basal requirement in infant's is approximately 55 Kcal/kg/24 hr. A gradual decrease takes place during childhood until maturity, when it is 25-30 Kcal/kg/24 hr.[2] The increased metabolic rate of infants is due to their greater proportionate surface area, growth needs and relatively larger viscera and brain.*[5] Body surface area of an infant is proportionately two to three times greater than that of an adult. It is not until the child is 2 to 3 years of age that the relatively greater surface is no longer present.[7] This increased metabolic rate accounts for the rapid rate of water turnover. In the event of no water intake it would take a baby five days to lose the amount of water contained in his extracellular compartments; it would take an adult about 10 days to lose an amount equal to his extracellular fluid.[7] The homeostatic mechanisms of the body are less mature in infants and small children; thus when they become ill they are more vulnerable to imbalances.

Gains and Losses

Gains and losses are more rapid during infancy and childhood, but in conditions of health this rapid turnover of water is of little consequence. It is when fluid and electrolyte losses are compounded by illness that infants and young children can quickly develop extracellular fluid volume deficit and suffer from electrolyte and

---

*The viscera and brain are the most metabolically active organs in the body.[5]

Acknowledgement is given to W. D. Snively, M.D. for review of this section.

TABLE 17-7 APPROXIMATE TOTAL BODY WATER AND INTERNAL WATER DISTRIBUTION AT BIRTH, 1 YEAR, AND AFTER 2 YEARS OF AGE

	Percentage of Total Body Weight		
	At Birth	At 1 Year	After 2 Years
Extracellular (plasma and interstitial)*	40–45	30	20–25
Intracellular†	30–35	35	35
Total Body Water	75–80	65	55–60

*The plasma portion of extracellular fluid remains relatively constant. The major difference in the newborn is in interstitial fluid.
†Shows relatively small variation after birth and is essentially constant after 1 year of age.[13]

acid-base imbalances. Furthermore an infant or child cannot be persuaded to take fluids, whereas an adult will respond to explanation. Losses in a child on the other hand occur even more rapidly than in an adult. The losses in such common occurrences as fever, vomiting and diarrhea quickly deplete their supply of energy; thus imbalance results. The surface area through which these losses occur (skin, lungs and gastrointestinal tract) is proportionately greater in children than in adults. The kidneys, which regulate excretion, are less mature and cannot effectively conserve fluids and electrolytes to compensate for the energy depletion and electrolyte imbalances. More water is thus needed to excrete a given amount of solute.[7]

The gastrointestinal tract is of particular significance in the fluid and electrolyte balance of children. Under normal conditions there is a larger exchange of fluid in children as opposed to adults within the gastrointestinal tract whereby water and sodium are reabsorbed and potassium is excreted. Any illness that affects intestinal absorption thus seriously endangers the life of a child because of the rapid and great losses that can occur through the gastrointestinal tract.

The major system that regulates gains and losses is the renocardiovascular mechanism (kidneys, blood vessels, and heart). Although there are no major differences in the functioning of this system between children and adults, except for immaturity, a discussion on fluid and electrolyte balance is hardly complete without a brief explanation of the renal mechanisms of regulation.

The primary regulating hormone is the antidiuretic hormone (ADH) excreted by the posterior pituitary gland. ADH is manufactured in the hypothalamus but stored in and released from the posterior pituitary gland. When the plasma sodium level is high, ADH is secreted in response to a stimulus from the hypothalamus, and the kidney in turn conserves water. When plasma sodium levels are low, the system is reversed, with ADH secretion being inhibited, resulting in diuresis. Thus ADH decreases urine volume and lack of ADH increases urine volume.

Additional renal regulation is accomplished through the renin-angiotensin system and aldosterone. The renin-angiotensin system is a feedback system whereby reduced blood flow to the kidney stimulates a specialized area in the glomerulus to secrete renin. Renin in turn generates angiotensin (angiotensin is produced from the plasma globulin angiotensinogen) within the blood vessels. Angiotensin constricts vessels and restores blood pressure and blood flow. The release of the adrenal hormone aldosterone is also stimulated by angiotensin. Aldosterone promotes increased blood pressure by enhancing sodium and water reabsorption from the renal tubules.

Internal Transport of Fluids and Electrolytes

When a concentration gradient for water develops across a membrane, osmosis takes place. Water diffuses from an area of lesser concentration of solutes to an area of greater concentration of solutes. In other words, "water goes where salt is."[7] The pull or pressure gradient that is created by the particle concentration is called osmotic pressure. Each unit of osmotic pressure is an osmol. Osmolality (particle concentration) is measured in milliosmols (mOsm). When osmolality in one fluid compartment is altered, the resultant concentration gradient for water causes osmosis to take place.

Shifts Between Cellular and Extracellular Fluid Fluid shifts between the cellular and extracellular fluid compartments occur when concentration of sodium in the blood is either higher (hypertonic, or hypernatremia) or lower (hypotonic, or hyponatremia) than normal. Fluid will shift from the extracellular to intracellular in the event of hyponatremia and from intracellular to extracellular in the presence of hypernatremia.

Sodium is primarily extracellular and potassium intracellular. It is by active transport that sodium and potassium ions pass through the cell membrane from areas of lesser ion concentration to areas of greater ion concentration. Sodium and potassium are both cations and when there is a loss of potassium in the cells, sodium enters the cell. This shift of sodium into cells is a slow process. Potassium is continually moving in and out of the cells and is excreted by the kidneys.

An important clinical consideration is that electrolytes are primarily evaluated by serum levels. In normal states of health serum evaluation gives a relatively accurate assessment of other body fluid compartments. In the presence of illness and trauma these values must be carefully assessed with regard to the likelihood of fluid and electrolyte shifts between body fluid compartments.

Shifts Between Vascular Fluids and Interstitial Fluids Osmolality of plasma is slightly higher than that of interstitial fluids because of the concentration of plasma proteins. The difference between the pressures of the plasma and interstitial fluids is oncotic pressure. Transport of fluids from plasma to interstitial fluid occurs at the arterial end of the capillary bed. Oncotic pressure of the plasma proteins holds the water and electrolytes in the plasma compartment, whereas hydrostatic pressure pushes them out. (Hydrostatic pressure is a force produced by the pumping action of the heart, which favors movement of fluids and electrolytes out of the capillaries.) Under normal conditions these pressures are balanced so that almost all of the fluid and electrolytes that are pushed out at the capillary end are reabsorbed at the venous end. In certain conditions of infants and children these pressures are altered, resulting in accumulation of fluid (edema) in the interstitial spaces. This fluid shift from plasma to interstitial fluid is frequently referred to as third-spacing.[12] Also, when capillary permeability is increased, as in allergy, fluid follows protein into the third space.

It is important for the nurse who cares for infants and children to recognize tht there are two phases to third-spacing: the loss phase and the reabsorption phase. Extensive fluid shifts from plasma to interstitial fluid can cause hypovolemic shock during the loss phase and shifts from the interstitial fluid to plasma can cause circulatory overload during the reabsorption phase. A child is highly vulnerable to both of the phenomena, making both fluid loss and rehydration potentially life-threatening.

BODY EQUILIBRIUM AND IMBALANCES

Fluid and electrolyte imbalance results from numerous common conditions occurring in children. Neonates, infants and young children are highly vulnerable to a critical condition, acidosis. In neonates acidosis most commonly is the result of hypoxia, whereas in older children its usual cause is fluid loss.[3] Electrolyte imbalance typically occurs in association with fluid loss. The types of disturbance the pediatric nurse should be prepared to deal with include acid-base imbalances, fluid disturbances and electrolyte derangement.

Acid-Base Balance

The concentration of hydrogen ions determines whether a solution is neutral, acidic or alkaline (basic). Hydrogen ion concentration is expressed on a pH scale from 1 to 14. A pH of 7 is neutral, less than 7 is acidic, and higher than 7 is alkaline. Ordinarily plasma pH is between 7.35 and 7.45. Hydrogen ion concentration of extracellular fluid is maintained by the kidneys, the lungs and chemical buffer system (primarily bicarbonate-carbonic acid). It is largely the maintenance of a 20:1 ratio between bicarbonate ion and carbonic acid* concentrations that keeps the body in acid-base balance. Buffers reduce the degree of pH shift in the body by neutralizing excess hydrogen or base ions. Carbonic acid concentrations are regulated by the lungs. When carbon dioxide is blown off as a gas, water is left; thus the hydrogen ion of the carbonic acid is no longer present. The result of the blowing off of carbon dioxide thus is a decrease in acidity. Regulation of serum bicarbonate takes place in the kidneys. Renal response to acid-base imbalance is much slower

---

*Carbonic acid is in equilibrium with dissolved carbon dioxide; therefore measurement of partial pressure of carbon dioxide (pCO_2) can be used as a clinical estimate of carbonic acid concentration.[9]

TABLE 17-8 ACID-BASE IMBALANCES: CLINICAL CAUSES, COMPENSATORY MECHANISMS, AND CLINICAL MANIFESTATIONS

Classification	Clinical Causes	Compensatory Mechanism	Clinical Manifestations and Blood Gases
Respiratory acidosis: Impaired respiratory function with CO_2 retention	Disturbance of respiratory center (drugs, head trauma); disease affecting respiratory muscles; airway obstruction; pulmonary disease; cardiac failure; right-to-left cardiac shunts	Renal compensation: increased urinary excretion of hydrogen ion; makes and reabsorbs more bicarbonate	Respiratory distress, including tachypnea and use of accessory muscles. Hypoxemia often present due to underlying cause. Hypoxemia can lead to metabolic lactic acidosis* • Arterial pH low • pCO_2 elevated • Plasma bicarbonate moderately elevated
Respiratory alkalosis: alveolar hyperventilation results in blowing off CO_2 in excess of its production	Acute anxiety states; hyperactivity of respiratory center in association with infection (encephalitis, meningitis); salicylate ingestion (early stages); improper use of mechanical respirators; increased sensitivity of the respiratory center to pCO_2	Renal compensation: less hydrogen ion is excreted so that less bicarbonate is produced (each time a hydrogen ion is excreted by the kidney a bicarbonate ion is produced and reabsorbed); decreased conservation of filtered bicarbonate	Tetany due to decreased ionized calcium in the presence of alkalemia. • Arterial pH high • pCO_2 low • Plasma bicarbonate low
Metabolic acidosis • Increased production of hydrogen ions	Ketone acids (starvation, diabetes); lactic acids (usually secondary to tissue hypoxia); salicylate poisoning	Respiratory compensation: Increased respirations to blow off CO_2 Renal Compensation: • Acidosis also stimulates kidney to produce ammonia so that hydrogen ion can be excreted with it • As hydrogen ion is excreted new bicarbonate is generated	Deep, rapid respirations (Küssmaul breathing); severe acidosis can reduce peripheral vascular resistance and cause decreased function of the ventricles of the heart. Hypotension, pulmonary edema, and tissue hypoxia may result. • Arterial pH low • pCO_2 low • Plasma bicarbonate low
• Excessive loss of bicarbonate ions (hyperchloremia due to resulting elevated chloride level)	Via GI tract† (diarrhea, vomiting, suction, fistula drainage); via kidney (renal tubular acidosis)		
• Decreased hydrogen ion excreted and decreased formation of new bicarbonate	Occurs due to low glomerular filtration rate secondary to acute dehydration. Reduced tubular mass (chronic renal insufficiency) limits amount of ammonia kidney can produce. Excretion of hydrogen ion with ammonia is thus decreased		

348 FAMILIES WITH CHILDREN

Metabolic alkalosis
- Loss of hydrogen ion resulting in the presence of comparatively too much base
- Gain of bicarbonate.

1. Loss of hydrogen ion (gastric aspiration, persistent vomiting, e.g., pyloric stenosis).
2. Loading with bicarbonate as by:
   - Increased renal reabsorption of bicarbonate as in a potassium cellular deficit (reasons not clear).
   - When chlorides are lost as in vomiting the body releases more bicarbonate to keep the total number of anions equal.
3. Administration of a diuretic.

- Reduced extracellular fluid volume with a greater NaCl loss than bicarbonate loss.

Respiratory compensation: Compensation is not effective, therefore the problem must be eliminated.

Depressed respiration. Hypertonic muscles due to decreased ionized calcium in the presence of alkalemia‡
- Arterial pH high
- pCO_2 elevated
- Plasma bicarbonate elevated

---

*Hypoxemia can result in metabolic acidosis due to accumulation of lactic acid in presence of reduced oxygen supply to tissues. Exercise, trauma and infection are common causes of tissue hypoxia that can result in metabolic lactic acidosis.

†Large amounts of bicarbonate are present in gastrointestinal tract from a point distal of pylorus to anal sphincter.

‡In acidosis there is a high ionization of calcium and in alkalosis a decreased ionization.[7]

Sources: N. W. Metheney and W. D. Snively. Nurse's Handbook of Fluid Balance, J. B. Lippincott Co., 1979. V. C. Vaughn et al. Nelson Textbook of Pediatrics, W. B. Saunders Co., 1979. R. A. Hoekelmen et al. Principles of Pediatrics, McGraw-Hill Book Co., 1978.

than that of the lungs: hours and days compared to seconds and minutes are required to restore balance. The kidney can conserve or excrete bicarbonate ion to re-establish a 1:20 ratio between carbonic acid and bicarbonate.

In a primary metabolic disorder the respiratory system compensates.[9] Acid-base disturbances are summarized in Table 17-8. Laboratory methods of evaluation can provide measurements of pH and Pco_2 and an approximation of bicarbonate ion concentration in the form of total carbon dioxide content. If two of these three are known the other one can be calculated.[10] (See Appendix VI for normal blood gases.)

The most common clinical entity that leads to metabolic acidosis in children is diarrhea. The relationship between diarrhea and acidosis can be explained by reviewing how the hydrogen ion concentration in the body is affected when large amounts of fluid losses occur via diarrhea stools. Hydrogen ion levels increase because (1) the bicarbonate content of stool may be high; (2) ketone body* production increases as a result of fat being metabolized for energy; (3) dehydration increases anaerobic metabolism, resulting in release of acids (lactic, pyruvic, and acetoacetic), free hydrogen ions, and carbon dioxide; and (4) reduced blood volume causes the kidneys to function less effectively with a reduced excretion of hydrogen ions.[3]

Fluid and Electrolyte Imbalances

Fluid and electrolyte imbalances occur when there is a total body deficit or gain in fluids and electrolytes or when an alteration exists within a body fluid compartment. In many instances an alteration exists both in total amount and in position within body compartments. Third-spacing and dehydration are two common imbalances that occur in children.

Third-Spacing (Edema) The processes and diseases common to children that cause third-spacing are (1) lowered plasma proteins (nephrotic syndrome and malnutrition); (2) interference with cardiac function resulting in increased capillary pressure (congestive heart failure); (3) an increase in capillary permeability (burns, allergy, cellulitis); and (4) obstruction of venous or lymphatic flow (tumors). The imbalance that results in these conditions is discussed in the section of this text that deals with the particular alteration.

Dehydration Dehydration occurs when body fluids are lost in excess of fluid gain. Common alterations that result in dehydration are due to disturbances in: (1) the gastrointestinal tract (vomiting, diarrhea, malabsorption, pyloric stenosis); (2) the skin (burns); (3) metabolism (fever, diabetes mellitus); and (4) the lungs (hyperventilation as in tracheobronchitis). Dehydration also results from injury or surgery. Management of specific problems that result in dehydration and associated electrolyte imbalance are discussed with the various conditions throughout the text. A general discussion of dehydration follows, including isotonic dehydration, hypertonic dehydration and hypotonic dehydration.

Isotonic Dehydration This occurs when fluids and electrolytes are lost in approximately the same proportion as they exist in the body (normal osmotic concentration). In this type of dehydration there is no fluid shift because body fluid osmolality is not affected. This is the most common type of dehydration encountered; it is seen in about 70 per cent of children with acute dehydration due to diarrhea.[4]

Hypertonic Dehydration (Hypernatremia) When there is a proportionately greater loss of water than electrolytes this type of dehydration results, producing a state of hypernatremia. This condition occurs in about 20 per cent of dehydrated infants who have either received insufficient water or a hypertonic solution. The proportionate excess of solutes results in a fluid shift from intracellular to the extracellular spaces. The result of this fluid shift is that intracellular dehydration is present, causing early neurological symptoms (marked lethargy and irritability on stimulation) but circulatory disturbances are absent.[4]

Hypotonic Dehydration (Hyponatremia) This occurs when electrolyte losses are greater than fluid losses. This can occur when in the presence of diarrhea losses are replaced with large amounts of water rather than a variety of clear

---

*Ketone bodies include acetoacetic acid, B-hydroxy butyric acid and acetone.

TABLE 17-9 CLINICAL MANIFESTATIONS OF IMBALANCE OF SODIUM, POTASSIUM, AND CALCIUM

Electrolyte Imbalance	Clinical Manifestations and Laboratory Findings
Hypernatremia: due to a water deficit or sodium excess.	Dry, sticky mucous membranes and flushed skin. Excessive thirst in the older child. Nuchal and muscle rigidity. Irritability with stimuli, with possible tremors and convulsions.* Edema (visible on examination). Skin turgor may be fair due to cellular-to-extracellular fluid shift. Specific gravity (SG) of urine above 1.030.
Hyponatremia: due to sodium depletion or water overload in relation to sodium.	Rapid fall in sodium causes severe symptoms of shock. Skin is clammy and cold, and child may have twitching and convulsions*). A slower fall in sodium causes milder symptoms of nausea and vomiting, apathy, and weakness. SG of urine below 1.010.
Hyperkalemia: due to an increased intake of potassium, an inadequate excretion, or a shift of potassium from within the cells to the extracellular compartment.	Malaise, nausea. Muscle weakness. Hyperreflexia. Shallow breathing. Bradycardia. Oliguria progressing to anuria. Flaccid paralysis. Intestinal colic and diarrhea. Cardiac muscle failure. ECG changes (T-wave elevation, depressed S-T segment, and flat P wave). Cardiac changes may be lethal.
Hypokalemia: due to an inadequate intake of potassium, an excessive loss of potassium, and a shift of extracellular potassium to intracellular fluid.	Apathy, drowsiness. Abdominal distention and ileus. Muscular weakness, hyporeflexia or flaccid paralysis. Shallow breathing. Hypotension. Tachycardia. Cardiac arrhythmias. Flat T wave with prolonged ST segment on ECG.
Hypercalcemia: due to excessive administration of vitamin D, hyperparathyroidism or prolonged immobilization.	Abdominal or flank pain. Nausea, vomiting. Dryness of mouth. Muscle hypotonicity. Stupor and coma. Cardiac arrest.
Hypocalcemia: due to cow's milk with high phosphorus/calcium ratio and during the period when acidosis is corrected. (Calcium returns to bone.)	Tingling and numbness. Tetany. Muscular cramps. Laryngospasm. Convulsions.

*Changes in body fluid tonicity occurring abruptly cause central nervous system disturbances. In hypertonicity (hypernatremia) it is from "desiccation of the brain" and in hypotonicity (hyponatremia) it is from "cerebral edema."
Sources: N. W. Metheney and W. D. Snively, Nurse's Handbook of Fluid Balance, J. B. Lippincott Co., 1979. M. J. Sweeney. Fluid Therapy, In Principles of Pediatrics, R. A. Hoekelman et al., McGraw-Hill Book Co., 1978. G. M. Reed, Confused about potassium? Here's a clear concise guide, Nursing '74, March, 1974, p. 20.

liquids. In this type of dehydration water shifts from the extracellular spaces of low solute concentration to an area of greater solute concentration, the intracellular. This condition is present in only about 10 per cent of dehydrated children.[4]

Electrolyte Imbalances The specific electrolyte imbalances that accompany specific disease states are discussed elsewhere in the text. A general discussion of electrolyte imbalances as they pertain to children follows.

Sodium Imbalance Sodium imbalance occurs when the sodium level is either excessive (hypernatremia) or is deficient (hyponatremia). Normal concentration of plasma sodium ranges from 137 to 147 mEq/L.

Hypernatremia This may be the result of water depletion (decreased intake or increased output) or both. Thus any clinical condition that depletes the body of water has the potential to result in a state of hypernatremia.

The administration of hypertonic intravenous fluids or hypertonic tube feedings may also result in hypernatremia. A high solute intake (protein) in the presence of insufficient water results in a water shift from tissues to the vascular fluid to facilitate urinary excretion of the excess solutes.[7] Eventually hypernatremic dehydration occurs. Table 17–9 lists clinical manifestations of hypernatremia.

Hyponatremia When there is an excessive loss of sodium or an overloading of water, hyponatremia results. Excessive losses of sodium result from gastroenteritis, losses through the skin (fever, cystic fibrosis, burns), nasogastric suction, or adrenal insufficiency. Water overloading occurs when electrolyte-free intravenous solutions are administered to children. Repeated administration of tap water enemas (electrolyte-free) can also eventually cause a hyponatremic state; therefore, enemas for children consist of normal saline, especially when it is necessary to give repeated enemas.

Another cause of water overload is oversecretion of the antidiuretic hormone (ADH). Conditions that may result in excessive ADH secretion are meningitis, hydrocephalus, pneumonia and bronchogenic neoplasms. Head injuries and some medications (morphine or barbiturates) and extreme stress can also cause excess ADH. This syndrome of inappropriate antidiuretic hormone secretion (SIADH) is being increasingly observed. It is necessary that all health team members recognize the importance of having electrolyte values tested for the child who might possibly be susceptible to this syndrome. Table 17-9 lists clinical manifestations of hyponatremia.

Potassium Imbalance Potassium imbalance in the body is a serious condition to which infants and young children are particularly vulnerable. Potassium imbalance occurs when the potassium level is either excessive (hyperkalemia) or deficient (hypokalemia). Normal plasma potassium level ranges from 4.0 to 5.6 mEq/L.

The potassium gradient between the intracellular and extracellular compartments is influenced by various factors, one of which is pH changes. Because infants and children are especially vulnerable to acid-base imbalance, the nurse should be aware of this relationship. Plasma potassium increases about 0.6 mEq/L for each 0.1 unit fall in blood pH and it decreases 0.6 mEq/L for each 0.1 unit rise in blood pH.[1] Potassium imbalance in infants and children is a serious condition and requires immediate attention by the nurse. Constant surveillance is warranted whenever potassium imbalance is in question.

Hyperkalemia This results from increased intake of potassium, inadequate excretion of potassium or a shift of potassium from within the cells to the extracellular compartments. An increased intake most commonly occurs in children as a result of too-rapid administration of intravenous potassium chloride. Inadequate excretion of potassium occurs in the event of renal failure, adrenal insufficiency or metabolic acidosis. (In metabolic acidosis there is a reduced excretion of hydrogen ion; potassium excretion depends on excretion of hydrogen.) A shift of potassium from within the cells to extracellular fluid occurs when there is severe dehydration in the early phase of burns or in massive crushing injuries (potassium is released from the cells because of cellular injury) or in the event of hemolysis due to sudden excessive water intake. See Table 17-9 for clinical manifestations of hyperkalemia.

Hypokalemia Hypokalemia occurs when there is inadequate intake of potassium, an excessive loss of potassium and a shift of extracellular potassium to intracellular fluid. Poor food intake over an extended period or administration of intravenous fluids without added potassium may result in hypokalemia. Excessive losses also occur in vomiting and diarrhea or nasogastric suctioning, and when potassium-losing diuretics or corticosteroids are administered. A shift of potassium from extracellular compartments to within the cells occurs under numerous circumstances: (1) on about the third day after a burn (healing stage), (2) during intravenous administration of insulin in ketoacidosis and (3) in the presence of metabolic alkalosis. Table 17-9 lists clinical manifestations of hypokalemia.

Calcium Imbalance Calcium imbalance occurs when the calcium level is either excessive (hypercalcemia) or deficient (hypocalcemia). Normal plasma calcium concentration ranges from 4.5 to 5.8 mEq/L.

Hypercalcemia This may result from excessive administration of vitamin D or hyperparathyroidism, but more importantly in children, from prolonged immobilization. Disuse of bones (absence of weight bearing) causes calcium to be resorbed from the bone into extracellular fluid.[7] Hypercalcemia may be more common in the presence of acidosis. Ionization of calcium is increased in metabolic acidosis and depressed in metabolic alkalosis. Table 17-9 shows clinical manifestations of hypercalcemia.

Hypocalcemia This condition occurs in infants and children for a variety of reasons.

Sometimes a disorder called tetany of the newborn is seen early in infancy when cow's milk formulas with a high ratio of phosphorus to calcium are given. Because a reciprocal relationship exists between calcium and phosphorus, an increase in phosphorus results in hypocalcemia.[7] Hypocalcemia may also occur when acidosis is corrected. Some of the calcium that moves out of the bone matrix during acidosis (to buffer the acidity) is lost in the urine. Once the acidosis is corrected, calcium re-enters the bones, resulting in a state of hypocalcemia. The premature infant is particularly prone to the complication of acidosis.[3] Table 17–9 lists clinical manifestations of hypocalcemia.

NURSE'S ROLE IN MAINTAINING FLUID, ELECTROLYTE AND ACID-BASE BALANCE

Teaching Role in Prevention

One of the greatest responsibilities of the nurse is to teach parents how to prevent imbalances and how to detect early symptoms. Parents can be taught a few basic principles regarding fluid intake and output that in times of minor illness may help them to prevent their child from developing more serious problems. Overdressing for the environmental temperature causes increased perspiration, resulting in both fluid and electrolyte losses. When a child becomes ill parents should also be taught to check the child's temperature early in the illness and offer additional fluids if he has temperature elevation. Additional fluids should be offered to young children during hot weather, and attention should be given to the number and saturation of diapers as a guide to need for additional fluids. Parents should be taught to reduce solid and milk intake and give primarily clear fluids when vomiting or diarrhea occurs. It is important, however, that parents also understand how to gradually increase the child's food intake to avoid a condition of starvation. (See Chapter 23 for discussion of diet for diarrhea and vomiting.) Undiluted skim milk should not be used because of its high solute content; large quantities of water are required for excretion of solutes, further depleting the body of water.

Parents should be taught to identify early signs of imbalance so that treatment can be initiated. A change in a child's behavior and general appearance may be easily overlooked as a clue to illness. Frequently a child's eyes lack luster; he looks pale and is more irritable and demanding than usual in the beginning stages of imbalance. If a child's diaper is seen to be dry at the usual times of changing, the parent should also check the mouth, tongue and lips for dryness. Frequently the nurse can assist parents to prevent development of more serious problems if she takes the time to discuss these few early signs and encourages parents to seek professional assistance when their baby is ill. Families with infants under 6 months of age particularly should be cautioned to seek assistance early when their baby has vomiting and diarrhea.

Assessment

The nurse should collect data regarding intake and output. The type, frequency and amount of fluid and food given at home during the illness should be described by the parents. The nurse should ask the parents whether the child has had any vomiting and diarrhea, any appreciable weight loss and whether they have noted any recent change in behavior. Parents should be given the opportunity to describe any change that they have noted in their baby.

Information from parents and the nurse's observations are important for identification and management of imbalance in children. A child's condition can change rapidly so that assessments need to be made frequently and thoroughly. The nurse evaluates vital signs, body weight, skin color and turgor (tautness), mucous membranes, fontanels and eyes, intake and output and neurological status. Laboratory evaluation of the urine, serum electrolytes, hemoglobin, and blood gases provides important information that the nurse should review during her care of a child with potential fluid and electrolyte imbalance.

Vital Signs Frequent evaluation of vital signs is necessary to monitor the status of a child with potential imbalance. Evaluation of temperature is important because fever increases the metabolic rate. A heightened metabolic rate increases the amount of metabolic wastes, thus additional fluids are required for excretion of wastes via the kidneys.[7] Body fluids and electrolytes are also lost via perspiration and additional fluid is lost through hyperpnea, which commonly accompanies fever. In the early

TABLE 17–10. CORRELATION OF CLINICAL FEATURES WITH DEGREE OF ISOTONIC DEHYDRATION

Clinical Features	Mild Dehydration	Moderate Dehydration	Severe Dehydration
Loss of body weight	5%	10%	15%
Skin color	Pale	Gray	Mottled
Skin turgor	Decreased	Moderately decreased	Markedly decreased
Urine output	Decreased	Oliguria	Marked oliguria and azotemia
Blood pressure	Normal	Normal or slightly above or below normal	Low
Pulse	Normal or tachycardia	Tachycardia	Increased tachycardia and thready pulse

Source: S. K. Dube, Immediate Care of the Sick and Injured Child, C. V. Mosby Co., 1978.

phase of extracellular fluid volume depletion the body temperature is commonly elevated, whereas a subnormal body temperature may occur in the later stages of a volume deficit.[3]

Pulse is evaluated for rate, quality and regularity. When extravascular fluid volume is reduced the pulse is rapid, weak and thready. This can occur in either total body fluid deficit or when plasma shifts from intravascular to interstitial spaces. A bounding pulse is a sign of increased plasma fluid volume and occurs in hypertonic dehydration or when there is an excess of total body fluid volume during the recovery phase of third-spacing. Dehydration is frequently associated with loss of potassium-rich body fluids that results in hypokalemia. Either a severe potassium deficit or excess causes a weak, irregular pulse. The difference is that a potassium deficit generally causes a rapid pulse and potassium excess causes the pulse to slow.

Respirations are affected by fluid volume alterations, electrolyte imbalances and acid-base imbalances. (See Table 17–8 for respiratory responses in acid-base imbalance.) Dehydration is frequently accompanied by metabolic acidosis; therefore, there is an increased respiratory rate (hyperpnea) to compensate. However, hyperpnea in metabolic acidosis is not always as apparent in a child as it is in an adult.[7] Dyspnea and moist rales are additional signs that should be noted. These signs may be present when fluid shifts from interstitial to plasma, causing an increased intravascular load. Potassium alterations, either a deficit or an excess, result in shallow breathing caused by weakness or paralysis of the respiratory muscles.

Blood pressure is not a reliable sign in infants and young children because of the elasticity of blood vessels, but it does add valuable information when evaluated along with other data. Increased blood pressure occurs in fluid volume excess or in the early phase of interstitial fluid-to-plasma shift. Blood pressure is decreased in a fluid deficit or when there is a plasma-to-interstitial fluid shift.

Weight Weight loss or gain provides important data in the assessment of hydration. Weight loss can occur rapidly in children because of large fluid losses. Severity of isotonic dehydration is classified as mild, moderate or severe according to the weight that has been lost. (Table 17–10 presents a correlation of clinical symptoms with degree of dehydration.)

Weight gain during illness can be a sign of fluid retention resulting in pulmonary edema or generalized edema. When a dehydrated child gains weight suddenly the nurse should recheck the weight but also look for signs of fluid retention.

Skin Assessment The skin should be assessed for color, temperature, turgor and moisture. (Skin turgor is assessed by pinching the skin and allowing it to fall back to its original position. When the skin remains slightly raised for a few seconds this is called "poor skin turgor.") In the most common type of dehydration in children, isotonic dehydration, the skin is pale and dry and the elasticity is decreased. The peripheral blood flow is decreased; therefore, the extremities become cool and have poor capillary refill. The skin is a grayish color, and mottling, if it occurs, is an unfavorable sign.[7] In fluid volume excess there is pitting edema due to a shift of fluid from the plasma to interstitial spaces. In a fluid volume deficit the skin loses turgor; in hypertonic dehydration there is much less loss because of the fluid shift to the intravascular compartment. In hypernatremia the skin is flushed, whereas in hyponatremia the child approaches a shock-like state with pale, cool, clammy skin.

The mouth and tongue are dry, tearing and salivation are absent and in an older child thirst is pronounced in states of fluid deficit. Furthermore, in hypernatremia the mucous membranes are dry and sticky.

Anterior Fontanel and Eyes The anterior fontanel and the eyes should be assessed as routinely as are the vital signs when a child has a potential or actual imbalance. The fontanels (if still patent) are tense and bulging when there is a fluid excess and are sunken or depressed when a child is dehydrated; suture lines in the skull may become prominent in dehydration. The eyeballs are also sunken when a child is dehydrated and the eyeball tension is poor; that is, the eyeball is soft. In hypernatremic dehydration the eyeball tension is somewhat preserved.

Intake and Output and Urine Specific Gravity A nurse's accurate assessment and recording of intake and output are of prime importance in caring for children with fluid and electrolyte imbalances. *A physician's order is not required for a nurse to institute the keeping of an intake and output record if she deems it necessary.* The nurse can also check specific gravity without a physician's order and should do so if such data are required.

An infant's urine is normally dilute and so will show a low specific gravity. In the immediate newborn and neonatal periods it ranges from 1.001 to 1.020 and thereafter from 1.001 to 1.030. A fluid excess in the body is reflected in a low specific gravity (1.010 or less) and a fluid deficit is reflected in a high specific gravity reading. After a period of fluid restriction specific gravity is commonly greater than 1.025.

Oral fluid intake usually equals urinary output daily. Fluid that results from metabolism approximately equals that which is lost through the skin, lungs and stool. Normal range for 24-hour urinary output varies with age as follows: in the neonate 50 to 300 ml; in the infant 350 to 550 ml; in the child 500 to 1000 ml; and in the adolescent 700 to 1400 ml. When there is a markedly higher output of urine than fluid intake, it may be due to a shift of fluid from interstitial fluid to plasma or because of a high solute intake. The nurse should be aware that if a child with a known fluid volume deficit excretes large amounts of urine, it is likely that the child has renal damage.[7]

Common pediatric conditions that result in a high volume of urine are fever and infection. Due to the higher metabolic rate there are increased wastes for the kidneys to excrete; additional water is required to clear such wastes from the body.

Neurological and General Behavior Behavior changes are commonly reported by parents and should be regarded as an important aspect of the nurse's assessment. With a fluid deficit a child may be lethargic or irritable, and an infant's cry may be high pitched and weak. Most commonly a degree of irritability is first noted, followed by lethargy. In hypertonic dehydration an infant is usually lethargic with irritability on stimulation. Extreme restlessness in a child may indicate a potassium deficit. Potassium deficits also cause abdominal distention, hypotonia and in severe cases flaccid paralysis, whereas a calcium deficit may be the reason for a child's tendency for twitching, irritability and eventual convulsions.

Laboratory Assessment Laboratory findings in various states of pH imbalance are summarized in Table 17–8. Urine specific gravity and its significance in evaluating hydration has been discussed. Hemoglobin is an additional parameter that the nurse should include in her clinical evaluation of a patient's hydration status. As a child becomes severely dehydrated, hemoconcentration results in an elevated hemoglobin level.

Imbalances in various electrolytes have also been reviewed. Serum electrolyte levels represent only samples. If there is a fluid and electrolyte imbalance, the normal relationship of electrolytes within the various body compartments is altered. Serum potassium may not be lowered even though there is a cellular deficit of potassium. When potassium is lost from the body as in diarrhea, potassium leaves the cells and because of the extracellular fluid volume deficit, the childs' glomerular filtration is de-

PRINCIPLES AND SKILLS OF PEDIATRIC NURSING 355

creased. Thus potassium excretion from the body is inhibited. Young infants in particular must be closely observed for cardiac changes and impending cardiac arrest, which could occur as a result of an intracellular potassium deficit.[3]

It is important for the nurse to strive to gain an increased understanding of laboratory reports. However, laboratory findings must always be evaluated in conjunction with findings on clinical observation.

Management of Imbalances in Fluids, Electrolytes and Acid-Base

Administration of intravenous fluids and electrolytes to children is a highly specialized technique. The nurse who participates in such therapy requires knowledge and a high level of clinical competence to meet this responsibility effectively. A nurse involved in the administration of intravenous fluids and electrolytes should strive to increase her theoretical knowledge base as well as her technical skill. The care of these children and families traverses all aspects of pediatric nursing. The chemical and physiological processes are complex and the psychological effects on the child and parents are far-reaching. Starting and maintaining intravenous lines requires special skill and practice, and the mathematical calculations necessary to administer the prescribed fluid and electrolyte medication require precision and are of utmost importance. Under no circumstances should unsupervised novice practitioners have sole responsibility for such potentially life-threatening procedures. In the opinion of this author student nurses and newly practicing graduate nurses deserve the security, and the child deserves the right, of having another more experienced nurse check all calculations when electrolytes are added to an IV bottle.

Fluid and electrolyte therapy is employed under a variety of circumstances. The goal of therapy is to provide maintenance therapy to compensate for normal and abnormal losses and to replace pre-existing deficits. The type of solution and the rate of administration vary according to the condition being corrected and the metabolic rate of the child.

Although the nurse is not responsible for prescribing the required amount of fluids and electrolytes, she should have sufficient knowledge to be able to check by her own calculations and to decide whether the amount of fluid and electrolytes she is administering is indeed a reasonable and safe dose for the particular child and condition being treated.

Calculation of Maintenance Fluid and Electrolyte Dose The body is in a continuous dynamic state. Fluids and electrolytes are normally gained and lost and when the "intake equals the output, the balance is zero."[13] Maintenance therapy provides for fluids and electrolytes lost under normal conditions through insensible water loss (skin and lungs), sweat, urine and stool. When the child is ill ongoing losses must also be included in maintenance therapy. Thus maintenance therapy includes the normal and abnormal ongoing losses.[13] (Table 17–11 lists water losses under normal conditions.)

Calculation of maintenance therapy may be done on the basis of the patient's body weight, body surface area or caloric expenditure. The method most widely used now because of its accuracy and ease of calculation is based on caloric expenditure. Holliday and Segar's formula (Table 17–12) can be committed to memory for easy use in the clinical area.

Electrolytes must also be maintained on a daily basis to keep the body in balance. Maintenance requirements of electrolytes are: (1) sodium: 2.5 mEq per 100 cal; (2) chloride: 5.0 mEq per 100 cal; (3) potassium: 2.5 mEq per 100 cal.[13] In addition to electrolytes, glucose must be provided at 5 gm/100 cal metabolized. A solution of 5 per cent glucose* in 0.2 per cent sodium chloride† (may be written as

TABLE 17–11 WATER LOSS PER 100 CALORIES METABOLIZED UNDER NORMAL CONDITIONS

Route	Water Lost (ml/100 Cal)
Insensible water loss	45 ml
Sweat	0–25 ml
Urine	50–75 ml
Stool	5–10 ml

Usual loss in absence of sweating is 100 ml/100 cal metabolized.

Adapted from R. W. Winters. Maintenance Fluid Therapy in The Body Fluids in Pediatrics, Little, Brown & Co., 1973, p. 124.

---

*This solution contains 50 gm of glucose per liter.[13]
†Full-strength normal saline has 0.9 per cent sodium chloride; therefore one-half strength has 0.45 per cent and ¼ strength has 0.22 per cent or 0.2 per cent sodium chloride.

TABLE 17-12 MAINTENANCE REQUIREMENTS OF FLUIDS (IN ML) BASED ON CALORIC EXPENDITURE

Body Weight in Kg	Caloric Expenditure	Fluid Requirements*
3–10 kg	100 cal/kg/day	100 ml/kg/day
10–20 kg	1000 cal + 50 cal/kg for each kg of body weight above 10 kg	1000 ml + 50 ml/kg for each kg of body weight above 10 kg
Over 20 kg	1500 cal + 20 cal/kg for each kg of body weight above 20 kg	1500 ml + 20 ml/kg for each kg of body weight above 20 kg

*Water of oxidation provides a small daily source of fluid to the body. Water losses that must be replaced (insensible water loss and renal water loss) can be provided by 100 ml/100 cal/day; thus "Cal" can be replaced by "ml" as shown in last column above.

Adapted from M. A. Holliday and W. E. Segar, The maintenance need for water in parenteral fluid therapy, Pediatrics, May 1957, p. 823.

$D_5/0.2NS$ or $D_5/\frac{1}{4}NS$) with 20 mEq/L of potassium chloride (KCl) provides adequate maintenance therapy under normal conditions.

Potassium administration must be done with extreme caution. A commonly made mathematical error is incorrect placement of a decimal point. When such an error is made involving KCl, ten times the prescribed dose may be administered; this error, for a child, is lethal. Some general guidelines to use, in addition to calculations based on caloric expenditure, are: (1) the concentration of potassium chloride should not exceed 20 mEq/L (never give IV push); (2) no more than 4 mEq/kg/day should be given to correct hypokalemia; and (3) it should not be given in the presence of oliguria or anuria.

The nurse should also understand the principles of deficit therapy. It is beyond the scope of this text to discuss specific deficit therapy for pediatric illnesses. Included in this section is a discussion of some principles that will help the nurse to understand deficit therapy.

Principles of Deficit Therapy Deficit therapy is most frequently described in three phases: an initial phase in which the goal is to improve circulation and renal function, a repletion phase during which intracellular and extracellular deficits are replaced and the final phase during which the child's nutritional state returns to normal.[4, 11]

Initial therapy (emergency phase) is designed to rapidly expand the extracellular fluid volume. Ringer's lactated solution or 0.9 per cent saline solution equal to 20 to 30 ml/kg can be administered within the first hour. This usually restores normal circulation; however, if it does not, a second or in some cases a third infusion of 20 to 30 ml/kg may be necessary.[11] If normal saline (0.9 per cent) is used for an acidotic child it may be necessary to add appropriate amounts of bicarbonate. Only when shock cannot be reversed is blood or another plasma expander (10 mg/kg) administered to restore circulation.[11]

Repletion therapy (subsequent therapy) is aimed at correcting previous losses as well as providing therapy for normal and abnormal ongoing losses. This phase may last from 2 to 24 hours; however, the fluid deficit of hypertonic (hypernatremic) dehydration must be corrected slowly. This frequently takes up to 48 hours. Urinary flow must be established before potassium is added. Replacement of electrolytes is guided by serum electrolytes and varies according to the underlying problem.

The final phase begins when oral intake can be resumed. Reintroduction of oral feedings usually begins with small amounts of clear liquids. Milk and solids are then introduced gradually while careful observation is being made for the body's tolerance of oral feedings.

Fluid Therapy Related to Surgery

Preoperative parenteral therapy is not required unless there is a pre-existing deficit. Fluid administration during surgery varies according to the types of losses occurring during surgery. According to Sweeney, "The most common error in parenteral fluid administration during and after surgery is overadministration, particularly of dextrose in water."[11]

Postoperative fluids are provided by the parenteral route at least until the child has completely recovered from anesthesia and is

TABLE 17-13 NURSING GUIDELINES FOR PEDIATRIC IV'S AT VARIOUS STAGES OF CHILD'S DEVELOPMENT

	Developmental Characteristics Note: Each stage builds on the earlier ones, and during hospitalization many children regress to behaviors appropriate to earlier levels of development.	IV Placement (ideal sites)	Preparation of Child	Family Involvement
Infant (First Year)	Dependent on others for all needs. Needs to feel physically safe, through close relationship with one caretaking person (usually the mother). Trust develops through needs being met consistently. Mistrust and anxiety develop when needs are met inconsistently. "Stranger anxiety" begins at approximately 6 months.	Scalp vein (best site); foot, hand, forearm	Best not to feed infant immediately before IV insertion (vomiting and aspiration possible).	Prepare family as to need for IV therapy, insertion procedure, appearance of infant with IV, and fluid needs. Encourage family to continue providing baby with tactile and verbal stimulation, and TLC. Demonstrate safe ways to hold an infant with an IV. Encourage questions and clarify misconceptions.
Toddler (Ages 1–3)	Discovers and explores self and world around him. Enjoys new mobility skills. Develops egocentric thinking, and need for parallel play. Tolerates short separations from mother. Transitional objects (security blanket, special toy) provide some comfort. Oppositional syndrome ("no" stage). "Separation anxiety" an important problem in hospitalized toddlers separated from mother, ages 8–24 months.	Hand, arm, foot. Important: From this age group on, the less dominant extremity should be used for the IV whenever possible. Determine handedness prior to IV insertion.	Prepare child immediately before procedure (child has limited attention span, and is likely to become more anxious if prepared sooner). Give very simple explanation in concrete terms. Show equipment to be used. Do not offer choice. See preparation for preschool age (below) and assess ability of each child to understand.	Prepare family as to need for IV therapy, insertion procedure, and appearance of child with IV. Whether parents remain with the child during the procedure varies. If they stay with the child their role is to comfort him rather than to assist with restraining. Demonstrate to parents how to safely handle child with IV.
Preschool (Ages 4–6)	Magical thinking, based on what the child would like to believe. Cannot always distinguish fantasy from reality. Fears intrusive procedures. Castration fears common. Develops conscience (guilt), while asserting independence and mastering new skills. Learning to share.	Hand, forearm (less dominant)	Prepare child just prior to procedure. Using small bottle, tubing, and doll or stuffed animal, explain in literal terms the need for IV, and insertion procedure. Allow child to see and touch equipment. Explain how child can help with procedure by cleaning site, opening packages, taping, etc. Allow some degree of control in the situation. Tell child you will help him hold still, and that it's OK to cry.	As with toddlers, parents may or may not stay with the child during the procedure. If they stay, they should provide comfort and support, but should not be asked to restrain the child for IV insertion. Reinforce child's need for honest, simple explanations. Reassure parents that child can still play and be active, even with IV.
School Age (Ages 7–11)	Struggles between mastering new skills and failure. Enjoys school, learning skills, games with rules. Needs to succeed. Fears body mutilation. May feel need to be "brave." Can understand hospital rules. World now expanding beyond family. Peer group becomes important. Competitiveness.	Hand, forearm (less dominant)	Prepare child ahead of time, but same day of insertion. Carefully explain and demonstrate equipment and reasons for IV therapy, letting patient watch you or help set up equipment. Ask child for questions about need for IV and procedure. Give child choices and let him help in procedure whenever possible. Tell child crying is OK because needles hurt, and you will help him hold still.	Whenever possible, family and child should be prepared together, so that family can reinforce what the child has been told. Stress to family the child's need for some independence in ADL, even with an IV. Parental presence or participation in IV insertion may be appropriate, but child's preference should be considered primary.
Adolescent (Ages 12–18)	Vacillates between needs for independence and dependence. Adult cognitive abilities, deductive reasoning. Coping mechanisms: rationalization, intellectualization. Peer acceptance very important. Egocentric, rebellious at times, especially against parents and authority figures. Very concerned with body image, body changes, sexuality, and role. Searching for "who I am."	Hand, forearm (less dominant)	Prepare child several hours to a day before procedure, if possible. Needs time between preparation and insertion to absorb explanations and ask questions. For most adolescents, approach discussions on an adult level. Explain need for IV therapy and expected duration, and show equipment. May need much support for acceptance of therapy.	Explain therapy needs and duration as per patient. Decision regarding parental presence during procedure should be patient's, not parents'. Stress to family the patient's need for independence and participation in decisions affecting his care.

Reprinted with adaptations by permission from L. J. Guhlow and J. Kolb. Pediatric IVs: Special Measures You Should Take. March *RN Magazine*, 1979, p. 40.

TABLE 17-13 NURSING GUIDELINES FOR PEDIATRIC IV'S AT VARIOUS STAGES OF CHILD'S DEVELOPMENT (Continued)

Related Nursing Actions	Protection of IV Site	Mobility Considerations Note: No child should be restricted to bed simply because he has an IV!	Safety Needs
Restrain during insertion. Comfort and cuddle during and after insertion. Observe carefully during insertion for problems of vomiting, aspiration, etc. Firmly restrain extremity with IV (see next column). Use of pacifier diminishes stress, especially for NPO infants.	IV may be secured with tape only or by using a paper cup with bottom cut out or a plastic medicine cup to protect insertion site. Extremity may be restrained by using a board, a sand bag or wrist and ankle restraints.	Keep restraints as loose as possible to allow for motion. Release any restrained extremities hourly for ROM. Mitten hands with cotton and stockinette to prohibit infant's grasping IV. Restraining all extremities is *rarely* necessary. Remember infant's need for sensory stimulation.	Maintain strict I & O. Secure IV tubing out of range of kicking legs and flailing arms. Check restraints frequently for effectiveness and presence of adequate circulation.
Restraining the toddler for an IV usually requires more than one person. Reassure child through verbal and tactile stimulation during procedure. Provide toys to hit or throw, for therapeutic expression of anger, after procedure and throughout hospitalization.	See above (infant). A securely anchored IV is essential for the normally active toddler. Even the best site protection will not remain effective unless it is coupled with close nursing supervision, and with distracting activities for the child.	Toddlers cope with the world and learn about it through action. Therefore, minimal restraints should be used, and tying the child in bed is to be avoided. Parental presence during waking hours permits the child to be constantly supervised, and makes restraints unnecessary in many cases. However, be careful to avoid setting up a situation in which the child associates his parent's departure with "punishment" of restraint.	Child is unaware of danger at this age. He won't know that movement of IV causes pain. Constant supervision needed when out of bed. Remind frequently not to touch IV, but don't expect compliance. Distracting activities will accomplish much more than a scolding for handling the IV. Tape connections on tubing if child continues to handle tubing. Keep tubing clamps out of reach.
Tell child he's not being given an IV as punishment. *Never* bribe or threaten with IVs (e.g., "Drink, or you'll get another IV.") Praise for cooperation, or any efforts in that direction. Maintain patient privacy. Don't start an IV in view of other patients, visitors, or staff. Child needs support to cope with intrusiveness of this procedure. Show understanding.	See above (infant). As with toddlers, securely anchored IVs are essential, but inadequate unless coupled with food supervision and age-appropriate activities	As with infants, any restrained extremity needs hourly release for ROM. Preschoolers need maximum mobility to master surroundings. Provide a range of out-of-bed activities whenever possible.	Child will be curious about IV. Is capable of understanding instructions to not touch it, but needs frequent reminders. IV clamps should be out of reach or taped over. Constant supervision needed when out of bed. Child is liable to "take off" down the hall, heedless of pole, bottle, etc. Short attention span limits duration of cooperation with instructions.
Approach child expecting his cooperation (this age group likes to please adults), but expect that child will need help holding still. Allow the child to clean the site with alcohol swab, and to cut tape, prior to insertion. Praise cooperative efforts. Give child step-by-step explanation of procedure as it progresses. Child may like to take some responsibility in keeping I & O.	Will need less protection than younger children due to interest in making IV "work" correctly. May naturally protect extremity with IV. Some children will appreciate a warning sign, "Hands Off," on a piece of tape over the IV as a reminder. Utilize the child's natural curiosity and interest in learning. Tell him the "rules" of safe IV handling.	Show patient and family how to safely manipulate IV for out-of-bed activities (walking in hall with pole, keeping tubing out of wheelchair wheels, etc.).	Remind patient periodically about necessary caution with IV. Show patient the clamps, and caution against handling them. Teach patient signs of IV problems. Enlist child's help in the interest of good compliance, but do not entirely depend on it. Tape tubing connections. Child may forget about IV. Emphasize need for caution in some activities, especially if play includes other children.
Be aware of IV adding to patient's dependency status, and his need for some control. Encourage him to keep his own I & O, help in counting drip rate, etc. Privacy during insertion is very important.	See above (School Age). If patient is very active, will need well-protected, well-anchored IV, as his movements may be more forceful and his strength greater than younger patients'.	See above (School Age). Encourage mobility as much as possible as a means of independence for the adolescent.	Be aware of possibility of adolescent rebellion showing itself in lack of cooperation with therapy. These patients may rebel if feeling threatened, and may be very manipulative in "testing" behaviors. Consistent limits, clearly communicated to patient, parents, and staff, are needed. Instruct patient as to signs of infiltration, phlebitis, etc.

PRINCIPLES AND SKILLS OF PEDIATRIC NURSING

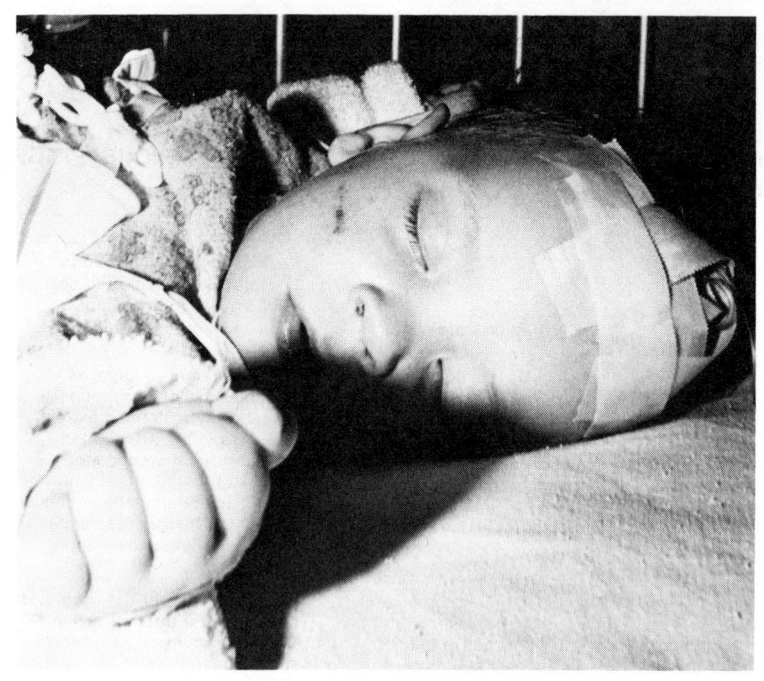

Figure 17–16 A scalp vein catheter inserted in a central position permits the child to be turned to either side.

free of nausea and vomiting. In many minor operations, fluids can be resumed gradually within the first 24 hours. Intravenous fluids are continued when the particular surgical intervention prohibits oral intake. A common postoperative solution used in pediatrics is $D_5/0.2$ NS. Potassium is not administered to the oliguric child because the kidney is the major organ of potassium excretion and therefore hyperkalemia can develop. Surgery frequently causes an excess of tissue loss of potassium owing to trauma and an increased level of ADH owing to stress. Consequently, potassium is not administered in the immediate postoperative period; after urinary function is established potassium can safely be added to IV fluids.

Administering Intravenous Fluids and Electrolytes

Once the parenteral solution has been ordered by the physician the nurse assumes the major responsibility for its proper, safe administration. After checking whether the dose prescribed (amount and rate of administration) is within safe limits, she starts the IV or assists another individual to do so.

Starting an IV Whether the nurse starts the IV or assists another person to do so she should (1) be aware of preferred sites, (2) prepare the child and family and (3) evaluate whether the child needs to be restrained, and if so, how restraint can most effectively be accomplished. Each of these interventions depends on the developmental characteristics of the child and are summarized in Table 17–13.

Choice of site varies according to the age of the child and the condition of veins. Scalp veins are used in infants because they are prominent and because of the difficulty in finding peripheral veins. Because veins in the scalp do not have valves, the needle can be inserted in either direction. A rubber band with an adhesive tag placed around the infant's head (across the forehead) assists to distend the scalp veins. The adhesive tag facilitates quick grasping and cutting of the rubber band after the needle has been inserted. The veins of the scalp communicate with the dural sinuses; therefore, careful cleansing of the insertion site is necessary.[7] Cleansing with Betadine or a similar solution is recommended rather than the traditional alcohol swab. Placing the needle in a vein positioned as far to the front of the head as possible reduces the amount of hair that must be shaved and allows the baby to lie on either side and on his back (Fig. 17–16).

Once the preferred site has been identified, an appropriate needle size is chosen. The needle size varies according to the size of the vein. In pediatrics butterfly needles gauged 25, 23 or

21 are most commonly used. The higher the number, the smaller the needle. Although the smaller needles are perhaps easier to insert, the IV can usually be maintained longer if either a 23-gauge or 21-gauge needle is used.

Regardless of the site used, the position of the needle in the vein, the manner of taping, and the effectiveness of the restraint largely determine the duration of the IV. The needle must be inserted well into the vein and the tape must be placed to stabilize the needle without covering the surrounding area needlessly.

The following guidelines can be used to keep the child restrained when unattended. First, when a hand is used for an IV, the opposite arm must be restrained to prevent the child from pulling out the IV. If the child is a young infant who cannot reach to the opposite hand, a jacket restraint is appropriate. Second, when a foot is used for an IV, the other leg must be restrained to keep the child from kicking the involved foot. Also, either a jacket restraint or a restraint device of both arms is necessary to keep the child from sitting up and pulling out the IV. Third, a scalp vein is frequently used on young infants who often require only mitts on their hands or positioning with a rolled blanket. Older infants may require restraint of all extremities to prevent their rolling over onto the IV (Fig. 17–17). Also, placing the tubing away from the infant's body is helpful.

To avoid overload of the child's cardiovascular system two special features in equipment are recommended. A special control chamber that holds a limited amount of fluid and provides for accurate measurement is recommended for pediatric use. The pediatric set delivers 60 gtts/* min (Fig. 17–18). Also, a special delivery pump system is used to ensure accurate, steady intravenous flow. The tubing is threaded through the machine and the dial is set for the desired rate of flow (Fig. 17–19). When the machine is not functioning properly, an alarm sounds. To prepare IV fluids and begin administration the following steps are suggested.

1. Prepare the IV fluids by connecting the fluid chamber to the main reservoir.
2. Put enough fluid into the fluid chamber to fill the IV tubing; (approximately 15 to 20 cc's plus fluid for one to two hours.)
3. Have pump and fluid set-up available *before* the needle is inserted.
4. Once the needle is inserted, connect the

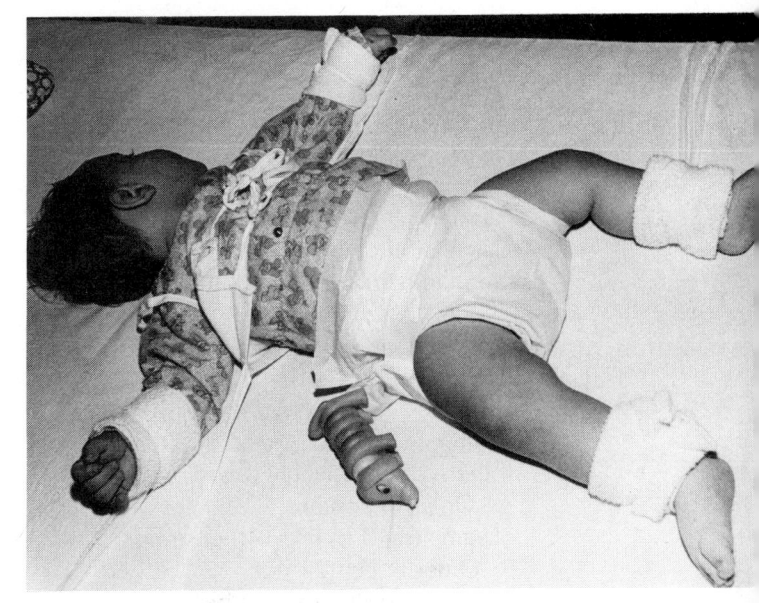

Figure 17–17 When a family member is not at the bedside, an active infant may require restraint of all extremities to prevent rolling over onto the scalp vein insertion site.

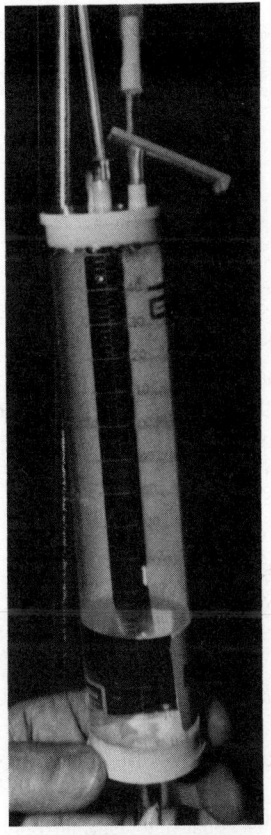

Figure 17–18 A special control chamber holds a limited amount of fluid and provides for accurate measurement of fluid administration.

---
*Drops.

PRINCIPLES AND SKILLS OF PEDIATRIC NURSING

tubing and check whether the IV runs by gravity, i.e., before threading it into pump. (This serves as a useful guide for comparison if difficulty with the IV is encountered later.)

5. Thread the tubing through the pump, set the desired rate and start the pump.

Calculation of the proper rate of fluid administration in pediatrics is simplified by the use of a system that delivers 60 gtts/min. Typical orders for fluid therapy are either ordered in cc's/hr or cc's/24 hrs. The following simple calculations will convert such orders into gtts/min.

If the system delivers 60 gtts/cc:
A. Order in cc's/hr:
  Example: 40 cc/hr = 40 gtts/min*
B. Order in cc's/24 hr.
  Example: 960 cc's/24 hr
  1. Change to cc's/hr
     960 ÷ 24 hrs = 40 cc/hr
  2. 40 cc/hr = 40 gtts/min*

The reason that cc's/hr = gtts/min is explained by the following:

Step 1:

No. cc's/hr ordered × no. gtts/cc delivered by system = no. gtts/hr
Example   40   ×   60   =   2400

Step 2:

No. gtts/hr ÷ no. min/hr = no. gtts/cc
    2400   ÷   60   =   40

In the first step one multiplies by 60 and in the second step one divides by 60; the beginning number of 40 remains unchanged. Thus, whenever the IV set is designed to deliver 60 gtts/cc the order of 40 cc's/hr can be immediately converted to 40 gtts/min without any calculations.

Maintaining the IV Maintaining an IV means that fluids will be administered accurately with maximum safety and benefit to the child. The machinery available to monitor IV's cannot be used to *replace* the nurse; they are used to *assist* the nurse. The pump system does not reduce the work for the nurse, but if used properly it

---

*cc's/hr can be equated to gtts/min *only if the system delivers 60 gtts/cc.*

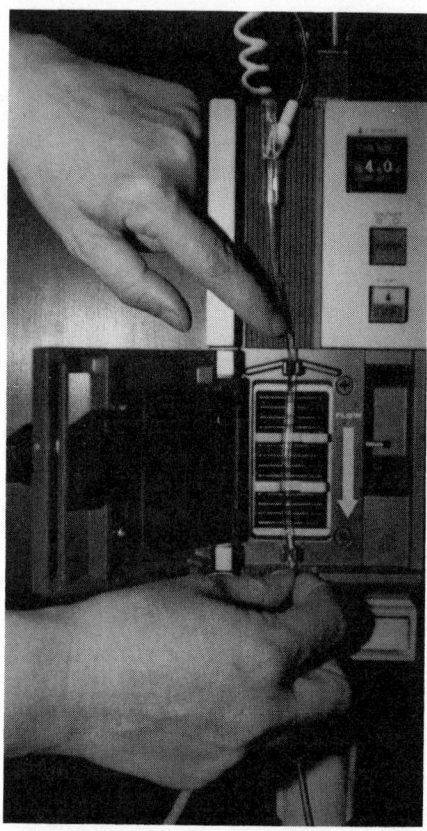

Figure 17-19 IV tubing is threaded through the pump, following the direction of the arrow on the pump. Pump designs vary; the placement of tubing through the pump may be vertical or horizontal, depending on the type of pump used.

increases the safety of parenteral administration.

At the beginning of each shift the nurse responsible for a particular IV must make a complete IV check. An important part of this assessment is to be sure that the proper solution is hanging and that correct electrolytes have been ordered. Also, the nurse should find out when the bottle and tubing were last changed. Most institutions have adopted the policy of changing solution and tubing every 24 hours. In pediatric practice, where IV rates are slow, small bottles of 250 cc's or 500 cc's are recommended to avoid unnecessary wasting of IV solutions. The nurse can make a quick assessment by checking the following:

1. Type of solution and electrolyte dose.
2. Date and time the bottle and tubing was hung.
3. Rate of the IV. Check the setting on the machine and *count the actual gtts/min.*
4. Check tubing for kinks or flattening and blood and air. This is done by following through the entire length of tubing to the insertion site.

5. Check that tubing is threaded into machine in the correct direction.
6. Check IV site for redness, puffiness and intactness of tape. Be sure tape is not too tight.
7. Check for blood return by pinching the tubing close to needle.
8. Check intactness and appropriateness of restraint. Check all involved extremities for warmth, color and general appearance.
9. See if a medication is running.
10. Verify that the amount is absorbed on schedule as prescribed.
11. Check general status of the child.
12. See if vital signs and urinary output are within normal limits.

The nurse should make this check in the presence of the nurse who was previously in charge of the child's care. It cannot be done without lighting; therefore, a flashlight must be used to make IV checks when children are asleep. A dim light from the hallway is not adequate. If there is any question regarding the site, overhead lights must be turned on even though the child and other children may awaken.

Special nursing care must be provided to all children with an IV. Hourly checks must be made including the following:
1. Check the setting on the machine and count the actual drops.
2. Check the entire length of tubing.
3. Check the site and restrained extremities.
4. Check the general status of the child.
5. Calculate the amount of fluid absorbed and enter it on an IV record sheet.

IV record sheets are used to monitor fluid administration. Types of forms used vary among institutions. Columns should be provided to show type of fluid being administered, rate of IV, amount of fluid actually absorbed hourly, and a running total to show total number of cc's absorbed per shift. A column should be provided for the nurse to write her comments about site, and each hourly check should be documented with the nurse's initials.

The nurse is also responsible for making ongoing assessments of the child's fluid, electrolyte, and acid-base balance whenever parenteral therapy (therapy by injection) is being administered. The previous discussion on assessment of vital signs, weight, skin, anterior fontanel and eyes, intake and output and urine specific gravity, and laboratory reports describes pertinent observations that must be made during intravenous therapy.

The nurse must also be aware of certain clinical situations that will affect fluid and electrolyte balance during fluid therapy. If a child is in a hot environment, has a fever or is tachypneic, insensible water loss is increased. For every degree of fever above 37.8° C 12 per cent of fluid maintenance is added. (For each degree of fever above 100° F 8 per cent of fluid maintenance is added.) Crying may double insensible water loss in a baby. Also, a newborn placed under a radiant heat warmer or in a phototherapy situation may have increased fluid loss through evaporation. Decreases in insensible water loss may also occur. Decreased insensible water losses occur in cool environments or if humidity is high. If these conditions exist when a child has renal disease or has a high concentration of antidiuretic hormone (ADH), water intake may need to be decreased.

A major responsibility of the nurse is to prevent the IV from clotting and to prevent infiltration (fluid collecting under the skin at the site). Clotting of IV's occurs when the fluid chamber becomes dry. Clotting can develop if the chamber remains dry only momentarily, therefore, it is essential to keep some fluid in the chamber at all times. An exception to keeping some fluid in the chamber occurs when medications are administered via the fluid chamber and it must be allowed to empty completely. In these circumstances the nurse can avoid clotting of the IV by being present to check it at about the time the chamber is expected to empty. As soon as the chamber empties the alarm rings, requiring an immediate response from the nurse.

Infiltration of IV's can best be prevented by use of secure restraints and proper insertion. In addition to providing for these, it is equally important for the nurse to be able to identify early infiltration of an IV. IV's must be checked by *looking at the actual insertion site* and then checking the surrounding area. Because infiltrated fluid collects in dependent areas, it is important to check underneath an arm or foot. Also, if tape appears to be becoming tighter, infiltration should be suspected. Fluid not only causes puffiness at the site but it also causes enlargement of the entire limb. When a scalp vein site infiltrates, a generalized fullness can be noted and slight asymmetry of the head may be apparent. Lack of blood return is not always proof of infiltration. The best test for infiltration is to take a "mental picture" of the site when the first IV check is made and carefully check its appearance hourly to compare it to its original appearance.

Any degree of infiltration causes discomfort to the child. The nurse's expertise in managing IV's is a skill that greatly contributes to the recovery and well-being of a child. Large amounts of infiltration are serious and may even require skin grafting. Infiltration during medication administration is particularly dangerous; thus before any medication is added to an IV, a thorough assessment must be made of the site. Also, the site should be checked *during* administration of the medication.

Providing Comfort to Child and Family During IV Therapy

A major responsibility of the nurse is to prepare the child and family effectively and keep them appropriately involved. Age-appropriate suggestions are offered in Table 17–13 for preparation of the child and involvement of the family.

Intravenous therapy, to the nurse, is a common pediatric procedure. However, to the child and family it has a variety of meanings and is the subject of numerous fears. The nurse must therefore approach IV therapy with a concern and recognition of the individuals' particular fears and questions. The need for an IV may mean to the family that their child's condition is more serious than it actually is. Responding to individual needs for reassurance and comfort is primary, even though for the nurse starting and maintaining an IV are common procedures.

A gentle, positive approach to the child will facilitate gaining the child's cooperation. Whether the parents should stay or leave when an IV is started is a decision that should be made with the child, the parent and the nurse taken into account. There is no prescribed rule to follow. Some parents wish to stay and are able to provide support to the child; the nurse's skill is not affected adversely by their presence. In such cases it may be beneficial for the child if the parent stays. However, if the parents' fears are communicated to the child, or if the nurse cannot work as effectively with parents present, they usually will agree to wait in a lounge away from the room.

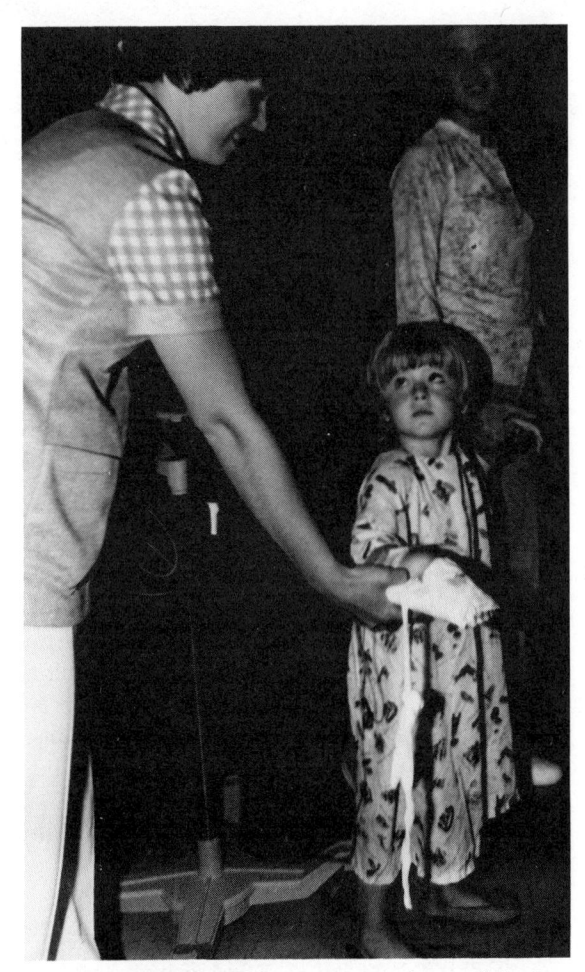

Older children should be encouraged to walk in the hospital hall and go to the playroom with proper assistance to prevent dislodging of the IV.

Children with IV's should not be immobilized unnecessarily. Young children with IV's require restraints when unsupervised, but parents and nurses can hold them, take them for a ride or take them to a play room. Older children can be up in wheelchairs can be allowed to walk in the halls and can go to the play area.

Age-appropriate independence to the degree the IV permits should be fostered. Parents can be taught how to care for the child or assist the child in self-care or do both. Too often parents fear dislodging the IV and defer to the nurse when care is required. The physical isolation that is imposed by an IV makes it particularly important that the nurse make every effort to assist parents to become involved to the degree they can be and desire to be. The child benefits by the comfort of feeling close to his parent and the parent derives a feeling of comfort by providing that closeness.

References

1. Abbott Laboratories. Fluid and Electrolytes: Some Practical Guides to Clinical Use. Abbott Laboratories, 1970
2. L. A. Barness. Nutrition and nutritional disorders. In Nelson Textbook of Pediatrics. V. C. Vaughn et al, W. B. Saunders Co., 1979
3. A. Burgess. The Nurse's Guide to Fluid and Electrolyte Balance. McGraw-Hill Book Co., 1979
4. S. V. Dube. Metabolic emergencies. In Immediate Care of the Sick and Injured Child. S. K. Dube, ed., C. V. Mosby, 1978
5. G. B. Forbes. Nutritional requirements. In Principles of Pediatrics, R. A. Hoekelman et al., McGraw-Hill Book Co., 1978
6. M. A. Holliday and W. E. Segar. The maintenance need for water in parenteral fluid therapy. Pediatrics, 1957, p. 823
7. N. W. Metheney and W. D. Snively. Nurses' Handbook of Fluid Balance. J. B. Lippincott Co., 1979
8. G. M. Reed. Confused about potassium - Here's a clear concise guide. Nursing '74, March 1974, p. 23
9. A. M. Robson. The pathophysiology of body fluids. In Nelson Textbook of Pediatrics. V. C. Vaughn et al., W. B. Saunders, 1979
10. W. D. Snively. Sea Within: Story of Our Body Fluids. J. B. Lippincott Co., 1960
11. M. J. Sweeney. Fluid therapy. In Principles of Pediatrics. R. A. Hoekelman et al., McGraw-Hill Book Co., 1978
12. M. T. Twombly. The Shift Into Third Space. Nursing '78, June 1978, p. 38
13. R. W. Winters. The Body Fluids In Pediatrics. Little, Brown & Co., 1973

TOTAL PARENTERAL NUTRITION (HYPERALIMENTATION)

by Anita Clavier, RN, BSN

Total parenteral nutrition (TPN) is the provision of all nutrients needed to sustain life through the venous system. This therapy is used either as a supplement to a regular diet or as the sole method of providing nutrition. To provide parenteral nutrition safely, the nurse must be aware of the child's nutritional requirements, the composition of the solution, the indications for TPN, the implications for nursing care and the potential complications.

NUTRITIONAL REQUIREMENTS

The goal of this therapy is to ensure that the patient is in an anabolic state. To accomplish this, the TPN infusate (the solution being administered) must meet all the patient's nutritional requirements. Enough calories and protein must be supplied not only to meet the child's needs to maintain life but also to promote growth. In conjunction with maintenance and growth, the requirements are based on the child's age and weight. For example, the newborn and the infant require 90 to 120 calories/kg/day and 2.0 to 3.5 grams protein/kg/day.[1] The adolescent requires 30 to 60 calories/kg/day and 1.0 to 1.7 grams protein/kg/day.[1] These energy requirements are increased by surgery, sepsis, each degree of fever and the degree of burn.[5]

COMPOSITION OF TPN SOLUTIONS

TPN consists of giving the child the required protein, carbohydrates, fat, electrolytes, vitamins and trace elements. Protein is most commonly provided in the form of crystalline amino acids.[3] Adequate carbohydrates and fat must be the source of calories so that the amino acids provided are utilized for protein synthesis, not for energy. The amount of dextrose to be infused is limited by the child's tolerance to the dextrose and location of the intravenous catheter. The child's tolerance is measured by serum and urine glucose levels. Hypertonic TPN is initiated slowly and the rate and concentration of dextrose are gradually increased to allow the pancreas to respond to the increased demand for insulin.[1] The hypertonic solution, which has a high osmolality, must be infused in a large vein, in which there is a more rapid blood flow, to decrease the irritation to the vein. A child with the catheter tip in a large vein, such as the superior vena cava, can receive as high a final concentration as 25 to 47 per cent.[1] If the child is receiving the infusion through a peripheral vein, the maximum final concentration of dextrose is 12.5 per cent.[1]

For additional calories, a fat emulsion may be infused. The calories provided by fat are especially important in peripheral TPN because the carbohydrate source of calories is decreased. The fat emulsion is nearly isotonic so it may be infused in either peripheral or central veins. By infusing the fat emulsion simultaneously with the dextrose and amino acid solution, the osmolality of the total infusate is decreased. Fat emulsions are also given to prevent essential fatty acid deficiency.

Electrolytes, vitamins and trace elements are also included in the parenteral nutrition infusate. Electrolytes include potassium, sodium, chloride, calcium, phosphorus and magnesium. Electrolyte requirements are determined by the serum levels. Daily basic electrolyte requirements must be met along with the additional needs resulting from such factors as the particular disease process, surgery or both. Water- and fat-soluble vitamins are given to the child routinely. Some of these vitamins may be added to the TPN infusate. Trace element requirements for infants are still being determined; school-age children and adolescents usually receive trace elements in the solution two or more times a week. The trace elements commonly added are zinc, copper, iodide and manganese.[1]

The dextrose, amino acids, electrolytes, vitamins and trace elements are mixed in one container by a pharmacist. This is done under a laminar air flow hood to decrease the risk of contamination. The fat emulsion is administered from a separate container because the addition of any other solution could disrupt the stability of the emulsion.

INDICATIONS FOR TPN ADMINISTRATION

TPN is indicated when the patient is unable to take any nourishment by mouth, or if what he can take is inadequate. The patient may be malnourished or prolonged starvation may be expected. The indications for each child must be weighed against the potential life-threatening complications related to TPN infusion before TPN is chosen. The child's age, current nutritional status and clinical status are considered when deciding if TPN is indicated. For example, the newborn, especially the premature newborn, has minimal nutritional reserves, so parenteral nutrition may be given sooner than in the older child.[1]

Clinical conditions in the newborn and infant that generally are indications for parenteral nutrition include major anomalies (congenital or acquired) of the gastrointestinal tract, chronic intractable diarrhea, necrotizing enterocolitis, and very low birthweight (less than 1200 gm).[2, 4] Indications for toddlers and older children are similar to adults. Inflammatory bowel disease, short bowel syndrome, fistulas, severe burns, major trauma, acute pancreatitis, renal failure and hepatic failure are some conditions in which TPN is commonly used.

NURSING RESPONSIBILITIES IN TPN ADMINISTRATION

Nursing care is very important in preventing or monitoring complications that can occur with total parenteral nutrition. Table 17–14 lists common complications. Nursing care to prevent complications includes careful administration and monitoring of the TPN solution and meticulous catheter care. A description of these aspects of care follows.

TPN Administration The TPN solution must be administered at a constant rate to avoid po-

TABLE 17–14 COMPLICATIONS OF TOTAL PARENTERAL NUTRITION

Metabolic
Hyperglycemia
Hypoglycemia
Imbalance of fluids, electrolytes, vitamins and trace elements
Acid-base disorders
Hepatic disorders
Mechanical
Air emboli
Infiltration/sloughing
Thrombosis
Occlusion
Septic
Localized infection
General sepsis

tential metabolic complications. The infusion rate must never be adjusted to "catch up." Whether a pump or a Buretrol system is used to assist with controlling the rate, it is still vital that the nurse check the rate by counting the drops every 30 to 60 minutes.

The bottle, IV administration tubing and filter (if used) must be changed every 24 hours to prevent infection. Frequently the practice is to place the sterile extension tubing partly under the dressing so it is changed only with the dressing change. All connections in the tubing system must be cleaned with Iodophor solution to prevent yeast and bacterial growth. The connections are then taped to prevent accidental separation.

Whenever a fat emulsion is being infused, it must be added aseptically below the filter because the fat particles are too large to pass through the filter. It should be added as close to the intravenous site as possible so there is minimal mixture of the two infusates.

Since drug compatibilities with parenteral nutrition have not been established, medications should not be added to either the dextrose and amino acid solution or the fat emulsion. Also, with the high risk of infection due to the concentrated dextrose solution, additions to the central intravenous line must be restricted to the fat emulsion. To prevent hypoglycemia a hypertonic dextrose solution must be administered IV whenever hypertonic TPN must be suddenly discontinued.

Catheter Care A child may receive parenteral nutrition through either a central or a peripheral vein. For a hypertonic solution the tip of the catheter must be placed into the superior vena cava. In the newborn and infant this is accomplished by inserting a silicone rubber catheter through the internal or external jugular vein to the superior vena cava. The catheter is then tunneled subcutaneously to an exit site two to four inches away from the vein insertion site. In the newborn and infant this exit site is usually on the scalp; in the young child the site may be in the neck or chest wall.[1,6] School-age and older children may have a catheter inserted into the superior vena cava via the subclavian vein. (This is also commonly used in adults.[7]) To avoid potential complications resulting from infusing the hypertonic solution outside the superior vena cava, an isotonic solution must be infused until the placement of the catheter tip is confirmed by x-ray.

Proper nursing care of the catheter is vital to decrease the risk of infection, both local and systemic. The dressing should be changed every 48 hours and whenever it is wet or loose, using sterile standardized technique. The site should be cleaned with an acetone and alcohol solution followed by Iodophor solution, cleansing from the site in an outward direction. After the antibacterial and antifungal ointment is applied, the site is covered with a small sterile dressing. Then the extension tubing is changed while the child performs, or someone simulates, the Valsalva maneuver* to prevent air embolus. The connection between the catheter and Luer Lok extension tubing is then covered with part of the sterile dressing. With hypoallergenic tape, the dressing is taped occlusively, then dated and signed. Part of the extension tubing should be looped and taped on top of the secured dressing to prevent direct tension on the catheter. The physician should be notified if erythema, edema, drainage or any change in catheter placement (i.e., catheter kink or loose sutures) is noted.

If the final glucose concentration of the solution is 12.5% or below, it may be given through a peripheral vein. In infants, the site is commonly a scalp vein; in the older child frequently one of the larger arm veins is used. The site must be checked at least every 30 minutes for the possibility of vein irritation or infiltration. If infiltration is suspected, the site must be changed immediately because of the risk of sloughing. Care of the intravenous site is the same as for any peripheral intravenous site.

Monitoring The nurse must carefully monitor the child receiving parenteral nutrition, whether it is a peripheral or central venous infusion. The child should be weighed daily to assess the fluid balance and the effectiveness of the nutritional therapy. In addition, a daily strict intake and output record must be maintained to assess the fluid balance. The record must show a breakdown of the total intake and output, so the calorie intake, nitrogen intake and output may be accurately determined. After the condition of

---

*The Valsalva maneuver involves forcible exhalation against the closed glottis. The child may perform this maneuver by taking a deep breath and bearing down as if having a bowel movement. This may be simulated by applying pressure to the abdomen, if this is not contraindicated.

the newborn or the infant has been stabilized on parenteral nutrition, a diaper count may be obtained for the urine output. Blood pressure, pulse, respirations and temperature must be checked at least every eight hours. Also, urine fractionals are checked at least every eight hours. It is very important to continue to check urine fractionals because stress, infection, pain and major trauma can affect glucose tolerance. Glucosuria of 2+ or greater must be corrected to prevent eventual development of hyperosmotic nonketotic coma.[7,8] Dextrostix should be used to check the blood sugar for possible hypoglycemia whenever the infusion is suddenly decreased or stopped. In the newborn or the infant the urine pH, protein, ketones, specific gravity, head circumference and length are also regularly checked.

Oral Hygiene Oral hygiene is a very important, but often forgotten, part of nursing care. Oral hygiene must be performed at least three times a day to prevent such complications as oral lesions and parotitis. Brushing teeth to prevent tooth decay is important for all children and especially for these children who are allowed hard candy as the only oral intake.

Exercise Exercise is important to maintain or regain muscle strength and for the proper utilization of the nutrition the child is receiving. Unless otherwise contraindicated, the child should be allowed and encouraged to move as freely as possible with proper protection for the IV line. Frequently, physical or occupational therapists are involved to assist in the promotion of proper exercise.

Emotional Needs The nurse must be aware of the emotional impact total parenteral nutrition can have on the child and his family. Information and support given to the child depends on the child's age and level of understanding. The family must be kept informed about what is happening to the child.

The newborn or infant who is receiving nothing by mouth (NPO) needs a pacifier so that his sucking needs are met. Also, the baby should be held at regular intervals since the child will not routinely be held for meals. The importance of remaining NPO and avoiding dislodgement of the intravenous needle must be explained to both the older child and the family. Different flavored mouthwashes may be offered to the child to give him some taste sensations. Since some children still feel hungry even when receiving adequate parenteral nutrition, they will need extra attention or distraction during mealtimes and when they see food or food advertisements. The reasons for the monitoring done by the nurses and physicians must be explained to the child and family so that their understanding will enhance their acceptance and cooperation.

Many of these children have chronic illnesses and consequently are hospitalized for a long time. Since family members are not always able to be present, the children will need extra love and attention from the nursing staff.

Adequate nutrition for weight maintenance and growth is vital for children. Rapid healing and immune competence depend on nutritional status. For the malnourished or potentially malnourished child, parenteral nutrition can satisfy all nutritional requirements if dietary intake is contraindicated. However, before enteral nutrition can be initiated, it must be determined that the risks of starvation are greater than the risks of parenteral nutrition. Informed nursing care will greatly decrease the risks of parenteral nutrition.

References

1. A. Coran. Nutritional support of the pediatric surgical patient. In Pediatric Surgery by T. Holder and K. Aschcraft. W. B. Saunders Co., 1980.
2. D. Feliciano and R. Telander. Total parenteral nutrition in infants and children. Mayo Clinical Proceedings, October 1976, p. 648
3. W. Heird and R. Winters. Total parenteral nutrition: The state of the art. Journal of pediatrics. January 1975, p. 3
4. J. Keating et al. An experience with total parenteral nutrition. American Journal of Clinical Nutrition, September 1977, p. 1508
5. J. Kinney. Energy requirements for parenteral nutrition. In Total Parenteral Nutrition, E. Fischer, ed., Little, Brown & Co., 1976
6. C. Muttart. The role of the pediatric nurse in total parenteral nutrition. Presented at the 2nd Annual Clinical Congress of the American Society of Parenteral Nutrition, Houston, February 1978
7. K. Phillips. Nursing care in parenteral nutrition. In Total Parenteral Nutrition, G. E. Fisher, ed., Little, Brown & Company, 1976
8. J. Ryan. Complications of total parenteral nutrition. In Total Parenteral Nutrition, G. E. Fisher, ed., Little, Brown, & Company, 1976

NURSING CARE OF CHILDREN REQUIRING ANESTHESIA

by Mary Jean Yablonky, BSN, CRNA

Anesthesia is but one part of the total hospital experience of the pediatric surgical patient. It has been reported, however, that children can suffer tremendous emotional consequences as a result of their anesthetic experience. How a child responds to his anesthetic experience depends on the preparation that he has been given for anesthesia and surgery.

Table 17–15 summarizes care of children requiring anesthesia.

PREANESTHETIC PREPARATION TO MINIMIZE STRESS

Children's fears concerning anesthesia are age-related. Young children from 6 months to 3 years of age fear separation from their parents. This has been demonstrated by behavioral disturbances caused by fears that occur after hospitalization: fear of strangers, fear of the dark and fear of separation from parents. Allowing the child to bring a favorite toy or blanket to the operating room and encouraging his parents to be with him in the immediate preoperative period and as soon as possible in the postoperative period help allay some of the fears of separation.

The preschooler has fears that stem from an inability to understand the rationale for specific treatments and procedures. Preschool children are egocentric and their reactions to illness, anesthesia and surgery are directly related to this stage of their development. Hospitalization forces the preschooler into a state of dependence while developmentally he is trying to assert his independence. Every effort should be made to explain procedures to the preschooler in language he can understand and, when possible, he should be permitted active participation in his care (holding the anesthesia mask while breathing himself to sleep.

School-age children fear the anesthesia itself. They are curious as to how they will go to sleep. "What if I'm not tired?" is an often-asked question. Explaining to these children that "anesthesia sleep" is a special kind of sleep caused by "medicines" that work even when the child is not tired will help to dispel some of these fears. Some children at this age have been told by their families, upon the death of a relative or the loss of a pet, that the person or animal is "sleeping." To this child, sleep is equated with death; anesthesia, when explained in terms of sleep, is viewed as being permanent. These children need to be reassured that anesthesia is a special type of sleep, and that, at the completion of their surgery, they will wake up. Adolescents fear what will happen to them while they are under anesthesia. They are concerned about body image and what they may do while in a state of unawareness. They need to be reassured that only what is supposed to be done will occur and that they need not fear doing or saying anything that will injure their self-image while under anesthesia.

All children scheduled for surgery should have a preoperative visit by the person who will be administering their anesthetic. Besides to gather pertinent medical data, the visit is an opportunity for the anesthetist to establish rapport with the child and his parents and to communicate with the nurses who are caring for the child. As parental anxiety is often transmitted to the child, every effort should be made to gain their confidence by explaining the anesthetic procedure to them. The anesthetic procedure should also be explained to the child in language he can understand so as to dispel some of his fears and misconceptions. The

TABLE 17-15 SUMMARY OF PREANESTHETIC AND POSTANESTHETIC CARE OF THE PEDIATRIC PATIENT

Expected Outcome	Intervention	Rationale
Child will suffer minimal psychological trauma as a result of his anesthetic/surgical experience	Explain pre- and postanesthetic routines and procedures to child and parents.	Parental anxiety is transmitted to child. Adequate information on routines, procedures and outcomes helps decrease anxiety.
	Encourage child to express his concerns and fears of the anesthetic and surgery.	Children have age-related fears about anesthesia.
	Encourage parents to visit with child in the immediate preanesthetic period.	Parental presence increases child's security and decreases anxiety.
	Allow child to bring a favorite toy or object with him to the operating room.	Security items help decrease some fears of separation.
The child will be physically prepared for his anesthetic/surgery.	Maintain NPO status.	A potential risk during anesthesia induction is aspiration of gastric contents. Length of preanesthetic fast is determined to provide adequate time for stomach emptying.
	Remove make-up, nail polish, jewelry and prosthetic devices.	Make-up and nail polish camouflage normal skin and nailbed color, parameters used to assess adequacy of tissue oxygenation during anesthesia. Jewelry and prosthetic devices can become lost or damaged if removed in operating room.
	Check that child has on a proper identification bracelet.	Provide operating room personnel with a means for properly identifying child.
	Instruct the child to void before receiving premedication.	Anesthetics diminish and/or abolish normal bladder-emptying reflexes. Assuring that the bladder is empty before surgery decreases risk of bladder distention during anesthesia.
	Administer premedication(s) at the appropriate time.	Premedication(s) help sedate before surgery or act as an adjunct to a planned balanced anesthetic technique. Premedication(s) given at appropriate time assures that child will derive desired response.
Child will have an anesthetic induction that is appropriate for his physical condition	Anesthetic technique and anesthetic agent(s) used will be chosen by the anesthetist/anesthesiologist assigned to child.	
Child will emerge uneventfully from his anesthetic and have a safe postoperative course.	Monitor vital signs every 15 minutes or more often if child's condition is unstable.	Vital signs reflect changes in child's condition. A decreasing blood pressure, increasing heart rate, weak, thready pulse, and cool, clammy skin indicate shock.
	Assess adequacy of ventilation.	The child's tracheal anatomy makes him more susceptible to laryngeal edema after tracheal intubation. Respiratory depression may indicate inadequate reversal of drugs used as part of anesthetic.
	Restrain child during his emergence from anesthesia	Children may become delirious during their anesthetic emergence and need to be restrained to protect them from harm and prevent them from dislodging IV lines, chest tubes, drains, etc.
	Observe operative site for drainage and/or bleeding.	The physician should be notified of increased bleeding and/or drainage on the dressing.
	Initiate reunion of child and his parents as soon as possible in the postoperative period.	Parental presence in the recovery area decreases separation anxiety for both parent and child and increases child's security.

nurse should be present whenever possible for at least part of the anesthetist's visit so that she can accurately reinforce the explanations that have been given.

In situations in which an inhalation induction is planned, the anesthetist may show the child the mask that will be used and explain to the child how he will breathe the anesthetic gases through the mask. Upon completion of the preanesthetic visit, the anesthetist will be better prepared to administer a safe and appropriate anesthetic to a child with whom he has established rapport, and the child will be better prepared for his anesthetic by having a better understanding of what to expect.

PREANESTHETIC PHYSICAL PREPARATION

All children who are to receive an anesthetic must undergo a period of fasting before surgery to eliminate the risk of aspiration upon induction of anesthesia. The length of the fasting period is determined on the basis of the child's age and should be specified in the preoperative orders. The nurse should explain to the child and his parents the reason for the fast, and she should see to it that the child remains NPO as ordered. If oral intake inadvertently occurs, the nurse should notify the anesthesia staff immediately as this may necessitate the postponement of the child's surgery rather than risking aspiration.

Premedication is ordered by the anesthetist for some children to help sedate them before receiving anesthesia or it is ordered as an adjunct to a planned balanced anesthetic technique. Before administering the premedication, the nurse should instruct the child to void. This is necessary to eliminate the risk of having a sedated child attempt to get out of bed to go to the bathroom and possibly fall and injure himself. Voiding at this time also decreases the risk of bladder distention occurring during anesthesia. Once the child receives his premedication he should be placed in bed with the side rails up for safety, and he should not be unnecessarily disturbed so that he may derive maximum benefit from the sedative effects of the medication. Therefore, it is important for the nurse to be sure that the child is properly prepared for the operating room before the time he receives his premedication. This preparation includes seeing to it that the child is properly attired, that he has an identification number on either his wrist or ankle, and when applicable, that jewelry, make-up, nail polish and prosthetic devices have been removed.

Once prepared for surgery, the child will be transported to the operating room. If the child is asleep from his premedication, his parents should be discouraged from awakening him to give him a kiss or to say goodbye, because the child may be disoriented from his medication and arousing him will only add to his anxiety.

ANESTHETIC MANAGEMENT OF THE PEDIATRIC PATIENT

Parents and older children have many questions about the period of anesthesia. Although the nurse on the unit is not required to participate in management of the patient during anesthesia, she should be familiar with what will occur so she can answer questions accurately. An understanding of the period of anesthesia also provides the nurse with information that is needed to give safe postoperative nursing care.

Once the child is brought into the operating room, he is under the constant care of an anesthetist. Unnecessary conversation and the opening of instruments should cease with the child's arrival into the operating room. Everyone's attention should focus on the child and every effort should be made to eliminate stress before and during the induction of anesthesia.

Anesthesia is induced by one of four routes: inhalation, intravenous, intramuscular and rectal. The most commonly used routes are intravenous and inhalation. The method for the intravenous route consists of inserting a needle or catheter in an extremity vein. The anesthetic medication is then administered through this site. The most frequently used intravenous induction agents are the very short-acting barbiturates thiopental, thiamylal, and methohexital. They have the advantage of a rapid onset of amnesia and unconsciousness. Ketamine is used as an intravenous induction agent in certain situations, but its use is limited by its pharmacological effects.

The inhalation method of anesthesia induction consists of the child "breathing" himself to sleep by inhaling a mixture of oxygen and the anesthetic agent. The agents used are gases (nitrous oxide) or vapors of liquid agents (Fluothane, enflurane, methoxyflurane), or a combination of the two. The anesthetic mixture is delivered through a mask that is attached to an anesthetic circuit. Some children prefer to hold the mask themselves during the induction. This gives them a sense of control as well as a feeling of participation in their anesthetic administration. Throughout the inhalation induction, the anesthetist should talk to the child, reassuring him that he is doing well and explaining that the dizziness and floating sensation he is experiencing are normal for a person breathing an anesthetic mixture. During the induction, the child should be reassured that at the completion of his surgery he will wake up in the recovery room.

Methods for the intramuscular and rectal routes of anesthesia induction are used when the inhalation agents are inappropriate for the patient's known pathophysiology and an intravenous line cannot be inserted without causing the child tremendous trauma and pain. The agents used for the intramuscular route are ketamine or a 5 per cent solution of methohexital. A specially prepared suspension of thiopental is used for rectal induction. The route selected for induction of anesthesia should be appropriate for the child's condition, and the method should be executed with skill so as to minimize both physical and psychological trauma to the child.

Once the induction is completed, anesthesia is maintained with one of the inhalation agents, intravenous narcotics and sedatives or a combination of inhalation agents and intravenous medication. When indicated by the operative site or surgical position, a muscle relaxant may also be used as part of the anesthetic. Throughout the surgical procedure the child's physiological response to the anesthetic is assessed. He receives appropriate glucose and electrolyte therapy and, when indicated, blood replacement. Upon completion of the surgical procedure, the anesthesia is discontinued and the child will be transferred to the postanesthesia recovery area.

POSTANESTHESIA RECOVERY

In the recovery area the anesthetist transfers the care of the child to a nurse experienced in caring for children recovering from anesthesia. At the time of transfer, the nurse is given a report on the surgical procedure that was performed, the child's physical and psychological preoperative state, the type of anesthetic that was administered and the child's response to the anesthetic agent.

This nurse's responsibility is to see that the child safely emerges from his anesthetic. The nurse should monitor the child's vital signs frequently, immediately alerting the physician of any signs and symptoms of shock (decreasing blood pressure; increasing heart rate; weak, thready pulse; cool, clammy skin). Children are prone to laryngeal edema, especially after endoscopy and tracheal intubation.

Children with stridor should be placed in a mist tent and carefully observed for signs of respiratory obstruction. If a muscle relaxant or narcotic was used as part of the anesthetic, the child should be watched for signs and symptoms of respiratory depression, which may be caused by inadequate reversal of these drugs. The operative site should be checked for bleeding and any increased or continual bleeding reported to the child's physician. Some children may become delirious during their emergence from anesthesia. These children need to be restrained in order to protect them from harm during this period. Parents should be reunited with their children as soon as possible in the postoperative period. This helps to relieve parental anxiety caused by the operation and helps to increase the child's sense of security as well as decrease his separation anxiety. Once the child's condition is stable and he is fully awakened from his anesthetic, he will be discharged from the postanesthesia recovery area by an anesthesiologist.

References

1. T. Brown and B. Fisk. Anesthesia for Children. Blackwell Scientific Publications, 1979
2. J. Eckenhoff. Relationship of anesthesia to postoperative personality changes in children. American Journal of Diseases of Children, November 1953, p. 587
3. B. Korsch. The child and the operating room. Anesthesiology, August 1975, p. 251
4. D. Levy. Psychic trauma of operations in children and note on combat neurosis. American Journal of Diseases of Children, January 1945, p. 7
5. R. Smith. Anesthesia for Infants and Children. C. V. Mosby Co., 1980
6. K. Whitt et al. Children's conceptions of illness and cognitive development. Clinical Pediatrics, June 1979, p. 327

PREOPERATIVE AND POSTOPERATIVE NURSING CARE

by Mabel Hunsberger, BSN, MSN

Parents look to the nurse to answer their questions and to assist in the effective management of their child's preoperative and postoperative experience. To meet these expectations satisfactorily the nurse must be skilled in handling the unique responses of a child and family, making adaptations for the age of the child and the particular circumstances within the family. She must also be knowledgeable in caring for a child undergoing anesthesia and provide the specialized care required for the various surgical procedures.

Specific age-related approaches to prepare children for procedures and surgery are discussed in the age-specific chapters on hospitalization. Specialized nursing care for the various surgical problems is discussed throughout the text as applicable. The following is a general discussion on preoperative and postoperative nursing care when a child requires surgery.

PREOPERATIVE NURSING CARE

Usually the child is admitted on the day before surgery; this allows time for orienting him to the unit and preparing him for the events of the following day. Parents are encouraged to stay with their child during this period of preparation; their presence is comforting to the child and provides an opportunity for the nurse and the family to become acquainted.

A history and nursing assessment is completed on admission. Special attention is given to gathering information about the child's and family's understanding of the operation. The order of events should be explained; the parents are encouraged to see their child on the morning before the operation. In many institutions parents may visit on a 24-hour basis and may stay the entire preoperative night. When this is not the practice, parents must be told what time the surgery will be; usually they are advised to arrive at least an hour before the scheduled operation to see their child, but this varies.

Psychological Preparation The nurse reviews with the child and family any preoperative restrictions related to food and drink intake, activity and so forth. The child must also be forewarned that he will receive a "shot" before surgery. An opportunity to play with hospital equipment acquaints him with his environment and the events that will follow. Children should be prepared for the scrub gown and masks worn by operating room personnel.

Drawings or demonstrations can be useful in answering the older child's questions about the operation. Some institutions give a slide or movie presentation to prepare children preoperatively. Also, the child and family are prepared for postoperative care as the nurse explains the IV, the need for monitoring vital signs frequently and the placement of a dressing. She adds that medicine is available for the discomfort that may be experienced. Whether these explanations are given to the child the evening before or the morning of surgery depends on the child's age. Older children who can cooperate in coughing and deep breathing should be assisted to practice the evening before surgery. Usually the anesthetist visits and prepares the child in an age-appropriate way for anesthesia. The parents need to be given an explanation and an opportunity to ask questions regarding anesthesia. After the anesthetist has talked to the parents, the consent form can be signed and witnessed.

A preoperative psychological checklist can provide an organized method of preparation.

Pediatric Psychological Checklist for Surgery	
Patient's Name: **Unit #:** **Rm #:** **Service:**	**Directions:** 1. The following items will be covered before surgery or procedures. 2. All explanations will include parents or some other responsible person(s). 3. All explanations will consider the child's developmental level.

ITEM	INITIAL
1. Explain operation or procedure. Have patient verbalize understanding.	
2. Explain and get return demonstration of coughing, deep breathing, and using blow bottles. Emphasize importance and rationale.	
3. Explain dietary limitations, if any.	
4. Explain postoperative use of equipment, bandages, tubes, restraints. Use pictures if they are necessary.	
5. Inform child of preoperative injections. Be honest. It will hurt.	
6. Explain about the "stretcher man" who wears green and will take the child to the operating room on a stretcher. Explain that O.R. personnel also wear green suits and that someone will be with the child at all times. Allow the child to play with O.R. hats, masks, gloves, etc.	
7. Let child know that parent will wait closeby for his return.	
8. Explain about the "special sleep" (anesthesia) for the operation or procedure and the method of inducing it. Emphasize that the doctor will wake the child up only when the operation is over. For those seven years old and younger anesthesia is administered via face mask. Let child play with demonstration mask. For those 8 years and older intravenous medication is used.	
9. Explain about the recovery room and how the child will stay there until awake. Emphasize that the child will be cared for by special nurses in green.	
10. Allow child to select gift from the Toy Chest.	
11. Answer questions.	

Comments:

_____

_____

_____

This checklist is a guideline that can be adapted to the specific needs of a particular institution. As each phase of preparation is completed the checklist is initialed to avoid repetition when more than one nurse is involved in this preoperative stage.[6]

Physical Preparation The nurse also is responsible for physical preparation of the child. A complete blood count and urinalysis are routinely done on admission. The nurse should check the chart to be sure that these tests have been done. Any abnormal laboratory results or unusual clinical findings (especially elevated temperature) should be reported to the surgeon and documented in the chart.

On the evening before surgery the child is prepared for bed and offered a drink, as all fluids will be removed from his room during the night or early morning. This should be explained to the child and the parents. He is bathed either at bedtime or early in the morning before he receives his preoperative medication.

On the morning of surgery he is given mouth care and again reminded that he is not allowed to have water. Because children are frequently ambulatory before surgery, it is necessary not only to place identification on the child but also on the bed and the door of his room. Placing a broad piece of tape across the front of his gown with "I may not eat or drink" usually ensures that another uniformed adult will not give the child anything to eat or drink. It is helpful if, during breakfast, the parent or a nurse can engage the child in an activity in an area away from the vicinity where other children are eating.

A preoperative checklist is placed on the front of the child's chart. This list contains the basic preoperative care that must be done before the child is released from the unit. These lists vary in their content. Table 17–16 lists nursing responsibilities that are commonly performed preoperatively. As it is completed the item on the list is initaled or checked off.

The preoperative medication is given either at a specified time or when a call is received from the operating room (on-call). All the preparations in Table 17–15 should be completed

(From D. Treloar. Ready, set—No: Something is missing from pediatric pre-op preparation. Copyright 1978, American Journal of Nursing Company. Reprinted with permission from MCN, The American Journal of Maternal Child Nursing, Jan/Feb 1978, p. 51.)

TABLE 17-16 PREOPERATIVE CARE CHECKLIST

1. Vital signs are taken and recorded on the chart. Preferably they should also be recorded on the preoperative checklist. Temperature, pulse, and respirations are always recorded; blood pressure is usually taken on any child over 3 years but this varies with condition of the child and policy of the institution. Any abnormal findings are reported to the surgeon and a note should be attached to the front of the chart drawing attention to such findings. The nurse should also record in the chart that she has notified the surgeon, including the time.
2. The child's height and weight are recorded on the chart and checklist.
3. All preoperative laboratory tests are completed (including blood type and crossmatch, if ordered). Any abnormalities have been reported to the surgeon and the chart marked accordingly.
4. The child has been assessed for allergies and these are clearly marked on the chart.
5. All external objects such as ribbons, barrettes, glasses, contact lenses, jewelry have been removed. Long hair is kept in place by a rubber band. Nail polish is removed.
6. The mouth has been checked for braces and loose teeth. Braces were removed and given to parents Loose teeth have been brought to the attention of the anesthetist.
7. The ID band is correct and secure, and the crib or bed is marked correctly if child is to be transported in a crib or bed.
8. The consent form (anesthetic and operative) are on the chart and correctly signed and witnessed.
9. All surgical preparation procedures have been completed (e.g., skin prep, enema, NPO maintained, nasogastric tube inserted).
10. The child has voided.
11. The child has been bathed and has clean gown and underpants or diaper.

---

before the preoperative medication is given. The medication is brought to the room, the child is told that it will hurt a bit and it will make him sleepy. After the preoperative medication is given the child is kept in bed with the side rails up or is quietly held in the parent's arms, whichever is most soothing to the child. Just before the child is taken to the operating room, the nurse should again be sure that the names on the chart, on the child, and on the bed coincide. The nurse must also ensure that the young child has a needed source of comfort to take with him, such as his special blanket, teddy bear, or other security object.

POSTOPERATIVE NURSING CARE

The nurse's responsibility in caring for a child postoperatively is multifaceted. She must be knowledgeable about the effect of anesthesia, the type of surgery performed and the effect of the experience on the child and family. She must also be skilled in the various nursing procedures that must be performed and in observing for postoperative complications.

Before the child returns to his room the nurse should have received a thorough report on his status. This report should contain information regarding:

1. Type of operation performed and anesthesia and medication received.
2. Amount of blood loss.
3. Stability of vital signs.
4. Presence of drains, dressings or appliances.
5. Whether the child has voided.
6. The presence, rate and site of the IV.
7. Presence of cough and gag reflex.
8. Level of consciousness.
9. Any difficulties encountered during surgery.
10. Any concerns expressed by the child or parents just before or since the operation.
11. What the family has been told by the surgeon regarding the success of the operation.
12. Need for any special equipment such as mist tent, oxygen tent or suction machine.

When the child returns to the unit the nurse should attend to him immediately. The person transporting the child cannot leave until the nurse is in attendance. An immediate general assessment is done, observing the IV site, the child's color and respirations, dressings, any tubes or drains and the tightness of any restraints. Preferably the nurse has immediate access to the postoperative orders and can review them at the bedside before beginning a more detailed assessment. Vital signs are then taken and the nurse checks that the IV has the proper solution and is being delivered at the proper rate. The patient is assessed every 15 minutes for vital signs, level of consciousness, condition and intactness of dressing and functioning of any other tubes or appliances. The frequency of checking vital signs varies according to the surgeon's orders or the policy established within the institution. A general guideline is every 15 minutes for one hour, then every half hour for two hours, then every two hours until bedtime. During the first postoperative night vital signs are typically taken every four hours.

Although specific postoperative care varies according to the age of the child and type of surgery, many aspects of care are similar. Children are especially vulnerable to fluid and electrolyte imbalances. Potassium should not be added to the IV until the child has voided (see preceding section on fluid and electrolytes). Accurate intake and output records should be kept while an IV is infusing even if there is no specific order to do so.

Assessment and management of pain in children is another important aspect of postoperative care. The conclusion that children require proportionately less pain medication than adults may be erroneous; the difference may be that the child is less able to communicate that he is in pain.[3] The most reliable indicator that the child is experiencing pain is irritability and a lowered frustration tolerance.[3,4] The child may also respond physiologically with elevated vital signs or pallor.[3] Pain may also be manifested by facial grimacing, crying, muscle rigidity, clenching of fists and twisting and turning away from the painful stimulus.[2,3] In some cases pain may cause enough fatigue so that the child finally goes to sleep.[3] The nurse should observe for these signs of pain in addition to asking a child who can communicate about his sensation of pain.

The goal of the nurse is to keep the child comfortable. The nurse must recognize that the child's perception of pain is affected by environmental factors such as the presence or absence of parents and the degree of familiarity with the environment.[2] The child's cultural heritage may affect how pain is expressed. The nurse can attempt to alleviate pain through distraction, change of position or other comfort measures, but pain medication should be given as needed to keep the child comfortable. It must also be recognized that a child who appears to be in pain but verbally denies pain may fear the injection more than he does the pain he is expressing nonverbally.

Painful procedures and activities can be done in conjunction with the administration of pain medication. Coughing and deep breathing, change of position and early ambulation are common postoperative activities that may cause pain. Giving medication 10 to 15 minutes before carrying out these procedures may increase the child's ability to cooperate. Pain medication is not given every time a procedure is performed, but nursing care is adapted whenever possible to allow procedures to be done around the time that pain medication is given.

As soon as the nurse has read the postoperative orders, she should explain the required care to parents and to the child. Parents can assist in watching the child so that restraints for the IV may be unnecessary. They can also assist with coughing and deep breathing, turning and helping their child to ambulate. Care by parents is a great asset to the child, therefore parents should be given adequate explanations immediately postoperatively to make them feel comfortable in assisting with care.

Regardless of the type of operation, the nurse plays an important role in coordination of postoperative care. Parents frequently ask questions that must be answered by the surgeon. The nurse can reduce the parents' anxiety by telling them how to contact the surgeon or making a telephone call for them. Those questions that can be answered by the nurse should be answered promptly. Involvement of the parents throughout the postoperative course prepares them for an easier transition when it is time to take the child home.

Reactions to hospitalization and the experience of surgery vary with the age of the child. The nurse should prepare the family for some behaviorial changes when the child returns home. The nurse should also give explicit instructions to the family and child (when appropriate) on follow-up care and care at home. It is preferable that discharge instructions be given both verbally and in writing. A system that provides for continuity of care and a method of follow-up is to use a discharge form in triplicate — one copy stays on the chart, one is given to the parents and one is sent to the physician's office. The nurse should always clarify when the child should return to the physician's office or a clinic, how to give medications and their major side effects, how to perform any procedures to be done at home, and what restrictions in activity or diet, if any, should be followed. The nurse should assess the type of care and support that is needed at home and make referral to agencies that may assist the family as she deems necessary.

References

1. T. Kenny. The hospitalized child. Pediatric Clinics of North America, August 1975, p. 583
2. M. McBride. Assessing children with pain: Can you tell me where it hurts? Pediatric Nursing, Jul/Aug 1977, p. 7
3. M. McCaffery. Pain relief for the child: Problem areas and selected nonpharmacological methods. Pediatric Nursing, Jul/Aug 1977, p. 11
4. P. Chinn. Child Health Maintenance: Concepts in Family-Centered Care. C. V. Mosby, 1979
5. M. Petrillo. Emotional Care of Hospitalized Children. J. B. Lippincott, 1980
6. D. Treloar. Ready, Set — No: Something is missing from pediatric pre-op preparation. American Journal of Maternal Child Nursing, Jan/Feb 1978, p. 50

Additional Recommended Reading

Daily Care Considerations

V. Brown. Providing a safe environment for children. American Journal of Maternal Child Nursing, Jan/Feb 1978, p. 53
N. Dison. Clinical Nursing Techniques. C. V. Mosby, 1979
V. Jensen. Better techniques for bagging stomas. Nursing '74, August 1974, p. 30
K. Jeter. Reality therapy: a realistic approach to enterostomy rehabilitation. Nursing Forum, 1978, Vol. I, p. 72
J. Kaler and H. Kaler. Michael had a tracheostomy. American Journal of Nursing, May 1974, p. 852
K. Keenan, et al. A trial of a new ostomy system. Nursing Times, July 29, 1979, p. 1283
H. M. Kukuk. Safety precautions: Protecting your patient and yourself. Nursing '76, July 1976, p. 45
G. Leifer. Principles and Techniques in Pediatric Nursing, 3rd ed. W. B. Saunders Co., 1977
S. Lindensmith. Body image and the crisis of enterostomy. Canadian Nurse, November 1977, p. 24
J. Mahoney. What you should know about ostomies. Nursing '78, May, 1978, p. 74
E. A. McConnell. All about gastrointestinal intubation. Nursing '75, September 1975, p. 30
R. D. McCormick et al. Patient and Family Education. John Wiley & Sons, 1979, p. 244
M. Ziemer and J. Carroll. Infant gavage reconsidered. American Journal of Nursing, September 1978, p. 1543

Fluid and Electrolyte Balance

E. Beaumont. The new IV infusion pumps. Nursing '77, July 1977, p. 31
M. Dreszer, Fluid and electrolyte requirements in the newborn infant. Pediatric Clinics of North America, August 1977, p. 537
L. J. Guhlow and J. Kolb. Pediatric IVs: Special measures you should take. RN, March 1979, p. 40
J. Kee. The ABC's of fluid balance. Nursing '74, June 1974, p. 28
B. McGrath. Fluids, electrolytes and replacement therapy in pediatric nursing. American Journal of Maternal Child Nursing, Jan/Feb 1980, p. 58
K. Shake, The ABC's of ABG's — or how to interpret a blood gas value. Nursing '79, September 1979, p. 26

Total Parenteral Nutrition Hyperalimentation

J. Benner et al. The importance of different calorie sources in the intravenous nutrition of infants and children. Surgery, September 1979, p. 429
R. Colley et al. Providing hyperalimentation for infants and children — meeting patients' nutritional needs with hyperalimentation. Nursing 79, July 1979, p. 50
R. Colley and J. Wilson. How to begin hyperalimentation therapy — Meeting patient's nutritional needs with hyperalimentation. Nursing 79, May, 1979, p. 50
A. Conway and T. Williams. Parenteral Alimentation. American Journal of Nursing, April 1976, p. 574
D. M. Parfitt and V. Thompson. Pediatric home hyperalimentation: educating the family. American Journal of Maternal Child Nursing, May/June 1980, p. 197
J. Sherman, Pediatric Hyperalimentation. Contemporary Surgery, July 1978, p. 55

Anesthesia and Preoperative and Postoperative Nursing Care

A. Bothe and R. Galdston. The child's loss of consciousness: a psychiatric view of pediatric anesthesia. Pediatrics, August 1972. p. 252
C. B. Drain and S. B. Shipley. The Recovery Room. W. B. Saunders Co., 1979
B. Ferguson. Preparing young children for hospitalization: A comparison of two methods. Pediatrics, November 1979, p. 656
L. Francis and R. Cutler. Psychological preparation and premedication for pediatric anesthesia. Anesthesiology, Jan/Feb 1957, p. 106
K. Jackson. Psychologic preparation as a method of reducing the emotional trauma of anesthesia in children. Anesthesioloy, May 1951, p. 293
E. Meyers and S. Muravchick. Anesthesia induction technics in pediatric patients: a controlled study of behavioral consequences. Anesthesia-Analgesia, Jul/Aug 1977, p. 538
R. Smith. Children, hospitals and parents. Anesthesiology, Jul/Aug 1964, p. 461
D. Steward, Manual of Pediatric Anesthesia. Churchill-Livingstone, 1979
D. Vernon, and W. Bailey. The use of motion pictures in the psychological preparation of children for induction of anesthesia. Anesthesiology, January 1974, p. 68
D. Vernon et al. Changes in children's behavior after hospitalization. Some dimensions of response and their correlates. American Journal of Diseases of Children, June 1966, p. 111
M. Visintainer and J. Wolfer. Psychological preparation for surgical pediatric patients. The effect on children's and parents' stress responses and adjustment. Pediatrics, August 1975, p. 187
J. Wolfer and M. Visintainer. Prehospital psychological preparation for tonsillectomy patients: effects on children's and parents' adjustment. Pediatrics, November 1979, p. 646

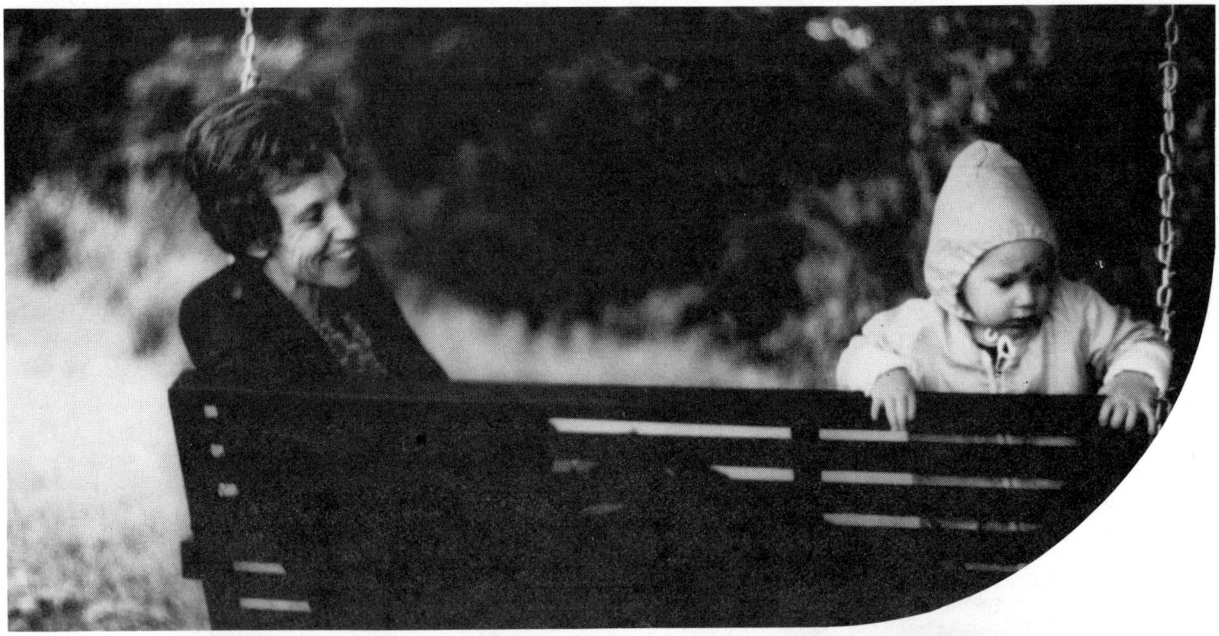

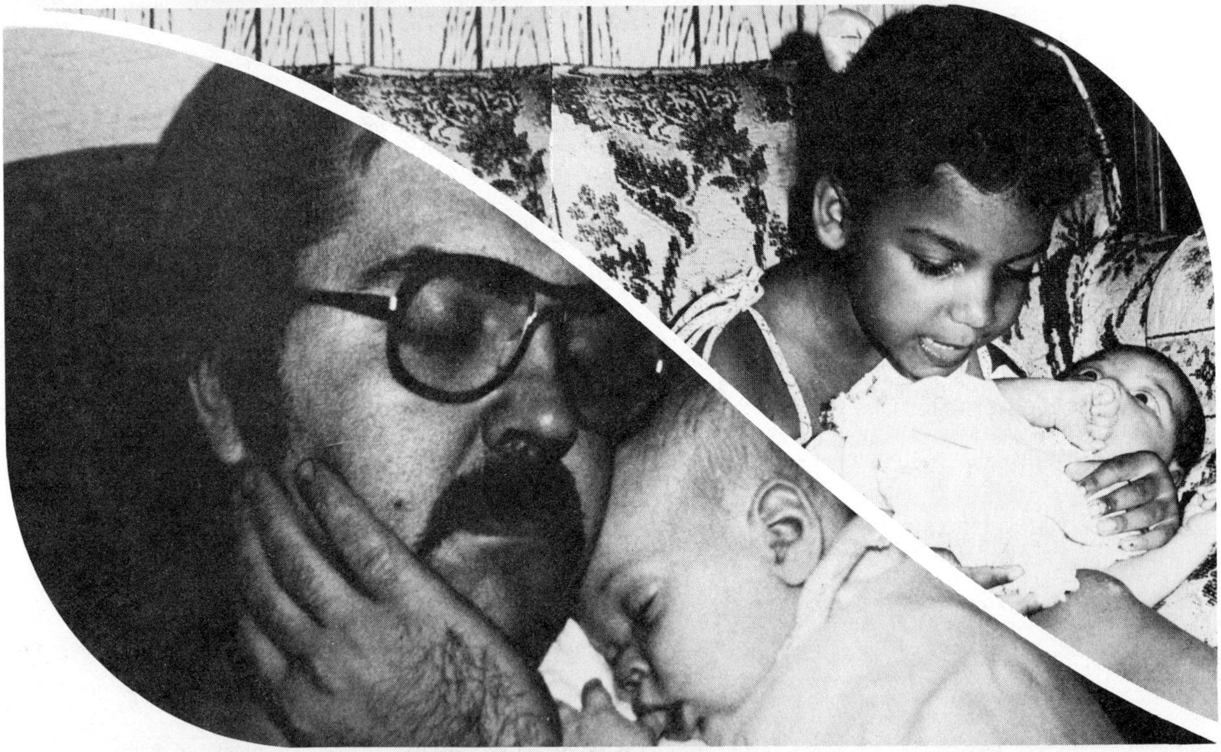

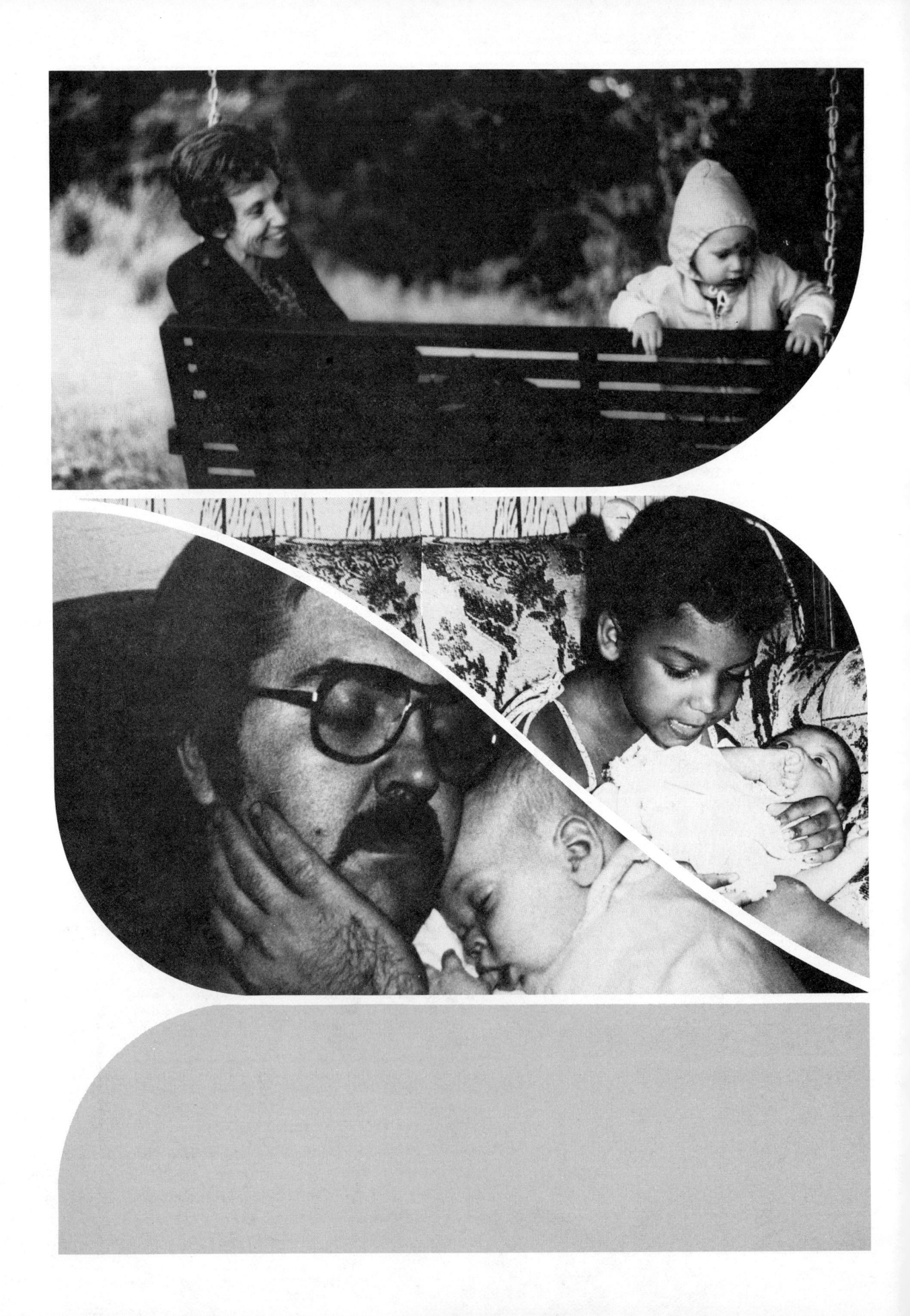

PART 4

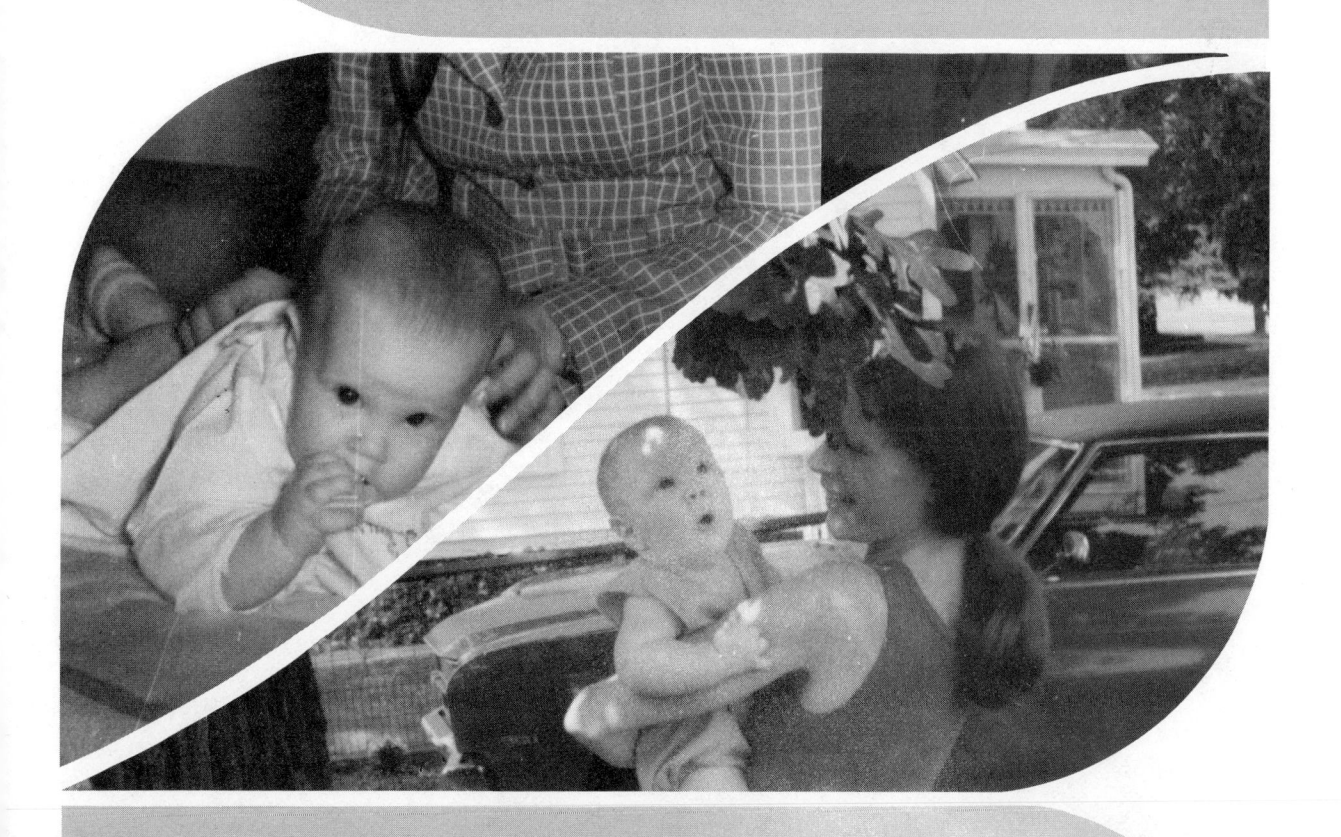

FAMILIES WITH INFANTS

18 GROWTH AND DEVELOPMENT NEEDS OF THE FAMILY WITH AN INFANT: MAINTAINING WELLNESS

by Anne Krabill Hershberger, RN, MSN

It is at the birth of a first baby that the woman becomes a mother, the man becomes a father and the newborn infant starts a completely new life cycle. They all are sensitive and vulnerable at this time. In this vulnerable period new developmental tasks face each person in the family. Each family member's developmental tasks and the nurse's role in assisting the family in the healthy mastery of these tasks are discussed in this chapter.

The major task of a family with an infant is the healthy incorporation of a new person into the existing family. This process requires that the family (1) internalizes the infant's existence, (2) makes necessary adjustments, and (3) establishes a stable family unit.

INTERNALIZING THE INFANT'S EXISTENCE

The baby is an unknown, unreal concept to the family until the birth occurs. One mother's response upon first seeing her baby illustrates this: she exclaimed repeatedly, "It's a baby! It's a baby!" She needed to internalize the fact that the baby really existed. According to Mercer, after the baby's birth, the mother establishes a realistic image of her infant and absorbs the infant into her self and social systems through an acquaintance-attachment process. Inherent in this process is maternal identification and claiming of her infant.[13]

Identification

The identification and claiming process is an important first step in the family's incorporation of the "real" baby into their family. Rubin has described the typical manner in which a mother identifies and claims her infant.[17] She examines the baby's soft and tiny features first by touching them with her fingertips and then with her palms and finally she enfolds the baby in her arms and looks directly into the baby's eyes — an *en face position*. Klaus and Kennell define en face as the position in which the mother's face is rotated so that her eyes and those of the infant meet fully in the same vertical plane of rota-

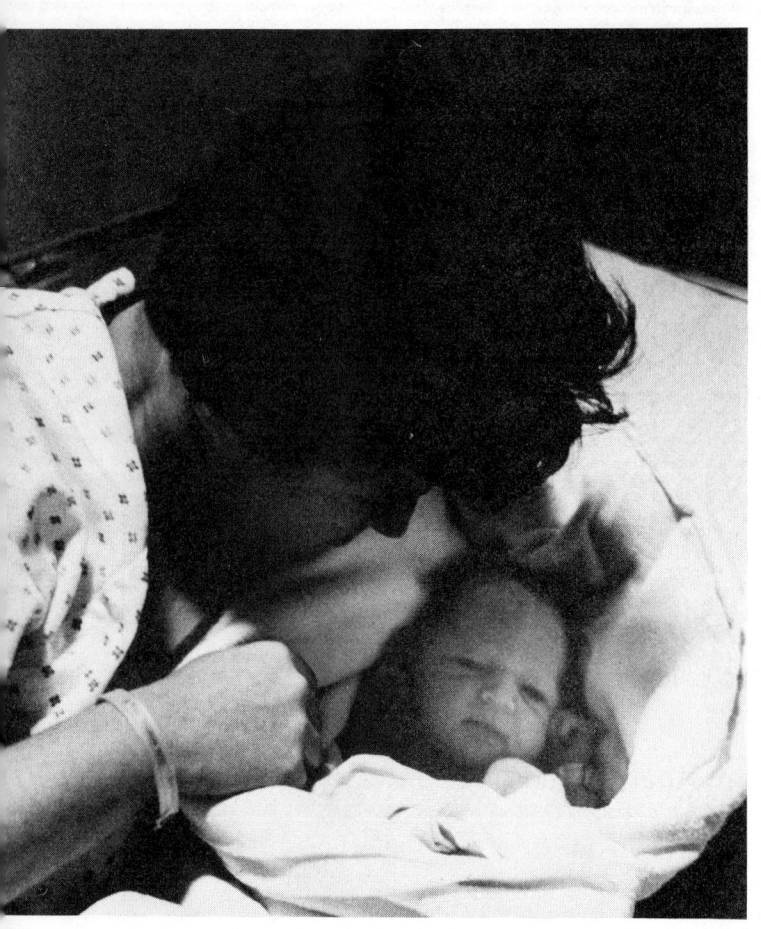

The en face position indicates progress in the identification process.

tion.[9] This entire behavior pattern proceeds gradually, perhaps over several days. In some instances the process is delayed longer and the mother's inability to enfold her infant and focus en face may indicate maladaptive behavior. The tactile identification process confirms the existence of a separate person and an object to which attachment can be made. Eventually the touch progression evolves into snuggling the infant up against the chest. This progression can be used as an index of how the mother feels about herself and her relationship with her child, says Ludington-Hoe.[12]

Reaching is another indication of identification work. At first the mother may receive her baby passively, but over the next few days most mothers progress toward active reaching for the baby. Active reaching indicates a desire to take the infant into the mother's personal body space — to get closer.[12]

The father of a newborn infant also must identify the infant as a real person joining his family. Greenberg and Morris in their research on the engrossment of fathers with their infants found fathers typically expressing these feelings: "... that they could easily distinguish their baby from the others ... that their child was perfect; that they were strongly attracted to their infant and focused their attention on him or her; and that they felt extreme elation and increased self-esteem because of their child. There was, however, a trend that fathers who were present at their infant's birth felt more comfortable in holding their baby."[16] If the father is given opportunities to be with his infant he will increase his involvement with it. This will involve him, with the mother and the baby, as part of the family unit.

When the newborn comes to a family with other children, the older children must adjust their fantasized concept of "baby" to a realization that this baby is theirs. Furman says, "To the children, and to young children in particular, this baby was not looked forward to as a cherished newcomer — it was a potential rival without whom they could have easily gotten along happily in life."[7] Even though a young child cannot verbalize these feelings, it is logical that he might be thinking, "Where have I failed? Mommy and Daddy wanted to have another baby. They must not have been satisfied with me." A child's excitement at meeting a new brother or sister is often tempered by these negative feelings. As children have opportunity to examine, touch and interact with their new sibling, their negative feelings can be altered and finally replaced by feelings of protectiveness and love.

This family process of identifying and claiming the infant can be facilitated by nurses who recognize the significance of this initial step in incorporating the new member of the family. The nurse present at the birth and afterward can provide opportunities for all family members to relate to the newborn.

Traditional hospital practices often interfere with the process of identification and claiming by isolating the baby from some family members. Fortunately, these practices are changing in many places to allow more total family interaction shortly after the birth.

The nurse also can model methods of interacting with the baby. She can point out characteristics of the baby that resemble family traits. She can encourage the unwrapping and examination of the whole baby and can talk to the baby and respond to his or her behavior. This behavior by the nurse will give permission and endorsement for the family to proceed with their developmental task of identifying and claiming this baby as theirs.

Accepting Responsibility for the Infant

Another task that is a part of internalizing the infant's existence is the acceptance of new or added responsibilities associated with the infant. For some people, having a baby may satisfy a need for purpose and responsibility. For others, the responsibility for another's survival is overwhelming. The feeling of being overwhelmed by the new responsibilities is emphasized when parents first realize that the parent role is irrevocable. The realization of irrevocability comes relatively soon after the birth of the infant.

The nurse can provide support to parents of infants as they try to accept their new respon-

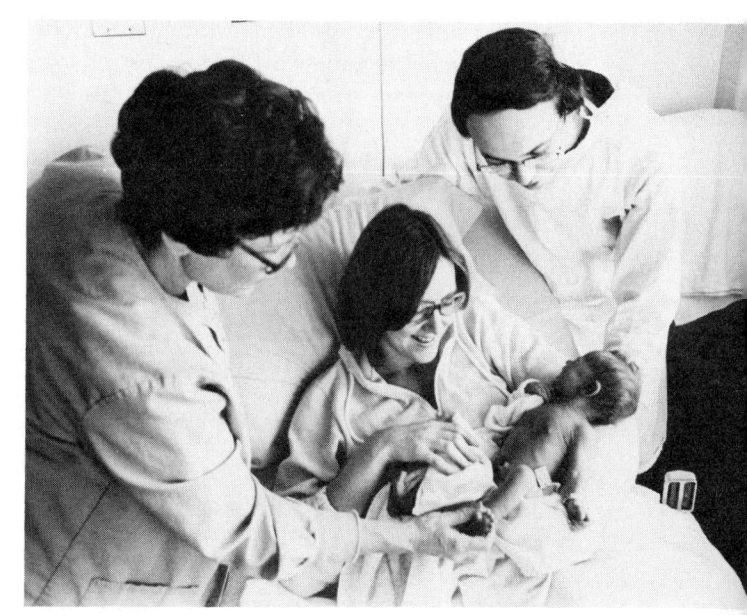

The nurse can point out characteristics that will help the family claim their baby.

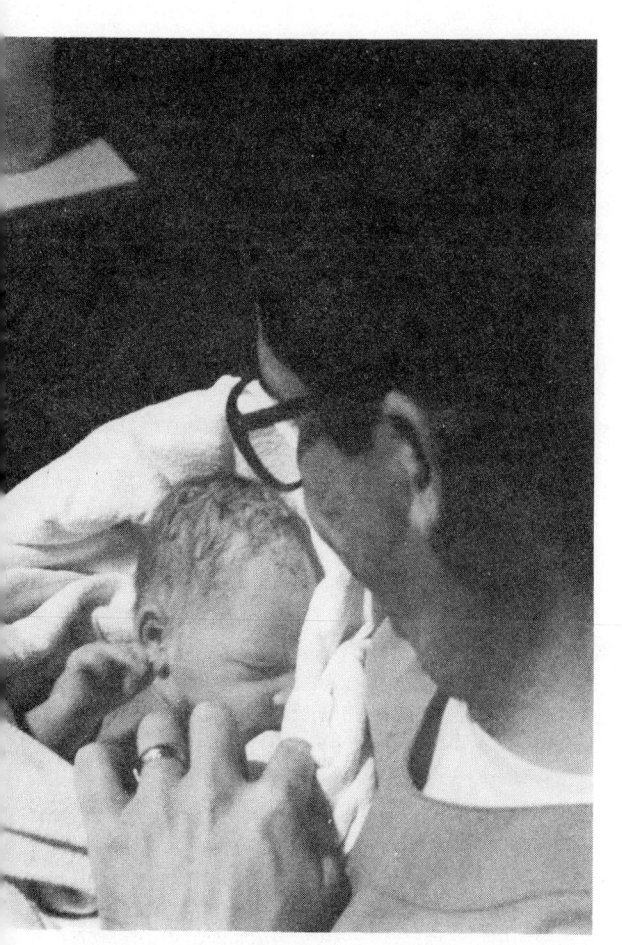

sibilities. Not only is she in an ideal position to teach parents about their new tasks, but she can help parents make the transition to parenthood successfully by providing the opportunities they need to express their concerns and feelings and to explore ways of maximizing their role. This type of professional support should facilitate the parents' acceptance of their new and added responsibilities.

Assuming New Roles

The new responsibilities associated with the infant require that all members in the infant's family assume some new roles. The addition of parental or sibling roles creates critical role transition periods while each family member works out an accommodation among new and old roles. Making a transition from husband-wife to father-mother requires development of several new interrelated roles. What these new roles are perceived to be and how they are internalized varies according to the individual's own experiences, feelings and needs. Parents who have been only children and youngest children have had fewer opportunities for exposure to infant and child-care responsibilities and are therefore unprepared for what to expect in the way of infant behaviors.

Father's identification with his baby requires his involvement.

GROWTH AND DEVELOPMENT NEEDS OF THE FAMILY WITH AN INFANT: MAINTAINING WELLNESS

Mother Role The mother in the family of an infant usually experiences the greatest change in her position. Her maternal roles usually require at least temporary interruption of her occupational role and often most of her other extrafamilial responsibilities.

A need that mothers display as a preface to assuming a mothering role with the infant is to discuss their labor and birth experiences in detail. Only after they process this experience can they focus on caring for the infant outside the womb.[19] During the postpartum period, women undergo three definite phases in assuming the maternal role. Rubin identified these phases as the taking-in phase, the taking-hold phase and the letting-go phase.[18] Luddington-Hoe notes: "The first three days postpartum is the taking-in phase. New mothers are generally passive in regard to their own care as well as their infant's.... During the next ten days, women pass through the taking-hold and then the letting-go phases of assuming the maternal role. These are the phases of task execution and letting-go of predelivery expectations."[12]

Nursing interventions during the taking-in phase incorporate meeting the mother's dependency needs. However, during the taking-hold phase the nurse may be most helpful by contributing to the mother's self-esteem by praising her efforts in mothering. This can be done by verbally identifying her maternal behaviors and the baby's positive responses to those behaviors as well as by giving her instruction and opportunities to experience successful infant caretaking. The nurse's reassurance of the mother will help to build her self-confidence. At no time should a nurse's behavior communicate that she is better able to care for the baby; instead she must grasp every opportunity to foster feelings of adequacy within the mother.

When the mother is experiencing the letting-go phase of assuming her maternal role, the nurse can make assessments of the mother's adaptive or maladaptive behavior. Early detection of maladaptive behavior can alert the health care team to begin therapeutic intervention before further harm is done.

Father Role Just as the mother must gradually become oriented to her parent role, so must the father assume his. A whole series of myths has developed about fathers and their involvement with newborn and older infants. Some of the myths project the ideas that fathers are uninterested and uninvolved with newborn infants; fathers are less capable of nurturing than mothers; fathers prefer to assume noncaretaking roles and leave the caretaking to the mother; and fathers are less competent than mothers to care for newborn infants.[14] A number of research studies have shown most fathers to be highly involved participants in the family context who either equalled or excelled the mothers in stimulating and nurturing the infant.[15] These studies reveal that most fathers do have the potential for caretaking, because they can be competent, sensitive and able to read baby cues. Aside from his role in actual caretaking, the father has a special role that complements the caretaker role of the mother — the role of a playmate.[14] Whereas the mother's caretaking interactions with the infant tend to produce dependency behaviors in the infant, the father's communication and play patterns encourage more independence in the infant.

The father's role is complementary to the mother's role in another way as well. The father's presence during the mother's interactions with their baby tends to increase the amount of positive affect the mother displays toward the baby. When she is alone with the baby, she handles and observes him more but she smiles more when the father is also present, probably because of conversation between them.[14]

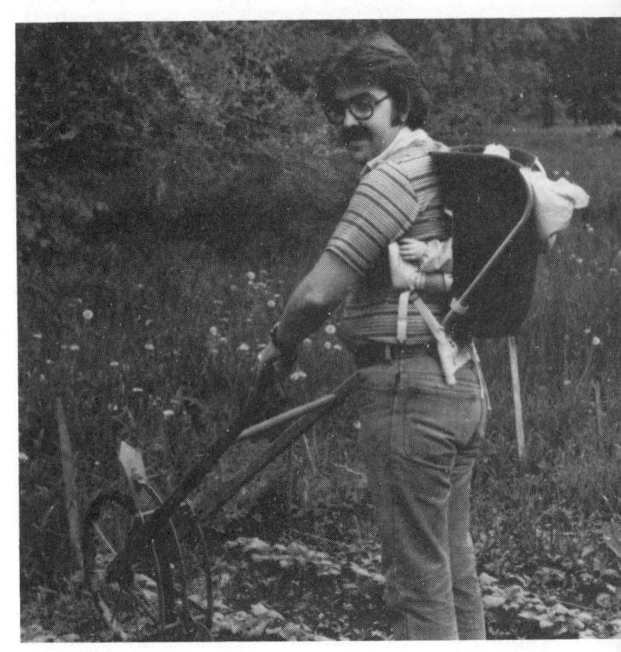

Many fathers want to be responsible for some of their baby's care.

Not only are fathers able to be involved with their infants, many want to be and all should be helped to have this involvement as a parent. Their involvement makes a difference to the baby's well-being. It behooves nurses in contact with the families of infants to provide unlimited opportunities for fathers to be with their infants in the hospital and to encourage their family involvement at home.

The father's involvement in the home may call for the development of sociocultural support systems such as paternity leaves from employment after the birth of a baby. This type of social change may be hastened by nurses who recognize the importance of the father's involvement with his infant to the baby, himself and the total family. Such nurses can seek opportunities to increase community awareness of this and make contacts with persons in positions of power to help bring about changes in policies.

The foregoing discussion about the assumption of parental roles may lead one to think that the response of parents to each child as it is born is similar. This is not so. The baby actually molds or triggers adult behavior. It is the individual characteristics of the child that set up specific parental responses and influence their feelings and nurturing. The mother's and father's orientation to their parental roles surely will be influenced by this particular baby as they learn to communicate and to stimulate the baby's further development.

Sibling Role Just as parents must assume new roles in relation to the newborn, an older child in the family has the sibling role thrust upon him by the baby's arrival. The need to assume this developmental task comes at a time when support structures are not as available and predictable as usual. If the birth occurs at a hospital, the older child likely will be separated from his mother for several days and nights. As the father tries to establish an early relationship with his infant, he too will be separated from the older child for extended periods of time. Some attempts are being made by hospital maternity units to reduce the older child's stress at being separated from his mother by promoting sibling visitation at the hospital. According to Trause, "Children do show difficulties when separated from their mothers for the birth of a second child, and children who visit show no more, and possibly less, distress than those who do not."[20]

Some changes have been observed in the nature of the relationship between the mother and the older child when a new baby arrives. A new baby's arrival seems to stimulate higher expectations by the mother for her other children, as she pressures them to master additional developmental tasks without as much maternal encouragement. The children may resent the family newcomer whose presence seems to have prompted these changes in their mother's behaviors.[1]

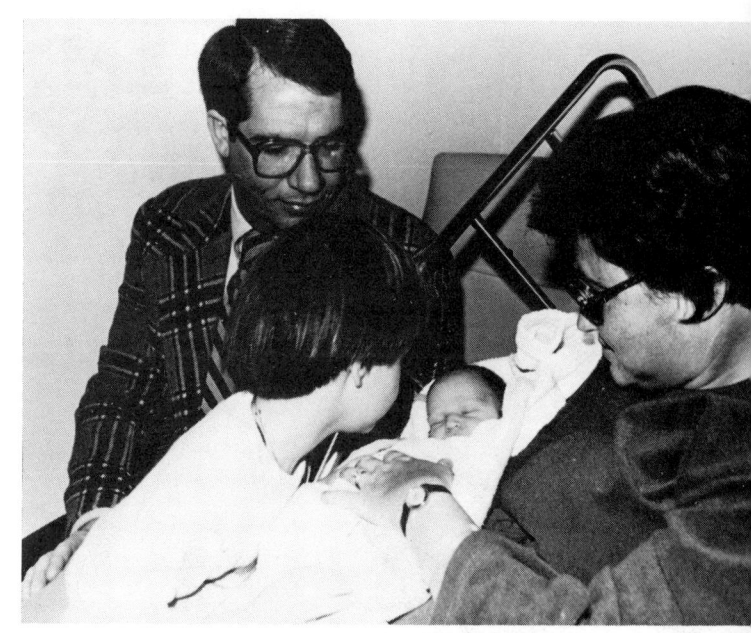

Hospital visitation helps the sibling claim his new role.

The older child will be able to assume the sibling role in a healthier way if he can express his honest feelings about the changes he is experiencing to an understanding person — preferably his parents — and also can have his personal needs for affection and security met.

The nurse in contact with the family before the baby arrives is in a good position to help parents anticipate the adjustments that the infant's siblings will need to make when the baby is born. She also can help the parents to understand the importance of their attitudes and responses to the older children and can offer concrete suggestions for easing the child's transition into a sibling role. Examples of such suggestions follow: (1) Do not assume that the siblings will be overjoyed upon meeting the infant. Their more immediate concern is the well-being of the mother. (2) It is helpful to have the father or another person carry the new baby

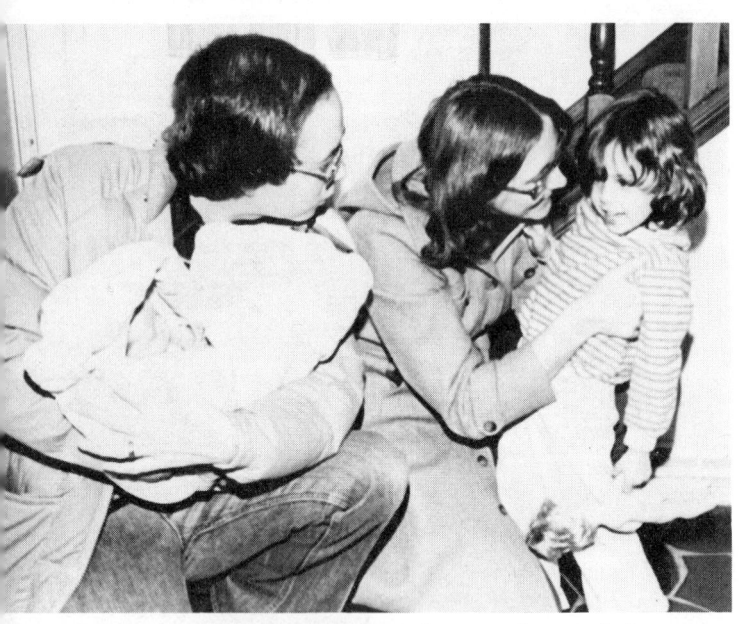

Mother's attention at homecoming wisely focuses on the new infant's siblings.

into the house when mother and baby return home from the hospital. This allows the mother to give her undivided attention to the older children from whom she has been separated. (3) Expect some negative reactions or jealous responses from the infant's siblings and express understanding about how they are feeling. (4) If an older child needs to give up his bed for the new baby, make the transition to a larger bed at a time well in advance of the arrival of the baby. This can be a very positive "graduation" experience in which the child takes pride rather than a negative experience in which the older child might feel that he is being pushed out of his bed. (5) Expect from the older child some regressive behavior more typical of an earlier stage of development when no baby was around to interfere with his relationship with his parents. (6) Express interest in the older child's activities and ideas and try to spend time with each child away from the baby. (7) Allow the siblings to enter into baby care and interaction as much as they care to, but set clearly understood limits as to what is safe behavior with an infant. (8) Recognize that negative feelings about the baby may be expressed months after the baby's arrival.

When the siblings are school age and older the responses of their peers to the baby's birth are significant to them and affect their own responses to the sibling role. If the newborn is more than 10 years younger than the sibling, some embarrassment about the sexual connotations of birth may be a part of the sibling's response. Frequently, older siblings prove to be delighted to have a baby in the home. Parents should be alerted, however, not to expect parental behavior of older siblings; parents should protect the privacy of the older siblings and the safety of their possessions from the infant's explorations when the time comes.

Forming an Attachment

Along with identifying and claiming the newborn as theirs, accepting new responsibilities and assuming new roles in relation to the baby and each other, members of the family of an infant need to form a bond or attachment to the newborn. This is critical to the survival and development of the infant.[9]

Mother-Infant Bond A healthy mother-child relationship does not spontaneously occur at the birth of a child. It has to develop as the mother and child learn to respond to each other. A mother may not always feel the enormous happiness that she expected to feel at the birth of her baby. Instead she often feels disoriented and tired. However, many internal processes are activated to promote bonding during the first days of life. According to Klaus, "Keeping the mother and baby together soon after birth is thus likely to initiate and enhance the operation of many behavioral, hormonal, physiological, and immunological mechanisms that probably 'lock' parent and infant together.... It may be this cascade of interactions... which insures the further development of attachment."[8]

A synchronization occurs as the mother and baby react to each other's affective, psychophysiological and attentional rhythms. If this interaction is prevented or disrupted, the baby literally curls up and withdraws.[3]

Luddington-Hoe reports on the findings of Brazelton, who has researched mother-infant interactions by studying videotape recordings.[12] He found that infants exhibit a cycle that is characterized by eight stages of interaction:

1. Initiation — The infant's attention is attracted by the mother and he looks back at her.
2. Orientation — The infant orients his body to face the mother.

3. State of attention — The infant alternately sends and receives cues.
4. Acceleration — There are fewer oscillations of attention and inattention.
5. Vocalizing — The infant whirls his arms and kicks his legs.
6. Peak of excitement — The infant exhibits jerky activity.
7. Deceleration — There is a gradual decrease in activity, eye contact and vocalizations.
8. Withdrawal — The infant withdraws from looking and interacting.

The infant's overtures must be perceived and reciprocated by his mother if the interrelationship between them is to occur. It is clear that both mother and baby are active participants in the attachment process.

The term *maternicity* has been used to mean the characteristic quality of a woman's personality that supplies her with the emotional energy for feeling that her infant occupies an essential part of her life as determined by bonds of affection.[21] These bonds include feelings of warmth, devotion and protectiveness toward the infant, concern for the infant's well-being, and pleasant anticipation of continuing contact. Maternicity develops as the mother and infant are in close contact, and it indicates a high probability for the successful development of a healthy mother-child relationship.

The nurse should remember in assessing the development of maternicity in the mother of an infant that observation of eye-to-eye contact between mother and infant is of primary importance. To establish eye-to-eye contact, mother and infant must be in the en face position. This presupposes the opportunity for close contact.

The mother's style of feeding and bathing her infant are reliable indicators of maternal behavior. Thus bathing and feeding periods afford the nurse reliable opportunities to evaluate maternal adaptive behavior. Ludington-Hoe suggests parameters to observe in mothers for the development of maternicity.[12] Absence of these behaviors strongly suggests a retarded mother-infant attachment.

1. Initial identifying behaviors prior to and after delivery.
2. Active and passive reaching behavior.
3. Touch progression: fingertip to palm or to hand; hand to arm embrace.
4. Positioning of the infant to the left of sternum; en face positioning.
5. Eye-to-eye contact.
6. Verbal identifying behaviors: association and pronoun identification.
7. Developmental phases: taking-in phase of dependency; taking-hold phase of task execution; letting-go of predelivery expectations.
8. Rhythm-reciprocity patterns.
9. Cooing behaviors.

Prompt assessment of deviations and early therapeutic intervention when maladaptive maternal behaviors exist support the prevention of child abuse, mental illness and many psychosomatic and learning disorders.

Father-Infant Bond Although mothers require a period of time to separate from the image they have developed of the baby as an integral part of them, the father's image of his baby is one of separateness. Greenberg and Morris found that of a sample of 30 first-time fathers from three British maternity hospitals, all manifested "engrossment" in their newborn infants, a sense of bonding, absorption and preoccupation in their child. The researchers interpreted this as an innate potential "released" in fathers by exposure to the infant.[16] Releasing this potential in fathers may be of even greater significance today than previously. The importance of early bonding of father and infant is accentuated today because the extended family is seldom readily available to new parents; thus fathers need to contribute to the early emotional and physical care of new infants in the nuclear family. Early parent-child attachment facilitates normal development in the child and also makes the demands of child nurturing more palatable to both mother and father.

Sibling-Infant Bond The attachment experienced between the infant and his siblings is less explored and documented than parent-infant attachment. When an older child is prepared to expect a new baby in the family, he will be able to handle with less stress his jealous feelings at the time of his displacement. The older child's attachment to a new sibling seems to be facilitated when parents help him to understand what is happening, explain that this is his baby as well as theirs and reassure him of their continuing love by verbal expressions and by demonstration. The infant's responses to the older sibling may be influential in establishing a bond between them as well.

Supporting and reinforcing parents and siblings during the early infant acquaintance process is an important nursing function. To do so we observe the quality and progress of interactions between parents and children, offering reinforcement when they observe their infant, talk to him, comment about his behaviors. The nurse can also teach family members to interpret their infant's behaviors appropriately.

The immediate period after birth is crucial in terms of developing attachment behaviors between parents and infants. Nurses in contact with these families can do much to provide extensive opportunities for parent-infant interaction. In every contact nurses can reinforce parents' strengths and their capacity to cope, thereby improving parents' self-images and increasing the self-confidence they pass on to their babies.[3]

ADJUSTING FAMILY LIFE TO INCORPORATE A NEW BABY

Perhaps no single event in human growth and development requires the number of adjustments that the birth of a baby requires in the life of a family. Adjustments in relation to maintaining morale, realigning division of labor, providing family financial support and establishing daily routines will be discussed.

The period after the birth of a baby frequently is referred to as a period of crisis in the family. The family must learn new coping mechanisms to meet the demands brought on by this event. Edwards says, "When the family equilibrium is upset by the addition of a member... the parents reach a turning point where they must learn to operate within a new time structure centered around the child's demands."[5] Both mothers and fathers face major adjustments at the birth of a baby. The mother especially must reorganize her life to meet the needs of the infant in addition to her usual responsibilities. Reorganization of the household is simple; reorganization of a woman's identity from woman and wife to woman, wife and mother is considerably more complicated, as Luddington-Hoe notes.[12]

For the father, the new role also involves self-image changes and added responsibilities.

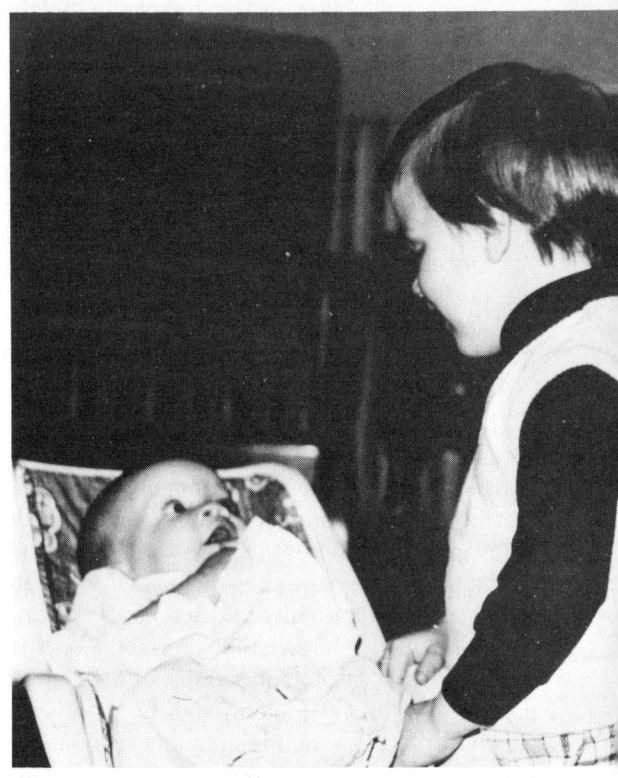

The infant's responses to siblings influence sibling-infant bonding. (Photograph by David Trainor.)

As described by Edwards, "The new father brings home his baby and a wife who needs lots of babying. Some men can nurture; others feel scared when called upon to parent their wives. They want to be cared for themselves, particularly sexually."[5]

Maintaining Morale

The effect of the physical and psychological upheaval experienced by families in the transition to parenthood often takes the form of mood swings and low morale. More specific identification of the stresses encountered is discussed in the next chapter, but here it is important to note that new coping mechanisms are needed to maintain the family's morale.

Duvall lists five attitudes or behaviors that help families living at the childbearing stage to cope and maintain good morale:[4]
1. Seeing beyond the drudgeries to the fundamental satisfactions of parenthood.
2. Valuing persons above things.
3. Resolving the conflicts inherent in the contradictory developmental tasks of parents and young children, and of fathers and mothers.

4. Establishing healthy independence as a married couple.
5. Accepting help in a spirit of appreciation and growth.

These attitudes and behaviors help to keep priorities in proper perspective for the family.

Edwards has identified some questions that the new mother might explore, ideally with her husband, in the attempt to promote good morale in the family during this period of transition:[5]

> Am I doing important things as a mother?
> What is my fantasy mother asking me to do?
> Is it possible and helpful to me and my family to do them?
> If I'm important, then how can I get some sleep and eat better?
> Did my fantasy mother have fun?
> Do I want to be like her?
> What can I do for fun everyday? Can I dance alone, listen to music, read while I nurse?
> What did I decide to give up for fourth trimester: ironing, working on a business at home, cleaning rooms that are seldom used?
> What did I decide I wouldn't give up for fourth trimester: massages, playing the piano, reading to my two-year-old?
> How can I feel better now with my dirty house and demanding baby?

The nurse can be of service to the mother by helping her to identify the unrealistic demands she may be placing on herself. These demands come from her concept of what a mother ought to be and ought to do (her fantasy mother). Exploring answers to the questions listed can help the mother to clarify her real priorities.

Many parents are ill prepared for the total dependency upon them of their infant. This total dependency, plus the uncompromising and demanding nature of the infant's expression of need, yields an inevitable irregularity of schedule and a sense of fatigue for the caretakers. The nurse can be helpful to new parents in this situation by suggesting that they realign their priorities as to what must be done and what can be ignored for the initial adjustment period. As a neutral third party, the nurse can facilitate the couple's identification of which tasks can be shared or shifted to others in order to reduce fatigue and promote rest. Research done by Russell revealed that there was less sense of crisis in the postpartum families she studied when the husbands got up at night with the baby.[1] This activity conveys concern for the wife's well-being, which helps to maintain good marital relations and encourages a common interest in the child that strengthens the marital bond.

Realigning Division of Labor

The actual division of labor with its strains and benefits is something that parents often wish to work out for themselves and not have prescribed for them.[16] The division of labor will likely change from one day to the next to meet demands of changing schedules and energy levels.

Nurses would do well to give fathers instruction and practice opportunities in the care of the infant during the prenatal period and in the hospital, because when the mother comes home she must have help.[11] Infant care is a major concern at this time, but the parents must also realign their division of labor in regard to care of older children, household chores and community responsibilities.

Older children may be expected to assume more self-care or helping roles when the new baby arrives, but it is important that parents provide adequate emotional support for the siblings and affirmation to accompany their expectations of what the older children can do. Regardless of how the family assigns and carries

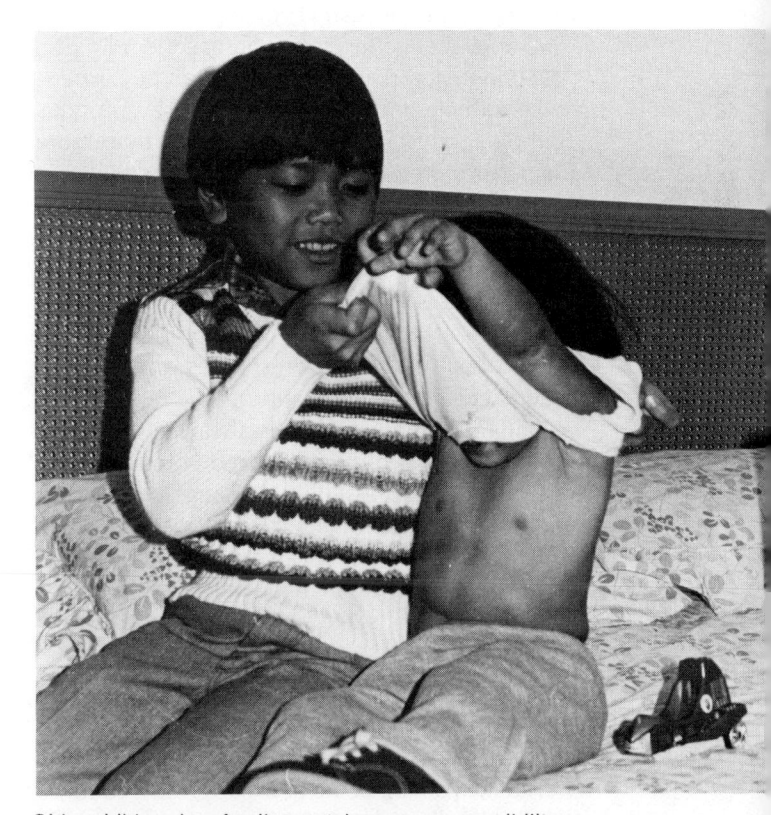

Older children in a family can take more responsibility for their own care when the infant arrives.

out its various tasks, hopefully family members can feel good about their roles. With this comes a sense of contributing to the welfare of the family and thus each achieves a sense of belonging, importance and self-esteem.

Financial Adjustments

Another significant adjustment that many families face upon the birth of an infant is in the financial realm. Frequently the mother has been employed outside the home prior to the birth of at least the first baby. Although expenses multiply at this time, income is often lessened significantly, at least temporarily. If the father works extra hours to compensate for his wife's unemployment, then his role at home may need to be curtailed somewhat to allow him to get adequate rest.

In this perinatal period when the father needs to accept the total provider role, the nurse can help the couple to see the benefits of well-chosen and simple baby supplies. She can also point out when improvisations or substitutions for more expensive items are possible. For example, parents can (1) choose larger sizes of infant clothes so the baby can use them longer; (2) choose to breast-feed rather than buy expensive formula and equipment; (3) use nutritious simple foods for family meals rather than more expensive prepared convenience foods; (4) improvise a box, basket or dresser drawer for a baby bed. (The bed should have a firm mattress and be made so that the baby cannot fall from it.) If there is insufficient income in the family with an infant, the nurse must be knowledgeable about community resources and governmental funds and make appropriate referrals.

Financial management is always a challenge that requires self-discipline and some maturity to handle successfully. Although the nurse cannot provide financial security for any family, she should be aware of and sensitive to the importance of financial resources as a family adapts its life style to include a new infant.

Reorganizing Family Routines

With the coming of the new baby, daily routines must be adjusted to incorporate the new family member. Initially, all routine seems shattered as the infant expresses needs unpredictably and as parents are first trying on new roles. However, very soon a daily routine, although flexible, should be established for the welfare of all family members. Since the baby's needs are somewhat unpredictable at first and since meeting his needs promptly is significant in his development of basic trust, other family members will need to be flexible enough to allow for the baby's needs to be met as they arise.

Routines that promote basic trust in infants not only allow their needs to be met promptly, but also allow their needs to be met usually by the same person. Having the same person meet the baby's needs routinely should not be interpreted to mean that this person must give care each and every time, but rather care should be given in a general pattern in order for the baby to develop a specific relationship with the main caretaker and to be able to predict responses.

Older children, too, have grown to expect certain responses and behaviors from their parents and each other. These routines are inevitably altered with the coming of an infant to the family. Parents should try to continue the most significant parts of the older children's routines if at all possible so that they can identify some areas of sameness and consistency from their life before the baby came. This will contribute to a greater sense of security and assurance that their parents have not forgotten what has been important to them. Examples of significant routines to continue with older children might be a regular story hour after lunch or specific bedtime activities. The times for these activities may shift because of infant demands, but continuing to include them each day seems important.

Perhaps the biggest challenge for the parents is to find time for personal interests and for each other. How much effort is exerted to provide personal and couple time is related to how highly it is valued. The nurse can make a significant contribution to the family with an infant by impressing upon the parents the importance of their feeling good about themselves, their new roles and the ways they spend their time. The nurse can help them to identify when their concept of "the good parent" is making unreasonable demands on them and how they can incorporate new "parent models" that are more lenient and that permit them to enjoy themselves as parents.[5]

It is possible to meet the needs of various family members simultaneously. For example, play time with older children may involve imitating mother as she does her postpartum exercises. The mother may read a novel while breast-feeding the infant. Time alone with her husband may not always need to wait until she is exhausted at the end of a day, but might be possible during a favorite children's TV program — if the infant is cooperative then.

The coming of a new baby does bring the need for major adjustments within the family. The nurse in contact with family members before the baby's arrival can help them gain a realistic concept of changes that will be necessary so that they can plan for these changes. After the baby arrives, the nurse can provide reassurance and support, teach needed skills and help parents set priorities and realistic expectations for themselves and their family.

ESTABLISHING A STABLE FAMILY UNIT

As orientation to new roles and family adjustments proceed in relation to the arrival of a new family member, the characteristics of the family unit become established. The creation of a stable family unit will depend upon the family's ability to adapt resources to accommodate the infant, re-establish relationships to include the infant but retain spouse intimacy and rework the family philosophy.

Adapting Resources

The adaptation of resources to accommodate the infant cannot be prescribed generally because the resources available to families vary extensively. However, some basic considerations in the decision making include individuals' needs for privacy, personal attention and finances as well as the need for family planning.

Providing space for individual and couple privacy may be difficult in some settings. During the early days at home with an infant, parents often find it convenient to keep the infant's bed near their own because of his need for care at night. However, when the baby begins to sleep through the night, it is advisable for parents to get some distance from the infant. Physical distance means that parents are not disturbed by normal baby noises and movement and the baby is not disturbed by parental voices and movements. Psychologically, the distance provided by moving the baby's bed outside the parents' room gives the parents a sense of privacy for intimacy and for a respite from the demands of the family. When separate rooms are not possible, portable screens or dividers may be useful.

Each family member should be allowed to have some space that is his own to arrange, keep "treasures" in and go to for time alone. This may not necessarily be an entire room, but some section of a room would be useful.

For the mother who regularly is at home caring for the infant and possibly other children, the greatest sense of privacy may come when she is relieved of all household and child care responsibilities for a period of time to go outside the home and do what she pleases. Time away from home may also provide the best arrangement for the couple to have some privacy if child care is available from others. Recognizing the need for time alone and a place for each individual to call his own can stimulate creative planning and be one factor in establishing a stable family unit.

Finding a time and place for each family member's privacy may be difficult, but equally difficult is finding time to give attention to each family member. Older children often experience some change in the parental attention they receive when a newborn arrives. Aldous reports on an earlier study done by Baldwin in which he found that the amount of warmth mothers showed their first children, as indicated by such variables as affection-giving approval, dropped significantly with the arrival of another child, as did the amount of contact they had with the older child or children. At the same time, there was an increase in maternal restrictiveness with these older children and in severity of penalties used in disciplining them.[1]

The nurse can serve the enlarging family well if she informs parents about this tendency to lessen their attention given to older children. When they become conscious of this tendency, they can plan ways to prevent it from happening. Parental behaviors such as touching, hugging, kissing, and smiling and expressing interest, sympathy and patience as well as spending time with the child communicate that each child is vitally important to the family.

Parents can expect some regressive behavior in older children as they share their parents' attention with another baby. Accepting this behavior as understandable and not cause for punishment likely will bring about the return of the child's normal behavior.

Mobilizing the energies of children to help with some of the household tasks or infant care may help them to feel important to the family as well as to learn respect for their parents as people with needs for help.

Attention given by spouses to each other frequently takes low priority among the demands on parental time. However, planning for this on a daily basis may make the difference between one spouse or both feeling overwhelmed and depressed by new responsibilities and roles or feeling that the new challenges are exciting and bring fulfillment and a sense of unified effort. The kinds of attention desired by each spouse relate to the need to feel good as a person, spouse and parent. Reassurance that each is still attractive and important to the other can be communicated by the expression of physical love and by arranging for times to talk alone. Actual courtship-like "dates" occasionally may be useful in meeting the attention needs of spouses. When parents take time to "refuel" their affectional relationship, this seems to have the effect of providing them with new energy and motivation to fulfill their other responsibilities. Their positive relationship with each other bolsters the self-esteem of each.

In addition to adapting resources for assuring privacy, attention and financial security for each member of the family, the parental resource itself must be protected to accommodate the infant. If this baby is followed by another infant within a year or so, he will not receive the intense parental attention that is important to him during infancy. Before a subsequent baby is born, the parents should feel physically and emotionally ready for the baby. If the previous child is less than a year old and still very demanding, it is difficult for the parents to meet his many demands for nurturing as well as those of a new baby.

The nurse can be an important source of information to parents regarding family planning services. The postpartum period is a particularly appropriate time to provide this. Specific information that new parents should be made aware of at this time includes the facts that a woman can become pregnant even though her regular menstrual periods are not yet re-established and that methods of contraception other than oral contraceptives are usually recommended during the period of lactation. The progesterone content of the oral contraceptive tends to inhibit the production of prolactin from the anterior pituitary gland, which is responsible for milk production. Securing reliable aids for the desired spacing of children is an important way to establish a stable family unit.

Re-establishing Relationships

Another important aspect in achieving a stable family unit is the re-establishing of relationships to include the infant but retain spouse intimacy. The marital relationship is the base upon which all other family relationships are shaped. The mates are the "architects" of the family. A disturbed marital relationship tends to foster dysfunctional parenting. Affectional and intimate relations seem to be the single most important factor in family relationships. Affection is something family members value, invest much energy to preserve and seek to replace promptly if family ties are broken.[1] A new baby competes with spouse affectional bonds to become a recipient of affection within the family system. This competition forces reorganization of family relationships to include the new member.[1]

In the early postpartum period each family member has a somewhat egocentric focus. The infant, of course, knows only his own comfort or discomfort and demands care at the time he senses his needs. The new mother has just experienced a dramatic upheaval of her physical and emotional self, which tends to make her focus on herself and the changes she is experiencing. The new father, facing new responsibilities and concerned about finances, is called upon to support his wife emotionally and help care for the baby when he wants to be cared for himself. Older children are trying to determine who they are in the family now that a new member has arrived. An older child may feel that he has been replaced by the infant.

While the family members are experiencing this egocentric focus, their external social relationships also are being altered. If this is a first baby, the parents will not be able to leave home as spontaneously as before to engage in activities with friends. If the mother was employed previously and is no longer employed, her contacts at work will no longer occur. Many couples find that the birth of their first child brings them in touch with their own parents in a new way. Whether the grandparents live near or distant, an identification with the parental role provides a common interest that causes a new bond between the generations.

The family social relationships will need to allow for the inclusion of the infant or they will cause dependence on babysitters. The baby's presence in a group of adults may or may not be welcomed. Social planning and interaction inevitably becomes more complex with the arrival of an infant.

The nurse can be influential in assisting family members to regain a sense of equilibrium for themselves and for the family unit. She can assess each member's response to the new family member and identify areas in which help is needed in adjusting to the changes brought about by the infant. The nurse's clarification or reassurance on a number of issues will smooth the couple's transition to parenthood. For example, she can assure the parents that meeting the baby's needs will not "spoil" the baby. Meeting the baby's needs and interacting with him will not cause manipulative behavior but rather will cause development of a sense of trust and well-being.

The nurse should help the mother to understand that her husband may feel left out of the special closeness between the infant and herself, especially if she is breast-feeding. The mother may need help to realize that sexual activities short of intercourse, if she is not physically ready to resume intercourse, may help to ease her husband's feeling. Edwards notes that the "pleasuring" described by Masters and Johnson is appropriate for mothers not ready for intercourse. Pleasuring consists of sensual interchange such as stroking, massage, stimulation for the fun of it rather than as a prelude to intercourse.[5] Each spouse must be reassured that the baby has not replaced him or her in the other's heart.

The nurse can facilitate the return of family equilibrium by helping the father to recognize the significant role he has in providing emotional support to the family. He is usually the one who gets away from home each day, so he can bring a perspective of the larger world to the family. His lower voice, different touch and sense of humor can reduce tensions among children — even the infant — and his wife as he relieves her of some of the interacting and caretaking. If, however, he refuses to enter into the life of the family, tension and discord are likely to build and become serious problems. His expressions of love and demonstration of caring are especially needed by his wife now.

She needs to feel that she is still attractive to her husband even though she may have a sore perineum, protruding abdomen and leaking breasts, and though she is feeling tired.

A tired mother may resent the infant who prevents her from sleeping or even taking a bath. Unconsciously she may even plot to get rid of the demanding baby.[5] The nurse can urge her to talk about these feelings with her husband or a woman who also has experienced them and take action to remedy the situations that distress her. This will stimulate a better self-image and greater ability to cope. Appropriate actions the nurse might suggest include: (1) sitting in a warm bath for at least 20 minutes a day, (2) doing postpartum exercises regularly, (3) wearing Netsy cups (made in Sweden but available in some United States hospitals and pharmacies) or breast pads inside her bra to collect leaking milk and protect clothing, and (4) napping whenever possible. Napping should take priority over many household tasks because tensions will become less debilitating and tasks will be easier if the mother is well rested. When she is feeling good about herself and is assured of her husband's love, she will be able to foster a sense of equilibrium in the family as well.

The father's personal sense of well-being is facilitated by a wife who has interest in his life outside the home, expresses love and appreciation for him, engages in sexual "pleasuring," and tries to make the home a pleasant place for him, although it may not be as neat and clean as usual. The mother's support of her husband's beginning attempts at fathering will encourage his future involvement with the baby.

The most urgent issue needing to be resolved in the mind of an older child is whether or not his mother and daddy can be parents to both him and the baby and have love enough for two children. Fear of losing his parents, not the presence of a new baby, motivates the older child's resentment.[2] The child will regain his personal sense of equilibrium only when he is convinced that his parents love and care for him as much or more than ever.

The birth of a baby requires a redefinition of family relationships and thus affects family balance. The sooner family balance can be reestablished, the sooner individuals within the family can feel good about themselves and their role within the family. Family stability supports the stability of each individual member.

Altering Family Philosophy

In the effort to establish a stable unit after the birth of a new member, the family philosophy will need to be reworked. According to Aldous, "In assessing how well they are meeting their goals, families examine how well members are performing certain tasks. The tasks are based on members' needs, and their accomplishment enables the members to perform their family roles, to reach family goals and to meet the requirements of societal agencies."[1]

The examination of family members' performance of developmental tasks will inevitably reveal the presence of some conflicts. There are some very logical reasons for conflicts to occur in the family of an infant. These families have conscious or unconscious goals toward which they strive. While the parents work toward meeting these goals, their efforts will be thwarted at times by the relentless demands of the infant. When behavior is goal oriented, conflict is inevitable. However, conflict in itself is not the problem. It is the manner in which conflicts are resolved that affects the health of the family and the individuals within it.

Three common sources of conflict within families with infants in our society include: the lack of parental communication about roles expected of each other, lack of knowledge of infant developmental norms and lack of knowledge of parenting skills. In the research of Knafl and Grace, parents usually admitted to use of division of labor that had evolved rather than one that had been negotiated. Task allocation was discussed only when one partner felt that the existing arrangement was intolerably unbalanced and the other partner failed to notice the nonverbal cues given and to adjust his or her behavior accordingly.[10]

Openly recognizing the feelings and differing expectations of each family member will make it possible to begin working at the resolution of the conflicts that arise. Verbalization, along with efforts to maintain a sense of humor, is the basic ingredient in healthy family relationships. The functioning of many families has been lubricated by members' ability to identify problem areas and laugh about their stereotyped responses, the irony of events or the unreasonable expectations set.

Parents' lack of knowledge about child growth and development can cause them to have unrealistically high expectations of their children. It is common for parents to expect babies to smile, sit up or be toilet trained much earlier than is usually possible. Parents may thwart a child's normal curiosity and need to explore because of their own concept of "good behavior." Unrealistic expectations will cause conflicts.

The lack of knowledge of parenting skills makes the parent role less enjoyable and less successful than it could be. Just because one is biologically capable of having children or because one has been a child and had parents does not necessarily equip one to parent well.

Nurses who are in contact with parents early in their parental careers need to be aware of the sources of conflict within families. This awareness can lead to perceptive assessments and creative nursing interventions to help parents in their parental roles. The nurse can inform parents of the resources available to them and be instrumental in creating new resources appropriate for people of diversified educational levels and cultural and language groups.

The resolution of conflicts in roles and developmental tasks among family members represents one area in which the family philosophy must be reworked. Another area is in relation to the development of parenting attitudes that respect the individuality of each child.

With a family philosophy that takes into account the differences in people, parents will be less likely to compare one child with another and expect similar responses and behavior. Hopefully, they will encourage each child's development of his special interests. Parents can be urged to help older children recognize the developmental achievements of the infant and realize that the expectations placed on the infant are different from those placed on him.

A new philosophy of the family with an infant must emerge because of the irrevocable change that the baby's arrival brings to each family member. Furman notes: "Just as the child remains a part of the parent's self, the parent for a long time remains an essential part of the child's self. This is what makes the parent-child relationships unique and different from all other relationships. It consists of the double processes of loving or caring for the other as a separate person and loving and caring for the other as the self, even when the child is grown up."[7]

References

1. J. Aldous. Family Careers: Developmental Change in Families. John Wiley & Sons, 1978
2. A. Bernstein. Jealousy in the family. Parents, February 1979, p. 47
3. T. Brazelton. Future care of the infant. Birth and the Family Journal, Winter 1978, p. 242
4. E. Duvall. Marriage and Family Development. J. B. Lippincott Co., 1977
5. M. Edwards. The crises of the fourth trimester. Birth and the Family Journal, Winter 1974, p. 19
6. M. Erickson. Trends in assessing the newborn with his parents. American Journal of Maternal Child Nursing, Mar/Apr 1978, p. 99
7. E. Furman. The death of a newborn: care of the parents. Birth and the Family Journal, Winter 1978, p. 214
8. M. Klaus. The biology of parent-to-infant attachment. Birth and the Family Journal, Winter 1978, p. 200
9. M. Klaus and J. Kennell. Maternal-Infant Bonding. C.V. Mosby Co., 1976
10. M. Kanfl and H. Grace. Families Across the Life Cycle: Studies for Nursing. Little, Brown & Co., 1978
11. J. Lind. The family in the Swedish birth room. Birth and the Family Journal, Winter 1978, p. 249
12. S. Luddington-Hoe. Postpartum: development of maternicity. American Journal of Nursing, July 1977, p. 1171
13. R. Mercer. Postpartum illness and acquaintance-attachment process. American Journal of Nursing, July 1977, p. 1174
14. R. Parke. The father's role in infancy: a re-evaluation. Birth and the Family Journal, Winter 1978, p. 211
15. R. Parke et al. The father's role in the family system. Seminars in Perinatology, January 1979, p. 25
16. R. Rapoport et al. Fathers, Mothers and Society. Basic Books, 1977
17. R. Rubin. Basic maternal behavior. Nursing Outlook, November 1961, p. 683
18. R. Rubin. Puerperal change. Nursing Outlook, December 1961. p. 753
19. L. Swendsen et al. Role supplementation for new parents: a role master plan. American Journal of Maternal Child Nursing, Mar/Apr 1978, p. 84
20. M. Trause. Birth in the hospital: the effect on the sibling. Birth and the Family Journal, Winter 1978, p. 207

Additional Recommended Reading

K. Barnard. The family and you. American Journal of Maternal Child Nursing, Mar/Apr 1978, p. 82

L. Barnhill and D. Longo. Fixation and regression in the family life cycle. Family Process, December 1978, p. 469

H. Biller and D. Meredith. Father Power. Anchor Press-Doubleday, 1975

A. Brenner. The blues: how postpartum depression affects both mother and child. American Baby, March 1979, p. 50

F. Cline. Lack of attachment in children. Nurse Practitioner, Jan/Feb 1979, p. 35

J. Funke and M. Irby. An instrument to assess the quality of maternal behavior. Journal of Obstetric, Gynecologic and Neonatal Nursing, October 1978, p. 19

S. Goodman and P. Taylor. Bonding and attachment: theoretical issues. Seminars in Perinatology, January 1979, p. 3

S. Hersh and K. Levin. How love begins between parent and child. Children Today, Mar/Apr 1978, p. 2

M. Klaus. Future care of the parents. Birth and the Family Journal, Winter 1978, p. 246

H. Marano. Breastfeeding: new evidence it's far more than nutrition. Medical World News, February 1979, p. 62

M. Moore. Realities in Childbearing. W. B. Saunders Co., 1978

V. Satir. Conjoint Family Therapy, revised edition. Science and Behavior Books, Inc., 1967

J. Segal and H. Yahraes. Protecting children's mental health. Children Today, Sept/Oct 1978, p. 23

P. Taylor. Introduction. Seminars in Perinatology, January 1979, p. 1

19 POTENTIAL STRESS IN FAMILIES WITH INFANTS

by Anne Krabill Hershberger, RN, MSN

Family life cycle transitions are important because all families experience them and because they frequently are associated with family crisis. The life cycle transition to beginning parenthood, however, is generally looked forward to by prospective parents as a period of emotional enhancement rather than crisis. Therefore new parents frequently are unprepared to experience the variety of stresses that may accompany the arrival of their infant.

In this chapter, six areas of potential stress experienced by families with infants are presented in relation to the impact they have on family members and the family as a unit. The nurse's role in preventing potential stresses is discussed, as well as in intervening when the stresses occur. The six causes of potential stress discussed are (1) lack of family support structures, (2) fatigue, (3) unsatisfactory division of labor, (4) lack of knowledge of infant care, (5) problems generated by family relationships, (6) financial problems.

An analysis of the normal development of the infant's early social relations and discussion of the breakdown of attachment are in Chapter 22.

POTENTIAL STRESS RELATED TO PARENTS' LACK OF SUPPORT STRUCTURES

In the United States, the ease of mobility and general availability of jobs have been at least partially responsible for young couples moving away from the communities in which their parents live. This independence is desirable for exposing them to new experiences and ideas. However, great geographical distances between these couples and their parents remove a usual family support structure that operates when an infant is born to the young couple. Loving relatives have cushioned the stress associated with the transition to parenthood in many homes.[5]

When an extended family support structure is not available, friends and neighbors can provide some help to the family with a new infant. Forty-six per cent of the thirty-nine couples studied by Williams stated that they turned to their physician or friends for assistance.[13] One out of four had not sought the help of others.

Those without sufficient emotional support from outside their nuclear family will expect most of this support to come from within the family. At a time when transition to new roles is occurring among nuclear family members, this support for one another may be limited. A couple with self-esteem is able to trust one another. When a couple lacks this trust based on self-esteem, each feels he has barely enough to sustain his own life, let alone help the other. The mother and father in such a family not only lack emotional support at a time when it is sorely needed but this lack of support brings a sense of social isolation as well. Lack of adult companionship and stimulation from outside relationships produces stress.

The mother and father who feel alone with their new responsibilities may develop resentment toward the infant, whom they see as having brought about this situation, or they may become so totally involved with the infant and his needs that their own personal development and self-confidence suffer. This decreasing confidence actually may cause them to withdraw from opportunities for social interaction.

The father usually is able to maintain some contacts outside the home through his employment even though support from the extended family is lacking. It is the mother who usually needs special planning to meet her personal needs for support and social interaction. Otherwise she may resent her confinement and her husband's freedom.

When older children are present in the home, they too will suffer from the family's lack of outside support, but they may not be able to identify the source of their suffering. What they feel is their parent's frustration communicated in many ways and possibly some lack of personal attention.

When friends or relatives are available, they frequently are very helpful to families with an infant and older children by giving the older child special personal attention. This eases his jealousy of the attention being devoted to the baby. If this special attention is given to him when away from home, he has unique experiences to share with his family upon returning. His time away from home also temporarily gives his parents some lessened responsibility. When these opportunities do not exist, some potential richness is lacking from the older children's lives. As individuals within the family find support outside the family, the whole family benefits because of greater personal fulfillment of its members.

The nurse in contact with families with an infant may find herself in a good position to fulfill a strong nurturing, supportive role. Her beginning goal should be to establish a helping relationship with the mother and concentrate on her needs. Identifying strengths she observes in the family rather than focusing on problems will contribute to the support they feel.[8] Parents' strengths are the qualities that can be relied on as they cope, and for which they do not need the professional's help. What the professional can offer is support and encouragement for their strengths.[2]

Nurses in many communities are recognizing the need for supportive follow-up of families after an infant's birth because of the lack of family support structures. This is referred to as *fourth trimester follow-up*. The fourth trimester is the first three months after a baby's birth or the fourth trimester of the childbearing cycle — the period of transition to parenthood.

The fourth trimester follow-up program carried out by the nursing department at Hoag Memorial Hospital Presbyterian in Newport Beach, California, includes a bedside visit and interview with the mother and an initial telephone call by a maternity unit nurse during the first week after she and the baby return home from the hospital. Repeat telephone calls, a home visit and referral to community agencies take place if necessary.[4] In this program 50 to 60 per cent of the families need more than the initial phone call.

When the nurse makes the initial follow-up phone call, she has the maternal and infant Kardex care plans, plus the postpartum follow-up care plan, in front of her. She assesses the mother's psychosocial adjustment; knowledge of health concepts including nutrition, hygiene, sexual matters, rest and activity; understanding of basic infant care, feeding, hygiene, safety, growth, and nurturing; maternal attachment;

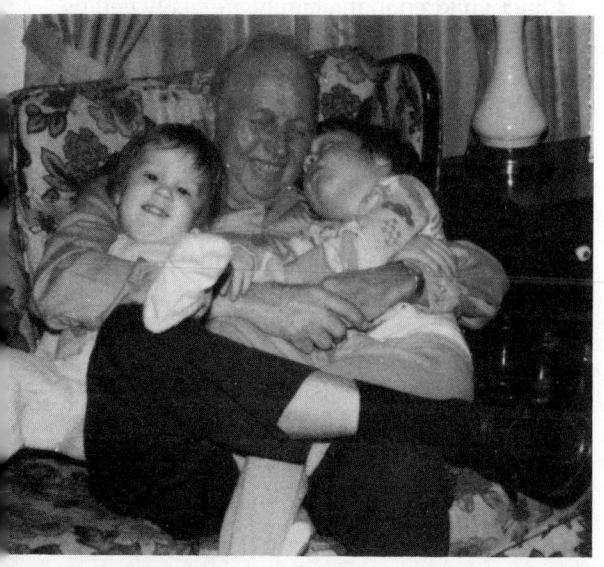

Having grandparents near helps ease the adjustments that must be made when the new baby arrives. (Photograph by Dave Trainor.)

paternal engrossment;* and the nature of parental expectations for this baby. During follow-up the nurse is committed to promote confidence, competence and independence among families in the fourth trimester. This is done by nurturing their growth and strengths.[4] This type of program provides much support and professional help to new parents.

Another innovative community project in which nurses have a role for supporting families with infants is the Young Family Resource Center in San Antonio, Texas.[7] This program offers parenting services to young families in need through the efforts of professionals and volunteers. According to Miller and Baird, "The center has provided a new role for nursing, a place in which parent volunteers can help those who are less knowledgeable about parenting, a learning site for physicians and nurses, and most of all, an opportunity for young parents to share and increase their knowledge of parenting the young child."[17]

Since family support structures are less available to families with infants today, professional and community resources should provide some of the supportive care needed.

POTENTIAL STRESS RELATED TO PARENTAL FATIGUE

No one is at his best when he is tired, and the parents of infants have many reasons for their chronic fatigue. The mother recently has had a dramatic change in her physiological and psychological status due to the baby's birth. The unpredictable nature of the baby's needs in the early weeks of life causes an irregular "schedule" to which the parents must adjust. This irregularity in schedule is responsible for parental loss of sleep as well as a sense of disorientation. The pressures inherent in the transition to new roles cause a certain degree of physical and emotional exhaustion. The inability to finish tasks that are begun plus the sheer number of new tasks added to the daily schedule cause a demoralization of spirit, which adds to the feeling of fatigue.

It is not difficult to understand why postpartum depression and a general disenchantment with the parenting role might afflict the parents of an infant, particularly during the early weeks after the birth. As the infant develops, he usually sleeps longer between feedings and establishes a more predictable and regular schedule that allows the parents to get more rest.

For the mother, chronic fatigue lessens her enjoyment of the maternal role, her self-confidence, her feeling of attractiveness to her husband and her patience with the infant's siblings.

The father may resent the fatigue he feels from needing to earn the living and then assuming heavy family responsibilities upon his return home, plus having his sleep interrupted by the baby's crying. Tensions are likely to build between the parents in such an atmosphere. His wife's inability to resume sexual intercourse or her temporarily diminished interest in sexual activity contributes to the tensions felt. Sexual communication short of intercourse would seem appropriate until both partners are ready for sexual intercourse again.

The infant can sense tensions in the parents by the way in which he is held and spoken to. When he senses tension, he often responds by crying or being fussy and irritable, which in turn causes more tension in the parents. This cycle must be broken by getting some distance between parents and infant for a brief period. This is another indication of the family's need for support persons to relieve them of child care responsibility occasionally.

Older children in the family are likely getting sufficient rest but sense parental fatigue. If the siblings are old enough to assume some of the household responsibility and infant care occasionally, the parents may not experience extreme fatigue.

The nurse can help parents to prevent extreme fatigue by helping them to think through how they will set priorities, during the fourth trimester particularly. The nurse's help in determining which tasks must be done and which can be ignored temporarily gives professional reassurance that parents should not try to do everything they did before the baby came plus the many new tasks associated with the baby. A top priority for the fatigued mother may be to take a nap at the time the baby sleeps rather than to do a lot of needed housework. The most pressing housework will be done better and more quickly after she has rested; the less pressing tasks can wait. The nurse might also

---

*Process of father identifying and claiming the infant as his; focusing attention and investing emotionally in the baby.

> **NURSING ACTIONS TO FACILITATE COPING WITH STRESS IN FAMILIES WITH INFANTS**
>
> Assess the family's support structure, financial resources, and level of knowledge of infant care
> - Obtain a family history. Find out specifically whether the couple (or single parent) has relatives or friends available for help with the infant and for emotional support.
> - As early in the pregnancy as possible, discuss the costs of medical care and the costs of taking care of an infant. Refer to sources of financial aid if necessary.
> - Establish a helping, nonjudgmental relationship with the parents, so that they feel free to ask questions.
>
> Provide an opportunity for parents to express their emotions about the infant's care. Sometimes just the acknowledgment by another person that the baby's crying and the parents' interrupted sleep are problems can help the parents cope. Reassurance by the nurse (who may be viewed as an "authority figure") that it is common to feel irritated, frustrated or angry can help relieve parents' guilt at having such emotions.
>
> Discuss with parents their own needs for rest, a sexual relationship and adult stimulation. Reassure parents (especially the primary caregiver) that needing relief from caregiving occasionally is OK.
>
> Keep informed about formal and informal helping groups in the community. Among possibilities are continuation of prenatal classes, informal mothers' groups organized in apartment complexes or neighborhoods and formal groups such as LaLeche League or babysitting cooperatives.
>
> Investigate possibilities for establishing parents' support groups or fourth trimester followup programs in practice settings, whether hospital, clinic or private practice.

inform the parents of a crisis day care center in the community to which they may take the baby and older children without prior notice when they are too fatigued to parent well.

POTENTIAL STRESSES RELATED TO DIVISION OF LABOR

In some families the division of labor is not equitable; so one spouse experiences greater fatigue. The nurse as a neutral third person might be helpful to the couple as they assess and renegotiate their division of labor.

In a study of 38 mothers and their infants, Friedemann and Emrich found that mothers seemed ill-prepared for the infant's total dependence on them and the resultant demands.[7] A common surprise expressed by mothers of first babies is, "I had no idea one little baby could keep one so busy." Feeding, diapering, bathing and holding the infant plus doing additional laundry, possibly preparing formula and performing self-care tasks such as postpartum exercises and sitz baths on top of usual household tasks create a busy schedule. The baby's unpredictable needs divert the parents from keeping a regular schedule, so a sense of disorganization adds to the busy feeling.

Each couple needs to determine the appropriate division of labor for themselves. The decisions will not be appropriate, however, until they are satisfactory to both members of the couple. These decisions frequently are not discussed openly, so one spouse's feelings of unfair distribution of duties may not be known by the other. The older children in the family who may assume some responsibility for certain household tasks should not be required to sacrifice all of their personal time for family tasks, because such demands may foster the development of resentment toward the baby and their parents.

The nurse's greatest contribution to relieving stress related to the family's division of labor is the promotion of open communication. If the family members are not able to discuss their feelings on this topic, the nurse can help by asking questions, interpreting feelings and facilitating decision making.

POTENTIAL STRESSES RELATED TO PARENTAL LACK OF KNOWLEDGE OF INFANT CARE

One of the most crucial needs felt by parents of an infant is based on their sense of insufficient knowledge. Basic infant care is taught both before and after the baby is born in prenatal classes and in the hospital following the baby's birth. However, two factors make this teaching less effective than it might be at a different time. The baby care in prenatal class is taught before the baby is born, and parents tend to forget this information becuase they cannot relate it to their baby until they can see and hold him. The teaching done in the hospital following the birth comes during the mother's "taking-in" phase of restoration. At this time she feels very dependent and is not yet ready to think in terms of caring for her baby. She has a need for care herself. Much of what a mother is taught in the first days after the birth of her baby is not retained after discharge. In the couples studied by Williams, 74 per cent said they would like to have included in postnatal classes information on the physical care of infants such as bathing and feeding. These topics had been taught in the postpartum units of each hospital in which these women delivered.[13]

A group of 14 baccalaureate nursing students at Goshen College in Goshen, Indiana, visited 28 families in their homes in the early days and weeks after their babies were born. This was designed to be a learning activity in a nursing elective course on the fourth trimester. One goal of the students in visiting the families was to identify the knowledge needs expressed by the parents or observed by themselves. The knowledge needs they identified were in the areas of baby care and feeding; mother's self-care; infant characteristics, growth and development; family planning; and sibling adjustments and discipline. Some representative questions raised by the parents in relation to baby care were:

"How can I tell if the baby is dressed warmly enough?"
"He sleeps such a short time. Why is he so fussy?"
"Is she constipated if she has no bowel movement one day?"
"Am I spoiling the baby by picking him up every time he cries?"
"What should I do for diaper rash?"
"She's so yellow. Should I take her to the doctor?"
"Is one kind of pacifier better than another?"
"What should I do about hiccoughs?"
"May I lay the baby on his abdomen if the cord is not off? When will it come off?"
"Are cloth diapers better than disposable diapers?"
"When may I give a tub bath to the baby?"
"Should I be giving sugar water to the baby?"
"Is it OK to let the baby sleep seven hours at night without breastfeeding?"
"May I diet while I breastfeed?"

At least some of the information asked for in this list is routinely included in the postpartum teaching done in the hospitals in which these women delivered, but the questions remain when the parents have sole responsibility for the baby at home.

In the Williams study, in which parents were asked for suggestions for content in a postnatal class for parents, couples commented on the usefulness of including such topics as changes in family life, roles of grandparents, dependence and independence of the baby, learning to pick up cues from the baby, physical care, and child care literature. They cited the value of having the opportunity to hear how other new parents handle their difficulties.[13]

The major stresses that result from parents' lack of knowledge are feelings of insecurity and fear and a lowering of self-esteem. Because their feelings of inadequacy leave them vulnerable, the parents may not follow their own judgment but rather may take the advice of others — anyone. Well-meaning friends and relatives may give conflicting advice, which adds to the parents' frustration in not knowing what to do.

The mother's self-esteem is lowered because she may feel that she ought to know the answers to her questions: "All mothers do." If her husband communicates to her that he thinks she ought to know more, she again loses self-respect. The husband may be less chagrined by his lack of knowledge about babies; society does not expect fathers to know as much as mothers about baby care. He may, in fact, be more experimental and innovative than the mother in trying to find answers to his own questions. Some mothers indicate that when they are at a loss to know what to do, their husbands seem to be able to think of the right thing.

The infant probably will not suffer severely from the experimentations of his parents (within reason, of course) as long as their basic attitude is one of love for the baby and concern for his safety. However, he will be better cared for if the parents can act from a base of knowledge rather than from instinct only.

Siblings will feel the impact of their parents' lack of or forgotten knowledge about babies through the frustration they communicate in their interactions with the older children.

The nurse's role in preventing parents' stress related to lack of knowledge is to anticipate their needs and provide the opportunities for them to learn what they need to know. Prenatal nurse-educators, postpartum nurses and community health nurses can present a picture of the newborn infant that more accurately reflects his inability to respond to his parents as older infants do. Aspects of the infant's dependency could be pointed out by nurses both prenatally and especially postnatally. Mothers would then have an improved knowledge base that would perhaps lessen their initial problems on taking their baby home.[7]

Some instructional opportunities for nurses are (1) making parenting literature and bibliographies available; (2) teaching prenatal classes and postnatal parenting classes; (3) capitalizing on teaching opportunities in hospitals, pediatrician's offices and well-baby clinics; (4) organizing parent coffees and functioning as a resource person in the discussions; (5) implementing fourth trimester follow-up by phone or home visiting and (6) becoming involved in community education programs. In facilities in which such arrangements are feasible, the nurse can give the phone number of the hospital maternity unit to the parents for a knowledge resource, since nurses are on duty 24 hours a day.

When the parental stresses of insecurity, fear and low self-esteem already exist, the nurse's major intervention is one of reassurance and of identification of the parents' strengths. Parents' need for reassurance is poignant even in those families in which the knowledge base is strong. They frequently ask, "What am I doing wrong?" "Do other mothers feel this way?" "Do bottle-fed babies cry this much?"[9]

Brazelton believes that traditional hospital maternity care is reinforcement for parental insecurity, failure and for ambivalence exemplified by young parents' questioning of their abilities, as well as for reinforcement of detachment rather than attachment.[3] Nurses in hospital settings need to evaluate the effects of their practices on parents' sense of personal security and plan appropriate changes.

Parents' security and self-esteem as parents will be enhanced by actively participating with the nurse and other health care professionals in the assessment process. This can be done by giving mothers and fathers more opportunities to define their concerns, to state what they believe to be effective solutions to their problems, to describe actions they have tried and what they want to do next. Erickson states: "Mothers and fathers are creative and resourceful. More importantly, by including them we encourage them to feel more personally responsible for their child's care."[6] The nurse can help parents to become problem-solvers rather than merely help-seekers.

POTENTIAL STRESS RELATED TO FAMILY RELATIONSHIPS

Friedemann and Emrich offer a formula for the number of interpersonal relationships within a family, in which x equals the number of interpersonal relationships and y equals the number of persons:[5]

$$x = \frac{y^2 - y}{2}$$

Therefore in a family of four persons, six interpersonal relationships exist: husband-wife, mother-child, mother-infant, father-child, father-infant and child-infant (Fig. 19-1). The potential for the development of stress when new relationships are established with the arrival of the infant is understandable.

Duvall says that husband and wife must re-establish effective communication as they become parents. They have new feelings to share in the pride, joys, anxieties, annoyances and insecurities of early parenthood. The danger, she adds, is that their marriage may be eclipsed by their new family roles.[5] Duvall reports some findings from Feldman's research, which show that parents of infants talk less with each other, especially about personal things, than they did before their babies came. They tend to have fewer joyous times, to laugh less, to have fewer stimulating exchanges of ideas and to feel resentful more often. Generally, the coming of the first baby has a sobering effect on the parents and a depressing effect on the marriage.[5] This situation can and likely will produce stress in the husband and wife.

Other stresses affecting the husband-wife relationship include:[14]

1. The spouses no longer belong only to each other.
2. The power relationship and division of labor are affected drastically.

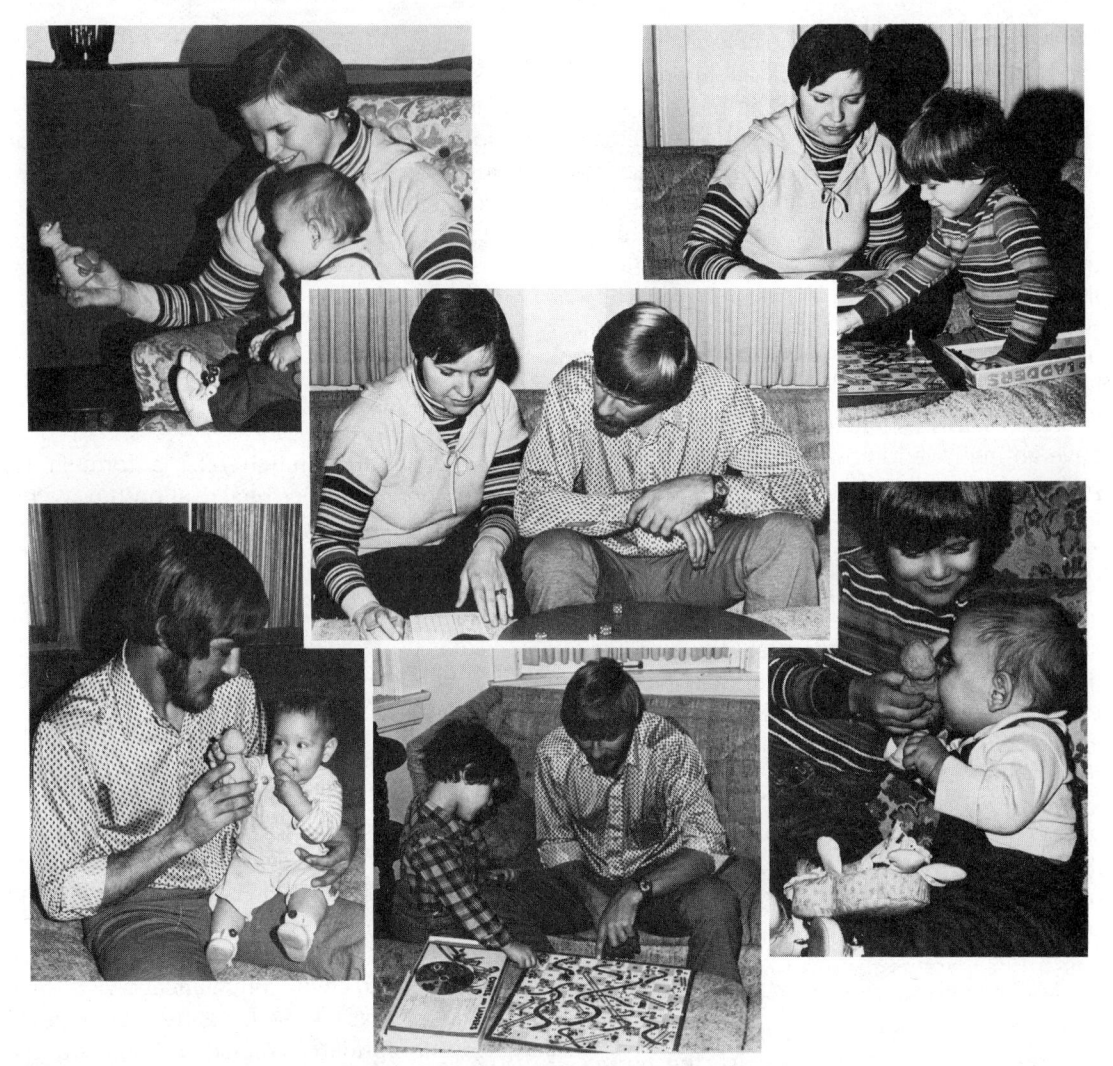

Figure 19-1 In a family of two persons, one relationship exists; in a family of three, three relationships. Adding one more family member increases the number of relationships to six.

3. Each spouse may discover another person in their marriage partner.
4. A sharp increase in role differentiation and specialization may occur.
5. The sexual relationship must be adapted to the new family situation.
6. Both partners may have difficulty balancing the needs of the child or children with marital and personal satisfaction.
7. Opportunity for communication may be cut severely.
8. Couples may stop enjoying each other.
9. Mothers may resent their confinement and their husbands' freedom.

Perhaps the most sensitive area for the husband and wife to deal with is the changes in their sexual relationship brought about by the birth of an infant. It is usual for the couple to decrease their sexual interaction during the pregnancy, childbirth and postpartum periods. However, re-establishing sex relations is not merely a physiological problem; there are many psychological features for both the wife and her mate.[5] The wife may be so absorbed in infant care that she invests less time in the marital relationship. She may also feel that the physical changes she has experienced and her frequent feelings of fatigue make her less sexually attractive to her husband. She may face the dilemma of needing reassurance of her husband's continuing sexual interest in her but not yet being ready to resume sexual intercourse. The husband also often faces the dilemma of

402 FAMILIES WITH INFANTS

desiring resumption of full marital relations but being hesitant to take sexual initiative before his wife is interested.

After the couple has resumed regular sexual intercourse, it is not unusual to find that the infant's call for attention may interrupt lovemaking at the most inopportune times. Duvall notes, "It is at such times that the couple's communication systems and philosophy of life stand them in good stead as they meet the baby's need and return to each other in good humor without the overtones of frustrated, disgruntled impulses spoiling their relationship with one another."[5]

The nurse can be helpful to couples who identify problems and seek help with their marital relationship. She may interpret the dynamics of how the two spouses may be feeling and promote open communication between them. Serious disturbances in the relationship may require referral to a marriage or family counselor. The marriage relationship is so paramount to the family's well-being that needed resources should be sought to protect it.

The relationship between mother and infant also has far-reaching implications, as has been discussed in the previous chapter. But a close mother-infant relationship, while desirable, may cause some negative responses from other family members. The husband may feel excluded by his wife and baby and somewhat deprived. He is expected to help care for his wife and infant and receive less attention himself. Older children may experience some sense of exclusion as well, particularly while the mother is breast-feeding the infant.

When the infant is about 6 to 8 months of age, he may be very possessive of his mother and refuse to allow others to hold or care for him. This may be stressful to the mother, who needs to leave the baby occasionally to pursue her own interests; however, it does represent a strong maternal-infant attachment.

An intimate father-infant relationship, again very desirable, may cause stress for some mothers. Bernstein comments that the mother may have a hard time making room for an intimacy between father and child that excludes her even temporarily. Seeing a child who has turned to her for all his primary needs turn to another can stir up feelings of loss.[1] Through the course of pregnancy, childbirth and the postpartum period an older child in the family often spends more time with his father and the father assumes more caretaking activities for the mother. Therefore, the older child may become jealous of the attention the father shows the new baby.

The relationship of the older child with his mother may need some reconstructing after the birth of the infant. The older child may feel that his mother is not to be trusted because she decided to have another baby. Now some of her attention is taken away from him. She went away from him to have this baby. She now expects him to be more grown up than ever before at a time when he does not feel like growing up — babies get more attention. With all of these thoughts in mind, the older child may be slow in developing a warm sibling relationship with the infant. The older child will be fascinated with observing and eliciting responses from the infant, but for some time the infant will represent an intruder or unnecessary family addition for the older child. When the older child acts out his feelings of jealousy or anger toward the baby, the parents will experience stress. They face the dilemma of preventing the sibling's unsafe behavior toward the baby while trying to be patient and understanding of his needs and his behavior. The parents' patience and sensitive treatment of the child at times when he acts out negative feelings about the baby can lead to his developing a meaningful relationship with his sibling.

A sibling relationship is good preparation for life outside the family. With siblings children learn how to relate to peers, to share skills and support, to negotiate, cooperate and compromise, to win with grace and lose with dignity, to make friends.[1]

What can the nurse do to help the family of an infant reduce the stresses in family relationships produced by the infant's arrival? A first step is for her to gain some understanding of the complexity of the relationships and the nature of potential stresses in these families. With this knowledge she should be able to assess carefully the stresses present in a given family and, with the family members, plan ways to reduce or alleviate the stress. Her identification of the strengths that the family members bring to the situation may mobilize them to make the needed changes in behavior.

It is a perceptive nurse who can identify family relationship stresses in the brief contacts she may have with families during fourth trimester follow-up visits to the well-baby clinic or pediatrician's office. The most effective role for

> In San Francisco, the Kaiser-Permanente Medical Center offers a Family Centered Perinatal Program that begins with prenatal courses for both parents. A team of obstetricians, pediatricians and nurse practitioners work with the family throughout the birth period. The father attends the delivery and stays with the mother directly afterward. The mother and child are examined 12 hours after birth and are permitted to return home if all is well; in some cases they remain 24 hours, then are released. The nurse practitioner who was originally assigned to the mother makes daily home visits for four days afterward and is available for two weeks to assist the family in caring for the infant. Besides being economical and safe, the program provides concentrated and personalized care. But most important, it expedites parent-child attachment. — Hersh and Levin[10]

the nurse may be to educate families as to the importance of positive relationships, what the potential problems are and how they can try to prevent these from occurring. To fulfill this role the nurse needs a knowledge base in human growth and development, human behavior and psychology. Much of the success of reducing family relationship stresses will depend upon the maturity of the parents and their willingness to try some behavior changes or their ability to help other family members to do so. The nurse's positive support and attitude can facilitate their efforts.

POTENTIAL STRESS RELATED TO FINANCES

In an inflationary economy as in the United States, there are few young families that can escape the burden of needing to plan very carefully for adequate funds for their needs. The many expenses that accompany the birth experience and the needs of the infant often put a strain on the family budget.

The father, usually the chief family provider of income during this period, may experience the most stress in relation to finances. The increased responsibility of providing for a new, totally dependent family member will have an impact on him. Some men may feel that assuming this responsibility should exempt them from home duties. A nurse can help fathers understand the significance of their involvement with the family and with their infant.

The impact of limited finances on the mother generally affects the type of management decisions she must make. What criteria will she use to set priorities for spending? What kind of discipline can she apply in her decision-making?

Children get accustomed to the life style of their parents and consider it "normal." They may not feel the stress of limited income directly, unless it is extreme. The parents' attitude and degree of stress affects the children more directly than does the fact that they have fewer things in the home.

If the infant's birth requires major life style changes for the family, they may become resentful toward the baby and serious relationship problems may emerge. The nurse can help to prevent problems related to finances by listening and assessing the situation carefully. Then she can help the family to think of all possible resources for funds, to set careful priorities for spending, and to plan management strategies. She can make referrals to community agencies that can help meet their needs.

Families experiencing increased responsibilities with a new infant plus financial concerns are generally interested in learning about family planning. The nurse should be prepared to meet their need for information and be able to suggest additional resources such as a family planning agency or their physician. She should be particularly alert to misconceptions they may have about the effectiveness of various contraceptive methods and clarify their understanding of the facts.

Most families with infants are vulnerable to the potential stresses that have been identified in this chapter. Some circumstances such as the birth of twins or of a premature, ill or malformed baby add significantly to the degree of stress experienced by the family. There are, in addition to such circumstances, maternal and family characteristics that make some families particularly prone to develop stress when a new baby arrives. (See Chapters 5 and 22 for a full discussion of these families.) The stresses derived from these situations may have devastating effects on the infant and his family.

The suggestions for nursing interventions with the families of infants indicate that a significant contribution can be made by a well-prepared, perceptive and supportive professional nurse. However, her role in working with these families will depend upon her opportunities to have contact with them.

Typical points of nurse-family contact today are in the hospital after birth, in physicians' offices and clinics, in parenting classes, in community health department channels, in informal neighborhood contacts and in fourth trimester follow-up (given in a few communities).

The postpartum nurse is in an ideal position to meet parents and share their initial experiences with the infant. However, new parents who have not yet taken their baby home do not know what their concerns will be at that point. As was noted before, the nurse's teaching is not retained well while the mother is in the taking-in phase of restoration, and the trend to earlier discharge limits the time available for teaching. Office and clinic contacts by the physician with the parents are usually very brief. Parenting classes are not available in all communities and may have a structured format that does not facilitate in-depth individual family assessment. Contacts through the community health department frequently involve the nurse in situations in which major problems already exist, diminishing the opportunity to provide preventive teaching and care. Informal neighborhood contacts may not occur, and if they do, the nurse carries no official authority to back her nursing intervention. The fourth trimester follow-up after hospitalization seems to offer the best opportunity for nursing intervention with the families of infants.

Nurses will need to prove the value of their role in the fourth trimester, just as they have needed to do in the development of prenatal education programs, if demand for their services and funding is to occur. If innovative nurses in a given community can begin to serve some families with infants after they bring their babies home from the hospital, the families' satisfied, word-of-mouth advertising will be the most convincing evidence that such intervention is helpful and needed.

Fourth trimester nursing follow-up might be made a part of a package of services offered by a group of physicians or a clinic. The package could include prenatal medical care and classes, intrapartum and postpartum medical care, parenting classes and fourth trimester nursing follow-up.

It is rarely mother alone, father alone, schools alone, friends alone — any one factor alone — that shapes the destiny of the child. Children from birth onward are affected by a mosaic of forces.[12] However, the most significant influences on a child's life are his parental relationships and family experience. It is for this reason that nurses who are prepared to assess the needs of families and to plan and intervene to meet these needs can have a significant role in identifying stress within families of infants and can initiate care to alleviate or reduce this stress.

In this chapter some potential stresses in the families of infants are identified and discussed. It is apparent that nurses have a significant role to play in relation to alleviating or reducing these stresses. One of the important new frontiers in the nursing of families is to bring the nurse in contact with the families of infants after they return to their homes and establish new family patterns.

References

1. A. Bernstein. Jealousy in the family. Parents, February 1979, p. 47
2. T. Brazelton. Future care of the infant. Birth and the Family Journal, Winter 1978, p. 242
3. T. Brazelton. The remarkable talents of the newborn. Birth and the Family Journal, Winter 1978, p. 187
4. N. Donaldson. Fourth trimester follow-up. American Journal of Nursing, July 1977, p. 1176
5. E. Duvall. Marriage and Family Development. J. B. Lippincott Co., 1977
6. M. Erickson. Trends in assessing the newborn and his parents. American Journal of Maternal-Child Nursing, Mar/Apr 1978, p. 99
7. M. Friedemann and K. Emrich. Emergence of infant sleep-wake patterns in the first three months after birth. International Journal of Nursing Studies, 1978, p. 5
8. J. Funke-Furber and C. Roemer. Failure to thrive. Canadian Nurse, December 1978, p. 30
9. J. Harris. When babies cry. Canadian Nurse, February 1979, p. 32
10. S. Hersh and K. Levin. How love begins between parent and child. Children Today, Mar/Apr 1978, p. 2
11. D. Miller and S. Baird. Helping parents to be parents — a special center. American Journal of Maternal-Child Nursing, Mar/Apr 1978, p. 117
12. J. Segal and H. Yahraes. Protecting children's mental health. Children Today, Sept/Oct 1978, p. 23
13. J. Williams. Learning needs of new parents. American Journal of Nursing, July 1977, p. 1173
14. J. Wit and C. Bernard. The fourth trimester. Continuing Education Conference sponsored by the Nurse's Association of the American College of Obstetricians, Gynecologists, and Neonatologists, March 1979

Additional Recommended Reading

L. Barnhill and D. Longo. Fixation and regression in the family life cycle. Family Process, December 1978, p. 469

J. Block. Impaired children: helping families through the critical period of first identification. Children Today, Nov/Dec 1978, p. 2

V. Satir. Conjoint Family Therapy (Revised edition). Science and Behavior Books, Inc., 1967

20 THE NEWBORN INFANT

by Carolyn Pedigo DeLoach, BSN, MSN
and Mary Lou Moore, BSN, MA, FAAN

The newborn period is defined as that from birth to one month of age. A synonymous term for newborn is *neonate*. The terms will be used interchangeably in this chapter.

The first section of the chapter focuses on the appraisal and care of the normal full-term newborn. "Normal" refers to the absence of physiological, pathological or neuromuscular conditions or all three. Minor deviations are common and considered normal; therefore they are included. "Full-term" refers to gestational age. The full-term newborn is one who is born following 38 to 42 weeks of gestation in utero.

Nursing appraisal and care is best learned first with the normal full-term newborn. Working from a normal base, the nurse can begin to recognize deviations from normal as minor or major and instigate appropriate nursing interventions.

The second section of the chapter focuses on identification and care of the dysmature neonate. Dysmature includes newborns who are preterm (less than 38 weeks of gestation at birth), small for gestational age, and large for age, and neonates with low birth weights. These newborns are at risk for morbidity and mortality; therefore, early identification and initiation of medical and nursing management is of utmost importance.

THE NORMAL NEWBORN

by Carolyn Pedigo DeLoach, BSN, MSN

"It's a girl!" "It's a boy!" A baby has been born. The whole gamut of emotional response might be compressed into this exclamation. After nine months of waiting, the momentous event has occurred. Parental adaptation to the birth may be influenced by many factors: whether or not the pregnancy was planned, whether or not the pregnancy was normal, the length of time and degree of difficulty in labor and delivery; the medications administered during labor and delivery, and the sex and appearance of the newborn. Nursing interventions are geared toward identifying those factors — parental or neonatal or both — which might interfere with a positive adaptation.

The birth transition from intrauterine to extrauterine existence may enhance or interfere with neonatal adaptation. In the neonate born at term, all systems are considered mature enough to adapt and support life outside the uterus. Following a nine-month existence in an environment that is totally protected and nurturing, the fetus is suddenly and sometimes painfully propelled through a narrow constricted passage into the bright, cold and noisy environment of the delivery room. In order to facilitate extrauterine adaptation, the neonate's nose and mouth are suctioned with a bulb syringe to remove mucus, which may obstruct respiratory passages. Once the umbilical cord is clamped and cut, the child is forced to establish independent life-sustaining functions. At no other time in an individual's life are greater physiological adjustments required than during the first hour after birth.[4]

INITIAL ASSESSMENT OF THE NEWBORN

Assessment of the newborn includes the initial Apgar scoring and comprehensive physical assessment, including gestational age and size (weight and length), and assessment of behavioral characteristics. Assessment is done to determine how satisfactorily the newborn is adapting to extrauterine life and to rule out any risk factors that might compromise growth or life or both.

Apgar Score

Dr. Virginia Apgar developed this tool for evaluating the infant's condition at birth.[2] Assessment is done at one minute and again at five minutes, using five standardized observations (heart rate, respiratory effort, reflex irritability, muscle tone and color). The one-minute assessment is valuable because it provides a rapid method of determining the infant's ability to adapt to extrauterine life. With the one-minute Apgar score, one can identify specifically the resuscitative measures that should be taken. The purpose of the five-minute score is to re-evaluate the newborn's condition, particularly his response to resuscitative measures.

As soon as delivery is complete a timer is started, so that the newborn can be assessed at exactly one minute. The *heart rate* is the first and most important observation made, providing the most useful diagnostic and prognostic information. It should be counted for a full minute either through auscultation of the precordium or palpation of the umbilical cord pulse located at the junction of the umbilical cord and the abdominal wall.

The second most important observation is *respiratory effort*. Only the newborn's unassisted respiratory rate is counted. Respiratory rate should be assessed by counting the number of

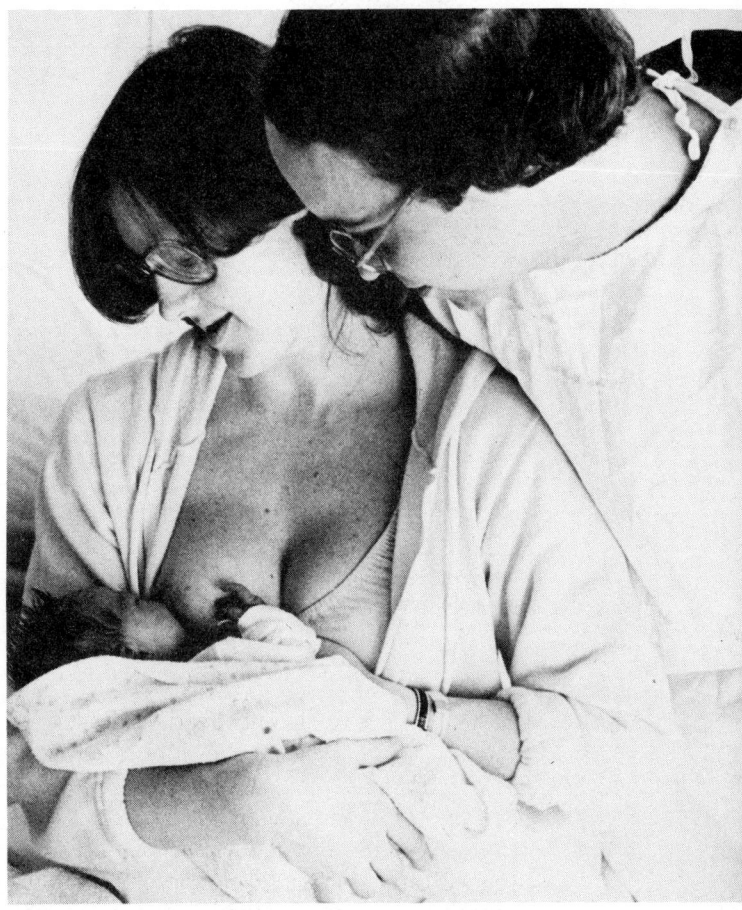

Parents and baby derive pleasure and form bonds of attachment during feeding.

inspirations within one full minute in order to note any delays in inspiratory effort. The rate may be determined by auscultation of the chest or observation of chest wall excursions.

Reflex irritability is assessed by stimulating the newborn in order to evoke a response. Suctioning the nares, gently rubbing the back or lightly flicking the sole of the foot are examples of stimuli used. The more alert the newborn, the more easily one can evoke a response.

Muscle tone is assessed by observing the infant's spontaneous return to a state of flexion, that is, when limbs are extended, they should return rapidly to their original position when released. The examiner should attempt to extend the extremities, noting the presence or absence of resistance and the rapidness of return to flexion. The infant's appearance in flexion is discussed later under the heading "General Appearance."

Color is the last observation, and according to

TABLE 20-1 APGAR SCORE CHART*

Observation	Score 0	Score 1	Score 2
Heart rate	Absent	Slow (below 100)	Over 100
Respiratory effort	Absent (apneic)	Slow, irregular, shallow	Good, sustained cry; regular respirations
Reflex irritability	No response	Grimace, frown	Sneeze, cough, cry
Muscle tone	Limp, completely flaccid	Some flexion of extremities; some resistance to extension of extremities	Active motion, good muscle tone, spontaneous flexion
Color	Cyanotic, pale	Body pink, extremities pale	Completely pink

*From V. Apgar, A Proposal For a New Method of Evaluating the Newborn Infant. Current Researches in Anesthesia, July-Aug 1953, p. 160.

Dr. Apgar, of least significance. All babies are cyanotic at birth. With the onset of respirations the skin becomes pink, except for the extremities, which may remain slightly cyanotic (*acrocyanosis*) for the first few hours of life. Acrocyanosis is due to insufficient circulation to the extremities, a condition that becomes reversed with adaptation to extrauterine life.

The Apgar Scoring Chart is found in Table 20-1. Each of the five observation areas should receive a score of 0, 1, or 2 according to the descriptions found in the score chart. When each of the five areas is scored, the sum total equals the Apgar score. A score of 10 is the highest possible and 0 is the lowest. An infant who has a score of 7 to 10 is in good condition and will only need suction of the nose and mouth and routine care and observation. A score of 3 to 6 indicates a moderately depressed infant who will need some form of resuscitation along with close observation during the first 24 hours of life. An infant who receives a score of 0, 1, or 2 is considered severely depressed and will need ventilatory assistance and intensive care as part of resuscitative measures.

Physical Assessment

Gross physical assessment should be performed immediately after delivery to identify risk factors that could potentially interfere with life or growth. Within the first 24 hours of life a thorough physical examination, including assessment of physical, neurological and behavioral characteristics, should be performed to provide a normal data base for comparison as the newborn progresses through life.

Dubowitz Assessment for Estimation of Gestational Age A standard set of criteria should be utilized for estimation of gestational age (GA) as an indicator of maturity. GA is defined as the number of weeks spent in utero to the time of birth. Dr. Lillian Dubowitz[7] and her colleagues developed a standardized tool, using 11 external signs and 10 neurological signs for estimating the gestational age of the newborn.

External physical characteristics should be assessed as soon as possible after birth. These physical characteristics are external signs of progressive tissue development. They provide data for evaluating the degree of physical maturity of the newborn.

The neurological signs provide data for evaluating neurological development and maturity through passive and active muscle tone. The newborn should be alert and quiet during the neurological testing in order to obtain valid results. Any signs that deviate from normal should be reassessed within 24 hours. The gestational age of the newborn is estimated by combining the score from the physical maturity chart (Table 20-2) and the score from the

TABLE 20-2 SCORE SHEET FOR EXTERNAL PHYSICAL CHARACTERISTICS*

External Sign	0	1	2	3	4	Score
Edema	Obvious edema of hands and feet; pitting over tibia.	No obvious edema of hands and feet; pitting over tibia.	No edema.			
Skin texture	Very thin, gelatinous.	Thin and smooth.	Smooth; medium thickness. Rash or superficial peeling.	Slight thickening. and peeling especially of hands and feet.	Thick and parchment-like; superficial or deep cracking.	
Skin color	Dark red.	Uniformly pink.	Pale pink; variable over body.	Pale; only pink over ears, lips, palms, or soles.		
Skin opacity (trunk)	Numerous veins and venules clearly seen, especially over abdomen.	Veins and tributaries seen.	A few large vessels clearly seen over abdomen.	A few large vessels seen indistinctly over abdomen.	No blood vessels seen.	
Lanugo (over back)	No lanugo.	Abundant; long and thick over whole back.	Hair thinning especially over lower back.	Small amount of lanugo and bald areas.	At least 1/2 of back devoid of lanugo.	
Plantar creases	No skin creases.	Faint red marks over anterior half of sole.	Definite red marks over > anterior 1/2; indentations over < 1/3.	Indentations over > anterior 1/3.	Definite deep indentations over > anterior 1/3.	
Nipple formation	Nipple barely visible, no areola.	Nipple well defined; areola smooth and and flat, diameter flat, diameter <0.75 cm.	Areola stippled, edge not raised, diameter < 0.75 cm.	Areola stippled, edge raised, diameter > 0.75 cm.		
Breast size	No breast tissue palpable.	Breast tissue on one or both sides, < 0.5 cm. diameter.	Breast tissue both sides; one or both 0.5–1.0 cm.	Breast tissue both sides; one or both > 1 cm.		
Ear form	Pinna flat and shapeless, little or no incurving of edge.	Incurving of part of edge of pinna.	Partial incurving whole of upper pinna.	Well-defined incurving whole of upper pinna.		
Ear firmness	Pinna soft, easily folded, no recoil.	Pinna soft, easily folded, slow recoil.	Cartilage to edge of pinna, but soft in places, ready recoil.	Pinna firm, cartilage to edge; instant recoil.		
Genitals Male	Neither testis in scrotum.	At least one testis high in scrotum.	At least one testis right down.			
Female (with hips 1/2 abducted)	Labia majora widely separated, labia minora protruding.	Labia majora almost cover labia minora.	Labia majora completely cover labia minora.			

EXTERNAL TOTAL:

*From L. Dubowitz et al. Clinical Assessment of Gestational Age in the Newborn Infant, Journal of Pediatrics, July 1970, p. 1.

neurological maturity chart (Fig. 20-1). The final score is then compared with the maturity rating scale (Table 20-3) in order to determine estimated gestational age. The full-term infant is 38 to 42 weeks of gestation.

The sections following are designed to provide experience in actual evaluation of an infant.

Physical Maturity With the newborn on an examining surface and using the scale in Table 20-2, assess each of the following physical characteristics: edema, skin texture, skin color, skin opacity, lanugo, plantar creases, nipple formation, breast size, ear formation, ear firmness and genitalia. The descriptions for each area range from 0 to 4 beginning with less mature development and progressing to mature tissue. After assessing the presence or absence

NEUROLOGICAL SIGN	SCORE 0	1	2	3	4	5
POSTURE						
SQUARE WINDOW	90°	60°	45°	30°	0°	
ANKLE DORSIFLEXION	90°	75°	45°	20°	0°	
ARM RECOIL	180°	90–180°	<90°			
LEG RECOIL	180°	90–180°	<90°			
POPLITEAL ANGLE	180	160°	130°	110°	90°	<90°
HEEL TO EAR						
SCARF SIGN						
HEAD LAG						
VENTRAL SUSPENSION						

Figure 20-1 Score sheet for neurological characteristics. (Reprinted by permission from L. Dubowitz et al. Clinical assessment of gestational age in the newborn infant. Journal of Pediatrics, July 1970, p. 1.)

flexion as possible. Measure the angle between the base of the thumb and the anterior aspect of the forearm. Full flexion = 4.

Ankle dorsiflexion–at the ankle, flex the foot onto the shin with sufficient pressure to provide maximum flexion ability. Measure the angle between the dorsum of the foot and the anterior aspect of the leg. A 20 degree angle = 3.

Arm recoil–with the baby in a supine position, fully flex both arms, hold for five seconds, fully extend and rapidly release arms. Recoil to a state of flexion should occur instantly. A brisk return to full flexion = 2.

Leg recoil–with the baby in a supine position, fully flex both legs without lifting the hips up from the surface. Hold flexed for five seconds, fully extend and rapidly release. Recoil to a state of flexion should occur instantaneously. A brisk return to full flexion (less than 90 degrees at knees and hips) = 2.

Popliteal angle–with the newborn in a supine position, flex one thigh on the abdomen. Be certain to keep body alignment straight and hips flat on the surface. While maintaining flexion of the thigh, attempt to straighten the leg toward the head until resistance is met. Measure the popliteal angle and score. Less than 90 degrees = 5.

Heel to ear–with the newborn in a supine position, pelvis flat on examining surface, attempt to pull the feet toward the head. When resistance is met, determine the distance between the heels and the ears and score according to distance.

Scarf sign–with the newborn in a supine position, place the arm across the chest so that the hand touches the opposite shoulder. The elbow may be lifted across the body. The score is determined by the location of the elbow. If the elbow does not reach the midline of the thorax, the score = 3.

Head lag–with the newborn supine, grasp both arms and slowly pull the infant up to a sitting

of edema, find the description in the scale that best describes your observation and give the newborn the appropriate score. Proceed in the same manner with each characteristic until you have completed the assessment, then add all the scores for a sum total of physical maturity.

Neuromuscular Maturity Using the scale in Figure 20-1, assess each of the neuromuscular signs using the following guide and assign the score that is closest to your observation.

Posture–with the infant quiet and in a supine position, observe the degree of flexion in the arms and legs. Muscle tone and degree of flexion increase with maturity. Full flexion of the arms and the legs = 4.

Square window–without rotating the wrist, flex the hand with enough pressure to get as great a degree of

TABLE 20-3 DUBOWITZ SCORE SHEET OF GESTATIONAL AGE

Total Score	Gestational Age (in weeks)
0–9	26
10–12	27
13–16	28
17–20	29
21–24	30
25–27	31
28–31	32
32–35	33
36–39	34
40–43	35
44–46	36
47–50	37
51–54	38
55–58	39
59–62	40
63–65	41
66–69	42

*From L. Dubowitz et al. Clinical Assessment of Gestational Age in the Newborn Infant, Journal of Pediatrics, July 1970, p. 1.

position. Observe the relationship of the head to the trunk during the procedure. If the newborn has sufficient muscle tone to hold his head slightly forward of the body, the score = 3.

Ventral suspension– with the newborn prone, place the palm of your hand supporting the chest. Raise the infant off the examining surface and observe the infant's independent postural change. Straightening of the back with slight hyperextension of the head = 4.

The sum total of these observations will yield the score for neuromuscular maturity. Find the sum total of the physical maturity scale and the neuromuscular maturity scale. Using Table 20–3, compare the newborn's score with the maturity rating scale to determine the newborn's estimated gestational age. This score is accurate within two weeks of the neonate's actual gestational age. After five days of life, the scoring becomes less accurate due to neurological and tissue maturing.

Appropriateness of Size for Gestational Age Once the gestational age (GA) has been determined, the examiner can assess the newborn's size in relation to the estimated gestational age (EGA). In their research, Dr. Lula Lubchenco and co-workers[10, 11] developed standardized tools for assessing weight, length and head circumference related to GA in order to determine if the newborn is appropriate for gestational age (AGA), small for gestational age (SGA), or large for gestational age (LGA). According to Figure 20–2, the AGA newborn has an average gestation of 40 weeks and a birth weight of approximately 3200 gm (7 lbs, 1 oz), which places the neonate at the 50th percentile. The average AGA newborn at 40 weeks has a length of 49 cm (19.3 in). The average head circumference of the AGA newborn at 40 weeks is 34 cm (13½ in).

LATER PHYSICAL ASSESSMENT

The initial assessment of the newborn is done immediately after birth, with the Apgar score and a gross assessment to rule out any life-threatening anomalies or major anomalies that are not life-threatening. Within the first 24 hours of life a second, more thorough assessment should be performed to provide a total comparative health data base for future assessment.

Before this examination is performed, a complete chart review should be done. Important areas to review are maternal and paternal age, family history, previous obstetrical history, whether or not the pregnancy was planned, course of pregnancy, labor and delivery, medication administered during labor and delivery, intrusive procedures (e.g., internal monitoring), and Apgar scores with appropriate resuscitative measures. Identification of any deviations from normal gives the examiner specific indicators to evaluate and hopefully rule out anomalies or provide data for immediate medical and nursing intervention.

For the examination, the newborn should be placed in a well-lighted, warm area that is free from drafts. Clothing should be removed as needed. Placing a hand on the newborn's abdomen provides a sense of safety and security for the newborn. The examination may need to be interrupted several times to cuddle and soothe the newborn. Be aware that examination results obtained when the newborn is quiet may be different from those when he is actively crying. Deviations from normal do not necessarily mean an abnormality exists; therefore, findings that deviate from normal should be reassessed within 24 hours. Allowing the parents to be present during the examination provides an excellent opportunity for teaching, reassuring and assessing parental interaction with the newborn. Parents must be able to see their newborn as an individual in order to progress through their developmental stages of adjustment. Utilizing the examination time to point out the unique characteristics of the newborn will provide parents with an increased awareness of their infant and facilitate their adjustment.

Growth and development is evaluated cephalocaudally (head to foot) and from gross motor to fine motor. A systematic examination carefully follows this sequence so that no area is missed. However, it may be necessary to assess those areas of observation requiring that the infant be in a quiet state first, or at a point when he becomes quiet, to assure accurate findings.

General Appearance The newborn assumes a posture similar to that in utero. If the fetus was in a vertex position, the newborn readily assumes a posture of flexion. The head is flexed with the chin on the chest, arms are flexed and held close to the chest with hands fisted, the back is slightly bent, the knees are flexed with thighs on abdomen and feet are dorsiflexed

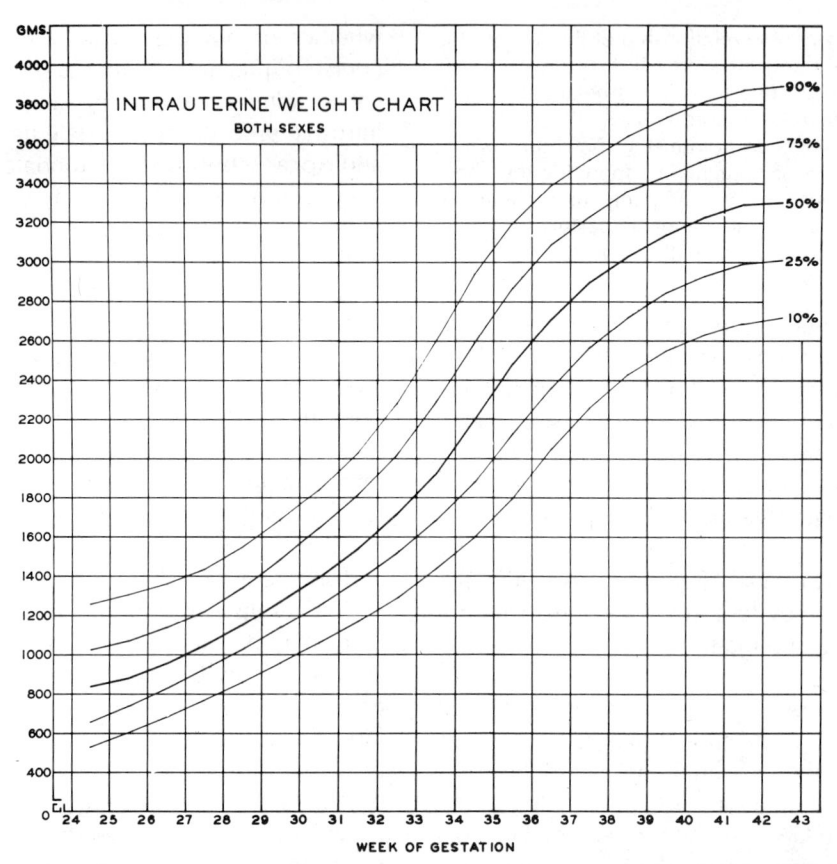

Figure 20–2 Intrauterine length, weight and head circumference charts. (Reprinted by permission from L. Lubchenco et al. Intrauterine growth as estimated from liveborn birthweight data at 24 to 42 weeks of gestation. Pediatrics, October 1963, p. 793.)

Illustration continued on opposite page

on the anterior aspect of the leg. This is the position of comfort for the newborn and is indicative of normal muscle tone. A decrease in muscle tone may be associated with trauma, sedation or preterm gestation. The newborn's size appropriateness for gestational age is as outlined in Figure 20–2. Flexion decreases the amount of body surface area exposed to the environment and thereby interferes with the rate of heat loss for the newborn. Swaddling the newborn loosely or covering lightly with a blanket will allow him to assume a position of flexion, yet not interfere with freedom of movement.

Respirations The neonate must rapidly initiate and maintain inspirations and expirations of sufficient depth and regularity to replace the terminated placental source of oxygen and carbon dioxide exchange. The normal term neonate takes his first breath within 30 seconds after birth (Fig. 20–3). A key factor in the initiation of respiration is the cooling and clamping of the umbilical cord with a resultant drop in arterial oxygen or hypoxemia (low PO_2). Cold, pain, touch, movement and light are all considered somatic (body) sensory stimuli that also affect the respiratory center to stimulate breathing.[5] Normally, fetal lungs are filled with fluid to at least the functional residual capacity (the amount of air still left in the lungs following normal expiration). Once the head is delivered during a vaginal, vertex (fetal head first) delivery, pressure from maternal vaginal muscles and tissue actually compresses the fetal thorax, squeezing out almost half of this lung fluid so that it can be suctioned from the nose and mouth. Following delivery, the chest reflexively expands, drawing in 20 to 40 ml of air.[8] Suctioning of the nose and mouth following delivery of the head is important, because without it any fluid remaining in the nose and trachea will also be pulled back into the lungs during reflexive chest wall expansion, interfering with effi-

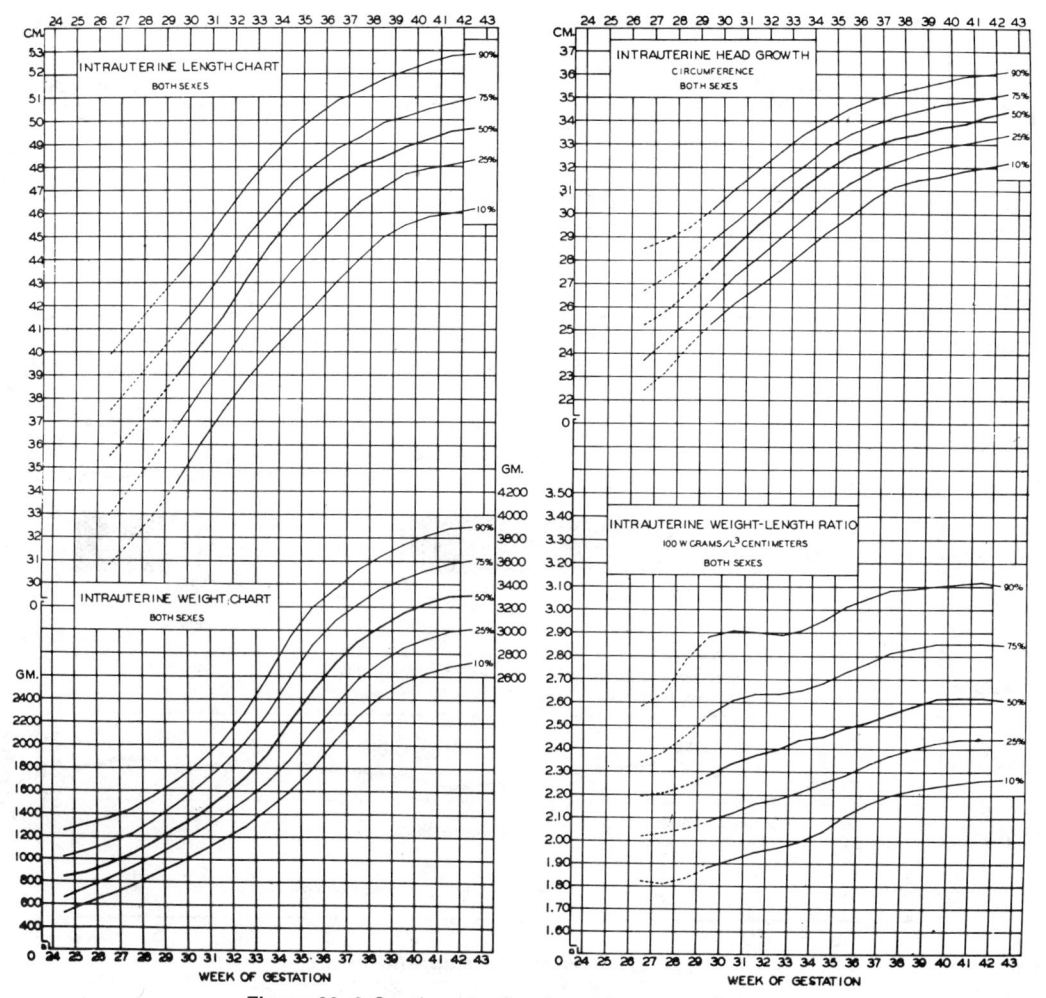

Figure 20-2 Continued. See legend on opposite page

cient gas exchange. The remaining lung fluid is rapidly absorbed within 6 to 24 hours. It moves from the lungs into the pulmonary capillaries and lymphatic system, then into the main circulation for excretion through the kidneys.[1]

The baby delivered by cesarean section does not have the benefit of vaginal compression of the thorax; therefore, considerable lung fluid remains and must be cleared for maximum gas exchange to occur.

Respirations (Fig. 20-3) may be irregular and should be assessed by counting the number of expirations for a full minute. The normal respiratory rate following successful adaptation to extrauterine life is 35 to 50 breaths per minute.

Circulatory Changes Fetal circulation and the changes that occur after birth are shown in detail in Chapter 24 (p. 530-531).

The newborn's peripheral circulation may be somewhat sluggish, accounting for transient cyanosis of the hands and feet and around the mouth (*circumoral cyanosis*).

At the time of birth, if the cord is allowed to cease pulsating before being clamped and cut, the baby will receive an additional 50 to 100 cc of blood from the placenta. The appropriate time to cut the cord is debatable. Some authorities think that the newborn can benefit from the additional volume of iron-rich oxygenated blood. Others believe that the additional volume is an overload for the newborn's system.

Assessment of the heart is done by auscultating the apical pulse at the fifth intercostal space, where it crosses the midclavicular line. This is also where the *point of maximum impulse* (PMI) can be palpated or observed or both. The first and second heart sounds should be clearly

THE NEWBORN INFANT   413

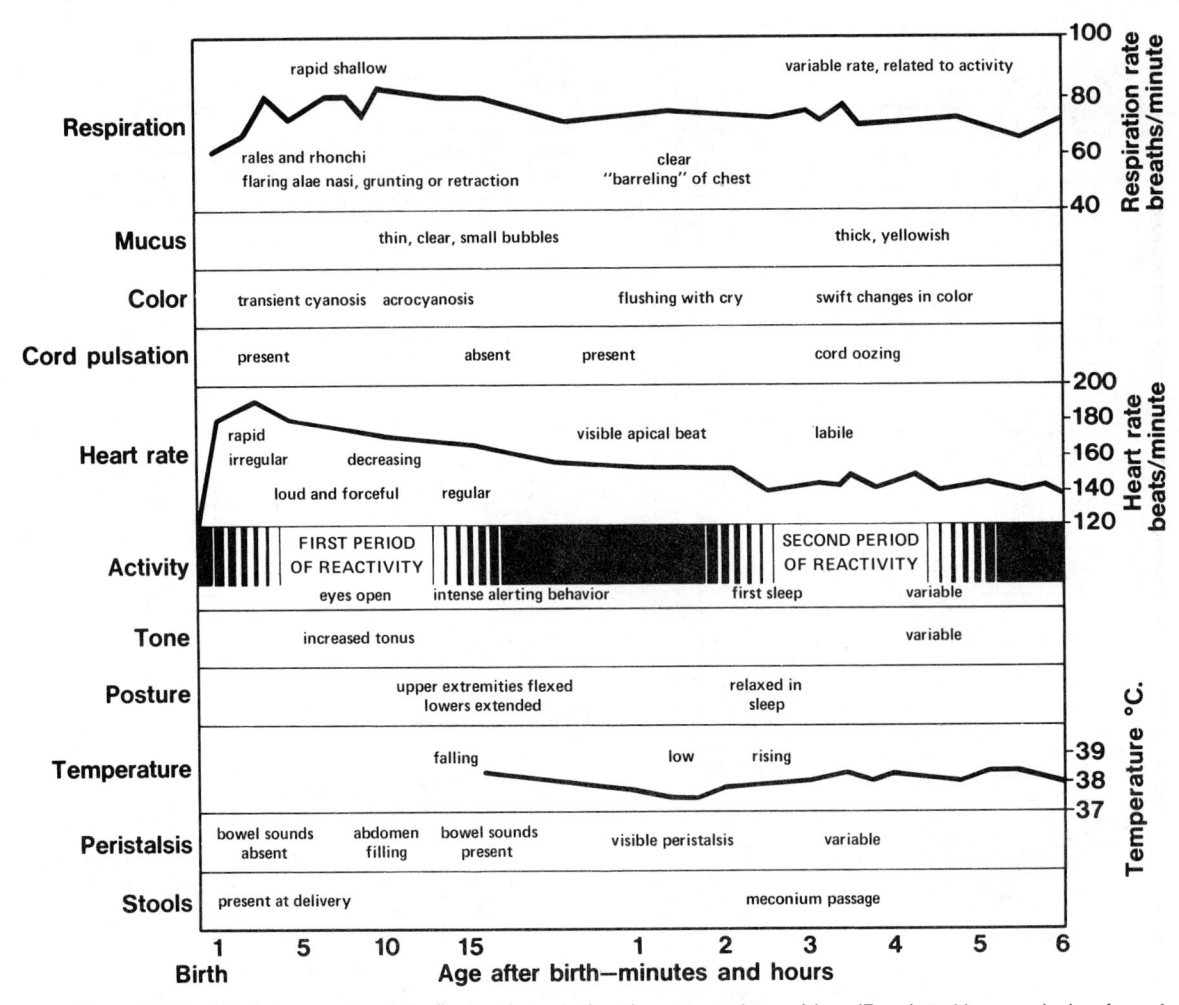

Figure 20-3 Vital signs and activity fluctuations during the neonatal transition. (Reprinted by permission from A. Clark and D. Affonso. Childbearing: A Nursing Perspective., 2nd ed. F. A. Davis, 1979.)

distinct. The rate may be rapid but should be regular, between 120 and 150 beats per minute (Fig. 20-3). Since activity influences the heart rate, the baby should be quiet for an accurate assessment.

Skin Assessment The skin of the newborn provides an index of growth. Well-nourished newborns have well-defined layers of subcutaneous fat over their bodies, which provide thermoregulation and a barrier against infection. Lack of subcutaneous fat may indicate prematurity or malnutrition. The skin should be observed closely for breaks as this may be a portal of entry for bacteria.

Skin Color Immediately after birth the term newborn's skin is erythematous (beefy red), then fades to its normal color within a few hours (Fig. 20-3). Acrocyanosis is a normal transient phenomenon caused by vasomotor instability, capillary stasis and high hemoglobin. Persistent generalized cyanosis is indicative of underlying distress.

Although skin pigmentation and darkening begins at birth, cyanosis may be difficult to assess in the non-caucasian newborn by simply looking at the skin. Careful inspection of the mucous membranes of the mouth and eyes and nail beds of the hands and feet will provide more accurate assessment.

Harlequin Color Change When the newborn is placed in a side-lying position, the side next to the mattress will turn pink while the upper side remains pale. This is known as harlequin color change and has no known significance. However, color distribution should remain even in supine or prone positions.

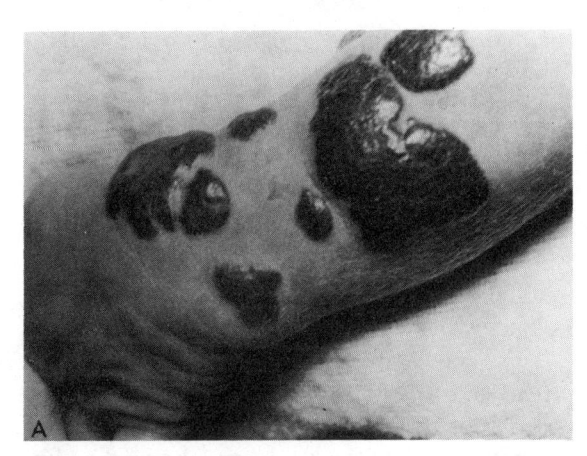

Figure 20-4 Strawberry hemangioma. (From M. Moore. The Newborn and the Nurse. W. B. Saunders Co., 1972, p. 104.)

Telangiectatic Nevi (Stork Bites) These are common on the upper eyelids, back of the neck and occiput. They are flat, localized, reddened areas created by capillary dilation and should disappear during the first year of life.

Strawberry Hemangiomas These may be present at birth or appear up to two weeks following birth. They resemble strawberry clusters and consist of dilated capillaries in the dermal and subdermal layers (Fig. 20-4). They are elevated and may continue to grow up to one year of age. Absorption and shrinkage takes place slowly and usually requires 7 to 10 years for completion. Although hemangiomas are unsightly and may be disturbing to parents, they are best left untreated.

Icterus Neonatorum Jaundice (yellowish color of the skin and sclera) is a normal physiological occurrence between the second and third day of life, appearing in about 50 per cent of all newborns.[12]

The normal breakdown of hemoglobin in fetal red blood cells produces bilirubin, which is conjugated by the liver. Bilirubin must be conjugated in order to bind with albumin for excretion. Unbound (indirect) bilirubin cannot be excreted from the body and is absorbed into fatty tissue and the brain. *Kernicterus* (permanent brain cell damage) will occur if the indirect bilirubin rises above 20 mg/100 ml of blood.

Phototherapy treatment may be instituted if the indirect bilirubin rises above 15 mg/100 ml.[3] Phototherapy involves continuous exposure of the naked neonate to fluorescent white light. It is important to keep the newborn's eyes covered at all times to prevent corneal and retinal damage. Parents should receive a full explanation of why their baby's eyes are being covered.

Once phototherapy is instituted, daily monitoring of bilirubin levels is necessary. Common side effects of phototherapy include overheating of the body, loose stools, skin rash and alteration in activity. Extra fluids should be given to prevent dehydration.

Mongolian Spots Bluish-gray or purple patches of pigmentation are seen across the sacrum or buttocks (Fig. 20-5). The pigmentation begins at birth in the basal layer of the epidermis and is prevalent among children of Asian, Southern European and African descent. These spots disappear by school age without treatment.

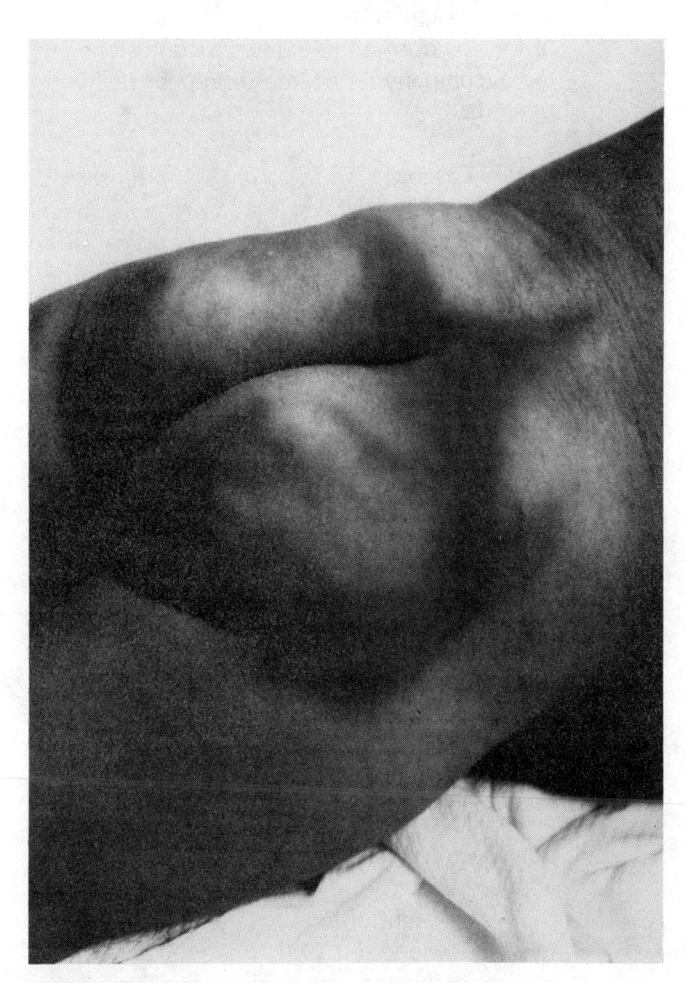

Figure 20-5. Mongolian spots. (Photo courtesy of Mead Johnson & Co., Nutritional Division.)

Erythema Toxicum This is a transient pink papular rash that may contain purulent vesicles. It occurs in 30 to 70 per cent of all normal newborns between the first and fourth day of life. The cause is unknown, although it may be a reaction to air, sheets and clothing. It disappears spontaneously within the first week.

Milia Small white papules commonly appear on the chin, cheeks, nose and forehead. They are caused by immature, distended sebaceous glands and disappear by two to four weeks of age. The nurse can teach mothers to clean the baby's face with clear water. Milia should not be squeezed or punctured.

Forceps Marks Contusions matching the rim of the forcep blade may appear on the newborn's face. Although this may be frightening to parents, it indicates correct placement and use of forceps during the delivery. Contusions and the accompanying edema disappear in two to three days.

Vernix Caseosa This is a cheesy, whitish substance that covers the skin as a protective agent in utero. It is usually caked in the folds of the skin. Some of the vernix is gradually absorbed by the skin, some dries and flakes off, and some is washed off with each bath. If vernix is allowed to remain caked in the skin folds after 24 hours, it can become a breeding place for bacteria. Excessive vernix may indicate prematurity; absence of vernix may indicate postmaturity.

Lanugo The presence, in varying amounts, of fine, downy hair over the shoulders, back and upper arms is a common newborn characteristic. It is indicative of gestational age (Table 20–2) and usually rubs off within two weeks.

Skin Texture At birth, the epidermis is thin, smooth and soft to touch. Within 24 hours, normal desquamation (scaling) occurs as the skin becomes extremely dry. Lotion may be applied to these dry areas, mostly for the mother's benefit. If lotion is used, excess lotion must be wiped off and the area should be washed before the next application. Skin texture at birth is important in assessing gestational age (Table 20–2).

Skin Turgor Turgor is related to tissue hydration and is present in the normal newborn. Transient edema may also be present around the eyes and dorsal aspects of the extremities due to birth trauma. Lack of skin turgor may indicate malnutrition in utero or metabolic disorders. To assess turgor, grasp the skin with thumb and forefinger and gently turn. The skin should feel elastic and return to a smooth surface when released.

Head Assessment The head of the newborn is proportionately large (approximately one fourth the total length of the newborn). The forehead is prominent and the chin recedes.

Head circumference (Fig. 20–2) is measured by placing the tape above the eyebrows and around the most prominent aspect of the occiput. Measurement may need to be repeated several times for accuracy. Accurate assessment of circumference provides a baseline for future assessment of cephalic development.

Molding With a vaginal, vertex delivery, the newborn's head molds to fit the birth canal more easily by gradual overlapping of the calvarium bones and narrowing or overriding of the sutures. Molding is usually not present following a cesarean birth. Parents may be anxious about the presence of molding; they need reassurance that it will disappear in a few days.

Fontanels and Suture Lines The fontanels are soft membraneous spaces where the skull bones join (Fig. 20–6). The anterior fontanel (soft spot) is diamond shaped and lies between the sagittal and coronal sutures. It is approximately 2 to 3 cm wide and 3 to 4 cm long. It closes at about 18 months of age. The posterior fontanel is triangular and lies between the sagittal and lambdoidal sutures. It is approximately 1 cm long and closes at about 2 months. The nurse should feel and measure the fontanels. Bulging fontanels are indicative of increased intracranial pressure; depressed or sunken fontanels are indicative of dehydration. Parents are sometimes afraid to touch the "soft spot" for fear of causing brain damage. Actually it is as tough as canvas and needs the same amount of stimulation as the rest of the scalp. The suture lines denote the separation of the cranial bones and are either closely approximated or overriding. They should never appear or feel separated; this is indicative of increased intracranial pressure.

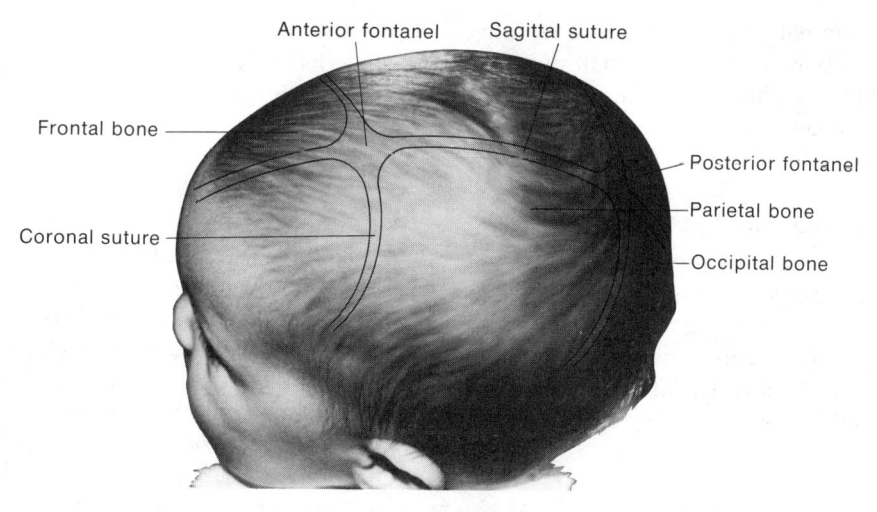

Figure 20-6 Location of the anterior and posterior fontanels.

Caput Succedaneum This is the result of diffuse (margins of swelling are indistinct) edema of the soft tissues of the scalp which may extend across suture lines (Fig. 20–7). It is caused by continuous pressure on the scalp during labor and is most pronounced following prolonged labor. It is gradually absorbed and disappears within a few days. Ecchymotic coloration (black and blue bruises) may be present; this may cause feelings of guilt and anxiety in parents. Nursing intervention should be directed toward helping parents resolve these feelings.

Cephalhematoma A collection of blood from ruptured blood vessels forms between the skull bone and the periosteum because of trauma to the head during the birth process (See Fig. 20–8). It does not cross suture lines because it is confined to one bone. Obvious swelling develops within 24 to 48 hours after birth. The area may be ecchymotic due to the presence of coagulated blood. Absorption of a cephalhematoma may take two to three weeks or longer. As with caput succedaneum, parents may experience guilt. The nurse should help absolve them of this feeling.

Scalp The nurse should palpate and inspect the scalp for lesions, bleeding or coarse, brittle

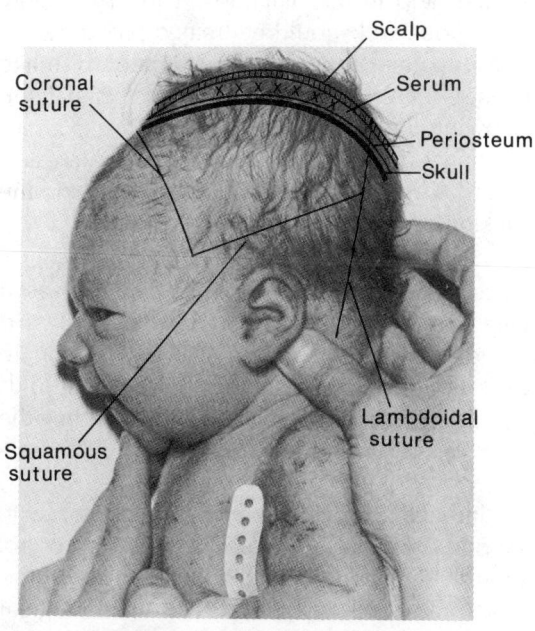

Figure 20-7 Caput succedaneum.

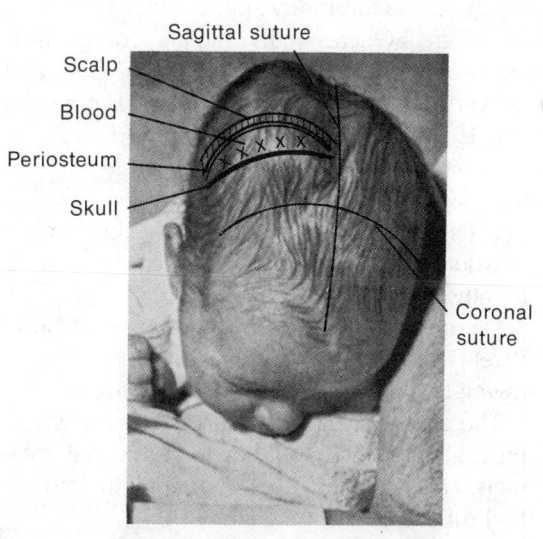

Figure 20-8 Cephalhematoma.

THE NEWBORN INFANT 417

hair. If an internal monitor was used during labor, the newborn will have a small puncture wound in the occipital area of the scalp. This area should be kept clean and dry and inspected for signs of infection.

Face The face should be inspected for symmetry of parts and symmetry between the left and right sides. Some asymmetry may be due to position — that is, resuming a position that was maintained in utero. This will disappear within a few weeks or months. Facial asymmetry may indicate facial nerve palsy due to birth trauma.

Eyes The eyes should appear clear without redness or purulent discharge. Occasionally, the eyelids are puffy with a purulent discharge during the first 24 hours. This is a transient chemical conjunctivitis due to silver nitrate (AGNO$_3$) drops administered to prevent ophthalmia neonatorum (gonorrheal conjunctivitis).

The eyelids are closed most of the time. Attempts to force the eyelids open will meet with resistance. Holding the newborn in an upright position and gently rocking the head back and forth will usually stimulate opening of the eyelids. Bright lights, loud noises and touching the eyelashes will cause the newborn to promptly close his eyes.

The sclera has a slightly bluish tint. When jaundice is present, the sclera becomes yellowish; this may be the first indication of jaundice because the ruddy skin color may mask it elsewhere. Occasionally, small conjunctival vessels rupture during the pressure of labor and delivery, causing a bright red streak near the iris. This is a subconjunctival hemorrhage and will disappear spontaneously within two to three weeks.

The iris is usually dark or grayish-blue in most newborns. Final eye color is present by 6 to 12 months of age.

Lacrimal gland ducts are immature at birth. Parents should be told not to expect tears with crying until one to three months of age.

The pupils should be observed for any whiteness or opacities that indicate congenital cataracts. This is particularly important if the mother had rubella during pregnancy.

Incoordinate eye movements, "setting sun" eyes, and the doll's eye phenomenon are transient reflections of neuromuscular immaturity. They usually disappear after 10 days. However, setting sun eyes may also be indicative of hydrocephaly.

Ears Cartilage formation is present in the ears, although not complete. This allows the pinna to bend easily, but it should rebound. It is important to assess the position of the ears. The top of the external ear should be slightly above the level of the eyes. Low-set ears are seen in infants with chromosomal abnormalities; these abnormalities include other physical defects and mental retardation. Low-set ears may also be associated with renal disorders.

Nose The newborn's nose may appear large or slightly flattened. This discrepancy will disappear as the newborn's face grows. Remember that newborns are nose breathers; therefore, nasal obstructions should be prevented. (Mucus should be removed by suction; breast tissue should be held away from the baby's nose during breast feeding.)

Mouth The mouth can be visualized during crying. The mucous membrane is pink and moist. Thrush, a candida infection transmitted during the birth process, may be identified as white or gray patches on the tongue, gums and entire buccal mucosa. Occasionally, milk curds are mistaken for thrush. Irrigating with sterile water or gently wiping with a tongue blade should help in the diagnosis. Thrush is highly contagious and should be treated promptly.

The palate should be examined to make certain there is no separation (cleft palate). Allowing the newborn to suck on the examiner's finger is a good way to assess the palate and at the same time assess the strength of the sucking reflex.

Neck The neck is short, chubby and creased with skin folds. It should be flexible enough to rotate from side to side and from flexion to extension. The nurse should visualize the folds by raising the shoulders and hyperextending the neck. Excessive folds (webbing) may be associated with pathological conditions.

Although the neck is not strong enough to support the head, some degree of head control should be evident. Hyperextension (*opisthotonus*) may be associated with pathological conditions. Decreased muscle tone (*hypotonia*) is manifested by inability to lift the head. This may be indicative of prematurity, pathology or hypoxia.

Chest The overall appearance of the chest should be symmetrical. Breast engorgement may occur in both males and females due to circulating maternal hormones. Occasionally, a thin, watery fluid may be secreted from the nipples. Engorgement and fluid will disappear within two weeks. Fluid should not be expressed from the breasts.

Abdomen The abdomen of the newborn is slightly protuberant. The nurse should observe it for signs of distention such as tight skin that makes subcutaneous vessels visible.

The umbilical stump is bluish, moist and shiny. It should contain two arteries and one vein. An umbilical cord containing only one artery may be associated with congenital anomalies. The cord stump begins to dry, darken and slough off by the sixth to tenth day.

The cord stump should be inspected for bleeding and signs of infection. Swabbing the cord stump with alcohol facilitates the drying process. Bellybands should not be used, since they interfere with drying and provide a dark, warm, moist environment conducive to bacterial growth.

Anogenital Area The anus should be inspected for patency. An imperforate (closed) anus interferes with the passage of stools. The first stool should be passed within 24 hours. This condition may also be diagnosed when it is found impossible to insert a rectal thermometer.

The female genitals consist of the *labia majora*, the *labia minora*, the *clitoris* and the *vaginal opening*. The labia majora covers the labia minora. The hymenal tag is a fleshy pink tag protruding from the base of the vagina. It is present in nearly all female newborns, but gradually atrophies and disappears by the end of the fourth week. The labia may be engorged due to the influence of circulating maternal hormones. Hormones are also responsible for a milky vaginal discharge tinged with mucus or blood or both. Both the edema and the discharge should disappear as soon as the hormones have cleared from the newborn's system. The urinary meatus is diffuclt to visualize; therefore, the number of voidings should be observed and recorded.

In male newborns, the scrotum is edematous and covered with rugae. Both testes can be palpated in the sac. Occasionally, one or both testicles may recede temporarily into the body cavity through the inguinal ring when the baby is exposed to cold. *Cryptorchidism* is a condition in which one or both testes has not descended. This condition requires referral to determine the cause and treatment.

The *glans penis* (head of the penis) is covered by the *prepuce* (foreskin). The foreskin is not retractable and cannot be displaced until four to six months of age. The foreskin should never be forcefully retracted, not even for cleansing purposes. The prepuce should be examined to rule out stenosis. The external *urinary meatus* (a small slit) is located near the tip of the glans penis and should be easily visualized. Occasionally, the meatal opening is located on the ventral portion of the glans penis (*hypospadias*) or dorsal portion (*epispadias*).

Circumcision (surgical removal of the prepuce) is a common practice today, although the necessity for this operation is debatable. Only rarely is it required to correct a defect, as when the foreskin is so constricted that it interferes with voiding or circulation (phimosis). Circumcision is contraindicated in the presence of *hypospadias*, because the foreskin will be used during surgical reconstruction of the meatal opening at a later time.

Extremities The arms and legs of the newborn appear short. They should be symmetrical in shape and movement. The nurse should observe the position (flexion) assumed at rest and inspect fingers and toes for extra digits, clubbing of fingers, fusion or webbing. The hands are examined for palmar creases. A simian crease (single line crease across the palm) is associated with Down's syndrome. The feet are inspected for area of sole creases and clubbing.

Hip dislocation is determined by placing the newborn in a supine position and testing for Ortolani's sign. Both legs are flexed and abducted (away from the body) to nearly touch the examining surface. A click may be felt or heard if a dislocation is present. On turning the newborn to a prone position, the nurse should note the creases of the buttocks and thighs. They should be symmetrical and the legs should be the same length. Movement should be noted, as

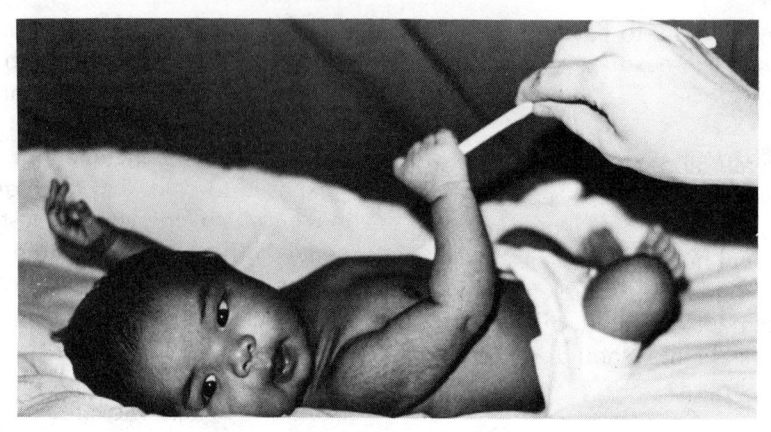

Figure 20-9 Palmar grasp reflex.

fine tremors of the extremities may indicate hypoglycemia.

Back The back is examined and palpated for spinal defects and curvature. Tufts of hair may indicate *spina bifida*. The coccygeal area (base of the spine) should be examined for pilonidal dimples, or cysts.

NEUROLOGICAL EXAMINATION

Reflex responses provide important data on the status of neurological functioning. Abnormal signs that are present in the first days or weeks of life may disappear and be followed by abnormal findings months or years later. Therefore, every physical examination should include assessment of reflexes. Since this may be a tedious, tiring experience for the newborn, the total examination may have to be performed in stages. Also remember that neonatal central nervous system function may be decreased by narcotics administered to the mother during labor.

Rooting Reflex Lightly stroking the cheek at the side of the mouth will stimulate the newborn to turn his head in that direction in order to find food. The rooting reflex disappears at about six weeks, when it is no longer needed. If the mother grasps both cheeks in an effort to turn the newborn's head in the direction of breast or bottle, she creates confusion for the newborn with this double stimulus. Absence, weakness or asymmetry of responses may indicate CNS depression or dysfunction.

Sucking Reflex The sucking reflex is stimulated by touching the newborn's lips or placing an object in his mouth. Sucking should be rhythmic and strong enough to obtain nourishment from breast or bottle. If the sucking reflex is unstimulated it will disappear rapidly. Ordinarily it begins to diminish at about 6 months of age. This is a good time to begin weaning.

Swallowing Reflex The swallowing reflex is stimulated by food on the posterior portion of the tongue. Swallowing is spontaneous, but the newborn may need a little time to coordinate sucking and swallowing effectively. Gag, cough and sneeze reflexes are protective methods of maintaining a clear airway. These are particularly evident during early feedings when the newborn has to handle mucous in addition to nursing.

Grasp Reflexes: Palmar and Plantar Exerting pressure on the palmar surface of the hand will stimulate curling or grasping of the fingers (Fig. 20-9). The grasp is so strong that the newborn can be raised momentarily by the examiner's finger. This reflex disappears at 6 weeks to 3 months of age.

Placing an object on the plantar surface (sole) of the foot will stimulate curling or grasping of the toes (Fig. 20-10). This reflex disappears at about 8 to 9 months of age.

Traction Response Placing the newborn in a supine position and slowly pulling him to a sitting position by holding the wrists demonstrates this. Response should be extension of the arms with some degree of head control.

Moro Reflex (Startle Response) The Moro reflex is the single most significant response denoting CNS status. This response can be elicited

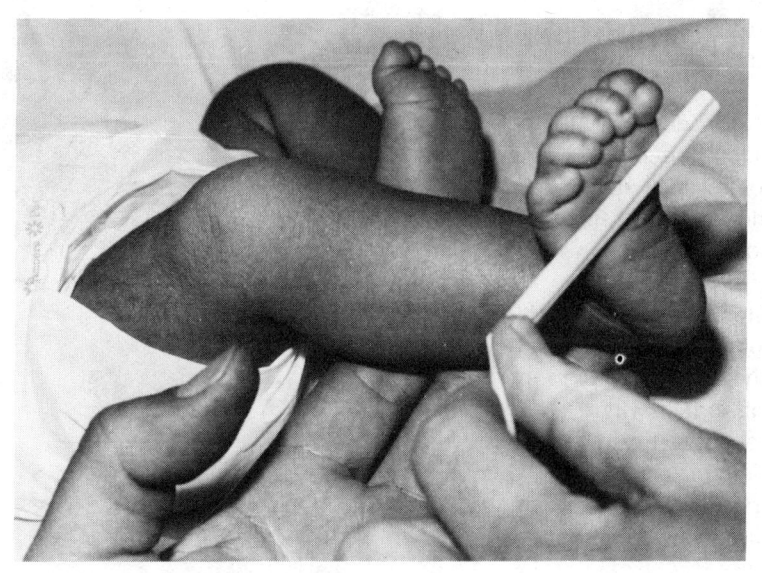

Figure 20-10 Plantar grasp reflex.

by startling the newborn with a loud noise or by bumping his crib. The nurse can place the newborn in a supine position, grasp both arms, allow the head to remain on the exam surface, and raise the shoulders by gentle traction on the arms: release arms, allowing shoulders to drop to the surface and observe the newborn's response. A normal response includes two phases: (1) Quick flexion at elbows is followed by abduction (away from the body) of the upper limbs at the shoulders, extension of the forearms at the elbows and extension of the fingers and legs; (2) Subsequent adduction (toward the body) of the arms at the shoulders and the legs against the abdomen (Fig. 20-11). Observe the completeness and symmetry of the response and the degree of difficulty in eliciting it.

The Moro reflex is strong during the first eight weeks of life and fades by the end of the second or third month.

Yawn, Stretch and Hiccough Reflexes These reflexes are demonstrated spontaneously by the newborn and have been related to increasing oxygen intake and elimination of gas. Parents generally express concern and want to know how to intervene when the newborn develops hiccoughs. The nurse can reassure them that this hiccoughing is normal. Increased yawning, sneezing and hiccoughing are frequently ob-

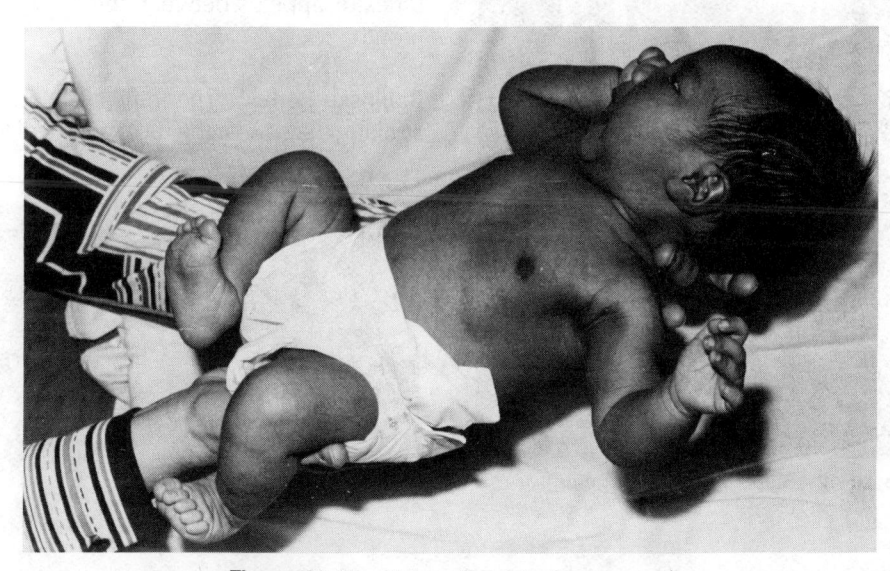

Figure 20-11 Moro reflex (startle response).

served in newborns of heroin-addicted mothers as they experience withdrawal syndrome.

Trunk Incurvation Reflex With the newborn in a prone position, touching along one side of the vertebral column will elicit curvature of the spine toward the stimulated side. This is a good test of spinal cord integrity.

Placing and Stepping Reflexes Holding the infant in an upright position and allowing the dorsal part of the foot to lightly touch one edge of the examining surface will result in spontaneous lifting of the foot by flexion of the knees and hips. The newborn looks as though he is *placing* each foot alternately on the examining surface. This reflex disappears after three to four weeks.

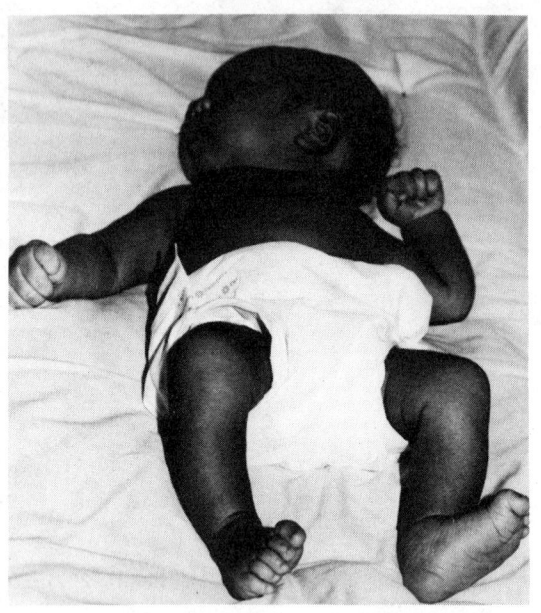

Figure 20–13 Tonic neck response (fencing position).

The stepping reflex is stimulated with the newborn in an upright position. When the soles of his feet touch a hard surface he will take a few quick alternating steps (Fig. 20–12). The stepping reflex disappears by 3 months.

Tonic Neck Reflex (TNR) TNR is known as the "fencing position" because it simulates the position assumed by someone preparing to fence. Place the newborn in a supine position and turn his head to one side or the other. Observe extension of the arm and leg on the side to which the head is turned and flexion of the opposite arm and leg (Fig. 20–13). This reflex disappears between the second and third month.

Babinski Reflex The reflex is stimulated by stroking the sole of the foot from heel to toe. The

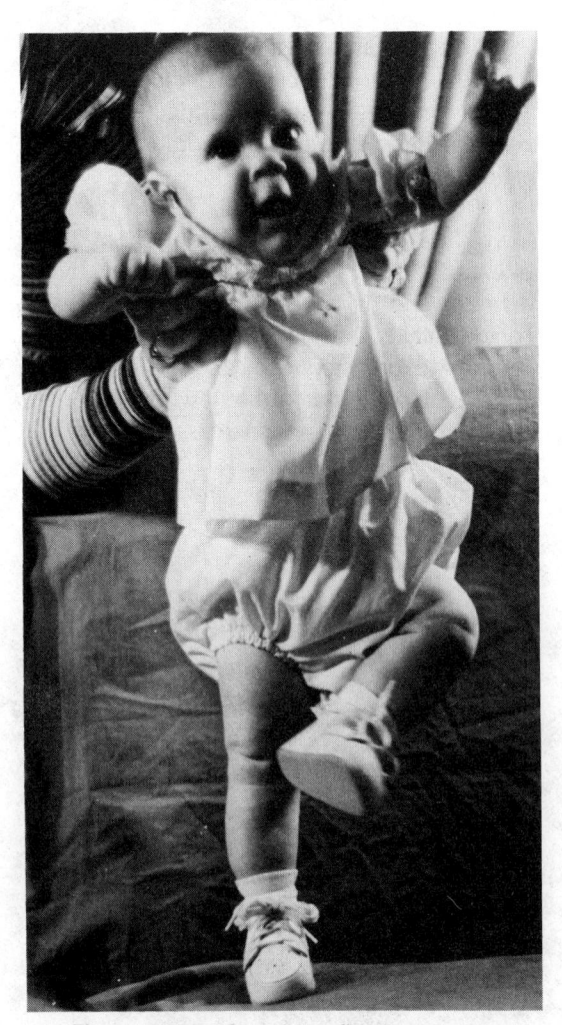

Figure 20–12 Stepping reflex (dancing).

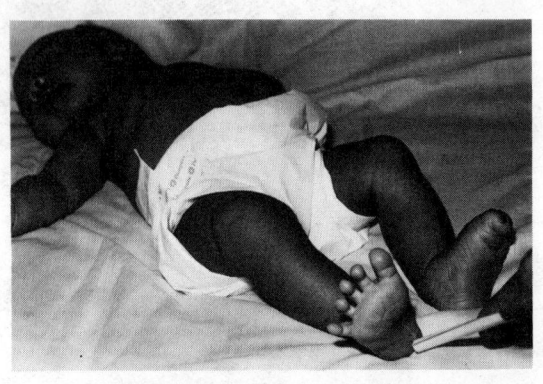

Figure 20–14 Babinski reflex.

response is dorsiflexion of the big toe and fanning or spreading of the other toes (Fig. 20-14). The Babinski reflex is present until three months of age but may persist until the child walks, at which time an adult response of flexion is elicited.

There are many other reflexes to include in a thorough neurological examination. However, the ones discussed here are of greatest importance in performing a nursing assessment of the central nervous system of the newborn.

Senses

Vision Visual behavior is present at birth. The neonate is farsighted, so that near vision is unclear. Fixation is present immediately at birth. The newborn seems to have a preference for the human face and will follow a moving object with his eyes. If the face or object moves past his midline of vision, it no longer exists for him and he is unable to actively seek the object of fixation. Parents need to be encouraged to engage in frequent face-to-face contact with their infants.

The eyes are sensitive to light and the newborn will blink or squint in response to light. The newborn has the ability to see details of forms such as the human face and to see contrast and color. Parents need to be informed of the newborn's visual capacity so that they may provide visual stimulation.

Hearing Hearing is present at birth, although temporarily hindered by amniotic fluid in the middle ear. Within a few hours after birth, the fluid is absorbed and replaced by air. Behavioral manifestations of hearing include *alerting* (seems to stop and listen), eye movements, startle reaction and crying. The newborn's ability to determine the cause and direction of sound does not develop until weeks later.

The newborn will respond to various sounds in a reflexive manner (Moro, blink). An actively crying newborn will respond to a soothing voice by abruptly ceasing all activity as though alerting to the sound. From 3 to 14 weeks of age, eye response to noise includes opening the eyes or squinting. Some head movement may also occur.

Taste The newborn can differentiate between bitter and sweet tastes. Pleasurable flavors will elicit active sucking, whereas bitter or unpleasant flavors will cause the newborn to protrude his tongue and turn away.

Smell The sense of smell is present as soon as the nose is clear of amniotic fluid and mucus, although the degree of development is unclear. Some researchers speculate that the newborn learns to differentiate his mother by recognizing her own particular body scent.

Touch Tactile sensation is well developed at birth, particularly in the facial area (rooting, sucking). Sensitivity to pain and extreme temperatures seems to be present, but not distinct, at first. By the tenth day, a definite reaction to painful stimuli is observed.

Assessment of Behavioral Patterns

Brazelton was instrumental in bringing to focus neonatal behavioral states as part of the overall assessment. Cortical control, responsiveness and eventual management of the environment can be more accurately predicted through evaluation of behavioral responses of infants. Interaction of parents and newborn, in which the newborn shares some responsibility, is of primary importance. Through his behavioral responses, the newborn can either facilitate or interfere with attachment and caretaking responsibilities. Fostering attachment must begin with helping the parents become aware of the unique behavioral responses of their newborn.

Sleep/Wake Patterns The first six to eight hours after birth are termed the *transitional period* from intrauterine to extrauterine existence. Phases of physiological instability are identifiable during this period.[6]

First Period of Reactivity This period lasts up to 30 minutes after birth (see Fig. 20-3). The newborn is awake, alert and active. His eyes are open, he looks around and may even appear hungry. (This is the best time for first introductions between parents and newborn.) The prophylactic use of silver nitrate drops should be slightly delayed so as not to cloud the newborn's vision during this phase. Respirations are rapid and irregular. Some grunting and barreling of the chest may be present. The heart rate is rapid with some irregularity. The body temperature falls.

Recent studies reveal that newborns held close to the mother's body during this period experience no significant heat loss as compared to those placed under a warming light.*

The nurse should use this first period of reactivity to encourage parents to hold, touch and observe their newborn. Face-to-face contact is particularly important. The newborn's alertness begins to fade, his activity level gradually decreases and he sleeps. Air enters the gastrointestinal tract and bowel sounds can be heard by the end of the first hour.

Second Period of Reactivity This period occurs at about four to eight hours of life (see Fig. 20-3). The newborn awakens and is alert. He usually experiences a gagging episode with regurgitation of mucus and debris from the birth canal. The sucking reflex is present and he again appears hungry. Passage of the first meconium stool occurs.

All neonates experience this sequence of events regardless of gestational age or type of delivery. However, the amount and kind of stress experienced by the neonate will cause some variation in the length of time the periods last. Once the periods are completed, the infant's behavior becomes stabilized, with predictable waking periods every three to four hours.

PHYSICAL CARE OF THE NEWBORN

Thermoregulation

Thermal balance is maintained by regulation of heat loss and heat production. The environment plays a major role in heat loss; therefore maintenance of an optimal thermal environment is one of the most important aspects of neonatal care. Heat exchange (loss) between the body and the environment occurs by evaporation, conduction, convection and radiation.

Evaporation Immediately after delivery the newborn is covered with amniotic fluid (liquid), which is converted to a vapor utilizing thermal energy. Evaporation with heat loss is increased when the environmental humidity is low. Drying the newborn thoroughly with warm towels will interfere with heat loss through evaporation. Bathing the newborn may also contribute to evaporative heat loss. Therefore, bathing should not be performed until the body temperature is normal and stable. In many institutions vital signs (especially temperature) are taken before a bath is begun. This is a good way to determine the appropriateness of the planned bath.

Conduction Loss of body heat through conduction occurs when the skin is in direct contact with a cooler surface. Body heat rapidly moves to the cooler surface to equalize the different temperatures. The naked newborn should always be placed on a padded, warm surface to prevent conductive heat loss. This is important to remember when performing bathing and examining procedures.

Convection Loss of body heat via convection occurs when the surrounding air is cool. Heat moves from the body surface to the cooler surrounding air. Temperature, air movement and humidity all contribute to the rate of convection. Convective heat loss can be reduced by maintaining an ideal environmental temperature and humidity (72 to 76° F; 40 to 60 per cent humidity); however, air temperature will have no significant effect on heat loss by radiation or evaporation.

Radiation Radiant heat loss occurs by transfer of body heat to a cooler solid object that is not in direct contact with the newborn. If the warmer or incubator has a warm padded surface and the environmental temperature is warm and the newborn is dry, heat loss may still occur if the newborn unit is placed in close proximity to a cold window or wall or other sources of coldness. The amount of heat loss through radiation is directly related to the distance from a cold surface. The implications are obvious for placement of the newborn in the delivery room, newborn nursery and home nursery.

Discussion of the four modalities of exchange of heat between the body and the environment has focused on heat loss for the newborn. However, body heat gains may occur in the same manner from external sources. Precau-

---

*C. Britton. Early mother-infant contact and infant temperature stabilization. Journal of Obstetrical, Gynecological and Newborn Nursing, Mar/Apr 1980, p. 84
S. Hill and L. Shronk. The effect of early parent-infant contact on newborn body temperature. Journal of Obstetrical, Gynecological and Newborn Nursing, Sept/Oct 1979, p. 287.

tions should be taken to prevent excess heat loss or heat gain when caring for the newborn.

Heat Production The newborn who is exposed to a heat-loss environment will compensate by increasing his heat production through increased metabolic activity. The full-term infant who is exposed to cold can increase his thermogenic rate two and one-half times over the resting state to a level that almost equals that of the adult.[9]

The newborn exposed to cold stress increases his heat production through a mechanism called *nonshivering thermogenesis*. This refers to heat that is produced by an increased metabolic rate in a cold environment. This in turn requires increased oxygen consumption. The type of body fat known as brown fat seems to be the major source of heat that is produced by nonshivering thermogenesis. Brown fat comprises 2 to 6 per cent of the newborn's body weight. It usually disappears some weeks after birth when it is no longer needed. Exposure to cold will deplete stores of brown fat. If the depletion is severe, as with prolonged cold stress, it is hypothesized that effective thermogenic capacity is eliminated.[9] The cold-stressed newborn is also at risk for developing hypoxemia, metabolic acidosis, rapid depletion of glycogen stores and reduction of blood glucose levels (*hypoglycemia*).

Thermal Management All newborns lose some body heat immediately after delivery. Physiologically, cold stimuli are probably essential to the initiation of extrauterine respirations; however, too much is hazardous. The temperature of the newborn's skin signals the presence of a metabolic response to heat loss. A drop in skin temperature indicates a heat loss environment that requires warming. The metabolic responses to cold stress will be triggered before core (deep tissue) temperature changes occur. Rectal temperature may be normal in the cold stressed newborn in the beginning. Axillary temperatures may be falsely high due to the presence of brown fat padding. During the first few hours after birth, when the newborn has difficulty regulating and maintaining body temperature, a heat-sensitive probe taped to the abdomen is the most accurate method of continually assessing body temperature status. The probe should remain uncovered to assure accuracy of skin temperature recordings. Once the newborn's temperature has stabilized, rectal temperature readings are sufficiently accurate.

Parents should be taught how to use a rectal thermometer on their newborn: lubricate the tip with petroleum jelly and gently insert the tip (about ¼ inch) into the rectum. The thermometer can be held in place with one hand while the infant's legs are grasped at the ankles with the other hand. This prevents kicking, which may cause the thermometer to be inserted deeper. Hold the thermometer in place for three minutes before reading.

A good basic understanding of the modalities of heat loss, heat production and thermal regulation is extremely important in giving care to the newborn.

Bathing

The purpose of bathing is to provide skin stimulation and maintain cleanliness while allowing inspection. Newborns do not perspire; therefore they do not need to be bathed daily. The face, chin and neck should be cleansed after each feeding, and the perianal area is cleansed with each diaper change. The condition of the skin and the environmental temperature are good guidelines in assessing the need for a bath. During the summer when it is hot and humid a daily bath may be refreshing, whereas during the winter, bathing the newborn three to four times per week is sufficient.

During the first few days after birth, the vernix gradually disappears and the skin becomes dry and scaling. There may even be slight bleeding where the skin becomes cracked around the hands and feet. This is normal, but to bathe the infant daily will increase this drying process. Parents express concern about dryness and generally wish to apply lotion to the dry skin. The use of lotion is of benefit only to the parents. However, it will cause no harm if the excess lotion is removed and the area is washed before reapplication of lotion. Allowing layers of lotion to remain on the newborn's skin provides a warm, moist environment for bacteria to breed and grow. A newborn should not be immersed in a tub of water until the cord has dropped off and the stump has healed (approximately 10 days maximum). During that time, sponge bathing is appropriate.

Parents should be told that bath time should be planned sometime before a meal and when the baby is not fussy. Bathing right after a feeding may cause the newborn to spit up. Bath time should be fun for the parents and the baby. Teaching parents to bathe their infant while still in the hospital is an important part of discharge preparation.

The newborn can be bathed in a baby bathtub or placed on the kitchen table or a bed. The bath area should be warm, without drafts and at a comfortable height so that the parent does not become overly tired (stretching and bending). The area should also be big enough to work in comfortably. Some parents enjoy using the kitchen sink. If the sink is used, a few safety factors must be kept in mind:

1. Clean the sink thoroughly.
2. Place a folded towel in the bottom of the sink for padding.
3. Prepare the water and then turn the faucet away from the baby before placing the baby in the water. Accidental burns could occur if the temperature should change while water is allowed to flow directly over the newborn.

The bath water should be comfortably warm. Feeling the water with the elbow is a good way to test the water. Other articles needed are a clean towel and washcloth, a bar of mild soap, a comb or a soft brush and clean clothing. Everything should be arranged in the bathing area before beginning. *Once the procedure is begun, the newborn must not be left unattended for any reason.* One hand should be kept on the baby at all times. This is an important safety rule to be applied in all areas of infant care.

Place the newborn on a padded surface and wash his eyes and face gently with clear water. Use a different portion of the washcloth for each eye and clean by wiping from the edge of the nose outward (inner canthus to outer canthus). Some babies do not like to have their faces covered. Gentle, soothing touch and speaking or singing quietly will help the newborn learn to enjoy the experience. The ears and nose should be cleaned with a wisp of cotton or the end of a washcloth. A Q-tip should never be inserted into these areas; damage to the delicate tissue may result.

The head should be lathered and the fontanel area (soft spot) should be washed as well. There is no need for the parents to be afraid to touch this area.

Cradle cap, a desquamation that may occur on the scalp (particularly over the fontanel area) can be prevented by daily washing and rinsing. If scales do occur, they can be softened with baby oil and removed with a fine tooth comb or brush after washing. The newborn should be picked up and the soap rinsed off the head. The "football carry" is a comfortable and safe way to hold the newborn. This also gives good face-to-face contact during the procedure.

Further instructions for the mother bathing the baby are: place the newborn back on the padded surface and dry his head. Proceed to undress him and gently lather his front; turn him on his abdomen and lather his back. It feels nice to lather the infant's head and skin with the hands; the skin-to-skin contact can be very satisfying to parents and baby. After lathering, remember that the baby is very slippery. Pick him up gently, supporting head and back, and gradually lower him into the water. Supporting the baby's head out of the water with one hand, use the other hand to gently swirl the water over his body. As the baby learns to enjoy the water, he will enjoy kicking and splashing. Allow enough time for this form of play.

Cord Care

The cord should be kept dry until it falls off and the stump has healed. The process generally requires 5 to 10 days. There should be no active bleeding at the site. A few drops of blood are not uncommon when the cord begins to separate. The nurse should inspect the area for signs of infection (redness, edema, drainage).

A drying agent may be used. Some physicians recommend applying triple dye once a day or swabbing the cord and base with alcohol at each diaper change. The use of bellybands is contraindicated. They do not prevent umbilical hernias and may cause infection by delaying or preventing the drying process. Diapers and rubber pants should be folded down to keep the cord area dry.

Circumcision Care

Circumcision is the surgical removal of the foreskin. Care following a circumcision is based on general principles of postoperative care: keep the wound clean and dry, and observe for signs of bleeding or infection or both.

Following the circumcision, a sterile dressing with petroleum jelly is applied to the area. This should be changed with each voiding unless the physician wishes for it to remain securely in place to serve as a pressure dressing for 24 hours. Keep the newborn off his abdomen for the first 12 hours to eliminate discomfort, pressure or friction rubbing. The penis should be observed for bleeding at least every hour during the first six hours postoperatively.

The newborn may be fussy. Crying is due to the restrained position during the procedure and a small amount of pain. Taking the baby out to his mother as soon as possible for nursing, comforting and cuddling is reassuring and helpful for both.

Clothing

Parents have a tendency to overdress the newborn. They mistakenly conclude that cool, slightly bluish hands and feet mean that the baby is cold. The newborn who is overheated must activate heat-loss physiological mechanisms. Conversely, room temperatures that are comfortable for the adult will cause the newborn to initiate heat production. The nurse should explain to parents the importance of sufficient, but not excessive, clothing. Generally, the newborn will be comfortable when dressed in the same amount of clothing as the adult, with one additional layer. The extremities will feel slightly cool, while the trunk is warm to touch.

Feeding

Feeding is one of the first tasks the new parents must accomplish in learning to care for their newborn. The method of feeding (breast or bottle) is a choice that must be made with guidance and without undue pressure. Information should be provided as needed and the decision supported rather than judged. Parents not only must learn to successfully feed their infant, they must also learn to assess his hunger. Readiness for feeding can be determined by observing the infant's behavior. Rooting and sucking, hand-to-mouth activity, crying and alertness are clues that the baby is hungry. These behaviors should be explained and demonstrated to both parents. The nurse can ensure a happy, satisfying feeding time for both newborn and parent by showing the parent how to hold, feed and burp the newborn successfully and by providing positive feedback to strengthen healthy interaction and feeding activity.

Parents should be urged to hold their baby for his feedings and to spend a few minutes talking with and stroking him before feeding to facilitate both their own and the baby's relaxation. Prefeeding relaxation reduces the incidence of vomiting and colic and encourages bonding.

Body Composition The newborn can survive for several days without fluid because 75 per cent of his body weight is composed of water. The normal weight loss of up to six ounces after birth represents fluid loss. Parents can be assured that this weight loss is normal and harmless.

Fat constitutes about 12 per cent of the body weight, giving the newborn a somewhat thin appearance. The total protein is similar to that of other ages. The newborn has a high hematocrit and hemoglobin concentration, plus large stores of iron in the liver. This provides an iron concentration that is approximately double that of the adult. Calcium and phosphorus are present in low concentrations. The newborn's bones are flexible and poorly mineralized; this facilitates the birth process. Both fat-soluble and water-soluble vitamins are present in adequate amounts.[13]

The supply of vitamin K (fat-soluble) is commonly less than adequate. Vitamin K deficiency may cause uncontrollable bleeding; therefore, an injection of vitamin K (Aquamephyton) is routinely given shortly after birth. Bacterial synthesis in the intestinal tract leads to the production of vitamin K. However, at birth, the intestinal tract of the newborn is sterile. Breast-fed babies experience more vitamin K deficiency because human milk has only one-fourth as much vitamin K as cow's milk does.

The digestive tract is somewhat immature, with a scant production of saliva. "Spitting up" is common until the digestive system matures. This needs to be differentiated from vomiting, which indicates that pyloric stenosis (stricture of the pyloric sphincter between the esophagus and the stomach), or other illness may be present.

Due to immaturity of the kidneys, there is limited production of concentrated urine. Therefore, in order to excrete solutes (urea, uric acid, creatinine, minerals), a large volume of water must be excreted. Improper formula preparation, excess sweating, diarrhea or insufficient fluid intake may cause dehydration.[13]

Nutritional Needs Sips of sterile water are generally given at the first feeding (four to six hours after birth, when the baby's condition is stable). Water is given first to assess sucking and swallowing coordination and to help liquefy mucus secretions that may still be present. Choking and gagging are not uncommon; therefore, if aspiration occurs, water is less irritating to the lungs than milk.

Parents should be informed of the importance of placing their baby in a position that reduces the likelihood of regurgitation or aspiration of food after feeding. Placement in an infant seat or laying the infant on his side or abdomen are all acceptable positions in which to place the baby for 30 minutes to an hour after each feeding.

Some babies are allowed to nurse immediately after birth, during the first period of reactivity. This can be a very meaningful experience since the newborn is alert and interested in sucking.

The first milk intake usually occurs about four hours after the first water feeding. Newborns require 120 Kcal/kg of body weight every 24 hours. Approximately three to four minutes sucking time at the breast, or 30 - 50 cc of formula per feeding, will meet this requirement for maintenance of body weight and growth. The newborn averages six to eight feedings per day. In addition to formula or breast milk, the newborn also needs water. The total fluid requirement is 160 to 200 ml/kg of body weight per 24 hours.

Fluid loss through the skin and kidneys needs to be replaced, especially if the environmental temperature is high. Feeding formula to a thirsty newborn will only increase the thirst and may cause overfeeding. Parents must learn to differentiate between cries of thirst and cries of hunger.

Elimination

The first stools of the newborn are called *meconium*. They are dark greenish to black, sticky and odorless. Meconium stools are present during the first three days of life. Then the stools change to a greenish-brown, becoming greenish-yellow about the third or fourth day. This is called transitional stool. Subsequent stool patterns are dependent upon the type of food the baby receives.

Breast-fed babies have bright, golden-yellow stools that are soft (mushy) and unformed, but not watery. They are sometimes a light greenish color. The odor is sweet smelling. Initially, a breast-fed baby will have one to two stools per day, increasing to more than four per day by the second week.

Formula-fed babies have pale yellow or yellow-white stools that are firmer and more formed. The odor is foul smelling. Initially, a bottle-fed baby has more stools per day than a breast fed-baby, but these decrease to about three per day by the second week.

Green, watery stools indicate diarrhea, and a physician should be notified. Stools should be observed for blood indicative of intestinal bleeding.

Most newborns void during the first 12 hours of life. The number of voidings should be assessed. Occasionally, urate crystals are passed with the urine. These appear as pink (brick dust) staining on the diaper. Urate is not significant but should be differentiated from blood. Urates dissolve and disappear when the diaper is placed in water; blood does not.

Keeping the newborn clean and dry will prevent diaper rash. If the baby's skin is so sensitive that rash does occur in spite of diligent efforts, short periods of exposure to air during the day can be beneficial. Petroleum jelly applied to the clean skin can serve as a protective barrier against skin breakdown from urine and stool.

Safety

All persons involved in handling or caring for the newborn should participate in good handwashing measures both before and after handling the baby.

Safe handling techniques should be demonstrated, taught and practiced by all who handle the newborn. These are: firmly supporting all body parts, especially the head; keeping a controlling hand on the infant while weighing him or giving care on any surface without protective straps; placing a hand between the baby's skin and the diaper when pins are used; placing the infant on his side or abdomen or in an infant seat for at least 30 minutes after feeding to prevent aspiration of regurgitated fluids; and carrying the newborn in a protected, secure manner.

The nurse should discuss the use of infant car seats with parents before the newborn leaves the hospital. If an infant car seat has not been purchased, the nurse should encourage the family to do so. If the family feels that a car seat costs too much, the nurse can suggest options such as borrowing one or purchasing one second hand (good sources include garage sales or posting a notice on a bulletin board in a local supermarket or even the clinic or physician's office). In some cities, local service club organizations have rental programs. The nurse should be aware of such resources in the community.

Nurses and physicians recognize their responsibility to counsel parents about a newborn's health in regard to immunizations and nutrition. *It is time that all health care personnel recognize their responsibility to encourage the use of proper newborn and child car restraints.* Automobile accidents are a prime cause of death and injury in children. Use of a car seat — from birth — is an important health measure. Consistent, regular use will establish an early pattern for the child of being restrained while riding in a car and will make it easier to later restrain the active toddler and preschooler.

References

1. F. Adams et al., The disappearance of fetal lung fluid following birth. Journal of Pediatrics, May 1971, p. 837.
2. V. Apgar. A proposal for a new method of evaluating the newborn infant. Current Researches in Anesthesia and Analgesia, Jul/Aug 1953, p. 260.
3. S. Babson et al. Management of High Risk Pregnancy and Intensive Care of the Neonate. C. V. Mosby Co., 1975.
4. V. Chernick. Epilogue to the development of the lung and the onset of respiration. In Perinatal Medicine, J. Goodwin et al., eds. Williams and Wilkins, 1976.
5. A. Clark and D. Affonso. Childbearing: A Nursing Perspective. F. A. Davis, 1979.
6. M. Desmond et al. The transitional care nursery. Pediatric Clinics of North America, August 1966, p. 651.
7. L. Dubowitz et al. Clinical assessment of gestational age in the newborn infant. Journal of Pediatrics, July 1970, p. 1.
8. P. Karlberg et al. Alteration of the infant's thorax during vaginal delivery. Acta Obstetrics and Gynecology of Scandinavia, 1962, p. 223.
9. S. Korones et al. High-Risk Newborn Infants. C. V. Mosby Co., 1976.
10. L. Lubchenco et al. Intrauterine growth in length and head circumference as estimated from live births at gestational ages from 26–42 weeks. Pediatrics, March 1966, p. 403.
11. L. Lubchenco, et al. Intrauterine growth as estimated from liveborn birth-weight data at 24 to 42 weeks of gestation. Pediatrics, October 1963, p. 793.
12. A. Pillitteri. Nursing Care of the Growing Family. Little, Brown & Co., 1976.
13. T. Runyan. Nutrition for Today. Harper and Row, 1976.

Additional Recommended Reading

F. Battaglia and L. Lubchenco. A practical classification of newborn infants by weight and gestational age. Journal of Pediatrics, August 1967, p. 159.

J. Clausen et al. Maternity Nursing Today. McGraw-Hill Book Co., 1977.

D. Grimes. Routine circumcision reconsidered. American Journal of Nursing, January 1980, p. 108.

M. Jenson et al. Maternity Care: The Nurse and the Family. C. V. Mosby Co. 1977.

G. Lipkin. Psychosocial Aspects of Maternal-Child Nursing. C. V. Mosby Co., 1974.

M. Moore. Newborn, Family, and Nurse. W. B. Saunders Co., 1981.

S. Reeder et al. Maternity Nursing. J. B. Lippincott Co., 1976.

F. Robert and J. Chapman. Perinatal Nursing. McGraw-Hill Book Co., 1977.

VARIATIONS IN GESTATIONAL AGE OR WEIGHT OR BOTH

by Mary Lou Moore, BSN, MA, FAAN

Some infants are at high risk for survival because of their altered ability to adapt to extrauterine life. Except for birth injuries and congenital malformations, most of the complications the dysmature infant faces in adapting result from chemical disturbances or the inadequate functioning of organs and systems due to immaturity or postmaturity, or to both.

Earlier in this chapter the Dubowitz assessment of gestational age and the relationship between the infant's gestational age and weight were discussed. Thus every infant may be described as *preterm* (gestational age of 37 weeks or less), *term* (gestational age of 38 to 42 weeks) or *post-term* (gestational age of greater than 42 weeks). Moreover, every infant may also be described as small for gestational age (SGA), appropriate for gestational age (AGA) or large for gestational age (LGS). Infants in each group have unique needs.

The nurse must have a general understanding of the characteristics of the term newborn to use as a baseline for comparison of dysmature infant. (A description of the term infant is presented and the complete physical examination of the newborn is discussed earlier in this chapter.)

The initial appraisal of any newborn should begin at the moment of birth, with particular attention to the first several breaths and the ease of respiration. After respiration is well established, a careful examination of the newborn baby should be completed. This examination is important to rule out the presence of major abnormalities and to determine whether or not birth injuries and minor anomalies exist.

The special needs of babies who are other than healthy term infants frequently necessitate an increased period of hospitalization, and perhaps transfer from a community hospital to a regional center, with a separation of the infant from parents and family within the first minutes or hours of life. Therefore, families as well as babies require nursing intervention and support. The needs of other family members are as important as the needs of the infant and deserve equally meticulous attention from nurses.

THE PRETERM INFANT

Preterm infants differ from term infants in a number of ways that will be described, but it is important to remember that they also differ markedly from one another. Although individual exceptions may be cited, infants born before 27 to 28 weeks' gestational age do not usually survive. The physical characteristics, the behavior and the needs of infants of 28 weeks, who weigh 1000 grams or less, are obviously different from those of infants of 32 weeks, who average 1500 grams, or those of infants of 36 weeks, whose weight is usually between 2000 and 2500 grams. Preterm infants may be SGA, AGA or LGA.

Known causes for preterm deliveries are uterine malformations, incompetent cervical os, multiple gestations, and premature rupture of membranes. Another variable, low socioeconomic status, has also been correlated with preterm births and intrauterine growth retardation (IUGR). It is not entirely clear how this variable relates to the development of a preterm infant and IUGR. Infants severely affected by Rh incompatibilities are often delivered preterm. Approximately 60 per cent of infants born to narcotic-addicted mothers are also preterm.

Differences Between Term and Preterm Infants

General Appearance Differences in the general appearance of term and preterm infants are evaluated in the Dubowitz assessment (see Newborn Assessment). Preterm infants have less flexor muscle tone (Fig. 20–15), so that extremities are frequently extended rather than flexed (Fig. 20–16). The younger the gestational

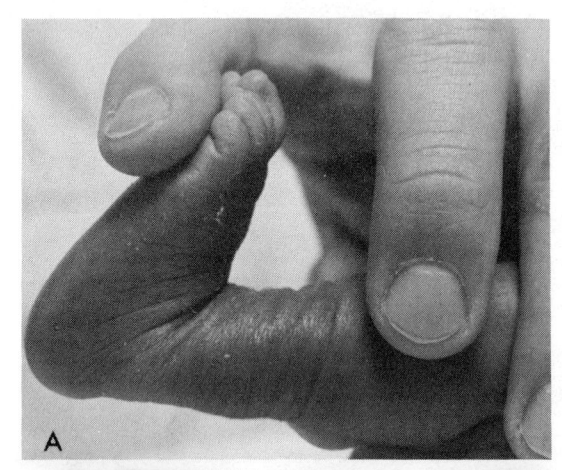

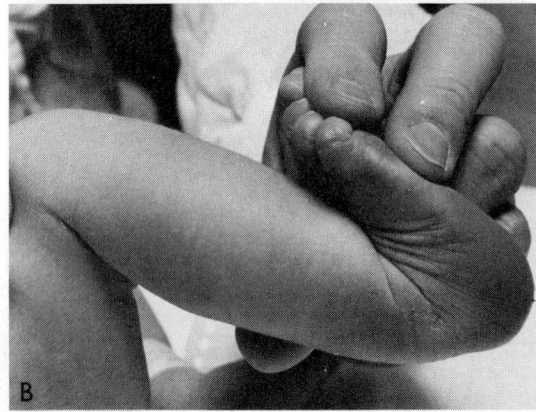

Figure 20–15 Ankle flexion in the premature (A) and the full-term (B) infant. The foot is pushed onto the anterior aspect of the leg. Enough pressure is applied to get as full flexion as possible. The angle between the dorsum of the foot and the anterior of the leg is measured. In a premature infant there is an angle of 45-90°. In the full-term infant it is possible to flex the foot until it touches the leg. (From R. Sullivan, J. Foster and R. Schreiner. Determining a newborn's gestational age. Copyright © 1979, American Journal of Nursing Company. Reprinted with permission from MCN, The American Journal of Maternal Child Nursing, Jan/Feb 1979, p. 44.)

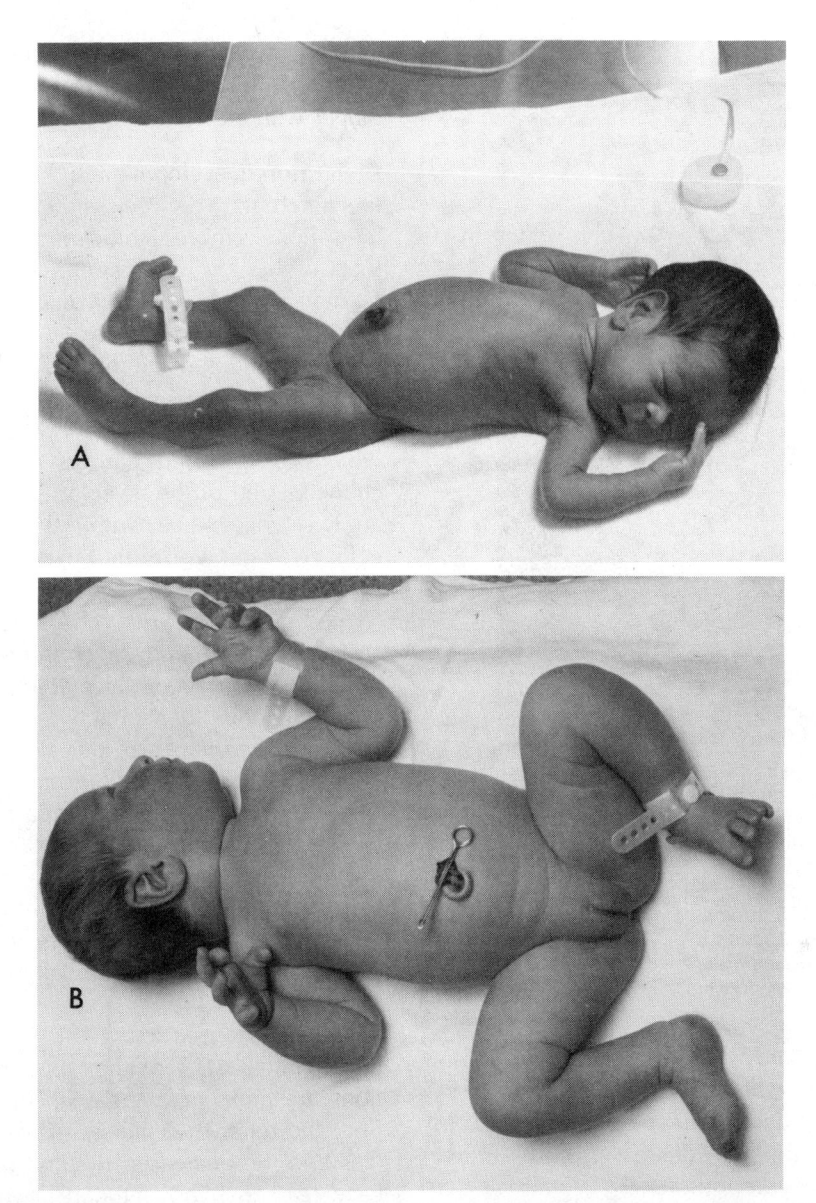

Figure 20–16 Resting posture in the premature (A) and the full-term infant (B). The premature infant is characterized by little, if any, flexion in the upper extremities and only partial flexion in the lower extremities. The term infant shows flexion in all four extremities. (From R. Sullivan, J. Foster and R. Schreiner. Determining a newborn's gestational age. Copyright © 1979, American Journal of Nursing Company. Reprinted with permission from MCN, The American Journal of Maternal Child Nursing, Jan/Feb 1979, p. 42.)

age of the baby, the larger his head will be in proportion to his body, because of the cephalocaudal progression of development. Genitalia are less well developed in preterm infants; boys' testes do not descend until the eighth month of life. In girls, the labia majora do not cover the labia minora until their age approaches that of a term baby. Lanugo is abundant on the body of an immature infant. The preterm infant's head hair is in wooly bunches, while the term baby's hair is silky and flat, with individual strands (Fig. 20–17).

Skin is thin, with blood vessels visible; even infants as old as 34 weeks' gestational age have relatively little subcutaneous fat because that layer is deposited chiefly in the four weeks before term. The lack of subcutaneous fat is important in planning care. Energy is stored in the body as glycogen and fat. Because the preterm baby has very little fat and his glycogen stores are practically nonexistent, those stores will be quickly utilized, and the baby will rapidly become hypoglycemic if a source of

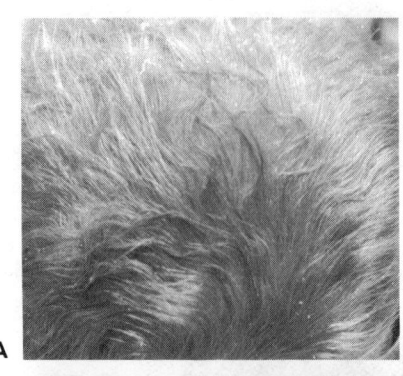

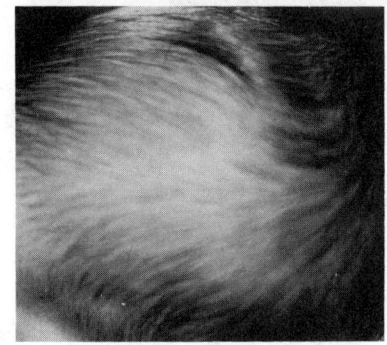

Figure 20–17 Hair of the premature (A) and full-term (B) infant. The premature infant has fine wooly hair occurring in bunches. The full-term has silky hair in single strands, which lies flat. (Hair must be thoroughly cleaned of vernix or appearances may be deceptive in this observation.) (Top photograph from R. Sullivan, J. Foster and R. Schreiner. Determining a newborn's gestational age. Copyright © 1979, American Journal of Nursing Company. Reprinted with permission from MCN, The American Journal of Maternal Child Nursing, Jan/Feb 1979, p. 42.)

glucose is not provided. For the preterm infant that source must be intravenous fluids.

Thermoregulation is increasingly affected as the weight of the baby decreases; body surface area becomes proportionately greater as the body mass (weight) decreases. Constant effort is required to keep a preterm baby at that temperature which is *thermoneutral,* that is, at which he requires the least amount of oxygen to meet metabolic needs.

The thin skin of preterm infants is easily broken in the course of everyday care through the use of tape, urine bags and other devices that come in contact with the baby's skin. Great care must be taken to protect the baby's skin, because breaks serve as a port of entry for infection as well as being uncomfortable for the baby. Small amounts of "paper tape" can be used. Solvents are available to facilitate the removal of adhesive tape. Diapers can be weighed to measure urine output, thereby avoiding the use of urine collection bags. Many times specimens can be extracted from the diaper with a syringe.

Respiratory Development and Function Of all the differences between preterm and term infants, none is more significant than the development of the respiratory tract. Respiratory development is the crucial difference between viability and nonviability. Before 26 to 28 weeks' gestational age there is limited development of the alveoli (the tiny air sacs at the terminal end of the respiratory system through which oxygen and carbon dioxide are exchanged) and of the alveolar capillaries. There are two types of cells within the alveoli; Type I cells give structure to the alveolus and Type II cells produce several compounds collectively termed *surfactant.* The most abundant of the surfactant compounds, accounting for 50 to 70 per cent of surfactant, is *lecithin.* The function of lecithin and other surfactant compounds is to prevent the collapse of the alveoli on expiration. Surfactant production may be inadequate because of the immaturity, impairment or death of the surfactant-producing cells that line the alveoli. Fetal and neonatal stress also diminishes the production of surfactant. When surfactant production is inadequate, *respiratory distress syndrome* (RDS, hyaline membrane disease) results.

Preterm infants also differ from term infants in the characteristics of their breathing; respirations are more irregular, with periodic apnea. Both the relative weakness of respiratory muscles and the decreased rigidity of the thoracic cage lead to hypoventilation, which, in turn, results in the retention of carbon dioxide and subsequent acidosis. Respiratory complications may occur because of the weak cough and gag reflexes of preterm babies, which increases the possibility of aspiration. The treatment of respiratory distress in preterm infants is directed to the correction of these problems (see Special Needs of Preterm Infants discussed later in this section).

Gastrointestinal Development and Function The gastrointestinal tract in preterm infants differs from that in the term infant in several ways. Gastrointestinal motility is decreased; stools may be infrequent, with abdominal distention. Glycerin suppositories will usually stimulate defecation. For a preterm infant a small piece of a suppository is shaped in the nurse's warm hand before insertion.

Before 34 weeks' gestation, the sucking and swallowing reflexes of the preterm baby are not sufficiently coordinated to allow direct feeding from breast or bottle, so alternate feeding methods are necessary (gavage, intravenous feedings).

The immature digestive system of the preterm baby makes certain dietary adjustments necessary. Not only must the type of carbohydrate, fat and protein be adapted to the special needs of the preterm baby, but factors such as renal solute load must be considered.

Lactose is the carbohydrate of human and cow's milk and of many commercially prepared formulas. The enzyme *lactase* is necessary for lactose digestion. Since lactase enzymes do not attain maximal activity until nine months' gestation, preterm infants may have impaired lactose tolerance.

Fats, even those digested rather easily by term infants, are not believed to be well assimilated by preterm babies. Medium chain fatty acids however are readily absorbed into the blood. MCT (medium chain triglyceride) is an example of a fat often added to preterm infant formulas. In addition to providing essential fatty acids, added fats provide nine calories per gram in contrast to the four calories per gram provided by proteins and carbohydrates, making them a valuable source of energy.

Preterm infants with respiratory distress syndrome have higher caloric needs because of an increased respiratory rate and thus an increased metabolic rate. When glucose alone is supplied to meet caloric needs, negative nitrogen balance results. Thus, protein breakdown is very high at a time when the body's need for protein for brain development is high.

Provision of minerals is also a major problem. Lack of calcium can lead to undermineralization of the skeleton; however, it is not clear whether calcium supplementation is of any value. Since iron is stored by the fetus during the last trimester of pregnancy, preterm infants have minimal iron stores. Iron supplementation usually is given before the baby leaves the hospital, either in the form of an iron-fortified formula or iron drops. Vitamin supplements are also frequently given to preterm babies, including vitamin E when the baby is believed to have a vitamin E–dependent anemia.

In view of the differences between the digestive capabilities of preterm and term infants, we may well wonder what the ideal feeding for preterm infants might be. In spite of a great deal of research, the answer to this question remains unclear. The use of human milk is again coming into favor in some preterm nurseries; the advantage of giving the mother an opportunity to participate in her baby's care by providing milk if she chooses to do so is obvious. Formulas with added oil, along with vitamins and iron, are also used. Researchers continue to search for an "ideal" preterm feeding.

Liver Function The liver of a preterm infant is less mature than that of a term infant. In relation to the infant's care, this increases the likelihood of hyperbilirubinemia in preterm infants and also means great care must be taken when drugs are administered that must be excreted through the liver.

Bilirubin is a product of red blood cell destruction. Indirect bilirubin, which is fat soluble and cannot be excreted by the kidneys, is converted to direct bilirubin, which is water soluble and thus can be excreted by the kidneys, by the hepatic enzyme *glucuronyl transferase*. It is the unconjugated, or indirect, bilirubin that may cause *kernicterus,* a form of serious and nonreversible brain damage in newborns.

When the liver is immature, there is a decreased ability to conjugate bilirubin (convert indirect bilirubin to direct bilirubin), and this is one factor in the increased hyperbilirubinemia of preterm infants. Another factor that may be as significant or even more important is the decreased number of Y and Z carrier proteins in the cells of the liver to which bilirubin must bind in the conjugation process. There is a danger of kernicterus if (1) the level of protein is low, such as when blood volume is decreased, or (2) if other substances are competing for binding sites, such as when the baby is acidotic or receiving certain drugs. This danger of kernicterus exists even when total bilirubin levels may not be excessively high, because of the higher level of unconjugated bilirubin free to enter brain cells. An increased susceptibility to bruising in preterm infants leads to increased red blood cell destruction, increasing the risk of hyperbilirubinemia. Delayed feeding, which may allow reabsorption of bilirubin from the bowel, also increases the risk of hyperbilirubinemia. For all of these reasons, serum bilirubin is monitored very closely in preterm infants.

Treatment of Hyperbilirubinemia The treatment of hyperbilirubinemia is by phototherapy and, if necessary, by exchange transfusion.

Phototherapy It was the careful observation of a nurse at a hospital in England in the late 1950s that led to the use of phototherapy in the treatment of hyperbilirubinemia. The nurse, whose name unfortunately is not recorded in the published report, noted that jaundice faded after babies had been in direct sunlight for a short time. As a result, the use of phototherapy lights has become a common practice in the care of newborn infants with jaundice, particularly preterm infants. Light causes bilirubin to break down into water-soluble products that are rapidly excreted in the bile and to a lesser extent in the urine. Because of the mode of excretion, the stools of a baby who has been under the lights are brown or dark green; the urine may be a dark golden brown.

Blue light is more effective than white light in causing bilirubin breakdown. However, it is difficult to detect changes in the baby's color, particularly cyanosis, under blue lights. They must be turned off frequently for observation of the baby. The baby will also appear "strange" to his parents under blue lights. Even white lights are frightening and should be carefully explained. Blue lights should be turned off occasionally so the parents can see what their baby looks like.

Nurses caring for babies receiving phototherapy must understand several aspects of care for these babies:

1. Because photodegradation of bilirubin takes place in the skin, the baby should be fully undressed while he is under the lights.

2. His temperature must be monitored; overheating with subsequent dehydration is a possibility. If the skin temperature is being monitored by placing a heat-sensitive probe on the baby's abdomen, the probe should be covered with opaque tape, because phototherapy lights produce radiant heat. The uncovered probe may become heated and the servo-mechanism subsequently may respond to temperature of the probe rather than the skin temperature of the body.

3. Fluid intake should be increased because of increased insensible water loss, which may be increased by as much as 300 per cent in the preterm baby (approximately 40 per cent in the term baby). The baby should be weighed twice a day and fluid intake further increased if weight loss exceeds 2 per cent of body weight.

4. Both of the baby's eyes should be shielded completely. There is no human data concerning eye damage, but some retinal damage has been produced in experimental animals.[2]

5. Lights should be turned off and eyes uncovered to allow eye contact between family members and baby at intervals during the day.

6. Skin color is not an adequate guide to levels of serum bilirubin; bilirubin level in the blood must be measured.

7. Babies under the bilirubin light may develop a rash from ultraviolet radiation. There should always be a plexiglass shield between the baby and the light to filter out this radiation and to protect the baby from possible explosion of the light bulb.

8. Light emission may decay over a period of time. Specific instructions for various types of lights are contained in instruction manuals and should be reviewed periodically.

9. Because the rate of bilirubin excreted by the liver is increased, stools frequently are dark green or brown and urine may be darker in color. Parents may be concerned if they see their baby's stool when they observe a diaper change or change the diaper themselves.

In using any modality of treatment, there is concern for possible hazards. Lucey[4] suggests that sunlight is a more important source of radiant energy than phototherapy lights in some nurseries. Although research data on the possible long-term effects of phototherapy is currently insufficient, there is suspicion that phototherapy may be associated with minimal brain dysfunction and hyperactive behavior.

Exchange transfusion. A second method of treatment for hyperbilirubinemia is exchange transfusion. When bilirubin levels are rising rapidly, exchange transfusion rather than phototherapy is indicated. The most common reason for exchange transfusion is Rh incompatibility, although hyperbilirubinemia for any reason may be treated by exchange. The wide use of phototherapy has made exchange transfusion rare for babies with no problem other than the hyperbilirubinemia of prematurity.

Cardiovascular Function. The transition from fetal circulation to neonatal circulation is a response to the increased level of oxygen in the baby's circulatory system following initial respiration. When levels of oxygen are low, fetal circulation may persist. (Fetal circulation is shown in detail in Chapter 24, p. 530.) Particularly frequent in the small preterm infant is the persistence of a patent (open) ductus arteriosus (PDA), or an intermittent PDA. A distinct murmur due to the rush of blood through the PDA can be heard on auscultation and should be followed, along with monitoring of vital signs. If the ductus arteriosus continues to remain open, the baby's condition will usually deteriorate. The medication indomethacin may lead to closure of a PDA in some instances. Surgical clamping of the PDA is frequently necessary.

Renal Function. Because of a reduced glomerular filtration rate, preterm infants are more likely to retain fluid and to excrete drugs poorly. Moreover, when blood pressure is low, kidney perfusion and therefore urinary output will be diminished. When body water is diminished, however, the kidneys are not able to concentrate urine in order to conserve water, so the baby may become easily dehydrated.

Within the renal tubules themselves both reduced tubular absorption and reduced tubular secretion may occur. Reduced absorption of glucose and amino acids means that glucose and protein may be spilled into the urine at lower serum levels than in more mature infants or older children. Metabolic acidosis is more likely because of the decreased ability to retain bicarbonate. Reduced secretion in the tubules, like the reduced glomerular filtration rate, limits drug clearance. The doses of medication given to preterm infants are very small, but nevertheless they may accumulate in the body.

Immunological Competence Immunological competence refers to the ability of an organism to resist infection. Immunologic competence involves cellular factors such as white blood cells, factors that enhance the ability of white blood cells to destroy bacteria, and immunoglobulins such as IgG, IgM and IgA. For a variety of reasons white blood cells are less effective in their action in these babies. The immunoglobulin IgG crosses the placenta and provides the newborn with immunity to certain infections to which his mother is immune (diphtheria, measles, tetanus). In the preterm infant there is a deficit of IgG because transplacental passage of IgG occurs primarily in the third trimester. IgA, the primary immunoglobulin of colostrum, is not available to the baby who does not receive breast milk; many preterm babies do not.

SPECIAL NEEDS OF PRETERM INFANTS

Though his basic needs are similar to those of any newborn, with such variance from the norm in the characteristics of preterm infants, nursing care necessarily becomes highly specialized. The main nursing considerations are related to: (1) maintaining warmth, (2) maintaining gas exchange, (3) providing suitable nutrition and hydration, (4) preventing infection, (5) providing sensory stimulation and (6) handling gently to provide physiological and psychological comfort.

Warmth

The basic need of all newborns for warmth has been described earlier in this chapter. Thermoregulation for a preterm infant, especially an infant weighing less than 1000 grams, requires placing him in a unit that provides external warmth.

The baby's temperature is maintained at a constant level by a heat-sensitive probe that is taped to his abdomen. Like the thermostat of a furnace, the warmer turns on when the baby's own temperature falls below the desired level of thermoneutrality (36.5° C; 97.8° F). If the warmer is functioning properly, temperature lability should not be a problem. The baby's axillary temperature should also be monitored at regular, frequent intervals as a check of the accuracy of the probe.

For very small babies, it may not be possible to maintain warmth. A device such as a K-pad beneath the baby can assist in temperature maintenance. Great care must be taken not to cause burns either from the radiant warmer, *which must never be used without the skin probe in place,* or from any other heating device. In many nurseries an open bed with a radiant warmer is now preferred to an isolette, particularly for the sickest babies.

The open bed has several advantages. Because the baby is in an open bed, he is more accessible for care. Moreover, care does not interfere with thermoregulation as it may in an isolette. Each time the "port holes" of the isolette are opened, environmental temperature within the isolette drops to some extent. If the baby requires prolonged attention, such as the starting of intravenous fluids, he can become hypothermic.

Another advantage of an open bed with radiant heat is the removal of a barrier between the baby and his parents. The importance of early touching of the baby by his parents is widely recognized. Yet many parents are hesitant to reach into the "box" (isolette). They seem less reluctant to hold the baby's hand or stroke him in the open bed.

There are also disadvantages to care in an open bed. Infection control may be more difficult. There is sometimes a tendency to touch the baby without the proper preliminary handwashing; this can be overcome with proper teaching.

Preterm babies who are larger and less critically ill may be cared for in "isolettes." Many babies "graduate" from open beds with radiant warmers to isolettes and subsequently to open beds without radiant heat. When the baby can maintain a temperature of 97.6° F (36.4° C) in an 87° F (30.5° C) environment, he is ready for an open bed.

Gas Exchange

The neonate tends to have an accumulation of mucus and amniotic fluid in the airway during the first several days after birth. The dysmature infant's immature reflexes make it difficult for him to rid his airway of these secretions without assistance. Suctioning of mucus from the air passages is achieved with a soft rubber catheter attached to a bulb syringe or with a rubber-tipped medicine dropper. By gently rotating the catheter during aspiration and squeezing gently, trauma to the fragile mucous membranes can be avoided. Mechanical suction equipment is not recommended, since the dysmature infant's membranes do not withstand the pressure well. However, if this is used, more than 16 mm of negative pressure should never be used.

Frequent change of position (every two or three hours) from side to abdomen to other side helps prevent pooling of secretions in the pharynx and stagnation of secretion within the lungs.

Periodic apnea, reflective of the immature neurological, chemical and respiratory mechanisms, is also typical of the dysmature neonate. Usually these infants are positioned over mechanical apnea monitoring devices to alert nursing staff of any apneic spells. Gentle tactile cutaneous stimulation for 5 minutes every 15 minutes helps prevent or reduce apnea. If apnea occurs, gentle tactile stimulation over the face and trunk or movement of the infant that stimulates the Moro reflex will stop apnea if begun promptly. Suctioning or blowing of oxygen across the infant's face may also be required to halt the apneic spell. If apnea persists, manual or mechanical resuscitative measures must be taken. (See Chapter 17 for a discussion of manual infant resuscitation.)

Every nurse who cares for preterm infants must be thoroughly familiar with the signs of respiratory distress. Physical signs include cyanosis (which may be due to cardiac disease rather than respiratory distress), grunting, retractions, nasal flaring and a respiratory rate greater than 60 breaths per minute. Blood gas determinations show low or decreasing levels of oxygenation with increasing retention of carbon dioxide, resulting first in respiratory acidosis and then in metabolic acidosis. A chest x-ray shows a characteristic "ground glass" appearance (white areas) representing collapsed, nonfunctioning alveoli.

The provision of oxygen is a basic part of care. While neither oxygen nor any form of assisted ventilation is a cure for the respiratory distress syndrome, treatment may enable the baby to survive until he is able to begin surfactant production on his own. The amount of oxygen given to the baby (the FIO_2, or fraction of inspired oxygen) is dependent upon the arterial oxygen concentration (PaO_2) of the baby. If the PaO_2 is greater than 90 to 100, there is a risk of retrolental fibroplasia or bronchopulmonary dysplasia or both. At PaO_2 levels of less than 50, pulmonary blood vessels constrict, further hindering gas exchange in the alveoli. Brain damage may occur at PaO_2 levels below 40. The level of FIO_2 necessary to maintain PaO_2 above 50 and below 90 will vary not only from baby to baby but from hour to hour within the same baby. Oxygen therapy is risky in hospitals that cannot monitor oxygen levels in the blood, preferably through an umbilical artery catheter. A transcutaneous oxygen monitor, which records oxygen concentration through an electrode placed on the skin, offers continuous monitoring of oxygen levels.

Oxygen given to a baby (or to any patient)

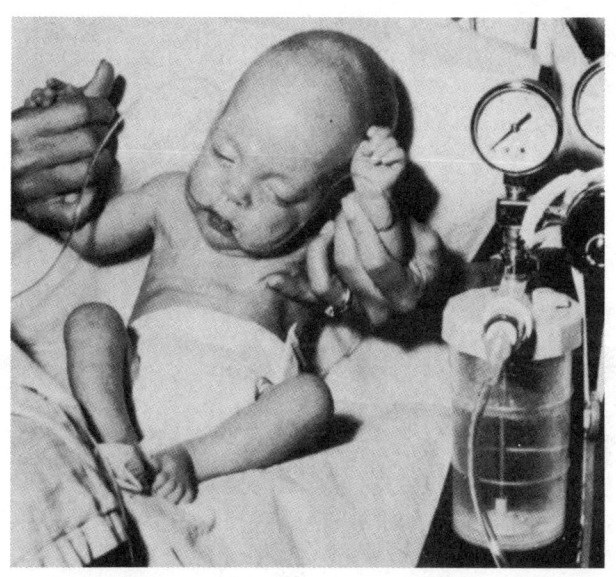

Figure 20–18 A new technique for administering oxygen — a feeding tube inserted into the nares and taped — allows oxygen-dependent infants to go home sooner. (From M. Glassanos. Infants who are oxygen dependent — sending them home. American Journal of Maternal Child Nursing, Jan/Feb 1980, p. 43.)

must be delivered in combination with humidity and warmth. Humidity is necessary to prevent oxygen from drying out the respiratory mucosa. Drying of the mucosa leads to crusting, which impedes the normal function of the respiratory cilia and not only makes suctioning the baby difficult, but increases the chance of airway obstruction. Moreover, the crusted mucosa affords a medium for bacterial growth.

Methods of Oxygen Administration Oxygen may be administered by cannula, by hood, by continuous positive airway pressure (CPAP) or through the use of a mechanical ventilator.

Oxygen by Cannula Cannula oxygenation (Fig. 20–18) is a practical innovation that permits oxygen to flow into the nares. A No. 8 feeding tube (6 mm) is inserted into the nares and securely taped. The tube is changed to the opposite nostril daily to minimize nasal irritation. Liter flow is used to regulate the oxygen, making delivery less precise than by hood when oxygen concentration can be measured with an analyzer. Oxygen by cannula is most useful in infants who have survived severe respiratory distress syndrome but have not been successfully weaned to room air.[1] This method may be alternated with hood oxygenation. Several advantages exist in this method for the infant not requiring precise oxygenation. Sensory stimulation is improved, since there is no hood to create visual distortion. When not confined by a hood, the child is more easily handled and cared for.

Oxygen by Hood If the baby's need is simply to breathe air with a higher concentration of oxygen, FIO_2 levels from 80 to 90 per cent can be achieved with a head hood (Fig. 20–19). The hood does not correct CO_2 levels, nor does it assist ventilation. Oxygen concentrations in the hood should be checked and charted every 30 minutes. Blood gases should also be checked frequently. Temperature within the hood should be monitored every 30 minutes, since the area can become quite warm. Constant observation of the baby's respiratory effort is essential. The symptoms described as the initial symptoms of respiratory distress syndrome are those with which to be particularly concerned.

Continuous Positive Airway Pressure (CPAP) Positive pressure during expiration can prevent the collapse of alveoli that occurs in the absence of surfactant, making the work of breathing easier. CPAP has no effect on carbon dioxide levels, however. If levels of carbon dioxide (determined by blood gas evaluation) are high, periodic bag and mask ventilation may remove excessive carbon dioxide. If this technique is not successful, mechanical ventilation will be required.

Mechanical Ventilation If the baby is unable to breathe for himself, a mechanical ventilator may assist him. Unlike the modalities just discussed, in mechanical ventilation levels of car-

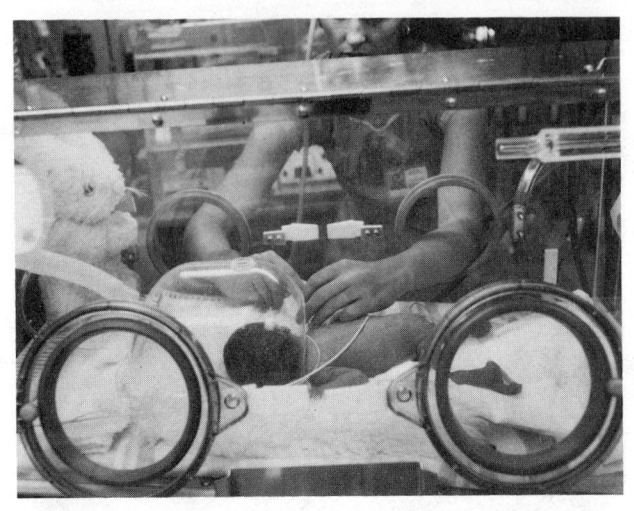

Figure 20-19 Constant observation and frequent monitoring of the environment inside the hood is essential when oxygen is delivered by oxygen hood.

bon dioxide as well as oxygen are controlled. On most mechanical ventilators used with newborn infants, there are three possible breathing patterns: assist, assist-control and control.

On *assist* the baby initiates every breath himself. The *assist-control* pattern, probably the one most frequently used, allows the baby to initiate his own breathing as often as he is able; if he stops breathing the ventilator will give him a programmed number of breaths per minute. On the *control* setting, the baby has no role in his own respiration; the ventilator breathes for him.

Hazards of Oxygen Therapy The two chief hazards of oxygen therapy are retrolental fibroplasia and broncho-pulmonary dysplasia. Pneumothorax, pneumopericardium and/or pneumomediastinum may occur when oxygen is given under pressure (CPAP or ventilator).

Retrolental fibroplasia The basis of retrolental fibroplasia is in the development of the blood supply of the retina. Until the fourth month of gestation no retinal vessels are present; vascularization of the retina is not complete until after the eighth month. A baby born at 30 weeks' gestation, for example, has no blood vessels in much of the retina. The incompletely vascularized retina is susceptible to oxygen damage. Damage to the retina by oxygen may lead to retinal detachment and blindness.

The severity of retrolental fibroplasia is related to the concentration of oxygen, the length of time during which oxygen is administered, and the degree of immaturity of the eye.

The American Academy of Pediatrics recommends the following guidelines for oxygen therapy for newborns:[9]

1. Oxygen tension of arterial blood should not exceed 100 mm. Hg and should be maintained between 50 to 70 mm Hg.

2. Inspired oxygen may be needed in relatively high concentrations to maintain the arterial oxygen in the normal range.

3. If blood gas measurements are not available, a mature infant (gestational age greater than 36 weeks) who is not apneic but who has generalized cyanosis may be given oxygen for a short period of time in a concentration just high enough to abolish the cyanosis. However, if supplemental oxygen is necessary for an immature infant, he should be taken to a center where inspired oxygen concentration can be regulated by blood gas measurements.

4. The ideal sampling sites for arterial oxygen tension studies are the radial or temporal arteries, but this is technically difficult. In most circumstances a sample from the descending aorta through an indwelling umbilical arterial catheter is satisfactory.

5. Equipment for the regulation of oxygen concentration (as provided by some incubators and respirators) and devices for mixing oxygen and room air may not function properly. Therefore, when an infant is placed in an oxygen-enriched environment, the concentration of ox-

TABLE 20-4 PROBLEMS AND INTERVENTIONS IN MAINTAINING THE PRETERM INFANT'S NUTRITION

Problems	Interventions
Small energy stores Relatively higher energy needs	Early provision of adequate calories

Glucose intolerance
    Hypoglycemia
    Hyperglycemia
	Careful monitoring of blood glucose and glucose intake

Immature gastrointestinal system
    Impaired lactose tolerance
    Relative inability to digest fats
    Increased nitrogen catabolism with respiratory distress syndrome
	Feedings adjusted to the special needs of the preterm baby

Immature sucking and swallowing reflexes	Alternate routes of feeding, including gavage, intravenous feedings
Treatment for respiratory distress may interfere with oral or gavage feeding	Intravenous feeding

ygen must be measured with an oxygen analyzer every hour. The performance of the oxygen analyzer must be checked and recorded every eight hours by calibration with room air and 100 per cent oxygen.

6. Oxygen should be warmed and humidified, except in an emergency.

7. A person experienced in recognizing retrolental fibroplasia should examine the eyes of all infants born at less than 36 weeks' gestation or weighing less than 2000 gm (4.2 lb) who have received oxygen therapy. This examination should be made before the baby is discharged from the nursery and again at four to six weeks and six months after discharge.

Bronchopulmonary dysplasia Bronchopulmonary dysplasia refers to a second condition that may occur in newborns exposed to high concentrations of oxygen. It has been recognized even more recently than retrolental fibroplasia, being first described by Northway and his associates in 1967.[6]

Bronchopulmonary dysplasia is related to the concentration of oxygen, the amount of pressure in the oxygen delivery system, and the length of time during which oxygen is given. If oxygen levels above 70 per cent are given for longer than four to five days, severe pulmonary disease may result. Concentrations of 100 per cent oxygen for 36 hours can lead to pulmonary changes. The principal changes occur in the alveolar epithelium and in the endothelium of the blood vessels around the alveoli. As a result there is progressive thickening of the blood-air barrier. In some babies these changes appear to reverse themselves over a period of two to three months. Other babies do not recover and eventually die.

Nutrition

Babies born before 34 to 36 weeks will have inconsistent coordination of their sucking and swallowing reflexes and must usually have their nutritional needs met through feeding methods other than breast or bottle. Moreover, the nutritional needs of the preterm infant are specialized. Preterm infants also have increased fluid losses that must be considered in meeting their nutritional needs. Major nutritional problems of preterm infants are summarized in Table 20-4.

Lubchenco's studies show that a fetus in utero gains approximately 18 gm per day from 28 to 32 weeks' gestation and 38 gm per day from 32 to 36 weeks' gestation.[5] Lubchenco suggested that similar gains may be appropriate for the preterm baby of the same gestational age. However, providing the nutrients for such a weight gain in a properly balanced form is difficult.

Calories must be provided to the preterm infant as quickly as possible after birth. Unlike the term baby, the preterm infant has little glucose reserve, and he has an increased need for energy. Intravenous glucose, along with evaluation of blood glucose, should be begun immediately. Blood glucose should be maintained at or above 40 mg per cent. *Hypoglycemia*, that is, blood levels below 30 to 40 mg per cent, can lead to brain damage. *Hyperglycemia* from inappropriate administration of glucose may also cause brain damage.

When the baby's condition is stable, formula or breast milk may be given via oral gastric tube. Nasogastric feeding tubes are used in some hospitals; irritation of the nares is a possible complication. Also, because all newborns are able to breathe only through the nose, the ease of inserting the oral feeding tube makes that route seem preferable.

Mothers of preterm infants are encouraged to provide breast milk for their babies. In addition to some possible nutritional advantages, the opportunity for the mother to participate in her baby's care in this unique way can enhance her attachment to the baby. She can be taught to express her milk manually or with a hand or electric pump. There is controversy as to whether human milk can meet all of the nutritional needs of a preterm infant, but it is clear that human milk can be a part of preterm feeding.

Some preterm babies may be unable to tolerate any feedings into the stomach regardless of the route. For these babies intravenous glucose, protein and fat solutions are available.

Protection from Infection

The preterm infant is deprived of the transplacental transfer of immunoglobins from the mother, which are normally stored in fetal tissues during the last few weeks of gestation. These provide the infant passive immunity to a myriad of infectious agents. Thus the preterm infant is extremely susceptible to most of the common infectious organisms. In addition, this infant's immature immunologic system allows him only meager anti-inflammatory response when exposure to infectious agents does occur.

Since this infant's ability to ward off infection is minimal, great responsibility lies upon his caretakers to prevent neonatal sepsis. Several simple measures can be taken to diminish the likelihood of exposure of this infant to infectious agents. The most obvious and yet most frequently ignored measure is through handwashing (using a bacteriocidal solution) by personnel giving care to these infants both before and after handling each infant, upon entering the nursery, and after handling any equipment not belonging to a specific infant. Persons who enter to work within the nursery should either wear a gown during the time they are in the nursery or don scrub clothes to wear in the nursery and cover these with a gown any time it is necessary to leave the nursery.

Cleanliness of the infant's immediate environment is also very important. Nursery linen should be sterilized. The isolette should be damp-dusted daily with sterile water and cloth. Using the proper service exit on the isolette to remove soiled articles and using the sleeved portholes to place clean articles within the isolette canot be overemphasized.

Caring for the preterm infant in a separate nursery and limiting access to essential authorized persons (parents, nurse, physician) helps restrict the amount of infectious organisms entering the nursery. No one who is ill should be given entry to the nursery regardless of their authorization to be there. Scrupulous cleanliness of the nursery and its equipment should be maintained on a daily basis. If concentrated exposure of this dysmature infant to organisms is known or suspected, prophylactic medication may be prescribed. When infants have specific infections, appropriate isolation measures are utilized, as they are with older children.

Signs of infection in preterm infants are more general than specific. Traditionally, clinical signs such as vomiting, failure to feed well, inability to maintain body temperature, and gray or mottled skin color have been recognized as the first evidence of sepsis. However, by the time these signs appear, the infection may be generalized. And in spite of all the antibiotics developed in recent years, there has been little change in infant mortality due to generalized sepsis.

Although we need to carefully observe and record the aforementioned symptoms the current emphasis is on detecting earlier signs of infection. These signs may be: (1) changes in blood count, particularly white blood cells and platelets; (2) hypoglycemia or hyperglycemia (glucose intolerance); (3) metabolic acidosis; (4) decrease in blood pressure; (5) hyperbilirubinemia.

Treatment of Infection

In addition to the supportive treatment that all sick newborns need, babies with infections require parenteral antibiotics. Because drugs are excreted more slowly by the immature kidney of newborns, blood levels of antibiotics remain high for a longer period of time than in older children and adults; a 12-hour schedule is usually satisfactory. Dosage is calculated on the basis of body weight.

Antibiotics given most frequently to preterm infants include ampicillin (50 to 100 mg/kg/day), the aminoglycosides kanamycin (15 mg/kg/day), and gentamycin (5 mg/kg/day). Ampicillin is active against many gram-positive as well as gram-negative organisms; kanamycin and gentamycin provide broad-spectrum activity against gram-negative organisms. Nafcillin (100 mg/kg/day) given every eight hours is active against penicillin-resistant staphylococci.

Four antibiotics have been found to be highly toxic to newborn infants: the sulfa drugs, tetracycline, chloramphenicol, and potassium penicillin. The sulfas compete with bilirubin for albumin-binding sites and can thus cause kernicterus and death at levels of serum bilirubin that would generally be considered safe. Tetracycline inhibits the growth of infants and also causes permanent yellow-green staining of the enamel of the baby teeth (as does the ingestion of tetracycline by the mother during late pregnancy). Chloramphenicol, because it is poorly excreted by newborns, can lead to sudden collapse and death, a condition known as the "gray baby" syndrome. Potassium penicillin can cause heart block in infants.

Sensory Stimulation and Gentle Handling

The manner in which the preterm neonate is handled influences his progress in growth, development and overall health. Special attention must be offered this hospitalized infant to ensure that his need for a balance between stimulation and rest and his need for comfort are not overlooked and that specific planned measures are taken to meet these needs.

While our understanding of the sensory needs of preterm infants remains limited, research indicates that sensory stimulation can be significant in the baby's development, both in the first weeks of life and later during the first year.

Regardless of the newborn's gestational age or size, he needs and thrives on basic human interaction. The hospitalized preterm infant needs the stimulation of objects that offer variation in color, brightness, contour and movement in his visual field (9 to 10 inches from his eyes). The infant also needs auditory variety to offset the monotonous hum of the isolette. He particularly prefers rhythmical, soft and high-pitched sounds such as music boxes, records and humming of the human voice. Tactile stimulation may include warm, gentle and rhythmical stroking or rocking (during holding, or on a water mattress); this is soothing to the infant. The following report is an example of the potential benefit that may be derived from a coordinated program of sensory stimulation for preterm infants.

Scarr-Salapatek and Williams randomly assigned a group of 30 infants weighing less than 1800 gm to experimental (E) and control (C) groups.[8] By chance, the infants in C group were heavier and experienced fewer complications. The E group received a program of stimulation, which consisted of (1) suspending nursery birds in a focal plane about nine inches from the baby's eyes inside the incubator; (2) 30 minutes of rocking, fondling and talking to the baby at each feeding period (eight times in 24 hours); and (3) holding the baby in a ventro-ventral position for burping. C Group infants received minimal handling, which was generally believed most appropriate for low-weight infants at the time of the study (1968 to 1969).

Following discharge, infant stimulation at home for the E group included (1) a weekly home visit by a child guidance social worker; (2) provision of a mobile and infant seat so the baby could be out of his bed while awake, wall posters to hang near the baby's crib, rattles and other appropriate toys and books; and (3) demonstrations and instructions of games and various forms of stimulation by the social worker. Major differences between the two groups were significantly greater weight gain at four weeks and significantly higher developmental status at one year by the E group.

Importance of Rest A balance between stimulation and rest is essential to the dysmature infant's total well-being. Sensory deprivation and sensory overload can both cause fatigue and diminish the infant's capacity for learning.

Many times the baby being cared for in the neonatal intensive care unit has little opportunity for uninterrupted rest: either the physician needs to examine him, it is time for obtaining vital signs and giving a gavage feeding, or the respiratory care therapist has come to give him his needed chest physical therapy. Because the baby's condition is precarious and demands constant and careful watching, his sleep and rest are interrupted at frequent intervals 24 hours a day.

The habit of regular sleep is best established by waking the newborn for his daytime feedings and allowing him to sleep as long as possible during the night. It has been found that the infant may be helped to establish a day-night cycle by covering his eyes or by turning out the lights at night. The infant may also rest better in the prone position. Rest is also fostered when noise levels are kept to a minimum. The power unit in incubators and isolettes produces a constant humming noise, and babies placed on open warmer beds are continuously exposed to the noises from ventilators, mist units, monitors and infusion pumps as well as general noises common to neonatal intensive care units.

If the newborn cannot be allowed to have an uninterrupted nighttime sleep with a minimum of exposure to noises, periods for quiet rest should be planned at specific times throughout the day. Although the duration of sleep in newborns is usually between two and four hours, the sick neonate being cared for in the neonatal intensive care unit rarely has more than an hour of uninterrupted rest at one time if his routine care is not organized in such a way as to conserve his energy and ensure planned rest periods.

The preterm infant should be handled in a manner that gives full appreciation to his physical characteristics. He should be touched and moved in a smooth, slow manner with sufficient support to his immature spine, head and extremities. When he is grasped or held, the touch should be firm but gentle, and he should be held near to the caretaker's body so that he feels both comfortable and secure.

SIGNIFICANCE OF PREMATURITY FOR LONG-TERM DEVELOPMENT

What does being born premature mean for the infant as he becomes a toddler . . . an older child . . . an adolescent? As technology has enabled us to sustain life at an earlier gestational age — first at 36 weeks, then at 34, now at 28 to 30 weeks — there has been a growing concern about the quality of life that is the lot of the tiny babies who survive these first weeks.

Early studies of babies born in the 1950s found that a large percentage of preterm infants had major neurological damage.[5] However, more recent reports indicate that major neurological problems are far less likely. Reynolds studied preterm babies who had respiratory distress syndrome requiring mechanical ventilation.[7] After following these babies for seven years after birth, he found that only 2 per cent had a major neurological defect or slowed development. Long-term studies of preterm babies are needed to identify problems that may not be obvious until the child is of school age. Many major perinatal centers are involved in follow-up studies to assess the "quality" of their survivors.

POST-TERM INFANTS

Approximately 4 to 5 per cent of newborns have a gestational age of more than 42 weeks and are therefore considered post-term. Some of these infants have a characteristic appearance that may include absence of the vernix caseosa; dry, cracking skin; a long, thin body with wasting muscles which suggests weight loss; and yellow to yellow-green staining of the umbilical cord or skin or both, while others appear no different from term infants (Fig. 20-20). Post-term infants frequently have an alert expression.

When physical symptoms are present, the cause is considered to be an inability of the "aging" placenta to adequately nourish the baby in utero; the term *placental dysfunction syndrome* is used to describe the problems of these infants.

As gestational age is prolonged, the likelihood of intrauterine passage of meconium into amniotic fluid increases. Placental dysfunction, with associated intrauterine respiratory distress, also is a factor in meconium passage. Thus the major problem of post-maturity is meconium aspiration and neonatal asphyxia. Thick meconium, if present, must be carefully suctioned from the oropharynx and tracheobronchial tree. The baby may need mechanical ventilatory support for days to weeks.

Hypoglycemia is a frequent problem in infants who have been malnourished in utero; blood glucose is closely monitored with Dextrostix and intravenous glucose is provided if adequate oral intake is impossible.

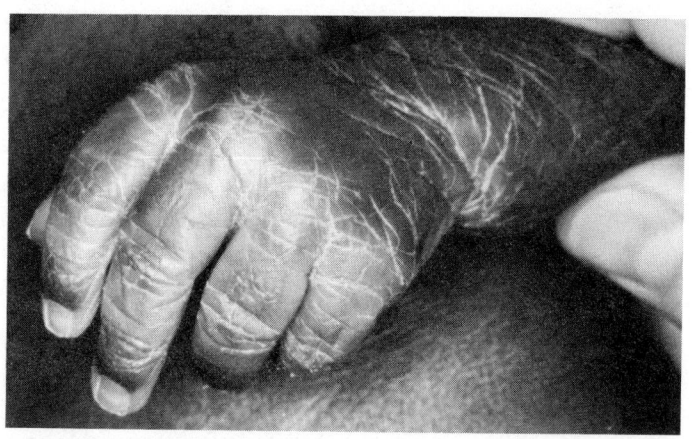

Figure 20-20 The skin of a postmature infant is thick and pale, with marked desquamation over the body. It is meconium-stained; no vernix is seen. (Copyright 1979, American Journal of Nursing Company. Reprinted with permission from R. Sullivan, J. Foster and R. Schreiner. Determining a newborn's gestational age. American Journal of Maternal Child Nursing, Jan/Feb 1979, p. 42.)

Traumatic deliveries and birth injuries which may produce neurological insult are mechanical difficulties prompted by the oversized baby. Consequently, prenatal detection of overgrown fetuses is necessary to help prevent neonatal deaths related to excessive fetal size.

Because of the high mortality and neurological morbidity in many post-term infants, it has become increasingly common to induce labor in women who are approaching 42 weeks' gestation.

THE INFANT WHO IS SMALL FOR GESTATIONAL AGE

At any gestational age, an infant's weight may fall below the 10th percentile for his age. This baby will be termed small for gestational age (SGA). Approximately one-third of all babies weighing less than 2500 grams are SGA rather than preterm; these babies comprise about 2 per cent of all births.

The reasons for low birth weight in SGA infants are multiple — inadequate weight gain by the mother during pregnancy, maternal smoking during pregnancy, intrauterine infection (rubella and cytomegalic inclusion disease), congenital anomalies, and placental dysfunction (as in the mother with hypertension).

Because SGA infants have small reserves of both glycogen and fat, hypoglycemia can be a significant problem. If glucose is not supplied from the time of birth, central nervous system damage can result.

Polycythemia (an excess of red blood cells) is frequent, probably an intrauterine response to chronic fetal hypoxia. When the hematocrit is greater than 65 per cent, the blood becomes sufficiently viscous to reduce its flow. If hematocrit exceeds 75 per cent, a partial exchange transfusion may be required.

Because the incidence of congenital malformations is increased in infants who are SGA, particularly meticulous inspection is indicated.

If congenital infection is suspected, blood from both mother and baby is examined for the presence of antibodies to the TORCH group of infections (toxoplasmosis, syphilis, rubella, cytomegalic inclusion disease, herpes simplex). One clue to possible infection is a disproportionately small head circumference.

THE INFANT WHO IS LARGE FOR GESTATIONAL AGE

When an infant's birth weight exceeds the 90th percentile for gestational age, that infant is considered large for gestational age (LGA). Infants of diabetic mothers comprise a majority of large-for-gestational-age infants, although with excellent maternal control during the last trimester of pregnancy the birth of an LGA infant to a diabetic mother should be less likely.

Hypoglycemia is a major concern in infants of diabetic mothers because of the following sequence: increased maternal blood glucose means a higher level of glucose crossing the placenta; fetal insulin production increases to metabolize the glucose that is stored as glycogen (hence the increased infant size); at birth, maternal glucose is no longer available but fetal insulin production remains increased, leading rapidly to hypoglycemia. In infants of diabetic mothers intravenous glucose is started as soon as possible after birth and gradually reduced so that a precipitous drop in blood glucose is avoided.

The other major problem involving LGA infants is the possibility that prematurity and the problems asociated with prematurity may be overlooked unless gestational age is carefully assessed.

INFANTS EXPERIENCING INTRAUTERINE GROWTH RETARDATION

Any infant, regardless of gestational age, may experience intrauterine growth retardation (IUGR). Common causes of IUGR are: (1) inadequate length of intrauterine life such as occurs in the preterm (premature) infant, (2) inadequate placental function that hinders nourishment of the fetus, (3) inadequate nourishment or health problems in the mother that prevents adequate placental nourishment to the fetus, and (4) intrauterine life of a length that surpasses the placenta's capacity to provide sufficient nourishment or to function adequately, such as may occur in the post-term (postmature) infant.

The clinical picture of retarded intrauterine growth is related to the duration, severity and time of initial onset. With *proportionate* IUGR the infant will not appear wasted, since growth in body weight stopped weeks before birth, prior to the development of adipose tissue. Length, weight, and, at times, head circumference are all below normal for gestational age in this type of chronic fetal distress. However, with *disproportionate* IUGR, the newborn will appear wasted. Weight diminishes a few days or weeks before birth, with soft tissue wasting, a reduction in muscle mass, a scaphoid abdomen and thin and peeling skin. Infants who survive the birth process usually do well; those having suffered antepartum or intrapartum asphyxia exhibit the effects of these insults.

FAMILY OF THE INFANT WITH PROBLEMS OF GESTATIONAL AGE OR BIRTH WEIGHT

When a baby needs specialized care because of gestational age or birth weight, the reactions and needs of the family are like those of families when an infant with a congenital defect is born (see discussion in Chapter 24). Parents must grieve for the lost baby of their fantasies so they can then accept their baby as he really is. When the infant is critically ill, this grief may be compounded by an anticipatory grief by which parents try to prepare themselves for their infant's death. Sadness, denial, guilt, diminishing of self-esteem and anger are some of the emotions parents express before reaching a stage at which adaptation to the reality begins.

Just as parents of babies with anomalies look within themselves for possible reasons for the defect, parents of preterm infants and infants small for gestational age search for reasons. The diabetic mother of a large-for-gestational age infant may feel particularly guilty if her infant has more than transient problems because she sees a direct link between her own condition and the baby's problems.

Attachment is essential for babies and parents, including those very immature infants with a high statistical likelihood of dying. Approximately one-third of all infants who are battered or "fail to thrive" in the absence of physiologic disease are either preterm or babies who are ill following birth.[3] When an infant dies, having a specific tangible baby, rather than a vague unknown baby, to grieve for promotes the grief process. Without this, resolution of grief is delayed, often for months or years. Understandably, parents are often reluctant to allow themselves to become attached to a baby who may die.

Providing around-the-clock opportunities for visiting and telephoning, careful explanation about day-to-day changes in the baby's condition and treatments, and opportunities for participation by parents in care contribute to attachment. Significant also is the opportunity for parents to discuss their feelings, particularly their negative feelings. Many intensive care nurseries sponsor group discussions in which parents can share feelings with one another as well as with staff members. Before their first visit they should be prepared for their infant's appearance, the equipment involved in his treatment and how it is contributing to his recovery and what they may expect to do to help with his care. The nurse should stay near during the parents' visits but allow them some degree of privacy. Most parents require some direction and reassurances that they may interact with and touch their baby. The nurse can take each opportunity available to point out the infant's positive features and progress. As the parents indicate readiness and the infant's condition warrants, they may be taught how to perform their infant's basic care. When discharge becomes imminent, contact of a community health nurse with the family should be initiated.

In caring for parents and their infant with gestational age or birth weight problems it is easy to overlook the siblings of that infant. Parents, too, are frequently so involved with their own feelings that they are unable to think about the needs of their other children or to give them adequate support. Preschool children, with their limited understanding of cause and effect and a focus which is primarily self-centered, are especially likely to feel responsible for the baby's illness. Nursery assessment includes checking with parents about what siblings have said or what the parents may have observed in sibling behavior. One could say, "Brothers and sisters often have worries about their baby brother (sister). Has _____ asked about the baby?" Many intensive care nurseries provide opportunities for children to briefly visit with siblings.

The parents' division of time between children who need them at home and their own need to be with their baby in the hospital can be discussed in groups as well as individually. There is no one satisfactory answer, but helping parents recognize the issue is a beginning. We can assure parents that their absence from the hospital to be with other family members is not neglect of their baby.

FAMILY CARE AFTER DISCHARGE OR DEATH

The nursing care of families does not end with the baby's discharge from the hospital or even with the death of the baby. When the infant returns home, communication between hospital and community health agency nurses should facilitate continuity of care. If referrals are made before discharge, the community health nurse can begin to establish a relationship with and provide support to the family before discharge.

When the baby dies, it is equally important to provide an opportunity for assessment of and support during grieving. This may be done through community health agencies or return visits to the medical center where the baby received care. What is important is that "out of sight" does not become "out of mind" and that this significant aspect of care is not overlooked.

References

1. M. Glassanos. Infants who are oxygen dependent-sending them home. American Journal of Maternal Child Nursing, Jan/Feb 1980, p. 42.
2. R. Kalina and G. Forrest. Ocular hazards of phototherapy. Journal of Pediatric Ophthalmology, August 1971, p. 116.
3. M. Klein and L. Stern. Low birth weight and the battered child syndrome. American Journal of Diseases of Children, 1971, p. 15.
4. J. Lucey et al. A flux day — observations on factors influencing the light environment of infants (abstract). Pediatric Research, July 1973, p. 169.
5. L. Lubchenco et al. Long-term follow-up studies of prematurely born infants. II. Influence of birth weight and gestational age on sequelae, Journal of Pediatrics, March 1972, p. 509
6. W. Northway et al. Pulmonary disease following respiratory therapy. New England Journal of Medicine, 16 February 1967, p. 357
7. E. Reymonds and A. Taghizadek. Improved prognosis of infants mechanically ventilated for hyaline membrane disease. Archives of Disease in Childhood, July 1974, p. 505
8. S. Scarr-Salapatek and M. Williams. The effects of early stimulation on low birth-weight infants. Child Development, March 1973, p. 94
9. Standards and Recommendations for Hospital Care of Newborn Infants, 6th ed. American Academy of Pediatrics, 1977

Additional Recommended Reading

S. Babson et al. Management of High Risk Pregnancy and Intensive Care of the Neonate, 3rd ed. C. V. Mosby Co., 1974.

L. Barness. Nutrition for the low birth weight infant. Clinical Perinatology, September 1975, p. 345

M. Barnard. Supportive nursing care for the mother and newborn who are separated from each other. American Journal Maternal Child Nursing, Mar/Apr 1976, p. 107

S Boros and J. Reynolds. Prolonged apnea of prematurity. Clinical Pediatrics, February 1976, p. 123

C. Bresadola. One infant/one nurse/one objective. American Journal of Maternal and Child Nursing. Mar/Apr 1977, p. 287

J. Brown and R. Hepler. Stimulation: a corollary to physical care. American Journal of Nursing, April 1976, p. 578

R. Dingle et al. Continuous transcutaneous monitoring in the neonate. American Journal of Nursing, May 1980, p. 890

L. Dubowitz et al. Clinical assessment of gestational age in the newborn infant. Journal of Pediatrics, July 1970, p. 1

S. Ennis and T. Harris. Positioning infants with hyaline membrane disease. American Journal of Nursing, March 1978, p. 398

L. Finnegan and B. Macnew. Care of the addicted infant. American Journal of Nursing, April 1974, p. 685

R. Flores. Necrotizing enterocolitis. Nursing Clinics of North America, March 1978, p. 40

S. Fomon. Human milk in premature infant feeding. American Journal of Public Health, April 1977, p. 361

B. Hancock. Clinical assessment of gestational age in the neonate. Archives of Disease in Childhood, February 1973, p. 152

W. Heird and J. Driscoll. Newer methods for feeding low birth weight infants. Clinical Perinatology, September 1975, p. 309

L. James and J. Lanmon. History of oxygen therapy and retrolentil fibroplasia (supplement). Pediatrics, April 1976, p. 591

M. Klaus and A. Fanaroff. Care of the High Risk Neonate, 2nd ed. W. B. Saunders Co., 1979

S. Korones. High Risk Newborn Infants: The Basis for Intensive Care Nursing, 2nd ed. C. V. Mosby Co., 1976

L. Kress. Transporting the sick neonate. Issues in Comprehenisve Pediatric Nursing, January 1977, p. 8

J. Long et al. Excessive handling as a cause of hypoxemia. Pediatrics, February 1980, p. 203

L. Lubchenco. The High Risk Infant, W. B. Saunders Co., 1976

R. Martin et al. Effect of supine and prone positions on arterial oxygen tension in the preterm infant. Pediatrics, April 1979, p. 528

F. McLean. Significance of birthweight for gestational age in identifying infants at risk. Journal Obstetric and Gynecological Nursing, Nov/Dec 1974, p. 19

C. Miller. Working with parents of high risk infants. American Journal of Nursing, July 1978

A. Philip et al. Transcutaneous PO_2 monitoring in the home management of bronchopulmonary dysplasia. Pediatrics, April 1978, p. 655

S. Pierog and A. Ferrara. Medical Care of the Sick Newborn, 2nd ed., C. V. Mosby Co., 1976

C. Porth and L. Kaylor. Temperature regulation in the newborn. American Journal of Nursing, March 1979, p. 453

N. Rancilio. When a pregnant woman is diabetic: postpartal care. American Journal of Nursing, March 1979, p. 453

M. Robert et al. Association between maternal diabetes and the respiratory-distress syndrome in the newborn. New England Journal of Medicine, 12 February 1976, p. 357

J. Schwartz and L. Schwartz, eds. Vulnerable Infants. McGraw-Hill Book Co., 1977

C. Smith, ed. The Critically Ill Child: Diagnosis and Management. W. B. Saunders Co., 1972

R. Sullivan et al. Determining a newborn's gestational age. American Journal of Maternal Child Nursing, Jan/Feb 1979, p. 38

M. Vogel. When a pregnant woman is diabetic: care of the newborn. American Journal of Nursing, March 1979, p. 458.

D. Whiteside. Proper use of infant radiant warmers. American Journal of Nursing, October 1978, p. 1694

M. Ziemer and J. Carroll. Infant gavage reconsidered. American Journal of Nursing, September 1978, p. 1543

21

GROWTH AND DEVELOPMENT OF THE INFANT: MAINTAINING WELLNESS

by Linda Upton, RN, MS

Infancy is a period of rapid growth and development. The infant and his family have many adjustments to make as each develops competencies in their changing roles. The nurse must incorporate many interrelated aspects of growth and development as she promotes the health of the infant within his family. The nurse provides information to parents and reinforces their self-confidence in providing care of their infant. Table 21-1 contains a summary of infant growth and development.

PHYSICAL COMPETENCY

The development of physical competency in the infant covers many aspects of his life. It is this competency that many people use to judge the infant's health and, indirectly, the competence of the family as caregivers. Although physical competency is not the only measure of health, it is useful to explore this competency in some depth, since it does significantly affect the infant's total functioning.

Height and Weight

From birth of the infant throughout the first year of life, one of the first questions asked is "How much does the baby weigh?" The rate of growth of the infant is usually more important than his actual height and weight (see height and weight charts, Chapter 13). Birth weight is generally doubled by 4 to 6 months and tripled by 1 year of age. Height increases about 50 per cent in the first year of life. No accurate predictions can be made about the infant's ultimate height and weight from the absolute or percentile height and weight figures of infancy.

Anticipatory Guidance: Height and Weight Height and weight charts are most valuable when used at each periodic health assessment. The nurse should share infant growth charts with the parents, taking into account the multiple factors that can affect an infant's height and weight as she assists the family in evaluating the appropriateness of their infant's growth. Sharing this information with the family can be a useful teaching tool in pointing out some of the factors affecting growth. She can clearly identify their infant's pattern of growth as well as his actual height and weight. Reassurance that their infant is growing at an appropriate rate, if such is the case, is an important nursing intervention. Further assessment is indicated if there has been

TABLE 21-1 SUMMARY OF INFANT GROWTH AND DEVELOPMENT

Approximate Age in Months	Physical Competency	Emotional-Social Competency	Intellectual Competency	Nutrition	Play	Safety
1–2	Holds head up when prone; Moro reflex to loud sound; follows objects; smiles	Gratification through sucking and basic needs being promptly met; smiles at people	Reflex activity; vowel sounds produced	Breast fed or fortified formula	Variety of positions. Caretaker should hold and talk to him; large, brightly colored objects	Car carrier; proper use of infant seat
2–4	Turns back to side; laughs; reaches for objects; follows object through midline; drools; begins to localize sounds; prefers configuration of face	Social responsiveness; temperament characteristics; awareness of those who are not primary caregiver; smiles in response to familiar face	Reproduces behavior initially achieved by random activity; imitates behavior he has previously done. Studies objects; makes cooing sounds; does not look for objects removed from his presence		Talk to and hold. Musical toys; rattle, mobile. Variety of objects of different color, size and texture; mirror, crib toys, variety of settings	Do not leave unattended on couch, bed, etc. Remove any small objects that he could choke on
4–6	Birth weight doubled; teeth eruption may begin; sits with stable head and back control; picks up object with palmar grasp	Prefers primary caregiver; sucking needs decrease	Some intentional actions; some sense of object permanence, looks on same path for vanished object; recognizes partially hidden objects; more systematic in imitative behavior; babbles	Introduction of solids; begin use of cup; store of iron depleted	Talk to and hold. Provide open space to move and objects to grasp	Keep environment free of safety hazards; check toys for sharp edges and small pieces that might break
6–8	Turns back to stomach; sits alone; crawls; transfers objects hand to hand; turns to sound behind him	Differentiated response to non-primary caretakers; evidence of "stranger" or "separation" anxiety	Continued development as in 4–6 months		Provide place to explore. Stack toys, blocks; nursery rhymes	Check his expanding environment for hazards
8–10	Creeps; pulls to stand; pincer grasp	Attachment occurs	Actions more goal directed; able to solve simple problems by using previously mastered responses. Actively searches for an object that disappears; begins to imitate behavior he has done before but not seen himself do. Understands words being said to him; words emerging		Games: hide and seek, peek-a-boo, pat-a-cake. Beginning reading	Keep: electrical outlets plugged, cords out of reach, stairs blocked, coffee and end tables cleared of hazards. Do not leave alone in bath tub.
10–12	Birth weight tripled; cruises; stands by self; may use spoon	Begins to explore and separate briefly		More solids than liquids; use of cup; begin to wean	Increase space; read to him. Name and point to body parts. Water; sand play; ball	Keep poisons out of reach and locked. Continue use of safety seat in car

significant change in the usual weight percentile or a slower consistent change upward or downward. An infant who is consistently above the ninety-seventh percentile in weight or below the third percentile needs to be assessed more fully.

Body Proportions

The body proportions of the infant are also changing. The head is most developed at birth. The trunk and legs are not as fully developed as the head but begin to slowly catch up with head growth during the first year. By six months of age the thorax circumference may be larger than the head circumference, although there is great variability in this ratio.

Head Circumference Brain growth occurs at a faster rate than growth of other tissues and organs during infancy. Rapid brain growth results from both an increase in cell number and in cell size. The cranial bones have not completely fused, so fontanels and cranial sutures are still open. This allows for growth of the skull as the brain expands. In fact, the growth of the skull is mainly determined by the growth rate of the brain. Growth of the skull, as determined by increasing head circumference, is a much more accurate index of brain growth than is the presence or size of fontanels.[29] The anterior fontanel normally closes between 10 and 18 months and the posterior fontanel usually closes by 2 months. The size and shape of the fontanel may be affected by conditions other than the rate of brain growth, such as hydration and intracranial pressure.

The head circumference is an important measurement in the physical assessment of the infant. The circumference of the head increases from an average of 35 cm at birth to 47 cm at one year.[29] The use of head circumference charts is valuable in determining the absolute growth as well as the rate of growth of the skull. Deviations from the normal pattern need to be assessed in detail by a physician.

Anticipatory Guidance: Head Circumference As the nurse is measuring the head circumference, she has an opportunity to point out to the family why this measurement is being taken. This is also a good time to reiterate the information that the fontanel is covered by a very strong membrane, so there is no substance to the common belief that the brain can be damaged by touching the area. It may be washed. Since the young infant's skull is pliable, the skull may be flattened if the infant spends a great deal of time in the same position. This flattening does not cause damage to the brain and usually is gradually corrected as the skull continues to grow and the infant spends more and more time with the head erect. If the infant's head has become flattened and his hair has rubbed off in one spot, the nurse should explore in more detail the infant's daily routine. These signs may be a clue that the infant is spending a majority of his day in the same position. The nurse should offer suggestions about positioning the infant on his abdomen, sides and in a sitting position. Placement of colorful stimuli in a variety of locations could stimulate the infant to turn himself.

Mouth Mature sucking, which occurs at about 16 weeks of age, is an acquired function of the orofacial muscles with the tongue moving back and forth and is not a continuous process. The oral cavity is growing larger so that the tongue no longer fills the mouth. The tongue is growing differentially at the tip. These two features allow the tongue more mobility. The longer tongue can be protruded to receive and pass food between the gum pads and erupting teeth, allowing mastication.[27] Around 24 to 28 weeks the up-and-down movement of the jaw occurs.

Teeth Another landmark that nurses and families readily observe as an index of physical competency is the eruption of teeth. This often begins about 4 to 6 months of age, although the time of the first tooth eruption varies. It is not unusual for the first tooth not to appear until the end of the first year. For the usual pattern of tooth eruption see Chapter 13, p. 217.

Anticipatory Guidance: Teeth Parents have many questions about teething. The nurse should discuss the general pattern of tooth eruption with the family when the infant is about 3 months old. Drooling occurs at about this time. Saliva is now being produced, but the infant has not learned to swallow it. This drooling at 3 months is not directly associated with teething. There are many myths about the supposed responses of the body to eruption of the teeth (e.g., fever, diarrhea, vomiting). It has not been proved that there is a cause-and-effect relationship between teething and these symptoms. Since teething usually extends over quite a long period and infants have frequent minor illnesses, teething has probably been unjustly blamed for at least some of these illnesses. Many parents remain firmly convinced that there is a cause-and-effect relationship between teething and these illnesses. Further research is needed on this topic. Parents need to be encouraged to consult with health care providers about the same signs and symptoms that they would if the infant were not teething.

Teething causes discomfort to many infants. These infants are irritable, rub at their gums, and may display a desire to bite. Their gums are often red and swollen. Chewing on hard, clean objects such as teething rings, hard rubber toys or zwieback toast may bring some relief. Some parents find that rubbing whiskey or a teething lotion on the infant's gums helps relieve his discomfort. Some teething lotions contain a high percentage of alcohol. The nurse can point out the need for caution in the amount used and frequency of use of these alcohol-containing products; absorption of the alcohol could have systemic effects on the infant.

Nurses can provide guidance to prevent a tragic and needlessly occurring condition—*milk bottle syndrome*.* Milk bottle syndrome occurs in older infants and toddlers who fall asleep with a bottle of milk or other sweetened fluids in their mouth. These fluids pool in the oral cavity, particularly around the upper front teeth. Frequent feedings of fermentable carbohydrates, especially sucrose, have been documented as a caries-producing practice. These carbohydrates are acted upon by mouth bacteria, particularly streptococci, and metabolic acids are produced. These acids decalcify the tooth's enamel and destroy its protein structures, resulting in total destruction of the tooth. Early severe dental caries of the deciduous teeth result (Fig. 21–1). The lower front teeth are less involved, probably because they are protected by the tongue and the nipple of the bottle.

Treatment consists of prevention. Children

---

*The discussion of milk bottle syndrome was contributed by Ellen Christian and Judith Clark.

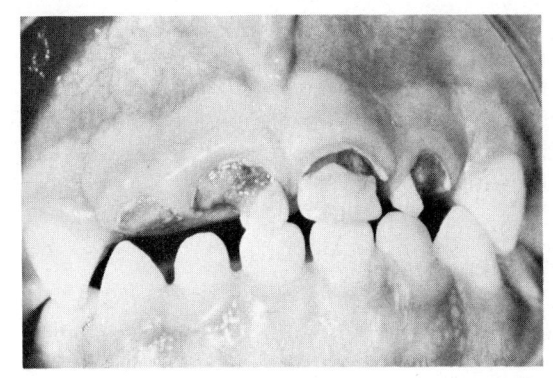

Figure 21–1 Clinical photograph of a three year old suffering from "baby bottle syndrome." The four upper anterior teeth are severely decayed, while the rest of the mouth is caries free. This child went to sleep at night with a bottle containing Kool-Aid. (From R. C. Caldwell and R. E. Stallard. A Textbook of Preventive Dentistry, W. B. Saunders Co., 1977.)

over 10 to 12 months of age should not be permitted to sleep with a bottle in their mouth. Anticipatory guidance given to parents to avoid this practice when the infant is young is a nursing responsibility. If the older infant is accustomed to going to sleep with a bottle, plain water may be substituted for the milk or sugar-containing liquids. Eventually, if untreated, the rampant decay may cause alterations in the permanent teeth as well as great discomfort to the infant.

Motor Development

The rapid development of neuromuscular control is an extremely important aspect of physical competency. The maturation of the central nervous system provides progressively better control and integration of muscular movements throughout the first year of life. The sequence of development of motor skills is much more consistent than the specific age at which the skills are achieved. Numerous complex factors affect motor development. However, in this discussion the focus is on motor skills.

TABLE 21–2 STAGES OF HEAD CONTROL

Age	Behavior
Birth	Turns head when prone
	Holds head up momentarily while prone
	Holds head 45–95 degrees when prone
	Holds head in fairly good control in a variety of positions
	No head lag when pulled to sit
4 months	Sits with stable head and back control

TABLE 21-3 STEPS IN LEARNING TO SIT

Approximate Age in Months	Behavior
4	Sits with support
6	Sits alone momentarily with own hand support
7	Sits alone briefly
8	Sits without support

Head Control One of the major motor tasks of early infancy is head control. This skill is necessary for the infant to sit and eventually to walk. See Table 21-2 for the stages in development of head control.

Sitting Another important skill is sitting alone. The infant must achieve head control before he can sit alone. Table 21-3 lists steps leading to the infant's ability to sit alone.

Locomotion During this same period the infant is learning a variety of locomotion skills that will prepare him for walking (see Table 21-4 for stages of rolling over). Many infants will use this rolling ability to get from one place to another. Another means of locomotion is hitching or scooting (moving along while sitting up), which appears at about 6 months. Crawling (wriggling on abdomen, pulling with arms) usually appears by 8 months. Creeping (on hands, knees, with trunk off floor) usually appears by nine months. Individual infants may use hitching or crawling as a substitute for creeping and progress to walking without creeping. At about 10 months of age the infant begins to pull himself to a standing position and soon stands with assistance. The infant then begins to cruise around furniture (walking sideways while holding onto supporting object). Once the infant is able to stand by himself it is usually not long (about 1 month) before he attempts to walk by himself. The average infant can walk alone well by 15 months. Throughout the first year of life the infant has mastered many incremental steps in learning to walk.

TABLE 21-4 STAGES OF ROLLING

Approximate Age in Months	Behavior
2	Side to back
4	Back to side
7	Back to stomach

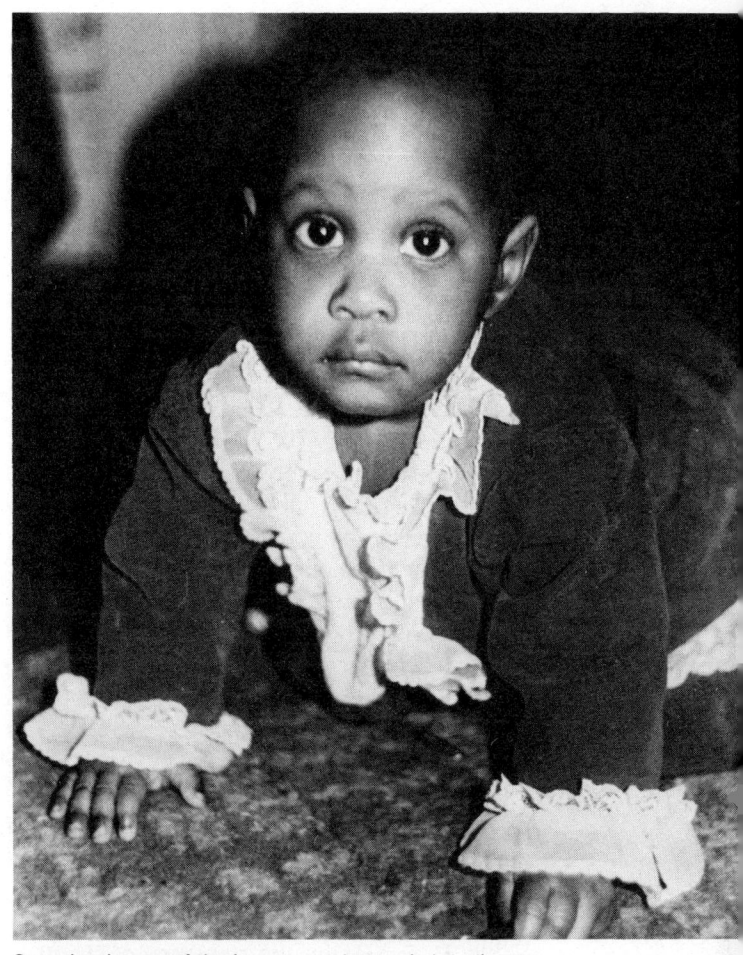

Creeping is one of the incremental steps in learning to walk that the infant masters.

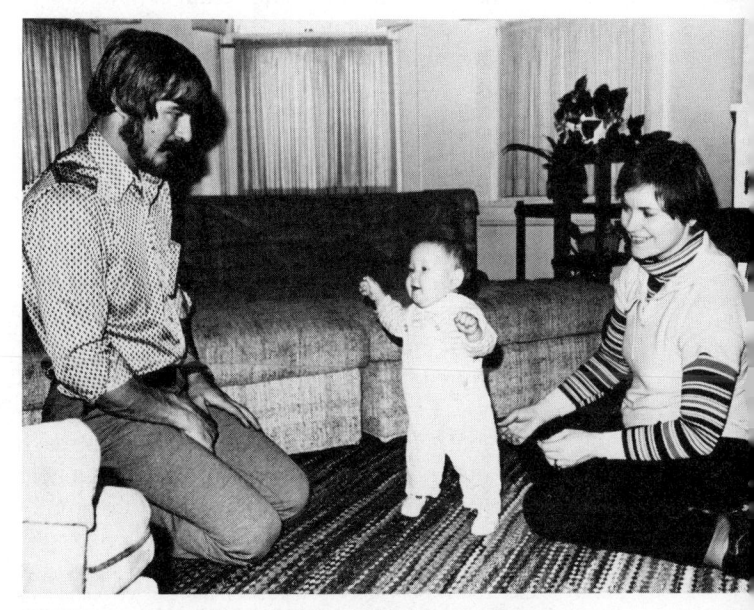

Infant and parents alike delight in those first steps taken alone.

TABLE 21-5 STEPS IN LEARNING TO GRASP AN OBJECT

Approximate Age in Months	Behavior
3	Object placed in hands retained briefly
4	Reaches for objects and picks them up with raking action
6	Picks up objects deftly with palmar grasp
6–7	Transfers objects hand to hand Bangs objects together
8–9	Pincer grasp developed

Fine Motor Manipulation The infant is also rapidly developing fine motor skills that greatly assist him in manipulating his environment. Fine motor development is complex and involves eye-to-hand coordination. Fine motor skills, as with other aspects of physical competency, seem to occur in an orderly sequence.

One of the fine motor skills to be developed is that of grasping an object. The newborn has a grasp reflex that gradually gives way to an intentional grasp. Before this skill has developed it may appear to the parents that the infant actually has lost a skill he once had. The normal sequence of events needs to be pointed out to parents even for such an apparently simple task. Table 21-5 contains the sequence of events in development of the infant's ability to grasp.

The infant develops the visual skill to follow objects past midline by 2 to 3 months. He is usually able to follow objects through 180 degrees by the age of 3 to 4 months. This skill, in combination with his increasing skill of grasping objects, gives the infant ever-increasing ability to manipulate his environment.

Anticipatory Guidance: Motor Development From the preceding discussion it can be seen that much information about motor development can be shared with parents. They need to know the sequence of development and the fact that the exact time of appearance of each skill depends on the individual. Nurses can help parents explore ways to promote the motor development of their infant.*

---

*See *The Washington Guide to Promoting Development in the Young Child* Appendix III (Reference 4) for useful suggestions.

Specific suggestions can be made as to how to promote head control. The infant can be periodically placed in a prone position; he will be able to more easily lift his head in this position. This assists development of the necessary muscles for head control. He also needs to have an opportunity to be placed in a sitting position and to practice holding his head erect. Once his head is fairly steady in the sitting position, pulling the infant to a sitting position will promote further development of head control and his ability to sit. In order to further develop the ability to sit by himself, the infant needs the opportunity to practice with gradually decreasing support as he becomes more stable.

As locomotion is developing, the infant again needs the opportunity to try out and practice these skills. Placing the infant on the floor and allowing space for him to move will promote development of the various locomotion skills. Keeping the infant confined to a playpen or walker does not allow sufficient opportunity for turning, rolling and eventually creeping. As the infant progresses in his readiness to pull to a standing position he needs opportunities to do so. The playpen can provide this opportunity, as well as safe, sturdy pieces of furniture that have no sharp edges. The infant needs the opportunity to practice the skills of cruising around items and eventually walking. There is some controversy over the use of "walkers" in this period. Used for short periods several times a day, the walker may assist the infant in some skills, such as use of leg muscles and balance. However, walkers can limit the developing locomotion and exploratory skills of the infant if used in place of opportunities for crawling, cruising and walking on his own.

There are a variety of ways that parents can promote fine motor development in their infant. In order to develop the infant's grasp, attractive objects can be presented within his reach by 3 to 4 months. Small objects such as rattles, cups, and cubes are good choices. Items that can be attached to the crib or playpen within the infant's reach are also appropriate. A variety of colors, patterns and textures are fascinating to the infant. These small objects also encourage the infant to develop the skill of banging objects together and transferring them from hand to hand. To encourage the pincer grasp as the infant approaches 9 months, smaller objects need to be provided, but with supervision. Giving the infant dry cereals to feed himself can be one mechanism to promote the pincer grasp.

At the same time, the infant can be given activities to stimulate development of the ability to follow objects and further increase eye-hand coordination. The placement of mobiles and brightly colored objects within the infant's range of vision is useful. Many of the same objects that promote grasp also can be used to promote hand-eye coordination. Placing the infant in a variety of settings and positions stimulates him to look at and reach for new objects. Expensive toys are not necessary; items commonly found in the home can be used, such as plastic cups, spoons or bowls.

Hearing and Vision

The senses of hearing and vision are another aspect of physical competency that significantly affect the infant's growth and development. Much research has been done recently which shows that the newborn has greater development in these areas than was once thought.[1, 21] The newborn's auditory system is functioning and is developed well enough to detect differences in sound.[25]

Assessment of an infant's hearing, although important, is quite difficult. Careful family and prenatal histories are important. Factors in the family and prenatal histories that indicate a high risk of hearing impairment are family members with hearing loss and maternal infections during the first trimester.

Developmentally associated observations can be made to roughly evaluate an infant's hearing. If a loud sound is made close to an infant up to 3 months of age, a Moro reflex should be seen.* By about 3 months of age an infant begins to try to localize sounds. By 8 months the infant should turn his head to seek out a sound behind him. Suspicion of hearing impairment should be aroused if the infant has babbled normally until 6 months and then gradually decreases his sound production.

Assessment of the infant's vision is also essential. Again, evaluation of this sense is difficult in the infant, but a number of observations give clues to visual acuity. At 2 months of age the infant should follow bright, shiny objects. By 4 months his eyes will focus on small objects and

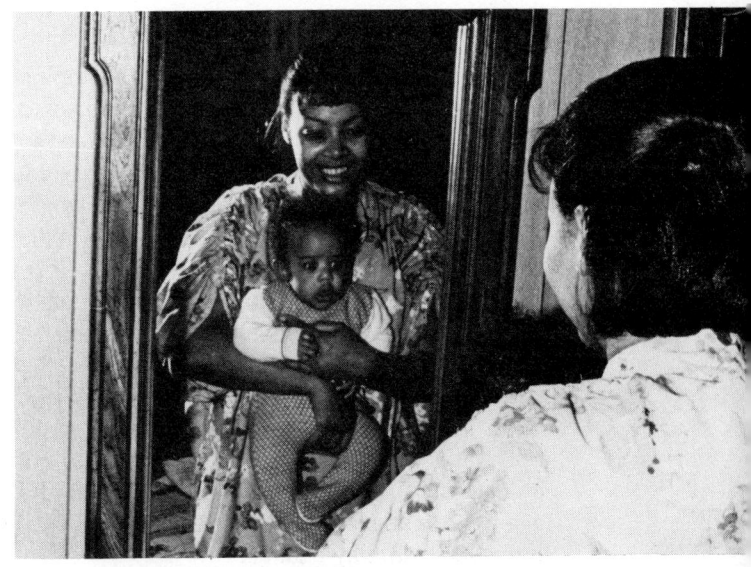

---
*When the infant is placed on a table and the table is forcibly struck on either side of the child, his arms are suddenly thrown out in an embrace attitude; also called *startle* reflex.

A large mirror provides the infant with exciting opportunities for discovery.

he will smile at a mirror image by 5 months. By 4 months of age infants have visual preference for the configuration of the human face. Hand-eye coordination problems might indicate a visual deficiency. An infant will generally turn to a source of light. Muscular control of the eyes will also give clues to the visual ability of the infant. The muscles of the eyes should be balanced to allow the infant's eyes to focus together. Many infants will have intermittent crossing of the eyes. This can be normal until 6 months of age. If it persists after the baby is 6 months old, he should be referred for further evaluation. The parents can assist the nurse in assessing the infant's ability to hear and see. The parents should be asked if they believe their infant can hear and see.

Anticipatory Guidance: Vision and Hearing The nurse can point out the visual and auditory capabilities of the infant to parents, and his fascination with human faces. The infant needs to be exposed to a variety of visual and auditory stimuli. The importance of a variety of colors and shapes in the infant's environment can be stressed. The human voice is an important and readily available sound stimulus. The infant also responds well to musical toys and toys that make different sounds. Stimulation needs of individual infants will vary. Infants do need periods of rest during which they are not bombarded by visual and auditory stimuli.

Sleep

Sleep as an aspect of the infant's developing physical competency is of special interest to parents. The developmental changes in sleep in the first year are not so much in the total number of hours spent sleeping but in length and timing of the sleep periods, as well as in the type of sleep. Individual differences in sleep patterns for infants are significant. All too often a long sleep pattern becomes equated with "a good infant." The average amount of time the infant sleeps is 14 to 16 hours at 6 weeks of age, 12 to 16 hours at 6 months of age and 12 to 14 hours at 1 year. The total hours of sleep do not change substantially in the first year for the average infant. However, a specific infant's total hours of sleep may change.

Paemalee and associates[26] found that by about 4 months of age the average longest period of sleep was 8.48 hours, which is double that of the second week of life. The ability to sustain long periods of wakefulness does not increase as rapidly, going from an average long period of 2.39 hours in the first week to 3.56 hours in the 16th week. At 16 weeks, along with gaining length in periods of sleep, the infant is establishing diurnal cycles, with more sleep at night than in the daytime. Thus the infant's sleep pattern is becoming more similar to that of the adult.

Sleep reflects, among other things, the maturity of the central nervous system. Research has been done about relationships of electrical activity of the brain to sleep.[30, 31] REM* (active) and NREM† (quiet) have been identified as two distinct sleep types. During development REM sleep gradually diminishes from about 8 hours a day in the newborn to 1 hour and 40 minutes a day in the adult.[30] REM sleep in the newborn is different from that of the adult.[30] It changes to an adult-like form at about 3 months of age.[30]

Anticipatory Guidance: Sleep Parents can be assisted to understand sleep patterns and the individual needs of their infant. The nurse can point out that sleep patterns (longer periods of sleep and diurnal cycles) are signs of maturation in the infant. Parents need not be left with only the general impression that infants sleep a lot.

Sleeping arrangements for the infant vary from family to family. It is usually recommended that sleeping space be provided for the infant in a place separate from the parents' bedroom, to minimize disturbance to the infant and to the parents. During the first few weeks of the infant's life, while he is waking as often as every 2 to 3 hours during the night, parents may wish to have him closer to them than when he begins to sleep for longer periods at night.

Around 4 to 8 months of age the infant may again begin to awaken at night, even though he has been sleeping through the night since 2 to 3 months. The parents need to be aware that this is a normal occurrence. Often the infant will go back to sleep without any action by the parent. Once the parents have determined that there is no specific cause for these awakenings, such as the infant being ill or cold, a consistent approach is needed. Often parents find that if they ignore this behavior of the infant, it soon stops. Some parents report that a brief reassurance to the infant, but not picking him up or feeding him, is all that is needed. Parents need to recognize that there are limits to their ability to alter the sleep pattern of their infant. However, this does not mean that the infant will not respond to some routines established by parents. Rituals for the infant (being rocked, being put to bed at a specific time) related to naps and bedtime are often useful, especially after 6 months. These rituals help him know what to expect and give him comfort. Throughout the first year the infant is establishing regularity of basic body processes, including sleep.

Elimination

Another area of physical competency that becomes somewhat regular in the first year is the timing of elimination. Both breast-fed and bottle-fed infants progress to a pattern of fewer number of stools per day after the first month or two. Stools of breast-fed infants remain less formed than those of bottle-fed infants. Stool color varies, especially with the introduction of solid food. The timing and number of stools per day tends to be stable by 6 months of age, although a large number of infants remain unpredictable. The kidneys are continuing to mature. Rectal and urethral sphincters are not mature enough for control in most infants until after a year of age.

---

*Rapid eye movement.
†Nonrapid eye movement.

Anticipatory Guidance: Elimination Parents often need help to understand that even though the infant's voiding and stooling patterns have become more regular, he is not developmentally ready to achieve self-control. Also, the young infant often strains during a bowel movement, and some parents assume that this straining means the infant is constipated. This straining may be due to the immaturity of muscle coordination rather than constipation. If the bowel movement pattern is regular for that infant (may range from several per day to one every four to five days) and the stool is not hard, no intervention is necessary.

Nutritional Requirements

There have been many opinions expressed about the nutritional needs of the infant. As research in this area continues, recommendations and opinions will change; however, some basic facts about nutritional requirements remain fairly consistent. Infant nutritional requirements are based on what is considered necessary to support life, to provide for growth and to maintain health. Components to meet the nutritional needs of the infant include water, nutrients (protein, fat, carbohydrates), vitamins and minerals. Since the first year of life is a period of rapid change, the nutritional requirements of this period also change.

Water The percentage of body weight provided by water is greater in the newborn infant than after a year of age, going from 75 per cent at birth to 60 per cent at 1 year.[27] Water requirements average between 125 and 150 ml/kg/day in the first six months of life to 120 and 135 ml/kg/day in the second six months. The infant has a relatively greater need for water than do children and adults, and he is therefore more vulnerable to water imbalance. Water lost by evaporation in infancy is 60 per cent of that needed to maintain homeostasis compared to 40 to 50 per cent in the adult.[27] The young infant has functionally immature kidneys. The faster rate of the infant's metabolism also is a factor in his need for relatively more fluid than is needed by the adult. Also, the young infant is unable to let adults know when he is thirsty. The usual diets of most infants meet this basic water requirement.

The sources of water are fluids (mostly milk) and food. Most strained foods are 75 to 85 per cent water. Difficulties may occur in meeting the water requirements if formulas are improperly prepared, if infants ingest a limited amount of milk (especially with illness), if fever exists during hot weather, or if diarrhea and vomiting are present. Dehydration results much more rapidly from these difficulties in the infant because of the factors previously outlined.

Nutrients Infants must take in adequate nutrients to promote growth as well as to provide fuel. The infant's body size and composition, physical activity and rate of growth all affect the amount of energy expended to maintain life. The energy requirement for infants is much greater per unit of body weight than for adults. There is a gradual decrease in energy requirements per unit of body weight throughout the first year of life from 120 Kcal/kg/day at birth to 100 Kcal/kg/day at 1 year. There are several reasons for these changes in energy requirements of infants. The higher basal metabolic demand in early infancy is thought to be due to a larger loss of heat because of relatively greater body surface and a larger proportion of metabolic tissue.[27] Decreasing rate of growth throughout the first year results in decreasing energy requirements per unit of body weight.

The energy requirements due to physical activity are as variable in infants as in other age groups. Some infants are much more active than others. Some fuel for energy is lost in stools. Thus precise requirements are difficult to predict for a specific child. However, the recommended energy amounts meet the needs of the average infant and can be used as a basis for adjustments for a specific infant.

Protein Recommended protein requirements for infants are based on amounts of protein provided by the quantity of milk needed to ensure a satisfactory rate of growth. The requirements gradually decrease from 2.2 gm/kg/day during the first 6 months to 2.0 gm/kg/day for 6 to 12 months of age. Protein of high quality is available in human milk and modified cow's milk formulas.

Fat No specific requirements for fat can be recommended. It has been suggested that 30 to 50 per cent of total calories in the infant's diet should be derived from fat.

Carbohydrates There are no specific recommendations for carbohydrate intake. It has been

TABLE 21-6 SUMMARY OF INFANT'S NUTRITIONAL REQUIREMENTS

Component	Daily Requirements 1–6 Months	Daily Requirements 6–12 Months
Water	125–150 ml/kg	120–135 ml/kg
Calories	117 Kcal/kg	108 Kcal/kg
Protein	2.2 gm/kg	2 gm/kg
Fat	30–50% of total calories	30–50% of total calories
Carbohydrate	50–100 gm	50–100 gm
Vitamins		
A	1400 IU	2000 IU
D	400 IU	400 IU
E	4 IU	5 IU
C	35 mg	35 mg
Thiamine	0.5 mg/1000 Kcal	0.5 mg/1000 Kcal
Riboflavin	0.6 mg/1000 Kcal	0.6 mg/1000 Kcal
Niacin	8 mg/1000 Kcal	8 mg/1000 Kcal
Pyridoxine	0.3 mg	0.3 mg
Folate	50 µg	50 µg
Minerals		
Calcium	360 mg	540 mg
Phosphorus	240 mg	400 mg
Magnesium	60 mg	70 mg
Iron	10 mg (1.5 mg/kg)	15 mg
Iodine	35 mcg	45 mcg
Zinc	3 mg	5 mg
Fluoride	0.25 mg	0.25 mg

suggested that minimum intake might be 50 to 100 gm/day, or approximately 50 per cent of total calorie intake during infancy. In the breast-fed or formula-fed infant the primary source of carbohydrate is lactose, found in human and cow's milk.

Vitamins Vitamins are essential components in the infant's diet, although there is still much to be learned about how they function and how much of each is required. Breast milk or prepared fortified formula consumed in appropriate amounts generally meets the infant's needs for vitamins. Infants who are receiving only breast milk may need vitamin D supplement.

Minerals The Food and Nutrition Board of the National Research Council has established recommended allowances for six minerals. Some of the other minerals found in the body are extremely abundant; there is not sufficient information about some minerals to suggest how much is required. For the most part it appears that minerals are consumed in adequate quantities in a normal infant diet. The main exception is iron.

From a review of the nutritional requirements for the infant it can be seen that milk (human or fortified formula) meets most or all of the nutritional needs of the infant through most of the first year of life if consumed in appropriate quantities (Table 21–6). Especially in the first six months of life there have been no data to support the theory that solid foods are needed in order to meet the nutritional needs of the infant. Breast milk provides necessary nutrients, except possibly for vitamin D, iron and fluoride, although there is no consensus on this point. Formula-fed infants may need no supplements, depending on the formula used. Labels of formula need to be checked carefully for information on its nutritional adequacy.

There has been a consensus that breast-fed infants need supplements of vitamin D.[11] However, the rarity of rickets in breast-fed infants opens this practice to question. A water-soluble form of vitamin D has been found in human milk.[22] Recommendations for vitamin D supplementation for breast-fed infants may change.

The Committee on Nutrition of the American Academy of Pediatrics says that the optimal dosage of fluoride for infants is 0.25 mg/day.[12] Supplementation is necessary when the diet does not contain sufficient fluoridated water. There is a difference of opinion about when to begin giving fluoride supplements to breast-fed infants. The committee on nutrition recommends that fluoride supplements be started shortly after birth in the breast-fed infant.[12]

Normal infants of well-nourished mothers are

born with adequate stores of iron to meet their needs for 4 to 6 months. Small and preterm infants' neonatal iron stores meet their needs for two months. In the past, iron supplements have been recommended for the breast-fed infant and still are by some professionals.[17] It has been discovered that the trace quantities of iron found in breast milk are extremely absorbable, so that iron supplementation is not believed to be needed by term infants until their weight triples.[23,28] Iron-fortified formulas are recommended for the first year of life.[11]

INTELLECTUAL COMPETENCY

Intelligence

Another major competency area that undergoes rapid change in the infancy period is intellectual development. There are a number of factors in intellectual development that are essential for the nurse to be aware of as she assesses the growth and development and total health status of the infant.

The Swiss psychologist Piaget has made significant contributions to what is known about the intellectual development of the infant. His theory is discussed in Chapter 10. The infant is in the sensorimotor stage as described by Piaget. The infant progresses from responding primarily through reflex activity to beginning to organize his sensorimotor activities in relation to the environment.

The concept of the *permanent object* is an important achievement of the sensorimotor period. The permanent object has a reality of its own and continues to exist even though the infant cannot see, hear, feel, taste or smell it. Within the sensorimotor stage Piaget outlines six substages in the development of the concept of object permanency.[3] Four of these substages are usually developed in the first year of life. The first substage (0-1 month) is one of basically reflex activity by the infant that allows him to adapt and survive. Learning occurs in this substage but is confined to the sphere of reflexes. Chapter 20 contains further information about neonatal reflex activity. The second substage (1 to 4½ months) is characterized as that of *primary circular reactions*. At this time the infant makes an active effort to reproduce a behavior that he initially achieved by random activity. The behavior must have some value to him, such as the pleasure produced by placing his thumb in his mouth. Another example is when the infant accidentally shakes a toy, producing an interesting sound. He can be observed actively trying to reproduce both these behaviors. The infant can be observed studying objects, including faces, during this period. He is beginning to develop hand-eye coordination. The activities of looking and grasping begin to extend the infant's environment and his interaction with it. As the infant becomes familiar with objects in his environment, he is attracted to objects that are moderately novel. Piaget believes the curiosity of the infant at this stage is stimulated by an object that is not too familiar to him. However, an object that is completely foreign to the infant does not seem to attract him as readily. This may be because he cannot relate it to anything with which he is familiar and therefore it has little meaning to him. The infant (1 to 4½ months) has not developed a true concept of object permanence. When an object is removed from his presence he does not look for it. It is as if the object no longer existed. This clearly can be seen when the infant is being held and is attracted to the eye glasses of the adult. If the adult removes the glasses and places them behind a book on the table the infant does not look for the glasses. He moves on to some other activity.

The third substage (4½ to 9 months) is described as that of *secondary circular reactions*. The infant is beginning to show evidence of intentional action. His horizons are expanding and his reactions involve events in the external environment. The infant is becoming interested in the results of his actions. He has perceived an interesting external result from an accidental movement and connected the results to his actions, and he desires to repeat the result. One can note this particular sequence as the infant accidentally knocks over a tower of blocks, expresses pleasure and repeats the action over and over, given the opportunity. He learns to prolong an interesting activity. The infant has become interested in his external environment and is beginning to have an impact on it. He is gradually differentiating between means and ends. Secondary circular reactions do have limitations in that they are not fully intentional; with them the infant does not attempt to invent new behaviors. For instance, in the block episode the infant does not build the tower initially for the purpose of knocking it over.

During this substage (4½ to 9 months) the infant makes progress in the formation of the concept of object permanence, but it is far from the mature concept. The infant indicates that he has some sense of object permanence by various behaviors. He begins to look for objects that have disappeared, but he only looks under special conditions. His searching behavior must lead to early discovery of the lost object, or it ceases. He does not pause and renew his search for the object. This behavior seems to relate to the infant's own actions rather than to the independent individual existence of the object. Another indication of some progress in the concept of object permanence is the infant's ability to recognize and seek objects that are partially hidden. A favorite toy partially covered by a blanket will now attract his attention.

Substage four (9 to 12 months) is that of *coordination of secondary schemata* and their application to new situations. The infant's actions are becoming increasingly goal directed. He is able to solve simple problems by using responses he has previously mastered. If an obstacle arises that prevents the infant from attaining his goal, he must develop new means for removing the obstacle so he can achieve his ends. The new means developed by the infant have limitations. He is able to generalize patterns of previously learned behavior, modify them slightly and coordinate two secondary behaviors to achieve his ends by removing the obstacle. An example of this kind of activity is seen when an older sibling grabs a toy away from the infant. The infant may initially just try to grab randomly for the object. Soon, however, he will first push aside his sibling's hand and then grab the toy. He has not invented new means (behaviors) but has coordinated two previously learned behaviors, those of pushing aside a hand and grasping a toy. He has removed an obstacle (the hand) to achieve his end of holding the toy.

The infant is also making great strides in his developing concept of object permanence. His improved manipulatory skills contribute significantly because he can more readily explore the objects. As the infant explores and moves the object, he becomes aware that it remains the same even though his visual perception of it changes. He thus begins to recognize permanence and substance of the object. At this point the infant will actively search for an object that vanishes. Hiding the eye glasses behind a book on the table no longer works. There are some limitations to the infant's concept of object permanence at this stage. If the movement of the object becomes too complicated (number or complexity of movements), the object again takes on subjective qualities and becomes related to the infant's past actions. He thus searches for the object in the place where he was successful in discovering the object previously rather than looking for it where he last saw it. This concept can be illustrated by hiding a cracker in the presence of the infant who is at this stage of development. If a cracker is hidden under a napkin while he watches, the infant will search for the cracker, push aside the napkin and retrieve the cracker. Then, while the infant still watches, the cracker is placed under the napkin, taken out and shown to the infant and then placed under a bowl. The infant will look for the cracker under the napkin.

The infant has made significant progress in his intellectual development in the first year of life, moving from primarily reflex activity to more goal-directed behavior. Much learning has occurred. His developing sense of object permanence greatly affects his interaction with the environment, including human interactions. Many factors affect the intellectual development of the infant, including environment, physical competency, social-emotional competency and the unique qualities of the infant.

A number of types of learning are a part of the infant's developing intellectual competency. *Imitative learning* seems to be one of the most important types during infancy. A number of investigators, including Piaget and Uzgiris, have explored the steps in the development of imitative behavior and have arrived at similar sequences.[25] By about 3 months the infant imitates certain behaviors, but only those such as cooing that he has previously spontaneously performed himself. Around 4 to 8 months the infant becomes more systematic in his imitative behavior. He is more interested in the actions of others. As the infant develops more behaviors of his own he is capable of imitating more behaviors. He still imitates only those acts he has previously been able to watch himself do, such as clapping his hands. At times it appears as if the infant will imitate only enough of the behavior to get the other person to repeat the behavior.

By 10 to 12 months the infant has made

progress in his use of imitation. He begins to imitate actions that he has done before but never watched himself do, such as forming facial expressions. He is able to make a connection between what he sees and the corresponding movement of his own body parts. He may begin to imitate new actions. There are limitations in the accuracy of the infant's imitations and his ability to imitate new actions. Research evidence has been gathered to support the concepts of classical conditioning and operant learning, and a combination of these two, as well as imitation, as means of learning for the infant.[25]

Anticipatory Guidance: Intelligence Many of the activities that stimulate development of the physical competency of the infant also promote his intellectual competency, since this is the sensorimotor period. The infant of 1 to 4 months needs a variety of objects to study. Parents need to know that they should introduce new objects into the environment to stimulate his curiosity. He needs objects to manipulate in order to associate his random activities with specific results. The infant needs the opportunity to fully explore objects. These activities will promote development of his sense of object permanence.

He also needs the opportunity to explore and get to know his environment. Between 4 to 8 months of age, his parents can initiate games with the infant in order to assist him in developing the concept of object permanence. Hiding and recovering objects, dropping and recovering objects and hide-and-seek with people are all appropriate activities. As the infant progresses to the next stage at 8 to 12 months his actions become more goal-directed. Stacking, nesting and ring games are interesting and challenging to the infant. This allows him to perceive connections between events such as placing a certain block on top of another and building a tower. Toys or household items that can be placed in containers and taken out easily also contribute to his goal-directed abilities and development of the concept of object permanence. By this time the infant does imitate new actions, so demonstration by the parents may assist him to learn activities. The infant enjoys imitating facial expressions and body movements. Throughout discussion with the parents the nurse should include the rationale for the suggested activities.

Questions are often raised about the feasibility of measuring infant intelligence. Intelligence is a difficult concept to define and measure, especially for infants. Since the infant does not have command of language he cannot be tested for thinking or reasoning. The infant's range of behaviors is limited. In addition, his motivation cannot be controlled. There is almost no predictability between an infant's score on various infant intelligence tests and his scores on intelligence tests given later. This may be because tests for infants and tests for older individuals are measuring two different things. The infant intelligence tests look at behavior. Tests such as the Bayley Scales of Infant Development[6] are useful in finding deviations from normal development.

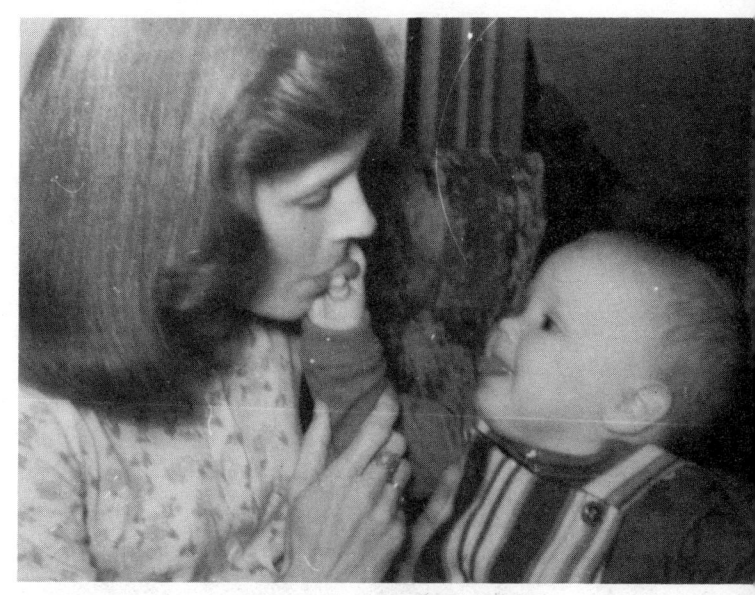

By 10 months the infant can imitate actions she has done before but never watched herself do, such as forming facial expressions. (Photograph by David Trainor.)

Language

Language development is an important aspect of intellectual competency. It has been repeatedly noted that children throughout the world go through the same basic stages of language acquisition. Language development is affected by intellectual development, maturation of the central nervous system, development of the organs of speech and by exposure to human language. Receptive language (what a person understands) and expressive language (what he says) are both important to consider. The infant appears to be especially attuned to the types of sound needed for language development. It can be observed that by about 10 months of age infants understand some of the words being said to them, such as "bye-bye" and "peek-a-boo."

Vocalization in infancy follows a definite sequence. During the first two months most of the sounds produced are vowels and are made mostly in the front part of the mouth.[30] Crying is a means of communication during this period. Cooing sounds are noted at about 2 to 3 months; they consist of a variety of simple vowel-like sounds. These sounds are usually produced when the infant is happy and is responding to an adult's social smiling and vocalizing. Around 2 to 6 months babbling appears, which consists of sounds of vowels and consonants resembling syllables. The most common sounds are *ma, mu, da, di*. By 9 to 10 months these sounds are repeated as two syllables. The infant is attempting to imitate sounds at this point. Sounds are mixed with play such as bubble-blowing or gurgling. By 12 months words such as mama and dada are emerging. All normal children learn their native language and show similarities in this learning.

Anticipatory Guidance: Language The nurse, in order to most effectively assist the parents, needs to make sure they understand the process of language development in their infant. There are a number of activities that are appropriate to promote language development in the infant. Keeping in mind the receptive abilities of even the very young infant, parents can be encouraged to talk to their infant while holding or handling him. They can be encouraged to observe the response of the infant to adult vocalizations. Incorporating smiling and eye-to-eye contact while talking with the infant can make this type of interaction positive for adult and infant. As the infant starts making sounds, the parents can imitate the sounds and vocalize in response to the infant. Infants seem to enjoy vocalization during activities such as eating, bathing and dressing. Toys and household items that produce sounds also elicit response from the infant. As the infant approaches 9 to 10 months it is helpful to accompany simple verbal directions with gestures, to repeat the directions and to have the infant participate in the activity. Continued vocalizing with the infant during activities remains important. Parents can make sounds such as tongue clicking or lip smacking that the infant can imitate.

The infant at 1 year of age has made enormous strides in his intellectual competency. This competency is consistently influencing and influenced by the development of other competencies.

EMOTIONAL-SOCIAL COMPETENCY

The emotional-social competency is another essential and rapidly changing competency in the infancy period. A number of theories have been devised to explain this phase of infant development. No one theory adequately explains all that is happening in the emotional-social area.

Talking to the infant encourages vocalizations that lead to his first words.

Freud described infancy as the oral stage of psychosexual development. Through sucking, the infant receives gratification that appears to be more than just satisfaction of hunger. Erik Erikson takes into account the cultural and societal influences on development. The crisis of conflict he describes for the infancy period is that of basic trust versus basic mistrust. If the infant's physical and emotional needs are met through sensitive care, a state of trust is created. This forms a foundation for further development. According to Erikson, the mother-infant relationship is an important factor in the infant's sense of trust. Erikson and Freud emphasize the importance of the feeding experience in the infant's development of a sense of trust. Erikson states that the nature of the interpersonal contacts during feeding (physical and psychological comfort) determines the infant's feeling about his early social life. Through his oral development the infant acquires experiences with satisfaction or nonsatisfaction of his basic needs. He associates a sense of well-being with consistent behavior of a caring person. Erikson believes the actual skill used in handling and caring for the infant is of little importance when compared with underlying motivation of the caretaker. The infant must learn that those who care for him can be relied upon to satisfy his basic needs for survival and comfort.

Attachment Bonding of parents to their infant and beginning attachment of the infant to his parents has been discussed in an earlier chapter. These processes continue to be an important component of the developing emotional-social competency of the infant. Keep in mind that infant-to-parent attachment and parent-to-infant bonding are two different processes.[1] The process of the infant becoming attached to parents occurs later and is a sequential process that develops over time.[1]

The initial phase is *social responsiveness*. The infant responds to all humans with little or no discrimination. At about 3 months the infant becomes aware of those people who are not mother (or the primary caregiver). In the second phase the infant progresses to discrimination in his social responsiveness. By 6 months his responses clearly indicate that the primary caregiver is preferred. By the third phase at 9 to 10 months of age most authorities believe the infant is truly attached.[1] He actively initiates proximity-seeking, contact-seeking behaviors and maintains contact with his parents (primary caregivers). He may relate easily to others, but with discrimination. The attachment behaviors of smiling, gazing, vocalization and motor approach are of a different quality and intensity toward people to whom the infant is attached. He does not seek the same kind of contact with people to whom he is not attached.

A number of studies have clearly indicated that formation of a secure attachment to at least one parent (person) is necessary before the 9- to 12-month-old infant will explore and start to separate from his parents, as he begins the process of developing autonomy.[1] A strong attachment serves as a secure base from which to explore. Infants do form attachments to more than one person, although not to large numbers. Once the infant is attached to one or both parents, attachment behaviors, rather than autonomy behaviors, are likely to increase following separation from parents.

Anticipatory Guidance: Oral, Trust and Attachment Needs The nurse can assist parents to understand the developing emotional-social competency of their infant and their role in promoting his sense of trust and attachment. She can give support to the parents as they respond to the needs of their infant. She can discuss the reciprocity between bonding of the parents to their infant and his attachment to them. Parents bond earlier and quicker to their infant; later the infant attaches to the parents. In addition, she can point out the specific attachment behaviors of the infant to his parents and stress the importance of promptly responding to these behaviors. Reinforcement should be given to the parents for responding to attachment behaviors of their infant. The nurse can encourage parents to provide periods of close contact with their infant. The infant needs to be held, cuddled and carried. The use of infant carriers that allow the infant contact with his parents could be encouraged, instead of the exclusive use of baby carriages or strollers.

Discussion about meeting the basic needs of the infant for survival and comfort is appropriate. The prompt meeting of the infant's basic needs in a consistent manner helps to give the infant a secure and trusting view of his environment. The technical skill of the parents is not the key factor in meeting these needs. It is the manner (warm, consistent, caring) in which these needs are met that is the key factor. The infant is not concerned with how neatly the diaper is secured or how few wasted motions the parents use in giving his bath. What is important in these interactions is the fact that the parents responded to his need to be clean and dry in a social, caring manner. Parents need to feel positive about their ability to meet the needs of their infant.

The importance of the oral sense to the infant should be discussed with parents. Sucking is an important way for the infant to meet his nutritional needs. The mouth is also used as an organ for touch. In addition, sucking in itself seems to be an important need for the infant. Some infants have greater needs related to sucking than do other infants. Parents may need assistance in determining if their infant is hungry or has a non-nutritive sucking need. Overfeeding can result if sucking needs are interpreted as hunger needs. Non-nutritive sucking need is greatest in the first 4 to 6 months of life. Satisfying the need for sucking provides comfort to the infant and does not lead to dependency on sucking.

Many parents, professionals and family members and friends have strong positive or negative feelings about use of a pacifier. The nurse can provide information about its appropriate use and can assist parents to determine if their infant needs this mechanism to meet his sucking needs. If the pacifier is used, the infant can be held and cuddled while he uses it. It should not be used constantly or to substitute for holding and other ways of meeting the infant's needs. Use of the pacifier should be eliminated at about 4 to 5 months of age, when the infant evidences a diminishing need to suck. Pacifiers do not become a habit when used in this manner. Use of pacifiers beyond infancy or as a substitute for caretaking may lead to a habit that is difficult to overcome. Some infants may substitute use of a thumb for use of the pacifier. The type of pacifier used (size, shape) does not justify its prolonged use. Parents may choose the shape of pacifier that corresponds to the type of nipple that is used during feeding.

Parents may want to discuss coping with the changing needs of the infant as he progresses in the stages of attachment. In the first few months of life the infant needs opportunity to interact this information. The questionnaire developed press the idea that it does not seem to matter to the infant who takes care of him. He seems to respond in the same way to all caretakers. These parents need assistance in understanding that discrimination in response and ultimate attachment is a process that is enhanced by these early opportunities for interaction.

Parents often ask how much time is actually necessary to allow attachment to occur, or what effect the fact that both parents work outside the home has on the infant, or both questions. The nurse must realize that there are no specific answers. In light of what is known about attachment, the nurse can assist parents to arrive at a satisfactory plan to promote attachment of their infant as well as meet the family's needs. It is certainly clear that there is flexibility in the amount of time needed for interaction between parents and infant.

Parents need assistance in anticipating that as an infant becomes attached to one or both parents, he will respond differently to other family members and friends and caretakers. Parents can then help others (such as grandparents) not to feel rejected. It may help to suggest a little distance in these persons' interaction with the infant until he gives clues he is ready for more interaction with them.

Parents need opportunities to discuss their feelings as the infant begins to demonstrate exploratory and independent behaviors. All of a sudden their infant seems not to want them as much or to be as close to them. In reality, of course, the infant needs them as much as ever, but in a slightly different way. As he explores, he needs them as a secure, consistent base to come back to for support. In this period, if he has been separated from his parents for even a few hours he may demonstrate more contact-seeking attachment behaviors, such as clinging and wishing to be held. Parents need to understand that this is not regressive or spoiled behavior. The infant still needs the close contact with his parents and is not capable of functioning in an independent manner. He uses attachment behaviors to maintain the support from his parents. This period can be confusing to parents as they try to meet the attachment needs of their infant as well as his beginning needs for independence.

Temperament A number of people have reviewed Thomas and Chess's temperament studies to determine how to make practical use of this information. The questionnaire developed by Carey to assess the temperament profile of the infant is discussed in Chapter 14. This tool can be an excellent one for the nurse as she works with parents to promote optimal health of children and families. Carey discusses two goals for the use of the tool: (1) achievement of balance between parental attitudes and practices and the child's temperament traits and (2) alleviation of inappropriate parental guilt and anxiety when the child shows certain behavioral patterns that deviate from what is considered normal. The tool is useful in general discussion of the differences in infant temperament. It assists the nurse and family to better understand and meet individual infant needs.

Anticipatory Guidance: Temperament Whether or not the nurse incorporates a specific tool such as Carey's Infant Temperament Questionnaire into her practice, she has to take into account the effect the infant's temperament has on his family, friends and health care providers. In order to more fully understand an infant's behavior the parents and nurse need to be aware of the specific characteristics of the infant. If the family and nurse are aware that an infant has intense reactions and slow adaptation to change in his environment, they will not approach the issue of changing the location of the place of sleep in the same way for him as for an infant who has low-intensity reactions and readily adapts. This does not mean the parents cannot change the infant's place of sleep. Rather the best or least disturbing approach can be sought. Families need assistance in recognizing that infants, even within the same family, may have very different temperaments. The infant's temperament characteristics will affect how family members and others respond to him. The characteristics and responses do not indicate that either the infant or parent is good or bad. The nurse can assist the family to look at approaches to childbearing, taking into account the temperament of this infant and their response to his temperament.

Emotions There has been much controversy over the time at which emotions appear in the infant. It does appear that infants have a range of emotions from an early age. However, they cannot express emotions as adults do, nor are infant emotions likely to be exactly like those of adults. The smiles and cries of infants seem to give evidence of differentiation at an early age and are definite means of communication.

Parents and professionals must be cautious in interpreting these clues (cries and smiles) just as they would adult cries and smiles.

The smile of the infant is considered an important developmental milestone. Many emotional connotations are placed in the powerful smile of the infant. It certainly plays an important role in promoting contact between the infant and adults. Initially the smile of the infant is spontaneous, but by 1 month of age the infant directs the smile toward people. By 2 to 3 months the smile is in response to the face of a familiar person. The smile often occurs in conjunction with the gratification and comfort associated wtih these interaction experiences. These experiences help the infant to develop the association between pleasure and smiling.

Another evidence of the developing differentiation of emotions is the temperament characteristics of the infant that were previously discussed. The overall regularity in patterns of functioning of the infant also influences how adults view his emotions. For example, an infant with a slow-to-warm temperament might be viewed as displaying the emotion of fear. In reality we are unable to assess this emotion in the infant. Physiologically the infant may not have progressed to regularity in sleep, elimination and so forth, and his unpredictability might be interpreted as emotions of anger or unhappiness.

Wolff has identified a variety of infant cries:[33] (1) basic rhythmical cry, (2) mad or angry cry, (3) pain cry and (4) cry of frustration. Infants do develop certain individual crying patterns. Parents need assistance in understanding crying as one of the methods of communication available to the infant. Although there are no scientific bases for saying that certain amounts of crying are "good" for the infant, families may have strong opinions on this subject. At times, crying does seem to allow the infant to release some of his tension. Crying is discussed in detail in Chapter 22.

Anticipatory Guidance: Emotions Nurses need to assist parents to understand behaviors of infants and our limited ability to adequately assess the emotional state of the infant. Infants do show different behaviors that indicate a range of emotions, but we do not know if the emotions differ in degree or substance or both from adult emotional responses. Parents need opportunities to discuss their particular infant and his behaviors that have emotional connotations. It is important to respond promptly to an infant's behavior (smiling or crying). The nurse can assist parents in trying to understand their infant and their responses to him.

Cultural Influences Cultural influences are important considerations in the developing emotional-social competency of the infant. Culture influences a family's view of their infant. The values of the family and their definitions of roles are influenced by culture. In today's world cultural values are undergoing change. These changing values usually result in changing childrearing methods. Certain cultures seem to be more clear about their childrearing goals. For instance, in China, the Soviet Union and Israel there is much emphasis on learning to love and help one's peers, with the goal of placing society's needs ahead of one's own.[30] This emphasis starts in infancy. Some societies and cultures provide more parental support than others.

Subcultures within the same society may hold different views of infants and childrearing methods. For example, a study compared American middle and lower socioeconomic class mothers and their 10-month-old infants.[25] The middle class mothers talked more to their infants, tried harder to entertain them, gave them more toys and responded more to their fretfulness. It has been noted in a number of studies that black American infants appeared more advanced than white American infants in motor development. It is unclear whether this results from differences in physical development or emotional-social factors or both. Genetic factors, method of handling the infant and encouragement of activity all have been considered as possible reasons for these differences.

A number of studies have been done that compare Chinese and Caucasian infants. These studies have shown striking differences in temperament and behavior among ethnic groups.[18] The Chinese infants were more amenable and adaptable during testing, while the Caucasian infants were annoyed and complained. Another study compared Navaho and Anglo mothers and infants. The mothers used very different methods to get the attention of their infants and the infants responded differently.[18] Despite the different methods, both groups of mothers were equally successful in getting their infants' attention.

Anticipatory Guidance: Cultural Influences In order for the nurse to work effectively with the infant and his family she must be aware of the cultural influences and values of the particular family. Assumptions based on names or physical appearance may be very misleading. Chapter 2 further discusses cultural influences.

GUIDING PARENTS TO PROMOTE THEIR INFANT'S DEVELOPMENT

As was indicated throughout discussion of the growth and development of the infant, parents' perceptions, characteristics, needs and developmental level greatly influence the development of the infant and vice versa. Broussard explored the assessment of maternal perceptions of infants.[14] Broussard held the conviction that an infant who is not perceived by his mother as being better than average is at a much higher risk for development of subsequent emotional difficulty. In a 1963 study Broussard found the critical variable approach to be the mother's perceptions of her infant at 1 month of age. In addition to their perceptions of their infant, parents are influenced by the special concerns of being parents of an infant. They are becoming acquainted with and bonded to a new member of the family who has unique needs. The interaction patterns within the family have been increased. The parents are just beginning to sort out their roles as parents with this particular infant and to deal with childrearing issues and their expectations of the infant. They are dealing with an individual who is dependent on them and limited in his ability to express his needs. In addition, the infant is changing so rapidly that it is difficult for parents to establish a pattern of anticipating and meeting the infant's needs. The addition of this new member to the family calls for adjustments in the life of all family members.

Parents need a great deal of support for the difficult but rewarding task of raising an infant. They may have been given little information about developmental expectations for the infant. Parents need an opportunity to discuss their concerns with a knowledgeable nonjudgmental person. The nurse must acknowledge the parents as people with their own needs and concerns. The nurse will find it useful to get some sense of how parents view the health of the infant, including growth and development, so she can begin to recognize how the parents view health and development. (Do they believe they can affect their infant's health?) Also, the nurse can assess how competent parents seem to feel. She can then gear her counselling to the unique needs of this particular family. The parents may need assistance in recognizing they still have needs of their own. The nurse can assist them to look at their pattern of communication with each other now that an infant is part of the family. She can also assist them to look at the impact of an infant on their total situation.

The parents will be the people providing most of the health care for the infant. The nurse should assist parents as they care for their infant to promote his optimum growth and development without neglecting their own developmental needs. Throughout this chapter growth and development knowledge and issues have been discussed that are pertinent to the nurse as she provides assistance to parents through education, discussion of concerns, guidance and counselling on the needs of their developing infants. If the parents know what to expect in the process of healthy growth and development of their infant, they will be better prepared to meet these needs and feel more capable as parents. In addition to providing anticipatory guidance on the developing competencies of the infant, the nurse can help parents see their infant's needs in the areas of nutrition, play, safety and immunizations. Included should be an emphasis on the individual differences between infants.

Nutrition

Introduction of Solids Introduction of solid foods to the infant's diet is an issue of interest to parents and health professionals. Current information supports the view that the infant does not need solid foods for adequate nutrition until at least 6 months of age.[5] Previous recommendations had been for early introduction of solids, from 2 to 6 weeks of age. Solids were introduced at this early age because of developmental expectations and several beliefs: that the infant needed the solids to grow, that he was hungry, that he needed to practice feeding skills, and that solids would help him sleep through the night. None of these beliefs has been supported by sound research data. However, parents and professionals have used this pattern of early introduction of foods and found satisfaction with it, and some see no need to change.

Those persons advocating later introduction of foods do so primarily on the basis of three assumptions: (1) infants do not require solids for adequate nutrition, (2) in allergy-prone infants food allergies are more likely to occur early because of the incomplete digestion of food, and (3) the tendency is to give too many calories, producing an overweight infant. All these assumptions have some research data to support them.[5]

Developmental skills give some guidance for the introduction of solids. Maturation of the central nervous system controls motor skills that influence the infant's ability to eat and drink. Illengsworth and Listen point out that an infant learns to chew at about 6 to 7 months of age and therefore is ready developmentally to consume food.[27] The sucking pattern of the infant changes in the first year as maturation alters both the form of the oral structure and the way the infant takes liquid from a nipple.[27] By 4 to 6 months the oral cavity has grown, mature sucking and jaw motion have developed and these indicate the readiness of the infant to start solid foods. At the same time the infant has achieved other developmental skills that affect feeding: ability to grasp, hand-to-mouth movements, and ability to sit. The infant is truly ready to handle solid foods, including finger foods. At this age the tongue is still better able to handle spoon feeding than drinking from a cup.

Taking into consideration all the variables discussed, the introduction of solid feeding recommended by Barness is a logical one: introduce solid foods between 4 to 6 months; finger foods can be started for the infant who is able to sit; table food can be introduced by 1 year.[5]

The nurse can assist parents by relaying information about the nutritional requirements of infants and developmental skills that aid feeding, and the rationale for current recommendations about introduction of solids. Parents often have many questions about the sequence and methods of introducing solids. No one sequence is consistently recommended. However, some concepts that will aid the nurse in helping parents establish the pattern they will use in introduction of solids can be identified. The addition of food to the diet should be individualized to the infant and should never be forced. The infant will need some practice as he learns the new skill of eating solids, changing gradually from a sucking to a chewing motion. One new food should be introduced at a time, and a number of days (two to seven) should intervene before another new food is introduced, so that an allergic response could be more easily identified.

It has been generally recommended that the first food offered to the infant be rice cereal, as it is considered to be the least allergenic of the cereal grains and because most cereals are fortified with iron. Parents should give only cereals that are fortified with iron. Labels on the numerous cereal products available need to be read carefully. These products vary significantly in their nutritional value. Fruits are often the next solid introduced. It is thought that infants find fruits better tasting than some other foods; this may be an adult bias. Vegetables are introduced next and meats last.

It appears that infants find the texture of meat (sticky, granular) less appealing than the taste of meat itself. Some parents find it useful to mix the meat with another food. However, mixing of foods should be done with caution. Parents should be encouraged to give the meat alone a number of times to allow the infant to get accustomed to the taste and texture. Vegetables might be the food of choice if parents do decide to mix the meat with another food. Mixing meat with fruit only tends to bias the infant toward only sweet food. Another order of introduction of solids that some parents have used is vegetables, fruit, cereal and meat.

Frequently parents ask about the merits of using commercially prepared strained food as opposed to making their own strained foods. Either method can safely meet the nutritional needs of the infant. Some parents prefer to use a combination of these methods. If using commercially prepared foods, the parents should be encouraged to read the labels carefully. An item to look for is the amount of sugar and salt contained in the product; foods containing less of these are preferred. A number of companies in the last few years have altered the additives in their baby food products. The nurse should also point out that the mixed dinner labels should be especially carefully examined. There is usually substantially less meat in the dinner labeled

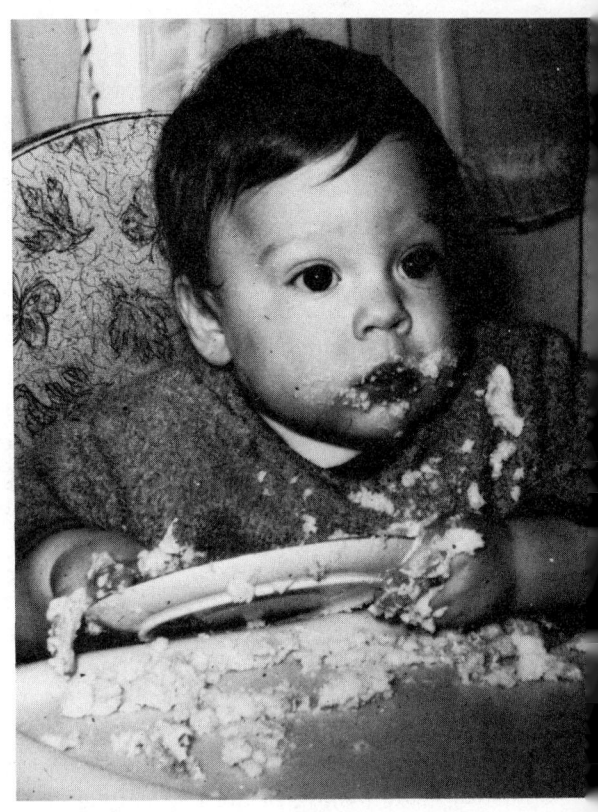

Feeding time can become messy as the infant's drive to explore includes his food. (Photograph by David Trainor.)

"vegetable and meat" than in the "meat and vegetable" dinners. Even the latter type of dinner may not contain an adequate amount of meat relative to cost. Many of the commercial dessert items have a high content of starch filler and add little to the diet other than calories.

If parents are preparing the strained food themselves, they must be sure to prepare a well-balanced diet. They may prepare just enough food to be fed immediately. If they prepare extra food, it can be mixed with a little water or milk, frozen in ice cube trays, placed in storage bags and kept frozen until immediately before use. There are a number of books available with helpful suggestions on preparing strained foods.[10] The nurse needs to keep up to date on what books are available to the public as well as suggesting that the parents explore current literature.

At about the same time or soon after strained foods are introduced, table (finger) foods also may be given. Much chewing can be done with the gums, so a large number of teeth are not necessary. The infant can feed himself such items as melba toast, crackers and zwieback. As the infant gains skill in chewing with teeth or gums or both, other bite-sized finger foods may be gradually added, including cereals, chicken, vegetables, cheese and canned fruits. Parents need to be aware of the dangers of some food items that are small and hard and easily aspirated, such as nuts, popcorn and kernels of corn. These food items should not be given to infants. Developmentally the infant enjoys exploring the food he is eating and the ability to begin to feed himself.

Parents need to be aware that feeding time can become quite messy. However, this is normal as the infant explores food as well as everything else. Near the end of the first year the infant is beginning to exert his independence, self-control, and mastery of skills that include feeding himself. Coordination of skills needed to finger-feed himself eventually becomes transferred to skill in using utensils. By the end of the first year infants have begun to feed themselves and in the next year will perfect the skills.

Type of Milk and Use of Cup Along with learning the skills associated with feeding himself, the infant is also developing the ability to drink from a cup. As indicated by the earlier discussion related to developmental skills achieved because of neuromuscular maturation, the infant can begin to drink from the cup by 6 months of age. Most infants can drink from a cup by 12 months. Introduction of the cup usually raises issues of when to wean the infant and when to change to whole cow's milk. Also of interest is whether to use 2 per cent milk or skim milk. There is no consensus on this question. The nurse needs to be aware of information currently available as she assists parents to make decisions in this area.

The rationale for not using whole cow's milk in the first 6 months of life is discussed in Chapter 20. For the most part the infant over 6 months is able to tolerate whole cow's milk quite well. The kidneys have matured to tolerate an increased solute load. There is decreased frequency of allergic reactions. Gastrointestinal disturbances seem to be fewer at this time. Whole cow's milk does not have the vitamin and mineral content of either breast milk or fortified formula. For this reason a number of authorities, including the American Academy of Pediatrics, recommend that infants remain on breast milk or iron-fortified formulas for the first year of life. Concern has been voiced about the relationship between whole cow's milk and iron deficiency anemia. There is some speculation about whether whole cow's milk might actually impair the absorption of iron by contributing to malfunction of duodenal villi.[32] However, this mechanism is not clearly understood. More data are needed about the relationship between whole cow's milk and iron deficiency anemia before practical implications can be made. If a switch is made to whole cow's milk, the total nutritional needs of the infant must be met with either food or supplements of vitamins and iron.

Questions about the use of 2 per cent milk or skim milk are often raised, especially if the infant is overweight. Some authorities believe that even at 6 to 12 months the extra solute load from either of these preparations could be too much for the infant.[5] This is more likely to be true in the case of 2 per cent milk or skim milk than with whole cow's milk, because often these preparations are fortified with nonfat milk solids that increase the protein and mineral content of the milk. Fatty acid requirements may not be met with the use of 2 per cent milk or skim milk. Fatty acid deficiencies have been demonstrated in infants. Dermatitis was the most frequent finding in infants receiving low levels of linoleic acid.[24] The infant's caloric needs for growth may not be met if a large amount (more than one quart) of low-calorie low-fat milk is consumed instead of a reasonable amount of milk and a balanced solid food intake.

Consumption of skim milk may eventually lead to a tendency to overeat in an infant. He comes to rely on volume rather than calories to determine satiety. A number of professionals believe that 2 per cent milk or skim milk consumed in reasonable amounts after 6 months of age will do no harm and may be good for control of weight and cholesterol levels. No official group has recommended restriction in dietary intake of cholesterol in normal infants.[17]

Weaning occurs as the infant moves from primarily a liquid to a more solid diet. As he increases his solid intake and begins to drink from a cup, he will need less from the bottle or breast. The issue of when to fully wean a particular infant often arises when he is 6 to 12 months of age. There is no one right time or way to wean an infant. The nurse must assist parents in their individual approach to weaning their infant. Factors to be considered as she discusses this process with the parents include developmental readiness of the infant, his sucking needs, parents' beliefs and feelings, environmental pressures (family, job), finances, nutritional requirements and past experiences of family and nurse.

Meeting nutritional needs of the infant certainly contributes significantly to his attainment of maximum physical competency. Conversely, the infant's current level of physical competency affects his ability to develop the necessary skills to begin to meet his own nutritional needs. However, more than physical competency is involved in an infant's nutritional needs. Parent-infant interaction and developing emotional-social competency are intimately involved in the infant's nutritional status. Intellectual competency becomes important as the older infant begins to develop abilities to feed himself and make his individual needs clearly known. The nurse must keep all competency areas of the infant in focus, as well as parent-infant interaction, as she assists the family to meet the nutritional needs of their infant.

Play

The needs of the infant for play are implicit throughout the discussion regarding promotion of infant growth and development. Play provides opportunities for the infant to learn and develop many skills. The importance of a variety of play opportunities can be pointed out to parents. Play is not just an extra activity that serves no purpose (see discussion in Chapter 12). It is the way the infant learns about himself and his environment. As the reader reflects on the discussion of the activities that promote development of physical and intellectual competencies, it becomes clear that many of these activities are usually classified as play activities. Expensive toys are not necessary for play; articles commonly found in the home are perfectly adequate. The nurse can assist the family to creatively use the resources available to them. Play activities promote emotional-social development of the infant as he separates himself from his environment. Many such activities foster interaction of the infant with other people. Play can stimulate the attachment of the infant to parents and his eventual ability to separate. It can provide many pleasurable experiences for the infant as he learns to trust and adapt to his world.

Safety

Safety is another key issue implicit in the discussion of infant growth and development. As the nurse discusses the developing competencies of the infant, she can help parents look at the environment in terms of the hazards these developing skills may introduce.

Parents need to recognize that even the very young infant soon will be turning and rolling over (Table 21–3). Thus it is not safe to leave the infant unrestrained on any object he might roll off of, such as a bed or change table. As the infant becomes able to reach items and grasp and bring them to his mouth, parents must be even more alert to what is within reach. Small objects such as coins, buttons and pins must be removed from his territory. Nothing should be tied around the infant's neck, including pacifiers on strings.

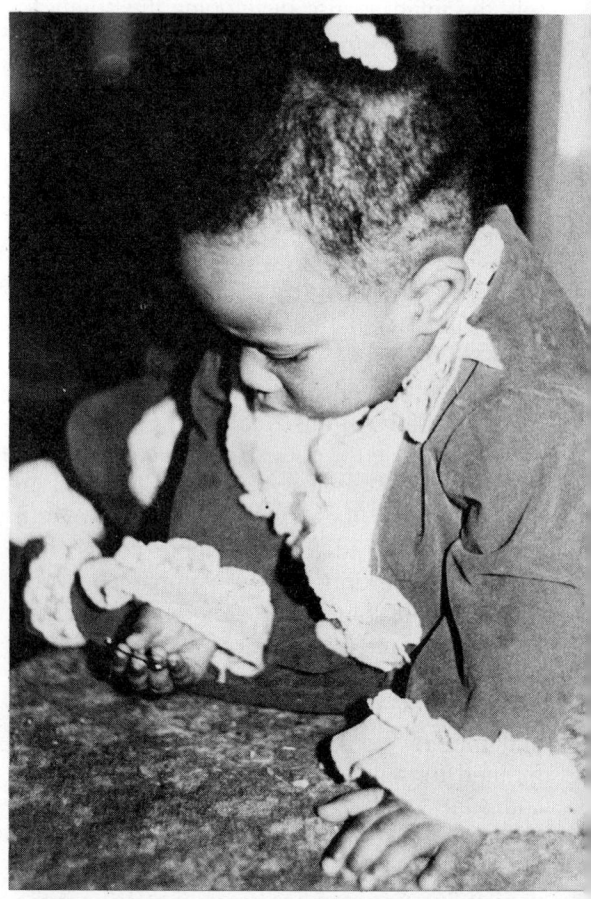

The infant's developing mobility makes child-proofing mandatory for her safety. This infant has discovered an open safety pin lying in the carpet.

As the infant becomes mobile, the parents or any caretaker must learn to anticipate his ability to creep and crawl farther and faster than they think he can. An infant's ability to explore his environment increases every day. The parents must anticipate that he will soon be able to pull himself to standing and begin to walk around objects. Safety hazards are covered in more detail in Chapter 30 in discussing growth and development of the toddler; however, the infant too must be protected from the risks of his ever-widening environment. Particular dangers include chewing on electric cords, being burned by too-hot bath water, and poisoning from household items such as laundry soap and detergents, bleach, cosmetics and even some household plants.

Parents should be instructed to have the nearest Poison Control Center telephone number clearly displayed, preferably on the telephone itself. In the event of poisoning, the Poison Control Center should be called for specific instructions before any measures are taken at home. Syrup of ipecac is not usually recommended for children under 1 year of age because of the potential danger of aspiration when vomiting is induced. Although syrup of ipecac is not recommended for the infant, parents should be advised to buy it as soon as the baby is born so that it is available if needed.

Falls are common accidents for infants. When in a highchair, the infant should be securely fastened and watched carefully. Parents need to be reminded that an infant in an infant seat can easily tip it over. He should not be left unattended when in this seat and placed on a table, chair or similar surface. As the infant becomes mobile, stairways need to be closed off with doors, gates or some other safety device.

Another major safety concern relates to automobile travel. A large percentage of infants are not properly restrained in cars, even though it is known that restraints can reduce death and injury. Infants held on laps or placed in open baskets (car beds) in the car can become flying missiles in the event of a sudden stop or collision. The infant should always be restrained in an infant car seat that is properly installed and that meets federal motor vehicle safety standards. Parents need to choose carefully from the many infant car seats on the market. Not all meet safety standards, especially used ones being passed on from friends or sold second hand. Using a car seat correctly and consistent-ly *every time* the infant is in the car will make it easier to restrain the active toddler later (see Chapter 30).

> The abundance of anticipatory guidance required in the promotion of growth and development of infants makes it important that the nurse see families periodically throughout the first year of the infant's life. This amount of information is too overwhelming to be shared in one or two visits. Dealing with childrearing concerns and reinforcing parental efforts are part of an ongoing process. The nurse working with infants and their families must remember that what is standard practice to her may be totally unfamiliar to new parents. She must be careful not to give merely routine advice but rather to assess each family individually and to provide advice according to their needs. She must work with parents as they provide care to their infants rather than telling them what to do.
>
> The first year of life is one of rapid changes. It is an exciting time as infant and parents learn and grow together. The nurse can work with these families to assist them to make this unique period one of optimal growth and development for them and their infant.

Immunizations

Immunizations are an important component of anticipatory guidance. Parents need to be informed about the benefits of immunization procedures and the rationale for the procedure. Parents must be informed of the risks as well as the benefits of immunizations. The Committee on Infectious Disease of the American Academy of Pediatrics recommends immunization schedules. These are revised periodically as new information arises. Table 21–7 gives the current recommendations for normal infants.

The nurse should consult current resources such as latest editions of AAP's *Report of the Committee on Infectious Disease* (Red Book) for detailed information about immunizations. The nurse also needs to help prepare parents for possible reaction of the infant to certain immunizations and related interventions. There may be a local reaction to an immunization injection, including redness or induration at the site and/or a nodule. Discomfort from a local reaction may be relieved by placing the infant in a

TABLE 21-7 RECOMMENDED IMMUNIZATION SCHEDULE FOR NORMAL HEALTHY INFANTS*

Schedule	Diphtheria-Tetanus-Pertussis	Polio	TB Test
2 mo	X	X	
4 mo	X	X	
6 mo	X		
1 year			X

*Recommended by the American Academy of Pediatrics, October 1980. From Standards of Child Health Care, 3rd ed. Copyright American Academy of Pediatrics, 1977.

warm bath or using warm soaks on the involved area. Mild systemic reactions may occur, including irritability and temperature elevation. Proper use of acetaminophen or aspirin should be reviewed with parents at the time immunizations are given. The nurse must recognize the importance of immunizations, but not overlook other equally important areas of anticipatory guidance.

References

1. M. Ainsworth. The development of the infant-mother attachment. In Review of Child Development Research 3 by B. M. Caldwell and H. N. Riccuiti. University of Chicago Press, 1973
2. American Academy of Pediatrics. Standards of Child Health Care. Evanston, Illinois, 1977
3. A. Baldwin. Theories of Child Development. John Wiley & Sons, Inc., 1967
4. K. Barnard and M. Powell. Teaching the Mentally Retarded Child. C. V. Mosby Co., 1972
5. L. Barness. The feeding transitions in the first year. Dialogues in Infant Nutrition, July 1977, p. 1
6. N. Bayley. Comparisons of mental and motor test scores for 1–15 months by sex, birth order, race, geographical location and education of parents. Child Development, June 1965, p. 379
7. S. M. Bell and M. Ainsworth. Infant crying and maternal responsiveness. Child Development, September 1972, p. 1171
8. T. Brazelton. Infant and Mothers: Differences in Development. Delacorte Press, 1969
9. W. Carey, Clinical application of infant temperament measurements. Journal of Pediatrics, October 1972, p. 823
10. S. Castle. The Complete Guide to Preparing Baby Foods at Home. Doubleday & Co., Inc., 1973
11. M. Chow et al. Handbook of Pediatric Primary Care. John Wiley & Sons, 1979
12. Committee on Nutrition, American Academy of Pediatrics. Fluoride as a nutrient. Pediatrics, January 1979, p. 150
13. C. DeAngelis. Pediatric Primary Care. Little, Brown & Co., 1979
14. M. Erickson. Assessment and Management of Developmental Changes in Children. C. V. Mosby Co., 1976
15. Food and Nutrition Board, National Research Council. Recommended Daily Dietary Allowances. National Academy of Sciences, 1974
16. S. Fomon. Infant Nutrition. W. B. Saunders Co., 1974
17. S. Fomon. Nutritional Disorders of Children. USDHEW Publication No. (HSA) 77–5104, 1977
18. D. Freedman. Ethnic differences in babies. Human Nature, January 1979, p. 36
19. H. Ginsberg and S. Upper. Piaget's Theory of Intellectual Development. Prentice-Hall, Inc., 1969
20. M. Kenda and P. Williams. The Natural Baby Food Cookbook. Avon Books, 1972
21. M. Klaus and J. Kennell. Maternal-Infant Bonding. C. V. Mosby Co., 1976
22. D. Lakdawala and E. Widdowson. Vitamin D in human milk. Lancet, 22 January 1977, p. 167
23. J. McMillan, S. Landau and F. Uski. Iron sufficiency in breast-fed infants and the availability of iron from human milk. Pediatrics, November 1976, p. 686
24. H. Mitchell et al. Nutrition in Health and Disease. J. B. Lippincott Co., 1976
25. D. Papalia and S. Olds. A Child's World: Infancy Through Adolescence. McGraw-Hill Book Co., 1975.
26. A. Paemalee, W. Wenner and H. Schultz. Infant sleep patterns from birth to 16 weeks of age. Journal of Pediatrics, October 1964, p. 576
27. P. Pipes. Nutrition in Infancy and Childhood. C. V. Mosby Co., 1977
28. U. Saarinen and P. Dallman. Iron absorption in infants: high bioavailability of breast milk iron as indicated by the extrinsic tag method of iron absorption and the concentration of serum ferritin. Journal of Pediatrics, July 1977, p. 36
29. H. Silver, C. Kempe and H. Bruyn. Handbook of Pediatrics. Lange Medical Publications, 1975
30. M. Smart and R. Smart. Infants: Development and Relationships. MacMillan Inc., 1978
31. E. Stein et al. Sleep characteristics in infants. Pediatrics, January 1969
32. E. Waitrowski et al. Dietary fluoride intake of infants. Pediatrics, April 1975, p. 517
33. P. Wolff. The natural history of crying and other vocalizations in early infancy. In Determinants of Infant Behaviors. F. Foss, ed. Methuen and Co. Ltd., 1969
34. C. Woodruff. The role of fresh cow's milk in iron deficiency anemia. American Journal of Disease in Childhood, July 1972, p. 18

Additional Recommended Reading

M. Alexander and M. Scott Brown. Pediatric History Taking and Physical Diagnosis for Nurses. McGraw-Hill Co., 1979

J. Bowlby. Attachment and Loss, Vol. 1. Basic Books, 1969

E. Charney et al. Childhood antecedents of adult obesity. New England Journal of Medicine, July 1976, p. 6

S. Chess, A. Thomas and H. Birch. Your Child is a Person: A Psychological Approach to Parenthood without Guilt. Viking Press, 1972

E. Erikson. Childhood and Society. Norton, 1950

A. Gesell and C. Amatruda. Developmental Diagnosis: Normal and Abnormal Child Development. Haber Press, 1947

M. Lamb. Father-infant and mother-infant interaction in the first year of life. Child Development, March 1977, p. 167

H. Maier, Three Theories of Child Development. Harper & Row, 1969

L. Murphy and A. Moriarty. Vulnerability, Coping and Growth from Infancy to Adolescence. Yale University Press, 1976

C. Snow. The development of conversation between mothers and babies. Journal of Child Language, May 1976, p. 1

S. Trotter and E. Thomas. Social Responsiveness of Infants. Pediatric Round Table 2, Johnson and Johnson Baby Products Co., 1978

POTENTIAL STRESSES DURING INFANCY: THE GROWTH OF HUMAN BONDS

by Michael Trout, MA

The author wishes to acknowledge the guidance, support and wise counsel of Bette Chapman, LPN, without whose assistance this chapter would not be.

Interest in postpartum parental behavior has been heightened by the discovery — over the past 40 years or so — that even unremembered infant experiences may have a dramatic effect on character growth, that infancy may be a "critical period" in personality development. The quality of early parenting has thus taken on new significance for those interested in the optimal development of children and the prevention of emotional disorder. And, since the quality of that parenting has appeared to be deeply rooted in the kind of relationship a baby and his parents have, we have become observant about what parents and their babies do with each other from the beginning.

Only recently, however, have we begun to come to grips with how it is that babies and their parents get on together. If parental love of the newborn were the automatic, perhaps even hormonally inspired, overture from active parent to passive infant that we have always assumed it to be, then such early and extended contact would be unnecessary. Parental love would flow "naturally" to the baby, whenever baby happened to be around.

NORMAL DEVELOPMENT OF EARLY SOCIAL RELATIONS

The Process of Lovemaking

Observations of mothers and fathers with their newborns,[12, 13, 17] and careful listening to the reports of new parents about their earliest experiences with their babies,[4, 14, 22, 25] reveal that the "falling in love" of latency and early adolescence may constitute a remarkably apt analogy to growth of attachments between parents and infants. It appears, in other words, as if we *learn* to love our babies, and our babies *learn* to love us. The process is as vulnerable, and as subject to disappointment, ambivalence, fear and regression, as any human growth process.

A couple of discoveries have been critical to the construction of this view of the development of social relations in infancy. Of extreme importance has been the research literature of the past 20 years, which has demonstrated the reflexive, visual, auditory and affective capabilities of the human neonate. Armed with these research data, one can begin to consider each particular infant (behavior, cueing systems, irritability, re-

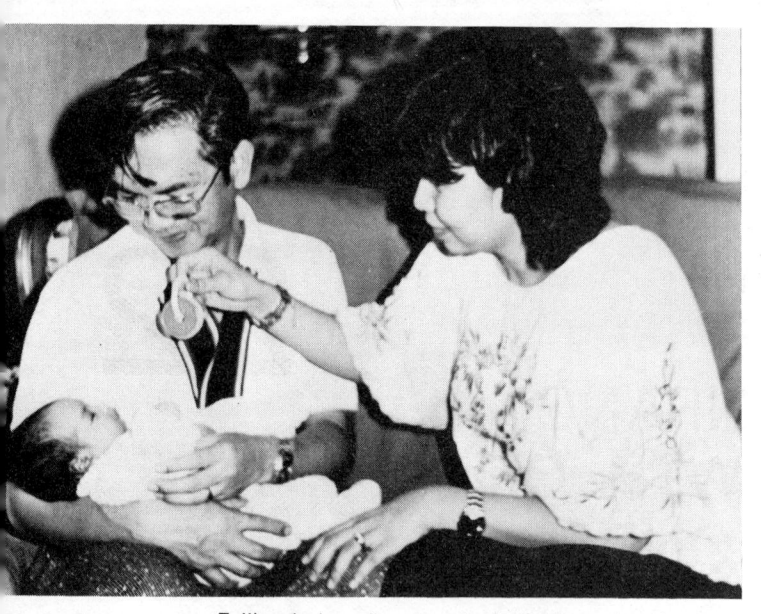

Falling in love (human attachment) requires frequent and regular interaction between parents and their baby.

sponsiveness, reflexive precocity, attractiveness) as *part of the equation* in the caregiver-infant dyad.

Another discovery critical to this view of the growth of human love bonds is that not all parents and babies get on well together. These serious caregiver-infant relationship struggles were overlooked by health care professionals partly because we were not clinically sophisticated enough to know what it looked like when a baby and a parent were failing to attach to one another. Words such as "spoiled" and "colicky" were invented so we could talk at arms' length about babies who were struggling to communicate with us. We had made too many assumptions about the "innate" capabilities of parents to love their babies and were left wondering why parents were messing up so often, why they were failing to take our advice, and why our advice was so often failing to help when it was taken. We found ourselves outraged at the child abuse statistics, angry at parents who were finding excuses not to visit their sick newborns in the neonatal intensive care nursery, dismayed when mothers had obvious preferences for one twin over the other. And we did, finally, the most constructive and scientifically useful thing we had done in some time — we began to watch and to listen.

We began to observe that parents who were having trouble with their babies — who were ambivalent about taking baby home with them from the hospital, who were bringing baby back to the hospital with too-frequent diarrhea and complaints of chronic feeding problems —were also *not* talking about their babies' smiles or their babies' visual discriminative capacity as parents were who had thriving relationships with their babies. When we watched the troubled families, we noticed that sometimes the babies really *were* different, they really failed to smile or to respond with the rhythmic body movement and affect that is recognized as typical. Sometimes these appropriate infant behaviors were present, at least for a while, but the parents seemed unable to notice or to be touched, and the infant grew less responsive over time.

It is now apparent that parents are affected deeply by the particular qualities of their babies, by the circumstances of the pregnancy and delivery and the postnatal period, and by the elements of their own character brought to childbearing and rearing. Human attachment can now be seen as something parents accomplish cooperatively with their babies. The growth of love bonds between an infant and his primary caregiver is now viewed as a delicate and vulnerable interplay of elements that each have an impact on the nature of the relationship and, as a secondary effect, the chances for the baby's optimal development.

Dynamics of Attachment

Human attachment is an emotional link created between two individuals when they invest emotional energy in each other. Among the most obvious and significant features of the growth of love bonds between a caregiver and a baby is the tendency for an attached caregiver to be both physically and socially available to the baby. Because the relationship is a reciprocal one, the caregiver's behavior is oriented toward increasing the frequency of such experiences as feeling competent, being smiled at, being nuzzled, being "picked out" by the baby's differential response. This tendency toward increasing social availability and physical proximity behaviors in the caregiver has a number of ramifications for the caregiver-infant relationship.

First of all, there is a circular effect in being near to, and responsive to, the baby. For example, infant crying as a signal tends to decrease over the second quarter of the first year of life when the caregiver's response to early crying is consistently prompt. At the same time that the frequency and duration of crying episodes are decreasing, there is an increase in other social signals that are thought of as less noxious, and that are finally replaced by direct communications focused specifically on the caregiver. Being responsive to the baby has the tendency, then, to reduce an infant behavior (crying) that is often upsetting to a new parent and often difficult to understand, and to replace it with a more enjoyable and clearer set of communications. Even during the immediate postpartum period, the physical proximity and social availability of the mother made possible by rooming-in allows a more consistently prompt maternal response to infant crying and a concomitant decrease in such crying. Neonates have shown a tendency to stop crying in less than five seconds when the mother responds within 90 seconds of the commencement of a crying episode. An average of 50 seconds of maternal attention is required, however, to soothe a newborn left to cry more than 90 seconds.[14] An interesting side effect of this reduction in infant crying and the development of other social signals between baby and caregiver is the tendency for mothers who have experienced the phenomenon to report feeling more self-confident and to call for medical advice less frequently.[14] Early lovemaking behavior between caregiver and infant, then, has a self-perpetuating nature: behavior that has need-gratifying qualities is repeated by both partners,

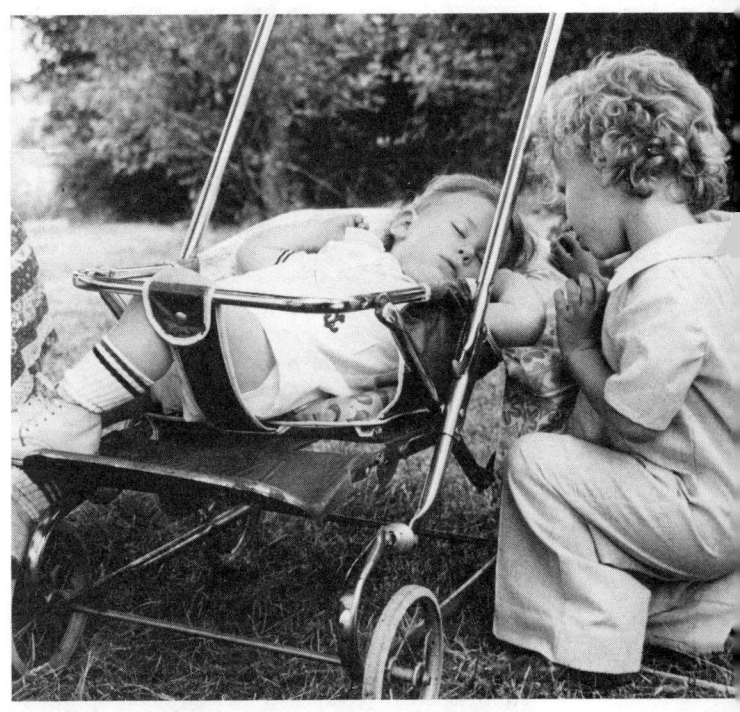

Children can teach us much about watching and listening. (Photograph by Michael Trout.)

and they soon develop remarkably sophisticated and specific means for signaling their needs even though the kinds of needs that are met may change substantially over time.

Physical proximity and social availability on the caregiver's part create more opportunities for gratification (of both caregiver and infant). However, proximal and responsive parental behaviors have other ramifications for early child development. An infant's capacity for self-regulation and his capacity to control or organize behavior and to gain a mastery of events and of developmental challenges are deeply rooted in the predictability, stability and consistency of his early experience.

There appears to be a link between the acquisition of object constancy — a critical milestone in development and a preliminary to other achievements — and the infant's experience with response expectations and with predictability in caregiving. Interestingly, the capacity of the child to conceive of the existence of things when he cannot see them (object constancy) is part and parcel of learning the concept of "other" and then the concept of "self." When the human infant is able to distinguish himself from people and things around

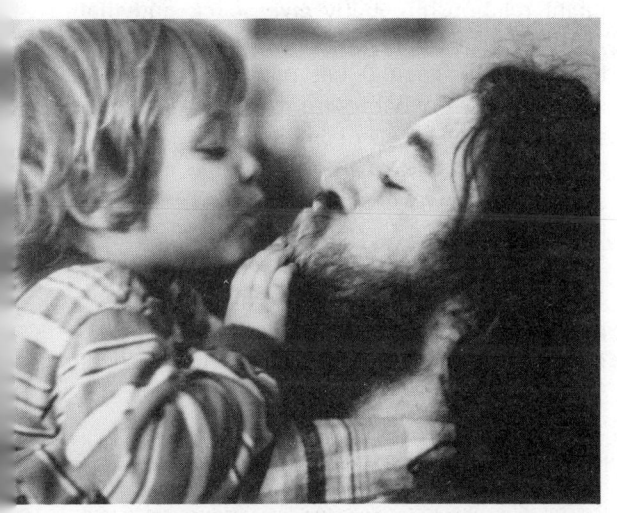

The lovemaking behaviors of attachment have a self-perpetuating quality that persists, although the needs they meet change substantially over time. (Photograph by Michael Trout.)

SPOILING ISN'T WHAT IT USED TO BE

Silvia Bell and Mary Ainsworth have conducted one of the most organized studies into maternal responsiveness to infant crying while doing longitudinal research with 26 mother-infant pairs.[2] They conclude: "Those infants who are conspicuous for fussing and crying after the first few months of life and who fit the stereotype of the 'spoiled child' are those whose mothers have ignored their cries or have delayed long in responding to them.... Infants whose mothers have given them relatively much tender and affectionate holding in the earliest months of life are content with surprisingly little physical contact by the end of the first year; although they enjoy being held, when put down they are happy to move off into independent exploration. In contrast, those held for relatively brief periods during the early months tend to be ambivalent about contact by the end of the first year; they do not respond positively when held but yet protest when put down and do not turn readily to independent activity .... In short, those infants in our sample who are fussy, demanding and difficult to control are those whose mothers have been unresponsive to signals and generally insensitive or interfering in their efforts to mold their babies to their routines, wishes and expectations."[2]

him, he is able to slowly move away, with the assurance that the world will remain intact even when he does not keep an eye on it. Such a child is on his way to becoming independent and social, and that has become possible because of the intimate, responsive relationship he has had with a stable caregiver.

This discussion would be incomplete without a reminder that physical proximity — even parental "doting" behavior — is not equivalent to parental responsiveness and predictability. *The physical availability of a socially unavailable mother* is a recurrent and devastating experience for some children and frequently accompanies the object-avoiding syndromes of infancy.[21]

In addition to the ramifications of parent-infant attachment, and the accompanying behavioral manifestations of touch, smiling, looking and responsiveness already discussed, we must consider the greater tendency on the part of a well-attached parent to protect the baby from harm. Not only does this set of parental behaviors result in the obvious increase in the likelihood of the infant surviving, but parental protective behavior gives important messages to the baby. Infants grow up protecting themselves as a direct extension of the value they place on their own protection — a value learned by being cared for again and again, by being restrained from danger, by seeing adult concern for the comfort and integrity of the infants' bodies.[19]

Among the more interesting features of families in which reciprocal love bonds with the infant are growing and flourishing is the apparent protection of parental sanity, and encouragement of the parental role, afforded by the loving parent-infant relationship. Unquestionably, being a parent is one of the most anxiety-provoking, physically exhausting and emotionally draining series of events imaginable. Mothers (and in a different sense fathers) are giving up some of their gilded myths about parenthood and admitting that they are something less than thrilled about getting up at 2 a.m. (and 4 a.m. and 6 a.m.!) for feedings; that some days they feel very much like chucking their little one right out of the upstairs window. But most continue getting up, and most leave the window closed. The reason, we can now see, may lie in the reciprocal nature of the parent-infant relationship. Baby *gives back* and that giving (the nuzzling, the differential smile, the touching, the gazing) has probably served to keep a number of babies from unplanned excursions into the sky. On some days it may seem that baby will drive us crazy very soon; at the same time, however, it will be baby who will keep us sane.*

Finally, and perhaps most importantly, an attachment with a primary caregiver in infancy provides baby's first experience with the pleasures (entirely narcissistic and self-centered at

---

*This is, of course, an important lesson for the infant mental health intervener. As therapists, we haven't a prayer in *convincing* parents that they should be better parents, that they must be more responsive, that they really ought to stop hitting. Our only hope is in attracting parents to their own babies, in "hooking" them to the remarkable capabilities of, and the possibilities for a relationship with, their babies.

first, of course) of human social contact. Through the earliest relationships a child has the opportunity to learn trust as he sees that his caregiver reliably takes care of him, responds to him and protects him. In the strictest behavioral sense, he learns to participate in social relationships in a manner that will later be seen as "loving." He will control himself, gratify others and engage in socially attractive behaviors at first because those behaviors encourage the incoming of narcissistic supplies. The links between giving and getting eventually become blurred, however, as the child begins to enjoy pleasing others, making affectionate overtures to them and responding warmly to them, because those behaviors have gained inherently pleasing qualities for him. Baby and caregiver have conspired to create a child who understands how to signal adults about his needs and who feels reasonably assured that most of those needs will be met; a child who enjoys human social contact and who guides his behavior in such a way as to maximize the frequency and pleasure of such contact; a child who trusts and can be trusted; a child who values himself and who will slowly take charge of (and pride in) mastering his body. Out of the framework of this social experience he will begin to make choices about his own behavior and will demonstrate the development of conscience and self-control.

THE ELEMENTS OF A BREAKDOWN IN ATTACHMENT

A careful look has just been taken at how human attachments grow in infancy, what the process is like for infant and for caregiver. To understand breakdowns in early attachment, one needs to maintain a holistic view of parent-infant relationships and examine the same elements that support a healthy attachment: qualities and experiences of the *baby*, qualities and experiences of the *parents*, and the *circumstances* of the pregnancy, birth and postnatal period. The flourishing of love bonds is contingent on a positive interplay of these three elements. When the relationship breaks down, one usually finds a destructive mix of the same elements. Potentially disruptive examples from each of the three elements are discussed here; it should be remembered that no one feature alone causes breakdowns in early social relations. A baby who is physically unattractive or who is unusually demanding is not necessarily a baby in social trouble, any more than is a parent who was abused as a young child. It is the *interplay* of forces that is critical.

The Baby as a Factor in Attachment Breakdown

Potentially disruptive features of the baby include neonatal illness, anomalies, premature delivery (particularly when a separation between the parents and their newborn ensues), irritability, appearance, "incorrect" sex, tactile hypersensitivity, motor depression, unresponsiveness and affective blandness. When mixed with certain circumstantial elements, or parental factors, or both, these act to disrupt parent-infant bonding.

Neonatal illness is sometimes problematic for a number of reasons. First of all, many parents with sick newborns feel that they are at fault for the infant's illness. Their memories flip back through the pregnancy, thinking about the mother's problem in giving up cigarettes, the father's job loss and their subsequent poverty that may have left the mother (and the fetus) malnourished. Particularly when the illness is severe or life-threatening, one or both parents may blame their own body systems. When one of the parents may already feel vulnerable or worthless, or both, the thought that he or she has contributed to the birth of a sick baby may reinforce these feelings of incompetence and worthlessness. It has been the unfortunate experience of a number of families to break up after the discovery that the baby was seriously ill. The causative factor is not, of course, baby's illness per se, but often the interplay of the illness and the father's vulnerability and extreme fear for his own safety.

Neonatal anomalies, perhaps even more than illness, are sometimes viewed by parents as punishment for some real or imagined misdeed. Attachment with the anomalous child may then be blocked, and associated depression may be complicated by agitation and an inability to find any joy whatsoever in caring for the new child. In addition, some minor anomalies or reparable major anomalies may appear to parents as more devastating than they actually are, because of parental experience with similar problems. A father whose younger sibling died early in life with a lung disease may be terrified at relatively simple respiratory distress in his own newborn.

Other aspects of normal physical appearance in the newborn may compound already-present parental fear or vulnerability, producing an early problem in attachment. Sometimes the heart of the matter turns out to be the incongruity between parental expectations (the child fantasized about during the pregnancy) and the infant's real appearance. It is often most useful to give parents an opportunity to speak of the physical characteristics they had hoped for, and to clarify with parents why a particular feature was important to them. Physical size seems especially culturally significant in the United States, and great support is given to parents who produce large, robust babies. In addition, infant smallness may generate parental fears that the baby will always be frail or that they will be unable to care for such a helpless child. Other physical characteristics (the length or color of hair, the nose shape) may remind a parent of another person. If that other person is despised (the boyfriend who disappeared in the last trimester) or feared (the mother's mother, who abused her), or yearned for (a sibling who died), the relationship with the baby may be disturbed.

There is, of course, nothing inherently abnormal about parents hoping for a baby of a particular sex. Problems arise principally when the baby's sex has a specific meaning for a parent and acceptance of a particular sex is blocked. It is not uncommon for unwed adolescent mothers who have decided to keep their babies to be quite ambivalent about the delivery of a male child. Initially, the mother may be quite pleased that her offspring is a male, perhaps because she assumes male babies have a higher social value, thus increasing her acceptability to her boyfriend or to others. However, particularly when the boyfriend/father has departed during the pregnancy, a male child may become an object of abuse or rejection when he begins to crawl and become mobile. At this point, some unwed adolescent mothers begin to imagine that their male child is going to leave them, just as other boys have done. It is not really the baby who is being psychologically rejected but another person of the same sex who is represented by the baby.

Prematurity is a significant variable to consider here, particularly since it raises the spectre of separation, illness, infant smallness, and parental disappointment. Many parents of premature infants have reported a uniquely troubling dimension to the particular kind of separation that sometimes follows a premature delivery. When babies do come home (for the *first time,* we should remember), parents sometimes experience their offspring as strangers, as intruders who do not belong.

Even without the additional burden (for parents *and* for baby) of a separation, a significantly premature delivery may inspire feelings of disappointment, grief and loss (over not having the perfect child fantasized during the pregnancy). As with neonatal illness, anomalies and unattractive physical characteristics, parents of a significantly premature child may feel ashamed, may blame themselves or each other, and may burden themselves and their marriage with anger and guilt at a time when they most need their own inner resources and the support of each other.

Some babies who have spent long periods in neonatal intensive care units experience tactile hypersensitivity. What some parents have reported is an extreme aversion to human touch observed in their babies who have been poked, prodded, tested, surgically cut, had tubes inserted and who have lain bare in an incubator or on an "island" under bright lights for weeks on end.[18] When such hypersensitive babies come home, they often scream upon being picked up by their parents, they fail to mold comfortably or cuddle and they generally make the already overwhelmed and worried parents feel helpless, incompetent or even hated by their own baby. Without reassurance and guidance about what is happening, some parents begin to initiate less contact with their hypersensitive babies. Careful attention to this phenomenon by hospital staff (including a discussion with parents about it before the baby goes home) and a great deal of regular caressing by a primary-care nurse on the unit have been helpful in reducing the devastating impact of this phenomenon on the parent-infant relationship.[18]

Similar infant tactile hypersensitivity has been noted when baby is blind or deaf or both.[15] Here the critical feature seems to be not the child's early experience with touch as hurtful, but rather the child's lack of control over incoming stimuli due to sensory deprivation. An approximation of what the experience of touch is like for a deaf-blind infant may be made by imagining oneself awakening in a completely darkened room in which one has never been before and to which one was brought during sleep. Because entry was made during sleep, the size, shape and limits of the room are unknown. It also cannot be known whether there are doors or people in the room, or giant holes in the floor. To add to the sense of complete disorientation and terror, it is not possible to move about the room to explore; one must simply sit and wait. Out of this frightening bleakness, a hand suddenly touches one's shoulder! Assuming that this otherwise normal human greeting did not result in immediate cardiac arrest, one might certainly expect to do a bit of screaming or trembling. For the deaf-blind infant, experiences of human touch without warning may seem just as frightening and just as invasive. An uninstructed parent may find most upsetting the screams of the infant that greet attempts at affectionate touching. Parents may decide that the infant does not love them, that he wishes to be left alone, that this baby "hates to be loved." In all likelihood, of course, none of these is the correct interpretation of baby's screamed message. Carefully guided and nurtured parents have learned to signal their blind or deaf-blind children with voice or vibration and have continued to gently stroke and rock their babies until the screaming stops. The potential threat to the development of warm social relations between a deaf-blind baby and his parents is painfully clear, however.

There is a group of other infant characteristics that may, in combination with certain parental characteristics or life circumstances, threaten the normal growth of attachment. A newborn delivered when the mother is heavily sedated may be considerably less responsive and show less reflexive maturity than a baby delivered with less medication. Under most circumstances parents may not notice the difference, or they will understand that the effect is temporary. In a family in which a high premium is put on intelligence, however, or in which a mother may be secretly terrified that her drug use during the early stages of pregnancy may have made her baby retarded, parents' feelings about a relatively flaccid and unresponsive newborn may be powerful. Nicknames such as "Deadhead" and jokes about the baby being "burned out" may barely mask parental guilt and worry. If, in fact, the parents turn away from their baby and fail to stimulate or interact with this living symbol of their felt worthlessness as parents, then a partially self-fulfilling prophecy may have been created.

If an infant is unusually irritable, or unusually demanding of physical contact, or relatively uninterested in physical contact, or a bit bland, or sleeps much less than the parents have known to be normal, these qualities may also join with particular parental vulnerabilities to create a barrier to attachment. To the busy hospital nurse or family physician, the repeated parental questions or remarks about the baby being dumb or never liking to be held may seem routine and only related to the child's current developmental level. It is probably a worthwhile medical or nursing practice, however, to look a bit further; the stakes may be, after all, rather high.

Parents as a Factor in Attachment Breakdown

There are characteristics or experiences of *parents* that may, in combination with certain features of the baby and of the family's life circumstances, serve to threaten the normal growth of social relations. A history of loss is a particularly troublesome element for parents to carry into childbearing and rearing. One or more spontaneous or induced abortions, a close experience with sudden infant death syndrome or earlier neonatal death or the earlier loss of a child or sibling by accident or disease may each make parents feel a bit defective as babymakers, or guilty about their earlier failures. Miscarriages have long been ignored by both professionals and other family members (by everyone except the parents, in fact), but are often experienced as very real deaths by parents. The healthy child delivered after one or more miscarriages may be one that parents protect too much (out of fear for his safety), or the one that parents turn away from (particularly if the newborn's sex or other characteristics make it difficult for him to play the role of "the replacement baby"). If a lengthy depression has followed the previous miscarriage, the subsequent child may find himself with a parent who is notably understimulating or who is unfinished with the earlier loss (a manifestation of which may be the subsequent pregnancy itself).

An earlier loss of a child who was relinquished for adoption may have an impact on a subsequent child. Particularly if the relinquishing parent has unresolved feelings about whether or not the action was justified, he or she may find that the delivery of a new baby who will be kept makes the relinquishment seem like a terrible thing to have done. Parents in these circumstances have reported being burdened with dreams about an older child harming their new baby, fantasies about being suddenly visited by the relinquished child and terror about someone taking away the new child.

An earlier neonatal death or the loss of a previous child from sudden infant death syndrome (SIDS) may create difficulties in attaching to the new baby, with extra features of extreme parental guilt and chronic anxiety about a repetition. SIDS leaves parents without the kind of medical explanation that will help them move on without fear to the care of the next child. Parents are nagged by doubts about the adequacy of their earlier care of the child who died and are sometimes haunted by suspicions that their perfectly normal ambivalence (some days enjoying the baby less than others, sometimes daydreaming about the freedom of the pre-baby days) may have caused the death. Ambivalence then becomes something to be feared, and attempts are made to immediately resolve (or deny) all ambivalent feelings about the subsequent pregnancy and the subsequent child. Denied the normal psychological process of having a number of different feelings at the same time (about the pregnancy, about the baby, even about the marriage), some parents find themselves enormously agitated or depressed or both, simultaneously, and their interaction with the new baby becomes inconsistent and chaotic.

Neonatal death often inspires similar feelings of helplessness and guilt, as well as anxiety during the next pregnancy that the loss will be repeated. An important difference between the loss of a child who has lived with the parents for a while and neonatal or fetal death is the absence, in the latter case, of the availability of a clearly separate person who can be properly mourned. To remove a dead fetus or to deliver a baby who dies is to tear away from the mother something that was quite literally a part of her.

This part of the mother's grief may be poorly understood by other family members or by nurses or physicians in attendance. It is significant, however, because it may be the part of mother's grief that she is least able to resolve and that is, therefore, most likely to affect her next pregnancy. She may experience a "phantom baby" in her uterus after the death of her newborn or may wake up in the night feeling pregnant (much as an amputee can sometimes "feel" a phantom limb). Certainly the loss of self-esteem and the depression that often accompany the loss of body parts threaten the mother's adjustment and her readiness to attempt pregnancy and childbearing in the future.[11]

Another kind of parental experience that can have important ramifications for the building of a healthy attachment with a new baby is an early history of separation or loss in the family of origin. A parent who as an infant experienced losing a parent or sibling because of death or frequent or lengthy hospitalizations, or circumstances that required frequent and unstable caregiver changes, may experience dramatic shifts in feeling about the baby. Sometimes these shifts appear to have an "anniversary" quality; that is, a parent may suddenly experience a change in feeling at a point that is related in time to his or her own infant experience. A father who was the second child in his family of origin, and whose next-younger sister fell ill and died while he was still young, may find himself being unduly protective — with his own third child. He may seek to slow her motor development (and therefore her imminent growth into a child who will die, as his sister did) and may accuse his wife of purposefully trying to harm their daughter when she allows her to move freely about the house or to play outside. If the second child in the family is a male, the father may find his relationship with this son deteriorating as the third child approaches the age of the father's sister when she died. Under these circumstances, it is likely that the father felt a bit responsible when his sister died, and his own son — acting as a transference object representing himself as a young child — catches some of the blame the father put on himself when he was young.*

Another element brought by some parents to

---

*When a person acts as a transference object, he temporarily represents to another a person from the other's own past about whom he still has repressed, and probably conflicting and ambivalent, feelings.[3]

their childrearing job is a tendency to drape over the baby a mantle he cannot possibly wear. The baby may be seen as the mother's hope for her own reformation from promiscuous sexual behavior or drug abuse that she was unable to change alone. The baby may be viewed as "someone who will finally love me," or as "something that will finally be mine, all mine." He may be used as a means for a young parent to demonstrate maturity or competence to his or her own parents (from whom the mother or the father may have felt hopelessly estranged for some time). A pregnancy may represent a last-ditch effort on the part of either partner in a troubled relationship to hold things together, or it may be used as a means to draw back home an errant lover. The pregnancy may be an unconscious ploy to teach someone a lesson (perhaps the parents of the parent-to-be) or to flaunt independence. In any of these circumstances, it is easy to see that the parents will have a difficult time divorcing their *actual* new baby from the symbolic meanings that have surrounded his conception or his presence in the world. Parents will not actually be building a relationship with *this particular* infant, but principally with the significant (and perhaps imaginary) features of the infant that have the most symbolic power. Problems arise, of course, when the baby is simply unable to fulfill these symbolic functions and parents begin to realize that they have a real live baby on their hands. If a parent wants a baby so that the effects of many years of feeling unloved can be reversed and the baby fails to be cooperative by being consistently and publicly demonstrative, then the parent's outrage will create a considerable over-reaction. If a parent is looking for a friend and discovers that the newborn is really quite clinging and dependent and hardly gossips at all, the parent's disappointment may be striking.

Earlier we discussed the anniversary phenomenon with respect to a history of loss or separation in a parent's family of origin. There are other kinds of parental histories that may have dramatic impact on the quality of the parent-infant relationship. Fraiberg speaks eloquently of these bits from the past: "In every nursery there are ghosts. They are the visitors from the unremembered past of the parents; the uninvited guests at the christening ... even among families where the love bonds are stable and strong, the intruders from the parental past may break through the magic circle in an unguarded moment, and a parent and his child may find themselves re-enacting a moment or a scene from another time with another set of characters."[8]

Such ghosts may affect the overall development of attachment between a parent and child or may be a problem only at certain vulnerable times, with certain developmental areas or with respect to certain kinds of infant behavior. And it may well be that only certain children — the timing of whose entry into the family or whose characteristics mesh most completely with the ghost — will be affected. A mother may suddenly fly into an abusive rage when the large, beautiful eyes of her daughter look for an instant like the "bug-eyes" her father got when he was angry at her and was chasing her with a belt. A father who was the first child in his family of origin and whose normal feelings of jealousy and displacement when a sibling was born made his parents furious, may find himself mysteriously angry about his wife's second pregnancy. He may have a real struggle attaching to the second baby, even after experience in loving and caring for the first, because of the ghosts: he was displaced and no one understood, and now his first child must be protected from the hurt he experienced as a baby. A parent who was enuretic until an advanced age may be inordinately demanding that the baby be toilet trained early, tolerating no mistakes, and may introduce a significant conflict in an otherwise positive relationship. The impact of these "intruders from the past" can rarely be blunted by attacking them head on: by giving more "education" about toilet training, for example, or by informing a parent that her daughter's big brown eyes are really quite lovely. We do not banish ghosts by denying their existence, but by joining parents in an alliance to discover the links between past and present.

Family Circumstances as a Factor in Attachment Breakdown

The third category in our consideration of elements that may affect the development of normal social relations in infancy is that of the *circumstances* surrounding the pregnancy, delivery and early life of an infant. The overwhelming number of circumstantial elements that can impinge on the early social life of a baby makes impossible more than a cursory mention of a few of them. As has been the case in our discussion throughout this section, we will take a holistic approach to understanding both normal and pathological early social relations. No one circumstance, then, shall be seen as causative; rather, circumstances are part of a matrix that also includes strengths and vulnerabilities in the parents and in the baby. Were this not our approach, we would be at a loss to explain why so many families in poverty have such loving attachments among their members, why so many children of abused parents remain unabused or why so many irritable babies are loved anyway.

Certainly a key circumstantial element is the delivery itself. Just as at any other crisis point in life, many things that happen or are said at the time of delivery have lasting impact. To certain especially vulnerable mothers or fathers, the kinds of messages attending medical and nursing staff give — about the vitality or appearance or intelligence or capabilities of the baby, about the capabilities or "parenting sense" or competence of the parents — may powerfully affect the attitudes parents develop about themselves and their baby. Hospital practices and staff attitudes that seem to clearly award "ownership" of the baby to his parents may dramatically improve the chances of the occasional highly vulnerable parents who may otherwise have had a harder time with attachment.[12, 13, 17]

The type of delivery may be significant as a variable in those cases in which the family's vulnerability means they need every possible break. A mother who doubts her worth and her ability as a baby-maker, a childbearer and a mother may be especially devastated by an emergency cesarean section. Having gone to childbirth preparation classes and armed herself with every possible tool to prevent "failure" in this singularly important job of childbearing, she is "cheated" out of proving herself worthy as a mother. This mother's first contacts after the surgical recovery period may be tainted with her sadness and her inward-turned anger, and she may be less interested in or responsive to her newborn. If the unfortunate happens, if the baby responds to mother's mood by fussing and failing to mold comfortably, a cycle may begin that the mother will be hard pressed to reverse alone.

The support systems surrounding new parents may also be a critical variable, having major impact on how well the new family binds together. The support system needed is one that protects mother and baby from intrusion, affords them many early hours together, and minimizes concern about the well-being of the other children or the household. The support that many families receive today is often unreliable and contingent. (Friends may say "Call me if you need anything," but fail to follow through with help.)

The important thing to consider when assessing the potential impact of any circumstance on the ability or opportunity for parents and their baby to attach to one another is not whether a certain circumstance exists, but how that circumstance meshes with other family strengths and vulnerabilities. This is, of course, also true when assessing apparently "high-risk" characteristics of parents or babies. It is the interplay of the elements that is prognostically most significant.

Researchers have referred to the specific interplay between parental and infant behaviors or characteristics as "mutual adaptation,"[19] or mother-infant "fit."[11, 28] They have noted that even relatively minor characteristics of parent or infant can dramatically affect a relationship if those characteristics directly exacerbate a "fit" problem. The etiology of an early feeding disturbance, for example, is fairly clear in a home in which a fidgety mother who dislikes sitting still during feedings and who detests getting baby food on herself insists on feeding her highly distractable but cuddly infant in a baby seat instead of in her arms. Neither partner's characteristics are abnormal, and neither would be readily identified as "high risk." But the baby is failing to gain weight and is beginning to ruminate as he watches his mother get up and down from her chair and as his 2-year-old sibling races about the room in play. The problem is in the failure to achieve an adaptation at feeding time that meets the baby's needs for closeness and protection from excessive stimulation and the mother's need for freedom of movement and personal hygiene. Only careful observation of this dyad, probably in the home, would reveal the nature of a potentially serious problem, since the family is quite normal in most easily visible respects.

Manifestations of Attachment Breakdown

For the past 40 years our understanding of the social development of young children has increased immensely. However, there are still answers that elude us: What is the exact nature of the connection between early social experience and emotional and developmental pathology? When we feel close to an answer to this question, we are forced to confront another one: If there really are causal links, then why do so many children survive so well whose early social experience appears so destructive? And if there are connections, how stable are the effects of early experience over time? How much can we say about the later emotional health of a baby in trouble? None of these monumental questions can be answered clearly, and that is simultaneously most frustrating, most exhilarating and most humbling. The fact that our questions outstrip our capacity to answer may, at least, keep us undogmatic and empirical, and force us to stay close to the source: listening and watching babies and their families do their work together.

In this chapter we cannot discuss all the categories of infant behavior that appear to be most directly affected by early social experience. Those pathologies that have been repeatedly observed in babies who have negative early experiences in common with each other are mentioned.

Prugh has examined the symptomatic reactions of infants and toddlers to stress (psychological and interpersonal) and offered five categories of affected infant behavior:[20]

1. *Disturbances related to bodily functions,* such as eating (as in food refusal, rumination, pica, vomiting, and failure to thrive); sleeping; bowel and bladder control; speech; patterns of motoric activity: rhythmic patterns (such as rocking, head rolling and head banging); various habit patterns (such as thumb sucking, nose picking, and masturbation); and sensory disturbances.
2. *Disturbances related to cognitive functions,* including learning failure of various types, distortions of perception and disorders in thinking.
3. *Disturbances in social behavior,* as in over-aggressive patterns, negativistic or oppositional behavior; disturbed sexual behavior; isolated or withdrawn behavior; and overly dependent or overly independent behavior.
4. *Disturbances in emotional behavior,* as in chronic anxiety, marked fears, acute panic states, depression, and feelings of inadequacy.
5. *Disturbances in integrative behavior,* as in repeated tantrums, impulsive behavior, or disorganized behavior.

While this fairly comprehensive overview could be written in 1963 with confidence in the notion that babies are fully human creatures who respond quickly and observably to stress, the first observational data only 25 years earlier came to us in raw form, without a theoretical base for understanding. Freud and Burlingham[9] could hardly have imagined that they were doing a deprivational study when they reported observing in their wartime nurseries in London breakdowns in habit training (especially toilet training), development of nervous tics, refusals to eat or be comforted and monotonous repetitions of words used to identify the mother among the infants and young children. Only later, when dramatic improvement was observed in these same children after substitute mothers were provided for them, did it become known that these family-reared infants had been reacting powerfully to the loss of their mothers and the social relationships that had been central to their lives. During the same period in another country, Spitz[23] observed infant responses to a breakdown in early social relations when the babies' unwed mothers left them (after providing maternal care for about six months) in the hands of constantly changing shifts of personnel at an institution. Spitz labeled the observed syndrome "anaclitic depression" and reported symptoms including weight loss, insomnia, susceptibility to colds, decline in developmental quotient, apprehensiveness, weepiness, lack of initiative contact, withdrawal, developmental retardation, slowed movements, stupor, refusal to eat, screaming at forced contact with people, averting of the face upon approach, and a "physiognomic expression . . . which would in an adult be described as depression."[24]

For several years after the war, research focused on "maternal deprivation" that at the time referred principally to actual physical loss of or separation from the primary caregiver. We are now fully aware, of course, that infants can be seriously "deprived" (of the kind of social relationships they seem to require for optimal development) even when the mother and father are present. The elements of breakdown in attachment have been described earlier in this chapter. Such breakdowns have been examined for a number of years by Selma Fraiberg and the staff at the Child Development Project, University of Michigan Medical Center. She uses the term "diseases of nonattachment"[7] to describe basic character problems that are rooted in social relationship deficiencies of the ego developmental period (from birth to 18 months). As older children or adults, people with such "diseases of the ego" are characterized by an "incapacity of the person to form human bonds . . . . The life histories of people with such a disease reveal no single significant human relationship . . . . There is no pain in loss . . . . There is no joy, no grief, no guilt, and no remorse. In the absence of human ties, a conscience cannot be formed; even the qualities of self-observation and self-criticism fail to develop."[7] Fraiberg further reports that the age at which a person suffers deprivation of human ties "is closely correlated to certain effects in later personality and the capacity to sustain human ties . . . . The period of greatest vulnerability with respect to later development is in the period under two years of life. When, for any reason, a child has spent the whole or a large part of his infancy in an environment that could not provide him with human partners or the conditions for sustained human attachments, the later development of the child demonstrates measurable effects."[7] These effects are principally in the areas of disorders of impulse control (particularly with respect to aggression), impairment of intellectual function (with irreversible effects in conceptual thinking), and impairment in the capacity to attach intimately to anyone (except to fulfill an immediate need).[7]

Robson identifies "maternal response failure"[21] as a contributing factor in idiopathic failure to thrive, anaclitic depression and infantile autism. He also described "object-hungry infants"[22] who, because of a disturbance in early attachment, "exhibit neither fear of strangers nor separation reactions, and smile indiscriminately . . . . As children or adolescents they often present the exploitative (need-fulfilling) and impoverished interpersonal relations of the psychopath."[21]

ASSESSING PROBLEMS IN PARENT-INFANT ATTACHMENT

Assessment of attachment requires careful examination of the elements (specific vulnerabilities in the baby, the parents, the circumstances) that may contribute to an experience of early social deprivation for an infant. At the very least, families are ambivalent about inviting professionals inside to hear a clear and concise account about "how it is going with the baby." Particularly at a time when they feel on the firing line, catching the blame for the rebelliousness of adolescents and the brattiness of 4-year-olds from every article they read and every expert they hear, most parents are a bit reticent. They have no reason to believe that they will be treated with respect or even that their pleas will be heard. So parents do not come to us and, since everyone knows babies cannot talk, the family in trouble is ominously silent.

Or is it?

Perhaps there is another side to parental ambivalence; a side that knows something is not right about life with this baby, a side that wants very much what is best for the baby, a side that once had a fleeting awareness of the basically unconscious material that is making itself so painfully felt in daily caregiving.

Perhaps this side makes itself heard in a language system that is different from — but just as powerful as — the system of speech upon which we usually rely so heavily for our diagnostic work. At one level, then, a mother may declare to the nurse at the well-baby clinic that all is well with baby, that her only real problem is money. If the nurse *wants to avoid hearing the full message from this mother,* she may joke about how no one seems to have enough money these days, or she may even make a routine referral for financial assistance. If the nurse is prepared and willing to care for the whole family, however, she will look beyond the mother's words and notice a somewhat more subtle communication: as the mother mentioned her money problem, she moved her infant son from a position on her lap where he was facing her and resting against her chest, to a position in which he was facing away and sitting on her knees. The position change was accomplished so deftly that only an unusually observant person would ever notice. If the clinic nurse *did* notice, however, she might put away her jokes and her referral form and ask about the money problem. Mother may then pretend it is unimportant, and wave her hand as if to dismiss the subject, but not before she makes reference to "that creep, Leon," who turns out to be the baby's father *and* his namesake, who denied paternity and left the mother a few days

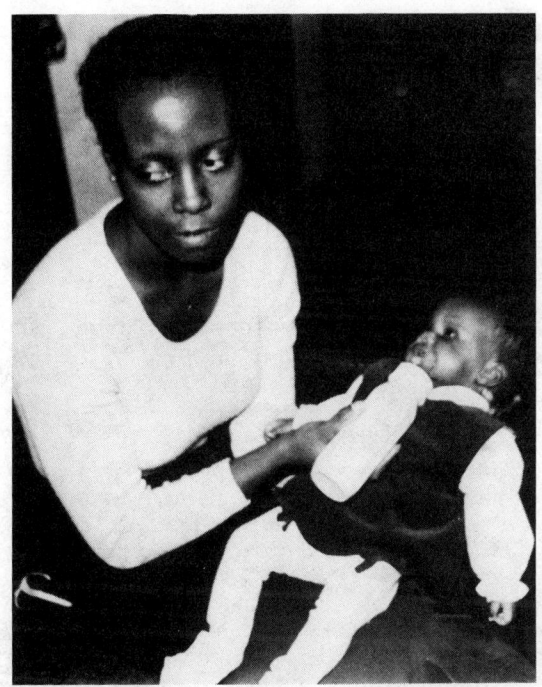

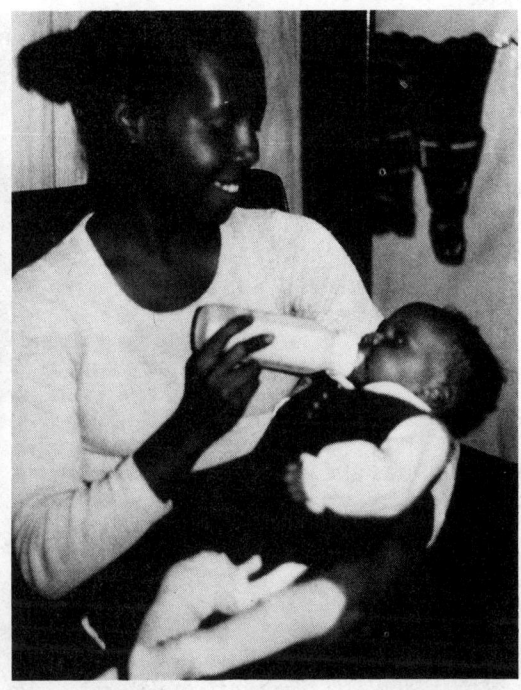

Subtle messages convey the conflict (left) or health (right) of parent-infant interaction (posed photos.)

before the baby was born. The nurse also notes that the placid infant begins to squirm and whimper in his newly uncomfortable position on mother's lap. Is he participating in this subtle "second-level" of communication, which so clearly underscores the problems in this family? He certainly is, since as an alive and responsive part of a *reciprocal* relationship with his mother, he *reacts* when stress enters the picture. As the baby fusses, the mother starts to avert her gaze from the baby *and* from the nurse, and the family situation is clear. All is *not* well with the baby, and the problem may be rooted in the rage and grief the mother may be feeling about being abandoned in her time of great need. She named the baby after Leon anyway — perhaps in hope of enticing him back, perhaps in hope of giving herself a substitute — but the baby cannot give her what her boyfriend did. Sometimes when she thinks about the baby's father she becomes very angry at the baby. So far, she has protected the baby from herself by simply leaving for a few hours to "cool off" (and, being without a support system, she leaves her child alone). The *language of parent-infant interaction* alerted us to the message that neither baby nor mother could speak about in words. The family in trouble was not silent, after all!

The nurse's diagnosis requires the use of systematic instruments to assess risk and the taking of a social history as a means to assess family problems. To understand the "second level" communication system referred to as the language of parent-infant interaction, one must be aware that the covert nature of this communication system is there for a specific psychological purpose. If a parent or baby were *able* to speak clearly and cogently about their attachment struggles, they would probably do so. They are hamstrung, however, by any of a number of factors: baby's inability to speak with words, parents' fears of displaying their parenting failures to professionals they suspect are too critical of them, the unavailability of basically unconscious material to parents who may be deeply troubled but who are not aware of (or have an abiding interest in protecting themselves from an awareness of) the roots of the matter. The message is given in code, then, and parents may not even be consciously aware of their own communication.

While the nurse must listen to the communication carefully, she must also listen covertly. If she responds to the mother's movement of her baby to the end of her lap while talking about money by immediately informing her about the existence and meaning of her behavior, then she has violated the nature of this privileged subtle communication. She has dragged too

A GUIDE FOR ASSESSMENT OF PARENT-CHILD INTERACTIONS

Touch and Movement Interaction

What sort of synchrony is there in posture and postural adjustments? Are postural adjustments (scooting baby closer, moving an arm to make him more comfortable) in response to infant cues, or are they chaotic, too late, too abrupt? Does the parent's posture give the baby access to the parent's "inner circle" or does it serve the function of keeping the baby physically isolated? Does the baby seem to "fit" during holding? Does he do any postural stiffening or back-arching?

How often do baby and parent touch each other? Does the baby seek physical proximity?* Does he cling? How does he seem to be using touch and proximity?

What is the quality of touching? Are the parent's hands open or closed? Does the parent use only fingertips, or the whole hand? What parts of the baby's body are touched most often? When does the parent touch? What is the parent saying to the nurse when touching? Is there ventral-ventral contact? How satisfying does touch seem to be to each partner? Is this a cuddly or more isolated baby? Does the parent seem "tuned in" to baby's wish for physical contact? Is there intrusiveness in the parent's demand for contact? With a newborn, does the parent have a tendency to move to an *en face* position with the baby.

Visual Interaction

Is there mutuality to the gaze patterns between parent and baby? That is, do they respond to each other's looks? Do they look at *each other*, or is the looking usually one-way? Is the parent visually aware of the baby's whereabouts and safety even while the parent is doing other things?

---
*Interpretations about this behavioral area will vary as a function of baby's age and developmental level. For example, infant seeking of physical proximity means something different at 7 months than it does at 24 months.

Does either partner ever avert his or her gaze? If so, what does the aversion seem to be in response to, and what does parent say about it?

Does looking sometimes elicit a smile from either partner?

Does the baby visually check* for parent? Has he learned to rely on looking as a means for maintaining contact with parent, even when they are out of proximity?

Vocal Interaction

How much does the baby cry? What is the persistence, pitch, intensity and duration of crying? How does crying behavior change when the parent approaches or intervenes or both?

Does baby "coo" and babble to parent while maintaining eye contact?

After the baby has acquired language: what sorts of adult-sounding phrases are repeated? What is the nature of the baby's talking to dolls or playmates or both? (Does he threaten them, provide comfort to them, repeat parental gestures that have originally been made to himself?) Can the baby state his needs clearly (as if a timely and helpful response is expected from the parent)?

What sorts of references does the parent make to past events or to other persons in conversion with the baby? ("You look just like your Aunt Margaret when you do that!" "You're not going to grow up spoiled like my brother Ralph did!")

What sort of threats or (even joking) allusions does the parent make with respect to hurting, selling or giving away the baby?

What sort of comments does the parent make about the baby's behavior (admiring, critical, supportive, blaming)?

Does the baby seem to be blamed for family problems for which he is not responsible? Is intentionality ascribed to baby's behavior inappropriately? ("You know I hate for you to do that! You do it just to upset me!")

---

quickly to the surface a communication that was offered in code because mother could offer it in no other way at the moment. By the time parents are able to decode their own subtle messages and present them in clear words, the conflict is probably very close to resolution. In the beginning, the nurse must tread lightly and respectfully.

The principal elements of the language of parent-infant interaction are in the areas of touching and movement, looking and speech.[27] The nurse might consider the questions listed in the box as she watches parent and baby interact.

Parents' teasing of and games with the baby appear to constitute a special kind of interactional sequence therefore and, should be a part of the nurse's assessment. These games offer a stylized way to express affection and tenderness (with repeated versions of "I'm going to get you," for example, a game that often ends, to the delight of both partners, with the child being vigorously chased, caught, picked up, cuddled and kissed). Games with the baby offer other psychological opportunities to families, however, and may offer diagnostic information to an observer. They may offer a "safe" opportunity for parents (and even baby, at a later age) to bring up worrisome topics, to express anger, to "play act" safely a hidden feeling. Fraiberg comments about the meaningful but safe nature of such games: "If we grant ambivalence to all parents . . . we might also expect that the invented games of our parents would reflect these conflicts, rendered 'harmless' in play."[6] She goes on to alert us to the diagnostic significance of baby games, which "regulate, through ritual and through the conventional disguises of play, the discharge of forbidden impulses."[6] A father, disappointed over the developmental slowness of his year-old son, may give him a "pretend" spanking during play, while adding "You know, we spank little boys around here who are too lazy to walk!" A mother may "throw away" her 5-month-old in the safety of the swinging-through-the-air ritual. A 30-month-old may even have the opportunity to "shoot" his father during play. In none of these three examples does the game behavior constitute the whole of the story. The child does not really want his father dead, least of all by his own hand. The mother does not really want to throw her baby completely away. But the games they have created offer each of them a useful opportunity to express a side of their ambivalence that usually is tucked away. Impulses are discharged in a manner that prevents them from being taken too seriously by the game partner, and the impulses are regulated by the game boundaries.

From an assessment viewpoint, the nurse is not just interested in a mother's "throwing away" behavior. Chances are excellent that many parents have this impulse, and this mother's unconscious is merely doing her the favor of offering a regulated means of discharge. The nurse should also be interested in the manner in which the impulses are held in check during play, the points at which the hostility expressed in tickling or shooting is prevented from turning into aggression. This tells her some things about the self-regulating capacities of each family member, as well as about the volume and relative weight of unconscious material that may be struggling to the surface during play.

There are times, of course, when the defenses that normally regulate impulse discharge during play break down. The scene then becomes dangerous, as one observes a parent losing in the battle to gain control. Under the weight of rage or disappointment or despondence, play may suddenly turn into a chance for a parent to act out feelings about his child. The nurse must watch carefully to understand at exactly which point the defense system began to crumble. (What was baby doing at the moment? What was the parent talking about just before the facial expression began to change and the danger signals began to flash about the room?)

Although she must be prepared to do so, the nurse does not want to intervene too soon. Parent and baby have probably been through this before and made it, and it is critical for her to see if, and how, they can pull themselves back together. If they are able to do it without controls being exerted from without, then the nurse, the parent and the baby have all learned some extraordinarily important information. Sometimes, the mere presence of an observer serves to mirror to the parent the crossing of the boundary into aggression, as he angrily jams the spoon too far into baby's mouth in a feeding game, or as she pulls to hard and too long on baby's penis during a diaper-changing game, or as both parents hide too long in the next room from their terrified, screaming infant in a hide-and-seek game. In these — as well as in the safer baby games — the nurse is being invited in to see how the family really works, and the information should not be missed.

Another important part of the assessment work involves careful attention to parent's *stories* about their child, even when they appear irrelevant. (It should be emphasized here that very *little* of what parents say in the presence of someone who is helping them with their baby is irrelevant. Although neither the parents nor the nurse may understand why certain things are said at the moment, they should not be ignored. Parents rarely bother with meaningless chatter; if they seem to be, doing this then the chattering itself may be the message.) The telling of stories about apparently unrelated topics may be a safe means selected (probably unconsciously) to turn the nurse's attention either to or away from

Research Form

AIDS SCALE

THE MASSIE-CAMPBELL SCALE OF MOTHER-INFANT ATTACHMENT INDICATORS DURING STRESS

For Use During the Pediatric Examination and Other Stressful Childcare Situations

Infant's Behavior During Stress Event

	(1)	(2)	(3)	(4)	(5)	X
GAZING	1 Always looks away from mother's face.	2 Rarely searches out mother's face. Fleeting looks at mother's face.	3 Occasionally looks at mother's face.	4 Frequently long & short gazing at mother's face.	5 Rivets gaze on mother's face for long periods.	6 Behavior not observed.
	1	1	1	1	1	1
VOCALIZING	1 Quiet. Never vocalizing.	2 Rarely vocalizing or whimpering.	3 Occasionally vocalizing or mild crying.	4 Frequently vocalizing or intense crying.	5 Uncontrollable, intense crying much of time.	6 Behavior not observed.
	2	2	2	2	2	2
TOUCHING (a)	1 Never touches or reaches toward mother.	2 Rarely touches mother.	3 Occasionally touches mother.	4 Frequently reaches toward & touches mother.	5 When close, always touching mother.	6 Behavior not observed.
	3	3	3	3	3	3
(b)	1 Always pulls away from mother's touch.	2 Frequently pulls away from her touch.	3 Occasionally pulls away from her touch.	4 Rarely pulls away from her touch.	5 Never pulls away from her touch.	6 Behavior not observed.
	4	4	4	4	4	4
HOLDING	1 Violently resists holding; always arches away from mother.	2 Does not relax in mother's arms. Frequently pulls away.	3 Rests in mother's arms and against her shoulder. Occasionally pulls away.	4 Body molds to mother's. Rarely pulls away.	5 Actively turns & arches body toward mother's. Clings strongly. Never pulls away.	6 Behavior not observed.
	5	5	5	5	5	5
AFFECT	1 Always intensely anguished and fearful.	2 Frequently irritable & fearful.	3 Largely unclear, constricted or bland expressions.	4 Frequently content & smiling.	5 Always full smile & content.	6 Behavior not observed.
	6	6	6	6	6	6
PROXIMITY	1 Never follows mother bodily or with eyes; goes to far corner or out of room.	2 Rarely follows mother bodily or with eyes; often at far corner of room from mother.	3 Intermittently follows mother bodily or with eyes.	4 Frequently follows mother bodily or with eyes.	5 Always follows mother bodily or with eyes.	6 Behavior not observed.
	7	7	7	7	7	7

Mother's Response to Infant's Stress

	(1)	(2)	(3)	(4)	(5)	X
GAZING	1 Always looks away from child's face.	2 Rarely looks at child's face. Fleeting looks at child's face.	3 Occasionally looks at child's face.	4 Frequently long & short gazing at child's face.	5 Rivets gaze on child's face for long periods.	6 Behavior not observed.
	1/8	2/8	3/8	4/8	5/8	6/8
VOCALIZING	1 Quiet. Never vocalizing.	2 Rare words, cooing or murmuring.	3 Occasionally vocalizing to child.	4 Frequently speaks, murmurs, coos.	5 Intense vocalizations throughout exam.	6 Behavior not observed.
	1/9	2/9	3/9	4/9	5/9	6/9
TOUCHING (a)	1 Never touches or reaches toward child.	2 Rarely touches child.	3 Occasionally touches child.	4 Frequently reaches toward & touches child.	5 When close, always touching child.	6 Behavior not observed.
	1/10	2/10	3/10	4/10	5/10	6/10
(b)	1 Always pulls away from his touch.	2 Frequently pulls away from his touch.	3 Occasionally pulls away from his touch.	4 Rarely pulls away from his touch.	5 Never pulls away from his touch.	6 Behavior not observed.
	1/11	2/11	3/11	4/11	5/11	6/11
HOLDING	1 Pushes upset child away, or holds away from body.	2 Holds child stiffly & awkwardly. Not relaxed.	3 Supports child relaxedly against her chest or shoulder briefly.	4 Body molds to child & maintains contact until child quiets.	5 Body inclines toward child, followed by prolonged holding with molding.	6 Behavior not observed.
	1/12	2/12	3/12	4/12	5/12	6/12
AFFECT	1 Always intensely anguished & fearful.	2 Frequently irritable & fearful.	3 Largely unclear, constricted or bland expressions.	4 Frequently content & smiling	5 Always full smile & content.	6 Behavior not observed.
	1/13	2/13	3/13	4/13	5/13	6/13
PROXIMITY	1 Leaves examining room.	2 Frequently out of reach of child; or at far corner of room from child.	3 Intermittently standing or seated within arm's reach of child.	4 Frequently holding or touching child.	5 Always holding or touching child.	6 Behavior not observed.
	1/14	2/14	3/14	4/14	5/14	6/14

Growth and development: 1 normal 2 abnormal   Explain: _____
                        1/15   2/15

Social behavior appears: 1 normal 2 abnormal   Describe: _____
                         1/16   2/16

Unusual circumstances today: 1 No 2 Yes   Describe: _____
                             1/17 2/17

Infant Sex: 1 Boy 2 Girl   Birthdate: _____   Infant's Name: _____
            1/18 2/18   month day year

Ethnic Group: 1 Cauc. 2 Black 3 Asian 4 Hispanic 5 Other   Economic   1 $0–10,000 2 $11–20,000 3 $21–30,000 4 $31,000+
              1/25   2/25   3/25   4/25   5/25   Group: 1/26   2/26   3/26   4/26

Observation Date: _____   ID or Chart Number: 33 34 35 36 37 38   Observer: _____
                  month day year
                  27 28 29 30 31 32

Firstborn: 1 No 2 Yes   Mother's Age: 40 41   Marital 1 single 2 married 3 other   Lives: 1 alone 2 with   3 other
           1/39 2/39   Status: 1/42   2/42   3/42   1/43   2/43 partner 3/43

Reproduced with permission from Henry N. Massie, M.D. and B. Kay Campbell, Ph.D., © 1977. Children's Hospital and McAuley Neuropsychiatric Institute of St. Mary's Hospital, San Francisco, CA.

AIDS Scale Instructions

INTRODUCTION

The Attachment Indicators During Stress Scale is to be used with infants from birth to 18 months of age to detect aberrant mother-infant responsiveness in stressful situations. The Scale quantifies the reciprocal process of mother-infant attachment while the infant is under the stress of an ordinary physical examination. The Scale can also be used in other situations which produce tension in mother and baby. When stressed, infants normatively seek out their mothers; mothers normatively seek out their infants when they perceive them to be in danger or suffering. Such interactions fall within the general category of attachment behaviors. The Scale includes six basic attachment modalities: gazing, vocalizing, touching, and holding, affect and proximity. These modalities are subdivided into component behaviors and correspond to mother and infant responses clinically seen in stressful situations which arouse tension and anxiety in mother and/or infant. The responses in each attachment modality are graded from 1 to 5 to indicate the increasing intensity of mother-infant involvement that may occur during a stress episode. Generally, behavior at the low end of the Scale (1) indicates abnormal isolation or avoidance of attachment, and responses at the high end (5) indicate abnormally anxious attachment behavior or clinging. The top half of the single-page Scale quantifies the infant's behavior with its mother, and the bottom half quantifies the mother's behavior with her infant during the stressful situation.

APPLICATIONS

The AIDS Scale is for use during the pediatric examination as well as other situations where a relatively standardized stress occurs for parents and babies. For example, it can be used by mental health or childcare workers to assess mother-infant attachment at the moment of reunion following the stress of a brief separation between mother and child. In whatever setting it is used it may serve some or all of the following functions:

1) To record the clinician's assessment of the adequacy of maternal infant dyadic responsiveness.
2) To document the need for developmental and psychological care to prevent the crystallization of pathological modes of social interaction.
3) To document the efficacy of early intervention efforts by registering improvement in the clinical indicators of attachment when used longitudinally during the first 18 months of life with deviant mother-infant pairs.
4) To teach by heightening the clinician's awareness of parameters of mother-infant interaction central to psychological development.

INSTRUCTIONS FOR ADMINISTRATION AND SCORING

The clinician conducting the examination or an independent observer can administer the AIDS Scale. Generally, the mother should not be alerted to the details of the observation so that she does not modify her usual style; and for the same reason the examiner should not suggest to the mother that she either hold the baby or place the baby on the examining table, but instead leave the decision with the mother.

To use the Scale, observe the interaction between mother and infant WHILE the infant is being physically examined (the *stress episode*) and IMMEDIATELY AFTERWARD (the *reunion and recovery episode*). In many pediatric examinations the final phase is the inspection of the head, eyes, ears, nose and throat. This usually takes about 3 minutes and is often the most difficult for mother and infant. The period immediately following this (about 3 minutes) is the time when mother and infant reunite and tension subsides. Similarly, in non-pediatric settings there is a corresponding rise and fall of tension around a stressful event. Assessment is made by focusing on the period of most heightened stress (the first 3 minutes of the physical examination) and the period of tension decline (the first 3 minutes of the recovery phase). IMMEDIATELY AFTER THE OBSERVATION OF THE RECOVERY EPISODE circle the behavior description that best fits the mother's and infant's response in each attachment modality during both stress and recovery episodes. If a particular attachment modality, such as holding, has not occurred circle "not observed" so that an entry is made in every category.

OPERATIONAL DEFINITIONS

Holding: the mutually reciprocated posturing of the infant and mother while the infant is supported in the arms of the mother.
Gazing: the eye-to-face contact within a dyad and the maintenance of this contact.
Vocalizing: the making of vocal sounds for the benefit of the partner in the mother-infant dyad. The infant's crying is considered a vocal signal of dismay during stress which alerts the mother to its tension.
Touching (a): the making of skin-to-skin contact initiated by either the mother or the infant.
Touching (b): the withdrawal from skin-to-skin contact initiated by either the mother or the infant.
Affect: the facial expressions signaling emotional states. A bland expression is considered typical of the individual under stress and is appropriate.
Proximity: the state of being near, close to, or beside another. In the context of the AIDS Scale it refers to the infant maintaining either physical or visual contact with the mother, and to the mother maintaining physical contact or being immediately accessible to her infant.
Rarely: the behavior occurs once in a while, or seldom; it doesn't happen often during the observation period.
Occasionally: the behavior occurs from time to time, now and then during the observation period.
Frequently: the behavior happens often but not all the time during the observation period.

INTERPRETATION OF SCORING

Normal behaviors will usually rate at 3 and 4. When an infant or a mother rates at 1 or 2 it suggests that the infant or mother may be either avoiding contact or not responding to the other's display of tension or attempts at attachment. When there are scores of 5 it should raise concern that there is an over-anxious intense attachment or an unusually strong reaction to stress. Further, in dyads where one member rates at 1 or 2 and the other at 5, there is a dissynchrony of interaction which may also have pathological significance. To derive a single or "correct" score is *not* the proper use of the Scale. The most productive way to interpret the ratings is to use the attachment indicators as a guide to the adequacy of interaction in a given mother-infant pair. Studies indicate that deviant attachment is associated with subsequent psychomotor developmental delays, pathological intrapsychic management of tension and aggression, and the inability to postpone gratification—all with their attendant behavioral disturbances. When behaviors of 1, 2, or 5 occur in 2 successive episodes, there should be a diagnostic workup, for, once established, unhealthy patterns of mother-infant interaction show little change without therapeutic intervention. The exception occurs with some very young or premature infants who show a normal dampened responsiveness. They may rate 2 for gazing, vocalizing, touching (a), and proximity in the first weeks of life. Mother-infant affect at 5 at any age is not necessarily clinging but is aberrant.

VARIABLES

Relatively standardized stress situations may be affected by several variables. An infant's ability to tolerate tension or respond to comforting may be affected, for example, by concurrent illness or hunger. Likewise, a mother's capacities may be affected by concurrent disturbances in her life. History taking should elicit this; and the AIDS Scale can then assist in assessing the capacity of the mother and infant to compensate for additional stress, or their liability for decompensation and the traumatic behaviors that follow. Additionally, a disturbing examining situation or other unusual circumstances can intensify the stress of customary events. If there are unusual occurrences when the rating takes place explain briefly in the space provided at the bottom of the Scale.
Fathers accompany infants less frequently than mothers, but the AIDS Scale can be appropriately used to assess father-infant interaction. When infants are older than 18 months their behaviors have become so increasingly complex that the AIDS Scale is less useful.

certain topics, to explain something discussed earlier, to introduce a new concern or to enlist the nurse's aid in rapping on the door or more deeply buried material. A parent may, for example, tell a long and detailed story about a neighbor child who is retarded "because his mother never fed him anything regular, and ignored him most of the time." On the surface, it might appear to the nurse that the parent is trying to change the subject or to avoid talking about himself by talking about a neighbor. In fact, parents may be choosing the only safe way available to speak about a powerful worry or a problem in the family: an overpowering fear that their own baby is developmentally delayed or sick, a wish to go back to work, a barely repressed impulse to put baby away in a room (like the neighbor who "ignores" her child).

By nature, such stories may be remarkably devoid of appropriately matched affect. After all, if the parent were able to come face-to-face with the problem being hinted at in the story and to allow feelings about the problem to surface, then probably the story mechanism would not be needed.

The taking of a careful social history is also of great significance in the assessment process. At the least, the history should include the following (not necessarily collected in this order):

1. Parents' descriptions of their families of origins;
2. Parents' histories of pregnancy and parenting;
3. Parents' descriptions of their first feelings upon discovering they were pregnant with the present infant;
4. Parents' descriptions of the course of the pregnancy, including family changes, health changes, job changes, marital changes;
5. Parents' descriptions of their wishes for this baby during the pregnancy, including preferred sex, appearance, physical attributes, character traits, infant personality, what baby would do for the family;
6. Parents' descriptions of the labor and delivery, including length and difficulty of labor and delivery, preparation for labor and delivery, disappointments, wish fulfillments, feelings upon first seeing the baby, early postpartum experience with the baby, first responses of staff and friends to the baby;
7. Parents' descriptions of life at home, including what homecoming was like for the mother (responses of the older children to her); what sort of support the parents had; how the baby has changed family life (sleeping, sex play and lovemaking, family rituals); how caregiving responsibilities are handled;
8. The baby's growth and development history, what others say to parents about how their baby is doing;
9. The baby's nutritional history and current state (how is the baby fed, by whom, when, occurrence of recent dramatic slowing of weight gain, etc.);
10. Parents' descriptions about what the baby is like: temperament, cuddliness, attractiveness, soothability, intelligence, independence/dependence, how he behaves under stress or in public or when tired;
11. Parents' descriptions about the situation that brought them to the interviewer;
12. Parents' descriptions of their belief systems about dependence or independence, "spoiling," caregiving, discipline.

In addition to this core history, a careful assessment will use objective instruments to look at parental and infant behavior and infant development. The AIDS (Attachment Indicators During Stress) Scale (Fig. 22–1) is useful in coherently examining parent and baby behavior with each other during high-stress events (a medical examination of the baby, for example). A number of scales offer helpful information about the temperament, capabilities and characteristics of the child, including Brazleton's Neonatal Behavioral Assessment Scale (NBAS)[5] (useful principally in the first two to four days of life), Murphy's Vulnerability Inventory,[16] and the Hampstead Baby Profile.[10] To gain an overall view of the developmental level of the baby, a useful instrument is the Bayley Scales of Infant Development,[1] which offers information about how the infant's mental development, psychomotor development and behavior compare with those of other infants his age. Developmental information about highly specific areas (object permanence, for example, which might be of interest when parents whose baby has been in a series of unstable care settings complain that he seems too clinging) may be obtained by borrowing items for standardized profiles. A highly trained diagnostician may also use a play session with baby and parents to gain information about the baby's developmental level and personality. Provence suggests a format that looks at activity-inactivity, perception, cognitive development, affective behavior and development, interaction with toys, interaction with people, language, coping behavior and reactions to stress, aggressive behavior, capacity to delay and self-stimulating behavior.[19]

Regardless of the setting in which the family assessment is accomplished, the purpose for which the information is being collected or the instruments used, great care and unusual skill are required when one approaches a family troubled about their baby. As nurses — or teams of nurses, psychologists and physicians — begin to use the principles of observation and assessment described in this chapter, it is crucial that support systems for the staff be established. The kind of diagnostic and intervention work described here is often upsetting, even to an experienced specialist in infant mental health. Staff need an opportunity to check out their observations with each other, to establish plans for the assessment and intervention work with each family (so that each family is not being torn by the eager overtures of several staff persons), to turn to each other with questions, to comfort each other when the repetition of similarly dismal stories from different families becomes too much to bear.

Unquestionably, excellence in practice, backed by sound training and staff support, must be the watchword as nurses begin to expand their roles to become observers and helpers of families in trouble with their babies. Nurses are more often where babies are than those in most professions, and when a family is ready to let someone in on the problem, the nurse selected by the family should be ready. "If there were not a part of a caregiver that wanted to protect the baby, the unconscious motivation to speak about what is wrong would go away. We are clearly being invited to hear. If we do not hear the first time, the parent and baby are likely to show us again. If we do not hear at all, however, we must be aware that we have made a *choice* to be deaf. The side of parental ambivalence that is frightened of the ghosts and wants to hide them away will applaud our deafness. The side of parental ambivalence that wants to tear at the walls that are preventing attachment with baby, the side that wants to stop generational cycles of shallowness or abuse, the side that longs to love the baby and be loved back — that side will resent our choice."[28]

References

1. N. Bayley. Bayley Scales of Infant Development. The Psychological Corporation, 1969
2. S. M. Bell and M. Ainsworth. Infant crying and maternal responsiveness. Child Development, 1972, p. 1171
3. G. Blanck and R. Blanck. Ego Psychology: Theory and Practice. Columbia University Press, 1974
4. T. B. Brazleton. Early parent-infant reciprocity. In The Family: Can It Be Saved? Yearbook Medical Publishers, Inc., 1975
5. T. B. Brazleton. Neonatal behavioral assessment scale. In Clinics in Developmental Medicine. J. B. Lippincott Company, 1973
6. S. Fraiberg. The clinical dimension of baby games. Journal of the American Academy of Child Psychiatry, 1974, p. 202
7. S. Fraiberg. The origins of human bonds, A Commentary Report, 1967. (Available as a monograph from The American Jewish Committee, 165 East 56th Street, New York)
8. S. Fraiberg, E. Adelson and V. Shapiro. Ghosts in the nursery. Journal of the American Academy of Child Psychiatry, Summer 1975, p. 387
9. A. Freud and D. Burlingham. War and Children. Medical War Books, 1943
10. W. Freud. Assessment of early infancy: problems and considerations. Psychoanalytic Study of the Child, Vol. 22, 1967, p. 216
11. E. Furman. The Death of a Newborn: Care of the Parents. Unpublished manuscript presented at the International Conference on Parent-to-Infant Attachment, Cleveland, November 1977
12. M. Klaus et al. Maternal attachment: importance of the first post-partum days. New England Journal of Medicine, March 1972, p. 460
13. M. Klaus et al. Human maternal behavior at the first contact with her young. Pediatrics, August 1970, p. 2
14. B. Lozoff et al. The mother-newborn relationship: limits of adaptability. The Journal of Pediatrics, July 1977, p. 1
15. S. Mouchka. The Deaf-Blind Infant in the Family: Early Crisis Intervention. Unpubished article
16. L. Murphy. Assessment of infants and young children. In Early Child-Care: The New Perspectives. L. Dittman, ed. Atherton Press, 1968
17. N. Newton and M. Newton. Mother's reactions to their newborn babies. Journal of the American Medical Association, 21 July 1962 p. 206
18. Personal communication with the staff of the Neonatal Intensive Care Unit, Butterworth Hospital, Grand Rapids, Michigan, 1978–1979
19. S. Provence. Psychoanalysis and the treatment of psychological disorders of infancy. In Handbook of Child Psychoanalysis: Research, Theory and Practice. B. Wolman, ed. Van Nostrand Reinhold Co., 1972
20. D. Prugh. Toward an understanding of psychosomatic concepts in relation to illness in children. In Modern Perspectives in Child Development. A. J. Solnit and S. Provence, eds. International Universities Press, 1963
21. K. S. Robson. Development of object relations during the first year of life. Seminars in Psychiatry, April 1972, p. 301
22. K. S. Robson. The Role of Eye-to-Eye Contact in the Development of Early Object Relations. Unpublished manuscript. The majority of the author's points are also presented in K. S. Robson: The role of eye-to-eye contact in maternal-infant attachment, Journal of Child Psychology and Psychiatry, August 1967, p. 13

23. R. Spitz. Hospitalism: An inquiry into the genesis of psychiatric conditions in early childhood. Psychoanalytic Study of the Child, January 1945
24. R. Spitz with K. M. Wolf. Anaclitic depression: an inquiry into the genesis of psychiatric conditions in early childhood. Psychoanalytic Study of the Child, February 1946, p. 313
25. M. D. Trout. Maternal Separation in Infancy: An Examination of Temporary Object Loss in Children 0–30 Months of Age and a Case study of Differentially Separated Infant Twins. Master's thesis, Central Michigan University, 1978
26. M. D. Trout. Implications for Parent-Infant Attachment of the Birth of a Sick or Malformed Baby. Presented at the Annual Conference of the Illinois Teachers of the Hearing Impaired, Peoria, Illinois 1977
27. M. D. Trout. The language of parent-infant interaction: a tool in the assessment of jeopardized attachment in infancy. In The Special Infant. J. Stack, ed. Human Sciences Press, 1981
28. L. J. Yarrow and F. A. Pedersen. Attachment: its origins and course. Young Children, June 1972, p. 302

Additional Recommended Reading

J. Bowlby. Attachment and Loss. Basic Books, 1973

J. Bowlby. Maternal Care and Mental Health. Schocken Books, Inc., 1966. The original manuscript was published as a World Health Organization paper in 1951

R. R. Homan and S. Kanwar. Early life of the battered child. Archives of Disease in Childhood, January 1975, p. 78

M. Klein and L. Stern. Low birth weight and the battered child syndrome. American Journal of Diseases of Children, July 1971, p. 15

M. Lynch. Risk factors in the child: a study of abused children and their siblings. In The Abused Child. H. D. Martin ed. Ballinger Publishing Co., 1976

H. P. Martin and P. Beezley. Prevention and the consequences of child abuse. Journal of Operational Psychiatry, January 1974, p. 68

23 POTENTIAL STRESSES DURING INFANCY: TEMPORARY ALTERATIONS IN HEALTH STATUS

by Jo Joyce Tackett, BSN, MPHN

The infant is susceptible to several ailments of a temporary nature primarily due to his immature physiologic development. While most of these conditions do not have serious consequences, they can be worrisome and frustrating to parents who have primary responsibility for trying to resolve such ailments.

Some of these ailments, such as the skin disorders, may also create embarrassment for the parents and school-age or older siblings because of their unsightliness. The infant does not perceive these unsightly features as a part of himself and responds only to the discomforts those manifestations pose. He will, however, react to any rejection or repulsion he senses in his caretakers that result from his physical appearance or his behavioral responses to the discomfort.

The nurse who is conscious of these potential reactions by family members can appreciate the importance of encouraging parents and older siblings to express their feelings regarding their infant's illness, even though it is only temporary. Continued positive contact with their ill infant is important for perpetuation of the attachment process and to maintain the infant's developing sense of security. The infant's caretakers need to feel comfortable with the infant during his altered health status. This is facilitated by the continued contact required to carry out the prescribed treatment at home. The nurse's role, therefore, becomes one of conveying her confidence in the parents' abilities to perform the necessary management regimen and teaching them the skills and facts they need to employ treatments safely and comfortably.

Three facets of care must be communicated to the infant's caretakers. First, the treatment regimen must be explained and, as indicated, demonstrated and practiced by the caretakers until they master the tasks. Strict adherence to the treatment orders should be stressed; however, compliance with the plan will occur only if the child's routines and the family's life style are considered. Teaching should include management of symptoms at home and clear guidelines as to when symptoms should be reported because medical intervention or hospitalization is desirable. Parents should be provided with a resource person with whom they may confer if they forget anything they have been taught, if questions arise, or if changes in symptoms occur. (Written instructions should always accompany verbal teaching.) Typical resources are the doctor's office nurse, the pediatric nurse practitioner or the community health nurse.

Second, the parents need to be urged to watch closely for any changes in their infant's condition and to be assured that they need not hesitate to contact their resource person if any changes are noted.

Third, parents need reassurance that their infant's ailment is temporary, and that they should attempt to deal with it patiently and cheerfully so that he continues to feel secure despite his discomfort and to feel accepted and loved despite his unsightly symptoms.

In conditions with a hereditary predisposition, preventive measures should be incorporated in the nurse's anticipatory guidance teaching. Changes in the home environment are often a significant aspect of preventive action. Home visits by the nurse may be needed to assist the family in identifying necessary changes and defining how they can be made with minimal disruption to family living.

ALLERGIES IN INFANCY

Allergy can be described as a hypersensitivity of certain body tissues or organs to some ordinary substance or environmental condition (antigen) that causes no response in most persons. The antigen may be inhaled, ingested, injected or contracted from direct contact with the foreign substance and can involve any part of the body, although the respiratory tract and skin are most frequently reactive. Table 23–1 contains a listing of common antigens. The degree of body tissue response to an antigen (a substance to which it has been sensitized) depends on the frequency and duration of exposure to the antigen, the amount of other stress being experienced at the time of exposure, the body's state of health at exposure, age and existence of a genetic predisposition for allergic reactivity to the antigen.[6]

One in five children under age 15 will suffer from an allergy. Although allergy can develop at any age, for some unknown reason infants and children at age 5, 10, or 15 are most susceptible to allergic reactions.[6] If intervention is initiated, 80 per cent of these children gain relief from allergic symptoms.[20] Untreated, the allergy can worsen or become chronic, causing immeasurable physical, emotional and social distress as the child grows and develops.

TABLE 23–1 COMMON ALLERGY-PRODUCING SUBSTANCES

Inhalants
Pollen
Mold
House dust
Animal dander
Fabric fiber
Feathers
Dyes
Chemicals

Injectants
Vaccines
Injected drugs
Animal serum
Animal saliva
Animal venom
Insect stings

Bacterial Infectants

Ingestants
Food
  Cow's milk
  Eggs
  Wheat
  Chocolate
  Cola products
  Fish, pork, chicken, legumes
  Corn
  Citrus fruits, strawberries
Drugs
  Aspirin
  Antibiotics
  Barbiturates
Food additives

Contactants
Plants
Topical drugs
Resins
Metals
Cosmetics
Dyes
Chemicals

Other Environmental Factors
Sunshine
Temperature changes
Air pollution

Pathophysiology of Allergy

Allergy develops because the body's immune system overreacts to foreign substances. Normally when a foreign organism (usually protein; antigen) invades, the body mobilizes antibodies to disarm and paralyze them. In the allergy victim, a first-time invasion of the antigen stimulates the production of a special antibody (im-

TABLE 23-2 DIAGNOSTIC LABORATORY TESTS INDICATED IN SUSPECTED ALLERGIC DISEASE

Test	Significant Results	Obtaining Specimen
CBC	7–25% eosinophils	Peripheral blood smear from finger, heel or ear lobe prick.
Mucus cytology	10% + eosinophils	Infant–aspirate nasal secretions in bulb syringe. Older child–blow nose into wax paper
Conjunctival cytology	10% + eosinophils	Swab (sterile) inner canthus of conjunctiva
Bronchial secretion cytology	10% + eosinophils	Infant–aspirate bronchial secretions by suctioning; seldom done. Older child–rinse mouth several times with mouthwash, then cough sputum into sterile container

mune globulin E, or IgE.). A small number of these IgE antibodies adhere to mast cells somewhere in the body (lung, nose, gastrointestinal tract, skin) and "sensitize" them. The next time a large enough dose of the same antigen enters the body, these sensitized cells release a group of chemicals (mediators, of which histamine is only one) that are the real villains in allergy. These chemicals cause muscle contraction and dilate blood vessels, resulting in tissue swelling. They also stimulate production of mucus by the mucous membranes. Nerve endings are irritated by these chemicals, and sometimes shock occurs because the heart's pumping efficiency is disturbed by this nervous irritation. The allergic reaction may be immediate (as it most commonly is in infants) and related to circulating antibodies, or it may be delayed and related to cellular antibodies. Allergic responses are also either atopic (ectopic), meaning there is a hereditary predisposition, or nonatopic, in which case there is no known hereditary factor.[6]

Clinical manifestations of allergies vary depending upon whether the reaction is local or systemic and which specific body tissues are affected.

Diagnosing Allergies

Establishing that an allergic disorder exists and specifically identifying antigens requires patience, time and skill, particularly in history taking. The history, laboratory test findings and physical examination findings are adequate to determine some antigens. However, in some circumstances, skin testing (rarely done in infancy and never before 6 months of age) or elimination procedures* are also needed for a definitive diagnosis. A thorough history is the first and most significant aspect in diagnosing an allergy. It should include a description of the signs and symptoms observed, including their onset and facts documenting exposure to environment factors or activities just prior to their onset. Additionally, the history should document any present or past history of the following: (1) bronchial manifestations; (2) nasal and sinus symptoms; (3) dermatoses; (4) gastrointestinal symptoms; (5) recurrent periods of inactivity or lassitude; (6) genitourinary, cardiovascular or glandular disturbance; (7) colicky, irritable behavior; (8) dietary history; (9) drug reaction history and (10) environmental reaction history.[26] The presence or absence of symptoms in any of these areas should be noted in the history and if present, their duration, frequency, variation from one time to the next, and degree of severity. The source of this information (usually parents) is important because valid recall of times and events associated with symptomatology is critical in providing clues to the causal antigen as well as in establishing the diagnosis.

Laboratory tests on blood as well as nasal, conjunctival and bronchial secretions are conducted to check for elevated levels of eosinophils (Table 23–2). X-rays of the paranasal sinuses may be done when symptomatology suggests their involvement. A radioallergosorbent test (RAST) may be employed to measure the quantity of IgE in blood serum and to identify increases in antigen specific IgE. This test is expensive and is less sensitive, resulting in a higher incidence of false-negatives than skin testing. However, in young infants, especially those under 6 months, it may be used

---

*Elimination procedures involve controlling the environment or diet to establish antigen sources and are discussed more thoroughly later in this chapter.

TABLE 23-3 DRUGS USED IN TREATMENT OF PEDIATRIC ALLERGY

Drug Group	Route	Treatment Action	Side Effects
Antihistamines	Oral; give with meals. Not used with other CNS depressants.	Antagonist to most actions of mediator chemicals (histamine), thus decreasing severity of allergic reaction. Antispasmodic effect on respiratory muscles. Decreases edema by vasodilation and reducing capillary permeability. Prevents pruritus by suppressing stimulant action on nerve endings.	Common but with marked variation in individual child. Drowsiness, sedation, headache, tinnitus. GI complaints. Dry mouth. Dizziness, blurred vision. Depression, nervousness. Orthostatic hypotension. Polyuria, dysuria.
Bronchodilators (adrenergics)	Topical; nebulizer. Oral (after meals and h.s.). Rectal	Relaxes bronchial smooth muscles. Vasoconstriction of mucosal blood vessels, reducing congestion of mucous membranes. General relief of allergic symptoms.	Palpitation, hypertension. Nervousness, tremors. GI complaints. Headache, pallor.
Corticosteroids	Oral or topical. Administered on alternate days in early morning.	Anti-inflammatory; antiallergic effect; reduces eosinophils in blood.	Suppression of linear growth with long-term therapy. Electrolyte imbalance. Cushing's syndrome symptoms. Depression of immune response to infections.

since it is much less risky than skin testing at this age and may diagnose antigens in acutely allergic infants.[6] The parents and older child (age-appropriate explanation) should be told what will happen during each diagnostic test or procedure, including what they may expect to see and feel and what they may do to help.

Physical examination is invaluable in identifying symptoms of allergy. Special attention should be given during the examination to body parts involved in the symptomatology.

When ingestants, drugs or contactants are suspected antigens, elimination procedures may be used to establish diagnosis. Removal of suspected objects (frequently toys, clothing, bedding, or drapery fabrics) or avoidance of suspected drugs is initiated. Disappearance of the allergic symptoms after removal helps diagnose causation. Elimination or rotary diets may be tried to establish the villain substance in suspected food allergy.

General Management of Allergy

Prompt and early treatment of allergy is extremely important to prevent secondary complications and emotional and social consequences. Carty stresses that treatment of allergic disease is based upon five steps: (1) proper diagnosis of the ailment as allergic disease; (2) discovery of the causative antigens; (3) elimination of those antigens (environmental control) as far as possible; (4) increasing resistance to unavoidable antigens through immunotherapy or desensitization; and (5) maintenance of the child in a state of physical and emotional and social health that accommodates normal growth and development through supportive management of symptoms and health promotional actions.[7]

Whenever possible, the most logical and most successful principle of allergy treatment is removal of the cause. For example, if the antigen is a pet or mattress stuffing or a food substance, removal or avoidance of it will eliminate or relieve the allergic symptoms.

Symptomatic relief during the course of allergic disease primarily involves the use of antihistamines, bronchodilators and steroids. Table 23-3 describes the functions of these drugs in the relief of allergy symptoms. Antibiotics are also employed during bouts of secondary infection to maintain general good health.

Health promotion is extremely important, since stress increases the likelihood of allergic reactions to smaller doses of antigen; that is, it lowers the threshold (antigen resistance). Of particular significance is immediate attention to even minor infections or illness. A balanced diet and adequate amounts of both rest and stimulation are of obvious value. The allergy-prone infant also benefits from a predominantly calm, routine environment that facilitates stability of his emotional well-being. Parents are a very significant part of the management team, since overanxiousness or overprotectiveness aggravates the child's allergic condition by increasing his emotional tension.

Impact of Allergy on the Family

The management efforts taken to reduce or eliminate an antigen from an infant's environment often affect all family members. Aesthetic features of the home (carpets, drapes, overstuffed furniture) often have to be removed to accommodate the allergic child's health state. Members may also have to deprive themselves of habits such as smoking or pleasures such as pets. The frequent, time-consuming medical attention, costly testing and treatment, and expensive but necessary visits to allergy specialists create a financial strain for many families. Such limitations to family living often cause anger or resentment toward the affected child and the eventual development of guilt feelings in the child himself.[3]

Health professionals have a responsibility to help these families cope effectively with this anger and guilt. Sharing as much information as exists about the allergy helps family members to understand the reasons for the limitations imposed. They also need to know that feelings of anger are natural but that there are healthy ways to ventilate that anger such as talking about it (the listening ear may belong to a spouse, parent, sibling, the nurse), seeking substitute pleasures for those given up, and using extended family or community resources to relieve financial pressures.

Preventive Actions in Allergy-Prone Families

Families with a history of allergy are usually willing to comply with prophylactic measures to decrease their infant's chances of developing allergy, since they are likely acquainted with the consequences and sacrifices involved in managing allergic disease. Prophylaxis can begin prenatally when a strong family tendency for allergy exists. The pregnant woman can limit her intake of potential antigens such as milk, eggs and chocolate. Before and after the infant's arrival, "allergy proofing" of the home (Table 23–4), or at least the infant's room, can be done.

When the child is born into such a family, prophylaxis can continue by either breastfeeding or using soybean formula rather than

TABLE 23–4 HOME ALLERGY-PROOFING TECHNIQUES

Potential Antigen	Proofing Actions
House dust (leading cause of respiratory allergy)	1. Restrict use of bedroom to sleeping. 2. Use shades instead of blinds or curtains. 3. Place washable plastic over mattresses. 4. Use no carpeting or wool scatter rugs. 5. Damp dust daily with child out of room. 6. Allow no stuffed animals or knickknacks. 7. Have minimal furniture; if stuffed should be foam rubber. 8. Either close off heat ducts or cover with cheesecloth. (Wash often.) 9. Keep doors and windows closed. 10. Avoid storing wool in closets or use of wool blankets.
Mold, mildew	1. Eliminate plants and aquariums from child's bedroom and play area; keep to minimum throughout home. 2. Avoid use of cellars as play or living area. 3. Clean bathroom and tile areas with antimold agent (Lysol) regularly. 4. Cleanse vaporizers or humidifiers frequently. 5. Use dehumidifier in humid or damp areas.
Danders, feathers	1. Use Dacron or foam rubber pillows and mattresses. 2. Get rid of pets or limit to outdoors. 3. Allow no stuffed animals or furniture and no clothing stuffed or insulated with feathers (down).
Contactants	1. Buy no wool clothing. 2. Wash all new clothing and linens before using. 3. Double-rinse infant's clothing and diapers. 4. Wash baby articles in mild soap. 5. Use mild soap to bathe baby and rinse well. 6. Avoid use of perfumed lotions, powders, oils.

milk, especially during the first six months of life. Once solid food is introduced (preferably after six months for infants at risk for allergy), one food should be tried at a time so that the source of any reaction is immediately recognizable and can be eliminated from the diet. Eggs should not be given until at least one year in allergy-prone infants.[14] All foods should be thoroughly cooked for ingestion by infants and toddlers under 3 years of age. When diarrhea occurs in these children, foods should be reintroduced simply and gradually.[14]

NURSING ACTIONS

During Diagnosis The thorough history required to diagnose allergic disease usually takes more than an hour. Most parents appreciate the nurse's suggestion that they bring along a relative or friend to help manage the child during this time. They should also be given an estimation of the time that the evaluation will take.

If the parents have documented (for example, in a baby book or home medical guide) any of the infant's previous illnesses or episodes of symptomatology, the nurse should ask them to bring this. This may help them to recall in a more chronological and seasonal order any previous symptomatic periods and will often help them recall more accurately any potential precipitating factors or events.

Parents also experience less anxiety when they are told how they may assist during the physical examination and diagnostic tests. When parents are less anxious, the child also feels more at ease in this stressful situation. The nurse may suggest that parents bring along a few of the baby's favorite toys and security objects (blanket, pacifier, doll). The parents can then be instructed to use these items to distract, entertain or soothe the infant during the examination. The parent can also help by undressing the infant as needed and assisting in restraining him during ophthalmic and otoscopic examinations or while culture specimens are obtained, since most infants tolerate these intrusions better from their caretakers. The parents' participation in the examination makes them feel more useful and the infant more secure.

During Treatment Parental attitudes are crucial to the management of childhood allergy. It is important that they be helped to understand the pathogenesis of allergy and the interrelationship between antigens and stress in causing symptoms. Teaching should cover a description of the specific allergy — why it occurs, what happens to cause symptoms, how the allergy and its treatment will affect the infant and family life. The parents should be encouraged to keep a diary of symptom episodes so that any pattern or predisposing factors might be recognized.

The course of infant allergy poses multiple stresses for the family. Common concerns they express about allergy are:
1. Their part in transmitting the condition if there is a positive family history of allergy,
2. How to manage the infant's irritable behavior,
3. Their negative reaction to the lesions,
4. Their difficulties in setting limits and being consistent about expectations,
5. Their ability to carry out the treatment regimen.

Effective nursing interventions are preventive and supportive.

The infant with allergy may be irritable and fretful, particularly if pruritus is involved. This intense itching makes him very uncomfortable and difficult to soothe. Many such infants do not sleep well at night. Some scratch their irritated skin when they are angry or frustrated instead of crying. Keeping the infant from scratching is a difficult task; coupled with the knowledge that scratching leads to exacerbations and infection, the situation may result in added parental frustration and guilt. An explanation that the infant's irritable behavior is related to his physical discomfort, not to the fact that he is "ill-tempered" or "spoiled," is helpful in minimizing parental anxiety. Encouraging parents to play with the infant at times when he is comfortable and is not undergoing soaks or other treatments and to provide extra physical contact in the form of rocking, cuddling and stroking promotes emotional-social development. Removal of restraints allows active play that relieves frustration and encourages expression of feelings. A pacifier may be used to meet infant sucking needs that become accentuated by use of restraints and by physical discomfort. Mealtimes should be relaxed, and infants who are ready for finger foods should be encouraged to feed themselves.

Washable, soft toys appropriate to the infant's developmental level provide outlets for frustration and opportunities for exploration. If the infant's hands must remain covered, large balls with bells inside, big cloth blocks, and other similar large toys can be offered for play. *Environmental stimulation must be increased during periods of exacerbations necessitating restraint in order for normal development to progress.*

The physical appearance of the infant with allergy may repulse parents. They can be reluctant to touch or hold their infant because of these feelings, placing him at risk for bonding disorders and sensory deprivation. All of these factors contribute to parental fatigue. Overwhelmed parents feel that their efforts to help their infant are ineffective and that they have little control over the disease process. These factors can lead to expressions of rejection or to patterns of overprotection and restriction. The inconsistent environment produced by this alternating rejection and overprotection may have devastating effects on the infant's emotional and social development. His needs for love and attention are probably greater than those of a normal child because of his discomfort and the restrictions of his treatment regimen.

Allergy-imposed limitations should be kept minimal to avoid adverse effects on the infant's development. Parents should not allow the child to use his symptoms to manipulate. (Infants learn very early to do this if parental responses sanction it.) The nurse should emphasize the infant's healthy features and encourage the parents to do likewise.

Treatment of allergy is usually done in the home, leaving the major responsibility for the management regimen to the parents. Supervision by a community health nurse is often supportive to the family as they attempt to comply with regimen requirements and cope with the frustrations of a special diet, frequent medication administrations, allergy-proofing their home, tolerating the infant's general irritability and juggling financial resources to make environmental changes. Parental self-confidence is enhanced by developing skill in managing the infant's treatment regimen. Demonstration by the nurse and return demonstration by the parent is most effective. A nurse can be supportive by acknowledging to the parent that the treatments are time consuming and that the constant vigilance needed to prevent scratching is wearing. Ventilation of feelings is therapeutic for parents.

Parents also need to be informed of the importance of keeping key people (baby sitters, relatives) in the infant's environment informed about his allergy management. All instructions regarding medications for symptomatic relief should be written as well as explained verbally. If a drug is involved, instruction should include when the drug should be used, proper administration, side effects to watch for and report, appropriate antidotes, and avoidance of non-judicious use of prescribed or over-the-counter medications.

The cycle of exacerbation and remission is frustrating to parents, who invest large amounts of time and energy following the treatment regimen. If the infant is hospitalized during an exacerbation, the allergy often improves quickly because environmental allergens are more carefully controlled and the stress resulting from parental frustration is reduced. This rapid improvement contributes to the parents' sense of failure. Counselling to help in dealing with these feelings should be available to them. Parent support groups are also an effective source of strength in helping parents manage their reactions.

Continued reassurance and support that the negative feelings they may have about the infant and his care are normal and worthy of discussion is a critical nursing action. If parents can lower their anxiety levels and respond to the infant's needs related to health as well as those pertaining to his illness, family stress is often reduced and the allergy improves. Above all else, parents need to understand that this infant's first need is the same as any other infant's — to be loved for who he is and the fact that he is.

DERMATITIDES OF INFANCY

In infants, the epidermis is thin, particularly the stratum corneum, and the immunological system is immature, resulting in increased susceptibility to irritations and infection. Sweating is scanty or absent and the sebaceous glands that supply the skin with lubrication are virtually inactive. Lacking lubrication, the infant's skin is more susceptible to drying and chapping. These factors make the infant susceptible to a number of inflammatory skin conditions that can be differentiated primarily on the basis of which body surface areas the rash covers and where it began. The more common dermatitides of infancy are discussed here, including contact dermatitis, diaper dermatitis (intertrigo or diaper rash), seborrheic dermatitis (cradle cap) and atopic dermatitis (infantile eczema).

Allergic Contact Dermatitis

This dermatitis involves skin inflammation as a result of direct skin contact with an antigen,

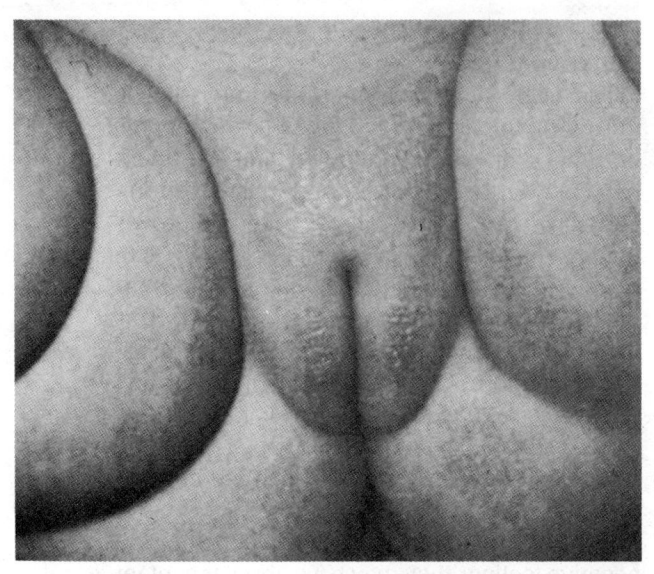

Figure 23-1 Primary irritant contact dermatitis (ammoniacal). Note involvement of convex surfaces but not the folds. (From A. H. Jacobs. Eruptions in the Diaper Area. Pediatric Clinics of North America, May 1975, p. 212.)

usually a nonprotein. Males show a greater tendency for this allergy. It occurs more often in infants and toddlers, usually beginning around 3 to 4 months of age.[24] Susceptible children tend to have very dry skin from birth and a family history of atopy. The most common antigen sources are plants, soap or detergents, plastics or metals, adhesive tape and medicated ointments or lotions.[2]

Clinical Manifestations and Diagnosis A delayed response (cellular antibodies) to antigen contact is typical, with symptoms appearing 12 to 72 hours after exposure. The inflamed area usually has the configuration of the area of contact. The exposed skin area is erythematous, edematous and pruritic. The pruritus intensifies during emotional stress and with temperature changes. Papules form and, if scratched, begin oozing. Lichenification (hardened, leathery skin) eventually develops as the area heals.

A history of dry skin, family atopy and ready skin blanching (tendency toward vasoconstriction of cutaneous vessels) coupled with localized inflammatory configuration and distribution is adequate to establish diagnosis.

Management This allergic disease is self-limiting, so treatment is primarily symptomatic and preventive. Preventive management involves keeping the skin lubricated, clean and healthy to increase its resistance and to minimize infection secondary to allergic response. Daily tepid baths without soap and lasting no more than five minutes, followed by application of a bland lubricant (Alpha-Keri, Cetaphil or Shepard's Lotion) while the skin is still wet is usually sufficient to maintain general integumentary health.[5] Use of a humidifier in the home during dry months also helps combat the infant's dry skin condition. Once the antigen is identified, its elimination, if possible, prevents further bouts of contact dermatitis. Desensitization therapy is hardly ever successful in managing this dermatitis, although it may decrease the severity of reaction if the antigen is a plant source that cannot be eliminated.[2] In these cases it is usually used preseasonally for a few weeks. Inflammatory discomfort and pruritus may be relieved with the use of antipruritics, corticosteroid creams or ointments, or wet soaks of 1:20 Burow's solution.[5]

The nurse must demonstrate to the parents how to mix the Burow's solution in the correct concentration and how to apply the compresses. Compresses are usually applied at room temperature with a thoroughly soaked cloth one layer thick. They remain on the affected areas for 20- to 30-minute periods and are resoaked every 10 to 15 minutes to prevent drying and sticking. This routine is repeated three to four times a day. During the soaks, parents can divert the infant with brightly colored toys or music. Wearing a plastic apron for protection will enable the parent to also hold and rock the baby. These actions facilitate emotional-social development by encouraging pleasant interactions between parent and infant. Discomfort severe enough to disturb sleep should be controlled with temporary use of antihistamines or hormone ointments administered at bedtime.[2]

Emotional distress increases suceptibility to allergic response and intensifies reaction severity. Once the dermatitis is present, such distress increases the pruritus experienced. Therefore, a calm environment void of as much friction and emotional pressure as possible is of utmost importance to this infant. Parents need assistance to understand this relationship so that they are more likely to comply with this most valuable aspect of management. Despite their infant's irritability due to his discomfort and his unappealing appearance caused by the dermatitis, parents must be urged to continue communicating love and acceptance so that his attachment needs and developing self-concept are not jeopardized.

Diaper Rashes

The diaper rashes involve inflammatory response in areas normally covered by a diaper (Fig. 23–2). They are extremely common in infants. Table 23–5 describes the most frequent diaper eruptions, their characteristic appearance and specific treatments.

Diagnosis is readily made by inspection of the rash characteristics and area involved. The history often reveals inadequate hygiene of the diaper region, insufficient laundering of diapers or a tendency to overdress the infant. General treatment of any of the diaper rashes requires basic diaper and skin care. Prompt, thorough cleansing of the diaper region with a mild soap and water after each defecation or voiding is imperative to rid the skin of irritant byproducts and reduce the pathogen population. The caretaker should be instructed to check every hour for elimination. Compliance is more likely when the caretaker(s) understands the reasons for the diaper rash and is given a clear explanation of how adequate skin hygiene and cleansing of diapers will help prevent or eliminate diaper rash. The region should be air dried and exposed to the air at additional frequent intervals to promote faster healing. In severe cases use of a heat lamp may be prescribed in addition to the air exposure.* A protective ointment such as Desitin or zinc oxide is used after inflammation is reduced or prophylactically. An antibiotic may also be prescribed if secondary infection exists. Suggesting that the diaper and ointment be removed when the infant is resting or sleeping and that ointment and a loosely applied diaper be put on when he is up or being held may be helpful to the caretakers. Rubber pants and disposable diapers should be avoided during bouts of diaper rash or continuously in very susceptible infants. Parents need explanations that the rubber and plastic prevent evaporation, thereby increasing maceration from urine breakdown. Even though disposables are advertised to reduce wetness by pulling the urine toward the liner and away from baby's skin, the urea and ammonia salts that cause the breakdown are left behind as a residue on the diaper surface touching the baby's skin.

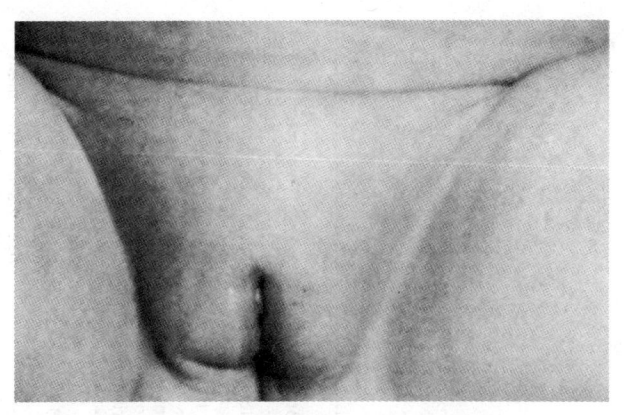

Figure 23–2 Early intertrigo. Note the erythema in the folds with sparing of the convex surfaces. (From A. H. Jacobs. Eruptions in the Diaper Area. Pediatric Clinics of North America, May 1975, p. 213.)

Healing of diaper rashes involving skin folds is facilitated by frequent applications of cornstarch or unmedicated powder. The previous application should be completely washed off before each new application. A new application should be applied at each diaper change. If diaper laundering has been inadequate or the mother has never used cloth diapers before, instruction should be given to launder them separately, using a mild soap and a double rinsing. Soaking rinsed, soiled diapers in a quaternary ammonium compound such as Diaparene or diluted chlorine bleach (1 cup in 1 gallon of water) helps sterilize them.

The procedures described here to treat existing diaper rashes may also be used to prevent recurrences. During acute stages of eruption, regardless of the cause, application of intermittent cool wet compresses, using saline (1 level tsp salt per pint of water) or Burow's (1 tablet of commercially available Burow's to 1 qt of water) solution for two to three days is helpful in reducing rash severity.[16]

Seborrheic Dermatitis

Seborrheic dermatitis (cradle cap, seborrheic eczema) is an inflammatory skin disease of unknown origin. It usually appears shortly after

---

*In some hospitals lamps are used only if ordered by a doctor. They should be used with great care. Never use a lamp until any medication or ointment has been completely removed, because moisture causes burning. Never leave the infant unattended while the lamp is on. The lamp should not be left at the bedside when not in use.

TABLE 23-5 DIFFERENTIAL DIAGNOSIS OF DIAPER RASHES

Diagnosis	Rash Characteristics	Area Involved	Source	Age of Occurrence	Treatment	Remarks
Primary irritant contact dermatitis	Parchment-like erythema (similar to scald)	Convex area of buttocks, medial thighs, mons pubis and scrotum but *not* the folds	Ammonia (urine) and putrefactive enzymes (feces) interact to create irritant by-products. In older infants the contact dermatitis may be an allergic response to enzyme detergent or rubber	3 months or older	Topical glucocorticoid cream (1% hydrocortisone or triamcinolone); add 1 cup of vinegar to last diaper rinse and let soak 1/2 hr before spinning (acidifies urine); daily oral feedings of 2–3 oz cranberry juice also acidifies urine; basic diaper and skin care	Allergic contact dermatitis of diaper area is similar but does not usually occur in infancy
Intertrigo	Red macerated area of sharp demarcation	Areas where skin surfaces are in opposition, particularly groin folds	Heat, moisture and sweat retention combine to irritate and macerate the skin	Any age	Basic diaper and skin care	Bacterial populations grow with maceration, increasing risk of secondary infections
Seborrheic dermatitis	Intertrigo type rash but greasy looking; non-pruritic (differentiates it from eczema)	Presence of intertrigo in groin and in other skin folds (neck or axilla) plus cradle cap indicates seborrheic dermatitis	Inborn physiologic trait	3 weeks to 4 months	Same as for contact dermatitis	May spread to entire diaper region after initial appearance in folds; highly susceptible to secondary yeast or bacterial infection; subsides spontaneously
Miliaria (heat rash)	Small, sterile, clear vesicopustules	Anywhere that heat and moisture accumulate, especially diaper area	Reaction to concentrated heat and humidity	Any age	Basic diaper and skin care	
Primary candidiasis	Small red papules with peripheral scaling	Perianal involvement with satellite lesions; will become generalized over trunk if untreated	*Candida albicans* from GI tract or an untreated infected caretaker	Any age; usually after 2 weeks of age	1% hydrocortisone or .01% triamcinolone lotion followed by nystatin powder after lotion dries; basic diaper and skin care	Often secondary to seborrheic dermatitis; usually occurs following oral thrush

birth when hormone levels are high, disappears after several weeks even without treatment, then reappears at adolescence when hormone levels again rise.[17] Fifty per cent of all infants have it at some time before 6 months of age.[14] This dermatitis occurs most often on the scalp (cradle cap) (Fig. 23-3), although it may also involve the eyelids and eyebrows (blepharitis), the external ear canal (otitis externa), the postauricular region (behind the ears), the axillae and neck folds (Fig. 23-4) and the inguinal region (seborrheic diaper dermatitis). The lesions appear as thick, greasy crusts of a salmon color or as waxy yellow plaques with large scales. Transient alopecia may be present over the area of the crusty or scaly patches.

Seborrheic dermatitis is similar to eczema in appearance and is, in fact, frequently referred to as seborrheic eczema, but it differs in several recognizable ways. Unlike eczema, cradle cap can and usually does occur in the first month of life. The lesion surfaces of seborrhea are pink or yellow as compared to the obvious red lesions of eczema. Seborrhea is not necessarily accompanied by a positive family history of allergy. Lichenification of lesion areas does not occur in cradle cap. While eczema almost always begins on the cheeks, seborrhea usually presents on the scalp, eyelids, or ear folds. Although contact dermatitis also sometimes begins on the cheeks, the pruritus is much less severe than in eczema. Seborrhea also responds rapidly to treatment. The most significant difference, however, is the fact that seborrhea is not pruritic, while eczema produces extreme pruritus. Diagnosis is based upon the characteristic appearance of the crusts and the absence of pruritus.

Preventive and symptomatic intervention is essentially the same. The most important aspect is adequate and frequent scalp hygiene measures. The scalp should be shampooed vigorously and thoroughly every other day. Parents usually have some reservations about vigorous scalp hygiene because of misconceptions about the durability of the "soft spots," or fontanels. They should be informed that these spots are as durable as the skin anywhere else on the body and will not be punctured by the pressure required for vigorous scrubbing. For some families, a demonstration shampoo may be more convincing than verbal descriptions. The "no tears" shampoos or those containing salicylic acid or coal tars are most effective, with two applications of shampoo used each time.

If seborrheic lesions exist, measures may be taken to soften and remove some of the crusts prior to shampooing. Sulfur or coal tar ointments, salicylic acid preparations or resorcinol may be massaged into the scaly or crusty patches and left intact for 5 to 15 minutes before shampooing. Before and just after shampooing a fine-toothed comb run through the hair helps remove some of the softened crusts from the scalp surface and hair strands. If lesions are extensive or inflamed, topical corticosteroids are extremely effective in producing remission. Secondarily infected lesions, although infrequent, may require treatment with either topical or systemic antibiotic or antifungal therapy. Fre-

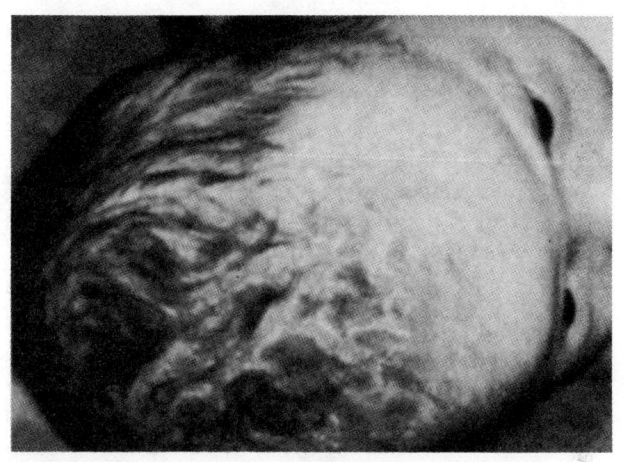

Figure 23-3 Cradle cap, a seborrheic dermatitis of the scalp, is extremely common in young infants. (From A. H. Jacobs. Eruptions in the Diaper Area. Pediatric Clinics of North America, May 1975, p. 214.)

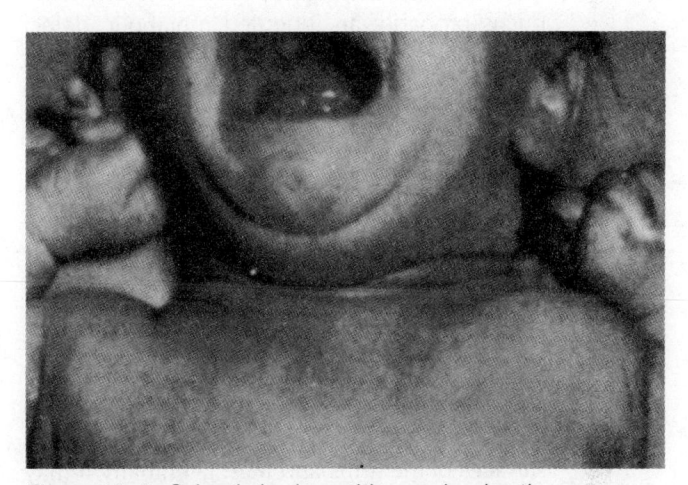

Figure 23-4 Seborrheic dermatitis may involve the axillae and neck folds. (From A. H. Jacobs. Eruptions in the Diaper Area. Pediatric Clinics of North America, May 1975, p. 214.)

quent changes of bed linens and clothing that touches the affected area helps prevent secondary infection. Parents should be cautioned to avoid getting any ointments or medications into the infant's eyes during treatment.

Although the lesions are unsightly and the crust softening techniques somewhat bothersome, the child's behavior is generally unaltered by the disease, since it produces no sensory discomfort. Parents are generally able to institute the desired treatment without difficulty once given adequate instruction. However, in families in which attitudes exist that do not emphasize hygiene, a community health nurse or nurse practitioner referral may be desirable to help the family maintain adequate treatment.

Atopic Dermatitis

Atopic dermatitis (infantile eczema)* is a relatively common inflammatory response in infants after 3 months of age; but, unlike the other dermatitides presented in this chapter, it is not always temporary. A significant number of infants with eczema have only a temporary remission, with recurrences in their preschool years and again during adulthood.

Pathophysiology The skin of an infant with atopic dermatitis is abnormally dry and sensitive to heat, humidity and external irritants. It reacts to these with intense pruritus. The exact mechanism of this pruritic reaction is unknown but is probably an inherited metabolic defect involving IgE humoral antibodies. The skin of affected children has been shown to release twice as much histamine as that of normal children. Vasodilation from this histamine release aggravates the itching by causing erythema and edema. Exacerbations are common in the winter and summer.

Clinical Manifestations Infantile atopic dermatitis appears within the first year of life, seldom before 3 months of age. A red, papular rash appears first on the cheeks and spreads to the forehead, scalp and down the extensor surfaces of the arms and legs. Eventually it may cover the whole body. Vesicles quickly form as fluid, caused by the histamine release, escapes into the tissues. The pruritus is intense and the infant scratches the lesions, rupturing the vesicles and causing excoriation. The trauma of scratching plays a major role in the occurrence and progression of the dermatitis. Much of the clinical picture is related to the results of the scratching.

Weeping, followed by crusting, appears next. As the crusts heal they fall off, leaving healthy new epithelium. Secondary infection occurs frequently and is usually staphylococcal or streptococcal in origin. There is no scarring involved unless infection is severe.

Etiology and Diagnosis As the word atopic implies, 70 per cent of infants with atopic dermatitis have a positive family history of allergy. The mode of inheritance has not been established, but the genetic predisposition definitely exists. Therefore, the prenatal and postnatal preventive measures discussed in this section on allergy and the methods of management of contact dermatitis are important in preventing the development of infantile atopic dermatitis, or minimizing its severity.

If atopic dermatitis develops, the parents are usually concerned about the facial rash and seek medical attention as it spreads and becomes excoriated by the infant's scratching. The diagnosis is made based on the positive family history, the character and distribution of the lesions, the intense pruritus and the pattern of exacerbation and remission of the condition. Atopic dermatitis must be differentiated from seborrheic dermatitis. (See the discussion on differentiating these two dermatitides in the description of seborrheic dermatitis in this section.) As with all the dermatitides, a thorough history is imperative to an accurate diagnosis. (See history-taking discussion at the beginning of the allergy section.)

Physical examination of the eczema victim often reveals an array of several types of dermatitides in varying stages of healing. The child's discomfort and fatigue are usually apparent in his forlorn, sallow appearance. Accentuated skin folds under the eyes (Dennie's lines) or excessive numbers of crosshatched palm markings are positive signs of eczema and are present in some children. Local lymphadenopathy is often present.

If pustular or vesicular areas are inflamed or crusted, scrapings should be cultured for sec-

---
*The discussion of atopic dermatitis was contributed by Ellen Christian and Judith Clark.

ondary infection organisms and for eosinophilia. Elevated serum IgE levels with the presence of Prausnitz-Küstner antibodies is found in many infants with eczema.

Management The mainstay of management in atopic dermatitis is topical therapy to control the symptoms. The primary goal of treatment is the control of itching, since scratching may lead to excoriation, secondary infection and scarring. Specific antipruritic drugs such as hydroxyzine hydrochloride (Atarax), diphenhydramine hydrochloride (Benadryl) and cyproheptadine (Periactin) are most effective when used at bedtime. Arm and hand restraints may be needed to prevent scratching. Fingernails should be kept short and clean. The young infant's hands can be wrapped in soft cotton gloves, which are then pinned to his shirt sleeves. Elbow restraints are also effective, and they have the advantage of allowing more movement of the arms. Any restraint should be removed frequently to permit skin care and to allow supervised, unrestricted movement that is crucial to optimal development.

Consideration of the adverse effect of increased environmental temperature and humidity on itching is important. In particular, overheating aggravates itching. Dressing the infant in lightweight cotton garments will help minimize this effect. He should wear the same amount of clothing that is comfortable for an adult.

Care of the skin is important in minimizing itching. In the acute exudative phase, a carefully followed topical skin regimen as described for the management of contact dermatitis can control the symptoms.

Inflammation is controlled by the application of a steroid cream following Burow's solution soaks. A fluorinated steroid cream is never used on the face because it causes permanent, unsightly acne-like eruptions and capillary dilation. A 1 per cent hydrocortisone cream or desonide (Tridesilon) is most often used on the face. Other local steroids often used on the rest of the body include Kenalog Cream 0.1 per cent, Cordran Cream 0.05 per cent, Synalar Cream, 0.025 per cent, and Valisone Cream 0.1 per cent. During the acute exudative phase, a cream or lotion base is used to avoid the occlusive effects of an ointment. Applied to large areas, steroids may be absorbed in quantities sufficient to depress adrenal function. Parents are taught that several thin applications of steroid cream are more effective than one thick application and that small areas may be wrapped with a plastic film (Saran Wrap) to enhance the effectiveness of the medication. Since this practice increases the risk of adverse systemic effects, large body areas should not be wrapped. Another teaching point related to topical therapy is that steroids have a tendency to mask infection. The skin must be inspected carefully for subtle signs of bacterial and yeast infection. Increased inflammation, pain or pruritus may be indicative of infection. Usually, systemic antibiotics such as erythromycin are prescribed. The antibiotic dosage and administration schedule should be thoroughly discussed with parents to promote compliance with treatment.

Elimination of identified or common allergens is an approach often used in treating infants with atopic dermatitis. Allergy-proofing the home is recommended (Table 23–4). The results, however, are often disappointing. Many authorities now believe that unless a specific allergy to a specific food can be demonstrated, the trial elimination diet (see description of this diet in management of gastrointestinal allergy, next section) is of questionable value. Sometimes a caretaker can date the onset of rash exactly to the time of a change in formula or addition of a new food to the child's diet. (Eggs, milk and wheat are the leading food offenders.)

Prognosis Atopic dermatitis can be controlled but not cured. By 2 years of age most children undergo permanent remission. They have little scarring and the changes in pigmentation that occur after inflammation are temporary. Not reassuring is the fact that half of infants with atopic dermatitis develop asthma or hay fever later in life. For those in whom there is not a permanent remission, a childhood stage of atopic dermatitis usually appears during the preschool years. It is characterized by less redness and beginning lichenification (thickening of the dermal and epidermal skin layers). The third stage, the adult stage, is characterized by dermatitis on the face, neck and flexural spaces such as the antecubital and axillary areas, and popliteal lichenification is common.

GASTROINTESTINAL ALLERGY

Nutritional allergy is a common disorder that can occur at any age but has a particularly high incidence during infancy, especially the first six months of life. This is because the infant's digestive system is immature, absorbing larger amounts of incompletely catabolized proteins, which can be antigenic. Herein also lies the explanation for why infants frequently outgrow food allergies as they mature. Another reason why food allergy is common in infancy is because that is the time when the child is introduced to many new potentially antigenic foods.

The most frequent nutritional offenders are milk, egg white, wheat, citrus fruits, chocolate and corn. Fish and legumes are also possible offenders, and allergy to these is less often outgrown. Occasionally an inhalant or a drug, especially vitamins and antibiotics with lactose filler, may cause gastrointestinal allergic responses.

There are two distinct reactions in gastrointestinal allergy. An immediate response, with appearance of symptoms within minutes after food ingestion, is usually to the food substance itself. A delayed response, with symptomatic appearance occurring hours or days after ingestion, is usually caused by some product formed during the digestion of the food. There is thought to be a congenital transmission in some infants, which explains why those children display explosive allergic reactions with their first exposure to the causative food.[1]

A wide variety of symptoms is possible in nutritional allergy, as is a wide range of intensity of reaction. Clinical manifestations may be oral, most commonly resulting in allergic inflammation of the lips (cheilitis) or mouth (stomatitis), canker sores, or geographic tongue. Gastrointestinal disturbances frequently occur, including nausea and vomiting, intestinal cramping associated with spastic constipation or diarrhea containing abundant mucus, distention and eructation, painful bowel muscle spasms (colic), intestinal bleeding, or mucous colitis.[1] Occasionally systemic responses such as hives or palmar or anal pruritus accompany the gastrointestinal reaction.

Diagnosis of food allergy is based on disappearance of symptoms once the suspected food is removed from the infant's diet (trial elimination diet). Confirmation may then be made by reintroducing the food (elimination-challenge diet) on a trial basis to determine if symptoms reappear. X-ray study may also be used to confirm such suspicion. The suspected food is ingested and x-rays are taken to determine if a spasm response occurs along the gastrointestinal tract. Although skin testing may reveal the antigen if the allergic reaction is to a food substance, suspected antigens are more readily identified through a careful family history and nutritional history, including having the caretaker keep a food diary of foods ingested, the date and time, how foods were prepared, and any untoward reactions in the infant. This diary is then analyzed for clues to the antigenic substance.

The diagnostic process requires the cooperation of the parents and other regular caretakers. Verbal and written instructions should be given concerning the food diary or any of the elimination diets to all involved in food purchase, food preparation and feeding of the infant. Caution about scrutinizing food labels for contents of the suspected antigen should be emphasized. If parental cooperation is not forthcoming, the child may have to be hospitalized to establish the diagnosis.

The antigenic food is often very hard to identify, particularly if a delayed reaction occurs. Also, the food may be eaten often but only occasionally cause a reaction, such as when it is ingested in the raw form or served cold. Sometimes certain food combinations produce the reaction, or the food may produce a reaction only when ingested during certain seasons.[1] In infants on cow's milk who have a history of colic, nasal congestion and irritability, the milk should always be suspected first as the probable antigen. Milk should also be suspected if the infant shows repeated bouts of respiratory illness.[9]

Intervention is at three levels. Preventively, certain foods should be avoided during the first year in infants with a substantial family history for allergy. Those foods include the ones that predispose to allergic responses mentioned at the beginning of this discussion and any foods for which there is a family history of reaction. Carefully and gradually introducing new foods to these susceptible infants helps to promptly identify any offending food. Foods should be introduced one at a time, allowing at least four days before an additional food is introduced.

Foods should be well cooked and offered in small quantities (½ to 1 tsp).

Any food that causes even a local reaction should be avoided for at least six months before it is reintroduced on a trial basis. If reaction occurs again, another six months should elapse before another trial is done. If milk is the offender, milk substitutes in the form of soybean preparations (Isomil, Prosobee, Neo-Mull-Soy), predigested synthetic milk preparations (Pregestimil, Nutramigen) or a meat-base formula may be used.

If a specific food has been implicated as a cause, a trial elimination diet may be employed. Raw foods are avoided since heating reduces the antigen properties of foods. The suspected food is eliminated from the diet for four weeks during which time the allergic response should improve measurably or clear if the food is the real cause.

If a specific food is not suspected but food is the probable antigen, the child is placed on a hypoallergenic diet. A typical diet includes a milk substitute such as soy formula, a nonwheat cereal such as rice cereal, one or two noncitrus fruits such as apples and apricots, nonlegume vegetables such as green beans and carrots, beef and a multivitamin supplement. The child is restricted to this diet for 10 days. If the rash recedes or clears, new foods are added to this basic diet one at a time at intervals of four to seven days until the antigenic food(s) is identified because of a recurrence or worsening of the rash. If the hypoallergenic diet does not alter the rash status, food is not the antigenic substance and other aspects of the infant's environment must be investigated.

Parental education is crucial to successful intervention through preventive or corrective diet management. Supervision by a community health nurse who can further clarify educational factors to management helps the family to implement management measures and provides regular reinforcement for management efforts. This supervision and support may be desirable in some situations. Community financial assistance may also be necessary for the family to afford expensive food substitutes, as is often the case in milk allergy.

Symptomatic relief of gastrointestinal reactions may be initiated until the reaction subsides or the causative food is identified and eliminated. An antihistamine may be used to control intestinal spasms or abdominal pain (colic). Reducing the spasms and pains usually results in eliminating other complaints such as nausea, diarrhea or constipation.

Prevention of allergy by beginning appropriate teaching before the child is born, especially when strong family history for allergy exists, cannot be overemphasized. Informing such families of the significantly reduced incidence of allergy when an infant is breast-fed is a nursing responsibility. Avoiding introduction of solid foods until after the infant is 6 months old also helps reduce the likelihood of food allergy. These actions by the nurse can aid significantly in reducing the incidence of food allergy in infancy.

CONJUNCTIVITIS

Conjunctivitis is an inflammation of the eye that may be the result of an allergic response to an environmental irritant such as pollen (atopic conjunctivitis), a reaction to chemicals or medication (dermatologic conjunctivitis) with typical eyelid involvement as well, or a result of bacterial or viral infection (nonallergic conjunctivitis, or pink eye). Sometimes specific etiology is unknown.

The degree to which symptoms are manifested varies, but several symptoms are characteristically present. The conjunctivae are erythematous and edematous. Extreme pruritus exists and there is usually photophobia, increased lacrimation and scanty, thick exudate. The exudate may result in the eye matting shut during sleep, in which case when the child wakes the eye should be cleansed with warm water and cotton balls to soften and remove crusts.

Diagnosis is made on the basis of a thorough history relevant to the inflammation and other symptoms and a culture of the discharge. This reveals viral or bacterial growth if it is associated with infection and eosinophilia if related to an allergic response.[21]

Treatment is based on etiology.[21] If related to bacterial infection, the conjunctivitis is treated with an ophthalmic antibiotic or sulfanilamide. Viral infection is unresponsive to treatment and is self-limiting within two to three weeks.[14] Dermatological conjunctivitis is typically treated with optic cortisone drops or other steroid. Atopic conjunctivitis is usually treated with equal parts of steroid and antihistamine in optic form, 1:1000 epinephrine and 0.5 per cent Pontocaine being a common choice.

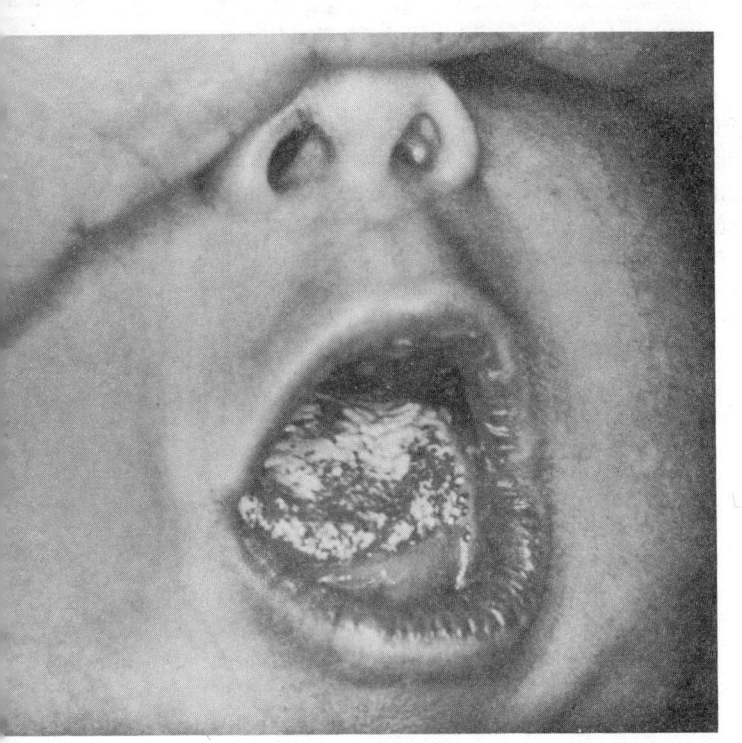

Figure 23-5 Thrush is characterized by white patches in the mouth that resemble curdled milk. (Photograph courtesy of Mead Johnson & Co. Nutritional Division.)

COMMON INFECTIONS

Thrush (Moniliasis)

Thrush involves a stomatitis, particularly of the tongue, buccal membranes, and pharynx, caused by a yeast-like fungus, *Candida albicans*. Five per cent of all newborns contract thrush during descent through an infected birth canal, evidencing symptoms 7 to 10 days later. Infection with Candida may also result from prolonged antibiotic therapy or be transmitted by contaminated hands, bottles or nipples. The incidence is greater in females, in infants with immunologic deficiencies, in infants of diabetic mothers, and in infants with oronasal anomalies. It is much less common after the neonatal period.

Candida is normally present in the mouth, gastrointestinal tract and vagina. However, the circulating anticandidal factor present in normal serum that keeps most individuals asymptomatic is reduced or virtually absent in the serum of newborn infants and exists in reduced serum levels during the first six months of life and in persons with hematopoietic disorders.[14, 24]

Clinical Manifestations Moniliasis is characterized by white or gray-white patches in the oral cavity, which are slightly elevated and closely resemble curdled milk (Fig. 23-5). When an attempt is made to scrape off the patch, the underlying mucosa is seen to be raw and may bleed. Inspection alone is usually adequate to diagnose thrush, although the plaque may be cultured for *Candida albicans*.

Management Thrush is eventually self-limiting, but it should be treated with good hygiene and application of a fungicide to prevent spread into the upper respiratory or gastrointestinal tracts. Three fungicides are commonly effective in treating thrush. One treatment is to apply gentian violet to the patches three to four times daily. Placing the infant on his abdomen after application prevents swallowing of the fungicide, which is irritating to the trachea and esophagus. Caution should be used in application, since gentian violet stains anything it contacts.

Nystatin is another fungicide effective against Candida when applied to the oral cavity four times a day for one week. It can be swallowed to treat any moniliasis of the gastrointestinal tract and should be applied after feedings. It must be given slowly, with some applied to each side of the mouth before it is swallowed to ensure adequate exposure of the oral mucosa to the medication. Parents should be directed to complete the seven-day regimen even if the lesions have cleared.

Application of 3 per cent hydrogen peroxide may also be effective treatment and promotes debridement of the affected membranes.

Boiling bottles and nipples for 20 minutes before use, following feedings with plain water, and use of good handwashing technique by the infant's caretakers are preventive measures.

Blennorrhea

Blennorrhea, or inclusion conjunctivitis, is a communicable conjunctival disease, primarily of the newborn. It appears about the 5th to 15th day of life, following exposure to the richettsia *Chlamydia oculogenitalis* (bedsonia) during passage through the birth canal. It may also be transmitted after birth by the genito-eye route if infected persons do not practice good hand hygiene before handling the child. Since the infection is communicable, there is obligatory reporting of cases in the neonate.[12]

Symptoms are those of any conjunctivitis — edematous lids, hyperemia, mucopurulent discharge from the eye and fever. Diagnosis is confirmed when conjunctival scrapings stained with Giemsa stain reveal cap-like cytoplasmic inclusion bodies near the nuclei of host epithelial cells, indicating invasion by bedsonia.

Proper management requires isolation up to 48 hours after treatment is begun, using sulfonamide or chloramphenicol ophthalmic drops four to six times daily for one week. The mother is treated simultaneously with an oral sulfonamide for her genital infection. Unlike other forms of conjunctivitis, blennorrhea does not respond to penicillin. The mother must be taught proper handwashing technique to prevent recurrence of this or other transferable infections to her child. Blennorrhea will resolve spontaneously, with the acute phase lasting 10 days to two weeks in newborns and six to eight weeks in older infants or children. The chronic phase of minimal exudate lasts three to four months.

Roseola Infantum (Exanthem Subitum)

Roseola is a slightly contagious communicable disease that may appear in children from 6 months to 3 years of age, with a peak incidence before 1 year of age.[14] Although it occurs sporadically throughout the year, a concentration of cases occurs in the spring. The disease has an incubation period of 7 to 18 days. Although etiology is not definitely known, roseola is suspected to be viral and transmitted by airborne droplets.

Onset is sudden, with a high fever of 40° to 41.1° C (104° to 106° F) that lasts three or four days and then has a precipitous drop to normal. This is followed by the unexpected appearance of a pinkish-red, maculopapular rash. The rash is discrete, fades on pressure, favors the trunk and neck and spontaneously fades in one or two days. The child does not appear as ill as his temperature suggests. The course may include anorexia, mild malaise and some irritability.

Management is symptomatic to reduce the fever and prevent irritation of the rash that could invite secondary infection. The child should be isolated until symptoms subside.

The Common Cold

The common cold is a mild illness that does not include bacterial superinfection of the upper respiratory tract.[15] There are typically three epidemic waves of the common cold annually. The greatest incidence seems to occur during the fall months, while the more severe cases with greater tendency for complications tend to occur in midwinter. Another round of mild cases occurs in the spring. The common cold is, in fact, the most prevalent infectious disease among all ages, with older children and adults averaging two colds per year, while children under four years average eight colds per year.[15] Boys are more affected during infancy and toddlerhood, whereas girls have the larger proportion of colds after age 3.[15] Infants and toddlers have severe responses to upper respiratory infections (URI) out of proportion to the local manifestations experienced.[14] This age group also more frequently develops complications.

Viral invasion of the mucous membranes of the upper respiratory tract causes swelling and hypersecretion of mucus. Symptoms are preceded by a 24- to 48-hour incubation period, which is why isolation is ineffective in preventing spread of this disease. There are approximately 100 different cold-causing viruses; however, about 35 per cent of children's colds are caused by rhinovirus.[15] These viruses are transmitted directly (air droplets) and indirectly (fomites).

Clinical Manifestations Symptoms usually last two to 10 days and begin with a fever. Infants and toddlers frequently show a rapid temperature elevation (39.5° to 40.5° C [103° to 105° F]), occurring in the presence of even mild infection. Neonates and premature infants often have no fever or may even show a reduction in temperature during cold infections. Older children and adults usually run a low-grade fever under 37.8° C (100° F). Mucous membrane irritation by the virus results in rhinorrhea, stuffy nose and generalized nasopharyngeal congestion. The obstruction these symptoms pose to respirations causes the child to experience restlessness, malaise and anorexia (because of the difficulty sucking poses to adequate oxygenation). The irritation to membranes also causes sneezing, increased lacrimation and a raspy sensation in the back of the throat. Hyperexcretion of mucus causes coughing, especially at night when secretions pool in the nasopharyngeal cavity. The excess mucus, containing virus, that is swallowed may produce diarrhea. Bacterial superinfections of the tonsils, ears, sinuses or lower respiratory tract are not infrequent, especially in infancy. Secondary dehydration is also a potential problem in infants or toddlers with colds. Diagnosis is based on history and clinical manifestations. A culture of nasal discharge may be made to determine if bacterial involvement exists. The common cold is self-limiting and, although it affects millions each year, its cure eludes medical science. Treatment is therefore symptomatic in nature, focusing on (1) general comfort measures, (2) procedures to relieve local irritation and (3) relief through use of medication.[8]

Treatment

General Comfort Measures Keeping the infant's exposure to family members minimal for the duration of his fever may help control the cold's spread. It also helps minimize external stimuli during this phase when stimuli irritate the infant. This action also serves to decrease the child's exposure to other viruses or bacteria that might cause superinfection.

Rest in bed until the fever subsides helps reduce the likelihood of secondary complications. Raising the head of the bed up on blocks helps the infant to breathe easier. Placing the infant on his stomach facilitates the drainage of nasal secretions. Bed rest is hard to achieve in the older infant but a satisfactory compromise is quiet play in a playpen.

Anorexia is often frustrating to the parent. Urging food often leads to vomiting or diarrhea, while forcing it may cause food aversions. Parents should be reassured that a brief interval without normal intake will not create malnutrition. Allowing the child to establish his own intake is usually best, provided nourishment is offered at fairly frequent intervals. Diluting or temporarily eliminating formula, providing a liquid diet and suctioning the nose with an ear bulb syringe to remove excess secretions prior to feedings are helpful suggestions to help maintain adequate intake.[19]

Relief from the discomforts caused by fever is achieved by dressing the child in light clothing, keeping room temperatures somewhat cool and sponging with tepid water when temperatures reach 39.5° C (103° F) or higher.

Local Symptom Relief Several measures may be taken to help relieve nasal congestion. Saline nose drops (1 tsp of salt in 1 pint of warm water) are usually satisfactory to clear secretions in young infants. Vasoconstrictive decongestant nose drops such as Neo-Synephrine 0.25 per cent shrink congested nasal membranes, making breathing much easier for the older infant. They are not effective if abundant thick exudate is occluding the nares.

To administer nose drops, the child's head should be lowered and turned to the side. Several drops should be injected into the lower nostril and the position maintained for one minute; then the procedure is repeated in the opposite nostril. Nasal drops should not be administered longer than two days, since danger of rebound engorgement exists after that time.[15] Postural drainage facilitates loosening and drainage of secretions from the upper airway. A cold steam vaporizer also liquifies and loosens secretions of the upper airway as well as soothing irritated membranes and relieving coughing. Gentle removal of excessive mucus exudate with an infant aspirator or ear bulb syringe four to five times a day (especially before feeding) increases the effectiveness of nasal drops or vaporizer. Petroleum jelly applied regularly to chapped lips and irritated nose both soothes and prevents further excoriation.

Medication Antipyretics may be employed, such as aspirin or acetaminophen (Tylenol), to reduce fever. If aspirin is used to reduce fever, extra special care must be taken in handling and disposal of nasal secretions since its use increases the viral content of those secretions. A decongestant may be prescribed to help reduce congestion of the nasal passages. An antitussive may be desirable if coughing is paroxysmal or if necessary at bedtime to facilitate adequate rest. Vitamin C is highly debated as an effective agent in treating a cold, but some evidence exists that it aids in reducing its severity and slightly shortens it course.[15] Bacterial superinfections may be treated with antibacterials, but this may result in some increase of the cold symptoms since antibiotics destroy bacteria that are functionally helping to control the cold virus.[15] Research is currently being conducted to develop an antiviral drug that would be effective against the common cold as well as other viral disease. (See the box for a discussion of interferon.)

When a child under 4 is being treated for a cold at home, phone follow-up by the nurse is wise to ascertain whether the cold is resolving or complications are developing, since colds in young children often are a precursor to streptococcal infections. Parents should also be told to seek medical help if their child develops retractions, nasal flaring or grunting; if nasal discharge becomes purulent, foul smelling, thick or bloody; when fever persists beyond 48 to 72 hours; or if the child has a cold without fever and fever occurs after three or four days, indicating bacterial involvement.

Otitis Media

Otitis media is the most common complication of upper respiratory infections. Infants and children under 3 years are particularly predisposed because of their shorter, more horizontal, wider and more distensible eustachian tube that more readily allows passage of foreign matter up the tube. The infant's humoral defenses are also less developed. His usual lying position also increases his susceptibility because fluid pools in the pharyngeal cavity, hindering tube drainage.

Obstruction of the eustachian tube from enlarged adenoids, URI with mucosal edema, nasal allergy or cleft palate — all of which are common in young children — results in nonpurulent middle ear effusion referred to as *serous otitis media*. *Suppurative otitis media* results from accumulation of bacterial or viral exudate (usually *Hemophilus influenzae*, streptococci or pneumococci) in the middle ear.

Normally the eustachian tube is closed and flat, opening only long enough to permit drainage of middle ear secretions. With blockage drainage is impaired, causing retention of secretions (serous otitis media). Trapped air is absorbed during circulation and a vacuum is produced (negative middle ear pressure). If the tube opens, infectious organisms are swept into the middle ear owing to the pressure change (suppurative otitis media).

Clinical Manifestations Since otitis media is often associated with upper respiratory infections, respiratory symptoms are usually present. An upper respiratory infection with persistent fever always suggests otitis media. Table 23–6 describes the otologic symptoms that exist in serous and suppurative otitis media. If persistent or recurrent otitis media infection occurs, the tympanic membrane (eardrum) becomes stretched enough so that retraction or bulging does not create pain. Table 23–6 also describes the typical behavior or complaints and systemic signs that suggest otitis media.

Diagnosis Physical examination will reveal edematous, erythematous nasal cavities with clear (viral) or greenish-yellow (bacterial) exudate present. Otoscopic examination also reveals varying degrees of change from normal. The tympanic membrane (eardrum) is usually easily visible, but its appearance varies. Table 23–6 describes the usual otologic manifestations. Nasopharyngeal cultures are worthless in diagnosing suppurative otitis media organisms, as the infectious agent of the ear is most often not the same one that is causing nasopharyngeal symptoms.[14] If purulent ear drainage exists, it should be cultured for specific organisms.

Tympanometry is considered one of the most reliable indicators of otitis media.[23] It involves the placement of a soft rubber cuff over the external ear canal to achieve an airtight seal at which time air pressure registers on an attached hand-held probe. Decreased tympanic membrane mobility, indicated by a negative air

---

INTERFERON

Researchers have isolated an antiviral agent, interferon, that effectively prevents new viral growth and limits the spread of existing organisms. Interferon is made up of a class of soluble small proteins manufactured in small quantities within the body; therefore, it causes minimal side effects or toxicity. Ingested intranasally, interferon does prevent colds when large dosages are used.

So far interferon can be extracted only from human leukocytes (those of other species are not effective), which makes it a rather scarce commodity and very costly. Scientists are attempting to develop interferon inducers that will stimulate the body to increase its own interferon production to prevent viral infection.[15]

TABLE 23-6 A COMPARISON OF SEROUS OTITIS MEDIA AND SUPPURATIVE OTITIS MEDIA

	Pathology	Etiology	Otologic Manifestations	Indicative Behaviors or Complaints
Serous otitis media (fluid ear)	Nonpurulent middle ear effusion	Blocked eustachian tube causes retention of middle ear secretions	May not be any. Light reflex obscured. Varying degrees of hyperemia, redness of tympanic membrane (eardrum). Bony landmarks are visible with handle of malleus prominent and more horizontal, and umbo is stark white. Fluid level (miniscus) sometimes visible through the eardrum. Membrane retracted, usually in posterosuperior region.	May be none. Fullness in ear. May feel some pain in early stage. Snapping sensation when swallow or yawn. Diminished hearing expressed by listlessness and general inattentiveness to voice in infant. Rolling motions of head. Tugging or digging at ear. Restlessness.
Suppurative otitis media	Purulent accumulation of exudate in middle ear	Bacterial or viral invasion of middle ear secretions often secondary to middle ear effusion (negative pressure draws infectious organisms in)	Light reflex obscured or absent. Vivid (angry) red tympanic membrane. Fluid miniscus or bubbling visible through membrane; obscuring of bony landmarks. Membrane bulging—spontaneous rupture possible.	Discomfort expressed when ear touched. Fever. Pain acute (earache). May have purulent ear drainage if eardrum ruptures. Inconsolable irritability and restlessness. Persistent crying. May have cervical lymph node involvement.

pressure, reveals serous otitis media. Treatment of this can prevent development of suppurative otitis media.

Management Vigorous antibiotic therapy for 10 to 14 days is essential to get suppurative otitis media under control. Ampicillin is often the drug of choice. Since symptoms usually subside in 24 to 48 hours, the nurse must give adequate explanations to parents so they understand that the full course of drug therapy is necessary to eradicate the infection, despite the child's apparent early improvement. A phone follow-up in two to five days after therapy is initiated is appropriate to determine if the drug seems to be taking effect and relieving symptoms. The child should be re-evaluated at the end of the therapy course to determine if the infection is resolved. Ideally, another checkup is done in two to three months to ensure that a chronic condition does not exist.

A decongestant may be prescribed for suppurative otitis media to reduce membrane edema and improve eustachian tube function. Analgesic and antipyretic drugs may also be used to relieve earache and fever. Application of heat or cold to the affected ear region may also relieve discomfort. Young children should be watched closely for signs of secondary mastoiditis, meningitis (especially under 4 months of age), or hearing loss.

Serous otitis media is treated with a four-week course of antihistamines and decongestants to shrink membranes and improve eustachian tube function. If hearing loss persists or treatment does not resolve the problem, myringotomy or aspiration is indicated. Aeration of the middle ear can be taught to the older child and is achieved by pinching the nose then closing the lips and forcing air into the ear by blowing up balloons or chewing sugarless gum.[18] When a child has recurrent serous otitis, parents should be instructed to initiate drug treatment prophylactically at the first sign of upper respiratory infection. If allergy is contributing to serous otitis, its evaluation and treatment is important to prevent recurrent otitis involvement.

If the accumulated fluid of either type of otitis media has not begun to subside in two to five days after therapy is initiated, aspiration of fluid by surgical incision of the eardrum (myringotomy) or placement of myringotomy tubes to facilitate drainage may be indicated. The procedure is performed under general anesthesia in children. Suppurative complications may also require myringotomy. The incision allows for removal of the accumulated fluid. If tubes are placed, they function as accessory eustachian tubes, allowing air exchange between the middle and outer ear. The tubes are made to work their way out in two to nine months. A small amount of bloody drainage and slight pain is normal when the tubes work their way out.[13]

Draining exudate should be cleansed from the external ear canal frequently with sterile cotton swabs soaked in hydrogen peroxide to prevent excoriation. The ear canal is straightened for cleansing by pulling *down* and *back* on the ear lobe of children under 3 years or *up* and *back* for older children. If myringotomy tubes are placed, parents need instruction to plug the ears lightly with sterile cotton coated with petroleum jelly during baths or shampooing to keep water from entering the ear canal. Swimming is best avoided until they are removed.

Mastoiditis

Acute mastoiditis, a frequent complication of suppurative otitis media, has become rare since the availability of antibiotics. It does still occur in children with untreated otitis media or when the antibiotic course was inadequate in dose or duration of administration. The anatomical communication between the mastoid process and middle ear invites infectious exchange.

Clinically mastoiditis presents with pain over the mastoid process, erythema, edema and tenderness to pressure. Diagnosis may be difficult if the infection has been partially suppressed by antibiotics.

Once the condition is diagnosed, antibiotic therapy should be begun immediately. Sedation may be necessary to allay restlessness until pain subsides. Pain is lessened by application of a cold compress or ice bag to the mastoid process. Fever is relieved with antipyretics.

Mastoidectomy is indicated only if subperiosteal abscess occurs or if antibiotic therapy fails.

GASTROINTESTINAL DISTURBANCES

Constipation

Some infants have recurrent or chronic constipation during which stool is passed infrequently or, if passed daily, consists of hard, small masses. Often the cause is a diet that contains too much cow's milk or insufficient amounts of fluids or bulk-forming foods. Prevention and correction require that parents receive instruction in the diet needs of their infant. When an infant is on solids, parents should be taught to offer cereals, vegetables, fruits and meat before offering milk. The infant also needs plenty of fluids besides milk. After he reaches 6 months of age, he can have some foods that are finely chopped rather than pureed to increase bulk. Honey or molasses may be added to milk for infants who are prone to constipation. Prunes or prune juice should be offered regularly to infants with a tendency to hard stools.

Conditions that make defecation painful may also promote constipation, as the child withholds feces to avoid pain. The most common condition is anal fissures that have developed during the previous passage of hard stool. Inspection of the anus to identify fissures is done by placing a thumb on either side of the anus and retracting the anal tissues laterally. Fissures are cauterized with full-strength silver nitrate. Until healing is complete, an anesthetic ointment and stool softener may be prescribed to relieve defecatory distress. Another condition that makes defecation painful, rectal prolapse, is discussed in Chapter 24.

Mechanical obstruction may also precipitate constipation. Rectal stenosis and Hirschsprung's disease are often etiological factors. Rectal stenosis can be confirmed by digital examination. The little finger will be difficult to insert into the anus, and will seem to meet with resistance in the presence of stenosis. The stenosis is corrected by frequent dilation of the anal canal with the finger regularly until the stenosis is eliminated. Hirschsprung's disease is discussed in Chapter 24.

In older infants and children constipation may be due to a chronic misuse of laxatives by apprehensive parents or a psychological response to faulty toilet training, producing poor bowel evacuation habits.

Regardless of the etiology of constipation in infancy, certain measures may be taken to promote adequate defecations while the etiological factor is being remedied. The first of these measures is use of a mild laxative. However, laxatives should not be used for longer than two weeks (milk of magnesia is not used in infants except in severe constipation). Second, a stool softener may be given until normal bowel habits are established, especially when lesions are involved. Third, if impaction exists, an isotonic (1 level tsp salt to a pint of water) enema solution may be administered to clear the bowel. It should be stressed, however, that most constipation in infancy is readily managed by diet alone.

Parents need reassurance that their child does not absorb toxic substances from the bowel during constipation. They also may need orientation to the normal variations in bowel habits among children. Both verbal and written instruction should be given the parents regarding treatment measures to be conducted at home. One or two demonstrations should also be a part of instruction when parents seem unsure of instructions or if nursing judgment establishes the need.

Mild Diarrhea

Diarrhea is very common in infancy, and as a general rule the younger the infant is, the more susceptible he is and the more severe the diarrhea is likely to be. It is a symptom that accompanies a variety of childhood illnesses. (See Chapter 24 for a discussion of gastroenteritis, a more severe form of diarrhea.) Fluid and electrolyte imbalance poses the greatest hazard in diarrhea of the infant. Diarrhea is the consequence of increased motility and decreased absorption within the intestine for whatever reason and results in looser, more watery and more frequent bowel evacuation than is normal. Particularly in the infant, this can lead rapidly to dehydration, metabolic acidosis or shock.[10] Mild diarrhea is described as the evacuation of a few loose stools of a mucous or greenish nature or both without any other symptoms other than perhaps a low-grade fever and transient anorexia. The diarrhea ends after two to five days.[10]

Noninfectious diarrhea can result from several etiologies. (1) Teething. This is probably because of the increased amounts of saliva swallowed during that time. (2) Overfeeding. This is the most common cause of mild diarrhea and usually is accompanied by vomiting. (3) Food intolerance. Most often this is an allergic reaction to milk in infants. (4) Antibiotics. The normal floral balance of the bowel is disturbed, interrupting normal digestive function. (5) Parenteral (not gastrointestinal related) disease. Most often this is the common cold. (6) Unexplained etiology. Some infants have periodic bouts of mild diarrhea without any apparent reason.[10]

Diagnosis of mild noninfectious diarrhea is established from a history that portrays the characteristic diarrhea stool without any change in the infant's behavior or eating habits. Urinary output is normal, coloring is good, and no vomiting or fever exists. History also will usually reveal one or more of the typical etiological factors.

Mild diarrhea is usually treated at home by parents under the indirect supervision of the nurse practitioner, community nurse or physician. Once mild diarrhea is diagnosed, management involves continued observation and dietary measures until normal bowel patterns are re-established.

Nursing management involves evaluating the caretaker's knowledge of normal stool characteristics. Proper dietary management of the diarrhea must be taught. Parents also need instruction about the symptoms of dehydration or bacterial involvement and how these are evaluated. That the onset of these symptoms should be reported immediately if they occur must be emphasized. See Chapter 24 for a discussion of these teaching points in the gastroenteritis section. Any changes in fecal characteristics other than a return to normal should be noted and reported promptly also. If stool specimens of the affected infant or of other family members are desired, the parent(s) is given oral and written instruction in how to collect and dispense with them and is provided with the appropriate specimen containers. If the diarrhea worsens or does not resolve within five days, the child should be seen again and re-evaluated.

Diet management is aimed at a temporary decrease in oral intake to rest the bowel, coupled with adequate fluid and electrolyte replacement. How long oral intake is withheld (NPO) before intake is gradually reinitiated and the types of fluid to be initiated depend upon the philosophy of the physician. Although many variations exist, two main approaches characterize the usual diet management for mild diarrhea. Table 23–7 describes these two approaches. Both approaches decrease solid foods to rest the bowel while increasing fluids to

TABLE 23-7 TWO BASIC APPROACHES TO MANAGEMENT OF MILD DIARRHEA

| Starvation Method | | Feeding Method | |
Duration	Diet	Duration	Diet
First 2–6 hours	Nothing by mouth.	First 2–6 hours	Nothing by mouth. (Skip 1 or 2 feedings.)
Next 12 hours	No solid foods or formula. Offer small amounts of clear liquids often, such as boiled water, sugar water, Jello water (1–2 bl. jello per 8 oz of water); weak sweetened tea; flat coke, ginger ale or root beer, Gatorade, half-strength bouillon, apple juice, or grape juice. Continue breast-feeding if usual feeding method.	Remainder of first 24 hours or until stools return to normal	Half-strength formula or milk and clear liquids (offer every 4 hours). See other column for clear liquids. If fluids do not satisfy infant's hunger, offer foods with high pectin content, such as mashed ripe banana, scraped apple, rice cereal, jello. After 12 hours, if stools are progressing toward normal character and frequency, begin gradually increasing strength of formula or milk.
Remainder of first 24 hours	Increase quantities of clear liquids offered.		
Second 24 hours, if stools are nearing normal character and and frequency	Add high pectin content foods (see other column for list), saltine crackers and dry toast.	After 24 hours with normal stools	Return to full-strength formula or milk and continue clear liquids.
After 24 hours with normal stools	Return gradually to full-strength formula or milk and continue clear liquids.	After 48 hours with normal stools	Return to usual solid food diet.
After 48 hours with normal stools and for next 48 hours	Gradual progression to usual solid food diet, beginning with bland, low residue foods, such as hard boiled or scrambled egg (no butter), custards and puddings, well cooked ground hamburger, baked potato (no butter).		

ensure adequate fluid and electrolyte replacement. The feeding method should not be utilized if the infant's diarrhea is accompanied by vomiting.[10] As a general rule fluids are tolerated best if offered at room temperature, since cold increases intestinal activity. Many infants also do not tolerate feedings more frequently than every two hours because too frequent feedings activate their gastrocolic reflex. In some instances an antispasmodic is temporarily prescribed.

Colic

Colic is characterized by vigorous crying and drawing of the legs up to the abdomen. It occurs in infants under three months of age and rarely persists past that time, although parents cannot be guaranteed of this. It usually begins several days after birth and is suspected to be the result of paroxysmal abdominal cramping, although specific etiology is rarely uncovered. Colic is often a symptom of gastrointestinal allergy. Many children who experience colic in infancy later evidence allergic disease of some type. Occasionally colic can be connected with improper feeding techniques or inadequate burping, but this etiology is not nearly as prevalent as was once thought, since change in diet or burping and feeding methods rarely eliminates colic.

Despite the fact that colic disappears spontaneously and is often given only minor attention by medical personnel, any family — especially the main caretaker — that has lived through only a few days of the crying episodes of an infant that is unresponsive to any efforts to comfort or console feels the extreme emotional impact. The disruption that a crying, irritable infant causes to family relationships and routines produces a vicious cycle of fatigue, frustration, anger and helplessness that can be destructive to family unit functioning if sympathetic intervention is not initiated early and continuously until the colicky period is outgrown.

Intervention should have three foci: (1) emotional support to family members, especially the primary caretaker; (2) efforts to maintain healthy attachment development; and (3) efforts to reduce or prevent colic episodes. A detailed history of daily events to establish any pattern to the colic attacks or any precipitating factors and to document caretaker reactions and efforts taken to relieve the crying facilitates colic management. Colic associated with improper feeding methods, although rare is readily halted by improvement in technique achieved through teaching. Caregivers should be asked to demonstrate the feeding process to rule out this possible source of colic.

Emotional support involves reassurances to the caregiver that despite the crying and pain, the infant is gaining weight and developing normally. Regular emphasis should be placed on the fact that colic is not the result of poor mothering, and that maternal feelings of inadequacy, anger or periodic dislike of the baby and mothering are universal. The caretaker should be offered regular opportunities to talk about her feelings and be encouraged to do so. Some communities have parental stress hot lines (COPE, CALM), which parents of colicky infants should be informed of. They should be encouraged to keep the number available even if they never need to use it.[25] Some parents find solace just in knowing the resource is there in case the stress becomes too much.

The caretaker should be urged to spend time away from the colicky infant on a fairly regular basis. Some relief from constant full responsibility makes most caretakers better able to handle themselves when they are "on duty." Some parents need help to overcome guilt feelings associated with "getting away" awhile.

There is no reason why a caretaker should have to listen to the noise if this can be avoided. Radl comments: "It is far less heartless to close the door of the baby's room, to use ear plugs, stuff cotton in your ears, or turn up the stereo full blast, than it is to become so frustrated and angry that you lose control and resort to hitting or shaking. If the weather is nice and you can go outside, so much the better. And remember that people who may criticize you for such practices generally aren't subject to this particular situation."[25]

Recognizing those times when it is harder to cope helps some parents achieve better control or think of ways to circumvent total responsibility for infant care at those times. Situations commonly identified as more stressful include the dinner hour, premenstrual days, holidays, and days when routine is disrupted.

Fostering attachment is important, since frequent negative feelings can eventually disrupt development of healthy parent-child attachment. Pointing out the infant's desirable features and signs of normal development regularly helps the parent(s) focus on more pleasant aspects of the child that encourage attachment feelings. Acknowledging and praising positive interaction between parent and infant as well as helping the parent notice how the infant responds to parental overtures also nurture healthy bonds.

Efforts to prevent or reduce colic episodes require experimentation, since success of a given method is highly individualistic. Some infants respond to measures that stimulate peristalsis. This may be achieved by carrying the infant close,* placing him prone over a warm towel, hot water bottle or heating pad or by offering the infant a couple of ounces of warm diluted tea. Much caution should be used with a heating pad or hot water bottle, as severe burns can occur with too much heat. The infant's skin does not tolerate as much heat as does that of older children or adults. The hot water bottle should be securely closed. Either appliance should be covered with a towel before placing the baby on it. A heating pad should never be set above the medium temperature for an infant. The infant's skin should be checked frequently when these appliances are used to ensure that overheating of the skin does not occur.

Other infants show improvement when their position is changed often, when they are burped using the shoulder method and massaging rather than patting, and when smaller feedings are offered more frequently. Taking time to

---

*An infant carrier allows the caretaker to keep the infant close in either a chest or back position while giving freedom of the hands to carry out activities.

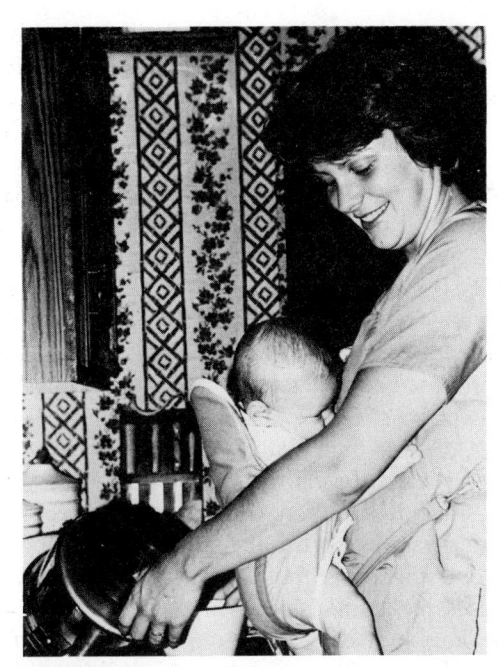

An infant carrier allows the caretaker to keep the infant close while giving freedom of the hands to carry out other activities.

relax and play with the baby before beginning feeding and placing the baby in an infant seat for at least 30 minutes after feedings is sometimes effective in reducing colic episodes. Glycerine suppositories (child size) or digital stimulation of the rectum with the little finger to relieve flatus may be effective in infants whose colic episodes seem to be associated with abdominal distention.[27, 29]

Some infants can be successfully distracted from their colicky episodes with brightly colored wrapping paper, pictures of varying complexity and depth, or music of varied rhythm and loudness. Some colicky infants respond to the rhythm of an automatic infant swing or to being placed on top of a running clothes dryer. Use of sedatives is sometimes prescribed but it is wise to reserve these for bedtime so that adequate rest of both infant and caretaker is insured. It is preferably used as a last resort measure rather than as a routine intervention.

Esophageal Chalasia

Esophageal chalasia involves failure of the cardioesophageal sphincter mechanism to prevent reflux of gastric contents into the esophagus, resulting in regurgitation of foodstuffs even when the patient is supine or prone. Forceful or projectile vomiting rarely occurs. This inappropriate relaxation of the lower esophageal sphincter occurs in infants during the first month of life, usually in the first days or weeks of life.

Physical examination reveals nothing unless vomiting is severe enough to prevent adequate hydration or normal weight gain. Barium swallow reveals normal gastrointestinal structures and passage but the cardia remains open, allowing reflux.

Esophageal chalasia tends to be self-corrective within a few weeks or months, but measures can be taken to facilitate correction and to discourage regurgitation.[14] Offering this child frequent small feedings of formula thickened with cereal and placing him in a sitting or semi-sitting position for an hour after feedings is easily explained to parents, along with the rationale for these measures. Antispasmodics and mild sedatives are sometimes helpful in more severe cases, particularly if vomiting is impairing growth and hydration. Positional treatment, which consists of placing the infant in a head-up supine position while on a 45 degree angle 24 hours a day, is indicated for severe cases (see Fig. 24–26). Reassurances about the brevity of this condition help parents to cope with this temporary problem.

NEUROMUSCULAR DISORDERS

Peripheral Nerve Injuries

The bracheal nerve palsies (Erb-Duchenne paralysis and Klumpke's palsy) and facial palsy are injuries that result from the trauma of birth causing peripheral nerve damage.

Erb-Duchenne paralysis is most common and involves a temporary paralysis of the upper arm following forceps or manual breech deliveries. The condition is obvious at birth and results from a stretching of the anterior roots of the fifth and sixth cervical nerves. The affected arm is held close to the chest, is not flexed at the elbow and is internally rotated with forearm rotation. Abduction and external rotation of the shoulder are impossible. Correction involves placing the paralyzed muscles in a position of rest by tying the arm to the head of the crib in a position of abduction, with external rotation of the shoulder and forearm supination. Sometimes a Statue of Liberty splint or cast is applied. It must be changed frequently due to the rapid growth of infants. Passive range of motion is important to maintain circulation and muscle tonus in the affected arm. Careful support is essential when the child is moved to prevent shoulder dislocation.

Lower arm palsy (Klumpke's palsy) is less common and results from pulling and stretching the arm while the trunk is essentially immobile during delivery. The compression on the eighth cranial nerve and first thoracic nerve from hemorrhage and edema creates paralysis of the wrist and hand. Obvious at birth, the hand falls limp in the flexor position. Wrist movements are not possible and the grasp reflex is absent. Treatment requires supporting the hand and wrist by binding them firmly to a flat splint under the palm and forearm. Passive range of motion is important to recovery.

Unilateral facial paralysis (facial palsy) is common after rapid spontaneous or forceps deliveries. It is caused by pressure of the mother's sacrum on the posterior cheek as the head moves through the birth canal. The affected side appears smooth with no forehead wrinkling on that side, the eye does not close firmly and the mouth droops at the corner. These characteristics become more obvious during crying.

Recovery from peripheral nerve injuries depends on the degree of nerve damage. Mild paralysis spontaneously disappears in one to three months. Injuries of moderate degree improve more slowly, and reconstructive surgery may be needed if recovery is not complete within two years. Severe injuries involving tearing or neural cell death do not improve, and wasting of the part increases with age.

Parents must learn how to properly position the affected extremity and how to do range of motion exercises. Since compliance is very important to recovery, community health nurse follow-up is usually wise.

Neonatal Myasthenia Gravis

A transient form of myasthenia gravis occurs in infants born of mothers with myasthenia gravis. At birth or within a week the infant displays generalized weakness, hypotonia, a decreased Moro response, and ptosis, and has difficulty swallowing and sucking. Symptoms usually disappear within a month.

Febrile Seizures

One of the most common pediatric neurological problems, febrile convulsions, occurs in response to acute, benign febrile illnesses, particularly respiratory and gastrointestinal infections in which the temperature rises above 38.8° C (102° F). The seizure occurs at the onset of the fever. This transient disorder is twice as common in boys, occurring more often in children between 6 months and 3 years of age, with a peak incidence before 18 months of age.[4] Febrile seizures rarely occur after 5 years of age but may occur in children up to age 8. There seems to be a family predisposition, suggesting inheritance as a factor.

Two possible explanations of pathogenesis exist. One is that a rapid rise in fever reduces body sodium levels, which lowers the seizure threshold in children with pre-existing predisposing factors, precipitating a convulsion. A second theory is that the rapid rise of fever causes the convulsion owing to immatuity of the brain in infants and young children. Febrile convulsions will cease when the child is older and the brain has matured.

Regardless of the underlying pathogenesis, several predisposing factors do seem to contribute to the occurrence of febrile seizures.[4, 11, 28] These include a genetic predisposition; family history of allergies, especially to aspirin or penicillin; cerebral trauma at birth; a threatened abortion or cesarean section delivery; a history of fetal distress; and rapid rises in fever with infection.

Clinical Manifestations The convulsion usually occurs the first day of the fever. Neonates display focal seizures that may appear as a transient reduction in tonus or activity, focal motoric movements, oral or facial twitching, ocular deviation or an apneic spell. Infants and children usually show generalized tonic-clonic movements similar to grand mal seizures, manifested by generalized body stiffness, eye rolling and loss of muscle tonus. The lethargy following a benign seizure is less pronounced than in grand mal seizures. Febrile seizures most often last less than five minutes and seldom longer than 20 minutes.[4] This feature is the most significant in differentiating benign febrile seizures from those due to brain pathology.

Febrile convulsions may be benign or nonbenign (indicating brain pathology) with later development of epilepsy more likely in the nonbenign form. Table 23–8 characterizes both types of febrile seizures.

Diagnosis Authorities differ widely on the criteria for diagnosis and on signs that suggest

TABLE 23-8 CHARACTERISTICS OF BENIGN AND NONBENIGN SEIZURES

Benign	Nonbenign (Pathology Involved)
Brief, under 20 min duration, usually 5 min	Longer than 20 min duration
Generalized tonic-clonic seizure	Focal or psychomotor seizure
Neurologic evaluation normal prior to seizure	Suggestive of pre-existing neurological abnormality
No family history of epilepsy, may be history of febrile seizure	Family history of epilepsy
A single seizure associated with fever (>38.8° C); seizure occurs during first day of fever	Two or more seizures associated with fever with recurrence within 24 hours
Seizure occurs by 8 years of age, usually not before 6 months of age	Seizure occurs before 1 year of age
Normal EEG in 2 weeks	EEG may remain abnormal after 2 weeks
Often unresponsive to anticonvulsant therapy	Responds to anticonvulsant therapy

future seizures or interference in intellectual development. Physical examination focuses on identification of the source of infection and of any neurological abnormalities. History should cover familial predisposition to febrile or epileptic seizures and to allergy, the child's developmental progress, and details of any known allergy in the child. Any medications he has taken recently, any history of head injury, and labor and delivery details are also ascertained. A description of the manifestations of the fever and accompanying illness and a thorough description of present and past seizure activity are imperative data. Seizure documentation must include descriptions of the length of the seizure, when it occurred in relation to fever onset, the type of movement and body parts involved, behavior or symptoms just before the seizure and, if unconsciousness occurred, how long it lasted after the seizure. Table 23-9 lists laboratory tests and x-rays done to help establish diagnosis. Evaluation of cerebral spinal fluid is always conducted. Other tests are usually done only if long-term anticonvulsant therapy is being considered or if the seizure was nonbenign.[11]

The nurse has some responsibilities during the diagnostic phase besides preparing the older infant and parents for diagnostic tests and attending during procedures to either assist or to support the infant. One is to obtain a thorough nursing history, including facts surrounding the seizure, predisposing factors and details of any existing febrile illness. The nurse is involved in collecting diagnostic data regarding vital signs, hydration status, level of consciousness and observable signs and symptoms of febrile illness she assesses from the child. The nurse will consider in her history that parents cannot always accurately recall the details of the seizure.

Management Treatment focuses on care during seizure activity, control of fever, resolution of infection and chemotherapy.

Most febrile seizures are brief and require no specific intervention beyond measures to protect the child from injury and general support measures to maintain the airway. See the management of epileptic seizures in Chapter 52 for appropriate nursing intervention during seizure activity.

Measures taken to control fever depend on how elevated the temperature is. Encouraging drinking of fluids, keeping the child dressed in light clothing (diaper or panties), and alternate administration of acetaminophen (Tylenol) and aspirin (dosages of 60 mg/year of age) effectively manages fever under 39.5° C (103° F). Higher fevers may require vigorous sponging with tepid water 15 minutes of every hour or use of a cooling mattress. Infection resolution

TABLE 23-9 DIAGNOSTIC TESTS CONDUCTED TO ESTABLISH BENIGN FEBRILE SEIZURES

Diagnostic Test	Purpose (Rules Out (R/O) Cause of Seizure)
CSF (cerebrospinal fluid)	R/O meningitis
Blood electrolytes	Determine Na level, R/O electrolyte imbalance
Blood glucose	R/O hypoglycemia
Blood calcium	R/O hypocalcemia
Urine checked for blood	R/O glomerulonephritis
Blood urea nitrogen (BUN)	R/O glomerulonephritis
Chest x-ray	R/O Pneumonia infection
Skull x-ray	R/O head injury
EEG 7 to 14 days after seizure	If normal, was a benign febrile seizure

TABLE 23-10 CHEMOTHERAPEUTIC REGIMENS IN MANAGEMENT OF FEBRILE SEIZURES

No Therapy	Initial Therapy	Intermittent Therapy
Fever and infection control measures only	Immediately: IV Valium to control seizure (0.3 mg/kg to a maximum of 10 mg/24 hrs) IM or IV phenobarbital (6–15 mg/kg to a maximum of 120 mg/24 hrs as a loading dose), then 5 mg/kg oral doses till fever subsides, then 3–5 mg/kg/day orally for 2 to 4 years as a maintenance dose.)	Same as initial therapy until fever subsides; then the phenobarbital is tapered to none but prescribed to be given with onset of any fever.
Main argument against this method is that 50–60% of infants have at least a second febrile seizure, with 25% eventually developing epilepsy.	Blood levels of 15 micrograms/ml of blood must be maintained to prevent seizure; blood levels monitored every 3 months, dosage adjusted to growth changes. After 2–4 years if EEG is normal phenobarbital is decreased over 2 months and discontinued.	This method has not been proved effective. The main problem is that 48 hours is required before phenobarbital levels become adequate to control seizure. Another is that parents often neglect to get dosage altered as child grows.

will depend upon the disease but antibiotic therapy is usually indicated.

Prophylactic chemotherapy is controversial, with three regimens (Table 23–10) currently popular.[4, 11, 28]

Monitoring of vital signs and frequent evaluation of neurological status and hydration status are always appropriate nursing interventions when febrile seizures are suspected. The nurse has other responsibilities when febrile seizures are diagnosed. In addition to gathering the history and assisting with diagnostic tests, she must help parents cope with their fears, teach them how to prevent recurrence of seizures and how to manage them if they do recur. Many of the parents' fears are allayed by verbal reassurances that the febrile seizure does not mean that their child is epileptic. This is better understood if they are given explanations regarding the cause of febrile seizures. They should also be encouraged to verbalize their fears and talk about their reactions. Preventing recurrence requires that parents be taught how to take a temperature, how to use measures to reduce fever and how to safely administer antipyretics. (See Chapter 52 for instructions parents need in order to manage a seizure if it recurs.) The importance of seeking medical care any time a seizure occurs should be stressed. If prophylactic anticonvulsant therapy is begun, parents need to know how the medication works and how to administer it, the side effects to watch for and report, and the significance of having blood levels of anticonvulsant evaluated every three months.

DACRYOSTENOSIS

Dacryostenosis is a congenital lacrimal stenosis that creates an obstruction of the lacrimal duct and is often accompanied by dacryocystitis. This condition is relatively common in infancy. It is suspected in infants with purulent discharge (dacryocystitis) but without any conjunctival injection or irritation. Infants who have prompt recurrence of purulent discharge after cessation of ophthalmic antibiotics are also suspected. If pressure over the lacrimal sac produces an outpouring of mucopurulent material, diagnosis is confirmed. Excessive lacrimation (tearing) during the second month of life is a sign that suggests dacryostenosis which may be readily noticed by the nurse during infant examinations.

Nonsurgical correction involves forcing the

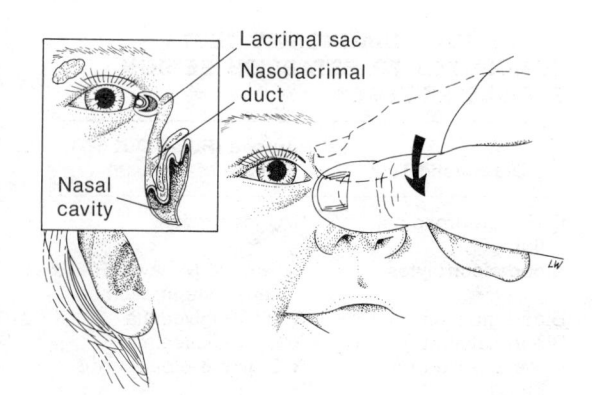

Figure 23-6 Massage of the lacrimal drainage tract to force fluid in the lacrimal sac through the obstructed drainage tract. The tip of the thumb is placed above the sac at the medial angle of the eye. Slowly and steadily the thumb is rolled downward. (Redrawn from J. McMillan et al. The Whole Pediatrician Catalogue, W. B. Saunders Co., 1977.)

fluid collected in the affected lacrimal sac through the obstructed duct by placing the tip of one thumb over the sac at the medial angle of the eye and slowly, steadily rolling the thumb toward the duct opening, thereby increasing pressure on the stenosis to gradually open it (Fig. 23-6). This is done four times daily for a month. The parents should be instructed in the procedure and should demonstrate its use satisfactorily. If this procedure does not open the duct within a month, an ophthalmologist can open the duct by probing the lacrimal tract. An ophthalmic antibiotic may be prescribed to control infection until the obstruction is cleared.

References

1. The Allergy Foundation of America. Food allergy. Pamphlet L-483, 1976.
2. The Allergy Foundation of America. The skin and its allergies. Pamphlet D-375, 1974
3. M. Bergner and C. Hutelmyer. Teaching kids how to live with their allergies. Nursing 76, August 1976, p. 11
4. R. Bindler and L. Howry. Nursing care of children with febrile seizures. American Journal of Maternal Child Nursing, Sept/Oct 1978, p. 270
5. M. J. Brakl. Atopic dermatitis. Patient Care, 15 August 1977, p. 69
6. S. Bridgewater et al. Allergies in children: recognition. American Journal of Nursing, April 1978, p. 613
7. R. Carty. Some facts about allergy. Pediatric Nursing. Mar/Apr 1977, p. 7
8. J. Cormier et al. Treating the common cold. Pediatric Nursing, Jan/Feb 1978, p. 7
9. W. Crook. Food allergy: the great masquerader. Pediatric Clinics of North America, Feb 1975, p. 227
10. A. Eden. Visit with a pediatrician: diarrhea. American Baby, November 1979, p. 10
11. R. Gorman and C. Snead. Febrile seizures. Academy of Family Practice Journal, January 1979, p. 101
12. D. Heffelfinger. Inclusion blennorrhea of the newborn. Clinical Pediatrics, July 1978, p. 579
13. H. Huber, Draining the "fluid ear" with myringotomy and tube insertion. Nursing 78, July 1978, p. 28
14. J. Hughes. Synopsis of Pediatrics. C.V. Mosby Co., 1979
15. R. Hutchinson. The common cold primer. Nursing 79, March 1979, p. 57
16. A. Jacobs. Eruptions in the diaper area. Pediatric Clinics of North America, May 1978, p. 209
17. G. Kahn. Eczematoid eruptions in children. Pediatric Clinics of North America, February 1975, p. 203
18. J. Kass and M. Beebe. Serous otitis media, Nurse Practitioner, Mar/Apr 1979, p. 25
19. I. Librach. Layman's guide to common complaints: common cold, stomach upsets. Part I. Nursing Mirror, 2 August 1979, p. 18
20. Mead Johnson & Co. Facts about allergy. Pamphlet 101, 1970
21. National Society for the Prevention of Blindness, Inc. Vocabulary of terms relating to the eye. Publication P-607, April 1973
22. M. C. Neal. The child with diarrhea. Nursing Care Plan Guide 3:17, NURSECO, 1977
23. J. Northern et al. Tympanometry: a technique for identifying ear disease in children. Pediatric Nursing Mar/Apr 1976, p. 32
24. J. Parrish. Dermatology and Skin Care. McGraw-Hill Book Co., 1975
25. S. Radl. Mother's Day Is Over. Warner Books, 1974
26. A. Rowe, Food Allergy: Its Manifestations and Control and the Elimination Diets. Charles C Thomas, 1972
27. P. Rowell. Infantile colic: reviewing the situation. Pediatric Nursing, May/June 1978, p. 20
28. J. Willis and E. Oppenheimer. Children's seizures and their management. Issues In Comprehensive Pediatric Nursing, 1977
29. L. Whaley and D. Wong. Nursing Care of Infants and Children. C.V. Mosby Co., 1979

Additional Recommended Reading

C. Beirman and C. Furukawa. Medical management of serous otitis in children. Pediatrics, May 1978, p. 768
C. Bertholf. Protocol: acute diarrhea. Nurse Practitioner, May/June 1978, p. 17
S. Bridgewater and R. Voigner. Allergies in children: teaching. American Journal of Nursing, April 1978, p. 620
M. Brown et al. Otitis media. Comprehensive Pediatric Nurse, August 1978, p. 35
J. Caldwell. A new look at colic. American Baby, August 1979, p. 24
S. Cohen and G. Glass. Skin rashes in infants and children. American Journal of Nursing, June 1978, p. 104
B. Dudding. Problems related to the common cold. Comprehensive Pediatric Nurse, August 1978, p. 1
C. Eng et al. Brachial plexus palsy in neonates and children. Archives of Physical Medical Rehabilitation, October 1978, p. 458
N. Gonzalez. What's eating you? Family Health, November 1977, p. 22
E. Hawkins-Walsh and C. Pettrone. Drugs used in the treatment of pediatric allergy and asthma. Pediatric Nursing, Mar/Apr 1977, p. 12
Investigation and treatment of allergy: Part 2. Nursing Times, 23 March 1978, p. 506
D. Kasanof. Office pediatrics: managing recurrent otitis media. Patient care, 30 May 1978, p. 158
M. Jones and T. Tuppett. Assessment of the red eye. Nurse Practitioner, Jan/Feb 1980, p. 10
C. May. Food allergy: a commentary. Pediatric Clinics of North America, February 1975, p. 217
C. McAdams. Interferon: The penicillin of the future. American Journal of Nursing, April 1980, p. 714
J. McMillan et al. The Whole Pediatrician Catalog. W. B. Saunders Co., 1977
Myringotomy. Patient Care, 15 September 1979, p. 141
H. Orgel. Genetic and developmental aspects of IgE. Pediatric Clinics of North America, February 1975, p. 17
C. Parker. Food allergies. American Journal of Nursing, February 1980, p. 262
R. Reisman and J. Bernstein. Allergy and secretory otitis media. Pediatric Clinics of North America, February 1975, p. 251
S. Todd et al. Allergy to food and chemicals: the scope of the problem: Part 1. Nursing Times, 16 March 1978, p. 438
M. Wessel. Allergy in infancy: early care can prevent future problems, Parents, December 1977, p. 18
J. Zapha et al. Self care for colds: a cost effective alternative to upper respiratory infection management. American Journal of Public Health, August 1979, p. 814
M. Ziai. Pediatrics. Little, Brown and Co., 1975

24 POTENTIAL STRESSES DURING INFANCY: REVERSIBLE ALTERATIONS IN HEALTH STATUS

THE NURSE'S ROLE WITH THE FAMILY

by Mabel Hunsberger, BSN, MSN

Reversible alterations in infant health status may be apparent at birth or may occur later. Regardless of the type of alteration, the nurse must recognize that the family of the affected infant needs continued understanding and support from the entire health team. The nurse's own interactions with the infant and the family are a primary contributing factor to the well-being of these families. Furthermore, the nurse can function in the capacity of coordinator and facilitator of health care. To function effectively, the nurse must have an understanding of (1) the reactions of a family when their well infant becomes ill, (2) her own reactions and those of the family when an infant with a defect is born and (3) her responsibility to support the parenting role when an infant's health status is altered.

Family Reactions When a Well Infant Becomes Ill: Nurse's Role

The complete dependency of an infant makes parents feel overwhelmed when their baby becomes ill. Even those parents who have developed confidence in their ability to parent suddenly feel helpless and anxious when their infant is sick. The nurse's actions can either help to compound their insecurity or restore their confidence. Questions asked during the initial interview frequently are threatening to parents. The parents may feel that the nurse is blaming them for the illness. For example, questions such as "How long has your infant been ill?" or "How have you treated the illness at home?" may mean to the parents that they should have sought treatment earlier or that they have done something wrong at home. The family with an infant is particularly vulnerable to these insecurities because the family members are still learning to respond to the cues of the baby. The nurse can avoid compounding the already-present guilt feelings of the parents by beginning the interview with a simple explanation of its purpose. Most important is that the nurse not be judgmental in her attitude.

It can be very difficult for a nurse to cope with her feelings if, in fact, she learns that the parents did neglect to seek treatment early enough. The nurse's first goal at this time is to restore the parent's confidence with her accepting attitude. At a later time, when the infant is recovering and the parents have re-established their own self-confidence, the nurse should attempt to help the parents identify those signs and symptoms that in retrospect were clues to their baby's illness. This will help the parents develop skill and confidence in caring for their baby in the event of future illness.

If the baby shows physical signs of illness such as high fever, paleness, listlessness or respiratory difficulty, parents may fear losing him. The nurse must, of course, give immediate attention to the baby. While she is busy suctioning, preparing IV's and giving oxygen, parents are haunted with the thought that their baby is dying. At a time when parents have a need to hold their baby to ward off the fear of losing him, it is often necessary to release him to a stranger who rushes him off for diagnostic procedures. Once the baby has been cared for, the nurse can ease the stress parents are feeling by providing a time for them to express how they feel. Often they feel stunned and in a state of shock and it is only by verbalizing their feelings that they and the nurse can begin to identify what they need most from the health team at this time. A basic need of all parents is to be made to feel welcome; the nurse must be sure that their guilt is not compounded by tactless communication from the health team.

During the course of an infant's illness each family member is affected by the increased attention needs of the infant. Parents become exhausted and siblings may regress or engage in aggressive attention-getting behaviors. A parent may be short-tempered in response to an older child's whining plea for attention, only to be rebuked by his or her spouse. The drain on the family's emotional resources is acute and the usual joys within the family are muted by the stress that each member is experiencing.

The nurse can intervene by helping family members to maintain optimal relationships. Parents frequently need the nurse to help them recognize that their own resources are being exhausted and that they need the assistance of relatives, neighbors or friends. The siblings of an infant are likely to be of toddler or preschool age and cannot cope well with a change in routine or the absence of parents. The nurse should encourage parents to ease the stress of siblings by having one parent available to them most of the time. Help can be sought from support persons to prepare meals and do laundry and other household chores, but a parent should be available to provide such securities as reading to siblings at bedtime and being there when they awaken. With some outside help, the couple's own relationship can also be maintained as some of the household duties are taken on by others.

The nurse can also intervene by encouraging parents to continue to provide the usual comforts and physical contacts for their infant even though he shows a reduced response. The smiles and softly spoken words of his parents may seem to have less meaning now. The baby may hardly notice the mobile or the carefully placed teddy bear. However, the nurse should encourage parents to continue to provide these necessary stimuli to enhance the baby's development and to maintain the infant-parent relationship.

Reactions When An Infant With a Defect is Born: Nurse's Role

The defects discussed in this chapter can be corrected. Some are visible at birth and others are not detected until later in infancy. The nurse who cares for these children and their parents should (1) understand her own reactions to the crisis, (2) have an idea of what the event means to the parents and (3) be able to deal with the family's response to the crisis.

Response of the Nurse Whether a defect is apparent at birth or discovered later in infancy, there is no time for the nurse or the family to prepare for this occurrence. The nurse may feel stunned and helpless, wishing to escape, and may initially look for ways to avoid any involvement with the baby or the parents. These are normal reactions and should be acknowledged as a beginning step toward understanding how the parents probably feel. If the nurse can accept these feelings within herself, she can seek assistance from other staff members to direct those feelings into effective communication with the family. It is when the nurse does not acknowledge her feelings and does not allow herself to react like other human beings that her feelings of anxiety and helplessness interfere with her effectiveness.

If she does not master her feelings, the parents may mistakenly sense the nurse to be disinterested and uncaring. Parents watch closely how the nurse responds to their baby. The way the nurse handles their baby, her facial expression, and even where the baby is placed in the nursery are interpreted by the parents as signals of acceptance or rejection.

Meaning of Having an Infant with a Defect Some people view the birth of an imperfect child as punishment for wrongdoing. Even though the parents may be able to accept their baby eventually, adjustment is difficult if friends and relatives are judgmental or begin avoiding contact with them.

Personal values will determine the meaning the defect will have for family members. No family can easily accept the birth of a baby with a defect, but a family who has a high acceptance of values of beauty, perfection and physical prowess characteristic of United States culture may have particular difficulty coping with the birth of their imperfect baby. The *appearance of the infant* and *whether or not the defect is correctable* have been reported to greatly influence the reactions of parents and their future attachment difficulties.[6, 16] Visible anomalies of the head have been reported as causing the greatest stress to parents.[16] However, Lampe and others studied parental visiting patterns and interactions between parents and their sick infant and found no significant differences between the reactions of parents who had an infant with a visible anomaly and those who had an infant with a hidden anomaly.[9] The important element for the nurse to recognize is that what she views as a minor defect may bring about intense reactions in parents because *they* perceive the infant to be imperfect and must cope with the stigma of producing a baby with a defect.

When a newborn requires surgery immediately or soon after birth, there are additional stresses on the family. The father must cope with visiting the infant and the mother in two separate hospital locations. Because the mother and infant are separated, it is important for the father to bring frequent reports to the mother regarding the baby. For this situation it has been recommended that a photograph be taken of the infant and be given to the mother during this period of separation.[8] Also, taking a picture before the separation helps to make the family feel more united.[3]

In many instances the functioning of the home is totally disrupted by the transfer of the infant to a distant regional center. In these situations siblings most often live with relatives. The father is torn between staying in close proximity to his wife or going to the center in which the baby is being treated. If the mother's recovery is prolonged because of delivery by cesarean birth or postpartal complications, the father frequently makes the decision to drive long distances for the sake of keeping in touch with his wife and the baby. Thus he has the opportunity to form a relationship with the baby before the mother does. This may result in differences of attachment experienced by the parents later.[13]

Benfield and others studied the attitudes, feelings and behavior in 101 mother-father pairs after their critically ill newborn was transferred to a regional center.[1] In the majority of these parents transfer of the newborn to a distant hospital brought about reactions similar to those in parents whose infants had died in the neonatal period. Those parents who experienced the most pleasure during their pregnancy also grieved more intensely. These findings have important implications for the nurse who works with these families. These families feel as if their baby has died, and they need the support of the nurse during the process of grieving. The intense grief which is expressed is not a sign that they are adjusting less well, but it is an expression of the disappointment they feel because of the loss of their hoped for normal, healthy child.

A defect that will require frequent hospitalization for staged repairs and long periods of recuperation is likely to cause additional family stress. One parent may be required to quit his or her job, resulting in loss of income. At the same time the high cost of specialized care may exhaust health insurance policies. Under these circumstances the nurse must refer the family to available resources that can help them to obtain assistance through special programs. A family with older children needs to cope with planning for the care of the other children while the baby is hospitalized. This may mean additional expenses for the family such as babysitting, eating out, and transportation. When a family's support systems are few, they will feel overwhelmed with the crisis of extensive or repeated surgery or both. The nurse should serve these families by helping them to find available support systems and financial assistance through referral to social service and public health agencies.

Parent's Response: Nurse's Role The way parents are told about their baby's problem can affect the adjustment period that follows. Any delay in showing the infant or telling them specifically what is wrong when they know that a problem exists leaves them to use their own imaginations. Parents tend to formulate extreme distortions or even assume the baby is dead when they are told nothing. Drotar found that parents who saw their infants later reported that the infants actually appeared less abnormal than they had imagined.[2] In fact, seeing the baby promptly after birth seems to help reduce the parents' anxiety.

When a baby with a defect is born, parents are faced with a complex psychic task. They have no time to work through the loss of the fantasized perfect child before they are faced with the demand to adapt to their real infant who has a defect.[15] This overwhelming task is encountered at a time of physiological and psychological depletion.

The reactions of parents tend to occur in several identifiable stages. Drotar interviewed 20 mothers and 5 fathers and found the adjustment process to consist of a series of five stages, which overlap and vary in intensity and duration.[2] In the initial stage of shock parents feel helpless, engage in much crying and at times behave irrationally. This is followed with a period of denial, when parents avoid information about the defect and generally wish to be free of the situation. Feelings of sadness, anger and anxiety compose the next stage. Parents may cry for long periods and fear that they will lose their baby. Their reluctance to become attached and interact with their baby results in feelings of estrangement and isolation. During this phase they also may direct their feelings of anger toward themselves, the baby, their family or the hospital staff. As they work through their feelings and become less emotionally upset, they begin the phase of adaptation. During the phase of adaptation, they demonstrate an increased interest in caring for their baby and confidence in their ability to care for him, and they begin to verbalize feelings of close attachment. The final stage of reorganization is a time of dealing with the question of what caused the defect. Some accept that it "just happened," but others look to themselves for possible causes.

The nurse encounters the family at various phases of adjustment. Her goals are to support the family during the process of mourning and to facilitate the attachment process. During both the mourning process and the attachment phase parents can be helped by other parents who have had a similar experience. The benefits of parent-to-parent support when an infant is sick cannot be equaled.[3,4]

The nurse can be supportive during the mourning process by listening to parents repeatedly rehearse the wishes and expectations they had for their fantasized perfect child. It is through this process that the psychic energy invested in the idealized baby is reduced.[15] Providing opportunities for parents to express their intense involvement with their idealized child is the most important function of the nurse during this phase. At times the nurse may feel compelled to forceably redirect the parents' thinking into the here and now, but it is crucial that she understand the significance of mourning and have the patience to facilitate the process.

The nurse should also be alert for the family who has never mourned the loss of their longed-for child. Solnit and Stark describe two extreme patterns of reaction that compose pathological adjustment.[15] The one extreme is manifested by a "mother's exclusive and unremitting dedication" to her child; the other extreme is an intolerance of the child with a near denial of having any relationship with the child. If a nurse recognizes either a pattern of extreme overprotection or of rejection, she should seek the assistance of those in other disciplines to effect a team approach that can facilitate a healthy attachment.

It has been emphasized that the nurse should take an active role in supporting the family through the grieving process. During her contacts with the family the nurse can also encourage attachment behaviors by her own gentle handling of the baby and by pointing out the baby's positive features. Touching and holding the baby and talking about him should be done in a natural way. It is apparent to parents when the nurse is trying to convince herself that she accepts the baby. Mercer suggests that the nurse relieve her own tension by spending time alone with the baby before she attempts to help the parents care for him.[11]

The nurse can best facilitate attachment if she sensitively responds to the readiness of the parents to interact with their baby. As they begin to ask the same questions over and over, the nurse can repeat some of the earlier explanations that were blocked out of their consciousness during the shock phase. Signals for more information include direct questioning of what the nurse is doing and requests for further explanations of something the doctor has told them.[17] As parents begin to show these signs of interest, increased participation in the care of their infant should be encouraged.

The quality of the attachment is dependent on the relationships within the family. The crisis of producing a child with a defect can effect long-term changes in family functioning. Some families experience a degree of persistent sadness that has been referred to as *chronic sorrow*.[12] (See Chapter 25.) The nurse's goal is to help each family achieve its maximum potential in adaptation. If there are older siblings, the nurse will want to help the parents develop approaches that are consistent with each child's developmental level. The nurse can also discuss with parents the particular problems they can expect to encounter. For example, the parents should be advised that sibling rivalry is common and that any rejection of the baby is probably unrelated to the baby's particular problem. If the baby has a visible defect that will be repaired immediately, toddlers will only be confused by any attempted explanation. Preschoolers and particularly school-age children should be given an explanation of why the baby is not coming home. They will hear discussions by friends and family, and they deserve an accurate, simple explanation.

Drotar's findings suggest that positive adaptation to the baby is facilitated by a satisfactory relationship between the parents. Although there is the potential for parents to develop a closer relationship as a result of this experience, some find that the demands of the baby's care bring about feelings of isolation and estrangement.[2] An important phenomenon for the nurse to observe is what Drotar and others describe as "asynchronous parental reactions." In this situation, parents pass through the stages of adjustment at different rates, resulting in absence of shared feelings and in "temporary emotional separation." According to Drotar, these asynchronous parental reactions "may be a significant factor in the incidence of parental separations following family crisis."[2] The nurse can support parents throughout their stages of adjustment and thereby encourage reintegration of the family.

The nurse's responsibility as described is demanding and emotionally taxing. She cannot overlook the importance of dealing with her own feelings so that she can effectively support parents through the stages of adjustment with patient understanding. Her ultimate goal is to help each family reach their maximum level of functioning so that their baby has the best possible chance to grow and thrive in an environment of love.

Support of the Parenting Role When an Infant Is Sick

When an infant is sick and requires a period of intensive care, the parents need special consideration from the nurse as they seek to fulfill their roles as parents. The forced temporary separation of an infant from his parents interrupts the normal development of the parent-infant relationship. In some instances the infant is physically separated only briefly for immediate emergency care, but tubes and equipment may continue to create a barrier between the parents and their baby. In other cases an infant may be ill for several months or may require repeated serious operations before he is returned to his parents and the comforts of a home environment. In the interim, the nurse has an important responsibility to encourage and support parents in their parenting role.

Major stresses for parents when a child is admitted for intensive care revolve around three areas: (1) fears about their child's condition, (2) anxiety resulting from the environment and (3) concern about their role as parents.[10] Information provided to them on a day-to-day basis helps parents to begin to understand their baby's condition and makes them feel more in control of what is coming next. Encouraging parents to participate in the care of their baby is another way that the nurse can foster the parent-infant attachment process. The nurse must, however, recognize that parents vary in the way they respond to the stress of having a sick infant. Many parents are reported to be hesitant to touch their child who is in an intensive care unit

TABLE 24-1 STAGES OF PARENTING BEHAVIORS DURING LENGTHY CARE OF ILL INFANTS*

Stage I Touching	**Stage II** Care-Taking	**Stage III** Identity
Uses fingertips	Provides clean clothing, toys, grooming aids	Brings linens from home
Uses whole hand	Performs activities of daily living (bathing, diapering, feeding, dressing)	Takes photographs
Strokes child	Performs care-taking tasks with proficiency and expresses pleasure in meeting infant's needs	Brings individualized toys
Holds and studies child "en face"	Able to comfort child when distressed or crying	Can make personalized observations about child
Spontaneously lowers crib rails to fondle, hold or talk to child	Able to meet child's special health needs (suctioning, cleaning stoma sites, treatments)	Offers suggestions and makes demands for personalized care
		Demonstrates "advocacy" behavior
		Feels he or she can care for child better than anyone else
		Demonstrates consistent visiting or calling pattern or both
		Questions focus on total child, not only physiological parameters

*Adapted from S. S. Jay. Pediatric intensive care: involving parents in the care of their child. Maternal Child Nursing Journal, Fall 1977, Vol. 6. No. 3, p. 195; B. Schraeder. Attachment and parenting despite lengthy intensive care. American Journal of Maternal Child Nursing, Jan/Feb 1980, p. 37; R. Rubin. Maternal touch. Nursing Outlook, November 1963, p. 829; R. Rubin. Binding in the post-partum period. Maternal Child Nursing Journal, Summer 1977, p. 67; R. Rubin. Attainment of the maternal role: Part I. Processes. Nursing Research, Summer 1967, p. 237; R. Rubin. Attainment of the maternal role: Part II. Models and referrants. Nursing Research, Fall 1967, p. 342.

because they fear hurting him or disconnecting tubes or equipment.[7] The appearance of a baby amidst the cumbersome and awesome equipment brings varied responses of fear and shock. While some parents only need to be told that they may touch their baby, others may need to watch the nurse handle their baby for a period of time before they even feel ready to touch their child.[7] If the nurse is not prepared for these varied responses, she may misinterpret the reticence of such parents and mistakenly assume that they are not interested in their baby.

The nurse can facilitate parenting behaviors in various ways. First, the parents must clearly understand that they may and should touch their baby; they need to be shown how to hold the baby when this is permissible. Parents can also be encouraged to observe the nurse care for the baby and to begin helping in small ways in the presence of the nurse. Eventually parents are able to learn how to care for their infant independently. When prolonged specialized care is necessary it is particularly important for the nurse to foster the parent-child relationship. Parents can easily feel displaced when the health team members take over the baby's complete care and the required procedures appear too complicated for them to learn. The nurse must not overlook that parents by and large feel incompetent to care for their sick infant.[5] Parents need the support of the nurse to help them feel competent in the care of their baby and in their role as parents. These children belong to their parents and although there is a tremendous investment by members of the health care team in these infants, their role must not be confused with the unique role of parents.[14]

Even though an illness is eventually reversible, a lengthy period of illness requires that the nurse give parents special support. Schraeder reports on stages of parenting behaviors through which parents are supported when lengthy intensive care is required.[14] These stages of parenting represent a continuum from touching to care-taking to a period during which parents "incorporate the child into their family," called *identity*.[14] Table 24–1 describes the parenting behaviors of each stage. The nurse can be more effective in her support of parents if she recognizes that parents may need time to gradually become involved with their baby who is sick. These stages of parenting involvement can serve as a guide for the nurse in her assessment of parents. In the program described by Schraeder,[14] parents are placed on the continuum as both verbal and nonverbal cues are assessed. The nurse can then formulate goals that are congruent with the demonstrated level of parenting and that promote the progression of parenting to the next level.

The nurse's goal is to "parent the parents" so that the infant can be returned to parents who feel comfortable in their parenting role.

References

1. B. G. Benfield et al. Grief response of parents after referral of the critically ill newborn to a regional center. New England Journal of Medicine, 29 April 1976, p. 975
2. D. Drotar et al. The adaptations of parents to the birth of an infant with a congenital malformation: a hypothetical model. Pediatrics, November 1975, p. 710
3. M. Eager and R. Exoo. Parents visiting parents for unequaled support. American Journal of Maternal Child Nursing, Jan/Feb 1980, p. 35
4. D. Erdman. Parent-to-parent support: The best for those with sick newborns. American Journal of Maternal Child Nursing, Sept/Oct 1977, p. 291
5. E. Goldson. Parents' reactions to the birth of a sick infant. Children Today, Jul/Aug 1979, p. 13
6. N. Irvin et al. Caring for parents of an infant with a congenital malformation. In Maternal-Infant Bonding, M. H. Klaus and J. H. Kennel, C. V. Mosby Co., 1976
7. S. S. Jay. Pediatric intensive care: involving parents in the care of their child. Maternal Child Nursing Journal, Fall 1977, Vol. 6, No. 3, p. 195
8. M. H. Klaus. Caring for parents. Perinatal Care, March 1978, p. 28
9. Lampe J., et al. Parental visiting of sick infants: the effect of living at home prior to hospitalization. Pediatrics, November 1977, p. 294
10. M. H. Miles. Impact of the intensive care unit on parents. Issues In Comprehensive Pediatric Nursing, December 1979, p. 72
11. R. T. Mercer. Crises: A baby is born with a defect. Nursing '77, November 1977, p. 45
12. S. Ohlansky. Chronic sorrow: A response to having a mentally defective child. Social Casework, April 1962, p. 191
13. G. J. Opirhory. Counseling the parents of a critically ill newborn, Journal of Obstetrical, Gynecological and Neonatal Nursing, May/June 1979, p. 179
14. B. D. Schraeder. Attachment and parenting despite lengthy intensive care. American Journal of Maternal Child Nursing, January/February 1980, p. 37
15. A. J. Solnit and M. H. Stark. Mourning and the birth of a defective child. Psychoanalytic Study of The Child, Vol. 16, 1961, p. 523
16. E. H. Waechter. Bonding problems of infants with congenital anomalies. Nursing Forum, Vol. 16, No. 3, 4, 1977, p. 298
17. R. K. Young. Chronic sorrow: Parents' response to the birth of a child with a defect. American Journal of Maternal Child Nursing, Jan/Feb 1977, p. 38

CONGENITAL HEART ANOMALIES

by Mary Burkhart, RN, MA CPNP
and Marianne Glassanos, RN, MS CPNP

If an infant is born with any type of birth defect, the parents' coping abilities are challenged. Because the heart is vital to human existence and is viewed by many as the "life force" of the human body, a defect of the cardiac structure may have heightened significance to the parents and family. The nurse caring for the child with a cardiac defect must help the parents cope with their feelings of grief so that they are able to deal with the facts related to their infant's illness.

Incidence and Etiology

It is important to examine the incidence of congenital heart disease in order to understand the implications it has for nursing. Approximately 1 of every 100 babies born alive has one or more congenital cardiovascular abnormalities.[11] The chance of occurrence of a congenital heart defect in the newborn sibling of an affected child is approximately 2 per cent, or 1 per 50 live births.[11] These parents need genetic coun-

> **CONGENITAL HEART ANOMALIES: NURSE'S ROLE IN PREVENTION**
>
> **Assessing for children and families at risk**
>   Genetic counselling for parents with one child with CHD or if a parent has CHD.
>   Screening infants of mothers with maternal rubella or diabetes.
>   Screening of premature infants.
>   Screening of infants with congenital scoliosis, with other congenital anomalies, or with chromosomal aberrations.
>
> **Implementing preventive measures**
>   Rubella vaccine by 15 months of age.
>   Rubella titer on women with questionable history of rubella.
>   Genetic counselling of women over 35 years of age.
>   Maintaining a positive maternal environment:
>   • adequate nutrition, rest and exercise
>   • prevention of illness during pregnancy
>   • no self-prescribed drugs
>   • no cigarette smoking
>   • no alcohol ingestion

selling and referral to appropriate resources for help.

The incidence has been shown to be two to three times greater in premature infants than in term infants. Both male and female children are affected equally; however, specific defects show a tendency toward sexual differences. Patent ductus arteriosus and atrial septal defects are more common in females. In males coarctation of the aorta, transposition of the great vessels, and tetralogy of Fallot are more common.

The actual cause of congenital heart disease is not known. Heart defects result from a failure of a part of the heart structure to develop beyond the early stage of embryonic development. Etiology appears to be related to maternal environment and genetic makeup. Some examples of factors compromising the maternal environment are diabetes, rubella, drugs and hypoxia. Down's syndrome is an example of a genetic condition that is frequently associated with cardiac defects.

Anatomy and Physiology of the Circulatory System

It is helpful to be familiar with the development of the heart and fetal circulation in order to understand congenital cardiac defects. The critical period for development of the heart is from about 20 to 50 days' gestation. During this period the heart is especially vulnerable to the effects of the intrauterine environment.

Heart development is first apparent at about three weeks of intrauterine life when the developing embryo's need for nutrition and oxygenation can no longer be met by diffusion alone.[19] At this time the heart is a single tube that consists of two layers of tissue, the endocardium and the epimyocardium. The midportion of the tube grows and bends rapidly and by the fourth week partitioning of the chambers of the heart begins. The valves of the heart are usually developed and partitioning is complete by the seventh or eighth week of gestation.

Cardiac problems are not evident in utero. Because of the fetal structures of circulation and oxygenation (placenta, umbilical vein, ductus venosus, foramen ovale, ductus arteriosus, and umbilical arteries), blood is not oxygenated in the lungs. Throughout the life of the fetus, oxygenation occurs via the placenta. (Figure 24–1 shows fetal circulation.) Fetal blood in the placenta receives oxygen, along with other nutrients, by osmosis across the placental villi. Well-oxygenated blood returns from the placenta via the umbilical vein, which joins the portal vein within the liver. About one-half of this blood is circulated through the portal vein system in the liver. The other half is shunted directly to the inferior vena cava via the ductus venosus in order to retain a high level of oxygenation to the fetus. The blood in the inferior vena cava thus contains both unoxygenated blood from the lower limbs, abdomen and pelvis and highly oxygenated blood from the ductus venosus. After a short course in the inferior vena cava, the oxygenated blood enters the right atrium.

Most of the blood from the right atrium is directed through the foramen ovale, an opening in the atrial septum, into the left atrium. Here it mixes with a small amount of blood returning from the lungs via the pulmonary veins. The blood then passes into the left ventricle and

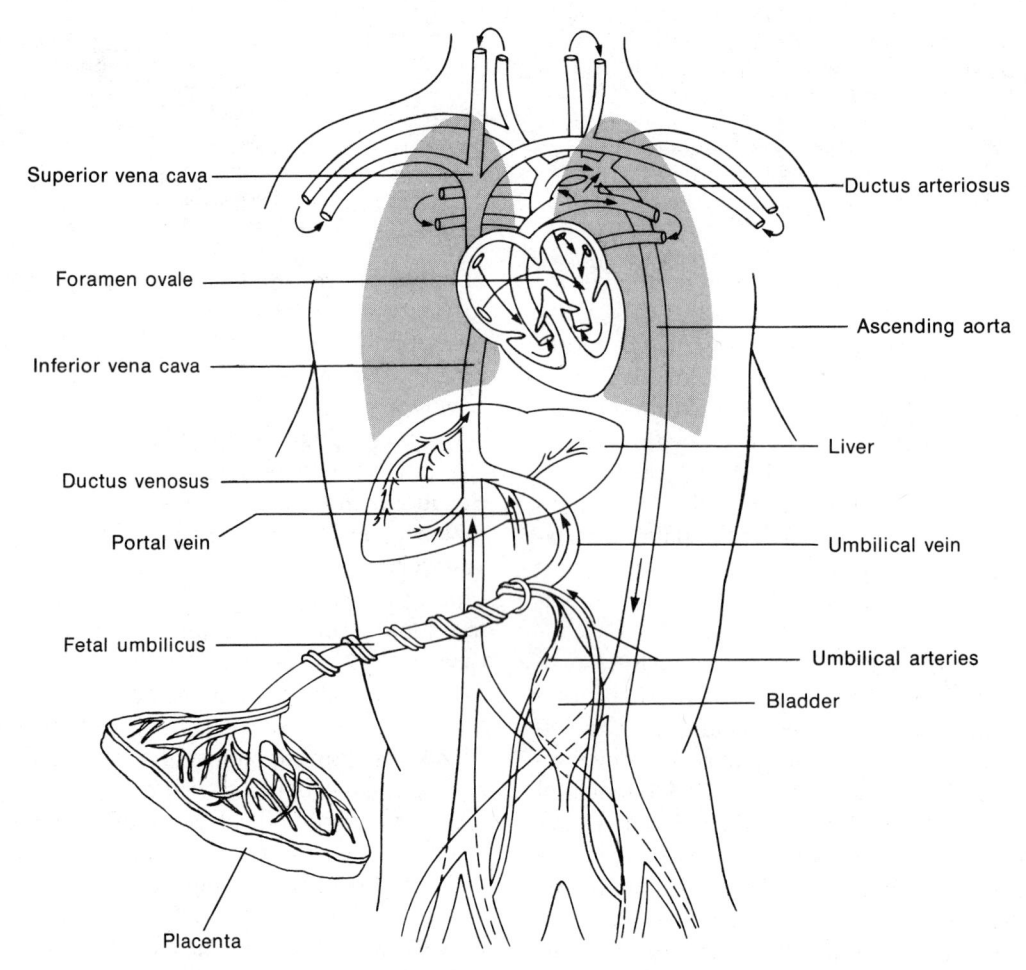

Figure 24–1 Fetal circulation.

leaves via the ascending aorta. Thus the vessels to the heart, head, and neck and upper limbs receive rather well-oxygenated blood.

Simultaneously with the circulation just described, a small amount of oxygenated blood from the inferior vena cava remains in the right atrium. This blood mixes with unoxygenated blood from the superior vena cava and passes into the right ventricle. The blood then leaves by the pulmonary artery, most of it passing through the ductus arteriosus (a structure joining the pulmonary artery and the aorta), bypassing the lungs and going directly into the aorta. Very little blood goes to the lungs, as in the fetus they are nonfunctional. Most of the blood in the descending aorta passes into the umbilical arteries and is returned to the placenta for reoxygenation. The remainder circulates through the lower part of the body and eventually enters the inferior vena cava.

Changes in the Circulation after Birth Shortly after birth many changes occur in the infant's cardiorespiratory systems that allow for adaptation to the external environment. (Figure 24–2 shows neonatal circulation.) Oxygenation now occurs in the lungs. With the first breath the

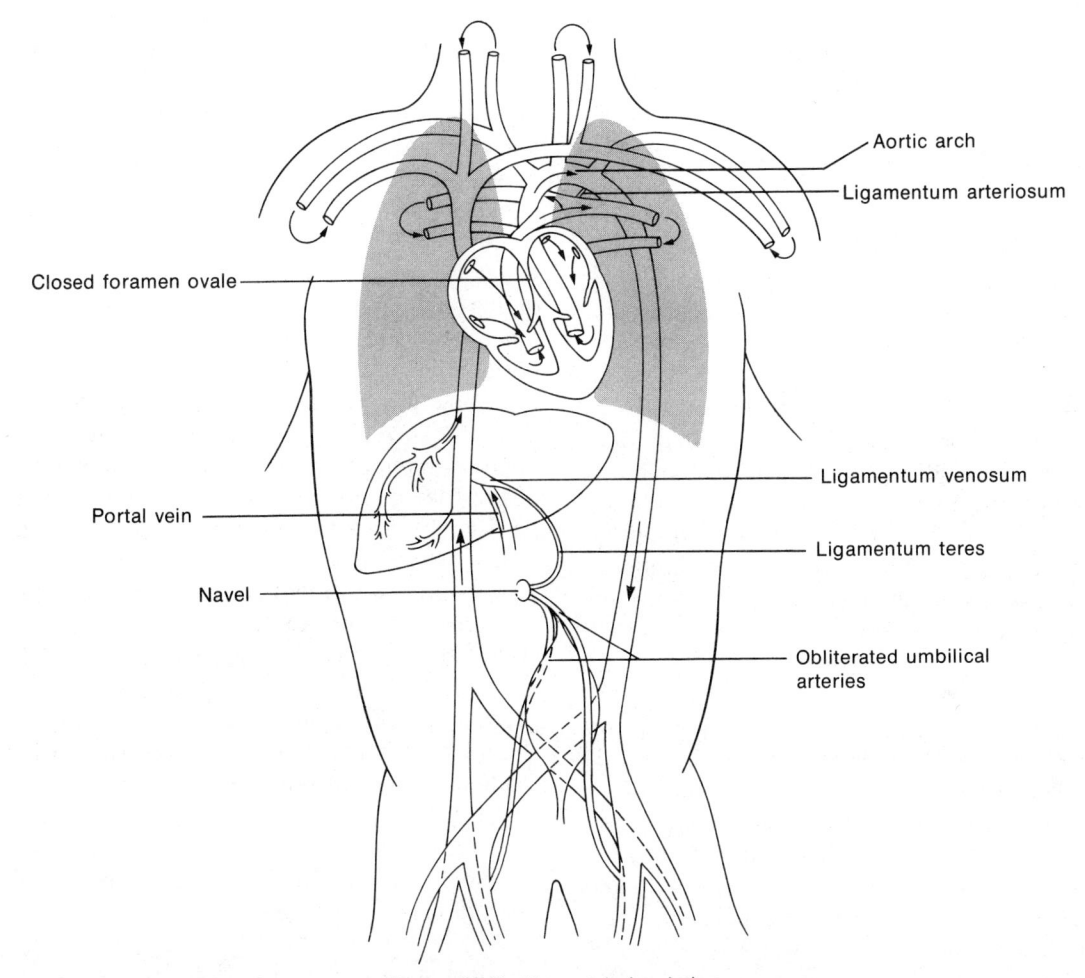

Figure 24-2 Neonatal circulation.

alveoli expand and more blood flows through the lungs. With an increase in the volume of pulmonary blood flow and a decrease in pulmonary vascular resistance, there is an increased return of blood to the left atrium. This causes a rise in left atrial pressure and a drop in right atrial pressure. These pressure changes, in addition to loss of umbilical circulation, increased peripheral vascular resistance, and the structure of the foramen ovale permitting flow only from right to left, cause the closure of the foramen ovale. The foramen ovale functionally closes after birth and disappears during childhood.

Increased oxygen content and decreased pulmonary vascular resistance play a major role in closure of the ductus arteriosus. In the ensuing weeks it becomes obliterated and the remaining ligament becomes the ligamentus arteriosum. The umbilical vein, two umbilical arteries and the ductus venosus no longer carry blood, so clotting and atrophy of these structures occur.

Now unoxygenated blood returns from the body via the superior and inferior venae cavae and enters the right atrium. The blood passes through the tricuspid valve and enters the right ventricle. Passing through the pulmonic valve, the unoxygenated blood enters the pulmonary artery and is transported to the lungs. Oxygenation occurs in the alveoli of the lungs and the blood is carried back to the left atrium via the pulmonary veins. The well-oxygenated blood leaves the left atrium through the mitral valve to the left ventricle. This oxygen-saturated blood enters the systemic circulation by passing through the aortic valve into the ascending aorta.

Recognizing a Problem in Neonatal Circulation

Vital to the diagnosis of congenital heart disease is a thorough history and physical examination. A variety of other diagnostic procedures and tests may also be ordered.

History The earlier an infant develops cardiac disease, the greater is the potential for a sudden downhill course. Because congenital heart disease may not be discovered while the infant is in the hospital, parents may bring the infant to the physician's office with a number of concerns. Often the chief complaint seems apparently unrelated to a heart problem. During the history the parents may mention that the infant is having feeding problems. These problems may include difficulty in swallowing, regurgitation of uncurdled milk, having to be awakened for feedings, and falling asleep during feedings. A poor weight gain may result. Feeding problems are usually due to tachycardia and tachypnea, which fatigue the child and are signs of a decompensated cardiopulmonary system. The parents should be asked to describe the infant's feeding behavior in detail. How often does the infant eat? How long does it take to feed him? How does the child act during a feeding? How much formula does he take at one feeding? How much formula does he take in 24 hours? How does he respond after a feeding? Is there any vomiting?

Respiratory difficulties such as fainting, difficulty in breathing, "blackouts" (anoxic spells), "sighing," stridor or frequent respiratory infections may be reported by the parents. Some parents may relate that the infant's difficulty in breathing is relieved by slightly hyperextending his neck. Parents should be asked to elaborate on any respiratory problems. Does the baby ever make strange noises when breathing? Does he cough or choke? Has the baby had any respiratory infections? Does he have difficulty breathing, or does he breathe very rapidly? Has he ever stopped breathing?

A bluish cast to skin, mucous membranes, lips and conjunctivae, either persistent or intermittent, and pallor are manifestations of cardiac problems that should be explored with parents. Does the baby's color change when crying? When feeding? When defecating? When position is changed suddenly? Has the baby ever turned blue?

Activity level or activity intolerance must be investigated. Parents may complain that their infant is continuously restless, fatigues easily during feedings, or is lethargic and sleeps all the time. Parents should be asked to describe the position the infant usually assumes when asleep or resting. Often infants with cardiac problems favor the knee-chest position or sleep with the upper extremities flaccidly extended above the head. The mother may say that the infant is persistently "sweaty," even while at complete rest.

It is important to explore any other parental concerns at a time when full attention can be given to the parents. After information is collected about these concerns, a history related to the pregnancy, birth and the neonatal period should be elicited. Special inquiry should be made as to the maternal health history during the first trimester of pregnancy: rubella, viral infections, medications, x-rays and threatened abortions. Family history related to congenital heart disease must be ascertained.

Physical Assessment In addition to the concerns expressed by parents there are signs indicative of congenital heart disease that the nurse must assess.

Skin In assessment of the infant's color it is important to observe for cyanosis, both centrally and peripherally. Cyanosis is a purplish-blue cast to the skin, mucous membranes, lips and conjunctiva. With central cyanosis there is at least 5 gm per cent of reduced hemoglobin in the circulating blood. This is best observed in the mucous membranes, but it affects the entire body.[12] Central cyanosis is caused by circulation of deoxygenated blood in the systemic circulation. This is usually associated with those lesions causing right-to-left cardiac shunts.

Peripheral cyanosis does not usually affect

the mucous membranes but is best demonstrated in the fingers, toes, ears and nose. The cyanosis results from deoxygenated capillary blood flow; it may be seen with vasoconstriction.[12] Peripheral cyanosis is usually associated with obstructive cardiac lesions: aortic stenosis, mitral stenosis and pulmonic stenosis. It usually occurs in extremities farthest from the heart, hence the name peripheral cyanosis.[12]

Cyanosis may be the only evidence of a cardiac lesion during the first weeks of life. Cyanosis that increases with crying suggests a cardiac lesion because the infant's circulatory system is unable to meet the increased demands on it. Accurate assessment of color requires good lighting. Also, the infant should be kept warm and assessed both while at rest and during activity. Observation of the lips, tongue, and mucous membranes should be made first for central cyanosis and then the skin should be observed. In dark-skinned infants peripheral cyanosis is more difficult to assess; thus these infants should be assessed primarily by checking for central cyanosis.

Cyanosis can also be identified by checking the nail beds. Normally the nail beds are pink; however, with cyanosis the nail beds may have a blue or purple hue. The nail beds should also be checked for capillary refill by pressing lightly with the finger on the infant's nails then releasing the pressure. Capillary refill normally occurs immediately.

Moistness of the skin should be observed. Diaphoresis (excessive perspiration) may occur in children with left-to-right shunts.

The infant or child is observed for edema. This may be generalized; often it is noticed around the eyes (periorbital edema) and is a late sign of congestive heart failure.

Vital Signs (See Chapter 13 for normal values.) Respiratory status must be assessed. Respirations are counted for one full minute with the infant at rest. The child's activity level is observed and documented when assessing respiratory status. Tachypnea (a respiratory rate greater than 60 respirations per minute while at rest) may be indicative of congenital heart disease. Any grunting, stridor, nasal flaring, retractions (between and below the ribs) and labored respirations are noted. Nail beds are examined for clubbing (Fig. 24–3). A problem of persistent poor oxygenation leads to clubbing of the fingernails and toenails.

The pulse must be carefully assessed. A resting heart rate that is over 200 beats per minute is a sign of congenital heart disease. Activity level of the child must be taken into account, along with fever and other existing illness, when evaluating heart rate. The apical pulse should be assessed for one full minute, with its character, regularity and rate noted. Peripheral and apical pulses should be assessed simultaneously and any pulse deficit should be noted.

Blood pressure is another parameter that must be assessed. The usual spread between diastolic and systolic pressures is 20 to 50 mm Hg. In a child with suspected heart disease the blood pressure should be taken in all four extremities and recorded. Normally the pressure is about 20 mm Hg higher in the thighs.

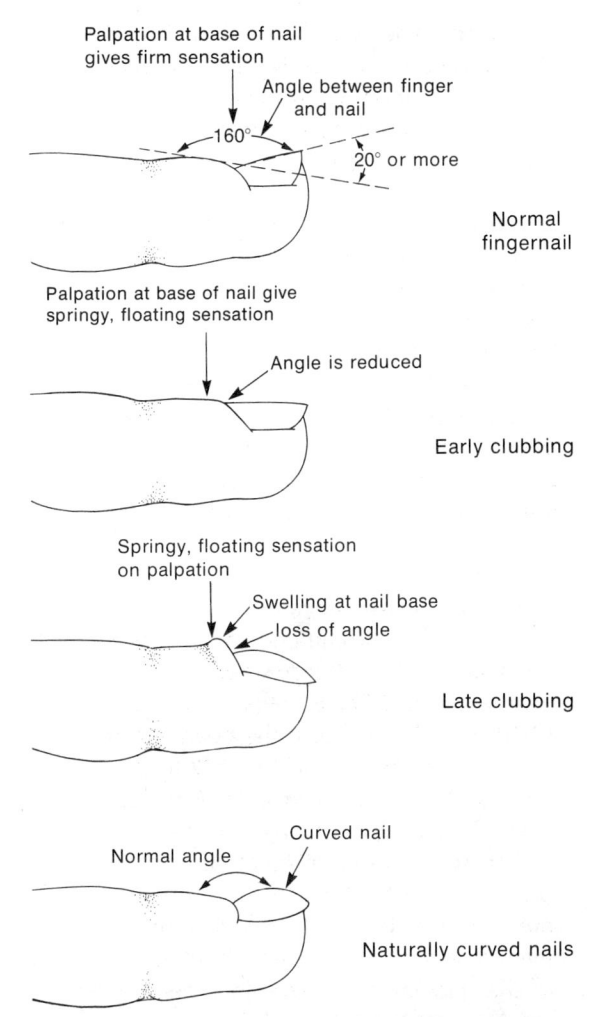

Figure 24–3 Clubbing in infant's fingers, caused by poor oxygenation. (Redrawn from J. Luckmann and K. Sorensen. Medical-Surgical Nursing: a Psychophysiologic Approach. W. B. Saunders Co., 1980.)

Abdomen The abdomen should be palpated. Hepatomegaly, which is enlargement of the liver greater than 3 cm below the right costal margin in a neonate, is indicative of congestive heart failure.

General Appearance The infant's position is observed during sleep. "Cardiac infants" may sleep in the knee-chest position or lie with the upper extremities flaccidly extended above the head. Growth of the child is assessed by comparing height, weight and head circumference to standardized growth charts. Plotting this information helps to determine any lag in physical growth. Many children with congenital cardiac lesions demonstrate some degree of growth failure.

Chest The chest is examined to see if there is any bulging or prominence on the chest wall, especially on the left side where the apex of the heart is situated. The point of maximum impulse (PMI) is the area where the heartbeat is heard the loudest. Sometimes the PMI is visually apparent as a pulsation in children with thin chest walls or with enlarged hearts.

Palpation is done to locate the PMI and the presence of a thrill. In infants and young children the PMI is usually palpable in the fourth intercostal space on the left chest just to the left of the midclavicular line. In older children it can be palpated at the fifth intercostal space at the midclavicular line (Fig. 24–4). A thrill (a vibration caused by turbulence of blood in the heart) may be felt by placing the tips of the fingers on the anterior chest wall. The vibration that may be felt has been described as feeling like a purring kitten. This may be due to the passage of blood through a narrowed opening such as a stenosed value.

Auscultation of the heart using a stethoscope is done to check the quality, rate and rhythm of the heart sound and to identify murmurs. Murmurs are the most common means of identifying congenital heart disease. A murmur is a sound created by turbulent blood flow through the heart. When assessing a murmur it must be described in terms of several parameters: its position in the cardiac cycle and its duration, configuration, pitch, intensity, quality, and response to exercise and movement. There are two categories of murmurs: innocent and organic. Innocent murmurs are not associated with any underlying pathology. Organic murmurs are associated with either acquired or congenital heart disease.

Heart murmurs are classified according to their loudness and presence or absence of a thrill. Murmurs graded from I (least severe) to VI (most severe) are described as follows:[1]

Grade I–Very faint, difficult to hear unless child is very quiet; may be heard faintly after a period of attentive listening.
Grade II–Soft though readily heard; louder than Grade I.
Grade III–Moderately loud; no thrill.
Grade IV–Loud with a thrill.
Grade V–Loud enough to be heard with a stethoscope barely on the chest wall; thrill is present.
Grade IV–Can be heard without having the stethoscope on the chest wall; accompanied by a thrill.

Diagnostic Tests Electrical conduction stimulates the muscular contraction of the heart. Disease processes and surgery may disrupt this system, producing a variety of results. In the normal heart, the impulse originates in the right atrium from the sinoatrial (SA) node located near the opening of the superior vena cava. The SA node functions much like a pacemaker, releasing impulses at a regular rate that produce contraction of the atria. Nerve centers in the brain control the release of impulses, with sympathetic fiber stimulation increasing the rate and vagus nerve fiber stimulation decreasing it. The impulse travels through the right and left atria to the atrioventricular node, located at the atrial septum. The impulse then passes along

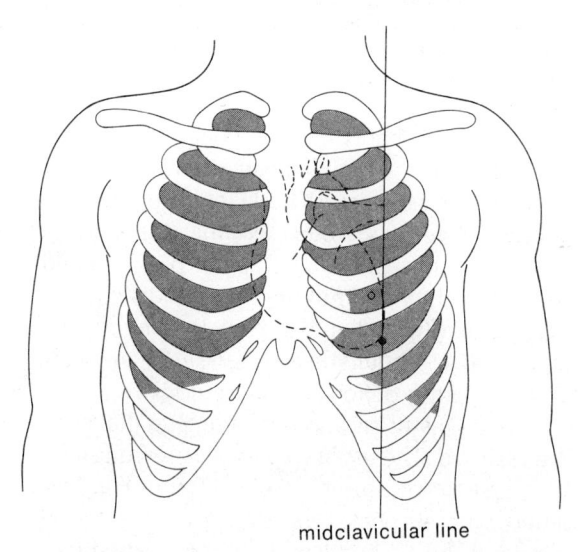

Figure 24–4 The point of maximum impulse (PMI), where the heartbeat is heard the loudest. ○ in older children and adults; ● in infants.

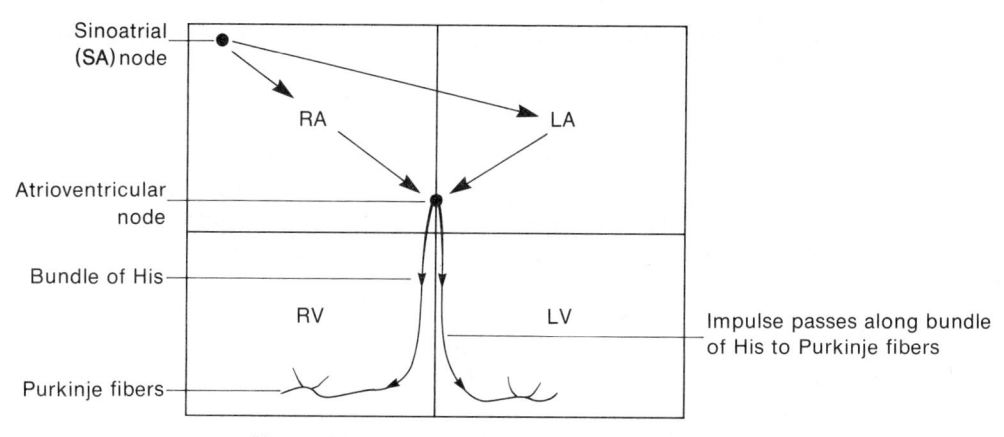

Figure 24–5 The conduction system of the heart.

the bundle of His to the Purkinje fibers and stimulates ventricular contraction (Fig. 24–5).

An electrocardiogram (ECG or EKG) is a graphic tracing of the electrical activity produced by the heart muscle. (The heart action that accompanies each phase of electrical activity is described in Figure 24–6.) An ECG tracing shows the contraction of the atria and ventricles as stimulated by the sinoatrial node, the atrioventricular node, the bundle of His, and the Purkinje fibers. The P wave represents the electrical activity associated with the impulse from the sinoatrial node and its subsequent spread through the atria. The PR interval is the period from the start of the P wave to the onset of the QRS complex. The PR interval shows the time for the original impulse to reach the ventricles and initiate ventricular contraction. The QRS complex represents the contraction of the ventricular muscle. The QRS complex reflects the time necessary for the impulse to traverse the bundle of His and the Purkinje fibers to complete ventricular contraction. The ST segment interval describes the period between the com-

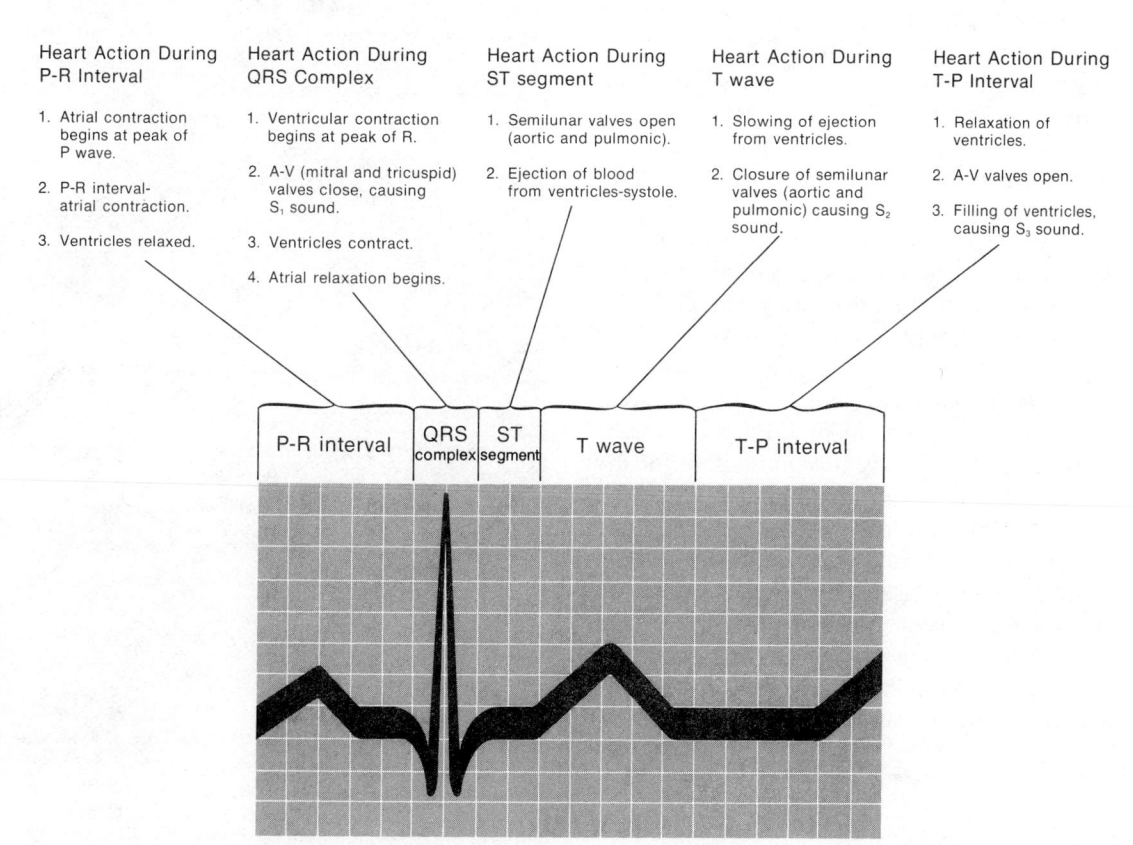

Heart Action During P-R Interval	Heart Action During QRS Complex	Heart Action During ST segment	Heart Action During T wave	Heart Action During T-P Interval
1. Atrial contraction begins at peak of P wave.	1. Ventricular contraction begins at peak of R.	1. Semilunar valves open (aortic and pulmonic).	1. Slowing of ejection from ventricles.	1. Relaxation of ventricles.
2. P-R interval-atrial contraction.	2. A-V (mitral and tricuspid) valves close, causing S_1 sound.	2. Ejection of blood from ventricles-systole.	2. Closure of semilunar valves (aortic and pulmonic) causing S_2 sound.	2. A-V valves open.
3. Ventricles relaxed.	3. Ventricles contract.			3. Filling of ventricles, causing S_3 sound.
	4. Atrial relaxation begins.			

Figure 24–6 Electrocardiogram (ECG) with description of heart action in each phase of electrical activity.

pletion of contraction and recovery of the ventricular muscles. The T wave illustrates the recovery phase after contraction.

The ECG shows the sequence of electrical events in the heart, the heart rate and rhythm, and any damage to the heart muscle and conduction disturbances. Leads are placed on the limbs and the chest for recording of the ECG; this is a noninvasive technique.

A vectorcardiogram is a type of electrocardiogram that is helpful in the diagnosis of congenital heart disease. Three leads placed on the chest record electrical activity of the heart simultaneously and demonstrate a precise time relationship between electrical impulses and response of the myocardium. Echocardiography is a noninvasive technique used for localizing the origin of heart sounds, especially murmurs. Ultrasound (high frequency sound waves) is directed toward the heart and an image is produced of the sound waves within the heart. Movements and dimensions of cardiac structures can be studied. A phonocardiogram is a graphic recording of sounds produced within the heart and great vessels. It records sounds that occur too rapidly to be detected by the human ear with a stethoscope.

Although all these diagnostic studies are noninvasive techniques and are not painful, careful explanations of each test must be given to the parents and to the child. The strangeness of the environment and the equipment is frightening; therefore nursing interventions aimed at informing the parent and patient help to lessen their anxiety.

Hematologic tests are done to help in the workup and diagnosis of congenital heart disease. A complete blood count is ordered. The child with a cyanotic defect will usually show an increased hemoglobin and hematocrit. This is due to an increased number of red blood cells, known as polycythemia. Polycythemia is a response of the body to compensate for the circulation of unoxygenated blood in the arterial system. This may lead to problems of clotting owing to the increased viscosity of the blood.

Arterial blood gases may also be ordered to determine the oxygen saturation of the arterial blood. Normally this is between 92 and 100 mg per cent. A saturation below 92 mg per cent may be a sign of cyanotic heart disease.

Cardiac Catheterization: The Nurse's Role

A diagnostic test that requires special nursing care is cardiac catheterization. Cardiac catheterization is an invasive, definitive procedure used to diagnose congenital heart disease. It involves passing a thin, flexible radiopaque catheter (Fig. 24–7) into the chambers of the heart via a peripheral vessel, usually the femoral vein or artery. The catheterization is usually done in combination with angiocardiography. In this procedure a contrast medium is injected into a chamber of the heart and a video recording of the x-rays is made. This allows for later replay and examination of the cardiac catheterization.

The objectives of cardiac catheterization are to (1) measure the pressures within the different chambers; (2) measure cardiac output and function; (3) measure oxygen saturation within the chambers of the heart, (4) visualize the structures of the heart to determine any anomalies and (5) evaluate the flow of blood through the heart.

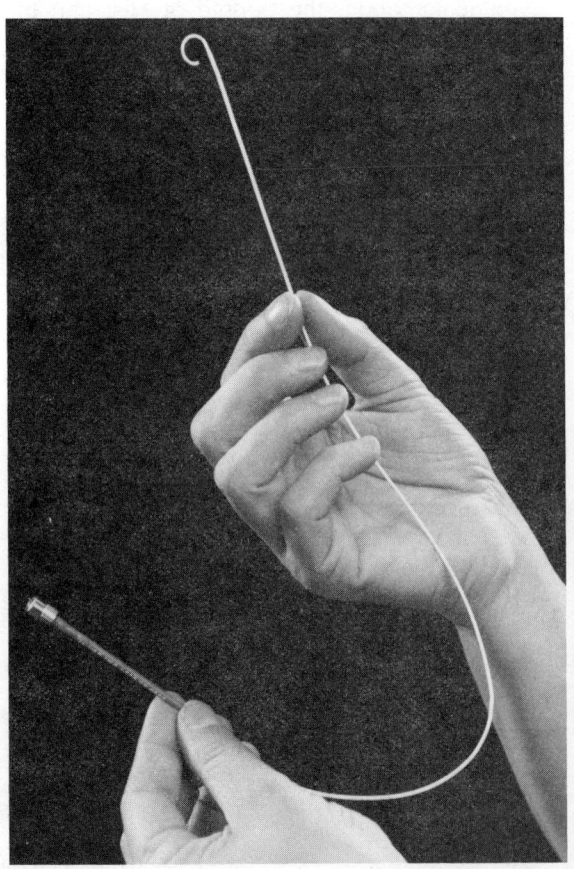

Figure 24–7 Catheter used for cardiac catheterization of an infant. This is called a pigtail catheter because of the curled end. This end has small holes out of which dye is injected into the heart chamber.

Preparation of Child and Family Psychological preparation of the child and the family is an integral part of nursing care for the catheterization procedure. It is important to explain the procedure to parents and keep them informed of what will take place next. For cardiac catheterization the infant or child is usually admitted to the hospital for a 48-hour stay. The child is admitted the day before the procedure, during which time the physical examination, chest x-ray, ECG, and laboratory work are performed.

Laboratory work done will include a type and cross match for blood to have available should any bleeding occur during or after the procedure. Blood should not be drawn from the potential catheterization site.

The following day the catheterization is done; it lasts from two to five hours. The child is not allowed to eat or drink for 4 to 6 hours immediately before the procedure. Preoperative medications include Benadryl and morphine, which are administered approximately 30 to 45 minutes before the catheterization to help the child relax. The morphine dose for a cyanotic child is usually one-half the dose used for an acyanotic child. After the catheterization the child is observed closely overnight and is discharged the next morning.

Little can be done to prepare an infant psychologically for the procedure. Consistency of care from a primary nurse can facilitate feelings of security. Some security object such as a favorite blanket, toy or pacifier can provide comfort, but the presence of parents provides the most security for an infant undergoing such a procedure. Comfort measures that may soothe the infant during the procedure are singing and talking to him, providing music and stroking him; the presence of the infant's primary nurse can be soothing. The parents are encouraged to hold and cuddle the infant and participate in his care as desired, before and after the procedure. Older children can understand explanations, but young children require special approaches to prepare them for this procedure.

For the child 2 to 3 years of age, a simple explanation should be given on the morning of the procedure. He should also be told that he will not receive breakfast. Diversions such as play, carrying the child for a walk down the hall, or reading to the child to keep him occupied during mealtime should be done by the parents and, in their absence, by the nurse. If the mother will be there waiting when he returns, explain this to the child. Sitting with a toddler briefly and talking to him gives him a sense of security and warmth. Even though the child may not understand the full implications, the nurse's warmth and concern are communicated. He will feel safer than if someone abruptly came in and took him from his crib.

The child 3 to 7 years of age is capable of understanding something of what the inside of the body is, and it is appropriate to give him simple explanations with a diagram or a doll. Fear of the unknown is reduced by allowing the child to play with a cap, mask, gown and stethoscope and by taking the child for a ride on a stretcher. If possible, the child should be taken to the cardiac catheterization laboratory the day before the procedure and should meet the nurses and physicians who will be caring for him.

The child 3 to 7 years of age is able to understand why he cannot have breakfast; this should be explained to him. It may be helpful for the nurse to tell the child that she will have a favorite drink waiting for him when he returns or that he will find a special treat on his afternoon tray.

When discussing the actual catheterization the nurse can show the child on a doll or on himself where the catheter will go, and can explain the warm, tingling feeling of the medication going in. She should explain to the child that on his return from the procedure he will have a dressing on his thigh and that he will have to keep his leg straight. She should tell him that the nurses will be taking his blood pressure frequently and, if applicable, that his parents will be there with him. This allows the child to maintain control when he goes for the actual procedure because he knows something of what to expect.

Nursing Care During and After the Procedure Complications to be watched for during and after the procedure are conduction disturbances, perforation, bleeding, and vessel thrombosis or spasm.

During the procedure the child is restrained very securely to prevent movement that could result in injury. The arms and legs are strapped down and electrodes are applied to monitor for any arrhythmias that could occur during the procedure. The groin area is prepared with an antimicrobial solution; after the administration of a local anesthetic a cutdown is done on the femoral vein or artery. Catheterization of the right side of the heart is done by feeding the catheter into the femoral vein and advancing it through the inferior vena cava and on into the right atrium, the right ventricle and the pulmonary artery. Pressure measurements are recorded and later evaluated. If the foramen ovale is patent or an atrial septal defect is present, the catheter may be advanced into the left atrium through this opening. The left side of the heart may be catheterized by passing the catheter into the femoral artery and into the descending aorta to the left atrium. In either approach, after the pressure readings and blood samples have been taken, dye is injected (angiocardiography) into the heart to produce a more specific view of the heart structures.

From the moment the procedure is over and the child returns to the unit the nurse begins immediate, careful, systematic observations. After the catheterization the child returns to his room with a pressure dressing over the cutdown site (entry site of catheter) and possibly with IV fluids being infused. The child must be observed closely for any complications. When the child is moved from the stretcher to the bed, his color and level of consciousness are noted. The pressure dressing over the cutdown site is checked to see that it is snug and that no bleeding is present. The diaper should be unfastened to allow for complete examination of the dressing on each assessment because blood can pool under the child. The pulse, color, temperature and capillary refill of the extremity distal to the cutdown site should be checked, because arterial thrombosis and spasm of the vessel are the most frequent complications of the cardiac catheterization procedure. All the vital signs are checked immediately on return from the procedure and monitored closely for several hours. The patient may have a transient temperature elevation due to physiological dehydration from being without fluids for four to six hours before and during the procedure. If the temperature persists after fluid intake, the fever may be due to the introduction of pathogens during the procedure. The patient must be observed closely for signs of bradycardia, apnea, dyspnea with retractions, or hypotension. If any of these occur the physician must be notified. The extremity distal to the site must remain extended until the pressure dressing is removed, usually six hours after the catheterization. To keep the infant's leg extended, a piece of Kerlix as a clove-hitch restraint may be used or the parents may hold the child on a pillow on their lap, keeping the leg straight. For infants the dressing may need to be waterproofed with plastic to prevent contamination by stool or urine.

CLASSIFICATION OF DEFECTS

Congenital heart defects can be classified into four groups: (1) acyanotic defects with normal pulmonary vascularity, (2) acyanotic defects with pulmonary vascular involvement, (3) cyanotic defects with increased pulmonary vascularity and (4) cyanotic defects with decreased pulmonary vascularity. Each defect is presented here as if it were the only anomaly present, which is often not the case. Therefore, the description may vary depending upon the individual circumstances.

The easiest way to approach the study of cardiac defects is to gain an understanding of levels within the heart. The pressure within the chambers, arteries and veins of the heart will determine the direction of its blood flow: blood will flow from an area of high pressure to one of lower pressure. Normally, the left side of the heart is a high pressure chamber because it must maintain systemic flow. The pressure of each ventricle is higher than the pressure of their respective atria, since the ventricles must pump blood through either the pulmonic (right ventricle) or systemic (left ventricle) systems. Therefore, when a septal defect is present, one would expect blood to flow from the left to right side of the heart, i.e., from an area of higher pressure to an area of lower pressure.

A shunt exists when blood flows from one chamber, artery or vein to another, resulting in the mixing of oxygenated and deoxygenated blood. Left-to-right shunts are usually acyanotic, since oxygenated blood flows to the right side and is recirculated through the pulmonic system. Right-to-left shunts usually produce cyanosis because deoxygenated blood from the right side flows to the left and is pumped into the systemic circulation.

Acyanotic Defects with Increased Pulmonary Vascularity

Atrial Septal Defect Atrial septal defects (ASD) comprise about 15 per cent of all congen-

> **THE NURSE'S ROLE IN IDENTIFICATION OF CONGENITAL HEART DEFECTS AND SUPPORT OF THE FAMILY DURING DIAGNOSIS**
>
> **Carefinding and Early Identification**
> History findings
> Feeding problems
> Respiratory problems
> Cyanosis
> Activity intolerance
> Hyperhydrosis
> Failure to thrive
>
> Physical examination findings:
> Color–dusky, blue, pale
> Respiratory rate–more than 60/minute, labored respirations, retractions, grunting, stridor
> Pulse–more than 200/minute bounding or absent peripheral pulses
> Blood pressure–increased or decreased pressure, lower in thighs
> Hepatomegaly–liver more than 3 cm below right costal margin
> Hyperhydrosis–excessive perspiration
> Growth failure–below 5% weight on growth charts
>
> **Facilitating the Diagnosis**
> Offer support to parents and child by preparing them for diagnostic procedures (ECG, echocardiography, phonocardiography, x-ray, blood work, cardiac catheterization). Allow parents to be with child as much as possible before, during and after procedures. Provide for consistency of care by allowing primary nurse to be with child during painful procedures.
>
> *Infant*
> Provide security object (blanket, toy, pacifier). Have primary nurse and parents present if possible. Playing music, singing, talking and stroking may soothe infant.
>
> *Toddler*
> Explain to toddler in simple terms what to expect just before procedure. If it is true, tell him "Mommy will be here waiting for you when you return." Use diversion, such as play, reading to toddler.
>
> *3–7 year old*
> Give simple explanations of procedures. Use doll and/or diagram to show child what the procedure will be like. (For example, for cardiac catheterization show what catheter looks like; tell where it will go; tell how dye will feel, where dressing will be afterward.) Allow the child to play with mask, cap, gown and stethoscope and take him for a ride on the stretcher. Allow child to meet nurses who will care for him during and after procedure (catheterization or surgery). Explain to child what will be expected after procedure (dressing will be in place, he must keep leg straight, nurses will take blood pressure often; he can have something cool to drink).
>
> *Parents*
> Explain objectives of surgery or procedure to parents. Tell them that child will be NPO before the procedure. Tell them medication will be given to make child drowsy and to relieve pain. Explain what child will experience during procedure using diagram or doll. Assure parents that child will be well cared for. Tell them what to expect after procedure: child may be drowsy, fluids should be encouraged, dressing will be present on groin, frequent blood pressure, pulse and respiration and dressing checks, leg used for procedure must be kept straight.

ital cardiac defects.[18] These defects are classified as either secundum defects or primum defects. Secundum defects are located higher in the septal wall, whereas primum defects occur closer to the endocardial cushion. This section contains a discussion of the secundum variety, since it is the most common type (Fig. 24–8).

In utero communication between the atria exists via the foramen ovale. After birth, with ventilation of the lungs, there is an increase in circulatory flow through the lungs and an increase in pulmonary venous return to the left atrium. The increased pressure of the left atrium, along with the decreased velocity of flow from the inferior vena cava, results in closure of the foramen ovale. In the initial hours of life a small amount of blood may shunt from the right to the left atrium. The foramen ovale usually seals off at 2 to 3 months of age, but a small opening may persist into adulthood without symptomatology.

Clinical manifestations of atrial septal defects depend on their size and location and the outflow resistances of the ventricles. The average size of an ASD is 2 to 3 cm. Since the atria are low-pressure chambers, a defect must be quite large to permit a large left-to-right shunt.

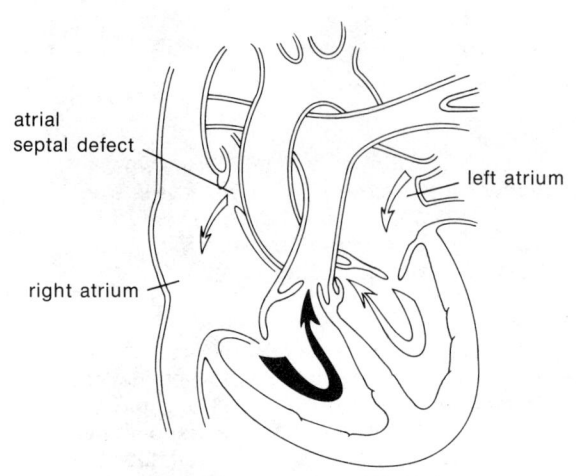

Figure 24-8 Atrial septal defect.

When large amounts of blood are permitted to shunt from left to right, pressures eventually equalize between the right and left atria. Thus the final result is little or no shunting as pressures equalize.

Shunting is dependent upon pulmonary vascular changes as well as pressure in both pulmonic and systemic systems. A decrease in systemic pressure or a rise in pulmonic pressure will decrease the left-to-right shunt. Therefore, other defects such as pulmonary stenosis or obstructive lung disease (which increase right-sided pressure) will decrease the left-to-right shunting and may even precipitate right-to-left shunting with the development of cyanosis.

Right atrial and right ventricular enlargement may occur with these defects, yet the development of cardiac failure is quite rare in infancy unless a large shunt exists. In fact, most atrial septal defects are not diagnosed until after the neonatal period and may not be detected until the school-age years. At birth the muscle thickness of the ventricles is roughly equal. Gradually the right ventricular wall thins and the left ventricular wall thickens. It has been hypothesized that no shunt will occur until the compliance of the ventricles improves and thus no murmur is heard and diagnosis is delayed.[18] Most often a heart murmur is the first clue.

Unlike ventricular septal defects (VSD), the increased blood flow to the lungs through an atrial defect is less likely to cause pulmonary vascular disease and there is usually no pulmonary hypertension. The lower ejection pressure within the right ventricle amounts for this difference between ASD and VSD. The pulmonary circulation may dilate to accommodate this increased flow. Secondary vascular changes (intimal proliferation, gradual occlusion of small vessels) are a risk, but they are slow to develop and may not be evident until adulthood.

Infants and children with atrial defects are usually asymptomatic. There may be exercise intolerance and recurrent infections because of increased workload of the right ventricle. Right-sided congestive heart failure occurs only in those with significant left-to-right shunts. Cyanosis is rare, especially after infancy. There may be some enlargement of the heart.

Management is usually surgical correction at age 3 to 7 years for moderate or large defects. The defect is surgically closed by suturing, or for very large defects a Dacron patch is used. Since small defects do not pose problems and may even close spontaneously, surgery is not recommended. Operative risk is usually minimal but postoperative complications, including cardiac enlargement, arrythmias and mitral valve prolapse can occur.[16] Continued antibiotic prophylaxis for certain procedures (dental work, surgery) is necessary to prevent bacterial endocarditis. Cardiology follow-up is required for the patient with a repaired defect at one- to three-year intervals, since mitral valve prolapse may not occur until adolescence or adulthood.

Patent Ductus Arteriosus The ductus arteriosus is a large channel connecting the descending aorta and the pulmonary artery (Fig. 24-9). Its diameter is roughly the same size as the descending aorta. In utero, the ductus allows most of the fetal blood to bypass the lungs. This bypass is compatible with fetal life since the placenta provides for oxygenation of blood. Before birth, blood flows from the pulmonary artery via the ductus to the aorta, from an area of high pressure to an area of lower pressure.

Closure of the ductus usually occurs spontaneously during the first 24 hours of life. Permanent closure occurs within 5 to 7 days in most infants but may take up to 21 days. The remnants of the ductus gradually disappear during the first few months of life. The exact mechanisms of closure of the ductus are still not well defined. One of the major effects on closure is exposure of the infant to the constricting effect of the high oxygen content of the extrauterine environment immedi-

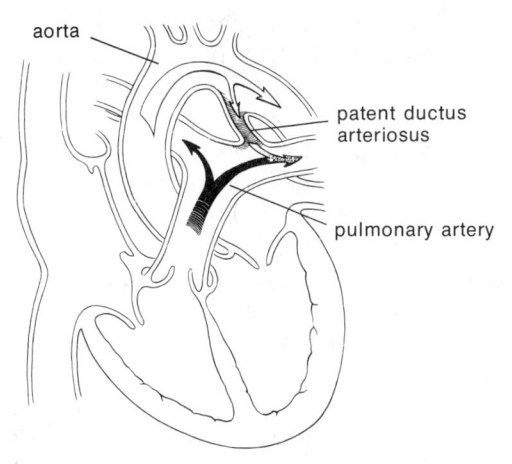

Figure 24-9 Patent ductus arteriosus.

ately after birth. Parasympathetic stimulation may also play a part in closure. Bradykinin, a vasoactive peptide that is released into circulation after birth, also has a constricting effect on the ductus.

In some infants, both full-term and preterm, the ductus fails to close spontaneously. This patent ductus arteriosus, as a solitary defect, accounts for about 15 per cent of congenital heart defects.[17] Patent ductus may occur in association with other heart defects.

In preterm infants the ductus may remain open for several months before beginning to close spontaneously. Lower oxygen levels, especially in relation to respiratory distress, may foster this patency (increased oxygen stimulates closure).

With the first breath of life, pulmonary arteriolar resistance decreases, systemic resistance increases (due to cutting of the cord and low environmental temperature), and left-sided pressure increases. When the ductus remains patent after birth the blood flow is reversed, with blood shunting from the aorta to the pulmonary artery. With this left-to-right shunt, the pulmonary circulation receives an increased volume of blood while the systemic circulation is deprived of blood flow. The left atrium receives increased pulmonary venous return and cardiac output increases in order to meet the needs of the systemic circulation. The pulmonary circulation may not be able to tolerate this increased blood volume and therefore pulmonary hypertension and pulmonary vascular obstruction may develop, especially with a large ductus. Aortic diastolic pressure is low because of left-to-right shunting, and the systemic pulse pressure widens. With continued increase in output, the left ventricle hypertrophies and cardiac failure may develop.

Cardiac failure usually occurs early in the preterm infant with patent ductus, whereas in the term infant it may not occur until 6 to 12 weeks. The earlier onset of symptoms in the preterm infant may be due to the more rapid decrease in pulmonary vascular resistance. In the preterm infant with hypoxia or respiratory disease the pulmonary vessels will constrict and increase the pulmonary resistance, offsetting the left-to-right shunt. Once respiratory distress decreases, the pulmonary resistance decreases and left-to-right shunting through the ductus occurs.

Any conditions that put extra demands on the heart for increased systemic flow will exaggerate the symptoms of cardiac failure. Such conditions include infection, poor nutrition, decreased hemoglobin, increased environmental temperature and increased activity.

The clinical manifestations of a patent ductus depend on the size of the ductus as well as the age of the infant. Frequently infants are asymptomatic and are referred to a cardiologist only after a murmur is auscultated during a routine physical examination.

Infants with a small ductus usually show no evidence of cardiac failure. There may be some widening of pulse pressures along with a continuous murmur. Peripheral pulses may be abnormally strong or bounding. The ductus may close spontaneously or require surgical intervention, usually around 12 to 18 months of age. Closure is indicated in order to prevent later risk of subacute bacterial endocarditis.

Infants with a moderate-sized ductus may appear asymptomatic or may exhibit tachypnea and tachycardia. At about 6 to 12 weeks of age signs of left ventricular failure begin to become apparent: poor feeding, irritability, lethargy, diaphoresis, tachypnea and dyspnea. Growth delay may also occur due to poor feeding. These infants may respond well to medical treatment or may require immediate surgical correction. Some may even survive without any treatment, but life expectancy decreases without surgical correction.

Infants with a large ductus will most likely show symptoms of cardiac failure earlier. Left ventricular failure with pulmonary edema is followed by eventual right ventricular failure. Cyanosis may appear with exertion. Symptoms of severe pulmonary obstruction may continue to develop through late adolescence if surgical repair is not performed.

A patent ductus creates a continuous murmur that begins just after the first heart sound. It is often described as a "machinery-like" murmur originating from the turbulent flow through the ductus. It is heard best at the left intraclavicular area. A systolic murmur may be auscultated in the neonate, especially if pulmonary hypertension has developed, altering flow through the ductus. Diagnosis is confirmed by echocardiogram or cardiac catheterization.

Surgical closure of a patent ductus is done by multiple suture ligation (sutures are tied at each end of the ductus) or complete division (the ductus is excised). The presence of a ductus is indication for surgery, since operative risk is low compared to the risk of endocarditis in later years. Recannulization (reopening) of the ductus is possible after surgical correction, necessitating close follow-up for assessment of any murmurs. Prophylactic antibiotics should be administered during the first six months after any invasive procedures.

Medical management has two components. The first involves management of cardiac failure in order to allow the infant time to grow before surgery is performed. Medical treatment consists of diuretics and digitalization. Diuretics decrease the blood volume and thus the burden on the left ventricle. Digitalization may be instituted in order to increase the cardiac stroke force. Electrolytes need to be monitored during diuretic and digitalis therapy, as do the digitalis levels. Since infancy is a period of rapid growth, these doses may need to be increased as the infant grows.

Recently indomethacin has been used experimentally in preterm infants to induce closure of patent ductus arteriosus.[6, 10] Indomethacin inhibits prostaglandin synthesis, and in some infants has induced spontaneous closure, thus avoiding surgical intervention.

Endocardial Cushion Defect The endocardial cushions are large projections of endomyocardial jelly that separate the atrioventricular canal into the atria and ventricles during fetal development. There are four cushions arising from the sides of the canal, with the posterior and anterior cushions contributing to most of the division. These two cushions also contribute to formation of the mitral and tricuspid valves. Endocardial cushion defects result from arrested or abnormal embryologic development of these cushions in utero. These defects are often classified as complete or partial, each having varied clinical manifestations that depend upon the size of the defect as well as the involvement of the atrioventricular valves.

Partial defects are usually atrial septal defects of the ostium primum variety, in which there is a large atrial septal defect and an intact ventricular septum, with or without mitral or tricuspid valve involvement. The manifestations are similar to those of atrial septal defects of the secundum variety, although mitral regurgitation may also be present. Complete endocardial cushion defects present with more severe clinical manifestations and it is these defects that are discussed.

Complete defects involve a large atrial septal defect, a ventricular septal defect of varying size (the earlier in utero the anomaly develops, the larger the defect), and involvement of the mitral and tricuspid valves. Cushion defects are the most common heart anomaly associated with trisomy 21 (Down's syndrome). Congenital heart lesions associated with cushion defects include pulmonary stenosis, patent ductus arteriosus and aortic isthmus narrowing.

Hemodynamics resulting from this defect depend on the size of the septal defect as well as the degree of involvement of the atrioventricular valves. Essentially, there is a large central hole in the heart. Mitral regurgitation, tricuspid regurgitation and shunts, either left to right or right to left, may exist. The direction of the shunt is determined by pulmonic and systemic resistance and compliance of each chamber of the heart. As pulmonary resistance increases, shunting will occur from right to left and cyanosis will develop.

Most frequently, there will be a left-to-right shunt at the atrial and ventricular defects along with regurgitation of the involved atrioventricular valves. If a large ventricular septal defect exists, pulmonary vascular obstruction and pulmonary hypertension may develop, causing the shunting to be bidirectional. In both partial and complete defects the atrioventricular node and the bundle of His may be interrupted or displaced, creating conduction problems.

Clinical manifestations of complete endocardial cushion defects are usually quite severe. If the atrioventricular valves are not involved to a great extent, the symptoms may differ but most complete defects involve these valves. Symptoms develop in early infancy and include tachypnea, dyspnea, poor weight gain and diaphoresis. Congestive heart failure develops early, as does cardiomegaly. Cardiac failure may become chronic owing to pulmonary vascular changes. Cyanosis may result from bidirectional shunting. Usually these infants are pale and prone to recurrent respiratory infections. Arrhythmias may develop because of alteration of the conduction system.

Palliative procedures have been attempted in infancy with poor success. Pulmonary artery banding is done to increase right ventricular pressure and thus decrease the left-to-right shunt through a VSD. Corrective surgery consists of patch closure of the septal defects and repair of the mitral and tricuspid valves. This operation carries with it a high mortality. Postoperative complications include heart block that is usually fatal and residual mitral regurgitation. These children all need close cardiology follow-up as well as prophylactic antibiotic therapy for certain procedures.

Ventricular Septal Defect Ventricular septal defects (VSD) are among the most common heart lesions, comprising 20 per cent of all congenital heart defects.[17] Often these defects are one part of other more complex defects such as truncus arteriosus, tetrology of Fallot, endocardial cushion defects, double outlet right ventricle and transposition of the great arteries. The size of a VSD varies, as does the location, with these factors determining clinical manifestations. After birth pulmonary vascular resistance begins to decrease and systemic vascular pressure rises. With these hemodynamic adjustments blood will flow from the left ventricle through the defect to the right ventricle, from an area of high pressure to an area of lower pressure (Fig. 24–10). The symptoms that develop depend on the size of the defect, the age of the child and the amount of pulmonary vascular change that occurs.

Small defects are usually located in the muscular portion of the septum. Most often there are few clinical manifestations and closure usually occurs spontaneously, within the first two years. A heart murmur is usually not audible at birth because of the still equalizing pressures of the

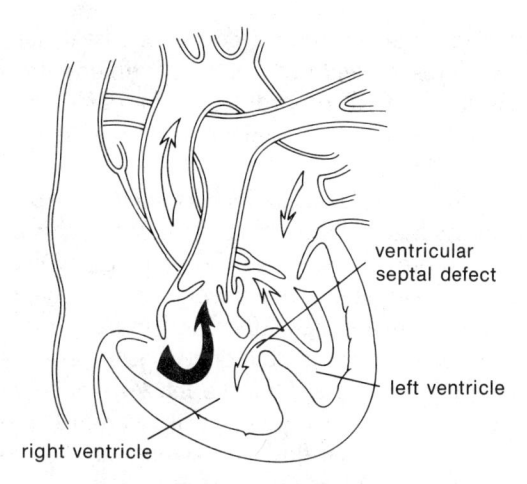

Figure 24–10 Ventricular septal defect.

pulmonic and systemic systems. Once the systemic resistance increases and pulmonary resistance decreases, only a small amount of shunting from left to right remains. This places a small increased volume load on the left ventricle due to the increased blood return from pulmonary circulation. In these small defects, there are usually no pulmonary vascular changes. Symptoms, if any, would include exercise intolerance, recurrent respiratory infection, fatigue and dyspnea. Management includes routine follow-up by a cardiologist and prophylactic antibiotics for invasive procedures.

Moderate-sized defects vary in symptomatology also. Some will close spontaneously, while others may persist indefinitely. There may be pulmonary vascular changes owing to an increased flow through the pulmonary system. Since a greater amount of blood is flowing from the left ventricle to the right ventricle, the chance of overload and congestive heart failure (right- and left-sided failure) increases. Exercise intolerance, dyspnea, fatigue and recurrent infections increase in severity, although growth usually is not delayed. These symptoms begin around two months of age. If pulmonary vascular resistance begins to increase in response to overload, flow of the blood may be reversed due to increased right-sided pressure and a right-to-left shunt develops. Mild cyanosis will be evident because of mixing of unoxygenated with oxygenated blood. Management of moderate-sized defects includes close cardiology follow-up, medical management of congestive heart failure if present, and prophylactic antibiotic therapy for invasive procedures. If the defect fails to close spontaneously, surgical intervention may be indicated.

With a large defect, defined as a defect the size of the diameter of the aorta or greater, infants will show more obvious signs of cardiac involvement. The pressures in both ventricles will begin to approximate each other and initially there may be no shunting. Pulmonary vascular resistance may increase if a large left-to-right shunt exists. The pulmonary system is overburdened with the increased flow and symptoms of congestive heart failure develop.

As pulmonary resistance continues to increase and ventricular pressures equalize, shunting may develop from right to left with resulting cyanosis. Pulmonary vascular changes usually develop by 1 year of age and are quite advanced by the age of 2 to 3 years. If pulmonary resistance increases rapidly, total correction may not be feasible. Increased pulmonary resistance results in an increased pressure in the right ventricle, with a right-to-left shunt through any residual defect and the right ventricle hypertrophies. Symptomatic treatment may be indicated in these cases.

Treatment of ventricular septal defects includes medical management of heart failure, palliative surgery or total corrective surgery. Palliative surgery (surgery that alleviates symptoms but does not correct the defect) is aimed at decreasing the burden of increased blood flow through the pulmonary system and thus decreasing return to the left atrium and ventricle. This is accomplished via banding of the pulmonary artery, a procedure that constricts the artery, decreasing pulmonary blood flow and decreasing the left-to-right shunt. One problem encountered is necrosis of the artery beneath the banding. This usually requires replacement at the time that total correction is performed. Banding is only a temporary, palliative procedure.

Current literature describes a preference for early total correction in large defects when possible, in order to prevent long-term complications of the defect such as pulmonary vascular obstruction, early left ventricular hypertrophy and damage, growth delay and complications from banding.[2, 16]

Surgical correction consists of closure of the defect by a Dacron patch. Total correction is not without its complications. The major postoperative complications involve conduction defects and residual ventricular defects. Conduction defects occur with great frequency and may result in sudden death. These defects are the result of scarring and injury to the proximal conduction system during surgery. Continued antibiotic prophylaxis for invasive procedures and indefinite cardiology follow-up are recommended after surgical correction.

Acyanotic Defects with Normal Pulmonary Vascularity

Coarctation of the Aorta Coarctation, a narrowing of the lumen of the aorta, constitutes 7 to 8 per cent of congenital heart defects.[17] This narrowing is often classified as preductal or postductal (Figs. 24–11 and 24–12). Preductal coarctation occurs in the area between the left subclavian artery and ductus arteriosus and is often associated with major intracardiac lesions. It is this type that occurs most commonly in neonates. The ductus remains patent and shunts blood from the pulmonary artery to the aorta. Postductal coarctation is a constriction of the aorta in the area just beyond the ductus arteriosus. Although this type occurs more frequently, it is less commonly associated with other cardiac anomalies and more frequently produces no symptoms until later childhood.

There appear to be two groups of patients with coarctation: (1) those who are symptomatic in infancy and (2) those who remain asymptomatic and are diagnosed during routine physical exam-

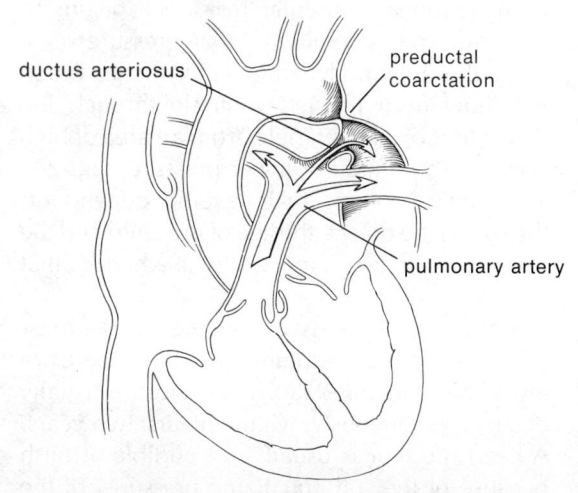

Figure 24–11 Preductal coarctation of aorta.

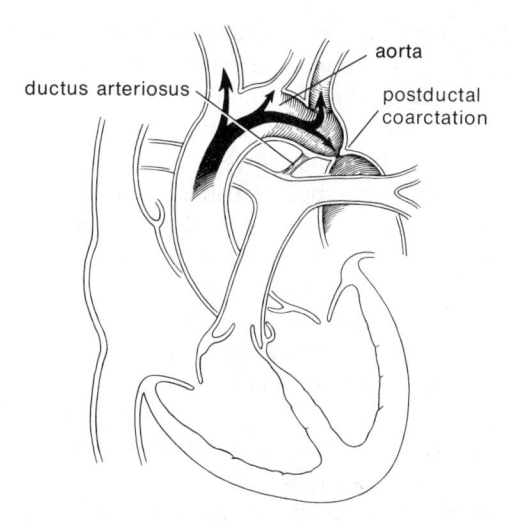

Figure 24-12 Postductal coarctation of aorta.

ination in later years. If symptoms do not develop during infancy the child will most likely grow normally and remain asymptomatic until later childhood, when upper extremity hypertension or diminished femoral pulses are noted.[2] Infants usually become symptomatic once the ductus arteriosus closes. The left ventricular workload suddenly increases and unless adequate collateral circulation develops, the left ventricle hypertrophies and cardiac failure ensues. Symptoms include respiratory distress, poor weight gain, feeding problems, irritability and tachycardia. With medical management, consisting of digitalis and diuretics, the infant's symptoms may subside and surgical correction can be delayed.

More commonly children exhibit few, if any, symptoms. The aorta is narrowed, decreasing blood flow to the lower part of the body. Blood flow to the upper part of the body is maintained via the innominate and subclavian arteries. Since the pressure in the left ventricle and ascending aorta is increased from the coarctation, the upper part of the body will display hypertension. Flow to the lower part of the body is maintained by the development of collateral circulation due to the increased systolic pressure in the proximal aortic segment. This collateral circulation provides enough blood for the body to survive, yet growth in the lower extremities is often slightly impeded.

Clinical manifestations of coarctation include absence of or decrease in femoral pulses, increase in blood pressure of upper extremities along with a substantial difference between blood pressure in upper and lower extremities, and decrease in growth of lower extremities as compared with upper body growth. There may be claudication (pain in muscles due to inadequate blood supply) in lower extremities or complaints of leg pain on exertion.

If the coarctation is symptomatic it can be repaired at the time of diagnosis. Even if there are no symptoms it is usually repaired when the child is between 3 and 5 years of age. The narrowed portion is removed and the ends of the aorta are anastamosed. A graft is rarely needed unless the area of coarctation is unusually large, since the aorta remains fairly pliable during childhood. Surgical repair of coarctation is not without risk of postoperative complications. Residual hypertension exists and there is risk of re-stenosis, mitral valve disease, cardiovascular disease and premature death. Continued antibiotic prophylaxis for certain procedures is necessary, as is cardiology follow-up at least every one to two years.

Without correction, coarctation can pose life-threatening dangers. Cerebral vascular accidents, aneurysms and rupture of the aorta occur as a result of the increased pressure and formation of collateral circulation. If left untreated, calcification of the aorta, changes in the eye grounds and left ventricular hypertrophy develop.

Pulmonary Stenosis Pulmonary stenosis is an obstructive, acyanotic heart defect that interferes with right ventricular outflow. Most often the defect is at the valvar level where the cusps are either fused into a membrane with a small orifice or the leaflets are thickened to varying degrees. Pulmonary stenosis exists in 10 to 20 per cent of all patients with congenital heart disease and is often associated with other anomalies such as tetralogy of Fallot, transposition of the great arteries, double outlet right ventricle defects and endocardial cushion defects.[17] This section deals with pure pulmonary stenosis, which usually consists of valvar stenosis with an intact ventricular septum. Patency of the foramen ovale as well as atrial septal defects may occur. The pulmonary artery is usually large as a result of a separate malformation of the artery that is not secondary to the pulmonary obstruction. Pure pulmonic stenosis symptomatology varies according to the degree of obstruction.

Hemodynamically, as obstruction increases,

right ventricular pressure increases and hypertrophy develops. If right ventricular hypertrophy is severe, right atrial pressure and hypertrophy may develop. With obstruction, pulmonary blood flow is decreased. Hypertrophy of the right ventricle develops as the ventricle tries to compensate for the pulmonary constriction by increasing its effort. Cyanosis develops only when communication between the left and the right sides of the heart exists and stenosis is severe. Since right ventricular pressure increases with stenosis, if a communication exists blood will flow from right to left, causing cyanosis.

Clinical manifestations depend on severity of obstruction. With severe pulmonary stenosis, cardiac failure may develop early in infancy. The ductus arteriosus, if patent, will provide for some pulmonary blood flow, but once closed, symptoms increase. If the foramen ovale remains patent, cyanosis will be evident. The stenosis causes a resistance to right ventricular outflow, which increases right-sided pressure enough to cause a right-to-left atrial shunt. If cardiac failure does not develop by 6 to 9 months of age, it probably will not develop. In some infants there exists adequate growth of muscle in the right ventricle to maintain increased pressure for increased flow and thus failure does not develop.

Most children with mild to moderate pulmonary stenosis remain asymptomatic until childhood or adolescence. Some never have symptoms and may progress through the fourth or fifth decade of life without problems. Research findings remain limited as to the long-term effects of mild pulmonary stenosis.

Symptoms usually include dyspnea on exertion and a decrease in exercise tolerance, since exercise increases the blood return to the right atrium, adding more stress. Cyanosis is an infrequent, late occurrence and results from decreased cardiac output or from existence of a right-to-left shunt.

Treatment of pulmonary stenosis consists of surgical repair. Infrequently, palliative treatment of severely cyanotic infants may be necessary. Corrective surgery is not indicated until there is evidence of increasing right ventricular pressure and hypertrophy. These children are followed closely by cardiologists, who have specific criteria for the need of surgical repair.

For valvar stenosis, a valvotomy is performed through the pulmonary artery and incisions are made along the fused commissures of the valve. In subvalvar stenosis, excess muscle is removed from the right ventricle. Operative mortality depends on age but is usually quite low.[16] Long-term postoperative complications include mild to moderate residual stenosis that is common but usually not progressive, murmur of pulmonary insufficiency, risk of subacute bacterial endocarditis and impaired right ventricular function. Conduction defects are rare because surgery is performed through the pulmonary artery instead of through the wall of the right ventricle. Cardiac follow-up every one to three years and antibiotic prophylaxis for certain procedures is necessary.

Aortic Stenosis Aortic stenosis constitutes 3 to 5 per cent of all congenital heart disease.[17] Aortic stenosis in infants and small children is always regarded as a congenital defect, whereas adults may develop aortic stenosis following rheumatic fever or from progressive atherosclerotic disease. Males are affected more with congenital aortic stenosis, especially the valvar type, than are females. Other congenital heart defects associated with aortic stenosis are ventricular septal defects, endocardial cushion defects and coarctation of the aorta.

Aortic stenosis is divided into four types: (1) valvar, (2) supravalvar, (3) discrete subvalvar and (4) diffuse subvalvar. Diffuse subvalvar stenosis, classified as a cardiac myopathy and also termed idiopathic hypertrophic subaortic stenosis (IHSS), bears little resemblance to the remaining three types. Supravalvar aortic stenosis occurs above the aortic valve. This type of stenosis is fairly uncommon and is usually associated with other defects such as mental retardation, defective dental development, abnormal facies, infantile hypocalcemia and pulmonary stenosis. Discrete subvalvar stenosis results from a thin membrane or thick fibrous ring in the subvalvar region of the aortic valve. Valvar aortic stenosis is the type most frequently encountered. The aortic valve may be unicuspid, bicuspid or tricuspid. In most cases the valve is bicuspid and thickened.

The clinical manifestations of aortic stenosis vary according to the type and extent of stenosis, yet all forms do have some points in common. Most children do not have any symptoms and are referred to a cardiologist only after a murmur is heard during a routine physical examination. This murmur may be detected during infancy or may not be detected until the preschool or school-age period. Physical development is normal. Symptoms would include mild fatigue, dyspnea and precordial pain.

Aortic stenosis affects the left ventricle. The left ventricle has an excess workload and it hypertrophies. This results in a decreased output in accordance with the degree of decreased compliance of the ventricle. This is determined by the severity of the stenosis. In severe cases, pulmonary edema may ensue as a result of increased left atrial pressure that may cause a backflow of blood into the lungs. Often infants with severe aortic valvar stenosis do poorly even after surgical correction because the left ventricle has already undergone extensive changes.

Some infants may develop cardiac failure in the first few months of life as a result of the increased demands on the heart. As growth continues and hemoglobin decreases, the left ventricle is required to increase output to meet these demands, but adequate compensation may not be possible in severe cases. If cardiac failure does not develop during infancy it is unlikely that symptoms will develop before the school-age years. The left ventricle, if able to maintain adequate cardiac output during infancy, will continue to adapt and sufficiently increase cardiac output.

Syncope and sudden death are complications related to the inability of the left ventricle to maintain adequate output. Sudden death occurs in diffuse subvalvar stenosis and to a lesser degree in the remaining types. Syncope and sudden death are not commonly seen in the child under 6 years of age. Bacterial endocarditis is another complication most frequently encountered in children over age 3. Even in children with mild aortic stenosis, follow-up is crucial. This is because the stenosis may progress, especially during the adolescent growth spurt, when the resting output increases and athletic activities are prominent.

Treatment of aortic stenosis entails surgical correction, when possible, although postoperative complications are numerous. The valve will never be completely normal; some degree of stenosis will remain. The likelihood of progressive stenosis and calcification exists and these patients may eventually require valve replacement. Arrhythmias result from progression of the disease. It is imperative that prophylactic antibiotics be continued for certain procedures; cardiology follow-up must continue at least every year. Children who do not undergo surgical correction must be restricted from the strenuous physical activity that increases the risk of ischemic attacks and sudden death.

Cyanotic Heart Defects With Increased Pulmonary Vascularity

Transposition of the Great Vessels Transposition of the great vessels is a cyanotic defect that accounts for 10 to 18 per cent of congenital heart defects.[17] It may take several forms, the most common consisting of normal positioning of the four heart chambers with the great vessels transposed (Fig. 24–13). The aorta arises from the right ventricle and the pulmonary artery leaves the left ventricle, resulting in two separate parallel circulatory systems. The pulmonary artery delivers blood to the lungs for oxygenation; this returns to the left atrium and left ventricle and is recycled again through the pulmonary circulation. The aorta delivers unoxygenated blood to the systemic circulation. This blood then returns to the right atrium and ventricle and instead of being oxygenated is circulated via the aorta again.

Transposition is always diagnosed in infancy since it is usually incompatible with life. There is greater frequency in males and these infants tend to be full-term and large. Some islet hypertrophy in the pancreas exists; this suggests one reason for the large size. A family history of diabetes is sometimes found. Associated anomalies are

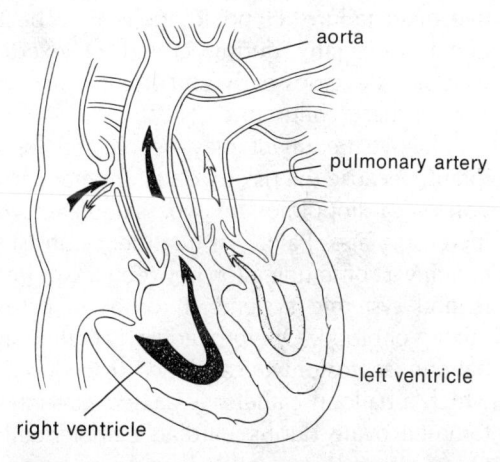

Figure 24–13 Transposition of great vessels.

quite common, since communication between the pulmonary and systemic systems is necessary for survival. These defects include ventricular septal defects, atrial septal defects and patent ductus arteriosus. Pulmonary stenosis is a common finding, especially in those children with large ventricular defects. Other less commonly associated defects include tricuspid atresia or stenosis, mitral atresia or stenosis, dextrocardia, levocardia, single ventricle, single atria and coarctation of the aorta.

Hemodynamically, two separate circulatory systems exist. Blood in the right side of the heart is oxygenated yet never reaches systemic circulation. The pulmonary oxygen saturation far exceeds that of systemic circulation. Life is possible only with the existence of communication between these two systems. Patency of the ductus arteriosus and foramen ovale at birth provides such communication only temporarily. As systemic resistance increases, the force of the right ventricular contraction must increase to pump blood out of the aorta and into the systemic circulation.

Clinical manifestations develop according to the type of transposition. Without any other defects that allow mixture of blood, cyanosis is marked and congestive heart failure develops rapidly. The right ventricle is not constructed to handle the workload of pumping to the systemic circulation. In transposition with a ventricular septal defect, the clinical manifestations are similar to those of a large ventricular defect. Congestive heart failure occurs (see discussion of VSD) with mild cyanosis. With a ventricular defect and pulmonary stenosis, the infant will have early cyanosis and, less frequently, congestive heart failure. Hypoxic spells may be frequent, especially during crying or exertion. Clubbing develops early and squatting may be seen in these children.

Palliative treatment may be elected for the infant, because the risk involved in total correction via cardiopulmonary bypass decreases with increasing age. Palliative treatment consists of creating a communication between the pulmonic and systemic systems in order to provide mixing of blood. One procedure is that of atrial balloon septostomy (Rashkind procedure), in which a balloon catheter is passed through the foramen ovale during cardiac catheterization. Once inflated, it is pulled back to create an opening between the two atria. The procedure may or may not be successful, but with it thoracotomy may be avoided. Creation of an atrial septal defect surgically is termed a Blalock-Hanlon procedure. This is done through a thoracotomy (incision into chest wall). Pulmonary vascular disease remains a complication after creation of an atrial defect, and total repair is indicated when the infant can better tolerate the surgery.

Corrective surgery has been possible only since 1964 with the development of the Mustard procedure. A new atrial septum is created by using pericardium to make a baffle. This baffle alters the blood flow by redirecting unoxygenated blood from the right atrium through the mitral valve to the left ventricle and out to the lungs via the pulmonary artery;* oxygenated blood from the left atrium is redirected through the tricuspid valve to the right ventricle to systemic circulation via the aorta.† Mortality for this procedure is still relatively high. Ideally it is performed at 2 to 3 years of age, although successful repair has been done on infants less than six months old. Corrective surgery should be performed before pulmonary vascular changes develop. Since this is a relatively new procedure, long-term outcomes are unknown. Complications postoperatively include rhythm and conduction disturbances, baffle leaks, and tricuspid regurgitation. Whether the right ventricle can continue to function as the systemic ventricle is another question that is raised. These children need cardiac follow-up at least every 6 to 12 months and will require prophylactic antibiotics for certain procedures.

Total Anomalous Venous Drainage Oxygenated blood is carried from the lungs to the right atrium or vena cava (superior or inferior) via the pulmonary veins instead of into the left atrium. Frequently an atrial septal defect exists that allows mixing of blood. This defect is classified according to entry into venous circulation above the level of the diaphragm or below the diaphragm. Prognosis is poor for those defects below the level of the diaphragm.

Truncus Arteriosus A large single vessel arises from both ventricles over a ventricular septal defect. This results from failure of normal septa-

---

*The pulmonary artery is transposed; therefore it comes off the left ventricle.
†The aorta is transposed and comes off the right ventricle.

tion and division of the trunk into an aorta and a pulmonary artery. The entire pulmonic and systemic system is supplied through this vessel, and as a result cyanosis develops, especially as pulmonary vascular disease develops. Prognosis is poor because the mortality is high for surgical repair.

Cyanotic Defects With Decreased Pulmonary Vascularity

Tetralogy of Fallot Tetralogy of Fallot accounts for 15 per cent of all congenital heart disease in patients less than 2 years of age.[17] Described by Fallot over 100 years ago, the anomaly is composed of four defects (pulmonary stenosis, right ventricular hypertrophy, ventricular septal defect and an over-riding aorta) (Fig. 24-14). Cardiologists now believe that two main defects exist and the anomaly is often termed pulmonary stenosis with ventricular septal defect rather than tetralogy of Fallot. This defect is the most common cyanotic defect and may also be associated with patent ductus arteriosus, atrial septal defects and aortic regurgitation.

The two major defects that occur in tetralogy are a ventricular septal defect and right ventricular outflow obstruction. The septal defect is usually large and located high in the septum. The obstruction to outflow results from pulmonary atresia or stenosis (most commonly the latter) located in the infundibular region of the right ventricle, although the pulmonic valve and pulmonic artery are sometimes involved. The third defect is that of right ventricular hypertrophy, most likely a result of outflow obstruction. Lastly, dextroposition,* or over-riding of the aorta, is present. This was once thought to be the main reason for cyanosis, but the degree of outflow obstruction actually determines the degree of cyanosis.

Clinical manifestations of tetralogy may be noted in the neonatal period, although they more commonly become apparent either at 3 to 6 months or after 2 years of age. Symptoms are a result of the shunting of blood from the right ventricle to the left ventricle. Normally, pressures are much higher in the left side of the heart, but the obstruction to flow out of the right ventricle causes an increase in pressure and thus a flow from an area of higher to lower

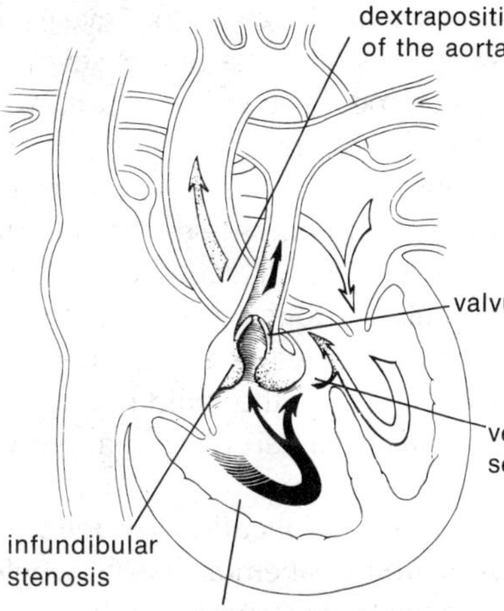

Figure 24-14 Tetralogy of Fallot.

pressure. Unoxygenated blood then passes to the systemic circulation, resulting in central cyanosis. The degree of cyanosis depends upon the size of the septal defect and the degree of outflow obstruction.

The obstruction decreases pulmonary blood flow. If the ductus arteriosus remains patent, blood will shunt from the aorta through the ductus to the pulmonary artery, then to the lungs for oxygenation. Thus, symptoms are rarely seen at birth or while the ductus is patent. Depending upon the degree of obstruction, some blood will circulate normally through the pulmonary artery. Collateral bronchial circulation may also develop in response to decreased pulmonary artery pressure, affording the body another means to oxygenate blood.

Symptoms commonly seen result from hypoxemia and include central cyanosis, clubbing, dyspnea on exertion, poor dental development and delayed growth. Cardiac failure and pulmonary edema are rarely seen as a result of tetralogy, since the presence of a large ventricular defect decreases pressure in the right ventricle, protecting it from failure. The neonate that exhibits symptoms usually has a severe form of tetralogy. Symptoms most commonly are seen at 3 to 6 months of age when the ductus closes and increased demands are made on the heart with increased growth, decreased hemoglobin and increase in activity. Prolonged crying decreases the pulmonary blood flow, causing an increase in symptoms. Some patients may not

---

*Dextroposition, or over-riding, is the placement of the aorta to the right of its normal position resulting in the aorta being positioned directly over (over-riding) the VSD.

develop symptoms until age 3 to 5 years or later. Their symptoms are usually less severe.

Squatting is commonly seen in children with tetralogy, especially during and after physical activity. Squatting relieves some strain on the heart. When the child compresses the muscles in the lower extremities in squatting, arterial and right ventricular systolic pressures increase. As the child grows, squatting becomes less acceptable socially. Often the child must avoid many activities that are a part of normal growth and development.

There are several complications of tetralogy of Fallot. Hypochromic anemia (low hemoglobin) results from the low oxygen saturation. This low oxygen saturation stimulates production of more red blood cells, resulting in polycythemia, hypervolemia and increased viscosity of blood. The polycythemia may be a factor that contributes to thrombus formation. Hemiplegia may result from cerebral thrombosis, embolism or anoxia. Cerebral vascular accidents are more common with severe cyanosis. Brain abscess is also a complication of this defect, but the actual mechanism for this is not well understood. Bacterial endocarditis remains a threat, owing to the large ventricular defect. Hemorrhagic disorders and gout have also been associated with tetralogy.

Treatment of this defect is either palliative surgical intervention or complete surgical repair. Palliative measures are performed in infancy to provide the child with a means of oxygenating more blood. These procedures consist of creating shunts that allow partially oxygenated blood to enter the pulmonary artery for additional oxygenation by the lungs. The Potts and Waterston procedures were used most frequently in years past. The Potts shunt connects the descending aorta to the left pulmonary artery; the Waterston shunt connects the ascending aorta to the right pulmonary artery. The danger of these shunts, especially the Potts, is creation of a shunt that is too large, sending a volume of blood to the lungs that cannot be handled, resulting in pulmonary edema. Another complication of shunting is thrombosis, which is promoted by polycythemia and hypotension. The Blalock-Taussig procedure is used more frequently today. It connects the right or left subclavian artery to the ipsilateral (on the same side) pulmonary artery. With this procedure there is less possibility of a large communication. In each of these palliative procedures (Potts, Waterston, and Blalock-Taussig) complete repair is done at a later time.

Corrective surgery consists of repair of the ventricular septal defect and pulmonary stenosis using cardiopulmonary bypass. Corrective surgery can be done in infancy, but the mortality rate increases as age decreases. All children with tetralogy need complete repair, ideally at age 5 to 8 years when toleration of this procedure is improved. Repair may be done even later in those children who have mild symptomatology.

Corrective surgery can involve complications that include residual pulmonary stenosis, right bundle branch block, cardiomegaly and residual ventricular septal defect. Lifelong cardiac follow-up is necessary, as is prophylactic antibiotic treatment for certain procedures. Total repair often alleviates so much of the symptomatology that previously affected children feel and act completely different. Parents need to be cautioned about the complications and the need for close follow-up.

Ebstein's Malformation Obstruction to filling of the right ventricle develops owing to malformation of the tricuspid valve, which causes tricuspid regurgitation. A right-to-left shunt develops along with cyanosis. The prognosis is better with milder tricuspid regurgitation. Several methods of correction are currently being utilized.

Tricuspid Atresia Closure of the tricuspid valve, an atrial septal defect, and hypoplastic right ventricle exist. Cyanosis develops because blood can only enter the pulmonary circulation via shunting through a ventricular defect or patent ductus. The prognosis is poor and a palliative shunt may be required before total correction can be attempted.

CONGESTIVE HEART FAILURE

Congestive heart failure is often a result of congenital heart defects. Failure results from several factors, which include decreased cardiac output, inefficient emptying or overloading of the pulmonary system, or inefficient emptying of the heart ventricles. As blood supply to the kidneys decreases, glomerular filtration decreases and excess sodium and water are retained by the body. Pulmonary engorgement inhibits respiratory function. When venous blood becomes backed up venous pressure increases.

Failure can occur on the right side or the left side or it may involve both sides, depending upon the underlying defect. With left ventricular failure, the ventricle weakens and blood backs up into the pulmonary system — pulmonary edema may ensue. In right-sided failure the right ventricle weakens and blood backs up into the systemic circulation. When failure develops, either right- or left-sided, the remaining side will eventually fail unless treatment is initiated.

Signs and symptoms of congestive heart failure are different in infants from those in older children. In infancy there may be tachypnea, feeding difficulties, poor weight gain, perspiration, irritability, weak cry and labored respiratory effort. Liver enlargement is present, as is cardiomegaly (enlargement of heart seen on x-ray). Edema is difficult to determine in the infant. Older children may exhibit anorexia, fatigue, exercise intolerance, cough and abdominal pain. The liver may be enlarged owing to venous congestion and edema is present from decreased glomerular filtration. Rales that indicate pulmonary congestion are heard in the lungs. Cardiomegaly is present.

Treatment of failure includes rest, low sodium diet, oxygen (if needed), and diuretic and digitalis therapy. Diuretics relieve the pulmonary congestion and edema. It is important to monitor electrolytes closely when diuretic therapy is utilized, since hypokalemia (decreased potassium) and hypochloremia (decreased chloride) may develop from rapid diuresis. Potassium supplements may be indicated. This is especially important if the child is on digitalis preparations, because hypokalemia exaggerates the signs of digitalis toxicity. Digitalis strengthens the heartbeat and has a diuretic effect. Parents need to be instructed to recognize signs and symptoms of digitalis toxicity, which include anorexia, vomiting, nausea, diarrhea, dizziness and headache.

SUBACUTE BACTERIAL ENDOCARDITIS

Subacute bacterial endocarditis is a disease of the endocardium (inner lining) of the heart. This infection develops at the site of congenital or acquired defects of the heart. Organisms responsible for the infection include streptococci, enterococci, staphylococci and fungi. The infecting organisms usually settle at the site of the defect. These organisms can be introduced during dental procedures, invasive diagnostic procedures (urinary catheterization) or during surgery.

Symptoms include anorexia, weight loss, malaise, pallor, fever and chills. Heart failure may develop along with splenomegaly (enlargement of the spleen). Blood cultures are done to determine the organism and its sensitivity to antibiotic therapy. Penicillin is the drug most frequently used both for treatment and prevention.

CARDIAC SURGERY

Preoperative Preparation

The child is usually admitted a few days before surgery for physical and psychological preparation. Physical preparation includes a complete history, thorough physical examination, laboratory studies (complete blood count, hemoglobin, hematocrit, determination of clotting times, electrolyte levels, type and cross match for two to three units of blood and urinalysis), chest x-ray, ECG, phonocardiogram, and results of a recent cardiac catheterization. The infant will be kept NPO after midnight the evening before surgery. It is important to post a sign on the door to the child's room and on the crib so that he is given nothing by mouth before surgery. Preoperative medications include morphine and Seconal given intramuscularly 30 to 45 minutes before surgery.

In the case of an older child psychological preparation for surgery must include both the parents and the child. It is ideal if the parents and the child can visit the hospital and the intensive care unit (ICU) before the operation to meet the nurses who will be caring for him and to become more familiar with the environment. At this time a description of the equipment used postoperatively will be helpful. In some hospitals the nurses in the ICU visit the patients and their parents the evening before surgery to explain the care the patient will receive while in the unit.

It is most important that parents be prepared for the appearance of their child postoperatively because all the equipment can be frightening. It is helpful to use some type of visual aid such as

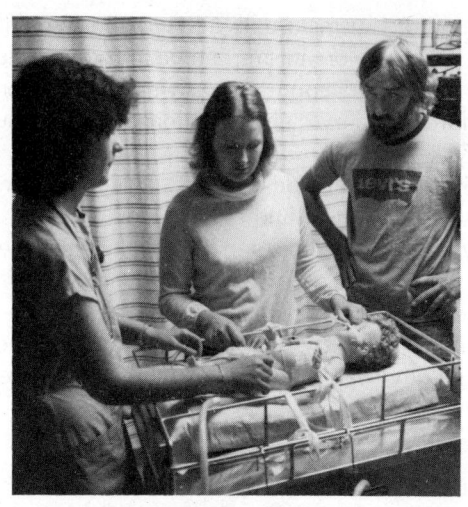

Preoperatively, a doll can be used to prepare parents for the appearance of their baby after his operation. This gives parents an opportunity to discuss their fears and concerns about the numerous machines and tubes.

a doll or a diagram to explain the purpose of the equipment and of nursing interventions. Parents also need reassurance that the nurses will be watching the infant or child closely and that medication will be given for pain. When teaching parents it is necessary to proceed slowly and discuss one aspect of care at a time. Parents should be told specifically how their child will appear postoperatively and forewarned that he will be asleep or heavily sedated. Specific things to tell parents preoperatively and to review again immediately upon the child's entering the intensive care unit follow:

1. An endotracheal tube is placed into the throat to aid the child's breathing. (An infant is unable to cry and an older child unable to talk.)
2. A tube (nasogastric tube) is placed through the nose into the stomach to keep the stomach empty and free of air and stomach juices until digestive function is restored.
3. Two or three intravenous tubes may be present to replace fluids and blood and to provide a means of checking pressures within the heart.
4. A dressing or tape (Steri-strips) is placed across the chest covering the incision.
5. Two tubes (chest tubes), one on either side of the chest, are required to remove air and blood that enters the chest during surgery.
6. A small plastic bag may be applied to the perineum to collect urine or a small tube may be placed into the bladder to drain the urine.
7. Discs with wires (cardiac leads) are put on the infant's chest to monitor the heart rate and observe the pattern of how the heart beats.
8. The nurse will be checking the status of the infant every 15 minutes until his condition stabilizes.

Open heart surgery is an extremely invasive procedure that requires opening the thoracic cavity and use of an extracorporeal cardiopulmonary bypass machine. There are four approaches to opening the chest: median sternotomy, anterolateral thoracotomy, posterolateral thoracotomy and transverse sternotomy.[12] Open heart surgery is usually very lengthy. Following the cardiac repair the infant is taken directly to the intensive care unit rather than to the recovery room. Constant observation by the nursing staff is done to monitor the child's vital functions: circulatory status, respiratory status, level of consciousness, and fluid and electrolyte balance.

On return from cardiac surgery the child will be heavily sedated. The level of consciousness should be noted frequently during the first 24 hours postoperatively. The infant will usually be without clothing for maximum observation and may be placed on a radiant heated table or Aqua K pad to maintain the body temperature. If hypothermia* has been used during cardiac surgery the child's temperature may be unstable for a period of time. Vital signs should be checked every 15 minutes for the first 24 hours. Signs of distress such as tachycardia, tachypnea, retractions, stridor, nasal flaring, expiratory wheezing and grunting should be reported to the physician. The infant's skin should be observed for color, temperature and diaphoresis. Cyanosis may be circumoral or circumorbital. The mucous membranes and tongue should always be checked for central cyanosis.

A monitor is attached to the infant to note the rate and rhythm of the heart. The central venous pressure (CVP) is monitored via two atrial catheters. Cardiac output is measured in this way. Pacemaker leads may be left in place in case arrhythmias develop in the postoperative period. An intra-arterial line is placed to moni-

---

*Hypothermia is used to reduce oxygen needs during surgery.

tor blood pressure. This should be compared with the blood pressure reading obtained at the extremity.

To maintain a patent airway, an endotracheal tube will be in place. Percussion of the chest and application of suction via the endotracheal tube should be done every hour. If no endotracheal tube is in place, stimulation of a cough can be achieved by placing a suction catheter to the back of the pharynx. Suction return, amount, color and mucus plugs should be noted and recorded. Oxygen concentration should be carefully assessed by use of an analyzer to ensure delivery as ordered. The infant may require the assistance of a respirator to maintain ventilation.

The nasogastric tube in the stomach is usually placed on straight drainage to keep the stomach decompressed. Normally the nasogastric tube is not irrigated; if plugged, the tube is replaced.

A dressing is in place over the chest incision. The incision site should be checked every 15 minutes during the first 24 hours for bleeding or hematoma formation. Two to three chest tubes are placed for drainage or suction or both to remove fluid and air that entered the thoracic cavity during surgery. The chest tubes should be checked frequently for patency and should be stripped (milked) every hour. The connections of the chest tube and every inch of the tubing should be checked and all connections taped. The tubing should be carefully examined regularly from the site of insertion in the chest to the chest bottle to ensure that it is not kinked under the infant. Color, amount and viscosity of the drainage is noted every hour.

The infant will have a urine bag on or a Foley catheter in place. Amount, color and specific gravity of the urine is noted hourly. If the infant is not catheterized, the bladder may need to be emptied by the Credé maneuver (see Fig. 25–3). Renal function may be depressed following open heart surgery. The infant should void within two to three hours postoperatively. The expected urinary output of an infant is 0.5 cc/kg/hour.

Accurate intake and output must be monitored every hour. Intravenous solutions and blood are being given to make up for the blood lost during surgery. The hourly output includes chest tube drainage, urine, stool, nasogastric drainage, blood drawn, suction return from the airway, and drainage from the dressing.

Usually the child will have morphine ordered for pain, prophylactic antibiotics and heparin to prevent clotting. His weight is checked daily and a daily chest x-ray is done. Usually the infant will be given nothing by mouth until he is alert and no longer requires assisted ventilation, and the bowel sounds are active. These children require good oral hygiene at least every four hours with either sponge-tipped applicators or lemon glycerine swabs.

Ideally parents are allowed to visit frequently during the child's stay in the intensive care unit. The nurse can help the parents ventilate their feelings and can provide a supportive environment during this stressful period. Keeping the parents informed of how their child is doing and explaining the care helps to create confidence in the nursing staff. It is helpful if one nurse on each shift is assigned to the patient and family to provide for continuity of care. The primary nurse can facilitate a supportive climate by taking time to sit with and talk to the parents to assess their needs and concerns about their child. This assessment needs to be done daily to promote and maintain a healthy family environment.

After two to three days in the intensive care unit, the child will be returned to the unit where he was before surgery. The child is hospitalized for an additional five to seven days, during which normal daily activities are gradually resumed. Usually infants and toddlers resume activity on their own, whereas older children

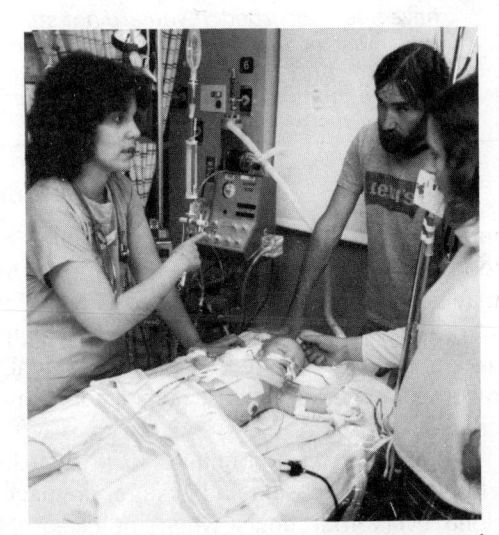

Keeping the parents informed of how their child is doing after the operation and explaining the care helps to create confidence in the nursing staff.

> **ANSWERING PARENTS' QUESTIONS ABOUT DIGOXIN ADMINISTRATION**
>
> 1. If dose is missed
>   Give the next dose on time. Do not double the dosage to make up for the missed one.
> 2. If more than one dose is missed in a row or one dose is missed for several days in a row
>   Notify your physician of the number of doses missed and the times they were missed.
>   It is helpful to make the administration of this medication part of your child's daily routine so that it will not be forgotten and to help with the child's acceptance of it.
> 3. How often is the medication given?
>   Digoxin is usually given every 12 hours. It takes about one hour to take effect. It reaches its peak between one and two hours after it was given. The effects decrease over 24 to 35 hours.
> 4. What is the best time to give the digoxin?
>   Digoxin is best absorbed when the stomach is empty because food may interfere with its absorption. For this reason it is best to give the digoxin one hour before or 2 hours after eating.
> 5. What if my child vomits after receiving the medication?
>   If your child vomits within 15 minutes after the medication has been given and you feel most of the medication has been lost you may repeat the dose once. If more than 15 minutes has elapsed the dose should not be repeated because some of the digoxin will have been absorbed. If you are not sure that most of the medication has been lost it is best not to repeat it. If your child continues to vomit notify your physician because this may be the sign of some other problem.
> 6. What shall I do if the child has the flu with vomiting, diarrhea and fever?
>   Your physician should be notified immediately. If your child becomes dehydrated through loss of fluid the effects of digoxin on the body may be altered. Continue to give the digoxin as prescribed and encourage fluids. The type of fluid will vary with the degree of illness.
> 7. Where should digoxin be stored?
>   Digoxin, like any medication, should be stored in a secure place out of the reach of children. An accidental ingestion of digoxin could be fatal so it should not be kept at the bedside or in the child's room.
> 8. What should be done if a child accidentally swallows digoxin?
>   A call to your poison control center immediately. Have the bottle with you when you call. They will ask for age and size of the child who took the digoxin, when the incident occurred and approximately how much digoxin was in the bottle. If you have ipecac (a medication which induces vomiting) they may recommend that you give one dose before going to your nearest emergency room. Time should not be wasted. If you do not have a car the police or fire department should be called or an emergency ambulance sent. Take the digoxin bottle with you to the emergency room.
>
> ---
>
> Adapted from P. L. Jackson. Digoxin therapy at home: Keeping the child safe. American Journal of Maternal Child Nursing, Mar/Apr 1979, p. 105

may need some encouragement. Fluids and foods are introduced gradually; fluid restriction may be necessary to prevent overloading of the cardiovascular system. The intake and output are carefully monitored and daily weight is recorded. Accuracy in these nursing functions is crucial.

Respiratory status continues to be watched closely and percussion and postural drainage is done every four hours while indicated. Nasopharyngeal suctioning will be done after postural drainage to remove secretions and to stimulate coughing. It is important for these children to cough and breathe deeply to fully aerate all lobes of their lungs.

For an infant or toddler who has had a thoracotomy, it is important not to pick him up under his arms because this puts stress on the suture line and may be painful to the child. The nurse should put her arms under the child's shoulders and buttocks and lift him in this manner.

The incision should be carefully inspected for infection; intactness of the suture line should be ascertained, and redness, swelling, heat, tenderness and presence of drainage should be checked for.

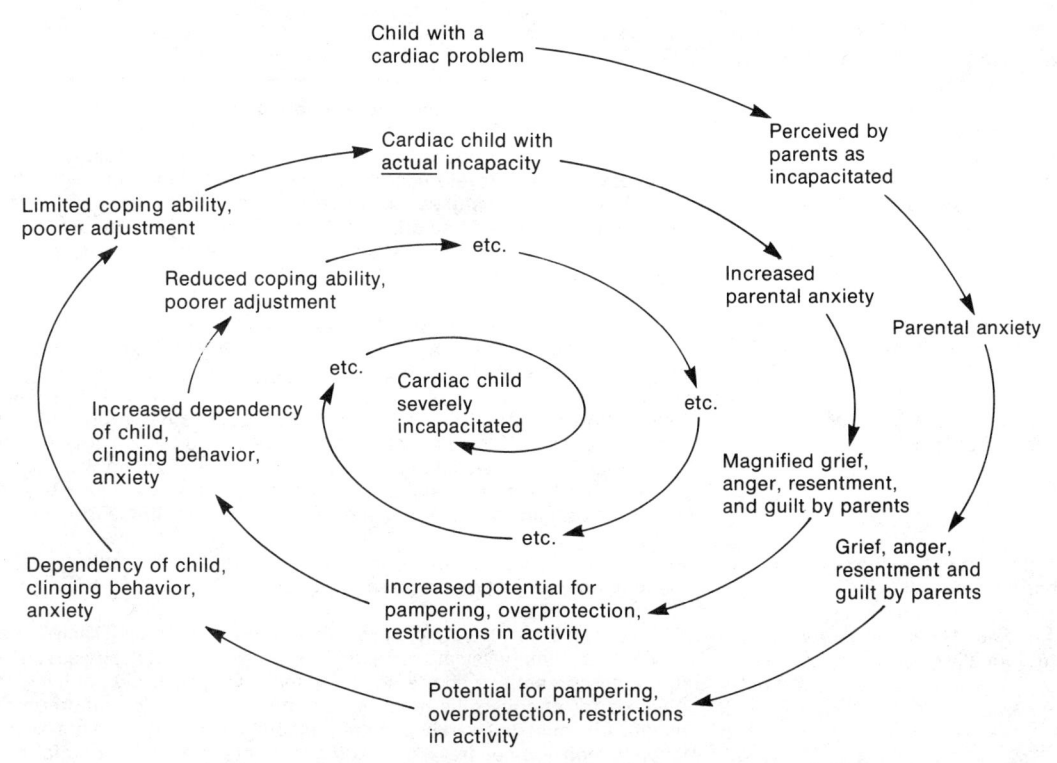

Figure 24–15 Cyclic pattern of parental responses in cardiac problems.

Medications ordered during the postoperative period are usually digoxin, a diuretic and an antibiotic. Before administering digoxin the apical pulse must be taken for one full minute. It is important to teach the mother or primary caretaker how to take an apical pulse so that she is prepared to care for the child at home. If the apical pulse is below 100 beats per minute in an infant, digoxin is usually withheld until the physician is notified. Digoxin strengthens the force of the heartbeat but it also slows the rate.

Parents need instruction in how to accurately weigh their child daily. The same scale should be used for each weighing and the infant should be weighed without clothing. The parents should be given a written list of danger signs that will alert them to cardiac difficulty. This list should include the signs of congestive heart failure: labored or rapid breathing, feeding difficulties, perspiration, swelling around the eyes and irritability. The parents should be given a number to call for assistance should any problems arise. A referral to a community health nurse is essential and provides the added support a family needs in such a stressful time. These infants require close follow-up and are usually seen for a return visit at the cardiology clinic or their private physician's office two weeks after discharge.

IMPACT OF HEART DISEASE ON THE INFANT AND FAMILY

Emotional and Social Impact

The diagnosis of congenital heart disease in an infant has a tremendous impact on the family unit and those individuals involved in caring for the child in the community. These children not only must adapt to the physical stress or hospitalization, evaluative testing and palliative and corrective surgery but also may have to contend with an altered psychological, social and emotional environment.

Parents of the child with a congenital heart defect usually experience extreme stress, which may be compounded by guilt feelings and many fears. The family of this child requires support and practical guidance at the initial diagnosis and throughout the management of the disease to maintain and promote a healthy life style for the child and the family's other members.

Studies have shown that parental anxiety is related to the presence rather than to the severity of the cardiac lesion.[13] Anxiety directly affects how the parents relate to their children and rear them. In instances in which the parents

TABLE 24–2 CONCERNS PARENTS HAVE ABOUT THEIR INFANT WITH A CARDIAC CONDITION*

Concerns	Nursing Interventions
What caused my child's heart defect? Am I responsible?	Tell parents: You are not responsible for the defect — we do not know the exact cause. Heart development occurs in the first 2 months of gestation. Part of the heart sometimes fails to develop beyond this early stage. Many factors may be related, including maternal rubella during pregnancy, prematurity, chromosomal aberrations. The condition is not related to a family history of heart attacks.
Why did it take so long to diagnose the problem?	Often a murmur is not heard until 6 weeks of age and it may not have been apparent at birth. Therefore, to identify problems early it is necessary to examine infants frequently in the first months of life.
What causes the murmur? What is the defect?	Review flow of blood through normal heart. Using a diagram, explain the defect to parents. (This may have to be done 2 or 3 times.) Use the same terminology the physician has used (and explain it). Explain that the murmur is caused by abnormal flow of blood through the heart. Give diagram, name and definition of defect to the parents to keep at home for reference.
What will my child look like when he gets sick?	Provide parents with a list of signs: cyanosis, difficulty breathing, difficulty feeding, edema, perspiring, easy tiring, exhaustion.
What does it mean to treat him normally?	Tell parents: Treat this child as you do your other children. Discipline and set limits for him. Physical education is ok unless physician advises against it, but *no* competitive sports. Infants usually limit their own activity. Prophylaxis for endocarditis must be adhered to. Give information on diet, usually a normal diet, rarely a salt restriction diet. Instruct parents how and when to feed — small frequent feedings may prevent fatigue of infants and parents. Allow parents ample time to feed and handle baby while in the hospital. Instruct parents not to allow baby to cry for prolonged periods. See that they have vitamins and iron for the baby as anemia causes a strain on the heart. Reinforce child's normal, desirable features: for example, remark on all normal aspects of the child when doing bath demonstration for parents.
What is my child's future?	Outline the long range problems so that surprises in treatment are kept to a minimum: hospitalization, cardiac catheterization, surgical repair. Explain medications to be given, their purpose, name, dose, time and side effects.
What should I tell my child and my other children?	Explain that the child has a heart defect. Be honest with the other children. As the child grows older, explanations can go into greater depth.

*Adapted from A. Garson et al. Parental reactions to children with congenital heart disease, Child Psychiatry and Human Development, February 1978, p. 86.

demonstrate a high level of anxiety about their child's heart defect, the children have shown poor adjustment to their condition. For example, the anxious parent may exhibit overprotective behavior and increased pampering, which fosters anxiety and dependency in the child (Fig. 24–15).

It has also been observed that parents may experience difficulty with their infants who have congenital heart defects.[8] This may be due to parental perceptions of the infant's behaviors — poor feeding, lethargy, restlessness. The parents may interpret these as reflections of poor parenting.

Parents of a child with congenital heart disease go through the grieving process. They must mourn the loss of their fantasized normal child before they are able to accept this child. Many parents block these feelings of loss and cope by denying the problem. Denial is especially prevalent in parents of asymptomatic children. Parents' anger and resentment may be expressed toward these children by overprotective behavior leading to infantilization of the children.[7] Parents may go through a second grieving process after the repair of the cardiac defect. During this grieving they mourn the loss of the defective child who now may be essentially normal. This is usually apparent in the children who are quite symptomatic and who, after repair, improve remarkably.[7]

Table 24-2 summarizes the common concerns of families with children who have a congenital heart defect.[9] Often parents are uncomfortable asking questions of health professionals and do not want to take up their time. These unanswered questions can add to the stress that parents experience. By giving parents some concrete and factual answers to their questions, the nurse can alleviate some of their anxiety and help them cope with the stress of the situation. Also, by supplying parents with factual information we aid them in becoming informed participants in their child's care and promote their increased self-esteem and competence as caretakers.

There are many things to keep in mind when teaching and working with parents of children with congenital heart disease. Parents and other family members will be shocked when they first hear the diagnosis and the two-way process of communication may suffer during this time of crisis. Parents must be allowed to grieve before they are taught to care for the child. Terminology used in explanations should be consistent with that used by other members of the health care team. Explanations of care must be built on current knowledge the parents have; therefore, ongoing assessment of parental knowledge is necessary. Information may need to be shared with parents repeatedly before they are able to take in and absorb the facts. Sharing information with parents makes them feel an integral part of the health care team. Referral to a community health nurse and school nurse while the child is hospitalized will supply some of the added support that is needed once the family returns to the community. Encouraging parental participation with a group of other parents with similar problems often is beneficial and allows for sharing of feelings, concerns and common problems.

Physical Impact

Children with congenital heart disease often demonstrate retardation of physical growth or growth failure from a variety of causes.[3, 14, 15] This growth failure affects weight more than height. Children who are sicker and demonstrate the symptoms of cardiac incapacity (cyanosis and congestive heart failure) often show greater degrees of growth retardation. Delayed pubescence often accompanies the more severe degrees of cyanosis. Puberty may begin three to four years after the expected age; this may cause concern for the patient and family.[13]

Children with the highest percentage of growth failure are those with VSD and a history of congestive heart failure in infancy. If surgical correction occurred before puberty, most patients experience increased growth postoperatively.[4] Improvement in growth occurs within months after surgical correction in patients who previously exhibited growth failure.

Cognitive Impact

Intellectual development may be affected by congenital heart disease. In tests of intellectual function, children with congenital heart disease score lower than normal children. This is most evident in children below the age of 3 with cyanosis.[4] Impaired physical activity or limited developmental opportunities due to illness may have an effect on the results of these tests because they are primarily tests of gross motor function, especially in younger children.

Motor milestones such as sitting, crawling and walking may be delayed in those children with limited exercise tolerance as occurs in severe cyanosis and congestive heart failure.[15] Other measures of development — fine motor movements, speech adaptive and social behavior — may progress normally.

References

1. L. A. Barness. Manual of Pediatric Physical Diagnosis. Yearbook Medical Publishers, 1976
2. A. Coran et al. Surgery of the Neonate. Little, Brown & Co., 1978
3. K. H. Ehlers, Growth Failure in association with congenital heart disease. Pediatric Annals, November 1978, p. 750
4. R. H. Feldt et al. Growth of children with congenital heart disease. American Journal of Diseases of Children, May 1969, p. 573
5. R. H. Feldt et al. Children with congenital heart disease: motor development and intelligence. American Journal of Diseases of Children, March 1969, p. 281
6. W. E. F. Friedman et al. Pharmacologic closure of patent ductus arteriosus in the premature infant. New England Journal of Medicine, 2 September 1976, p. 526
7. A. Garson et al. Parental reactions to children with congenital heart disease. Child Psychiatry and Human Development. February 1978, p. 86
8. S. Gundermuth. Mother's reports of early experiences of infants with congenital heart disease. Maternal-Child Nursing Journal, March 1975, p. 155
9. J. Hendry and J. Mitton. Childhood cardiac anomalies: a review. Canadian Nurse, September 1976, p. 28
10. M. A. Heymann et al. Closure of the ductus arteriosus in premature infants by inhibition of prostaglandin synthesis. New England Journal of Medicine, 2 September 1976, p. 530

11. J. D. Keith et al. Heart Disease in Infancy and Childhood. Macmillan, Inc., 1978
12. O. M. King. Care of the Cardiac Surgical Patient. C. V. Mosby Co., 1975
13. L. M. Linde et al. Attitudinal factors in congenital heart disease. Pediatrics, January 1966, p. 92
14. L. M. Linde et al. Physical and emotional aspects of congenital heart disease in children. American Journal of Cardiology, June 1971, p. 712
15. L. M. Linde and S. D. Linde. Emotional factors of pediatric patients in cardiac surgery. American Operating Room Nursing Journal, January 1973, p. 95
16. A. Moss. What every primary physician should know about the postoperative cardiac patient. Pediatrics, February 1979, p. 326
17. A. Nadas and D. Fyler. Pediatric Cardiology. W. B. Saunders Co., 1972
18. A. Rudolph. Congenital Disease of the Heart. Yearbook Medical Publishers, 1974
19. S. Sacksteder. Congenital Cardiac Defects: embryology and fetal circulation. American Journal of Nursing, February 1978, p. 262
20. University of Iowa. Pediatric Nurse Practitioner Syllabus, January 1978

CONGENITAL ANOMALIES OF THE RESPIRATORY TRACT

by Mabel Hunsberger, BSN, MSN

CHOANAL ATRESIA

Each nasal cavity communicates with the nasopharynx by posterior nasal openings (choanae). Choanal atresia is an obstruction of one or both of these openings owing to the presence of a membranous or bony septum located between the nose and the pharynx. Congenital obstruction of the choanae is relatively common, with twice as many females being affected as males.

Most newborns are unable to breathe through their mouths; therefore when this anomaly is present an infant develops varying degrees of respiratory distress depending on the degree of obstruction and whether it is unilateral or bilateral. Unilateral choanal atresia can be overlooked because the infant may be asymptomatic until the time of a respiratory infection. Signs of unilateral choanal atresia are nasal obstruction and nasal discharge from the involved side. Both of these signs may be pronounced during a respiratory infection, giving the first diagnostic sign of choanal atresia.

Infants with bilateral choanal atresia usually develop severe signs of respiratory distress after the initial cry at birth. When the infant quiets and attempts to breathe through his nose, cyanosis and severe retractions follow. Vigorous attempts to inspire air are made by a sucking-in motion of the lips.[1] This distress can be relieved by opening the infant's mouth. Bilateral nasal discharge is noted. Sucking is almost impossible in the presence of bilateral atresia. Prompt treatment is required to prevent death by asphyxiation.

Nurse's Role

During Diagnosis The clinical signs of severe respiratory distress are cause to suspect bilateral choanal atresia and should be identified by the nurse. Unilateral choanal atresia should be suspected if during suctioning of the nares, the nurse observes excessive discomfort and cyanosis. As the uninvolved side is being suctioned the only open airway is being blocked by the catheter; therefore signs of respiratory distress may be manifested. Diagnosis of choanal atresia is considered if the dyspnea is increased by holding the infant's mouth closed and if a firm catheter cannot be passed through the nostril. It is the nurse's astute observations in the first moments of life that can lead to early recognition and management of this condition.

During Treatment and Course of Illness Prompt provision of an adequate airway is essential. An oral airway must be inserted; gavage feedings are administered until the infant learns to mouth breathe (two to three weeks). Surgical correction of the anomaly can be deferred until much later, although some surgeons advise immediate operation for bilateral choanal atresia.[1] If it is postponed until the child is a year of age or older, cautious bottle and spoon feeding can be introduced after the initial period of gavage feeding.

Surgical correction is accomplished by approach through the nasal cavity. The obstruction is removed and the new airway is splinted with tubing that is brought out through the nose and stabilized with a safety pin. The tubing is left in place for six weeks, during which time it may need to be rinsed with normal saline and suctioned if it becomes obstructed.[4]

Parents are under a great deal of stress during the treatment process. The nurse must recognize that the severe respiratory distress manifested by the infant with bilateral obstruction is frightening for parents to see. The early feelings of closeness and satisfaction that feeding brings are delayed because of the need for gastrostomy feedings and surgical intervention. These circumstances have the potential to seriously alter the early bonding and attachment process between the parents and child. The nurse can intervene by providing opportunities for the parents to have physical contact with their baby and participate in his daily physical care, including holding him for gavage feedings.

CONGENITAL LARYNGEAL STRIDOR (LARYNGOMALACIA)

The larynx is the organ of voice; it includes the upper end of the trachea. It is a musculocartilaginous structure that is normally flaccid in infancy. When the laryngeal cartilage is especially soft and flaccid, the supraglottic structures are not well supported and collapse into the airway, causing a partial obstruction. The term *laryngomalacia* is used to describe this excessively flabby larynx, which results in stridor (noisy breathing). When stridor is caused by laryngomalacia there is no underlying structural anomaly but rather it is an exaggeration of the normally flaccid infant larynx.[2]

The most characteristic symptom is a noisy crowing sound on inspiration. Noisy breathing may be accompanied by retractions and is usually compounded by a supine position. When the child is in the prone position, the supraglottic structures fall away from the airway, causing less obstruction. The infant's cry is usually normal, cyanosis is uncommon and weight gain is within normal limits.

Nurse's Role

Congenital laryngeal stridor caused by laryngomalacia is a self-limiting condition and symptoms usually subside by 1 to 2 years of age. However, stridor during the first year of life may indicate a serious condition and requires the attention of the nurse and physician for early identification. The nurse should take a thorough history regarding the baby's feeding and respiratory patterns when symptoms of stridor are reported. Diagnosis of laryngomalacia can be made on direct laryngoscopy. Although no treatment is necessary if laryngomalacia is the cause of stridor, direct laryngoscopy is carried out to rule out other anatomical abnormalities that may require treatment.

The nurse is an important resource to the family when their infant is a noisy breather. Parents are apprehensive about their baby's symptoms and need reassurance that the condition will resolve as their baby develops. The nurse should be prepared to answer repeated questions about the baby's symptoms and offer suggestions for increasing the baby's comfort and reducing the parents' anxiety. Stridor may be more pronounced during crying or feeding;[3] therefore the nurse should discuss these aspects of infant care with the parents. The prone position can be suggested as a means of easing the baby's respirations. Feeding slowly, allowing time for the baby to breathe between sucking, should be recommended. Parents need to be encouraged to call for assistance if they note any changes in the respiratory status of their infant because these changes may indicate an infection or other problem requiring treatment.

References

1. T. F. Boat et al. Upper respiratory tract. In Nelson Textbook of Pediatrics, V. Vaughan et al., eds. W. B. Saunders Co., 1979
2. J. D. Norante. Congenital lesions of the head and neck. In Principles of Pediatrics, R. A. Hoekelman et al., eds. McGraw-Hill Book Co., 1978
3. A. L. Quinn-Bogard and W. P. Potsic. Stridor in the first year of life. Clinical Pediatrics, October 1977, p. 913
4. W. S. Schley and A. N. Krauss. Diseases of the Upper Airway. In Pulmonary Disease of the Fetus Newborn and Child, E. Scarpelli et al., eds. Lea & Febiger, 1978

URINARY TRACT ANOMALIES AND RELATED CONDITIONS

by Stephen Koff, MD
and Mabel Hunsberger, BSN, MSN

Correctable urinary tract anomalies occur frequently in infancy and are commonly associated with abnormalities in other organ systems. Some anomalies are readily detected at birth, while others remain occult. It is those abnormalities that are not easily detected but cause progressive damage to the urinary tract that present the greatest challenge for diagnosis. The nurse plays an important role in facilitating early identification of urinary tract anomalies and in the care of the child and family throughout the entire course of illness.

RECOGNITION OF URINARY TRACT ANOMALIES IN INFANCY

The nurse should focus on three main areas in assessing the infant's urinary tract: (1) collection of a complete history of the infant and his birth and the family; (2) recognition of symptoms that indicate or suggest urinary tract anomalies; and (3) identification of the actual anomaly by physical examination. Because many signs and symptoms of urinary anomalies are not manifested in early infancy, the search for these defects must be ongoing. The nurse cannot, therefore, assume that a specific infant is free of urinary tract pathology in spite of numerous previously negative historical and physical examinations.

The history may provide useful clues to the presence of urinary tract abnormalities. The occurrence of genitourinary tract disease in siblings and parents should be documented. Although most urinary tract anomalies are not strictly genetically transmitted, a positive family history must not be disregarded. The birth history is significant when there is an abnormality in the amount of amniotic fluid (oligohydramnios or polyhydramnios) or in the number of umbilical cord vessels.

Because of the relative paucity of clinical symptoms in the newborn infant, the nurse must be alert to any subtle alterations from normal that may suggest urinary tract disease. The urinary output in the neonate must be carefully scrutinized for quantity because failure to void is perhaps the most serious urologic problem in this age group. Occasionally, a normal infant may not void for 24 hours after birth but may have done so, unnoticed, during delivery. Delay in micturition must arouse a suspicion of serious urinary tract pathology; the situation becomes urgent after more than 24 hours.

For the infant voiding normally, the urinary volume is generally considered adequate if the diapers are found to be damp each time they are changed for bowel movements. The urinary stream in the male infant must be observed for forcefulness, as a consistently weak and dribbling stream may be the only early clue to posterior urethral valves and urinary obstruction. Although hematuria is rare in infancy, its presence may indicate serious and potentially lethal abnormalities such as renal vein thrombosis, hydronephrosis, or polycystic kidney disease. However, the nurse must be aware that certain benign conditions can simulate hematuria, such as red urate crystals, discoloration of the diapers by chromobacteria residing in the intestines, and contamination of urine by uterine bleeding from estrogen withdrawal. Urinalysis can usually distinguish true from spurious (superficially like but morphologically unlike) causes of hematuria. The nurse should also recognize that non-specific symptoms such as poor feeding, failure to thrive, fever of unknown origin, convulsions and diarrhea may be the only symptoms accompanying a serious urinary tract abnormality.

Several urinary tract anomalies can be detected by direct physical examination of the newborn infant. However, a complete assessment should include a search for physical manifestations such as low-set malformed ears, an absence of abdominal muscles (prune belly syndrome), spina bifida or widely spaced nipples that are frequently associated with urinary tract anomalies. Palpation of the abdomen, especially with the infant quiet and feeding, may identify a distended bladder or an abdominal mass. Likewise, genital defects such as cryptorchidism, hypospadias, epispadias and hydrocele are readily diagnosed by direct inspection.

SPECIFIC GENITOURINARY TRACT ANOMALIES

Ureteral duplication is probably the most commonly occurring urinary tract anomaly and is more frequent in females. Duplication may involve the renal pelves and calyceal systems that collect urine from functionally separate but anatomically attached renal halves: the upper and lower renal segments. Duplication may be complete with both ureters entering the bladder separately or incomplete with the duplicate ureters joining into one ureter before entering the bladder (Figs. 24-16 and 24-17). Incomplete duplication is usually inconsequential, but complete duplication may become problematic when it predisposes to vesicoureteral reflux or obstruction.

When two separate duplicate ureters enter the bladder through a common opening (hiatus), the upper pole ureter usually penetrates the bladder mucosa closer to the urethra than does the lower pole ureter. This results in a shorter-than-normal submucosal tunnel for the lower pole ureter, which reduces the effectiveness of the valve mechanism that prevents reflux. The resultant reflux of urine permits bladder bacterial infection to gain access to the upper urinary tract. Correction of reflux by ureteral reimplantation is required in certain instances depending on the degree of reflux, the condition of the kidneys and the tendency for

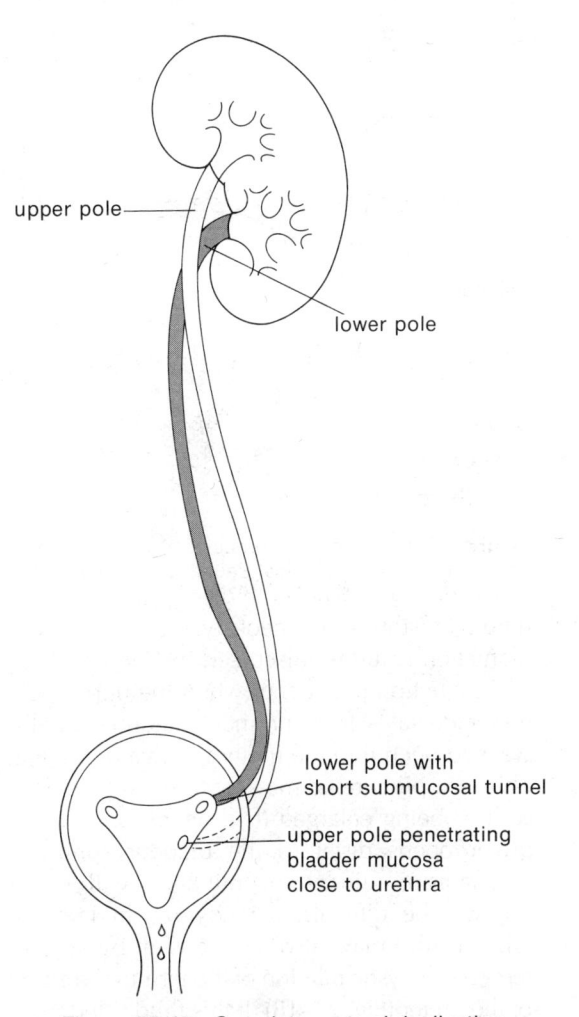

Figure 24-17 Complete ureteral duplication.

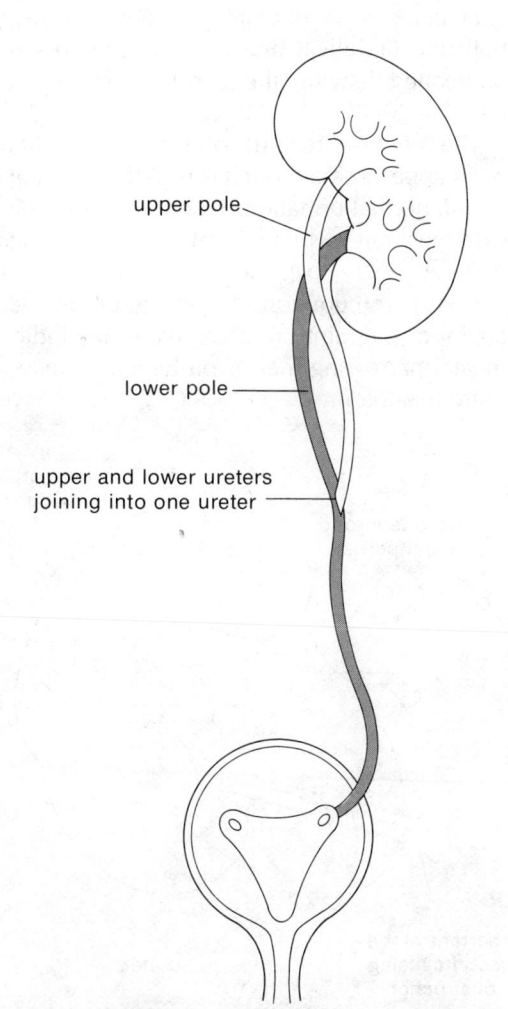

Figure 24-16 Incomplete ureteral duplication.

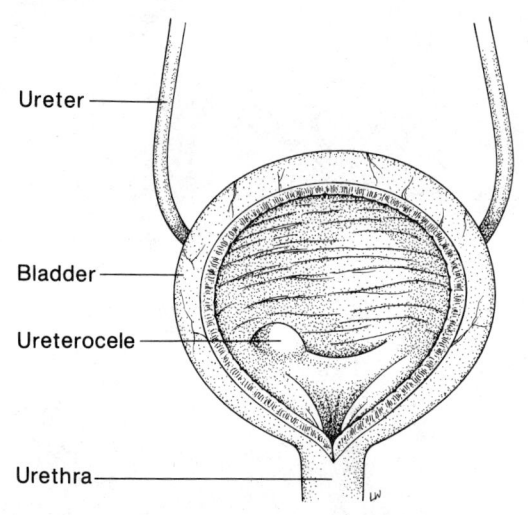

Figure 24-18 Simple ureterocele. (Redrawn from P. Kelalis and L. King. Clinical Pediatric Urology, Vols. I and II. W. B. Saunders Co., 1976.)

reflux to stop spontaneously. (Ureteral reimplantation is further discussed in Chapter 42.)

Obstruction may occur when the upper pole ureter deviates from normal anatomical pathways to open into the urethra, vulva or vagina. This ectopic ureter may become infected as well as being enlarged (hydronephrotic). If the ureter opens distal to the bladder sphincter mechanism, urinary incontinence will occur but will be difficult to recognize in infancy. Obstruction may also be caused by a ureterocele, a cystic dilation of the terminal portion of the ureter (Fig. 24-18). If this fluid-filled mass enlarges within the bladder it may interfere with bladder emptying; at times it will be forced through the female urethra during voiding, appearing as a mass in the perineum. Corrective surgery for both these anomalies usually requires their removal and often necessitates removal of the upper pole renal segments as well.

The most common site for obstruction in the upper urinary tract is at the junction of the ureter and the renal pelvis (Fig. 24-19). In most cases of ureteropelvic junction obstruction, there is a defect in the intrinsic muscular function of this region that may be associated with external compression caused by constricting fibrous bands or anomalous blood vessels. In its most severe form a total anatomical blockage with nonpatency (atresia) of a segment of ureter is seen. Renal function is negligible in these cases and the kidney appears as a dysmorphic (abnormal in form) collection of fluid-filled cysts. This multicystic kidney is often palpated as an abdominal mass; the condition is probably the most common cause for such a mass in the neonate. Less severely obstructed kidneys will manifest variable degrees of hydronephrosis (collection of urine in kidney pelvis) and functional impairment. Treatment of ureteropelvic junction obstruction involves excision of the diseased muscular segment and reanastomosis of the ureter and pelvis. Nephrectomy is rarely performed in the neonate, except for the multicystic kidney, because of the great potential for recoverability of renal function in this age group.

Urachal anomalies may be present at birth if the tubular structure that extends from the bladder to the umbilicus fails to undergo normal obliteration. Patent urachus is identified by urine draining from the umbilicus; this indicates a direct communication with the bladder. Before surgical excision, careful urological testing is required to diagnose an occult bladder outlet obstruction that may be perpetuating the urachal patency. A urachal cyst develops when both the umbilical and bladder ends become obliterated leaving the central portion intact (Fig. 24-20).

The urethral meatus of the male neonate often appears small, but it is usually sufficient to permit normal urination. True meatal stenosis is extremely rare, while meatal narrowing or scarring secondary to postcircumcision inflammation is more common. A deflected (downward angle) or pinpoint urinary stream may indicate meatal narrowing that, if problematic, may require meatotomy.

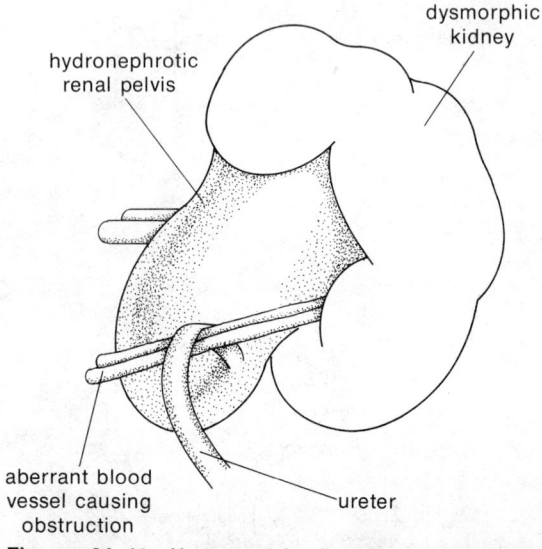

Figure 24-19 Ureteropelvic junction obstruction. (Redrawn from Kelalis and King.)

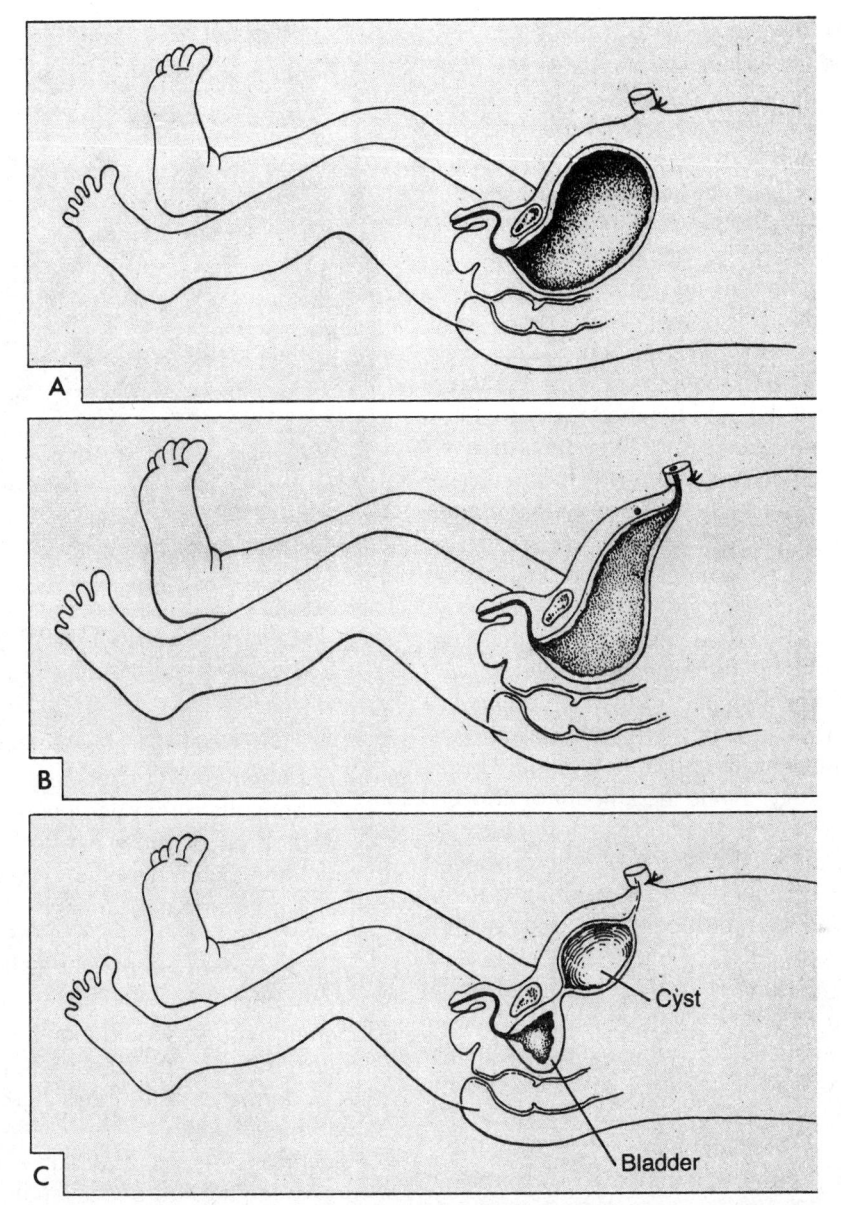

Figure 24–20 Midline abdominal masses. A, distended bladder. B, patent urachus. C, Urachal cyst. (From S. Koff. Clues to neonatal genitourinary problems. Postgraduate Medicine, September 1977, p. 95.)

NURSING CARE FOR THE INFANT UNDERGOING UROLOGICAL SURGERY

A young infant swathed in bandages and having multiple urinary catheters is an upsetting sight to parents. They will need a great deal of support and help to cope with a difficult situation. Successful postoperative nursing care for the infant undergoing urological surgery begins with preoperative preparation of the parents. The nurse can ease their anxiety significantly by describing for the parents the appearance of their child after surgery and by outlining the care required to ensure a speedy recuperation. Because urological nursing care depends so heavily upon the proper maintenance and management of multiple tubes and catheters, the nurse must have considerable knowledge of these systems.

Basically, there are three types of tubes employed in pediatric urological surgery: catheters, stents and drains. Catheters transport urine from any portion of the urinary tract to a drainage bag and are named according to the organ they drain: nephrostomy tube (kidney), ureterostomy tube (ureter). Because the bladder can be drained in several ways, bladder catheters are named according to the route of drainage: (1) urethral catheter, (2) suprapubic cystostomy catheter and (3) perineal urethrostomy catheter that is inserted through an incision in the middle portion of the urethra.

Stents are tubes that serve as internal splints to ensure the patency of an anastomosis and thereby permit proper tissue healing. Stents can have a dual function, also serving as catheters to carry urine past a surgical site without leakage. The diminutive size of the infant's urinary tract requires that stents be delicate and of very small caliber. Drains are placed outside of the urinary channels to provide an avenue for leaking or extravasated urine to reach the body exterior. This prevents a buildup of urine around the surgical site that, undrained, could become either infected and form an abscess or lead to fibrosis and impaired tissue healing.

The catheters and drainage tubes permit a direct measurement of the individual urinary outputs of each kidney or the bladder or all of these. The volume from each catheter should be recorded separately. While the amount of urine output collected from each tube may fluctuate considerably, the total absence of output from any catheter for over an hour may indicate obstruction. The tube must be checked to see if movement has produced a kink or if the child is lying on it or twisting it. In the absence of an external obstruction, the physician must be notified immediately. If the tube is blocked, the physician may need to irrigate it with sterile saline.

After surgery, the infant must be carefully positioned to prevent tube kinking or external compression. To protect the tubes from the innocent grip of an infant's hand, restraints or gauze mittens may be needed. The presence of drainage tubes and the care needed to ensure their patency should not prevent parental contact, and the nurse should instruct the parents in careful handling and holding of the child and in observing for kinks or twists in the tubes.

Changes in the color of tube drainage will be confusing and anxiety-provoking to parents. This anxiety can be alleviated by explaining the expected patterns of postoperative urine drainage following major pediatric urological surgery. Immediately after surgery, the urine color is often bright red but of a watery consistency.

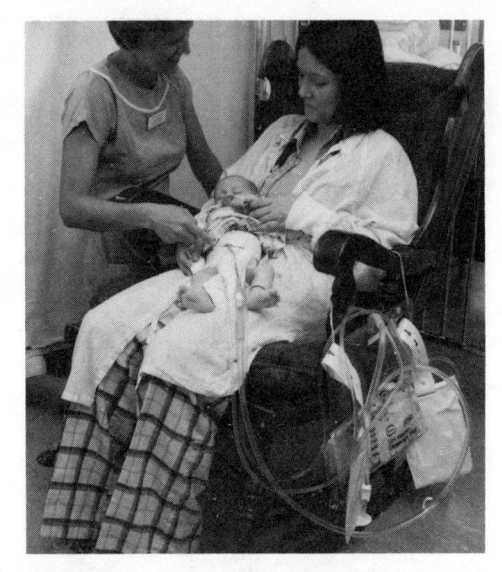

An important role of the nurse after an infant has urological surgery is to help parents to become comfortable in holding their baby in spite of the cumbersome tubes and urinary bags.

This reflects the fact that it takes only a small amount of blood to visibly discolor urine. After 12 to 48 hours the urine will become progressively darker red or brownish, indicating that old or clotted blood is dissolving. Within four to seven days, the urinary drainage will become progressively more yellow in color. Small blood clots may be seen periodically in the catheter and are normal. However, at no time in the postoperative course should there be significant red drainage having the consistency of blood. This is abnormal and the physician should be notified immediately.

An accurate assessment of pain after urological surgery requires an understanding and recognition of bladder spasm. The surgical trauma or a catheter within the bladder may produce uncontrolled bladder contractions (spasms) and pain. This discomfort is usually short-lived but severe and may be repetitive. The infant may be seen to writhe and strain to void while the older child complains of needing to urinate and having abdominal or suprapubic pain. Small amounts of urine may pass through the urethra during these spasms even if a urethral catheter is in place. The most common correctable cause for bladder spasms is a kinked or obstructed catheter. Therefore, before medication for discomfort is administered, the tubes must be inspected to be sure they are not kinked. Although narcotic drugs will allay restlessness, they are not effective against bladder spasms. Spasms are treated with anticholinergic, antispasmodic agents such as belladonna, belladonna and opium suppositories, or oxybutynin.

Because of the wide variability in the type and significance of urinary tract anomalies, the nurse must gain a clear understanding of the treatment options and their implications in order to counsel the parents properly and prepare them for the child's discharge. The nurse has an important role in the discharge instructions by encouraging parents to ask questions and to express any fears or concerns they may have. The goal of these interactions is to transform those appropriate parental apprehensions related to surgery into warm and binding infant-parent relationships that will promote optimal infant growth and development.

References

1. P. P. Kelalis and L. K. King. Clinical Pediatric Urology, Vols. I and II. W. B. Saunders Co., 1976
2. S. A. Koff. Clues to neonatal genitourinary problems. Postgraduate Medicine, September 1977, p. 93
3. M. Ravitch. Pediatric Surgery, 3rd ed., Vols. I and II. Yearbook Medical Publishers, 1979.

FACIAL ANOMALIES

by Deborah Braunstein, RN, BSN

CLEFT LIP AND PALATE

Cleft lip and cleft palate and the combination of these are the most common facial anomalies. Cleft lip (harelip) with or without cleft palate is more common in males. Cleft palate alone is more common in females. The incidence also shows a variation in races, with a higher incidence in the Japanese (twice that of the white population), and a lower incidence in the black population (less than half as many as the white population).

It is generally thought that there is a hereditary factor in the formation of both cleft lip and palate, but sometimes the family history reveals no previous occurrence. Nonhereditary factors may cause similar defects but research on fetal environmental factors has been done primarily with laboratory animals. Few hard data are reported in the literature on environmental factors in the etiology of human orofacial clefts.[1] Suggested maternal factors include (1) malnutrition, (2) vitamin A in excess or deficiency, (3) cortisol therapy, (4) insulin therapy, (5) rubella or other viral infections, (6) toxemia of pregnancy, (7) pernicious anemia during pregnancy, (8) anoxia and (9) radiation.[6]

Physiology, Pathophysiology and Clinical Manifestations

Development of the facial structures occurs between five to nine weeks after conception; the lips form at seven weeks, the hard and soft palate at nine weeks. Cleft lip and cleft palate may occur together or either defect may occur separately, because even though their embryological development takes place around the same time, it occurs independently.

Cleft lip and palate result from failure of fusion of the facial maxillary and premaxillary processes that normally form the lip and palate. The cleft lip can be unilateral or bilateral (Fig. 24–21). Midline clefts are rare. The extent of the cleft can vary from a slight indentation (incomplete) to a widely opened (complete) cleft. Varying degrees of nasal distortion usually accompany the cleft lip, and the defect may also involve supernumerary, deformed or absent teeth.[3]

The degree of deformity of the cleft palate also varies. Because it is less obvious than the cleft lip, the cleft palate may not be detected without a thorough assessment of the mouth. It can be identified by placing the fingers directly on the palate. The defect may involve only the uvula (incomplete) or may extend to both the soft palate (the posterior portion) and hard palate (anterior portion), which is complete.

The isolated cleft palate occurs in the midline and may involve the uvula only or extend to the soft and hard palates. When cleft palate is associated with a cleft lip it presents in a variety of forms. It may involve the uvula and midline of the soft palate, and if it extends into the hard palate it may involve one or both sides (unilateral or bilateral cleft palate) (see Fig. 24–21).

CLEFT LIP

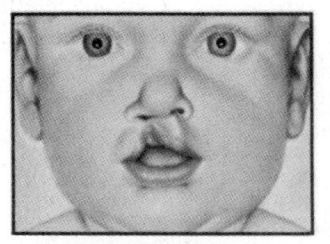

Unilateral Incomplete **Unilateral Complete** **Bilateral Complete**

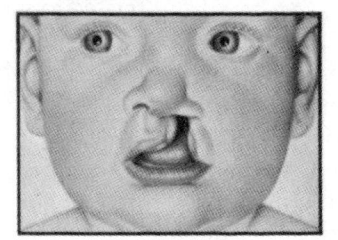

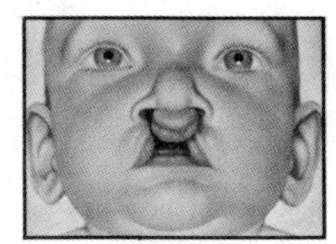

CLEFT PALATE

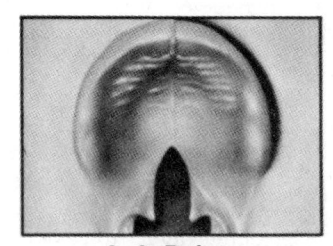

Soft Palate Only **Unilateral Complete** **Bilateral Complete**

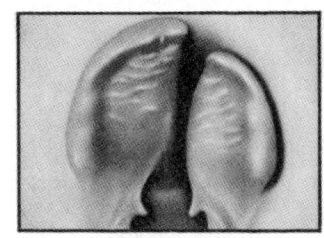

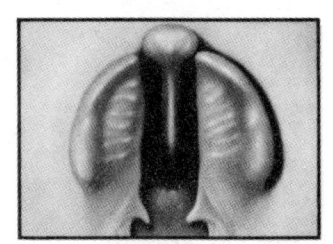

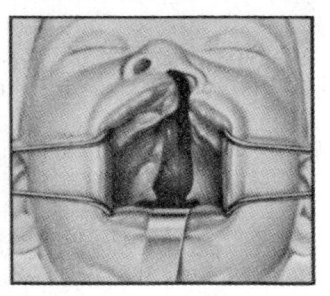

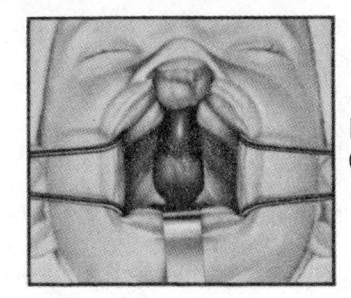

CLEFT LIP AND CLEFT PALATE

Unilateral Complete **Bilateral Complete**

Figure 24–21 Variations in cleft lip and cleft palate. (Courtesy of Ross Laboratories.)

Nursing Care

Treatment of the child with a cleft lip or cleft palate or both requires a multidisciplinary team approach. A complete program of habilitation for such a child may require years of special medical, surgical and dental care in combination with speech therapy.

The most immediate nursing care problems of a cleft lip or palate or both involve the infant's ability to feed, the prevention of aspiration, and the parental reaction to having a baby with a defect.

A cleft lip can be very disfiguring; therefore it is especially important for nurses to emphasize the positive aspects of the infant's appearance, along with optimism with respect to surgical correction. The infant is at home with his parents for one or two months before repair work begins. Parents usually adjust fairly well to this cosmetic defect if they have been given reasonable explanations of the cause of the deformity, are supported by a nurse who maintains phone or home visit contact during this interval, and are shown evidence of the improvement that surgery will make in their child's appearance and functioning. Photos of successful repairs are often more impressive and reassuring than verbal assurance that improvement will be significant. An opportunity to talk with other parents who have been through the expe-

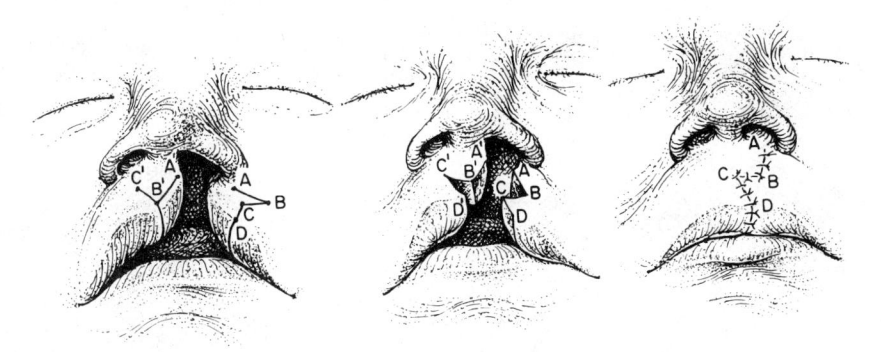

Figure 24-22 A procedure for cleft lip repair. The surgeon makes several incisions, then sutures the lip together. (From D. Fochtman and J. Raffensperger. Principles of Nursing Care for the Pediatric Surgery Patient, 2nd ed. Little, Brown & Co., 1976.)

rience is the most useful intervention the health team can offer the parents. Parents who have cared for their infant and gotten used to his deformity generally have a greater appreciation for and satisfaction about the surgical results than those whose infant's repair is done shortly after birth.

An infant with a cleft lip or palate cannot maintain closed suction around a nipple; this often makes breast feeding or bottle feeding difficult. Fluid taken into the mouth tends to escape through the cleft and out the nose. Therefore the usual bottle nipples frequently cannot be used for these infants. Large soft nipples with large holes or long soft nipples (lamb's nipples) seem to be most effective. The nurse should be aware that the infant will naturally cough and tend to choke during feedings. An upright position decreases the likelihood of aspiration and in this position the natural cough reflex can more readily clear the airway. The nipple should be firmly positioned into the baby's mouth and removed only to burp him or when the coughing warrants removal. Continually removing the nipple each time the baby has a slight cough frustrates a hungry infant and increases his distress. However, burping should be done frequently because these babies tend to swallow air readily.

If the infant has trouble with nipple feeding, a rubber-tipped medicine dropper or an Asepto syringe with a rubber tip can be used. The rubber piece should reach to the back of the mouth. Small amounts of formula are squirted on the back of the tongue to reduce the possibility of leakage through the nose. With some infants, spoon feeding may also work well.

Children with cleft palates have impaired functioning of their eustachian tubes. Under normal conditions the muscles of the soft palate facilitate proper functioning of the eustachian tube. In the presence of a cleft palate involvement of these muscles results in inefficient drainage of the middle ear, resulting in a greater susceptibility to ear infections. Since ear and upper respiratory infections are frequent, precautions against infection should be taken. Since the pharyngeal opening of the eustachian tube is often in an abnormal position, the infant should not be fed in a lying-down position, nor should he be confined to a supine position for long periods. Successful breastfeeding of an infant with a cleft of the soft palate has been reported, indicating that it reduced the risk of ear infection.[2] Good mouth care is also important in reducing infections. A milk feeding should be followed with a small amount of clear water to rinse the mouth. If an infection occurs and fluid accumulates, movement of the ear drum is inhibited and a hearing loss may occur.[3] Thus, when a child has a cleft palate, language acquisition may be hampered by inability to hear if careful attention is not given to early treatment of middle ear infections.

The parents of the infant should start feeding the baby as soon as possible. With the nurse's assistance, the feeding method that is most suited to the infant and his parents should be determined during hospitalization. If this is done early the parents will be accustomed to feeding their infant by the time of discharge.

Surgical repair of the cleft lip precedes repair of the palate and is done within the first three months of life (usually at one month) if the infant is gaining weight and is free of infection. Z-plasty, the most commonly used surgical technique, utilizes a staggered Z-shaped suture line (Fig. 24-22). The goal is to approximate the vermilion border and minimize notching. A

POTENTIAL STRESSES DURING INFANCY: REVERSIBLE ALTERATIONS IN HEALTH STATUS

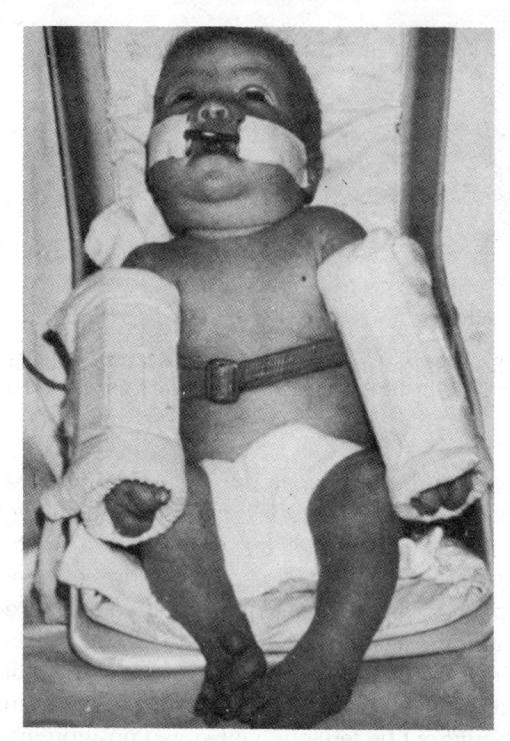

Figure 24–23 Infant restrained after cleft lip repair. Lateral tension on suture line is prevented by use of the Logan bow. Elbow restraints are in place to help prevent injury to the suture line. (From A. Ingalls and M. Salerno. Maternal and Child Health Nursing, 4th ed. C.V. Mosby Co, 1979, p. 248.)

Logan clamp (a curved metal bow taped down on both sides of the suture line over the lip) or a butterfly adhesive restraint is applied immediately after surgery to prevent tension on the suture line (Fig. 24–23). The cosmetic results of the surgery will depend on the extent of the original defect and the absence of infection or trauma. Revisions on the initial surgery may be needed at a later age.

Cleft palate surgery is usually done later, between the ages of 6 months and 5 years (usually when child weighs 20 pounds, has 2 front teeth, and is about 14 months old). The repair may be done in one operation, as in the case of a soft palate defect, or may require several stages of repair, depending on the severity of the defect. Most surgeons prefer to close the palate before the age of 3 in order to prevent the development of faulty speech habits.[4] If surgery is delayed further, an appliance (a contoured speech bulb) can be used to occlude the cleft and help the child develop normal speech. Without this appliance the child with a cleft palate may develop a speech defect.

The three major physical problems that may lead to this are: (1) hearing loss, (2) dental problems, and (3) palate insufficiency (the soft palate consists of muscles that move to effect swallowing and produce normal speech sounds).[5]

The major emphasis in nursing care following cleft lip repair is on protecting the operative site. Arm restraints should be used to prevent the child from rubbing or otherwise disturbing the suture line, such as by thumbsucking or putting objects in the mouth. The child who is old enough to roll over will also need a jacket restraint to prevent him from rolling onto the abdomen and rubbing his face on the bed. The arm restraints should be removed periodically to exercise the arms and to check for skin irritation. Also, since the child should be only on his back or side after repair, periodically sitting him up in an infant seat will allow for a change in position, comfort and increased stimulation.

The watchfulness required to maintain the surgical repair of a cleft lip is demanding of the nurse and the parents. The parents require assistance in understanding the importance of keeping the baby's hands away from his face. Parents also need to be shown how to hold their baby safely and provide physical contact even though restraints are in place. Mobiles and toys with various sounds, colors and textures are essential for these babies' developmental progress. Parents should be encouraged to participate in the provision of an appropriately stimulating environment.

The respiratory status of the infant after surgery should be observed closely in order to prevent aspiration or other respiratory complications. Gentle suctioning of the mouth and nasopharynx and placing the infant in a side-lying position will aid in the handling of secretions. Mist tents are also frequently used to help in this respect.

Feeding methods postoperatively are similar to those used before surgery. A medicine dropper or Asepto syringe may be used. These should be placed in the mouth from the side to avoid the suture line and care should be taken to prevent the infant from sucking. Initial feedings should be of clear liquids as tolerated and then advanced according to the physician's orders. The mouth should be gently rinsed with water after each feeding. Also, the suture line should be cleaned with gauze or a cotton-tipped applicator and half-strength hydrogen peroxide. Protection and astute care of the suture line is essential to provide for optimum healing and cosmetic results.

As with a cleft lip repair, care of the child who has had a cleft palate repair is directed mainly toward protection of the operative site and prevention of respiratory complications. The child should be protected against putting any objects into his mouth. This may require restraints of the elbows in the child who is too young to understand explanations. Feedings can be done with a cup or by gentle pouring of liquids into the mouth with a spoon, but the spoon should never actually enter the mouth. Straws should not be used as they may poke the surgical area.

The child who has had a cleft palate repair can be placed on his abdomen to help facilitate the drainage of secretions following surgery. A mist tent is also often used to aid in liquifying secretions. Although there is oozing of blood for several hours after surgery, oral or nasal suctioning should be avoided.

Aside from surgical repairs, the complete program of habilitation for the child with a cleft lip or palate will require long-term care, particularly with respect to dental corrections and the development of normal speech. A speech pathologist can help the child develop normal speech early in life and can assist parents in early speech training as needed.

Remarkable progress in the management of children born with a cleft lip or palate or both has made it possible for these children to look like other children, speak like other children and essentially live a normal life. The team approach provides the supportive care and coordinated treatment that is needed by these families. The nurse has an important role in helping families cope with the stress of having a baby with a defect and assist them to understand and participate in the treatment and management program for their child.

References

1. S. Fletcher et al. Cleft lip and palate research: an updated state of the art. Cleft Palate Journal, July 1977, p. 261
2. E. Grady. Breastfeeding the baby with a cleft of the soft palate: success and its benefits. Clinical Pediatrics, November 1977, p. 978
3. F. M. Parkins. Developmental abnormalities of the palate and soft tissues of the mouth. In Nelson Textbook of Pediatrics, V. Vaughan, et al., eds., W. B. Saunders Co., 1979
4. C. Shah and D. Wong. Management of children with cleft lip and palate. Canadian Medical Association Journal, 12 January 1980, p. 19
5. G. B. Snyder et al. Your Cleft Lip and Palate Child — A Basic Guide for Parents. Mead Johnson Laboratories
6. D. K. Wicha and M. L. Falk. Advice to Parents of a Cleft Palate Child. Charles C Thomas, 1970

GASTROINTESTINAL TRACT ANOMALIES

by Terry Sarahan, BSN, PNP and Mabel Hunsberger, BSN, MSN

Anomalies included in this section are reversible by surgical intervention, with the type of procedures ranging from simple repair of an inguinal hernia to complex staged repairs of the intestines. In most instances of gastrointestinal surgery there is a period when the infant's greatest source of gratification — eating — is interrupted. When an infant requires surgery that necessitates that no fluids are taken by mouth, other sources of comfort must be provided. The use of a pacifier may be resisted by some parents, but it is an appropriate option to suggest during this time, especially in an infant under 3 months of age, whose need to suck is particularly great.

The nurse should also recognize that surgery on the gastrointestinal tract may influence the child's response to toilet training. Because the majority of operations are done during infancy, the potential for normal bowel control remains in question for several years. These children may need extra time and support from parents to achieve this task.

The nurse has an important role in the early

Acknowledgement is given to John R. Wesley, MD, Assistant Professor of Surgery, Pediatric Surgery, University of Michigan Medical Center, for consultation and review of this section.

identification of gastrointestinal tract anomalies, most of which cause some degree of obstruction. Obstructive anomalies of the gastrointestinal tract cause characteristic signs and symptoms that vary according to the level of the obstruction. Important observations to make are: (1) presence of excessive secretions from the nose or mouth; (2) character of and color of vomitus, if present; (3) presence of abdominal distention and character of bowel sounds; (4) absence or diminished amount of meconium; and (5) character and color of stools.

PYLORIC STENOSIS

In this condition there is an overgrowth (hypertrophy and hyperplasia) of the circular muscle of the pylorus, which results in obstruction of the pyloric sphincter. The cause of this alteration is unknown. It is more common in first-born males.

The pylorus is an opening through which food passes from the stomach to the intestines. This opening is surrounded with a muscular ring called the pyloric sphincter. In pyloric stenosis the sphincter is in a state of spasm that causes hypertrophy of the muscle, resulting in a narrowed opening (Fig. 24–24). The stomach's peristaltic movements do not effectively move contents through the obstructed pylorus, consequently the overworked stomach musculature hypertrophies. The stomach contractions increase in frequency and force as they attempt to push stomach contents through the elongated, partially obstructed pyloric canal.

Although the history may vary, it is typical that at about 3 weeks of age the infant begins to regurgitate small amounts of milk immediately after a feeding. Within a week, the pattern and type of vomiting can change dramatically. It becomes projectile in character (vomitus propelled distances of several feet) and occurs with almost every feeding. It usually occurs during the feeding or shortly thereafter, but in some instances may occur several hours later.[24] The infant is hungry in spite of the vomiting and will usually eat again if offered milk. The vomitus contains no bile because the constriction is proximal to the ampulla of Vater.

Gastritis may occur owing to the irritation caused by stomach contents remaining in the stomach for prolonged periods. Gastritis causes the vomitus to be blood-tinged (brownish discoloration).

The initial pattern of regurgitation after feedings may not be reflected in the baby's weight, nutritional state or fluid and electrolyte balance, but with continuous, progressive vomiting some serious alterations eventually develop. If untreated, the infant will lose weight — with eventual nutritional depletion he will show signs of dehydration and become alkalotic. With excessive loss of gastric juices, the electrolytes sodium, potassium and chloride are lost. Gastric juice contains more chloride than sodium; therefore hypochloremic alkalosis develops.[9] As hydrochloric acid is lost there is an increased pH and increased carbon dioxide content. The fluid and electrolyte imbalance that results from excessive vomiting must be corrected before surgery is attempted.

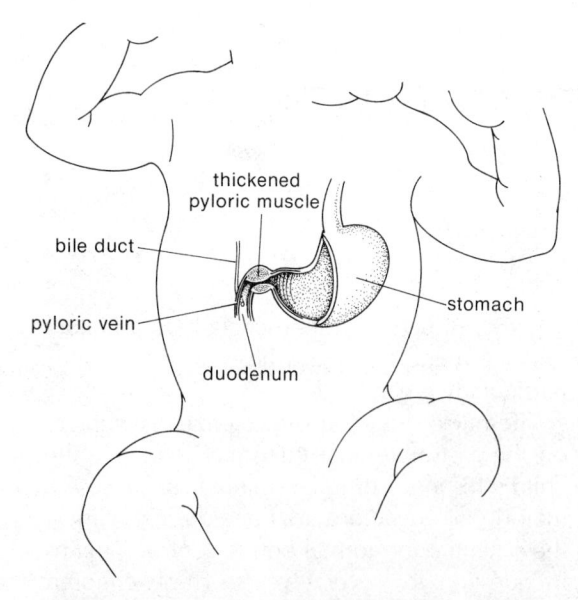

Figure 24–24 Pyloric stenosis. Hypertrophy, or thickening, of the pyloric sphincter blocks the stomach contents, causing the infant to regurgitate forcefully. Serious electrolyte imbalances ultimately occur and surgery is necessary to correct the condition.

Nurse's Role

During Diagnosis The nurse in a clinic or similar primary care setting may be the first to hear parents' account of an infant who shows the beginning signs of pyloric stenosis. A careful history must be taken to differentiate this infant from the one who is vomiting owing to a poor feeding experience such as an overly anxious caretaker or inadequate bonding. In 90 per cent of the infants with pyloric stenosis a mass (the hypertrophied pylorus) can be palpated in the right epigastrium under the edge of the liver. The mass feels hard and is movable and shaped like an olive. Successful palpation requires a relaxed abdominal muscle and an empty stomach. A nasogastric tube is passed and placed on continuous suction to facilitate palpation. Abdominal muscle relaxation can be achieved by holding the infant to quiet him and offering a pacifier with sugar or a bottle of warm sugar water, and elevating the baby's feet.[9]

X-rays are indicated only when the mass cannot be palpated after several examinations. If pyloric stenosis is present, contrast media ingestion reveals delayed gastric emptying and an elongated, narrow pyloric canal (string sign), which may appear as a small or double streak of barium. In the event that the x-rays are normal, other conditions must be considered. However, the infant should be examined again in a week or 10 days because it may take some time for the typical x-ray findings to develop in the presence of pyloric stenosis.[9]

During Treatment If an infant is dehydrated with electrolyte imbalance it is imperative that this condition be corrected before surgery. There may be a delay of 24 to 36 hours while the infant receives intravenous fluids with potassium. During this period the nurse must carefully administer IV fluids and help the family cope with the news that surgery is necessary. The baby may be irritable and crying because he is not being given oral fluids. It is disturbing to parents to see their tiny baby restrained and distressed; they should be allowed to discuss their feelings. Parents should be taught how to protect the IV site while holding their infant and should be encouraged to be present during this period to hold, comfort and talk to him. They should also be prepared for the surgery and the postoperative period. The surgery is a short procedure (15 to 30 minutes) and the infant will probably return from surgery with an IV. Parents should be prepared for vomiting, which is likely to occur in the immediate postoperative period. The nurse should also discuss the reintroduction of fluids postoperatively and clarify when the breast-feeding mother may resume feeding.

The stenosis is corrected by the Fredet-Ramstedt operation, which involves splitting the hypertrophied muscle down to the mucosa so that the mucosa bulges between the split muscle. Introduction of oral feedings varies. Coran and others[10] recommend giving 15 cc of dextrose and water two hours after surgery and again two hours later. Formula or breast-feeding can then be introduced gradually. For a bottle-fed infant, diluted formula is given in small amounts and gradually the quantity and strength of formula is increased. An infant who is breast-fed can be allowed a gradual increase in the length of time at the breast.

The nurse has a special role to play in the postoperative progress of these infants. Postoperative vomiting may occur for various reasons, and the nurse must make every effort to ensure that improper feeding technique is not the cause. These infants need to be fed using a firm nipple with a hole small enough so that milk is not taken too quickly. The nurse should emphasize that the nipple must be kept full of milk at all times to minimize swallowing of air and the infant should be burped at any sign of discomfort. Also, these infants are often hungry and should not be allowed to suck on an empty bottle. Positioning after feeding is not thought to be a critical factor affecting vomiting.[24] If the infant must be disturbed after feeding, he should be handled gently.

Helping parents to feel at ease by staying with them, helping them feed correctly, and reassuring them that they are playing an important part in the recovery of their infant gives them support and courage during this sometimes difficult period. Parents may easily become upset when vomiting recurs and may feel it is their fault. It is particularly discouraging if they have not been prepared preoperatively to expect this.

Usually these infants can be discharged on the morning of the second postoperative day on an unrestricted diet. The incision is often sealed with collodion, so that no dressing changes are required. Parents can resume their usual infant care routine and should be encouraged to plan their responsibilities in a way that will allow for a relaxed quiet feeding environment. It is important that parents feel positive about the feeding experience at discharge, otherwise the preconditioned feeling of failure may again make feeding an unpleasant and unsuccessful experience.

The mortality rate is well below 1 per cent in infants whose condition has been identified early and who have been properly prepared for

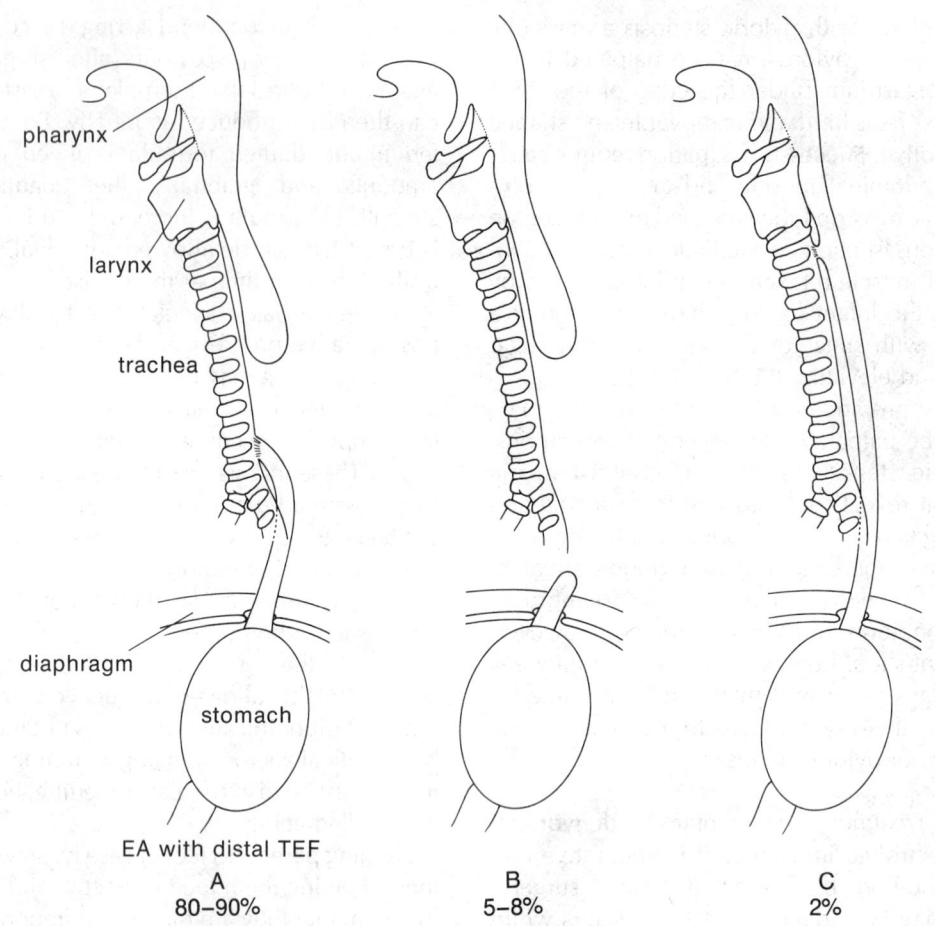

Figure 24-25 The three most common types of esophageal atresia and transesophageal fistula. A, esophageal atresia with a distal fistula constitutes 80 to 90 per cent of all cases. B, atresia without a fistula—5 to 8 per cent. C, isolated tracheoesophageal fistula without esophageal atresia (H type) — 2 per cent.

surgery. The nurse, as a member of the health team, has an important role in both of these areas.

ESOPHAGEAL ATRESIA AND TRACHEOESOPHAGEAL FISTULA

Esophageal atresia and tracheoesophageal fistula can each occur as a single entity, but usually they occur together. The reported incidence of atresia (with or without tracheoesophageal fistula) is approximately 1 per 3000 live births. There are numerous types of esophageal atresia with or without tracheoesophageal fistula. Atresia with a distal fistula comprises 80 to 90 per cent of all cases (Fig. 24–25A). In this type the upper (proximal) esophagus ends in a blind pouch and the lower (distal) esophagus exits from the stomach and joins the trachea instead of forming a continuous tube with the upper esophagus. The second most frequent type (Fig. 24–25B) is atresia without a fistula, accounting for 5 to 8 per cent of all cases. In this type there is a proximal dilated pouch and the distal end of the esophagus is narrowed and short. The third type, an isolated tracheoesophageal fistula without esophageal atresia, comprises about 2 per cent of all cases. It is sometimes called the H-type because a fistula connects the trachea and esophagus in a way that resembles the letter H (Fig. 24–25C). Rare types occur in varying combinations of fistulas and atresia but will not be discussed here.

The Nurse's Role During Diagnosis

Aspiration of secretions into the lungs is a major determinant of prognosis.[16] Aspiration can be prevented or diminished by early diagnosis and placement of a nasogastric sump tube in the proximal pouch to remove secretions.

There are only a few clues that the nurse can rely upon for early identification of an infant with esophageal atresia and tracheoesophageal fistula. Prematurity and hydramnios (excess amniotic fluid) are two conditions that should alert the nurse to make further assessments. There is a maternal history of hydramnios in 85 per cent of infants with atresia accompanied by fistula.[2] This suggests that effective swallowing and absorption of amniotic fluid in utero is prevented. Approximately one-third of the affected infants are premature. In addition to being alerted by prematurity or hydramnios or both, the nurse should look for signs of excessive pharyngeal secretions such as drooling, or in a classical case, bubbling from the nostrils. Unfortunately, atresia is often first suspected when an infant coughs, chokes, regurgitates or becomes cyanotic on feeding. In the H-type fistula, drooling does not occur and choking and coughing on feeding are the first signs. When the fistula is small, the symptoms are not so obvious, but repeated pneumonia in the first few months of life should raise the suspicion of an H-type tracheoesophageal fistula.[12]

When atresia is suspected, the presence of a blind pouch of the proximal esophagus is confirmed by the inability of a nasogastric tube to pass into the stomach. Curling of the tube in the proximal esophagus is shown on x-ray. If a fistula is present, the x-rays will show air in the stomach and intestines because of the esophageal connection to the trachea. In 30 per cent of cases of esophageal atresia additional anomalies are present, especially cardiac anomalies; therefore a thorough physical examination and appropriate diagnostic studies in search of other anomalies is also done.

The parents are under a great deal of stress during the diagnostic period. If they witness the choking, coughing and cyanosis produced by feeding, they may be particularly frightened; they need careful explanation of what the existing problem is and why their baby cannot be fed by mouth. Once the diagnosis is established, the family must be prepared for the necessary procedures and surgery that will follow.

Nursing Care During Treatment

Esophageal Atresia with Tracheoesophageal Fistula In the most common type of esophageal atresia (with fistula) the goal of immediate care is to prevent aspiration of the secretions in the proximal esophageal pouch and prevent regurgitation of stomach contents through the fistula into the trachea. The latter condition is the more serious in that it causes chemical pneumonitis.

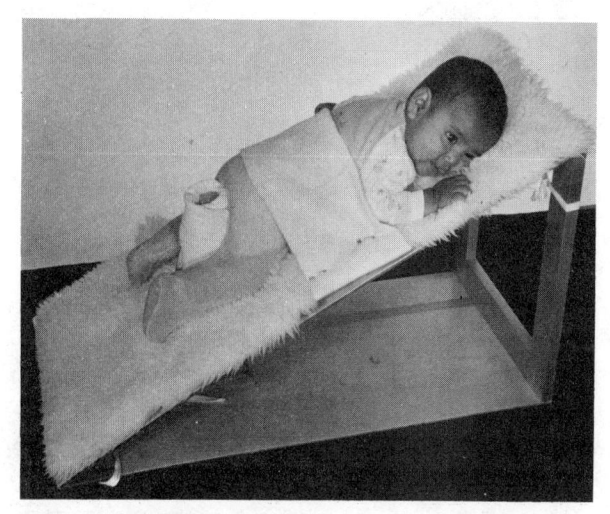

Figure 24-26 Positional treatment for esophageal atresia. The child is straddled on a padded peg on the board and restrained in this position. (From V. Vaughan et al., eds., Nelson Textbook of Pediatrics. W. B. Saunders Co., 1979.)

Immediate nursing care includes allowing nothing by mouth, and performing suctioning* of the nasopharynx until a sump tube (Replogle) can be inserted into the proximal pouch and placed on constant suction. This tube requires frequent irrigation or cleaning and reinsertion to ensure its patency. The infant should be placed in an upright position with head and chest elevated 30 degrees (Fig. 24-26). This accomplishes two goals: (1) secretions are pooled in the bottom of the esophageal pouch, facilitating withdrawal by constant suction and (2) gravity counteracts gastric reflux into the trachea and lungs. In spite of this position, distention of the stomach during crying causes gastric regurgitation. Therefore, keeping the baby quiet by stroking and gentle handling are important measures during this period of constant stimulation that is the result of the required emergency care. Although use of a pacifier may increase salivation, once the Replogle tube is in place the mucus is easily removed and the use of a pacifier diminishes crying and helps to satisfy the infant's need to suck.

These infants are usually placed in an incubator with oxygen and humidity as necessary. Constant observation and assessment is required to maintain an open airway and prevent aspiration. Under local anesthesia a gastros-

---

*May be necessary every 10 to 15 minutes but must be done gently to avoid traumatizing of the mucosa, which can cause edema.

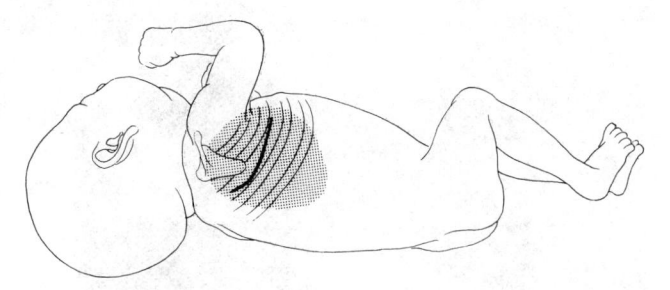

Figure 24–27 Incision for primary repair of TEF. (From A. Coran. Surgery of the Neonate. Little, Brown & Co., 1979, p. 48.)

tomy tube is placed immediately to allow escape of air from the stomach, lessening the possibility of gastric reflux into the fistula. This tube is placed on gravity drainage and should not be irrigated preoperatively. The appearance of an infant awaiting primary repair may be so overwhelming to the family that they hardly hear what is being said about the surgery to follow or about the postoperative period. The nurse can ease this stressful period for parents by keeping them informed of the status of their infant and answering questions about the surgery, which may have been answered before but which they have forgotten.

Primary repair constitutes ligation of the fistula and anastomosis of the upper and lower segments of the esophagus. This is done through a right posterolateral thoracotomy[10] (Fig. 24–27). When the anastomosis is completed, the Replogle tube is removed and the gastrostomy tube remains on gravity drainage. At the end of the operation a retropleural chest tube is placed through a stab wound. The nurse should be prepared to answer questions that the family has regarding the purpose and care of the tubes when the baby returns from the operating room.

Postoperatively, two of the nurse's most important goals are to maintain a patent airway and prevent trauma to the anastomosis. To meet both of these goals a suction catheter is marked by the surgeon showing the maximum length that can be inserted when suctioning through the nares. The nurse should place this premeasured catheter in a clearly visible location with careful instructions so that each person suctioning the infant will measure the catheter used against the premeasured catheter. The nurse must carefully observe the infant for early signs of airway obstruction. An anxious expression on the infant's face is often the first sign, followed by an increase in respiratory rate, and, in serious trouble, the onset of retractions.[14]

Suctioning technique is extremely important. It must be done gently to avoid traumatizing the tissue, quickly to avoid oxygen deficit, and frequently to maintain the airway. The nurse must use judgment regarding frequency of suctioning, realizing that suctioning increases the edema that already exists from the operation.

The preferred position of placing the infant postoperatively varies. Coran et al. recommend that the infant be placed semierect in an infant seat.[10] Regardless of the position, hyperextension of the neck must be avoided to prevent pull on the sutured esophagus. In the immediate postoperative period, the upright position and placement of the gastrostomy tube on gravity drainage prevents gastric regurgitation, thereby protecting the anastomosis from the pressure of such regurgitated materials. The infant's position should be changed from back to either side at least every two hours to prevent pneumonia and provide comfort. Percussion and postural drainage are also employed as preventive measures.

Fluid and electrolyte balance is maintained by an IV, and prophylactic antibiotics are administered. For some infants peripheral hyperalimentation is indicated. Usually by the third day postoperatively, the gastrostomy tube is elevated and kept open. The goal is to allow secretions to enter the duodenum from the stomach and minimize regurgitation. The open tube allows air to escape; thus during crying stomach contents are forced up the tube rather than refluxing into the esophagus. Gastrostomy feedings are begun cautiously by administering small amounts of water and gradually increasing volume and strength of formula. Before each feeding the stomach is gently aspirated to determine how much additional feeding can be given without distending the stomach. The aspirate is measured and refed. The amount of aspirate and the amount of additional feeding must not exceed the ordered amount. Gastrostomy feeding is continued until the tenth postoperative day, when a Hypaque esophageal swallow is done under fluoroscopy. Clear liquid oral feedings are started if no leak from the anastomosis is seen.[10] The nurse should constantly observe for saliva in the chest tube, which signals an anastomotic leak.

When oral feeding is begun, the nurse should

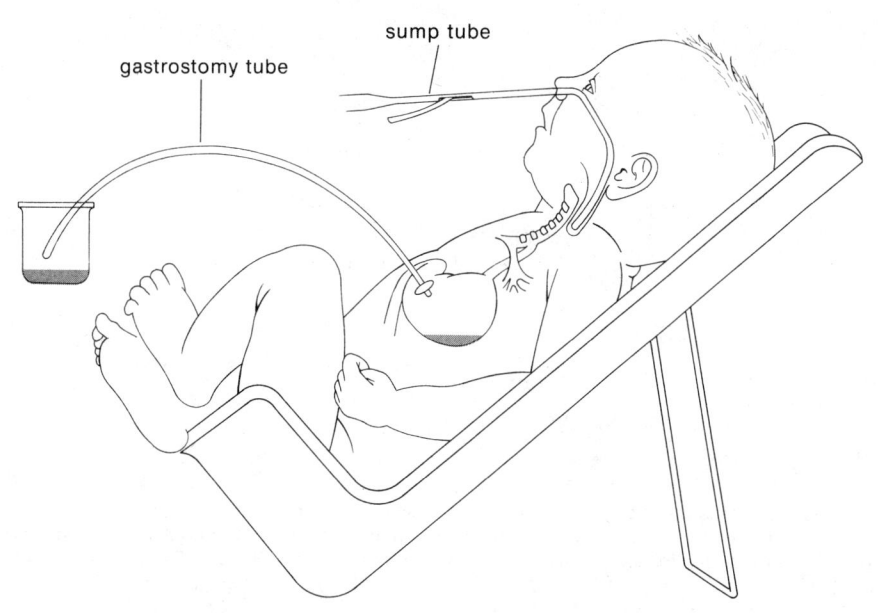

Figure 24-28 Preoperative care is administered with the child in the semi-Fowler's position with proximal sump drainage and gastrostomy decompression.

immediately begin teaching the family effective feeding techniques. The first feeding is clear (glucose water) and must be given slowly in a slightly elevated position. Extreme care must be taken to prevent the baby from swallowing large amounts of air that would potentiate regurgitation. If the feedings are tolerated and there is no sign of a leak, the chest tube is removed the following day.

The amount of family involvement at this time varies with each institution and family situation, but nurses in support of holistic care must take the stand that families be allowed and encouraged to participate in the care of their infant and give them the support and help to do so. In many cases parents can be helped to feed their baby after oral feedings have been given for 24 hours. If the family has been included in the infant's care during hospitalization, discharge preparation requires very little additional time by the nurse.

When the infant is discharged, the family should have had several experiences in feeding, positioning and handling him. The gastrostomy tube is usually left in place for four to six weeks after surgery until oral intake is well tolerated. Care of the gastrostomy tube requires minimal alteration in daily care. The skin is kept clean with soap and water, the tube is clamped, and it should be protected from the infant's grasp. Parents should also be familiar with signs of respiratory distress and be instructed to report any pronounced coughing, gagging or dysphagia that may indicate anastomotic stricture.

Parents should also be informed that their infant will have a raspy cough.

Esophageal Atresia without Fistula In the event there is esophageal atresia without a fistula (see Fig. 24-25) the nurse should expect to encounter some variations in treatment and care from that described for esophageal atresia with tracheoesophageal fistula. The presenting symptoms are similar but x-rays demonstrate absence of gastrointestinal gas. It may be necessary to stage* the surgical correction because there is too great a distance between the two esophageal ends for an anastomosis. A gastrostomy tube to gravity drainage and a sump tube to constant suction are employed as in esophageal atresia with fistula.

The next step of treatment varies considerably, depending on numerous circumstances. A cervical esophagostomy (opens on the neck above the left clavicle) may be done to prevent aspiration of secretions from the blind pouch (Fig. 24-28). During this period the infant is fed by gastrostomy tube, and sham† oral feedings

---

*Staging means that two or more surgical procedures are required for complete correction.
†Sham feedings are any fluids given orally. These feedings immediately drain from the opening on the neck (esophagostomy) but provide a sucking experience for the infant. When given at the time of a gastrostomy feeding, the act of sucking is associated with the comfort of satiety.

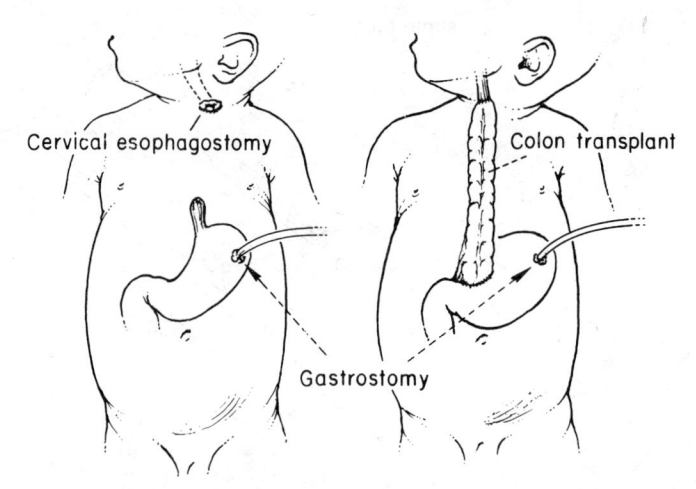

Figure 24-29 Stages in treatment of esophageal atresia. Cervical esophagostomy and gastrostomy, which are performed on newborns, and colon interposition between the esophagus in the neck and the stomach. (From D. Fochtman and J. Raffensperger. Principles of Nursing Care for the Pediatric Surgery Patient, 2nd ed. Little, Brown & Co., 1976, p. 39.)

are offered to maintain swallowing reflexes and meet the infant's need to suck. These feedings take additional time and do not provide any nutritive value, but a nurse should not make the mistake of overlooking the importance of meeting these normal developmental needs. Parents should be encouraged to give these feedings with an explanation of their purpose. The skin around the esophagostomy becomes easily excoriated from secretions. A protective ointment can be applied or a pad of soft, absorbent material can be placed over the area and held in place by the infant's shirt. Tape should be avoided as it increases skin breakdown. The pad must be changed frequently and the ointment removed daily to allow for thorough cleansing and drying of the skin.

The infant is maintained by gastrostomy feedings until a colon interposition is performed. A segment of the colon is mobilized from the abdomen and interposed in the chest to connect the proximal and distal ends of the esophagus (Fig. 24-29). This procedure is usually done after 6 months and before the child reaches 24 months of age.

Coran and associates recommend that cervical esophagostomy be done only in extreme cases and that instead the upper pouch be dilated and stretched over a period of three to five weeks.[10] After primary repair by anastomosis, postoperative care is the same as that described for esophageal atresia with fistula.

H-Type Tracheoesophageal Fistula The fistula is ligated and the openings into the trachea and esophagus are closed through a supraclavicular incision. The infant receives intravenous feedings and by the fifth day a Hypaque swallow is done.[10] Clear liquids are then begun cautiously.

The family of a child with esophageal atresia experiences stress because of the immediacy and intensity of the care required. When special care is needed, such as gastrostomy feeding, sham feeding and care of the incision and surrounding skin, the nurse must help parents during the course of the hospitalization to gain confidence in their ability to care for the infant. On discharge the nurse should give the parents written instructions about when to return for a clinic appointment or to visit their primary physician. Frequently, public health referrals are necessary for the optimal care of these infants, especially when special procedures are necessary. The parents should also be made to feel that they can contact the hospital nurses even for the smallest problem.

Almost all full-term infants with esophageal atresia survive if no other serious anomalies are present.[12] Pneumonia is a frequent complication in patients with tracheoesophageal fistula. Other complications are a leak at the anastomosis, recurrent fistula and gastroesophageal reflux, but the most common late complication is stricture at the anastomosis.[10] Coran reports that 50 per cent of patients with fistula repair require from one to several dozen dilations until the esophagus is wide enough to permit passage of food. These dilations may be required over a period of weeks, months or years.[10] Therefore, the help that the family needs from the professional team varies with the occurrence of complications and the type and length of follow-up treatment required.

OMPHALOCELE

An omphalocele is a herniation of variable amounts of abdominal viscera into the base of the umbilical cord. Movement of the midgut into the umbilical cord around the sixth to tenth week of embryonic life is a normal developmental process. The intestines thus grow outside of the abdominal wall for a portion of fetal life. Re-entry of the intestines into the abdominal cavity takes place around the eleventh week of fetal life, but when this fails to occur, an omphalocele exists and the abdominal cavity remains small. (It is the presence of abdominal contents within the cavity that causes the cavity to grow and develop, consequently the larger the omphalocele the smaller the abdominal cavity.) The herniated viscera are enclosed by a translucent membrane with the umbilical cord extending from its surface. A small sac may contain only one or two loops of bowel but a large sac may contain the liver, spleen and most of the bowel (Fig. 24–30).

Nursing Care During Treatment

The nurse has an important role in protecting the infant from the danger of a ruptured sac. The omphalocele must be immediately wrapped with warm, moist sterile normal saline gauze to prevent it from drying. The moist gauze should then be covered with dry sterile towels or plastic wrap to retain warmth and prevent contamination. This procedure must be done with sterile gloves and without placing undue pressure on the omphalocele. A nasogastric tube must be inserted and placed on suction to prevent distention of the stomach and intestines. The infant is kept in an incubator and prepared for immediate surgery.

The family will be shocked by the appearance of their infant. When the omphalocele is large the parents may feel repulsed by the gross abnormality. It may be difficult for them to comprehend that an anomaly of this magnitude can be corrected with excellent results when there are no associated anomalies.[10] They may be pessimistic about the surgery and show little interest in their infant. It is the nurse's role to encourage parents to talk about their infant and help them express what they are experiencing. The nurse needs to be patient with the parents who do not seem to hear or believe that their child can be helped. The appearance of the infant cannot be overlooked as an influential deterrent in this early phase of bonding.

The nurse should be familiar with the goals of treatment so that she can keep the family informed and answer questions pertaining to the daily care of the infant. When the sac is small,* it is excised and the intestines are placed back into the abdominal cavity and the abdomen is closed. Most omphaloceles are too large to fit back into the abdominal cavity; therefore, a staged repair is necessary.

In a staged repair the omphalocele is encased in a Silastic mesh sac. The mesh is sutured in place all around the defect to create a tall cylindric silo, which is then tied with umbilical tape to form a pouch over the defect (Fig. 24–31). The contact area between the skin and the mesh is susceptible to infection and can be protected by wrapping the abdomen and silo with Kerlex gauze that has been saturated with one half strength Betadine solution. The top of the silo is loosely supported by attaching it to a flexible device suspended from the top of the incubator. This is done to prevent it from falling to one side. With a large omphalocele it is also necessary to perform a gastrostomy.

The goal of the procedure that follows is to move the viscera gradually into the abdominal cavity without causing undue pressure on the vena cava or diaphragm. Gradually the surgeon

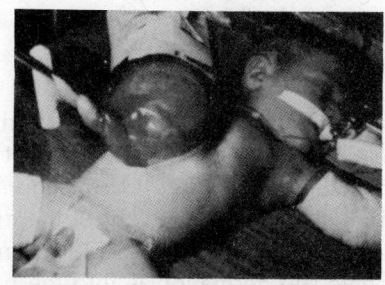

Figure 24–30 A large omphalocele containing liver. (From S. Kim. Surgical Clinics of North America, April 1976, p. 368.)

---

*The size of the defect can vary from 2 cm to the entire breadth of the anterior abdominal wall.[10]

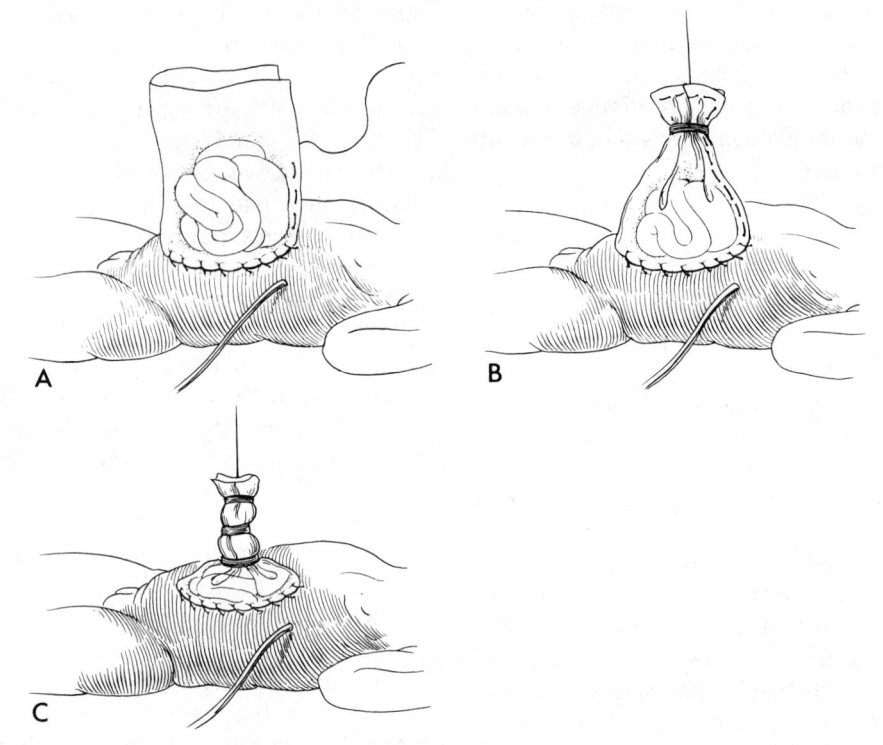

Figure 24-31 Silastic mesh is used to creat a silo and the viscera are gradually pushed into the abdominal cavity using a system of lower levels of ties. (From A. Coran. Surgery of the Neonate. Little, Brown & Co., 1979, p. 193.)

gently pushes more of the viscera into the abdomen and ties a new tape at the lower level (Fig. 24-31). Within 5 to 10 days the viscera are usually reduced into the abdominal cavity.

During the postoperative period the infant needs supportive care. Peripheral hyperalimentation is recommended the day after creation of the silo. Gastrostomy feedings of water are given when ordered; volume and strength of the formula is gradually increased. Atelectasis is common after the repair of large omphaloceles and must be prevented by position changes and maintaining a clear airway. As the intestines are gradually pushed back into the abdominal cavity, there is increased pressure on the inferior vena cava. This can result in circulatory overload problems manifested by edema in the lower extremities, and the incision must be carefully inspected for signs of dehiscence. After reduction of the viscera is complete, the infant must be returned to surgery for closure of the abdomen. The infant is then gradually advanced on oral feedings.

Even with explanation and encouragement parents may be distressed by the appearance of their infant. The nurse should be available to help them make contact with their infant by touching and holding him when possible. As the silo becomes less awkward increased contact can be encouraged and these parents can experience increased physical closeness with their infant.

Prognosis depends on whether there are associated anomalies present. Approximately 50 per cent of children with an omphalocele have associated anomalies. When there are no associated anomalies, the results should be excellent. The use of Silastic sheeting and total parenteral nutrition has made it possible to repair even severe omphaloceles.

GASTROSCHISIS

Gastroschisis differs in appearance from omphalocele, but the operative management of the two anomalies is similar. Gastroschisis is a herniation of bowel to the right of the midline beside the umbilicus (Fig. 24-32), whereas in an omphalocele herniation is into the base of the umbilical cord. In gastroschisis the bowel is not protected by a sac as in omphalocele.

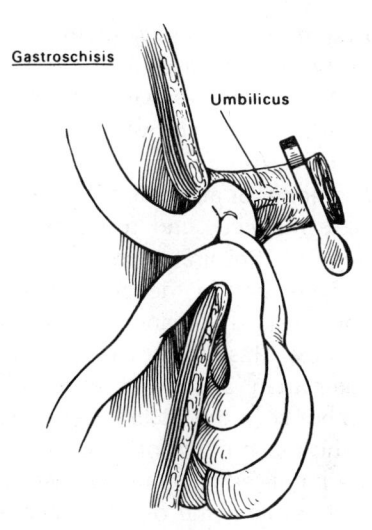

Figure 24-32 Gastroschisis: a defect in the abdominal wall that allows the intestines to protrude from the abdomen in utero. (From S. Schwartz et al. Principles of Surgery. McGraw-Hill Book Co., 1979, p. 1653.)

Consequently, the bowel is irritated by amniotic fluid and there is considerable inflammation and edema that interferes with normal bowel activity after surgical repair.

Treatment varies with the amount of bowel outside the abdomen. In some cases, the intestines can be placed into the abdomen without the use of the silo technique, discussed in repair of omphalocele. However, often the bowel is too edematous, prohibiting primary closure. The silo technique then used for repair of gastroschisis is similar to that used for repair of omphalocele.

Postoperatively, the infant will have a gastrostomy tube and receive hyperalimentation. Hyperalimentation is almost always necessary because these children have delayed intestinal tract function.[11] The silo can be reduced quickly (four to six days) as the edematous fluid of the bowel returns to the circulatory system. After the silo is reduced and the abdomen has been closed, intestinal motility returns within about three weeks.[11] Associated anomalies in these infants are uncommon and most of them survive and lead a normal life.

DIAPHRAGMATIC HERNIA

Normally, the strong musculature of the diaphragm prevents entrance of abdominal viscera into the chest. When defective embryonic development occurs, an aperture persists in the posterior lateral segment of the diaphragm (foramen of Bochdalek), located most often on the left side. Abdominal contents protrude through the defect and cause a group of symptoms that the nurse should be proficient in recognizing as indicative of diaphragmatic hernia. Abdominal contents in the left thorax compress the lung on the left and displace the heart to the right (dextrocardia). This results in some compression of the lung on the right side (Fig. 24-33). Congenital hypoplasia of the lung is usually present on the affected side; it has also been observed on the opposite side.[3] The severe respiratory embarrassment that results from compression and hypoplasia of the lungs causes

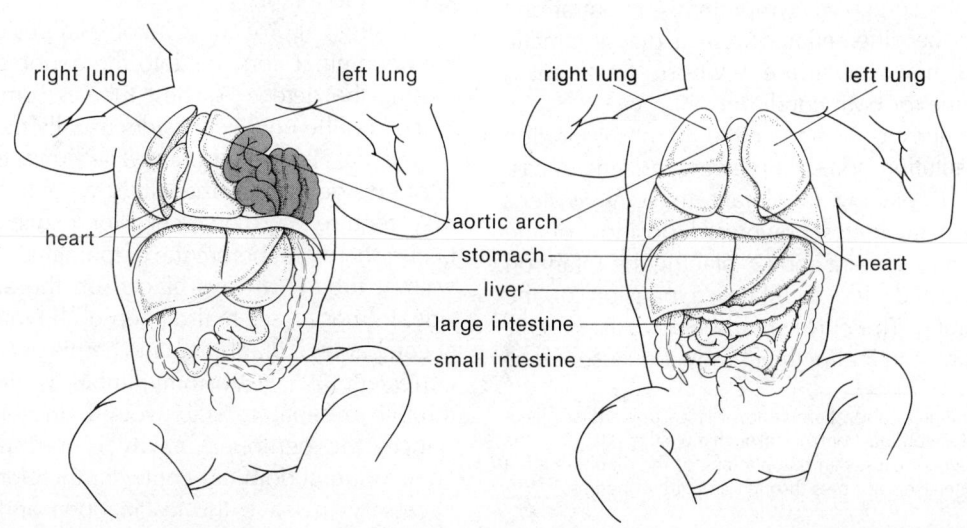

Figure 24-33 Diaphragmatic hernia; on the right is shown the normal relationships of the heart, lungs and diaphragm. When an abnormal hole exists in the diaphragm (left), abdominal contents can crowd the lungs. Respiratory embarrassment can result, with severity of symptoms depending on the amount of bowel displaced into the thorax.

dyspnea, cyanosis, nasal flaring, tachypnea, and chest retraction that may constitute an acute emergency. These symptoms vary with the amount of bowel that is displaced into the thorax and the degree of lung hypoplasia that is present.

A knowledge of the physiological alteration that exists will help the nurse contribute to identification of this condition and care of these infants.

On assessment the nurse should expect to find diminished or absent breath sounds on the affected side and carefully listen for bowel sounds that may be audible over the chest. The apical heartbeat will be heard at a point to the right of the usual position owing to dextrocardia. A barrel chest and scaphoid abdomen result, depending on the amount of abdominal viscera that have been displaced into the thorax.

If the hernia is less severe and symptoms are not present at birth, they usually appear soon thereafter. Common symptoms are vomiting, severe colic, distress after eating, constipation and dyspnea.

Nurse's Role During Diagnosis and Treatment

A typical x-ray shows fluid and air-filled loops of the intestine in the chest and a shift of the mediastinum to the unaffected side. The presence of bowel sounds in the chest, a scaphoid abdomen, and a typical x-ray film are indications for surgery.[10] Symptomatic eventration* cannot be differentiated from a diaphragmatic hernia; however, in the newborn, treatment is the same for both conditions.[10]

The nurse can improve the infant's condition by instituting some immediate nursing measures: (1) placing the infant in semi-Fowler's position facilitates downward position of the abdominal viscera and (2) placing the infant on the affected side facilitates expansion of the good lung. The nurse should also assist parents to quiet and calm their baby because air is swallowed during excessive crying. This further distends the stomach and intestines, resulting in increased respiratory embarrassment.

Nasogastric intubation with intermittent suction is begun as soon as the diagnosis is suspected. The amount of air getting into the intestines is thereby reduced, and respirations are less compromised. Respiratory assistance by positive pressure may be necessary and must be done cautiously by means of a mask or endotracheal tube. (Inspiratory pressure should not be greater than 20 cm of water to prevent pneumothorax in the contralateral chest.[10]) Although the nurse may not be directly responsible for administering ventilatory assistance, she should understand the overall management of this infant and intervene if the necessary precautions are not being taken. The respiratory acidosis (increased P_{CO_2}) and metabolic acidosis (decreased tissue oxygenation)[10] caused by severe respiratory embarrassment must be corrected preoperatively; therefore, intravenous sodium bicarbonate must be administered during this early phase of treatment. Acidosis is further complicated by a lowered body temperature; therefore, the infant should be kept warm.

The nurse must be attentive to the stress that the parents are experiencing during these emergency procedures. Although little time is available to explain the emergency treatment to parents, briefly telling them what is being done while the baby is being treated is appreciated. Before surgery the family should be told about the procedure and the postoperative appearance of the infant.

The surgical procedure involves repositioning the abdominal contents into the abdomen and closing the defect. A chest tube is sometimes placed on the unaffected side (usually the right) to prevent pneumothorax. The lung on the affected side (usually the left) is hypoplastic and may require days or weeks for expansion to occur; therefore, before the diaphragm is closed a chest tube is always placed on the affected side. In most cases malrotation of the intestines accompanies a diaphragmatic hernia and is also corrected. A gastrostomy tube is inserted through a separate stab wound. In some instances the peritoneal cavity is too small to contain the abdominal contents; therefore, it is necessary to leave the fascia open and close only the skin. This results in a ventral hernia that is repaired several months after the initial surgery. The family should be prepared to see their

---

*Eventration is not a herniation; it is an upward displacement of abdominal contents through a weakened area in the diaphragm. It causes an outpouching of the diaphragm but the contents do not pass through an actual opening.[3]

infant with bilateral chest tubes, a gastrostomy tube, IV apparatus, in some instances an endotracheal tube, and perhaps a ventral hernia.

In the postoperative period, parents will continue to feel anxious because of the constant threat of respiratory complications and the equipment needed to maintain their infant. Early physical contact with the infant is encouraged to foster bonding and reduce parental anxiety. The nurse can also intervene by helping the parents understand the purpose of her actions and by explaining expected results. For example, parents need to be informed whether drainage is expected through the various tubes and the meaning of changes in drainage. They also must be kept informed of the general status of their infant.

Postoperatively the gastrostomy is allowed to drain by gravity. Intravenous fluids are continued until gastrostomy feedings are tolerated. If mechanical ventilation is necessary the same precautions regarding inspiratory pressure must be taken as preoperatively. The nurse is responsible for maintaining the chest tubes for drainage and observing for any signs of malfunction. They are usually required for two or three days. Poor lung function continues to be a threat during the postoperative period. Therefore, the nurse must focus on maintaining clear respiratory passages and institute care to prevent pneumothorax. Frequent position changes, nasopharyngeal suction, endotracheal suction if the child is intubated, and chest physiotherapy require constant nursing attention.

The family should feed their infant at least several days before discharge. After surgery the infant may be lethargic and coaxing him to eat may cause vomiting or gagging. Parents should be taught to burp their infant frequently and not force-feed him when he shows disinterest in feeding. They must also be taught gastrostomy care and how to feed via gastrostomy because these infants are often discharged with a gastrostomy tube in place for four to six weeks in the event of difficulty with oral feedings.

About half of these infants survive.[10] When resuscitation and surgery have been managed optimally the prognosis still depends on three factors: (1) the size of the defect, (2) the degree of hypoplasia of the lung, and (3) the condition of the lung on the unaffected side. In general, the earlier symptoms appear, the poorer the prognosis. The final determinant of success is the total amount of pulmonary function available for gas exchange.[18]

HIATAL HERNIA WITH GASTROESOPHAGEAL REFLUX

Hiatal hernia is the intermittent or constant displacement of the proximal segment of the stomach through the esophageal hiatus of the diaphragm. This protrusion causes a displacement of the esophagogastric junction and portions of the proximal part of the stomach through the esophageal hiatus into the mediastinum, resulting in the regurgitation of food and fluid.[21] As a consequence, the child may experience recurrent emesis severe enough to result in failure to thrive, aspiration pneumonia or septic esophagitis with anemia due to gastrointestinal bleeding. Hiatal hernias are rare in the neonatal period, but the incidence increases after the first few months of life.

The existence of a hiatal hernia should be suspected if the child's caretaker notes persistent emesis. Documentation of the frequency, volume, and bile- or blood-staining of the emesis and respiratory symptoms such as coughing, wheezing or short apneic periods facilitate diagnosis. It is important to determine the adequacy of weight gain by referring to the child's placement on a growth chart.

Beyond the history, diagnosis involves a barium swallow. This demonstrates reflux of barium into the esophagus from a segment of the stomach situated above the diaphragm.

Nurse's Role in Management

Medical management of the infant with a hiatal hernia is aimed at reducing the likelihood of reflux and its consequences. This is done by use of cereal-thickened formula and maintenance of the infant in an upright position during feeding and for one-half hour afterward. An infant seat is most commonly used to maintain the baby in this position. If positional therapy is required for longer periods, infants are usually more comfortable when prone (see Fig. 24–26). Symptoms and weight gain are carefully monitored during this trial period of conservative medical management. If the latter is deemed unsuccessful after about two months, surgical intervention (e.g., Nissen-Hill fundoplication) is indicated. In this procedure the distal esophagus is surrounded by the adjacent gastric fundus with plicating sutures to create a new gastroesophageal junction and thereby curtail reflux.

During the procedure a gastrostomy tube is inserted for alimentation.

The major focus of postoperative care is the preservation of good respiratory function. The child is usually unable to cooperate in coughing and deep-breathing, thereby necessitating frequent suctioning and repositioning every two hours. An additional important measure is postural drainage if the child becomes febrile secondary to atelectasis or pneumonia.

Postoperatively the gastrostomy tube is placed to dependent drainage until bowel motility resumes as evidenced by the presence of bowel sounds and the passage of flatus and stool. (See Chapter 17 for discussion on care of the child with a gastrostomy.)

Gastrostomy feedings are begun slowly, with gradual increase in their volume and strength and with variation in the type of diet. It is important to document residuals (the amount in cc's of stomach contents remaining in the stomach just before a feeding) and any episode of vomiting. For older children, when they are allowed to eat it is essential that they be encouraged to chew their food thoroughly. Parents should be advised that the child may complain of a bloated sensation after eating. Although bloating may occur because of transient impairment of the child's ability to burp, this can be easily remedied by opening the gastrostomy tube for a short period of time.

The gastrostomy tube is usually removed approximately four weeks postoperatively when the child has a documented weight gain. This is done during a clinic visit and does not require an anesthetic. Parents are advised to place 4 by 4 dressings over the opening until the tract for the gastrostomy tubes closes. This prevents leakage of fluid onto the child's clothes.

Although the surgery can alleviate many altered health states for the child, it also presents new challenges for the parents. They will need support and education in the proper care of the gastrostomy tube and the administration of the tube feedings. A community health nurse referral can help to provide support for the family after discharge.

UMBILICAL HERNIA, INGUINAL HERNIA AND HYDROCELE

A hernia is the protrusion of a part of the bowel, ovary or testis through an abnormal opening in the containing walls of the abdomen. It consists of three parts: the sac or outpouching of the peritoneum, the coverings of the sac that is derived from the abdominal wall and the contents of the sac — bowel, ovary or testis. The most frequent locations for hernias are the umbilical and inguinal regions. Although congenital, the hernia may not appear until the infant is several months of age.

An umbilical hernia is a protrusion of the intestine at the umbilicus. Diagnosis is made by observation and palpation of the defect. Parents should be advised that 90 per cent of these hernias resolve on their own.[23] It is rare for an umbilical hernia to incarcerate. (If the hernia has not resolved by age 2, surgery is scheduled, usually on an outpatient basis.) Parents should be advised not to use binders, tape or other materials to compress the hernia. It has never been documented that these remedies aid in the closure of the defect, and they can cause infection.

The hernia is repaired through a transverse incision, which is made within the fold of the inferior aspect of the umbilicus. The incision is then carried through the subcutaneous fat and areolar tissue to the linea alba at the inferior rim of the umbilical ring. A plane is dissected around the ring at the level of the linea alba and the sac is dissected away from the umbilical skin. The sac is then transected and closed along with the fibrous umbilical ring in one to two layers.[3] The incision is coated with a protective sealant, and a compression dressing is applied for seven days.

The child is ready for discharge from the recovery room within two hours. The parents are requested to sponge bathe the child and to maintain the compression dressing for a week. It is important that the parents attempt to limit the child's physical sports activities for several weeks, although this is not easy to accomplish. Otherwise, the child has no dietary or activity restrictions. The child is seen one week after surgery and the dressing is removed. The parents should be advised that edema is still present and that this will decrease over time.

An inguinal hernia is the protrusion of bowel into the groin region (Fig. 24–34B). In the male, the testis descends from the abdominal cavity into the scrotum. The testis carries the parietal peritoneum with it, thus forming a tube (processus vaginalis) from the abdomen to the scrotum. Normally, the processus vaginalis will close spontaneously during development; if

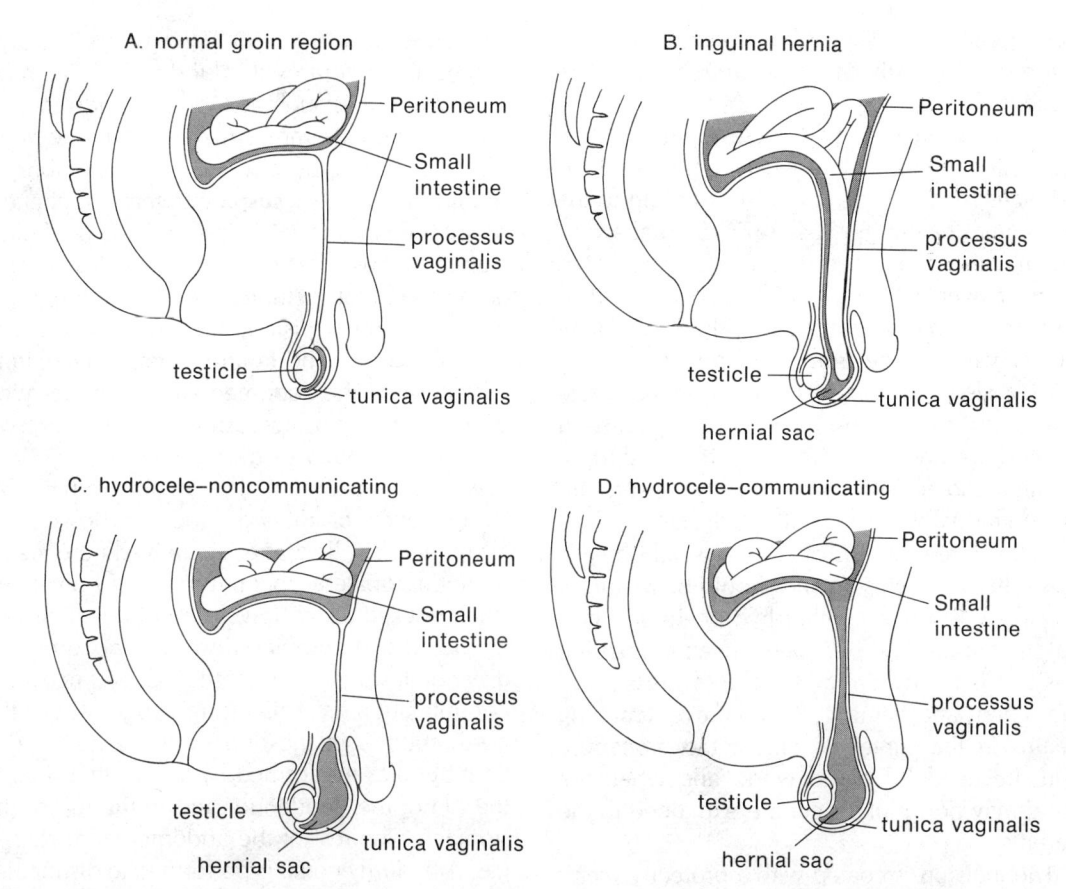

Figure 24-34 Hydroceles and hernias. A, Groin region of the normal male infant. An *inguinal hernia* (B) is the protrusion of bowel into the groin region. A *hydrocele* is a collection of fluid within the processus vaginalis. In a *noncommunicating hydrocele* (C), the scrotal swelling does not change in size or shape because there is no connection with the abdominal cavity. In a *communicating hydrocele* (D), the processus vaginalis remains open from the scrotum to the abdominal cavity, and scrotal swelling may vary in size during the course of an infant's day.

not, the descent of the intestine into the patent processus produces an inguinal hernia.

In the female, the round ligament extends from the uterus through the inguinal canal to its attachment in the labia majora. Weakness of the tissue around the round ligament together with increased abdominal pressure produces an inguinal hernia.

Diagnosis of a hernia is made by observation and palpation of a bulge in the groin area. Frequently, the diagnosis must be made on the basis of a history of a bulge in the groin that a reliable parent has noted while the infant was crying or straining to defecate. During the examination, it is important to check that both testes are in the scrotal sac and to determine the presence or absence of a scrotal or cord hydrocele (a collection of fluid in the tunica vaginalis of the testicle or along the spermatic cord).

The hernia causes the infant little discomfort unless it incarcerates. There is a high incidence of incarceration of an inguinal hernia in the first three months of life. Parents must be advised to watch for redness in the area of the hernia, increased swelling of the hernia and an inability to reduce the hernia. Under any of these circumstances they should be advised to contact their pediatrician immediately.

A hydrocele is a collection of fluid within the processus vaginalis. Hydroceles are most commonly seen in males. The type seen at birth presents as a soft scrotal swelling. In this type the upper portion of the processus vaginalis is obliterated but the portion within the scrotum (tunica vaginalis) remains open. Peritoneal fluid is trapped within the tunica vaginalis. There is no communication with the peritoneal cavity — thus it is referred to as a *noncommunicating hydrocele* (Fig. 24-34C). The scrotal swelling is painless and does not change in size or shape when the baby cries or when his position is changed. It is not reducible but can be easily transilluminated. The fluid is gradually absorbed and usually this type does not require surgery.

A communicating hydrocele is more often associated with a hernia because the processus vaginalis remains open from the scrotum to the abdominal cavity (Fig. 24–34D). Scrotal swelling may not be noticed until a few weeks after birth or even later in infancy. When a hydrocele communicates with the abdominal cavity it may vary in size from one time to another. During sleep decreased intra-abdominal pressure and a supine position effect a decrease in scrotal swelling by morning. With an upright position and activity during the day the scrotum again gradually enlarges. If a hydrocele is present after three months of age, it usually means that a hernia is present and should be repaired.

Surgery to correct either hydrocele or inguinal hernia or both is done on an outpatient basis. It is believed that this is less stressful for the child and family. Preoperative teaching begins in the surgeon's office: the procedure and the need for blood work, and when the child may not drink or eat are explained to the parents.

The incision is coated with a protective sealant and no dressing is applied. Parents should be advised that the scrotum may become edematous and appear bruised. This is due to the manipulation of the testis during the operation and should resolve in one to two weeks after the operation. No additional care is required. The procedure should cause the child no discomfort.

Parents are requested to sponge bathe the child for one week. In an older child, parents should attempt to limit physical activities for several weeks. Otherwise, the child has no restrictions.

Although the surgical treatment for umbilical hernia, inguinal hernia or hydrocele is a minor procedure, it is usually the family's first experience in the hospital and they need frequent reassurance that their child is doing well.

INTESTINAL ATRESIA

Intestinal atresia is the complete obliteration of the intestinal lumen. The most common site of intestinal atresia is the ileum, followed by the jejunem, then the colon. It is believed to be the result of a vascular accident in utero. It occurs about once in 1500 to 3000 live births.[10] A large number of children with duodenal atresia have other anomalies such as Down's syndrome.

Although hydramnios (excess amniotic fluid) may be caused by a variety of conditions, it should raise one's suspicion that esophageal or duodenal atresia is present. The clinical manifestations of atresia are signs of intestinal obstruction that include bilious vomiting, jaundice, abdominal distention (more pronounced in ileal atresia), and failure to pass meconium. Distention of the abdomen causes an elevation of the diaphragm, necessitating close observation for respiratory distress.

Atresia is documented on an abdominal x-ray by evidence of dilated loops of bowel and air-fluid levels. Ileal atresia can be differentiated by noting dilated proximal loops of bowel and small unused distal bowel. In duodenal atresia, an upright abdominal film will document a distended stomach with the appearance of a "double bubble." This strongly suggests that the obstruction is in the duodenum. The two distinct bubbles are formed by the air that rises to the top of the duodenum and to the top of the stomach. The rest of the abdomen is devoid of gas. A barium enema is performed to distinguish between small and large bowel distention, to determine if the colon is functional or nonfunctional and to locate the position of the cecum in order to rule out the presence of a malrotation (abnormal rotation of the cecum and duodenum).

It is important to obtain results of these tests quickly. The infant is at risk of developing a volvulus (a twisting of the bowel onto itself). Many times the parents are able to see the infant only briefly before he is taken to the operating room or is transferred to another hospital. It is essential to spend time with the family, to answer their questions and to encourage involvement in the infant's care. If the mother was planning to breast-feed her infant, she should continue with her attempts. She can pump her breasts so that when the infant is ready to feed, she will have an adequate supply of milk. In this way, the parents can become involved in their child's care.

Nurse's Role During Treatment

Preoperatively the infant is maintained in the incubator and a nasogastric tube is inserted through his mouth or nares in order to decompress the abdomen and prevent further vomiting

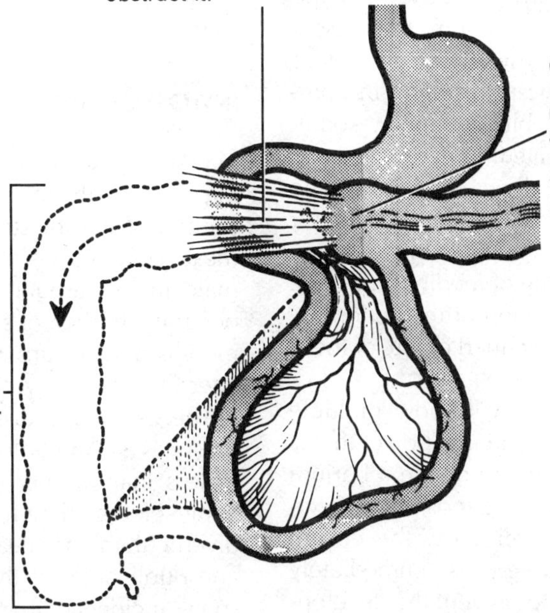

Figure 24–35 Malrotation of the intestine. (From H. Nixon and B. O'Donnell. The Essentials of Pediatric Surgery. J. B. Lippincott Co., 1961.)

and gaseous distention. It is essential that this tube remain patent — this may require irrigation with air or water once or twice a shift. Baseline laboratory studies (complete blood count and electrolytes) are obtained and the infant is maintained on IV hydration. Broad-spectrum antibiotics and vitamin K are administered.

During the surgical procedure the entire bowel is inspected for evidence of malrotation, volvulus and atresia. The dilated proximal segment is resected and then an anastomosis is performed between the proximal and distal segments of the bowel. A gastrostomy tube is inserted at this time.

Postoperatively the infant is maintained on IV hydration until stooling occurs. If this does not occur within three to four days, parenteral hyperalimentation should be considered. When stooling does occur the infant is gradually started on gastrostomy feedings. The feedings are increased in volume and strength gradually. It is important to document the consistency and number of stools per shift. As the infant increasingly tolerates gastrostomy feedings, he is slowly weaned from his incubator. The infant is then encouraged to take his feedings orally, but the gastrostomy tube is utilized if necessary. The parents are taught to wash the area around the gastrostomy tube with soap and water and then to tape the tube securely in place. (See page 574 for further discussion on care of the child with a gastrostomy.)

The parents must be encouraged to become involved in the infant's care. This can be accomplished by supporting the mother if she desires to breast-feed the infant. Also, times should be scheduled for the primary nurse to contact the family to let them know how the infant is progressing. In this way, the prolonged separation and its effects on the family can be diminished.

MALROTATION AND VOLVULUS

In fetal development, the abdominal cavity is unable to accommodate the rapidly developing intestine. The intestinal loops return to the abdominal cavity in the tenth week of fetal life. The final fixation and rotation of the intestine occurs at this time. The cecum is fixed in the right lower quadrant of the abdomen and the duodenum is in the right upper quadrant.

A volvulus is the twisting of the intestine upon itself (Fig. 24-35). Malrotation is the abnormal rotation of the cecum and duodenum. If the cecum remains in the epigastrium, the mesentery (blood supply) is narrowed and the entire midgut will volvulate (twist), resulting in compromise of the bowel's blood supply, sometimes leading to life-threatening necrosis.

The symptoms are usually evident during the first postnatal week. The nurse should watch for any signs of intestinal obstruction: bilious vomiting or increased vomiting of feedings, passage of bloody stool and distention of the abdomen. The physician should be notified of any of these signs.

A film of the abdomen will show multiple distended bowel loops and a large bowel that is devoid of gas. It is essential to obtain a barium enema study as soon as the diagnosis is suspected. The barium enema will show the cecum abnormally placed. Surgery is immediately scheduled. This is done to prevent the development of intestinal gangrene.

It is important to explain this anomaly to the family. It is a stressful period because the parents initially have perceived the infant as being healthy. The parents will have questions concerning the cause of the anomaly, the operation and postoperative care.

The infant is given broad-spectrum antibiotics intravenously, vitamin K is administered and a nasogastric tube is placed in the stomach as a means of decompressing the abdomen. During the operation the bowel is inspected for areas of obstruction. The intestine is untwisted to relieve the vascular obstruction. The bands of tissue (Ladd's bands) between the cecum and abdominal wall are divided. The duodenum is then positioned vertically on the right side of the abdomen and the cecum is placed in the left lower quadrant. An appendectomy is also performed. If a large portion of the bowel is compromised, it will be necessary to perform a bowel resection and a jejunostomy or ileostomy (a portion of the small bowel is brought onto the skin to provide an outlet for defecation).

The child is maintained on IV hydration postoperatively. If stooling does not occur by the third or fourth postoperative day, parenteral hyperalimentation should be considered. Once the infant has begun to defecate, gastrostomy feedings are initiated. The feedings are increased slowly in volume and strength. Parents are encouraged to hold, feed and care for their infant during this period. In this way, they will continue or begin the infant-parent relationship.

INTUSSUSCEPTION

Intussusception is an invagination or telescoping of part of the intestine into an adjacent distal portion of the intestine. (Fig. 24-36). It occurs most commonly in healthy, well-nourished male infants around 6 months of age. It can occur in children of any age but is rare before 3 months and occurs with decreasing frequency after the age of 3 years.

The cause of intussusception is unknown in most cases. An etiological factor is determined in less than 10 per cent of afflicted children. Some of the identifiable causes are Meckel's diverticulum, an ileal polyp, lymphosarcoma and duplication of the bowel.[8] There is a seasonal incidence that has been linked to the prevalence of adenovirus infections in the early summer and early winter months.

During an infection there is hypertrophy of the Peyer's patches (configuration of lymph nodules, single or in groups, in the ileum near its junction with the colon). It is thought that the presence of the resultant swelling may stimulate peristalsis.[24] The ileum, with its greater number of Peyer's patches, thus has greater potential to become the lead point for invagination into adjacent bowel.

The most common type of intussusception begins at or near the ileocecal valve, pushing into the cecum and onto the colon (referred to as ileocecocolic or ileocolic). The lumen of the bowel is compromised and vascular flow is obstructed. The involved intestine becomes inflamed and edematous with eventual bleeding from the mucosa. The initial incomplete obstruction progresses to a state of complete obstruction, producing distention and vomiting. Strangulation of the bowel can result, although this does not usually occur in the first 24 hours.[24] Intussusception, if untreated, can lead to intestinal gangrene, peritonitis and death.

The infants with intussusception presents with symptoms that are frightening and disturbing to parents. A healthy infant suddenly shows symptoms of severe abdominal pain, which recurs at frequent intervals. The infant draws his legs up sharply with a sudden piercing cry. The infant usually vomits, becomes extremely restless and often appears diaphoretic and pale. Normal stool may be passed during the initial

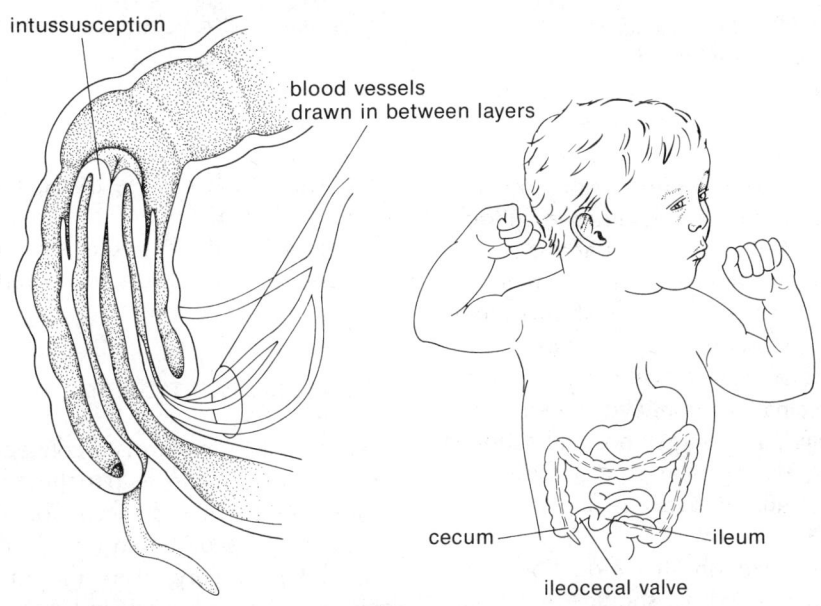

Figure 24–36 Intussusception. The most common type begins at or near the ileocecal valve, pushing into the cecum and onto the colon. At first, the obstruction is partial, but as the bowel becomes inflamed and edematous, complete obstruction occurs.

phase. The attack then subsides and the infant shows no abnormal signs between the severe attacks of abdominal pain.

As the condition worsens, the infant becomes lethargic and progressively weaker. Vital signs reflect a shock-like state, vomitus may now be biled-stained and abdominal distention is apparent. There will be either no stool or a stool characteristically described as being like currant jelly in appearance owing to the blood and mucus it contains. Blood usually appears in the stool within 12 hours from the onset of symptoms. Between attacks of pain, in some cases a sausage-shaped mass can be palpated in the right upper quadrant of the abdomen. A barium enema confirms the diagnosis and in many cases successfully treats the intussusception by hydrostatic reduction.

The nurse needs to be prepared to give accurate guidance when parents initially report symptoms. Because the infant may sleep and is comfortable between attacks, the seriousness of the symptoms can be overlooked by the nurse if she is not familiar with the characteristic pattern of their onset. She must advise the family to seek immediate medical attention and explain to them that, even though the baby seems normal between attacks, his condition may change rapidly.

Nurse's Role During Treatment

There are three types of treatment for intussusception: (1) reduction by the hydrostatic pressure of a barium enema, (2) reduction by surgical manipulation, and (3) surgical resection of the nonreducible involved intestine.

Reduction by Barium Enema During the first 24 hours of symptoms the intussusception can usually be reduced by hydrostatic pressure. Contraindications for reduction by barium enema are: (1) a complete mechanical obstruction and (2) a high temperature, vomiting, and signs of peritonitis, sepsis or shock.[30]

The infant must be prepared for a barium enema as though surgery will follow, because if barium enema reduction is unsuccessful, the infant undergoes operation immediately. The family must understand the purpose of the barium enema and must realize that surgery may be necessary. Preparation for the barium enema includes giving the infant nothing by mouth, insertion of a nasogastric tube to prevent aspiration during the barium enema, and administering intravenous fluids. Preparation for such treatment occurs rapidly and may leave parents stunned. They can be helped to calm their infant if the nurse attends to their need for a description of the problem and frequent explanations of what is occurring. (The nurse can use a rubber glove or tube gauze to describe telescoping of the bowel. By inverting a finger of the glove or the gauze into itself, intussusception is illustrated.) The parents may have numerous questions about the meaning of reduction of the bowel and how the procedure is done. The nurse can provide some basic information to the family if she is familiar with the barium reduction procedure: A nonlubricated catheter is placed into the rectum; the buttocks are pulled together and taped. Barium is then allowed to flow into the rectum from a height of 90 to 100 cm and the pathway of the barium is observed by fluoroscopy. The pressure caused by the flow of barium results in extension of the bowel to its normal position. Even when reduction is successful, 48 hours of hospitalization is recommended, during which nasogastric suction, antibiotics and intravenous fluids are provided.[30]

During hospitalization after reduction of intussusception, the nurse should encourage parents to hold their infant. They can be taught to handle their infant so that the IV will not be dislodged and the nasogastric tube will function properly. Parents must be forewarned that stool will contain grayish-white barium and that each diaper should be checked by the nurse. Parents should be encouraged to change diapers and care for their infant, but the nurse must record and describe the stools accurately. The infant must be observed by the nurse and parents for any signs of recurring obstruction.

Surgical Treatment Surgical intervention is necessary in cases when the barium enema is not successful and when there is clinical evidence of intestinal obstruction with abdominal distention. The intussusception is surgically reduced by milking the intestine (distal to proximal) to move the invaginated portion back to its normal position. (Attempts lasting longer than 10 minutes are not recommended.) If this is not successful, intestinal resection may be necessary. Postoperatively the nurse must help the family cope with the stress of caring for their infant, who is not allowed to eat, requires frequent position changes and needs to be restrained to prevent dislodging of the nasogastric tube and IV needle. Also, the nurse must frequently assess the infant's vital signs (particularly a high fever), blood pressure, bowel sounds, and sutures and dressing, proper functioning of the nasogastric tube, and accurate infusion of IV fluids.

Spontaneous reduction occasionally occurs. When an intussusception is reduced by barium enema there is a recurrence of 5 to 10 per cent. Recurrence is also possible after surgical reduction; it is least common after intestinal resection. The length of time that elapses between onset and reduction of the intestines affects prognosis. Prognosis is excellent if the condition is treated within 12 to 24 hours, and grave in the event of strangulation.[28]

MECKEL'S DIVERTICULUM

Meckel's diverticulum is a congenital anomaly characterized by an outpouching of the ileum. The condition may be asymptomatic for many years and may be found only in the course of abdominal surgery. It is the most common gastrointestinal anomaly and is present in 1 to 2 per cent of the population. It may manifest itself at any age but the majority of symptomatic cases become apparent before the child reaches 2 years of age. Its importance is that it can cause intestinal obstruction, massive bleeding, perforation and peritonitis.

Intestinal obstruction can be caused by a strand of obliterated vessels that connects the diverticulum to the umbilicus. The band may compress another loop of intestine and cause obstruction or it may be the focal point of a volvulus (twisting of the intestines). The outpouching ileum can act as a lead point for intussusception with symptoms.

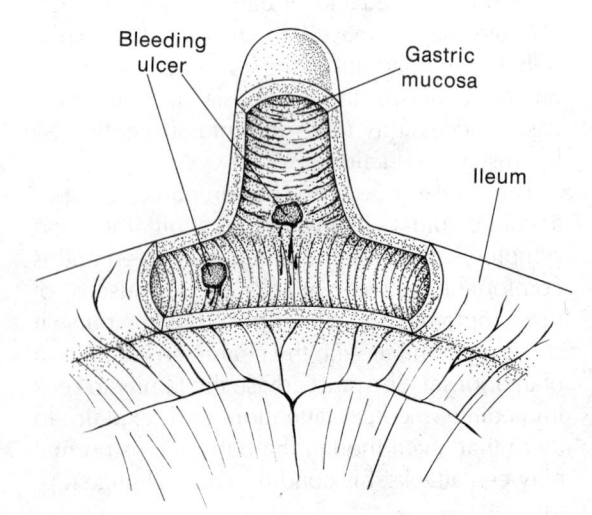

Figure 24–37 Meckel's diverticulum is an outpouching of the ileum. This congenital anomaly may remain asymptomatic for years, or it may become a source of intestinal bleeding, it may become inflamed and lead to perforation, or it may become the focal point for intussusception, obstruction or volvulus.

Bleeding occurs because the tip of the outpouched ileum frequently contains ectopic gastric mucosa rather than ileal mucosa (Fig. 24–37). The gastric secretions are an irritant to the surrounding tissue. Eventually there is severe ulceration of the ileal mucosa at the base of the diverticulum or within the adjacent ileum to which it is connected. The eroded area hemorrhages, resulting in painless rectal bleeding, the most common sign in children. Blood is dark red in color or bright red and is usually passed without stool. Less frequently the diverticulum becomes inflamed and may progress to perforation.

Meckel's diverticulum is generally not demonstrated on x-ray. Diagnosis is made by the history and a technetium scan, which shows an area of radioactivity suggestive of gastric mucosa in the diverticulum.

The immediate concern is to surgically remove the lesion to prevent shock. When a peptic ulcer is present in the adjacent ileum, excision of the involved bowel is necessary. Postoperatively the child has a nasogastric tube and requires the usual postoperative care indicated for bowel surgery. Postoperative nursing responsibilities are to maintain patency of the nasogastric tube, administer IV fluid, check vital signs and bowel sounds, calculate intake and output until eating is resumed and provide for the early resumption of a normal level of activity.

It is frightening to parents when their otherwise healthy child develops massive rectal bleeding and requires immediate surgery. The family needs frequent reassurance that the child is recuperating satisfactorily. The nurse should recognize the stress the child and his family have experienced. The nurse can reduce that stress by keeping parents informed, and ensuring that their questions are answered. Especially when the child is being prepared for surgery, parents feel bewildered and are worried about their baby.

HIRSCHSPRUNG'S DISEASE (CONGENITAL AGANGLIONOSIS OR AGANGLIONIC MEGACOLON)

Hirschsprung's disease was first described in 1691, but the appropriate surgical intervention and management was not developed until 1948. Hirschsprung's disease occurs in 1 in 5000 live births. It is an anomaly of the full-term infant and predominantly affects males. It has been associated with other anomalies such as Down's syndrome and with genitourinary anomalies. Although usually it is diagnosed in infancy, there have been many documented cases of the diagnosis first being made in childhood and adolescence.

Hirschsprung's disease can be referred to as a congenital megacolon (large colon since birth). The anomaly is characterized by "partial to complete obstruction associated with the absence of intramural ganglion cells in the distal alimentary tract"[10] (Fig. 24–38). The absence of intramural ganglion cells (nerve cells) involves both the submucosal and intermuscular nerve plexuses. This may involve as small an area as the lower rectum (short-segment Hirschsprung's) or as large a one as the entire colon (long-segment Hirschsprung's). The lack of ganglion cells prevents the bowel from transmitting the coordinated peristaltic waves that normally enable fecal material to pass through the alimentary tract. The internal sphincter is unable to relax; evacuation of solids, liquid or gas is prevented. Thus the infant has a mechanical intestinal obstruction.

The onset of symptoms is usually noted in the first 24 to 48 hours of life. The nurse should consider Hirschsprung's as a possible diagnosis for any infant who does not pass meconium within the first 24 to 48 hours of life. The nurse should watch the infant closely for passage of meconium or for bile-stained vomitus and abdominal distention.

The nurse's history should include a detailed documentation of family members with stooling difficulties. A genetic familial factor has been associated with Hirschsprung's disease in 3 to 5 per cent of all cases. There is an 18 per cent incidence for brothers of females with long aganglionic segments and 0.6 per cent incidence for sisters of males with short segments.[26] This is an important consideration for genetic counselling.

The rectal examination may raise the suspicion of Hirschsprung's disease. A tight sphincter is frequently felt and the examination produces explosive, watery, foul-smelling diarrhea. During the diagnostic period, the nurse must be aware of any signs of enterocolitis, an inflammation of the small intestine and colon. The physician should be notified of fever, bloody diarrhea and vomiting.

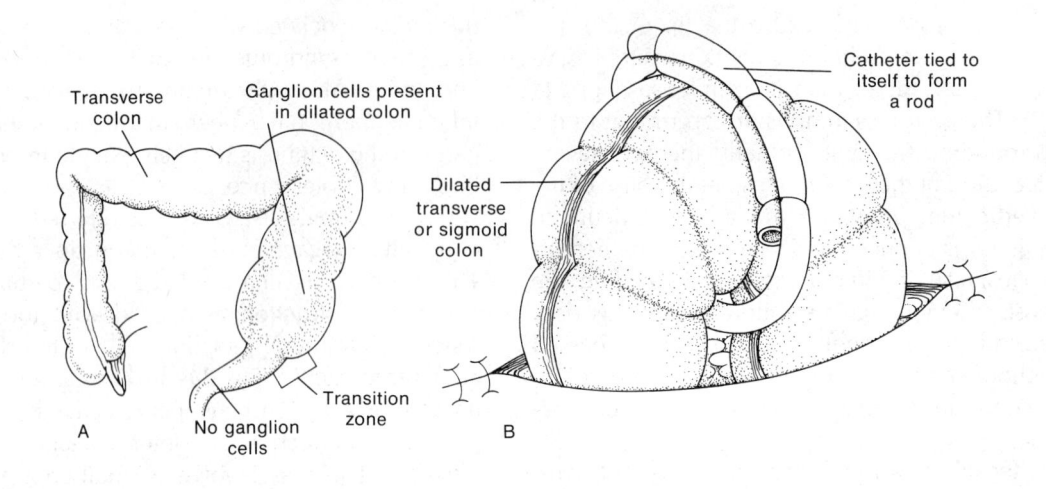

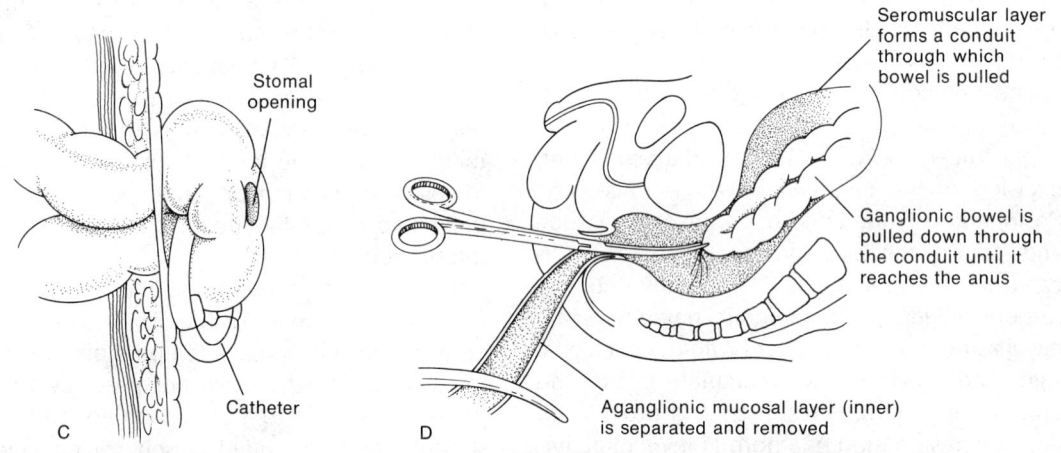

Figure 24-38 The cause and surgical correction of Hirschsprung's disease. A, a lack of ganglion cells in a segment of the colon prevents the transmission of normal peristaltic waves and results in an intestinal obstruction. B, the surgical procedure for correction involves bringing out a loop of the colon and encircling it with a catheter to prepare for creation of a stomal opening. C, the ostomy is maintained until the infant reaches 20 pounds or 1 year of age. D, corrective surgery involves separating the aganglionic mucosal layer of the transition zone from the outer seromuscular layer, removing the aganglionic layer, and suturing ganglionic bowel to the anal opening.

A barium enema radiologically documents the retention of barium and any evidence of a transition zone. The transition zone represents the abrupt change from dilated proximal intestine (ganglionic bowel) to narrowed and frequently spastic-appearing bowel (aganglionic bowel) (Fig. 24-38A). The dilation of the proximal intestine is due to the edema and hypertrophy of the bowel.

A suction rectal biopsy is also performed to histologically document the lack of ganglion cells. The procedure can be done in the treatment room without anesthesia. A section of rectal mucosa and submucosa is obtained. The nurse must emphasize to the parents that this procedure can result in a small amount of rectal bleeding that disappears in a day.

Nurse's Role During Treatment

Initial Phase: Temporary Colostomy If the submucosa does not contain ganglion cells, surgery is scheduled. The infant is prepared for surgery by insertion of a nasogastric tube and administration of broad-spectrum antibiotics and vitamin K. Once the infant has been anesthetized, the surgeon must determine the exact level of aganglionic bowel in relationship to ganglionic bowel. This is accomplished by obtaining multiple pathological specimens for histological evaluation. It is important to explain to the parents that this can be time-consuming, thus lengthening the time of the operation. A colostomy (temporary opening of the colon through the abdominal wall) is created just above the determined level of ganglionic bowel.

The colostomy is created to provide the infant with the means to defecate and to allow the distended bowel to become normal in size. The colostomy is referred to as a leveling colostomy (because it is created at the level of aganglionic-ganglionic bowel) or as a transverse or sigmoid loop colostomy (a loop of sigmoid or transverse colon is brought to the abdominal surface). To prevent retraction of the stoma into the wound, a small segment of a No. 16 French Robinson catheter is brought under the section of intestine that is brought onto the skin and tied to itself as a rod. (Fig. 34-38 B and C). The colostomy is then opened by electrocauterization. An appropriate ostomy appliance is applied.

The infant remains on IV hydration and antibiotics for three to five days. The nasogastric tube is discontinued after defecation through the colostomy has begun, usually on the third postoperative day. It is important to allow the parents the opportunity to hold and comfort the infant during this period to begin to develop a relationship with him.

The rod (French Robinson catheter tied to itself) is taken out 10 days after the operation. The parents should be advised that the stoma will decrease in size. It is also essential for them to understand that their baby will pass mucus and small amounts of stool (sometimes daily) through the anus. This occurs because there is communication between the proximal and distal loop that allows for spillage of stool into the distal loop. Furthermore, parents need to be given an explanation about the stoma of the colostomy. The bowel has a good vascular supply and few nerves, so parents can be assured that they will not hurt their infant when they touch the stoma. The infant can be placed on the abdomen and can be held on the shoulder without pain.

Postoperative teaching of ostomy care is the primary responsibility of the nursing staff. Many hospitals have enterostomal therapists who can aid the nurse and family in selection of the appropriate equipment for proper care of the ostomy. Parents should be given time initially to adjust to the physical appearance of their infant with an ostomy, and then to become more involved in the actual care of the ostomy. The fact that the stoma is temporary and will be closed at 1 year of age should be stressed to the parents.

Parents must be taught to empty, cleanse and change the ostomy bag. Skin care is essential because the stool is irritating. (See Table 17-3 for a care guide for parents.) These goals can be accomplished by establishing a discharge teaching plan cooperatively with the parents. Because ostomy equipment is expensive, in appropriate cases parents should be referred to a social worker for financial assistance. A community health nurse referral provides continued help for the family after discharge.

Through the establishment of a trusting relationship, the nurse can aid parents in voicing their perceptions of their infant and in working toward an acceptance of him and his condition. An important consideration is that although body image is not an issue for the infant, it is for the parents who must care for an infant with an ostomy. Also, provided with an atmosphere of support, participation and understanding, the family will be prepared when the infant is medically ready for discharge.

Final Phase: Corrective Surgery The ostomy is maintained until the infant weighs 20 pounds or reaches one year of age. The Swenson, the Duhamel and the Soave procedures are operations done for the definitive treatment of Hirschsprung's disease. Today the majority of pediatric surgeons choose to perform a modification of the Soave procedure.[6, 7, 11]

The infant is admitted three days before the date of the operation so that adequate cleansing of the bowel can be accomplished. It is essential that the bowel be cleansed of stool to prevent contamination during the operation. The child is immediately placed on a clear liquid diet. The day before surgery, the child is given four doses of oral neomycin and erythromycin. In conjunction with oral antibiotics, the ostomy is irrigated with an appropriate amount of neomycin-based irrigation solution. This is done to cleanse the bowel of bacteria. (See Chapter 17 for a discussion of colostomy irrigation.)

The physician will designate whether the distal loop, the proximal loop or both loops of the ostomy should be irrigated. The physician may also order rectal irrigations. This is done to dislodge any stool in the distal limb of the intestine. Intramuscular antibiotics are administered at midnight and again just before the operation.

Once the child is anesthetized, a Foley catheter is inserted into the bladder. This is done so that the bladder will not become distended with urine. The colostomy is then surgically taken down (excised). Unless the transition zone (level of aganglionic-ganglionic bowel) has been predetermined, biopsies are done at this time. Once the transition zone is determined, the inner aganglionic mucosal layer is separated from the outer seromuscular layer of the rectum and removed. The outer layer of the rectum forms a conduit through which the aganglionic bowel is then pulled until it reaches the anus (Fig. 24–3D). The ganglionic bowel is then sutured to the anal opening. In this way the sphincters (muscles of continence) in the rectal region are preserved. A Penrose drain is placed between the anus and the pulled-through bowel to prevent any collection of serous fluid in that area. This is helpful in reducing the possibility of infection. After the peritoneal cavity has been irrigated with saline, the abdomen is closed.

Postoperatively, the child is fed intravenously, a nasogastric tube is inserted to prevent distention of the abdomen,* urinary output is measured through the use of a Foley catheter, and the Penrose drain provides for drainage of serous fluid through the rectum. The child is restrained enough so that he is unable to pull out the various tubes. The nasogastric tube is placed to Gomco suction (intermittent suction) in order to decompress the stomach. It should be irrigated routinely (every four hours) with air or saline to ensure its patency. The Penrose drain is removed by the physician within the first 48 hours postoperatively. The child should be turned every 2 hours and should be encouraged to cough. This can be done in conjunction with postural drainage, with cupping and clapping or nasopharyngeal suctioning. These nursing measures are important to prevent pneumonia. It is essential that rectal temperature not be taken or rectal examinations not be done postoperatively.

---

*The stomach and upper gastrointestinal tract continuously secretes digestive juices. The nasogastric tube allows these juices to be drained, which reduces the child's feeling of nausea and prevents vomiting. It also prevents pressure of the distended abdomen on the new suture line.

When the child begins to pass flatus (usually on the third postoperative day), intermittent suction of the nasogasttric tube is no longer necessary and the nasogastric tube is placed on dependent drainage (drained by gravity). Once the child has begun to pass stools, the nasogastric tube is removed. The Foley catheter is removed on the third to fifth postoperative day. It is important to obtain a urine culture after removal of the catheter to identify any possible source of infection. Diet is slowly advanced from clear liquids to full liquids and eventually to a regular diet. Intravenous antibiotics are given for five days.

On the tenth postoperative day, the surgeon performs a rectal examination to assess the sphincter tone and the site of anastomosis. The child is then medically ready for discharge. The parents must understand that the child may have 5 to 15 stools per day. Excoriation of the skin of the buttocks is the major concern before and after discharge. The stool lacks consistency and is very acidic, causing excoriation.

The reason for the excoriation should be explained to the parents before discharge. They should be encouraged to apply an ointment (Desitin, Mycostatin or another similar agent) with each diaper change and to air-dry the area whenever possible. A lamp is usually used during the hospitalization to dry the excoriated area. It is essential that the parents be advised not to place the lamp too close to the skin as this will cause burning. It should be about six to eight inches away from the skin. Ointment should always be removed before the lamp is used. The excoriation can be a persistent problem for two to three months after the operation. Parents need to be supported and their diligent care of the skin acknowledged.

After discharge the child is seen in the clinic on a weekly basis. A rectal examination is done at each clinic visit. The purpose of this is to dilate and assess the patency of the anastomosis site. The segment of intestine that has been pulled through may undergo stricture, and it is essential that it remain patent and functioning. The rectal examinations are upsetting and uncomfortable for the child. There is usually a moderate amount of bloody discharge from the rectum for about 24 hours after the examination.

After the initial postoperative period, the child has rectal examinations in the clinic every six months. It is important to emphasize to the parents that the child may be difficult or slow to toilet train. They are encouraged not to attempt this process until the child is over 2 years of age. Once toilet trained, the child is followed on a yearly basis to monitor his stooling patterns.

This disease process affects the functioning of the family primarily for the first year or two of the child's life. It is important to provide support through community health services. It is essential to emphasize that the infant will defecate normally after the definitive operative procedure is performed.

NECROTIZING ENTEROCOLITIS

Necrotizing enterocolitis is defined as "a condition in which there is diffuse or patchy necrosis of the mucosa or submucosa in the large and small bowel."[13] The disease affects 1 to 7 per cent of all newborns admitted to the nursery[22] and 3 to 8 per cent of all premature infants.[5] It was not until the late 1960s that researchers were able to correlate the many components of the disease. Although its specific cause is unknown, many studies demonstrate that the disease is secondary to vascular ischemia of the intestinal tract. According to Flores, "Hypoxia leads to bowel ischemia, ileus and stasis which leads to bacterial proliferation and severe damage to the wall of the intestine."[13]

The onset of symptoms usually occurs on the fourth or fifth day of life, after the infant has had his initial feedings. At greatest risk of developing necrotizing enterocolitis are premature infants weighing less than 1500 gm who also have respiratory distress syndrome. Other contributing factors are jaundice, sepsis and congestive heart disease.

Nurse's Role

During Diagnosis The nurse daily assesses the infant at risk for developing this condition. Many of the signs and symptoms center on the infant's ability to tolerate feedings. One must be concerned if the infant develops difficulty with feedings, has increased residuals before feedings (if he is gavaged*) or has decreased interest in feedings and decreased energy to feed. The infant may also have bilious vomiting and an inability to defecate, which may indicate a developing ileus (intestinal obstruction).

Stools are tested for occult blood, which would document ongoing disease and irritation of the bowel. Other signs are increased listlessness or irritability, bradycardia with an increased number of apneic episodes and an inability to maintain temperature. Other signs of necrotizing enterocolitis are increased abdominal girth with shiny erythema of the abdominal wall, increased rigidity of the abdominal musculature, and a change in breathing pattern (an infant uses abdominal muscles to breathe).

The infant can be tolerating feedings and requiring decreasing amounts of oxygen and then unexpectedly develop this disease. The changes can occur quite rapidly and must be dealt with immediately; however, it is essential that explanations and support for the parents not be forgotten. The physician and nurse should spend time explaining to the family what is going on with their infant and should inform them of the options and possibilities for the future.

The nurse should explore with the mother the possibility of breast feeding for infants at risk of developing necrotizing enterocolitis. Fresh breast milk contains lymphocytes, macrophages and lactoferrin that aid the infant's natural defense against bacterial invasion of the intestinal mucosa. Many hospitals have breast pumps that can be utilized during the infant's long hospitalization to aid the mother to continue to breastfeed. Resource groups such as La Leche League may be supportive referrals. In this way, the mother is given an opportunity to participate actively in the care of her infant.

During Treatment Management of necrotizing enterocolitis may be accomplished through medical means. A Replogle tube, a type of nasogastric tube that is attached to intermittent suction, is inserted in an attempt to decompress the abdomen. The infant is given nothing orally; hydration and nutrition are maintained intravenously. After blood, urine, stool and spinal fluid cultures are taken, antibiotics are administered, both intravenously and orally. Oral antibiotics are administered in an attempt to alter the bacteria in the intestine. A thorough blood workup is carried out to monitor the infant's electrolytes, blood gas levels, complete blood count and platelet count. Intubation of the infant may be necessary if respiratory compromise develops.

Abdominal x-rays are taken every 8 to 12 hours to look for distention of bowel loops, pneumoperitoneum (air in the peritoneum) or

---
*Forced-fed, especially through a tube.

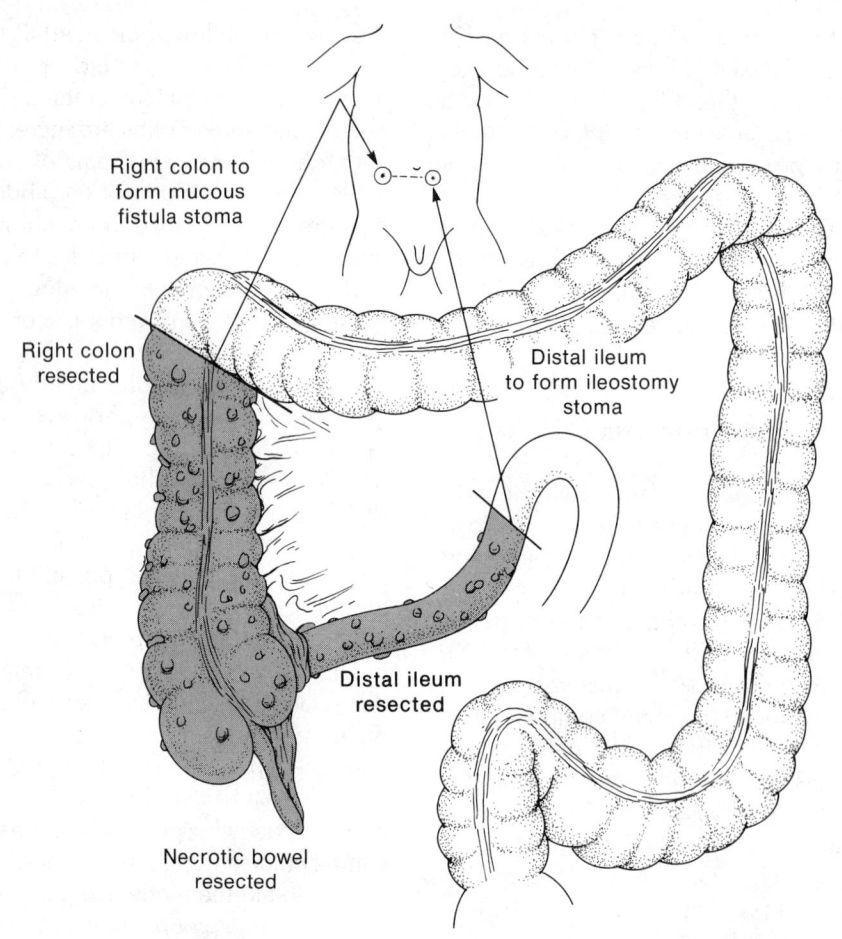

Figure 24–39 Necrotizing enterocolitis can be corrected in the majority of cases by surgery. The right colon is resected and a colonic mucous fistula is created. The distal ileum is resected to create an ileostomy stoma. Gastrostomy tube feedings are used until a second surgical procedure is carried out to remove the ostomies and reanastomose the two ends of the intestines.

pneumatosis intestinalis. Pneumatosis intestinalis is the presence of air pockets within the intestinal wall caused by invading bacteria that can result in the perforation of the bowel. This most commonly affects the terminal ileum and right colon, but can be much more extensive.

Medical treatment is reported to be adequate in 75 per cent of patients and there is no development of gangrene of the intestine.[10] The other 25 per cent develop necrosis of segments of the intestinal tract that requires surgical intervention.

During surgery the entire bowel is examined for perforations. Necrotic bowel, usually the distal ileum and right colon, is resected (cut out), leaving two free ends of bowel. The free ileum is brought out through the abdominal wall, creating an ileostomy to provide a means of defecation. The free colon is stabilized by bringing it to the abdomen to create a colonic mucous fistula stoma (Fig. 24–39). A gastrostomy tube is inserted at the time of the operation as a means of providing alimentation for the infant in the future.

Gastrostomy tube feedings are begun when the infant has passed feces through the ileostomy. Breast milk or predigested formula in small amounts and diluted strengths is used for gastrostomy feedings. The infant must be watched closely for residuals before feedings and for diarrhea and bloody feces, which would signify further irritation or necrosis of the bowel.

As the infant continues to improve, attempts are made to feed him via the nipple. The infant is given the opportunity to take a designated amount by mouth and the remainder is given via the gastrostomy tube. In this way, the infant can learn to feed without jeopardizing his progress.

The final stage of treatment is removal of the ostomies and reanastomosis of the two ends of

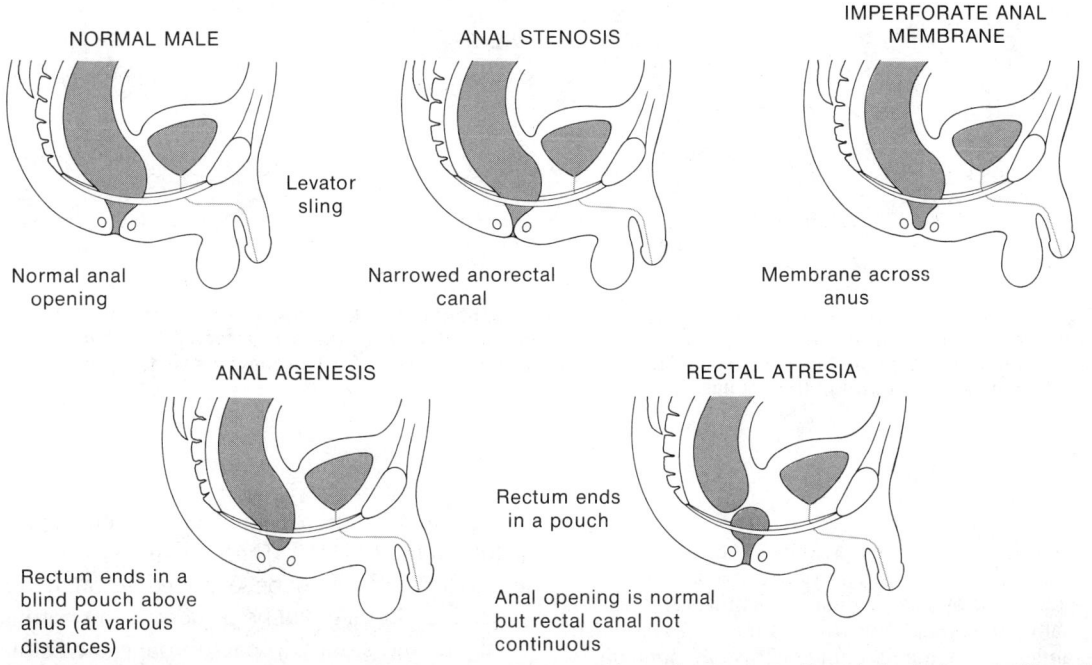

Figure 24-40 Normal anal anatomy and four main types of imperforate anus. Type I, Anal stenosis. Type II, Imperforate anal membrane. Type III, Anal agenesis (This is the most common type, occurring in about 80 per cent of cases of imperforate anus.) Type IV, Rectal atresia.

the intestines. It is becoming an accepted practice at medical centers to close the stomas before discharge, when the baby weighs 2.27 kg. (5 lbs). This should be explained to the parents because care of the ostomies is of great concern to them. Since the infant will be discharged with a gastrostomy tube, the teaching of gastrostomy care and use should be continuous throughout hospitalization.

Necrotizing enterocolitis is a debilitating disease that results in prolonged hospitalization with the potential of at least two major operative procedures for the infant. This places added stress on the family and on the bonding process between the infant and his parents. The nursing staff can minimize family members' anxieties by establishing a trusting relationship with them. This is done through honestly answering their questions and being available to hear their concerns. This relationship will foster the exchange of information and support the development of plans for discharge. These families have been under a great deal of stress and usually require referral to community resources such as a public health nurse to facilitate adjustment to home care of the infant.

ANORECTAL MALFORMATIONS

Congenital anomalies of the anus and rectum occur in various forms with or without fistulas. They occur in approximately 1:3000 to 4000 live births and are more common in males.[10] Whenever the passage of fecal material is obstructed by a structural anomaly of the anus and rectum, the anus is described as imperforate. There are four main types of imperforate anus: (1) anal stenosis, (2) imperforate anal membrane, (3) anal agenesis and (4) rectal atresia (Fig. 24–40).

Type I
 Congenital anal stenosis is a narrowing of the anorectal canal that may occur at any point or extend its entire length. Diagnosis can be established by digital and endoscopic examination. Manual dilatations can often correct this type of malformation.

Type II
 With imperforate anal membrane, a thin cutaneous membrane persists across the anal opening. Meconium fills the rectum and can frequently be seen as a discoloration of the membrane. Treatment consists of incision or excision of the membrane followed by anal dilatations until bowel function is normal.

Type III
 In anal agenesis the terminal end of the rectum ends in a blind pouch at variable distances above the anus. This type accounts for approximately 80 per cent of anorectal malformations. Most of these infants have associated fistulas of various types. Treatment is surgical and varies with the type of lesion and fistula.

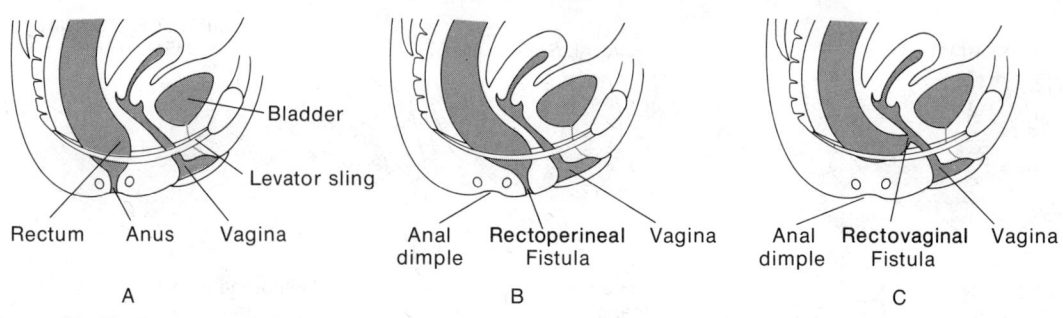

Figure 24–41 Anal agenesis in females. A shows the normal configuration. B is a low lesion in which the terminal end of the rectum opens in the perineum in front of the normal site of the anus (termed *rectoperineal fistula*). C is a low lesion in which the rectum is connected to the vagina (*rectovaginal fistula*). The openings are large enough for stool to be expelled through the fistulas.

Type IV

In rectal atresia there is a normal anus but the rectal canal is not continuous. The lower rectal pouch can be identified by careful digital examination. There is usually a complete block that is encountered when examining with the little finger. This rare anomaly is corrected by anastomosis through an abdominoperineal approach.

Because 80 per cent of anorectal malformations are type III (anal agenesis), the remainder of this discussion covers anal agenesis.

Anal agenesis is described as high if the blind pouch of the rectum lies above the levator sling. (The pubococcygeal and puborectalis muscles comprise the levator sling. For rectal continence to be accomplished, the rectum must be placed within the sling.) A line drawn from the tip of the coccyx to the symphysis pubis would approximate the level of the levator sling. If the blind pouch lies below this line it has theoretically transversed the levator sling and is referred to as a low lesion. Most males have high lesions, whereas most females have low lesions. Fistulas occur in 80 to 90 per cent of patients with anal agenesis.

The specific variations of anal agenesis are as follows.

Anal Agenesis in Females

Females usually have larger fistulas than males, therefore surgery need not be done immediately.

Low Lesions The terminal end of the rectum forms a fistula that opens in the perineum anterior to the normal site of the anus (rectoperineal fistula) (Fig. 24–41B) or a fistula connects the rectum to the vagina (rectovaginal fistula) (Fig. 24–41C). These openings are large enough for stool to be expelled through the vagina. A dimple may be present at the normal anal site and stool will pass through the fistula anterior to the dimple or through the vagina. These anomalies can be corrected by anoplasty (creation or enlargement of the anus) in the newborn period, but 3 to 6 months of age is recommended as the optimal time for repair.

High Lesions High lesions are not common in females, but when they exist a fistula is usually associated; this opens into the proximal portion of the vagina (rectovaginal). Anomalies of the spine are commonly associated with high lesions in females.[10] To correct the anomaly a sigmoid loop colostomy is done when the diagnosis is confirmed and a sacroperineal pull-through is deferred for 6 months to 1 year or until weight of 8 to 10 kg is attained.

Anal Agenesis in Males

Low Lesions Low lesions are not common in males but when they exist there is usually a fistula to the perineum, opening at a point anterior to the normal anal site (Fig. 24–42B). These lesions can be corrected by dilatations alone or perineal anoplasty followed by dilatations.

High Lesions High lesions exist almost exclusively in males and almost always have an associated urinary fistula (usually rectourethral) (Fig. 24–42C). These infants are initially treated by a sigmoid loop colostomy followed by a sacroperineal pull-through at 6 to 12 months of age.

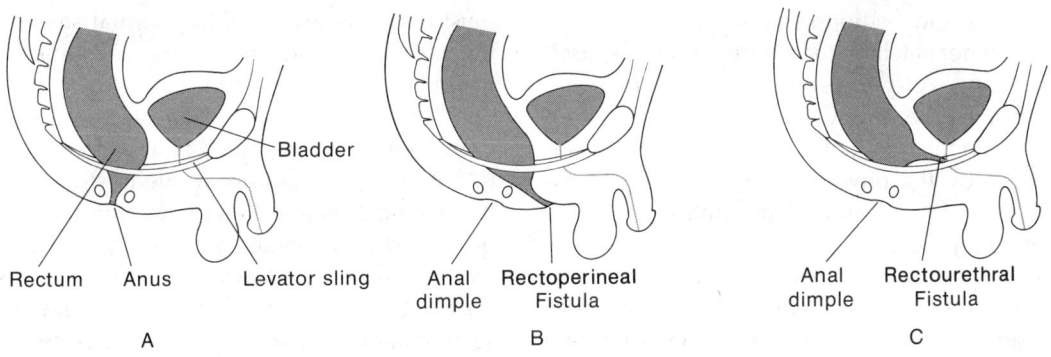

Figure 24–42 Anal agenesis in males. A shows the normal configuration. B shows a fistula to the perineum, with the opening anterior to the normal anal opening. C shows a high lesion in a male, in which there is a connection between the rectum and the urethra.

Clinical Manifestations and Diagnosis

When checking temperature rectally on a newborn the nurse should always inspect the anus to be sure the thermometer is being inserted into the anus and not into a perineal fistula. The anal area should always be inspected for a dimple as a clue to imperforate anus. The nurse must carefully check that there is a normal anal opening and that there is no membrane present.

An understanding of the various anorectal malformations assists the nurse to make accurate observations. If meconium is not passed she must inspect the perineum, urethra and vagina for a speck of meconium. Fistulas may not be apparent at birth but usually during the first 24 hours of life meconium is gradually forced through the fistula by peristalsis and is seen as a tiny speck at the opening of a fistula.[24] Each voiding must be inspected for meconium, which may have passed via a recto-urinary fistula (most common in males). Also, abdominal distention observed by the nurse could lead to the diagnosis of an undetected anorectal anomaly.

Definitive diagnosis is made by x-ray. The infant is placed prone in the Trendelenburg position to allow air to rise to outline the rectal pouch; this indicates whether a high or low lesion exists. A retrograde urethrocystogram will usually confirm the presence of a rectourethral fistula.[24] Other anomalies are common and the infant should be inspected for their presence. During the diagnostic period the nurse should be in communication with the physician about the various procedures to be done. It is a comfort to parents when the nurse is informed and can reinforce explanations given by the physician. Also, the fact of stool being expelled from any body orifice other than the rectum is difficult for many parents to accept. They may feel their infant is very abnormal and they need special attention from the health team to help them understand the available treatment.

Nursing Care During Treatment

Nursing care of patients with anorectal malformations varies according to the type of treatment required. To prepare an infant for surgery, oral feedings are withheld and IV hydration is maintained; the nurse continues to observe for any signs of abdominal distention. When stool is expelled it should be gently wiped from the opening of the fistula with cotton balls and soap and water.

The nurse must be available to parents as they begin to adjust to the fact that surgery is required. If a colostomy is to be done, they may have difficulty seeing beyond the immediate crisis. The nurse must be sensitive to their feelings and avoid discounting their concerns with the reply, "But it's only temporary." An opportunity to speak with the parents of a child who has had a similar procedure with subsequent closure of the colostomy is a great comfort to these parents.

Postoperative nursing care varies according to the type of lesion corrected. When an anoplasty is done for low lesions, the diaper is left off to expose the perineum to air to promote healing. The suture line should be kept clean by removing stool from the anoplasty with a soft cloth and mild soap and water. Care must be taken to avoid disrupting the sutures; a material that will not catch on the sutures should be used for wiping. After the stool has been removed, meticulous cleaning can be done with cotton-tipped applicators and water or a solution as ordered by the physician. In the event of excoriation of the skin, a bland ointment may be used to promote healing. Generally the baby is allowed to assume a position of comfort. Side-lying and prone positions prevent excessive spreading of the buttocks and also permit easy removal of stool. No rectal temperatures are to be taken and the nurse must make this known, by way of written and verbal communication, to the family and all team members who care for the infant. Regular diet is resumed as soon as peristalsis returns. Dilatations may be required for several months after anoplasty, and parents are taught to perform them daily.

When a colostomy is performed for high lesions, parents are taught how to care for the colostomy (see Chapter 17 for colostomy care). The nurse should recognize that although the colostomy is temporary it is necessary for approximately an entire year. This can be an overwhelming thought to parents; they may not adequately understand, in spite of careful explanation, about the care their infant requires. The nurse should not be judgmental of parents who have difficulty accepting the need for a colostomy, even though it is temporary.

Parents wait expectantly and with great hope for permanent closure of the colostomy. The nurse must be aware of the factors that affect prognosis to avoid making inaccurate extraneous remarks. It is irresponsible of the nurse to give false hope to these families. Fecal continence varies according to type of lesion and surgical technique; therefore, specific information should be given by the surgeon and reinforced by the nurse.

Normal or near-normal bowel control is achieved in 85 to 90 per cent of the infants with low lesions because the rectum has traversed the main muscle of continence, the levator sling.[10] When the rectum must be placed within the muscles of continence, a lesser success rate is achieved. In children with high lesions only 50 to 65 per cent will be continent at all times.[10]

Parents may need assistance in later years when toilet training is necessary. The parents must be made aware of the normal stresses of toilet training and should be encouraged to maintain a relaxed attitude. They must also be counseled truthfully about what they can expect from their child. Repeated failures may be due to physiological reasons or due to stress within the parent. This is a difficult time for the family because they are facing the ultimate question of whether their child will be able to achieve normal bowel control. The nurse should counsel the family regarding approaches to toilet training as she would for any other child.

References

1. P. Altman et al. Pediatric surgery. In Principles of Surgery, S. Schwartz et al., eds., McGraw-Hill Book Co., 1979
2. K. W. Ashcraft and T. M. Holder. Esophageal atresia and tracheoesophageal fistula malformations. Surgical Clinics of North America, April 1976, p. 299
3. R. E. Behrman and W. Speck. Peritoneum and allied structures. In Nelson Textbook of Pediatrics, V. Vaughn et al., W. B. Saunders Co., 1979
4. A. Bill. Malrotation of the intestine. In Pediatric Surgery, M. Ravitch et al., eds., Yearbook Medical Publishers, 1979
5. J. Bliss. Nursing care for infants with neonatal necrotizing enterocolitis. American Journal of Nursing, Jan/Feb 1976, p. 37
6. S. J. Boley. An endorectal pull-though operation with primary anastomosis for Hirschsprung's disease. Surgery, Gynecology and Obstetrics, August 1968, p. 353
7. S. J. Boley et al. Endorectal pull-through procedure for Hirschsprung's disease with and without primary anastomosis. Journal of Pediatric Surgery, April 1968, p. 258
8. J. Chang. Malrotation of the intestine. Pediatric Nurse, Jan/Feb 1980
9. A. H. Colodny. Pyloric stenosis and antral web. In Principles of Pediatrics, R. A. Hoekelman, et al., eds., McGraw-Hill Book Co., 1978
10. A. G. Coran et al. Surgery of the Neonate. Little, Brown & Co., 1979
11. A. G. Coran and W. H. Weintraub. Modification of the endorectal procedure for Hirschsprung's disease. Surgery, Gynecology and Obstetrics, August 1976, p. 277
12. R. M. Filler. Esophageal atresia and tracheoesophageal fistula. In Principles of Pediatrics, R. A. Hoekelman et al., eds., McGraw-Hill Book Co., 1978
13. R. Flores. Necrotizing enterocolitis. Nursing Clinics of North America, March 1978, p. 39
14. D. Fochtman and J. G. Raffensberger. Principles of Nursing Care for the Pediatric Surgery Patient. Little, Brown & Co., 1976
15. J. Grosfield. Atresia and stenosis of the jejunum and ileum. In Pediatric Surgery, M. Ravitch et al., eds., Yearbook Medical Publishers, 1979
16. J. J. Herbst. The esophagus. In Nelson Textbook of Pediatrics, V. Vaughan, et al., eds., W. B. Saunders Co., 1979
17. S. H. Kim. Omphalocele. Surgical Clinics of North America, April 1976, p. 361
18. W. Oh. Extrauterine life: The newborn infant. In Principles of Pediatrics, R. A. Hoekelman, et al., eds., McGraw-Hill Book Co., 1978
19. H. B. Lynn. Duodenal obstruction: atresia, stenosis and

annular pancreas. In Pediatric Surgery, M. Ravitch, et al., eds., Year Book Medical Publishers, Inc., 1979
20. J. Morton. Abdominal wall hernias. In Principles of Surgery, S. Schwartz et al., eds., McGraw-Hill Book Co., 1979
21. W. S. Payne, and F. H. Ellis. Esophagus and diaphragmatic hernia. In Principles of Surgery, S. Schwartz, et al., eds., McGraw-Hill Book Co., 1979, p. 1097
22. A. Philliphart and F. Rector. Necrotizing enterocolitis. In Principles of Surgery, S. Schwartz, et al., eds., McGraw-Hill Book Co., 1979
23. S. Schuster. Omphalocele, hernia of umbilical cord and gastroschisis. In Pediatric Surgery, M. Ravitch, et al., eds., Year Book Medical Publishers, 1979
24. B. Shandling. Congenital anomalies of the gastrointestinal tract and intestinal obstruction. In Nelson Textbook of Pediatrics, V. Vaughan et al., eds., W. B. Saunders Co., 1979
25. R. M. Shannon. The gastrointestinal system. In Comprehensive Pediatric Nursing, G. M. Scipien et al., eds., McGraw-Hill Book Co., 1979
26. W. Sieber. Hirschsprung's disease. In Pediatric Surgery, M. Ravitch, et al., eds., Year Book Medical Publishers, 1979
27. E. Storer. Colon, rectum, and anus. In Principles of Surgery, S. Schwartz, et al., eds., McGraw-Hill Book Co., 1979
28. E. Wasserman and L. B. Slobody. Survey of Clinical Pediatrics. McGraw-Hill Book Co., 1974
29. W. Weintraub et al. A simplified approach to diagnostic rectal biopsy in infants and children. American Journal of Surgery, August 1977, p. 307
30. K. J. Welch. Intussusception. In Principles of Pediatrics, R. A. Hoekelman, et al., eds., McGraw-Hill Book Co., 1978
31. M. Woolley. Inguinal hernias. In Pediatric Surgery, M. Ravitch, et al., eds., Year Book Medical Publishers, Inc., 1979

MUSCULOSKELETAL ANOMALIES

by Stephanie Wright, RN, MSN

There are numerous congenital anomalies involving the musculoskeletal system. Three common ones are congenital clubfoot, metatarsus adductus (a type of clubfoot), and congenital dislocation of the hip. Early diagnosis is the critical factor that determines whether these conditions can be corrected. The nurse's recognition of each is extremely important in increasing casefinding. When the condition is recognized early, the treatment period is also dramatically shortened. Although the prognosis is good, the treatment course brings some special stresses on the family. In many cases, the majority of the physical care and the implementation of the treatment regimen will be the parents' responsibility. Their education will ensure good treatment results and greater comfort for the child. The nurse's ability to communicate with the parents concerning all aspects of treatment and care is her primary tool.

CLUBFOOT

Clubfoot is a congenital anomaly involving bones, muscles and tendons of the foot. The most common form of clubfoot is talipes equinovarus, in which the forefoot is adducted, along with inversion and equinus (plantar flexion). A typical clubfoot is shown in Figure 24–43. Congenital clubfoot occurs about once in every one thousand live births and is more common in males. It can occur unilaterally or bilaterally.[5]

The etiology of congenital clubfoot remains unknown. Whether it is a primary germ plasm defect originating in either bones or muscles or whether the intrauterine environment contributes to the development of this problem is unclear.

The true clubfoot has an anatomical deformity that prevents the foot from being manipulated into a normal position. It varies in severity. The severe forms are easily recognized, but the milder forms can go undetected. Some infants are born with a positional deformity of the foot resembling clubfoot. If the foot can be manipulated into a normal position, there is no bony deformity. Positional deformities, usually treated with a passive exercise program, are readily corrected.

The diagnosis is made by examination, manipulation and x-ray. Since the defect is often quite apparent at birth, parents become aware of it in the delivery room. Usually some explanation of the nature of the problem and the usual methods of treatment is given to them at this time. The retention of this information varies considerably, since the parents are experiencing considerable stress at this time.

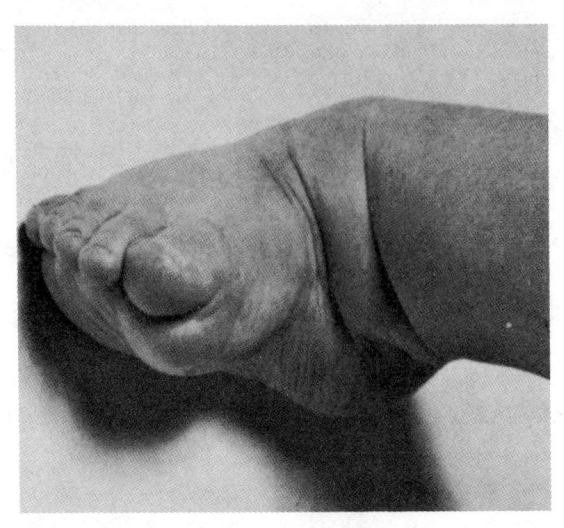

Figure 24-43 Typical clubfoot deformity. (From M. Delp and R. Manning. Major's Physical Diagnosis. W. B. Saunders Co., 1975.)

The meaning of the defect to the parents must be ascertained as part of the initial nursing assessment. Medical personnel often view clubfoot as a minor health problem to be resolved. The parents, however, may see only a very nonfunctional-appearing foot and may be thinking about long-term repercussions for the child. In some families, physical prowess and athletic ability may be highly valued; for them, this type of physical anomaly will be more difficult to accept.

Treatment and Care of a Child with Clubfoot

Treatment is usually begun within a few days after birth. The longer treatment is delayed, the more pronounced the soft tissue changes become, and correction becomes more difficult. Serial casting is the usual method of treatment. The foot is gradually manipulated toward a normal anatomical position and a short leg cast is applied to hold this correction. Casts are usually changed at weekly intervals. With each cast removal, the foot is manipulated and recasted. With this method the foot is gradually corrected over a period of several months. Once correction is obtained, some method of maintaining correction is used in conjunction with stretching to be performed by the parents. Bivalved (split) casts may be used to maintain correction or corrective shoes attached to a Denis-Browne bar. This is a metal bar attached to the soles of the shoes that maintains the shoes and feet in a prescribed position. Whichever splinting method is used, it is worn continuously until the child is ready for walking and then only at naptime or bedtime. Exercises may need to be continued for a period of years. Unless surgery is required, treatment is completed on an outpatient basis.

For the child, the treatment course is not a painful one. Children are often frightened by cast removal and application, but this is a reaction to the noise of the cast cutter, the physical restraint, and the wetness and warmth generated by the plaster application. Distraction with a pacifier or some visual stimulus will often work well to quiet the infant. The parents should be present to provide comfort during cast changes and should be reassured that it is not painful.

Two problems are encountered by the family during treatment: caring for the child in a cast and dealing with the reactions of others to the child's deformity and subsequent treatment. Parents need instruction in caring for the cast and checking neurovascular status after it has been applied. A cast must be kept dry and intact if it is to serve its therapeutic purpose. It requires about 24 hours to dry completely but is firmly set within a few minutes after it has been applied. Normal handling will not damage it. The cast should remain uncovered to allow for moisture evaporation. All surfaces should be exposed to air so that complete drying can occur. If the cast becomes softened by water or cracks, it should be reapplied so that correction is not lost. With a small infant, keeping a short leg cast clean is usually relatively easy. The main change in routine will be the bath. A tub bath will not be possible until after the cast has been removed.

With each cast change, there is the possibility of circulatory compromise or neurological impairment or both from the manipulation involved or pressure from the cast itself. The neurovascular status of the extremity should be checked hourly for the first four to six hours following application and then several times a day. Neurovascular checks generally include an assessment of amount of swelling, skin color, skin temperature, color return on blanching, sensation, motion and pain. If there is circulatory compromise from the cast, the first signs to appear will be swelling, cyanosis, coldness and sluggish color return on blanching. Pain, numbness and loss of motion are usually later signs.

Neurovascular status should be checked by the nurse immediately after cast application and before the family takes the child home. Checking neurovascular status can be easily demonstrated to parents; this should be followed by a return demonstration. Extremities are commonly cool to touch following cast application owing to contact with the wet cast. This can be expected until the cast dries thoroughly. Any unusual or extreme fussiness on the part of the child is an indication to have the cast checked. Written instructions for parents should be supplied on cast care and checking of neurovascular status.

The skin proximal to the cast edges needs special attention. After the cast is applied and before the child is taken home, obvious rough cast edges should be trimmed away. The finishing of cast edges with adhesive petals cannot be done when the cast is wet, but this can be done at home. The skin around the cast edges should be checked daily for redness. With a short leg cast the most common area for skin abrasion is behind the knee. The cast edge can be padded with gauze or smoothed with adhesive or moleskin petals to prevent or alleviate this problem. When the cast is removed for cast change, the skin surfaces under the cast should be inspected for signs of pressure or abrasion.

The cast is heavy and may limit normal kicking of the infant and impede his early efforts to turn over. Since major treatment is often completed within the first few months of life, any effects on physical development are rapidly corrected as the child develops normally.

Acceptance by the Family

An infant with a cast has a very visible problem and one that will be inquired about by people who see the child. Siblings usually accept a simple explanation of the difficulty. A cast is simply "a hard bandage used to hold the foot until it is better." The acceptance of the infant in a cast by grandparents and other family members is often extremely important to the parents. The ability of the family to hold and fondle the child despite the impediment of a leg in plaster reinforces the parents' acceptance of the infant and the defect. Parents may be somewhat reluctant to take their infant to public places. It is wise to inquire whether the cast is causing any such problems for the family.

The vast majority of infants with clubfoot will have good correction with serial casting and will develop a normal foot without limitations. Some clubfeet are more resistant to treatment and will require surgical intervention in the form of tendon transfers or releases and a longer treatment period. This may be apparent at the outset of treatment or may not become apparent until treatment is in progress.

METATARSUS ADDUCTUS

The most common congenital foot deformity, this condition occurs in both sexes and is usually bilateral (Fig. 24-44). It is one of the three deformities present in clubfoot and is frequently associated with internal tibial torsion and flatfeet. Abnormal intrauterine position is the most frequent etiology. Mild cases will resolve spontaneously by midinfancy. When the deformity is rigid (resists being turned to normal position) or severe, it is likely to persist into adulthood if untreated.

CARING FOR YOUR CHILD IN A CAST

First Day

HANDLE THE CAST WITH REASONABLE CARE. It cannot perform its intended function if it is cracked.

KEEP THE CAST EXPOSED TO AIR TO DRY. Turn the child from front to back if necessary to allow all sides to dry.

CHECK THE FINGERS OR TOES BELOW THE CAST. Swelling, blueness, coldness, numbness or pain should be reported to the nurse or doctor. Check this every few few hours.

CHECK THE SKIN AROUND THE CAST EDGES FOR REDNESS.

After the First Day

Check for swelling, coldness, blueness or numbness in the fingers or toes twice a day.

Check the skin around the cast edges each day. Try to smooth or pad any sharp cast edges with gauze or small pieces of adhesive tape placed over the cast edges in this fashion.

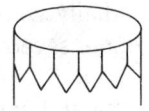

Keep the cast clean and dry. If the cast becomes wet, soft, or should crack, it should be replaced as soon as possible.

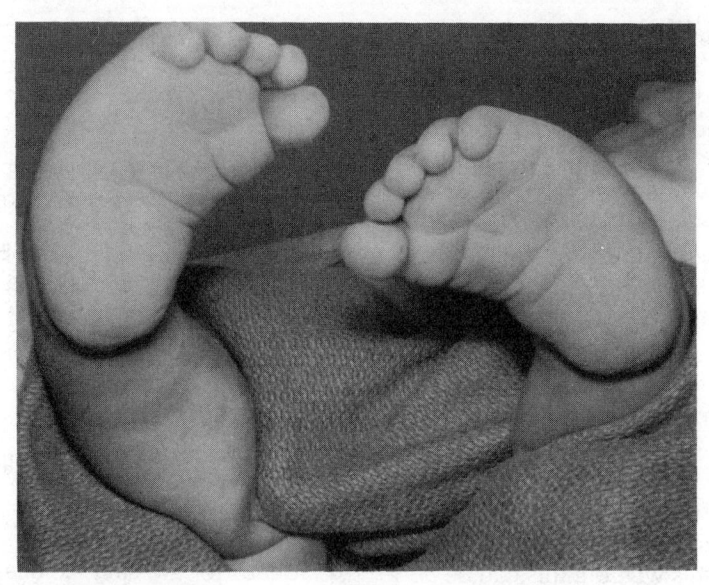

Figure 24–44 Infant with a metatarsus adductus deformity. (Photograph courtesy of Mead Johnson Nutritional Division.)

If the deformity is mild or is apparent at birth, parents can be taught to manipulate the foot by stabilizing the heel with one hand and massaging the forefoot medially with the other hand. This should be done several times at each diaper change. In addition, parents should be encouraged to place the infant on his side or back to sleep. If correction is not achieved by four months, a cast that immobilizes the foot in a corrected position is applied for two to six weeks.[7]

While their child is casted, parents should be encouraged to hold him frequently and provide him with extra sensory and motor experiences, since his own ambulatory exploration is temporarily interrupted. They will also need instruction in cast care, skin care and in how to monitor neurovascular status. (See Chapter 51.)

Some orthopedists prescribe that casting be followed by use of reverse (outflared) shoes for a few months to maintain correction. If internal tibial torsion accompanies the metatarsus adductus, a Denis-Browne night splint may be needed.

CONGENITAL DISLOCATION OF THE HIP

Congenital dislocation of the hip is one form of a group of hip problems often described collectively as congenital hip dysplasia. Hip dysplasia includes hips that are unstable or capable of being dislocated, subluxed (the femoral head has moved upward and laterally in the hip socket), or actually dislocated (out of the hip socket). At birth the hip joint is largely cartilage. As ossification of the hip structures proceeds during infancy, the head of the femur must be properly located within the acetabulum for the correct configuration of the hip to develop. If the head of the femur is outside the acetabulum or improperly located within it, the hip joint will develop abnormally. As ossification proceeds, correcting the deformity becomes more and more difficult. Once the child begins walking, the added stresses to the hip joint will worsen the deformity that occurs.

The etiology of this disorder is not clearly understood. There is a familial tendency. The condition is more prevalent in females; approximately 70 per cent of diagnosed infants are female.[5] There appears to be some relationship between relaxation of the hip capsule associated with increased estrogen levels and hip dislocation. Position in utero also has some effect upon this problem. Congenital hip dislocation is much more prevalent in babies carried in the breech position. Rapid or forceful extension of the hips immediately following birth may precipitate dislocation in an unstable hip. Infants should be allowed to hold their legs in the normal partially flexed position.

Early diagnosis is the greatest problem encountered when dealing with congenital dislo-

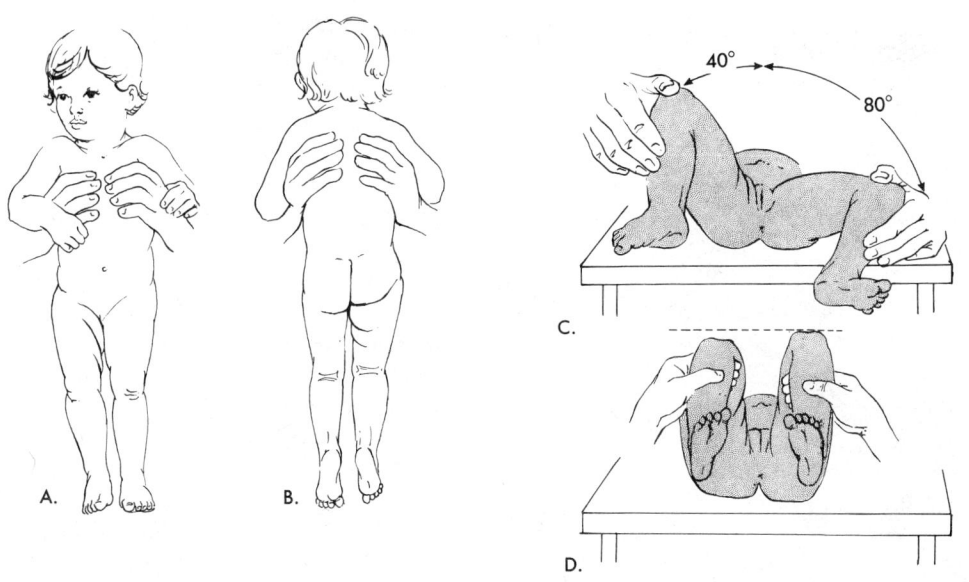

Figure 24–45 The three "classic" signs of CDH: (A and B) unequal skin folds, (C) limitation of abduction, and (D) unequal knee height. (From M. Tachdjian. Pediatric Orthopedics, W. B. Saunders Co., 1972.)

cation of the hip. Every newborn must be carefully checked for signs of dislocation or instability of the hip joint. The three commonly described signs of dislocation are unequal skin folds on the thighs or buttocks, limitation of abduction on the affected side and unequal knee height. These three signs are illustrated in Figure 24–45. These signs can be easily checked as part of a newborn assessment and on each subsequent visit for infant health care. Although these signs are easily assessed, they are often not present in newborns because their presence depends upon muscular changes that usually do not occur until the hip has been dislocated for a period of time. Therefore, these three "classic" signs are more likely to be seen in an infant who is several months old.

A more accurate diagnostic method involves an attempt to either reduce or dislocate the hip manually. One hand grasps the femur and, with the hip and knee flexed, abducts and lifts the thigh. The hip can be felt or heard to reduce as the head of the femur enters the acetabulum (Ortolani's sign). If this procedure is reversed and the leg is adducted and some downward pressure applied, the hip may be felt to dislocate as the femoral head leaves the acetabulum (subluxation provocation test of Barlow). This is an examination that is not difficult to perform but requires some practice and training. Most unstable hips in newborns will be diagnosed with these two maneuvers. X-rays may or may not confirm the diagnosis. The newborn hip is largely cartilage and not radiopaque. X-rays are more likely to be diagnostic in infants several months of age. Once diagnosis is made, parents need a thorough explanation of the problem at hand. Their child's condition is not visible and presents no current difficulty for him. A thorough understanding of the repercussions of neglect of the problem is necessary to ensure that the proper treatment regimen will be followed.

Treatment With Early and With Later Diagnosis

No matter what degree of dysplasia exists, treatment should begin immediately. Treatment in early infancy (up to 2 to 3 months) consists of placing the head of the femur within the acetabulum and keeping it there by maintaining the legs in a position of flexion and abduction. There are a variety of methods to accomplish this. For infants in whom the hip is not actually dislocated, triple diapers or a Frejka pillow (Fig. 24–46) may suffice. In infants in whom the hip is capable of being dislocated, diapers or pillow will not be satisfactory because they will be removed at each diaper change and the hip may dislocate at this time.

Various splints (abduction devices) are used to maintain proper placement of the hip, including during diapering. The length of time an infant will have to wear an abduction device

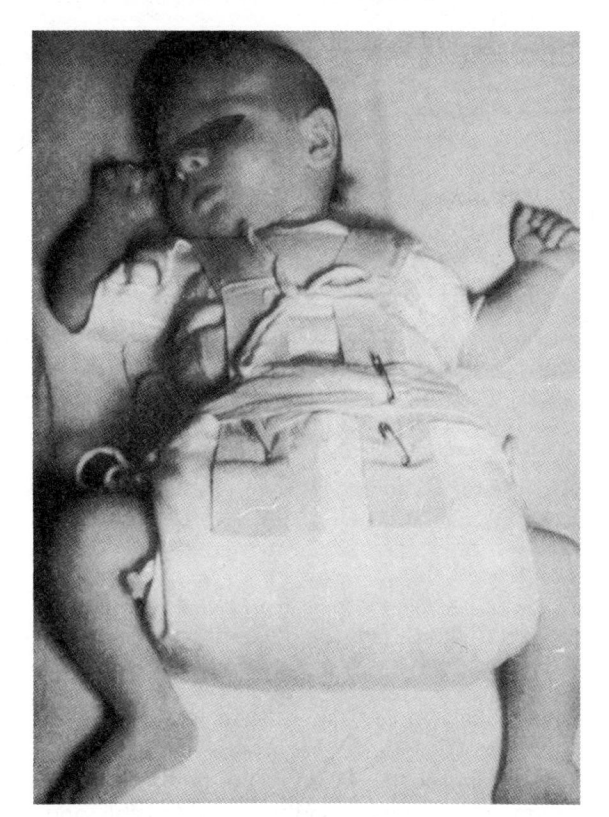

Figure 24-46 A Frejka pillow splint. (From C. Larson and M. Gould. Orthopedic Nursing. C. V. Mosby Co., 1978.)

depends upon the age at which diagnosis is made. When diagnosis is made in a newborn, treatment may be completed in two to four months. Treatment is continued until the hip is stable and can often be completed on an outpatient basis.

When congenital hip dislocation is not diagnosed until after 2 or 3 months of age, changes in hip structure may have occurred that prevent the hip from being reduced. Traction, either skin or skeletal, may be used to pull the head of the femur down to a position where it is opposite the acetabulum. This may require several weeks of hospitalization. Caring for children in traction devices is described in Chapter 51. Traction is followed by a reduction of the hip, usually with the child anesthetized, and the application of a hip spica cast. The cast maintains the proper position of the hip for the period of treatment. The child is usually cared for at home and returns to the hospital periodically for cast changes.

Care of a Child in a Hip Spica Cast Caring for a child in a hip spica cast requires the same careful attention to skin care and neurovascular status as in caring for a child with clubfoot. With a spica cast, keeping the perineal area clean and dry becomes an important goal. It is not difficult but requires diligence.

Commonly used for hospital care is a split Bradford frame (Fig. 24–47). The frame is metal covered with canvas. The child is positioned either prone or supine on the frame with the perineal area over the split and secured with a drawsheet or other restraining device. Several pieces of heavy plastic sheeting are tucked into the cast perineal opening so that all the cast edges are covered. The plastic sheets are funneled into a bedpan on the bed under the frame. Urine and feces drain into the bedpan without soiling the cast edges. It is important that the head of the frame be elevated slightly so that urine cannot run up inside the cast. The perineal area needs to be washed several times a day and the plastic sheeting changed to minimize odor and prevent skin problems.

Bradford frames are available for rental by parents taking home a child in a spica cast. At home the frame may be used in the crib or placed in a wagon so the child may be wheeled from room to room. When the child is not on the frame, a disposable diaper may be tucked inside the cast opening. These are rapidly saturated and must be changed frequently in order to keep the cast dry. A combination of a sanitary napkin and a disposable diaper may be used effectively for more absorbency.[1]

While traditional infant seats will not accommodate a baby in a spica cast, an upright position can be maintained by using a baby swing (with some modification of the leg openings), or a "beanbag" chair.[8] A canvas baby carrier may be adapted to accommodate the cast and allow for mobility and body contact with parents. Parents are often extremely creative in finding ways to normalize the infant's life and in solving problems imposed by the cast or other devices. Older infants may be active despite the cast and may attempt to bear weight. This is usually contraindicated.

Surgical Treatment When traction and closed reduction cannot reduce the hip, surgery may be required. This may take the form of an adductor tenotomy to allow for more movement of the hip. An open reduction of the hip may be required to correct some problem that is preventing the head of the femur from entering the acetabulum. These surgical procedures will be

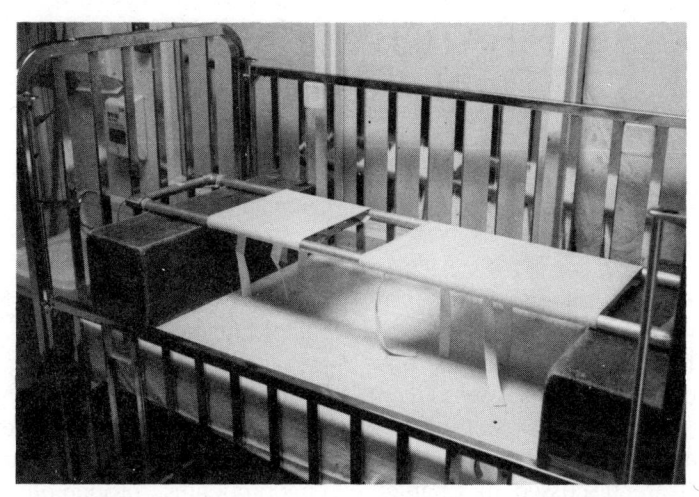

Figure 24-47 A split Bradford frame being set up in a crib. (Photograph by Stephanie Wright.)

followed by immobilization in a hip spica cast. The infant or child with an open hip reduction requires the usual postoperative monitoring of vital signs. The operative area will be less accessible for inspection, since the dressing is covered with plaster. Drainage from the surgical site may penetrate the plaster and some staining of the cast with blood is usual. The size and appearance of the stain should be noted as it would on any dressing. The stained areas can be covered with clean plaster before discharge to improve the appearance of the cast.

Surgery and the associated swelling increases the likelihood of impairment of neurovascular status. Neurovascular checks should be made every hour for the first 6 to 12 hours following surgery and then every 4 hours.

Family Involvement

Parents need to be involved in the care of the child as early as possible so that, upon discharge, they have confidence in their ability to care for him at home. Alterations of home care routines should be thoroughly discussed before discharge so that any necessary physical adaptations in the home can be anticipated.

Parents should be encouraged to prepare siblings for the appearance of their brother or sister in a cast and the adaptations in family routines that will be necessitated. As always, participation of siblings in preparation of the home or in the care of the child lessens their feeling that they are somehow less important than the child who is necessarily the subject of a great deal of attention during treatment.

With proper care and early diagnosis and treatment, children with congenital dislocation of the hip have an excellent chance of developing a hip that is functionally normal.

References

1. Y. Black. Spica cast care in the infant with a congenital dislocated hip. Orthopedic Nurses' Association Journal, November 1979, p. 439
2. A. Ferguson. Orthopedic Surgery in Infancy and Childhood. Williams and Wilkins Co., 1975
3. R. Gross and E. Hitch. Screening newborn infants for hip dysplasia. Orthopedic Nurses' Association Journal, May 1979, p. 186
4. R. Hensinger. Congenital dislocation of the hip. Clinical Symposia, #1, 1979
5. W. Lovell and R. Winter. Pediatric Orthopedics. J. B. Lippincott Co., 1978
6. L. Staheli, Torsional deformity. Pediatric Clinics of North America, November 1977, p. 799
7. M. Tachdjian. Pediatric Orthopedics. W. B. Saunders Co., 1972
8. American Journal of Nursing, Volume 78, No. 1, January 1978, p. 54

RESPIRATORY INFECTIONS IN INFANTS

by Mabel Hunsberger, BSN, MSN

Respiratory infections of infants can cause serious illness requiring hospitalization and intensive therapy. The respiratory illnesses discussed in this chapter are viral or bacterial in origin and usually require some specific interventions. Acute pharyngitis and nasopharyngitis (the common cold) are discussed in Chapter 23.

Infants and children have an increased susceptibility to infection of the respiratory tract for four reasons: (1) immunological immaturity, (2) an airway that is relatively small from the trachea down to the end of the bronchioles; (3) accessory muscles that are not well developed and (4) ineffectual coughing efforts.[3] The net result is that even small amounts of secretions and edema within the lumen of the respiratory tract can cause obstruction.

The nurse has a primary role in the prevention of respiratory illnesses. Counselling families in proper nutrition, rest and personal hygiene is an important preventive role of the nurse. When an infant has repeated respiratory infections the nurse should take a careful history in search of underlying problems such as cystic fibrosis, foreign body aspiration, immunodeficiency or allergies.

Clinical manifestations of respiratory infection vary according to the causative agent. Typical manifestations of respiratory infections and the significance of each is shown in Table 24–3.

An infant that has any combination of these signs and symptoms can cause parents to become extremely anxious and, in severe cases, parents may be in a state of panic. The onset of symptoms may be abrupt, often following a minor upper respiratory infection. This kind of situation has the potential to make parents feel guilty for not having sought treatment earlier. The nurse can reduce the stress felt by parents by encouraging them to express their feelings. Although immediate life-saving and comfort measures are frequently necessary, the nurse should encourage parents to stay with their infant and hold him as soon as his condition permits.

The infectious respiratory alterations discussed in this chapter are retropharyngeal abscess (an upper respiratory tract infection), tracheobronchitis, bronchiolitis and pneumonia (lower respiratory tract infections).

UPPER RESPIRATORY TRACT INFECTION

Retropharyngeal Abscess

A retropharyngeal abscess develops when lymph glands located behind the posterior pharyngeal wall become infected. This may result from pharyngitis (group A hemolytic streptococci) in which the infection extends to the lymph nodes via the lymphatic system. Purulent infection of contiguous areas (sinuses, adenoids, nasopharynx), causes the nodes to become infected, with resultant swelling and suppuration.

The illness usually follows an upper respiratory infection and produces an abrupt onset of fever, dyspnea, and difficulty swallowing. A typical response of the nurse may be to suction the nasopharynx to maintain the infant's airway. This imprudent action could have disastrous results: rupture and aspiration of the contents of the abscess. If suctioning is necessary to prevent aspiration of oral secretions, it should be of the mouth only.

The diagnosis is established by a lateral x-ray of the neck and by digital palpation of a fluctuant mass on one side of the posterior pharyngeal wall.[6] The infant is placed in the Trendelenberg position for the digital examination to prevent aspiration. The nurse should ensure that a suction apparatus is immediately available in the event of rupture of the abscess during the examination. A fluctuant abscess is treated by incision and drainage in conjunction with preoperative and postoperative antibiotic administration.

Postoperatively the nurse must observe the

TABLE 24-3 CLINICAL MANIFESTATIONS OF RESPIRATORY INFECTIONS

Signs and Symptoms	Cause and/or Significance of Signs and Symptoms
Tachypnea	A sign of impaired gas exchange
Dyspnea	Occurs with involvement of lung parenchyma
Fever	Occurs in both viral and bacterial infections and is often higher with bacterial infections
Tachycardia	Is a means of increasing ventilation and is common with fever and dehydration
Chest retractions: (substernal, suprasternal, intercostal, and subcostal)	Accessory muscles used when there is resistance in the airway due to secretions (airway may be narrowed or obstructed)
Flaring of nares	Accompanies retractions and dyspnea
Cough	Caused by irritation of the trachea; is a protective mechanism to clear excessive secretions; should generally not be suppressed by medication in presence of infection (especially when cough is productive). In infants a cough may or may not be present; it is a more common symptom in late infancy and childhood
Cyanosis	Appears when there is an increased amount of reduced hemoglobin (when the absolute amount of reduced hemoglobin is 5 g/dl); therefore, cyanosis appears less often in an anemic infant. Cyanosis appears first where the epidermis is thin and capillaries are numerous: nail beds, ear lobes, tip of tongue or nose, lips and around mouth
Restless, irritable and an anxious look on face	Occurs as a response to being unable to get adequate oxygen into system
Wheeze	Occurs when there is partial airway obstruction (e.g., bronchiolitis)
Stridor	A high-pitched inspiratory sound caused by obstruction of the upper airway
Rales	Produced by air bubbling through fluid or by a "snapping open of approximated airway walls"[13]
Rhonchi	Produced by air rapidly passing a fixed obstruction
Diminished breath sounds	Occur in lung consolidation, pneumothorax and with pleural fluid
Dehydration	Occurs owing to decreased intake of fluids, insensible fluid loss by tachypnea, and with fever.

infant for signs of respiratory distress and frequent swallowing (a sign of bleeding), and must keep the infant in a prone position to facilitate drainage of secretions. Parents should be kept informed of the infant's condition and be given explanations of how they can participate in his care.

LOWER RESPIRATORY TRACT INFECTION

Lower respiratory tract diseases are the single most frequent cause of death before 1 year of age.[4] A viral infection can cause bronchitis and tracheobronchitis, bronchiolitis or viral pneumonia. Table 24-4 contains a summary of viral infections of the lower respiratory tract.

Bronchiolitis

Bronchiolitis, an inflammation of the bronchioles, is most frequently caused by respiratory syncytial virus. It rarely occurs after 2 years of age and has a peak incidence at 6 months of age. It occurs most commonly during the winter and early spring months. Boys are affected more frequently than girls. It is primarily a condition treated on an outpatient basis with only one out of five children requiring hospitalization.[10]

Inflammation of the bronchioles results in edema of the airway passages and eventual accumulation of mucus and exudate from cellular destruction. The bronchioles consequently become occluded; some are partially obstructed and some may become totally obstructed. The alveoli are usually normal except those in the immediate vicinity of the inflamed bronchioles.

Under normal circumstances expiration is an entirely passive process whereby relaxation and upward movement of the diaphragm moves air out of the alveoli. Normally the bronchial passages narrow during expiration but when the lumen is further compromised by edema and exudate, air enters the alveoli and becomes trapped. Hyperinflation of the lungs and obstructive emphysema result. When the obstruc-

TABLE 24-4 VIRAL INFECTIONS OF THE LOWER RESPIRATORY TRACT

	Bronchitis* and Tracheobronchitis	Bronchiolitis	Viral Pneumonia
Definition	Infection of upper bronchi and lower trachea	Inflammation of bronchioles	Inflammation of lung parenchyma
Organism	Usually viral agents (paramyxovirus, respiratory syncytial virus, and adenovirus)	Respiratory syncytial virus (RSV)	Respiratory syncytial virus, parainfluenza and adenoviruses
Age	Occurs most frequently during the first 4 years of life	Peak incidence at 6 months of age. Rarely occurs after 2 yrs of age	Can occur in any age group; most of the pneumonia caused by RSV occurs in the first 3 years of life
Onset	Usually preceded by a viral upper respiratory infection but it can also follow illnesses such as croup or pneumonia	Begins as a mild upper respiratory infection	Insidious or acute symptoms usually precede pulmonary illness
Clinical manifestations	Persistent nonproductive, hacking cough that becomes loose and productive in a few days; rhonchi and rales can be heard as illness progresses; cough subsides in 7–10 days	Tachypnea, chest retractions and a paroxysmal wheezy cough; patient may be irritable, dyspneic, and have prolonged expirations. Rhonchi, wheezes or rales throughout lungs. Diminished breath sound where obstructed. X-rays show diffuse hyperinflation of lungs and peribronchial infiltrates suggestive of interstitial pneumonia. Scattered areas of consolidation are due to atelectasis or inflammation of alveoli	Cough, wheezing, coarse rhonchi and frequently a high fever. Headache, malaise, and myalgia are present in older children

Treatment	Cough suppression by medication is generally avoided (sometimes given in severe cases when sleep is interrupted by cough). Expectorants can be given. Mask inhalations of nebulized solutions and chest physiotherapy help raise secretions. Humidification of inspired air must produce small droplets to be effective. Hydration by increased oral fluids or intravenous fluids	Treated with rest, fluids, and humidified oxygen. Bronchodilators, sedatives and corticosteroids not recommended. Antibiotics usually not indicated. Intravenous fluids for hydration, electrolytes, and pH balance are often necessary. Mist-therapy delivering large droplets does not affect lower airway; therefore, ultrasonic nebulization is recommended	Symptomatic treatment. Antibiotics not used. Bed rest, analgesics and antipyretics with adequate fluid intake and increased humidity. In severe illness postural drainage and oxygen may be indicated. Ventilator assistance may be required.
Nursing considerations	Counsel family against use of over-the-counter drugs to suppress cough; a vaporizer that produces a sufficiently small droplet is recommended	Most critical phase is the first 48–72 hrs. RSV highly contagious — isolate from other infants. Infant needs to be observed closely. Parent-infant contact extremely important because of infant's anxiety. Stress of parents must be reduced by frequent explanations of status of infant	RSV highly contagious — isolate from other infants
Complications and/or prognosis	Complications of otitis media, sinusitis and pneumonia may occur in children who are undernourished or in poor health[12]	Most improve within 3–4 days and in 2 weeks respiratory rate is normal but in some instances illness is prolonged	Most recover in 7–10 days. Otitis media is common in children with RSV infections. Adenovirus can cause severe and fatal pneumonia in infants. There is some evidence that chronic lung disease in adulthood may be caused by viral pneumonia in childhood

*Bronchitis is usually accompanied by some degree of tracheitis.

tion is complete the air is absorbed by the blood flowing in the pulmonary capillaries and the walls of the alveoli are pulled together, resulting in atelectasis. The impaired ventilation can result in hypoxemia and hypercapnia (carbon dioxide retention),* leading to respiratory acidosis.

Clinical Manifestations After a few days of mild rhinorrhea, diminished appetite, sneezing, coughing and a low-grade fever, an acute phase begins. The infant's condition worsens rapidly with tachypnea (up to 80 per minute), chest retractions, and a paroxysmal wheezy cough. The infant may be irritable and appear anxious and have some cyanosis, flaring of the nares, and wheezing,† with a prolonged expiratory phase. Fine rales may be heard, especially on deep inspiration. When obstruction of the bronchioles is nearly complete breath sounds are diminished.

Feeding is often a problem because of the difficulty of breathing experienced by the infant while sucking. The pulse rate is usually increased and body temperature may range from normal to as high as 41° C (105.8° F).[4]

Diagnosis Chest x-rays may be normal or may show segmental collapse or hyperinflation. Areas of consolidation on chest x-rays are thought to be due to atelectasis or inflammation.[10] Certainty of diagnosis requires the use of virus isolation techniques. Immunofluorescent techniques applied to nasal aspirates are highly reliable.[14] Routine laboratory tests are not specific for the diagnosis of bronchiolitis. The age of the infant and the clinical manifestations in the face of an epidemic of respiratory syncytial virus in a community are highly suggestive of bronchiolitis.

Nursing Care Most infants can be treated conservatively with rest, fluids and humidified oxygen. Antibiotics are generally not indicated, the use of corticosteroids is not warranted, bronchodilators are contraindicated (they increase restlessness and oxygen requirements), and sedatives that depress respirations should be avoided. If antibiotics are used it is in the case of small, acutely ill infants when there is uncertainty about the causative organism. Also, the fact that viral infection predisposes an infant to secondary bacterial invasion is sometimes used to justify administration of antibiotics.[14]

The nurse should give careful attention to placing the infant where he can be easily observed and where other infants are not readily exposed. Constant surveillance is necessary to monitor respiratory status. Frequent assessment for tachypnea, retractions, flaring of the nares, cyanosis and restlessness are necessary. A sudden increase in respiratory and cardiac rates and a dramatic increase in audible rales are signs of cardiac failure. These findings should be reported immediately to allow for initiation of rapid treatment by digitalization.

The major consequence of inadequate ventilation is hypoxemia. Humidified oxygen is delivered via an isolette or oxygen tent. An inspired oxygen concentration of 35 to 40 per cent is usually adequate to correct the hypoxemia.[14] The environment within the device used for oxygen administration must be controlled to avoid increased oxygen consumption by the infant due to chilling or shivering.

The administration of oxygen to infants with carbon dioxide retention is usually not associated with further carbon dioxide retention; however, those infants who have a history of respiratory distress syndrome during the newborn period may suffer increased carbon dioxide retention when their hypoxic drive for respiration is blunted by increased concentrations of inspired oxygen.[14]

Mist therapy has not been proved to have a beneficial effect on the pulmonary problem. If mist tent therapy is used, a small particle mist delivered by an ultrasonic nebulizer is desired to aid in thinning secretions. (A large particle mist does not reach the lower respiratory tract.) These secretions can then be more readily removed through suctioning and postural drainage.

Some infants present with dehydration and mild metabolic acidosis. Intravenous fluids may be required to correct electrolyte imbalance. Intravenous fluids should be administered cautiously because unresolved bronchiolitis can eventually lead to heart failure.

Nursing care should provide maximum comfort to the infant and his parents. Care should be organized to avoid unnecessary disturbance of

---

*Carbon dioxide retention is usually not present unless respirations exceed 60 per minute.[12]
†When air exchange is severely compromised a wheeze may not be heard because insufficient air is being exchanged.

an infant who is already experiencing an energy deficit. Although infant-parent contact is hampered to some degree by an isolette, oxygen tent or mist therapy, touching, holding and cuddling by parents should be encouraged as tolerated by the infant. When these anxious infants are extremely ill, it has been suggested that the best sedative for them is provided by cuddling from their parents.[4] It is the nurse's responsibility to help the parents feel sufficiently calm to provide that comfort.

Parents are often anxious and fearful throughout the course of the illness. Therapy is supportive and they may need help to understand that antibiotics and other medications are not indicated. The anxious appearance and respiratory difficulty of their infant is distressing to parents. The nurse cannot overlook the importance of frequent explanations and encouragement to parents during this difficult period.

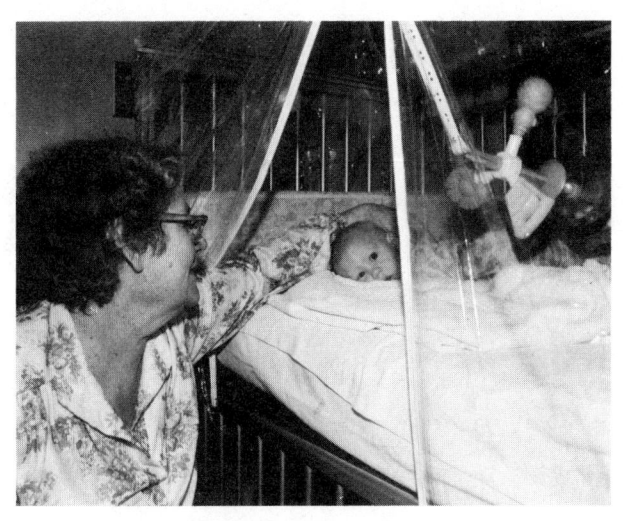

When an infant with respiratory illness requires a tent for mist or oxygen, brief periods of touching and holding are encouraged as tolerated by the infant. Here a grandmother takes pleasure in retaining a relationship with her hospitalized grandchild.

Prognosis Most infants improve within three to four days if given adequate supportive care, but usually two weeks is required to attain normal ventilation. However, in some cases the clinical course is longer. Approximately 20 per cent of these infants develop persistent wheezing and hyperinflation of the lungs with abnormal gas exchange that may last for many months.[14] Abnormalities in respiratory function have been found in some children many years after an infection of the bronchioles. Also, there is a high incidence of asthma in children who have had bronchiolitis in infancy.[14] It is unclear whether damage to the lungs from bronchiolitis predisposes these infants to asthma or whether the diagnosis of bronchiolitis was made when the first attacks of asthma were experienced.[14]

Pneumonia

Pneumonia is a term used to describe the presence of an acute inflammation of the lung parenchyma (tissue) including the smallest airways and alveoli. The lungs are involved in varying degrees depending on the type of organism and the severity of the infection. The various forms of pneumonia are:
1. Lobar–consolidation of all or part of a lobe; exudate is chiefly within the alveoli.
2. Disseminated lobular–a patchy distribution of infectious areas in both lung fields surrounding and involving the bronchi.
3. Interstitial–a diffuse bronchiolitis and peribronchiolitis in both lung fields; exudate is in the alveolar walls but not in the alveolar spaces.[3, 9]

Bronchopneumonia is a loose term used to describe a combination of disseminated lobular and interstitial pneumonia.[3] Lobar and lobular involvement are characteristic of bacterial pneumonia, whereas viral pneumonia is characterized by an interstitial inflammation.

Pneumonia may be viral (Table 24–4) or bacterial (Table 24–5) in origin. Certain causative organisms are more prevalent in certain age groups than others. Also, the same organism can result in varied clinical responses depending on the age and general health of the child. The neonate and young infant are particularly vulnerable to suffer serious consequences from pneumonia.

Etiology and Clinical Manifestations Pneumonia of the fetus and newborn has been classified into categories according to time and mode of acquisition as follows: (1) pneumonia acquired transplacentally, (2) congenital or intrauterine pneumonia, (3) pneumonia acquired during birth, and (4) pneumonia acquired after birth.[5] Pneumonia acquired transplacentally presents as one aspect of a congenital disease (e.g., rubella, cytomegalovirus disease (CMVD) or toxoplasmosis). Congenital or intrauterine pneumonia is an inflammation of the lungs that is seen at autopsy. These infants are stillborn or

TABLE 24-5 BACTERIAL PNEUMONIAS MOST COMMON IN INFANTS

	Streptococcal	Staphylococcal	Pneumococcal	Hemophilus Influenza
Organism	Group B beta-hemolytic streptococcus*	Stahylococcus aureus	Streptococcus pneumoniae	Hemophilus influenzae type B
Age	Occurs in newborns less than 5 days old (early onset) as in intrapartum infection or in infants up to 6 weeks of age (late onset). In early onset pneumonia is more common; in late onset meningitis predominates[2]	Occurs in infants more frequently than in older children. 30% of patients under 3 months of age; 70% under 1 year	Children under 4 years have a higher incidence than older ones. Children under 3 with sickle cell disease have an attack rate of 20%[9]	Most frequent in children under 1 year. Gram-negative organisms account for only a small percentage of pneumonia in infants and children (after the neonatal period) but they are becoming increasingly prevalent
Onset	History of prolonged rupture of membranes and low birth weight	History of mild upper respiratory infection (varies in duration from a few days to a week or sometimes longer)	In infants onset is abrupt, with a temperature of 39.5–40.1° C (103–105° F) and generalized convulsion; sometimes vomiting and diarrhea	Similar to pneumococcal but often with a more insidious onset. Most are preceded by a mild upper respiratory infection
Clinical findings	Apnea and shock within 24 hours of birth; hypoxia and hypercapnia. Pulmonary lesions may be patchy or extensive. Difficult to differentiate from respiratory distress syndrome of newborn	Extremely variable. Usually cough, high fever, abdominal distention, rapid grunting respirations. In more severe cases cyanosis and shock may occur. Chest auscultation may be misleading. In infants breath sound may be heard even with serious pneumonia. Progresses from a bronchopneumonia to consolidation of an entire lobe within hours. Pneumatocele, empyema and pyopneumothorax are common	Rapid, shallow respirations with grunting, tachycardia, and circumoral cyanosis. Cough not usual. Abdominal distention and nuchal rigidity. Auscultatory findings not reliable. Patchy bronchopneumonia is most typical in infants. Lobar consolidation more common in older children.	Cough almost always present (can be productive or nonproductive). Rales, fever, tachypnea, retractions and nasal flaring; dullness to percussion. Can be either lobar or disseminated (bronchopneumonia). Empyema is often present. Pneumatoceles have been seen (difficult to differentiate from pneumococcal)

Treatment	IV penicillin G and intensive supportive therapy	A penicillinase-resistant penicillin (Methicillin) is used. If organism sensitive to penicillin G then Methicillin is not used because of its nephrotoxicity. (Methicillin-resistant strains have also been reported.)[9] Chest tube drainage of fluid or pus from pleural cavity. Blood transfusions for anemia may be necessary. Supportive therapy.	Penicillin G is usual. Ampicillin is used for young children because it is effective for both pneumococcal and *H. influenzae*. If pneumonia is complicated by otitis media, medication is prescribed for a longer period than the usual course	Ampicillin and chloramphenicol. Ampicillin is required in large doses. Ampicillin-resistant strains occur; therefore, simultaneous chloramphenicol therapy is recommended
Specific nursing concerns	Avoid inaccurate encouraging remarks about an illness with an extremely high mortality rate. These newborns are seriously ill; the mother is likely to be hospitalized in the obstetrical department. Nurse caring for infant should facilitate communication with both parents.	Nephrotoxicity of Methicillin. Observe infection control procedure strictly. (Handwashing, gown and mask are required.) Long duration of hospitalization places entire family under severe stress	A pneumococcal vaccine is available that is recommended for persons 2 years of age or older who are especially vulnerable to high morbidity and mortality from pneumococcal infections	Observe for chloramphenicol side effects
Complications and/or prognosis	Mortality rate is 60–90%	Septic lesions outside the respiratory tract. Mortality rate is 10–30%	Meningitis, otitis media, sinusitis and purulent conjunctivitis. Empyema and pneumatoceles may develop. Mortality rate below 1%	Frequent complications include bacteremia, pericarditis, cellulitis, empyema, meningitis and pyarthrosis[10]

*Since the early 1970's incidence of Group B beta-hemolytic streptococcus has increased as a cause of mortality and serious morbidity in neonates. Group A beta-hemolytic streptococcal pneumonia occurs most frequently in children between 3 and 5 (chapter 42).

die usually within 24 hours after birth. The pathogenesis of congenital pneumonia is not well understood. Although there are inflammatory changes in the lungs, many do not contain bacteria. Pneumonia acquired during birth (perinatal) is thought to be due to aspiration of infected amniotic fluid or secretions from the birth canal. Sources of infection of pneumonia acquired after birth (postnatal) include human contact and contaminated equipment.

Pneumonia due to perinatal and postnatal infections usually is manifested by nonspecific signs of illness. Initially an infant has signs such as poor feeding, lethargy and fever. Respiratory distress may develop at the onset of the illness or sometime later. When the pneumonia is acquired perinatally, illness manifests itself during the first several days of life, whereas pneumonia acquired after birth manifests itself during the first month of life.[5]

After the neonatal period, pneumonia in infants and children is predominantly of viral origin. Although the vast majority recover without sequelae, viral pneumonia cannot be viewed as a benign illness. Adenovirus can cause a particularly serious illness with potential fatality. Many infants and children can be treated at home, but severely ill patients should be hospitalized for intravenous fluids, oxygen, or in some cases ventilator assistance.

Bacterial pneumonia is often preceded by a viral respiratory disease. The lower respiratory tract is made more susceptible to bacterial pneumonia in the presence of a viral respiratory disease in the following ways: (1) secretions are increased, therefore aspiration of bacteria-laden fluid is more probable; (2) there may be temporary disruption of the ciliary activity, causing less efficient clearing of bacteria from the respiratory tract; (3) phagocytosis and bactericidal activity of alveolar macrophages may be decreased; and (4) the immune response may be reduced.[11]

Nurse's Role During Diagnosis X-rays have limitations in their usefulness in establishing a diagnosis; they establish the location of involvement but do not verify etiology. However, certain findings are suggestive of specific organisms. For example, pneumatoceles suggest staphylococcus, pleural effusion signifies a bacterial pneumonia (usually pneumococcus or group A streptococcus) and the presence of empyema early in the illness is suggestive of pneumonia due to *Hemophilus influenzae* or staphylococcus.[1,4] Consolidation of a lobe or segment is suggestive of pneumococcal pneumonia. (Consolidation is also seen in pneumonia caused by klebsiella, but pneumococcal infections occur more frequently.)[1] Chest x-ray reports can be used by the nurse to identify the lobes that need particular emphasis when chest physiotherapy is performed.

White blood counts are variable in the presence of pneumonia. In viral pneumonia the white blood cell (WBC) count is usually less than 20,000/mm^3. Bacterial pneumonia is generally associated with more extreme WBC elevations and the presence of many immature cells. The elevated WBC is due primarily to an increase of polymorphonuclear cells. In the case of severe illness leukopenia may occur. Leukopenia, a poor prognostic sign, occurs when white cells leave the circulation faster than they are being produced by the bone marrow.[4]

The nurse has a primary role in facilitating early identification of the organism by assisting with specimen collections. It is important that she place priority on having the necessary equipment available and assisting the physician in diagnostic procedures so that antibiotic therapy can be instituted. She must also explain to parents that various specimens must be collected immediately because antibiotics must be initiated. Parents who do not understand this may feel that these procedures should be done at a later time when the infant is in a less acute state.

New approaches are being used to identify the causative organism in pneumonia.[11] Throat cultures have been found not to correlate well with blood cultures and autopsy findings. A technique called countercurrent immunoelectrophoresis (CIE) is used on serum, urine, pleural fluid and spinal fluid to detect specific bacterial antigens. The severity of the illness is suggested by the amount of antigen present, with an increased amount present in more severe illness. Lung punctures are recommended in some cases when immediate diagnosis is essential for prompt therapy.[11]

In addition to x-rays and white blood counts with differential, the physician takes into account the child's age, the clinical manifestations and existence of an epidemic in establishing a diagnosis.

Nursing Care During Course of Illness and Treatment Caring for the infant and family during the crisis of pneumonia requires that a nurse understand the nature of the illness and the treatment plan. Respiratory efforts are supported by providing humidified oxygen via an age-appropriate technique. For infants an oxygen hood or oxygen tent can be used. Oxygen concentrations are checked with an oxygen analyzer. Vital signs are checked frequently (initially every two hours) and in serious illness respiratory and cardiac monitors should be used. When assessing vital signs the nurse should check the infant's color, respirations and breath sounds, and observe for retractions, nasal flaring and restlessness. An acutely ill infant is also monitored by assessment of blood gases. Changing the position of the infant every two hours facilitates pulmonary drainage, helps to prevent skin breakdown and keeps the infant comfortable. Respirations are generally eased by placing the child in a semi-Fowler's position with the neck slightly hyperextended. Raising the head of the mattress 30 degrees and placing a small folded blanket or towel under the shoulders straightens the airway and facilitates respiration. Older infants assume a position of comfort. Suction should be available whenever secretions are not being handled effectively by the infant's respiratory system.

Fever is closely monitored and treated to prevent convulsions. Antipyretics, fluids and a cool mist environment are provided to reduce fever. A sponge bath with tepid water is recommended by some physicians for a temperature of 39.4° C (103° F), although extended cooling is controversial. Cool mist moistens the airway and helps to reduce fever, but chilling must be avoided. The nurse must also assess for dehydration that is caused by high fever, insensible water loss from tachypnea, and poor fluid intake due to dyspnea. The nurse should monitor intake and output, check specific gravity of urine and make ongoing assessments of hydration status. Oral fluids are encouraged, but intravenous fluid therapy may be indicated when intake is poor. Infants in particular have difficulty maintaining an adequate intake because of dyspnea while sucking.

A combined ultrasonic mist therapy and chest physiotherapy regimen loosens and removes secretions from the respiratory tract. Ultrasonic nebulizers are capable of producing a dense mist of small particles that are more likely to reach the lower respiratory tract than are the large particles produced by a croupette nebulizer. Percussion, vibration and postural drainage are usually done every four to six hours; times vary with the severity of the pneumonia. Parents should be taught to do percussion and postural drainage while their infant is hospitalized. They should be given the opportunity to participate in the treatment and should be able to demonstrate the entire procedure at least once before the infant is discharged. (See Chapter 17 for discussion of chest physical therapy.)

In the event of fluid accumulation in the pleural cavity, drainage is accomplished either by continuous drainage by chest tube or numerous thoracenteses. This is most common when pneumonia is caused by *Staphylococcus aureus*. Antibiotics are administered in bacterial pneumonia but are not indicated in viral pneumonia. Antibiotic regimens (types and dosage) change rapidly as resistant strains of organisms emerge; therefore, a formulary should be consulted for current information.

The nurse should also respond to the stresses that parents experience because of the nature of the illness. The need for oxygen, mist, chest physiotherapy, intravenous fluids and antibiotics is distressing to parents, especially when it interferes with their ability to hold their infant. When an infant can tolerate brief periods out of the oxygen tent or isolette the nurse can show parents how to properly handle the baby to prevent IV infiltration or dislodgement. Parents should also be shown how to support and cradle their infant while feeding him inside a tent. Providing for an infant-parent contact during all phases of the illness helps parents to feel prepared to take their infant home when he is discharged.

Before discharge the nurse should discuss the use of antipyretics, antibiotic administration and side effects, percussion and postural drainage, and review signs of respiratory distress. A discussion of adequate fluids, rest and diet for age will help parents to take preventive measures in maintaining the health of their infant.

References

1. H. F. Eichenwald. Pneumonia syndromes in children. Hospital Practice, May 1976, p. 89
2. L. A. Glasgow and J. C. Overall. Infections of the

newborn. In Nelson Textbook of Pediatrics. V. Vaughan et. al., eds., W. B. Saunders Co., 1979
3. S. Gordon. Infectious diseases. In Survey of Clinical Pediatrics, E. Wasserman and L. B. Slobody, McGraw-Hill Co., 1974
4. R. A. Hoekelman. Diseases of the lower respiratory tract. In Principles of Pediatrics. McGraw-Hill Book Co., 1978
5. J. O. Klein and M. Mavey. Bacterial infections. In Infectious Diseases of the Fetus and Newborn Infant. J. S. Remington and J. O. Klein, eds. W. B. Saunders Co., 1976
6. S. Krugman et al. Infectious Diseases of Children. C. V. Mosby Co., 1977
7. M. D. Lough. Pediatric Respiratory Therapy. Year Book Medical Publishers, 1979
8. A. E. Organ. Lower respiratory tract infection in childhood. Issues in Comprehensive Pediatric Nursing, August 1978, p. 13
9. S. A. Price and L. M. Wilson. Pathophysiology: Clinical Concepts of Disease Process. McGraw-Hill Book Co., 1978
10. W. S. Schley and A. N. Krauss. Bronchitis and bronchiolitis. In Pulmonary Disease of the Fetus, Newborn and Child. E. M. Scarpell et al., eds., Lea and Febiger, 1978
11. M. H. P. Smith. Bacterial pneumonias: gram-positive. In Disorders of the Respiratory Tract in Children. E. L. Kendig and V. Chernick, eds., W. B. Saunders Co., 1977
12. R. C. Stern. Lower respiratory tract. In Nelson Textbook of Pediatrics, V. Vaughan et al., eds., W. B. Saunders Co., 1979
13. W. W. Waring. The history and physical examination. In Disorders of the Respiratory Tract in Children. E. L. Kendig and V. Chernick, eds. W. B. Saunders, 1977
14. M. E. B. Wohl. Bronchiolitis. In Disorders of the Respiratory Tract in Children. E. L. Kendig and V. Chernick, eds. W. B. Saunders Co., 1977

NEUROLOGICAL AND RELATED INFECTIONS OF THE INFANT

by Judy Coltson Moyer, BS, MS

BACTERIAL MENINGITIS

Bacterial meningitis is a serious central nervous system infection caused by an invasion of the meninges by bacteria. Bacterial meningitis is a significant health problem for infants and children because of a moderate mortality rate associated with the disease and because of the high incidence of severe long-term neurological sequelae.

The majorty of cases of bacterial meningitis occur in children under 1 year. The disease is caused by one of three organisms: *Hemophilus influenzae* type B (H. flu meningitis), *Neisseria meningitidis* (meningococcal meningitis), and *Diplococcus pneumoniae* (pneumococcal meningitis).[7, 11] A higher incidence exists among low socioeconomic populations and minority ethnic groups.[11] In addition, the incidence of the disease resulting from *Hemophilus influenzae* has increased greatly over the last 25 years.[11]

In neonatal meningitis the causative agents are often of enteric origin, most commonly *E. coli*. Since the early 1970s an increasing number of serious neonatal infections have also been caused by Group B streptococcus.[4]

Pathophysiology and Clinical Manifestations

The disease frequently occurs following an upper respiratory infection caused by exposure to one of the common etiologic agents. The most common route of infection is via the venous channels that drain the upper respiratory tract. These vessels are in close proximity to the meninges.[12] Another way of entry into the meninges is through direct extension from an infection of the sinuses, or from a skull fracture. Organisms also reach the meninges in the presence of generalized septicemia. No immunization against meningitis is currently available. A preventive measure is prompt attention to respiratory infections.

Inflammation of the meninges is responsible for nuchal rigidity (stiff neck), the most striking sign of meningitis in older infants and children. Classically these children have a stiff neck, high fever and appear very ill. Kernig's sign (the inability to fully extend the legs) and Brudzinski's sign (flexion of the hips when the neck is flexed) are frequently present. An infant may have less striking symptoms. The parents may notice only a resistance by the child to being cuddled or being diapered, and mild fever and irritability. In addition, the child under 6 months may have a high-pitched cry, a transient vacant

TABLE 24-6 CEREBROSPINAL FLUID FINDINGS
(MEAN VALUES IN PARENTHESES)*

	Cells mm³	Glucose (As percentage of blood glucose)	Protein (Mg/100 ml)
Normal			
Child	0–1	≥60	<30
Full-term neonate	0–32 (8)	≥60	20–170 (90)
Premature	0–29 (9)	≥60	65–150 (115)
Viral meningitis	2–2000 (80)	≥60	30–80
Bacterial meningitis	5–5000 (800)	≤45	>60

*Adapted from D. W. Smith. Introduction to Clinical Pediatrics, W. B. Saunders Co., 1977, p. 147.

stare and anorexia. A bulging or tense fontanel is a frequent symptom and is a significant indication of cerebral edema. Meningococcal meningitis is associated with rapidly spreading petechiae. Any parent inquiring about a purple rash, especially if associated with other symptoms, should be told to have the child seen by a physician immediately.

Nurse's Role

During Diagnosis The only means of making a definitive diagnosis is by a lumbar puncture. A lumbar puncture is done by introducing a needle into the lumbar space and withdrawing a small amount of spinal fluid. The procedure is relatively safe but frightening to both the child and the parents. The nurse's major technical responsibility is to hold the patient in the correct arched position. Cloudy fluid indicates pathology but the source is not determined until further testing is completed. The fluid may appear grossly clear, but upon microscopic examination it shows the presence of white cells and organisms. Glucose is usually lowered and protein is elevated. (see Table 24–6 for cerebrospinal fluid findings.) The fluid is also cultured in order to identify the specific organism so that appropriate antibiotic therapy can be promptly initiated. In addition to the lumbar puncture, laboratory tests include a blood culture to identify septicemia, electrolyte determinations to identify imbalances that are commonly concurrent and a CBC to observe the body's response to the infection.

The period of diagnosis, although usually brief, is very frightening to families. They are aware that the child is seriously ill; the possibility of meningitis is real. Keeping the parents informed of the status of the child, explaining the diagnostic procedures and allowing the child to be with the parents as much as possible will alleviate some of this anxiety.

The child diagnosed as having meningitis is hospitalized and placed in respiratory isolation. Isolation is usually continued for 24 to 48 hours following the beginning of antibiotic therapy.[1] The risk of hospital personnel developing meningitis after exposure to a child with the disease is slight. The chance of a young family member who has had intimate contact with the patient being infected is a greater risk; the young sibling has a 1 to 3 per cent chance of developing the disease.[3, 12] The use of prophylactic antibiotics for these children is controversial; in any case parents should be advised to seek medical help promptly if other young children develop symptoms.

During Treatment and Course of Illness During the early stages of the disease, careful nursing assessment is vital. Complications frequently occur insidiously. Cerebral edema is one potential complication: a change in consciousness from alertness to irritability to stupor is a sign of this. Reactions to pain stimuli change from a normal response to lack of response. Pupillary response should be checked frequently and deviations from the norm reported. Other parameters signaling possible cerebral edema are an increase in fontanel fullness and changes in respiratory rate and rhythm. Seizures occur in about 60 per cent of all meningitis patients.[10] These occur in response to cerebral edema, the fever or the disease itself. Usual seizure precautions should be taken to assure the maintenance of an adequate airway. Obstructive or communicating hydrocephalus is a complication of meningitis in small infants. A daily record of head circumference and frequent checks of the fontanels will alert the nurse to the onset of this problem.

The child will be on intravenous antibiotic therapy. Length of time of this antibiotic therapy varies, with 7 to 10 days being an average. The dosage is much higher than the dosage in other infections because the antibiotic in this disease must cross the blood-brain barrier. Intravenous therapy necessitates restraining the child. During the first 72 hours this usually does not present a problem because the child is most comfortable when undisturbed. When the first critical days have passed, the child should be allowed to move about with the parents and staff as much as possible while the intravenous line is maintained.

Accurate intake and output recordings are maintained. These children are not usually dehydrated and require only maintenance fluids. Caution is needed to avoid overloading the circulating system, since overload may compound the problems of cerebral edema. In addition, the intravenous solution is chosen with respect to electrolyte balance because imbalance is a frequent complication. Measures to reduce the temperature in a febrile child are taken. Methods used to treat fever vary but may include tepid sponging, and use of a cooling mattress and antipyretics.

Nursing care of the family members during the acute phase of meningitis includes a complete explanation of procedures, the methods and rationale of isolation, and provision of opportunities for them to ventilate their feelings regarding the seriousness of the disease. It is frustrating for parents to see their child in obvious discomfort, unable to be soothed by holding and cuddling. It is helpful to assist these families to find other means of comforting their child such as pacifiers, talking quietly with the child and assisting in routine care.

Prognosis   Major factors in predicting the outcome of bacterial meningitis are the age of the child and the interval between onset of the disease and the initiation of therapy. The mortality rate nationally is 5 to 10 per cent for treated cases of bacterial meningitis for all ages.[12] Neurological sequelae have been found to be common when children who have had meningitis are compared with siblings. The sequelae from meningitis may vary considerably, ranging from mild learning disabilities to severe physical handicaps. Alterations in vision, hearing or mental ability may result. Alterations may not be evident at discharge or may improve significantly following discharge. As with mortality, the sequelae appear to be worse in very young infants or if there is a delay in treatment. These children should be closely followed with periodic developmental screening for a period of one year at three- to four-month intervals. If residual brain damage is identified the child is referred to appropriate remedial resources.

VIRAL MENINGITIS

Viral meningitis is frequently referred to as aseptic (without bacteria) meningitis. The organisms that most commonly cause viral meningitis are enteroviruses (coxsackievirus and ECHO viruses) and mumps. Inflammation of the meninges may also be associated with exanthematous conditions such as varicella (chickenpox), herpes, measles and roseola.

Viral meningitis is generally a benign self-limiting illness. The clinical manifestations are similar to those of bacterial meningitis but they do not progress as rapidly.[5] Initial symptoms in a neonate or young infant may be confined to lethargy and irritability when handled. Older children may have headache, fever, vomiting, general malaise, muscle aching and nuchal rigidity.

Diagnosis is made by clinical manifestations and findings in the cerebrospinal fluid (CSF) (see Table 24–6). Generally, the lumbar puncture shows elevated leukocytes (although not as high as in bacterial meningitis), normal or slightly elevated protein level, and a normal glucose level. Specimens of CSF and stool and secretions from the nasopharynx are collected for viral studies to isolate the causative agent.

Until a definitive diagnosis is made, antibiotics are frequently administered and isolation procedures instituted in the event the causative organism is bacterial. The nurse must be sensitive to the fear that parents harbor during this period of diagnosis.

Symptomatic treatment including fever control, analgesia, and positions of comfort comprise the usual treatment approach once the diagnosis of viral meningitis is established. Most children with viral meningitis have few complications, but the nurse must be careful not to assume that the illness is necessarily benign.

Deafness may follow mumps and some children who as infants have had enteroviral meningitis have been noted to have retardation and developmental delays.[5] The nurse's role is thus to work closely with team members to gain accurate information as a basis for her counselling with the family.

ENCEPHALITIS

Encephalitis is an acute central nervous system disease caused by a virus. The main site of infection is the brain tissue as opposed to the meninges, which are affected in viral (aseptic) meningitis. The clinical manifestations vary with the causative agent and the age of the child. Those causative agents included in this discussion are (1) enteroviruses, (2) arboviruses and (3) herpes simplex. Also some of the viral childhood illnesses, in rare cases, may result in the complication of encephalitis.

The most common etiologic agents are the enteroviruses.[8] In the past the enterovirus responsible for most cases was the poliomyelitis virus. The common causes now are coxsackievirus or ECHO virus. Encephalitis from these agents is most common during the summer or early fall. The symptoms initially are malaise manifested by headaches, lethargy, fever, anorexia, prostration and meningeal signs (nuchal rigidity, Kernig's and Brudzinski's signs).

Arboviruses are viruses transmitted by arthropods. These are most commonly transmitted by a mosquito from a mammal or bird to man. The disease occurs only during the months when mosquitos are present. California virus (most common in the Midwest) is the arbovirus that most frequently causes encephalitis in children. The symptoms of this form of the disease vary from mild neurological symptoms disappearing in a week to severe, abruptly occurring fever, headache, and seizures. This form is seldom fatal, but behavioral problems persisting for several months occur frequently.[8, 10] Western equine encephalitis is the type that most frequently affects young infants. The disease begins abruptly with a high fever and seizures. In this type, the mortality is reported in 20 per cent of cases, and neurological sequelae occur in 50 per cent of cases.[8]

Herpes simplex is a virus on the increase in the United States and now accounts for 10 per cent of all encephalitis cases.[8] Symptoms include fever, vomiting, convulsions and a decreasing state of consciousness. Encephalitis caused by herpes simplex has a high incidence of neurological impairment or death.[5]

Encephalitis is a rare complication of the viral childhood diseases such as chickenpox, measles, rubella and mumps. The occurrence of such sequelae is rare but should be recognized as possible when neurological symptoms occur during or after these communicable diseases. Encephalitis is also a rare response to the immunizations for these diseases.

Nurse's Role During Diagnosis and Course of Illness

Encephalitis is suspected when the child presents with the symptoms of headache, lethargy, fever and meningeal irritation, especially if other cases were recently identified in the locality. Blood culture and lumbar puncture are done to differentiate between encephalitis and bacterial meningitis, with the spinal fluid being clear in the case of encephalitis. Serologic tests are done to determine the etiologic agent, but many hospitals are not equipped to do these tests and it may take several days to receive results.

The abruptness with which the symptoms occur and the accompanying behavioral changes are confusing and frightening to parents. Explanations of the procedures and the usual course of the disease help to relieve some of the anxiety during the diagnostic period.

Care during the acute phase of the disease is mostly supportive. Seizure precautions should be initiated. Respiratory assistance is sometimes required. Intravenous fluid and electrolytes are given if the child is unable to take liquids orally. Antipyretics and use of supportive measures to reduce the temperature are required. Currently drug therapy to combat the viruses causing encephalitis is not widely available.

Prevention of encephalitis is based on the elimination of insect carriers and immunization of children to prevent the communicable diseases sometimes associated with encephalitis. In the event of occurrence of chickenpox and other communicable diseases for which there are no effective vaccines, patients affected should be isolated until their cases are resolved.

Following the acute phase of the illness, malaise may persist for several weeks or months. The family should be encouraged to provide stimulation for the child but should recognize his limitations. In the case of neurological sequelae involving behavioral changes, parents will need asistance in managing the new behaviors in a gentle and consistent manner. The type of disturbances that may be expected are sleep problems, headaches, inability to remember or concentrate, irritability and "dull speech patterns." These problems gradually subside, and the degree of permanent involvment is not established until one year after the acute episode.[2] The nurse has an important function in her role as a resource person to the family as they adapt to the new needs of their child. She must assist the family to attain comprehensive care to meet their child's health and education needs.

SEPTICEMIA

Sepsis and septicemia are terms used interchangeably that refer to bacterial invasion of the blood. Sepsis following a local infection is referred to as secondary sepsis; that which develops without apparent cause is primary sepsis. Neonatal sepsis is bacterial invasion occurring in the first weeks of life. Neonatal sepsis and meningitis are commonly referred to as a continuum of one disease entity because of the frequency with which the two occur simultaneously.

The major pathogens of neonatal sepsis are *Eschericha coli (E. coli)* and Group B beta-hemolytic streptococci (Group B strep). Together these organisms account for 70 per cent of the neonatal sepsis and meningitis.[7, 9] Both of these organisms are part of the normal flora of the human body. When host resistance is lowered or certain strains are outside of their normal environment the organism becomes pathogenic.

Nurse's Role in Prevention

Certain factors make an infant more prone to the development of sepsis. One factor is premature rupture of the membranes at birth. This exposes the fetus to infected amniotic fluid. Another is fetal hypoxia, which may cause the fetus to aspirate or swallow the fluid. A break in the fetal skin may provide bacteria a port of entry. Delivery through the birth canal, which has the organism as part of its normal flora, is another circumstance that potentiates the development of sepsis.

A secondary source of infection is through direct contact between an infant and someone who has the bacteria on his or her hands as part of their own flora or owing to handling an infected child. Nosocomial transmission is usually manifested in an onset during the first five days of life.[9] Most importantly, this disease can be minimized by diligent handwashing by all persons handling infants. The American Academy of Pediatrics recommends that Iodophor solution be used during the two-minute scrub that is required when entering the nursery.[9] Thorough washing between the handling of different infants with special attention to the nails and cuticles is also a requirement.

Clinical Manifestations and Diagnosis

The onset of sepsis is often very subtle and variable. The first signs may be lethargy, a poor suck reflex, a lowered or rising temperature or irregular respirations. The signs may be so subtle that the mother may be able to express only the thought that the baby "doesn't seem right." Any of these symptoms may be related to sepsis or a number of noninfectious diseases and should be regarded as significant until medically evaluated. In older infants one can expect chills, abrupt onset of fever and prostration.

Diagnosis is based on history, physical signs and symptoms and laboratory tests. A history of maternal infection, premature rupture of the membranes, difficult labor or concurrent symptoms in other infants in the nursery are significant. Laboratory tests include a blood culture to identify the specific organisms, urine culture to rule out urinary tract infection, lumbar puncture to identify possible meningitis, electrolyte studies to identify any imbalance and a CBC to identify the body's response to infection.

Nurse's Role During Treatment and Course of Illness

Treatment consists of intravenous or intramuscular antibiotics and supportive care. These infants are seriously ill and may require ventilatory assistance and therapy to correct electrolyte imbalance. Feedings may need to be completely replaced by intravenous fluids or nasogastric tube feedings. The infants are isolated within an isolette and meticulous handwashing technique is used. Close observation of other infants in the nursery is necessary and follow-up of discharged infants is recommended.[1]

The treatment of these infants has implications for the mother-infant bonding process. The baby is not allowed to be taken to the mother's bed for feeding and frequently is hospitalized after the mother is discharged. Efforts should be made to allow the parents to visit the nursery frequently. As soon as possible the parents are allowed to assist with daily care such as feeding, bathing and diapering. When isolation is discontinued the parents may assume more responsibility and may be provided a private area for time together as a family. Siblings should be allowed observational visits regularly. If frequent visits are not possible, phone contacts initiated by the infant's nurse can help to bridge the gap.

Breast-feeding mothers can be instructed on milk expression to establish and maintain lactation. If nasogastric feedings are used the breast milk may be expressed, refrigerated and used for feeding. Breast feeding can be resumed when oral feedings are begun. It is often a difficult task to maintain lactation without a suckling infant, but with support and accurate information it is possible.

Prognosis

The mortality rate for neonatal sepsis and meningitis is reported at 30 per cent.[6] The rate decreases with the age of the infant and promptness of diagnosis. Neurological sequelae are apparent in 50 per cent of the infants.[6] Careful follow-up with developmental testing and information regarding appropriate infant stimulation is advisable. Early detection of delays will allow for intervention for the infant at a young age and assist in minimizing the effects of such delays.

References

1. American Academy of Pediatrics, Report of the Committee on Infectious Diseases, 1977
2. B. L. Conway. Pediatric Neurologic Nursing, C. V. Mosby Co., 1977, p. 306
3. W. Bell and W. McCormick. Neurologic Infections in Children, Major Problems in Clinical Pediatrics. W. B. Saunders Co., 1975
4. L. A. Glasgow and J. C. Overall. Infections of the newborn. In Nelson Textbook of Pediatrics, V. Vaughan et al., eds., W. B. Saunders Co., 1979
5. C. B. Hall. Infections of the central nervous system. In Principles of Pediatrics, R. A. Hoekelman, ed., McGraw-Hill Book Co., 1978
6. G. H. McCracken. Neonatal sepsis and meningitis. Hospital Practice, January 1976, 1089.
7. G. H. McCracken. Neonatal septicemia and meningitis. In Pediatrics, A. M. Rudolph, et al., eds., Appleton-Century-Crofts, 1977
8. J. Menkes. Viral neurologic infections in children. Hospital Practice, November, 1977, p. 101
9. H. Mizer. Group B streptococci in neonatal infections. American Journal of Maternal Child Nursing, May/June 1978, p. 21
10. H. Moffet. Pediatric Infectious Disease, J. B. Lippincott Co., 1975
11. C. G. Ray. Severe life-threatening infectious diseases. In Introduction to Clinical Pediatrics, D. Smith, ed., W. B. Saunders Co., 1977
12. D. Smith. The challenge of bacterial meningitis. Hospital Practice, June 1976, p. 71

GASTROINTESTINAL INFECTION IN INFANCY

by Judy Coltson Moyer, BS, MS

GASTROENTERITIS

Diarrhea is a frequent symptom of illness in infants and young children. Causes of diarrhea include systemic disease, ingestion of poisons, food allergies and infectious gastroenteritis. It is estimated that 10 per cent of all children in the United States are at one time affected by infectious gastroenteritis.[2]

Gastroenteritis is an infection of the gastrointestinal tract resulting in increased motility and rapid emptying of the intestinal contents. This rapid excretion interferes with the absorption of necessary electrolytes and water. In addition it is thought that gastroenteritis may cause a temporary enzyme deficiency, particularly of the enzyme disaccharidase.[4]

The term nonspecific gastroenteritis has been

applied to gastroenteritis caused by a virus. The virus infects the gastrointestinal tract, causing congestion of the mucosa and dilation of the intestine. Viral gastroenteritis is highly contagious and can affect an individual at any age but is most common in young children and infants.

Bacterial gastroenteritis is caused by a number of agents. Infants are frequently infected by E. coli. This is a bacteria commonly found in the gut, but several strains are pathogenic. Salmonella gastroenteritis is caused by ingestion of milk, meat or eggs contaminated by the organism duirng preparation or storage. The contamination may occur in the home or in commercial preparation. Shigella gastroenteritis is transmitted from person to person through direct contact. A subclinical case in an adult may be transmitted to a child. Staphylococcal gastroenteritis is caused by ingestion of the staphylococcal bacteria. Frequently the foods affected are dairy products that have been improperly stored.

Nurse's Role in Prevention and Diagnosis

The disease may sometimes be avoided by instituting basic hygiene measures. The nurse functioning in a variety of settings is in an excellent position to teach families and children correct methods of storage and preparation of meat and dairy products. Discussing the importance of handwashing after diapering, after using the toilet and before food preparation and feeding is an important measure in decreasing the incidence of gastroenteritis. In addition, good handwashing and proper disposal of contaminated articles by personnel within institutions will discourage the spread of the disease.

Diagnosis is made largely by history. Parents report a large number of watery stools. These stools are frequently green from the excretion of bile and may contain pus and, infrequently, blood. The child often has a history of vomiting and a low-grade fever. An accurate history is important in differentiating normal stool changes, which occur with age and diet changes, from diarrhea, which reflects pathology. After obtaining an accurate history regarding the symptoms, a stool culture is done to identify the specific causative agent.

Clinical Manifestations

The major complication resulting from gastroenteritis regardless of cause is dehydration and accompanying electrolyte imbalance. Signs of dehydration are not always apparent to parents. These signs are depressed fontanels, sunken eyes, loss of skin turgor, oliguria or concentrated urine. Parents should know these signs and should report them. A decreased urinary output indicated by less than six wet diapers per 24 hours or a period of longer than four hours without urination is significant in an infant. Skin turgor can be checked by pinching the skin on the abdomen. If the skin returns to normal after being released there is no loss of skin turgor. Skin that remains elevated after being released signifies loss of subcutaneous fluid and is indicative of dehydration. Other signs for parents to watch for are the absence of tears, increasing lethargy or irritability and dry lips and tongue.

Potassium and sodium are normally lost through stool but replaced through oral intake. During diarrheal disease these losses are greater than can be replaced by normal oral intake. Sodium losses in turn create additional extracellular fluid loss, compounding the problem of volume deficit. Potassium losses cause muscle weakness, abdominal distention and possible electrocardiographic changes.

Nurse's Role During Treatment and Course of Illness

The management of infectious gastroenteritis has three components: (1) to maintain or restore fluid and electrolyte balance, (2) to restore the bowel to normal functioning, (3) to prevent the infection of others in contact with the child. Mild cases of the disease can be treated at home by the parents. Initially the child is given nothing by mouth for four to six hours. After this period of abstinence, which allows the bowel to become relatively inactive, clear liquids are started. Fluids recommended for parents to use at home are soft drinks and flavored gelatin water.* When using soft drinks the parents should be told to allow the drink to become "flat" by stirring until the carbonation is no longer present. The gelatin water is made by

---

*Pediatric electrolyte solutions such as Lytren or Pedi-Lyte may be recommended in some circumstances, but it is preferable to use these in a controlled setting such as a hospital to avoid hypertonic dehydration.

mixing two tablespoons of flavored gelatin powder in eight ounces of water. It is important to inform parents that the child's stools will be the color of the gelatin water and this is not cause for alarm. Liquids should be offered at room temperature because cold liquids increase bowel motility. After 24 to 48 hours on clear liquids, when stooling is less frequent and the consistency of the stool is becoming firmer, the child may be advanced to a low-residue and low-fat diet, most frequently consisting of bananas, rice cereal, applesauce and toast (BRAT diet).

Fluid intake should not be allowed to fall below 150 ml/kg per 24 hours.[4] The parents should be informed of specific minimal amounts necessary for the individual infant. Controversy exists over how to reintroduce the oral feedings. Most often small frequent feedings are given, yet larger quantities offered less frequently may be recommended due to the fact that frequent feedings have the potential to induce peristalsis.[4] Breast-fed infants with mild diarrhea are able to remain on breast milk. The diarrhea will usually resolve when the infant takes nothing orally for several hours and then continues with breast feeding.

Specific instructions are needed by parents who are managing gastroenteritis at home. Detailed dietary guidelines must be given. Other important information includes handwashing technique and proper disposal of soiled articles. Families should also be familiar with the signs of dehydration and instructed to seek additional assistance if these signs are present or if the diarrhea continues beyond a few days.

Infants and children with severe diarrhea, those with symptoms of dehydration, and those in whom vomiting accompanies diarrhea should be hospitalized for observation and parenteral fluid and electrolyte therapy. Medical treatment during hospitalization is aimed at restoring normal fluid and electrolyte balance and allowing the bowel to resume normal function. This is accomplished by the use of normal saline intravenous feeding with potassium added to the solution. Before potassium is added, kidney function is verified by the child urinating. The child is given nothing by mouth for 24 to 48 hours or until the frequency of stools lessens and the consistency becomes firmer.

The most accurate assessment of fluid loss is through body weight. Weight is the basis for assessing the success of management during the acute phase of the disease and weighing must be done on an accurate scale with the child completely undressed. The child is weighed on admission and all subsequent weighings should be done of the same scale. A precise record of oral and parenteral intake and of output is important. Stool and urinary output is most easily measured by weighing the diapers dry and again after soiling. This eliminates the difficulties associated with attempting to maintain a urine collection bag on a small child. Urine specific gravity (USG) is an accurate measure of the state of hydration; measurement can easily be done on the unit. The USG reflects the concentration of the urine: the higher the reading, the more concentrated the urine. USG of 1.025 or greater is indicative of dehydration. As intravenous fluids are begun, the USG will decrease. A reading of approximately 1.015 indicates normal hydration. During the acute phase of hospitalization USG should be measured every four hours.

As with the child treated at home, the hospitalized child is advanced to a low-residue and low-fat diet. The introduction of milk may cause the child's diarrhea to begin again because of possible disaccharidase deficiency. For this reason formula is introduced at a lower strength, with slow advance to full strength. In some instances it may be necessary to give the infant a soy formula until the deficiency is naturally corrected.[4]

During periods without oral feedings, the infant's need to suck is not decreased; not being given the means to suck is often a source of great frustration to the child. Offering a pacifier or allowing the child who normally sucks his thumb to continue to do so often relieves some of the frustration.

Although the child's activity is necessarily restricted to maintain a patent intravenous line, the child must be allowed frequent periods of free activity under supervision. Parents can be shown safe positions in which to hold the child without disturbing the IV.

Hospitalized children with gastroenteritis are in enteric isolation. Proper handwashing and disposal of soiled articles will prevent the spread of the disease. Parents need to be instructed in these techniques and the rationale for their use.

The stools during diarrhea are acidic and

irritating to the skin around the perineum. If the child is not promptly cleaned after defecation the skin quickly becomes excoriated. To prevent this, the area should immediately be gently cleaned with soap and water and thoroughly dried. Excoriation frequently responds quickly to air-drying; the area can simply be cleaned and then left uncovered to the air. A heat lamp used at a safe distance of at least 18 inches several times per day also helps to speed healing. The area is very painful and the child will be uncomfortable during diaper changes. Applying liberal amounts of zinc oxide, Desitin or other protective ointment to the area will keep the diaper from sticking to the skin area and also prevent contact of the skin with stool. Sometimes applying cornstarch after gently cleansing with soap and water provides sufficient protection. Cornstarch assists in drying the skin and is soothing.

References

1. L. Copeland. Chronic diarrhea in infancy. American Journal of Nursing, March 1977, p. 461
2. C. DeAngelis. Pediatric Primary Care. Little, Brown, & Co., 1979
3. I. Gray, ed. Acute Diarrhea in Children. Ross Laboratories, 1978
4. H. L. Hodes. Viral gastroenteritis. In Pediatrics, A. M. Rudolph et al., eds. Appleton-Century-Crofts, 1977

NUTRITIONAL ALTERATIONS

by Mabel Hunsberger, BSN, MSN

Malnutrition is most commonly used to describe a state of undernourishment resulting from insufficient food intake. Malnutrition in this text is used to describe both excessive and deficient intake of food. Whether an individual overindulges or has an inadequate source of food intake, the consequence is a state of faulty nourishment (malnutrition).

Severe deficiency states are now rarely seen in infants within the United States and other developed countries; however, many impoverished families do not have adequate food to meet their needs. As many as 15 per cent of families in the United States have been reported to have insufficient food.[17] While a segment of the population is being underfed, resulting in varying degrees of undernourishment, an increasing number of individuals in the United States are searching for the easiest solution to the problem of obesity.

While obesity and insufficient food intake coexist in the United States, third world countries are plagued with the tragic reality of starvation and death because of inadequate food. Insufficient food availability, contaminated food sources and inadequate distribution systems converge in the midst of the problem of political unrest. Overeating and varying degrees of undernutrition simultaneously persist as world health problems. Nutritional alterations discussed in this chapter are infant obesity, severe protein-calorie malnutrition, and vitamin D deficiency rickets.

INFANT OBESITY

Wide variations exist in infant feeding practices. The consequences of various feeding practices are not clearly established; therefore, recommendations regarding infant nutrition are speculative and must be considered tentative.[6] Infants fed in a variety of ways may appear equally healthy either because the consequences of a poor diet are too subtle or because differences can be verified only by long-term observations.[6] Some of the questions on the long-term consequences of early eating habits that remain unanswered are: (1) What is the relationship of intake of cholesterol during infancy to the later development of atherosclerosis? (2) How does salt intake in infancy affect blood pressure in later life? and (3) Are faulty eating habits of infancy and infant obesity an important determinant of obesity in later childhood and adulthood? (The theory that the critical period for the development of obesity is during the first year or two of life has been challenged.[4, 18]) While we wait for conclusive studies regarding the effects of infant obesity, infants at risk must be identified and families need assistance to establish healthful practices of feeding their infants.

Nursing Assessment

The practice of doing a thorough nutritional assessment will assist the nurse to identify those infants at risk for obesity. (See Chapter 13 for nutritional assessment.) Intake is evaluated in terms of the total caloric intake, amount of fluid intake and balance of nutrients.

The nurse should also assess the prevalence of obesity in the family. According to a 10-state nutritional survey, a child of obese parents is three times more likely to be obese than if his parents are not obese; if one child is obese, there is a 40 per cent chance that a sibling will also be obese.[4] The similarity of obesity patterns between parents and children cannot, however, be interpreted as having only a genetic base because there is considerable similarity between spouses in terms of obesity.[8] Family eating patterns and values placed on food are important factors to assess when parents and siblings of an infant are obese.

Obesity is an "excessive ratio of fat to fat-free body mass."[7] Estimates of total body content of fat are made by measuring skinfold thickness and by obtaining height and weight measurements. A general definition of obesity is (1) skinfold thickness greater than the 95th percentile and (2) weight for height greater than the 95th percentile.[7]

Height and weight measurements made at each health visit are the nurse's primary method of detecting infants at risk for obesity. Height and weight are plotted on a percentile chart to identify rapid or disproportionate weight gain. In some instances bone and muscle structure may give the erroneous clinical impression that an infant is obese. A more precise evaluation of fat disposition can be obtained by measuring skinfold thickness of the triceps and subscapular area. The triceps, the most widely advocated site for testing, is also the easiest site to use.[16] (See Chapter 13 for percentile growth charts and skinfold standards.) Use of calipers has some disadvantage in that when measurements are taken by various personnel a certain amount of error occurs due to varying techniques and subjective readings.

Prevention and Management: Nurse's Role

During infancy the goal in managing obesity is not to *reduce* the infant's weight but rather to *slow the rate* of weight gain. Management of obesity thus entails the same approaches as prevention: provision of a normal diet and sufficient exercise for the infant. Obesity results from a greater fuel intake than energy output. Prevention and management of obesity involve two approaches: (1) an increase in exercise and (2) a reduction in caloric intake. During infancy certain boundaries determine the type of interventions that are appropriate. The infant's developmental capabilities may limit the type of physical activity to only kicking, creeping, crawling, rolling and reaching. Parents should be made aware of the importance of providing adequate space and opportunity to engage in such developmentally appropriate exercise. Also, the infant's high nutritional requirements cannot be overlooked. It is necessary to maintain a level of caloric intake that supports growth and daily dissipation of energy.

Obesity in childhood has the potential to adversely affect a child's developing body image and self-esteem. The nurse can provide guidance and counselling to parents before obesity develops. It is during infancy that measures to prevent obesity must be taken. The nurse can make an important contribution in the prevention and management of obesity by helping parents to (1) avoid feeding practices that could contribute to infant obesity and (2) recognize and correct those patterns of interaction with their baby that potentiate the tendency to become obese.

Feeding Practices that Contribute to Infant Obesity The advantages of breast-feeding to infants are now sufficiently established to warrant active encouragement of mothers to breast feed.[2] Although studies do not consistently show that bottle-fed infants tend to become more obese than breast-fed infants, it has been observed that bottle-fed infants gain weight more rapidly.[3,5] It has been suggested that bottle-feeding invites the problem of obesity by a mother's tendency to encourage an infant to suck until the bottle is empty, whereas a breast-feeding mother no longer offers the breast when an infant stops sucking.[4] Thus a preventive role of the nurse is to support and encourage breast-feeding of infants, especially for the first three months and counsel parents who bottle-feed to avoid forcing their infant to empty the bottle at each feeding.[18]

Another practice that increases the potential

for infant obesity is the early introduction of solid foods. Parents need to be assured that infants before the age of 4 to 6 months do not need the additional calories that solid foods supply. They should particularly be advised against the addition of sugar and other sweets to the baby's diet. In counselling parents about solid foods for their baby, the nurse must recognize that parents start solid foods early for various reasons. Common reasons for beginning solids early are a belief that milk does not supply adequate nutrition, social pressure exerted by family and friends, and a belief that giving solid food will cause the baby to sleep through the night.[14] The nurse can help families to understand what constitutes normal infant nutrition and assist them to establish healthful feeding practices.

If an infant is particularly at risk for the development of obesity, the nurse can suggest to parents that when solid foods are added to the diet they may wish to prepare their own. Commercially prepared baby foods have a high content of carbohydrates; mixed dinners are particularly high in carbohydrates. Of the commercially prepared baby foods, plain vegetables and meats are higher in protein and lower in carbohydrates than the mixed dinners.[18]

Parental Responses That Contribute to Infant Obesity The stereotype that a fat baby is a healthy baby is still a prevalent myth that is transmitted from one generation to another. These beliefs are deeply rooted and not easily altered. Overfeeding babies thus can stem from a cultural or familial orientation on the part of parents to "fatten" their babies because it is believed that this is a sign of good parenting. The nurse can work with parents over a period of time, pointing out sufficient positive aspects of their parenting so that they eventually can give up the need to overfeed their baby.

The use of food to quiet and satisfy the infant can lead to obesity. To always offer additional breast or bottle feedings or solid food to quiet the baby can establish a pattern for him whereby food is used in response to anxiety rather than in response to hunger. This practice teaches an infant that internal needs can be satisfied by food and places him into a behavior pattern in which he interprets all internal tensions as indicative of the need for food.[11] The nurse can manage this problem by suggesting alternative methods of responding to the baby when he cries. Visual stimulation, cuddling, change of position, exercise or a drink of water may quiet the baby.

Counselling Role of the Nurse Severe dietary restrictions are not recommended during the first year of life, but the family may need assistance to calculate recommended dietary intake. Infants are particularly prone to become obese during the period from 6 months of age to a year. As solid foods are added, the nurse should teach parents to check the labels for caloric content and help them to feed according to the caloric need of their infant. (See Chapter 21 for a summary of infant nutritional requirements.) If the daily milk and food intake exceeds the required caloric amount,* water feedings can be used to replace excess caloric intake. Skim milk is not recommended in the diet of an infant under one year of age. It has been recommended by some nutritionists that 2 per cent fat milk may be used in the case of severe obesity in older infants.[18]

The question of whether frequent small feedings are better than three meals a day is not clearly answered. In adults, widely spaced large meals lead to increased serum concentrations of cholesterol and impaired glucose tolerance; the effects of feeding frequency have not been studied as they pertain to infants.[6] The dilution of formula to increase volume intake without increasing caloric intake may not be the correct approach. Moreover, Foman suggests that regular consumption of enormous volumes of calorically dilute food is not likely to achieve the goal of developing the habit of eating in moderation.[6]

Although many questions regarding infant obesity remain unanswered, the nurse can play an important role in prevention by using the information that is available. Assisting families to establish healthy feeding practices for their infants is a primary role of the nurse. If a family tends to overfeed an infant, the nurse must carefully assess the parents' values and cultural orientation to food, instituting a gradual teaching program whereby parents can learn to relate to their infant in a way that fosters eating in moderation.

---

*Daily requirements of calories: 1–6 months = 117 kcal/kg; 6–12 months = 108 kcal/kg.

SEVERE PROTEIN AND CALORIE MALNUTRITION

Marasmus and kwashiorkor are two serious forms of protein and calorie malnutrition. Both are rare in the United States and common in developing countries. A large proportion of children in the world do not get enough to eat, are subjected to poor hygienic conditions and have inadequate health care; these factors produce malnourishment. The incidence of protein and calorie malnutrition is markedly increased in these areas as a result of repeated bouts of gastroenteritis. Severe protein and calorie malnutrition typically results after an infant is weaned to a grossly inadequate diet.[10] Malnutrition can also result under other circumstances, including metabolic disturbances, chronic renal insufficiency and maladaptive parent-child relations (nonorganic failure to thrive). (See Chapter 5 for a discussion of failure to thrive.) There have also been reports of malnutrition occurring as a result of a prolonged clear liquid diet in the face of infantile diarrhea.[12] The nurse has a primary role in teaching families proper and safe administration of fluids typically prescribed for diarrhea to assist in the prevention of such an occurrence.

Marasmus is a condition of gradual wasting in the presence of grossly inadequate calories and protein. The caloric deficit is so severe that there is a marked reduction of subcutaneous fat, causing the skin to become wrinkled and loose. This results in an "old man" and "wasted" appearance. The marasmic infant is retarded in growth and development and appears restless, fretful and eventually becomes apathetic and listless. A starvation type of diarrhea or infectious diarrhea may further complicate the dehydrated and undernourished state of the infant.

Kwashiorkor is primarily a deficiency of protein resulting in severe muscle wasting. There is also a deficit in calories but it is the protein deficit that accounts for the principal symptoms.[1] The child is usually edematous; this varies in degree from a slight localized edema (primarily eyelids and feet) to a marked generalized edema.[9] When edema is generalized it may mask the muscle atrophy. Skin changes occur, beginning with erythema and progressing through a sequence of hyperpigmentation, desquamation (peeling), and finally depigmentation (loss of color). During the peeling stage the skin readily becomes infected; the risk of infection is increased by picking off the desquamating skin.[9] Another characteristic symptom is the fine, sparse, reddish-tinted hair. Alternating periods of adequate and inadequate dietary intake are mirrored in the streaked hair that results. When dietary intake is adequate hair is pigmented and when it is inadequate it is depigmented. The general depleted nutritional state is frequently further compromised by infections. Most commonly acute diarrhea, measles or parasitic infestations precede or accompany kwashiorkor in underdeveloped countries. Children suffering from kwashiorkor become irritable and apathetic and are typically sullen and withdrawn.

Management of Severe Protein-Calorie Malnutrition: Nurse's Role

These children are in a severe state of nutritional imbalance. The replacement of fluids, electrolytes and nutrients requires a highly specialized therapeutic approach. Furthermore, many infections either precede the undernourished state or occur as a result of it. Treatment consists of administration of fluids and electrolytes, antibiotic therapy to treat infections and a gradual dietary rehabilitation.

The nurse has a responsibility to care for the infant and to become actively involved in the process of identifying those factors that led to development of the condition. The nurse must try to prevent infection or reinfection of an already debilitated child, provide meticulous skin care in the presence of edema or skin desquamation, and carefully monitor dietary and fluid intake. While physical care of the infant is immediate, the nurse must simultaneously begin a careful collection of data and a relationship of sensitive interaction with the family to assist in identifying the cause of the malnutrition.

The nurse who cares for infants and families should also make every effort to identify those children with more moderate forms of malnutrition and especially evaluate the nutritional status of those children who show growth retardation and a developmental lag. Although many factors contribute to the problem of malnutrition, the one consistent finding is poverty.[15] The nurse's efforts to educate families in adequate nutritional intake can be most effective if equal importance is given toward increasing availability of food. Studies show a clear relationship between poverty and malnutrition so that it is safe to say "malnutrition when looked for will be found in the poor of every community."[15]

VITAMIN D DEFICIENCY RICKETS

Vitamin D deficiency results in poor mineralization of the growing parts of the skeleton leading to the disease of rickets. Vitamin D deficiency rickets is most common in children from 4 months to 2 years of age.[2] Vitamin D is required for (1) absorption of dietary calcium and phosphorus from the intestines, (2) conservation of phosphorus by the renal tubular cells and (3) mobilization of calcium from bone to maintain serum calcium levels when oral intake is inadequate.[2]

The vitamin is supplied by ingestion or through ultraviolet radiation. Sunlight converts a hormone (7-dehydrocholesterol) in the skin to vitamin D_3 (cholecalciferol). Vitamin D_3, whether ingested or synthesized in the skin, must be metabolized into an active form of vitamin D. Biochemical alterations called hydroxylations first occur in the liver, then in the kidneys.

Rickets may be caused by a poor dietary intake of vitamin D or because of lack of exposure to sunlight. Other circumstances that may produce rickets include (1) disorders of absorption in which vitamin D, calcium or both are not absorbed; (2) hepatic disease, which may decrease absorption of vitamin D or calcium or interfere with hydroxylation of vitamin D_3; (3) kidney disease, which interferes in the production of active vitamin D; (4) genetic factors as in familial vitamin D–resistant rickets with hypophosphatemia; (5) anticonvulsant therapy (the complication of rickets is a rare occurrence); or (6) administration of glucocorticoids.[1, 2] (Glucocorticoids appear to be antagonistic to vitamin D in calcium transport.[1])

Laboratory Findings A series of physiological processes account for the typical laboratory findings in rickets. Whether from faulty intake or absorption or inadequate sunlight, the vitamin D deficiency leads to impaired absorption of calcium and phosphorus, so that these minerals are lost in increasing amounts through urine and feces. Consequently, serum phosphorus concentration is usually lowered; serum calcium is usually normal* or slightly reduced. Children with rickets also have elevated serum alkaline phosphatase. Elevation of this enzyme reflects increased osteoblastic activity.[15] These laboratory findings are apparent before any histological bone changes.

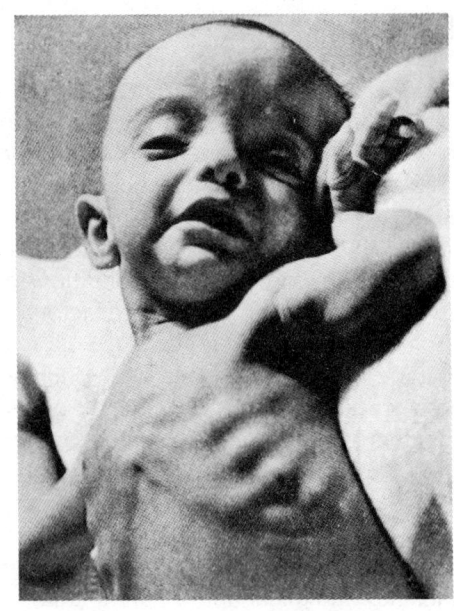

Figure 24–48 Rachitic rosary in an infant. (Lyons and Wallinger: Pediatrics and Pediatric Nursing. From V. Vaughan et al. Nelson Textbook of Pediatrics. W. B. Saunders Co., 1979, p. 231.)

Clinical Manifestations An early histological clinical manifestation of rickets in an infant under 6 months of age is craniotabes. Craniotabes results from a thinning or softening of the skull, usually in the occipitoparietal area. The thin skull bone can be indented by pressing it with a finger and, on the release of pressure, it rebounds with a "crackle like that of a Ping-Pong ball."[2] After the first 6 months it is more common to see frontal bossing (prominence of frontal and parietal bones) and delayed closure of the fontanels. Rachitic rosary (enlarged costochondral junctions) may be palpable in the early stages of rickets and in later stages may be seen as well as felt[1] (Fig. 24–48).

---

*The serum calcium may be normal because as serum calcium is lowered parathormone is secreted. Parathormone mobilizes calcium and phosphorus from the bone but it *increases* renal tubular calcium reabsorption. Thus the serum calcium may ultimately be maintained at a normal level.[20]

In later stages of rickets softening of the bones causes additional skeletal changes. The chest is pigeon-shaped (the sternum protrudes), and a depression is apparent along the lower border of the chest (Harrison's groove). This groove is produced by the pull of the diaphragm on the pliable rib structure.[11] Deformities of the spinal column, including scoliosis, kyphosis and lordosis, also occur in advanced stages of rickets. In children with lordosis, deformities of the pelvis frequently occur; in the past such deformities caused dystocia (difficult labor) in women who had had rickets in infancy.[1, 15] Also, epiphyseal enlargements at the wrists and ankles can be seen or palpated as a "thickening" in these areas in the early phase of rickets and later this enlargement becomes even more apparent. The enlarged epiphyses consist of cartilage and uncalcified bone tissue; therefore they do not show on an x-ray.[1] With weight-bearing, bending of the femur, tibia and fibula results in bowlegs (genu varum) or knock knees (genu valgum). (During development of the legs in infancy and early childhood a degree of genu varum and genu valgum is normal and should not be mistaken for rickets.) (See Chapter 25 for further discussion on assessment for abnormalities of the legs.)

Severe vitamin D deficiency can result in certain delays in growth and development. The appearance of the deciduous teeth may be delayed and out of normal progression. The quality of both the deciduous and permanent teeth may be affected, especially that of the enamel. Poorly developed muscles may be cause for the persisting pot belly (usually a child slims after toddler years), and delayed development in skills such as standing and walking.

Nurse's Role

Early Identification The nurse has an important role in the assessment of infants and children by contributing to the prevention and early detection of vitamin D deficiency. Although vitamin D deficiency may begin to have biochemical effects on the infant in the first few months of life, visible skeletal changes may not be identified until months later. Also, a newborn infant has some reserves of vitamin D that act as a temporary protection in the event of dietary deficiency, but a history of the early diet is essential to identify those children at risk. The nurse can play a preventive role by recommending vitamin D supplementation for premature infants, artificially fed infants who do not receive vitamin D–fortified formula, and infants who are breast fed. The premature infant requires vitamin D supplement much earlier than a full-term infant; vitamin D supplement at 5 to 10 days of age is recommended for the premature infant.[20]

The nurse should particularly assess for vitamin D deficiency in black children, who are more vulnerable to development of rickets than are nonblacks.[1] It has not been determined whether this is due to a reduced penetration of sunlight because of pigmentation. Data on environmental conditions provide significant information. Those children who live in heavy smog areas and who have limited opportunity to play outdoors, and those living in temperate zones, are more prone to vitamin D deficiency.

During Course of Treatment Vitamin D deficiency rickets is treated with the oral administration of vitamin D (1500 to 5000 IU daily).[1] Healing can be demonstrated on x-rays in two to four weeks after the beginning of treatment (except in vitamin D–resistant rickets).[1] Another method of treatment is to give a beginning single dose of 600,000 IU; this results in more rapid healing and the differentiation between vitamin D deficiency rickets and vitamin D–resistant rickets can be made more rapidly. In this regimen one more dose of 600,000 IU may be given two weeks after the initial dose if no healing has occurred.[1] Once healing is complete 400 IU vitamin D (normal daily requirement) is administered daily.

The nurse who cares for a child being treated for rickets must be on guard for various complications. Hypocalcemic tetany is a complication of rickets that requires the nurse to make provisions for the occurrence of seizures. If the large-dose (600,000 IU) vitamin D therapy regimen is used, calcium balance in the body is restored more quickly than when vitamin D is given in moderate daily doses. In any event, if hypocalcemic tetany does occur it is treated with 5 to 10 ml of 10 per cent calcium gluconate administered intravenously. The nurse involved in such therapy must assist in the careful monitoring of the heart rate required to prevent bradycardia and cardiac arrest, which can result from too rapid an elevation of serum calcium.[15] Also, children with rickets are more prone to respiratory infections such as bronchitis or bronchopneumonia, pulmonary atelectasis due to chest deformities, and chronic gastrointestinal disturbances of diarrhea or constipation.[1]

Some of the osseous changes that result from rickets may take months or years to disappear. In advanced cases some permanent alterations may persist. The nurse's role during recovery thus varies according to the severity of the disease but continues to be one of attempting to prevent those complications to which the child is vulnerable, assisting the child and family to a healthy recovery, and preventing a repetition of circumstances that make the child vulnerable to rickets.

References

1. L. A. Barness. Nutritional disorders. In Nelson Textbook of Pediatrics. Vaughan et al., eds., W.B. Saunders Co., 1979
2. J. M. Cooperman. Vitamins and metabolism. In Survey of Clinical Pediatrics, E. Wasserman and L. B. Slobody, eds., McGraw-Hill Book Co., 1974
3. A. S. Cunningham. Morbidity in breast-fed and artificially fed infant II. Journal of Pediatrics, November 1979, p. 685
4. L. J. Filer. Early nutrition: its long-term role. Hospital Practice, February 1978, p. 87
5. S. J. Fomon. Infant Nutrition. W. B. Saunders Co., 1974
6. S. J. Fomon et al. Recommendations for feeding normal infants. Pediatrics, January 1979, p. 52
7. S. J. Fomon and E. E. Ziegler. Prevention of obesity. In Nutritional Disorders of Children, U.S. Department of Health, Education and Welfare, No. (HSA)78-5104, 1976
8. S. M. Garn and D. C. Clark. Nutrition, growth, development, and maturation: findings from the ten-state nutrition survey of 1968-70. Pediatrics, August 1975, p. 306
9. G. G. Graham. Deficiencies of calories and proteins. In Pediatrics, A. M. Rudolph, ed., Appleton-Century-Crofts, 1977
10. G. G. Graham. Nutrition. In Pediatrics, M. Ziai, ed., Little, Brown & Co., 1975
11. H. Harrison. Vitamin D and the metabolism of calcium, phosphate and bone. In Pediatrics, A. M. Rudolph, ed., Appleton-Century-Crofts, 1977
12. D. J. Kallen and E. A. Seagull. Infant feeding and problems of parenting. In Problems Relating to Feeding in the First Two Years. Ross Laboratories, 1977
13. P. Kaplowitz and R. B. Isely. Marasmus-kwashiorkor in an 8-week old infant with prolonged clear liquids for diarrhea. Clinical Pediatrics, September 1979, p. 575
14. B. A. Markesbery and W. M. Wong. Watching baby's diet: a professional and parental guide. Maternal Child Nursing, May/June 1979, p. 177
15. A. M. Mauer. Malnutrition — still a common problem for children in the United States. Clinical Pediatrics, January 1975, p. 23
16. N. R. Rowe. Childhood obesity: growth charts vs. calipers. Pediatric Nursing, Mar/Apr 1980, p. 24
17. N. J. Smith. Nutrition in infancy and childhood including obesity. In Introduction to Clinical Pediatrics, D. W. Smith, ed., W. B. Saunders Co., 1977
18. L. S. Taitz. Obesity in pediatric practice: infantile obesity. Pediatric Clinics of North America, February 1977, p. 107
19. U.S. Department of Health, Education, and Welfare: Ten-State Nutrition Survey 1968-1970. DHEW Publication No. (HSM) 72-8130, Center for Disease Control, 1972
20. A. J. Vander et al. Human Physiology — The Mechanisms of Body Function. McGraw-Hill Book Co., 1980

ENDOCRINE ALTERATIONS IN INFANTS

by Kathleen U. Boggs, RN, MSN

The pituitary gland lies at the base of the brain in the sella turcica. Physiologically it has two sections: the adenohypophysis (anterior section) and the neurohypophysis (posterior section). The pituitary gland secretes a number of hormones controlling major organ functions (target organs) and body growth. Therefore the pituitary is referred to as the master gland. Changes in function of this gland lead to a number of unusual conditions (Table 24-7). These listed conditions occur as a result of a deficiency in one specific pituitary hormone. It is also possible for these hormones to be deficient in selected combinations. The term panhypopituitarism should be used to refer to a deficiency of all anterior and posterior pituitary hormones,[1] although some authorities confine this term to dysfunction of the adenohypophysis.[4]

PITUITARY DWARFISM (ANTERIOR PITUITARY HYPOFUNCTION)

Hypopituitarism is a rare disorder manifested most notably by growth failure (dwarfism). Decreased anterior pituitary function may also lead to symptoms of hormone insufficiency in

TABLE 24-7 ENDOCRINE ALTERATIONS IN INFANTS

Gland	Secretions*	Function	Hypofunction	Hyperfunction
Anterior pituitary (stimulated by hypothalamus)	Growth hormone (GH) also called somatotropic hormone (STH)	Influences protein synthesis in cells	Dwarfism: retarded growth, normal IQ, normal body proportions	Giantism: increased skeletal growth, increased weight gain (acromegaly in adults)
Thyroid (stimulated by TSH from anterior pituitary)	Thyroxine (T_4) and triiodothyroxine (T_3)	Regulate body metabolism of fat, proteins, carbohydrates, vitamins and calcium	Cretinism: failure in growth and development, mental deficiency (if in first 6 months). Altered facial appearance because bones grow less than soft tissue. (endemic goiter or myxedema in adults)	Graves' disease in adults that rarely causes transient neonatal hyperthyroidism in neonates of affected mothers.

*This table is not inclusive of all endocrine secretions; only those described in this section are included.

target organs. Dwarfism occurs when there is insufficient secretion of growth hormone. This hormone affects the metabolic processes of the body by increasing the rate of protein synthesis in all cells of the body, decreasing the rate of carbohydrate utilization throughout the body, and increasing the mobilization of fats and utilization of fats for energy.[4]

Causes of hypopituitarism are classified as congenital, acquired or idiopathic (unknown). The majority of cases are idiopathic. Intracranial tumors (primarily craniopharyngiomas) are the most frequently demonstrated acquired cause; other cases result from pituitary cysts and infectious or traumatic lesions. Surgical removal of the pituitary gland (hypophysectomy) may be necessitated by the presence of a malignancy. Cessation of growth hormone production may also occur secondary to radiation therapy directed at the sella turcica.

The nurse has an important role in early detection of delayed growth. It is vital for pediatric nurses to periodically assess height and weight gains on all children in their care. Data should be recorded on growth grids and compared with standardized growth norms. Most cases of delayed growth or growth failure will be attributed to factors other than pituitary deficiency. Consideration needs to be given to genetic factors, such as the stature of parents. The child's general state of health and past history of chronic illness is also considered. Growth recorded over a period of time gives the nurse a better indicator of disrupted patterns. Children demonstrating a consistent pattern of growth well below expected norms, without a discernible reason, should be referred for evaluation. Children with a history of surgery or radiation to the skull should be carefully and periodically evaluated.

Clinical Manifestations and Diagnosis

A noticeable characteristic of a pituitary dwarf is his short but well-proportioned stature. The face may be rather broad with a prominent frontal bone, small nose and underdeveloped mandible. Fine hair and a short neck are also characteristic. Delayed closure at the epiphyseal line occurs. Intelligence is normal.

In doing a diagnostic work-up, growth hormone serum levels can be evaluated by radioimmunoassay. X-ray studies are done to assess skeletal age, which is retarded in pituitary dwarfs. X-rays of the sella turcica may reveal enlargement or calcification; both are signs of a pituitary tumor. An initial screening test will rule out children with normal pituitary growth hormone reserves. In preparation for this test, diethylstilbestrol is administered orally for two or three days before testing. On the day of the test the fasting child's blood is drawn to check for growth hormone levels following a period of forced exercise. A level of GH above 7 ng/ml indicates normal pituitary reserves of growth hormone and eliminates the need for further testing.[1] Nonresponders are hospitalized so that two tests can be done: arginine tolerance test (ATT) and insulin tolerance test. These tests can be done separately or together. First a blood sample is taken on a fasting patient to obtain baseline measurements of GH, glucose and cortisol. Then an IV infusion of insulin is given (0.05 to 0.10 units/kg of body weight). Blood is drawn every 15 minutes until four samples are obtained to check GH and glucose levels; the last sample is used to check the cortisol level.

POTENTIAL STRESSES DURING INFANCY: REVERSIBLE ALTERATIONS IN HEALTH STATUS

The insulin induces hypoglycemia. A normal person responds by increasing his blood levels of growth hormone. This is a potentially dangerous test and should be terminated with a 50 per cent glucose intravenous solution, which should be kept at the bedside during the test to be administered if symptoms of significant hypoglycemia occur. A saline IV line should be kept open for the duration of the test.[1] Various other laboratory tests (thyroid function tests or adrenal function tests) may be done in an attempt to evaluate target gland function as an attempt to implicate pituitary function.

In the arginine test 0.5 gm/kg of L-arginine hydrochloride in an NaCl IV solution is given over 45 minutes. Blood samples are drawn every 15 minutes for 90 minutes to check GH levels. In pituitary growth hormone deficiency, the GH level generally will not exceed 2 ng/ml.

The nursing staff will be closely involved in the diagnostic workup of an infant with growth delay or growth failure. Nursing intervention may include information for parents to help clarify the complex issue of hormonal interactions. While tests are being done to evaluate hormone secretion, nurses will closely observe parent-child interactions, looking for disturbances in these relationships that might contribute to growth failure. Parents may be confused by the endocrine function tests. Parents may be even more concerned if they realize that their nurturing capabilities are being scrutinized. Making accurate observations of all parent-child interactions while providing tactful, positive support to parents requires skill and sensitivity on the part of the nurse.

Nursing Role During Course of Treatment

Treatment of pituitary hypofunction depends on the primary etiology. Tumors are removed surgically or by radiation if possible. The transsphenoidal microsurgery approach is often utilized to avoid the problems inherent in craniotomy. Dysfunction of the posterior pituitary can occur as a postoperative or postradiation complication. A major nursing responsibility is to observe for early symptoms of posterior pituitary dysfunction, diabetes insipidus. Both before and after these procedures the nurse will be responsible for administering endocrine supplementary hormones.

If pituitary function is permanently disrupted, the child will probably remain on hormone medications to correct target organ deficiencies. These may include one or more of the following: corticosteroids, thyroid hormone, sex hormones such as estrogen, and growth hormone. If posterior pituitary function is compromised, vasopressin may also be prescribed. Supplies of growth hormone are not readily available for all who need supplemental therapy, since this hormone can be derived only from cadaver donors. Administration of growth hormone will facilitate growth until the time of epiphyseal fusion.

Parents need to be aware that even though there is an early marked increase in height with growth hormone administration, the child's final height may still fall well below the norm. Ideally administration of this hormone should be started as early as possible, while the potential for growth is greatest. Androgen hormones are sometimes used to produce a growth spurt in older children but require large doses that produce virilizing effects. Corticosteroid doses need to be increased during times of stress, such as illness. Thyroid hormone should not be administered to a child with pituitary hypofunction unless he is also receiving corticosteroids.

In preparing parents for discharge some anticipatory guidance will help them be ready for possible difficulties stemming from their child's immature appearance. Even though the child remains small in stature or immature in appearance, people need to relate to him in a manner appropriate for his chronological age and developmental level. Since body image is an important part of self-esteem, remaining noticeably shorter than peers can be a potential problem, especially for boys. Emphasizing positive areas of achievement may help contribute to the child's developing sense of self.

GIANTISM (HYPERPITUITARY FUNCTION)

Hyperfunction of the pituitary is extremely rare in infants and young children. When there is hyperfunction of the anterior pituitary, increased amounts of growth hormone are secreted, producing a marked increase in tissue growth. If the increased secretion of growth hormone occurs while the child is young, before epiphyseal closure, there is usually an overall proportional increase in height called giantism. If the amount of growth hormone increases after epiphyseal closure, there will be a noticeable increase in growth of soft tissue and in the bones of the face, hands and feet, rather than a vertical gain in height. This is known in adults as acromegaly. Both giantism and acromegaly are rare. Oversecretion of growth hormone usually occurs as a result of a tumor of the anterior pituitary, such as an eosinophilic adenoma.

In addition to the increase in stature or the increased growth of face, hand and feet bones, the size of internal organs increases. Patients also complain of weakness and excessive diaphoresis. Postpubescent girls may have amenorrhea. If the hyperfunction is caused by a tumor, associated symptoms such as headache und visual field losses may be present. X-rays of the skull or a pneumoencephalogram may show evidence of an enlarged sella turcica. X-ray studies indicate normal bone age. Laboratory studies reveal an increase in serum growth hormone. Normally an elevation in serum glucose causes a decrease in serum growth hormone. If the serum level of growth hormone remains elevated after the child receives oral glucose (as in a three-hour glucose tolerance test) then hyperpituitary function may be suspected. Other studies may show glycosuria and a hyperglycemia that does not respond to insulin (insulin resistance), or they may show an increase in serum inorganic phosphorus, increased basal metabolic rate, and normal or decreased free thyroxin (a thyroid hormone).

A major nursing role is casefinding. This is similar to casefinding described for hypopituitary function in terms of the necessity for periodic nursing assessment of height and weight gains on all children. Children with unusual, inexplicable height gains should be referred for evaluation. The earlier the diagnosis is made and treatment begun, the better a child's chances are for a normal life.

No treatment or procedure for giantism or acromegaly is considered ideal. Radiation therapy has been less effective than surgery. A hypophysectomy may be done to remove hyperfunctioning tissue. Nurses need to be alert to possible signs of destruction of normal pituitary functioning as a complication of either radiation or surgery. Alternative treatments have recently been attempted, such as the administration of somatostatin, a hormone that inhibits release of growth hormone.

Symptoms associated with acromegaly and giantism develop over a period of years. Hypertension and organ enlargement may lead to complications such as congestive heart failure and diabetes mellitus. When an infant or child is hospitalized for diagnosis or treatment, the nurse should anticipate his need for increased caloric and fluid intake that occurs as a result of increased growth demands and increased fluid loss through diaphoresis. Urine should be checked for sugar and acetone, and observations for other symptoms of diabetes mellitus should be made. Vital signs should be monitored frequently, as well as other signs of impending heart failure. The nurse should monitor for signs of increasing tumor size, such as visual changes (diplopia, blindness) or headache. Information presented to the child or family can include specifics about scheduled radiation or surgery as well as standard preoperative and postoperative teaching. Since treatment measures may prevent continued further overgrowth but will not reverse growth anomalies already present, psychological support is an important area of nursing concern. Discussing with parents the interdependent relationship between extraordinary appearance and developing self-esteem may help them anticipate potential psychological or social problems.

HYPOTHYROIDISM

Hypothyroidism, occurring in infants and children, includes congenital cretinism and acquired juvenile hypothyroidism. The incidence of cretinism is about one in five thousand newborns.[6] It is probably the most common preventable cause of mental retardation.[3] Hypothyroidism is three times more likely to occur in females.

In the majority of cases of congenital cretinism the infant is born with only rudimentary thyroid tissue. Because of the thyroid's important influence on metabolic processes, the child will develop profound physical and mental retardation unless supplied with supplementary thyroid medication. Hypothyroidism classified as acquired usually does not occur until after the age of 2 years and is caused by damage or destruction of a previously functioning thyroid gland.

Physiology and Pathophysiology The thyroid is located below the cricoid cartilage at the base of the trachea and just lateral to it. This endocrine gland functions to regulate body metabolism by secreting and releasing the hormones thyroxin and triiodothyronine (see Table 24–7). A supply of iodine in the diet is essential for production of thyroxine. Iodine is absorbed from the intestine, circulates and is picked up by the thyroid. With the help of certain enzymes the iodine is converted to a usable form and then combined with tyrosine, an amino acid, to form hormones that are stored in the thyroid in the form of thyroglobin. This stored thyroglobin is acted on by the proteinases of the thyroid to release thyroxine and small amounts of triiodothyronine into the blood as needed. Thyroid activity is stimulated by the anterior pituitary through its secretion of thyroid-stimulating hormone (TSH), also called thyrotropin.

The thyroid hormones thyroxine and triiodothyronine have essentially similar functions but differ in rapidity and in intensity of action. On entering the circulation these hormones combine with circulating plasma proteins, eventually acting on individual cells to increase their metabolic activity. Specific effects of thyroxine are to increase the rate of protein synthesis and catabolism; accelerate growth rate, excite mental activity, excite the activity of other endocrine glands, increase the rate of glucose absorption and utilization, increase fat mobilization and utilization and promote rapid oxidation of fats and carbohydrates.[4] Certain thyroid cells also secrete calcitonin, which assists in regulating serum levels of calcium.

In the absence of thyroid hormones the infant's metabolic rate declines and there is less effective metabolism of fats, proteins, carbohydrates, and vitamins. Body heat control is affected, making the child less able to withstand cold temperatures. Cardiac function is affected; the heart rate, blood pressure and circulation time decline. There is decreased cardiac muscle tone and decreased oxygen requirements secondary to the decreased metabolic rate. Without treatment the hypothyroid infant will develop a markedly short stature (dwarfism), cretinoid facial features (wide anterior fontanel, depressed nasal bridge, open mouth, large protruding tongue), and significant mental retardation.

Etiology Congenital hypothyroidism (cretinism) may be caused by (1) hypoplasia of thyroid tissue due to embryonic defective development or possible autoimmune reaction, (2) metabolic inborn errors such as defective catalytic enzymes that result in defective synthesis of thyroid hormones, or (3) maternal ingestion of antithyroid substances or medications during pregnancy. Women who need to receive treatment for hyperthyroidism should be carefully screened for pregnancy before treatment. Nurses need to know that antithyroid medications can harm the fetus. Nurses working with infants with a family history of hypothyroidism or exposure to thyroid-inhibiting drugs in utero need to observe for symptoms of hypothyroidism.

Juvenile acquired hypothyroidism develops when the child's thyroid gland is damaged or destroyed through surgery, radiation or use of radioiodine or other antithyroid medications, as might be necessitated for treatment of cancer. Thyroid damage can also occur secondary to an autoimmune disorder, a chronic infection or excessive ingestion of goitrogens or iodine. Anterior pituitary dysfunction or hypothalamic dysfunction also leads to decreased thyroid function. Nurses can screen patients for goitrogen ingestion by inquiring whether large amounts of soybean or cabbage are included in the diet, or if there is any dietary supply of iodine such as is found in iodized salt. Excessive ingestion of iodide could occur, for example, when the patient takes iodide for the treatment of asthma. Goitrogenic substances ingested by an expectant mother may cause a transient thyroid depression in the infant but is not a lasting or serious problem.

Nurse's Role in Early Identification The effects of hypothyroidism are completely reversible if the condition is treated early enough. Fisher believes that detection and treatment must occur before the infant is 3 months old if the child is to retain normal intelligence.[3] Observing for early signs of hypothyroidism is a critical nursing function. The presence of three or more signs in the newborn from birth to four days should alert the nurse. These warning signs are:[2]

1. Gestation over 42 weeks and/or birth weight greater than 4 kg (9 lbs).
2. Large posterior fontanel.
3. Respiratory distress.
4. Hypothermia, 35° C or less.
5. Peripheral cyanosis.
6. Hypoactivity, lethargy, poor feeding.
7. Lag in stooling beyond 20 hours of age.
8. Abdominal distention or vomiting or both.

9. Jaundice beyond three days of age.
10. Edema.

Clinical Manifestations and Diagnosis In an older infant the nurse observes for delayed closure of fontanels, delayed appearance of teeth and decreased muscle tone, perhaps manifested by a protuberant abdomen and umbilical hernia. (These symptoms may be noted during the first three months of life.[2]) Because of the lack of thyroxine the muscles contract readily but relax slowly. This may be noted as depressed tendon reflexes. Sometimes the infant with hypotonicity is described as a "floppy baby." During the first three months of the baby's life parents might report that he is lethargic, cries little, sleeps more than usual and tires easily. The cry might be described as hoarse. Feeding problems and constipation persist and the baby fails to demonstrate interest in his environment. His skin may be dry, cool, gray or mottled or all of these. Prominent axillary and supraclavicular fat pads may be noted. As the child grows older more noticeable cretin characteristics appear. Since soft tissue growth proceeds more rapidly than skeletal growth, the young child appears short, obese, and a large tongue is noticeable. The nurse should assess for obvious retardation in growth and mental retardation, cold intolerance, diminished physical activity, poor muscle tone, bradycardia, low blood pressure, diminished pulse pressure, and sluggish circulation. Most of the obvious effects of congenital hypothyroidism are observable by 6 to 9 months of age. If the onset of the hypothyroidism occurs after 2 years of age brain development is less dependent on thyroxine and there will be less serious effect on the child's intelligence.

Because an early diagnosis of congenital hypothyroidism is essential to prevent mental retardation and because the early warning signs are vague, researchers have developed an inexpensive, effective screening test which could be used with the PKU test now legally required in many states. In the screening test for hypothyroidism a small drop of dried blood is spotted on filter paper and analyzed by radioimmunoassay to check for decreased serum thyroxine (T_4) or for an increased serum TSH. (This rises due to hypothalmic-pituitary feedback response to the thyroid hormone deficiency.[3, 6]) Unfortunately this test is not currently in widespread use.

In establishing the diagnosis, tests must be done to differentiate primary thyroid failure from a hypothalamic or pituitary dysfunction.* Basic diagnostic lab tests include tests that indicate low serum thyroxine levels (the T_4 serum concentration) and low erythrocyte T_3 binding. These findings, along with elevated TSH levels, establish a diagnosis of hypothyroidism. In addition to laboratory studies, x-rays are used to evaluate for delayed epiphyseal development (delayed bone age) and epiphyseal dysgenesis (the presence of stippled, fragmented centers of ossification).

The Nurse's Role During Course of Treatment Treatment consists of administration of levothyroxine or desiccated thyroid. Serum T_4 and TSH studies are used as a guide to check the adequacy of the dose. Nurses need to let parents know that results cannot be expected immediately but that they can expect to note an increase in their child's activity level and alertness in 2 to 21 days. As the hypothyroidism begins to respond to exogenous administration of thyroid, the infant will lose his edema. His intake and output should be recorded for the first weeks of therapy along with a daily weight. The nurse must observe for symptoms of thyroid toxicity such as tachycardia, dyspnea, tremors, insomnia and nervousness. Before administering each dose of thyroid the nurse should check for toxicity by monitoring the infant's pulse rate. Parents also need to be taught to observe for signs of insufficient thyroid dosage or symptoms of toxicity. They need to understand that their child will have to take thyroid hormone every day for the rest of his life. Administration of this hormone is best done in the early morning before breakfast.

The nurse caring for children with hypothyroidism needs to carefully evaluate their cardiac status. Vital signs, including blood pressure, need to be monitored frequently. Vagal stimulation should be avoided in children with bradycardia, so enemas and rectal temperatures should be avoided. This child has an increased sensitivity to narcotics and barbiturates. Pulse rate and respiratory status should be monitored before administration of either drug. Nursing interventions to promote comfort include regu-

---

*For in depth discussion refer to the article Thyroid Disorders by Janice Hallal, American Jounrnal of Nursing, March, 1977, p. 422.

lating the temperature of the room and providing adequate clothing to avoid chilling. (Chilling raises metabolic rate and strains the heart.) The tired, weak child needs adequate rest but also needs to turn, to breathe deeply and to move with full range of motion to prevent stasis problems. Providing stool softeners and ample liquids may help reduce constipation. Irritability accompanies decreased thyroid function. Knowing this may help staff and parents cope with a child's behavioral changes.

The infant who receives early and adequate treatment should have a normal life. Parents should be told about the need for periodic, continued medical follow-up. If the diagnosis was delayed, resulting in a lowered IQ, nurses can refer parents to supportive services in the community. Even when the child is mentally retarded, thyroid therapy can achieve remarkable gains in linear growth and amelioration of other cretin characteristics.

References

1. G. Bacon et al. A Practical Approach to Pediatric Endocrinology. Year Book Medical Publishers, 1975
2. M. Chow et al. Handbook of Pediatric Primary Care. John Wiley & Sons, 1979
3. D. Fisher. Screening for congenital hypothyroidism. Hospital Practice, December 1977
4. A. Guyton. Textbook of Medical Physiology. W.B. Saunders Co., 1971
5. W. Hung et al. Pediatric Endocrinology. Medical Examination Publishing Co., Inc., 1978
6. New test to detect hypothyroidism. Public Health Reports, May/June 1977

Additional Recommended Reading

General

P. Butani. Reactions of mothers to the birth of an anomalous infant: a review of the literature. Maternal Child Nursing, Spring, 1974, Vol. 3, No. 1, p. 59

H. M. Farrell. Crises intervention following the birth of a handicapped infant. Journal of Psychiatric Nursing, March 1977, p. 32

E. Hawkins-Walsh. Diminishing anxiety in parents of sick newborns. American Journal of Maternal Child Nursing, Jan/Feb 1980, p. 30

M. J. Kupst et al. Helping parents cope with the diagnosis of congenital heart defect: an experimental study. Pediatrics, February 1977, p. 266

E. H. Waechter. Developmental consequences of congenital abnormalities. Nursing Forum, Vol. 14, No. 2, 1975, p. 108

Cardiac Anomalies

A. Altshuler. Complete transposition of the great arteries. American Journal of Nursing, January 1971, p. 96

K. Andreoli et al. Comprehensive Cardiac Care. C.V. Mosby Co., 1971

J. Apley et al. Impact of congenital heart disease on the family: preliminary report. British Medical Journal, January 1967, p. 103

C. Barnes et al. Measurement in management of anxiety in children for open heart surgery. Pediatrics, February 1972, p. 250

R. Carr. Psychological adaptation to cardiac surgery. In The Child with Congenital Heart Disease After Surgery, B. Kidd and R. Rowe, eds., Futura Publishing Co., Inc., 1976

S. Cassell and M. Paul. The role of puppet therapy on the emotional responses of children hospitalized for cardiac catheterization. Journal of Pediatrics, February 1967, p. 233

R. Cogen. Preventing complications during cardiac catheterization. American Journal of Nursing, March 1976, p. 401

D. Friedberg and L. Caldart. A center for pediatric cardiovascular patients. American Journal of Nursing, September 1975, p. 1480

W. E. Friedman et al. Pharmacologic closure of patent ductus arteriosus in the premature infant. New England Journal of Medicine, September, 1976, p. 526

J. Gildea et al. Congenital cardiac defects: pre- and postoperative nursing care. American Journal of Nursing, February 1978, p. 273

J. Gillon. Continuity in nursing care of cardiac infants. Nursing Clinics of North America, January 1969, p. 19

J. Gillon. Family stresses when a child has congenital heart disease. Maternal Child Nursing Journal, May/June 1972, p. 265

J. Gillon. Behavior of newborns with cardiac distress. American Journal of Nursing, December 1973, p. 254

B. Kidd and R. Rowe. The Child with Congenital Heart Disease after Surgery. Futura Publishing Co., Inc., 1976

M. Kupst, et al. Improving physician-parent communication. Clinical Pediatrics, January 1979, p. 27.

M. Kupst et al. Helping parents cope with the diagnosis of congenital heart defect: an experimental study. Pediatrics, February 1977, p. 266

D. Lloyd. Postoperative nursing care following open heart surgery in children. Nursing Clinics of North America, March 1970, p. 399

A. Moss et al. Heart Disease in Infants, Children, and Adolescents. Waverly Press, 1978

R. Posey. Creative nursing care of babies with heart disease. Nursing '74. October 1974

S. Redo. Principles of Surgery in the First 6 Months of Life. Harper and Row, 1976

F. Roberts. The child with heart disease. American Journal of Nursing, June 1972, p. 1080

A. Rudolph. Congenital Disease of the Heart. Year Book Medical Publishers, 1974

J. Sacksteder et al. Common congenital cardiac defects. American Journal of Nursing, February 1978, p. 266

V. Shor. Congenital cardiac defects assessment and case finding. American Journal of Nursing, February 1978, p. 256

S. Steele. Nursing Care of the Child with Long-Term Illness. Appleton-Century-Crofts, 1971

L. Swendsen. Nursing care of the infant with congestive heart failure. Nursing Clinics of North America, April 1969, p. 621

M. Tesler and C. Hardgrove. Cardiac catheterization: preparing the child. American Journal of Nursing, January 1973, p. 80

K. Uzark. A child's cardiac catheterization — avoiding the potential risks. American Journal of Maternal Child Nursing, May/June 1978, p. 158

D. Vince. Essentials of Pediatric Cardiology. J. B. Lippincott Co., 1974

E. Waechter. Developmental consequences of congenital abnormalities. Nursing Forum, February 1975, p. 108

W. Weidman. Growth, development, and habilitation after cardiac surgery. In The Child with Congenital Heart Disease. After Surgery, B. Kidd and R. Rowe, eds. Futura Publishing Co., Inc., 1976

D. Wise. Crisis intervention before cardiac surgery. American Journal of Nursing, August 1975, p. 1316

Urinary Tract Anomalies and Related Conditions

P. S. Cross. Ureteral reimplantation: nursing care of the child. American Journal of Nursing, November 1976, p. 1800

J. G. Keurnelian and V. E. Sanders. Urologic Nursing. Macmillan, Inc., 1970

Orofacial Anomalies

H. Cooper et al. Cleft Palate and Cleft Lip. W. B. Saunders Co., 1979

W. Grabb et al. Cleft Lip and Palate: Surgical, Dental, and Speech Aspects. Little, Brown & Co., 1970

M. McDermott. The child with cleft lip and palate on the pediatric ward. American Journal of Nursing, April 1965, p. 122

R. Millard. Cleft palate and communication disorders. Ear, Nose and Throat Journal, February 1980, p. 23

R. Millard et al. Nursing care of the patient with cleft lip and palate. Nursing Clinics of North America, September 1967, p. 483

J. Warkany. Congenital malformations. Year Book Medical Publishers, Inc., 1971

Gastrointestinal Tract Anomalies

J. Adkins and W. Kieswetter. Imperforate anus. Surgical Clinics of North America, April 1976, p. 379

A. Brueggemeyer. Omphalocele: coping with a surgical emergency. Pediatric Nursing, Jul/Aug 1979, p. 54

D. Dodgeon et al. Surgical management of acute necrotizing enterocolitis in infancy. Journal of Pediatric Surgery, October 1973, p. 607

A. Fanaroff and M. Klaus. The gastrointestinal tract-feeding and selected disorders. In Care of the High-risk Neonate, M. Klaus and A. Fanaroff, W. B. Saunders Co., 1979

S. Gernaro. Necrotizing enterocolitis: detecting it and treating it. Nursing '80, January 1980, p. 52

M. Guinan et al., Epidemic occurrence of neonatal necrotizing enterocolitis. American Journal of Diseases of Children. June 1979, p. 594

R. Higson. Types of hernias. Nursing Mirror, 24 February 1978, p. 14

K. Jeter. Reality therapy, a realistic approach to enterostomy rehabilitation. Nursing Forum, No. 1, 1978, p. 72

S. Jolley et al. Surgery in children with gastroesophageal reflux and respiratory symptoms. Journal of Pediatrics, February 1980, p. 194

P. K. Kottmeier and D. Klotz. Surgical problems in the newborn. Pediatric Annals, February 1979, p. 93

K. Jones. Love and lavage: the urgent needs of children with Hirschsprung's disease. Nursing '78, July 1978, p. 32

J. McFarland. Hiatal hernia. Nursing Mirror, 14 April 1977, p. 50

J. Mahoney. What you should know about ostomies. Nursing '78, May 1978, p. 74

T. D. Moore, ed. Necrotizing enterocolitis in newborn infant. In Proceedings of 68th Ross Laboratories Conference on Pediatric Research, 1975, p. 28

J. Morton. Abdominal wall hernias. In Principles of Surgery, S. Schwartz, ed., McGraw-Hill Book Co., 1979

S. K. Waggoner. Nursing care of the infant in surgery. American Operating Room Nursing Journal, November 1978, p. 827

M. M. Woolley. Congenital posterolateral diaphragmatic hernia. Surgical Clinics of North America, April 1976, p. 317

D. G. Young and B. F. Weller. Baby Surgery Nursing Management and Care. University Park Press, 1971

Musculoskeletal Anomalies

A. Greenwald and B. Head. Wearing a cast. Family Communications, 1977 Available from Blue Cross/Blue Shield

N. Hilt and E. W. Schmitt, Jr. Pediatric Orthopedic Nursing, C. V. Mosby Co., 1975

N. Hilt. Care of the child in a hip spica cast, RN, April 1976, p. 27

P. Meservey. Congenital musculoskeletal abnormalities. Comprehensive Pediatric Nursing, Nov/Dec 1977, p. 14

Respiratory Infections

B. Hall et al. Clinical and physiological manifestations of bronchiolitis and pneumonia. American Journal of Diseases of Childhood, August 1979, p. 798

M. Kattan. Long-term sequelae of respiratory illness in infancy and childhood. Pediatric Clinics of North America, August 1979, p. 525

E. King. Care of the child hospitalized for treatment of lung disease. In Current Practice in Pediatric Nursing, P. A. Brandt et al., eds., Vol. 11, C. V. Mosby Co., 1978

W. A. Tomlinson. Parents' knowledge of respiratory disease, a comparison of inner-city and suburban parents. Pediatrics, December 1975, p. 1009

Gastroenteritis

S. K. Dube. Metabolic emergencies. In Immediate Care of the Sick and Injured Child. S. K. Dube, ed., C. V. Mosby Co., 1978

G. Keusch. Bacterial diarrhea. American Journal of Nursing, June 1973, p. 1028

A. Silverman et al. Pediatric Clinical Gastroenterology. C.V. Mosby Co., 1975

P. Spitz and H. Sweetwood. Kids in Crisis. Nursing '78, March 1978, p. 70

Neurological Infection and Related Conditions

J. Babineau. Infection control in the neonatal intensive care unit. Issues in Comprehensive Pediatric Nursing, Vol. 2, No 1, May/June 1977, p. 49

D. S. Gaddy. Meningitis in the pediatric population. Nursing Clinics of North America, March 1980, p. 83

B. Langner and J. Schott. Nursing implications of central nervous system infections in children. Issues in Comprehensive Pediatric Nursing. Vol. 2, No. 2, Jul/Aug 1977, p. 38.

W. T. Speck et al. Neonatal infections. In Care of the High-Risk Neonate, M. H. Klaus and A. A. Fanaroff, eds., W. B. Saunders Co., 1978

J. Taylor and S. Ballenger. Neurological Dysfunctions and Nursing Interventions. McGraw-Hill Book Co., 1980

Nutritional Alterations

N. Buergel. Monitoring nutritional status in the clinical setting. Nursing Clinics of North America, June 1979, p. 215

E. Charney et al. Childhood antecedents of adult obesity. New England Journal of Medicine, 1 July 1976, p. 16

D. Craddock. Obesity in childhood and adolescence. In Obesity and Its Management. Churchill-Livingstone, 1978

M. S. Dine et al. Where do the heaviest children come from? A prospective study of white children from birth to 5 years of age. Pediatrics, January 1979, p. 1

A. G. Ferris. The effect of feeding on fat deposition in early infancy. Pediatrics, October 1979, p. 397

J. H. Himes. Infant feeding practices and obesity. Journal of American Dietetic Association, August 1979, p. 122

P. L. Pipes. Nutrition in Infancy and Childhood. C.V. Mosby Co., 1977

J. N. Udall. Interaction of maternal and neonatal obesity. Pediatrics, July 1978, p. 17

A. Whitelaw. Infant feeding and subcutaneous fat at birth and at one year. Lancet, 26 November 1977, p. 1098

P. Worthington. Infant nutrition and feeding techniques. Pediatric Nursing, Jan/Feb 1977, p. 9

Endocrine Alterations

P. Beeson and W. McDermott. Cecil-Loeb Textbook of Medicine. W. B. Saunders Co., 1975

J. Hallal. Thyroid disorders. American Journal of Nursing, March 1977

C. Kempe et al. Current Pediatric Diagnosis and Treatment. Lange Publications, 1978

J. Krueger and J. Ray. Endocrine Problems in Nursing: A Physiologic Approach. C. V. Mosby Co., 1976

M. Krupp and M. Chatton. Current Medical Diagnosis and Treatment. Lange Publications, 1979

25

POTENTIAL STRESSES DURING INFANCY: IRREVERSIBLE ALTERATIONS IN HEALTH STATUS

by Ellen Christian, RN, MS, and Judith Clark, RN, MSN

An irreversible alteration in infant health status consists of an enduring disease process that can be progressively debilitating or associated with a relatively normal life span despite impaired physical or mental functioning. Although each specific condition may vary in severity, collectively they have one common area of concern in relation to the goals of nursing management — *promotion of optimal levels of individual and family functioning.* The nursing interventions pertinent to the effect of irreversible alterations on family coping, infant growth and development and specific body system functioning are presented in this chapter.

IMPACT OF DIAGNOSIS: THE NURSE'S ROLE

All pregnant couples have fears concerning the health of their unborn baby. As the time draws closer to delivery, most parents replace their wishes regarding the sex of their unborn child with concern about its health. The question most frequently asked first at delivery is "Does the baby seem OK?" Considering the odds of producing a child with a defect (except for those couples with known genetic predisposition), all couples have the right to expect a healthy, perfect newborn.

When a baby is born with an identifiable irreversible condition, all people involved (health personnel as well as parents) are stunned by and feel helpless in the situation. Because of their discomfort, the medical and nursing personnel alter their approaches to the parent(s) by limiting conversation, avoiding eye contact and decreasing the frequency of physical interactions. These nonverbal clues suggest that something is wrong and leave the parent reluctant to ask for information and support. A sense of frustration and powerlessness can cause the nurse to feel immobilized and incompetent. For the parents, the diagnosis of a defective child is a loss — a loss of the perfect, healthy child they had every right to expect and anticipate. Whether the condition is minor and reversible or severe and irreversible, the parents need to grieve over the loss of the perfect baby. Understanding the tasks that parents must face in order to cope with their situation will improve the effectiveness of the nurse's attempts to help them.

To parents a child represents an extension of one's self and to produce normal offspring is psychologically important for a positive self-concept.[12] A loss of self-esteem is experienced at the birth and diagnosis of an imperfect child. Furthermore, producing a child with a defect is especially painful to families in a culture such as in the United States, where a high value is placed on success, beauty and perfection. When parents learn that their infant has a defect, they experience disappointment, despair and sorrow over the loss of their perfect child. The response is similar to the reaction parents have to the death of a child and will occur even when the diagnosis is made after the newborn period.

It must be emphasized that the manner in which individual parents and families grieve over their loss and manage subsequent adjustment is individually unique and must be viewed from that perspective. Their previous experiences in coping with stress, the stability of the husband's and wife's relationship, the developmental level of the family, the support from the extended family and community, and financial stability are factors that influence the ability to cope and thereby maintain family equilibrium.

The initial response in the process of grieving is shock and disbelief. Parents feel numb and unable to think clearly. They frequently do not hear, understand or believe what is being said. As awareness progresses, anger and bitterness may be expressed. Parental anger may be directed at the nurse or other health team members. It usually stems from the powerlessness parents sense at not being able to change the course of events. Parents may believe that a stigma has been placed on them and that life has dealt them an unfair blow. They may be envious of others with normal children.

Parents may begin to express feelings of helplessness, despair and anxiety. They also experience feelings of guilt and seek a rational explanation for why their child has a problem. This searching and "shopping around" is probably an effort to assume some control over an otherwise hopeless set of circumstances. Some grieving over the loss of the perfect child will continue indefinitely.

The parents of an infant with a long-term disabling alteration experience all phases of the grief process and at the same time must cope with the impact and reality of the chronicity of their child's condition. Such "chronic sorrow"[19] poses stresses on family functioning long after the crisis of diagnosis is resolved. It may be unlikely that this child will achieve the important life goals that family and society normally expect. There is no escape, and the commitment to the child with an irreversible condition is a lifelong stress. The realization that the infant will not have a normal life span or be able to procreate intensifies the parents' sorrow. In the face of such loss and incongruence, family members frequently respond by feeling individually alienated and powerless. The resulting disequilibrium causes distortions in family relationships that ultimately necessitate a permanent alteration in family roles and goals.

Chronic sorrow, however, does not imply that parents are unable to meet the needs of their defective infant or to receive satisfaction from him. Again, it must be stressed that the manner and success of coping is unique to each family. Many parents exhibit great strength, and they will struggle both to assimilate the facts and to gain control over their situation. In fact, given half a chance, most families will compensate in all kinds of ways to counteract the insult to their self-esteem and to establish equilibrium. "Half a chance" for many families may very well be the appropriate and skillful intervention provided by the nurse.

Supporting the Parents of an Infant with a Defect

The nurse can help families achieve the following goals:
1. Sustain the health and life of the child;
2. Promote development of the child's and the whole family's optimal potential;
3. Promote family equilibrium so that the child is a welcome and integral member of the family.[9]

While there is no recipe that guarantees success in helping parents to meet these goals, the following presentation offers some specific suggestions for the nurse to consider in the planning of care during the family's various stages of coping with loss and subsequent integration of the disabled child.

When the parents are first advised of the infant's condition, it is recommended that the parents and infant be present together and that the "telling" occur as soon as possible after delivery. Parents are quick to suspect a problem. When there is a delay in presenting the facts of the situation, parents frequently fantasize a defect in the child far more serious than the reality. The infant should be undressed in the presence of the parents so that they can view the total child, as normal characteristics and strengths as well as the defect are pointed out. Anticipating that the parents' response will be that of shock and disbelief, the manner in which the condition is explained is critical in determining future communication with health team members. Parents should be given only brief, clear, basic information at first and this will need to be presented slowly and repeated several times. Furthermore, it is imperative that no conflicting information be presented, since this only compounds the crisis by adding confusion. Ultimately, when parents ask for clarification or more information, it is an indication that they are ready to assimilate more. Probably the best way to prevent unnecessary confusion is to designate one nurse as the coordinator of the family's care. Preferably it should be a nurse who has experience in working with families going through the grieving process and who also has some background in the care of children with the particular defect.

The principle of one professional working as a primary intervener to whom the family can turn for counselling and coordination of planned services is particularly applicable when care is required on a long-term basis. Parents can understand, cooperate and participate in long-term goal planning when they can relate to one person in an atmosphere of consistency and acceptance.

Initially, parents may not feel comfortable enough to touch their baby and should not be rushed to move toward acceptance. What appears to be an initial lack of acceptance may be related to the parents' need to offset the enormous blow to their self-concept.[19] The nurse, on the other hand, may inadvertently suppress the emerging grief response and hinder the acceptance process. For example, on the inaccurate premise that they can "protect" a mother from emotional pain, some nurses might:

1. Separate the mother of the infant with a defect from mothers of normal infants;
2. Keep the baby at the back of the nursery away from the windows;
3. Make meaningless remarks such as: "You can always have another baby," "You have healthy children at home," "It's God's will," "You'll get over it,";
4. Tell parents that the grief they are feeling is due to the loss of an expected perfect infant;
5. Decrease the number and duration of interactions with parents so that they have an opportunity for "privacy."

These inappropriate and possibly detrimental remarks and actions demonstrate avoidance and withdrawal mechanisms, which come from the nurse's own feelings of grief, uncertainty and sense of helplessness. Inability to recognize one's own grieving process and its associated painful and threatening feelings may render the nurse unable to respond appropriately. Inadequate communication and intervention is an unfair load to impose on an already burdened family.

A nurse will learn that she often cannot share a person's grief and sorrow with words. Instead, just being near the grieving person(s), sharing moments of silence and allowing time for them to absorb the truth is most helpful. Usually the parents appreciate the nurse's presence and are grateful when she does not fill the silence with meaningless words. Further, the nurse must realize that when her own anxiety levels are high, she should take the time to replenish her energy and discuss her feelings with supportive colleagues. With self-understanding the nurse can then plan interventions that will facilitate

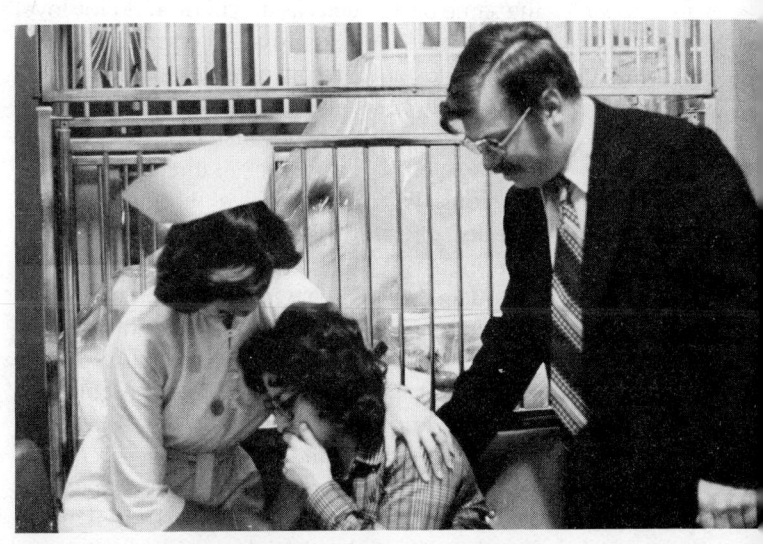

Just being near is often the most supportive nursing action for grieving parents.

> Nursing means being involved in relationships and making commitments to people. This involvement and commitment leaves the nurse vulnerable to the suffering of others. When caring for parents who are grieving, it is normal to share in the grieving process. It is hardly possible for the involved nurse not to feel angry or depressed, not to display emotions and not to experience sorrow and frustrations. Nurses need to understand that they may very well be dealing with their own grief along with that of the parents. Recognizing the process in one's self and accepting it as normal will permit the nurse to intervene in a more spontaneous, genuine and honest manner.

parental movement through the stages of grief following the initial shock of the diagnosis.

If the diagnosis occurs at birth, the nurse makes frequent visits to the mother's hospital room to lend her presence and support, offering a cup of coffee and a back rub, knowing that her presence gives the family the courage they need to manage grief. At the same time, the nurse looks for clues that the parents may be ready to reach out to their infant. The nurse should then institute steps to promote parental-infant bonding. When, in front of the parents, the nurse calls the infant by name, cuddles him and talks to him about his normal characteristics and strengths, she acts as a role model for the parents and communicates that this child has the same basic needs as all children do for love, security and room to grow. All efforts should be made to foster family involvement in child care. It is usually best to help parents begin to care for the infant's normal needs first and teach special care related to the defect as their confidence develops. Providing positive reinforcement of parents' efforts to participate in their infant's care increases their confidence, helps to foster adequate coping behaviors and promotes family satisfaction about caring for their child. When parents see that others are not repulsed by the infant, that they themselves have the ability to care for him and can accept the support of significant others, the prospect for successful bonding is enhanced. When the diagnosis occurs after the neonatal period, attachment may have been developed, providing a base for dealing with the grief reaction.

Sometimes, however, the parents' efforts at bonding are thwarted by the fact that the infant may be unable to respond to the interaction. This is particularly evident with infants who have visual, auditory and central nervous system disorders. The parents of these children will need a great deal of support and understanding in order to continue to reach out for their infant over and over again. These babies will eventually respond to their parents' efforts in their own unique ways, and once they are reached will begin to participate in the parent-child communication cycle in a more mutually satisfying way.[3]

Once parents become attached to their infant, they are then faced with the chronic fear of losing him. This becomes apparent each time the child is hospitalized or faces an upset in physical status. Nurses will observe that under these circumstances parents will again go through the grieving process. At such times parents will frequently feel the need for time and space to withdraw temporarily in order to regain courage.

HABILITATION: THE NURSE'S ROLE

In order to establish and maintain family equilibrium and develop the maximum potential of

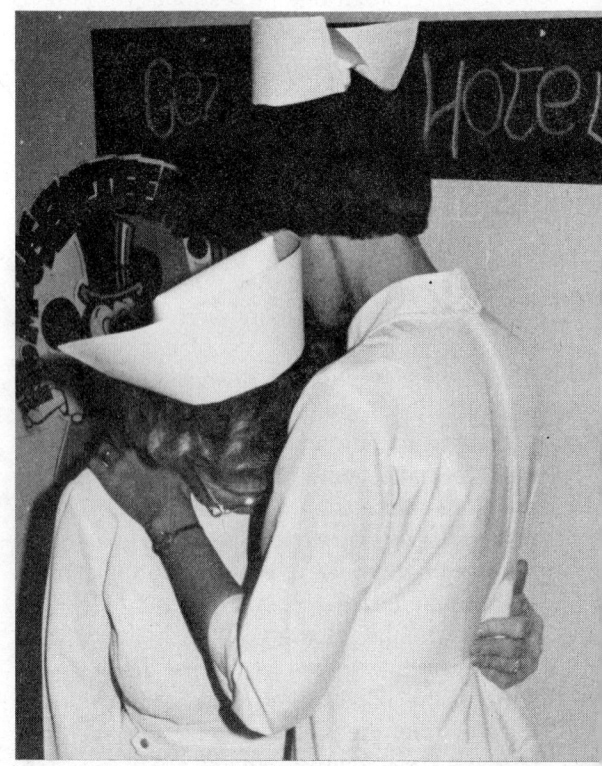

The nurse also grieves and needs the support of her colleagues.

the affected infant, the family will need information and various resources for a long time. In the past many families were left isolated with their problems. Today, it can frequently be just the opposite. There are so many available services and programs, each addressing a particular specialty area, that parents often find themselves overwhelmed in trying to decide which route to take. Again, one professional primary intervener helping parents sort and sift and feel competent to make satisfying decisions is important. Considering the fact that some families will be needing the professional services of physicians, nurses, social service workers, psychologists, nutritionists and others, a person to coordinate services and maintain interdisciplinary communication is a must. Parents cannot do it alone.

The crisis of prolonged childhood illness poses strains on the resources of the parents. Often it is difficult to find babysitters for their infant, particularly if there are feeding problems or visible alterations from the norm. Or the parents themselves may hesitate to leave their baby. This in turn will lead to isolation, which further strains the interaction of family members. These parents need time away from their handicapped infant and need to spend time with each other as a couple. Often the parents feel that there is little energy left for each other after caring for the affected infant. They may disagree over management of the child's care and about expectations they should have. These couples are in real danger of having marital problems. In addition, some parents have little awareness of their function in promoting positive infant growth and development. It is unlikely that such families can utilize professional services for maximum benefit of themselves or their child. A thorough family assessment is the basis for planning effective nursing care for infants with irreversible abnormalities.

Current literature has identified some specific characteristics of families that relate to their ability to adapt to chronic illness. Lawson has developed an assessment tool called the scale for detecting families at risk of adapting poorly to chronic illness in the child. (See p. 290 for this scale.) It is helpful in predicting which families are particularly vulnerable. Based on the collected data, the nurse can alter the priority ranking of services offered to these families to accommodate the need for early counselling. When parents' needs are adequately met, they are more able to seek and continue receiving services for the disabled child.

The nurse also gathers data about the infant's environment. Caldwell's HOME assessment tool is useful when measuring factors and relationships in the home environment that affect infant development. (See Appendix III for Caldwell's tool.) The information obtained from a home assessment is helpful in planning and implementing an early intervention program for the infant and his family.

Almost all parents of disabled children can benefit from involvement in a community support group. Being a member of a support group allows parents to understand and work through some of their ambivalence, confusion and anger in a nonthreatening environment. Family members are more able to understand each other's reactions and behaviors and verbalize their feelings. This in turn promotes a stronger basis for family members to support each other and work together. Many parents can also benefit from therapeutic family counselling services.

At this point it is well to consider that in some circumstances, preserving family integration means removing the affected child from the family system. Many nurses are quick to judge such action as heartless and unfeeling without stopping to consider that this difficult decision may be based on the family's recognition of the physical and emotional resources that are available for each family member. This family needs to be listened to and supported — not judged.

The child with an irreversible condition may be unable to perform age-stage related tasks. Subsequently, a younger sibling chronologically becomes an older one developmentally. Jealousy, insecurity, resentment and adjustment may be problems for them. It is important that the normal children be allowed to develop their own identity and abilities and be helped to understand the differences and similarities between them and their disabled sibling. Group sessions for siblings to get together to ventilate feelings about their roles and responsibilities are helpful. Often these sessions can be part of school health education and will usually incorporate the expertise of the school nurse.

Unfortunately, many children with irreversible alterations are reared in an overprotected environment that frequently imposes secondary handicaps and reduces the chances of the child to achieve independence. Instead, efforts to habilitate the child should be aimed at preventing interference of the disability and the associated treatment regimen with the child's social, mental, emotional, spiritual and physical development. Programs to foster optimal level of functioning in each of these areas must be started early — within the first five years — since this is the critical period of cognitive, emotional and social growth. The planning of an appropriate infant stimulation program depends upon accurate, ongoing assessments of the infant's developmental level. A variety of assessment tools is available to assist in conducting systematic evaluation of the infant's function. Periodic assessments must be done in the home as well as in the clinical setting. Some frequently used tools are:

1. The Denver Developmental Screening Test (DDST). This screening tool yields a developmental profile of an infant or child in terms of his gross motor, fine motor, adaptive, language and personal-social skills. If delays in these areas are identified, further specific developmental evaluation is indicated. The DDST is useful in evaluating the progress of a developmental stimulation program. (See Chapter 13 for DDST.)

2. The Brazelton Neonatal Behavioral Assessment Scale. This is an assessment scale that can be used to determine the newborn's developmental level as well as to demonstrate the infant's unique way of responding to stimulation, given by skilled workers. The emphasis of the scale is on the infant's neurological status, motor behaviors, states or moods and interactions with the environment. It is a valuable tool in that it helps parents identify the individuality of their newborn. There are many other tools available for developmental assessment.

The nurse in conjunction with other health professionals develops an individualized, home-centered plan for early intervention based on the developmental and family assessment. How the parents perceive their infant and his problems is an appropriate starting place. Asking what they believe is their most difficult problem in managing their baby at home and what they would like to be able to do for him gives clues to their goals. If parental goals are inappropriate, the nurse must devise a plan to help clarify and adjust these goals before attempting to initiate a developmental stimulation program. Parental understanding of their ability and role in influencing the infant's development is critical in promoting an optimal learning environment. Consistent stimulation is required for central nervous system development and function, and during early development there seems to be a critical period after which potential neural development is irretrievably lost.[4] Because of inadequate bonding or cultural views, some families cannot accept the explanation that they are vitally important in determining the nature of parent-infant relationships. They feel powerless to change their infant's behavior. Parents need to be given the opportunity to express and gradually work through these feelings before the nurse can expect their full participation in a program to stimulate infant development.

An early intervention program should emphasize social interaction and perceptual and motor experiences. All suggested activities should coincide with the family's life style. Family members are encouraged to carry out the program as it best fits into their schedules and not set aside specific stimulation times. Activities should be fun and not work.

Specific activities included in a developmental program should be chosen carefully. They should be experiences that elicit definite behaviors in the areas of gross motor, fine motor, language, social and self-help developmental skills.[29] In early infancy only one sensory mode should be stimulated at a time. The immature or abnormal nervous system has difficulty integrating more than one source of sensory input. Talking to the infant while dangling a bright toy in front of him is an example of a nonselective sensory overload. Both behaviors are appropriate but should not be offered at the same time. Each sensory mode (visual, auditory, tactile, proprioceptive) should be addressed in a stimulation program. Vestibular receptors that are stimulated by rocking should be included, also. Rocking inhibits crying and promotes visual alertness, a significant infant response that permits attending to other stimuli.[3]

The intensity of the stimulus should be sufficient to gain the infant's attention but not to overwhelm him. The infant paying attention is alert, inhibits his motor activity and displays changes in heart rate. Repeated stimuli must be altered slightly, since they tend to lose their impact. This novelty factor appears to be a primary component of successful interventions. Simple stimuli, frequently changed, are most important. Bright balls, stuffed animals, rattles, bells and the human face are inexpensive, readily available stimuli. Slow rocking, moving at different speeds and the use of front or back pack carriers provide important body contact for the infant. Natural stimuli that occur in the infant's environment should be incorporated into the stimulation program. Feeding provides a variety of exposures to textures, tastes and temperatures and an opportunity for motor patterning, which is an effort to promote development of motor coordination and skill through repetitive movements. The human voice saying the child's name can be effective in encouraging visual and social behaviors such as smiling. More complex stimuli, carefully introduced, promote further integration of sensory information. The Developmental Stimulation Suggestion Chart (Table 25-1) contains specific age-appropriate activities.

One of the nurse's tasks in planning an early intervention program is to identify not only the infant's current level of functioning but also cues that indicate readiness to accept new experiences that will promote higher levels of development. This approach dictates periodic reassessment of the infant and the family. Nurses should see that parents are provided with written as well as verbal instructions. Return demonstrations are helpful in developing parents' confidence and evaluating their competence in interacting with their infant.

It is understandable that parents can become discouraged by the lack of positive feedback they receive from their infants, even when they faithfully pursue the stimulation program. They need support and encouragement to recognize their infant's subtle but significant developmental gains. For the infant, the natural teachers are his parents, the natural place is his home and the natural tools for learning are toys. A commitment to that belief by all involved in the program is necessary for success.

Additional needs that parents and health care professionals must consider in the long-term planning are:
1. An appropriate health and education program, one that is part of the existing school and community so that they are not separated from their world;
2. Anticipatory guidance based on the fact that, like normal children, those with long-term disabilities have developmental crises and developmental lags;
3. Discipline, including reasonable and realistic restrictions and demands such as chores that must be done;
4. Development of independent functioning in relation to activities of daily living. Self-help tasks must be mastered one at a time.

Nurses can make a stronger effort to educate the public regarding disabling conditions in infants. Old wives' tales and myths cause many people in our society to react to handicapped children with pity. What is needed instead is a sense of acceptance of the total child as he is, regardless of an abnormality or defect, and an environment that supports realistic hopes and plans.

Parenting an infant with an irreversible alteration from the norm is a stress-producing situation, but it also has the potential for promoting growth. Children can and do learn to live with a disability, but they cannot develop to their fullest potential without feeling that significant others find them lovable. If the child feels loved and accepted as an infant, he can believe that others will also love him throughout his life. With this conviction he can live well today and have faith about the years to come.[12]

ALTERED HEALTH STATES

The specific irreversible alterations in health status presented in the following section illustrate the comprehensive nature of chronic disease and its management. Although the discussion is organized according to the major body systems that chronic diseases alter, their effects extend to the functioning of other systems, influencing both infant competency development and family adjustment. For example, an infant with exstrophy of the bladder has an alteration in urinary function. The anterior abdominal wall and bladder fail to fuse in the midline during fetal development and the defect results in exposure of the lower urinary tract, the ureters, bladder and urethra. Urine seeps continuously from the exposed ureteral outlets onto the abdomen. While primarily a defect of the urinary tract, the reproductive system is greatly affected because of its close proximity. The abnormal genitalia require surgical reconstruc-

TABLE 25-1 DEVELOPMENTAL STIMULATION SUGGESTION CHART

Area of Stimulation	1	2	3	4	5	6	7	8

Communication and Sound	Call child by name
	Use complete words and sentences, no baby talk
	Tell child what you are doing. Name objects used
	Parents should work together in all areas
	Leave with babysitter occasionally
	    Bells on wristlets and shoes (sew bells on with dental floss)
	  Sing to child
	    Encourage smiling. Encourage laughing
	Play radio in crib softly for short periods
	Introduce all kinds of sounds: running water, musical toys, household equipment, rattles, whistles
				Talk loud, soft, high pitch, low pitch and whisper
				  Pat-a-cake
				  Peek-a-boo
				  Repeat child's sounds to him
					Praise language attempts
					  Hide and seek (parent and toys)
					  With family at mealtime
					Toys to hold that make noise
					Finger and toe games
					Single objects scrapbook
					  Mother names pictures in book		

Touch and Smell	Cuddling, holding close, kissing, stroking
	Rub with different textures: cotton, silk, feathers, sandpaper, wood, yarn, etc.
	Introduce smell of fruit, vegetables, cereal, perfumes, soaps, flowers, spices, etc. Continuous experiences
	  Rub vigorously with towel after bath
				Warm, cold, hard, soft
				In kitchen during cooking time
				  Finger foods			

Sight	Feed and change from both sides
	Move crib around room
	Move infant to different rooms, by windows
	Single bright object mobile 8-9 inches from eyes
	  Change mobile weekly
	  Hand mitts
	  Move objects in air in arc and circle for eyes to follow
	Bright sheets, blankets, pillow cases, and clothing
				Multiple object mobile 12-15 inches from eyes
				Change mobile weekly
						Mirror play
						  Tie balloons on wrists and feet
							Alternate toy selection: divide toys into 2-3 groups. Change groups every 2-3 weeks

Gross Motor	Exercise arms and legs while bathing
	  Situps
	  On mat on floor
	On abdomen, hard surface
	  Stimulate to raise head
	Infant seat
	  Sitting position, short periods
				Outdoors daily as weather permits
				Rolling over and over
				  Tilting in all directions
				Swing in blanket
				Bounce on bed
					On beach ball on tummy; rock back and forth
					Support while sitting—sitting alone
					Work for objects out of reach
					  Rough housing with dad and family members
					  Swimming instruction if available
						Belly board	Ride on parents shoulders
							Large blocks
							Play airplane

Fine Motor	Objects of various textures
	  Bring hands together midline, around bottle
	  Bright objects and sounds for eyes to follow
				Hold objects in hands (grasp and release)
				Reach for small objects
							Banging blocks, lids, pans
							Kitchen items for toys

Feeding	Make mealtime relaxed and pleasant
	Bottle suck and swallow
	  Cereal
	  Strained foods
		Good variety of tastes
		Fruit
			Vegetables	Dinners, Egg yolk, Meats (Iron foods)
				  More coarse foods
				  Offer cup
					Finger foods: crackers, cereal, toast.
					Dip fingers into foods, bring to mouth		

Toileting								

Determine the developmental level of the child using the Denver Developmental Screening Tool or another tool. Use the stimulation suggestions appropriate for the child's level of development in each area.
*Use these suggestions according to the child's chronological age as much as possible.

*Reproduced with permission from C. Eddington and T. Lee. © 1975. American Journal of Nursing Company. Reproduced with permission from the American Journal Nursing. January, Vol. 75 No. 1.

TABLE 25-1 DEVELOPMENTAL STIMULATION SUGGESTION CHART (Continued)

9	10	12	14	16	20	24	30	36

- Toy phone
- Listen to real phone
- Single words for foods, toys, names
- Name and point to body parts
- Read simple stories
- Please, thank you
- Blowing games
- Use plurals
- Put two words together
- Games with others
- Say word for object desired
- Child names pictures
- Simple how, why of daily activities
- Puppet play
- Pretending other people, objects, animals
- Basic colors
- Opposites
- Learning to share

With family at mealtime

Animal sounds

Follow simple directions

Child points to pictures

Child fills in words in stories
Teach name, address

Feel and smell bushes, trees and flowers, grass, snow, etc.
Allow exploration within limits of safety

Encourage child to return affection

Floor objects in motion: cars, lawn mowers, planes, etc.

Alternate toy selection:
  Divide toys into 2-3 groups
  Change groups every 2-3 weeks

Hang bulletin board instead of pictures in child's room
Change board pictures often. Use large, single object pictures. Texture pictures, encourage touching

Concepts of shapes
Form box

Teach names of colors

Ride on parents' shoulders
Mirror on crib top
Outdoor swing— supported
Crawling on a variety of surfaces: floor, carpet, lawn, sand pile
Knee standing
Dropping and throwing games

Rocking horse, Sleigh rides, stroller, etc. In motion

Push and pull toys
Opportunities to help around house
Outdoor swing
Stair walking
Balance on one foot
Jumping games—imitate animals
Tricycle

Remove clothes

Fetch and carry
Encourage walking. Hold back of shirt
Walk on variety of surfaces: grass, mattress, sidewalk, etc.

Climbing
Play ball   Walking backwards

Broad jump
Wading pool with supervision
Somersaults

Stepping stones or similar

Walking games: well defined track
Follow the leader
Play with large cardboard box

Dresses self with help—without help

Staging blocks, lids, pans, kitchen items for toys
Tape on fingers to pull off

Cloth doll

Put things in and out of boxes, etc.
(helps with visual coordination)
Water play

Sand box with spoons, buckets, cars, strainers, etc.
Transporting objects

Opens, shuts, explores functions
Paper and crayons
Copy line
Finger paints
Put on shoes, not tied
Wash and dry hands

Tower with cubes
Quiet or busy book

Busy board   Setting table

Long, short, big, little
Copy circle
Bridge with blocks
Clay

Feels all kinds of food (raw and cooked) mush, dough, vegetables, fruit, liquids, etc.
Wants to know what everything will do splashing, stirring, pouring

Table foods
Attempt spoon feeding by child
Use bowl instead of plate
Offer cup often

Feed self and drink from cup
Brush teeth with help
Wean from bottle—omit one at a time till totally taking fluids from cup

Gradually learns neatness and table manners
Don't push
Drink from straw

Brushing teeth alone

See dentist

Watch for regularity in bowel movements
Put child on potty when BM expected
Praise for success, ignore failure
Use correct words for body functions
Use same words each time child goes to potty

Watch for readiness for urination training
1. Fairly regular urination
2. Holds urine 2½ hours
3. Bothered by wet diaper
Keep a written record of urination for 2-3 weeks
Put child on potty when urination is expected
Praise for success, ignore failure

Don't get child up at night to potty. Praise for staying dry at night

POTENTIAL STRESSES DURING INFANCY: IRREVERSIBLE ALTERATIONS IN HEALTH STATUS

tion and the child may never be capable of reproduction. Thus, a defect in one body system interferes with the functioning of another and inherently carries psychosocial alterations to which the child and family must adjust. Families whose infants have limitations affecting reproductive capabilities experience a high degree of loss and chronic sorrow.[12]

Amelia is an alteration from the norm in which the infant has absent or severely deformed extremities. It is primarily a defect of the musculoskeletal system. This highly visible defect affects physical competency — initially the development of hand-to-mouth exploration and later the achievement of locomotion. The family's reaction to this defect and the coping behaviors they display largely affect the child's adjustment to life with artificial arms or legs. Although these two conditions are very different in terms of the body systems affected, both exstrophy of the bladder and amelia produce long-term effects on every area of individual and family life.

Alterations in Central Nervous System Functioning

Spina Bifida Incomplete fusion of one or more vertebral laminae, with or without defective development of the spinal cord, is termed *spina bifida* (Fig. 25–1). It is a defect of neural tube development, occurring between the 3rd and 11th week of gestation. When the neural defect does not have external involvement it is called *spina bifida occulta*. *Spina bifida cystica* refers to neural anomaly that involves an external protrusion or sac. If the sac-like structure contains no spinal cord (will transilluminate with light), it is a *meningocele*. When spinal cord is present, a meningomyelocele (not translucent; also called *myelomeningocele*) exists that, left untreated, is incompatible with life. The location of the anomaly and the degree of neural involvement determine the long-term effects of spina bifida. Most of the spina bifida defects are located in the lumbar or lumbosacral region.

Etiology The actual cause of the neural tube's failure to close is unknown. Viruses, radiation and environmental factors have been implicated.

In 1972 Brock and Sutcliffe first described the relationship between elevated alpha-fetoprotein (AFP) levels in amniotic fluid and the presence of lesions of the cranium and spine. Mothers who have previously delivered a child with a defect such as spina bifida are considered at risk because the possibility of having another child with such an anomaly is considerably higher than in the general population. Since the presence of AFP can be ascertained at the 14th week of gestation, high-risk expectant parents should be aware that amniocentesis is available and, depending upon its results, may wish to consider elective abortion.[18]

Clinical Manifestations and Diagnosis Spina bifida occulta involves a failure of the spinal processes to merge posteriorly, usually in the lumbosacral area. There may be no obvious manifestations, resulting in no diagnosis unless it is discovered during a routine x-ray. Superficial signs may be present singly or in combination. They include a dimpling at the point where a dermal sinus tract outlet exists, dark tufts of hair in the involved region, port wine angiomatous nevi, and soft lipomas just under the cutaneous skin layer. Neuromuscular involvement occasionally exists that produces gait disturbances or bowel and bladder sphincter disturbances of varying severity, or both.

Spina bifida cystica deformities that result in permanent health alterations are recognizable at birth because of the herniation that produces a thin external cyst-like, membranous sac through which spinal fluid may leak and which may or may not contain neural roots, depending on the type of defect. Spina bifida cystica with meningocele results when the sac contains meninges and cerebrospinal fluid. Meningomyelocele is the form of spina bifida cystica that exists when a portion of the spinal cord and its neural roots have also protruded into the sac.

The majority occur in the lumbosacral region, producing motor dysfunction and sensory disturbances. With meningomyelocele, the spinal cord adhesions and subsequent traction results in paralysis below the level of the defect. The legs are most severely affected and appear either flaccid or spastic. Clubfoot is present as well as some flexion contractures of the hips and extension contractures of the knees. The bilateral roots of the pelvic nerves, which carry both motor and sensory fibers controlling micturition and anal sphincter function, are affected in varying degrees. In general, the lower

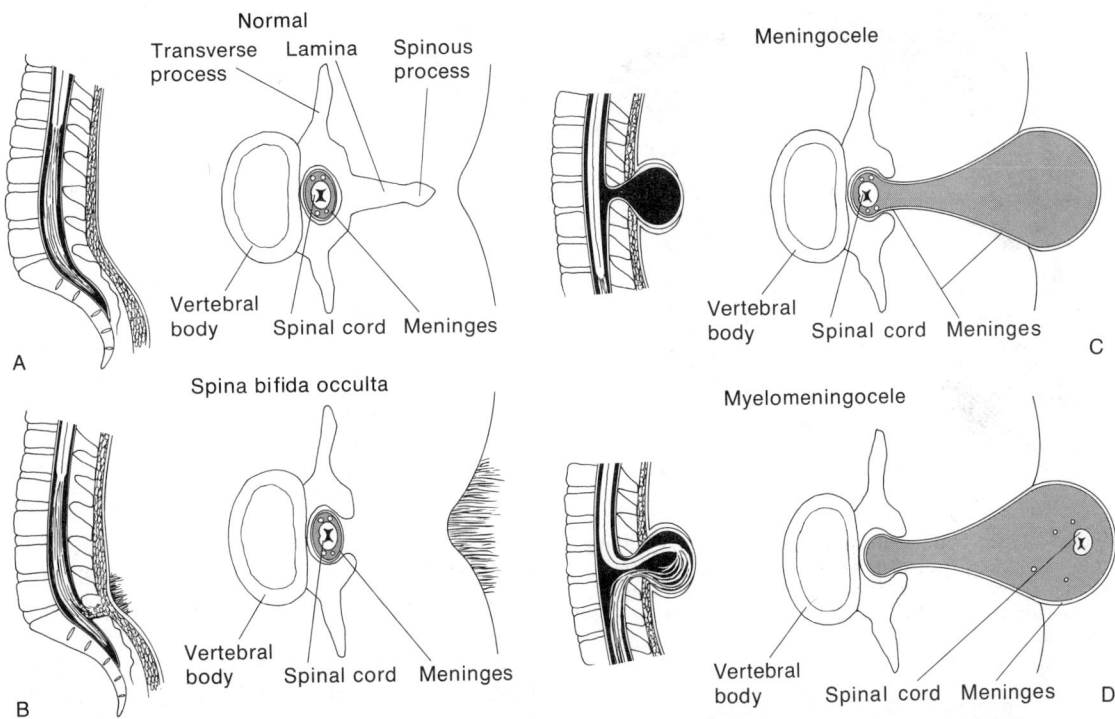

Figure 25–1 Spina bifida. *A*, Normal spinal and vertebral configuration. *B* illustrates spina bifida occulta, in which there is incomplete vertebral fusion but without external involvement. *C* is meningocele, in which there is external protrusion containing no spinal cord. *D* illustrates myelomeningocele, in which spinal cord is present within the sac-like protrusion.

extremities develop poorly and there is little or no protective sensation in the legs.

Diagnostic techniques are aimed at establishing the extent of neural involvement. For example, transillumination of the sac may reveal that only the meninges are protruding (meningocele) or may indicate that neural roots are contained in the sac (meningomyelocele). X-rays may be employed to more precisely identify the area involved in symptomatic defects and to verify diagnosis in suspected nonsymptomatic occult spina bifida.

Management of Spina Bifida Cystica Usually surgical intervention is indicated. How soon the surgery will be performed may vary. Early surgery will reduce the susceptibility to meningitis and prevent further neural traction. Later surgery, however, may allow for a better assessment of the neural function that can be preserved.

Preoperatively and immediately postoperatively the focus of nursing care planning is based upon prevention of infection (meningitis), prevention of trauma, maintenance of adequate hydration and electrolyte balance, observation of signs of increased intracranial pressure, implementation of appropriate passive exercises and encouragement of parental interaction.

In order to prevent infection and irritation of the defect and at the same time promote adequate observation, the infant should be left uncovered. Therefore, the child is placed in a temperature-controlled environment such as an incubator or warmer in order to maintain his body temperature at 36.5° C. Diapers are not applied to avoid contamination of the sac or operative site by urine and stool. Dry sterile dressings, sterile saline dressings or topical applications of antibiotic solutions or ointments are applied to the sac. Trauma to the sac is prevented by avoiding tension and pressure on the defect. Careful positioning and handling of the infant is necessary (Fig. 25–2). How large the myelomeningocele is and where it is located determines the options in positioning. The infant may be placed on his abdomen or in a side-lying position provided that the sac does not rest on the mattress. The use of a waterbed is helpful in reducing pressure and managing some positional restrictions.

When lifting the child, one of the nurse's hands should support the infant's buttocks and extremities while the other hand and forearm

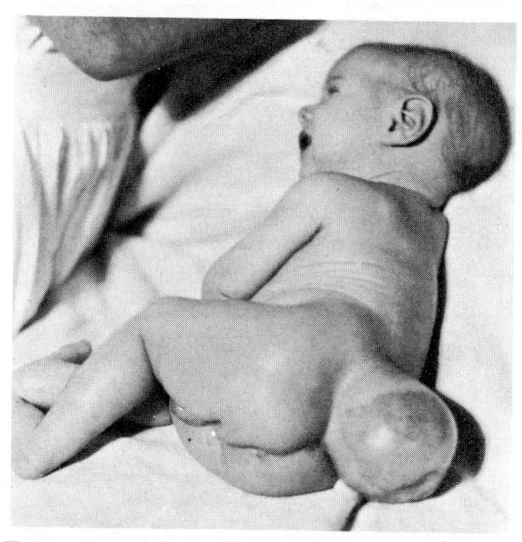

Figure 25–2 Infant with spina bifida cystica. Handling this infant requires extreme care so that the sac incurs no tension or pressure. The infant's head and the spine above the sac should be supported at all times as well as the lower extremities when the child is held.

supports the head and spine above the defect. When feeding or cuddling the infant outside the incubator, the buttocks and legs are supported on the nurse's lap. A small pillow is placed under the infant's head and spine above the level of the defect before resting the head in the en face position. At no time should the lower extremities be allowed to dangle.

The maintenance of adequate hydration and electrolyte balance is determined to some extent by the presence or absence of cerebral spinal fluid leakage. Without cerebral spinal fluid loss, the infant's nutritional needs are supplemented by intravenous therapy of 5 per cent dextrose in water. With loss of cerebral spinal fluid, electrolyte needs are determined by blood chemistries. In either case, the nurse must realize that any infant receiving parenteral fluids needs close observation, since fluid and electrolyte imbalance can occur easily. The nurse, therefore, must be able to keep accurate records of intake and output, understand and interpret normal serum chemistry values and understand how to use the equipment required to deliver intravenous fluids to infants, such as the infusion pump. Furthermore, when the infant is required to have nothing by mouth (NPO) before surgery, sucking needs should be met by providing a pacifier.

In order to provide early, appropriate passive exercises to the infant with spina bifida, the nurse can request the consultant services of a physical therapist to learn how vigorous exercise should be and which specific range-of-motion exercises should be carried out. To prevent deformity of the feet when the infant is placed on his abdomen, the ankles should be supported with padding so that the toes do not rest upon the mattress.

It is important that parents of the child with a spina bifida become involved with their infant. Teaching the steps of handling, exercising, caring for and stimulating their infant will promote parent-child interactions.

Once the infant has recovered from surgery, an extensive program of habilitation to include stimulation, physiotherapy and bracing, and bladder and bowel training should be begun to build a basis for later efforts to achieve the highest possible degree of independent functioning. Some unique considerations must be kept in mind when working with children with spina bifida.

The paralysis and insensitivity of the lower extremities leaves spina bifida children particularly vulnerable to burns, scratches and injury. Hot bath water, sharp objects or toys, tight garments and even wrinkles in the socks can result in trauma or ulcerations. The lack of sensations and bladder and bowel incontinence demand scrupulous attention to skin care.

Urinary incontinence is a threefold problem. The constant or intermittent dribbling of residual urine can lead to excoriation of the buttocks and perineal area. This same urinary overflow can reflux into the ureters and kidneys, causing urinary tract infections and nephritis. Incontinence is a source of psychosocial difficulties when the child is beyond the normal diaper-wearing years.

Use of the Credé method to manually empty the bladder is started early in infancy. The Credé maneuver consists of applying firm but gentle pressure beginning at the umbilicus and slowly progressing toward and under the symphysis pubis, thence moving toward the anus (Fig. 25–3).

In the infant, the fingertips of one hand are used to apply pressure; in the older child, one uses the palms of the hands. The Credé method yields best results, particularly in later infancy and in toddlerhood, if it is employed when the child is in a sitting position (ideally on a potty seat or commode).

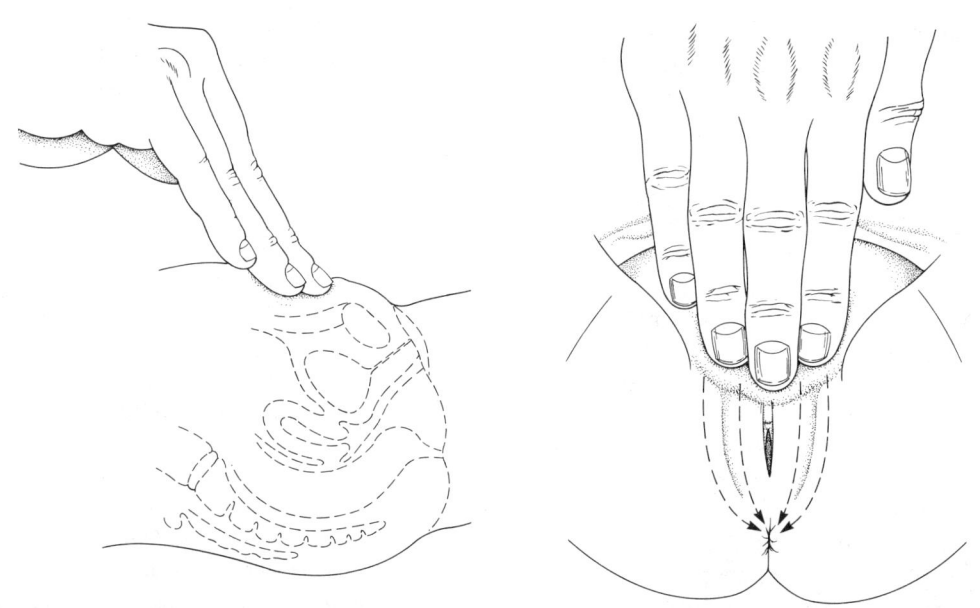

Figure 25-3 The Credé maneuver, in which external manual pressure is used, with the fingertips of one hand (for infants) pressing inward and downward over the abdomen starting over the umbilicus and moving down below the pubis as urine is eliminated. The Credé method permits manual emptying of the bladder and is an important part of the bladder training program.

During the daytime hours, the technique should be performed at two-hour intervals or more frequently if diapers continue to be wet. Parents should be closely supervised as they learn to apply the Credé maneuver, since incorrect technique can cause urinary reflux. Ultimately the child himself may be able to assume independent responsibility for this function. There are several external urinary collecting appliances that can be worn at night by the older male child. Unfortunately, similar devices for females have not been very satisfactory.

A program of bowel training must also begin in infancy. Constipation is more common than loose stools. In adhering to a pattern of regular, consistent evacuation, the goal of a bowel training program is to avoid chronic constipation yet keep feces firm enough to reduce involuntary elimination. A glycerine suppository inserted prior to the first feeding of the day helps to institute a pattern of regularity. Management of bladder and bowel incontinence depends upon a rigorous and consistent program.

Health care workers and parents may find that the greatest challenge in working with some spina bifida children is in motivating them to assume progressive responsibility for their own care. Allowing adequate time for the child to complete a task before assistance is given and providing consistent rewards for successful efforts will promote the development of desired behaviors.

Parents of spina bifida infants will require counselling as well as guidance from local support groups in order to make such an extensive commitment to the habilitation of one child and still allow for the healthy growth and development of each family member.

Hydrocephalus Ninety per cent of the cases of spina bifida with meningomyelocele are accompanied by hydrocephalus, a condition that has long-term implications in relation to cognitive functioning.[18] Hydrocephalus is an enlargement of the ventricular system from an imbalance in the circulation and absorption of cerebrospinal fluid.[18] The normal flow of fluid depends on the transfer of ions across the epithelial membrane of the choroid plexus. Water accompanies this transfer and circulates to the fourth ventricles via the aqueduct of Sylvius. Cerebrospinal fluid then flows into the subarachnoid spaces through the foramina of Luschka and Magendie and is subsequently absorbed into the venous circulation over the brain and to some extent over the spinal cord.

Etiology Any malformation of the brain stem that obstructs the normal flow and absorption of cerebrospinal fluid results in hydrocephaly. If the blockage is caused by an obstruction within the ventricles and therefore prevents cerebrospinal fluid from flowing to the subarachnoid space, it is termed *noncommunicating*. *Communicating hydrocephalus* indicates a patency of the ventricular system but an abnormal absorption of cerebrospinal fluid due to an obstruction located in the subarachnoid space. In the Arnold-Chiari malformation there is a meningomyelocele with displacement of the medulla and part of the cerebellum into the cervical canal. The resulting compression obstructs cerebrospinal flow and produces hydrocephaly.

The noncommunicating type of hydrocephalus may be the result of an inherited, sex-linked developmental defect, a fetal viral infection such as mumps, or a brain lesion or tumor. The etiology of the communicating type is often unknown. It can be a sequel to bacterial meningitis, toxoplasmosis, cytomegalic inclusion disease or subarachnoid hemorrhage.

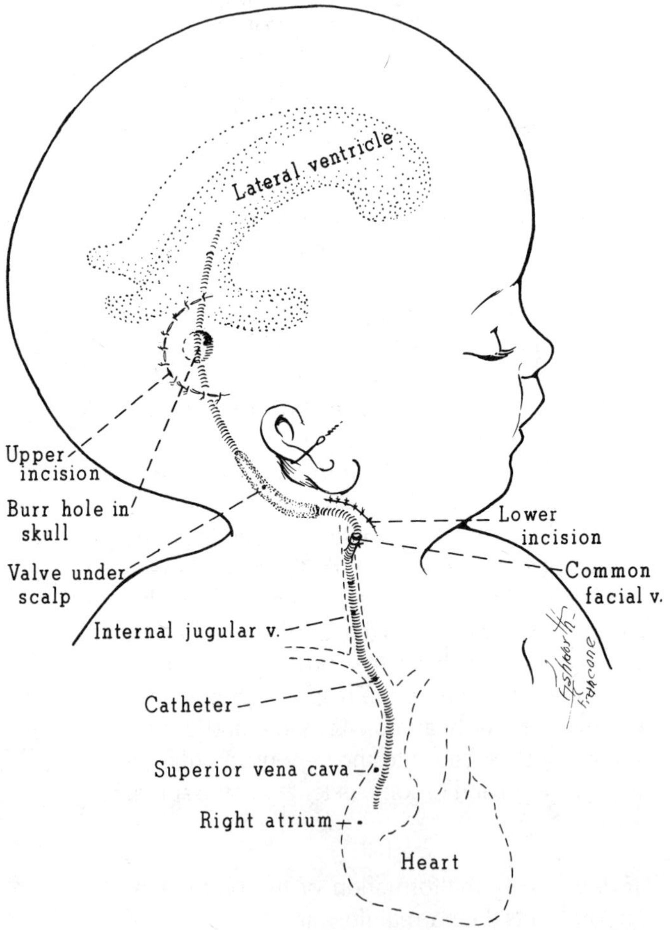

Figure 25–4 Operative treatment for hydrocephalus in which a catheter drains the ventricular system into the right atrium. (From S. Jacob et al., Structure and Function in Man, 4th ed. W. B. Saunders Co., 1978.)

Clinical Manifestations Conscientious prenatal maternal assessments may help identify those newborns who may be etiologically at risk. These infants and infants with spina bifida cystica will require careful observation of their neurological functioning. Since head enlargement is the primary sign of hydrocephalus in early infancy, the head circumference of the newborn infant at risk should be measured daily (average normal range is 33 to 35 cm). Neurological signs of increased intracranial pressure should be assessed, especially in older infants who are suspect. Such signs and symptoms include dilated scalp veins, separation of cranial suture lines (a "cracked pot" sound on percussion of skull), bulging fontanels, sunsetting eyes (upper sclera visible), shrill and high-pitched cry, listlessness, vomiting, irritability, fretfulness and delayed development. Severely affected infants seldom survive the newborn period.

Diagnosis Tentative diagnosis is based on progressive neurological signs and head circumference that increases one or more grid lines in less than one month. A definitive diagnosis and exact site of the defect can be determined by computerized axial tomography of the brain (CAT scan). The infant scheduled for a CAT scan needs no specific diet or dress. It is imperative, however, that the child remain motionless. In order to insure immobilization of the head during the procedure, it is necessary to sedate the child. General anesthesia or a combination of phenobarbital, Demerol, Phenergan and Thorazine is used for sedation.

Before the scan is done, the child's parents need a clear explanation of the procedure. They need to understand that because it is a noninvasive technique, there is no pain or discomfort involved. In addition, there are no aftereffects and no specific nursing care is needed as a result of the procedure itself.

Nursing Management Following a definitive diagnosis, treatment is instituted in order to attempt to establish an adequate flow of cerebrospinal fluid and promote a satisfactory balance between cerebrospinal fluid production and absorption. This is usually done by a surgical shunting procedure in which a bypass around the cranial obstruction is placed to carry cerebrospinal fluid to an extracranial site. In a ventriculo-atrial shunt, for example, a plastic tube allows cerebrospinal fluid to flow from the lateral ventricle into the vascular system at the right atrium via the jugular vein. A one-way valve inserted into the tubing prevents reflux of blood and allows cerebrospinal fluid to flow in one direction only (Fig. 25–4).

The nurse's role in caring for the infant preoperatively is to:

1. Monitor for signs of increasing intracranial pressure daily.
2. Ensure adequate fluid and nutritional intake through small, frequent feedings to reduce episodes of vomiting and accommodate diagnostic schedules. Extra time is usually required since many of these infants have difficulty sucking.
3. Prevent infection by following conscientious handwashing.
4. Prevent development of pressure areas by changing the infant's position frequently.
5. Provide adequate support of the head and neck to prevent neck strain from the oversized head.
6. Promote and support parental touching and cuddling since the child's enlarged head and altered facies frightens or repulses some parents. Model appropriate interaction with the infant and reinforce parents' positive responses toward the child.

Postoperatively, careful monitoring of the infant for signs and symptoms of increased intracranial pressure that indicate an obstructed shunt is imperative. The child should be positioned on his nonoperated side to avoid occlusion of the shunt valve (Fig. 25–5). Keeping the infant flat helps reduce the likelihood of a too-rapid decrease in intracranial pressure. The infant's parents will need to learn to observe for these same signs, since the shunt tubing is vulnerable to blockage or kinking and will need revision as the child grows. The nurse should also be alert for signs of infection, which is the greatest hazard of the postoperative period. The nurse in her teaching must emphasize that the child's future activities need not be limited, except for contact sports.

Improved diagnostic and management techniques provide a more optimistic outlook for the infant with hydrocephalus than was the case previously. With treatment, approximately 40 per cent of these children can achieve near-normal intelligence and functioning. The other 60 per cent, however, will suffer significant intellectual and motor limitations. The outcome for the individual infant is usually impossible to predict at the time of initial diagnosis and treatment. Therefore, in providing parental information and support, the nurse should communicate the importance of an infant stimulation program to promote optimal psychosocial-cognitive development. Referral to a community support group and follow-up by a community health nurse will aid parents in this. The parents will need positive feedback and encouragement in order to meaningfully invest in their infant's and thereby their family's outcome.

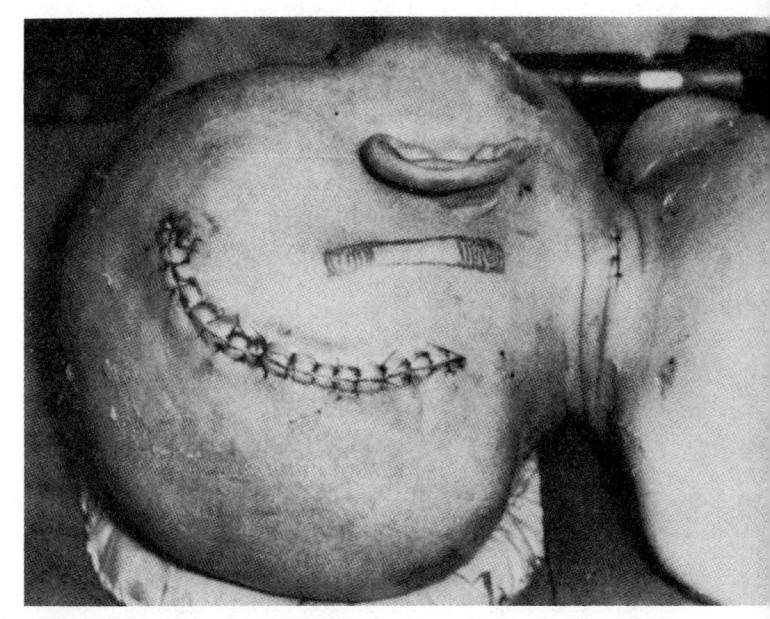

Figure 25–5 The closed incision in operative treatment of hydrocephalus. (From Mustarde, Plastic Surgery in Infancy and Childhood. W. B. Saunders Co., 1971.)

Neurocutaneous Syndromes

Neurocutaneous syndromes are conditions involving developmental defects of the nervous system, the eye and the skin. The alteration occurs between the 8th and the 24th weeks of gestation, when cellular proliferation is most active in the central nervous system. Sturge-Weber syndrome and neurofibromatosis are presented here as examples of neurocutaneous syndromes.

Sturge-Weber syndrome consists of focal motor seizures and a characteristic facial capillary hemangioma known as a *port wine stain,* or *nevus flammeus.* The port wine stain is flat and red to purplish in color. It varies in size, ranging from a small area to an area covering most of the face and neck, and may involve other parts of the body. It grows as the affected body surface grows. Intracranial vascular malformations cause atrophy of the cerebral cortex or calcification of cerebral blood vessels.[26] These cerebral alterations result in the seizure disorder, the mental retardation and the hemiparesis associated with Sturge-Weber syndrome. Eye involvement is common and is characterized by increased intraocular pressure resulting in congenital glaucoma in about one-third of affected infants. The diagnosis is usually made at birth on the basis of the port wine stain and seizures. Skull x-rays reveal a typical pattern of intracranial calcification.

The diagnosis of Sturge-Weber precipitates a family crisis that is compounded by the visibility of the facial lesion and the uncertainty of future manifestations, particularly in regard to the degree of mental retardation. The nurse encourages the family to express their reaction to the unsightly facial defect and supports them in their attempts to cope with the diagnosis. If suggestions for camouflaging the defect are sought by the parents, the nurse may suggest cosmetic cover-up creams. Attempts at surgical removal are delayed until school age or later, but they are generally unsatisfactory cosmetically.

Control of the seizures with anticonvulsant drugs is another treatment consideration of Sturge-Weber syndrome. In some instances, surgical removal of the affected portions of the cerebral cortex may be necessary if seizures cannot be controlled by medication. Nursing management of the infant with a seizure disorder, discussed later in this chapter, is the most appropriate framework for planning successful nursing intervention. Physical therapy is indicated to promote optimal motor function if there is paralysis of extremities. Parents require support in becoming actively involved in learning and carrying out the exercise program.

Ophthalmologic examinations at regularly scheduled intervals are essential because of the frequency of congenital glaucoma. If glaucoma develops, nursing measures to prevent visual sensory deprivation and to carry out treatment regimens are necessary. These are discussed in detail in this chapter under alterations involving the eye.

The most serious and disrupting long-term problem of Sturge-Weber syndrome is the associated mental retardation and its management.

The degree of developmental delay is difficult to predict, but early initiation of an infant stimulation program can promote optimal competency development. The prognosis depends on the extent of the cerebral involvement and the severity of the seizure disorder.

Neurofibromatosis (von Recklinghausen's disease) is a slowly progressive condition that involves a defect in supportive tissues and organs of ectodermal origin, mainly the central and peripheral nervous system, the skin and the eye. It occurs about once in every 3000 births and is caused by an autosomal dominant gene or as the result of a mutation.

About half of the affected infants have flat, irregularly shaped tan or brown skin discolorations called *café au lait spots*. Subcutaneous nodules also occur as part of the disease process. These are minute to large soft tumors found at varying depths below the skin or in various organs. They progressively increase in size and number as the infant grows. When found in the central or peripheral nervous system, they may cause deafness, dizziness, visual defects or compression of spinal nerves.[26]

Any infant with café au lait spots should be carefully assessed and a thorough family history obtained. Families with a known history of neurofibromatosis should be assessed during the prenatal period because of the genetic nature of the disease. The newborn is carefully examined for café au lait spots and subcutaneous nodules. More than six café au lait spots greater than 1.5 cm is diagnostic of neurofibromatosis. The size, location and number of lesions is recorded. A thorough neurological examination is performed and evaluation by electroencephalogram (EEG), CAT scan and other radiological procedures may be carried out. The nurse prepares the family for each procedure and assists them in understanding the results. Repeated explanations may be necessary because of the parents' high anxiety levels. If there are less than three lesions and the family history is negative, no further action is indicated other than follow-up assessment at regular intervals.

As the infant matures, the highly visible nodules on the face and neck may adversely affect the parent's interactions with him. Explanations that the nodules are painless and can be touched are reassuring to parents. Encouraging expression of feelings about the infant's disfigurement is supportive and helps with adjustment. The possibility of future hospitalization and surgery for removal of subcutaneous nodules that are painful or interfere with function should be discussed. The surgery is easily performed and gives good cosmetic results.

Parents often express concerns about the possibility of intellectual impairment in the infant. Neurofibromatosis is associated with mild retardation but severe impairment is rare. Anticipatory guidance that emphasizes normal patterns of infant development assists parents to realistically appraise their baby's growth. Appropriate stimulation activities for parents to use in day-to-day care can be demonstrated.

Genetic counselling is essential. The determination that the disease results from a mutation or is the autosomally dominant form of the disease has implications for future childbearing. If autosomally dominant, future children have a 50 per cent chance of inheriting the disease. Although many have a very mild form of neurofibromatosis and enjoy a normal life span, there is no way of predicting this. There is no cure for the disease itself and an increased incidence of malignant changes in the central nervous system or in the nodules may cause early death.

Infantile Spasms (Infantile Myoclonic Seizures) Seizure disorders are among the most frequently identified neurological disorders in childhood. Infantile spasms are, next to febrile seizures, the most common cause of seizures in the first two years of life.[17] They are twice as common in males as in females. Infantile spasms are almost always associated with major cerebral defects. Maternal infection, prematurity or birth injury may be identified during history taking as significant risk factors. A developmental lag may be identified before the onset of the spasms, but many infants appear to develop normally until about 3 to 6 months of age, when the seizures develop.[14] Mothers who receive good prenatal care and are in good general health are less likely to bear children with seizure disorders.

Infantile spasms are brief, lasting only a few seconds. They may recur frequently, 50 to 200 times a day, and massive spasms often occur just before sleep and immediately upon awakening. The infant may cry or laugh initially but does not lose consciousness during the seizure. The motor pattern is characterized by sudden flexor spasms; the head flexes on the chest, the arms thrust out and the thighs are drawn up on the abdomen. Seizures may be mistaken for colic in young infants. The myoclonic seizure pattern usually disappears by 4 years of age but is replaced by another major motor seizure pattern.

Diagnosis is based on a thorough family and pediatric history, skilled observation of seizure activity and physical and neurological examination. The EEG reveals a characteristic tracing indicating total disorganization of the electrical impulses in the cerebral cortex. The nurse carefully observes and records the infant's behavior immediately before the start of the seizure, noting changes in position, muscle tone or activity and the presence of a cry or laugh. The seizure activity itself and its duration are recorded along with the infant's behavior, appearance and level of consciousness after the seizures.

During the seizure the infant must be protected from harm. Padding the crib or playpen with bumpers and removing hard toys will maintain environmental safety. Parents are instructed to maintain these safety practices at home. Since jackknifing of the body is a prominent feature of infantile spasms, the infant should not be placed in an infant seat on a table or counter because of the danger of falling. As the infant becomes more mobile, usually toward the end of the first year, he may need a lightweight helmet to protect his head from trauma if he falls at the beginning of the seizure. When the infant is having a seizure, no attempt should be made to restrain him or place anything in his mouth. His head can be gently turned to the side to prevent pooling of secretions and subsequent aspiration. Any tight clothing around his neck should be loosened to allow uninhibited breathing. The nurse should teach the parents how to observe and record the pattern and frequency of the seizures in the manner described.

The course of infantile spasms is partially determined by the age at onset of the seizures. The older the infant when onset occurs, the better is his prognosis. Marked developmental alterations and deterioration leading to severe physical and mental retardation are soon observed in 90 per cent of the infants.[14] The drugs commonly used to control seizures are not effective in the treatment of infantile spasms. Occasional success in seizure control has been demonstrated with early administration of corticotropin (ACTH).[18] The treatment has little or no effect on developmental prognosis.

The nurse's role in supporting the physical,

intellectual and emotional-social adaptation of the child and his family focuses on establishing a supportive relationship. The family crisis is one of chronic sorrow associated with the rearing of a child with a progressive developmental deficit. Societal fears of seizures as related to mental deficiency are evident in the family's concerns about the future. The infant's progressive developmental delay may become increasingly difficult for the family to manage. Many infants with infantile spasms eventually require care in institutions because their needs overwhelm the family's ability to care for them at home. Thus the management of the seizures is only a small part of the nursing plan; the focus is on helping the parents cope with the crisis of caring for a mentally retarded child. A discussion of other types of seizure disorders and their management is included in Chapter 52.

At birth, the central nervous system is a quarter adult size, at 1 year of age it is half adult size and by age 7 it has attained 90 per cent of its total growth.[3] Thus it can be seen that the degree of developmental delay resulting from a central nervous system defect is difficult to predict in infancy. What will be predictable, however, is a parental response of chronic sorrow related to the fact that alterations in the central nervous system can limit cognitive and emotional-social growth, can impose developmental delays, can be accompanied by disfiguring lesions and can predispose the child to seizure disorders.

The concept that the infant and family are the primary rehabilitators and that the professional health team assists them with their task provides the basis for planning a successful habilitation program. The plan focuses on the infant's health needs and on the effect that the central nervous system defect has on his developmental level. The initial assessment is usually multidisciplinary and the nurse focuses on identifying the infant's and family's strengths. A thorough assessment of the infant's developmental level with special attention to neurological status is imperative. (See Chaps. 13 and 20 for a description of infant neurological assessment.)

Assessment of the family relationships is also important. Infants with central nervous system dysfunction are often irritable in the early months of life. They may be difficult to feed, and they may not suck well and demonstrate poor weight gain. Their signalling behavior may not be interpreted by the mother, or the infant may be unable to receive the mother's signals. The erratic patterns of basic functioning, coupled with feedback problems, lead to parental feelings of inadequacy because they seem unable to feed or comfort their own child.[2] These families are at risk for bonding disorders. (See Chapter 22 for a discussion of these.) The nursing role involves helping parents appreciate the unique characteristics of their infant and to develop realistic management routines based on his individual traits. The plan for habilitation, drawn from these assessments, encourages optimal competency development.

Infants with central nervous system conditions frequently have problems with physical competency. Locomotion is impaired by myelodysplasias and the neuromuscular involvement of infantile spasms. Skin integrity can be impaired if alterations in sensation exist or by use of assistive devises such as braces. Careful attention and protection of the skin is important to prevent breakdown. Teaching the use of assistive devices such as braces, crutches and wheelchair and working with the family to incorporate them into their daily routines are appropriate interventions to promote development of the child's locomotion.

Problems related to maintenance of adequate nutrition may occur, particularly if the infant sucks poorly or has difficulty coordinating sucking and swallowing. Dietary planning in consultation with a nutritionist is important to help the family develop skill and confidence in managing the infant. Special feeding techniques and postures may need to be taught to parents in order for them to be successful. For example, feeding adaptations such as enlarging the nipple hole or using compressible bottles may be necessary. Facilitation of sucking as an exploratory and adaptive response is encouraged to maximize the stimulation received during feedings. Alterations in elimination may require the development of special programs to promote optimal function. For success, bowel training programs especially require a long and concerted effort by the family.

The normal infant is increasingly responsive to and interested in novelty in his world. He explores further and further. He develops cognitive and language capacities that enable him to discover relationships. The infant with a central nervous system defect may be physically and cognitively unable to interact with his environment in the ways of the normal infant. He needs special structure to ensure opportunities for cognitive and emotional-social growth and development. A program that emphasizes sensorimotor stimulation appropriate to the infant's developmental level is devised. Infants with central nervous system dysfunction should begin the program as early as possible, by age 4 weeks if they are diagnosed at birth. The presence of central nervous system dysfunction dictates stimulation at a level that will not produce abnormal motor patterns, i.e., not result in a startle reaction. Activities to be stressed in the early months of life should encourage development of sucking, vision, hearing, grasping and the coordination of all of these skills. Coordination can be facilitated by helping the infant explore an object with his mouth or hand and encouraging head turning toward sound and touch. All activities are combined with as much pleasurable movement as possible. Active involvement in a home-base early intervention program hopefully will minimize the problem of sensory deprivation and secondary mental retardation often seen in infants with central nervous system abnormalities.

Community and state programs that provide services for infants are valuable aids in the habilitative process. Referral to birth defects clinics, often sponsored by the March of Dimes or the Easter Seal Society, helps coordinate multidisciplinary care for infants with central nervous system defects. This decreases the parental burden of planning multiple visits on different days, an extra expense in terms of money, time and transportation. Various government programs can provide financial support for surgery, physical therapy and equipment for eligible families. An awareness of current legislation and available health programs for infants with developmental alterations is part of the professional role of the nurse working with high-risk families and infants.

Alterations in Visual Functioning

Visual impairment poses a special threat to an infant's development. Deprived of visual cues, the infant must rely on other senses to learn about and relate to his environment. Visual impairment in infants can be caused by many factors such as inborn errors of metabolism, maternal infections and prematurity. Cataracts and glaucoma are two conditions appearing in infancy that cause alteration in visual competency.

Cataracts A cataract is an opacity of the crystalline lens of the eye that consists of precipitated lens protein. The lens is normally transparent to allow light to enter the eye and be refracted onto the retina. If a cataract is present, light cannot be refracted and visual impairment exists. Cataracts can be congenital or acquired. Congenital cataracts are formed during the sixth or seventh week of fetal life when the lens is being formed. Fifty per cent of congenital cataracts cannot be attributed to specific causes or associated with other anomalies. Trauma, anoxia or maternal systemic disease during the first trimester of pregnancy have a definite effect on their development. Infectious conditions, commonly maternal rubella, herpes simplex or inherited disorders such as Turner's syndrome or galactosemia, account for most of the other 50 per cent.[11] Acquired cataracts appear at different times after birth and are usually related to trauma, systemic disease and infections.

Pathophysiology Cataracts may be unilateral or bilateral, complete or incomplete. Visual acuity is determined by the density rather than the size of the cataracts. The longer the lens remains clear before the formation of the cataract, the better is the prognosis for vision when the cataract is removed.[8] Bilateral, complete cataracts are removed early, usually before the infant is 6 months old. Unilateral incomplete cataracts may not be removed. With other incomplete cataracts, the approach varies. Visual acuity is the essential factor in the decision about surgery.

Early Identification and Diagnosis Assessment and identification of prenatal high-risk populations is an important nursing role in prevention of cataracts. Prenatal factors such as inadequate immunization against rubella, systemic disease or vaginal infections caused by herpes simplex should be identified. Encouraging pregnant women to seek early and comprehensive prenatal care will positively influence these factors. Appropriate use of rubella vaccine for women in childbearing years decreases the risk of cataracts associated with congenital rubella syndrome. Genetic counselling should be made available for families with identified familial diseases. Encouraging compliance with medical regimens such as adherence to the prescribed diet when a child has galactosemia can be a factor in retarding the appearance of cataracts.

Early detection of visual problems is an important factor in determining visual outcome for a child. Visual deprivation in early life has profound effects on the development of normal emotional-social competency, which is dependent on eye contact with a significant other person.[25] Visual acuity can be assessed in the newborn period by testing the infant's ability to follow a slowly moving object.

When a congenital cataract is suspected, a thorough ophthalmologic examination is indicated. The extent of the cataract can be determined by ultrasonography (B-scan), a nonintrusive, painless diagnostic test that can be done through closed eyelids while the infant is sleeping. The nursing role during the stressful diagnostic period focuses on giving and repeating, if necessary, simple explanations of the diagnostic procedures and the proposed treatment plan. The use of terminology understandable to the family is critical to helping them cope. If surgery is decided upon, the nurse, along with other members of the health team, has a responsibility to help the family understand the life-long implications of cataract surgery. There is great emotional and financial stress for these families as they attempt to cope with repeated surgical procedures.

Nursing Management and Prognosis Preoperative preparation of the family should include discussion of eye patches and restraints used in the immediate postoperative period. The fact that vision will not be improved immediately, as corrective lenses are necessary after surgery, should also be explained.

Extraction of congenital cataracts is usually accomplished by aspiration of the lens material extracapsularly through a small incision in the corneal scleral wall. This approach differs from that used in adults, which is an intracapsular extraction. This difference in approach is necessitated by the immaturity of the infant eye. An intracapsular approach would result in aspiration of the vitreous humor, leaving only an empty shell. The newest procedure for lens removal is phacoemulsion. Ultrasonic waves are used to fragment the lens material into tiny particles, which are then aspirated.[22]

Postoperatively, the nurse is involved in physical support of the infant and in teaching the family to carry out his care. An eye shield is used for protection and kept on for about a week. If glasses are worn, the eye shield is used only at night and naptime after the first postoperative day. A combination of antibiotic and steroid drops is given for several weeks to prevent infection and minimize inflammation. Usually, there are minimal activity restrictions with current surgical techniques. The parents should demonstrate proficiency and ease with administration of eye drops before the infant is discharged from the hospital.

The fitting and wearing of corrective lenses or glasses is the next step in treatment. Infants may be fitted with contact lenses as early as three weeks after surgery. When contact lenses are prescribed, the nurse's teaching includes helping the family learn specific cleaning, insertion and removal techniques. The nurse also makes sure that the graduated schedule for wearing time is well understood so that corneal damage can be prevented. The importance of close medical follow-up must be stressed to ensure maximum benefits from the cataract surgery and prescribed lenses.

The prognosis for visual acuity after cataract surgery varies. The results are often poor because of other ocular defects associated with the cataracts. Visual acuity is also compromised by surgical complications, most commonly secondary glaucoma or, in later years, retinal detachment. The family's desire and ability to help the child wear suitable glasses or contact lenses is another determining factor. The real measure of success following cataract surgery is related to the child's ability to function at an optimal level in his environment.

Developmental Glaucoma (Congenital and Infantile) Developmental glaucomas are a significant cause of blindness in infants and children. Primary congenital glaucoma is an autosomal recessive disease that affects boys more frequently than girls. It is bilateral in 75 per cent of affected children and is present at birth. Infantile glaucoma develops during infancy. It is associated with hereditary disease such as Sturge-Weber syndrome and neurofibromatosis.[20]

Pathophysiology Glaucoma is a condition characterized by increased intraocular pressure. This pressure causes atrophy of the optic nerve and eventual blindness. Developmental glaucomas result from a deviation in the angle of the anterior chamber of the eye that interferes with drainage of the aqueous humor within the anterior chamber and causes increased intraocular pressure. As the elastic coating of the eye is stretched by the increased pressure, the globe enlarges and the optic nerve atrophies. Infants with developmental glaucoma have large, cowlike eyes (buphthalmos) as a result of this enlargement.

Clinical Manifestations and Diagnosis The nurse needs to be aware of the hereditary factor in identifying the population at high risk for primary congenital glaucoma. Genetic counselling should be available for these families. Early assessment of visual competency is an important component of case finding. Infants with developmental glaucoma tend to be irritable and have a history of poor eating patterns.[1] Frequent rubbing of the eyes, accompanied by redness and tearing, are symptoms associated with glaucoma. Twitching of the eyelids (blepharospasm) and increased sensitivity to light are also characteristic. The infant may burrow his head into the pillow to protect his eyes. Identification of these signs necessitates referral for ophthalmologic examination.

Diagnosis before 1 year of age is important to ensure adequate treatment and prevent visual loss. Diagnosis is made by measuring intraocular pressure with a tonometer, an instrument that, when placed on the anesthetized cornea, registers the underlying pressure. Corneal diameters are also measured and a complete ophthalmologic examination is carried out. The nurse assists the physician with examinations and provides support to the infant through her closeness and gentle touch. The family needs explanations of the various diagnostic tests in easily understood terms.

Management Initially, intraocular pressure can be lowered temporarily by oral administration of carbonic anhydrase inhibitors (acetazolamides), which suppress the production of aqueous humor. However, goniotomy, a surgical procedure, is the only definitive treatment for developmental glaucoma. This procedure consists of making a small incision into the tissue obstructing the angle of the anterior chamber. This incision facilitates drainage of the aqueous humor. Often two or three goniotomies in different locations are required to obtain normal intraocular pressure. Once the pressure is normal, the prognosis for control of glaucoma is good.

Eye patches are applied postoperatively and the infant should be observed closely for restlessness, which is indicative of rising intraocular pressure. Mydriatic medication is given to maximally dilate the pupil and encourage drainage. Dilating the pupil keeps the eye at rest and facilitates postoperative healing. Frequent tonometric readings of intraocular pressure and measurements of corneal diameters are used to detect increased pressure.

The infant is usually discharged from the hospital on the first or second postoperative day. In preparation for discharge, the nurse instructs the family in proper administration of eye medication. It is important to emphasize that the eye drops used for treatment of glaucoma in adults are not effective in children. The reasons for this are not fully understood; the drops have been tried clinically in children but do not lower intraocular pressure.

Provisions for adequate medical follow-up should be made and discussed with the family. Further surgery may be necessary if intraocular pressure rises again. With early diagnosis and treatment, the visual prognosis is good unless there is associated corneal haziness and/or increased ocular pressure had been present at the time of birth.

Management of Alterations in Visual Functioning The diagnostic period is a time of great stress for the family of an infant with suspected visual impairment. Fears of blindness, pain and disfigurement are common. If there is a hereditary aspect to the suspected condition such as in congenital glaucoma, feelings of guilt and responsibility may be experienced by family members. Blaming each other is not an unusual response. Relatives and friends often contribute to parental concerns by expressing pity and sadness about the infant's loss. The family's stress is heightened by the uncertainty of the treatment outcome and the difficulty of accurately predicting the degree of visual loss, even with early diagnosis and treatment.

The nurse identifies the grieving behavior of the family related to the infant's loss of sight and their loss of the perfect child. Encouraging them to express their feelings in an understanding environment is an important nursing intervention in helping them adjust to the loss.

Providing current, accurate information about diagnostic tests such as tonometry and ultrasonography increases parental understanding and sense of control during this time. It is important to convey to the family that infants with visual impairments, whatever the degree, are more like sighted children than they are different. They have the same growth patterns and variations in their developmental rates. Their major difference in development is in how they learn about themselves, others and the world around them.[16]

The treatment of the visual problem may provoke fears of pain and disfigurement related to the delicacy of the eye, the cutting involved in surgery and the need for corrective lenses. Frequent ophthalmologic examinations, tonometric testing and instillation of eyedrops several times a day can be a real burden on the parents. Adherence to these activities absorb a major share of the family's energies and resources and can disrupt family relationships.

Infants requiring surgical treatment need special nursing considerations. Preoperatively, the nurse must be familiar with the plans for surgery so appropriate explanations can be given to the family. Preparatory procedures should be discussed, expressions of concern about the surgery encouraged and the usual postoperative course interpreted. The nurse and physician collaborate to ensure that the parents are adequately prepared. The parents' participation in the infant's care both pre- and post-operatively develops their competence and confidence in managing his special needs.

Restraints are often necessary in the immediate period after surgery to prevent trauma to the operative site. Anxiety and activity increases with restraint so only the minimally effective amount should be used. Elbow restraints are less restrictive than wrist restraints and effectively prevent the infant from touching the eyes. Sandbags may be needed to keep the head from turning and a jacket type of restraint can be used to keep the infant in a desired position. The parents' presence can usually reduce the need for restraints and this should be encouraged.

The need for eye patches postoperatively varies with the procedure. The newer surgical techniques require a protective shield only in the period immediately after surgery. However, the physician will determine the length of time they are necessary. If both eyes must be covered simultaneously, prevention of sensory deprivation becomes a major nursing goal. The infant should be spoken to in a calm, soft voice before being touched so as not to frighten him. The parents are encouraged to be present around the clock to provide familiar auditory and tactile stimulation. Soft toys brought from home, music boxes and a radio are an especially effective means of providing tactile and auditory stimulation.

Close observation for vomiting and measures to prevent it are important because vomiting increases intraocular pressure that may damage the surgical repair. Excessive crying also raises intraocular pressure and is to be avoided. Prompt attention to the infant's needs, gentle rocking and mild sedation will minimize crying. A return to normal activity may occur as soon as the first day after surgery.

Families need instruction and actual experience in administration of eye medication and other treatment before attempting such procedures at home. The nurse teaches the correct procedure and evaluates the parent's readiness to manage the infant at home. (Points to emphasize when instructing parents about eye medication are discussed in Chapter 27.) Eye medications may be given frequently and for an indefinite period of time. Encouraging family compliance with the treatment is an important nursing intervention. Written instructions concerning the medications and their administration schedule are given to parents before the child returns home. Instructions about wearing times for eye patches, shields, glasses and limitation of activity are also written out. The need for community health agency involvement is assessed and appropriate referrals made before the infant returns home.

Counselling the Family with a Blind Infant
This infant and his family require early, aggressive intervention by a multidisciplinary health team to promote optimal competency development. Initially, nursing interventions are directed toward assessing and strengthening the parent-infant attachment process. Vision plays an important role in the establishment of the bonds between infant and caretaker and in early learning. The normal newborn is visually alert during the first hour of life and the eye contact that results with the parents provokes a powerful reciprocal response. The en face position assumed by new mothers with their infants during the early attachment phase is dependent on eye contact.[12] These early attachment experiences may be impaired when the infant's visual acuity is affected. Further, disruption of parent-infant attachment may occur if parents are not aware of

the infant's need for increased input via the other senses. Sensory stimulation of the visually impaired infant must be structured to support this early social interaction need.

Once visual alterations are identified, the problem of decreased sensory input must be considered. Unnecessary sensory impairment can be prevented if families are aware of the infant's special needs for stimulation. Experiences that encourage use of vision are extremely important. A common parental concern is that use of vision in a child with decreased acuity will adversely affect his future ability to develop sight. In fact, use of the eyes in a visually deprived child in no way affects the prognosis for visual acuity. Use of vision can be encouraged by providing toys that are colorful and involve movement, such as mobiles, and by playing games that require following a moving object, such as rolling a ball. Stimulation of the senses of smell, touch and taste is also necessary to compensate for reduced visual input. These sensations heighten the infant's ability to detect various subtleties and diversities while stimulating the reticular activating system in the brain to carry on the task of integrating sensory input with meaningful past experiences.[25] This integration is an important part of cognitive competency development. Story books that incorporate smell and touch are helpful in multisensory stimulation, as are toys of varied textures with musical components.

Auditory stimulation can be fostered by suggesting to parents that they talk to their infant frequently so he can recognize them by their voices and begin to make more vocalization by himself. The infant is kept near enough to his parent or caretaker to hear the sounds of working about the home and be talked to in order to be reassured about another's presence. Calling the infant by name fosters self-concept development. Also, encouraging parents to reinforce all actions with words, as with "Now I am putting on your shoes," helps with language development.

Playing simple lap games such as clap your hands encourages the infant to learn about his body while experiencing a sense of closeness with his parent. Holding, stroking and cuddling are among the most meaningful forms of communication between any infant and his caretaker but are especially important for the visually impaired infant. The effectiveness of these interventions can be evaluated by the infant's response — for example, the amount of his smiling, giggling, degree of muscular relaxation and ability to mold himself to his mother's body when held. Bodily changes such as decreased respirations, accelerated or decreased movement and responsive verbalizations also give evidence that the infant has his attention on the parent. Parents may need interpretation of these behaviors by the nurse to support their interactions with the infant.

Motor and perceptual skills basic to the development of spatial relationships and body image are also affected by visual impairment. The normal infant learns to voluntarily grasp an object by first seeing it and then reaching out for it. The visually impaired infant must have the stimulus reinforced through touch and voice. A brightly colored toy can be placed in the infant's grasp and then removed. He is encouraged to search and reach for it. Freedom of movement within limits of safety enhance an infant's balance, coordination and confidence. The motivation to move about can be provided by enticing him verbally and with toys. Scattering toys on the floor so that the infant comes in contact with them is an effective intervention. A walker can be used to provide experience with movement and contact with surroundings. Learning about himself and what he is able to do promotes development of a healthy self-concept. Taking him for short walks, playing with him outdoors and calling his attention to sounds, surfaces and smells increases sensory input. Parents tend to overprotect the visually impaired infant. They need support and encouragement to allow the infant to explore his environment, within appropriate safety guidelines. Keeping furniture in the same place as the infant becomes mobile and encouraging caution in unfamiliar places are helpful for maintaining a safe environment.

Another important nursing intervention consists of providing opportunities for parents to discuss feelings about their infant's response and to explore ways to develop pleasurable interaction patterns. The nurse's attitude toward the infant may influence the family's ability to interact with their child. An accepting attitude is conveyed when the nurse touches, holds and talks to the infant, pointing out normal aspects of development to the parents. Supporting parental attempts to provide sensory stimulation will facilitate early infant attachment.

The special needs of the visually impaired infant dictate use and coordination of a variety of educational and health services. The nurse's role may encompass both coordination of resources and referrals to ensure maximum use of available community resources. Ideally the infant should be enrolled in a structured infant stimulation program to develop age-appropriate skills. Community resources such as the state department of education, division of special education or rehabilitation services and services for the blind can be consulted for additional help. The goal of habilitation for a visually deprived infant is to emphasize to his parents his likeness to all children and to foster his growth and development. It is not the degree of visual acuity he possesses that determines his functional ability but how he uses his sight and senses.

Alterations in Metabolic Functioning

Phenylketonuria (PKU) and *galactosemia* are two inborn errors of metabolism that are irreversible. Both conditions are inherited as autosomal recessive genetic defects. PKU and galactosemia require an early diagnosis and the implementation of a rigid dietary regimen to offset irreversible central nervous system pathology. Table 25-2 is a comparison of the clinical aspects of these conditions.[23, 24, 31]

Management of Alterations in Metabolic Functioning Nurses have an important role in early detection of PKU and galactosemia. While all infants are usually tested for PKU before discharge from a hospital nursery, infants born at home must also be included in this screening program.

A screening program for metabolic disorders is usually a three-step process. A sample of umbilical cord blood is obtained at the time of delivery. A second blood specimen is taken from the heel of the infant no sooner than 24 hours after onset of protein ingestion and as close to discharge as possible. When the infant is 3 to 6 weeks old, a dried urine specimen is tested. Points to emphasize when instructing parents about obtaining this final specimen at home are as follows:
1. It is important that the filter paper not be soiled by the baby's stool or by such contaminants as baby skin creams or oils.
2. Soak the filter paper with the baby's urine. Take a wet but unsoiled portion of the diaper and sandwich the filter paper between two folds. Then blot the wet diaper into the filter paper until the paper is thoroughly wet.
3. Allow the specimen to dry in a clean, safe place.
4. Mail the filter paper specimen, with all requested information, to the appropriate laboratory.
5. Parents or physicians are not usually notified of results unless there are abnormal findings.
6. The metabolic screening program is tax supported and there is no charge for the specimen testing.

It is imperative that siblings of children known to have PKU and galactosemia be screened.

Since PKU and galactosemia cannot be diagnosed prenatally, parents who are carriers and do not want to risk producing a child with these alterations may need the nurse to teach contraceptive techniques and make referrals to counselling services if adoption is considered.

The impact of the diagnosis of PKU and galactosemia is traumatic and disorganizing to families. Parents initially react in an intense manner; they frequently suffer guilt and anxiety and sense a blow to their self-esteem related to the genetic aspects of these diseases. Skillful and intelligent nursing intervention as described earlier in this chapter is necessary to support and guide the family through the grieving and reintegration process.

The need for frequent medical checkups and laboratory testing and, in particular, the necessary dietary restrictions are a source of intrafamilial stress, and this can become an overwhelming burden. Maintaining an adequate nutritional intake while avoiding the food substances that would contribute to neurological dysfunction is the dilemma that parents of PKU and galactosemic children face over a long period of time. Understandably, parents get concerned about their infant's feedings; this may be manifested in tension at mealtime. In the case of low-phenylalanine foods, the parents may react negatively to the smell, taste and other characteristics of the special products. This negativism is readily communicated even to the very young infant.

Parent education is the key to clinical control of the disease process and is therefore the main focus of nursing intervention. First, the parents need to achieve a basic understanding of the condition. Second, the nurse must direct parental efforts toward reducing fear and anxiety.

TABLE 25–2 A COMPARISON OF PKU AND GALACTOSEMIA

Clinical Aspect	PKU	Galactosemia
Incidence	1 of 16,000 children born	1 of 30,000 children born
Enzyme affected	Absence of phenylaline hydroxylase	Absence of galactose-1-phosphate uridyl transferase
Normal enzyme function	Metabolism of the amino acid phenylalanine	Metabolism of galactose into glucose
Subsequent physiological alteration	Accumulation of phenylalanine and its abnormal metabolites in brain tissue	Accumulation of galactose-1-phosphate in erythrocytes, liver, spleen, lens of the eye, kidney, heart muscle, cerebral cortex
Resulting pathology (if untreated)	CNS dysfunction (seizures, microcephaly, mental retardation)	Mental retardation, cataracts, kidney dysfunction, cirrhosis, death
Onset of laboratory manifestations	24–48 hours following institution of milk feedings	End of first week of life, following institution of milk feedings. Manifestations most dramatic in breast-fed infants owing to higher levels of lactose in breast milk.
Presenting/associated symptoms	Musty odor, decreased pigmentation of hair and skin	Jaundice, anorexia, vomiting, diarrhea, abdominal distention
Laboratory findings	Elevated serum phenylalanine	Elevated galactose content in red cells
Case finding methods	Mass screening mandated by law in most states. Guthrie test—capillary blood samples. Urine test for ferric chloride at 3–6 weeks	Mass screening not routine-testing done on cord blood of infants of high risk families
Dietary management	Maintain minimal amount of phenylalanine (a protein) intake for healthy development while avoiding excessive amounts leading to neurologic dysfunction	Remove galactose from diet; involves milk, including breast milk and all milk products
Commercial preparations available	Lofenalac, special baking mixes, pastas, breads, cookies	Nutramigen, Prosbee, soybean products
Duration of dietary restrictions	Unknown, maybe indefinitely; more research needed	Unknown, maybe indefinitely; more research needed
Optimal serum maintenance levels	Serum phenylalanine level below 3–10 mg/100 ml	Below 3 mg/1000 ml of packed cells

Helpful activities would be to promote relaxation during feedings, to increase maternal-infant contact and to ensure that the mother is in a comfortable position for feedings. It is important that nurses primarily communicate enjoyment of the whole child rather than focus on the dietary regimen and infant feedings. Encouraging parents to joint a community support group will also help to reduce unnecessary worrying.

Another important role for nurses is in helping parents learn to prepare and manage an appropriate diet for their child who has PKU or galactosemia. Initially the infant's feeding needs can be satisfied by the special formula preparations available. A mother who had been breast-feeding before the diagnosis of either condition, however, will need to be instructed about formula preparation. In order to ensure an adequate nutritional intake, children with PKU or galactosemia may be given solid foods sooner than other infants. In this instance additional information and guidance will be needed. During a home visit the nurse can offer suggestions with menu planning and preparation. The nurse should observe that accurate measurements of ingredients are followed to keep nutritional elements at a prescribed level. In the case of a PKU diet, the use of a blender to dissolve the casein hydrolysate powder is helpful.

As the infant's growth rate fluctuates, so will his appetite. Mealtime can become stormy and anxiety-producing toward the end of infancy and on into toddlerhood. Suggesting that smaller meals be offered more frequently and that the method of preparation be varied may help these parents avoid mealtime tensions.

Children with either PKU or galactosemia need to participate in an appropriately planned stimulation program as discussed earlier in this chapter to promote cognitive and social-emotional function. With love, stimulation and dietary management children with PKU and galactosemia develop normally, although children with PKU tend to have lower IQ levels than their unaffected siblings.[31]

Alterations in Immunological Functioning

Agammaglobulinemia Agammaglobulinemia is a rare inherited immunologic defect. Immunoglobulins, also called gamma globulins, are serum proteins found in plasma, interstitial fluids and body secretions. They are produced by highly specialized cells called B cells and are responsible for the body's humoral immunity.* Gamma globulins are composed of five types: IgG, IgA, IgM, IgD and IgE. Each group possesses different antibody properties. IgG contains antiviral, antitoxic and some antibacterial antibodies, and it accounts for the greatest percentage of gamma globulins in the serum. IgA protects the mucous membranes, particularly in the gastrointestinal and respiratory tracts. It is a front line of defense against infection. IgM forms the antibodies of ABO blood groupings and of the rheumatoid factor and forms antibodies against gram-negative microorganisms. IgE provides atopic, allergic and anaphylactic antibodies.[5] It is the function of the B cells to rapidly manufacture gamma globulins for a swift defense against initial bacterial invasions and for prevention of repeated attacks by the same microorganism.

Pathophysiology and Etiology Congenital agammaglobulinemia is characterized by severe deficiency of all five classes of gamma globulins. The consequences of this defect in humoral immunity are an overwhelming susceptibility to bacterial infection and a lack of response to injected antigens such as DPT immunizations. However, the response to immunization may vary as it is related to the level of circulating gamma globulins and whether cellular immunity is also impaired. The decision to administer immunizations such as measles vaccine should be made in consultation with the infant's physician. Response to viral infections such as measles and chickenpox is usually normal.

The disease is transmitted as an X-linked recessive defect; therefore, affected infants are usually males. The exact defect is unknown but it is thought to be the result of a genetically determined abnormality of the lymphoid tissue. Apparently the mutant gene prevents the maturation of plasma cells.[30] All families with an affected infant should be referred for genetic counselling. Other females in the family may be carriers and their male offspring are at significant risk for the disorder.

Clinical Manifestations and Diagnosis Early identification of agammaglobulinemia depends on a high index of suspicion related to male infants who present with repeated severe bacterial infections. Common types of infection are pneumococcal or streptococcal in origin and include pneumonia, otitis media, sinusitis, meningitis and furunculosis (boils). These infections usually begin when the infant is 3 to 6 months old after transplacental immunity conferred by the mother has been depleted. The discovery on physical examination that the infant has decreased lymph tissue evidenced by the absence of tonsils and adenoids is indicative of immunologic deficiency. Referral for further diagnostic testing is appropriate with this observation.

Definitive diagnosis is shown by laboratory confirmation of low levels of gamma globulin in the infant's blood. IgG is less than 100 mg/100 ml and IgM and IgA are usually less than 1 per cent of normal adult levels. Parents need an explanation of the procedure for drawing blood and the approximate length of time until the

---

*The body has two categories of immunological response, humoral and cellular. Humoral immunity takes place in the body fluids and is concerned with antibody and complement activities. Cellular immunity involves a variety of activities designed to destroy cells recognized as foreign to the body and is primarily a delayed type of immune response. Agammaglobulinemia is a defect of humoral immunity.

results are ready. Frequent reinterpretation of these tests may be necessary for parents to grasp their significance owing to the complexity of the immunological system.

Management Medical treatment is aimed at maintaining protective levels of gamma globulin in the blood. A lifelong program of monthly injections of gamma globulin is necessary to achieve this goal. The intramuscular injections are painful and are given deep into the vastus lateralis muscle of the leg. The dose may be divided into two equal injections to reduce the amount injected into one site. The sites should be rotated and accurately recorded in the infant's health record. After the injection the mother is encouraged to hold and soothe the infant to minimize the discomfort. Frequent bacterial infections with their potential for life-threatening complications cause great family stress. Families often cope with this by isolating the infant from family, friends and normal social experiences. It is challenging to help families develop healthy patterns of interaction that are not overprotective and that encourage optimal competency development. Prevention of infection is vitally important for health maintenance of these infants. Anticipatory guidance to promote health involves stressing the importance of good general nutrition, especially since failure to thrive is associated with frequent infection. Conscientious infant hygiene practices are important in decreasing exposure to microorganisms. Discussion of appropriate safety measures to prevent trauma once the infant begins to play actively and move about on his own is indicated.

Signs and symptoms of inflammation and infection are reviewed with the family, as is the need to seek prompt medical attention when symptoms appear. Instruction related to techniques of administration of antibiotics to the infant and the scheduling of the medication are points to be stressed. The prognosis for normal life is good with the commitment to consistent medical management for treatment of infection and with the maintenance of adequate gamma globulin levels. Bone marrow transplants have proved to be somewhat successful in reversing the course of the disease. Throughout life the child is susceptible to chronic sinus and pulmonary infection and to rheumatoid arthritis.

Alterations in Reproductive Functioning

An alteration in infant health status primarily affecting the reproductive system is traumatic and disorganizing to families. Coping with the uncertainty of an ambiguous sexual assignment or the idea of the child's future inability to reproduce or both is an adjustment that many parents and growing children fail to make. These families have a particularly great need for counselling services. Confusion surrounding sexual identity and sexual matters threatens the individual child's and the family's self-concept. The term *hermaphrodite* is frequently applied to an individual who exhibits external genital characteristics of both sexes. A *true hermaphrodite*, however, is an individual who has both ovarian and testicular tissue (i.e., one ovary and one testicle or sex glands that contain mixtures of ovarian and testicular tissues). A true hermaphrodite usually has masculine genitals and feminine breasts. Less that 80 cases have been reported in the world medical literature of this century.[10] Individuals with adrenogenital syndrome and Turner's syndrome are referred to as *pseudohermaphrodites*. Occasionally diagnosed during infancy, these two conditions can alter reproductive functioning and contribute to psychosocial maladjustment.

Adrenogenital Syndrome Congenital adrenogenital syndrome is an inherited, autosomal recessive disorder. The incidence of the condition is approximately 1 in 15,000 births.[28] The disease stems from a deficiency in various enzymes such as 17-hydroxyprogesterone and 21-hydroxylase necessary to produce cortisol and aldosterone. The deficiency in turn causes a compensatory hypertrophy of the adrenal cortex. The pathological biochemical process results in a deficiency of aldosterone and an excessive production of androgen. Aldosterone is necessary to maintain electrolyte (particularly water and salt) balance and a substantial deficiency of it is responsible for salt losing and circulatory collapse, particularly during periods of stress.

Clinical Manifestations Excessive fetal exposure to androgenic hormones causes virilization of the urogenital system during the 12th to 20th weeks of gestation. A baby girl's clitoris can develop to the size of a penis and the fusion of the labia can resemble a scrotum without testes. The infant in many cases may be mistakenly identified as a boy, although female sex organs are present internally. The male infant will have enlarged genitalia with frequent erections.

If left untreated or undiagnosed, infants with adrenogenital syndrome will be excessively tall as children and will demonstrate precocious sexual growth, although breast development will be absent in the girl and spermatogenesis in the boy. Growth potential is exhausted at an early age and the patient will be very short in adulthood due to premature epiphyseal fusion.

Diagnosis Frequently, adrenogenital syndrome is suspected when there appears to be a congenital abnormality of the external genitalia. In the case of ambiguous genitalia it is imperative that the sex be determined as soon as possible, since parental-infant bonding is severely hampered when the infant's sex is uncertain. Sexual determination can be arrived at by chromosomal analysis from buccal smears and by noninvasive abdominal ultrasonography to visualize the presence of internal female organs.

While the technique of ultrasonography has speeded up the process of adrenogenital syndrome diagnosis and sex assignment, the sequence of events is painful and stressful for parents. Identity (our own and that of others) is an important aspect of our lives. Who we are, what we are and what we do determines not only our unique style of relating to others but also how they relate to us. When the infant's sex is ambiguous, the parent cannot comfortably address the child and has difficulty conjuring up images of the child's future. The genetic component of the alteration also adds to parental feelings of guilt. The loss of perfection in their child precipitates the grieving process described in detail earlier in this chapter. Parental guilt, grief and overall confusion surrounding the diagnosis of adrenogenital syndrome and possible ambiguous sexual identity demands that nursing intervention be carefully planned and skillfully executed.

Management The parents of a child with ambiguous genitalia must be informed immediately and adequate support for grieving and assimilation provided. The nurse can be helpful during the diagnostic period in the following ways:
1. By being certain that parents understand that the diagnostic tests are painless and noninvasive and will cause no aftereffects.
2. By role modeling for the parents to demonstrate a comfortable means of relating to the infant, i.e., calling the infant, "baby," not "it."
3. By using correct anatomical terminology to discuss the alteration. With repetition parents will eventually be able to explain the condition to their relatives and friends with confidence.

Once the sex genotype has been established, the nurse should encourage the use of the child's name and use the appropriate word, boy or girl, rather than continue the ambiguity implied in the term baby.

When sex determination reveals that an apparent male is in fact a female, the nurse may need to help parents select a girl's name. This process may be especially difficult for those parents who were anticipating a boy. Their sense of loss is further magnified.

Reconstructive surgery to separate the fused labia and widen the urogenital orifice yields good results. The surgical intervention is done in stages and before the child is old enough to be aware of the abnormality. With early diagnosis and treatment an intersex girl can develop into a woman with normal sexual functioning. It is helpful for parents to see "before and after" pictures of constructive surgery done for this condition in order to be reassured about its positive benefits.

In the case of a genotype female reared as a male in whom diagnosis and sexual determination is delayed until after age 2 it is preferable that the child continue to be reared as a male in order to prevent irreversible psychological trauma related to sex reassignment. Surgery to remove female organs and administration of hormones to stimulate male pubertal changes will be necessary. Obviously, parents will need a great deal of counselling and support to feel secure and confident about their approach to childrearing. Because the child is unable to reproduce, he will need advice in the future concerning alternate means of parenting.

In either case (sexual reassignment or genotype female reared as a male), it is extremely important to stress to parents that sexual role and functioning is not controlled by biological factors alone. Instead, it is heavily determined by environmental factors, psychosocial attitudes and societal expectations. Furthermore, parents need to realize that ambiguous sex in infancy and its eventual resolution need not

TABLE 25–3 A COMPARISON OF CONGENITAL SYPHILIS AND HERPES SIMPLEX II

Clinical Aspects	Herpes Simplex	Syphilis
Causative organism	Herpesvirus Hominis II	Treponema pallidum
Mode of transmission to fetus	Usually by direct contact; possibly transplacentally	Transplacentally
Incidence	Approximately 1 in 1500 pregnant women could be expected to have a herpes II infection	Approximately 1 in 5000 pregnant women could be expected to have a syphilitic infection
Consequences to fetus	Implicated as a cause of early abortion, prematurity and congenital malformations	Midtrimester abortion, stillbirths, prematurity
Consequences to infant	Localized or disseminated Herpes infection; possible CNS involvement and corneal ulceration	Severe rhinitis ("snuffles"); fissures at mucocutaneous junctions; painful, swollen joints; enlargement of spleen, liver, and lymph nodes; notching of permanent incisor teeth buds
Onset of symptoms	First week of life	Weeks or months after birth
Diagnostic methods	Viral culture of lesions	Serologic testing of infants of syphilitic mothers until age 1
Treatment	Symptomatic: new drugs being researched	Antibiotic therapy: 15,000 units aqueous procaine penicillin/kg/day, 10 days for child under 2 years old

relate to homosexual or bisexual activity in later life.

The long-term management of children with adrenogenital syndrome requires that cortisone be administered to suppress androgen production and that, in the salt-losing type, the sodium loss be prevented or replaced. The treatment and dose must be doubled whenever the child experiences stress such as illness or hospitalization. These aspects of the treatment regimen require that parents understand the signs and symptoms of dehydration and appreciate the need for immediate hospitalization in order to stabilize the infant's physiological condition. Realizing that these instructions may be misunderstood when parents are coping with high levels of guilt and grief, the nurse must remember to repeat them carefully and see that the parents have them written down.

Infants receiving treatment for salt loss are prone to hypertension. Regular medical checkups are necessary for children with all types of adrenogenital syndromes in order to promote health and maintain linear growth. A referral to a community nursing service for follow-up or supervision visits is important.

The prognosis for infants with adrenogenital syndrome is excellent if the alteration is recognized early, and hormonal therapy is instituted and readjusted as the child grows.

New tests are currently being explored to identify carriers of the adrenogenital syndrome. Identified carriers, parents who have given birth to a child with adrenogenital syndrome and children with the syndrome reared according to their sex genotype should all receive genetic counselling in order to make appropriate choices regarding future childbearing.

Maternal Infections Resulting in Long-Term Alterations in Infant Health Status

Congenital (fetal) syphilis and herpes simplex II are sexually transmitted infections that, when undiagnosed or untreated in the pregnant woman, may cause serious long-term alterations in an infant's health status. A comparison of the clinical aspects of both disease processes follows in Table 25–3.

Management Preventing the transmission of maternal syphilitic and herpetic infections to the infant and thereby avoiding the development of potentially grave consequences is the paramount focus of nursing and health care professional intervention. One can find few better examples for stressing the necessity of early and regular prenatal care as insurance for the birth of a healthy infant.

When diagnosed in the pregnant woman through serologic testing prior to the fourth month of gestation, syphilis can be treated before the fetus has mature cellular responses that are necessary for pathologic lesions to develop.[18] When the maternal disease is diagnosed after this time, the fetus may already be infected but may be cured, along with the mother, through antibiotic therapy.

A mother with genital herpes lesions who is near term can be scheduled for a cesarean section prior to spontaneous rupture of the membranes, thereby preventing the infant's contact with the virus either by viral ascension or direct viral contact. Unfortunately, the infant who does acquire a herpes virus simplex II infection has a guarded prognosis. Fifty per cent of exposed infants become infected, fifty per cent of infected infants die and fifty per cent of survivors have permanent sequelae such as CNS involvement (mental retardation and seizure disorders) or corneal scarring leading to blindness or both.[21] The reader is referred to previous discussions in this chapter of the nursing management of infants with CNS and visual disorders as a basis for providing appropriate care to infants and parents whose long-term adjustment to CNS and visual alterations stem from a herpetic viral infection.

Infants with syphilitic and herpetic lesions should be isolated. People caring for them should exercise conscientious gown and glove technique in order to prevent cross-contaminating others or contracting the disease themselves.

Alterations in Gastrointestinal Functioning

Biliary Atresia Biliary atresia, a congenital defect in which an infant is born with fibrotic or absent bile ducts, occurs once in every 10,000 live births. Normally, the liver secretes bile that passes through the bile ducts in the liver to the hepatic duct. The hepatic duct joins with the cystic duct from the gallbladder to form the common bile duct, which empties bile into the duodenum. Atresia may occur in any part or all of this duct system. Intrahepatic atresia occurs when the liver has no internal duct system. This is a defect for which there is no treatment other than supportive care for the infant with a terminal illness. Extrahepatic atresia involves defects of the hepatic or common bile duct and can be surgically corrected in many instances. Both types create backup of bile into the liver, which eventually causes cirrhosis.

The specific cause of biliary atresia is not known but it may be the consequence of in utero infection.[13] If so, proper prenatal care can lessen the possibility of its occurrence. There is no sex or familial tendency associated with the defect.

Diagnosis Diagnosis is based on the history of jaundice, the physical examination and laboratory tests. Conjugated serum bilirubin, serum alkaline phosphatase and cholesterol levels are elevated, indicating blockage of the bile ducts. The ^{131}I rose bengal test is a valuable diagnostic tool. Radioactive dye, which is rapidly taken up by liver cells and excreted in the bile, is injected intravenously. The amount appearing in the stool is a reflection of bile flow. In biliary atresia, the amount is less than 10 per cent. The accuracy of this test depends on careful stool collection for a timed period. The stool must not be contaminated by urine because in the presence of reduced bile flow, much of the tracer is excreted in the urine. If this urine mixes with stool, a falsely high excretion rate will be reported. Using a continuous collecting device for urine as well as a bed frame or mattress that allows for collection of stool helps maintain the accuracy of the test.

Liver biopsy provides the definitive diagnosis of biliary atresia. A core of liver tissue is obtained under local anesthesia by inserting a special needle (Menghini) into the liver. The tissue sample is sent for laboratory examination. Hemorrhage is the most frequent and serious complication of this procedure. Adequate immobilization of the infant's abdomen during the biopsy by holding the infant securely on the examining table is an important assistive nursing intervention. Moderate pressure is maintained over the biopsy site for five to 10 minutes after the procedure. Both of these nursing actions minimize the chance of hemorrhage.

Management The infant with biliary atresia has no chance for life without surgical correction. Parents are initially confronted with the news that their infant has a congenital defect that is usually fatal within 18 months. Then the chance for cure by surgical correction is offered to them. There is, however, the risk that the surgery will not be successful. Nursing intervention for the parents under stress during this time requires active listening and the development of a supportive relationship. Loss and grief are predominant themes expressed by the parents. (See section earlier in chapter on family reaction to an abnormal child for nursing management.) The surgical success rate is greatest when the surgery is performed within the first two months of life. After this time, the liver is permanently damaged by the trapped bile. The operation consists of using a portion of the small intestine to replace the blocked or fibrotic ducts. Part of the reconstructed bile duct is then brought out onto the infant's abdomen by way of a double-barreled enterostomy. Initially the bile flows from the liver into a collection bag on the infant's abdomen. It is then injected back into the intestine via the enterostomy. The enterostomy decreases the incidence of postoperative bile duct infection, a major surgical complication. Usually, within a year, when normal bile flow is established, the enterostomy is closed and bile flows from the liver into the intestine through the reconstructed bile duct.[13]

The preparation of the parents for the infant's surgery and appropriate support while they cope with his postoperative course are the mainstays of nursing care for the family. Preoperatively, the infant may be irritable and uncomfortable. The physical closeness of the parents will comfort the infant and will help the parents prepare for the reality of the surgery.

Questions concerning the surgical procedure and the anticipated postsurgical course should be answered by the health care team. Teaching parents is one of the most important aspects of nursing care during the postoperative period. Parents need to learn how to maintain skin integrity around the enterostomy and apply the collection device properly. Signs and symptoms of infection should be reviewed and parents should demonstrate competence in taking and interpreting the results of rectal temperatures. Vitamin K is frequently given by injection if the possibility of hemorrhage is great, so parents need to learn the technique of administering intramuscular injections to infants. A special diet, which includes predigested fats, is prescribed for 6 to 12 months after surgery. A formula such as Portagen, a medium chain fatty acid, may be used. Parents should feel comfortable with the dietary regimen before the infant returns home. Plans for the necessary long-term medical follow-up are made with the parents before they leave the hospital.

If surgical correction is not possible or is unsuccessful, liver transplantation has been carried out for infants with biliary atresia. At this time, the success of this approach is in doubt because of a high incidence of rejection and operative mortality.

References

1. M. M. Alexander and M. S. Brown. Pediatric History Taking and Physical Diagnosis for Nurses. McGraw-Hill Book Co., 1979
2. S. K. Campbell. Facilitation of cognitive and motor development in infants with central nervous system dysfunction. Physical Therapy, April 1974, p. 346
3. S. K. Campbell and J. M. Wilson. Planning infant learning programs. Physical Therapy, December 1976, p. 1347
4. P. L. Chinn. Child Health Maintenance. C.V. Mosby Co., 1979
5. M. Dharan. Immunoglobulin abnormalities. American Journal of Nursing, October 1976, p. 1626
6. C. Eddington and T. Lee. A home-centered program for infants. American Journal of Nursing, January 1975, p. 59
7. M. L. Erickson. Assessment and Management of Developmental Changes in Children. C.V. Mosby Co., 1976.
8. D. Hiles and A. W. Biglan. Indications for infantile cataract surgery. International Ophthalmology Clinics, Winter 1977, p. 44
9. D. P. Hymovich and M. V. Barnard, eds. Family Health Care, Vol. II. McGraw-Hill Book Co., 1979
10. H. Katchadourian and D. Lunde. Fundamentals of Human Sexuality. Holt, Rinehart & Winston, 1972
11. J. S. Kennerdel. Pre-operative evaluation of the juvenile cataract. International Ophthalmology Clinics. Winter 1977, p. 3
12. M. H. Klaus and J. H. Kennell. Maternal-Infant Bonding. C.V. Mosby Co., 1976
13. J. R. Lilly. Early surgery to correct biliary atresia. AORN Journal, October 1978, p. 718
14. S. Livingston. Comprehensive Management of Epilepsy in Infancy, Childhood and Adolescence. Charles C Thomas, 1972
15. A. McCollum. Coping With Prolonged Health Impairment in Your Child. Little, Brown and Co., 1975
16. P. Moor. Foster family care for visually impaired children. Children Today, Jul/Aug 1976, p. 12
17. J. N. Muehl. Seizure disorders in children: prevention and care. American Journal of Maternal and Child Nursing, May/June 1978, p. 156
18. V. Vaughan et al., eds. Nelson Textbook of Pediatrics. W. B. Saunders Co., 1979
19. S. Olshansky. Chronic sorrow: a response to having a mentally defective child. Social Casework, March 1962, p. 191
20. P. Paton and J. A. Craig. Glaucomas: diagnosis and management. Clinical Symposia, No. 2, 1976, p. 48

21. M. Philbrook, ed. Syphilis: now just a minor STD. Patient Care, February 15, 1978, p. 93
22. M. Pilgrim and B. Sigler. Phaco-emulsion of cataracts. American Journal of Nursing, June 1975, p. 976
23. S. Pueschel et al. Discontinuing the phenylalanine restricted diet in young children with PKU. Journal of the American Dietetic Association, May 1977, p. 5
24. K. Rothman and S. N. Pueschell. Birthweight of children with PKU. Pediatrics, December 1976, p. 842
25. B. M. Severtsen. Sensory impairment: its effect on the family. In Family Health Care, Vol. II. D. Hymovich and M. Barnard, eds., McGraw-Hill Book Co., 1979
26. L. Solomon and N. Esterly. Neonatal Dermatology. W. B. Saunders Co., 1973
27. B. H. Stone. Computerized transaxial brain scan. American Journal of Nursing, October 1977, p. 160
28. Test for early detection of adrenal hyperplasia is being developed. American Family Physician, January 1979, p. 224
29. M. Tudor. Nursing intervention with developmentally disabled children. American Journal of Maternal Child Nursing, Jan/Feb 1978, p. 25
30. L. Whaley. Understanding Inherited Disorders. C.V. Mosby Co., 1974
31. D. S. Wyatt. Phenylketonuria: the problems vary during different developmental stages. American Journal of Maternal and Child Nursing, Sept/Oct 1978, p. 296

Additional Recommended Reading

E. G. Chalhub. Neurocutaneous syndromes in children. Pediatric Clinics of North America, August 1976, p. 499

B. L. Conway. Pediatric Neurologic Nursing. C.V. Mosby Co., 1977

M. Edwards. Venereal herpes: a nursing overview. Journal of Obstetrics and Gynecology, Sept/Oct 1978, p. 7

A. B. Godfrey. A specialized program for public health nurses. American Journal of Nursing, January 1975, p. 56

M. Hill. The myelodysplastic child: bowel and bladder control. American Journal of Nursing, March 1969, p. 545

J. Parvin and G. F. Smith. Phenylketonuria. American Journal of Nursing, August 1975, p. 1303

S. Schid. Parents of children with PKU. Children Today, Jul/Aug 1972, p. 20

J. B. Stanburg and J. B. Wyngaarden. The Metabolic Basis of Inherited Disease. McGraw-Hill Book Co., 1972

S. Steele. Nursing Care of the Child with a Long Term Illness. Appleton-Century-Crofts, 1977

D. Vigliarolo. Managing bowel incontinence in children with meningomyelocele. American Journal of Nursing. January 1980, p. 105

POTENTIAL STRESSES DURING INFANCY: LIFE-THREATENING ALTERATIONS IN HEALTH STATUS

by Anita Spietz, RN, MSN
and Marcia Sheets, RN, MSN

This chapter deals with life-threatening alterations in the health status of the infant within the family unit. The text addresses the impact of life-threatening illness, grief associated with the birth of an infant with an infectious disease or genetic disorder and the impact on the family of the sudden and unexpected death of an infant.

THE INFANT WITH LIFE-THREATENING ILLNESS

When an infant is dying, the natural order of life is tragically reversed. It is hardly possible to view loss of life by someone who has barely begun life as anything but unnatural. Yet the unnaturalness of such an event cannot eliminate it as a real experience — one in which the nurse plays a vital role.

The Infant's Response

For the young infant, the experience of dying can be one of aloneness if his developmental requirement is not met for a consistently available, loving person to meet his needs, intensified by his dying state. The infant under 4 months primarily experiences his life-threatening health state through overwhelming physical sensations.[1] During infancy (4 to 12 months) he progressively experiences his dying as a fear of separation and a recognizable, hurtful sensation.[1] Since he does not perceive time, the infant cannot conceive of the irreversibility of death but rather equates it with abandonment: a sense of being left all alone. This infant's needs for a loving, consistent care giver are paramount.

Intervention, whether by the nurse or ideally by his own parents, should be focused on keeping his development as normal as possible through tactile, auditory and visual stimulation without overstimulation.

The most valuable stimulation to the infant is *touch*. This ill infant needs the comfort that contact with caring persons and gentleness in feeding, holding, rocking and cuddling offer. *Sounds* are part of the dying infant's environment. He should be spoken to before and during procedures. Anyone who approaches or provides care for him should use soft, soothing, reassuring voice tones that will provide a sense of security. Tapes of his parents' voices can have an especially calming effect during their absence or during periods when he appears anxious or restless. Singing softly or playing a music box is appropriate. The visual *stimulation* given any other child of this age should also be available to the dying infant. En face positions help him establish relationships with his caregivers, reducing his sense of being alone in his dying.

All these caring tasks may best be performed by his parents, who know and love him (or who may need to learn to know and love him before his death so that they can appropriately separate from him after his death). The nurse caring for the dying infant does not necessarily give direct care to the infant but rather by teaching, counselling and supporting the infant's parents with her presence, allows them to parent and reinforces their actions and decisions.

The Parents' Response

Typically the parents react with grief, fury and guilt that, while traumatic for them and those upon whom it is vented, is a necessary part of the anticipatory grief experience that prepares them for the finality of death. In Doyle's words, "The parents walk an impossible tight rope."[2] On one hand, it is crucial to their dying infant's developmentally intensified morale that they spend a good deal of time with him. On the other, family life, especially if there are other children, must go on. Depending upon the infant's age and the degree of bonding that has occurred, parents may display frantic closeness or emotional distance.[3] The frantic closeness tends to shut out spouse, children, job and friends, leaving the parent void of the support systems he or she desperately needs. Emotional distance involves a detachment from the infant in an effort to cope with the pain that being with him causes; with this response the infant is left without an essential support system. Most often parents fluctuate between frantic closeness and emotional distance.

Because of the disequilibrium created by the situation and since the parents' participation in their infant's care is crucial, the nurse often needs to be a sounding board as the parents work through their priorities. She needs to interpret the infant's need of and reactions to his parents. They may need assistance in explaining the situation to the infant's siblings. The nurse may have to redirect the parents' attention to their own individual needs and the periodic need they have of each other. By offering the parents emotional support when they are not with their infant, the nurse helps them be more effective in creating a secure, peaceful and calm environment for their infant when they are with him. They need frequent reassurances that they are doing all they can for their infant and that he knows they love him and are with him.

LIFE-THREATENING GENETIC DISORDERS OF INFANCY

The infant with a genetic disorder may be symptomatic during the first year of life. The parents have already been confronted with the possibility of a chronic or fatal illness and, in many cases, their most dreaded thoughts have been confirmed through diagnosis made by karyotyping or hemoglobin electrophoresis.

Riley-Day syndrome, Tay-Sachs disease, sickle cell anemia and thalassemia are examples of genetic disorders that are transmitted by the autosomal recessive mode of inheritance (see Appendix).

Autosomal recessive modes of inheritance pose unique problems to the family of an affected infant; often parents have terrible guilt feelings. "Genetic grief" is a term used for the process during which parents must deal with the guilt, anger and disappointment associated with having conceived a defective infant, the consequential death of that child, and also the fear of the threat of recurrence of the disorder in subsequent children. Unfortunately, the recurrence risk in autosomal recessive disorders is high (25 per cent).

Sickle Cell Disease (Sickle Cell Trait and Sickle Cell Anemia)

Sickle cell disease is an inclusive term for sickle cell trait and sickle cell anemia. It is a hematological disorder transmitted by an autosomal recessive pattern of genetic inheritance. An infant with *sickle cell trait* has inherited a recessive sickle gene from one of his parents (heterozygous disease) and a normal dominant hemoglobin gene from the other parent. The

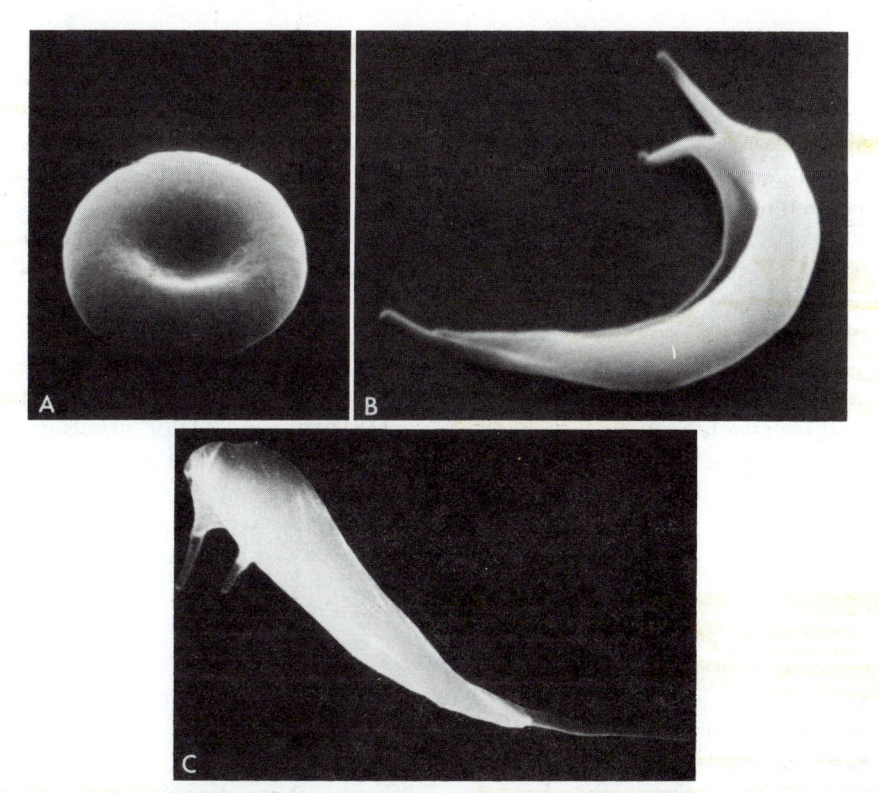

Figure 26–1 Scanning electron micrograph of erythrocytes. Comparison of a normal cell (*A*) and deoxygenated sickled cells (*B* and *C*). (Courtesy of Dr. James White, from H. F. Bunn, et al. Human Hemoglobins. W. B. Saunders Co., 1977.)

child with sickle cell trait is a carrier of the disease and almost always asymptomatic. *Sickle cell anemia* results when an infant inherits two recessive genes (homozygous disease). The child with sickle cell anemia is symptomatic with a potentially fatal consequence. Sickle cell anemia occurs predominantly in the black race and in one of every 625 births in American blacks.[8]

Hemoglobin of the full-term newborn is predominantly fetal hemoglobin (HgbF), which is rapidly replaced by adult hemoglobin (HgbA) during the first months of life. However, the infant who has inherited a sickle gene synthesizes abnormal hemoglobin (HgbS). The child who has inherited one recessive gene (trait) synthesizes both HgbA and HgbS, whereas the child who received two recessive genes (anemia) synthesizes only HgbS. This produces the anemic characteristics.

Pathophysiology and Clinical Manifestations of Sickle Cell Anemia As the postnatal decrease in HgbF occurs, the concentration of HgbS rises in infants with this anemia. Intravascular sickling and evidence of a hemolytic process may then occur. Sickling (sickle-like distortion of red cell shape) is the result of the precipitation of abnormal hemoglobin within the red cell causing crystal formation (clumping).[18] This precipitation results from the low insolubility of the HgbS at low oxygen concentrations. Because sickling of the red cells has occurred, impairment of flow through the capillary bed follows. Tissue hypoxia and necrosis ultimately occur if the condition is not reversed.

Symptoms in sickle cell anemia are associated with the decreased life span of the red cells and to the formation of thrombi in the small vessels of various organs as a result of sickling. The earliest symptomatology is often noted by the mother, who notes in her 3- to 6-month-old infant colicky behavior, swelling of the hands and feet (hand-foot syndrome), a failure to thrive or all of these. Hepatosplenomegaly frequently accompanies these symptoms in children under 5. If the condition is not diagnosed and treated at this time, these children soon begin having painful crises in one anatomical area or another.

Sickle Cell Crisis. A "crisis" is not a specific disease entity but rather more of an exacerba-

POTENTIAL STRESSES DURING INFANCY:
LIFE-THREATENING ALTERATIONS IN HEALTH STATUS

tion. There are several courses that these crises may take.

Hand-Foot Syndrome   The main type of crisis, involving bilateral and symmetrical swelling of the hands and feet, fever and irritability, occurs by 6 months of age. This inflammatory condition, called *dactylitis,* is noted in swollen, nonerythematous extremities. Soft tissue swelling and periostitis cause the symptoms.[20] An interference of adequate circulation to the hands and feet causes moderate to severe pain. This may be treated effectively with oral analgesics such as acetaminophen. Rigorous hydration, either orally or parenterally, should also be instituted.[18]

Thrombotic Crisis   This is the most common of the vaso-occlusive events. Sickled cells form infarcts in the small blood vessels. Bone marrow infarction and necrosis with subsequent new bone formation may occur. Some bony destruction of the cartilage may be noted by radiologic examination. In older children joints become painful and swollen and subsequently deformed. Hemarthrosis and splenic infarction may occur. Susceptibility to infectious processes such as septic arthritis and osteomyelitis may be noted, with the infectious agent most commonly being *salmonella* or *Staphylococcus aureus*.[18] Cerebral vascular accidents (CVA) may occur if the infarction leads to cerebral occlusion; hemiparesis or death may be the outcome.

Sequestration Crisis   At times large amounts of pooled blood are noted in the spleen or liver. Rapid enlargement of the spleen forms an acute build-up of red cells with resulting hypovolemia, severe abdominal pain, severe anemia and liver enlargement. Hepatosplenomegaly and splenic infarction are seen and circulatory collapse may develop rapidly. Death may be the outcome if sequestration crisis occurs during infancy.

Aplastic Crisis   During severe infections, aplastic crisis may occur. A sudden decrease in the rate of marrow red blood cell production is seen, resulting in a low reticulocyte count and a fall in the hematocrit. Treatment includes transfusion of packed cells.[18]

Hemolytic Crisis   Hemolytic crisis is likely the result of cellular fragmentation, which occurs as the relatively rigid sickled cell passes into the capillaries.[20] Other cells are phagocytized by macrophages in the spleen, causing hemolysis. Clinical features associated with chronic hemolysis such as pallor, jaundice, an increase in reticulocytes and hyperplasia of the bone marrow are noted.

Medical Complications.   Massive liver necrosis and kidney failure may develop as chronic damage occurs. Major insults to the central nervous system due to cerebral vessel occlusion are frequent, and severe sequelae including hemiparesis, seizures, disorders of consciousness and visual disturbances have been described in up to 43 per cent of reported cases.[20]

Nursing Care During Course of Disease and Treatment

Primary Prevention   *Genetic counselling* is available to the potential parents. Facilities such as the March of Dimes and various national sickle cell centers are available to provide genetic counselling for those who need and request it.

Maintaining the child's general health is an important preventive action. The nurse can provide adequate information that will assist parents to maintain their infant at his optimal health. This will help him weather the various clinical complications that may lie ahead. Utilization of nursing process with the family will help to define areas of strength and areas of need as the nurse and family formulate health care goals. (See Chapter 21 for further discussion of infant health maintenance.)

Secondary Prevention   In *early identification,* the nurse plays an important role in identifying children or families or both at risk for sickle cell anemia. In May 1972, Congress passed the National Sickle Cell Anemia Control Act. Under this act services for voluntary screening and diagnosis, counselling and education, medical referral and follow-up and research were mandated.[16] Because sickle cell screening is available upon request, and since sickle cell anemia and sickle cell trait are most prevalent in the black population, the nurse should discuss with the parents of a black infant the need for the test.

There is a certain amount of disapproval among blacks of the widespread use of testing by the Sickledex test (a solubility test) or sickle cell prep (the utilization of hemoglobin electrophoresis). This is because in some communities the black child identified as having the trait or as being a carrier of sickle cell disease may be treated differently and discriminated against. There is some thought that the knowledge that he has the trait may in fact be counterproductive to a positive self-concept for the developing child. If the presence of the trait is unknown and if no symptoms are evident, perhaps there is no need to perform the screening test. Perhaps the appropriate time to consider screening is when the individual has reached reproductive age and is more ready to make decisions regarding having children. In any event, the parents must provide informed consent prior to performance of the test, since the implications may be far-reaching for the infant. The nurse needs to respect the wishes of the parents in the setting of goals in health care planning for their infant.

Medical Management The nurse is usually responsible for carrying out the regimen prescribed by physicians in the management of sickle cell anemia.[18] During aplastic crisis, the transfusion of packed cells to a level of approximately 30 per cent is required. During splenic sequestration, vigorous replacement of blood volume with packed cells and a chronic transfusion program for two to three years to prevent recurrence is indicated.

Since sickling of the cells occurs in states of decreased oxygen tensions, the child's hematocrit level must be increased prior to surgery. Direct transfusion of packed cells can be performed to raise the hematocrit above 30 per cent. Preparation for surgery may require 10 days to two weeks. The process of transfusing packed cells every few days results in suppression of the production of sickle cells, causing an overall decrease in HgbS and a lower risk of crisis occurring due to the surgery.

Nursing Management Five major interventions can be instituted by the nurse to support the child in sickle cell crisis. They are analgesia, hydration, rest, prevention and detection of infection and siblings' involvement.

Analgesia Propoxyphene hydrochloride, acetaminophen or codeine-containing compounds may be useful for children during mildly painful episodes. Meperidine (Demerol) may be prescribed for children in more severe pain. The nurse is most often responsible for drug administration during the course of each crisis.[18]

The situation of an infant in pain can be extremely frustrating to caregivers and the nurse because of the difficulty posed in managing the pain. Holding the infant and providing a warm and caring environment will usually assist him in maintaining more control over his feelings of anxiety associated with the pain. Gentle, slow movements when handling the infant are essential. If the infant is immobilized for parenteral infusions, the nurse must provide for the physical, psychosocial and safety needs of the infant. Providing a comfortable infant seat may facilitate his comfort and safety. Restraints, if essential for safety, must be removed at least every 45 to 90 minutes, keeping in mind the infant's sleep patterns and the occurrence of REM sleep.

Hydration Since the sickling process is enhanced by dehydration, maintaining an adequate level of hydration is a primary intervention measure for the acutely ill infant. Both oral and parenteral fluids are used to improve the level of hydration. The oral route of hydration maintenance is preferable, if possible, since the infant's sucking needs may be increased owing to the stress and anxiety associated with pain and the trauma of hospitalization. Parents can identify for the nurse the child's receptiveness to various liquids. The administration of blood products may also be included in the immediate emergency care. The close monitoring of vital signs while the infant is receiving hydration is critical.

Rest The infant in crisis is likely to be hospitalized; every effort should be made to provide for the comfort needs of the infant and his caregivers. The infant must be kept as free from stress as possible. Rooming in is an essential component of basic care to the family. The caregivers' presence affords the infant more security and should be permitted and encouraged in a manner that does not place guilt upon the parent(s) who is unable to room in due to other family obligations.

Since increased anxiety can further complicate the crisis, the nurse must make every effort to anticipate and provide for the needs of the sick child within the family unit. Parents should be provided with adequate information regarding the latest episode and also should have their anxiety reduced so that they will be able to assist their infant during the crisis.

Prevention and Detection of Infection Immunizations will help protect the child from the usual childhood illnesses. The parents may also need information regarding common childhood illnesses and how to interpret the symptoms they may see. The nurse can help parents learn the proper method of taking their child's temperature. Changes in the infant's eating behaviors (refusal to eat) and changes in his disposition (irritability or lethargy) usually indicate the need for medical management.

Siblings' Involvement Siblings should play as active a role in caretaking of an affected infant as they would with any new brother or sister. Depending on the sibling child's cognitive level, explanations must be given for repeated admissions to the hospital and the other events surrounding the management of the ill infant's unique needs. The sibling may want to visit the pediatrician or the hospital with the infant to clarify the situation and to help him understand the infant's needs. Parents should be encouraged to set aside a special time each day to devote to the siblings so that jealousy or guilt will not predominate in the parent-child or sibling relationship.

Prognosis The infant with sickle cell disease has a better prognosis today than ever before. Although great variations are noted in the clinical course and progress of the disease through childhood, most infants now survive into adulthood and are able to lead productive lives. As adults, many must make decisions regarding parenting. Women with sickle cell disease have been able to conceive and deliver normal children. However, early prenatal medical and nursing management are essential to fostering a healthy outcome for both mother and newborn. Even though the prognosis has improved, no agent has been found that will prevent in vitro sickling without producing severe toxic effects.[18]

Thalassemia

The thalassemias (major and minor) predominantly occur in areas of Europe, Africa and Asia. In regions of wide occurrence of the gene that produces these, a frequency of more than 1 per 100 live births has been documented.[9] The thalassemias are hemoglobinopathies that cause symptoms similar to sickle cell disease. There appears to be a genetic defect that results in deficient synthesis of HgbA (adult hemoglobin). A severe hemolytic process may accompany the disorder.

Thalassemia minor (trait) is a heterozygous condition associated with mild anemia. A differential diagnosis from iron deficiency anemia can be made by the use of hemoglobin electrophoresis. Since this is basically a carrier form of the disease, severe symptoms do not occur.

Thalassemia major (Cooley's anemia) is a homozygous condition; in it progressive hemolytic anemia during the first year of life is common. Treatment is frequent blood transfusions.

The nursing care of the infant or child with Cooley's anemia or thalassemia minor is essentially the same as care provided to the child with sickle cell disease. Since thalassemia minor is a carrier state, the nurse must help the family to obtain genetic counselling to assist them in making important parenting decisions and also in providing the affected child with pertinent information as he becomes ready to make these life decisions for himself.

Although life-threatening crises and overwhelming infections may plague the child throughout his life, the prognosis of Cooley's anemia is favorable until early adulthood if the child has been successfully treated by use of blood transfusions.[9]

Tay-Sachs Disease

Tay-Sachs disease (also known as GM_2 gangliosidosis) is an inborn error of metabolism caused by a severe deficiency of the enzyme hexosaminidase A (HexA), a necessary enzyme in cellular function. The enzyme deficiency interrupts the breakdown of GM_2 ganglioside (lipid), causing it to be stored in large amounts in neurons throughout the brain, cerebellum and spinal cord.

The disease is inherited as an autosomal recessive disorder, occurring most frequently in populations of Ashkenazi (Eastern or Central

European) Jewish populations.* (See appendix for review of genetic transmission.)

Because the Tay-Sachs child experiences a progressive deterioration of the brain and nervous tissue (because of the accumulated lipid stores), seldom living beyond 3 or 4 years of age, effort has been concentrated on preventing the condition. Community-based mass screening efforts have been highly successful because the disease is common in a defined population. A simple, accurate, inexpensive test is available for carrier detection, and the enzymatic defect can be detected in utero (amniocentesis at 14 to 16 weeks of pregnancy) early enough to terminate the pregnancy. The nurse has a major role in prevention as the information giver, organizer, planner, public speaker, and coordinator of religious, community and medical efforts to eradicate the disease.

Clinical Manifestations The symptoms are neurological in nature; no enlargement of organs is associated with the condition. The most characteristic symptoms are a myoclonic jerk reaction to sound and a cherry red spot on the macula, caused by thickening of the retina due to the storage of gangliosides in the ganglion cells around the macula.

Effects of Tay-Sachs are seen early, usually becoming apparent during the first few months of the infant's life. Motor weakness may occur as early as the third to sixth months of life. Mental and motor deterioration are rapid and general. Few developmental milestones are met, although children generally learn to smile, reach for objects, and sit up. Some may crawl, but none walk. During the latter part of the first year, the infant becomes floppy and weak, although hyperactive reflexes, clonus and extensor plantar response are maintained. Seizures and myoclonus generally subside by the second year of life. Between twelve and fifteen months, the child has an enlarged head, begins to go blind, and has little spontaneous movement or reaction to the environment. By 18 months, the child leads a vegetative existence; progressive blindness, deafness, convulsions and motor spasticity appear. The child is often institutionalized and dies before 4 years of age, usually due to pneumonia.

Treatment and Nursing Care There is no cure or medical treatment for the child with Tay-Sachs disease. Enzyme replacement therapy has not been effective. The only therapy available for preventing this inborn error of metabolism is prenatal diagnosis of affected fetuses by amniocentesis (if the affected fetus is then aborted), carrier screening, and genetic counselling.

The nurse's role in caring for the Tay-Sachs child is limited. Since the disease is progressive, with rapid mental and motor deterioration between 6 and 12 months, the child needs to have a comfortable, supportive environment. Environmental stimuli should be kept to a minimum, as the child startles easily. His weakened condition and immobility require good skin care, adequate nutrition, and frequent turning to prevent pneumonia. Blindness progresses during the latter half of the first year; the nurse should attempt to orient the child through speech before touching him or providing care.

The parents of the child with Tay-Sachs particularly need an empathetic and understanding health professional. Not only are they dealing with feelings regarding their child's deteriorating condition but also are experiencing guilt because of the hereditary nature of the disease. These parents often have many questions regarding the course of the disease; therefore the nurse needs to be knowledgeable about it. They also need assistance in interpreting their child's behavior and may look to nurses for suggestions in how to manage new manifestations. The nurse may later help the parents arrange institutionalization for the child in the community.

Riley-Day Syndrome (Familial Dysautonomia)

Riley-Day syndrome is a rare hereditary disease with a spectrum of autonomic nervous system manifestations, the most common of which is insensitivity to pain. It occurs primarily in Ashkenazi (Eastern or Central European) Jewish families, following an autosomal recessive pattern of inheritance.

Although the basic mechanism of the disease is not known, several theories are under investigation. The features of the disease suggest a defect or deficiency in central nervous system neurotransmission involving acetylcholine. Another theory suggests that a biochemical defect of neuronal maturation or maintenance may be at fault, perhaps as a result of improper nerve

---

*Gene frequency in these families is 1 in 30, compared to 1 in 300 for non-Jews.)

development in utero. A deficiency of neuroreceptors is also being considered, since one set, the taste buds, has been proved absent.

The disease process presents a diffuse selective sensorimotor defect combined with autonomic nervous system dysfunction.[13] Not only do signs and symptoms vary, but they are manifested to various degrees and combinations in individual cases. The most common neurologic feature is an insensitivity to pain. Signs and symptoms may also include an absence of taste buds, absence of overflow tears, loss of vasomotor control, absent or hypoactive deep tendon reflexes, diminished temperature sensation, slowed motor and physical development and poor motor coordination.

Diagnosis and Treatment Delays in physical and motor development during the first year of life often alert parents and pediatricians to the diagnosis of Riley-Day syndrome. Four manifestations make it possible to confirm the diagnosis: (1) injection of histamine intradermally does not produce a wheal, (2) hypersensitivity exists to both cholinergic and adrenergic agents, (3) taste buds are absent, and (4) instillation of metacholine in conjunctiva causes prompt pupillary constriction.[13]

There is no specific treatment for the disease process. The nursing challenge lies in the unpredictable nature and variety of symptoms presented by the child with Riley-Day syndrome. Death generally results from complications of swallowing defects or secondary pneumonia. The rarity of the disease prevents health personnel from gaining experience in the care of the patient with Riley-Day syndrome. The most common causes of hospitalization during the early years include vomiting attacks, erratic temperature control, vasomotor instability, pulmonary disease, and the patient's relative indifference to pain, which allows him to experience major injuries such as fractures without immediately knowing about them. Each stage of development presents unique problems.

Treatment is principally symptomatic during the first year, aimed primarily at prevention of respiratory infection, corneal ulceration and injuries. Lack of overflow tears requires use of supplemental eye drops at least four times daily to prevent corneal ulcerations and abrasion, which often result from the child's insensitivity to pain. As the infant's teeth begin erupting, tongue sores may develop owing to decreased pain sensation coupled with tongue thrusting commonly seen in these infants. Treatment generally consists of filing sharp teeth and use of gentian violet to heal the ulcers.

As the child with Riley-Day syndrome grows and develops, the unpredictable nature of the disease and the frequency of illness, as well as the concomitant medical and psychosocial problems, require that the child and family make complex adjustments. A thorough understanding of the manifestations of the disease and life-threatening complications is vital for the nurse to be of assistance to the family. (Detailed information is available from the Dysautonomia Foundation.)

Prognosis for patients with dysautonomia varies. Approximately 25 per cent die from an acute crisis, usually in early childhood. Patients' adaptation to manifestations of the disease with increasing age, coupled with growing understanding of the disease by health professionals, may account for the number of adults with dysautonomia living fairly normal lives.

Impact of Genetic Disorders on the Family

Drotar's model (Fig. 26–2) depicting the sequence of normal parental reactions to the birth of a child with congenital malformation* is illustrative of the grief work of parents who have a baby with genetic disorder.[4]

The first stage, *shock*, is exemplified by parental crying and feelings of being overwhelmed, empty and helpless.

Following the initial shock the second stage, *denial*, occurs. The more physically apparent the disorder, the less denial or disbelief is expressed. Reality is more easily confronted when the parents are daily faced with the presence of an observable disorder.

Sadness, anger and *anxiety* follow. All three of these reactions are to be expected at this phase of grief work. All three also contribute to parental hesitance about becoming attached to their baby. Sadness arrives primarily out of the parents' disappointment in the child they produced. Anger may be directed toward the baby for not being perfect and toward the mother for creating an imperfect child, or toward whichev-

---

*Genetic disorder is one kind of congenital malformation. The anomaly may be visible, as with Down's syndrome, or basically invisible, as with sickle cell anemia.

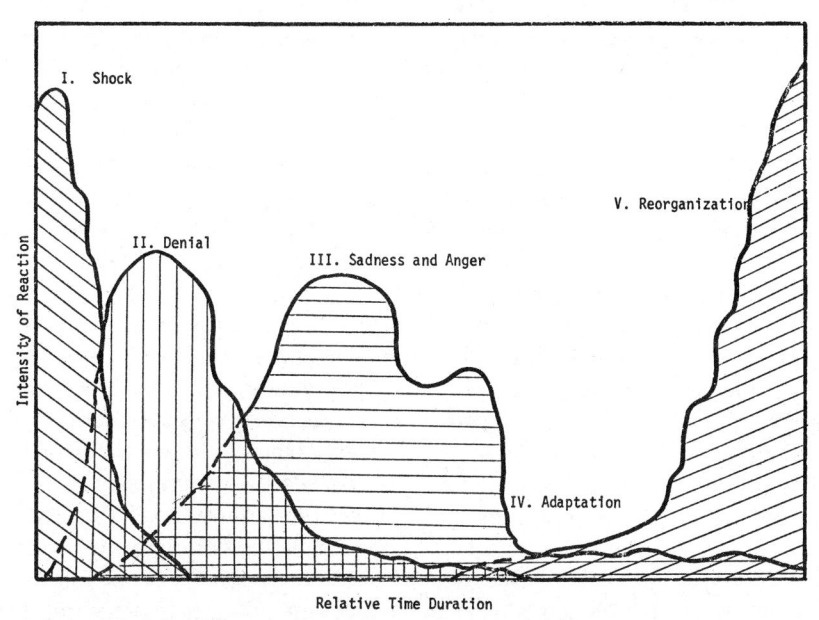

Figure 26-2 Hypothetical model of the sequence of normal parental reactions to the birth of a child with congenital malformations. (From D. Drotar, et. al. The adaptation of parents to the birth of an infant with a congenital malformation: a hypothetical model. Pediatrics, November 1975, p. 710. Copyright American Academy of Pediatrics 1975.)

er spouse is the carrier of the genetic defect. Anxiety is associated with the parents' fear that they will lose the baby because of the genetic defect.

During the fourth stage of grief work, *equilibrium*, parents tend to feel more in control of their reactions and their lives. Adaptation is continuing as the reality of the birth of the baby becomes a part of daily life. Parents begin to work toward helping the child develop, and they become more aware of the child's unique strengths, characteristics and personality traits as their attachment grows. A state of equilibrium is more difficult to achieve if the initial shock and emotional upset is intellectualized rather than emotionally experienced by the parents.

Reorganization is a period during which parents report dealing with the future goals for the child. A positive relationship has been developed with the child, the parents have accepted the child's problems and needs and they begin efforts to assist him toward a productive life.

Parents do not progress through this process at specific rates. The illustration clearly denotes a blending or meshing of stages with one another, and no time parameters are indicated.

In dealing with "genetic grief," the nurse must keep up with current information relative to specific genetic disorders. Once the diagnosis has been made, parents need information regarding the disease process. Parents are most concerned about the here and now, but they also need to be informed about possible developmental delays and the prognosis. There is currently some controversy regarding the timing of this information, as it may severely hamper the attachment process.

LIFE-THREATENING INFECTIOUS DISEASES OF INFANCY

The term TORCH, denoting the types of infections that a mother may transmit to her fetus or newborn that result in serious or long-term health problems, is discussed in Chapter 7. Two of these infections, *toxoplasmosis*, a protozoal infection, and *cytomegalic inclusion disease*, a viral infection, are discussed here, with specific reference to their effect on the infant and the family.

Toxoplasmosis

Toxoplasmosis is a parasitic disease that may be either congenital or acquired. Sources of infection are discussed in Chapter 7. Acquired infection is transient and only mildly symptomatic. Congenital infection is more common and has severe consequences, with 23 to 38 per cent of infected infants experiencing severe central nervous system impairment, ocular damage or death. Once infected, a woman has a lasting immunity, which means future offspring will not be affected.

Manifestations of acute active disease in congenitally infected infants include jaundice, petechiae, enlarged liver or spleen, chorioretinitis (inflammation of the choroid and retina), cerebral calcifications of damaged areas, encephalitis, and convulsions. These infants often die within the first month. Survivors are usually mentally retarded, with psychomotor impairment and varying degrees of blindness.

Third trimester infections result in subacute symptoms. Infants with the subacute form of congenital toxoplasmosis usually have no symptoms at birth, although chorioretinitis may be present. During the first year, subacutely infected infants may develop hydrocephaly, chorioretinitis, intracerebral calcification and psychomotor disturbances.

The presence of toxoplasmosis is diagnosed through serologic examination. Treatment of congenital toxoplasmosis is unsatisfactory, but daily doses of pyrimethamine (Daraprim) and sulfadiazine for four to eight weeks is sometimes effective. Folinic acid is given to stop adverse actions on the bone marrow by the sulfonamide drugs. Since Daraprim is an antifolic agent, leukocyte and platelet counts should be monitored biweekly to prevent leukopenia or anemia or both. In infants with the severe form of the disease, corticosteroids are often given to reduce inflammation, as in chorioretinitis. Once the inflammation has subsided the treatment is stopped.[6]

The progressive nature of the disease suggests that treatment should begin whether the infection is clinically apparent or not. Early treatment may prevent further tissue invasion and may arrest the disease. Treatment of asymptomatic infants is undertaken in order to prevent later sequelae.[6, 11]

In the severely affected infant with congenital toxoplasmosis, the nurse's role primarily consists of palliative treatment for the infant and support to the parents of this critically ill child. Infants with the subacute form of the disease are generally hospitalized for the duration of drug therapy due to the near toxic level of the dosages. Nursing care needs to consist of monitoring the child for signs and symptoms of drug toxicity, leukopenia, thrombocytopenia and anemia.

Cytomegalovirus Infection

Cytomegalovirus infection (CMV), cytomegalic inclusion disease (CID), cytomegaly, and salivary gland disease are synonymous. Cytomegalovirus belongs to a unique group of viruses, the Herpes family, in which the primary infection is followed by a latent form that may reactivate in the body at any time. All ages may be affected by CMV, beginning even before birth. It is the most common cause of intrauterine infection. Most infections take place during the childbearing years, between 15 and 35.[19]

There are three types of CMV infections: congenital, perinatal and other acquired forms. The congenital form is caused by a primary infection in the mother. The virus crosses the placenta and infects the fetus, causing inflammation and necrosis, especially of the central nervous system, resulting in brain damage and mental deficiency. Fetuses of mothers infected during the second trimester are most at risk for developing symptoms.

Clinical Manifestations Ninety per cent of congenitally infected infants are healthy and asymptomatic at birth. The other ten per cent of infants congenitally infected present symptoms. A small percentage of these infants present with "classical" newborn cytomegalic inclusion disease. Perinatally acquired CMV is transmitted at birth through contact with maternal cervical secretions, and the infant experiences mild transient illness. Other acquired forms of the disease are generally asymptomatic. During the early months of life the infection may be acquired from the mother's breast milk. Table 26–1 lists the clinical manifestations and prognosis of CMV.

Diagnosis and Treatment Both congenitally infected infants and those affected perinatally or postnatally excrete large amounts of the virus in the throat and urine, often for many months or years. Diagnosis of CMV is dependent on isolating the virus from the throat, body fluids or blood. In the congenitally infected newborn, an elevated IgM (specific CMV antibody) correlates with active disease. In acquired CMV, signifi-

TABLE 26-1 DESCRIPTION OF CYTOMEGALOVIRUS INFECTIONS

Classification			Clinical Manifestations	Prognosis
Congenital	90% asymptomatic		Normal development	Occasional mental retardation
	10%	Symptomatic	Transient jaundice Purpura Respiratory illness Hepatosplenomegaly Failure to thrive	High recovery Some with brain damage and mental retardation
		Symptomatic Classical	Severe jaundice Thrombocytopenia Chorioretinitis Hepatosplenomegaly Pneumonia Encephalitis	High mortality Survivors have severe brain damage, mental retardation, microcephaly
Acquired	Perinatal		Mild transient illness with symptoms similar to congenital symptomatic CMV	CNS damage may become evident at school entry
	Neonatal and early childhood		Asymptomatic Occasionally: Respiratory symptoms → pneumonia Hepatosplenomegaly Petechial rash	CNS damage may become evident at school entry
	Late childhood and adult		Mononucleosis-type symptoms	

cantly rising antibody titers are usually sufficient for diagnosis.

Other diagnostic signs that may be found on surface appraisal or in monitoring the child's health status include a petechial rash on the first day after birth, failure to thrive, or repeated respiratory infection with a high incidence of chronic interstitial pneumonia during infancy.

No effective treatment of CMV is known; therefore, preventive measures must be stressed. Recent attempts have been made to treat affected newborns with cytosine arabinoside and adenine arabinoside (metabolic inhibitors that interfere with in vitro synthesis of CMV), and although urinary excretion of the virus was suppressed, the long-term beneficial effects need further study before such drugs can become widely available.[10] Treatment with interferon inducers and various antiviral agents have to date produced minimal effects.[7]

A live vaccine is under active investigation. Research suggests that it is possible to prepare a vaccine that is well tolerated and antigenic[5] and that results in both neutralizing and complement-fixing antibodies.[17] Further work needs to be undertaken specifically in relation to mothers and infants. The safety of wide-scale use of this vaccine has not been established. Whether the vaccine would increase the potential for neoplastic disease, increase susceptibility to infection, and whether giving the vaccine to pregnant women will also afford immunity to the fetus are questions that remain unanswered.[10]

During the hospitalization of the child with CMV, isolation procedures are instituted, since infants excrete the virus in saliva for approximately six months and in urine for four months or more. The degree of thoroughness of isolation practices is controversial, varying from careful handwashing to strict isolation. Pregnant women and children are prohibited from rooms as a preventive measure.

Since the disease seems to occur more commonly in conditions of poor sanitation and overcrowding, the nurse may assist families to ensure adequate sanitation.

Complications of congenital CMV often result in spastic quadriplegia, mental retardation, obstructive hydrocephalus or acute respiratory problems. Therefore management of the child must be individualized and long term. The nurse is especially helpful in coordinating the efforts of the health team and community services involved. Most parental concerns result from the child's failure to attain developmental milestones. Support, understanding and proper referral to agencies designed to work with children with development delays is important.

The families of children with CMV may be socially isolated due to the stigma attached to the child who will be excreting the virus over many months. Although the virus is believed to be contagious only on intimate contact, encouraging good hygiene and proper disposal of diapers is imperative in such families. Discussing the rationale for protection of pregnant women and children may alleviate anxieties.

Impact of Infectious Processes on the Infant's Family Congenital infections are often transmitted unknowingly, since the disease and pregnancy are asymptomatic for the mother. Because the infant acquired the infection prenatally, the mother usually experiences guilt and may blame herself for the infant's affliction. Future pregnancies become a concern to both parents. The nurse needs to be aware of and communicate to these parents the fact that subsequent children are generally not affected.

If the infant survives beyond the first month of life, the nurse must assist the parents in meeting the developmental needs of the growing child. Child health maintenance become a focus of care. Since these infants need an individualized program of care, the nurse serves as a coordinator of treatment and as a child advocate to the interdisciplinary team working with the family. The nurse also interprets health care goals to the family, whether they be the goals of educational specialists involved or the health care specialists.

Since many crises affect the family and the child throughout the child's life, the nurse's role is to help parents move toward a response that will allow them to function and cope with their problems. Common problems include marital conflicts, sibling resentment, financial depletion and difficulty in finding adequate temporary care for the impaired child. A major contribution of the nurse is to help parents find services in the community to meet their needs.

SUDDEN INFANT DEATH SYNDROME (SIDS)

Sudden infant death syndrome (SIDS) has been defined by the Second International Conference on Causes of Sudden Death in Infants as the sudden death of any infant or young child, which is unexpected by history, and in which a thorough postmortem examination fails to demonstrate an adequate cause for death.[2] Although sudden infant death syndrome (also called crib death or cot death) has only in recent years been described as a specific disease entity, evidence of its existence has been noted since biblical times. That same conference declared that SIDS is, in fact, a disease: "It is a real disease every bit as much as cancer is a disease. We do not know the cause, but it can be readily diagnosed and the aura of mystery removed."[2]

Incidence

Approximately one-third of all deaths occurring in infants from the ages of one week to one year are the result of SIDS. During the third and fourth months of life the condition apparently accounts for more than one-half of all infant mortality. There are approximately 10,000 SIDS deaths each year in the United States.[1]

Epidemiological Data about Etiology

A variety of epidemiological factors have been investigated in relationship to the incidence of SIDS. Many theories emerge regarding the etiology of SIDS that are well publicized by the media — often prior to the completion of the scientific research. Parents of SIDS victims who are exposed to the publicity may grasp each theory as it comes along as an answer to questions regarding the death of their infant. It is essential that the nurse keep abreast of current research so that she can provide accurate information. The nurse must learn to discriminate between sensationalized reports that are essentially opinion sharing and sound, reproducible research findings. The etiology of SIDS remains unknown, but the various hypotheses that have been or are currently being investigated are discussed.

Relationship to Sleep Data show the SIDS event often occurs during the normal period of sleep. SIDS infants have been found in car seats or strollers, but most generally death occurs in the crib or parents' bed. There is no audible outcry at the approximate time of death.[1]

Even though death apparently occurs in silence, there is often evidence of activity prior to death. Often the parents find the infant face down or with blankets pulled over his head or wedged in a corner of the bed. Some infants are found face up with bedding clutched in their hands. These findings usually lead the caregivers to suspect suffocation and to feel guilty. The nurse must be aware of the developmental abilities of infants at various ages in order to reassure the parents and relatives of the unreasonableness of this hypothesis. The peak incidence of SIDS is 2 to 3 months of age, by which time the infant is able to reposition his head to maintain adequate ventilation. There is also evidence to indicate that ordinary bedding is incapable of causing hypoxia to the point of suffocation. The suffocation hypothesis is also refuted, because pathological findings at autopsy are identical in SIDS cases regardless of the position the infant was found in.[1]

Seasonal Variation Data have indicated that there are in fact seasonal variations in SIDS incidence. The peak incidence is during the fall-winter season, with the fewest cases occurring during the summer months.[1, 17]

Sex Almost every study has shown a male preponderance. The presumption is that this reflects the general male preponderance in mortality and infectious disease morbidity in infants, although there may be specific factors predisposing the male to SIDS.[1]

Multiple Births There is some evidence to suggest that simultaneous deaths in twins occur. Further research into this phenomenon must be conducted.[1]

Feeding History Early studies indicating that SIDS does not occur in breast-fed infants have since been refuted. Therefore, there apparently is no immunity to SIDS passed to the infant from breast milk.

Infectious Disease Because of the age distribution, the seasonal variations, and the autopsy finding of inflammation, researchers are involved in conducting studies into this area of possible causation.

Genetic Factors No evidence exists currently that would support the theory of SIDS as a genetic disease. However, due to the frequent occurrence of SIDS, families may unfortunately lose more than one infant to SIDS.

Signs and Symptoms Found During Autopsy

External examination of the infant reveals the typical victim to be in a normal state of nutrition and hydration. Over half exhibit frothy fluids in the mouth and nostrils, indicative of pulmonary edema.[1] Often this fluid is tinged with blood. The diapers usually are filled with urine and stool. These findings lead Beckwith to suspect that vigorous motor activity has occurred. Vomitus may be found on the face, and the hands may be clutching fibers of blanket materials.

Internal examination reveals intrathoracic petechiae. Typically, these dot the surfaces of lungs, pericardium and thymus, and frequently they also involve the parietal serosal surfaces of the chest. Beckwith proposes that these petechiae may be indicative of intrathoracic negative pressure during the final moments of life.[1] Typically, pulmonary congestion, edema and inflammatory infiltrates in the upper airway and lungs are discovered.

The theories of causation cover such possibilities as rickets, hypothermia, magnesium deficiency, infanticide, cardiac conduction defects, virus infections, apneic spells, collapse of the trachea, and conduction system abnormality.[1] Although many of these theories have been refuted in the literature, others are still under investigation. Current areas of investigation include sleep physiology, developmental neurophysiology and apnea. Dr. Bruce Beckwith, Seattle investigator, suspects the answer to the question of the cause of SIDS may lie in these areas. Figure 26–3 describes the hypothesized cycle.

The seemingly normal sleeping infant becomes hypoxic with positional narrowing of the airway and respiratory inflammation. Additional factors such as autonomic-neurologic instability and chemical factors such as pH balance, hypercalcemia and others then place the hypoxic sleeping infant on the path toward obstructive apnea. At this point the infant may either revert to normalcy after recuperating from the apneic episode or may die. When the reason for the reversible nature of obstructive apneic episodes in some infants and death in others is discovered, the answer to the cause of SIDS will be known. Detection of potential SIDS victims and prevention of sudden infant death syndrome will then be possible.

Impact of SIDS on the Family

Following the SIDS event, severe stress is experienced by all members of the family including parents, grandparents and siblings. Friends of the family, including the babysitter, will also be affected by the sudden unexpected death of an infant. This stress occurs without a noticeable precursor — the benefit of "anticipatory grief" is not experienced by the family.

The initial response to the child's confirmed death is extreme shock that produces varying degrees of confusion. This may be followed by outrage so intense that injury to self or to others may occur. Guilt is experienced either in the form of self-blaming or by projecting the blame onto another family member (often the spouse). These are the typical mixtures of responses experienced by all involved in the sudden death event. The nurse must be prepared to recognize these reactions.

During this critical period the parents of the SIDS infant need tremendous support. Reality orientation helps the family cope with their confusion and guilt. The first essential step in reality orientation is the physician's confirmation of the death to the family. This should not be done over the phone. Because of the extreme shock of sudden death, no family member should be told of the death without the presence of another family member, relative or friend. Family members have less difficulty accepting the death and resolving their grief when they are permitted to view or even hold their dead infant. The family should always be prepared prior to seeing the dead infant. Stressful as it is, seeing or holding their child facilitates the family's acceptance of the death; however, no family member should ever be forced to have this experience.

The family needs an opportunity to sort their feelings and to begin to cope with their outrage. A place for the family to be alone affords them privacy they need to regain composure and release feelings they do not wish to display publicly. An individual family member should never be left alone, nor should the family feel abandoned by the nurse. At this time the nurse can serve as a therapeutic person by listening to fears, answering questions about the death and

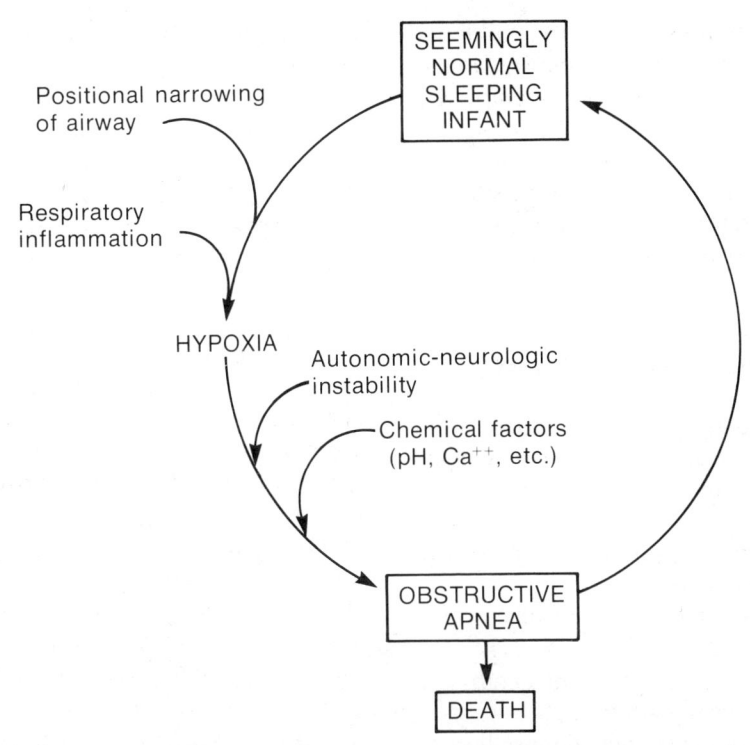

Figure 26–3 Proposed theory of SIDS showing the final common pathway terminating in death or reverting to a condition of normalcy. (Bergman, et al., 1970; revised 6/26/79 by Dr. Bruce Beckwith, Children's Orthopedic Hospital and Medical Center, Seattle, Washington.)

offering reassurance that the death was not preventable.

Some families find that this event draws them closer together, while other families are immobilized to the extent that they are unable to support each other. It is those families who are drawn apart that are more likely to project their guilt. Providing the family with printed information about SIDS helps allay some of the blame-making and guilt.

Inadequate parenting, the infant's suffocation by blankets or choking on vomitus, or inability to mouth breathe, as well as parents' failure to take the infant to the physician in time to cure a slight cold, are false explanations for the death often voiced by parents. These misunderstandings must be dispelled at the first visit with the family (in the emergency room or wherever the nurse first has contact with the family members). The crucial piece of information that parents and relatives must have is that *the death was not preventable.*

Impact of SIDS on Siblings

The inability of parents to cope with the needs of their other children during the initial period of shock and confusion can cause severe pain for the remaining siblings. They are often temporarily housed with relatives or friends to "protect" them from the pain of the mourning process and the funeral events. Such actions do not show recognition for the need of siblings to remain with their parents during this intense stress or work through their own grief. Only their parents can continue to provide the security needed by the surviving children through this stressful time.

The young child may also develop his own explanation for the baby's absence from the family. He may experience intense guilt or anxiety associated with the baby's absence. Children may associate their angry feelings toward the baby with the baby's death, especially if sibling rivalry has occurred. Sending the children away from home at this time further increases their anxiety, confusion and sense of guilt. Although the parents are having an extremely difficult time supporting one another, they must somehow share in their children's grief as well. The nurse's intervention centers on providing information about childhood grief to the parents and facilitating the family's unique grief work. The use of play therapy with siblings may assist the younger child to play out fears, guilty feelings, and anxieties. Older siblings may need time to talk about the death with the nurse or their parents. The nurse can facilitate their grief work by providing an opportunity for it to occur.

Intervention at the Time of SIDS Death

The National Foundation for Sudden Infant Death (NFSID) has advocated a management plan for SIDS. The four aspects of this program are as follows:
1. Performance of autopsies on all infants dying suddenly and unexpectedly;
2. Prompt notification of the results of that autopsy to the parents;
3. Use of the term *sudden infant death syndrome* on the death certificate;
4. Follow-up information and counselling for all families provided by a knowledgeable health professional.[12]

In the Home Paramedical personnel are frequently the first persons called to the home when the nonbreathing infant is found. Therefore it is imperative that they possess adequate information about SIDS. They must be trained to deal with the death in an empathetic and nonjudgmental manner. Local police, county coroner and other community officials must be informed by the community health care personnel about the special needs of SIDS families at the time of death.

In the Emergency Room Emergency room personnel may have an overwhelming reaction to the SIDS event. Because they are geared toward preservation of life, dealing with the family of a SIDS victim can be extremely difficult, so difficult that at times the family is left alone to deal with their grief and confusion. Emergency room personnel need assistance in dealing with their own feelings of grief so they can provide the kind of intervention needed by families at this critical time. Families need someone to stay with them and to reassure them that what has happened is not their fault. They need someone to listen to their pain, minister to their simple needs (get a cup of coffee for them), and help them make the important, immediate decision about whether or not to consent to an autopsy, and to make funeral arrangements and deal with the reactions of siblings.

At Autopsy According to Bergman,[2] autopsy serves two functions: in approximately 15 per cent of the cases a cause other than SIDS may be found, and the mysterious cause of death can be clarified. Otherwise, families are left with doubt for the rest of their lives. It has been suggested that the member of the health team who provides this immediate information regarding the results of the autopsy be the pathologist or family physician. Following this information (preferably in person and within the first 24 hours after the death of the infant), a letter summarizing the cause of death should be sent. This letter is often viewed by the family as an official statement of their blamelessness.[12]

Community Follow-up

A community outreach program, including counselling at three critical periods, has been advocated. This program would include three steps: (1) when the baby is found dead, immediate intervention must be provided; (2) during the year following the death counselling must follow either in the form of one-to-one intervention or group intervention and support; (3) counselling is again critical at the time of subsequent pregnancy and birth.

Every effort should be made to have contact with the family within the week following the SIDS event. Often a follow-up program involving community health nurses can be developed within the community health care network. Parents also need opportunities to draw support from other parents of SIDS infants if they so desire. During the first home visit the nurse must assess the family as to their level of understanding of the SIDS event. Information that has been misunderstood needs to be clarified at this time. Rather than an involved discussion of etiological theories, the nurse needs to focus attention on the family members' reactions to the SIDS event. During this time the nurse can provide continual reassurance that the parents could have done nothing to prevent, nor did they do anything to cause, the SIDS event.

During the next few months the nurse needs to be available to the parents through phone calls, letters or visits. Assisting the family in their grief work is her prime function. Throughout this period the nurse must be aware that special days within the year — the child's birthday, Christmas, Thanksgiving, Easter, the anniversary of the infant's death — have significance to the family members. The nurse should make every effort to prepare the parents for the extra stress that often exists on these days and see that they have support systems to lean on during these times.

Such support systems may be derived from a SIDS parents' group.* Films provided by these groups not only offer clarification of SIDS but also provide a focus for discussions about feelings and grief work. A unique relationship is shared among parents of SIDS infants. The strength of that relationship should not be underplayed by the health team.

References: The Dying Infant

1. R. Caughill, ed. The Dying Patient: A Supportive Approach. Little, Brown and Co., 1976
2. N. Doyle. The Dying Person and the Family. Public Affairs Committee, Inc. Pamphlet No. 485, November 1972
3. J. Gyulay. The Dying Child. McGraw-Hill Book Co., 1978

Additional Recommended Reading: The Dying Infant

G. Benfield et al. Grief response of parents to neonatal death and parent participation in deciding care. Pediatrics, June 1978, p. 171

P. Codden. The meaning of death for parent and child. Maternal-Child Nursing Journal, Spring 1977, p. 9

M. Coddington. A mother struggles to cope with the child's deteriorating illness. Maternal-Child Nursing Journal, Spring 1976, p. 39

B. Comerford. Parental anticipatory grief and guidelines for caregivers. Nursing Digest, Summer 1977, p. 64

J. Fischhoff and N. O'Brien. After a child dies. Journal of Pediatrics, September 1976, p. 140

J. Guimond. We knew our child was dying. American Journal of Nursing, February 1974, p. 248

J. Hagen. Infant death: nursing interaction and intervention with grieving families. Nursing Forum, April 1974, p. 371

T. Helmrath and E. Steinitz. Death of an infant: parental grieving and the failure of social support. Journal of Family Practice, April 1978, p. 785

P. Jackson. The child's developing concept of death; implications for nursing of the terminally ill child. Nursing Forum, February 1975

M. Keysen. At home with death; a natural child-death. Journal of Pediatrics, March 1977, p. 486

---

*Parents' groups are sponsored by the National Foundation of Sudden Infant Death (NFSID) or The Guild for Infant Survival (GIS). Films such as "You Are Not Alone" (a 16 mm 30-minute film) and "Sudden Infant Death" (a 16 mm film) are produced by the U.S. Bureau of Community Health Services and available through the National Sudden Infant Death Syndrome Foundation (318 So. Michigan Avenue, Chicago, Illinois); (312) 663-0650. These can be useful to SIDS parent groups.

M. Klaus and J. Kennell. Maternal-Infant Bonding. C. V. Mosby Co., 1976

K. Robson and H. Moss. Patterns and determinants of maternal attachment. Journal of Pediatrics, January 1970, p. 976

O. Sahler, ed. The Child and Death. C. V. Mosby Co., 1978

H. Schiff. The Bereaved Parent. Penguin Books, 1977

R. Zahourek and J. Jenson. Grieving and the loss of a newborn. American Journal of Nursing, May 1973, p. 836

References

1. J. Beckwith. The Sudden Infant Death Syndrome. U.S. Department of Health, Education and Welfare, DHEW Publication No. (HSA) 78–5251, 1978
2. A. Bergman, J. Beckwith and C. Ray, eds. Sudden infant death syndrome, Proceedings of the Second International Conference on Causes of Sudden Death in Infants. University of Washington Press, 1970
3. B. Conway. Pediatric Neurologic Nursing. C. V. Mosby Co., 1977
4. D. Drotar et al. The adaptation of parents to the birth of an infant with a congenital malformation: a hypothetical mode. Pediatrics, November 1975, p. 710
5. S. Elek and H. Stern. Development of a vaccine against mental retardation caused by cytomegalovirus in utero. Lancet, January 1974, p. 1
6. S. Gillis and B. Kagan, eds. Current Pediatric Therapy. W. B. Saunders Co., 1978
7. R. Hoekelman et al. Principles of Pediatrics: Health Care of the Young. McGraw-Hill Book Co., 1978
8. G. Honig and W. Borges. BDIS: birth defects information system REL.1.1, Information Retrieval Facility (National Foundation March of Dimes), Sickle Cell Anemia No. 836, 1 December 1978
9. G. Honig and W. Borges. BDIS: birth defects information system REL.1.1, Information Retrieval Facility (National Foundation March of Dimes), Thalessemia No. 939, 1 December 1978
10. S. Krugman et al. Infectious Diseases of Children. C. V. Mosby Co., 1977
11. J. Menkes. Textbook of Child Neurology. Lea and Febiger, 1974
12. M. Miles, ed. Mental Health Aspects of SIDS: Report of a conference sponsored by the National Foundation for Sudden Infant Death and the National Institute of Mental Health. U.S. Department of Health, Education and Welfare. (Kansas City), 30 July 1975
13. A. Osoff. Caring for the child with familial dysautonomia. American Journal of Nursing, July 1975, p. 1158
14. K. Robson and H. Moss. Patterns and determinants of maternal attachment. Journal of Pediatrics, January 1970, p. 976
15. G. Schneiderman, A. Lowden and Q. Rae-Grant. Tay-Sachs Disease and carrier screening programs: psychosocial aspects. Canadian Journal of Public Health, August 1977, p. 66
16. Sickle Cell Screening and Education Clinics: Model Protocol for Sickle Cell Counseling. U.S. Department of Health, Education and Welfare Publication No. (HSA) 77–5121, 1977
17. D. Smith. Introduction to Clinical Pediatrics. W. B. Saunders Co., 1977
18. J. Smith. Sickle cell disease. In Current Therapy, 1979. Latest Approved Methods of Treatment for the Practic-

ing Physician by H. Conn, ed. W. B. Saunders Co., 1979
19. H. Stern. Cytomegalovirus infection. Nursing Times, 10 February 1977, p. 190
20. M. Wintrobe et al. Clinical Hematology. Lea and Febiger, 1974

Additional Recommended Reading

Genetic Disorders of Infancy

B. Axelrod et al. Familial dysautonomia: diagnosis, pathogenesis and management. In Pediatrics, Volume 21. Year Book Medical Publishers, 1974

D. Fairweather et al. Antenatal diagnosis of thalassemia major. British Medical Journal, January 1979, p. 351

G. Karayalcin et al. Sickle cell anemia: clinical manifestations in 100 patients and review of the literature. American Journal of Medical Sciences, Jan/Feb 1975, p. 51

S. Martens, genetics associate, Children's Orthopedic Hospital and Medical Center, Seattle, WA. Personal Communication, Apr/May 1978

J. McFarlane. Sickle cell disorders. American Journal of Nursing, December 1977, p. 1948

G. McKhann. BDIS: birth defects information system REL.1.1, Information Retrieval Facility (National Foundation March of Dimes), Tay-Sachs No. 434, December 1978

R. Mercer. Mothers' responses to their infants with defects. Nursing Research, Mar/Apr 1974, p. 133

J. O'Brien. The gangliosidoses. In the Metabolic Basis of Inherited Disease by J. Standbury et al. (eds.). McGraw-Hill Book Co., 1978

G. Schneiderman et al. Family reactions, physicians' responses and management issues in fetal lipid storage diseases. Clinical Pediatrics, March 1976, p. 887

E. Schwartz. Hemaglobinopathies of clinical importance. Pediatric Clinics of North America, November 1972, p. 889

B. Westmoreland et al. Electrographic findings in three types of cerebromacular degeneration. Mayo Clinic Proceedings, June 1979, p. 12

R. Young. Chronic sorrow: parent's response to the birth of a child with a defect, Part 4. Maternal-Child Nursing, Jan/Feb, 1977, p. 38

Infections of Infancy

G. Desmonts and J. Couvreur. Congenital toxoplasmosis: a prospective study of 378 pregnancies. New England Journal of Medicine, 1974, p. 1110

J. Dudgeon. Viral infections. Journal of Clinical Pathology (Supplement), November 1976, p. 99

D. Greet. Toxoplasmosis: nursing care study. Nursing Mirror, December 1977, p. 53

C. Midgely. Neonatal and perinatal infections. Midwives Chronicle, July 1978, p. 251

J. Swartzberg and J. Remington. Transmission of toxoplasma. American Journal of Diseases of Children, July 1975, p. 777

Sudden Infant Death Syndrome

A. Bergman. Sudden infant death. Nursing Outlook, December 1972

A. Cleveland. Comment: sudden infant death syndrome (SIDS): a burgeoning medicolegal problem. American Journal of Law and Medicine, March 1975

J. DeFrain and L. Ernst. The psychological effects of SIDS on surviving family members. Journal of Family Practice, May 1978, p. 985

E. Hasselmeyer and E. Nox, eds. Research Planning Workshops on SIDS: Behavioral Aspects. U.S. Department of Health, Education and Welfare Publication No. (NIH) 74–577, 1972

J. Marx. Crib death; some promising leads but no solutions yet. Science, August 1975, p. 367

M. Pomeroy. Sudden infant death. Nursing Outlook, December 1969

THE HOSPITALIZED INFANT

27

by Linda Nicholson Grinstead, RN, BS, MN

For the infant hospitalized owing to illness, hospitalization can be a frightening experience. No longer is he secure in a familiar environment and surrounded by familiar people. Instead, he hears the strange sounds of children crying and machines beeping. He smells the unusual odors of medications and antiseptics. Even the food he eats is often different in some manner from what he is accustomed to. His orientation, once clarified by his senses, is now confused and overwhelmed. More importantly, his main supports, his parents, may be absent or responding to him differently because of their own anxiety in the situation.

EFFECTS OF HOSPITALIZATION

Chapter 16 discusses the common effects of hospitalization on children and ways in which the nurse can help parents and children cope. In infants, the primary factor that determines the effects of hospitalization is the infant's developmental level. Research has shown that younger infants respond differently from their older counterparts. It has been reported that infants as young as 10 days displayed a response to a change in caretakers. Schaffer found that the infant under seven months became subdued, no longer babbled and lost interest in his surroundings, whereas the child over seven months exhibited more outward signs of stress, such as crying and parental clinging.[6] Another researcher theorized that the major effect of hospitalization on the infant under eight months of age was a disruption of his routine, whereas the infant over eight months suffered more from anxiety over separation from the mother.[1]

Cooke found that the infant was primarily restricted in manner of dress and in regularity of feeding and postulated that, due to illness, the child is not as able to adapt as he would be if he was well.[3] The overall effect often is regression of the infant's development, or at least a delay in its progress.

The type of illness may also influence the infant's reaction to hospitalization. The infant who is not allowed to eat or suck because of oral surgery or for any other reason may react by persistent crying or thrashing about out of the frustration of not having his oral needs met. The infant with a problem of the central nervous system, on the other hand, may exhibit a wide range of behavior changes. An infant's instinctive need to move freely may be affected by restraints or other means of immobilization. Parents have reported incidents in which their children, when frustrated in later years, would assume the posture they were in during prolonged periods of immobilization. One needs to exert caution in assessing an infant's reactions, however. For example, the quiet, subdued infant in Bryant's traction may not attract the attention of his caretaker as readily as the crying, clinging child in the next bed. His

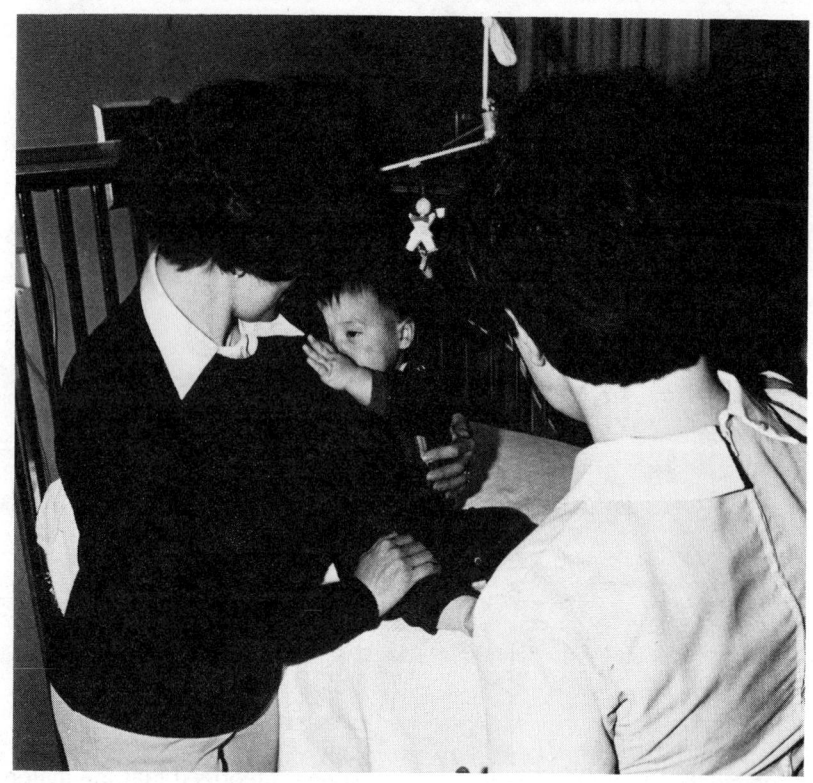

The infant over seven months of age exhibits outward signs of distress when hospitalized, such as crying and clinging to his mother.

means of coping, while less apparent, are equally important cues to the nurse.

Because infants are able to sense changes in their parents, such as anxiety or fear, parental attitudes toward the hospitalization experience can affect the infant. He may respond with expressions of abandonment if the parent is feeling overwhelmed and unable to meet his nurturing needs. The parent who is able to remain active and involved in the infant's care maintains the situation as near normal as possible and thereby reduces the anxiety.

It has been generally believed that the shorter the hospital stay, the less profound the effects on the infant. However, even with relatively short stays of two or three days, parents have reported changes in sleeping and eating habits of their infant. A more common statement by parents is that their child "wants to be held constantly" upon returning home. Restrictions in movement and bodily activity often accompany long-term hospitalization and thereby increase the demands placed on the infant's adaptive mechanisms.

The infant who has a warm, trusting relationship with his parents will be better able to withstand the changes in his routine associated with hospitalization. Positive home experiences aid him in his development of trust and assure him that his needs will be met wherever he may be. If his parents are able to continue to participate in his care, he should experience a relatively minor feeling of loss and will continue to be more outgoing and less anxious.

The infant, being small and physiologically immature, is in a particularly vulnerable position. Therefore, he requires intervention on his behalf. The nurse who has an understanding of the various aspects of infant development will be better able to utilize the nursing process for the benefit of both the infant and his family.

Parents, as part of the family unit, are also affected by this crisis. Their common feelings are anxiety, guilt and a sense of failure. Hospitalization may be a new experience for them. Fearing the unknown, they may react with a wide range of behaviors. One parent may appear concerned and overprotective, while another may seem to be apathetic and uncaring. Whether or not hospitalization is defined as a crisis is based on personal experience and will differ for each parent. If parents have had to struggle with the care of their infant at home, hospitalization may be viewed as a welcome relief from that burden.

Depending on their philosophical orientation, the illness may be seen as a punishment for something in the past. If the pregnancy was unwanted or if the infant interferes with career plans, the illness may be viewed as a just reward for these thoughts. Feelings of guilt may be inadvertently reinforced by members of the health team. For example, the parent who conscientiously treats the child at home for "flu" that later turns out to be meningitis may be given the impression by hospital staff that he or she was negligent in not seeking medical attention for the child earlier.

Parents may see the activities of the nurse, in particular, as a threat to their own abilities. Their prior responsibilities of feeding, administering medications and the like may now be taken over by persons unknown to them. Out of a sense of helplessness they may resort to criticism of their child's care. This means of coping on the part of parents must be understood by the nurse if she is going to be able to communicate effectively with them.

Siblings also feel the disruptive impact of the illness on the family unit and may exhibit an increase in somatic complaints, a decreased school performance or a change in attitudes.[7] Their initial jealousy of the infant and the attention he receives may have prompted wishes and fantasies about getting rid of him. With hospitalization, they may perceive themselves as responsible for the illness, and an intense feeling of guilt can result. As with the infant, the effects on the siblings vary, depending on their ages, family relationships and life experiences.

SPECIAL NEEDS DURING HOSPITALIZATION

The nurse in the acute care setting has the responsibility to provide nursing care that is developmentally oriented to the infant and his family. Only when she is able to recognize the coping behaviors and developmental level of each member of the family unit and plan her interventions accordingly will she be giving "total" care.

Initial contact is usually established through the admission interview. Most child care units have a structured guide to assist the process of data collection. It is at this time that the infant's routines, behaviors, preferences and special needs can be ascertained. This will form the basis for the plan of care that is fitted to the individual needs of a particular infant. Knowledge of the family, their socioeconomic status and the parents' understanding of their child's illness all assist the nurse in planning for the acute episode as well as for discharge. The interview is an excellent time to discuss and encourage parental visiting or rooming-in. It also serves as a time to share specific information regarding the routines and procedures of the child care unit. Many parents, although unable to room in, may wish to be present at feeding times, at bedtime or when procedures are being performed.

To reduce threat and anxiety, an infant's usual daily routine should be incorporated into his care as much as possible. For example, adherence to his usual feeding schedule should be given high priority, as well as following his established bedtime ritual. Primary nursing has been instituted on some units and has been found to be an effective means of meeting both staff and infant needs.

Because the infant does not comprehend the continued existence of objects when they are

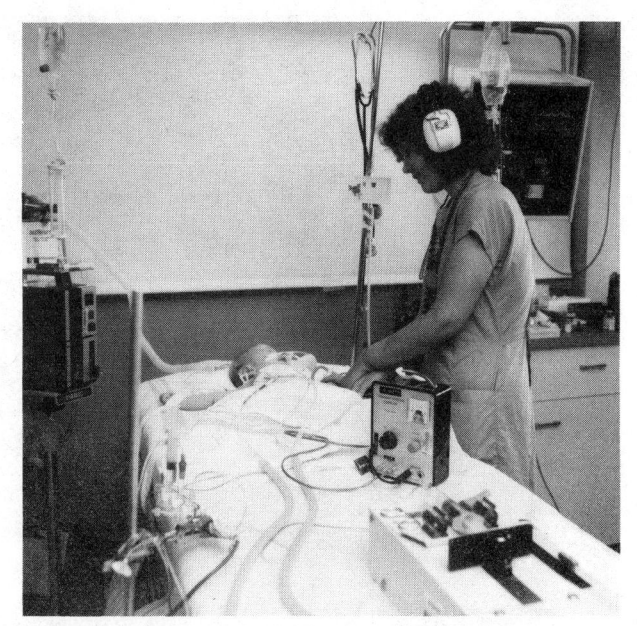

The infant, being small and physiologically immature, is vulnerable and needs close nursing observation.

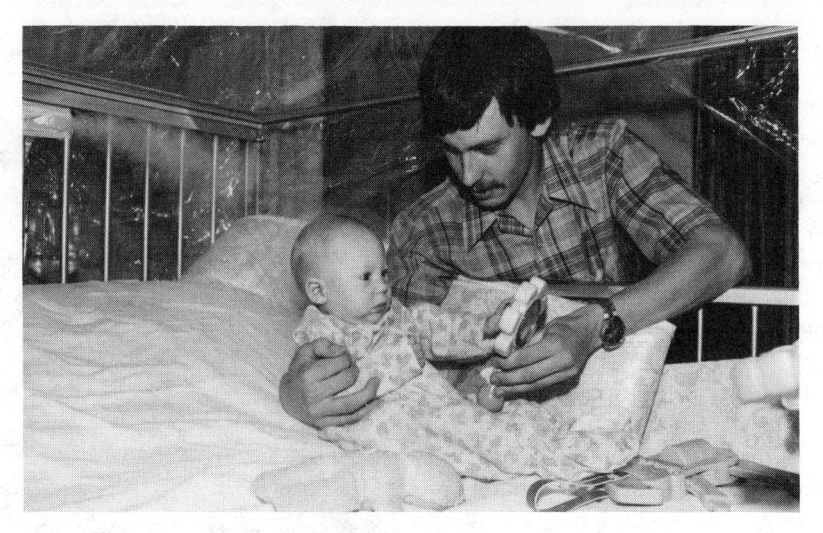

Hospitalized infants need the stimulation of play and toys to maintain their development.

no longer within his sight, it becomes important that the parents be present at regular intervals. This is not always so easily accomplished when parents have job and family responsibilities or are financially unable to make the trip to the hospital. At large referral centers the distance from home to hospital alone may prohibit frequent contact. Encouraging parents to telephone their infant's primary nurse or the child care unit is one way to facilitate continuance of the parent-child relationship.

Play

To assist in preventing regression in development and a delay in the attainment of developmental milestones, an organized play period or infant stimulation program is desirable. Plank recommends that infants who are more than 10 months of age be included in play programs.[12] Play is intellectually stimulating and provides opportunities for continued development of motor and social skills. Whether or not there is an organized program, the nurse can provide stimulation along with her other nursing care activities.

While feeding, dressing or diapering, the nurse should establish eye contact and speak to the infant. She should hold the child in a close, secure manner for all feedings. Bottles and pacifiers should not be propped. Until he has back control, an infant can be propped or placed in an infant seat at intervals if his condition permits, so that he can observe the activities about him. Mobiles, mirrors, baby gyms and music boxes provide additional auditory and visual stimulation. Every infant should have toys within his reach in his crib. Some hospital auxiliaries provide small soft toys for individual patients if none have been brought from home.

Activities can be planned away from the crib as well. Many units have strollers, swings and rockers. If these are not available, a mat or bath blanket can be placed on the floor to provide the older infant opportunities for crawling, rolling and reaching.

Restraints

Mobility is an important aspect of the development of the infant. When angry or frustrated, he frequently resorts to flailing of arms and legs. Occasionally, for his safety, he must be restrained during procedures such as intravenous therapy, nasogastric intubation, and following oral surgery. Unable to cope in his usual manner, his tension is increased. In one study Sibinga and Friedman[13] examined children who were restrained as infants and found a positive correlation between this restraint and later language delay and articulation problems.

Suggestions for nursing interventions include (1) providing stimulation to the infant while he is restrained (use of a suspended ball that could be kicked by the feet); (2) removing the restraints under supervision for 10 minutes every two hours to allow for random movement; and (3) changing the infant's position while unrestrained, and at the same time, talking to him and touching and holding him.[4] Infants with orthopedic anomalies often must undergo long periods of immobility and their need for stimulation is similarly acute.

Medications

One aspect of hospitalization that deserves special attention is the administration of medications to infants. Besides delivering the right dose to the right infant at the right time, the nurse must be able to administer the medication safely while using a developmental approach.

Oral Medications For security and comfort, the infant should be held on the nurse's or parent's lap when oral medications are being given. If this is not possible, the infant's head can usually be lifted off the bed and cradled in the nurse's hand. As a general rule, all medications should be crushed and mixed with a small amount of fluid. Depending on the medication and individual case restrictions, suggested fluids include water, flavored syrups and juices.

With many oral medications coming in syringes under unit dose medication administration systems, the medication can be administered directly into the infant's mouth. Since the infant's sucking reflex causes him to push out anything placed in the front of his mouth, the tip of the syringe should be placed in the back of the mouth and to one side and the medication given in small amounts. Medication given by dropper can be administered in the same manner. Small plastic medication cups bent to form a spout can also be used, but since the medication is delivered at the front of the mouth, it is easily pushed out and the administration process often must be repeated. Use of a nipple into which the medication is poured is recommended, as it best utilizes the infant's natural responses. The nipple method is not recommended, however, in those infants with sucking problems or when medication has a bad taste. If parents are present, they are often more effective than professionals in gaining the child's cooperation to give the medication.

Ormond and Caulfield, in their guide to giving oral medications to young children,[10] identify specific developmental tasks and behaviors and the attendant nursing implications.

Injections Although subcutaneous injections are given infrequently in many child care set-

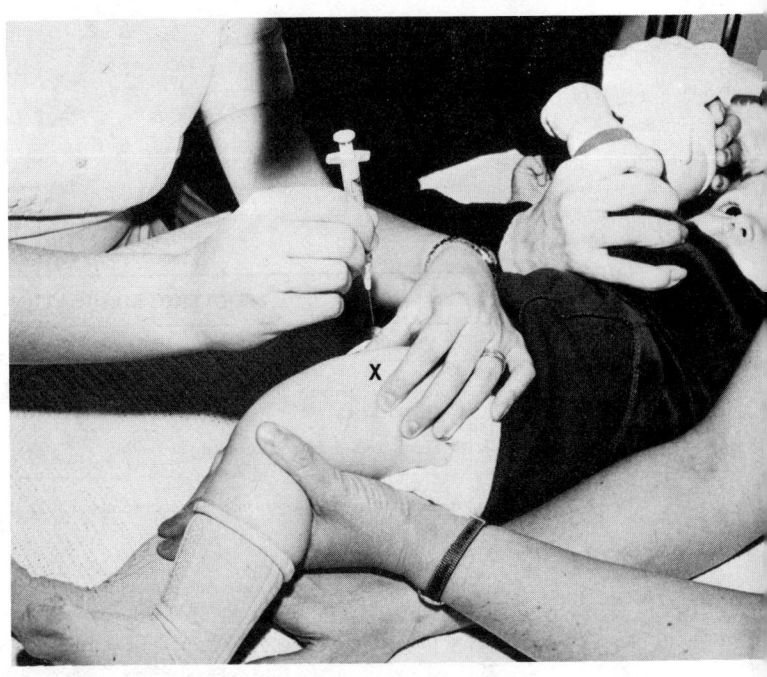

The desired site for injection is the vastus lateralis muscle (X on the photo indicates site). Safe administration is best achieved by two nurses; the parent should be free to divert the infant.

tings, some general guidelines are necessary. They include (1) Approach the infant with a positive attitude. (2) Always have another person help hold the infant. (3) Select an appropriate size needle and syringe. A 5/8 inch, 25 gauge needle can be used for most medications, and since the usual dose is 0.5 ml or less, a tuberculin syringe is most accurate. (4) Inject into the fatty layer underlying the skin, usually in the anterior or lateral aspects of the thighs, at a 45-degree angle (in some infants with adequate subcutaneous tissue, a 90-degree angle may be used. (5) Neither pinch nor stretch the skin but allow it to remain in its natural state.[10]

To give an infant an intramuscular injection, the following guidelines are suggested in addition to the first two just listed: (1) Select an appropriate size needle; usually a 1 inch, 22 or 23 gauge is best for most medications. (2) Pinch up the muscle tissue into which the needle will be inserted. (3) Inject at a 90-degree angle into the vastus lateralis muscle. To locate the injection site, draw a visual line between the trochanter and the lateral aspect of the patella on the outer aspect of the thigh. Determine the

PEDIATRIC MEDICATION GUIDELINES—1 to 3 MONTHS

	Developmental Tasks and Behaviors	Nursing Implications
MOTOR	• Reaches randomly toward mouth; shows strong palmar grasp reflex. • Head drops or exhibits bobbing control.	• Infant's hands should be monitored or controlled to prevent spilling of medications. • Head must be well supported.
FEEDING	• Sucks reflexively in response to tactile stimulation. • Corners of the mouth may not seal effectively and the tongue may be reflexively forced against the palate. • Tongue movement may project food out of mouth. • Sucking strength increases (3 mos.). • Stops taking fluids when full; progresses to fading of sucking reflex (3 mos.).	• Medication should be administered using this natural behavior: medication should be given via nipple. (See example.) • Correct position of the nipple, if used, must be assured for adequate sucking. • A syringe or dropper, if used, should be placed in the center back portion of the mouth. If placed along the gums, it must be toward the back of the mouth. • Amount of medication presented must be controlled. Infant may choke or drool because he can take in more medication than he can control. • Medication more easily given in small volumes and when infant is hungry.
INTERACTIVE	Basic Trust versus Mistrust Stage • Infant becomes socially responsible.	• Medication administration requires feeding behavior which establishes an easy, comfortable situation. This is part of the child's learning to form a trust relationship.

EXAMPLE: Jonathan, 2 months, has received 125 mg of ampicillin intravenously every 4 hours for 2 weeks and by mouth every 4 hours for 2 days. Irritable and febrile on admission, his status improves after the medication starts. He becomes alert and afebrile and orders for discharge are written. He is to continue the ampicillin for 5 more days and return to the clinic in 7 days.

Jonathan's mother is very nervous about "getting him to take medicine" at home. She explains that she herself "throws up" every time she tries to drink medicine.

The nurse helps mother prepare to give her son medication, which is available in a suspension. She teaches Jonathan's mother to draw the proper amount into a syringe and how to hold Jonathan in her lap so both her hands are free to hold the nipple and syringe. Then, touching the nipple to Jonathan's lips so his mouth opens and placing it well back in his mouth in a natural feeding position, the nurse drips the medicine into the nipple and follows it with some water to assure his getting full amount. For Jonathan this is like all feedings. Demonstrating this technique can help relieve the mother's fears and increase the likelihood of Jonathan's continued recovery as well.

From E. Ormond and C. Caulfield, A practical guide to giving oral medication to young children. American Journal of Maternal Child Nursing, Sept/Oct 1976, pp. 320–321.

PEDIATRIC MEDICATION GUIDELINES—3 TO 12 MONTHS

Developmental Tasks and Behaviors	Nursing Implications
MOTOR • Advances from sitting well with support (3-4 mos.) to crawling (10 mos.). • Begins to develop fine motor hand control. • Advances from lying as placed (3 mos.) to standing with support (12 mos.).	• Safety precautions regarding where medications are placed and kept become extremely important. • Child who does not want to cooperate has ability to resist with his whole body.
FEEDING Starting at 12-month-old level: • Smacks and pouts lips in act of shifting food in mouth and in swallowing. Lower lip active in eating. • Tongue may protrude during swallowing. • Learns to drink from cup. Generally has poor approximation of corners of the mouth when drinking. • Learns to finger-feed self. • Feeding behaviors become individualized.	• Child may spit out food and medicine he does not want. • Eating is inefficient, so medications may need to be retrieved and refed. A small medicine cup may be more effective than a spoon. • Feeding patterns and routines at home need to be considered.
INTERACTIVE Basic Trust versus Mistrust and Oral Sensory Stages • Communication skills develop from random social responses (3 mos.) to making simple requests by gesturing (12 mos.). • Is sensitive and responsive to tactile stimulation. Begins developing responsiveness to other stimuli. • Recognizes immediate family and, very important, may exhibit intense separation anxiety.	• One must be alert for child's indicating his own needs (12 mos.). • Physical comforting will be most effective with child. Verbal comforting secondary. • Exhibits early memory. May recall negative experiences, precipitating negative response in another similar situation.

EXAMPLE: Herman, age 8 months, has had recurrent otitis media, and his mother has given him medications from a syringe since he was 2 months. Currently admitted with fever, dehydration, and otitis media, he has received ampicillin intravenously. Herman's condition improves and oral fluids and medications are initiated. Knowing he drinks from a cup, the nurse pours his ampicillin suspension (200 mg) into a medicine cup. In his room she holds Herman, talks with him in a relaxed manner, then puts the cup to his mouth.

After a brief pause, Herman begins crying and reaching for his bottle. Herman's mother arrives to visit and explains that at home she uses a syringe and he does not seem to mind taking medicine. Leaving Herman with his mother, the nurse gets a syringe for the remainder of the dose, and Herman's mother then gives him a bottle of juice to drink. Familiar activities are very important to Herman. Six hours later the same approach works for the nurse. She describes Herman's familiar routine in the Kardex before going off duty.

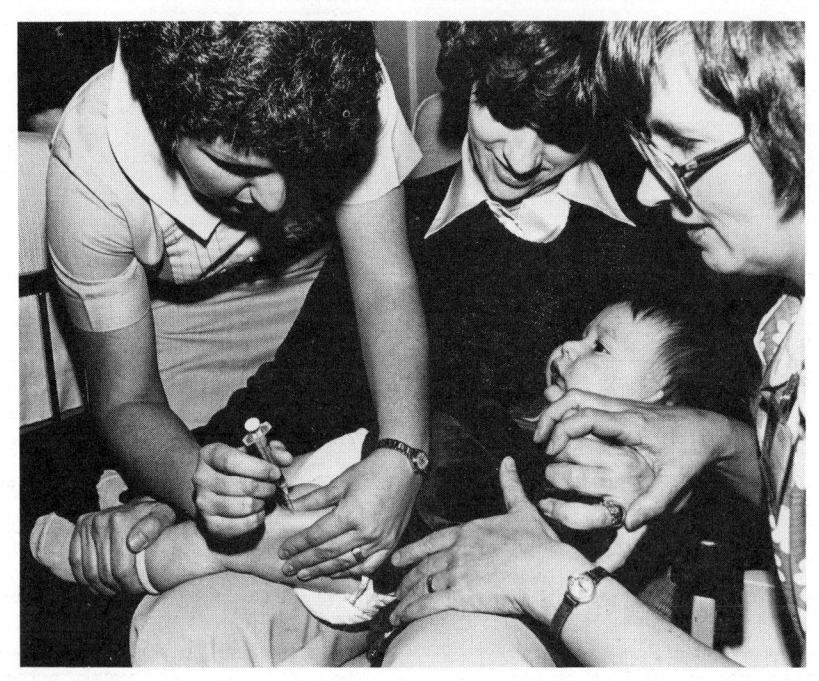

Infants tolerate procedures better in their parent's arms. Note the restraint and injection techniques.

middle third of the distance visually and follow the usual procedure for intramuscular injections.[2] As with any painful procedure, the infant should be held and comforted so that he does not come to associate the injection and pain with feelings of rejection.

Eye Drops When instilling eye drops, care must be taken to avoid pressure on the eyeball. With the infant lying supine, the head is steadied. The thumb and index finger of one hand are used to separate the eyelids and the other hand is used to administer the medication. The solution or ointment is directed into the sac formed by the lower lid or placed in the inner canthus, never directly onto the eyeball. When the infant subsequently blinks, the medication will then enter the eye socket. Ointments are applied along the inner margin of the lower lid from the inner canthus outward. The excess is gently wiped outward with a sterile cotton ball.

If the infant vigorously resists the eye medication, it may be necessary for two people to administer the treatment. One person holds the lids open properly and the other administers the medication. When the drops are instilled, the hand that holds the dropper should rest on the infant's head. The hand and head can then move together, reducing the possibility of trauma to the eye. If the medication causes burning, the parent should be prepared for the infant's crying after instillation and should provide cuddling.

DISCHARGE

Although a goal of any hospitalization is to avoid post-discharge behavioral disturbances in the infant, the literature cites numerous examples of such occurrences.[3,5,6,9] Withdrawal, sleep and eating disturbances, apathy, regression and increased clinging are just a few of the reported changes. These behaviors lasted from a few minutes to weeks in some instances. Separation of parent and infant appears to be a key precipitating factor, however. Since it has been shown that most parents do wish to participate in the care of their children, particularly in those activities seen as nurturing, they should be encouraged to do so.[8] This is the optimum situation for most infants.

If parents decide to room in, they need the support of the nursing staff. They may be hesitant to touch a seriously ill infant without the explanations and encouragement of a staff member. They should be given the opportunity to express feelings regarding hospitalization and their infant's illness. With the presence of the parents, teaching about home management of the infant's condition can be ongoing and not left until the day of discharge. Parents should also be prepared for the possibility of post-hospitalization behavioral changes. If the infant's needs are not met while he is hospitalized, his stay in the hospital, even for a short time, can interfere with his normal development.

References

1. L. Blackman. The infant in the hospital. In The Effects of Hospitalization on Children, E. Oremland and J. Oremland, eds. Charles C Thomas, 1973.
2. J. Chezen. Locating the best thigh injection site. Nursing 73, December 1973, p. 20.
3. R. Cooke. Effects of hospitalization upon the child. In The Hospitalized Child and His Family, A. Haller, et al., eds. The Johns Hopkins Press, 1967.
4. E. Dowd, et al. Releasing the hospitalized child from restraints. American Journal of Maternal Child Nursing, Nov./Dec. 1977, p. 370.
5. S. Droske. Children's behavioral changes following hospitalization—have we prepared the parents? Journal of the Association for the Care of Children in Hospitals, Fall 1978, p. 3.
6. A. Hales-Tooke. Children in Hospitals—The Parent's View. Priory Press Limited, 1973.
7. N. Issner. The family of the hospitalized child. Nursing Clinics of North America, March 1972, p. 5.
8. P. Jackson, et al. Child care in the hospital: A parent/staff partnership. American Journal of Maternal Child Nursing, Mar/Apr 1978, p. 104.
9. M. McGillicuddy. A Study of the Relationship Between Mother's Rooming-In During Their Children's Hospitalization and Changes in Selected Areas of Children's Behavior. Doctoral Dissertation, New York University Health Sciences, Nursing 1976.
10. E. Ormand and C. Caulfield. A practical guide to giving oral medications to young children. American Journal of Maternal Child Nursing, Sept/Oct 1976, p. 320.
11. M. Pitel. The subcutaneous injection. American Journal of Nursing, January 1971, p. 76.
12. E. Plank. Working with Children in Hospitals. The Press of Case Western Reserve Untiersity, 1971.
13. M. Sibinga and C. Friedman. Restraints and speech. Pediatrics, July 1971, p. 116.

Additional Recommended Reading

A. Ayer. Is partnership with parents really possible? American Journal of Maternal Child Nursing, Mar/Apr 1978, p. 107.

M. Blumberg. Depression in children on a general pediatric service. American Journal of Psychotherapy, January 1978, p. 20.

P. Brandt, et al. IM injections in children. American Journal of Nursing, August 1972, p. 1402.

C. Bresadola. One infant/one nurse/one objective: quality care. American Journal of Maternal Child Nursing, Sept/Oct 1977, p. 286.

C. Hardgrove and R. Dawson. Parents and Children in the Hospital. Little, Brown & Co., 1972.

S. Harvey and A. Hales-Tooke. Play in Hospital. Faber and Faber, 1972.

C. Isler. The fine art of handling a hospitalized child. R.N., March 1978, p. 41.

T. Kenny. The hospitalized child. Pediatric Clinics of North America, August 1975, p. 583.

L. Kunzman. Some factors influencing a young child's mastery of hospitalization. Nursing Clinics of North America, March 1972, p. 13.

H. Love, et al. Your Child Goes to the Hospital. Charles C Thomas, 1972.

D. Newton and M. Newton. Needles, syringes and sites for administering injectable medications. Journal of the American Pharmaceutical Association, November 1977, p. 685.

E. Noble. Play and the Sick Child. Faber and Faber, 1967.

J. Robertson. Young Children in Hospitals. Basic Books, 1958.

NURSING CARE PLAN FOR THE INFANT WITH RESPIRATORY ALTERATION
Kathy T. Edwards, RN, BSN
Amy L. Hofing, RN, MSN

Nursing Diagnosis	Expected Outcome	Nursing Interventions	Rationale
Respiratory Insufficiency	Immediate: A patent airway is achieved and/or maintained in the infant. Short term: Infant will begin to improve with treatment and will not suffer from oxygen deprivation. Long term: By discharge, infant will be free of any sign of respiratory distress.	Dx: 1. Obtain history from parents of infant's respiratory problems currently and before this time once the infant's respiratory stability is established. 2. Assess infant for signs of respiratory distress (varies with age and diagnosis): nasal congestion, sneezing, productive or nonproductive cough, pallor, cyanosis, mottling, flaring of the nares, grunting, retracting dyspnea, stridor, apnea or tachypnea, wheeze, inflammatory exudate, fever, restlessness, exhaustion. 3. Monitor vital signs (frequency varies with the degree of distress). Infant tolerates these procedures best when done while the infant is being held or cuddled by a parent or significant other. 4. Auscultation of breath sounds. Infants will cry less if they feel secure (are held, stroked or cuddled) during this assessment.	Dx: 1. To elicit all details of past and present respiratory symptoms that are essential to diagnostic and treatment process. 2. Accurate assessment and documentation are vital to the diagnosis and treatment of any respiratory problem. 3. Vital signs reflect the degree of distress. Interference with O_2 consumption will cause a change in vital signs. Apnea and bradycardia will occur in newborns; older infants have tachycardia and tachypnea. Fever is the body's response to some respiratory diseases. 4. Aids in determination of airway patency, and presence of rales, rhonchi, atelectasis, pulmonary edema, etc. Minimal discomfort during procedure to infant is essential because increased crying reduces available O_2 and complicates respiratory problem.

698 FAMILIES WITH INFANTS

Rx:
1. Suction gently as needed; stimulate cough reflex if possible.

2. Maintain constant air humidification, as indicated, with or without oxygen. Keep infant and bed dry to prevent chilling.

3. Place infant in semi-Fowler's position with slightly hyperextension of the neck.

4. Percussion and postural drainage as ordered.

- frequency and duration will depend on infant's problem and tolerance but should be performed before meals.

- position infant on the lap preferably of a parent, or with pillows.

Rx:
1. Suctioning enhances ventilation by removal of accumulated secretion. Infants have a weak cough reflex, so gentle suctioning to stimulate cough may be necessary to help loosen and move secretions upward.

2. Oxygen therapy is indicated for hypoxemia to be determined by infant's color and arterial blood gases. Humidification will soothe inflamed membranes, provide relief from distress and liquefy secretions. Humidification is always necessary when oxygen is administered to prevent drying of mucous membranes.

3. This position accommodates lung expansion and straightening of airway.

4. Percussion and postural drainage help facilitate drainage of the tracheobronchial tree, which is necessary for adequate aeration. This is indicated when fluid or mucus cannot be removed by normal activity or cough.

- necessary to prevent vomiting and aspiration.

- change in position will promote drainage from all major lung areas. A parent's lap is preferred because it allows opportunity for parent-infant contact and comforting.

Care Plan continued on following page

THE HOSPITALIZED INFANT 699

NURSING CARE PLAN FOR THE INFANT WITH RESPIRATORY ALTERATION (Continued)

Nursing Diagnosis	Expected Outcome	Nursing Interventions	Rationale
		5. Organize care to include frequent rest periods. Periods of age-appropriate stimulation for infant should also be provided.	5. Rest will promote the conservation of energy. A balance between rest and stimulation fosters return to wellness.
		6. Administration of medications as ordered by physician • antipyretics • decongestants • antibiotics • expectorants • bronchodilators	6. Medications will depend on age of infant and diagnosis.
		Parent Education: 1. Explain signs of respiratory distress and teach measures parents can take to prevent or relieve it.	Parent Education: 1. Since the infant cannot verbalize his distress, caretakers must be able to identify and intervene when the infant is in respiratory crisis.
		2. Explain procedures, treatments and equipment that will be involved in the infant's care.	2. Education about treatments or procedures to be done at home should begin early in baby's hospitalization. This will give the parents ample opportunity for practice in a supportive environment. If equipment will be needed it should be obtained early so the parents can use it before discharge.
Altered Nutrition	Infant will receive adequate calories and fluids to maintain good nutrition during illness.	Dx: 1. Obtain nutritional history from parents to include: • normal routine and feeding habits (type of nipple and pacifier, use of cup or bottle) • infants likes and dislikes • food allergies • effects of illness on eating habits: loss of appetite, difficulty sucking or swallowing, vomiting, diarrhea.	Dx: 1. Nutritional history provides information for nurse to plan for care of an infant. If the illness is brief, nutrition may not be compromised, but continual reassessment is necessary. Prolonged illness may be less stressful if infant's routines are maintained as much as possible.

2. Assess infant for signs of dehydration.
   - loss of skin turgor; skin dry and warm to touch
   - dry mucus membranes, lack of tears
   - decreased urine output; increased urine specific gravity
   - weight loss
   - sunken fontanel
   - tachycardia

Rx:
1. Nasal suction may be necessary.

2. Provide fluids and food frequently in small amounts using a soft nipple or cup. Choose types infant is familiar with and likes. Encourage those with high caloric content. Encourage parents to feed infant when possible.

3. Administer parenteral fluids if ordered.

Parent Education:
1. Explain how the infant's nutritional status will be maintained during illness (nasal suctioning; soft nipple or cup; high calorie foods, small, frequent feedings).

2. Children often refuse to eat or drink when not feeling well or when having difficulty breathing. This has special implications because the infant is especially susceptible to fluid and electrolyte imbalance. Assessment must be accurate and treatment immediate.

Rx:
1. Infants normally breathe through their nose, so clearing the passages will aid breathing and ability to feed. The procedure is done before meals to prevent vomiting and aspiration.

2. Small, frequent feedings through a soft nipple or cup will prevent tiring. An infant is more likely to take fluids he takes at home. High caloric feedings provide the energy needed by the body during illness.

3. May be necessary for infants with serious fluid and electrolyte imbalance. Also indicated for conditions such as tachypnea and vomiting.

Parent Education:
1. Parent involvement in infant's nutrition fosters bonding, relieves anxiety about child's intake, prepares them for home care of infant during respiratory illness.

Care Plan continued on following page

THE HOSPITALIZED INFANT 701

NURSING CARE PLAN FOR THE INFANT WITH RESPIRATORY ALTERATION (Continued)

Nursing Diagnosis	Expected Outcome	Nursing Interventions	Rationale
		2. Teach parents the signs of dehydration.	2. An infant can rapidly become dehydrated, requiring early and prompt recognition and intervention by parents.
Interference with intellectual, motor, and emotional-social development	Infant will have opportunities for development consistent with physical condition and developmental age.	Dx: 1. Assess degree of energy infant has available for developmental activities (activity tolerance).	Dx: 1. A severely distressed infant may not even have sufficient energy for eating. Appropriate developmental activities for energy-depleted infant are visual or auditory.
		2. If the baby has a long-term need for a higher O_2 concentration, periodically assess the need to alter the method of O_2 delivery in order to permit activities that promote development.	2. Delivery mode depends somewhat on O_2 concentration required. A tent provides some opportunity for baby to be mobile and gives him a larger visual field. An oxygen hood or an incubator distorts vision and creates a constant high noise level.
		3. If the infant is hospitalized for an extended time, plan for regular developmental assessments (e.g., monthly).	3. Developmental needs change quickly during infancy. Changes are not always readily apparent to nurses who do not consistently care for the baby.
		Rx: 1. Utilize other care-giving situations to provide developmental activities.	Rx: 1. Feeding or treatment times can be used for planned developmental activities (auditory stimulation) or encouraging midline behaviors by placing both of baby's hands on bottle during feeding. Follow-through will be more consistent if specific activities are included in care plan and listed at infant's bedside.

2. Provide variety of colors and textures of blankets and clothing to enrich environment.

3. Develop and maintain a list of specific developmental activities for the infant. Make regular changes based on assessment of development.

4. Provide as much as possible for variations in position and environment if infant is immobile because of treatments or respiratory distress.

Parent Education:
1. Include parents when developmental assessments are done and activities are planned.

2. These items are important, particularly for infants in more severe distress who cannot participate in other activities. Be sure that these items do not distort the nurse's color perception when assessing infant's color for signs of change in respiratory status.

3. List should emphasize activities in areas in which infant seems to be currently focusing. Emphasis will change, since development does not progress at the same rate in all areas.

4. Altering position of bed or infant seat can be helpful if more extensive alterations such as being carried about cannot be tolerated.

Parent Education:
1. May provide positive reinforcement for parents if baby has made some developmental progress or if some aspects of development are within normal limits. Parents can play an active role in developmental stimulation, particularly if they can be helped to identify specific activities or signs of progress.

Care Plan continued on following page

NURSING CARE PLAN FOR THE INFANT WITH RESPIRATORY ALTERATION (Continued)

Nursing Diagnosis	Expected Outcome	Nursing Interventions	Rationale
Altered parent-child relationship	Parents and baby will establish and/or maintain bonding and attachment.	Dx: 1. Record frequency of parental phone calls and visits. 2. Determine with parents if there is a need to establish a regular time when nurse will call to inform them about baby's condition and progress. Rx: 1. Initiate contact with parents of a newborn if neither of them have called to inquire about baby or visited within 24 hours of admission. 2. Encourage parents to gradually begin to participate in baby's care and treatments. 3. Encourage parents to bring clothes and toys for baby.	Dx: 1. Written record provides a mechanism for early identification of lack of contact or infrequent contact. 2. This is especially needed if parents live a distance from hospital and cannot afford frequent phone calls or visits. Giving them information that helps them identify baby as an individual will promote bonding of parents with newborn. An example would be telling the parents how much baby seems to enjoy feedings and kinds of facial expressions he uses to show this. Rx: 1. Parents of a newborn may have difficulty initiating contact because of grief and anxiety. They may need assurance that calling and visiting are appropriate. 2-3. Type and degree of parental participation indicates how bonding is progressing. Participation in care and learning special treatments is also part of early discharge planning.

4. Encourage touching and holding of infant and promote eye contact.

5. Provide opportunities for parents to express concerns and feelings.

6. Give clear explanations of equipment, symptoms and procedures to parents.

Parent Education:
1. On admission inform parents of visiting times, what care they may provide for baby, times they may call the unit, and unit phone number.

2. Develop a written teaching plan if parents will need to do any home treatments or procedures or take any preventive measures.

4. This may be limited to some degree by baby's physical condition and treatment. Both nurses and parents should be involved. By promoting these behaviors, especially eye contact, nurses can help baby remain emotionally accessible to parents. These behaviors are also part of the bonding/attachment process.

5–6. Seeing baby in respiratory distress may be particularly frightening for parents. Planned opportunities for communication help build trusting relationships and may prevent concerns from building up if the hospital stay is lengthy.

Parent Education:
1. Making parents feel welcome and helping them clarify their roles as parents of a hospitalized infant can help them develop regular visiting patterns.

2. A written plan shared with parents helps nurse and parents identify content and progress. It should be included as part of baby's permanent medical record.

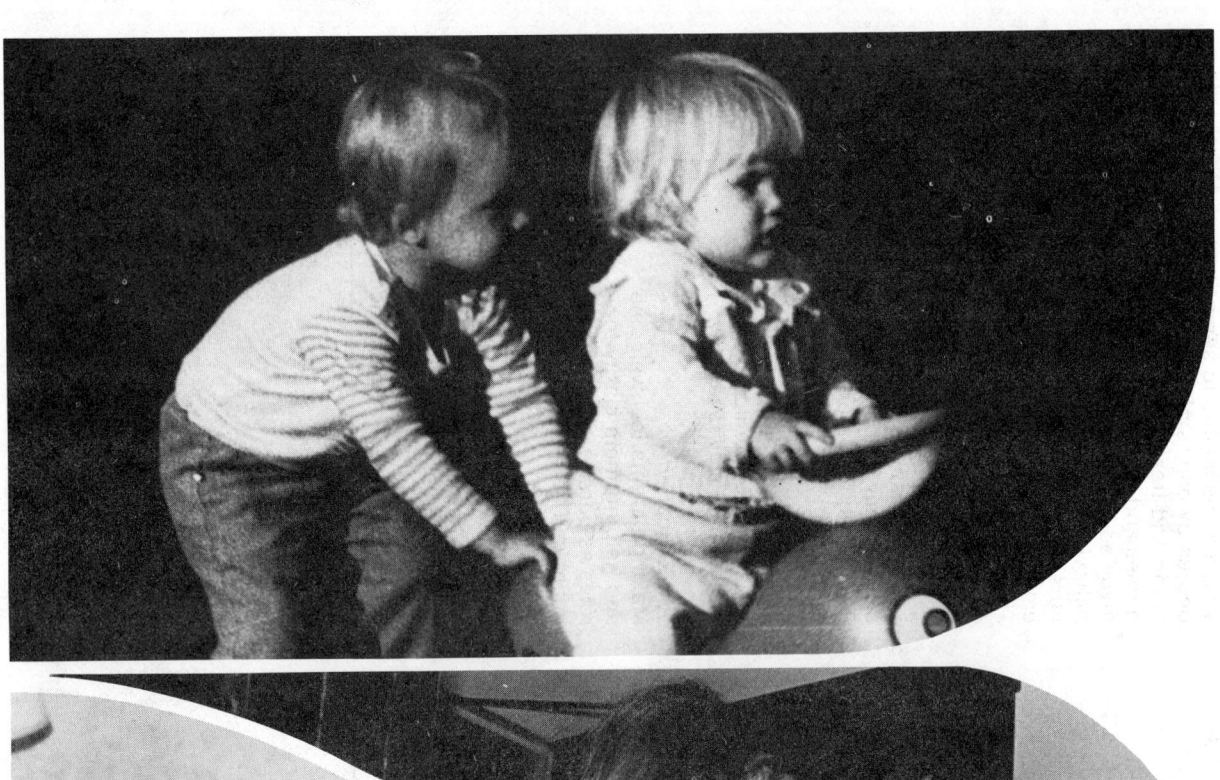

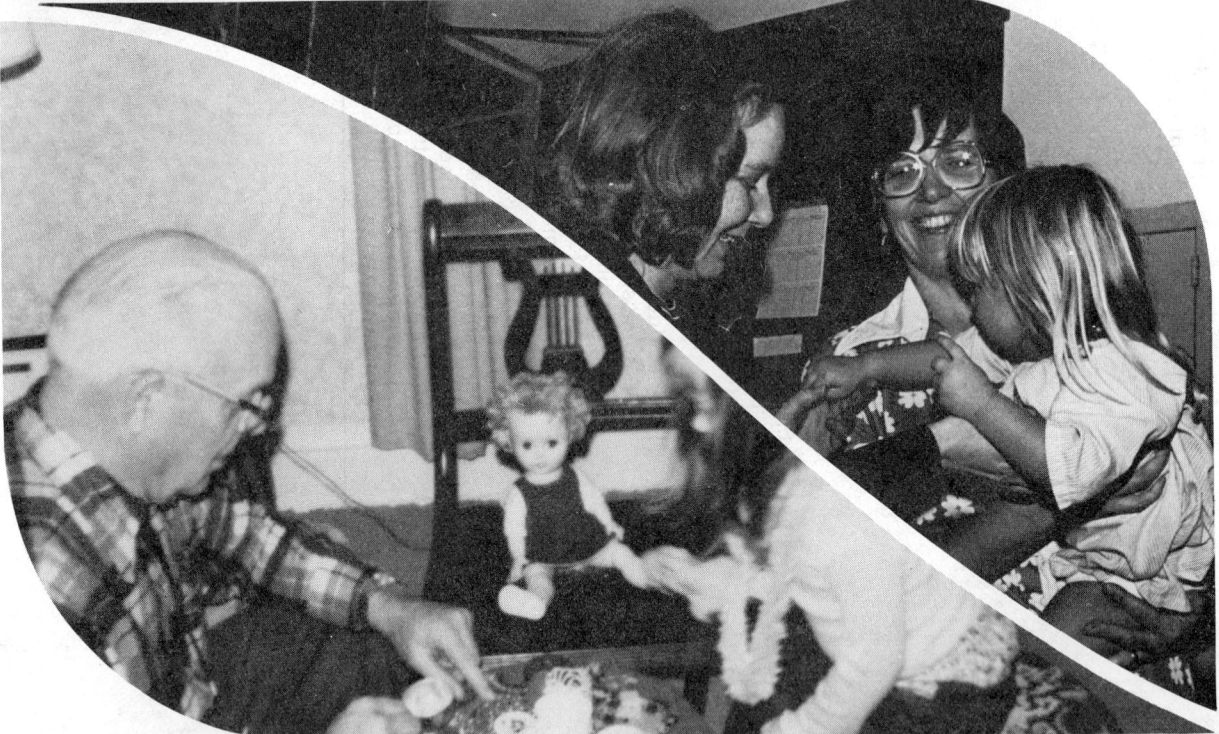

PART 5

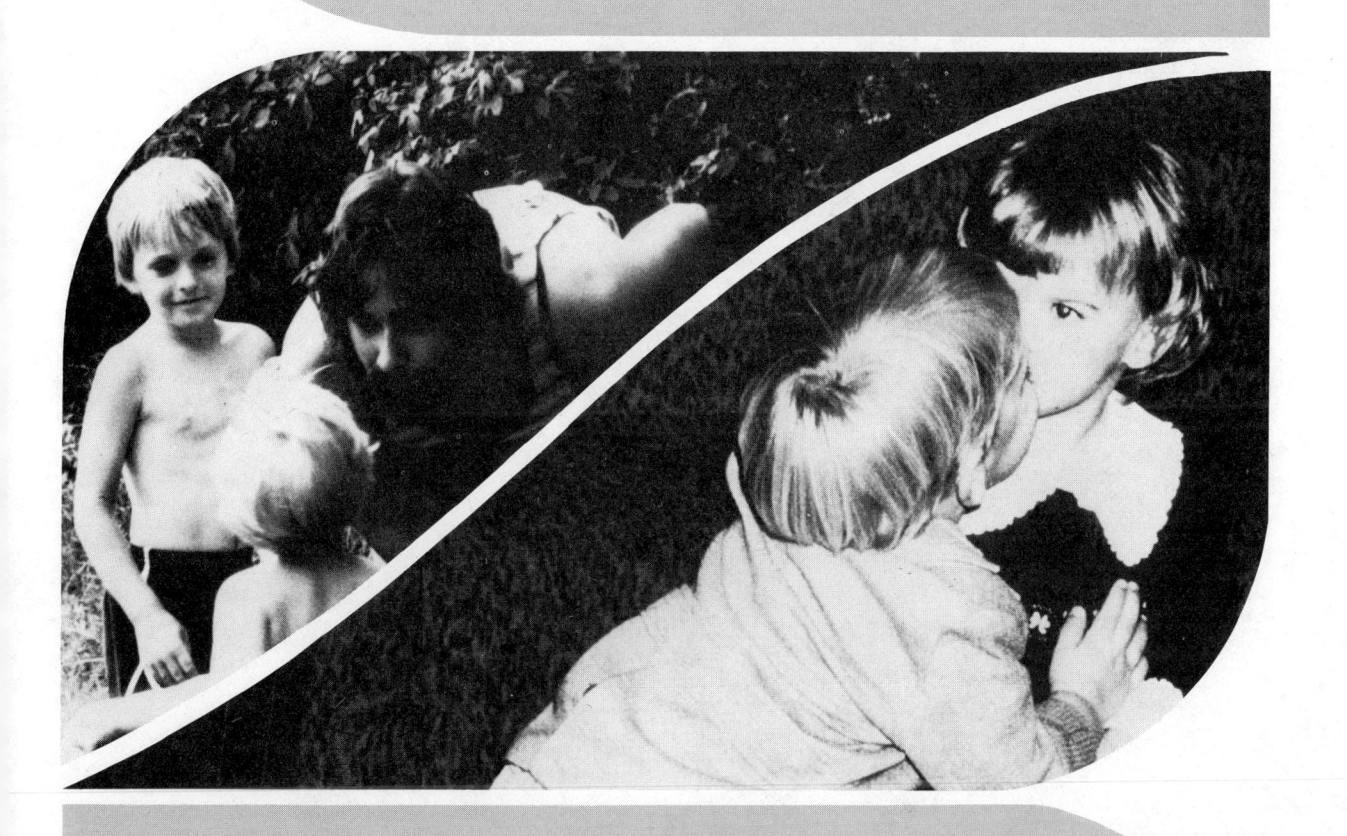

FAMILIES WITH TODDLERS

GROWTH AND DEVELOPMENT OF THE FAMILY WITH A TODDLER: MAINTAINING WELLNESS

by Jo Joyce Tackett, BSN, MPHN

The couple in the childbearing stage of their life cycle who now have a toddler rambling through their home, perhaps along with older children, find themselves faced with a revised set of family development tasks. This chapter looks at those tasks and their impact on each member, as well as each member's responsibility in accomplishing those tasks. The nurse's role in assisting families to adapt in healthy ways to these task demands is described.

The overall task of the family with a toddler is the establishment and maintenance of a stable home that values each member's contributions and responds to the changing needs of each. To accomplish this task the family must (1) successfully adapt its resources to accommodate an active child(ren), (2) reorganize relationships within and outside the home to include the child(ren) without disrupting intimate marital bonds and (3) rework the family philosophy to incorporate children and parenthood.

ADAPTING RESOURCES TO ACCOMMODATE CHILDREN

Managing this task involves reallocation of space and facilities within the home, making a decision about childproofing the toddler's environment, reprioritizing the family budget to handle new expenses, rearranging division of labor in the home so as to not overtax any one member and to consider new contributing potentials of growing members, and planning for future children.

Reallocation of Space and Facilities

Once a baby has taken the first steps that propel him into toddlerhood, his family quickly becomes aware of how much space this mobility requires. The baby who was satisfied to be contained in a crib or playpen where his small repertoire of toys could also be confined refuses to accept such limitations in space as a toddler. Furthermore, his selection of toys is expanding and he wants them to accompany him wherever he happens to meander in his world (home).

It is often at this point that families decide it is time to add another bedroom or invest in a larger home, or perhaps in their first home to get out of the small quarters. Other families decide to adapt happily to their limitations in space and to improvise as necessary to ensure private retreats for each family member. Whichever decision is made, the American norm is to provide children with some space of their own, separate from their parents, by the time the children approach toddlerhood. If the family's socioeconomic situation and values about privacy make it feasible, this means that each child has his own bedroom or at least one he shares with a same-sex sibling. If budget or values do not support such an arrangement, the toddler's private retreat may be a large closet renovated into his play and sleep area or a section of a room that can be closed off with folding doors or pull-around drapes.

Aside from his need for a space of his own, the toddler's demands for space to play and discover must also be reckoned with by the family unit. Again, depending on their attitudes about children and values about people and possessions, each family manages this situation differently. The more traditional family in terms of attitudes and values is motivated to manage this concern in a manner that keeps the child(ren) out of the adults' way but still considers the child's comfort. The modern family with a developmental orientation that places greater value on persons is motivated to manage the space dilemma so as to provide whatever is needed to help the child grow and develop at his best. Either approach can allow the toddler opportunities to move about, explore and manipulate; but the modern family approach tends to grant the toddler the range of the home. The traditional approach usually means confinement of toys and explorative activities to certain rooms or certain areas in rooms within the home.

Another alteration in space of a different form that families with expressive toddlers must make is with emotional space. A toddler's caretakers will foster his development of self-control by allowing him space for making choices and for emotional expression. For example, the toddler might choose the toys he will take to bed with him or which pajamas to wear. As long as the choices and emotional expressions are healthy, conducive to his development and will cause no one harm, as much choice as his age warrants should be given. But when his choices or emotional expressions breach these considerations, limits must be imposed, usually to the child's relief, because he is aware of his loss of control and it frightens him.

The parents' responsibility with regard to space and facilities is to make such allocations and, if limits exist in relation to the space provided, to make those limits realistic and clearly understood by the toddler.* Consistent enforcement of those limits is important so the toddler knows where the boundaries are and need not worry about whether he is inside or outside his limits "this time."

The toddler's responsibility in achieving this task is to learn to enjoy and discover his world within whatever space his parents can grant him, to incorporate a respect for whatever limits are imposed, and attempt to comply with them. The toddler's motivation to comply arises out of a desire to please his parents; therefore he is more likely to continue compliance if his cooperation is acknowledged and praised occasionally.

Childproofing

Each new move to independence in a child's life is an intrusion into his parents' life, and parents become especially conscious of this intrusion when their baby begins toddling after them at their every step and toward every precious possession in their home. His message — that this is his home, too — comes through loud and clear once he has achieved even amateur mobility (crawling and pulling himself up). This is the time for parents to make a careful study of the home for environmental hazards and possible relocation of precious possessions. They need to become aware that special vigilance and firm discipline can prevent accidental injury to their child.

Although some families choose to leave the home unaltered and teach their toddler what he may handle and what he must leave alone, most families opt for at least minimal childproofing. Ideally, every home with a toddler is child-

---

*Toddlers live in the present, having not yet developed the ability to recall the past or future conceptually. They need frequent reminders in simple terms, not a one-time discussion.

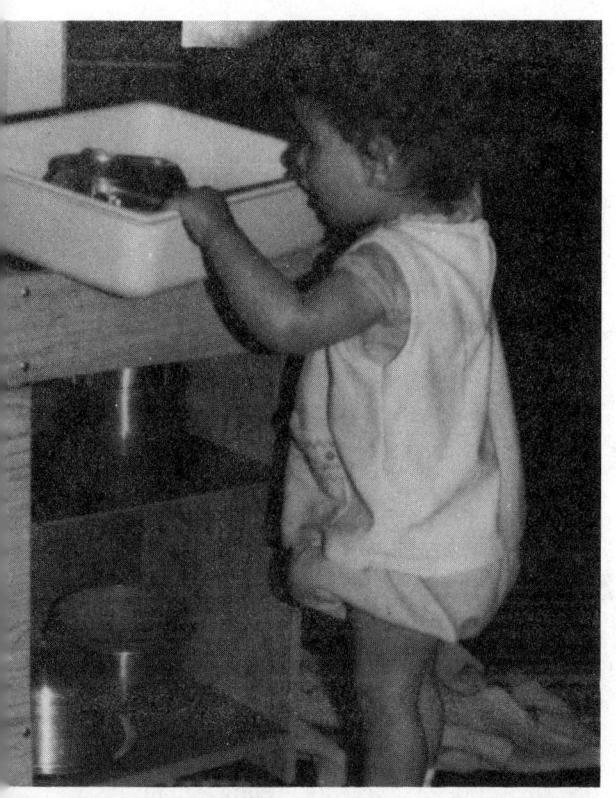

A thoroughly childproofed home provides nooks where safe household goodies are stashed especially for the toddler's discovery and creative play. In addition to these areas, authorities agree that children should have some space in the home to call their own, to the extent parents can afford. (Photograph by Dan R. Bruggeman)

proofed at least to the extent that medicines and poisonous or corrosive items are not available to the child. The less childproofing there is, the more continuous watchful surveillance is necessary to assure the toddler's safety.

Childproofing involves adapting the home so that the normal destructiveness of the toddler* will not violate the parents' values of a pleasant, comfortable home and will still give him the freedom to roam, explore and manipulate. The aims of childproofing actions are two: to prevent accidental injury and to minimize the destruction of property with a minimum of physical restraint to the growing toddler.

The more completely a home is childproofed, the freer a toddler is to absorb the facts of his investigations without the constant echo of "no-no" that inevitably means a "battle of the wills" and undermined self-confidence. In fact, a thoroughly childproofed home includes nooks and crannies where safe household goodies are stashed, especially for the toddler's discovery and creative play.

Parents must see that childproofing plans are carried out and periodically re-evaluated in light of their toddler's progressive motor skills (eventually he will climb, unscrew caps, open latches and unlock doors). Whatever limits are to exist must be communicated to all family members and to any caretakers of the toddler during parental absences. Enforcement of limits should be consistently enacted, especially since the child's safety may be at stake.

The toddler must internalize the limits set, to begin to comprehend concepts of safe and of dangerous (he can learn very early that "Hot, don't touch!" means unsafe), and to develop respect for things that belong to others (he is old enough to comprehend ownership).

Budget Reprioritizing

A toddler in the family inevitably places additional demands on the budget. During inflationary times when purchase power lessens, these new expenses are especially difficult to manage. While parents continue to pay off previous major purchases (furniture, car), they must absorb such toddler-associated expenses as new clothing, babysitter fees, medical charges* and

---

*More illness occurs during infancy and toddlerhood than in any other stages of childhood.

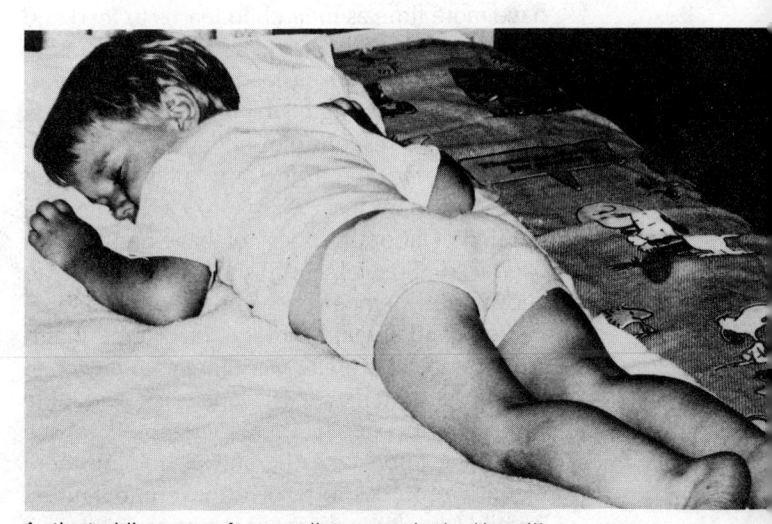

As the toddler moves from a crib to a regular bed he will need time to learn that the big bed has no rails to keep him from falling out. A safe approach is to place the bed mattress on the floor as a safety precaution against injury from falls until he learns to stay on the bed.

---

*Toddler destructiveness is not usually purposeful but arises out of his exploration, manipulation and immature motor coordination as he practices developing physical skills and satisfies his curiosity.

GROWTH AND DEVELOPMENT OF THE FAMILY WITH A TODDLER: MAINTAINING WELLNESS

life insurance premiums (usually either taken out or increased at this stage). Costs of home expansion or purchase of a home is another major expense for the toddler family.

Families resolve this "bulge of the budget" in various ways, depending on their skills, values, and many other variables. The husband may push for job advancement or a pay raise, or he may moonlight. The wife may supplement family income by a job at home or take a part-time job. Some modern families are splitting the financial and childbearing responsibilities by each working half-time. Today's parents are more amenable to borrowing money and installment buying. Many families simply "make do," adapting resources to multiple uses when possible and innovating in those areas of limited family resources of money, space or time.

The parents bear responsibility for accomplishing this task. However, if resolution involves the mother working at least part-time, then the toddler is required to adapt to these separations and learn to trust a surrogate caretaker.

Division of Labor

Just when parents have established a balance in the division of labor involving an infant, this is upset by the child's evolution into a toddler who requires an ever-watchful eye but seems to be everywhere at once. Parents think they will have more time as their child learns to feed and dress himself and go to the bathroom alone, but they soon discover instead how much *more* time it takes to engineer these small steps to independent, responsible self-care.

At no other time in the family life cycle is it more important for a couple to cooperate in a division of labor that does not leave one of them overtaxed. Special effort should be made to allow each member opportunity for individual interests and stimuli. Morale and energy maintenance are two areas that families often need assistance to achieve. The nurse is a valuable source to the family in helping them to see where the imbalances lie and in helping them identify resources to resolve those imbalances. A child's health assessment is not complete if it does not include an appraisal of the physical and emotional status of the people he relies on to care for him.

The toddler, too, discovers changes in the behavior expected of him as he emerges from infancy. He learns that certain demands and expectations are being made of him, especially from his parents, that require him to be increasingly self-sufficient, and that his world now demands that he "give" as well as "receive."

Many parents are hesitant about assigning responsibility to their toddlers. Some put off making such demands out of fear they will be accused by friends and relatives of passing their own duties along to the children. Others delay because they feel unable to find the time or patience that instruction for responsibility requires. But children are not born responsible, they have to learn responsibility.

There are some times when it is easier to teach responsibility than at others. The opportune time for teaching the toddler responsibility is when he first shows signs of willingness and readiness to do things for himself. Whether a youngster is 1 or 2 or 3, he should be given responsibility as he conveys his readiness — for dressing and caring for himself, for looking after his own possessions, for doing small tasks around the house. This is how he learns a healthy attitude toward doing his part.

The work a toddler does is not as important as the sense of responsibility he acquires. And learning this early helps him establish proper relationships with society as he matures. The toddler, like all of us, needs to feel the tasks he

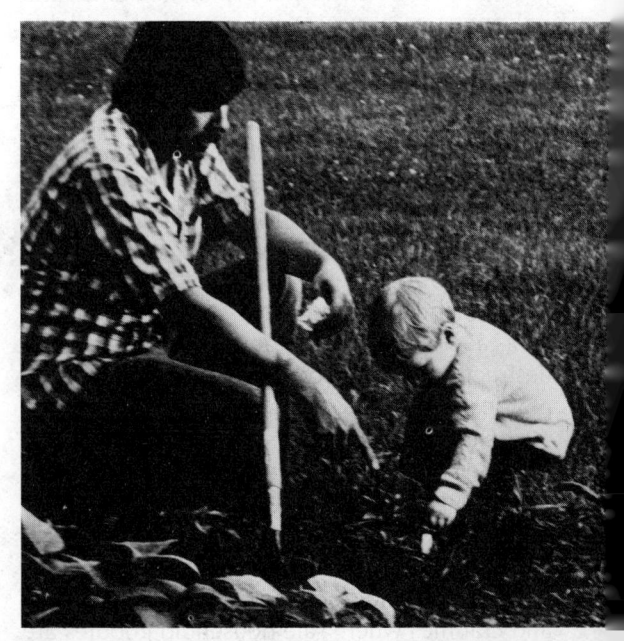

Many toddlers display an interest in helping Mommy or Daddy with work. Parents who respond to this interest encourage the development of responsibility in children.

is performing are necessary and helpful and not merely busy-work routines. To the toddler work is another form of play. Therefore, responsibility introduced in the toddler years helps him recognize early that work can be pleasant.

Many toddlers display an early interest in wanting to work with Mommy and Daddy. Parents should respond to this readiness for responsibility in home chores. The toddler is not too young to learn to put away his toys, empty trashbaskets, run simple errands inside the home, or put away papers and magazines. With assistance he can do a satisfactory job of dusting, watering houseplants, setting the table or drying unbreakable dishes. He finds the opportunity to help bake or fill the shopping cart a delightful experience. At this early age, of course, youngsters seldom do a perfect job; and they also tend to lose interest quickly. But parents who exercise tolerance with these early endeavors will find teaching much easier as the child grows older.

Toddlers need specific instructions when asked to do a task. "Clean up your room" means little to him so he will be unlikely to act. If he is asked to put his toys on the shelf and put the clothes he took off in the laundry basket, the toddler usually cooperates enthusiastically.

The toddler feels amply rewarded for his efforts if given a hug or a big smile and told "Thank you for helping me" or "You did a good job." Permitting him to take on responsibility at home makes him feel useful in an environment that accepts him for who he is, supports what he is becoming, and helps him cope with what he cannot be.

Being old enough to handle some responsibility in the division of labor at home should also entitle the toddler to opportunities to show his opinion — to make choices. He can learn to make big decisions later in life only if he is given opportunity to practice making smaller decisions as a youngster. However, the toddler needs a framework within which to make his choices. He cannot handle open choice, but rather manages to express his opinion when given two or three options to select from or some guidelines within which to make a decision. For example, he can help choose family activities or mealtime menus if given two or three alternatives from which to select. He can choose his own clothes to wear each day if told what kind are needed because of the weather or the type of activity planned for that day. The toddler's clothes should be kept where he can get to them easily. His combinations may not always be what his mother would match, but if praised for the pleasing combinations he makes, he will repeat those combinations often. However, if pleasing combinations are extremely important to a parent, choices of clothing can be made with limits by the parent so that selections are coordinated. Also, some clothiers today place tags with animals or colors inside the clothing to help with the matching process.

The toddler takes these choices seriously, and giving him these options communicates to him that he is a real person whose opinion matters. Nice side effects are that the child feels pride in himself, tantrums are reduced and he is more motivated to try other self-care tasks.

Planning Future Children

The family with a toddler has already made the decision for parenthood; the question before them now is how much parenthood. The best reason for having another child, in fact the only valid reason, is because it is truly wanted. However, the financial implications of another child are a crucial consideration. Other factors couples should weigh against their desire for another child are the amount of emotional and physical energy they have to offer another child; their career goals; their age, particularly the mother's; whether their life style would accommodate another child; their feelings about family size; and, if the toddler is presently their only child, the pros and cons of raising an only child.

If after serious evaluation of these factors a family decides it can accommodate another child and offer that child a good life, the next important consideration is spacing between children. It is best, from the standpoint of developmental needs of both the children and the parents, not to have children less than three years apart.[2, 10, 11] This three-year spacing makes a dramatic difference in the lives of the toddler and his sibling. The older toddler will have more maturity to cope constructively with his resentment of the tiny intruder, he will be developing more out-of-home interests (nursery school, peer play) with much less focus on his caretaker, which means displacement at home costs him considerably less than if he were younger. Studies have shown that significantly more rivalry exists when sibs have less than three years between them; that the closer the spacing is, the more excessive is the stress to the marital relationship; and that there is a much greater emotional drain on all family members with closer spacing.[2, 10, 11] Investigation has also shown that an age gap of at least three years between children allows more enjoyable experiences for all involved. And a mother whose children are happy is herself happier and vice versa. When she is happy she holds a more positive attitude about the marriage, which yields a happier husband, and a happy marriage means a happy home — a matter not to be taken lightly!

Most professionals involved with children believe that each child should be wanted before it is born, and this is most readily assured if parents are helped to plan their families without prohibition of marital sexual relations. The nurse is frequently the source first sought for information and guidance in this matter and, if parents do not initiate requests for assistance, the nurse has many opportunities to determine their need and offer her aid. This assessment is merited from the standpoint of its significant effect on the toddler, unborn children and the family as a whole. Whether the pediatric nurse offers assistance directly or through resource referral, her main concern is that the family understand the benefits of spacing and that the method of family planning chosen is congruent with the family's philosophy, attitudes and values.

If by decision or accident another child is expected in the home with a toddler, certain additional tasks are demanded of family members. Parents must consider how to realistically involve their toddler in preparation and planning for the new family member. According to one source, for the younger toddler, 12 to 18 months old, special preparations may not register at all. He may not react to the mother's absence but he will respond to being deprived, even unwittingly, of any accustomed privileges and even some necessities if the household has not been careful to consider him during this time.[3] The 2-year-old child can participate in simple ways in the physical preparations perhaps a month or so before the baby comes. The infant crib, the blankets, the baby clothes and doll play help to initiate him into the upcoming event. He will probably cleave to his mother as her due date draws near. He should have opportunity to become accustomed to his substitute caretaker before time of the hospitalization. He does best if kept at home during this separation and may be comforted if given some physical token of his mother. He is also comforted by frequent confirmation of where his mother is and by the daily homecoming of his father.

The toddler's adjustment to the new baby does not depend so much on advance information as on a thoughtfully planned protection of his sense of status and prestige by his parents. His status does change, however, and the toddler's task is to find ways to cope with his sibling status that reinforce rather than harm his fragile identity. Due to his immature emotional state, he will need his parents' guidance and love to be successful.

REORGANIZING RELATIONSHIPS TO ENCOMPASS A TODDLER

Three aspects of family relationships are particularly in need of attention during the toddler years. Marital maintenance, out-of-home environment and relative relationships are discussed in the following pages.

Marital Maintenance

Anything that strengthens the relationship between a husband and wife strengthens their children's health and happiness as well. Whether a child's parents live together or separately, he is most secure when his parents are healthy, well adjusted, mutually cooperative and have fulfilling life styles.

With children, a couple's lives are more structured and rigid. Problems begin to arise in their relationship if they unconsciously focus all their attention on the child(ren) and begin to neglect each other. A serious task of parents, then, is to continue to nurture their own relationship with each other. Dr. Wilson Grant, who emphasizes a close direct association in the effect that marital relationships have on the health of children, stresses that there are at least five actions spouses can take to ensure the continued health of their own relationship.[4]

1. Parents should avoid focusing all their shared time and interest on their child(ren)

so that he is not all they have in common. They need to share together the many little things that make life exciting for them aside from the child.
2. Parents should claim some time at home for themselves each day.
3. Parents should occasionally go out socially without their child(ren) and not feel guilty.
4. Both parents should pursue their own creative interests.
5. Parents should not hesitate to show their feelings in front of the child. Demonstrations of affection and peaceful working through of minor differences in front of a child helps him learn ways of expressing his own emotions.[4,5]

Although the state of a marriage affects the health and well-being of the family, the parental state also has its impact on the marital bond. A satisfying parental role is very important to maintenance of the marital bond, for disenchantment with that role usually produces friction and highly critical attitudes toward the spouse. This factor is reflected repeatedly in the behaviors that couples with toddlers identify as important to maintenance of their relationship during this period. Those behaviors include[2]

1. Each spouse allows the other time alone with their child(ren) on a regular basis;
2. Spouses make childbearing tasks a "family affair" that is shared by both;
3. They democratically make decisions that respect each other's needs and concerns;
4. They protect and respect each other's values;
5. They assure times to be alone as a couple;
6. They jointly participate in spiritual, recreational, intellectual and sexual activities; and
7. They accept without undue concern their heightened emotional and physical need for each other at various times.

Several of these behaviors are either directly or secondarily tied into parenting responsibilities.

During the nurse's interactions with the toddler's family she should attempt to ascertain whether the child's parents are being realistic in their expectations and demands on each other and evaluate whether either the husband or wife is becoming chronically or temporarily submerged in parenting responsibilities to the detriment of personal or marital development.

Relationships and Involvement Outside the Home

The couple with an infant tends to temporarily withdraw from activities involving social interactions away from home. But by the time that couple has a toddler, they are rediscovering the need to maintain relationships and involvements beyond their child and family. However, retaining some satisfying contacts with friends and personal interests away from home can be a rather complicated matter when there are small children. External activities, once spontaneously followed, now must be planned ahead and arrangements made for a babysitter. The trouble associated with getting the child cared for and paying for this service is so difficult for many

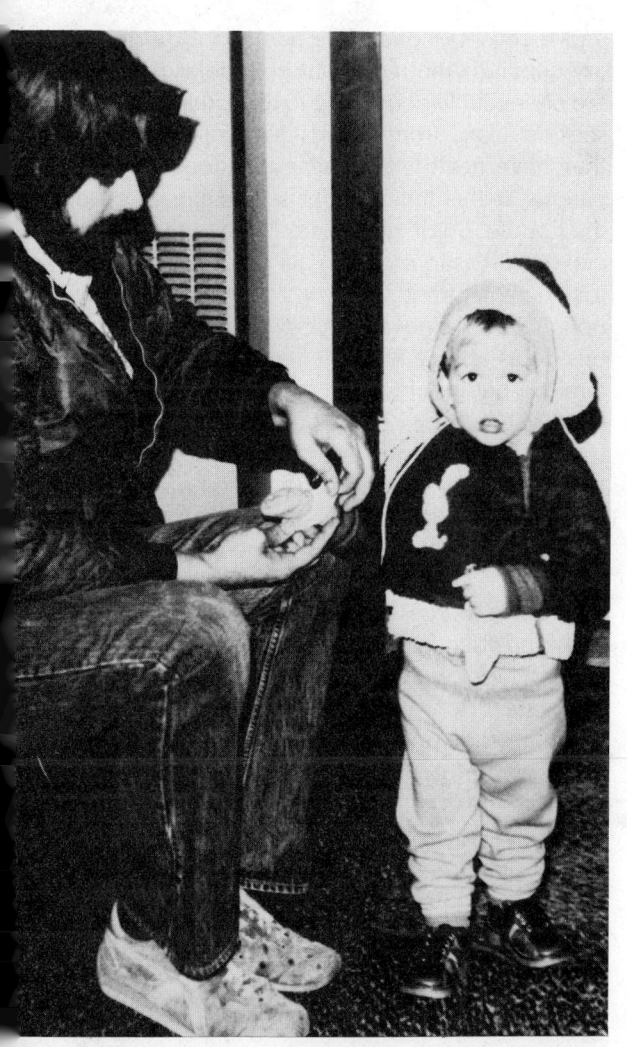

Each spouse needs to allow the other to have time alone, both with and away from their toddler. Such activity promotes the sharing of childrearing by both spouses.

couples that they tend to give up and stay home.

More innovative young couples have found numerous options available to them, with a little cooperation from others in the same circumstance as they. One option is to develop social relationships with other couples who have young children and take turns entertaining in each other's homes. These same couples might arrange a reciprocal child care agreement, whereby one couple watches the other's child(ren) so the couple can do something together and then the favor is exchanged at another time. Mothers (or fathers) who are full-time caregivers may arrange to "take turns" watching each other's child(ren) so that each can get away regularly to pursue personal interests or just enjoy a quiet morning at home alone. Such breaks in child care are refreshing, renewing energy for continued child care and for the spouse.

Some churches provide nurseries for small children during church services and social events. In those that do not, many parents have gotten together and agreed to take turns managing a children's nursery for these times, so that the other parents can participate without the interruptions of their infant or toddler.

Other young couples have formalized a child care cooperative in their community in which each spouse or couple contributes certain hours of child care supervision each week so that all families participating can benefit from these pre-established services at no or minimal expense on a regular basis.

Times away from home as a whole family can be an exhilarating break from routine, too. A trip to the zoo or beach, a family picnic, an outing to a movie or musical production can be a refreshing and uniting experience for even the youngster involved. Neighborhood get-togethers that include the whole family, church ice cream socials and other community activities suitable to the family's life stage are all feasible options to home confinement.

Relationships with Relatives

By the time there is a toddler in the family, his parents have gained a fair amount of confidence in their child care skills and are ready to accept the assistance and support that extended family

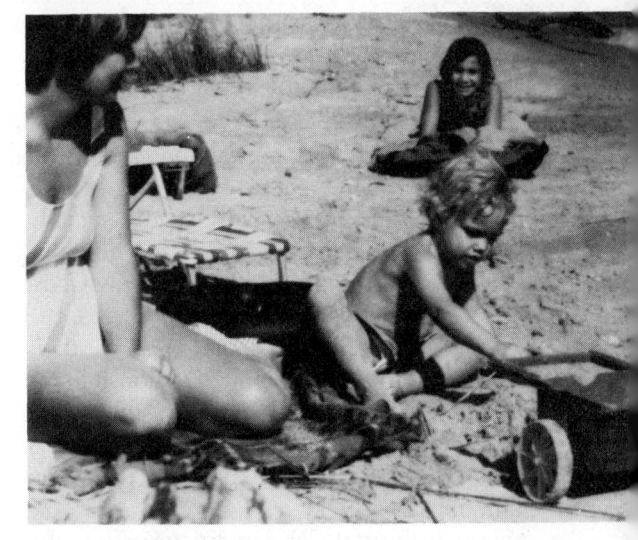

Time away from home as a family for a trip to the beach or zoo is an exhilarating break from routine. (Photograph by Dan R. Bruggeman.)

and friends can offer. The additional disciplinary demands the more mature toddler requires are often a little perplexing to his parents so they seek to learn from friends and relatives how they have dealt with similar situations. Grandparents at this time can be a valuable asset to the couple. Some grandparents have the financial resources to provide gifts of toys and clothing to their grandchild, with whom they can now have an enjoyable reciprocal relationship; this helps relieve some demands on the young family's budget. In some families grandparents may loan money to the young parents. Ideally, friends and relatives, especially grandparents if they live near enough, may become reliable, affordable (usually free) babysitters, allowing the couple to get away for the evening or even a weekend. Families who are able to enjoy the different resources available to them from relatives and friends are evidencing their ability to accept help with appreciation and maturity. They are discovering the satisfaction that can come from mutually serving each other's needs and they are permitting their toddler some very valuable relationships and learning experiences.

Grandparents hold a unique position in the toddler's life. He enjoys and thrives on the special position he has with them and with the indulgences they give — they, in turn, thrive on the admiration their affection and demonstrativeness gets them. The toddler learns through his experiences with grandparents and other relatives to know people of differing ages and to gain an inkling of the kinds of problems and reactions older people have. The grandparents are simultaneously revitalized by their toddler grandchild's exuberance and energy.

If parents tactfully communicate any major rules, concerns or limits they do not want breached, the majority of unnecessary conflict and misunderstandings that can occur with relatives and friends are eliminated, leaving everyone involved with the opportunity for fruitful and valuable relationships that enhance development at every age and reinforce familial and cultural values.

INCORPORATING PARENTHOOD AND CHILDREN INTO THE FAMILY PHILOSOPHY

The childbearing family finds original family philosophy incomplete once children enter the picture. The family with a toddler must, in particular, look for a philosophy that produces satisfaction in parenthood roles; reorganize goals to reflect the value of persons over things, establish means for the provision of healthy independence among members, resolve developmental task conflicts between members and learn to accept help in a spirit of appreciation and growth. The following is a discussion of the impact these tasks have on family members.

Deriving Satisfaction From Parenthood

Many parents today take parenthood seriously — they plan, they read, they keep their family size small so they can do a good job. They feel a stronger sense of obligation to do the parenting themselves. After a year they have begun to feel like parents and find that people perceive them that way. They have learned how to care for an infant and make some predictability of living with him. They have come to know their partner as a parent. And they have seen how society really treats families. Their parenthood is still fragile, a "work in progress," but it is more than they had before.

But now they have a toddler who changes faster than at any other time outside the womb. This series of developmental changes can provide a constant feast of fun for both parents and toddler — new words, new movements, new games, new self-care skills are an almost daily experience. The parents' satisfaction or frustration during this period depends largely on their confidence and the love, care and attention they can give the child. He can be a ticket back to fantasy and wonder if his parents pause and enjoy their child's new exploits. The child can now offer parents a reciprocal relationship of shared love and pleasure, bringing satisfaction in being together.

At no other time in their child's life will parents be a stronger influence than during the toddler years. It is about this time that the parents begin to recognize a need for direct, purposeful discipline. Many parents are hesitant about this task, unconsciously fearing that discipline will prove traumatic to the child. The important thing they need to realize is that discipline* is necessary to healthy growth and development. Certainly the child's image of his parents changes — the exclusively loving parent is gradually replaced by images of a parent who makes demands and punishes as well as loves — but the ambivalence toward the parents that this creates in the child is a necessa-

---

*Discipline, parenting, childrearing, socialization and training are all terms used in this book to refer to the process of socializing a child to become a responsible, productive and happy adult.

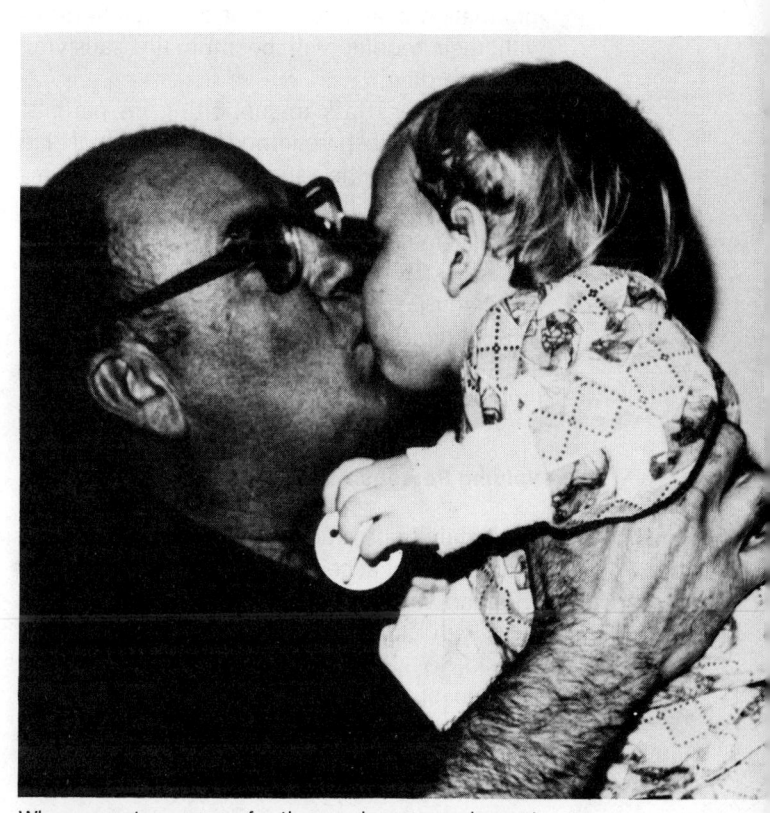

When parents are away for the evening, a grandparent can delight in babysitting the toddler, with whom he now enjoys a reciprocal relationship. The child thrives on the special position he has with his grandparents.

GROWTH AND DEVELOPMENT OF THE FAMILY WITH A TODDLER: MAINTAINING WELLNESS

ry step in the independence and separation process confronting him.

An important prerequisite for discipline based on love is that the child has learned to trust. His socialization is motivated by his desire to please, based on the love, warmth, and trust he experiences in his relationship with his parents, and his tendenccy to imitate.[1] The more positive the parent-child relationship, the less likely the toddler is to thwart his parents' disciplinary efforts.

But the parental task of realistically balancing the needs and demands of this active child and the expectations of a spouse and commitments to their own personhood can leave the best intentioned parent with some bouts of ambivalence toward parenthood. Some of the ambivalent feelings experienced by parents stem not from the fact that they sometimes do not like their child(ren) so much, but because they do not know how to cope with either the child or the whole juggling act just described. During this exciting but critical period of development, parents need all the help, reinforcement and information available so that their relationship with their toddler will be mutually satisfying and rewarding.

The toddler's task in supporting his parents' satisfaction with parenthood is instinctual. He will respond to the satisfaction he feels in his parents' care with unconditional love and a physical freedom timed to revive them from even their deepest doubts. His show of affection and enthusiasm for them is a mirrored reflection of what he senses he is receiving from them — for most parents there is no better reward for their efforts.

Valuing Persons Above Things

The family that values people over possessions and individual accomplishment over obedience will find satisfaction and stimulation in their years with a toddler around. The family seeking, instead, to gather in material success and to demand authority will find adapting to their toddler a stifling and frustrating experience. This issue of values is a prime concern in the family with a toddler.

When possessions are valued above people by one or both spouses, the work required to obtain those possessions becomes the dominant force in their life, to the detriment of personal, family and social relationships. Such persons need assistance to seek personal satisfaction in their marital and family situations, or the people in their life will suffer from the lack of the person's love, attention and presence.[1]

A stable family life is built with people, especially the spouse relationship, as the central value. A person-centered home nourishes the toddler's evolving, unique personality and makes it possible for him to incorporate a respect for himself and the people important to him. Parents who have developed a family philosophy that places prime value on the persons in it will respond to the unique personality of each child rather than treating the child and his siblings alike. Comparing siblings' achievements and forcing conformity to a parent-designed mold are not done in the family that values people as they are. These person-centered families will learn to share, to laugh together, and to stimulate each other rather than relying on possessions or status for their fulfillment.

Healthy Independence Among Members

Living together with enough harmony to allow expression of a variety of feelings, enough cooperation to permit each individual self-fulfillment in his developmental tasks, and enough open communication to condone each member's assertion of independence and selfhood or uniqueness requires a family to be in a continuous adaptive state.

Having established itself as a unit that can incorporate children and having accepted the entailed responsibilities, the family group with a toddler is now faced with the task of finding parenting patterns that meet the needs of both parents and active, mobile children and of establishing enough freedom for each member so that age-appropriate independence is possible.

This freedom for independent development in a family finds its origin in the spouse relationship. Spouses who are mature enough to allow each other independent social and recreational or hobby pursuits are much more likely to recognize and permit the individual endeavors of their children. Trust in the family member's motives is at the heart of such freedom. This trust provides the security necessary to "let go" of the family member and allow him to develop his uniquenesses. In his research, Kirkpatrick[5] found evidence that children are more independent in their activities when they can rely on (trust) parental affections. The same factor undoubtedly holds true in husband-wife independence. A spouse who knows he or she can count on a partner's affection is more likely to grant freedom in the relationship for pursuit of personal interests.

No parents at their child's birth would ever dream that within one brief year that child is already beginning to insist on "being on his way to his own fulfillment." But such is the case as the infant of about a year takes those first steps that bring him to the doorstep of toddlerhood. In conveying their respect for their toddler's selfhood or fulfillment activities, parents certainly want to let him be as grown up as he can be without pushing him too quickly out of babyhood. Parental respect for the developing toddler's individual efforts must be focused on three aspects of his activity: (1) his need to explore; (2) his need to learn self-control of body functions and emotional expression and (3) his need to develop an identity that will accommodate childhood rather than infancy.

Resolving Developmental Task Conflicts

Spouses in the family unit with a toddler are immersed in the task of maintaining intimacy while expanding their parental capacity to accept the growth and development of their child(ren), acknowledge his emerging selfhood and recognize his teachable moments. The toddler is working through the transition from babyhood to childhood by developing the autonomy necessary to control his body and his will.

This stage in the family life cycle seems full of paradoxes. Having just become settled in and comfortable as parents, the couple suddenly find themselves filling new, more difficult roles as limit setters, guides and teachers. These new parental roles involve much patience; the couple must accept their child's individual pace, let him make mistakes and learn from them, and accept roles as assistants to rather than directors of their child's activities. Some of the decisions to be made now are clear-cut, but most are not. The couple must agree on a form of discipline that is logical, consistent and comfortable without causing damage to the child's physical, intellectual or emotional-social development.

Another paradox involves the fact that while a husband is working on career consolidation, he is also confronted with a desire to invest time and energy in his marriage and family. Levinson's studies[6] showed that the man who works at stabilizing his marriage and helping raise his children during this stage is more likely to experiment with several different jobs, while the man who works at career establishment tends to have a less stable marriage and family structure.

The wife finds herself with a similar conflict of interests. While working at building a stable family life, she has a simultaneous urge to achieve self-actualization. For many women success as a wife, mother and homemaker is a gratifying source of self-actualization. But for others, especially those with career preparation, the urge for self-actualization has its gratification in activities outside the home — thus the paradox is apparent again.

Yet another paradox exists in families with toddlers. Most parents of toddlers are in their early to mid twenties. This stage in adult life tends to be a period of conformity. There is an urge to "do what one should do," to acknowledge and uphold the "rights" and "wrongs" of living.[7-9] For the toddler this stage is a period of rebellion — a testing time to find a healthy balance between cooperation and will assertion.

The ways in which his parents resolve their conflicts and the ways they interact with each other are imitated by the toddler. He uses these observations in a hundred ways to cope with his personal process of self-development. Parents best handle the conflicts of this stage when they (1) remember that their child's rebellion, expressed in his contrariness, is temporary and normal and that what often appears to be destructive behavior is simply the child's curiosity in action; (2) agree on democractic, shared parenting; (3) support each other in their role shifts; (4) work out realistic ways for each to fulfill some personal or career interests; and (5) learn to approach each other and their child(ren) positively, encouraging desirable actions through compliments and rewards for well-intentioned efforts. Daily family rituals are also invaluable means of providing a workable daily routine that eases conflict while giving family members a sense of order, security and satisfaction in living together.

Accepting Help With Appreciation and Maturity

The tasks of the family with a toddler are not easily achieved and, due to the rapidity with which the toddler develops, most families find themselves in an atmosphere of urgency during

FAMILY WITH A TODDLER: ESTABLISHING A STABLE HOME

I. Adapt resources to accommodate children
   A. Reallocate home space and facilities
      1. Provide private space for each family member
         a. Add more space
         b. Adapt existing space
      2. Manage play space
         a. Confinement to certain rooms or areas
         b. Freedom to range of house
      3. Emotional space allowed
         a. Allow choices by members
         b. Permit emotional expressions
   B. Decide about childproofing
      1. Determine extent environmental hazards and precious possessions will be eliminated
      2. Provide watchful surveillance for child's safety
      3. Provide firm discipline and limits for safety
   C. Reprioritize the family budget
      1. Pay off past purchases and other debts
      2. Absorb toddler-imposed expenses
      3. Save toward unexpected and future expenses
   D. Rearrange division of labor
      1. Share tasks so no one is overtaxed
      2. Assign realistic responsibilities to toddler
      3. Allow all members the right and respect to make decisions as capable
   E. Plan future children
      1. Decide how many children are wanted and affordable
      2. Determine spacing desired between children, if more than one is wanted
      3. Institute planning options that do not prohibit marital sexual relations
      4. If another child is expected, prepare all members according to age

II. Reorganize relationships to include children
   A. Marital maintenance
      1. Maintain common interests beyond those of child
      2. Establish some time together without children each day
      3. Socialize without children occasionally
      4. Pursue individual and couple creative interests
      5. Demonstrate feelings around children
      6. Allow each other satisfaction from the parenting role
   B. Provide out-of-home involvement
      1. Social relationships with other couples in each other's home
      2. Reciprocal child care among friends
      3. Neighborhood "take turns" arrangement
      4. Church: church nursery
      5. Child-care cooperatives
      6. Whole-family trips and outings
   C. Reaffirm relative relationships
      1. Seek guidance in parenting concerns
      2. Spend time with grandparents at least occasionally
      3. Enjoy gifts, assistance, reinforcement of family values they offer

III. Rework family philosophy to incorporate parenthood and children
   A. Seek satisfaction in parenthood
      1. Revel in the child's naiveté, fantasies and growth
      2. Maintain a positive parent/child relationship that supports cooperation
      3. Enact discipline needed for safety, order and harmony in family
   B. Align values to place people above possessions
      1. Confirm persons in family as central focus of life
      2. Respect unique personality of each member
      3. Depend on each other as family members for fun, learning and stimulation
   C. Provide healthy independence among members
      1. Establish realistic limits that allow freedom for growth but protect
      2. Allow each member time to pursue personal and social interests/hobbies
      3. Trust members' motives for their private times
      4. Convey affection for members
      5. Respect toddler's needs to explore, learn self-control and secure his own identity
   D. Resolve developmental task conflicts
      1. Accept members' adjustments to new roles with patience
      2. Spouses arrive at agreement on parenting plan
      3. Accept that conflict is inevitable, temporary, and can be managed democratically
      4. Use a positive approach to get members' cooperation
      5. Establish daily family routine and rituals
   E. Accept help in a mature manner
      1. Acknowledge needs that exist
      2. Use outside help that enriches what family offers
      3. Respect basic interdependence of human people

which time they feel a need for increased support and guidance, whether from relatives and neighbors (grandparents become important resources again), from health and child care professionals, or from all these sources. Most parents are willing to make use of any outside help that will enrich what they have to offer their child or the family group, but only if they are allowed to retain their parenting responsibilities throughout the helping situation. The acceptance of help is made easier if a family's philosophy recognizes the basic interdependence of all people.

The first step in accepting help is to acknowledge those areas of family life in which limitations exist. Then the family can draw on those outside resources that enhance existing strengths and those that will help strengthen weak spots (lack of knowledge, communication breakdown, chronic illness). Utilizing outside support systems such as relatives, helping professionals, government aid programs can help build and maintain internal support systems (members themselves, their skills, their caring), making life as a family with a toddler a happy, growth-producing experience.

Many parents at this stage need help anticipating their child's new skills, identifying his readiness for new experiences or responsibility, and learning how they can cope with his developing personality. These parents will be primarily interested in the teaching and anticipatory guidance a nurse can offer them in those areas. A nurse who is effective with children and their families will have learned that a parent so enlightened is more cooperative and will evidence that learning by affording parents every possible opportunity to question and to be taught. The nurse may also be involved in helping the family recognize their strengths and limitations in the management of the tasks of this stage. She can assist them to find ways to successfully accomplish the tasks causing them difficulty by offering them useful information that will help them move forward, by referring them to resources or support systems that can help them correct limitations to task achievement, and by reinforcing the efforts they are making to grow and develop as a family unit through praise, encouragement and advocacy of their needs and rights when necessary.

In some situations the nurse's relationship with the toddler will be as a parent surrogate. At such times she should reinforce those routines, parenting methods, affectional demonstrations, and self-care expectations that he is accustomed to from his parents. Knowledge of these factors should be learned from her assessment and integrated into her plan of care.

References

1. C. Deutsch. The workaholic spouse. Parents, March 1979, p. 36
2. E. Duvall. Marriage and Family Development. J. B. Lippincott Co., 1977
3. A. Gesell et al. Infant and Child in the Culture of Today. Harper and Row, 1974
4. W. Grant. The first goal of parenthood. Home Life, June 1976, p. 14
5. C. Kirkpatrick. The Family As Process and Institution. Ronald Press, 1963
6. D. Levinson et al. The Seasons of a Man's Life. Alfred A. Knopf, 1978
7. B. Schwarz and B. Ruggieri. Parent-Child Tensions. J. B. Lippincott Co., 1958
8. G. Sheehy. Passages. E. P. Dutton, 1976
9. G. Vaillant. Adaption to Life. Little, Brown and Company, 1977
10. B. White. The First Three Years of Life. Prentice-Hall Inc., 1975
11. L. Yarrow. Right and wrong reasons for having another baby. Parents, January 1979, p. 45

Additonal Recommended Reading

S. Ambron. Child Development. Holt, Rinehart & Winston, 1977

A. Craig. Ambivalent feelings of parenthood. Home Life, April 1977, p. 34

J. Ditzion and D. Wolf. Beginning parenthood. In Ourselves, Our Children: A Book By and For Parents by The Woman's Health Book Collective. Random House, 1978

J. Eicholz. Your children and chores. Home Life, February 1977, p. 44

C. Foster, Developing responsibility in children. Science Research Associates No. 5–939, 1977

A. Gabhart. Coping with the terrible two's. Home Life, April 1976, p. 50

S. Gilbert. Your child's first three years. In Parents Magazine's Self-Guidance Program To Successful Parenthood edited by Mary B. Hoover, Parents Institute Publishers, 1972

D. Helms and J. Turner. Exploring Child Behavior: Basic Principles. W. B. Saunders Co., 1978

D. Hymovich and M. Barnard. Family Health Care: Developmental Situational Crises, Volume II. McGraw-Hill Book Co., 1979

E. LeShan. A child needs tears as well as laughter. Woman's Day, May 1974, p. 120

E. LeShan. How to Survive Parenthood. Random House, 1965

J. Marzollo. Supertot. Harper and Row, 1977

D. Schulz. The Changing Family: Its Functions and Future. Prentce-Hall Inc., 1976

J. Segal and H. Yahroes. A Child's Journey: Forces That Shape the Lives of Our Young. McGraw Hill Book Co., 1978

J. Singer and D. Singer. Raising boys who know how to love. Parents, December 1977, p. 32

A. Skolnick. The Intimate Environment, Exploring Marriage and The Family. Little, Brown and Company, 1973

D. Winnicott. The Family and Individual Development. Harper and Row, 1969

29 POTENTIAL STRESSES IN FAMILIES WITH TODDLERS

by Jo Joyce Tackett, BSN, MPHN

Each of us is aware that some stress in any intimate relationship, such as those of a family, is normal and can be expected. How to live with stress, to develop healthy coping and problem-solving skills, is one of the most important skills we can learn, especially in today's world. Families who successfully manage stress have learned that, although it is normal, it is not inevitable and can be minimized.

In families with toddlers the most commonly encountered stresses are those related to parenting and either the threat of, or actual, breakdown in family relationships (husband and wife, parent and child, child and sibling). The family with a toddler is "ripe" for stress or crisis because of several developmentally associated factors. The toddler, in his first identity crisis or transitional state, is in disequilibrium much of the time; this puts extra stress on his relationships with family members. The parents are at a decisive point in the establishment of their childrearing goals and methods as their infant becomes mobile and self-realizing, an area in which they may discover that conflicting values exist. Siblings must now learn the lessons of sharing not only their mother and father but also toys, play space and perhaps even their bedroom or bed as a sibling moves into toddlerhood. Or, if the toddler is presented with a new baby brother or sister, he will find the demands on his immature coping skills quite draining.

And so goes the hotbed of potentially stressful situations and relationships in the home with a toddler.

Knowing about the potential stresses to families with toddlers is extremely valuable to the nurse who will interact frequently, and perhaps regularly, with this family. She can be involved in helping the toddler and his family manage stress in ways that will continue to foster healthy development of the family as a unit and of the individuals in it.

POTENTIAL STRESS: ENERGY DEPLETION

The family with a toddler is at particular risk for energy depletion in one or more of its members. (The mother or primary caretaker is by far the most frequent victim.) Any combination of the following dynamics is usually in play to cause energy depletion:

1. The toddler works hard to get what he wants; he is into everything. Exploring is his work and the more stimulated he gets, the more he likes it. He will pursue such stimulation to the point of exhausting his caretaker and himself, if not directed periodically into quiet activities.
2. When his routine is changed (friends visit and his nap is delayed) the ritualistic toddler finds it difficult to handle this breach in his

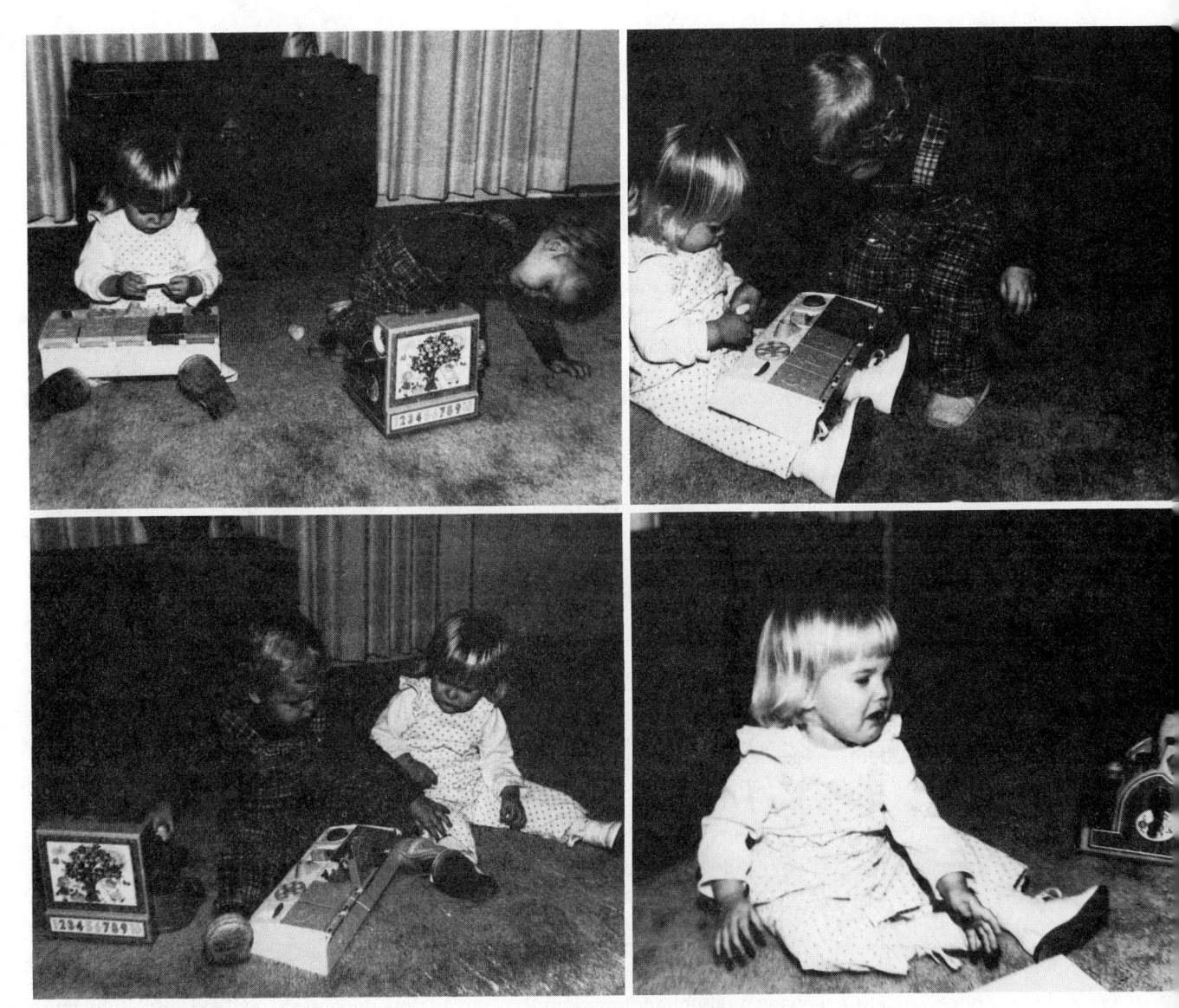

Siblings must learn to share not only Mommy and Daddy but also their toys and play space.

security. Family members around him can feel emotionally drained and exhausted just trying to satiate the frustrated child.
3. Because of the toddler's need to "check in" frequently with her, the mother has little opportunity for privacy or solitude, let alone opportunity to pursue her favorite pastimes or hobbies. Even being alone in the bathroom becomes a challenging accomplishment.
4. If family planning was ineffective or not practical, the mother may find herself pregnant again or caring for a completely dependent infant as well as her toddler.
5. If the mother is involved in bringing in income, she is carrying a double load. Even if division of labor has been equalized among family members, the toddler is still likely to make most of his demands upon the mother when she is around, especially during early toddlerhood when he has not completely separated his identity from his mother.
6. If the division of labor is not equalized among spouse and older siblings the mother's household responsibilities, along with the care of a busy toddler, may be quite heavy.
7. If family income is low, either or both parents may be undernourished or have other health problems because they cannot afford adequate food or medical attention for themselves.

8. If budget problems are being resolved by the husband's working overtime or holding two jobs, little time is left for rest or relaxation.
9. If the toddler and older sibling(s) share a room or even the same bed, the sleep patterns of one may interrupt or disturb the sleep of the other(s).*

If the family has not developed coping mechanisms that allow healthy adaptation to any one or more of these circumstances, some member(s) of the family will eventually become chronically fatigued. When physical or emotional energy is depleted, family relationships will inevitably suffer, with potentially serious consequences.

Obviously, a healthy toddler can emerge only out of a healthy family, so the nurse who works with children cannot neglect assessment of the energy status of all family members when promoting toddler health. Certainly the toddler is the most vulnerable family member and should be given first priority in terms of nursing assessment and intervention. But next in priority should be the caretaker (usually the mother), who is at greatest risk of energy depletion. Bishop[5] has developed the following assessment guidelines for determining the primary caretaker's physical and emotional energy status.

Physical energy status can be evaluated by investigating for any potentially debilitating conditions.† The caretaker's developmental status in relation to age should be investigated to determine if energy is being drained to handle more than one developmental level at once, such as a teenage mother handling simultaneous tasks of identity, intimacy and generativity. Sleep patterns should be checked to see if any sleep extremes (under four hours a night, over 10 hours a night) exist on a regular basis. Weight should be evaluated in relation to height and eating patterns assessed to identify any distortions (inadequate intake, unbalanced diet) which interfere with physical well-being and deplete energy. Medications the caretaker takes regularly, if any, should be determined as well as whether the caretaker is not taking prescribed, needed medication because of mass media scares or financial constraints. And an obvious, but frequently overlooked, assessment of the caretaker's general appearance should be made with particular attention to the eyes, posture and gaze.

Emotional energy status should include an evaluation of the caretaker's experience with his or her parents as a child. The question most likely to get a useful response is, "How were you punished as a child?" The caretaker needs to be evaluated for signs of postpartum or clinical depression,* such as listlessness, tense affect, body language suggesting anxiety or withdrawal, and negative body image. Just listening to the full meaning of the caretaker's comments gives the nurse a perspective on whether the caretaker's attitude is primarily positive or negative. The nurse should be alert, over time, to any deterioration in the caretaker's apparent level of understanding and comprehension. If the nurse's role takes her into the caretaker's home she should be alert to an environment there that is either chaotic or relentlessly clean, as both are danger signals of emotional energy depletion.

When the nurse suspects that energy depletion is developing in a family member or finds evidence that it already exists, she needs to help identify those dynamics in the family situation that are causing the problem. Rather than giving specific instructions as to what the family can do to help, she should expand their understanding of the dynamics involved and help them examine various alternatives to correct the situation and the likely consequences to the family unit of each alternative. The parents can then select the option that coincides with the unique needs, values and personalities of their unit and its members. The nurse may need to inform the family of community services such as homemaker services, visiting nurse, babysitting cooperatives and parent support groups.

All parents should be helped to realize that there will surely be bad days, even in the most smooth-running household, when there is a busy toddler around. And they should be helped to see that they have a number of options available to them when the bad days occur that they can select from without guilt.

---

*Toddlers sometimes display sleep problems in the form of waking and crying out at night or experiencing frightening dreams. They may require a night light to sleep. All these factors can interrupt the sleep of older siblings in close proximity.

†Elevated blood pressure; hemoglobin under 12 grams; pain of any intensity, or duration; bleeding of any type; acute or chronic infections; any generalized medical problem such as diabetes, asthma or a cardiac condition.

*Depression is clinical if the caretaker forgets to perform child care, essentially being so drained emotionally that she forgets that the baby or toddler exists.

For instance, when the mother is at her wits end, she could opt for any one of these solutions that best suit her situation and resources. She can get a sitter and leave for a time; forget about any tasks she planned to accomplish that day and indulge herself and her toddler in some unwinding, just-for-fun activities; take a walk with her toddler. Even in the rain this activity is refreshing to the spirit of most of us, especially with the delightfully curious toddler at our side to help us see the world from fresh, childish eyes. Or she can call a friend to come support her and share her day or select from any other options that will relieve boredom, change the scene or put embattled relationships into a different perspective.

The nurse whose focus is on the child *and* his family will see the significance of identifying families at risk for energy depletion of one or more members. She is motivated to help members of that family build their confidence and coping capacity by praising them in their healthy efforts and backing them in the options they choose. She will initiate a plan of care that has as its goal helping the family learn to problem-solve by focusing on their actual or potential stress, to recognize that options exist to resolve or minimize that stress, to select that option with which they are most comfortable and to carry it through.

POTENTIAL STRESS: DISAGREEMENTS ABOUT PARENTING PRACTICES BETWEEN SPOUSES

During a child's toddler years his parents are still learning to be parents. Thus the toddler can become a serious source of conflict between husband and wife. This conflict is most frequently centered around their differing attitudes and opinions about childrearing.

When a couple becomes parents to a toddler, they ideally would develop a comprehensive parenting "master plan" that takes into account the mutual rights, privileges, and responsibilites of every family member, arrived at out of consensus. The ideal master plan would cover the rewards and punishments allowable in that family, establish protective limits, and identify whether the parenting will be primarily the responsibility of one member or, ideally, a shared affair. Agreement about these issues may not be easy to achieve, especially if the parents have difficulty in communicating with each other. A nurse's assistance in developing such a parenting plan can be a true contribution to the well-being of the whole family.

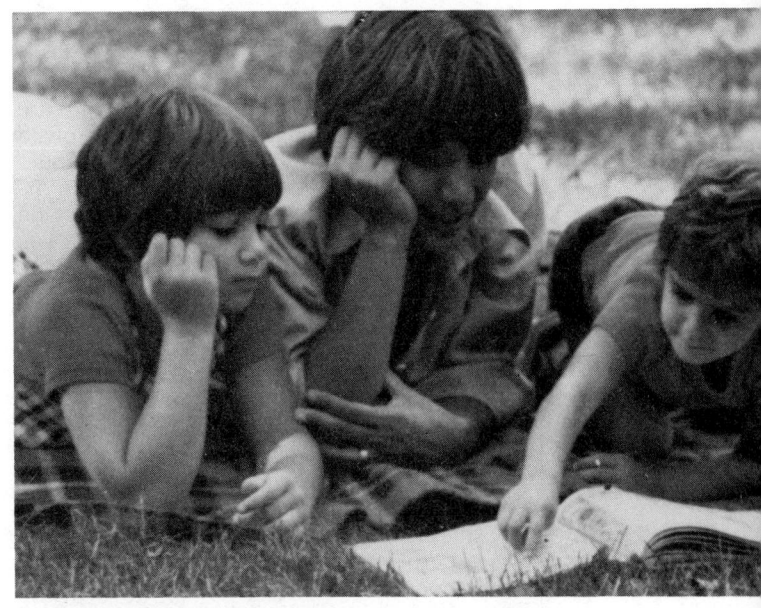

On a "bad day," forgetting about planned tasks and indulging herself and her toddler in some unwinding, just-for-fun activities can be good therapy for both mother and child as well as for their relationship. (Photograph by Daniel R. Bruggeman.)

If parents do not present a united front in their parenting, everyone loses. Since parenting is a daily responsibility, couples who do not stand together will become emotionally estranged due to the constant friction their disagreement presents, the toddler will learn very quickly how to play one parent against the other and all members will experience a high level of anxiety. In this circumstance the parents have progressively less control over their child's socialization. The child finds himself in the middle of a parental struggle that places more pressure on him than he can bear, causing him to lose respect for his parents and even to resent one or both of them. The toddler needs consistent limits, enforced with love, mutually endorsed by all caretakers.

The nurse's assessment in this area of potential stress in families with toddlers is especially important because couples usually will not seek professional help on their own unless their disagreement is pathologically intense or until their differences have existed for some time.[7] When a nurse identifies a family unit that is either at high risk for or currently displays conflicts related to childrearing attitude, she needs

> Volunteer, grassroots organizations exist in many communities, dedicated to lessening isolation of mothers who are full-time homemakers. Nurses involved with children and their families should make an effort to find out about such organizations in their own community. One example of such an organization is MOTHERS, which started in Austin, Texas, in 1976, and now has chapters in various cities and involves several hundred mothers. MOTHERS was formed as a support group for self-aware, middle-class mothers whose "physical environment, in many cases, consists of their lonely and isolated homes, their cars, and impersonal shopping malls." These mothers may especially lack opportunities for meaningful social interactions on an adult level. The following excerpt is from "One Mother's Thoughts" by Marilyn Holmes of MOTHERS, expressing what it can feel like to be alone at home.
>
>> I am a mother. I feel very isolated; isolated from my husband sometimes; isolated from my friends who aren't married; isolated from friends who don't have children; from people who work outside the home; from *all* people outside my home.
>> I need to be around people from diversified backgrounds, backgrounds other than those of the plumber, the TV repairman, the mailman. I need people to talk to, people like other mothers. I want to learn how other mothers think. I want positive, constructive conversation with other mothers. I want more than just an outlet to complain, but I need that, too.
>> I need to talk to other mothers about how motherhood has affected them as people. I need this so I won't feel so alone. I need new and stimulating relationships with women and men, too.
>> I want to know what other people are doing with their lives. I have a low self-concept. I don't feel that my job is seen as important. I need help in mothering. Often I don't know the answers. No one ever taught me how to be an effective parent.
>> My relatives are scattered throughout the country. They are so far away. I need their support, but how do I get it? Letters and long distance calls don't seem to bring them close enough to me.
>> I feel guilty about so many things; when I take time for myself, when I leave my children with my husband to go to a meeting at night, when I ask my husband for help with the children.
>
> Laraine Benedikt, founder of MOTHERS, says "Many experts indicate that abuse and neglect of children in middle and upper class homes occurs at least as frequently as in lower income families. It is widely assumed, however, that because these acts are not reported or are dealt with privately, nothing can be done about them. MOTHERS cannot claim to prevent child abuse, but we do offer a preventive support system to the middle-class housewife."
>
> Benedikt includes among the objectives of the organization: to provide a support group for women with children, to better understand the role of the mother in society and encourage dialogue between parents and professionals, to provide a forum for the discussion of common concerns, and to promote the role of the family in society by monitoring and reacting to public issues affecting the interests of children and families.

to help this couple talk out their childrearing differences honestly, calmly, and privately. (In extreme cases the nurse or a professional counselor may need to be present as an arbitrator in the early phases of these discussions.) The couple should be encouraged to try to understand each other's views and to work toward a satisfactory compromise in areas of opposition. Talking seldom hurts as much as silence and is essential to problem resolution in this situation. The nurse should also attempt to expand the parents' understanding of their toddler and the reasons for variations in his behavior so that they can select a comfortable parenting schema for their situation. The nurse may provide exposure by making appropriate reading materials available, through individual teaching, by involving the parents in parent groups, or by any other means that are appropriate and available within the community.

DEPENDENCE/INDEPENDENCE IMBALANCE IN PARENTING

A dependence-independence imbalance can involve either an overly dependent, indulged, overprotected child or an ignored, rejected child who is forced to a level of dependence or independence inappropriate for his age. The toddler is not comfortable with complete freedom to do as he pleases nor with demands that require developmentally unrealistic achievements. He wants protection, he craves security and consistency, and he needs realistic parental expectations to which he can successfully measure up.

The overly dependent toddler is playing out the script overprotective parents have structured for him.[2] This overprotection can be manifested in three ways and may carry over well beyond his toddler years if not identified and interrupted by a helping professional.[8] This can logically be the nurse since, of the helping professionals, she is most likely to have frequent, regular contact with the toddler and his family in the clinic, office or day care setting or through home visitation.

One manifestation of overprotection is *excessive contact*. In this situation the primary caretaker (usually the mother) never leaves the child, even encouraging the toddler to sleep with her. This mother often prolongs treatment for illness beyond the time the child is actually ill, a factor to which the nurse should be alert. A second form of overprotection is *encouraging infantilism*. The primary caretaker refuses to let her child grow up. She treats the toddler as if he were still an infant, incapable of doing anything for himself. The nurse should watch for the mother who prolongs doing for her child those functions he can do for himself. *Preventing independent behaviors* is the third type of overprotection manifested by some parents. The primary caretaker in this case restricts her toddler's social contacts (often even with his father) and will not allow him any risks, even though those risks are necessary to his development. This mother often expresses fears for her child's health or safety. The nurse can watch and listen for this repetitive and excessive concern about the child's well-being.

An overprotective mother may be either indulging or dominating.[10] The *indulgent* type yields to her toddler's every whim. Her toddler becomes rebellious and aggressive toward her because he is angry and frightened when he has no limits, though he may be socially civil toward others in his environment. He becomes unmotivated to master his developmental tasks because too much is done for him. This child learns that a persistent "I can't" gives him command over his caretaker and any others who will comply.[3]

The *dominating* overprotective mother demands strict obedience and dependence from her toddler. Feeling much guilt, he develops a highly active conscience. This child becomes inactive, submissive, and timid and as he nears preschool age, resentful of his peers with whom he cannot keep up because of his dependency needs. His creativity and curiosity are steadily dissolved by the dominance he experiences.

The overly dependent child is overtly honest, careful, polite and docile. He is highly suggestible and overly sensitive. Toddlers at special risk for overprotection are those with chronic or terminal disease, first borns, and those from a home that discourages independence in any of its members.[9]

Parents at special risk of becoming overprotective of their toddler are those who (1) see him as a type of personal adornment who must continually be a source of pride and reflect credit upon them, (2) those who want so much that he should have an easier childhood than they did that they pamper the child and cause him to believe all is free for the asking, or (3) those whose child has survived an illness or accident that the parents expected to be fatal.[2,3] Such overpowering forms of love damage both the giver and victim.

The toddler needs a constant supply of intelligent "neglect" so he has the chance to discover his world first hand, without adult interference, to the extent that it is safe and age-appropriate. If he is deprived of chances to take some risks and make mistakes he does not learn how to overcome difficulties by himself, he develops an inferiority complex and his further development is stunted and slowed.

The *rejected toddler* is harder to identify. The rejecting behaviors are often disguised because of the social stigma against such behavior toward children. The disguising efforts usually take one of two forms. Either the primary caretaker appears overprotective in an effort to hide or cope with the guilt feelings arising out of her rejection of the child, or the child is dressed exceptionally well and physical needs are meticulously met but without any of the acceptance and affection that toddlers directly need. The caretaker may give subtle verbal and nonverbal cues that the relationship is unhealthy. For example, there may be very little tactile contact and what does occur is abrupt and rough. Smiles between caretaker and child are few and appear forced. The caretaker seldom refers to the child by name, and references to the toddler are usually complaining or negative.

The rejective behaviors toward the child by his caretaker include excessive corporal and verbal punishment, continual demands for intellectually and developmentally unrealistic behaviors and persistent setting of standards for the toddler that he cannot possibly attain.

The mother's hostility and resentment toward the child, which are the basis for the rejecting behaviors, can arise from a number of causes. Some common underlying factors are (1) the child was not wanted; (2) the child, who was conceived to help patch up a shaky marriage, has instead been a source of the demise of that marriage; (3) the child, conceived as an object from which to get love, has not fulfilled the love needs his mother thought he would or should; (4) the child is perceived by the mother as being favored over her by her husband, arousing her severe jealousy; (5) some characteristic(s) in the child's temperament makes him distasteful or unlikable to the mother; (6) the child is perceived as a hindrance to the immature mother's life style or life goals and she feels trapped by his existence; (7) the birth of this child was exceptionally difficult or traumatic, resulting in strongly ambivalent feelings toward him.[2, 10] Most of these causes arise out of the caretaker's own immaturity and misconceptions about what a child is and what he is capable of, so that the child himself is an innocent victim of his own existence.

Rejected toddlers, if not identified very early, can suffer severe ego and self-concept damage due to the fragile status of their identity at this time. This damage is usually reflected in the child's behavior. For example, a rejected toddler frequently retains infantile speech or mannerisms, is overaggressive and hostile in all relationships, often appears hyperactive, expresses his jealousy toward his peers through sometimes radical attention-seeking behaviors, and is almost continuously rebellious and annoying, seemingly taking great pleasure in making others as miserable as he is himself.[10] If the weakening in the relationship with his caretaker is not recognized and appropriate intervention provided during toddlerhood or before, its breakdown accelerates and the child's acting out of his hurt becomes progressively more pathological. The alert nurse will include in her history taking and parenting assessment those questions and observations that evaluate the kind of relationship that exists between the toddler and his caretaker. She should listen for and watch for any of the factors just described, and if they are present, she should monitor the parent-and-child interactions closely to see if any maladaptive behaviors are occurring between them. Fortunately, toddlers themselves give direct clues as to whether they are being pushed too hard or being held back too much. Their behavior lets us know quite early, if we are watchful. Held too tight, the toddler will express rebellion and defiance beyond that typical of his age mates, either directly or subtly by being passive (a highly irregular behavior in the developing toddler). The toddler being pushed too hard will soon evidence anxiety and a reluctance to try new things (also atypical of the developing toddler).

Nurses, due to their opportunities for regular contact with toddlers and their families, are in a key position to recognize unhealthy balances in dependence-independence. Helping the parent to verbalize feelings about the relationship and the source of her resentment is important, or the situation will not improve. Expanding the parent's understanding of the realistic developmental capacities of the toddler is the second therapeutic step. A third step is to refer this parent and child to a professional counselor who can help them work through the unhealthy dynamics of their relationship. (See Chapter 31 for a more detailed discussion of interventions.)

POTENTIAL STRESS: UNHEALTHY TOILET TRAINING PATTERNS

Toilet training is often an early source of parent-child conflict, involving many emotional factors and psychological consequences. Chapter 30 discusses some of the practical techniques of toilet training. Here we look only at the effects that misdirected training attempts can have. There are three categories of unhealthy toilet training patterns: attempting to toilet train too early, placing undue emphasis on the product and cleanliness rather than the process of toilet training and being coercive and punitive during toilet training.[6, 11]

Attempting Training Too Early

The earlier toilet training is attempted, the longer it will take to accomplish and the greater

> **NURSING ACTIONS: FACILITATING COPING WITH STRESS IN THE FAMILY WITH A TODDLER**
>
> Energy depletion in family members
> - Assess parents and siblings for physical and psychological signs of energy depletion
> - Explain to family members that inability to cope can result from physical exhaustion
> - Encourage family members to get adequate food and rest
> - Explore alternative resources with family that lacks income or support system
>
> Disagreements between spouses about parenting practices
> - Assess parents for ability to communicate with each other
> - Help couple realize that this is an actual and common stress
> - Provide accurate information on what is "normal" behavior for toddler developmental stage
> - Encourage discussion between parents, provide reading materials, or refer to family therapist, depending on setting and needs of family
>
> Unhealthy toilet training practices
> - Assess parents' knowledge of and attitudes toward elimination
> - Provide parents with accurate information about developmental stage of child
> - Teach caretaker practical healthy toilet training techniques

the impact on the child's development and character.[4,11] Started in training before 18 months to 2 years, the child lacks enough muscular control to master voluntary "letting go," and he develops a sense of failure. Because he cannot intellectually connect the toileting sequence and involuntary sphincter relaxation with the product, he cannot understand what is being requested of him; instead he develops a fear of anger or loss of affection (sensed as abandonment) from his trainer and he fears a loss of self-control, since he perceives the product as having appeared magically or by some power in his trainer. A "battle of the pot" contest is likely to ensue because his physical mobility is restricted, the objects of his curiosity are removed, and for no apparent reason that he can perceive. There are indications that early training leads to some exaggerated character traits, including fearfulness, aggression, compulsiveness, obstinacy, and difficulty getting pleasure out of his experiences.[8]

Overemphasis on Product

The major problem with focusing on the product rather than the process of toilet training is that if there is no product (which can often be the case, especially if the parent rather than the child is prompting the visits to the bathroom), the parent's response shows annoyance, hostility, or even rejection, at least from the toddler's perspective. According to Freudian theorists, the child who attempts to meet these cleanliness (toileting) demands often over-responds to the point of becoming obsessed with an exaggerated need for cleanliness, orderliness, and punctuality, being scrupulous about very insignificant matters and confusing his body functions and sexuality with dirtiness. It is believed that such a person has a preoccupation with his bowel movements throughout life.

Strict, Coercive Training

This type of training leads to many emotional upsets in both the toddler and his trainer. The child has more accidents* and experiences more punitive measures, especially physical. This toddler learns to hate himself and his trainer. He is in a double bind, for if he complies with his parent's demands he loses autonomy and if he does not comply he experiences punishment and still does not feel autonomous because he cannot control this body function. He becomes a defeated child, full of frustration and undermined self-confidence. His frustration is often expressed in behaviors such as extreme shyness, night terrors, eating problems or outright rebellion during any interactions with his trainer. A research finding worth noting is that the parent who is coercive in toilet training almost always restricts other "messy" activities such as sand or water play, use of clay or finger paints, or play with food during meals.[1]

If conflicts are too great over toilet training, regardless of the method used or the child's age when it is initiated, the toddler may develop

---

*Perhaps a subconscious form of rebellion despite his fear of punishment.

difficulty in his relations with all persons in authority later in life, as a result of this disturbing experience with his mother (trainer) who was his first authority. He will face such relationships with either stubborn defiance or passive noncompliance.

The nurse who identifies actual or potential stress in the area of toilet training should immediately institute interventions to relieve the stress. Her teaching should emphasize that, given time, the toddler will himself indicate his readiness for training;* that there is no room in this matter for force or punishment, but rather the use of tactful suggestions and quiet flattery will gain the toddler's cooperation in the toileting sequence. She should teach that it is wise to wait until the child is at least 24 months of age so that training can be completed faster and easier by a toddler mature enough to perform the whole sequence alone. If a parent is patient enough (diapers do become a monotonous, bothersome feature of child care) to wait for the toddler's readiness, all she will have to invest in the training is an initial explanation of the toileting sequence in terms her child can understand. Then she can praise the successes and ignore the failures as her child masters for himself the task of toileting self-control.

---

*He develops distaste for wet or soiled diapers, recognizes when he has urinated or defecated and tells his caretaker. He searches out the potty chair if he has been acquainted with it.

References

1. S. Ambron. Child Development. Holt, Rinehart & Winston, 1977
2. M. Banks. A family's overconcern about a child in the first two years of life. Maternal-Child Nursing Journal, Fall 1977, p. 187
3. M. Beecher and W. Beecher. Parents on the Run. Grosset and Dunlap, 1967
4. A. Bernstein. Toilet training without fears. Parents, January 1979, p. 53
5. B. Bishop. A guide to assessing parenting capabilities. American Journal of Nursing, November 1976, p. 1784
6. F. Dodson. How to Parent. Signet Books, 1970
7. S. Gilbert. Your child's first three years. In Parents Magazine's Self-Guidance Program to Successful Parenthood by Mary Hoover, (ed.), Parents Institute Publishers, 1972
8. M. Herbert. Problems of Childhood. Pan Books Ltd., 1975
9. E. Hurlock. Child Development. McGraw-Hill Book Co., 1978
10. W. Martin and C. Stendler, Child Behavior and Development. Harcourt, Brace and Co., 1959
11. D. Shulz. The Changing Family: Its Function and Future. Prentice-Hall Inc., 1976

Additional Recommended Reading

N. Arzin and R. Foxx. Toilet Training in Less than a Day. Simon and Schuster, 1974

F. and T. Caplan. The Second Twelve Months of Life. Grosset and Dunlap, 1977

G. Fletcher. What's Right with Us Parents. William Morrow and Co., 1972

Dr. L. Salk. What Every Child Would Like His Parents to Know. Warner Paperback Library, 1973

I. Schleicher. Teaching parents to cope with behavior problems. American Journal of Nursing, May 1978, p. 838

B. White. The First Three Years of Life. Prentice-Hall Inc., 1975

GROWTH AND DEVELOPMENT OF THE TODDLER: MAINTAINING WELLNESS

30

by Mabel Hunsberger, BSN, MSN

The developmental changes that occur from 12 to 36 months in a child engage the entire family in a life full of drama. Within the first year of life the infant has developed attachments that serve as a secure base from which the toddler can wander to learn and explore. As his motor ability gives him access to new territory, his rapidly expanding intellectual and language abilities enable him to attach meaning to his discoveries. Because he has had only limited experience with people and objects, he is dependent on his family to rescue him from conflicts and protect him from danger. The imbalance between a toddler's motor skills and his mental capacity puts parents into the difficult position of protecting him from physical harm while nurturing his inexhaustible energy and curiosity toward the development of a creative human being.

The variations of a toddler test the family's ability to rapidly shift from scenes involving stressful conflict to those characterized by his irresistible charm. His physical, intellectual, and emotional-social development requires mutual adaptive behaviors between the toddler and his family. The nurses's role is to use herself, her knowledge and skills to promote healthy family functioning that allows each member to realize his full potential as the toddler grows and develops.

PHYSICAL COMPETENCY

To provide for the safety of a toddler without hindering development requires constant attention and ingenuity by the entire family. Assisting parents to identify expected physical development can contribute to their confidence and ability to cope with changes as they occur. In this chapter assessment parameters that reflect physical growth and development during the toddler years are discussed, with emphasis on the nurse's role with parents in promoting physical competency of their toddler.

Height and Weight

The growth *rate* slows in late infancy and continues to decelerate until 24 months of age. From 2 years of age through the preschool years growth remains relatively stable. A toddler gains about 2.5 kg (5.5 lb) a year and usually quadruples his birth weight by 2 to 2½ years of age. At 2 years a toddler's height represents approximately 50 per cent of his eventual adult height. During the 2 years of toddlerhood a child grows approximately 8 inches (20.3 cm) compared to 10 inches (25.4 cm) during the first 12 months of life.

Anticipatory Guidance: Height and Weight
Parents continue to have a keen interest in the physical growth of their child during the toddler years. They can best understand the characteristic slowed growth rate if the height and weight of their child is plotted on a graph to show them consistency in the percentile range. Parents need assurance that the decelerated growth rate is normal for this stage of development.

Head and Chest Circumference

Head circumference reflects the growth of the brain and is an important parameter to be assessed until at least 2 years of age. At 2 years of age the brain attains approximately 90 per cent of adult size. The posterior fontanel usually closes by 2 months of age and the anterior fontanel between 10 to 14 months, but there is a wide range of normalcy. In some normal children the anterior fontanel remains slightly open past 18 months of age. Head circumference increases approximately 3.5 cm (1.8 in) during the toddler years compared to a growth of 12 cm (4.7 in) during the first year of life.

In addition to measuring head circumference and palpating fontanels, one can evaluate growth by comparing head to chest circumference. At birth the head circumference exceeds the chest circumference, but during the second year of life the head and chest circumference usually become equal. The chest circumference continues to gradually increase and during childhood exceeds head circumference.

Anticipatory Guidance: Head and Chest The nurse should explain the expected progression of fontanel closure. It is important to explain the variability of fontanel closure that exists from one child to another because a parent may be comparing the child to a friend's child or to an older sibling.

General Appearance and Skeletal Growth

The general appearance of the toddler changes markedly between 12 and 36 months of age.

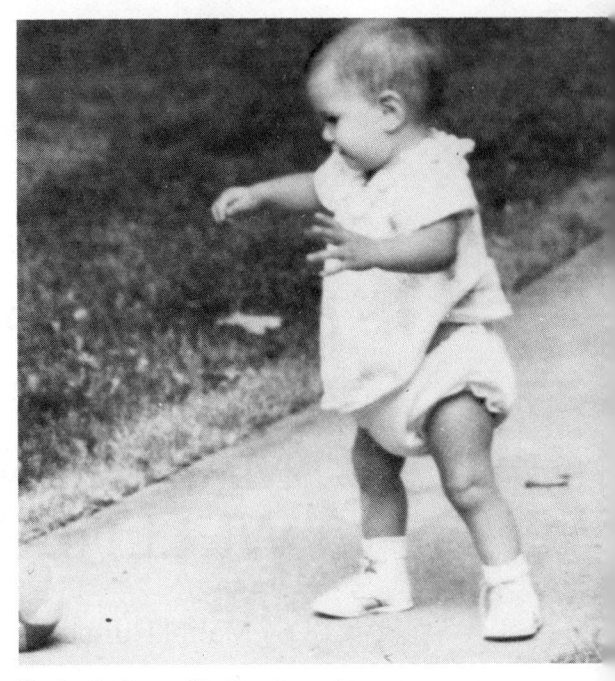

The beginning walker has a broad-based, toddling gait. (Photograph by Dan R. Bruggeman.)

When a toddler first begins to walk, the trunk is long, the legs and arms are short, and the head is proportionately large, giving him a top-heavy appearance. He walks with his feet spread apart to create a broad base, which helps to compensate for his weight distribution and immature musculoskeletal system. He also has a normal anterioposterior curvature of the spine (lordosis) and a characteristic pot-bellied appearance until the musculoskeletal system matures. Bowed legs (*genu varum*) and flat feet are common when a toddler begins to walk. The feet appear flat because of a plantar fat pad that gradually disappears by the age of 2 years. When a toddler first begins walking he tends to walk on the medial portion of the foot, and there is a slight external rotation that straightens with ambulation around 2 years of age.[11] These combined features account for the characteristic toddling gait of the beginning walker.

During the toddler years muscle tissue begins to replace the high proportion of adipose tissue characteristic of an infant, and bone ossification takes place. With increased ambulation and maturation a toddler's legs and arms lengthen, his body straightens, and the pot-bellied appearance disappears. The lordosis resolves as ambulation increases and muscle and bone develop. The legs retain a slightly bowed appearance until around 18 months of age. After the legs have shown a resolution of the genu varum,

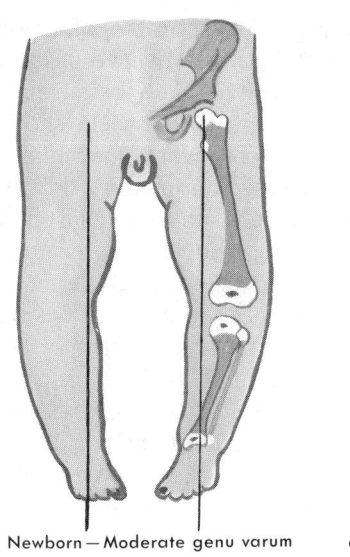

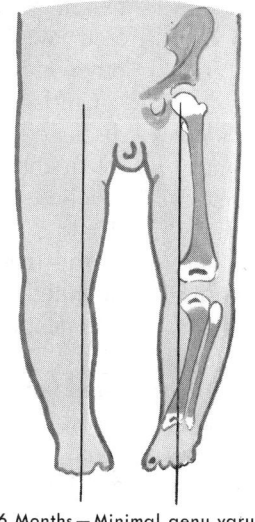

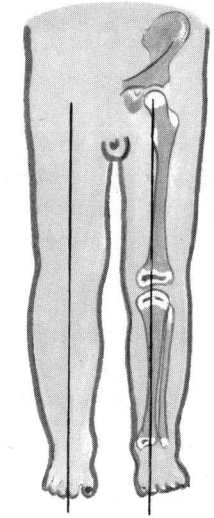

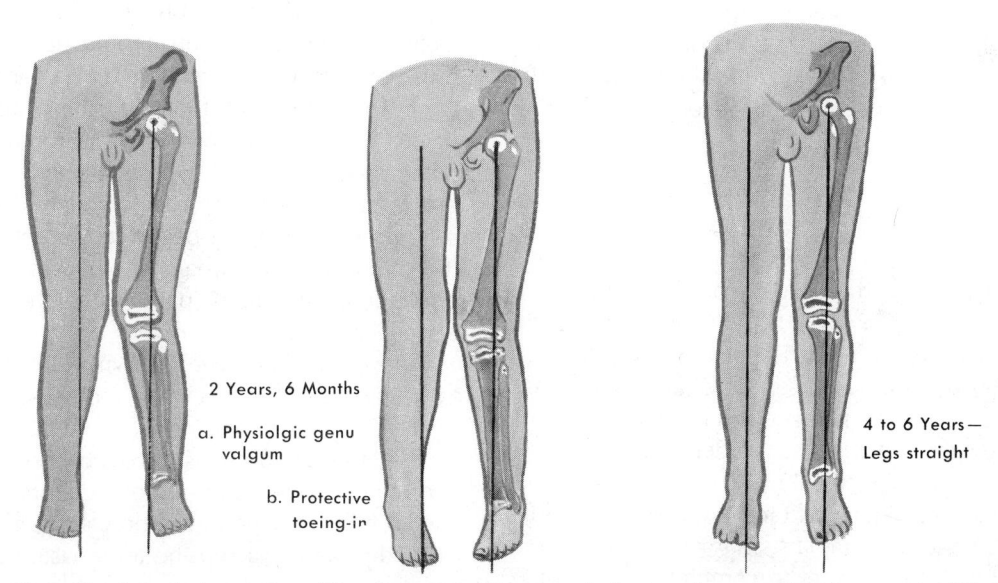

Figure 30–1 Physiological evolution of the alignment of the lower limbs at various ages in infancy and childhood. (From Pediatric Orthopedics, Vol. 2. M. O. Tachdjian, W. B. Saunders Co., 1972, p. 1463.)

a physiologic *genu valgum* (knock-knee) normally follows, lasting through the preschool years. This genu valgum is usually accompanied by a protective toeing in of the feet (Fig. 30–1).

Anticipatory Guidance: General Appearance and Ambulation The nurse should prepare parents for the normal changes that will occur in physical appearance. It is especially important for the nurse to inform parents regarding the normal changes that occur as the feet and legs mature. Nurses can often intervene to discourage parents from buying corrective shoes when it is unnecessary. If the genu varum and genu valgum is not within normal growth expectations, the nurse should refer the child for further evaluation and treatment.

Parents often ask what kind of shoe should be worn by a toddler. The function of shoes is to protect the feet from trauma and temperature changes. They should be comfortable and fit properly. Support to the foot and ankle is *not* a function of shoes unless an abnormality is present.[13] To meet the criteria of protection a toddler's shoes should have a firm sole and soft uppers. Sneakers provide adequate protection

GROWTH AND DEVELOPMENT OF THE TODDLER: MAINTAINING WELLNESS

and comfort if they fit properly and are worn with socks. Expensive shoes offer no added benefit to the proper development of a toddler's feet.

Because a child's foot grows rapidly, it is not uncommon for children to wear shoes that fit too snugly. Parents should be taught how to examine for proper fit of their toddler's shoes. When the toddler is in a standing position there should be three-fourths of an inch between the tip of the great toe and the front of the shoe and one-fourth of an inch between the edge of the fifth toe and the lateral edge of the shoe when the foot is pushed medially within the shoe.[13] Parents can identify shoes that have been outgrown because it becomes increasingly difficult to get the shoes on, and the toes can be felt pressing against the front part of the shoe. Parents should also be advised that while a toddler who constantly takes off his shoes may be practicing a new skill, they should also suspect that his shoes may be too small and may hurt.

Dentition

Although there is a great variation in the age at which teeth erupt, usually one tooth erupts for each month of age past 6 months up to 26 to 30 months of age. The age of a toddler in months minus 6 is used as an approximate guide to assess the expected number of teeth at a specific age. The usual order of appearance is shown in Chapter 13. At one year of age a child usually has eight teeth. During the toddler years four first molars, four cuspids, and four second molars erupt to complete the set of 20 deciduous teeth by about 30 months of age.

Anticipatory Guidance: Dentition Many parents are not aware that care of the deciduous teeth is important for the development of healthy permanent teeth. The nurse should explain to parents that ossification and formation of the permanent teeth take place during the toddler years even though the teeth are not visible.

Over 50 per cent of all children under the age of 2 have already experienced dental decay.[8] This presents a serious challenge to nurses to not only give information but also to spend the necessary time for explanation and follow-up that will help parents to provide early preventive dental care. The tedious care of a toddler's teeth requires that parents believe in its value, otherwise short-cuts will likely be taken.

Guidelines for care of the teeth should be discussed with parents when the child is an infant and readdressed during the toddler years. A toddler should be taken to a dentist between 2½ to 3 years of age. The visit for examination of the teeth should be preceded by a get-acquainted visit so that the toddler does not associate only unpleasantness with the dentist's office. As soon as the first teeth appear, the gums and teeth should be wiped with a soft, moist clean cloth after each feeding. A fluoride tooth paste can be applied to the cloth, and all sides of each tooth should be wiped. Tooth brushing is recommended by 18 months of age when the gingival tissue is no longer so easily damaged and a considerable number of teeth are present. Parents should be taught to brush their toddler's teeth twice a day and continue to assist with tooth brushing after he begins to brush his own teeth. A toddler will want to brush his own teeth by the age of 2 but needs supervision at least through the preschool years. Flossing begun by parents when the child is 2 to 3 years of age will have to continue to be done by parents until the child is about 7 or 8.

When a child brushes his own teeth he needs to be taught not to chew on toothpaste tubes, because many contain lead. An unsupervised toddler may eat toothpaste, possibly consuming excessive amounts of fluoride; therefore parents should be cautioned to use only small amounts of toothpaste and keep the toothpaste out of a toddler's reach.

The nurse should speak directly to the child when teaching proper brushing technique. Both the child and parents should be instructed to avoid a *vigorous* back and forth scrubbing motion, which a child of 2 is prone to use. Short back-and-forth or simple up-and-down brushing is easier for a child to learn than is the rotary motion. Effectiveness of brushing can be simply tested by use of disclosing tablets or by painting teeth with food coloring that stains the plaque, making it easier to locate and remove.

The nurse's role is not a one-time teaching event, but it is one in which dental care is stressed from various perspectives. Offering between-meal snacks of fruit, milk and crackers should be encouraged. Juice and milk should be taken from a cup rather than by bottle to avoid the disastrous dental trauma known as "bottle mouth syndrome'' in children between 1 and 3 years of age (see discussion, Chapter 21). Nighttime bottles, unless they contain water, are particularly hazardous to the toddler's teeth.

The nurse should be prepared to discuss up-to-date findings pertaining to use of fluoride. Excessive fluoride has been found to cause enamel fluorosis (mottling of enamel).[1] Therefore parents should be cautioned against using more than the prescribed dose of fluoride. Before 2 years of age the maximum fluoride supplement is 0.25 mg per day. From 2 to 3 years of age 0.50 mg per day is recommended if drinking water is unflouridated (below 0.3 ppm) and 0.25 mg per day if drinking water contains fluoride concentrations between 0.3 and 0.7 ppm.[1]

Lymphatic System

During early childhood the lymphatic tissue increases in size, accounting for the presence of peripheral nodes, enlargement of tonsils and adenoids, and a spleen tip that is more likely to be palpable.[29] Hyperplasia of lymphoid tissues is a phenomenon of normal physiological growth and is thought to occur as a response to the numerous infections of childhood. The excessive swelling and hyperplasia of lymphoid tissue in a normal child may persist long after the primary infection has resolved.[27] Lymphatic tissue shows progressive growth during the toddler years and attains maximum size by 10 to 11 years of age.

Anticipatory Guidance: Lymphatic System

The decline in use of surgical treatment of hypertrophied tonsils and adenoids is not always understood by parents. The nurse can gain the cooperation of parents to comply with the tedious task of repeated antibiotic treatment of upper respiratory infections if time is taken to explain the normal growth curve of lymphatic tissue. Parents are better able to cope with the stress of repeated visits to the practitioner's office if they understand that the hypertrophied tonsils and adenoids are thought to be a protective response to infection and a phenomenon of normal growth.

Motor Development

The significant advances in motor development during the toddler years affect his physical, mental and emotional-social development. A toddler employs new skills of locomotion and manipulation to satisfy his curiosity and experience new sensations. Physical maturation coupled with opportunities for practice fosters mastery of increasingly complex skills. He rapidly develops the motor skills that enable him to comply with socially accepted standards in his daily living.

Locomotion Important gross motor skills that are perfected during the toddler years are the ability to walk and run. The age at which these skills are perfected varies from one child to another and particularly from one culture to another. The advanced motor development that has been found to be present in black babies is thought to decrease and possibly level out during the second year of life.[28] Ethnic differences in locomotion observed during the first year are thus generally not as observable during the toddler years.

Most children are able to walk alone by the age of 15 months, although some normal chil-

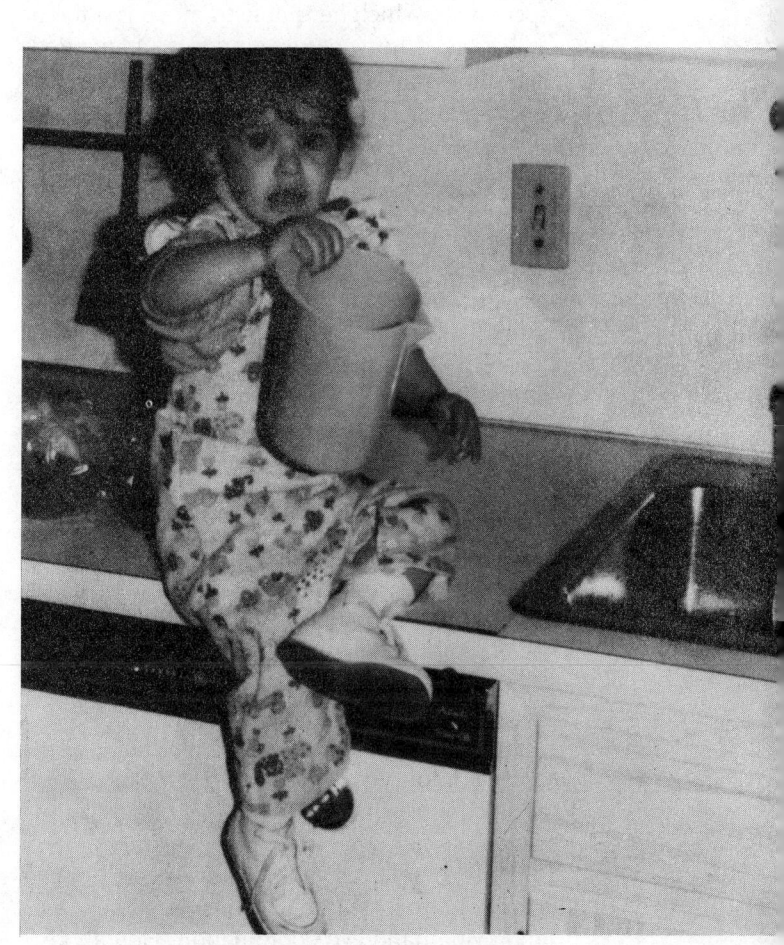

The climber. (Photograph by Dan R. Bruggeman.)

dren walk as late as 18 months and others as early as 10. At 15 months a toddler becomes an avid climber, climbing onto chairs, sofas and low tables, and may climb out of a crib, high chair or stroller. At this age a toddler can quickly disappear by climbing up a staircase on hands and knees. He can get down stairs by going backward and sliding from one step to the next, but he can still have an occasional accident and slip down the stairs too quickly.

At 18 months of age a toddler walks well. If he falls, it is usually because he tries to run too quickly. He now pushes chairs to cupboards and tables so that he can climb to higher, more intriguing destinations. He can walk up stairs one step at a time if someone holds onto one hand, but he still slides down the stairs backward. He likes to pull things while he walks and can even walk sideways while pulling a toy.

At 2 years of age a toddler has acquired a more steady gait and generally runs well with fewer falls but is not able to stop quickly. The speed with which he is able to move is a threat to his life if he ventures outdoors unattended. He can now go up and down stairs alone by holding onto a handrail but does so by putting both feet on each step rather than the more advanced method of alternating feet.

From a toddler's second to third birthday he becomes increasingly adept at all of his skills of locomotion. By 3 years of age he can walk downstairs alternating feet, can run and walk skillfully, and rides a tricycle. His skills of locomotion have progressed from the characteristic toddling gait to one of balance and control that qualifies him for the status of preschooler.

Motor Skills Affecting Play The toddler's play activities are affected by all aspects of development but are restricted to boundaries as prescribed by his motor abilities. At 15 months he is still highly engaged in gross motor activities, but he also enjoys the challenge of fine motor control.

At this age a toddler stacks two blocks, puts objects into a container and pours them out, and scribbles spontaneously if he is ingenious enough to get possession of a pencil.

At 18 months of age a toddler can build a tower of 3 to 4 blocks, which gives evidence of improving hand-eye coordination. He can also manipulate a pounding bench, although rather crudely. He will try to assist with turning the pages of a book but does so by turning two or three at a time. Although he cannot effectively kick a ball, he is able to clumsily catch and throw one without falling.

By 24 months a toddler can build a tower of six blocks and can line them horizontally to make a train. He now can turn the pages of a book one at a time and imitate vertical and circular strokes, but he still holds the crayon or pencil with a fist. By 30 months he can use his fingers to hold a pencil or a crayon and by 3 his hand is steady enough to build a bridge, an 8- to 10-block tower and a structure that resembles a house.

Motor Skills Affecting Eating A toddler makes it known that he wants access to eating utensils long before he can manipulate them efficiently. At 15 months of age the spoon is grasped, but because he rotates the spoon, he frequently loses its contents on the way to his mouth. At this age he spends a great deal of time practicing the skill of stirring his food during mealtime. He enjoys and is able to pick up pieces of food with his fingers. He can also hold a cup by grasping it rather clumsily with both hands, and as with the spoon, he spills the contents frequently because he tilts the cup before it reaches his mouth.

From 15 months to 2 years of age a toddler demonstrates remarkable advances in his eating skills. At 18 months of age he can use a spoon and drink from a cup or glass. He is able to partially feed himself but needs adult supervision because he easily gets engrossed in playing with his food. By 2 years of age he can feed himself, hold a cup with one hand and set it down after drinking without spilling. By 2 he has mastered the use of the spoon and spills little.

By 3 years of age a toddler can pour from a pitcher and prepare his own dish of milk and cold cereal. He feeds himself completely and has only occasional accidents of spilling.

Motor Skills Affecting Self-Care Activities At 15 months of age a toddler is dependent on his caretaker for most of his physical care. The toddler at this age has the fine motor skills to take off his socks and shoes and does so as a playful, experimental activity. By 18 months he assists in undressing more than dressing and may not necessarily be undressing when it is time for bed. He can unzip a large zipper and take off simple garments. He will also try to brush teeth at this age but has not acquired sufficient fine motor skill to perform this task. By 2 years of age he is able to assist in self-care by putting on simple garments but does not differentiate front from back. He is now able to zip and unzip zippers. He can put on his shoes but is not able to buckle or tie them. He washes and dries his hands, brushes teeth crudely and, if helped to reach the sink, can turn on a water faucet. He can also turn doorknobs and open doors without assistance. By 3 he dresses himself almost completely but still does not know front from back and cannot tie his shoes.

A toddler's physical development provides boundaries within which he performs increasingly complex activities of daily living. Although development of fine and gross motor skills determines when a child can perform a particular task, the emotional and social development of a child has tremendous impact on the accomplishment of these activities; thus activities of daily living are further addressed in the discussion on the emotional-social development of the toddler.

Anticipatory Guidance: Motor Skills The toddler years are a time when parents need special assistance from the nurse to provide adequate opportunity for the development of their child's motor skills. Parents need suggestions in how they can provide a safe environment without detracting from the toddler's opportunity to practice his motor skills. A toddler can be given the opportunity to practice stair climbing under supervision and to practice running outdoors on the grass, where a fall is less dangerous. The nurse should also encourage parents to allow their toddler to practice fine motor skills by permitting self-feeding, assistance in dressing and participation in other self-care activities.

Parents should be assisted in choosing play activities that promote fine and gross motor skills appropriate for the various stages of toddlerhood. If parents can regard the practice of motor skills as an essential component of their toddler's developing self-esteem as well as his physical development, the frustrations that eager toddlers pose to parents may be more tolerable. Encouraging parents to provide opportunities for the development of motor skills without undue emphasis on premature perfection builds an environment within which the toddler thrives.

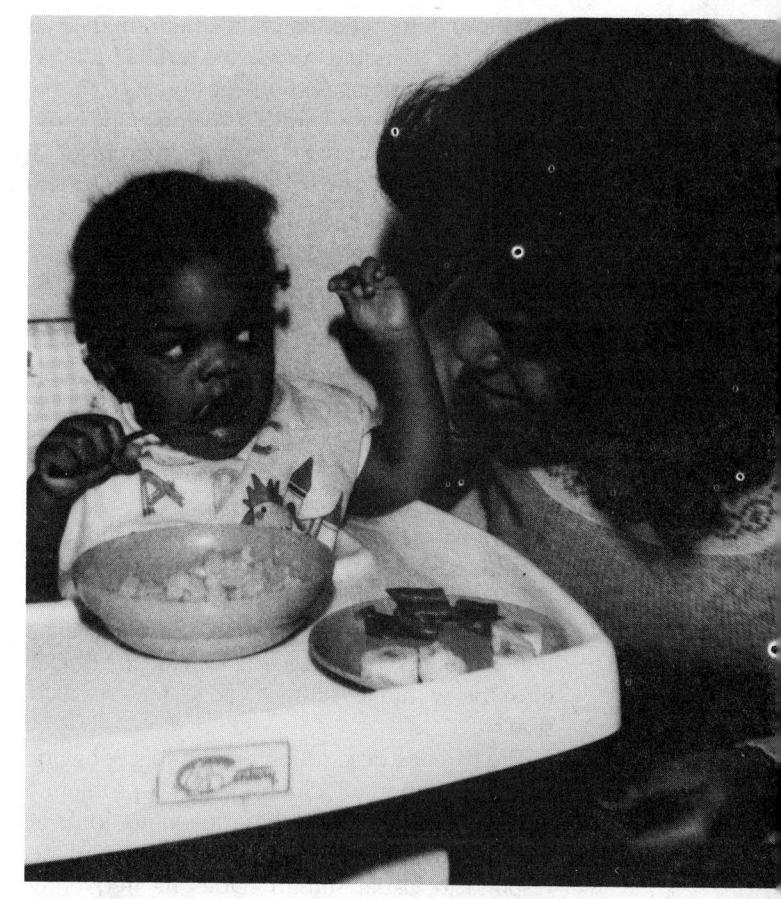

Toddlers need parental presence but prefer to tackle some tasks themselves.

Vision and Hearing

During toddlerhood the normal development of vision and hearing should be evaluated on each health care visit. Impaired hearing is difficult to detect if there is a unilateral or minimal hearing loss. However, it is crucial that hearing loss be detected because a toddler who cannot hear will not progress through the normal sequence of language development. A strong indication that the toddler's hearing is impaired is the case of an infant who babbled at 6 months and who does not progress to increased sound production but rather shows a marked decrease in vocalization and eventually does not produce any sounds.

To assess hearing the nurse should begin by asking the parents whether they think their child can hear. The ability to hear should be assessed by direct examination of the child's response to sounds, but the nurse should also question the parents to determine the child's performance at home: For example, does the toddler follow simple instructions without gestures? Can he point to familiar pictures in a book upon request? Does he turn his head to search for a sound presented behind him? Does he respond to his own name? If there is any delay or slowing of development pertaining to language, the child should be referred for audiometric testing. See Chapter 13 for further discussion on hearing testing.

Evaluation of visual acuity continues to be difficult during the toddler years. It is not until about the age of 3 that a child can cooperate sufficiently for use of the Snellen illiterate E chart. Before the age of 3 vision can be assessed by observing the child's eye-hand coordination and his response to bright lights and objects. Despite hyperopia (farsightedness), which is normal during the toddler years, distance fixation is not well developed, so that an object must be within a six-foot range for clear vision.[32]

The parent's description of a child's behavior can give important clues to visual problems. Does the toddler who has begun to look at books hold them close to his eyes? Does he respond to visual stimuli? Does he frequently rub his eyes, blink, squint or frown when looking at things? Does he bump into objects when walking?* The preference a child shows to sit close to a television set is not indicative of a visual problem. Many children with normal vision enjoy the stimulation of large images and sit close to a TV. Parents should always be asked for their evaluation of their toddler's vision.

The toddler should be assessed for *strabismus* and *amblyopia*. When strabismus (crossed eyes, squint) is present a child may alternate vision from one eye to the other or favor one eye to the exclusion of the other. It is when the one eye is not used that amblyopia develops and visual acuity decreases. The child learns to suppress vision in the deviating eye to avoid the diplopia (double vision), which is caused by the strabismus. Lack of use of the eye can seriously impair vision and if untreated can cause irreversible loss of vision. Careful assessment of the eyes is particularly important because the manifestations of strabismus may be intermittent and not easily detected by observation.

The Hirschberg test and the cover test are simple tests that should be routinely administered. (See Chapter 13 for test description.) Parents should also be consulted regarding their observations of any evidence of crossing of the eyes. Any findings suggestive of strabismus must be referred to an ophthalmologist for further evaluation so that loss of vision due to a secondary amblyopia can be prevented. See Chapter 43 for further discussion of strabismus and amblyopia.

Anticipatory Guidance: Vision and Hearing

The nurse should explain the relationship between hearing and language development. Parents should be taught the normal progression of language development as a preventive measure to detect hearing impairment. Parents should be encouraged to assess hearing and vision by observing their toddler's responsiveness to stimuli. The reports of parents can give the first clue to vision and hearing problems.

Nutritional Requirements

The amount of energy expended is determined by body size and composition, physical activity and rate of growth.

A toddler needs a greater number of total calories (1000 to 1500 Kcal/day) than during infancy due to an increase in body size, but the requirements *per unit of body weight* decrease. Two major factors affect energy requirements during the toddler years: slowed growth rate reduces energy requirements and increased activity increases energy requirements. The sum effect of these changes is only a slight decrease in requirements from 108 Kcal/kg/day in infants to 100 Kcal/kg/day in toddlers.

Although physical growth rate slows during the toddler years, protein requirements remain relatively high because of the rapid growth of muscle tissue. Protein requirements change from 2 gm/kg/day at 6 to 12 months of age to 1.8 gm/kg/day during the toddler years. In spite of a decrease in appetite, under normal circumstances the toddler's protein requirements are met if a balanced diet is consumed.

By about 2 years of age the percentage of total body water is similar to that of an adult, i.e., approximately 60 per cent of total body weight. The adult 40:60 ratio of extracellular to intracellular water is reached by about 1 year of age. Metabolic rate remains relatively high;

---

*Before 18 months of age a child with normal vision tends to bump into objects.

therefore a toddler's fluid requirement is 115 to 125 ml/kg/day.

A balanced diet including 16 to 24 ounces of milk supplies vitamin D, calcium and phosphorus in recommended amounts. Excessive amounts of milk may reduce a child's desire for intake of solid foods rich in iron, resulting in iron deficiency anemia. See Appendix V for recommended daily allowances for vitamins and minerals.

INTELLECTUAL COMPETENCY

A study of the intellectual development of a toddler offers some explanation of the increasing complexity with which the toddler relates to his environment. The toddler's fascination with practicing newly learned motor skills, his experimentation by poking, tasting and pushing, and his dramatic imitations are not simply explained. What are the mental processes accompanying this incessant activity? The question "What is he thinking?" becomes less of a mystery after he reaches the age of 2, when his remarkable advances in language development enable him to express his thoughts and make verbal requests. Stages of cognitive development identified by Piaget provide a theory base that the nurse can use to assess normal growth and development.

Stages of Cognitive Development

By 12 months of age an infant has progressed through four substages of development that have resulted in numerous important accomplishments. He now searches for an object that has vanished (object permanence); his actions show deliberate intention and he has a rudimentary concept of cause and effect.

The infant enters toddlerhood with a beginning understanding of spoken words and engages in prelinguistic formation of sounds. The imitative behaviors that were begun at about 3 months of age now become particularly noticeable as he imitates new actions daily. Things learned in the first four substages continue to be practiced, and new learning emerges during the next 12 to 36 months.

Substage five (12 to 18 months) is characterized by what Piaget has called *tertiary circular reactions*. This is a third type of circular reaction that differs from the other two (primary and secondary) circular reactions. In this stage a child knocks down a tower of blocks, helps to rebuild it and knocks it down again not for the sake of repetition (primary circular) and not only to observe the results (secondary circular). Now he is searching for new ways to bring about the same results and/or experimenting to see if he can produce new results. He may therefore push the blocks over gently one time, and the next time stand up and swing his arm to see if something new will happen. It is this "experimenting to see" that brings about new behaviors and results in trial-and-error as a predominant method of learning. Deliberate manipulation to find out what will happen fills the day of a busy toddler during this phase of development.

Substage six (18 to 24 months) marks the transition from predominantly trial-and-error behavior to thinking about solutions and consequences before carrying them out. This stage is characterized by a beginning ability to use mental images and words when referring to absent objects. He can also anticipate what will happen to the object as a result of a certain action and therefore solves problems by thinking about the results rather than always having to carry them out by trial and error. For example, during this stage a child is less fascinated with throwing a variety of objects from his high chair than he was earlier. He remembers that an object falls and makes a noise without doing it every day. He also can anticipate that if he throws a fork instead of a spoon, it will also make a noise; therefore it is not necessary to throw the fork on the floor. The breakthrough of being able to mentally try out alternate ways of accomplishing a goal has been described by Piaget as the stage of inventing new means through mental combinations.

The ability to retain an image of an object or action beyond immediate sensory experience is demonstrated when a toddler imitates a past event in the absence of the original stimuli. For example, when a child pretends he is shaving in front of the mirror hours after his father has gone to work, he is engaging in what has been described by Piaget as deferred imitation. During this stage a child imitates a model in his environment that has significance and meaning to him. The process of identification takes place as he takes on the behavior and values of those in his environment.

The concept of object permanence is now

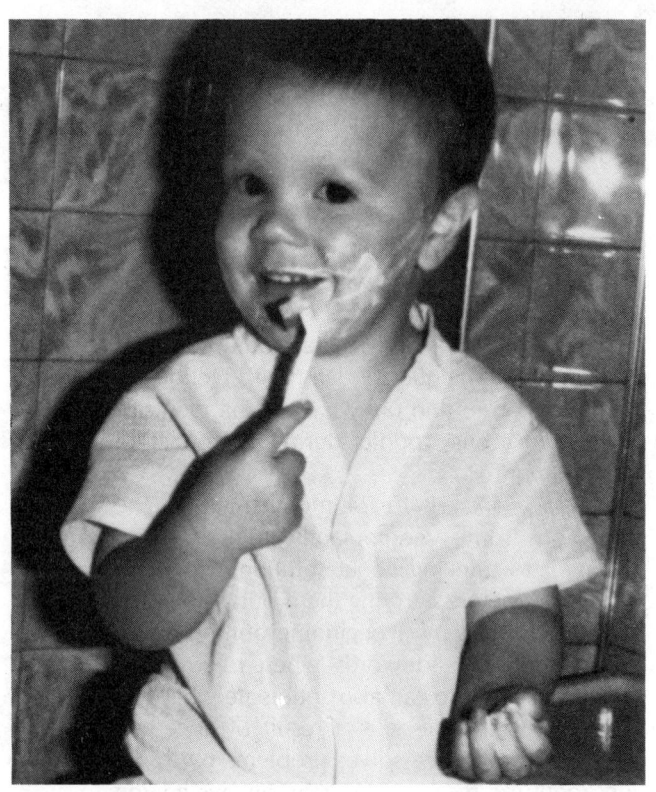

The toddler portrays deferred imitation when he pretends to be shaving after his father has gone off to work. (Photograph by David Trainor.)

fully developed. If a ball rolls under the sofa, he has a concept of the ball continuing to move even though he cannot see the movement. If he cannot find the ball under the sofa he will conclude that the ball has moved through to the other side and he will go around the sofa to look for the ball. It is the child's ability to retain a mental image of the ball and to think about the property of the ball that brings about this level of behavior.

Entrance into the preoperational period (2 to 7) is characterized by an increased internal representation of objects and the ability to engage in symbolic thought.* Piaget is not consistent in the use of the term "symbol," so that the difference in symbolism between the last phase of the sensorimotor period and the first stage of the preoperational period is not precise.[24] The preoperational child has greater ability to differentiate signifiers (blanket, pacifier) from significates (going to bed). For example,

---

*Symbolic thought is the ability to make something — a mental image, a word or an object — stand for something that is not present.

before 2 years of age the blanket and pacifier might be signs that symbolize going to bed (blanket-pacifier-bedtime are perceived as a single unit), whereas a preoperational child can differentiate the blanket and pacifier from the experience of going to bed.[24]

The preoperational period begins with a period described as *preconceptual*. The increased use of symbols permits the child to internalize what he sees and experiences, but his concepts are not as complete and logical as those of an adult, thus the term preconceptual. For example, all dogs will be called by the name of the child's dog. He is not able to comprehend that all objects within a class are not one and the same object; therefore his attempts at generalization result in cognitive errors.

Although pretending and imagination show their beginnings during the latter part of the sensorimotor period, *symbolic play* is at its peak in children from 2 to 4 years of age. Symbolization is greatly enhanced by rapidly developing language ability during this period. Egocentric thought also facilitates symbolic play. For imagination and pretending to ensue, assimilation must outweigh accommodation so that a distortion of reality takes place.[26]* A child distorts reality by taking into account only the characteristics of objects that meet his immediate needs. The greater the egocentrism, the greater the distortion of reality. At times there is almost no resemblance between the object and the symbol that it is representing in the child's mind (between the stick the child is using for a carrot and an actual carrot).

Over a two-year period a toddler's cognition progresses from a predominantly trial-and-error method of object manipulation to a beginning retention of mental images which allows him to think about alternate solutions, and finally, by the age of 3, internal representation of objects enables him to make a dish or a box become a hat or a shell a cup. Reality is first copied (imitation) and later (2 to 4 years) reality is distorted (symbolic play). Symbolism and imitation eventually disappear, but during the toddler period they represent his efforts to adapt to reality. Pulaski suggests that during this period a child's life is polarized around his attempt to adapt to reality by pleasing his parents (imitative accommodation) and his need to escape from parental demands and

---

*See Chapter 10 for further discussion of assimilation and accommodation.

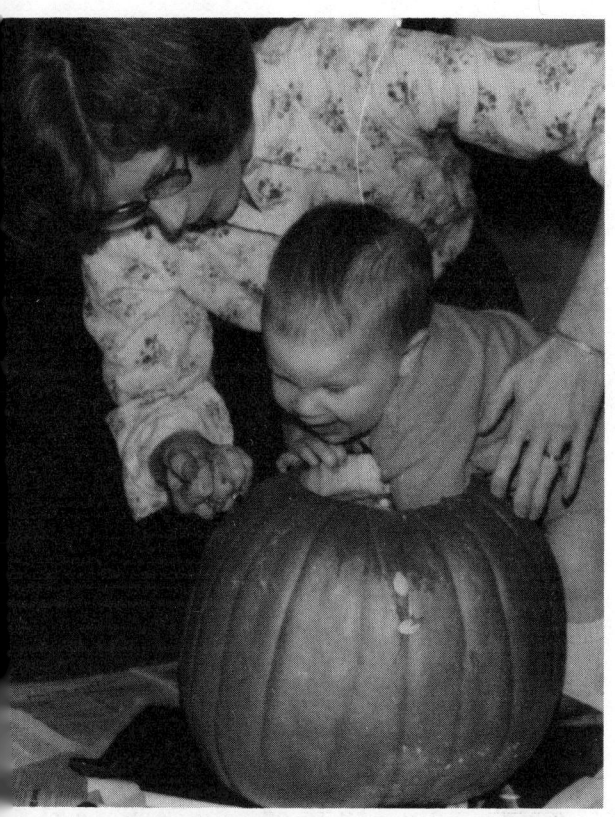

The toddler learns about his environment through exploration and sensory experiences. (Photograph by David Trainor.)

satisfy his own ego (assimilative symbolic play).[26]

Anticipatory Guidance: Intellectual Development The nurse can be in a position to evaluate how attuned the family is to their toddler's intellectual needs. A toddler needs a variety of experiences that allow him to make discoveries. Parents should be helped to understand that a toddler's intense examination and incessant manipulation of anything new is the way he learns. A toddler is growing intellectually when he insists on examining the contents of cupboards, drawers, boxes and anything he can reach. If a nurse will take the time to explain the meaning of such toddler behavior, a family is more likely to feel a sense of pride and even intrigue in their toddler's fascination with and scrutiny of everything and everybody he encounters.

The limit-setting and constant surveillance that is required by a family with a toddler is exhausting and often stressful. It is important for a nurse to explore with the family ways that encourage the development of their toddler without exhausting and immobilizing the rest of family life.

During the trial-and-error stage a toddler needs parents who can patiently stand by and watch his countless attempts to complete a task without reaching in and making the final move just as he is about to accomplish it on his own. Parents must maintain a delicate balance as they support the curiosity of their child (allowing him to make his own discoveries) while having the sensitivity to know when help is needed in order to avoid undue frustration.

It is important for the nurse to explain to families that their toddler's learning by experimentation is not restricted to planned play opportunities, but that dresser drawers, kitchen cupboards, and bathroom closets provide even a greater fascination to him. Making a special cupboard available with some kitchen utensils will please a toddler and may keep him out of the rest of the kitchen cupboards. In other areas of the house a similar approach can be taken.

As a child enters the preoperational period (around 2 years of age) parents need to be prepared for the symbolic play that emerges. A nurse can explain to them that games of pretending and creation of imaginary playmates are normal behaviors for a toddler from 24 to 36 months and continue through the preschool years. Nurses can encourage parents to listen to their toddler as he describes the contents of a box that has become a truck or the qualities of a plastic container that has become a rocket. It is appropriate for parents to carry on a conversation with a toddler about his imagined play and inappropriate to discourage the child's imagination with "But that is a box, not a truck."

In all phases of intellectual development during the toddler years many frustrations can be avoided if the nurse helps parents to be consistent in what is allowed and to avoid setting a child up for punishment. For example, knowingly leaving new and intriguing things within reach and then punishing him for destroying them is unreasonable. By observing the parent-child interaction and discussing activity of a normal day, the nurse can gather important clues regarding the family's encouragement of intellectual development of their toddler.

Language Development

It is the nurse's role to assess the appropriateness of the toddler's language ability and help families to provide an environment conducive to language development. Nurses must therefore be knowledgeable about (1) stages of language acquisition, (2) characteristics of toddler language and (3) factors that contribute to language development.

Stages of Language Acquisition By his first birthday the infant's language development has been influenced by the amount of reinforcement he has received. It has been noted that babies babble more when people talk to them. Also, when babies have been stimulated to practice babbling, they are likely to abandon babbling in favor of speech earlier than if no reinforcement was received.[14] The babbling stage (4 to 6 months) is followed by single-word utterances at about 1 year of age. A vocabulary of three words is common for a 1-year-old, typically including ma-ma, da-da, and bye-bye.

From 15 to 18 months of age an *expressive jargon* emerges that has rhythmic intonations, but no real words can be recognized. Expressive jargon is thought to be an expression of feelings or ideas, and it is a way to make contact with another human being.[28] Although expressive jargon does not seem to contain real words, a toddler uses it in conjunction with pointing and movement toward the object or person he is "talking" about, thereby communicating his wants.

Between 18 and 24 months of age one-word utterances are commonly used to communicate increasingly complex ideas. When one-word sentences are used to express whole ideas, the accompanying gestures give clues to the meaning. For example, saying bye-bye while standing at the door and hitting on it after playing indoors for several hours may mean "I want to go bye-bye," whereas standing at the door quietly as father is leaving for work and saying "Bye-bye" probably means "Da-da is going bye-bye." If, however, hitting of the door again accompanies the utterance "Bye-bye" as Daddy leaves, it now clearly means "I want to go bye-bye with Da-da." These one-word utterances that carry whole ideas are referred to as *holophrasic speech*. Giving careful attention to the situation surrounding one-word utterances and the accompanying gestures becomes an integral part of successful communication with a toddler.

By 18 to 24 months of age most toddlers have mastered locomotion reasonably well and can put more effort into expression through language. From 18 months to 3 years of age vocabulary growth and complexity of sentence structure progress rapidly and constantly. Although there is a wide variation in the number of words a toddler is able to say, a typical vocabulary at 18 months of age is 10 or more words; by 2 years of age he may easily progress to a phenomenal 300-word vocabulary, and by 3 he uses around 900 words. At about 2 years of age two-word utterances become increasingly common, by 2½ years of age an average sentence contains three words and by 3, complete sentences are constructed using all parts of speech.

Characteristics of Toddler Speech Around 2 years of age a characteristic pattern of speech emerges. There are a few words that seem to be used repeatedly and other less frequently used words are attached to them. The frequently used words have been described as *pivot* words and the less frequently used words as *open*. For example, "down" may emerge as a pivot word in "sit down," "put down" and "go down." Sit, put, and go (open words) are less frequently used than "down." Another characteristic is that when two words are combined it is usually a noun and verb. For example, "go outside" is a grammatically incomplete sentence containing only the words that carry meaning. Articles, prepositions, and adjectives are generally lacking as is typical in a telegram, which accounts for the use of the term *telegraphic sentences* to describe these phrases.

The egocentric thought that dominates in the preconceptual phase of the preoperational period (beginning at 24 months of age) is expressed in the content of a toddler's language. Toddlers in this stage engage in a monologue with little regard for a response of another child or adult who happens to be present. The function of this *egocentric speech* is that it meets the toddler's need to practice speech. This type of speech often accompanies the symbolic play which characterizes this period. As a toddler matures and is able to consider another's viewpoint, his speech becomes more socialized and he engages in increasingly more conversation with others and less monologue.

Anticipatory Guidance: Language Development The nurse's knowledge regarding the stages and characteristics of language development facilitates her own communication with children and serves as a guide in her counselling of parents. When parents have a concern that their toddler's language is not developing as rapidly as that of a sibling or other playmates, the nurse can help parents to understand the wide range of normal language acquisition and can explain the impact of other areas of their child's development. For example, pointing out that a toddler's language development is often delayed by his absorption in learning motor skills during the second year of life is reassuring to parents.

The nurse can also offer some practical suggestions on how parents can facilitate language development. The most frequently misunderstood element of relating to a toddler has to do with "baby talk." To shape the learning of speech a child should be given the opportunity to hear correct speech. A nurse can encourage parents to respond to their toddler's speech by using correct communication and by expanding and rephrasing what he says in a grammatically correct statement. They should not, however, correct the child's language by saying "No, its not wa-wa, it's water." If the parents avoid responding with "baby-talk" correct language is learned. It has been reported that young children are actually more responsive to adult forms of speech such as "throw me the ball" than they are to two-word commands of "throw ball."[19]

A nurse should also counsel parents to guard against giving a toddler what he wants in response to his crying and gestures. The incentive to learn to speak is dramatically hampered if a toddler's requests are granted in the absence of verbalization. A toddler understands much more than he can say, so he will understand "tell mama" or "tell daddy what you want." Most of the time it is quicker and easier to grant the request without asking the toddler to verbalize, but this practice establishes a pattern that discourages language development.

As a toddler progresses through the various stages of language development (holophrasic sentences, jargon, telegraphic speech) with its common characteristics (egocentrism, pivot and open words) parents need to be encouraged to be attentive to the situation as well as the actual words that are spoken. Parents may need help in understanding that the repetition of favorite words is a toddler's way of practicing language and is not necessarily a request or true expression of his desires. At all stages of language development a toddler needs a family whose members talk to him and respond to his language efforts. It is important for the nurse to stress that a toddler understands a great deal of what he hears. He certainly senses the tone and feeling of verbal language and is sensitive to the relationship that exists between family members. A toddler's language development thrives when he feels secure and loved and when warm, intimate relationships prevail within his family.

EMOTIONAL-SOCIAL COMPETENCY

The emotional-social development of a toddler is a dramatic unfolding of a person who has a sense of self, expresses feelings verbally and bodily and is struggling to become increasingly more independent without giving up the security and comfort that dependency affords. He is now able to differentiate the responses of those around him. He curbs those behaviors that result in disapproval and repeats performances that are given attention and approval. As he becomes increasingly aware of himself and the world around him, he experiments with a variety of ways to gain control over what happens to him without losing the approval of his parents and significant others.

The emotions expressed by a toddler become socially more obvious than during infancy. Young babies show discomfort and displeasure by crying or screaming, whereas a toddler adds

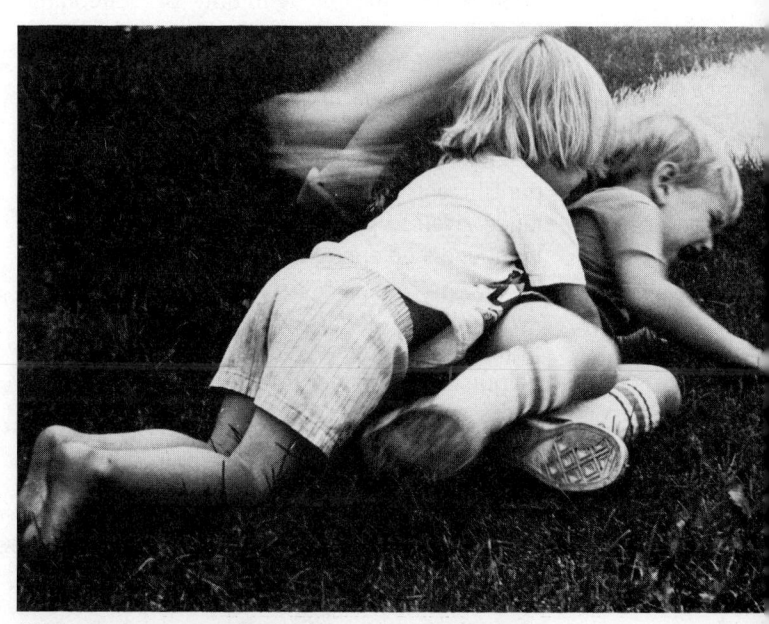

The toddler expresses his emotions physically through biting, hitting or pulling.

GROWTH AND DEVELOPMENT OF THE TODDLER: MAINTAINING WELLNESS 743

throwing, biting, hitting, stamping his feet and pushing or pulling to his repertoire. His pleasant emotions are also now expressed overtly. If he feels a need to be close to his parents he has the physical ability to pull on them and to hug them, and the verbal ability to say "love mama" or "love da-da." Expressions of both pleasant and unpleasant emotions elicit various responses from those in his environment. That which he experiences tends to encourage or discourage certain behaviors and in this way he begins to adapt to the social demands of his family and society. If a toddler can feel loved and accepted, with some sense of control over his own destiny, he is likely to develop a sense of worth and high self-esteem. As a toddler strives to master developmental tasks, his experiences within his family to a large degree shape his emotional and social development. Each family interprets the confines of acceptable behavior and has its owns ideals and expectations for its developing toddler.

There is much variation in how a family chooses to socialize its toddler. The decisions and choices that a family makes are largely a consequence of their own cultural values. Nurses must learn to relate to families from various cultures and seek to understand the ethnic differences in defining acceptable, socialized behavior for a toddler. Her own cultural orientation and family experiences will influence the nurse's definition of acceptable behavior. Areas of development in which cultural variations are particularly evident during the toddler years are: (1) time to begin toilet training, (2) handling of anger and aggressive behavior (temper tantrums), (3) use of corporal punishment, (4) tolerance for crying, (5) importance given to provision for play, (6) degree of independence encouraged and (7) age of weaning.

For a nurse to work effectively with families from various cultures she must recognize that unique cultural patterns persist and these differences affect socialization of a toddler. The tasks of the toddler are achieved in a way that is consistent with culturally defined family values. Expectations of the nurse may be inconsistent with those of the family, and it is important for the nurse to examine the impact that her own cultural values and beliefs will have on the guidance and counselling offered to families.

Temperament

By the time a baby reaches 1 year of age a pattern of interaction within the family has been established. The temperament* of the baby and of other family members is an influential determinant in the evolving pattern of communication. If relationships are tense and stressful, the toddler's behavioral style can be adversely affected. A toddler has so much learning and controlling of emotions to master during these years that his family may have difficulty adapting to the varied and new manifestations of the child's temperament. A toddler's emerging sense of self, his wish to control, and his insistence on having his own way are stressful to a family.

The temperament apparent during infancy tends to persist through toddlerhood and throughout later years but, according to Thomas and Chess, it is not immutable.[31] This view has particular meaning for the toddler years because of the numerous demands for socialization that are encountered. The way the developmental tasks are handled by parents may indeed bring about adaptations in the basic behavioral style. The environmental influences that a child experiences within his family may accentuate, modify or alter traits of temperament.[31]

Regardless of the temperament of the child and the expectations of parents, there is likely to be some stress and conflict between parent and toddler. The interactive process of temperament and environment has been described as being consonant or dissonant. Consonance, or "goodness of fit," between the temperament of the child and expectations of parents results in optimal development of the child. Dissonance, or "poorness of fit," between these two factors can result in behavioral problems and thwarted development.[31] During the toddler years numerous tasks are accomplished that have the potential to cause consonance or dissonance. Chess and Thomas have identified numerous areas in which consonance or dissonance between the child and his environment is elaborated. Areas identified are (1) establishment of regular sleep and feeding patterns; (2) mastery of self-care (feeding, dressing, toilet training); (3) compliance to family expectations; (4) response to masturbatory experiences and (5) the emergence and growth of interpersonal

---

*Temperament is the way a person behaves and can be equated with a *behavioral style*.[31]

relationships within the family.[31] The degree of consonance or dissonance between the toddler's temperament and capabilities and the demands and expectations of parents has a profound impact on his development.

Anticipatory Guidance: Temperament The nurse must first help family members to express their own frustrations and concern about the temperament of their toddler. Especially when there are older siblings, parents may feel baffled by the dramatic differences in behavior of their children. Using disciplinary approaches that they had found successful for an older child when he was a toddler may not be effective this time. For example, a highly adaptable toddler may comply if told to stop turning the TV knob, an easily distractible toddler may be readily diverted, but one who is persistent may have to be picked up and carried away from the TV. Parents need assistance to understand that these temperamental variations do not constitute bad or good behavior but that toddlers of certain temperaments need special responses from their family.

The way a child expresses normal toddler characteristics is consistent with his particular temperament. Parents of toddlers frequently compare their child's behavior with that of a friend's or relative's child in search of an answer to handling their toddlers' behaviors. The nurse can be of assistance by encouraging parents to identify those behaviors that are most stressful and then helping them develop approaches that are congruent with their own temperament as well as their toddler's. (See Chapter 3 for a discussion of parenting that considers temperament.)

Attachment and Separation

The interactions between infant and caretaker from birth gradually develop into an emotional tie described by Bowlby as an *affective bond*.[3] During the toddler years attachment behavior (seeking and maintaining proximity) is neither less intense nor less frequent than at the end of the first year. According to Bowlby, most children exhibit attachment behavior strongly and regularly until around their third birthday.[3] Typical toddler attachment behaviors are watching, smiling, following, calling, and listening. Crying and protesting at separation from their caretaker persists during the toddler years, but Bowlby reports a change in a toddler's ability to separate at about 2 years and 9 months.

By 3 years of age children are able to engage in play with other children in their caretaker's temporary absence. Although children before 2 years and 9 months may cry for only a short time when their caretaker leaves, they are likely to remain quiet and less involved in play, and constantly demand attention of the substitute caretaker.[3]

The need for a toddler to visualize his caretaker is frequently demonstrated when he momentarily wanders too far from his caretaker and frantically returns for contact, sometimes in tears, as though it was the caretaker who separated from him. As the toddler develops attachment and feels more secure, he is able to explore and play in his caretaker's presence with only occasional "checking back" for reassurance. The toddler who constantly seeks proximity with his caretaker cannot be assumed to be more attached, because the ability to separate is an outgrowth of a healthy attachment. It should be expected, however, that when a toddler is in a novel environment he will make contact with attachment figures more frequently than when in a familiar environment.

The quality of attachment in infancy has been studied to identify its relationship to competence and adaptation during the second year of life.[21] Matas et al. studied quality of attachment in infancy and quality of play and problem-solving behavior at 2 years of age. Infants who were assessed as securely attached at 18 months were, at 2 years of age, more enthusiastic, persistent and cooperative than insecurely attached infants. The competent 2-year-old boy in this study did not automatically comply with his mother's request, but demonstrated gradual cooperation (for example, on helping to clean up toys). These findings are in agreement with other studies that show securely attached infants to be more socially and cognitively competent.[21]

Anticipatory Guidance: Attachment and Separation The nurse needs to be aware of the particular lifestyle within a family, which will affect the toddler's ongoing development of attachment. If both parents are required to

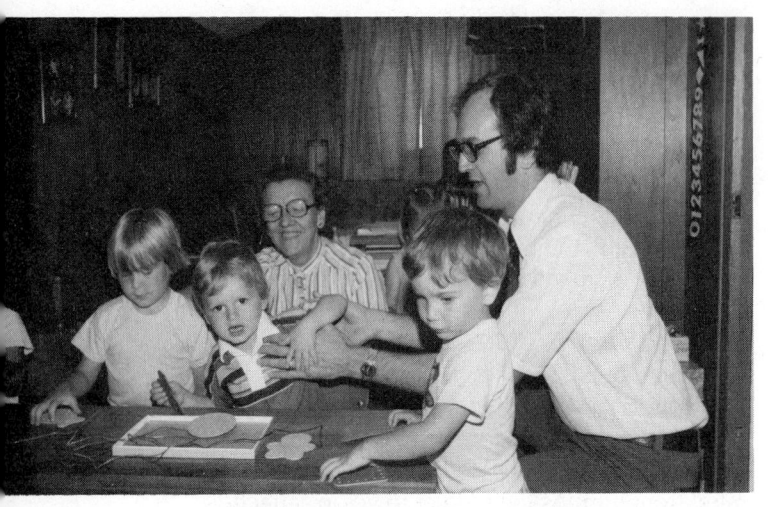

When the caretaker shares the toddler's day with his parent, the working parent feels more integrally a part of the child's development.

work, then the nurse should help the parents to feel comfortable with their child care arrangements. Parents need reassurance when their toddler momentarily seems more interested in continuing his play than returning home with his parent. If parents can be encouraged to take an interest in what has happened during the day — what their toddler has said, how he played, what he ate and what discipline was required — they can feel more integrally a part of his development and experience an ongoing attachment. The nurse might suggest that frequent conversations be held with the substitute caretaker so that parents will feel more in control.

The nurse should also provide some guidance in helping parents understand how a toddler perceives and responds to separation. A toddler learns from experience that parents reappear after a brief separation and that even though they are absent for short periods, they continue to exist. Learning to tolerate brief separations is a developmental task of a toddler that may cause some difficulty to parents. If parents understand the kinds of behavior that brief separations cause, their coping ability is enhanced. For example, a toddler, after being left with a babysitter, may become more clingy and show an increase in attachment behaviors. Parents need to respond to such behaviors by providing extra attention and affection and need to guard against demanding the level of independence that their toddler exhibited before the babysitting experience.

Fears

Each age seems to bring with it typical or characteristic *fears*. An increasing perception of his environment makes a toddler more alert to auditory, spatial and visual changes. The types of fears that result are fear of noise, sudden movement, an approaching object and unusual sensations (height, water). Fear of the water develops most frequently around 18 to 24 months of age in relationship to being bathed. A child typically suddenly refuses his bath and screams each time someone attempts to wash his face.[15] Fear of strange people and strange objects and places and of aloneness persists from the latter part of the first year until the third year, then tends to diminish.[4] Fear of the dark and of animals runs somewhat parallel and is not common before the age of 2.[15] The fear of being abandoned by parents persists as a continuous threat during the toddler years. It is experienced as a vague anxiety and heightened by separation from parents.

The fears of children under the age of 3 are usually not a problem. If parents can be sensitive to the normal fears of their toddler and provide the security he needs, he is likely to progress through this period experiencing only the normal fears. Chapter 31 discusses the development of extreme fears in toddlerhood and the effective management of normal and excessive fears of toddlers.

Anger, Aggression and Temper Tantrums

During the toddler years *anger* is commonly expressed through physical means. When one's goal is blocked by an obstacle frustration results, and aggressive behavior is a normal toddler reaction. For a toddler the obstacles encountered within a day are more frequent than many adults realize. Not only do adults interfere with a toddler's goals but his own ineptness leads him into one predicament after another. Toys get stuck, ice cream cones fall and balloons break, resulting in disappointment and frustration. Sometimes a toddler can be helped to accomplish his goal, but often he must learn to cope with his situation with little realization of the cause. Even though he caused his own dilemma he feels frustrated and angry. Expressions of anger are typically generalized and unproductive.

As the toddler develops in language and cognitive abilities he has other options for dealing with his feelings. However, for most of the toddler years his mode of expression of anger includes varied degrees of screaming, kicking, throwing things and even hurting himself by banging his head or biting himself. Sometimes a toddler will hold his breath when overcome with intense anger. When display of anger reaches an uncontrollable level it is typically referred to as a *temper tantrum*. One can hardly witness such an outburst without being impressed with its tone of desperation. It is as if the intensity of his feeling causes such internal distress that his only recourse is to release it all at once. The most common age for temper tantrums is 18 months to 3 years — the age of negativism and resistive behavior.[16] This developmental stage makes a toddler particularly vulnerable to physical demonstrations of anger. His struggle for independence is strong. Interference or thwarting of his self-determined course brings angry resistance, but his limited language and reasoning ability leave him little alternative but to have a tantrum.

Anticipatory Guidance: Anger, Aggression and Temper Tantrums Mismanagement of normal expressions of anger by a toddler can cause serious consequences to the child and his family. The nurse must be sensitive to clues that suggest developing conflict. Even before a pattern of temper tantrums develops the nurse can help parents cope with small annoyances caused by resistive behavior.

Nursing management begins by encouraging parents to express the distress and embarrassment they feel when their child has a temper tantrum. This period of "telling the story" is filled with clues for management. While hearing out a parent, the nurse should seek to answer the following questions: (1) How do the parents feel about how they handle temper tantrums? (2) Are they asking for help to change their behavior? (3) In the nurse's judgment, is there a potential for child abuse? (4) Are the parents making an attempt to control situational factors such as tiredness, hunger, excessive demands and insecurity? (5) Do the parents understand the developmental needs of a normal toddler? The goal of the nurse is to assist the family to cope with the normal developmental tasks that their toddler is mastering without making undue demands on individual family members.

When counselling parents, the nurse must also consider the varied cultural approaches to expressions of anger. There is a broad range of acceptable aggressive behaviors among cultures. That which is unacceptable behavior to the nurse may be encouraged by parents or vice versa. The nurse's concern then is to assist the family to handle the daily expressions of anger in a way that is consistent with their own pattern of behavior.

The goal for management of their toddler's normal expression of anger is that "tantrums must achieve nothing, and the cause of the tantrum — insecurity, faulty management or fatigue — should be looked for."[16] Although it is the nurse's role to help parents understand that temper tantrums are normal for this age, she should also assist the family to make every attempt to alter those circumstances that predictably result in a tantrum. The frequency, duration and intensity of tantrums can be reduced if situational factors are controlled. Situational factors affecting the toddler to be examined can be pinpointed with the following questions: (1) Is he tired and hungry? (2) Have excessive demands been made that are beyond his developmental capability? (3) Has his security been threatened? (4) Has he been excessively stimulated? (5) Is he suffering from boredom? (6) Does he lack physical exercise?

During the toddler years the most effective method of handling temper tantrums is to ignore the behavior. If a tantrum is to achieve nothing, parents are obliged to give nothing in response to it.

Two forms of ineffective responding are common, and in each case the tantrum has achieved something for the toddler. One response is to give in to the child and give him what he wants. This stops the tantrum at hand but breeds aggression because aggression has been rewarded. The most natural but ineffective response is for the parents to have a tantrum of their own.[7] Striking out at the child with violent verbal and physical aggression is just another form of reinforcement of aggressive behavior. When a child is treated violently he is likely to adopt these forms of behavior as a way to handle his own frustration. Any form of attention in response to a tantrum should be avoided if one hopes to break the inevitable cycle of repetition. A complete discussion of approaches to the handling of tantrums is presented in Chapter 31.

The nurse must realize that there is no foolproof method to handle temper tantrums. The counsel she gives must be given with an attitude of suggestions and options rather than solutions. Whenever temper tantrums become the pattern of behavior, the nurse should assist parents to carefully evaluate the circumstances surrounding the tantrums and correct any that predictably bring on a tantrum.

The Developing Person

Autonomy and Self-esteem To be autonomous is to see oneself as a separate being with a will of one's own. An infant develops a sense about the world by the way his needs are met. It is the caretaker's loving, attentive care that builds up the sense that the world is a pleasant place to be. This "sense of trust" as described by Erikson affects how a toddler views the world and how secure he feels to move away from the complete dependence he enjoyed in infancy to a more independent course dominated by his own will.

The toddler's central crisis involves the resolution of two opposing forces: that of "acquiring a sense of autonomy while combating a sense of doubt and shame."[20] He is in conflict because he wishes to exercise his own will but fears situations that extend his coping capacity.[20] This crisis of autonomy and doubt and shame is largely affected by how his family responds to his assertive behavior. If a toddler feels secure in his family, he is likely to venture farther in his exploration and take on unfamiliar tasks and territory. If a family encourages and rewards these expressions of expanding cognitive and motor development, he gains a sense of mastery and positive self-esteem. If a toddler's explorative behaviors are discouraged and repeatedly punished, the strivings for autonomy are thwarted. However, in the life of every toddler some punishment and interruption of intent must take place to ensure his physical safety, to maintain the integrity of personal belongings and to set limits that help him gain self-control and feel secure.

Independence, Negativism and Dawdling A toddler has attained numerous abilities that foster independence. His motor, language and cognitive skills combined with his developing sense of self have an additive effect toward independent behavior. Independence, however, does not exclude a toddler's need to be dependent. Much of a toddler's behavior is characterized by ambivalence. Although he is in constant battle to strive for his independence, he continues to seek attention, approval and physical closeness from his caretakers. When these goals are in conflict, a toddler needs the understanding of parents who are able to promote his independence and to respond flexibly to his periodic plea to be dependent.

Negativism and dawdling are manifestations of the noncompliant spirit that pervades the personality of a toddler. *Negativism* is the resistance a toddler displays around 18 months that lasts to about 3 years of age. This stage is characterized by a seeming delight in doing the opposite of what he is asked to do.[16] *Dawdling* is a form of controlling others by responding to demands in a self-determined way. If a child senses he is being hurried to perform or is asked to do something specifically, he may do it but prolong the activity unmercifully. Dawdling then controls to what degree he can be manipulated by others, whereas negativism is a decided resistance to being controlled by others.

The "no, no" of a toddler tells more about his ego development than it does about his desired course of action. Most of the time the firm assertion "no!" is little more than an affirmation of his power to decide his own course. The telltale feature of a toddler's "no" that means "yes" is that while repeating "no, no, no," he simultaneously carries out the very thing he is resisting as if his words have no relationship to his actions.

Dawdling is an expression of feelings similar to those reflected in the use of "no, no"; that is, he has the need to assert his power to control. There is no better way for a toddler to be in control than by showing others that he decides when and at what speed he will cooperate.

When one considers the unfolding toddler's sense of self and emanating drive to exercise his will, negativism and dawdling can be understood as constructive behaviors toward his developing autonomy and self-esteem. The nurse who works with a family of a toddler will probably, however, find that it is not so impressed with the constructive nature of these behaviors but rather finds the situation exasperating and frustrating. The assertion of the child's will to master self-control is difficult for the family to absorb.

Anticipatory Guidance: The Developing Person In an environment that fosters the attainment of a sense of autonomy and positive self-esteem, the family provides a graded independence with consistent application of limits. The nurse can help a family accomplish this goal by encouraging them to air their frustrations and describe those situations that cause difficulty. The nurse must understand that it is sometimes difficult for a family to adjust to their toddler who wants to do everything for himself and be held and cuddled at his convenience. Parents need to be assured that the strivings for independence are not a rejection of their love but are actually an index of the quality of their ongoing love and affection.

Family members can learn to cope with negativism and dawdling if the nurse informs them about the developmental significance of these behaviors, gives them an opportunity to express their own frustrations and gives suggestions to manage the behaviors. There are a number of consolations for parents with toddlers: these behaviors are normal, it is a stage that will eventually resolve, and other parents feel similar frustrations.

The following suggestions may be helpful if parents find their toddler's negativism and dawdling particularly stressful: (1) avoid questions that can be answered by no, (2) avoid requesting completion of tasks when he is tired or hungry, (3) help him finish when he dawdles (at his own pace), (4) pay special attention to him when there is excessive stimulation caused by the presence of many people and (5) avoid drawing attention to his negativistic and dawdling behaviors.

Forewarning a family of the activities that are potential battlegrounds is a preventive nursing function. Typical situations when a toddler is likely to exert his own will relate to eating, sleeping, elimination and dressing.

Becoming Social

The family is in a key position to influence the socialization of their toddler. The drive for autonomy needs to be molded for positive social development. A toddler who insists on his own way without modifying his behavior for the benefit of others clearly is not moving toward a socialized level of development. Social experiences can be described as those "designed to shape behavior in accordance with goals held by his family and society."[28]

During the toddler years many newly acquired skills affect the process of socialization. Increased perception, mobility, manual dexterity, language acquisition and mastery in self-care increase his self-esteem. With experience a toddler begins to realize that to feel accepted he must sometimes defer to the wishes of others rather than always have his own way. This conflict between the need for acceptance and the will to do as he pleases has been described as *growth ambivalence*.[7] Manifestations of growth ambivalence are prevalent; eating, sleeping, toilet training, playing, and self-care activities are all affected by a need to be dependent yet independent.

Becoming Social in Eating Behavior A toddler must move from a stage of relative dependence to one of almost complete independence in eating behavior. With practice he learns to manipulate eating utensils and show a beginning respect for the table manners adopted by his family. Socialized eating behavior is thus a standard determined within cultures and more specifically within families. A toddler within a traditional Chinese family may be fed longer than a child in Western culture because chopsticks are difficult to manipulate. Within some cultures utensils are not used and eating with hands is the social norm for adults. However, in western culture a toddler is taught to use fingers primarily for those foods prepared to be picked up.

Becoming social in eating behavior implies more than getting food into one's mouth. A toddler also must learn to control his behavior in the way he makes his likes and dislikes known. Impulsive throwing of food, demanding by screaming or pounding, or refusing to sit down to eat or to eat at all are typical toddler behaviors that must eventually be altered to a more acceptable level of behavior. A toddler's perpetual motion, his fascination with the varied textures of food and his clever experimentation of dumping, mixing and stacking are typical mealtime behaviors that eventually are given up for more acceptable table manners.

A toddler's developmental characteristics affect the gradual attainment of socialized eating behavior. At 15 months he may insist on trying to feed himself even though he lacks the physical skills to do so. From 18 to 24 months a toddler's physical skills have improved but now he becomes engrossed in playing with his food. He resists any interruption of his "game" and protests any infringement of his territory. By the age of 3 a toddler feeds himself with only occasional spills and less fascination with food manipulation. His imitative behaviors, increased motor skills and wish to be independent, coupled with his need for parental approval, brings about rapid social development in eating behavior during the toddler years. Reaching this level of independence gives him a sense of mastery and fosters his self-esteem. See Health Maintenance section for anticipatory guidance.

Developing Sleep Regularity and Routines A toddler requires approximately 10 to 14 hours of sleep. Most toddlers take an afternoon nap, and before 2 years of age some may need a morning and an afternoon nap. Keeping a toddler on a relatively consistent sleeping schedule reduces the frequency of irritable and cranky periods. He cannot tolerate losing sleep without showing changes in his behavior.

Developmental characteristics that are displayed in sleep behaviors of toddlers are ritualism, separation anxiety, and autonomy (they resist sleep). Beginning at 18 to 21 months and continuing until 3 years, he prepares for bed by performing several activities in a precise order (washing, brushing teeth, turning a light switch, putting shoes into a certain place and a variety of other time-consuming tasks). These rituals give the toddler a sense of security that he needs when he is learning to separate himself from his attachment figures. His autonomous nature is expressed in these rituals in that they give him a sense of control. Rituals can be viewed as a form of dawdling in which he goes to bed after he has done what he wants to and when he is ready to do so. At this stage it is also common to have a favorite toy or blanket (transitional object), which is taken to bed for security.

Sleep is also resisted by more obvious behaviors, especially as a toddler approaches his second birthday. A toddler may resist so violently that he has a temper tantrum or he may stand in his crib and cry for his parent. Such behaviors are eventually given up as he overcomes separation anxiety and as his intense need to control lessens.

Anticipatory Guidance: Sleep Behaviors Parents may need the assistance of a nurse as they try alternate methods of coping with normal bedtime behaviors of their toddler. Many bedtime crises can be avoided by planning approaches that take into consideration the developmental characteristics of a toddler. The incessant activity and curiosity so typical of this age leave a toddler irritable, overtired and highly stimulated if some effort is not made to provide a quiet period before bedtime. A toddler's engrossment in play and his need to have some control over his actions make it necessary to give him some warning before it is time for bed. To abruptly inform him that it is time for bed and he must put his toys away is certain to bring resistance and perhaps a tantrum, especially if he is tired. Forewarning and then helping him to put his toys away followed by reading a favorite book will more likely bring the desired result.

Helping parents cope with the bedtime rituals is another area for the nurse to consider. Parents should be advised to keep bedtime activities as simple as possible. Once a routine has been established a toddler will insist on following it; therefore it is easier to avoid adding additional rituals than it is to omit them after they have been started. It does not work to tell a toddler "just tonight you may turn the light switch off and on."

Bedtime can be a pleasant time if parents

A quiet activity such as reading a favorite book helps prepare the child for bedtime.

allow extra time for the rituals rather than altering them against the toddler's wishes. Once the usual rituals have been carried out, it is most effective if the parent says "good night" and does not return to the room. If a toddler can manipulate a parent to repeatedly return for minor requests, the behavior is likely to be repeated. If the child has a legitimate request it is only reasonable to grant it, but repeated requests are the toddler's way of postponing separation and is a form of sleep resistance. If a child stands in his crib and cries after the usual routines have been completed it is better to leave and usually the child goes to sleep. He may cry himself to sleep, but eventually he learns that his parents are in control of the sleep routine. It is not uncommon for a toddler to have particular difficulty separating from his mother at bedtime, in which case the father may have more success in getting him to bed.

A toddler's resistance to sleep can be exasperating to parents. It is helpful to point out that many of a toddler's fears are encountered when he goes to bed. His fear of separation, the dark and noises such as flushing the toilet and water rushing out of the tub all happen in relation to going to bed. Although fear of the dark is more common after 3 years of age, some toddlers show signs of such fear earlier. It is important for the nurse to help parents recognize that the child's fear is real and should not be ridiculed and that most bedtime fears can be dispelled with help and patience from parents. Although sleeping practices vary in cultures, it is generally recommended that a child not sleep in his parents' bed.

Toilet Training All areas of development are involved in the successful attainment of bowel and bladder control. Physical, intellectual and emotional-social aspects of development occur simultaneously and are interdependent with the completion of this task. Neuromuscular maturation, awareness of imminent elimination and the desire to please parents by staying clean and dry are necessary before toilet training can be achieved. Chapter 29 discusses the stress that can occur in families when parents do not understand the development necessary before a child can achieve elimination control.

Physical maturation of the sphincter muscles and myelination of the spinal cord are biological requirements for the control of elimination. By the time a toddler sits and walks well (12 to 18 months), the necessary physiological maturation has usually taken place to permit bowel and bladder control. The regularity of bowel movements is usually better established by 18 months than it was in infancy. Bowel movements are often associated with meals, with one after breakfast or one after supper or both times. However, there is a wide variation in when a toddler develops regularity and the pattern of regularity.

The awareness level that must accompany neuromuscular development comes later. The stages of awareness that most children go through are (1) an awareness that elimination has just occurred; (2) an awareness of the process of eliminating while doing it; and (3) an awareness that elimination is imminent.[7]

It is generally agreed that by 18 months of age a toddler has some awareness that a bowel movement is occurring and that some children even indicate by gestures that they know it is coming; however, it is usually not until closer to 2 years of age that he can give enough advance warning to be helped to the toilet. Waiting until closer to 2 years or 30 months of age to begin toilet training increases the success rate considerably.

Bowel control is usually attained before bladder control, and daytime dryness before nighttime dryness. By 2½ years there are few bowel accidents and by 3 few bladder daytime accidents. Sometime between 3½ and 4½ years of age nighttime control is possible. If training is not achieved by 5 or even later, it usually is not indicative of any pathology but rather of the individual variation that exists.

Anticipatory Guidance: Toilet Training By introducing the subject of toilet training early a nurse can prevent the conflict of too-early training. Soon after their baby is 1 year of age parents may be receiving toilet training advice from friends and relatives. The nurse should therefore discuss toilet training by the time the child is 12 to 15 months old so that parents have an understanding of the developmental factors affecting successful toilet training. If they have accurate information, they will feel less compelled to begin toilet training too early.

The readiness of the child and family are equally important when determining the best time to begin toilet training. The nurse should alert the family to the importance of a stable, nonstressed environment for successful toilet training. If certain stressful events can be predicted, it is better to wait until after the event has occurred and an equilibrium has been re-established. Events that cause a change in routine or environment interfere with the toddler's progress in accomplishing a new task. For example, birth of a sibling, parental change of jobs, an older sibling leaving for college, a family vacation, or geographical relocation would be felt as stresses by the toddler and the stress of toilet training should not be superimposed. If such events cannot be avoided during toilet training, the nurse has a responsibility to help the family understand and cope with the regression that such stresses cause.

The nurse should explain that there are no precise rules or schedules that can be applied to guarantee successful toilet training. From the beginning parents need to feel relaxed and confident that their toddler will achieve the task of toilet training without undue pressure and control from them. Some useful suggestions that the nurse can offer are: (1) avoid punishment for noncompliance, (2) do not force a toddler to sit on the toilet, (3) use praise as a reinforcer for positive results, (4) capitalize on a toddler's imitative behavior by allowing observance of adult elimination, (5) avoid creating a tense environment, (6) wait for readiness of the child and (7) do not begin when the family is experiencing undue stress.

Parents must be willing to wait for their child's readiness for toilet training and then accept his successes and relapses as he learns. In a positive, reinforcing environment a toddler actually "trains" himself.

Becoming Social by Participating in Self-Care
The increasing development of motor skills enables a toddler to participate in his own care. He participates in such activities in the spirit of play, but this is how he develops the necessary skills for independence. Toddlers are generally intent on doing things for themselves before they have the necessary gross and fine motor skills to complete tasks efficiently. They gradually become adept at self-care and from 1 to 3 years of age progress from almost total dependence to a remarkably high level of independence. Participation in self-care activities helps the toddler to feel positive about his own abilities, and the praise of his parents makes him feel loved and accepted, all of which contribute to his developing self-esteem.

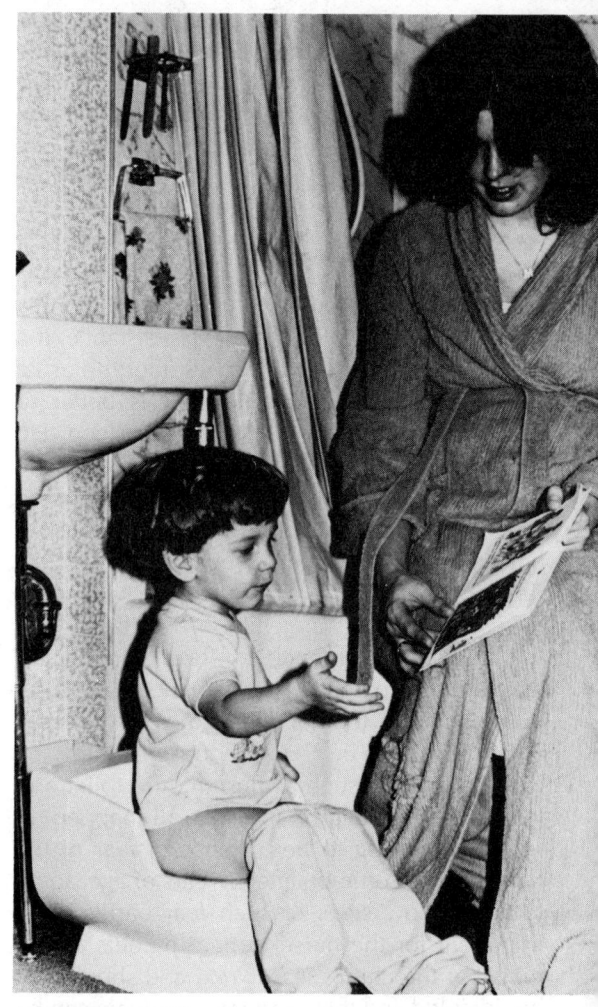

In a positive, reinforcing environment the toddler actually trains himself.

Becoming Social Through Play A toddler's play is affected by all aspects of development, and play influences his physical, intellectual and emotional-social development. A toddler has specific needs that can be met through play. He needs to be physically active and to explore and learn about objects, people, and unfamiliar territory, to experience a variety of sensations (movement, tactile), to practice small muscle skills, to identify with significant others by imitation, to develop language skills and to begin to relate to others through play. To facilitate a toddler's development it is important to provide a variety of play opportunities.

The characteristics of a toddler's play are determined by his developmental level. He remains primarily egocentric in play activities, showing little regard for the feelings of others. Egocentrism in play is characterized by a predominance of behaviors that prove his own power and central position. This is how he builds his self-image, which contributes to his rapidly developing awareness of himself as a person. The type of play coming out of these needs is *parallel play,* in which children engage in similar activities while playing beside each other but not together.

During this period a child learns a great deal by imitating his caretakers. He particuraly enjoys helping with household tasks. He will happily squeeze water out of a sponge, carry silverware to the table and fold clothes after a fashion. He also enjoys playing with real items that he sees his parent use. The classic example is the toddler's fascination with emptying a cupboard of pots and pans. To a toddler, manipulation of pots and pans is a form of helping by imitation. Although the help a toddler gives usually creates work for his parents, these imitative behaviors are an important step in development.

Another characteristic of a toddler's play is the love of active play and manipulation of objects. Exercise of both large and small muscles is necessary for a toddler to develop a sense of control over his body and his environment. A toddler's need to explore is facilitated by his gross and fine motor abilities that give him access to almost anything that intrigues him.

The toddler also learns about his environment through his sensory experiences. Anyone who observes a toddler at play will note that much of what he does provides sensory benefits. A toddler touches objects to see how they feel, runs his fingers over them, and still explores with his lips and tongue, although mouthing objects is now less frequent than during infancy. He is also fascinated by the various sounds he can make and experiments using his voice, tongue and lips to create new sounds or to imitate the sounds he hears.

Many toddlers enjoy activities of motion such as a ride on a bicycle, stroller, wagon or swing. A toddler is also fond of the game of roughhousing in which he is thrown or swung through the air, bounced on someone's back or rolled on the floor.

Some quiet, sedentary activities are also appropriate for the toddler and are especially useful before bedtime. Much of a toddler's encounter with books during the period from 12 to 24 months involves identification of objects, turning pages and imitating familiar sounds of animals and objects such as trains, cars and trucks. He also enjoys when parents read to him and repeat nursery rhymes. From 2 to 3 years of age, as his attention span increases, he becomes increasingly interested in listening to and imitating nursery rhymes and hearing short stories illustrated by pictures.

A child develops language through his play. His play experiences increase his encounters with the world, requiring him to attach labels to what he does and senses. For example, the toddler who wants the straddle toy that another child is using will pull on it and say "ride." He will likewise learn to say "bike-ride" if he wants his parents to take him for a ride. The raw material for thinking, imagination and language is experienced through the senses, and the more he can experience the more he has to express.[28]

The frustrations that a toddler experiences because of his struggle with developing autonomy can be directed into suitable play activities. Simple activities of running, throwing a ball and hammering on a peg board are ways to dissipate excess energy safely. Many sensory experiences have the added benefit of providing a means for expression of aggressive behavior. Pounding, splashing and hitting are harmless when directed at sand, water or soap bubbles. These energy-dissipating activities allow a toddler to express how he feels within the confines of social acceptance while gaining approval and increasing self-esteem and self-control. See Health Maintenance section for anticipatory guidance.

Gender Identity, Sex-Role Identification and Sexuality

Gender identity is one's subjectively felt sense at being male or female. *Sex role* (or gender role) refers to the behaviors that show appropriate male or female orientation. Awareness of gender identify begins around 18 months and is fully established by 5 years of age.[2] Although a 2-year-old is not aware of anatomical differences, he can distinguish between males and females by general appearance. Most toddlers know whether they are boys or girls by 3 years of age and have some notion of sex-appropriate behaviors.

During the toddler years gender identity and sex-role identification are primarily influenced by experiences within the family. When a toddler is consistently treated as being of a particular sex, the child internalizes that gender identity. For example, repeated expressions to him as a "big boy" or her as a "sweet girl" help a child learn this identity. Rewards for proper self-identification as male or female also help the child develop normal gender identity.

Sex-role identification during the toddler years is learned through imitation and involves differences in the way parents interact with boys and girls. A toddler imitates both parents but particularly the same-sex parent, adopting appropriate roles, attitudes, and values. From the child's birth, parents generally behave differently toward boys and girls, resulting in early socialization into male and female roles. Some of the differences are that mothers talk and respond more to infant girls than to boys, boys may be handled more roughly in play and more aggressive behavior is tolerated in boys than in girls.

A toddler learns which behaviors are appropriate for his or her sex by the responses received from parents. Such behaviors are referred to as *sex-typed behaviors*. Parents give different rewards for a certain behavior depending on whether the behavior is displayed by a boy or girl. Parents make such responses out of their own ideas of sex-appropriate behavior, resulting in a wide variety of responses from one parent to another and particularly from one culture to another. However, within most families and most cultures boys and girls behave differently.

Sexual behavior begins in infancy by random exploration of the genitals. Such contact with the genitals is not necessarily deliberate. During toddlerhood sexual activity of boys and girls takes the form of play. A toddler at 2 explores genitals more thoroughly than in infancy but, unless strictly inhibited or intentionally stimulated, a toddler does not become preoccupied with this activity. By 2 toddlers are likely to investigate playmates' genitals as well as display their own.[17] Masturbation and exploration of genitals among children becomes more predominant during the preschool years.

Anticipatory Guidance: Gender Identity, Sex-Role Identification and Sexuality A family may feel confused about what kind of behaviors to encourage regarding sex-role identification. The question of choice of toys may be brought to the nurse because parents disagree or because parents have read about the advantages of teaching all children the sex-role behaviors of both sexes. The nurse can be most helpful by encouraging parents to make traditionally sex-typed toys equally available to male and female children if this approach is consistent with their own philosophy. The nurse's own bias will certainly influence her stance, but it is essential that her counsel not pressure parents into feeling that they must strive either to enforce or discourage sex-typed behaviors. The nurse's role is to provide information so parents can make their own decisions according to their personal and cultural orientation.

The nurse can facilitate normal development of gender identity by encouraging parents to develop a close relationship with their toddler. Parents should be assisted to plan their responsibilities so that both can spend time with the child. If only one parent is present, the nurse should explore with the parent ways in which a substitute mother or father figure can be established. Often a relationship with a relative, friend or neighbor can play a significant role in a toddler's life and warrants the extra time and effort that a parent puts into providing such an opportunity.

It is during the toddler years that parents become aware of more deliberate genital self-exploration in their child. Also, parents begin to have concerns about their own nudity in the presence of a toddler of the opposite sex. The nurse should encourage parents to deal with these issues in a way that is comfortable for them, but they should not shame or punish a toddler for exploring his or her genitals. The way parents respond to these early sexual behaviors and interests forms the beginnings of the child's own sexuality.

HEALTH MAINTENANCE

Throughout this chapter counselling and guidance of parents has been emphasized as an important role of the nurse. Understanding and being prepared for developmental changes before they occur gives parents a feeling of security and eases the stress that the toddler years can bring. Counselling needs vary from one family to another. Concerns that a family might bring to a nurse are discussed throughout this chapter. However, during the toddler years there are four

TABLE 30-1 GUIDELINES TO PROMOTE SOCIALIZED EATING BEHAVIOR

Principles	Suggestions
To develop skill in manipulating utensils, a toddler needs the opportunity to practice but may need some assistance. He will often refuse assistance even though he needs it.	At 15 months: help by feeding with a second spoon, provide finger foods. At 18–24 months: be supportive by helping him get food onto spoon to mouth. Continue finger foods.
At mealtime a toddler should learn to associate mastery, pleasure, and acceptance with the experience of eating.	Avoid forcing of food. Allow self-feeding but assist on toddler's terms; avoid punishment for spills and messiness. Praise attempts at self-feeding even though many spills occur.
A toddler needs total concentration to accomplish the skills of self-feeding.	Provide a quiet place with minimal distraction; no loud music or television. Once the meal has begun, getting up from the table and returning by parents and siblings distracts a toddler.
Food intake is likely to decrease if a toddler has been involved in vigorous physical activity immediately prior to a meal, or if he has had to wait several hours past his regular mealtime. He also takes less interest in food if he is overtired (lacking sleep) or overfatigued (too much physical activity.)	A time of quiet before meals and regularity in mealtimes is conducive to a toddler's appetite. Keeping him on a balanced schedule of rest and activity improves his disposition and general eating behavior.
A toddler imitates eating behaviors of his family.	Parents need to provide appropriate role modeling and to discipline siblings in table manners.
A toddler finds security in following certain routines and rituals.	Use the same plate, cup and utensils, and consistency in the order of preparing him for eating (washing hands, sitting in chair, serving food).
A toddler's appetitie fluctuates, as do his moods. Variation from dependence to independence is prevalent in a toddler's eating behavior, as is a strong need to have his own way. A toddler cannot be forced to eat.	Do not try to force a child to eat. When a toddler refuses to eat and insists he wants to get out of the high chair or down from the table, let him miss a meal. Avoid snacks and he will probably eat the next scheduled meal. Over a period of a week intake is usually adequate.

areas of health maintenance that a nurse should discuss with each family: nutrition, play, safety and immunizations.

Nutrition and Development

Changes in each aspect of development affect nutritional intake during the toddler years. The nurse's counselling is based on a thorough assessment of (1) usual intake within a 24-hour period, (2) level of motor ability achieved in self-feeding skills, (3) effect of normal toddler development on eating behavior and (4) concerns that parents have about their toddler's food and nutrient intake.

The nurse's role is to prepare parents by reviewing developmental changes that influence the way their toddler eats. By 1 year of age many children have been weaned from the bottle, with the exception of a nighttime bottle. The eruption of additional teeth during the second year makes it possible for a toddler to eat most adult foods. His slowed growth decreases his requirement for food and is reflected in a decreased appetite. His increased motor ability enhances his eating skills and his

TABLE 30-2 BASIC FOOD GROUPS: PORTIONS AND NUMBER OF SERVINGS PER DAY FOR TODDLERS*

Food Group and Portion Size†		Number of Portions
Milk and Milk Equivalents		4
Milk	1/2–3/4 cup	
Cheese	1/2–3/4 oz	
Yogurt	1/4–1/2 cup	
Powdered skim milk	2 tbsp	
Meat and Meat Equivalents		2 or more
Meat	1 oz (2 tbsp) (liver once a week)	
Egg	1	
Frankfurter	1	
Peanut butter	1 tbsp	
Dried peas or beans	1/4–1/3 cup (cooked)	
Vegetables and Fruits		4–5 (to include 1 green leafy or yellow vegetable and 1 citrus fruit)
Vegetables	(1 green leafy or yellow)	
Cooked	2–4 tbsp	
Raw	2–4 pieces	
Fruit	(1 citrus fruit)	
Canned	4–8 tbsp	
Raw	1/2–1 small piece of fruit	
	3/4 cup strawberries	
Fruit Juice	3–4 oz	
Bread and Cereal		3–4
Whole grain or enriched white bread	1/2–1 slice	
Cooked cereal	1/4–1/2 cup	
Dry cereal	1/2–1 cup	
Spaghetti, macaroni, rice	1/4–1/2 cup	
Crackers	2–3	
Fat		3
Bacon	1 slice (not to replace a meat serving)	
Butter or vitamin A-fortified margarine	1 tsp	
Sugars	1/2–1 tsp	2

*Adapted from Pipes, P. L. Nutrition in infancy and childhood. C. V. Mosby Co., 1977.
†These portions represent the average amount of food a toddler eats and should not be used as rigid criteria that will cause parents to force a child to eat. Another general rule for determining appropriate serving size is one tablespoon per year of age.

emotional-social development markedly influences the eating behavior. Parents who know of and are prepared for these changes can more effectively prevent or cope with the stress involving eating during these years.

Parents should be told that a decrease in appetite is common, and that they can expect a pattern of fluctuation in the amount and type of food their toddler eats. It is difficult for parents to cope with a toddler who one day eats his meals eagerly and the next refuses to eat anything. A toddler's insistence on certain foods (food jags) can make it difficult for parents to ensure that he has a balanced diet. These food jags cannot be easily altered but often last for only a few days. During such time a toddler may refuse to eat anything if he is not given at least a small portion of the preferred food. Other foods can be offered in small portions and within a few days he will likely request a different food as his favorite. If the nurse can adequately inform a family and offer suggestions to handle normal developmental behaviors, mealtime and eating can be associated with pleasure and satisfaction in these early impressionable years (Table 30–1).

The nurse should also discuss nutritional concerns involving dentition, iron deficiency anemia and obesity. The major points to discuss with parents regarding nutrition and dentition are that sweets be avoided as between-meal snacks, that 16 to 24 ounces of milk be consumed daily, and that a bedtime bottle, if offered, does not contain juice or milk. Iron deficiency anemia is prevented if adequate iron-rich foods are consumed and milk is restricted to 24 ounces daily. This is recommended because toddlers may drink too much milk. This causes satiation that, in turn, decreases intake of solid foods rich in iron (liver, dark green vegetables, iron-enriched cereals, egg yolk). Obesity can be prevented by using skim or low-fat milk and by offering limited sweets (especially candy and sodas). Snacks should consist of small amounts of nutritious foods. Obesity in toddlerhood is also prevented by providing opportunities for physical exercise. The nurse should pay particular attention to how food is used by the parents. The practice of using food as a reward or to pacify may establish patterns that lead to obesity later.

A quantitative 24-hour dietary recall gives the nurse information to help her assess the need for additional nutritional counselling or referral for further evaluation and treatment. A toddler eats approximately half as much food as an adult and should be served foods from the basic four food groups. (Table 30-2 lists approximate portions and number of servings a toddler is likely to consume per day.) Vitamin and iron supplementation is unnecessary unless a well-balanced diet is not consumed. Parents should be encouraged to make a serious effort to provide a balanced diet to establish healthful practices of eating rather than relying on vitamins and iron preparations.

Play and Development

The nurse can increase a family's awareness and understanding of how play enhances the toddler's development. The motor skills that affect play (see chapter discussion on skills affecting play) can be discussed with parents, as well as the characteristics of a toddler's play, his developmental needs for play, and appropriate activities to meet these needs. Sharing this information helps parents to have realistic expectations regarding a toddler's interactions during play and prepares them to knowledgeably guide his development through play.

The nurse should encourage parents to play with their toddler. A toddler will play alone or beside another toddler for short periods, but he also enjoys the attention and interaction that play with adults affords. Special times set aside for play with a toddler are rewarding to both the child and adult. When siblings are present parents especially need to provide time for play for each child separately. Household tasks and work responsibilities can be arranged in such a way that each parent is free for at least a short time each day to provide opportunities for play.

There are certain circumstances that require special effort on the part of parents to provide adequate play opportunities. When a toddler is an only child some provision should be made for play with another child or children about the same age. When there are siblings close in age parents also have problems, such as arguments and fighting during play. Each family develops its own pattern of handling conflicts between children, but a basic rule is to let children solve their own problems as much as possible. When a babysitter cares for their toddler it is advisable that parents plan special activities such as drawing, water play or outdoor activities to guard against excessive use of television. Instructions can be given to the babysitter regarding play as one would for meal preparation.

A toddler is especially prone to injury because the excitement of play engrosses his entire being. He does not anticipate danger and is particularly vulnerable because of his insatiable curiosity and limited precision in gross and fine motor skills. The nurse should encourage parents to remove dangerous household objects and carefully evaluate the safety of toys before purchase.

The nurse should stress that a toddler needs a variety of play opportunities; however, it is unnecessary to buy expensive toys. Play with various-sized cardboard boxes, plastic containers and jar lids, access to pots and pans, permission to enjoy the sensations that nature offers, and encouragement to be his parents' helper give a toddler many of the experiences that foster development.

Suggestions for appropriate toys and play activities should be offered by the nurse for the age of the toddler. Children may play with the same toy throughout the toddler years, playing with it differently as they grow older. Therefore many of the same toys are appropriate throughout toddlerhood. There are certain toys and activities, however, that toddlers find particularly enjoyable at specific ages (Table 30-3).

TABLE 30-3 SUMMARY OF TODDLER GROWTH AND DEVELOPMENT AND HEALTH MAINTENANCE

Age	Physical Competency	Intellectual Competency	Emotional-Social Competency
General: From 1–3 yr	Gains 5 kg (11 lb) Grows 20.3 cm (8 in) 12 teeth erupt. Nutritional requirements: Energy 100 Kcal/kg/day Fluid 115–125 ml/kg/day Protein 1.8 gm/kg/day See Appendix for vitamins and minerals.	Learns by exploring and experimenting. Learns by imitating. Progresses from a vocabulary of 3 words at 12 months to about 900 words at 36 months.	Central crisis: to gain a sense of autonomy vs doubt and shame. Demonstrates independent behaviors. Exhibits attachment behavior strongly and regularly until third birthday. Fears persist of strange people, objects, and places and of aloneness and being abandoned. Egocentric in play (paralleled play). Imitation of parents in household talks and activities of daily living.
15 mo	Legs appear bowed. Walks alone, climbs, slides down stairs backwards. Stacks two blocks. Scribbles spontaneously. Grasps spoon but rotates it, holds cup with both hands. Takes off socks and shoes.	Trial and error method of learning. Experiments to see what will happen. Says at least 3 words. Uses expressive jargon.	Shows independence by trying to feed self and help in undressing.
18 mo	Runs but still falls. Walks upstairs with help. Slides down stairs backwards. Stacks 3–4 blocks. Clumsily throws a ball. Unzips a large zipper. Takes off simple garments.	Begins to be able to think. Begins to retain a mental image of an absent object. Concept of object permanence fully develops. Has vocabulary of 10 or more words. Holophrasic speech (one word used to communicate whole ideas)	Fears the water. Temper tantrums may begin. Negativism and dawdling predominate. Bedtime rituals begin. Awareness of gender identity begins. Helps with undressing.
24 mo	Runs quickly and with fewer falls. Pulls toys and walks sideways. Walks downstairs hanging on a rail (does not alternate feet). Stacks six blocks. Turns pages of a book. Imitates vertical and circular strokes. Uses spoon with little spilling. Can feed himself. Puts on simple garments. Can turn door knobs.	Enters into preconceptual phase of preoperational period: Symbolic thinking and symbolic play. Egocentric thinking, imagination and pretending are common. Has vocabulary of about 300 words. Uses two-word sentences (telegraphic speech). Engages in monologue.	Fears the dark and animals. Temper tantrums may continue. Negativism and dawdling continue. Bedtime rituals continue. Sleep resisted overtly. Usually shows readiness to begin bowel and bladder control. Explores genitalia. Brushes teeth with help. Helps with dressing and undressing.
36 mo	Has set of deciduous teeth at about 30 months. Walks downstairs alternating feet. Rides tricycle. Walks with balance and runs well. Stacks 8–10 blocks. Can pour from a pitcher. Feeds self completely. Dresses self almost completely (does not know front from back). Cannot tie shoes.	Preconceptual phase of preoperational period as for 24 months. Uses around 900 words. Constructs complete sentences and uses all parts of speech.	Temper tantrums subside. Negativism and dawdling subside. Bedtime rituals subside. Self-care in feeding, elimination and dressing enhances self-esteem.

Safety and Development

Accident prevention is one of the greatest challenges that faces health professionals who care for children. The stages of childhood development can be used to predict the type of accidents most likely to occur. By 1 year of age a toddler is very mobile, and as he pulls himself to standing position he pulls at whatever is within reach. Hanging table cloths, dangling cords and unstable furniture are hazards. From 1 to 2 years it is the child's curiosity without a sense of danger that makes him vulnerable to accidents. By the time a child is 2 his speed of mobility adds still another danger to which parents must be alerted. Types of accidents that parents should be alerted to as common hazards to toddlers are: (1) accidents while riding in a car; (2) being hit by a moving vehicle, (3) drowning; (4) ingesting harmful substances, (5) burns, (6) aspiration of a foreign body, (7) suffocation, (8) falls and (9) toy accidents.

Automotive Accidents Motor vehicle accidents are the leading cause of death in children

TABLE 30-3 SUMMARY OF TODDLER GROWTH AND DEVELOPMENT AND HEALTH MAINTENANCE *(Continued)*

Nutrition	Play	Safety	Immunizations
Milk 16–24 oz. Appetite decreases. Wants to feed self. Has food jags. Never force food; give nutritious snacks. Give iron and vitamin supplementation only if poor intake.	Books at all ages. Needs physical and quiet activities, does not need expensive toys.	Never leave alone in tub. Keep poisons locked. Use car seat. Have ipecac in house.	
Vulnerable to iron deficiency anemia. Give table foods except for tough meat and hard vegetables. Wants to feed self.	Stuffed animals, dolls, music toys. Peek-a-boo, hide and seek. Water and sand play. Stacking toys. Roll ball on floor. Push toys on floor. Read to toddler.	Keep small items off floor (pins, buttons, clips). Child may choke on hard food. Cords and table cloths are a danger. Keep electrical outlets plugged, and poisons locked away. Risk of kitchen accidents with toddler under foot.	MMR
Negativism may interfere with eating. Encourage self-feeding. Is easily distracted while eating. May play with his food. High activity level interferes with eating.	Rocking horse. Nesting toys. Shape-sorting cube. Pencil or crayon. Pull toys. Four wheeled toy to ride. Throw ball. Run and chasing games. Rough-housing. Puzzles. Blocks. Hammer and peg board.	Falls: from riding toy in bathtub because he runs too fast Climbs up to get dangerous objects. Keep dangerous things out of wastebasket.	DPT booster; oral polio booster
Requests certain foods, therefore snacks should be controlled. Imitates eating habits of others. May still play with food and especially with utensils and dish (pouring, stacking).	Clay and Play-Doh. Finger paint. Brush paint. Record player with record and story book and songs to sing along. Toys to take apart. Toy tea sets. Puppets. Puzzles.	May fall from outdoor large play equipment. Can reach farther than expected (knives, razors, and matches must be kept out of reach).	
Sits in booster seat rather than high chair. Makes known likes and dislikes.	Likes playing with other children, building toys, drawing and painting, doing puzzles. Imitation household objects for doll play. Nurse and doctor kits. Carpenter kits.	Protect from: turning on hot water. falling from tricycle. striking matches.	Tine test

after 1 year of age. Before 3 years most of the fatalities occur while the child is riding in a car; after 3 children are more often hit by a moving vehicle. The single most effective preventive measure to protect toddlers while riding in a car is to restrain them in a properly secured crash-tested car seat at all times.

The reasons for not using a car seat are varied. Cost may be the major reason for not using one. In this event the nurse's role is to provide both literature and counsel regarding its importance. When parents have a car seat and do not use it, the nurse should encourage them to discuss the particular difficulty they are having. Each situation is unique and requires individualized counselling, but some general principles can be shared with parents to encourage them to use a car seat. They are:

1. Toddlers are ritualistic and readily adapt to routine. If a car seat is comfortable and is consistently used, a toddler adapts more readily.
2. Providing toys and books may be sufficient to amuse a toddler for short trips. For longer trips bedtime security objects such as a blanket or

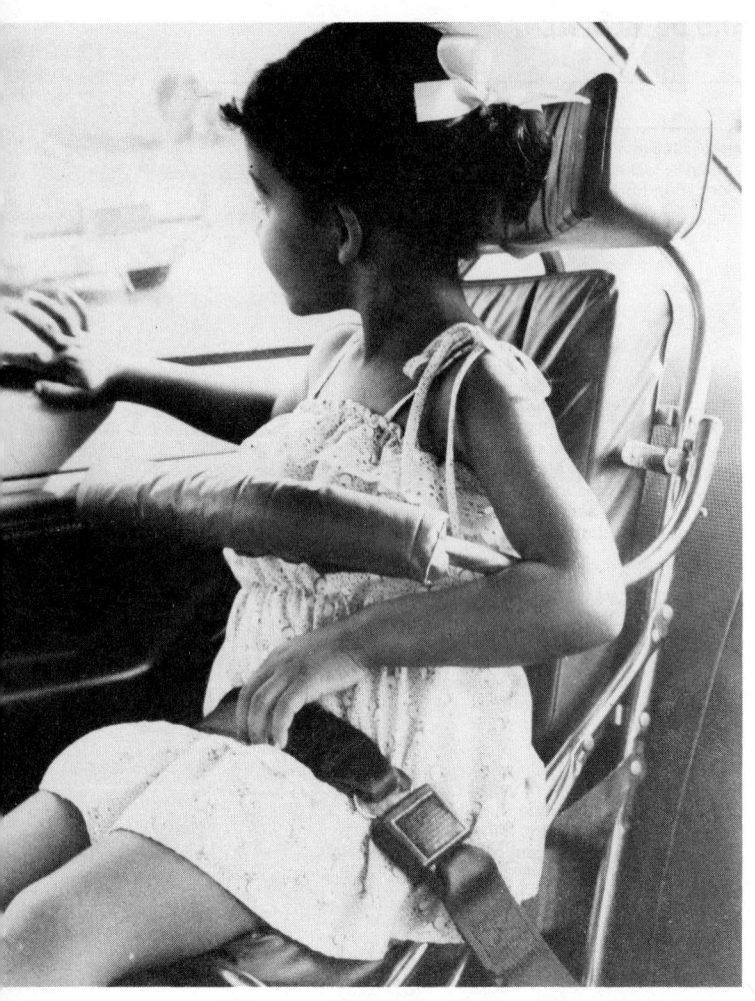

The nurse should encourage parents to restrain their toddler in a car seat at all times.

pacifier can make traveling relatively trouble free.
3. A toddler does not understand circumstantial differences, so he must be secured in a car seat even for very short trips.
4. A toddler's curiosity draws him into one danger after another inside a car. The distraction of a toddler on the move while the parent is driving can itself cause an accident.
5. Many toddlers are extremely eager to go for a ride in the car with a parent. The most effective method to get this child into a car seat is to leave him at home if he is not willing to sit in the seat. Invariably this brings prompt cooperation or willingness to ride in the car seat on the next outing.

In addition to sharing this information, the nurse should provide printed material that can be obtained from various sources.*

Constant surveillance is required to protect a toddler from the tragedy of being hit by a moving vehicle. A toddler is capable of dashing out of sight when this is least expected. Parents should use firm discipline and teach by example in an effort to keep their toddler off the street; however, he cannot be trusted during this active, explorative state. A nonclimbable, fenced-in play area is ideal to safely provide for the physical activity a toddler needs, but when this is not available he should never be left unattended near streets or driveways.

Drowning Drowning takes only seconds. Careful supervision of a toddler wherever water is cannot be overemphasized. Toddlers become excited when playing around water and resist restrictive measures such as holding their hand. They should never be left alone around wading pools or swimming pools nor be left unattended in a bath tub. Even shallow water is dangerous to a toddler. He may stand up, slip and fall face down. A swimming pool must be securely fenced in and the door locked at all times. A toddler should not be left in the care of a school-age sibling near deep water. The nurse is responsible for cautioning parents against having a carefree attitude about safe-guarding their toddler where water is accessible.

Ingestions The nurse can assist a family to provide an environment safe for a toddler. An awareness of the factors and circumstances contributing to accidental poisonings will serve as a guide in planning prevention. The most frequent error that parents make is that they underestimate the capability of their toddler. It is not only the height to which a toddler climbs but the speed with which he can move about that can catch parents off guard. The small-muscle abilities of toddlers can also give them access to containers parents do not anticipate they can open. It is the nurse's responsibility to help parents identify conditions that might contribute to incidents of poisoning. See Chapter 33 for further discussion of accidental ingestion of poisons.

Burns In the 1-to-4 age group burns are the second most common cause of accidental death

---

*Information can be obtained from (1) Physicians for Auto Safety, 50 Union Avenue, Irvington, N.J. 07111 (2) Consumers Union, 256 Washington St., Mt. Vernon, N.Y. 10550.

(motor vehicle accidents rank first).[22] A toddler's inquisitiveness and lack of judgment make him extremely vulnerable to burn accidents. The nurse can give parents practical suggestions to help them take the necessary preventive steps.

A child's thin skin increases his vulnerability to serious burns. A source of heat that would produce only a second degree burn in a middle-aged healthy adult may cause a third degree burn in a toddler.[22] The nurse needs to discuss the common sources of burns with parents. Table 33-2 summarizes the sources of burns that the nurse should include in such preventive teaching.

A child learns the meaning of the word "hot" early in the toddler years. He feels heat radiating from an oven and can feel the steam of boiling water, but he cannot be trusted to remember what "hot" means when his parents set hot coffee within his reach or when they turn their backs on an open oven door. Toddlers are always looking into containers and consequently spill their contents onto themselves. The simple act of drinking a hot beverage in a room where a toddler is on the run can easily end in disaster. A nurse should frequently remind parents of these daily precautions that need to be taken to protect their toddler from burns.

Aspiration of a Foreign Body A toddler can find the smallest object on a thickly carpeted floor. Objects such as nails, pins, paper clips, staples and any number of household items may be swallowed, aspirated or stuffed into a body orifice. Coins are attractive to toddlers but are frequently swallowed or aspirated and should not be treated as toys. Toys need to be inspected for removable parts that could be swallowed or aspirated. Dangerous objects cannot be put into an accessible wastebasket, as a toddler will discover even the most obscure item.

In a young toddler (12 to 18 months) the aspiration of food particles while eating can be prevented by refraining from giving hard foods such as nuts, carrots, corn and tough meats. Even though a 2-year-old has some molars, the ability to thoroughly chew food is not mastered until the preschool years.

Parents should be given some basic guidance to prepare them for an incident of aspiration. The following guidelines should be used when counselling parents:
1. If a child is breathing quietly even though a foreign object has been aspirated, every attempt should be made to rush the child to the nearest facility for treatment without disturbing the foreign body.
2. Do not suspend the child by the feet and pound on the back. This may dislodge a foreign body into the larynx, causing fatal obstruction.
3. Do not attempt to extract a pharyngeal or laryngeal foreign body by reaching into the mouth with one or two fingers. This is dangerous because the foreign body may be forced into the larynx more tightly, causing a partial obstruction to become a complete obstruction.
4. The Heimlich maneuver* has been successful in all ages and should be the first choice of emergency treatment for a life-threatening situation caused by aspiration of a foreign body.[9, 30]

The nurse should include these emergency measures in her counselling of parents with toddlers. Foreign body aspiration can cause panic and incorrect treatment by parents in the home. It is the nurse's responsibility to reduce the number of fatalities and injuries from foreign body aspiration by teaching parents how to prevent its occurrence and how to correctly apply first aid measures.

Suffocation A toddler is less likely to suffocate from plastic than an infant is, but thin plastic covers (used by drycleaners) should not be left where a toddler can reach it. He may crawl inside one or pull it over his head and be unable to free himself from it. Abandoned refrigerators and trunks are attractive hiding places and a toddler is capable of climbing inside and closing the door. Doors must be removed from such abandoned equipment and it should be disposed of as soon as possible.

Falls and Bodily Injury A toddler must be protected from dangerous heights and from areas that contain potentially harmful objects and equipment. Knives, scissors, and pointed objects within reach of a toddler can cause serious injury. A toddler should not be permitted near a power mower in operation, as it often propels missiles such as stones, pieces of metal or broken

---

*By approaching from behind a quick sharp thrust is given into the epigastrium with fist or clasped hand, causing forceful expiration.

> The nurse's role in promoting the development of a toddler lies primarily in her ability to motivate a family to use available resources to their fullest potential for healthful adaptation to the normal stresses of family living. A family that is stable is better prepared to absorb the additional stress a toddler brings to it. Parents need to be able to cope with the activity and exploration that helps a toddler learn but must be able to develop a consistent pattern of setting limits so that he can eventually gain a sense of confidence in his own ability to control himself. The family that has secure relationships among its members is best prepared to help a toddler grow.
>
> The nurse can provide information, counsel and encouragement to support a family in their task of learning what toddlers need and how to meet those needs. With the love and security of a family who provides for his needs, a toddler at 3 will have the characteristics of a preschooler.

glass. Gates leading to stairways and porches are necessary to protect a child from falling down steps that he has not learned to climb. Falling from open windows is a tragic accident in the toddler age that all families should be counselled to prevent. A crib should not be placed in front of an open window where a child can crawl up and push out the screen. It is advisable to open windows from the top when possible.

Toy and Play Equipment Accidents Toys that have removable parts or sharp edges are dangerous to a toddler. A toddler's fine motor skills enable him to pull off buttons, strings and yarn and his curiosity drives him to do it. Sharp or pointed edges are especailly dangerous to a toddler, who runs clumsily and falls frequently. A pencil can be a dreadful weapon if he runs and falls on the sharpened point.

Outdoor play equipment can be dangerous to a toddler if it is too large for him or if it is poorly constructed. Play equipment should be examined for bolts that protrude or S-shaped hooks that could catch tiny fingers. A toddler needs to be closely supervised in a play area where older children are playing to prevent him from being struck by a swing in motion. He also needs to be protected from being injured on large equipment, which he attempts to use by imitating older children.

A familiarity with what toddlers are likely to do is a parent's best defense. Safety should be discussed at each health care visit to keep the parents abreast of the rapid development that takes place during the toddler years. Parents need frequent reminders that toddlers are compelled by a constant drive to see "what would happen if . . ." but do not comprehend the danger involved. It is the preventive measures of their parents that keep toddlers safe, and it is the nurse's responsibility to provide the motivation and guidance required to help parents meet that obligation.

Immunizations

All children should have received immunization against diphtheria, pertussis, tetanus (DPT) and poliomyelitis during the first year of life. The nurse should evaluate the immunization status of a toddler and identify any missed doses. If one of the doses in a series was missed, it is not necessary to start the series over. That all children receive the required immunization is more important than following a rigid schedule, no matter how much time has passed since the previous dose(s).[12]

Immunizations to be received during the toddler years are MMR (measles, mumps, rubella) at 15 months of age given subcutaneously, DPT booster (diphtheria, pertussus, tetanus) at 18 months given intramuscularly and TOPV booster (trivalent oral polio vaccine) at 18 months. A tuberculin skin test is recommended at 12 months and every other year thereafter. In areas of high susceptibility, testing is recommended every year.

Some children who were immunized for measles before 12 months of age have contracted measles in spite of having received the vaccine. It is felt that persistent maternal antibodies can interfere with antibody production and inhibit immunity. For this reason it is now recommended that routine measles immunization be deferred until 15 months of age. In the event of a measles epidemic, measles vaccine should be given to children as young as 6 months of age. In these cases it is recommended that the immunization be repeated after 15 months of age.[23]

A tuberculin test should be done prior to or at the same time that the MMR vaccine is given. Measles vaccine is thought to alter the immune mechanism and may depress tuberculin sensitivity, producing a false-negative tuberculosis test. If a tuberculin skin test is done after measles vaccine has been given, a period of four to six weeks should be allowed from the time the vaccine was administered.[6] Administration of measles vaccine can cause exacerbation of tuberculosis and it is recommended that tuberculin testing be done prior to administration of measles vaccine when tuberculosis is endemic or suspected in an individual.[5]

References

1. American Academy of Pediatrics, Committee on Nutrition. Fluoride supplementation: revised dosage schedule. Pediatrics, January, 1979, p. 150.
2. J. Armstrong. Development of Sexual Identity. In Principles of Pediatrics. R. A. Hoekelman et al., McGraw-Hill Book Co., 1978
3. J. Bowlby. Attachment. Basic Books, 1969.
4. J. Bowlby. Attachment and Loss: Vol. II Separation Anxiety and Anger. Basic Books, 1973.
5. P. A. Brunell. Prevention of Disease: Immunizations. In Principles of Pediatrics, R. A. Hoekelman et al., McGraw-Hill Book Co., 1978
6. M. Chow et al. Handbook of Pediatric Primary Care. John Wiley and Sons, 1979.
7. J. Church. Understanding Your Child From Birth to Three. Pocket Books, 1976
8. D. J. Forrester. Preventive aspects of dental care. In Principles of Pediatrics. R. A. Hoekelman et al., McGraw-Hill Book Co., 1978
9. J. P. Frazer. Diseases of the ear, nose, and throat: Foreign bodies in food passages. In Principles of Pediatrics. R. A. Hoekleman et al., McGraw-Hill Book Co., 1978
10. C. Frazier. Children and poisonous plants. Pediatric Basics. Gerber Products Co., October 15, 1978, p. 10
11. J. H. Gundy. The pediatric physical examination. In Principles of Pediatrics. R. A. Hoekelman et al., McGraw-Hill Book Co., 1978
12. R. J. Haggerty. Preventive pediatrics: Prevention of specific diseases. In Nelson's Textbook of Pediatrics. V. C. Vaughan et al., W. B. Saunders, Co., 1979.
13. R. A. Hoekelman. Developmental variations of the legs and feet. In Principles of Pediatrics. R. A. Hoekelman et al., McGraw-Hill Book Co., 1978
14. E. Hurlock. Child Development. McGraw-Hill Book Co., 1978
15. F. Ilg and L. B. Ames. Child Development from Birth to Ten. Harper and Row, 1955
16. R. S. Illingworth. The Normal Child. Churchill Livingstone, 1975
17. H. A. Katchadourian and D. T. Lunde. Fundamentals of Human Sexuality. Holt, Rinehart & Winston, 1972
18. S. G. Kulig. School readiness: Screening for speech and language disorders. In Principles of Pediatrics. R. A. Hoekleman et al., McGraw-Hill Book Co., 1978
19. R. M. Liebert et al. Developmental Psychology. Prentice-Hall Inc., 1977
20. H. Maier. Three Theories of Child Development. Harper and Row, 1969
21. L. Matas et al. Continuity of adaptation in the second year: the relationship between quality attachment and later competence, Child Development. September 1978, p. 547
22. H. Mofenson and J. Greensher. Childhood Accidents: Burn Accidents. In Principles of Pediatrics. R. A. Hoekelman et al., McGraw-Hill Book Co., 1978
23. C. F. Phillips. Infectious diseases: Measles (rubella). In Nelson's Textbook of Pediatrics. V. C. Vaughn et al., W. B. Saunders Co., 1979
24. J. L. Phillips. Origins of Intellect: Piaget's theory. W. H. Freeman and Co., 1969
25. S. Piomelli. Screening Programs: Screening for Lead Poisoning. In Principles of Pediatrics. R. A. Hoekelman et al., McGraw-Hill Book Co., 1978
26. M. A. Pulaski. Understanding Piaget. Harper & Row Publishers, 1971
27. Ross Laboratories. Children are Different: Developmental Physiology. Ross Laboratories, 1978
28. M. S. Smart and R. C. Smart. Children: Development and Relationships, 3rd. ed. Macmillan Inc., 1977
29. D. W. Smith. Introduction to Clinical Pediatrics. W. B. Saunders Co., 1977
30. R. C. Stern. Diseases of the respiratory system: Foreign bodies in the larynx, trachea, and bronchi. In Nelson's Textbook of Pediatrics. V. C. Vaughan et al. W. B. Saunders, Co., 1979
31. A. Thomas and S. Chess. Temperament and Development. Brunner Mazel Publishers, 1977
32. I. H. Thorp. The toddler: 1 to 3 years: In Comprehensive Pediatric Nursing, 2nd ed. G. Scipien et al. McGraw-Hill Book Co., 1979
33. H. S. Toy. Poisoning: Epidemiology and Prevention. In Principles of Pediatrics. R. A. Hoekelman et al. McGraw-Hill Book Co., 1978

Additional Recommended Reading

T. Berry Brazelton. Toddlers and Parents. Dell Publishing Co., 1976
F. Caplan and T. Caplan. The Second Twelve Months. Grosset and Dunlap, 1977
E. H. Erikson. Childhood and Society. W. W. Norton, 1950
S. Fraiberg. The Magic Years. Scribner, 1959
J. Piaget. The Language and Thought of the Child. Translated by Majorie and Ruth Gabain, Latimer Trend and Co. Ltd., 1959
J. Piaget and B. Inhelder. The Psychology of the Child. Basic Books Inc., 1969
J. Smith. Promoting childhood dental health. Pediatric Nursing May/June 1976, p. 16
B. L. White. The First Three Years of Life. Prenctice-Hall, Inc., 1975

31 POTENTIAL STRESSES DURING TODDLERHOOD: MANAGEMENT OF TODDLER BEHAVIOR

by Jo Joyce Tackett, BSN, MPHN

INTRODUCTION

Temporary emotional dysfunction is commonly manifested in the toddler as a typical response to the emotional crises encountered as he moves through a new stage in his growth and development. If this temporary crisis and dysfunction is successfully handled by the child and his parents, the coping process and problem resolution strengthens the child and the relationship he has with his parents. Improperly resolved, the normal temporary emotional response becomes prolonged, excessive or otherwise abnormal and requires intervention.

EXCESSIVE FEARS IN TODDLERHOOD

No one experiences living without also experiencing at least some degree of fear along the way. Mild fear keeps one cautious in potentially dangerous situations, stimulates a sense of excitement and prompts the mind and body into maximum readiness in case action becomes necessary. However, extreme or excessive fear — terror, if it produces immobilization — serves no useful purpose at any age

An Altered Behavioral State

Fear is an anxiety state arising out of anticipated danger, pain or loss. Excessive fear (also called *irrational fear, phobia,* or *neurosis*) is an extreme and recurrent anxiety reaction out of proportion to the circumstance or object that produces it.[9] Fear is usually accompanied by a sense of helplessness, or loss of confidence that one is in control. The focus of the fear may be specific or generalized and either real or imagined. Examples of *specific fears* are fear of dogs, fear of men with beards and fear of strangers. The peak period for these fears is 2 to 6 years. *Generalized fears* could be of all horned animals because the child saw a bull chasing Grandpa, fear of the dark because of a scary experience that occurred while it was dark, or fear of separation because the child once awoke to find a stranger caring for him instead of his mother. *Real fears* are of actual objects (e.g., dogs) or situations that can actually be experienced. *Imagined fears* are of apparitions (monsters) or situations that cannot actually be observed or experienced.

Girls tend to express more fears than boys and usually display anxiety reactions at an earlier age.[9] Children of higher intelligence often have more fears than their less intelligent peers and are more likely to have generalized, imagined fears.[10] Socioeconomic status seems also to influence the incidence of fears in children. Children of lower socioeconomic classes experience more fears, and their fears are more likely to be associated with violence and a sense of danger.[10] Children who are extroverted and of easy temperament tend to have more fears, but their introverted counterparts of slow-to-warm and difficult temperaments tend to have more intense reactions to their fears and are at greater risk for developing excessive fears.[9,10] Children who have several siblings or who have many social contacts with other children experience more fears than children whose primary exposure is to adults, probably due to the imitative learning of each other's fears.[10] Fears are more easily learned by a child when he is tired or ill, and the anxiety state produced is likely to be more extreme than if the fear were learned under healthier circumstances.[10]

Statistical analyses have shown that children's fears tend to be interrelated and to fall in one of two categories: fears of loss or separation and fears of danger, hurt or pain.[9] A study done by David Bauer at California State University in the early 1970s classified the fears of children by incidence.[13] Twenty per cent of young (under 5) children's fears were of monsters, the supernatural or the occult intending them harm.* The second most frequent fear of children was fear of animals, the variety involved being adequate to fill a zoo. Third came the fears of danger associated with bad people, gestures suggestive of harm, and loud or strange noises. The most psychologically endangering but least common fears are those related to scolding, teasing, failure, losing possessions, or a near relative becoming ill or dying. More of children's fears tend to be imagined than real. Also, more fears are expressed at night than during the day, probably because of the added mysteriousness of darkness and the loss of control the child senses in falling asleep (equated with dreams).[13]

The three prominent fears of toddlers are of strangers, animals, and separation.[1] Children between the ages of 2 and 6 have a higher incidence of fears than any other age group. Children at greatest risk for excessive fear development are toddlers and preschoolers of difficult or slow-to-warm temperaments who are primarily introverted, especially girls.

Psychodynamics of Normal Fears

Most children's fears are transient and at most unsettling. Their fears are even predictable to some extent, since certain fears are more common at particular ages or stages, primarily due to the way the child perceives his world at that time in his life.[2] Toddler's fears are typically associated with animals, separation and the unfamiliar. Preschoolers tend to fear imaginary creatures and the dark. School-age children's fears center around fears of physical danger to self.[5]

The separation and animal fears of typical toddlers are evident in the separation anxiety behaviors of early toddlerhood, the security features of transitional objects ("Linus syndrone") in middle toddlerhood, and the imaginary animals and pretend animal play that corresponds with later toddlerhood. These behaviors subside as the fear is mastered.[7] This natural fading of these transient fears can in part be attributed to the child's increased experiences over time and his general maturation, especially intellectually.[9,14]

Disturbed Psychodynamics of Excessive Fears

Children whose fears are persistent, inappropriate or disabling may, unfortunately, succumb to pathological behaviors in their unsuccessful efforts to master these fears.[9] The behaviors

---

*In a study done by Arthur Jersild before the invention of television the types of fears cited were amazingly similar. Perhaps the oral fairy tales that television has largely replaced today conjured up as many thoughts of violence and harmful creatures as we today attribute to television exposure.

motivated by these excessive fears can be extremely persistent despite attempts to change them; in fact, the fear and its associated behaviors can increase with time even though they are not being reinforced by either exposure to the fear-provoking stimulus or parental overattention.[9]

Just which pathological behaviors are involved is largely dependent on the kind of fears motivating them. Fears that are associated with people, especially if the people to be feared are caretakers, are very difficult to combat. These children frequently develop a philosophy of life that requires them to be constantly defending themselves against a world perceived to be full of dangerous people.[7] Aggression, mistrust and numerous antisocial behaviors make up the repertoire of defenses against such a child's fears. Fears, particularly those associated with separation or loss, may be displayed in a wide variety of physical upsets (chronic fatigue, insomnia and gastrointestinal complaints), atypical obsessions, breathing disorders (asthma), or cardiovascular disorders (fainting, blushing).[9] (Because toddlers are naturally ritualistic, the category of behavior involving atypical obsessions must be evaluated carefully.) The pretending commonly used by children to master their fears tends to become a part of the personality of those children whose fears are excessive enough to have penetrated their real world. For these children, imaginary fears are so intense and real that a sense of danger permeates their lives.[7] The elaborate defenses they build against these imaginary dangers become a part of their personality.[7]

The child who is not allowed to behaviorally or verbally express his hostilities and hatreds or to whom such feelings are unacceptable is likely to experience a psychological reversal. The hatreds and hostilities that belong to the child are projected onto some imaginary creature or situation, creating in his mind a fear that something hates him and is after him. All children do this to some extent, but for a few the fear becomes an obsession.[13]

The responses produced by these excessive fears are under the control of the autonomic nervous system, not conscious control, and are therefore, involuntary.[9] For this reason, trying to reason with the child about his fear, demanding that he stop the resulting behaviors, or forcing the child to confront his fear (if it is real and can be confronted) are highly unsuccessful approaches to managing the situation.

Etiology of Fears

It is not really known why fears develop in children or why they become excessive in some, but certain contributing factors have been identified and are useful in helping to pinpoint children at risk so that preventive measures can be instituted. Most fears are not inherent to a child's development; they must be learned. The following is a list of contributing factors researchers have identified as supportive to the development of excessive fears.[9, 14, 15, 19] Fears:

1. Result from child having been hurt by an object or during certain circumstances, usually on more than one occasion;
2. Arise out of a child's sense of powerlessness, of not having any control over the fear stimulus (object or situation);
3. Are the product of extremely intense or prolonged exposure to a frightening situation;
4. Contagiously develop from imitation of parental, sibling or peer fears;
5. Are transferred to the child by regular verbal expressions from significant persons in his life; for example, the mother repeatedly tells relatives and neighbors her fear that the child will get lost if she is not with him every second he is outside, so the child develops a fear of going outdoors;
6. Derive from the positive consequences the child has learned follow his expressions of fear; for example, he gets to sleep with parents, a parent sits up with him, he gets carried when a feared object is around;
7. Emerge out of some experience used in the past as a punishment (put alone in dark room as a punishment, he now fears dark and/or being alone in a room whether it is dark or not);
8. Stimulated by observation of scenes of horror or violence (television shows and news, movies, abusive displays within family);
9. Assimilated vicariously by watching another child or adult experience pain, hurt or fear in the presence of the feared object or in a setting similar to the feared situation (child watches a sibling get shots and develops a fear of needles or people in white clothing or

rooms with beds; he may associate unpleasantness with the examining table that the sibling was sitting on when receiving the shots).

Children with an inherited high intensity of reaction to new experiences and the unfamiliar have a greater tendency to overreact with excessive fear. Some children seem to develop overactive imaginations that place them at special risk. Factors in the child's environment also can place him at higher risk of developing numerous or excessive fears. These include:[9, 13, 15, 19]

1. Children who live with overprotective parents incorporate an attitude that "the world is a dangerous place." They live in constant fear that someone or something might try to harm them.
2. Children whose parents make unrealistic demands on them or who expect perfection are placed in a position of continuous anxiety and tend to possess lower self-esteem and a sense of helplessness that can extend to other life experiences.
3. Parents who threaten a lot or give prolonged punishment place their children in danger of developing excessive fears.
4. Consistently heavy viewers of television are more likely to absorb a "mean world syndrome," making them more vulnerable to excessive fears.
5. If exposed repeatedly to adult problems, the toddler can become overwhelmed by the insecurities and burdens of life, making him more vulnerable to irrational fears.
6. Overpermissive parents subject their child to greater risk because of the insecurity unclear limits place on the child.

As the nurse interacts with the toddler and assesses his health status, she should be alert for any of these factors that place the child at greater risk for excessive fears. If risk factors exist she should include an evaluation of what, if any, fears the toddler displays and to what degree and frequency they are expressed. Preventively she can institute the following practices in her care of toddlers, especially those at special risk, and educate parents in preventive actions that will help decrease risk factors or help the child cope with fears so that they do not become excessive.

1. All children, but especially those at special risk, should be prepared for new situations or experiences that would otherwise be overwhelming. For example, if the family is adding a member, making a move or losing a member, the child should be prepared ahead in small increments and given opportunity to be involved in some way so the situation becomes familiar.
2. During exposure to situations or objects that are especially likely to create fear, adult reassurance and presence should be offered continuously. For example, a child receiving an immunization is less likely to develop associated fears if allowed to sit in his mother's lap and given continuous verbal reassurance and physical stroking by her or the nurse or both.
3. Comfort should be given promptly after any frightening experience or dream. However, parents should be warned against overdoing so that expression of fear becomes rewarding.
4. Others' fears, especially those of parents and older siblings, should be kept in tow as much as possible.
5. When a potentially fear-evoking object is expected to be encountered or a situation is to be experienced by the toddler, opportunity for play with actual or similar objects or for pretending in similar situations should be provided beforehand so the child has a chance to develop some control and coping skills. This is a basic premise for play therapy prior to and during hospitalization or treatment and diagnostic procedures.
6. Parenting methods that create an environment placing the toddler at special risk for excessive fears should be identified and corrected as early as possible.
7. Real situations that could reinforce a child's fantasied fears make the fears more difficult to overcome and should be avoided when possible.
8. Television viewing by toddlers should be kept light, since they do not have the maturity to cope with much of the violence and science fiction.

Clinical Manifestations of Excessive Fears

Differentiating excessive responses to fear from those common to toddlerhood is clinically a question of intensity and fixedness. If a toddler's fears persist over time, occur regularly or every night, or reach panic proportions so that he becomes very tense or immobilized by the fear-provoking object or situation, his fears are excessive and merit parental intervention or professional assistance.[13] The toddler may also be a victim of excessive fear if he prefers pretend creatures to real people and a pretend world to the real world and yet shows no increased ability to tolerate frustrations of the real world or master his fear.[7]

Toddlers who are working through the normal fears of their development use imaginary people or animals in pretend play, but this activity is not preferred over participation in the real world. They may respond to their fear by covering their face or hiding behind a person or large piece of furniture and they may cry, but they do not show evidence of terror or incapacitation.

Seldom do toddlers persist in expressing their fears through physical symptoms, although this may happen transiently due to the young toddler's limited command of language. These tension symptoms that may also become excessive are often seen in the child who is experiencing excessive fears. (Tension symptoms include physical complaints of headaches and gastrointestinal upsets, restlessness and fidgeting, daydreaming, body rocking, frequent urination, obstinacy, hysterical outbursts and a variety of nervous mannerisms, the most common in toddlers being thumb sucking, eye blinking or genital rubbing.)

The nurse's role at this stage is the early identification of behaviors indicative of excessive fear. Most parents will express some concern about those behaviors symptomatic of excessive fear because of their frustration in not knowing how to manage the behaviors and the fear that is motivating them. Therefore identification is not usually difficult if the nurse encourages toddlers and their parents to express any concerns they have and offers them opportunities to do so. When concerns are expressed by parents about their child's fears and his responses to those fears, or when the nurse directly observes behavior associated with fears, she should obtain a thorough data base relevant to the fears and associated circumstances. Based on her data, she can then help parents develop a plan of action to assist their toddler in overcoming the fear or refer them to a resource that can help them.

Management of Fears

Children need to know that the adults in their life understand that they are afraid and that those adults will help them to overcome their fear. During the time that a child is responding to a fear, there are several things that can be done to help him through the frightening situation.[1] The parent should try to find out the source of the fear. Throughout the frightening experience the child needs reassurance that he is not alone and that he will be helped through the experience. If possible, the source of the fear should be removed or else the child should be removed from the source. Someone should remain with the child until the fearful circumstance is over and the child has regained his composure. The adult with the child during the feared experience should model being unafraid in the situation. Once the frightening experience is over, the child should be encouraged to talk about his fear or, since many toddlers lack the language skills to communicate their fear or are hesitant to do so, to make up games to help him act out his fear through play.[13]

There are also some actions that should *not* be taken while a child is experiencing fear lest they aggravate or reinforce the fear.[15,19] The child should not be ignored, ridiculed or left alone while frightened. Nor should he be forced or coerced into confronting the source of his fear. The use of logic or reasoning to try to explain the situation or persuade the child there is nothing to fear is hardly ever successful and conveys to the child instead that his fear is not being understood by the adult he thought would help him.

Adults can help children to overcome their fears. Research by Jersild and Holmes[9,11] showed these mastery techniques to be most effective. The first is to help the child develop skills to gradually cope with the feared object or situation through imaginative play and by helping him discover things about the fear source that show it to be vulnerable; i.e., help him see that there are things he can do to have some control in the situation so he has less need to fear it.

Next, the child should be taken gradually into active contact with the feared object or participation in the feared situation. Confrontation should not be forced however; the child should be allowed to move into contact only to the extent that he appears ready. For example, a child who fears dogs might first be encouraged to pretend he is a dog. Then he might be read stories and shown pictures about dogs — puppies are less threatening and stories that reveal the friendly and people-controlled aspects of dogs are best. Next the child might be given a dog puppet to play with. A trip to a pet shop or some other place where puppies are kept caged may be acceptable exposure to the child by now. At another time the child may be ready to stand by while an adult holds and cuddles a puppy. Later the child may venture to touch the pup while it is caged or being held by an adult. Then the time may arrive when the child willingly, although cautiously, holds the pup himself. This is a good time to begin exposure to progressively larger dogs that are confined. At last, the child is able to cope with the experience of a loose dog of fair size without more than the cautious fear typical of toddlers.

As the preceding example illustrates, the child should be given opportunity to become acquainted with the feared object or situation under circumstances that at the same time give him the option to either inspect or ignore it.

Jersild and Holmes also listed methods adults can employ that are sometimes successful with toddlers but more often with older children or with toddlers who are bordering on excessive fear. Those methods include:

1. Verbal explanations by the adult that the object or situation cannot harm the child, coupled with reassurance that he will not be left alone.
2. Verbal explanation and practical demonstration that the feared object or situation is not dangerous.
3. Giving the child examples of siblings, peers or others who are not afraid of the fear source, i.e., offer the imitation of fearlessness.
4. Conditioning of the child to believe that the feared object or situation can provide pleasure for him rather than danger.

These two researchers verified that ignoring a child's fear, forcing him into contact with the fear source, or removal of the fear source are virtually useless methods in helping children overcome fears, regardless of their age. Removal of the fear source is helpful during the fright experience, however.

The nurse may be the adult who works with the child on mastery of his excessive fear using the aforementioned techniques, or she may teach these techniques to parents or other adults who can then work with the child to master the fear that constrains him from happier life experiences.

EXCESSIVE SEPARATION ANXIETY IN TODDLERHOOD

An Altered Behavioral State

Separation anxiety that is extreme or prolonged is a direct outgrowth of some disturbance in the attachment process involving a fear of being separated from someone or being left alone, out of reach of the persons who are the child's source of safety, familiarity and security.[1] Inappropriate or excessive separation anxiety tends to be cyclical, passing among generations.[4] The likelihood of disturbance in the separation process is greater when bonding or attachment has been disrupted with both parents. Fortunately, statistics reveal that only a very small number of children develop separation anxiety beyond that normal for the toddler stage.[9] It occurs more often in girls.[9]

Psychodynamics of Normal Separation Anxiety in Toddlerhood

A strong early attachment between a child and his parents or caretakers and the dependency that is a natural part of the attachment phenomenon pave the way for a child's development during toddlerhood as a separate being. Even with strong parent-child bonding in their favor, most children experience some degree of fear of being left alone or abandoned during late infancy and the early toddler years. This is in part due to the fact that children this age have no way of comprehending whether the separation will be brief, long or permanent. If the separation extends longer than the child finds tolerable, he often tries to punish parents or caretakers by ignoring or rejecting them upon their return and perhaps for a brief time afterward. The temporary "silent treatment" is usually followed by a transitory period of clinginess. Sleep or eating disturbances of a minor and passing nature are also common features of typical toddler separation anxiety reactions. The temporary and relatively benign characteristics of these behavioral responses to separation are the major factors that differentiate normal separation anxiety from the more disturbed separation responses of other toddlers.

Disturbed Psychodynamics of Excessive Separation Anxiety

The toddler who experiences excessive separation anxiety has developed an overly intense and dependent relationship with his caretaker that robs him of any self-confidence to function without her,[1] or, paradoxically, he has never developed adequate trust in his caretaker or felt her acceptance and approval of him, so that any experience of separation in his relationship with her further disrupts his capacity to depend upon her.[4] The anger that is the product of separation wells up inside the child and is vented any number of ways. It may be expressed in dreams or exaggerated fear of abandonment or vented on other people, causing a generalized over-fearing of people, especially those who resemble the source of his anger (caretaker); or the anger may be redirected onto himself through physical injury (head banging, hair pulling) or psychosomatic illness (asthma).[18] Dreams at this age are taken as real events; thus the initial frightening separation experience can be re-created repeatedly in dreams, reinforcing the child's fear and anger.[18] Occasionally the anger is directed toward the actual source and expressed through aggressive actions toward the caretaker, insensitivity and indifference toward her and her disciplinary measures, and waywardness.[8] This is much more common in boys.

Etiology of Excessive Separation Anxiety

Excessive separation anxiety is believed to be the result of either insufficient or overly intense bonding between child and caretaker (usually the mother).[4,9,18] How sharply the anxiety is experienced and how it is expressed depends on how intense or deprived the caretaker-and-child relationship is.[1]

Children whose temperaments cause them to overreact to new or different situations or people are at greater risk to develop excessive separation anxiety. Other factors in a toddler's environment, particularly factors related to parental approach and associated parent-and-child relationships, may place him at special risk to over-respond to separation experiences. Studies conducted in England[9] showed that two kinds of early separation experiences produced a higher incidence of excessive separation anxiety: (1) when a child was placed by his mother in substitute care daily before 2 years of age and (2) when a child's daily substitute care was unstable,* regardless of the child's age. Unstable care early on disturbs the child's equilibrium in his relations with parent figures, leading him to become either too clinging or too wayward, depending on the quality of their original attachment to each other.[9]

Another factor that places some children in a vulnerable state for excessive separation fears is extreme maternal overprotection ("smother love, momism") that involves indulgence, domination or a combination of both, and excessive maternal-and-child contact.[9] The parent who irritably rejects dependency demands from the toddler but eventually gives in to him is also placing the child at risk for development of extreme separation responses.[9] Separation is experienced more acutely by all children during family crises and at other times that foster insecure feelings (illness, moving), but the response is more extreme and prolonged in children at risk for excessive separation anxiety.

Questions concerning the toddler's response to separation should be included in any toddler's routine health appraisal, but particularly during the appraisal of those youngsters at special risk because of personality characteristics or environmental circumstances. Anticipatory guidance offered to families of high-risk toddlers should stress how important it is to avoid leaving the child with unfamiliar substitute caretakers or having frequent changes in substitute caretakers. When substitute caretakers are necessary it is best if the caretaker is someone familiar to the toddler and with whom he has had positive interaction. If the length of separation is to be very long, it is best to arrange for the toddler to be cared for in his own home. For toddlers with a normal separation response a long separation involves being away over-

---

*Unstable care includes different caretakers, sometimes being cared for at home and other times away from home, sometimes being cared for all day and at other times only a few hours or at night — any irregularity of pattern or persons.

night, but for the at-risk toddler any separation of more than a few hours merits such an arrangement.

Clinical Manifestations of Excessive Separation Anxiety

The degree of anxiety in children at separation from their primary caretaker (usually the mother) varies from mild to fairly severe. It is the behavior of the child with a severe or excessive response that is described here. The crying that is typical of most toddlers, at least initially, following separation turns to urgent and terrified sobbing of prolonged duration (often hours) in the toddler possessed by excessive anxiety. His *protest stage* of separation is louder, longer and accompanied by more aggressive motor activity than that of the typical toddler. His *despair stage* often shows more regressive activities, acted out more frequently and over a longer time. He feels complete helplessness and a host of negative feelings. His anxiety at this point may be expressed physically in an asthma attack,* nervous eczema, neurodermatitis, or nonbacterial gastroenteritis.[18] His *detachment phase* response is also more exaggerated that the typical toddler's responses. He may display absolute denial of any angry feelings, or submit to anyone's approach or any body intrusion with complete lack of response or acknowledgement, or evidence no mutual, genuine affection or respect in his relationships with all people including his mother and often even with his toys and transitional objects.

Children who experience intense separation anxiety have an acute compulsion to stay constantly near their caretaker. They possess a morbid preoccupation with their caretaker's health and whereabouts, seldom trusting the reassurances offered them. Their dependent behavior is revealed in their needless seeking of help even in routine tasks they are competent to carry out. They seem to be constantly seeking physical contact, have a persisting need to stay in close proximity to an adult and display a variety of attention-seeking ploys.[4, 8, 9]

The nurse's role, again, is early identification of behaviors suggestive of intense separational fears. Because parents hear constant reassurances from friends and parental guidance media sources that separation anxiety is normal and because they often find it difficult to determine if their child is over-reacting, they often are hesitant to bring up this subject with helping professionals, even though they may have much concern about their child's separation behaviors. Some parents find gratification in their child's behaviors that convey he needs and misses them and do not perceive it as maladjustive. Therefore, it is imperative that the nurse assess separation behaviors during toddler appraisals and encourage parents to discuss any concerns or questions they have about these behaviors.

Because attachment maladies are often involved, the nurse will usually refer families whose toddlers display over-reactive separation behaviors to psychological professionals. Hopefully, a team approach to treatment will keep the nurse involved so that she can reinforce the family's efforts to correct the disturbances.

Management of Separation Anxiety

Measures that help all toddlers cope with separation are applicable and even more imperative for the toddler with extreme separation reactions. Toddlers cannot really be prepared for separation experiences until they have developed some concept of time and permanence. However, arrangements on the parents' part can be made to preserve as much of the child's security as possible. The following actions taken by parents convey such consideration and help make the separation experience a little less traumatic:[4, 7, 8, 17]

1. Leave him at home where he is familiar with the environment and can see reminders of his primary caretaker's existence and possessions that, in his perception, assure her return.
2. Leave him with someone he knows and enjoys and who knows and will comply with his usual routines and allow for his unique quirks.
3. Give the child at least a half hour of time to interact with the substitute caretaker before the primary caretaker leaves, longer if the child is being cared for away from his own home. This has particular usefulness for the

---

*Nonseasonal or emotionally stimulated asthma is often associated with separation anxiety in early childhood.[18]

child who must be hospitalized under circumstances in which the mother cannot stay.
4. The primary caretaker should tell him in very simple terms that she is leaving, who will care for him until she returns, when she will return, and any other concrete facts that will reassure him of her return and what he can expect while she is away. Attaching her return to some routine the child experiences is most effective: for example, "I'll be back when you have eaten lunch."
5. The primary caretaker should make every effort to stay with her toddler when he must remain long in a strange environment (hospital) or during painful or intrusive procedures. Pediatric facilities whose policies reflect such consideration have contributed greatly to this type of child's mental health.
6. Lengthy separations or separations involving both parents should be avoided when possible during this toddler's peak period for separation anxiety developmentally (usually considered 6 to 18 months, but varies with the individual child).
7. Substitute caretakers should avoid pressure in developmental tasks (toilet training) during periods of separation.
8. It is extremely important to introduce separation experiences gradually to the toddler prone to excessive anxiety responses. For example, begin by leaving the child with the other parent (the one who is not the primary caretaker) for progressively longer periods of time. Once this child has learned to cope with these separations, introduce him to a nonparent substitute caretaker for a very brief time (half an hour) and gradually lengthen the time away. Unless absolutely unavoidable, this child should not be left with a substitute caretaker while asleep, but rather he should be awake when the substitute caretaker arrives and when the primary caretaker leaves. ("Sneaking out" only reinforces the child's belief that he cannot trust the primary caregiver.)

To help over-reactive children work through their anxiety of separation, they should be encouraged to participate in "going away" and "coming back" pretend play with the primary caretaker on a regular and frequent basis. Disappearing games (peek-a-boo, hide-the-handkerchief, who's under the blanket) for toddlers also help this child master his excessive feelings. These activities help this child learn some control over his reactions to separation without experiencing the trauma of the actual situation. They also allow the child to work through his anxieties while awake rather than through dreams.*

The primary caretaker should evaluate regularly whether plenty of unasked-for attention is being provided to the child. If it is, she should gently but firmly divert the child's interest toward his toys or the activities going on around him at those times when he is persistently seeking to cling or be held. Such action, preceded by a pat or hug, avoids reinforcement (positive or negative) of the anxiety behaviors while simultaneously conveying her approval of him and her confidence in his ability to function without her immediate presence.

EXCESSIVE OR INJURIOUS SIBLING RIVALRY

An Altered Behavioral State

Sibling rivalry and its associated unsettling behaviors can be a disruptive guest in any home with two or more children. The more siblings there are, the greater chance that at least one sibling will display excessive jealousy and accompanying rivalrous behavior.[10] The incidence is even greater when siblings are 3 years of age and younger.[10] The tendency for excessive competition for adult attention is greater when siblings are very close in age (under two years apart).[17] Middle children are more at risk, having both older and younger siblings with whom to contend and compete.[19]

Sibling rivalry is especially encouraged in a culture such as ours that values intense parent-and-child relationships, individuality and competitive self-assertion.[3] In the name of sibling rivalry, parents (in our society) tend to allow their children extraordinary license in cruelty and torment tactics designed to undermine each other's personalities.[7] Such tolerance means that nothing is being done to help these children

---

*Children with extreme separation reactions often display associated nighttime anxiety, awakening several times in great fright. Unless the child is unusually distressed by illness or other crisis, he should be kept in his own bed and diversions or entertainment should not be offered lest this behavior be reinforced.[7] He is usually not reassured simply from hearing his caretaker's voice, but seeing her and being patted until he falls back to sleep will usually calm him.

overcome their aggressive feelings, allowing potential damage to the personality development of the victimized sibling(s). No one, regardless of their age or whether the intent is purposeful or unconscious, should be allowed to ventilate his hostility in ways that come near barbarity, causing actual or potential hurt to others. Excessive sibling rivalry has been described as a reversion to antisocial behavior of one sibling toward another with the deliberate intent to hurt, embarrass or humiliate by physical or verbal means.[16] The harm may be purposely or unconsciously motivated.

Psychodynamics of Normal Sibling Rivalry in Toddlerhood

Although sibling rivalry is common, at least to some extent, in many families, it is not inevitable. Whenever there are changes in a family's structure (new baby, adoption of a child, new spouse or step-parent), a possible arena for competition between two members for the love and loyalty of the third is created. There is no such thing as a relationship between three people, only a shifting of two-person relationships with the third as an observer. Thus we must each learn to tolerate times of being left out.[3] How disturbing these experiences are depends on the child's age, how well he has been prepared for the changes in family membership, whether his needs are consistently met and his status in the family preserved, and how his parents handle his jealous or fearful feelings when they occur.

Disturbed Psychodynamics of Excessive Rivalry or Jealousy

When a child reacts toward his sibling(s) with aggressiveness and hostility his actions are usually prompted by one or several of the following feelings: (1) ambivalence toward the sibling. He is told to be loving and gentle with his sibling yet feels resentment because of the actual or perceived loss of status and attention the sibling has caused in his relationship to other family members, especially parents. (2) He fears that he will be replaced by the sibling, lose the affections of his parents or be an unequal match to the competition of his sibling. (3) There is an inadequate sense of approval from his parents, usually combined with the perception that the sibling is favored over him. (4) He has an actual or perceived belief that he is being unjustly compared to his sibling and the sibling comes out looking better in the comparison.

The toddler, still relying on his relationship with his primary caretaker for a portion of his developing identity, can find such feelings overwhelming. His natural instincts are to defend himself in two ways. One instinctual behavior is to regress, taking on the infantile behaviors that seem to win parental attention for the rivaled sibling. The other instinctual response is to get rid of the intruding sibling and, with that an impossible feat, to at least diminish the sibling's status in his parents' eyes or punish him for existing. At the toddler stage these responses are usually overt, in the form of direct aggression. The actual hurt inflicted on the sibling is usually not intentional, but unconsciously motivated. However, these unintentional aggressions can be just as dangerous as intentional ones.

Children with special vulnerabilities such as physical or emotional handicap, less attractive appearance, or an unstable or negative relationship with parent(s) tend to have lower self-esteem. This makes more difficult the tolerating of being temporarily left out (the observer) of interaction with his parents, and creates in this child an illusion of a scarcity of love.[3] When jealous aggressiveness is condoned or reinforced by parents, when limits are not set on unacceptable expressions of the associated anxiety and hostility, when parents do not acknowledge and satiate the child's affectional and attention needs, or when parents unwittingly promote a competitive relationship between siblings on a continuing basis, excessive or injurious rivalrous behaviors are the inevitable consequence. Thus the pathology of excessive sibling rivalry lies as much in parental response to initial rivalrous acts as it does in the child's own maladaptive psychodynamics.[18]

Etiology of Excessive Rivalry

The major cause of excessive rivalry involves a child's feelings of insecurity in his relationship with a significant person or loved one in his life, most often a parent.[10] Numerous factors in a child's environment can contribute to those insecure feelings and associated fears of loss, particularly of parental love and attention. A frequent factor is parental attitudes of comparison between siblings, usually unintentional. These comparisons contribute to normal sibling tensions by creating a competitive situation between the siblings. These comparative attitudes lead at least one of the siblings — usually the one who is less attractive, less talented or academically inclined, or less precocious — to believe his parents are expressing a preference or favoritism for the rival sibling, thus arousing in him a fear that he is less loved by them.[2,10]

The alert nurse will evaluate the interactions between siblings, particularly in their parents' presence, being watchful for parental attitudes that convey favoritism or comparative attitudes and for sibling behaviors that suggest excessive competition for parental recognition or affection. When counselling with parents who have a handicapped or chronically ill child, attention should be given to the parents' awareness of how their reactions to this child may foster rivalry between that child and his siblings. This would be particularly unhealthy since these children especially need the support and understanding of their siblings as they cope with their disability.

Birth order and space between children also can contribute to excessive rivalry. Children born too close together are forced to compete for similar need gratification and with similar developmental intensity. A toddler and his infant sibling are both very dependent upon their mother for care and for their developing identities. The oldest child often experiences jealousy more intensely because he once experienced the total attentions and affections of his parents, something his siblings will never know or experience. The middle child also has a more competitive situation, having to deal with both older and younger siblings.

The number of siblings in a family can contribute to excessive rivalry in one or more siblings. A toddler measures his parents' love in terms of the time spent with him and the subtle rather than verbal indicators of love and affection. When parents have several children to spread their time among, the deficiency their toddler perceives functions to stimulate development of excessive or aggressive rivalrous feelings, particularly toward younger or handicapped siblings who circumstantially reap more of his parents' time. Nurses working with families who have several children can help parents to periodically evaluate whether any of their children are unwittingly being left with a short supply of their undivided attention and to develop a plan that will ensure time for each child on a regular basis without compromising family functioning or life style.

Cruel, aggressive behavior toward siblings may be an imitation of parenting methods the toddler has observed or experienced. Parents who use corporal punishment or degrading verbal assaults to control antisocial behavior tend to see more aggressive acting out in their children's relationships.[16] Exposing parents to parenting alternatives is an important function of the nurse. Helping parents to see some of the consequences, including aggressive expressions of jealous feelings, of some parenting approaches may help them make more desirable choices.

The toddler does not have the inner control or knowledge of alternative ways to express hostile impulses; therefore his parents have a responsibility to help him discover productive ways to manage these impulses. More importantly, they can avoid creating situations that stimulate those hostile feelings toward siblings. The toddler constantly told to keep away from his baby brother or sister has justification for harboring resentful feelings. The nurse should encourage parents to involve their toddler in the infant's care, obviously under close adult supervision. Toddlers do not object to taking soiled diapers to the waste container or diaper pail. Coupled with praise for being a big boy who no longer needs diapers, the toddler may even find the experience ego-boosting. A toddler's pudgy hands are perfect sponge substitutes for soaping down the infant sibling's legs or back during bath time.

The toddler or older sibling who is frequently criticized for not being a good model for younger siblings or the toddler who is forced to imitate and obey older siblings is also involved in circumstances that breed excessive rivalry. Parents need encouragement and reinforcement from health professionals for allowing each child to develop his own unique personality and talents. They need help to realize that a toddler is not ready to be a role model, nor is he in any frame of mind to mimic older siblings at a time when his own selfhood is his primary concern.

Some toddlers are aggressive in their rivalry because they have found it to be a way to get the attention that they feel powerless to attain any other way.[14] Parents should be taught to recognize early signs of aggression or cruelty (biting, kicking, hitting or scratching, pushing or punching[10]) and to feel comfortable seeking help if signs of aggression toward siblings persist or grow more intense. They should also be advised against letting a toddler under 3 spend a great deal of time in unsupervised play with other children — he learns aggression instead of cooperation — because he does not yet have the maturity to recognize that others have needs too, nor does he curb his impulses to hurt others. (By 3 years most toddlers have enough moral maturity to recognize that hurting others is wrong, despite an urge to do so.) Around adults the young toddler is more likely to learn to be assertive but generous.[15]

Clinical Manifestations of Excessive Rivalry

Indirect reactions to jealousy are usually not vented toward the sibling but internalized or displayed through more generalized misbehavior. These reactions are considered excessive when they persist over a period of months or progressively increase in frequency or intensity. They include such behaviors as (1) regression to enuresis or thumb sucking; (2) bids for attention through new fears or food idiosyncracies, (3) general naughtiness and destructiveness, (4) tattling in an attempt to belittle the rivalled sibling in the parent's eyes, (5) unwarranted displays of affection or helpfulness toward either the sibling or parents, (6) venting of hostilities on toys or animals, (7) subdued or grief-like behavior or simulated helplessness in tasks previously accomplished unaided.[10]

Whether the attack against a sibling is covert and indirect or overt, with the infliction of direct harm or abuse, sibling battles that turn into consistent out-and-out warfare indicate that something is amiss in the family's relationships. Other signs suggestive of serious rivalry problems include (1) one child repeatedly having to gratify his own needs at his sibling's expense, (2) when a child derives pleasure from posing physical threat to or actually harming a sibling, (3) repeated failure of the aggressive sibling to show signs of guilt afterwards, (4) accompaniment of other antisocial behaviors, (5) habitual displays of excessive anger or violence when a sibling will not give in or go along with the other sibling, (6) habitual insensitivity to the victimized sibling's feelings or (7) regular efforts to humiliate or embarrass the sibling.[14] The significant factor in these behaviors is their habitual or excessive nature; they represent a plea for outside controls and help.

Management of Excessive Rivalry

In mild rivalry that primarily involves bickering but no cruel behavior, a hands-off approach is usually best. Letting siblings work out these minor conflicts helps them learn cooperation and how to manage interactions with peers. However, when the conflict between siblings involves cruel or demoralizing behaviors it should be stopped; both siblings should then be punished equally but without lecturing, nagging, or moralizing.[2, 7, 12] The parent should not participate in the quarrel, but merely stop it. The children involved should be told that such behavior toward each other is neither nice or acceptable. An older child who can verbalize should be asked how he thinks the other sibling would feel in his place. A clear description of the consequences if this behavior occurs again should be given. This approach gives the siblings a lesson in empathy and lays the ground rules of what is tolerable in the home and what is not.[16] Using this approach, parents convey to their children that excessive rivalry will not be supported or tolerated by them and that, in addition, they will make trouble for both siblings if such behavior persists or recurs. In these circumstances children learn that they are expected to live together in relative peace and that, whatever reasons they have for hostile or jealous feelings, they must find civilized solutions to their conflicts early on.[7] Labeling the behavior as bad or punishing aggressively only intensifies those feelings that triggered the incident.

The nurse is obligated to help parents who express a sense of concern or helplessness to develop effective means for ending the unhealthy aggressions between their youngsters. She may need to stand by them, encouraging and reinforcing their efforts to manage the disruptive behavior, until they are confident that they have control of the situation.

Parents also may express concern that one of their children is being bullied either by a sibling, his peers or both. In such instances the nurse can encourage them to see if the bullying incidents occur in situations that can be avoided or minimized. If so, parental action should be taken to eliminate or reduce opportunities for those situations to happen. Parents can also be assisted to evaluate whether there is anything about their child's appearance or personality that invites sibling or peer ridicule. If such conditions do exist and are remediable, action should be taken promptly to do so (clothing worn, hair style, color of glasses). If conditions exist that are not remediable (braces on teeth, need for thick glass lenses, some physical deformity), the child needs assistance to accept the situation and to develop an understanding of why children act that way* so he can learn to overlook their ignorance of his condition. Parents should also help this child discover his strengths and positive features and encourage him to develop those.

A bullied child should be backed when he feels he has handled a conflict situation well; this builds his confidence in himself, decreasing the likelihood that he will show signs of vulnerability that encourage further ridicule.[16] If the child is into a situation that he cannot handle, his parents should respond to help him gracefully out of it. For example, he can be called away to run an errand or for a snack, whatever disrupts the situation without requiring the parent to become involved in it.

Channeling excessive rivalry into peaceable directions also involves a set of do's and don'ts. It should be realized that parental management is the key to either the continuation or resolution of such rivalry. It is the nurse's role to help parents identify excessive or aggressive rivalry and then to assist them in developing a management plan that fits with their values and family life style. Each statement first presents the don'ts of management followed by do's.

1. Don't join the battle, stop it.
2. Don't convey, even indirectly, amusement or flattery from these jealous acts. Communicate instead that such acts are nonsense and will not be tolerated.
3. Don't take either child's side. If punishment is necessary, punish equally. Educate children involved to the fact that it is impossible for any of them to obtain exclusive rights to parental love.

4. Don't treat each child alike. This is unfair to the individuality of each child. Explain and demonstrate that each family member's needs are respected and responded to as they occur — not that each receives the same responses.
5. Don't compare siblings. Treat each child as a unique individual from his birth, expecting each to develop his own strengths and talents and to adapt to his own limitations.
6. Don't demand perfection. Acknowledge each child's efforts to achieve and his successes when he does. Ignore failures.
7. Don't force siblings to play together or to mutually own toys. Each child needs some toys, friends, interests and activities that are his own. Children should be encouraged to play primarily with others their own age. Allowing siblings independence from each other creates for each his own successes without a reason to compete or be jealous of the others. Be tactful in handing down possessions. It often helps to change them slightly for their new possessor (change color of buttons, paint the tricycle a different color).
8. Don't deny each child his negative feelings toward siblings. Do help him express these sociably by giving him resources to play them out, encouraging his verbalization of those feelings to parents who will listen seriously whether they agree or not. Help him gain insight into what is triggering the negative feelings. (Such a discussion helps the parent gain insight into the conflict, too.)
9. Don't overlook each child's need for some special time with parents. Spending 10 minutes a day with each child and doing something that is fun of the child's choice is a simple yet often effective way to dispel much rivalry. Offer frequent reassurances of parental love and of the child's place and position in the family, and help him to see the rewards and advantages of that position.

MALADAPTIVE TEMPER TANTRUMS

Children, like adults, are trying to learn the rules that will enable them to make sense out of life. A part of that learning is the discovery that life is not always fair, nor does life always go according to our personal desires. The child, whose first year of life most likely entailed relatively complete gratification of wants and needs, be-

---

*They feel uncomfortable or do not understand the situation.

comes acutely aware of these facts during his toddler years. Thus most young children experience at least one temper tantrum as a part of their development. But parents who manage this first outburst of emotional energy promptly and correctly can effectively discourage temper tantrums as a regular means of venting frustration or anger.

Altered Behavioral State

Temper tantrums are one of the most obvious displays of open defiance toward authority. Tantrums are a form of aggression indicating limited capacity for self-control. They are habit forming, continuing only because they are serving a purpose for the child — usually success at getting his own way.[14]

The peak age for temper tantrums, regardless of their frequency or severity, is between 2 and 4 years.[10] The child with a difficult temperament and predominately intense responses to experiences posing disappointment or frustration is at greatest risk for developing maladaptive temper tantrums.[9] Children who are teased a great deal are also more vulnerable to such behavior. Children with delayed language development tend to accumulate frustrations, placing them at greater risk for expression through excessive tantrum explosions.[20]

Disturbed Psychodynamics of Temper Tantrums

Emotionally maladaptive tantrum behavior is simply an exaggeration of behavior patterns common to all children. The concern arises out of the frequency, intensity or manner with which the behavior is expressed.[9] Temper tantrums are abnormal when the child responds violently to seemingly trivial circumstances on a repeated basis, when the child injures himself during tantrum episodes, or when his tantrum provokes excessively punitive or aggressive responses from his parents. Excessive tantrum behavior is at least partly due to the child's underdeveloped capacity to deal with relatively minor frustrations. Their repetition is almost always due to the fact that the behavior is being reinforced and maintained by parental response. If, in the end, he gets what he wants plus his parents' attention, even if it is negative, the toddler sees the behavior as a way to manipulate and control.

Etiology

Several factors have been identified that foster development or maintenance of inappropriate tantrum behavior. Such behavior is sometimes the result of parenting methods that disregard the child's capacity and temperament,[1] placing unrealistic demands on his coping skills.

Many children find excessive tantrum behavior is the only way they have to get needed attention from parents overinvolved in their own activities or who have a tendency to neglect their children. If a child experiences significant frustration* in his first year, he builds up a reservoir of aggressive feelings and his tolerance for frustration is diminished.[19]

Allowing children small degrees of freedom and exposing them to frustration in small increments helps them learn to manage frustration and disappointments appropriately. Nurses, in the preventive guidance to parents of children at special risk, should encourage parents to avoid making new or serious demands on this child when he is tired, ill, or during changes in family structure or life style. She can also explain to parents how allowing their child to exercise some control over his environment in allowable areas makes him more flexible and cooperative when social demands are placed on him in situations over which he has no control.[20]

Clinical Manifestations

Self-harming or destructive tantrum behavior includes head banging, self-biting, hair pulling, scratching, tearing or breaking or otherwise marring personal possessions during fits of anger and frustration.[1] Breath-holding and passing out is another extreme form of tantrum behavior that can be stopped with parental firmness. However, if fainting occurs, especially at times not accompanied by temper tantrums, medical evaluation should be done to rule out any physical cause.[18] Shrieking and hostile motor activity that is frequent, prolonged or seems to occur in response to even the smallest

---

*Examples are multiple prolonged separations from caretakers, frequent changes in caretakers, or frequent restraints on activity and emotional drains due to chronic illness, injury or anomaly.

provocation should be evaluated as it, too, is an indication of emotional maladjustment.

Early identification of children demonstrating such extreme behaviors on a regular basis is extremely important. The longer they persist, the more emotional problems they create. Most people, whether siblings, peers or adults, become steadily more intolerant of such acts in a very short time; thus there is risk of the child's relationships becoming negative. If these acts persist, the child is also not progressing in his development of more mature self-control and cooperation skills, which also serves to jeopardize his interpersonal relationships. The nurse's periodic health interview should include a question about how the child responds to frustration, particularly not getting his own way. How often the child is prompted to tantrum behavior should be asked and how the parents handle tantrum episodes should be discussed and evaluated.

Parents are often embarrassed by tantrum behavior, regardless of how severe it is, and are perplexed about the best way to manage it. Parents whose responses are predominately hostile, punitive or abusive are in immediate need of guidance to learn more effective measures for coping with this tantrum beavior. They need to be helped to realize that their child's aggressive response to frustration may, in fact, be an imitation of their own aggression toward him when he has frustrated them. Most parents eagerly cooperate in trying whatever methods are recommended to diminish or abolish extreme tantrum behaviors.

Management of Extreme Temper Tantrums

A debate has existed for many years over whether management should involve ignoring the tantrum behavior by isolating the child or intervening to help the child contain his antisocial impulses. Ignoring is based on reinforcement theory; this says that if the child's behavior receives no audience or any kind of reinforcement, positive or negative, nothing is gained by the behavior and it will disappear. Intervening is based on the belief that during a tantrum the child is temporarily out of touch with reality and at the mercy of the feelings going on inside him. Both methods are described here, as each approach has its merits and a substantial history of successes in managing extreme tantrum behavior. The nurse's responsibility is to educate parents in both approaches, then help them to select the approach with which they feel most comfortable and that seems more likely to have an impact upon their child.

The aim of both methods is to give the child a graceful, face-saving way out of a tantrum situation while simultaneously communicating its unacceptability and avoiding any reinforcing behaviors on the parent's part that would encourage or maintain this maladjustive behavior. If parents give in to the child or let him know that they are upset by the behavior, it has been reinforced and repeat episodes are guaranteed.

Both approaches also involve the same ground rule: when a request is made by the child, the parent should make a careful decision. If the decision is to deny the request, no tantrum behavior, regardless of how extreme, should be allowed to alter that decision.

The two approaches have in common the following parental actions: (1) praise the child whenever he makes an effort to maintain or successfully maintains control; (2) do not punish the child when he does lose control, as it will only serve to lower the child's already wavering self-esteem; (3) use a calm, firm, but unhostile tone of voice when communicating denial of the child's request; (4) answer the child's questions about why he is being denied in ways that satisfy rather than further frustrate the child ("Because I said so" is a frustrating response to receive at any age); (5) provide the child with some early gratifications during tantrum-prone times. (A box of raisins to munch from during a grocery shopping excursion, given when placing the child in the cart, may eliminate requests for all the goodies passed by on the shelves and the tantrums that would follow when requests were denied.)

Intervening Approach This approach advocates physical contact (firm hand on child's shoulder or clasping child's hand) accompanied by words: "Stop! I cannot understand what is bothering you when you are behaving like this." If the child is not flailing about, actually holding him sometimes helps him regain control; however, if the child is already flailing about he will most likely increase his frenzy under the restraint of being held. When the tantrum is over, parents or adults involved should communicate that although they understand the cause of the child's anger, behavior such as that just displayed is not acceptable. The child should be told why the behavior is unacceptable, how self-defeating it is (it didn't get him what he wanted, tired him out, gave him a sore throat), and how it only increases his unhappiness and disturbs all the other people around. (The parent should not admit to personally being disturbed.[20]) This approach is probably the wisest choice when tantrum behavior is self-injurious or destructive.

Ignoring Approach[6, 9, 19] This approach strongly stresses the avoidance of any semblance of condoning or reinforcing tantrum behavior. Ignoring the tantrum may be accomplished in several ways. The adult involved may just stand by, act as if nothing out of the ordinary is happening and wait the tantrum out. Or the adult involved can, without any hint of anger, disgust or embarrassment, simply walk out of the room. (Certainly this would not be the best option in a public place.)

The adult can apply "time-out from reinforcement" tactics. The child is told that it is acknowledged that he is mad but, if this is the way he chooses to display the anger, he will have to go to his room until he is done. This acknowledges the child's frustration but restricts the tantrum to an area with no audience; that is, it makes tantrum behavior costly. Some parents choose to add a distraction to the time-out directive by telling the child that something pleasant (being specific) awaits him when he is able to regain control (the parent will read him a story, take him for a walk, give him a snack, show him something new to him), thus reinforcing controlled behaviors. If the child does not go voluntarily to the specific time-out area, he should be placed there by the adult. It is important for the adult to maintain a calm tone of voice and convey no evidence of being upset or disturbed by the behavior.

To help parents identify which approach is most satisfactory for them and for the child involved, the nurse teaching these approaches may have them role-play both approaches. When role-playing an approach, one parent can take the parent role and the other the child's role; then they can exchange roles. This is repeated for the second approach. This gives each parent a perspective on their child's feelings and responses to the intervention and gives them a sense of their relative comfort or discomfort with each approach. The nurse can then point out to the parents any reactions she observed during the role-playing that the parents do not express awareness of having experienced. Her continued support of the parents' efforts to curb their child's tantrum behavior may be necessary until they begin to see change in the child's behavior.

References

1. S. Ambron. Child Development. Holt, Rinehart & Winston, 1977.
2. M. and W. Beecher. Parents on the Run. Grosset and Dunlap, 1967.
3. A. Bernstein. Jealousy in the family. Parents, February 1979, p. 47.
4. J. Bowlby. Attachment and Loss. Basic Books, 1973.
5. G. Carro. What frightens little children. Ladies' Home Journal, February 1979, p. 42.
6. F. Dodson. How to Parent. Signet Books, 1970.
7. S. Fraiberg. The Magic Years. Charles Scribner's Sons, 1959.
8. S. Gilbert. Your child's first three years. In Parents Magazine's Self Guidance Program to Successful Parenthood by M. Hoover (ed.), Parents Institute Publ., 1972.
9. M. Herbert. Problems in Childhood. Pan Books Ltd., 1975.
10. E. Hurlock. Child Development. McGraw-Hill Book Co., 1978.
11. A. Jersild. Child Psychology. Staples Press, 1957.
12. L. Katz. Sibling rivalry. Parents, January 1979, p. 78.
13. C. Lang. Children's fears. Parents, May 1979, p. 68.
14. R. McIntire. For Love of Children. Communications/Research/Machines Inc., 1970.
15. D. Papilia and S. Olds. Human Development. McGraw-Hill Book Co., 1978.
16. L. Salk. What Every Child Would Like His Parents to Know. Warner Paperback Library, 1973.
17. D. Schulz. The Changing Family: Its Functions and Future. Prentice-Hall Inc., 1976.
18. B. Schwarz and B. Ruggieri. Parent-Child Tensions. J. B. Lippincott Co., 1958.
19. M. Smart and R. Smart. Living and Learning with Children. Houghton-Mifflin Co., 1961.
20. M. Stewart. Temper temper: how to deal with tantrums. Parents, February 1979, p. 75.

Additional Recommended Reading

L. Bourne and B. Ekstrand. Psychology: Its Principles and Meanings. Holt, Rinehart & Winston, 1976.
L. Herson. Emotional disorders in childhood. Nursing Times, 9 June 1977, p. 864.
J. Marzolla. Supertot. Harper and Row, 1977.
M. Melichar. Using crisis theory to help parents cope with a child's temper tantrums. American Journal Maternal Child Nursing, May/June 1980, p. 181.
J. Ramsey. When children are cruel to other children. Family Circle, 31 May 1977, p. 28.
I. Schleicher. Teaching parents to cope with behavior problems. American Journal of Nursing, May 1978, p. 838.
A. Thomas et al. Temperament and Behavior Disorders in Children. New York University Press, 1968.
R. Turner. A method of working with disturbed children. American Journal of Nursing. October 1970, p. 2146.
B. White. The First Three Years of Life. Prentice-Hall Inc., 1975.

32 POTENTIAL STRESSES DURING TODDLERHOOD: TEMPORARY ALTERATIONS IN HEALTH STATUS

by Jo Joyce Tackett, BSN, MPHN

The toddler experiences even temporary illness as an intrusion on his need to be mobile, to investigate and to develop skills that make him independent. The hindrance to his developmental progress may result from symptomatology that leaves him lethargic or causes him to tire easily, or it may be a consequence of treatments that require confinement.

Parents of a temporarily ill toddler usually have primary responsibility for carrying out whatever treatment is prescribed and may feel anxious or inadequate in doing so if they have not been given sufficient instruction or reassurance that they can manage the tasks required. A typical fear of parents whose toddler has a temporary illness is that it may get worse or that the problem or its consequences may not be completely reversed. The nurse can prevent or alleviate this fear by providing a thorough explanation of the illness, its cause and how the prescribed treatments work to correct the problem. The nurse can also maintain contact with the family via phone calls or home monitoring visits and point out to family members the child's progress. This is also an opportunity to encourage or reinforce the parents' efforts to carry out the treatment regimen.

Parents often experience a sense of guilt when their toddler becomes ill. Many of the temporary problems of toddlerhood are familial in nature; that fact may serve to reinforce a parent's feeling that he or she is to blame. A variety of infections and iron deficiency anemia are common temporary ailments in the toddler. Such illnesses may cause the parents to feel that they are poor caretakers and that their parenting skills are inferior or else their child would not have contracted these conditions. The nurse must be careful as she explains etiology not to convey any blame or judgments of the parents or their parenting skills. Emphasis should, instead, be placed on positively reinforcing the parents' decision to seek treatment for the child; their parenting skills should be acknowledged and supported. Information that will help to prevent or reduce the likelihood of recurrence or continuation of the temporary health problem should be presented in a manner that does not hint of reprimand but rather focuses on how family members can work together to teach their toddler healthy behaviors and institute his treatment in a nontraumatic way.

TEMPORARY ORTHOPEDIC CONDITIONS

Torsional deformities of the tibia or hip or both, bowlegs (genu varum) and knock-knees (genu valgum) are common findings that affect the lower extremities of growing children and become particularly noticeable when the child begins walking. While a vast majority of these orthopedic problems are part of normal physiological development and are self-corrective as the child grows, it is important to differentiate the physiological conditions from those that may be pathological, requiring additional evaluation and treatment.[9] The nurse is often the first to suspect orthopedic problems during well-child assessments of the toddler. The following discussion is intended to help the nurse recognize when medical or orthopedic referral is advisable.

Torsional Deformity

Torsional deformity (malrotation or twisting of the hip or tibia) is the most common orthopedic problem in toddlers. The torsional deformity may occur anywhere between the foot and hip; identifying the location of the deformity becomes important in managing the problem correctly.

Physiology and Etiology Prenatally the fetal lower limbs rotate internally to bring the big toe to midline; therefore the newborn looks pigeon-toed. During infancy external rotation of the femur and tibia gradually occurs, steadily diminishing the child's pigeon-toed appearance. By adolescence the normal stance of slight external rotation of the tibia and femur is established.

If, owing to environmental or genetic factors, this gradual external rotation is restricted, an internal rotation deformity persists. Two major etiologies have been attributed to perpetuation of internal tibial rotation, producing intoeing. Sometimes internal tibial torsion is a consequence of the *intrauterine position*. A deformity with this etiology usually improves spontaneously unless a predominantly prone *sleeping posture* causes it to persist. Heredity is sometimes a factor in femoral torsion.

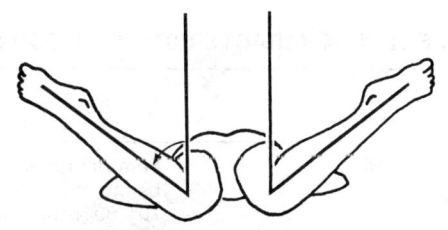

Figure 32–1 Assessment of internal hip rotation. (From L. Staheli, Torsional deformity. Pediatric Clinics of North America, November 1977, p. 803.)

Clinical Manifestations and Diagnosis Torsional deformities are primarily structural (resulting from bone position), although they may occasionally arise from abnormal abduction of the great toe muscle (*dynamic deformity*). Torsional deformities are almost always bilateral.

When a torsion deformity is suspected from routine physical examination or family history, a detailed medical history of the condition should be obtained that covers the progression of the deformity, any previous diagnosis and treatment, and parental response to the condition. Evaluation involves an estimate of hip rotation and tibial rotation.

Measurement of hip rotation is done with the child in a comfortable prone position. The lower legs are raised and permitted to fall outward; this puts the hip into full internal rotation. The angles formed by an imaginary line drawn vertically from the hip joint to the knee and a line from the knee to the great toe is measured to get an estimate of the degree of internal hip rotation (Fig. 32–1). The lower leg is then allowed to fall inward. This puts the hip into full external rotation while the examiner or parent holds the pelvis against the examination table. The angles formed by an imaginary line drawn vertically from the hip joint to the knee and a line from the knee to the small toe is measured to determine the degree of external hip rotation (Fig. 32–2). The angle of internal

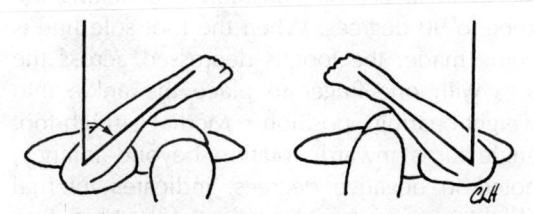

Figure 32–2 Assessment of external hip rotation. (From L. Staheli, Torsional deformity. Pediatric Clinics of North America, November 1977, p. 803.)

TABLE 32-1 CHARACTERISTICS OF TORSIONAL DEFORMITIES*

Level	Direction	
	Intoeing	Out-Toeing
Hip	Femoral torsion as estimated by internal hip rotation: 70°–80° rotation—mild 80°–85° rotation—moderate 85°+ rotation—severe	Normal physiologic position (i.e., internal hip rotation less than 70%)
Tibia	Internal tibial torsion indicated by thigh-foot angle: −10° — mild −20° — moderate −30° — severe	External tibial torsion (thigh-foot angle greater than +30°)

*From L. Staheli. Torsional deformity. Pediatric Clinics of North America. November 1977.

and of external hip rotation is measured for each leg.

The normal angle of hip rotation varies according to the child's age. External rotation of the hip is greatest (about 90 degrees) during early infancy. By the time the child is walking alone, internal and external hip rotation are about equal. External hip rotation supersedes internal rotation in the adolescent male, whereas internal and external hip rotation are still equal or internal rotation is slightly greater in the adolescent female.[13]

The sum of the internal and external hip rotation angles approximates 100 degrees normally, with the internal rotation angle comprising 70 degrees or less. Increased internal hip rotation is almost always evidence of femoral torsion. Table 32–1 correlates rotation with severity of a deformity when internal rotation exceeds 70 degrees.

Tibial rotation is determined by measuring the angular difference between an imaginary line drawn vertically down the back of the thigh and another line drawn vertically across the axis of the foot sole (Fig. 32–3), called the "thigh-foot angle." This is most easily done by placing the child in a prone position and flexing the knee to 90 degrees. When the foot sole line is being made, the foot is depressed across the toes with one finger to place the ankle into weight-bearing position. Medial (thigh-foot angle turns inward) rotation beyond infancy, noted in negative degrees, indicates internal tibial torsion; external rotation of the tibia (0 to +30 degrees thigh-foot angle) is normal by toddlerhood.

A profile of the factors just discussed distinguishes the presence of and type of torsional deformity, its severity and whether it is bilateral or unilateral. Correct diagnosis is critical in establishing the proper management.

Management The need for intervention and choice of management depend on the type and rigidity of the deformity. Although methods of management are still debated, most orthopedists today do not prescribe shoe modifications to correct any torsional deformities because this form of management most often proves expensive and ineffectual.[7] Because improvement usually occurs spontaneously except in severe cases, more orthopedists today merely observe the child over time to ensure progressive resolution of mild or moderate torsion deformity rather than prescribe a specific treatment. The nurse plays a major role in educating the family as to the pathophysiology and the physiological recovery typical of mild and moderate torsion deformities. Reassurance offered at each health

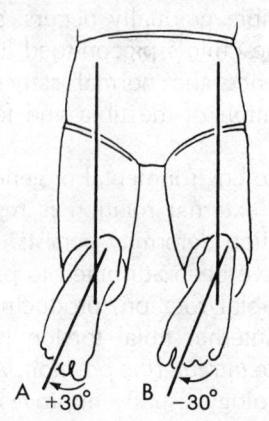

Figure 32–3 Assessment of tibial rotation. (A) external tibial rotation; (B) internal tibial rotation. (From L. Staheli, Torsional deformity. Pediatric Clinics of North America, November 1977, p. 809.)

visit as well as sharing of measurements indicating progress in resolution of the deformity helps to relieve parental anxiety.

Internal Tibial Torsion The most common torsional defect, this deformity is usually recognized at the onset of toddlerhood. Most of these deformities disappear by the time the child is 18 months old; if not, a corrective night splint may be necessary. The "clamp-on" splint consists of a bar the width of the pelvis (2 to 4 inches longer if the child is bowlegged) that is attached to the child's high-topped, stiff-soled shoes at night to maintain the feet in external rotation of 30 to 35 degrees.[13] If the deformity is unilateral, the normal foot is set at 10 to 15 degrees external rotation. Usually correction is achieved in a year; the child should be checked every three months and treatment discontinued when the involved foot shows a 10 to 15 degree external rotation.[4] Parents may need support to continue use of the night splint despite their toddler's obvious resistance. They should be reassured that, if they persist, their child will adjust to the splint and cooperate after a few nights. To help ensure the parents' cooperation in using the brace in spite of their child's rebellion, the nurse should make certain they understand the importance of the splint and how it works to correct the defect.

After age three, correction other than by surgery is seldom satisfactory.

Internal Femoral Rotation This is a common cause of intoeing in late toddler and preschool years. It is sometimes familial, is more common in girls and is rarely unilateral. Unless the internal hip rotation is severe, treatment is usually not recommended, since the deformity is eventually compensated and does not result in functional disability in adulthood.

Whatever treatment is prescribed, parents' involvement and cooperation in carrying it out is imperative if it is to be successful. The nurse must be sure the parents understand their responsibility in the treatment regimen by providing adequate explanations of the deformity and the purpose of treatment and by teaching them the skills required to carry out the treatment. Progress should be shared with the parents at each follow-up visit, and their efforts to comply with the regimen positively reinforced. If financial assistance is needed, the nurse may refer the family to a local crippled children's program for help. If parental compliance is doubted, the community health nurse is an appropriate adjunct to the treatment team.

The toddler will need age-appropriate explanations of the treatments and an opportunity to handle and investigate equipment used in the treatment. If his parents continue to relate to him in a positive and consistent fashion, he will feel secure and his cooperation is more likely.

Genu Varum and Genu Valgum

Bowlegs (genu varum) and knock-knees (genu valgum) usually are features of normal physiologic development that resolve as growth progresses. Studies of large numbers of children have shown that bowlegs are characteristic until 1½ to 2½ years of age, followed by knock-knees until around 4 to 6 years of age, at which time the lower extremities straighten to represent the normal adult stance.[5, 6] Physiological varus is accentuated by the internal tibial torsion that is characteristic of the infant and young toddler. Conversely, valgum also seems more extreme than it is because of the external tibial torsion characteristic of the toddler and preschool years. Sleep position, obesity and posture may also accentuate physiological varus and valgus.[15]

Physiological varus and valgus do not require any intervention other than periodic follow-up to assess the progressive resolution of each as the child develops. X-rays are not necessary, although the observations discussed earlier to determine the degree of femoral and tibial rotation may be conducted to ensure that lower extremity alignment is within normal limits for the child's age. A family history should be obtained at this time. Whether the deformity is bilateral or unilateral should be established, since unilateral deformities often require treatment. Likewise, leg symmetry should be determined so that asymmetrical deformities may also be treated. Parents may need reassurance that the deformity they perceive is normal and will resolve as the child grows.

Nonphysiological, or Extreme, Varus Bowlegs (Fig. 32-4) that are unilateral, asymmetrical, or that persist after 2 years of age are often pathological. Extreme varus has a greater incidence in black children. Etiologically it may be congenital or familial. It may also be associated

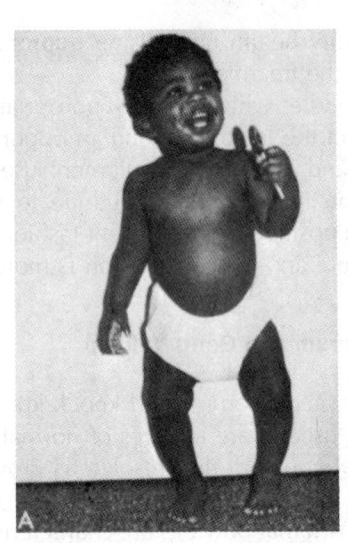

Figure 32–4 The "extreme variation," a 15-month-old boy with bowlegs. (From W. McDade, Bowlegs and knock knees. Pediatric Clinics of North America, November 1977, p. 833.)

with Blount's disease (a growth disturbance of the proximal tibia creating extreme internal tibial torsion) or rickets (a disturbance of calcium and phosphorus metabolism causing inadequate bone calcification during skeletal growth).

Any toddler in whom varus is not resolving by 18 to 24 months and who has a tibiofemoral angle (bowing of tibia and femur) on x-ray of 25 degrees or more of varus should be braced day and night for correction.[9] A brace is usually required for one to two years. If the brace has not achieved correction of the varus by 3 years of age, osteotomy may be recommended some time during the preschool years.[9]

The toddler and his parents will need explanations of the pathophysiology involved and the principles behind the use of a brace if their cooperation and participation are to be obtained. The nurse may need to maintain frequent contact with the family via phone calls or home visits initially to encourage and reinforce the family's compliance efforts. The brace may be removed twice a day for 30 to 45 minutes to relieve the pressure from the brace and provide skin care. Parents should be informed of the importance of daily skin care of the extremities to prevent skin breakdown from the pressure and tension exerted by the brace.

The toddler should be allowed and encouraged to participate in his usual activities to the extent possible to maintain his normal developmental progress. For example, consideration should be given to providing extra time for him to walk to reduce adults' temptation to carry him.

Nonphysiological, or Extreme, Valgus Excessive knock-knees (Fig. 32–5) as established by a tibiofemoral angle on x-ray of more than 15 degrees of valgus, by leg asymmetry or by a shortened stature requires intervention to achieve correction. Likewise, a severe valgus deformity that has not corrected to at least a mild valgus by age 10 will also need intervention.

Knock-knees may be congenital, familial, or associated with obesity, polio or rickets, or trauma or infection of the proximal tibial epiphysis. Girls tend to be more susceptible to extreme valgus deformity, probably because of their wider pelvis and more relaxed musculature.

Extreme genu valgum, left uncorrected, contributes to gait awkwardness, which increases the child's risk for sprains and fractures as he gets older, particularly during active or contact sports. The deformity also causes easy fatigability and joint pains.

If resolution of symmetrical knock-knees is not occurring by 7 years of age, day and night braces are usually prescribed to correct the deformity. Any correctable underlying etiology is also treated. When the valgus is asymmetri-

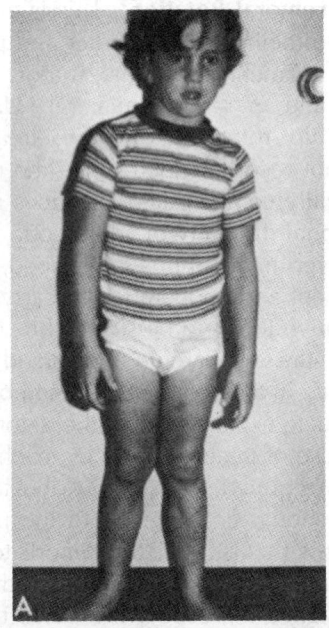

Figure 32–5 A 5-year-old boy with knock-knees. (From W. McDade, Bowlegs and knock knees. Pediatric Clinics of North America, November 1977, p. 831.)

cal, braces may be recommended earlier. If bracing is not successful by 10 years of age in girls or 12 years in boys, or if the condition is not diagnosed before this time, osteotomy is recommended to correct the angular deformity.[4, 9]

The prognosis for the torsional deformities and genu varum or valgum is excellent if the conditions are followed closely and treatment is initiated promptly when spontaneous resolution does not occur. The critical factor in treatment rests upon parental cooperation and compliance with prescribed interventions. The nurse has an important responsibility in helping parents understand the condition and its treatment sufficiently to cooperate and in providing the support and reassurance necessary to maintain that cooperation.

IRON DEFICIENCY ANEMIA

The most common nutritional deficiency in the United States, iron deficiency anemia in infants and young children is needless, since the cause is known. The condition is preventable and early detection is available with a simple blood test. This anemia results from an inadequate supply of iron to support the optimal formation of red blood cells.

The incidence of iron deficiency anemia peaks between 9 months and 2 years of age and again during the adolescent growth spurt. It is rare before 4 months of age because of the reserve of fetal iron the infant can utilize. Exceptions to this are premature infants, infants of teen-age mothers, and infants of mothers who had insufficient diets during pregnancy. These babies have earlier depletion or smaller fetal iron stores or both. If it occurs after age 2 it is more likely to be secondary to a slow, unsuspected blood loss, usually as a result of intestinal parasitic infections. The incidence after age 2, related to parasite infection, is greater in the southern United States, Mexico and the tropics.

The nurse can play a major role in prevention and early diagnosis by knowing facts about the incidence. She can provide nutrition counselling and information early to parents whose infants are at risk because of age, lowered fetal stores or geographic locale. The nurse can also see that a hematocrit evaluation is done every six months with well-child examinations during infancy and toddlerhood to identify iron depletion early.

Etiology

Infants and toddlers are especially at risk because of their rapid growth during this period and the greater likelihood of inadequate iron intake. The greater risk of inadequate iron intake is related to the fact that milk, still a major food and caloric source at this age, contains no iron. In addition, the phosphate in milk binds with iron, removing it from the body. A large amount of iron is needed (15 mg daily) owing to the rapid growth characterizing this period, yet the average mixed diet affords only about 6 mg/1000 Kcal* unless special effort is made to include one or two foods especially high in iron in each day's food intake. Many of the high iron content foods are not preferred by picky toddlers. The high bulk diet characteristic of some ethnic groups also reduces the body's utilization of iron because the foodstuffs are moved out of the gastrointestinal tract faster, resulting in less opportunity for iron absorption.

Causes other than dietary deficiency in toddlers are less common. Impaired iron absorption associated with conditions such as persistent or severe diarrhea or malabsorption syndromes may lead to iron deficiency anemia. This anemia may also be secondary to pica, lead poisoning or intestinal parasite infection, all of which have a higher incidence during toddlerhood. Intestinal bleeding from cow's milk allergy may also cause anemia. Unless iron supplement is given, children with chronic illness may have difficulty ingesting or utilizing adequate iron because of excessive need or poor absorption related to infection, the disease process, or iron absorption inhibiting affects of medications used to treat the chronic illness.

Physiology and Pathophysiology

Normally the body absorbs about 10 per cent of the dietary iron ingested daily. Regulatory sites in the intestinal walls determine the actual amount absorbed. The majority (60 to 70 per cent) of iron is stored as heme, which links with globin to form the hemoglobin portion of the erythrocyte. When the erythrocyte disintegrates

---

*1000 Kcal is the approximate caloric intake during late infancy and early toddlerhood.

after 120 days, the iron is recycled as long as adequate amounts exist. Another 20 to 30 per cent of absorbed iron is stored in the liver, spleen and bone marrow where red blood cells are made. Trace amounts are also present in muscle and blood serum and as transport iron in all cells. Another small store of iron, which is seldom depleted, is that combined with protein as an essential component of certain respiratory catalysts.

When iron deficit occurs due to dietary inadequacy, impaired absorption, blood loss or excessive demand, the production of hemoglobin is decreased, thereby diminishing the oxygen-carrying capacity of the blood. This reduced blood oxygen level is the primary factor in the clinical manifestations of iron deficiency anemia.

Clinical Manifestations

Children with slowly developing anemia (such as the dietary type) may show no clinical symptoms even though their hemoglobin may be as low as 6 gm/100 ml. Therefore, routine hemoglobin or hematocrit evaluation during well-child appraisals is critical to early identification of anemia. Pallor of the skin and mucosa is the predominant sign of moderate to severe iron deficiency anemia. The child may also be irritable, apathetic to his environment and display decreased exercise tolerance or weakness. These children are often overweight because of their large milk intake but display poor muscle development. These anemic children also experience more infections than other children their age. Characteristically the infant or toddler is described as pale, lacking energy and obese.

Diagnosis

The diagnostic process involves (1) a careful history and physical examination, (2) blood smear and red blood cell indices, (3) plasma iron and iron binding studies and (4) stool analysis. The nurse is often the first to notice symptoms suggestive of iron deficiency anemia and usually is responsible for gathering the history and conducting or participating in data collection, including physical examination and laboratory testing. The nurse should explain each procedure involved in terms the child and parent can comprehend. Parents should also be given enough information for them to understand the cause and meaning of data findings in a manner that tactfully avoids accusations about their child care skills or ridicule of their cultural beliefs or practices.

History and Physical Examination   The history should include information on the child's diet, his energy, stamina and any pica behavior. The physical should include evaluation of the child's oral, nasal and conjunctival mucosa; capillary refill of the nailbeds and hand creases;* general motor development; skin coloring; weight; and any evidence of infection. Mucosal and skin pallor and deficient capillary refill along with a history of iron deficient diet or pica are suggestive of anemia. Blood studies are indicated with the presence of these history and physical findings.

Blood Studies   Tissue anoxia, produced by the decreased supply of oxygen being carried by the blood as a result in decreased hemoglobin production, causes the bone marrow to continue producing red blood cells. Therefore the red blood cell (RBC) count is usually normal or only slightly reduced in anemia and typically is disproportionate with the decreased hemoglobin concentration. Hemoglobin is low because the iron required to form it is not available. The exact cutoff point between acceptable and low hemoglobin is controversial and varies with age. Testing of hematocrit is more accurate than of hemoglobin in evaluating the presence or severity of anemia. Since the red cells are not fully filled with hemoglobin when they are released into the blood, they are small in size (microcytic). This causes a low hematocrit level (below 33 per cent), and the concentration of hemoglobin is less than normal, causing the red cells to be pale (hypochromic).

The mean corpuscular volume (MCV) reveals the diminished size of a single RBC as a result of the decreased hemoglobin production. It is found by dividing the hematocrit by the number of RBC's. An MCV of 70 or less in infants and toddlers, 75 in preschoolers or 80 in older children and adults is indicative of microcytic anemia. Mean corpuscular hemoglobin (MCH) tells the concentration of hemoglobin in each

---

*With hand flexed dorsally, hand creases remain pink if capillary refill is adequate.

cell and will be low in anemia, again due to decreased hemoglobin production. The mean corpuscular hemoglobin concentration (MCHC) is also decreased, since hemoglobin is deficient. An MCH value under 27 $\mu\mu g$ or an MCHC value under 30 per cent indicates hypochromic anemia.

A definitive diagnosis may be made from a standard blood smear, which reveals microcytic and hypochromic red blood cells; however, additional studies may be done to determine the cause or severity of the anemia.

Plasma Iron and Iron-Binding Studies Serum iron studies help determine if the anemia is caused by deficient intake or absorption of iron, or insufficient utilization of the iron absorbed. The amount of circulating iron is determined by the serum-iron concentration (SIC) and is normally at least 70 μg/100 ml of serum. The amount of transferrin (iron-binding globulin) is measured by total iron-binding capacity (TIBC) and is normally around 250 μg/100 ml of serum. In iron deficiency anemia, as with no other condition, SIC is reduced while TIBC is increased to compensate for the circulating iron deficit. This finding differentiates iron deficiency anemia due to intake or absorption deficit from that due to insufficient iron utilization.

Stool Analysis Stool is analyzed to identify occult blood (guaiac test) or to identify parasitic organisms that may be causing the anemia.

Treatment: The Nurse's Role

Correction of iron deficiency anemia entails diet therapy, medication and treatment of underlying disease, if it exists. The response to treatment is usually immediate, with rises in hemoglobin by the third day, peaking by the ninth day after treatment begins.[12] However, unless permanent dietary changes are made, the child is in danger of repeated recurrence.

Diet Therapy Nutrition education of the child's caretakers is a significant nursing responsibility. The child needs iron-rich foods every day. Organ meats, dried legumes, shellfish and muscle meats are the richest sources of iron and have the highest iron absorption rate. Other good iron sources include nuts, green vegetables, unsweetened chocolate, dried fruits, and whole wheat or iron-enriched flours and breads, but the iron in these foods is less well absorbed than the iron is from meats and legumes. The iron in eggs is poorly absorbed unless these are eaten with a good food source of Vitamin C. Substantial sources of vitmain C are the citrus fruits, green vegetables and liver.

Protein intake, especially from animal sources, and vitamin C intake should also be increased, as both of these enhance the intestinal absorption of iron from foodstuffs. If the previous diet was high in bulk, bulk intake should be reduced. Milk intake should be limited to a maximum of one quart per day, allowing calories to be provided by other food sources and lowering phosphate levels, which inhibit iron absorption.

In presenting this nutrition education, the nurse must provide information that is realistic in terms of the family's economic resources, attitudes regarding food and cultural practices. For example, if beef is not a practical source of iron and protein because of the family's finances or religious and cultural beliefs, the nurse might instead encourage increased intake of dried beans, peanut butter or turkey, which also are iron-rich protein sources. The caretaker who plans meals and does the shopping may need the nurse's assistance to learn how to plan balanced meals rich in vitamin C, protein and iron or how to shop for low-cost foods high in these nutrients. Parents unfamiliar with food sources with high iron content may appreciate recipes and preparation guides for these foods. Positive reinforcement of the caretaker's efforts and successes in providing the child with the proper nutrition to prevent or correct an iron-deficient diet should continue until these diet measures become habitual food practices. Often parents need simple instruction in basic nutrition before being taught special diet measures. Instruction should always include the reasons for and intended effect of these foods on the child's health state.

Drug Therapy Daily administration of an oral iron supplement (usually Fer-In-Sol) is prescribed, initially in therapeutic doses, then in prophylactic doses. The elemental or ferrous form (ferrous sulfate) is usually used because it is absorbed better than the ferric form and is less likely to cause gastrointestinal irritation. Vitamin supplement is unnecessary and expensive. A therapeutic dose is usually calculated at

3 to 6 mg/kg/day, offered in three divided doses. The therapeutic dose is usually given for 6 to 12 weeks, followed indefinitely by a daily prophylactic dose (8 to 16 mg/day). It should be offered between meals when digestive acid concentration is highest to facilitate absorption. The supplement is given with a citrus fruit or juice to enhance its solubility and absorption.

Many parents are not aware of the differences between Fer-In-Sol Syrup and Fer-In-Sol Drops. Although both are forms of ferrous sulfate, the syrup contains only 6 mg/cc of elemental iron, while the drops contain 25 mg/cc. This significant difference in elemental iron content will obviously affect the amount of syrup as opposed to drops to be given. The nurse should make sure that the parents understand whether drops or syrup have been recommended and that they realize the differing iron content of each.

Parents should be cautioned that liquid iron preparations may stain if they come in contact with the child's teeth. Therefore, liquid iron should be taken through a straw or administered wtih a dropper to the back of the mouth. As an extra precaution, the child's teeth may be brushed after each administration. Parents should also be informed that the child's stool will turn a tarry green when adequate iron levels are reached. The nurse should assess for this occurrence periodically as an indicator of adequacy in administration or dose.

Parents should be urged to continue the iron over the entire prescribed course so the child can build up adequate iron stores, despite the tarry-appearing stools and the child's apparent improved health. Although side effects are rare in children, oral iron does sometimes cause gastrointestinal irritation, diarrhea or constipation, or anorexia. If side effects do occur, the iron should be given with meals or right after meals. Sometimes the iron is initially prescribed to be taken with meals so the intestinal mucosa has time to build up some tolerance to the drug; after three or four days, the iron is administered between meals so that absorption is greater. Another alternative is to initially give lower doses of the iron, gradually increasing to a therapeutic dose within three to five days in an effort to avoid the adverse effects of the drug. If hemoglobin and hematocrit levels do not begin improving within one month after oral iron is begun, parenteral iron (Imferon) is given daily by Z-track to keep skin irritation and discoloration minimal. Lack of improvement is often attributable to inconsistent or inaccurate oral administration. If this is the suspected cause, a community health nurse may be assigned to administer the oral supplement or to teach, supervise and support caretakers to gain their compliance with the prescribed regimen. Other times when parenteral therapy may be ordered are when the anemic child cannot take oral supplement, when gastrointestinal disorders exist that would interfere with intestinal absorption, when the anemia is severe such as during copious blood loss, or when surgery with anesthesia is required, or during serious systemic infection.

Iron poisoning has been known to cause death when children ingested as few as six iron tablets at once.[3] Therefore teaching parents to keep the medication out of the reach of children cannot be overstressed. If poisoning is suspected, treatment would include gastric lavage, sodium bicarbonate or exchange transfusion.

The nurse has a major responsibility in educating parents to carry out the treatment regimen. She must do this tactfully and within the framework of the family's income, customs and food preferences. The nurse also has a role in helping parents overcome their feeling that they are to blame for their toddler's anemia and to rebuild the wavering confidence they have in their parenting abilities. Positive reinforcement of even minor efforts to comply with the treatment regimen, frequent pointing out of signs of the child's improved health state, and support through regular phone calls or home visits help to restore feelings of parental adequacy. These feelings, in turn, yield greater cooperation for what needs to be done currently and on a long-term basis to resolve the child's anemia and prevent its recurrence.

PICA (GEOPHAGIA)

Pica is the voracious, compulsive ingestion of nonfood substances; eating of dirt is particularly common in children under 4. The peak incidence of pica is 18 to 24 months of age, predominantly in girls. It is also more prevalent in emotionally disturbed and severely mentally retarded children.

Etiology may be benign, resulting from the normal exploration of toddlerhood (hand-to-mouth explorative reflex). Continued or excessive pica, however, is pathological. The pervert-

TABLE 32-2 SUMMARY OF BASIC FEATURES OF FOUR HELMINTHIC INFECTIONS

Features	Roundworm	Pinworm	Tapeworm	Hookworm
Causative agent	*Ascaris lumbricoides*	*Enterobius vermicularis*	*Taenia saginata* or *solium*	*Necator americanus*
Mode of transmission	Ingestion of ova in dirt contaminated by human feces. Hand contamination from infested household dust.	Inhaled from infested air; ingested from hands that had contact with infested anal skin or fomites.	Ingested from handling or eating infested beef or pork.	Penetration of bare feet.
Clinical manifestations	May be asymptomatic. Fever and malaise; restless, disturbed sleep. Abdominal distention and discomfort; vomiting. Anemia. Infested stools; steatorrhea; intestinal obstruction. Peritonitis.	Perianal itch. Nose picking. Restless and irritable.	Varied symptoms: Abdominal cramping or pain, nervousness, insomnia, anorexia, weight loss. Sometimes asymptomatic.	Severe anemia. Occult blood in feces. Abdominal colic, malnutrition, intestinal or bile duct obstruction. Intestinal mucosa and liver damage.
Diagnostic findings	Positive stool culture for ova and parasites.	Microscopic viewing of parasite on scotch tape strip removed from perianal area.	Positive stool culture for ova and parasites.	Positive stool culture for ova and parasites.
Medical treatment	Piperazine derivative (Antepar).	Piperazine derivative (Antepar) or Povan.	Stabrine or Yomesan.	Tetrachloroethylene or Hexylresorcinal.

ed appetite may be a symptom of hookworm anemia, iron deficiency anemia or other dietary deficiency (usually protein or vitamin C). Pica is sometimes associated with emotional deprivation in children. The cultural practice of pica in adults is imitated by their children in some communities of the mideastern United States. The belief upon which this practice is based is that eating dirt protects one from some diseases, especially during pregnancy.[2]

The persistent practice of pica in children may result in lead poisoning, malnutrition, and visceral larva migrans, and other parasitic infection. Symptoms do not become apparent until the child has ingested dirt over several months. Symptoms appear as a "dirt-eating syndrome" that is characterized by retarded general growth, retarded bone development, hypogonadism and marked hepatosplenomegaly (in 50 per cent of cases).[2] Symptoms of associated disease may also be present.

A history that reveals pica behavior, anorexia related to food or any emotional distress should be thoroughly documented. Physical assessment findings will show skin and mucosal pallor, and red, irregular lines that are broad at one end and fade at the other (produced by larva migrans) may be present. Blood studies usually show hypochromic, microcytic anemia because the ingested dirt or clay interferes with iron absorption. A histological examination of an intestinal biopsy shows vast villous atrophy in most cases.

A diet high in protein, iron and calories usually results in prompt reversal of the dirt-eating syndrome, anemia and villous atrophy. It is essential that the child and parents be warned about the dangers associated with the diseases that are a consequence of continued pica practices. Any underlying etiological or secondary disease is also treated. If the etiology is psychologically based, psychotherapy (play therapy, essentially, with toddlers) is a significant intervention. A great deal of tact must be used by the nurse who explains pica, its consequences and its treatment to caretakers. Cultural factors in the etiology must be considered and the situation presented in a manner that does not judge or condemn the beliefs behind the practice but rather helps the parents see the serious consequences of continuing the practice.

PARASITIC INFECTIONS

Parasitic infections are much less common in the United States, because of better sanitation and the greater emphasis on hygiene, than in the third world countries. However, the nurse

Cycle of Parasitic Infection Between Child and the Environment

- Larvae feed and mature in the intestine
- Adult parasites breed and deposit ova in the intestine
- Ova, larvae expelled in feces
- House without running water, toilets, or sewage system
- Water from handwashing, containing parasites, poured to earth outside
- Feces deposited in earth near house
- Damp, warm earth contaminated by ova and larvae of parasites
- Children play in dirt, fail to wash hands, don't wear shoes
- Ova and larvae enter child via ingestion or skin penetration
- Larvae migrate through blood vessels and lymph to enter the lung, where they are coughed up and swallowed, to lodge in the intestine

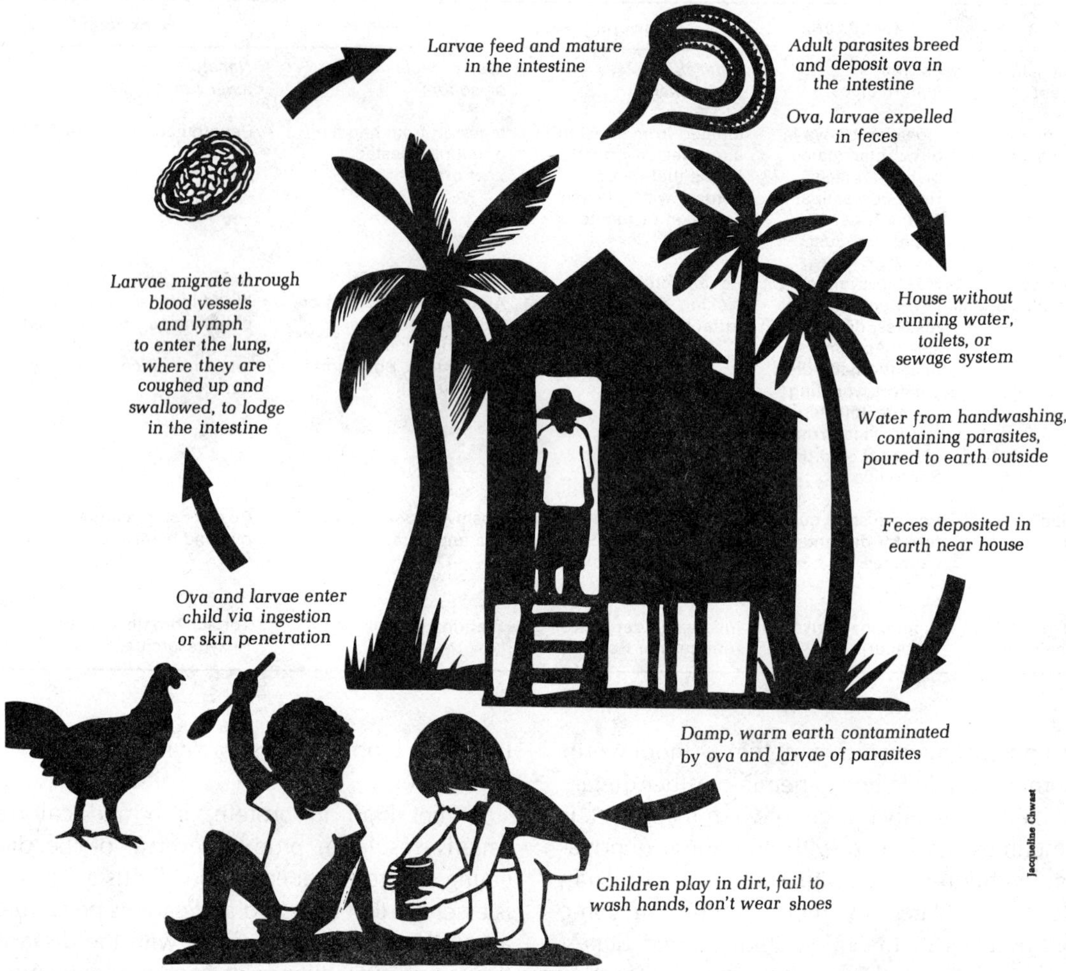

Figure 32–6 Cycle of parasitic infection between child and the environment. (From L. Malarky, Ridding School Children of Parasites—A community approach. Copyright 1979, American Journal of Nursing Company. Reprinted with permission from MCN, The American Journal of Maternal Child Nursing, Nov/Dec 1979. Drawing by Jacqueline Chwast.)

who works with migrants from temperate climates, with immigrants to the United States (Vietnamese, Cubans) or with impoverished Americans, especially in the southern states, is likely to have regular acquaintance with parasitic infections. Although these infections can occur in any age group with fairly equal incidence, this discussion is placed in the chapter on the toddler because of the greater tendency of the toddler for spontaneous hand-to-mouth activities without handwashing, his tendency to play on the ground and go barefoot,* and to investigate dirt with his hands, mouth and feet.

Helminthic Infections

There are a variety of helminthic infections, but this discussion will cover only four of the most common ones: roundworm, pinworm, tapeworm and hookworm. Table 32–2 describes the main characteristics, the definitive diagnostic findings, and the primary medical treatment of each. Figure 32–6 illustrates the typical cycle of transmission between the child and environment.

A careful environmental and economic history is helpful in establishing the diagnosis and in determining the most realistic approach to nursing intervention in treating and preventing recurrence of these infections. Nursing intervention in the helminthic infections requires strict

---

*Toddlers love to remove their shoes despite caretaker efforts to keep them on. Many times caretakers believe the toddler's feet develop better if he goes barefoot often, and if money is a problem, the use of shoes may be reserved for "going away" occasions, at least until school age.

adherence to enteric isolation and nursing measures to relieve accompanying symptoms. The nurse's more critical role, however, lies in educating the child and his family as to the cause of the infection and the measures that can be taken to prevent further infestations. Teaching about handwashing and personal hygiene is a first step. Community health nurse involvement to explore the family's environment and to identify the source(s) of infestation is usually essential to planning and motivating appropriate change so that the child is not reinfested. Because lack of sanitation facilities and overcrowding are frequently factors in the etiology, government involvement also becomes necessary and may require prompting from nurses and other health and social providers who can exert united political pressure.

Roundworm (Ascariasis) Occurring mostly in the southern United States, ascariasis can be a chronic infection of the small intestine. Ova are usually ingested from hands that have contacted contaminated dust or soil or from inadequately cleansed raw fruits or vegetables. The ova live in the small intestine and, when the larvae stage is reached, penetrate the intestinal villi and enter the portal circulation. Reaching the lungs, the larvae rise to the oropharynx and are swallowed, settling in the small intestine to mature to adult worms. Enough adult worms may accumulate to cause intestinal obstruction, or they may migrate to the appendix, causing perforation and peritonitis. Treatment includes antihelminthic drugs, enteric isolation and relief of symptoms. Prevention involves careful washing of raw fruits and vegetables, regular hygiene and handwashing and improvement of sanitation facilities or practices or both.

Pinworm (Oxyuriasis) Approximately 10 per cent of the American population is estimated to have pinworm infestation.[14] It occurs more in Caucasians.

Pinworms are a benign intestinal infection; the parasite is either swallowed (transfer of ova from hand to mouth after scratching anus or handling infected fomites such as undergarments, toilet seats, linens) or inhaled while handling infested clothes or linens. The adult worms inhabit the rectum and colon. They migrate to the perianal region to lay their ova during the child's sleep, causing intense itching. Treatment of each family member with an antihelmintic and disinfecting of clothing and linens is necessary. Prevention includes frequent changing of undergarments and bed linens, daily disinfection of public toilets and routine use of hygienic practices.

Tapeworm A nonfatal parasitic infection, tapeworm results from the ingestion of the tapeworm heads in improperly cared for or inadequately cooked beef or pork. The head settles in the small intestine and lengthens by generating segments. It is regurgitated to the stomach and migrates from there to the brain or eye to form cysts. Prevention involves careful handwashing after handling meat and thorough cooking of the meat before eating it.

Hookworm This worm thrives in the warm, sandy soil of the southern United States, especially where sanitation is inadequate. The worms penetrate the bare feet, causing a local dermatitis that may go unnoticed. Traveling through the lymph and blood systems to the lungs, the worm migrates to the throat, is swallowed and attaches to the walls of the small intestine. After sucking blood from the intestinal walls for several weeks, ova are produced. Although hookworms are seldom fatal, heavily infested children may show retarded mental and physical development.[1] Treatment is provided for the entire family and includes an antihelminthic, a diet high in protein and iron to correct the associated anemia, and improvement of sanitary conditions. Prevention includes routine personal hygiene, avoidance of going barefoot and adequate sanitary facilities and practices.

Fungal Infections

More than 60 fungi are known to be pathogenic in man. This discussion is limited to those causing ringworm and histoplasmosis. Permanent resistance is not developed to fungal infections; therefore the nurse is likely to see mycoses (fungal disease) often in her practice.

Ringworm Several different closely related fungi are known to cause ringworm, which is a general term for mycotic disease of the keratinizing areas (nails, scalp, skin) of the body. Tinea capitis and tinea corporis are described here.

TABLE 32-3 MANAGEMENT OF RINGWORM AND ASSOCIATED SYMPTOMS

Tinea Capitis	Tinea Corporis	All Ringworm Forms
1. Clip hair short and thoroughly wash daily. 2. Do not use towel more than once before laundering. 3. If a pillow is used, change pillowslip daily. 4. Avoid use of headgear till lesions healed. 5. Apply cold compresses to any oozing or swollen lesions.	1. Bathe thoroughly daily, removing scabs or crusts before applying medication. 2. Avoid heat, moisture and trauma during treatment, as these cause increased inflammation and pruritus. 3. Change towels, clothing and linens daily. 4. Wear nonocclusive clothing until lesions healed. 5. Distract child from scratching or picking at lesions.	1. Exclusion from gym, public showers and pools. 2. Apply an antifungal agent containing holoprogin, tolnaftate, or salicylic acid after shampooing or bathing (e.g., Tinactin or Viaform ointment). Do not apply to highly inflamed lesions, Usually prescribed for 1 to 3 weeks. 3. For extensive or topical resistant ringworm, give 6 wks. course of oral griseofulvin (antifungal antibiotic). Should be given after meals which should be high in fat content. Child should not be given phenobarbital. Blood anti-coagulating action is decreased by griseofulvin.

Tinea pedis (athlete's foot; ringworm of feet) is described in Chapter 50.

Tinea Capitis (Scalp Ringworm) Ringworm of the scalp is an ancient disease with worldwide incidence. The greatest susceptibility is in young boys (rare after puberty) from urban areas.[10] The fungus is transferred from infected animals or humans and from contaminated fomites (combs, hats).

The infection begins with a pimple and spreads to form a round sharply outlined area in which hairs exist but have dried and broken off just above the skin. One or several such lesions may exist. The scalp varies from being mildly erythematous and slightly scaly to being affected with a painful, deep, boggy and swollen inflammation called a *kerion*. The child's condition is communicable as long as the lesion(s) exists.

Diagnosis is positive if Wood's light shone on the scalp results in fluorescence of tinea capitis organisms or if a microscopic examination of scales or hairs treated with 10 per cent KOH reveals the fungi. A culture is required to determine the specific species of fungus causing the infection.

Table 32–3 describes the management of the infection and associated symptoms. The nurse's approach to the child and family is crucial to the feelings they experience. Careful explanation of the cause helps diminish parents' feelings that they have not kept their child clean enough. Their cooperation should be enlisted to help identify the source of the infection. Animals the child has contact with should be carefully inspected for evidence of ringworm lesions. The child's playmates and siblings should also be examined since children tend to share personal articles during play, making transfer more likely. The nurse and parents together can teach and reinforce that personal articles such as combs, brushes, barrettes and headgear are not playthings and should not be interchanged among siblings or playmates.

Tinea Corporis (Body Ringworm) Body ringworm also has a higher incidence in young boys and is more prevalent in rural, humid climates. This fungus infects nonhairy skin surfaces. The lesions are usually asymptomatic and appear in a flat, annular or arcuate shape. There is scaling and erythema of the border with a clear central area; the border may also contain vesicles. The lesions are contagious as long as they exist. Diagnosis is by microscopic examination and culture of scales or scabs. As with tinea capitis, parents should be approached in a nonaccusing manner that does not suggest they are inadequate parents, and their help should be solicited in finding the source. See Table 32–3 for a discussion of treatment.

Histoplasmosis Caused by *Histoplasma capsulatum*, a fungus found predominantly in soil with high organic content (e.g., chicken coops, composts) in the central United States, histoplasmosis can occur in persons of all ages. This fungus is not transmitted from human to human; airborne spores are inhaled in dust contaminated by the fungus and settle in the lungs. The disease may be (1) asymptomatic and benign, (2) symptomatic but benign or (3) acute, progressive and disseminated, producing serious systemic disease.

Asymptomatic Benign Histoplasmosis. This form of the disease is detected only by a positive histoplasmin test. The primary lung lesions created by the fungus calcify without causing any symptoms. No treatment is indicated.

Symptomatic Benign Histoplasmosis Symptoms are general and may appear as mild respiratory illness or temporary general malaise. The child may complain of some weakness and chest pain. A low-grade fever and dry or productive cough are usually present. Recovery is slow but spontaneous. Treatment involves symptomatic relief of fever and cough.

Acute Progressive Disseminated Histoplasmosis This form of the disease is most prevalent in infants and toddlers. The course is rapid and, left untreated, the disease is fatal. Symptoms include a high sepsis-related fever, prostration, hepatosplenomegaly, skin ulcers and mucosal purpura, atypical pneumonitis and often anemia.

Diagnosis is tentative when a serologic test for serum antihistoplasma antibody (histoplasmin test) is positive. Diagnosis can be made quickly when the fungus can be seen in Giemsa- or Wright-stained smears of sputum, bone marrow, blood or ulcerative exudate. Definitive diagnosis depends on culturing the fungus from these smear sources, but a longer time is required to learn the findings from culture than from the serologic test, so treatment is usually begun before the results of the report of the culture findings are known.

Management usually involves hospitalization so the course of the disease can be closely monitored. Wound isolation is initiated and amphotericin B (Fungizone) or a triple sulfonamide suspension or both is administered. All family members should be evaluated and infected members treated. Treatment of symptoms is also initiated. With prompt treatment recovery does occur. Parents will need emotional support as they learn the cause and potential seriousness of their child's disease. They should be educated as to the etiology of the disease and encouraged to take preventive precautions such as wearing a mask while inside chicken coops, periodically cleaning and spraying the coop and surrounding soil with 3 per cent formalin spray to reduce dust, and fencing in compost areas. Parents should be urged to keep their infant or toddler, who is more susceptible to the serious form of the disease, away from these sites of potential contamination.

Rickettsial Infections

Two fairly common rickettsial infections — Q fever and Rocky Mountain spotted fever — are discussed. These diseases can affect all ages; toddlers are susceptible because they tend to spend a lot of time crawling, sitting and playing on the ground, making them readily accessible to infected ticks, which are a major source of rickettsial disease.

Q Fever This is an acute febrile disease of sudden onset. Major reservoirs from which humans contract this disease are ticks, farm animals or raw milk from them, and dust. There is much variability in the severity and duration of symptoms, which include chills, diaphoresis, headache and malaise. Pneumonitis symptoms of cough and chest pain exist without any upper respiratory involvement. Diagnosis is made from a positive complement fixation or agglutination test. Oral tetracycline is given for this disease and is continued for 7 to 10 days after the fever dissipates. A person who has had Q fever develops permanent immunity. Immunization is also available and should be given to those at high risk for exposure. Prevention is an important aspect of nursing care in areas where Q fever seems to be prevalent. Preventive action should include education regarding sources of the rickettsiae and concerning the practice of appropriate hygienic measures in potential reservoir areas (e.g., animal barns and sheds). Parents should be cautioned not to give their children unpasteurized milk.

Rocky Mountain Spotted Fever This disease is caused by *Rickettsia rickettsii* and is transmitted to man via tick bite. The incidence is highest in the Kentucky mountains, the Carolinas and in the Cape Cod area during spring and summer.

However, in recent years as many as 15 or 20 cases have been documented in each of the midwestern states. Persons who contract this disease may be asymptomatic or seriously ill; there is a 20 to 50 per cent mortality in untreated cases. The clinical picture is a sudden onset of symptoms that include fever (lasts two to three weeks), headache, chills, conjunctivitis and severe myalgia (muscle pain) of wrists, ankles and forearms that precedes a rash by two to four days. The rash, if recognized, can be life saving. Typically it begins with macular and papular lesions that are pink and blanchable. These progressively cover the palms, soles, trunk and face within 24 hours. After 24 hours the rash turns red and is palpable, and petechiae are visible in the rash. By the fourth day the rash is no longer blanchable, has progressed to purpuric vesicles (small blood-filled sacs or wheals) and has extended to involve the scrotum or vulva. If treatment has not been initiated by this time, ulcers and gangrene can develop on the fingertips, nose and earlobes.

Aside from identification of the characteristic rash, diagnosis is made from a positive Weil-Felix test. However, this test requires 24 to 48 hours to obtain results. Treatment should be initiated if the clinical picture suggests this disease rather than waiting for test results, since waiting could prove fatal. Treatment involves five days of oral tetracycline or chloramphenicol or both. Penicillin is ineffective and sulfonamides worsen the symptoms. Begun early in the course of the disease, treatment favors a good prognosis; if extreme vasculitis involving the brain, heart or kidneys or of all these has evolved, treatment is unlikely to be effective.[10] Persons who survive the disease have permanent immunity.

Because of the critical factor of identifying this disease early, nurses should play a major role in educating the public regarding the clinical manifestations and the incidence in that locale. Preventing children from playing in high reservoir areas is a significant preventive action. When the disease is contracted, parents need much help from the nurse to work through the guilt feelings they are likely to experience and to cope with the potential seriousness of the disease. They should be kept continuously informed of their child's status and involved in his care as much as possible.

Amebiasis

Amebiasis, or amebic dysentery, is a disease of the large intestine as a consequence of mucosal invasion by pathologic protozoa. Reservoirs of transfer to humans include flies, contaminated water or raw vegetables and fruits, and hand-to-mouth transfer from contact with an infected person's stool. The disease occurs primarily in underdeveloped areas when sanitation is lacking and in temperate climates.

Symptoms vary depending on the degree of mucosal necrosis. The disease may be asymptomatic and resolve spontaneously after several days or remain at a carrier level. Carriers may fail to gain weight and be slightly anemic. Symptoms may be relatively mild, with diarrhea and mild cramping that alternates with constipation and bloating, accompanied by alternating anorexia and ravenous appetite, each lasting a few hours or days. A more severe picture appears in some children who experience an amebic enteritis characterized by colic and foul and watery stools containing blood and pus. If these stools reach a frequency of from 15 to 30 during 24 hours, true amebic dysentery exists. A serious complication of this disease is extension of the protozoa directly or via the bloodstream to cause abscesses of the liver, lungs or brain.

Diagnosis is made by identifying cysts in a fecal or lesion exudate smear. Various amebicides may be used to treat amebiasis, common ones being tetracycline, Milibis or Flagyl. The child is infective until the organism no longer appears in the feces, which is usually within 72 hours after therapy is initiated. Complete cure usually takes a couple of weeks; however, fecal smear should be repeated for three months to ensure elimination of the organism. Family members should also be evaluated and treated if infected. Enteric isolation is necessary until feces remain negative for the organism. The remainder of treatment is symptomatic and supportive. Preventive measures include personal hygiene education, pest control, adequate sanitation and chlorination of water supplies.

Shigellosis

Shigellosis, or bacillary dysentery, is an acute bacterial disease of the large intestine. Two-thirds of cases occur in children under 10; it is especially prevalent in toddlers. The incidence is greater in the summer. Persons from lower socioeconomic areas, in institutions or who practice poor personal hygiene are at greater risk.

Caused by any one of four groups of Shigella organisms, the disease is transmitted by the fecal-oral route, hence the lay term "hand-to-mouth disease." The organisms may be passed as a result of direct contact with an infected patient or carrier or indirectly from contact with flies or objects contaminated with infected feces, or by consuming fecally contaminated food or water.

The severity of symptoms varies widely, ranging from asymptomatic disease to serious illness. Mild disease results in daily passage of a few more stools than normal, lasting only a couple of days. The onset may be characterized by sudden fever, anorexia and gastrointestinal upset, followed hours later by diarrhea. The diarrhea is at first watery and green, then changes to bloody, mucous stools; their frequency increases to 10 or 20 a day. Dehydration and electrolyte imbalance can occur quickly, progressing to renal failure if not treated promptly. Untreated, symptoms persist two to three weeks, then subside. Severe cases are manifested by sudden high fever, convulsions and delirium, and meningitis-like symptoms. Stools contain blood, pus and mucus and are explosive.

Diagnosis is made from the symptomatic history, environmental history and culturing of the Shigella organism from a stool specimen. All cases must be reported to local health departments so that contact follow-up (epidemiological investigation) may be conducted.

Treatment involves killing the organisms with antibacterial drugs; ampicillin is usually given until the specific organism has been identified by culture. The drug is given orally in mild disease but intramuscularly or parenterally in more acute disease. Fluid and electrolyte replacement is necessary in all but mild cases of the disease. Oral intake of food and fluid is contraindicated for the first 24 to 48 hours, then gradually progressed through the typical diarrhea diet routine (see Chapter 23). Strict isolation is maintained until cultures are negative for the Shigella organisms, which is generally 5 to 7 days. Treatment of symptoms is also initiated.

This extremely uncomfortable, isolated child will need the supportive presence of his parents and a primary nurse. The toddler who has just mastered toilet training will need reassurance that his bowel incontinence is from the disease and is not his fault, and that it will eventually stop. If possible, the toddler should be able to observe his caretakers (parents, nurse, doctor) from a window before they put on isolation attire and watch them while they put on the gown, mask and gloves. This reassures him that they are not strange monsters, but rather people he knows.

Preventive education involves proper sanitary and hygiene practices and instruction in clean, safe ways to handle food. Environmental improvement of sanitary facilities, pest control and water purification are also necessary to prevent Shigella epidemics in communities.

References

1. A. Benenson, ed. Control of Communicable Diseases in Man. American Public Health Association, 1975
2. I. Dogramaci. Gastrointestinal disorders. In Pediatrics, by M. Ziai, Little, Brown & Co., 1975
3. W. Fletcher. The recalcitrant anemias. A paper prepared for nursing students, Goshen College, 1969
4. J. Hughes. Synopsis of Pediatrics. C.V. Mosby Co., 1979
5. M. Kadkhoda et al. Congenital dislocation of the hip: diagnostic screening and treatment: a comparative study of two populations of infants and children. Clinical Pediatrics, November 1976, p. 159
6. J. Kelsey et al. The incidence and distribution of slipped capital femoral epiphysis in Connecticut and Southwestern United States. Journal of Bone and Joint Surgery, January 1970, p. 1203
7. G. Knittel and L. Staheli. The effectiveness of shoe modification for intoeing. Orthopedic Clinics of North America, Jul/Aug 1976, p. 1019
8. H. Latham and R. Heckel. Pediatric Nursing. C.V. Mosby Co., 1977
9. W. McDade. Bowlegs and knock knees. Pediatric Clinics of North America, November 1977, p. 825
10. J. Parrish. Dermatology and Skin Care. McGraw-Hill Book Co., 1975
11. R. Pitkow. External rotation contractures of the extended hip. Clinical Orthopedics, 1975, p. 139
12. F. Porter. Anemia. In Pediatrics by M. Ziai, Little, Brown & Co., 1975
13. L. Staheli. Torsional deformity. Pediatric Clinics of North America, November 1977, p. 799
14. N. Welsh. Recent insight into the childhood "social diseases" — gonorrhea, scabies, pediculosis, pinworms. Clinical Pediatrics, April 1978, p. 318
15. M. Ziai, ed. Pediatrics. Little, Brown & Co., 1975

Additional Recommended Reading

S. Cohen. Skin rashes in infants and children. American Journal of Nursing, June 1978, p. 1041

L. Malarkey. Ridding school children of parasites — a community approach. American Journal of Maternal Child Nursing, Nov-Dec 1979, p. 363

J. McMillan et al. The Whole Pediatrician Catalog. W. B. Saunders Co., 1977

P. Meservey. Congenital musculoskeletal abnormalities. Comprehensive Pediatric Nurse, Nov/Dec 1977, p. 14

P. Pipes. Nutrition In Infancy and Childhood. C.V. Mosby, 1977

C. Reid, Pica — a common symptom of iron deficiency, the compulsive eating of substances. New Zealand Journal of Medical Laboratory Technology, March 1979, p. 1

L. Robinson et al. Iron therapy: helps and hazards. Pediatric Nurse, Nov/Dec 1978, p. 9

When you suspect iron deficiency anemia. Patient Care, 15 May 1979, p. 174

P. Wilson. Iron deficiency anemia. *In* Nursing of Children and Adolescents by A. O'Connor, ed., American Journal of Nursing Co., 1975

C. Woodruff. Iron deficiency in infancy and childhood. Pediatric Clinics of North American, February 1977, p. 85

POTENTIAL STRESSES DURING TODDLER YEARS: REVERSIBLE ALTERATIONS IN HEALTH STATUS

INTRODUCTION

by Linda Mowad, RN, BSN

Certain conditions during the toddler years occur with little or no warning, imposing physiological and psychosocial stress on the child and the family. Three of these potential stressors that are of particular relevance to the toddler are considered in this chapter: burns, ingestions and croup. The degree to which the toddler and his family are able to adapt to them determines the reversibility of these potentially life-threatening conditions. In its broadest sense the role of the nurse is to facilitate this adaptation.

During the toddler years there is a slowing down of the rate of physical growth. The child is stronger physically and is developing motor abilities that he uses to explore his world. He is discovering a separate identity and striving for autonomy. His curiosity and desire for independence are manifested in his continuous explorations and experimentations. Wanderings away from his mother increase in time and distance. He exerts his independence in a variety of ways, not the least of which is the characteristic negativism of the toddler.

Simultaneously parents are developing more security in their roles and are relaxing some of the constraints they imposed on the child as an infant. Without a clear understanding of growth and development, they may not realize that the toddler lacks the cognitive abilities and judgment needed to protect himself from accidents or illnesses originating from his explorations.

On the other hand, parents may be acutely aware of the potential hazards associated with the toddler's independence and may impose restrictions that could hamper his development. A balance is needed so that the toddler can exert his independence in order to achieve autonomy within an adequately structured environment so that his safety is not threatened.

Unfortunately, the nurse usually has few opportunities to assist parents in learning how to create this balance prior to an actual accident or illness. During toddler years the number of well-child visits declines, and community health nursing visits aimed at assisting the parenting process are the exception rather than the rule.

Once an accident or illness does arise the nurse's role is to decrease stress and facilitate adaptation. According to stress theory the physiologic response to stress occurs in three phases: alarm, resistance, which is when adaptation takes place, and finally exhaustion, when the organism can no longer adapt.[24] (Managing stress is discussed in Chapter 16.) Hence this period following an illness or injury, when the body is physically responding and adapting to stress, may be an excellent time to provide information that families need for psychosocial adaptation and prevention of future accidents. Following adaptation, there is some change in an organism. The nurse's goal for this change is to aid in developing a healthier life style.

DECREASING STRESS

The suddenness of the reversible conditions mentioned imposes much stress on the toddler and his family, disrupting the life with which they have grown to feel secure. Often emergency physical care must take precedence; this care can place severe restrictions on the toddler and possibly separate him from his family. Whenever possible, even during the emergency phase of treatment, every effort should be made to decrease this stress.

Parents should be encouraged to stay with their children and to participate in their care to the extent possible. They need to be encouraged to reassure their children by their presence and their touch and tone of voice, especially when the child is restrained. Toddlers become frustrated easily and tolerate restraint poorly. Every attempt should be made to minimize the amount of time they are restrained. Nurses should provide reassurance for the family. The nurse's soft, low-toned voice, eye contact and physical contact can do much to reassure an anxious parent and the child.

The toddler, because of his limited ability to express himself verbally, needs to have his fears put into words for him and responded to in an appropriate fashion. Some of the toddler's fears include fear of abandonment, the unknown, pain, and bodily invasion and restraint, especially in the back-lying position.[5, 23] His response to these fears will be varied; he may be cooperative, although more often he will attempt to resist interventions. Parents may blame themselves for the child's condition. They fear for their toddler's life, yet feel helpless to do anything for him. The nurse should avoid any statements of judgment or blame that would reinforce parental guilt, leaving the parents ineffective in supporting the child. Rather, the nurse can help relieve guilt by praising the parents for getting prompt help for their child and for any first aid measures taken before getting the child to the emergency room, clinic, or doctor's office. They should be informed that their presence, physical contact and familiar soothing voice and words are the most valuable therapy they can offer their child during emergency treatment and the period after. These simple measures taken by the nurse help immensely in relieving parental anxiety and helplessness.

Each procedure should be explained to the child immediately before it is done.[23] This explanation should be simple enough for the child to understand but brief and accurate. Parents should be instructed about procedures in the depth appropriate to their understanding. A conscious effort should be made to show respect for them and for their ability to make decisions for their child even when he is acutely ill.

FACILITATING ADAPTATION

After initial measures are completed and the child's condition is stabilized, the nurse's attention should turn to how she can facilitate adaptation to health, whether the child is sent home or admitted to the hospital. Specific aspects of care of the hospitalized toddler are discussed in Chapter 36.

After the initial shock of a child's sudden illness or injury, parents may feel anxiety, continuing fear and guilt, a sense of failure and insecurity. According to Jay,[13] parents need to go through a "role revision" when their children become ill suddenly. This is characterized by three stages: *grieving, mimicking* (sometimes of the nurse's behavior) and *identity*. Initially they may be afraid to see or touch their child, yet the child's dependence on touch increases at these times. The child is insecure, experiencing fear and frustration. He is in need of his parents' love and presence.

The nurse needs to help the parents express

their feelings and fears and to understand that these are normal. Individuals differ in their reactions, and care should be taken to accept these reactions in a nonjudgmental fashion. Parents should hold their child and participate fully in his care as soon as they feel ready. Instructions on what to expect and how to care for the child will help the parents adapt. Written instructions should be provided, since people under stress frequently forget what they are told.

The toddler needs to regain control of his world as soon as is reasonably possible. Even during emergency treatment he may be given simple choices.

Parent teaching and follow-up is essential to help counteract the tendency of the parents to withdraw the toddler's independence. They need to be encouraged to restructure the child's activities and environment. Home visits should be made by a community health nurse to individualize the teaching and assist parents with specific areas of concern, as well as in methods of teaching safety to their children. *Often accidents or illnesses are a manifestation of family dysfunction.* A home visit by a community health nurse or referral to a social welfare agency may help pinpoint sources of problems and provide alternatives, including encouraging the family to seek support and other resources to gain the knowledge necessary to maximize their child's growth and development.

THE CHILD WITH BURNS

by Claudella Archambeault-Jones, RN
and Irving Feller, MD

A severe burn — few other injuries happen so frequently to children or are as traumatic for everyone involved. Few other injuries are as debilitating or require such extended periods of hospitalization and extensive rehabilitation. However, few other catastrophic injuries offer the possibility of full recovery.

Burns and fires are the third leading cause of accidental death in the United States, exceeded only by motor vehicle accidents and falls. For children in the age group 1 to 14 years, burns are the leading cause of accidental death in the home. The highest incidence of burns in children occurs in 1- and 2-year-olds (Fig. 33-1); the incidence is closely related to the amount and adequacy of adult supervision and to the level of emotional stress in the home.

Sixty per cent of burns to children aged 4 and under are scalds, occurring in the home; 70 per cent of burns to children aged 5 and over are by flame. Any child who receives a significant burn must face, after recovery, a long series of rehospitalizations (to adulthood) for reconstruction procedures, both functional and cosmetic. Burned skin that has healed or been grafted does not grow at the same rate as underlying tissue and bone.[9]

The International Bibliography on Burns, published yearly from 1969 to 1980 by the National Institute for Burn Medicine, Ann Arbor, contains reference citations for all literature on burn medicine.

Care of the child with burns requires (1) sufficient knowledge and experience to identify the severity of the injury, (2) an understanding of the principles of burn care and (3) a close monitoring of all aspects of care. The nurse must also give special consideration to the child's place in a family and the family's role in the child's survival and quality of life thereafter.

In thinking of the care required to treat burns, we must first consider the primary body organ system involved, which is the skin. The skin is the body's largest organ, providing an intact anatomical barrier against infection and loss of body fluids. The skin also helps control body temperature. A vast capillary network is located in the skin, as are nerve endings, hair follicles, and sweat and sebaceous glands. Body image is also related to an intact skin covering.

The skin's functions are either diminished when the skin and its support systems are damaged (when there is a partial-thickness injury) or destroyed (when there is full-thickness injury). The trauma of the burn results in a decrease or complete loss of two of the most important functions of the skin: protection against infection and prevention of loss of body fluids. The nurse's role is to help protect the child until these functions of the skin can be regained. However, once the child has recovered physical function of the skin, the loss of

> ### TEACHING BURN PREVENTION TO CAREGIVERS: EFFECTIVE MEASURES
>
> **In the kitchen**
> 1. DON'T leave children unattended when you are cooking.
> 2. DON'T cook on front burners. Don't leave hot pans or food or liquids unattended on range, countertops or tables. Don't leave handles extending over the edge of a stove or countertop.
> 3. DON'T leave cords to electrical cooking appliances dangling. Children can grab them and receive severe burns from the spilled hot liquids and solids.
> 4. DON'T let young children pour or serve hot food or liquids. Keep them out of reach.
> 5. DON'T pour hot coffee, tea, soup or other liquids at the table and leave them unattended.
> 6. DON'T drink coffee, tea, soup, or other hot liquids with a child on your lap—one slip or a sudden darting hand is all it takes to cause a serious scald.
>
> **In the bathroom**
> 1. DON'T place a child in a tub of water until you have checked its temperature. The skin of a 1- or 2-year-old is tender and vulnerable to scalds. Use the back of your hand to check the temperture. The water should feel warm, not hot.
> 2. DON'T leave a child in the tub unattended. Many scalds occur when the child or his brother or sister turns on the hot water while playing.
>
> **In the bedroom**
> 1. DON'T leave a hot steam vaporizer close enough to a child's crib or bed so that it might be tipped or pulled over.
> 2. DON'T leave the cord of the vaporizer dangling where it might be tripped over and cause the child to be burned.
>
> **In general**
> 1. DO install smoke detectors.
> 2. DON'T store gasoline or other lighter fluids in open containers. Store these in proper receptacles high enough so children can't reach them. Better yet, don't store them at all; buy only in quantities you will use at one time and replace when needed again.
> 3. DON'T store matches and lighters where toddlers can reach them.
> 4. DO teach children 5 and older the proper use of matches.
> 5. DON'T allow lit candles to burn unattended.
> 6. DON'T store cleaning chemicals where children can reach them. Don't buy giant-size supplies; buy only enough for a one-time use and replenish as needed.
> 7. DON'T misuse extension cords or allow electrical appliances near water taps.
> 8. DO follow the recommendations of the local fire department for house checks and exit procedures, and teach these to children.

normal appearance and the pleasure-pain sensations and the change in body appearance can complicate rehabilitation.

Assessing the Severity of the Burn

All burns are not alike. Severity is influenced by five inter-related factors: (1) size of burn, (2) depth of burn, (3) age of the child, (4) medical history of the child and (5) part of the body injured and concurrent injuries. For example, a relatively minor burn (under 10 per cent total body area) in a child with a history of heart or renal problems would be serious enough for hospitalization.

Size of Burn Burn size is expressed as a percentage of the total body area. Two basic methods may be used to determine burn size. The *rule of nines* (Fig. 33–2) is frequently used because it is simple and quick, but it is not totally accurate, especially with small children.

The second method requires use of explanatory figures and tables and is more accurate because it takes into account the change in proportion of the head and lower extremities with age. For example, for an infant the head equals 19 per cent of the body; in an adult the head equals 7 per cent total body area. This method is referred to as the *estimation of size of burn by per cent* (Fig. 33–3). The nurse assessing burn size must refer to the diagram and to the burn wound to map out the injury accurately. Underestimation may result in inadequate treatment. Overestimation can result in overzealous therapy, especially in a child, in a person with cardiac problems or respiratory injury, or in an older person.

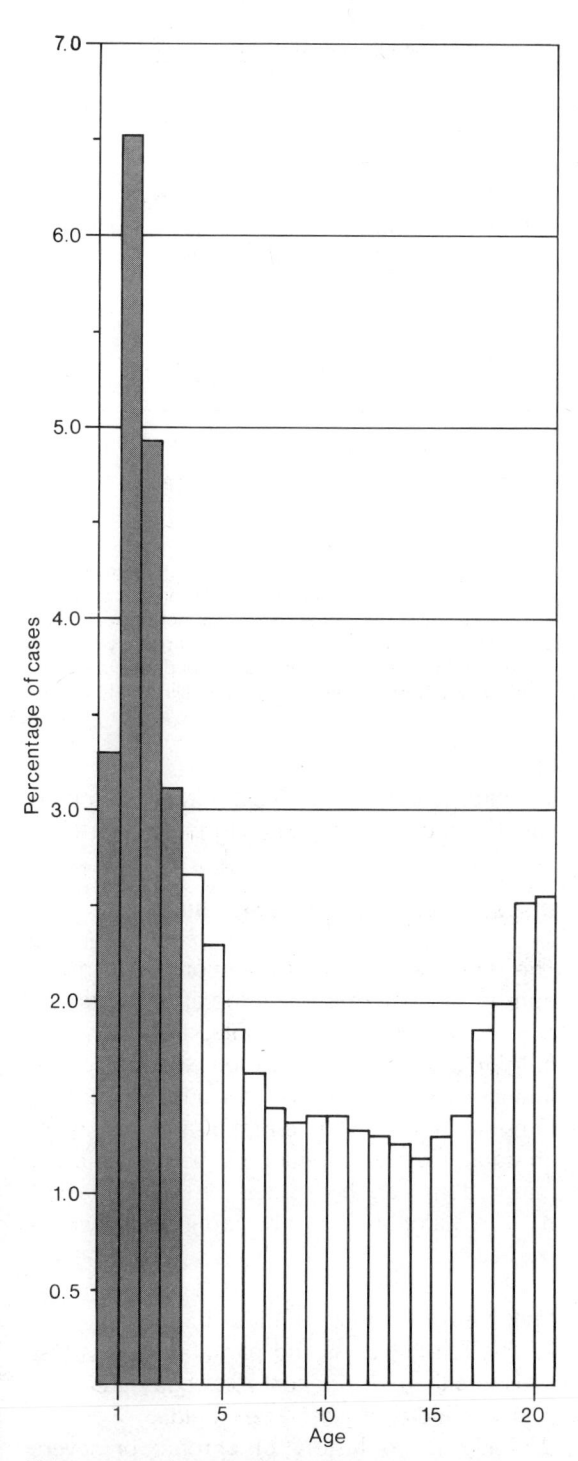

Figure 33-1 Age distribution of victims of severe burns. 45.6 per cent of all burns severe enough to require hospitalization in a specialized burn facility occur to young adults and children under 21. 14.8 per cent happen to toddlers and infants ages 3 and under. (Used with permission of the National Burn Information Exchange.)

Depth of Burn The depth of a burn is expressed in terms of full thickness or partial thickness. The term *partial-thickness burn* means that only part of the skin has been damaged or destroyed. Enough epithelial cells remain in hair follicles and sweat glands are left to grow new skin. This type of wound heals by itself if nothing in treatment causes further damage. The partial-thickness burn is equivalent to the first-degree (superficial epidermal injury) or second-degree (deep epidermal and some dermal injury) burn.

Full-thickness burns are defined as those in which all layers of the skin are destroyed and possibly subcutaneous tissue, muscle and bone, depending upon temperature of and duration of exposure to the burning agent. Regeneration of the skin is *not* possible when there is a full-thickness injury. These wounds must be grafted to provide cover and return normal skin function. They are serious wounds because the body has lost the life-preserving functions of the skin in the burned area. A full-thickness burn wound is equivalent to a third-degree burn. The deeper the burn, the more serious the problem.

The skin of the small child is slightly thinner than that of the adult; therefore a similar insult may result in a more severe injury to the child. The basic principles of evaluation of depth, however, remain the same. Depth of burn is difficult to determine visually. There are signs and symptoms that indicate the level of tissue damaged, but the exact depth of injury can be determined only when spontaneous healing has taken place or granulation tissue has appeared after eschar (dead tissue) removal. Figure 33-4 defines the differences between partial- and full-thickness injury.

Age of Child Age is an important factor in determining severity of injury. Children under 4 have a higher mortality than children of other age groups with similar size injury.[9] Essentially, the problem in the infant and toddler is poor response to infection, leading to septicemia. Infants and children up to age 4 have not developed a strong acquired immunity. In addition, their smaller body mass provides less protein and fat stores for metabolism. Their skin is thinner, so depth of burn is frequently greater than in older children and adults.

Medical History of Child The stress of a severe burn will exacerbate any existing disease process, which will in turn increase mortality. In a child, the presence of a major growth-retarding anomaly such as congenital heart disease, or

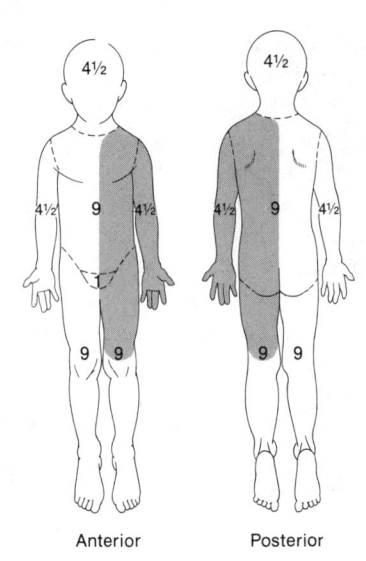

Calculation of Extent of Burn			
Body Part	Ant.	Post.	Total
Head	4½	4½	9
Rt. Upper Extremity	4½	4½	9
Lt. Upper Extremity	4½	4½	9
Trunk	18	18	36
Perineum	1		1
Rt. Lower Extremity	9	9	18
Lt. Lower Extremity	9	9	18
			Total 100%

Figure 33-2 Estimation of size of burn by rule of nines. The head and each entire upper extremity (shoulder to fingertips [glove fashion]) are each given the value of 9 per cent of the body surface. The anterior and posterior trunk are each valued at 18 per cent, as is each leg. The total of these parts is 99 per cent and the perineum is 1 per cent to make 100 per cent. This method may be used visually at the accident scene or in the emergency room to estimate the size burn quickly; however, it does not allow for the difference in proportion of head and lower extremities of the various ages. (Redrawn from I. Feller et al. Emergency Care of the Burn Victim. National Institute for Burn Medicine, Ann Arbor, MI, 1977.)

failure to thrive, complicates the burn. Unknown diseases may also complicate the burn; symptoms of these must be detected and the underlying cause treated simultaneously with the burn.

A dependable history for a child is best taken from the family or from the child's pediatrician. Information to be obtained and prominently recorded includes a history of (1) recent or past illnesses, chronic and severe; (2) dependence upon life-sustaining medication; (3) allergies to food or medicine (especially penicillin); (4) symptoms that may indicate latent and undetected diseases; and (5) events leading to the injury.

Part of Body Injured and Concurrent Injuries The part of the body injured is the fifth factor contributing to severity. Burns of the head, neck and chest lead to increase incidence of pulmonary problems. Burns of the perineum are prone to early infection. These areas are considered critical areas, making the burn affecting them more serious. Circumferential (all the way around) burns of the neck, chest and extremities also contribute to severity. A significant injury sustained in addition to the burn also increases severity (electrical injury, skull fracture, serious abdominal injury or compound fractures). Such injury must be found and treatment instituted during first aid procedures.

Diagnosis of Minor and Major Burns

The difference between a minor and a major burn is also determined by the aforementioned severity factors. For example, a 5 per cent full-thickness burn would be serious for an infant or a child with diabetes but may be only minor for a healthy child of the same age, or for an adult. Certain criteria must be met before a minor burn can be treated on an outpatient basis. A major burn must be admitted to specialized care.

Minor Burn A burn is minor if:
1. The full-thickness and partial-thickness loss is less than 10 per cent total body area.
2. The child is at least 4 years old.
3. There is no history of chronic or severe illness.
4. There are no significant concurrent injuries (e.g., respiratory damage, fractures).
5. The burn does not include the hands, face, feet or perineum, and/or no circumferential injury exists.
6. It is not an electrical injury.

Even when a burn is minor, the child is hospitalized if the family cannot cope with home care or if there is suspicion of abuse or neglect.

Figure 33-3 Estimation of size of burn by per cent. 1, Shade in the diagram to represent the extent of burn, as viewed anteriorly and posteriorly. 2, Circle age closest to that of the patient and use those percentages for the head, thigh and leg to calculate extent of burn. 3, The percentage of total body surface is printed on the diagram for those areas that do not vary with age. The areas that do vary with age are marked with H (head), T (thigh) and L (leg). The extent of the burn is calculated by adding the percentages of each affected area. If a portion of a body part is burned, an approximate fraction of the percentage should be used. (Redrawn from I. Feller et al. Emergency Care of the Burn Victim. National Institute for Burn Medicine, Ann Arbor, MI, 1977.)

Major Burns A burn is classified as major if any of the following conditions exist:

1. The wound covers more than 10 per cent total body area.
2. The wound is full thickness.
3. The child is less than 4 years old.
4. The medical history is positive for chronic or severe illness.
5. There are significant concurrent injuries (respiratory damage, fractures, and so forth).
6. There are burns of the face, hands, feet, or perineum, and/or circumferential injury.
7. It is an electrical injury.

Regardless of the severity of a burn, the child is hospitalized if the family cannot provide adequate home care or if there is suspicion of abuse or neglect.

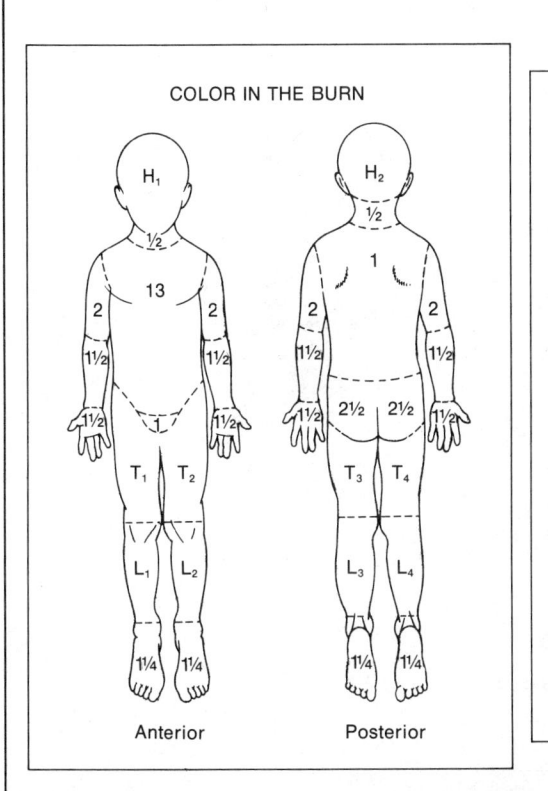

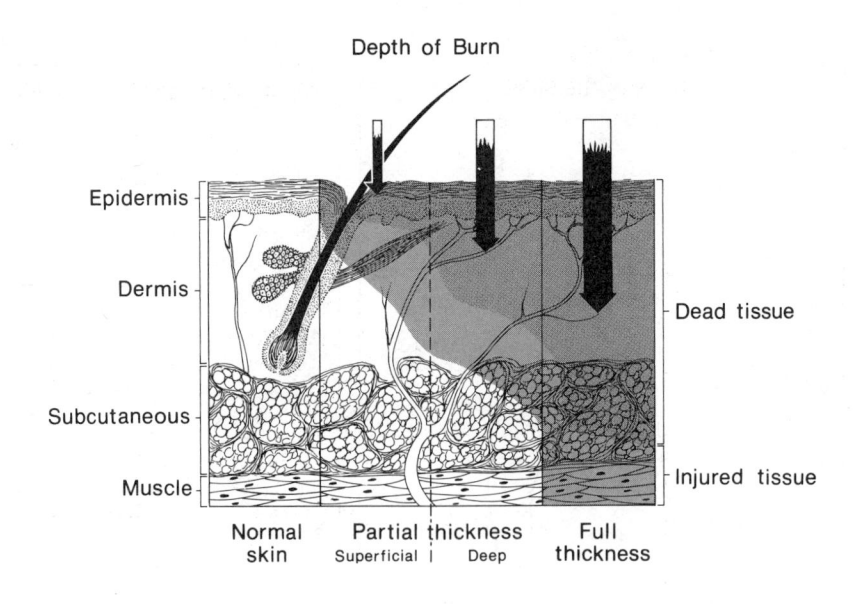

DIFFERENTIAL DIAGNOSIS

PARTIAL–THICKNESS BURN		FULL–THICKNESS BURN
Normal or increased sensitivity to pain and temperature.	Sensation	Anesthetic to pain and temperature.
Large, thick-walled, will usually increase in size.	Blisters	None, or if present, thin-walled and will not increase in size.
Red, will blanch with pressure and refill.	Color	White, brown, black or red. If red, will not blanch with pressure.
Normal or firm.	Texture	Firm or leathery.

Figure 33–4 Differential diagnosis of depth of burn. The arrows represent degree of heat or intensity of burning agent and the time of contact with skin. The darker shaded area represents dead tissue; the lighter shaded area, damaged or injured tissue that will heal with good care. When all tissue (epidermis and dermis) has been destroyed, this is termed full-thickness. Partial-thickness means only part of the skin has been destroyed. Damaged tissue can reheal with good care. (Redrawn from Feller et al. Emergency Care of the Burn Victim. National Institute for Burn Medicine, Ann Arbor, MI, 1977.)

National Burn Information Exchange
Burned Patient Survival By
Age Group - Percent Total Area Burned

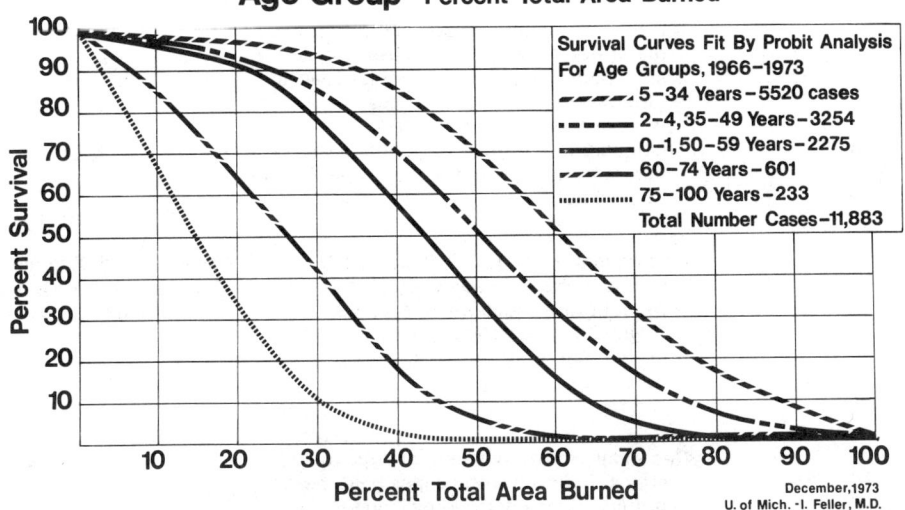

Survival Curves Fit By Probit Analysis
For Age Groups, 1966-1973
- 5-34 Years – 5520 cases
- 2-4, 35-49 Years – 3254
- 0-1, 50-59 Years – 2275
- 60-74 Years – 601
- 75-100 Years – 233
- Total Number Cases – 11,883

December, 1973
U. of Mich. - I. Feller, M.D.

Burn patient survival: age group vs. percentage of total area burned. The two severity factors (age and total area burned) greatly affect chance for survival. It is important, however, to keep in mind that these averages improve with excellence in burn care. (Taken with permission from the National Burn Information Exchange, I. Feller, M.D., Director, Ann Arbor, MI.)

Prognosis in Burns

A major burn requires admission to a hospital providing specialized burn care. This admission must take place as quickly as possible after the burn injury. To ensure proper treatment and a positive outcome, the nurse must be aware of the factors affecting severity and of the hospitals in her home area that provide specialized burn care.

The chances for survival of a particular patient can be affected by the size and depth of burn, the child's age, health status and medical history, part of the body injured and other injuries. Infants with 40 per cent total body area burns have a survival rate of 58 per cent, as contrasted with 2 to 4-year-old patients, who have a survival rate of 70 per cent. Children 5 and over with the same size burn have an expected survival rate of nearly 90 per cent.

The survival rate is lower when a given area contains all full-thickness burn than when the same area includes both partial-thickness and full-thickness burns. With age and area of burn held constant, the larger the percentage of body surface area affected by full-thickness burn, the more serious the injury.

Unlike in many other traumatic injuries, complications are the rule rather than the exception with most severe burns at present. Typically, a child with a severe burn may have four to six major complications, often at the same time, and one or a combination of several may be fatal. The most common complications seen in burn patients are also the most common causes of death.

Recent studies conducted by the National Institute for Burn Medicine and the University of Michigan Department of Biostatistics showed that survival is also related to the hospital in which the patient receives care; survival of children is improved when they are treated in children's hospitals providing specialized burn care.[7]

Basic Burn Care

For a full-thickness burn area, only grafting can decrease the negative metabolic processes and reinstitute skin functions. It is necessary to remove the dead skin and replace it with homografts or autografts as soon as possible, and at the same time detect complications early and treat them vigorously until the grafting can be accomplished. The nurse must be aware of the signs and symptoms of complications and then assist in their control. (See Table 33-1 for a list of complications, their etiology and the period when they typically occur.)

On the basis of the derangements that follow

TABLE 33–1 FREQUENT COMPLICATIONS OF MAJOR BURNS IN CHILDREN

Complication	Etiology	Period When Usually Present
Cardiovascular		
Hypovolemia	Normal inflammatory response to injury in major burns, results in a massive fluid shift from vascular to interstitial spaces (3rd spacing); if untreated, results in hypovolemic shock and death.	Emergent
Hypervolemia	Secondary to overzealous fluid therapy or failure to recognize diuretic phase of fluid replacement.	Emergent
Hypertension	Occurs in at least 1/3 of children with severe burns; etiology unclear, but thought to be secondary to stress. Treated prophylactically with reserpine in burns of greater than 40% total body area.	May occur during any one or all 3 phases; but usually seen in late emergent or early acute.
Renal		
Oliguria	Secondary to hypovolemia or hypovolemic shock. Relieved with proper fluid therapy. If fluid therapy delayed or inadequate, leads to anuria and renal failure. May be seen in acute period secondary to septic shock.	Emergent Acute
Hemomyoglobinuria	Secondary to massive deep full-thickness injury or electrical injury, causing release of myoglobin (muscle protein) and hemoglobin from RBC's. These free globins are then filtered by kidneys and can clog tubules. Sign of this is black urine. Immediate treatment with osmotic diuretic and increased fluids indicated to prevent tubular necrosis or failure.	Emergent
Pulmonary		
Carbon monoxide poisoning	Byproducts of combustion inhaled by burn victim; treatment with oxygen at the scene relieves symptoms.	Emergent
Upper airway obstruction	Secondary to absorption of heat and gases by upper airway; results in edema requiring early intubation. When edema subsides, endotracheal tube can be removed.	Emergent
Primary pulmonary damage	Secondary to lower airway and lung damage by noxious gases. Requires intubation by endotracheal tube. If unrelieved, then tracheostomy. Further treatment may require antibiotics, Aminophylline, cortisone, aerosol antibiotics. Humidified oxygen is indicated for all respiratory involvement.	Emergent
Pulmonary edema (Stiff, wet lungs)	May be secondary to primary pulmonary damage circumferential chest burn causing decreased chest movement,* overzealous fluid therapy and overload or immobility.	Acute
Pulmonary embolus	Usually a very late complication. Clot is released when mobility follows enforced immobility. Heparin used prophylactically.	
Bacterial pneumonia	Lowered resistance secondary to immobility,* decreased chest movement if circumferential chest burn, inhalation irritation. May be secondary to wound or tracheostomy, sepsis or pooled lung fluids.	Acute

*Early activity and turning, coughing, and deep breath exercise are *essential* preventive measures. Escharotomy of circumferential full-thickness burns of chest also indicated.

Table continued on opposite page

TABLE 33-1 FREQUENT COMPLICATIONS OF MAJOR BURNS IN CHILDREN *(Continued)*

Complication	Etiology	Period When Usually Present
Sepsis		
Wound infection	Infection during emergent phase is gram-positive usually staphylococcus as a result of autocontamination; usually treated prophylactically with penicillin. Infection during acute phase is frequently gram-negative *Pseudomonas aeruginosa* secondary to decreased vascular supply to wound, diminished overall immune response and the favorable medium the wound provides—heat, warmth, eschar. Prevention: The University of Michigan Burn Center developed a *Pseudomonas aeruginosa* vaccine and a hyperimmune serum; have been used successfully since 1963 (provide both active and passive coverage.)	Emergent and/or acute
Septicemia	Overwhelming systemic infection secondary to unsuccessful treatment of primary wound infection, or due to invading pathogens at indwelling catheter sites (central lines, urinary, etc.) Early detection is essential for proper therapy.	Acute
Metabolic and electrolyte disturbances		
Paralytic ileus (GI)	Normal response to initial hypovolemic state; usually lasts 2–3 days during which time oral intake is contraindicated. NG tube to intermittent drainage is used to decompress stomach.	Emergent
Weight gain	Secondary to fluid therapy. Child should gain no more than 10% of normal body weight or he risks overload, pulmonary edema or congestive failure.	Emergent
Weight loss	Secondary to catabolism. Requires high calorie, high protein diet. If greater than 20–30% of total body weight is lost, loss can be fatal.	Acute
Hypernatremia	As fluids return to vascular space at end of emergent period, salt also returns. Fluid therapy is changed to D5W or D10W (salt-poor fluids).	Late emergent
Acid-base imbalance	May be secondary to many other complications or result of treatment (e.g., some topical agents).	
Adrenal-cortical insufficiency	Stress response secondary to overwhelming injury; attempt to maintain body equilibrium. Steroids may be indicated.	Emergent and/or acute
Curling's ulcer	Twice as common in children. Stress response of body to overwhelming injury. Routine use of antacids in burn victims has decreased the incidence. If preventive antacid regimen not followed, GI hemorrhage may result. Once wound is healed, incidence is eliminated.	Emergent and acute

Table continued on following page

TABLE 33-1 FREQUENT COMPLICATIONS OF MAJOR BURNS IN CHILDREN (Continued)

Complication	Etiology	Period When Usually Present
Nervous system		
Personality change	Common in children; may be consequence of stress, fluid or electrolyte imbalance, septicemia, drug therapy. Usually resolved when systemic complications resolve and wound closes, unless there was preburn pathology.	Acute and/or rehabilitation
Post-burn seizures	Same as above; unique complication of children; full recovery is usual.	Acute
Peripheral neuropathy	Secondary to immobilization and certain antibiotics. Hearing loss and weakness in limbs (e.g., foot drop) are most frequent.	Acute or rehabilitation
Skin, bone, joint		
Scarring and contractures	Secondary to tissue injury, inflammation and healing. A good prevention program starting on admission involving splinting and activities by OT and PT is essential.	Acute and rehabilitation
Heterotopic bone	Calcium deposits in joint spaces, secondary to fluid and electrolyte disturbances, bed rest, inactivity. Cannot be removed until fully mature (i.e., 1–3 yrs. post-burn).	Acute and rehabilitation

an appreciable full-thickness skin loss, burn care can be divided into three definable but overlapping phases. They are the *emergent,* the *acute* and the *rehabilitation* periods. The terms for these periods of treatment were given in an attempt to clarify and explain the child's requirements during a long hospitalization. It is beyond the scope of this text to detail the role of the nurse in each of these periods of care. Following is a description of the derangements and a statement of the principles of each phase of care and the expected course and standard treatment. The bibliography lists sources for the nurse wishing to study burn care in more detail.[1,8]

The Emergent Period The emergent period of care refers to the first two or three days immediately following the burn. The life-threatening problems of the burn victim are similar to those of any trauma victim. Therefore, the first principle of care is immediate first aid. Attention should be given to *breathing, bleeding resulting from any concurrent injury,* and *shock.* Once necessary life-saving measures are taken, the treatment should be directed to combating shock through proper *fluid therapy* and to reevaluating the respiratory status. *Burn wound care* is considered only after systemic care is under way.

Respiratory Care Anticipation of and intervention in respiratory difficulties during the emergent period can reduce the severity of pulmonary complications. Lung involvement may not be apparent immediately post-burn regardless of the size of the burn, but impending pulmonary problems should be suspected and treated in the case of any or all of the following:

1. The child was burned by flame in an enclosed space and/or forced to breathe products of combustion (explosion, house fire).
2. Blackened oral and nasal mucous membranes or singed nasal hairs or both are present.
3. There are burns of the face, neck or chest, or all three.
4. The child is experiencing obvious respiratory difficulties.

Edema increases insidiously and within several hours after the burn, the patient may develop respiratory obstruction.

Upper airway involvement in those children with flame burns is due to absorption of heat and noxious gases, creating trauma to mucous membrane linings, edema and possible obstruction. Cold, moist steam (with oxygen) is administered to humidify incoming air. The oxygen

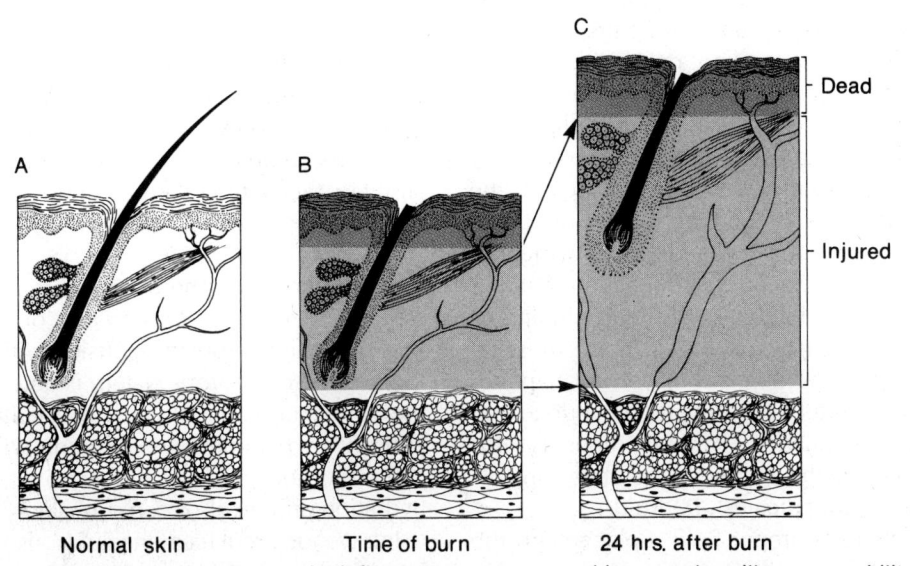

Figure 33-5 Edema formation. Due to the inflammatory process and increased capillary permeability following deep partial- or full-thickness burns, fluids lost from the vascular spaces enter the injured area. *A*, demonstrates normal skin; *B*, the depth of the injury at the time of the burn; and *C*, the amount of edema formed in this damaged tissue 24 hours after the burn. (Redrawn from I. Feller and C. Archambeault. Nursing the Burned Patient. National Institute for Burn Medicine, Ann Arbor, MI, 1973.)

also assists in correcting carbon monoxide poisoning. Insertion of an endotracheal tube is indicated for severe upper airway edema. As edema subsides (within a few days), the obstruction is relieved and the endotracheal tube can be removed.

Lower lung involvement, termed *primary pulmonary damage,* refers to injury at the alveolar level. Prolonged inhalation of noxious gases and chemicals traumatizes deeper lung tissues. Treatment of deep pulmonary involvement is difficult. Tracheostomy is performed if intubation will not resolve airway problems. Blood gas analysis is mandatory. Bronchodilators, steroids, and antibiotics may be used in the attempt to open the airways and to reduce the inflammatory process. Stiff, wet lungs* is a condition that may develop secondary to the injury or to overzealous fluid therapy. Another problem contributing to severe respiratory difficulty is a full-thickness circumferential burn of the chest. The thick eschar acts as a tourniquet and can constrict chest excursion to the point of diminishing air exchange. An escharotomy or release of the eschar is required.

Fluid Therapy Within a few hours after the burn, loss of circulating fluid causes hypovolemia that, if untreated, can lead to hypovolemic shock and death. Advances in technique of fluid therapy now make it possible to successfully resuscitate even the most severely burned victim. However, fluid overload can be an even greater danger than fluid losses and a complication of long-term care.

A major burn results in an outer layer of dead tissue and a deeper band or zone of injured or damaged cells (Fig. 33-5). The dead tissue is not important to fluid therapy. Fluid

---

*This term is used to describe atelectasis that develops into pulmonary edema.

does not leave the body but is leaked out of the bloodstream into the interstitial spaces. Fluid loss through dead burned tissue (eschar) is insignificant compared to this plasma shift. It is in the zone of damaged tissue that fluid shifts, causing hypovolemia (Fig. 33–5).

This inflammatory reaction is the body's normal response to trauma. It begins immediately after a burn and is profound for the first 24 hours. There is increased capillary permeability in the area of injury, upsetting the delicate balance of extracellular (interstitial and intravascular) fluid. In burns of less than 10 to 20 per cent total body area, depending on other severity factors, the child's body can compensate for this fluid shift by saving urine (oliguria) and vasoconstriction. In larger burns the fluid shift, if untreated, is life-threatening. Intravenous fluids similar to those shifted out of the bloodstream must be given in amounts sufficient to prevent hypovolemic shock, without causing fluid overload and electrolyte imbalance. Paralytic ileus is also seen owing to the hypovolemic state, and its presence contraindicates oral fluids.

When there is proper fluid replacement, the plasma shift gradually reverses. Within a few days the fluid that has leaked into interstitial spaces returns to the vascular spaces and a profound, spontaneous diuresis occurs, signaling successful resuscitation. (The term resuscitation is used in burn care to denote emergent period treatment that is life-saving, in this instance fluid therapy.) If excessive fluids have been given, the shift back to vascular spaces may cause hypervolemia, congestive heart failure and stiff, wet lungs.

In assessing the child with burns it must be determined if he needs fluid therapy and, if so, what type and how much fluid is needed. All victims of major burns require fluid therapy: Judicious fluid therapy must be considered for any child under the age of 4 (especially infants) with a burn of greater than 10 per cent of the total body area. Dehydrated children and those with concurrent injuries may also need fluid replacement even if burns are minor. Children with minor burns are monitored and given IV fluids only as needed; oral fluids often suffice. Keeping children with major burns NPO helps prevent vomiting, aspiration and electrolyte loss due to paralytic ileus from shock.

Fluid lost from the bloodstream in burn shock is composed of water, electrolytes and albumin and should be replaced in kind. Hartmann's solution (lactated Ringer's) is the fluid of choice because its electrolyte balance is similar to that of the blood. Albumin (human serum) may be added to provide colloid, although investigators who oppose its use during the first 24 hours of fluid therapy believe that the colloid becomes trapped during this time, adding to extravascular fluid retention. Red cell loss related to the burn injury is caused by hemolysis and generally approximates only 10 per cent of the total red cell mass. Whole blood is not necessary to resuscitate the victim of a major burn unless there is significant loss of blood from concurrent injuries.

Fluid therapy for the burn victim is based on titration. An adequate amount of parenteral fluids to maintain organ perfusion without overloading the circulatory system is determined by measuring urinary output and specific gravity and other parameters, including vital signs, central venous pressure, hematocrit, signs of hydration and level of consciousness.

Intravenous replacement fluids also leak into interstitial spaces. Until third-spaced fluids are expelled, no patient should gain more than 10 to 15 per cent of his preburn weight.* In an infant or child with a relatively small circulatory volume, close monitoring of IV intake and output is essential. Giving a 30 lb (13 to 14 kg) toddler a liter of fluid is replacing one-third to one-half of his total circulatory volume and represents a weight gain of 7 per cent of his normal weight. Vital signs and intake and output are measured hourly; a nude weight should be taken at least once a day.

Relative hematocrit values are a clue to the dilution of red blood cells, thereby suggesting the need for fluid replacement. Red cells do not shift; a concentrated hematocrit is due to burn shock. With proper fluid replacement hematocrit level returns to normal. The hematocrit is obtained in the emergency department as a baseline and then every six hours throughout the emergent period.

Monitoring of urinary output is essential in assessing the child's response to trauma. The amount, content and color of urine is a guide to fluid replacement. The amount of urine measured and recorded each hour is a guide to the amount of fluid to be infused the next hour. An

---

*One liter of fluid weighs 1 kg (2.2 lbs).

output of 10 to 30 ml of urine per hour for children (20 to 60 ml/hr for late adolescents) indicates adequate perfusion or organ systems without systemic overload. Amounts of output over 10 to 30 ml per hour for a child *do not* indicate "better" resuscitation but rather warn of impending fluid overload and stiff, wet lungs.

The emergent period ends when fluid resuscitation is successful. Third-spaced fluids return to the vascular space and are excreted by the kidneys. Fluid therapy is then re-evaluated and discontinued or continued, if indicated, for management of expected or apparent complication such as infection, weight loss or dehydration.

Deep tissue injury or massive burns damage circulating red blood cells (hemolysis), resulting in the release of large amounts of free-circulating hemoglobin (hemoglobinemia). When this free hemoglobin passes the basement membrane into the tubules of the kidney, there is the danger of acute tubular necrosis (ATN) and renal failure. Black urine (hemoglobinuria) seen on catheterization or in the immediate post-burn period indicates severe hemolysis. An osmotic diuretic is given immediately to flush the tubules. Intravenous intake is temporarily increased until the crisis is over. Obviously, hemoglobinuria will not be detected unless a urinary catheter is inserted as soon as the child arrives for treatment.

Other Elements of Care Other elements of emergent period care include (1) controlling pain, (2) obtaining baseline indices, (3) controlling infection and (4) treating the wound. Because the principles of wound care are the same during the emergent phase as in the acute phase, its discussion is included in acute period care.

Pain Control When the child is in burn shock (hypovolemic shock), pain control cannot be achieved with subcutaneous or intramuscular medication because the medication will pool, producing no relief. When circulation returns to normal, there will then be a possibly dangerous release of large, pooled dosages. For effectiveness, the analgesic must be given IV and in small enough dosages to prevent dulling of consciousness or respiratory centers. Routine tetanus coverage is also indicated but does not need to be given IV.

Baseline Values Baseline values for all vital signs, electrolytes, hemoglobin, and white cells are obtained, as are a chest X-ray, an electrocardiogram, and wound cultures. These should be obtained immediately to serve as a guide to assessing and planning care. Vital signs and laboratory tests are repeated at least daily and more often if indicated.

Infection Control The burn victim has lost the protective barrier of his skin — invasive infection can threaten his life. Septicemia or pneumonia accounts for about 50 per cent of burn fatalities. Burn patients are autocontaminated on admission by the bacteria that normally reside on the skin and in hair follicles and sweat glands, and the normal flora of the gastrointestinal tract. The role of the nurse is to aid in controlling infection, since it cannot be eliminated. Clean or isolation technique is needed to prevent cross-contamination (the spread of bacteria from one patient to another by staff and visitors). Aseptic technique is mandatory for any procedure in which an anatomical barrier is penetrated. Judicious antibiotic use and support of the body's natural immunological processes further serve to control infection.

The Acute Period The acute period of treatment begins at the end of the emergent period and lasts until all full-thickness wounds are covered with autografts. (Autografts are the patient's own skin transferred permanently to cover the wound.) If the burn is only a partial-thickness injury, the acute period is over within 10 to 20 days; the healing is spontaneous and grafts are unnecessary.

During the acute phase there are two main principles of management: The first is to remove the eschar as soon as possible to allow spontaneous healing or covering with autografts or homografts (temporary biological cover of skin from a donor of the same species). The second is to avoid, as far as possible, the complications that are known to occur with burns.

Complications Complications of every organ system may be encountered in care of the burned child. The key to successful therapy is anticipation and early detection of complications combined with rigorous therapy. Early detection is accomplished by close monitoring and a knowledge of proper management (basic nursing care) of each organ system. The tedious long-term care required for wound closure is balanced by the need for precise and exacting skill in preventing, detecting and treating the many possible complications.

The seriously burned patient remains acutely ill for a long time. The patient is not in a chronic state, as this prolonged, difficult period would suggest, but is instead acutely ill, continually in danger of developing complications. The patient may appear to be doing well one day only to be found to have developed a severe complication the next. Only when the full-thickness wound is reduced to less than 20 per cent of the body surface are these dangers past.

Minor Burn Wound Management Wound management is the main consideration for minor burns. There is generally no need for intravenous fluid therapy or prophylactic antibiotics. However, tetanus toxoid, tetanus antitoxin, or tetanus immune globulin (human) is used in all but small partial-thickness burns, on the basis of history of immunization. The basic principles of wound management are cleanliness and comfort. A partial-thickness burn is usually painful because pain fibers in the area of tissue damage are irritated. It may be necessary to give analgesics before cleaning the involved surface, but care should be taken to avoid oversedation because some reponse to pain during cleansing helps the nurse judge whether she is causing unnecessary trauma to the tissues. Rough handling of the burned area must be avoided. Partial-thickness wounds can be converted to full-thickness loss when mechanical trauma during cleaning further damages weakened tissues. This can easily occur with infants because their skin is delicate.

After the wound and surrounding areas have been gently but thoroughly cleaned of all debris (foreign matter and dead tissue) with soap and water and after any hairy area has been shaved to a two inch margin around the wound, the wound is rinsed thoroughly and a dressing is applied. One layer of a saline-moistened roll bandage is applied directly to the burned area and then covered with a moist Kerlix wrap, and then a dry one. This will provide a comfortable, occlusive dressing. (The type of dressing may be altered according to instructions of the physician in charge of care.)

The child and family are instructed to change this dressing daily by soaking it off with warm tap water, gently cleaning the wound with nonirritating soap and water and thoroughly rinsing. A new bandage is then applied in the manner just described. Parents should be informed that dressing changes remove exudate and products of infection, allowing the wound to heal spontaneously. Daily dressing changes and cleansing allow for detection of infection. If parental competence in following directions in dressing change is questionable, parents may be instructed to return to the nurse for daily dressing changes and observation of the wound.

Approximately two weeks are required for healing of a partial-thickness wound; the patient should be followed on an outpatient basis. Appearance of necrotic tissue* or granulation tissue† or both after the necrotic surface is cleaned indicates a full-thickness wound usually requiring hospital admission for closure with autograft.

The patient or family should be instructed to observe the unburned skin surrounding the wound for evidence of spreading infection (redness, purulence, fever) during the daily dressing changes. If cellulitis (intense redness, streaking, swelling, firm infiltration) appears, an immediate return visit is indicated for prescription of the proper antibiotic. In most instances, gram-positive organisms are responsible. Oral antibiotics are usually satisfactory, and more frequent dressing changes with increased soaking periods hasten the control of infection. Oral analgesics are used prior to dressing changes to minimize the child's discomfort during the treatment.

Ointments, other topical medications and expensive dressings are generally not indicated for minor wound management. There are no known chemicals that can restore vitality to dead tissue, nor do we now know of any that can speed the body's healing process. Many of the substances formerly used to coat burns actually increased the injury by their own chemical action on already weakened tissue. It is not so much what is put on the wound but how the wound is cared for that is important to healing. The attending physician should decide on topical therapy on the basis of the type and location of the wound.

---

*Necrotic tissue is dead cells that are in contact with living cells.
†Granulation tissue is newly formed capillaries filled with granulocytes mixed with fibrocytes; the spaces between capillaries are filled with an inflammatory exudate.

Major Burn Wound Management Care of a burn wound classified as major can be a time-consuming process. Full-thickness wounds cannot heal by themselves; all dead tissue must be removed and the area grafted with the patient's own skin for permanent coverage (autografting). The same donor site (site from which autografts are taken) may be used every 7 to 10 days if given proper care.

When the full-thickness wound is very large or the child's condition is such that he cannot tolerate surgical procedures, homografts (skin from another donor of the same species, such as cadaver skin) or heterografts (pig skin) may be used until autografts can be taken. This temporary skin coverage is rejected by the body.

Daily cleansing and debriding (removing dead tissue) are a time-consuming aspect of burn nursing. Frequently the patient is "tubbed" in a hydrotherapy tub, twice daily to assist with this process. Debridement can be accomplished in three ways. One is the *natural* process of proteolytic degradation of tissue by body and bacterial enzymes that loosen tissue. This process is enhanced by dressing changes and gentle cleansing. The second way, *sharp* debridement, is done with a scalpel (as in early tangential excision) or with sharp scissors and pickups; daily sharp debridement may be carried out at the bedside by the nurse or physician. (Early tangential excision is gaining favor among experts). The third method involves use of *enzymes* such as Travase, which destroy dead tissue. All of these methods may be used in a very large wound.

The human body can heal a partial-thickness wound if proper cleansing is done. In management of full-thickness wounds, bacteria must be controlled that can grow in or on the wound because of the optimal conditions present: body heat, body moisture and dead tissue. Bacterial growth is controlled by debridement, cleansing and use of topical agents. Debridement removes dead tissue, tubbing dilutes the bacterial population on the wound and softens eschar for debridement while providing body cleansing, and topical agents, when used properly, control bacterial growth in the wound. Systemic antibacterial therapy is also necessary.

Use of a dressing for major burns is dependent on the overall system of care and the condition of the patient's wound. Some burn centers use wet dressings (dressings impregnated with a particular topical agent), as described in the section on minor burns. Others use exposure therapy, which involves allowing the air to dry the wound. Usually exposure is utilized for minor wounds or for burns in areas that lend themselves to exposure therapy, such as the face or anterior areas of the body. A combination of methods also may be utilized. Once the wound is healed, no dressings are required.

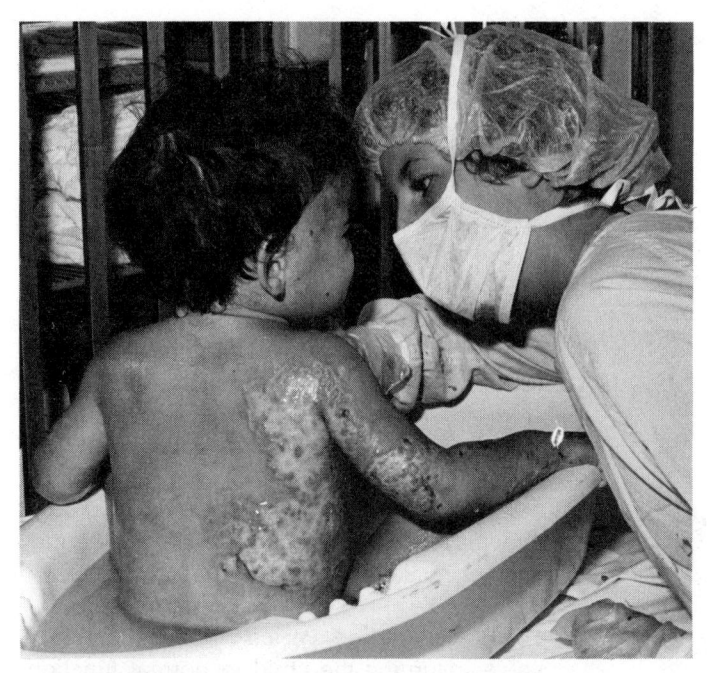

Hydrotherapy for the young child is best accomplished in a smaller tub, not the 100- to 300-gallon tanks. The smaller tub allows gentle, thorough cleansing as well as feeling of security and intimacy with the nurse. (Courtesy of the National Institute for Burn Medicine.)

As the size of the wound is reduced through debridement and autografting, the patient's chance for survival increases.

During wound treatment, nursing care must also deal with prevention of contractures and scar tissue as well as detection and early treatment of complications of other organ systems, as is true with minor burn care.

Nutrition The initial insult of the burn injury results in a hypovolemic state, which contributes to a paralytic ileus. Thus the patient is kept NPO for the first 36 to 72 hours or until normal bowel sounds return. Once the gastrointestinal tract is again normal, the child is taken rapidly from liquids to a full diet (as tolerated).

Because of the increased metabolism and catabolism as a result of the burn trauma, the child needs two or three times the normal amount of calories and protein. Caloric increases should be in the form of carbohydrates to spare protein breakdown. Vitamins and trace elements are provided to promote healing, as is iron to control anemia secondary to hemolysis and bleeding during debridement.

The nurse should be aware that burned children are often anorexic and that small, frequent feedings of the child's favorite nutritious foods may be necessary to achieve adequate intake. A list of favorite foods should be included in the care plan and families encouraged to bring in favorite foods from home. Nutrition for children who cannot tolerate oral feedings is provided through a combination of nasogastric feedings and intravenous hyperalimentation until they can again take nourishment orally.

The Rehabilitation Period Rehabilitation involves returning the child to normal functioning. Fortunately, most children who survive do very well even though they have been through a long and difficult hospitalization. A recent survey of 250 severely burned patients of all ages treated in the University of Michigan Burn Center revealed that 85 per cent returned to society as well as or better than they were before the accident.[7] This study took into consideration both functional and emotional factors. Children with an already good body image responded well to rehabilitation despite physical and cosmetic handicaps. Children who did not "feel good" about themselves prior to the burn accident had more cosmetic and physical problems. Adolescents especially had problems with adjustment, primarily because they were already going through an adjustment phase of their lives and the burn injury only served to compound their problems. With proper intervention, however, their adjustment improved as years passed.

There are two basic considerations during the rehabilitation phase: (1) restoration of function in joint surfaces that were scarred and (2) emotional assistance required by the child. Rehabilitation actually begins in the emergency room and must be kept in mind throughout the child's hospitalization. After the initial discharge, many readmissions may be necessary for reconstructive procedures as well as for emotional assistance and counselling. Children require long-term follow-up through their years of growth so that scarring over joints does not retard normal growth and development.

Impact of the Burn on the Child, His Family and Nurses

Remember that *the burn victim is an accident victim*. The child will have guilt feelings regarding the accident and most likely a fear of death, or at least a fear of the "unknown" concerning the injury and treatment. The shock and pain of the accident, the chaos and rush to the hospital, the unfamiliar surroundings and new people all produce emotional stress.

Supportive Nursing Care in the Emergency Phase An attitude showing confidence, genuine interest and concern are extremely important to the emotional welfare of the child and family. One simple act that provides an anchor in the storm is for the nurse to tell the child her name and to explain briefly what to expect of the staff, what sensations he will experience, and what will be expected of him. These instructions (a verbal contract) help reduce the inequality and inconsistency in the transition that the child makes from being healthy to being an accident victim to being a patient. Talking to the child also allows the nurse to evaluate his sensorium and orientation. The nurse should remember that no burn victim is ever rendered unconscious by the burn itself —a search for an underlying cause is imperative. The following nursing actions will help the child cope with his emotional stress and maintain some control:

1. Give the child your name and call the child by name.
2. Talk *to* the child, not just *about* him.
3. State what will be done and why and what he will feel, hear, and smell.
4. Request the child's cooperation and suggest possible ways he may participate.
5. Encourage the child to express his feelings and alter the contract to comply with his requests when possible.
6. If a parent does not accompany the child, you must, for legal reasons, take the time to notify a parent of the child to get his or her consent for what is being done or what must be done. Stay with the child during the treatment, acting as a surrogate parent, until the parent arrives. In the parent's absence, assure the child that his parents know about the accident and care about him.

Supportive Nursing Care During Hospital Management Children under school age pose a special problem because they likely cannot differentiate the various roles of an adult. They need their parents to provide an element of normalcy. Children will also regress due to the stress; the approach is to treat the child where he is and work toward age-appropriate behavior.

It is important to maintain a consistent plan of care, allowing the child to choose some options when they exist. Never ask the child if he wants to do something when you know he must do it anyway. Everything done to the child will make a difference. The burned child needs to be rocked, cuddled, taught and disciplined like any other child. Expectations for the child's behavior should be spelled out to him and maintained.

Maintaining a pleasant, supportive and loving atmosphere is essential to the child's emotional adjustment. The child should be encouraged to be out of bed as soon as possible and to participate in everyday activities (e.g., playing with toys, continuing with toilet training, eating in a high chair or at the table, and so forth).

The child should be allowed to talk, play and act out feelings of depression and hostility. The nurse should assess the need for help from other team members such as a social worker, a psychologist, or a play therapist and obtain their help.

Although the toddler is not as affected by his appearance as is the older child, he is sensitive to his body intactness and others' reactions to his appearance. To draw attention away from his overwhelming appearance, the nurse can ask parents to supply colorful pajamas and slippers and pretty decorations (jewelry, bows, badges) for the child to wear, and she can encourage good general grooming. Studies have also shown that all burned children are more comfortable and feel more "intact" when their dressings are on. Colorful pajamas or gowns can be worn over their dressings.

Nursing Care Note

Modern burn care — including frequent daily wound cleaning and daily body hygiene, use of topical agents, and good basic nursing care — eliminates the problem of *odor* associated with a burn patient. *Odors around the patient are a clear indication that he is not receiving proper care. Odors should not be tolerated or masked with air fresheners. The cause must be immedi-*

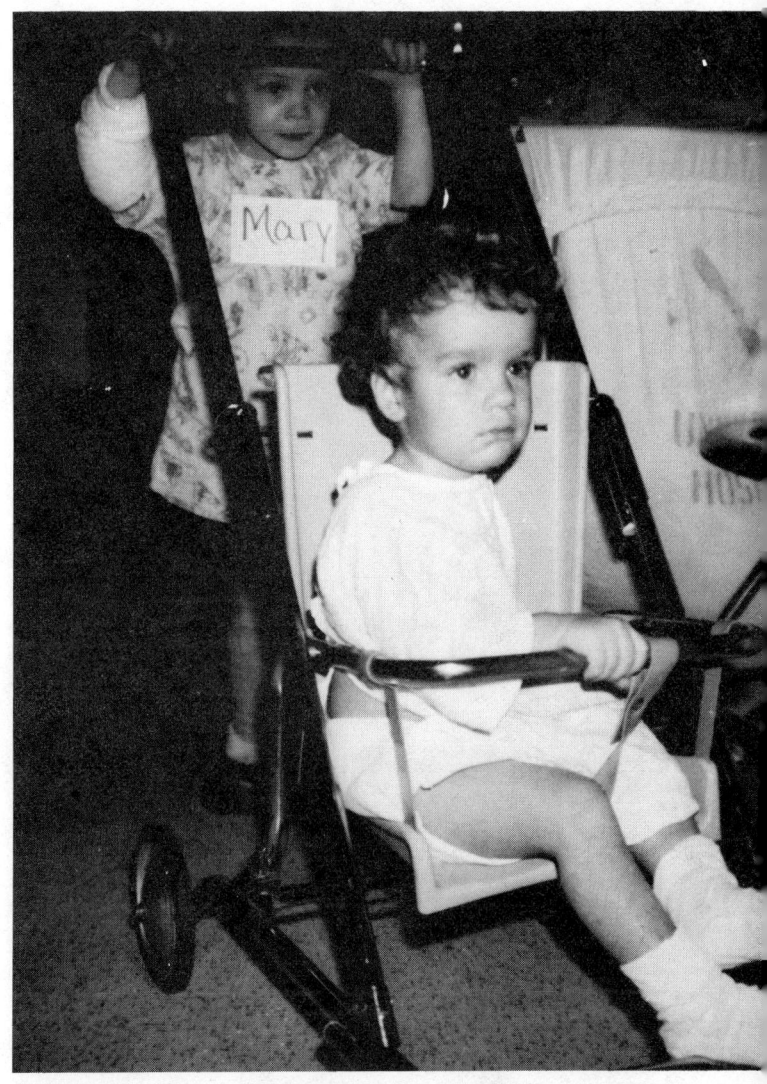

Children hospitalized with burns are encouraged to carry on normal activity. (Courtesy of the National Institute for Burn Medicine.)

ately identified and resolved. What is needed may be more aggressive or more frequent wound care; a change in topical agent; better oral or perineal hygiene, or other measures.

Impact on the Family Whether it is justified or not, parents usually experience extreme guilt and feel acute responsibility for their child's burns. These feelings are compounded by the fact that in many instances the accident could have been prevented if safety precautions or closer adult supervision had been initiated. The same feelings may be experienced by other family members. In addition, there is grave

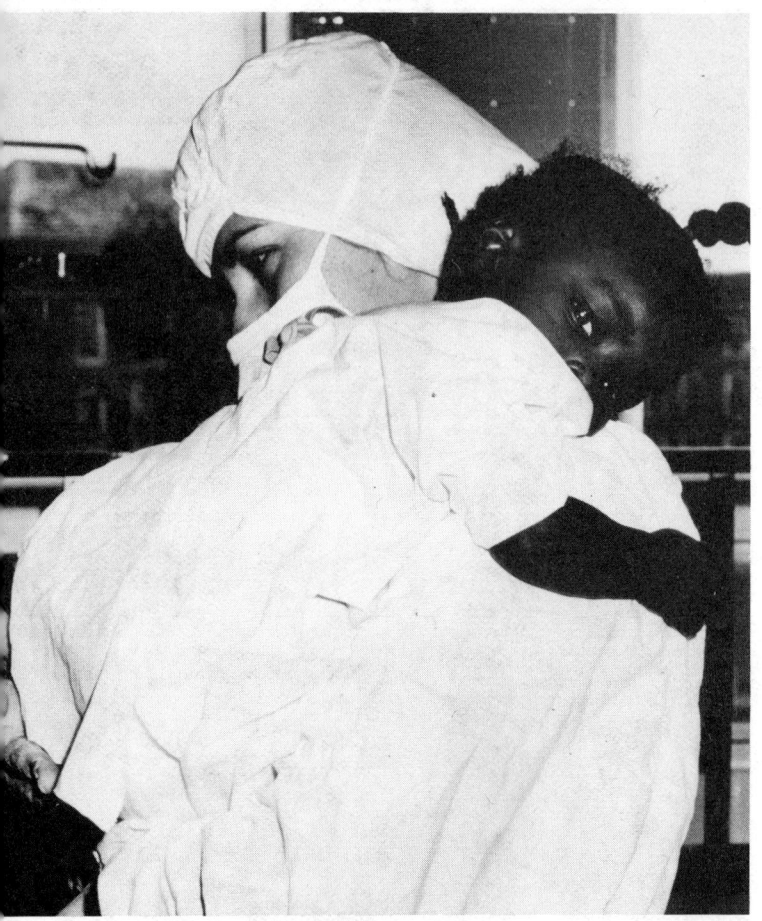

Cuddling and holding a child after dressing changes serves to comfort and reduce stress for both nurse and child. (Courtesy of the National Institute for Burn Medicine).

concern for the child's life and about his present and future appearance.

In an effort to handle these feelings, some parents may become oversolicitous and lenient with their burned child. Others refuse to look at or touch the child because of his appearance and the guilt feelings it produces. Neither reaction is therapeutic or conducive to the child's recovery.

Management of family members' needs and directing their activity toward supporting the burned child is another nursing responsibility. A system of family teaching should be instituted on admission; the family must have a clear explanation of what must be done and why. They must be prepared for what the child's appearance will be once dressings are applied and when dressings are removed and assisted to accept that treatments that inflict pain are essential to recovery, but that they will be as brief as possible. It should be explained that the consequences of not providing treatment are far worse. Also, the nurse should cuddle the child after painful experiences, not only for comfort of the patient but for her own emotional well-being.

The family should also be prepared for what to expect from the child behaviorally and encouraged to relate to the child in as supportive a fashion as possible. (Frequently the nurse may find a family problem that requires intervention by a social worker or a psychologist.) Reassurance that enforcement of normal routine, discipline and expectations (to the extent possible under the circumstances) is comforting and supportive to their child is often helpful to parents. Parents also benefit from contact with other parents who have recently been through the same ordeal. These contacts are helpful if all parents have been properly oriented. They can be harmful if parents pass along rumors or misinformation. Group time should be allotted on a regular basis for family members to verbalize their feelings and concerns to the nurse or another member of the burn team. Professional asistance for families is frequently required to help the child with a major burn and his family through the long months or years of rehabilitative care. In fact, studies show that this professional intervention is essential.[2]

Impact on Nurses Burn care of children can be especially difficult for the nurse. To remain calm when confronted by the child's appearance and the discomfort which he must suffer, while attempting to be efficient and effective during burn care activities, is extremely taxing for any nurse. In addition, the nurse must not only deal with a child who is in pain, she must also cope with the fact that she inflicts pain during treatments, dressing changes, and when positioning or holding the child.

The nurse caring for the burned child must confront her own feelings and anxieties before she can maintain therapeutic interaction with the child. It is important to recognize that behavior of the child or parent is neither good nor bad, but that by providing guidelines it can be guided to be "coping behavior." She must learn to respond in a manner that is firm but supportive and recovery-directed. Being well trained and knowledgeable in the intricacies of care relieves some of the nurse's stress and anxiety regarding the physical measures of care and allows her to concentrate on a therapeutic approach. The nurse also needs to be aware that a team of specialties is required to meet the patient's many needs; she cannot do it alone. She also should seek outlets (head nurse, social worker, physician) to express her frustrations, dismay, anger and anxiety created during care of the burned child. Burn care can be rewarding for all involved if properly managed.

Preventive Education

Nurses should take a major role in providing safety education to parents and children. Simple measures can be taken by parents in the home to prevent burn accidents. In addition, every individual should know how to respond if clothing or hair ignites. Likewise, proper immediate first aid for burns should be a part of preventive education so that burns that do occur are not aggravated by inappropriate measures.

IF A BURN ACCIDENT HAPPENS

Stop the Damage!
- Put out the fire the fastest way you can. Time is critical.
- Drop the victim and roll him, wrapped in a rug; cover him with water.
- Pull off burned clothes.
- Stop him from running.

Immediate Care of Burns
- When a scald burn occurs, flood with cold tap water and remove clothing carefully.
- If a chemical burn occurs, flood with water and remove clothing.
- If a large area is burned, wrap the victim in a clean sheet or towel and go immediately to the nearest hospital emergency room.
- If a small area is burned, wash it with cool water and soap. Do not use ice. Rinse thoroughly, dry gently and apply a bland ointment (e.g., A & D Ointment). Cover with a sterile gauze bandage.
- If you have *any doubt* about what to do, call your family physician or nearest hospital emergency room and ask for advice.

Later Care of Minor Burns
- Cleanse once or twice a day with soap and water; rinse thoroughly and dry. Cover with a thin layer of bland ointment and a sterile dressing.
- Do not break blisters; they provide a sterile cover over the wound. When blisters break, the loose skin should be removed.
- Watch for any signs of inflammation: redness, pain, heat or swelling. If they occur, call a doctor or take victim to the nearest hospital emergency room.

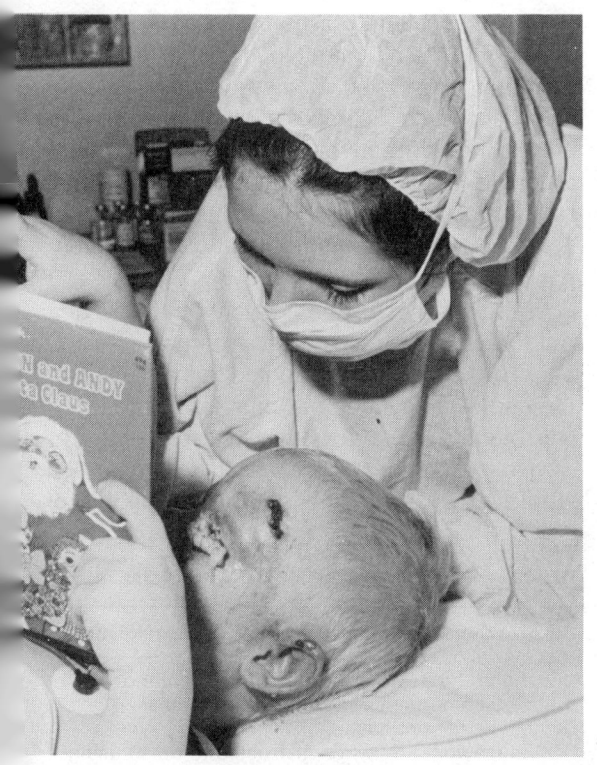

The presence of parents is a crucial aspect of the burned child's recovery. (Photograph by Dan Hill. Courtesy, National Institute for Burn Medicine.)

ACCIDENTAL POISONING

by Linda Mowad, RN, BSN

INGESTIONS

Ingestion is a broad term used to describe the process of taking substances into the body. In addition to food, toddlers can ingest many things, some of which are potentially harmful, including foreign bodies, contaminated food, medicine, various chemicals and plants. This section will cover the ingestion of poisons by toddlers. For our purpose, a poison is defined as any substance having the potential to produce functional impairment, permanent injury or death of cells or organ systems. The care of a child with food poisoning is similar to that of any child with gastrointestinal distress and is not discussed. Lead poisoning is covered separately.

Incidence Although its incidence is declining, accidental poisoning is the fourth leading cause of death in children ages 1 to 4 years. More boys are poisoned than girls and peak incidence is in the 2-year-old.[26] Poisoning is more common in lower socioeconomic groups, families with more than one child and, until recently, physicians' families.[4] Accidental poisoning in childhood may be higher in families with disturbed parent-child relationships, impaired childrearing potential or general psychopathology.[4]

The poisons that toddlers ingest are of many different types. The most common include household items, medicines, especially aspirin; vitamins and minerals; and plants.[15] Aspirin poisoning has been declining and acetaminophen poisoning is rising.[22]

Etiology Accidental poisoning in toddlers is the result of many factors. Toddlers are increasingly mobile and curious, seeking to increase their independence. While exploring the environment they can come in contact with many hazards. At this developmental stage in the child, parents are beginning to decrease some of the constant vigilance they kept for him as an infant. Family stress can contribute to preoccupation in parents and subsequently increase the risk of poisoning to the child. Numerous environmental conditions in a household contribute to poisoning, such as easy access to cleansing products. Generally, poisoning can be attributed to insufficient supervision or carelessness in childproofing the environment.

The role of the nurse is to identify children at risk and to educate parents in prevention. During the toddler years visits to a clinic or physician decrease and the nurse may not have contact with families whose children are at risk. In addition, the problems the nurse faces in evaluating the home environment and psychosocial family factors are apparent.

Potential solutions to these difficulties do exist, although some may be difficult to implement. Probably one of the most reasonable solutions is through involvement of community and social agencies in educational programs aimed at prevention. Community health nurses are in an excellent position to coordinate such efforts, but heavy case loads, massive paper work and restricted budgets do not usually allow for such activities. On a larger scale, nurses should be involved in legislation aimed at environmental safety. Safety packaging and labeling of some household items and medications are not yet required by law. While safety packaging alone will not prevent poisoning, it does help. The Poison Prevention Packaging Act of 1972 requires that aspirin be safety-packaged. This has contributed to the decline in the rate of salicylate poisoning in children.[18]

In addition to preventive measures, parents should be taught basic first aid for poisoning (Table 33-2) and to keep the phone number of

TABLE 33-2 FIRST AID DO'S AND DON'TS FOR INGESTION OF A POISON

DO give the child water to drink if he is awake and can swallow.
DO phone the nearest poison control center or hospital emergency room for instructions.
DO follow instructions explicitly.
DO induce vomiting when instructed to do so using 3 teaspoons of syrup of ipecac followed by a glass of water or by carefully stroking the back of the child's throat with a blunt object. Note: Be sure the child drinks water first.
DO save *all* containers and vomitus to take to the hospital.

DON'T use milk, vinegar, lemon juice, baking soda, carbonated beverages or anything other than water to dilute a poison.
DON'T induce vomiting without instructions from a poison control center or other reliable source.
DON'T follow instructions on commercial product labels—these are sometimes incorrect.
DON'T use your finger to stroke the back of a child's throat, as you may be bitten.
DON'T confuse syrup of ipecac with other medications.

TEACHING POISON PREVENTION TO CAREGIVERS: EFFECTIVE MEASURES

1. Never keep poisonous substances in food containers.
2. Discard all old food promptly.
3. Keep all medication and cleansing products out of reach in a cabinet with a child-resistant lock.
4. Avoid keeping excess medicine in the house.
5. Do not take medicine in front of small children.
6. Do not refer to medicine as candy. Similarly, avoid keeping pleasant-tasting medicine in the house.
7. Choose medicines and cleansing products with safety lids.
8. Discard any unlabeled substances or medicines.
9. Get in the habit of reading all labels.
10. Teach children about poisons.
11. Learn first aid for poisons, and keep a poison chart and poison control center number readily available.
12. Know what children are doing at all times.

---

the local poison control center accessible. Syrup of ipecac can be kept in the home.

Teaching toddlers to be safe is a continuous job. Parents need patience and guidance for this task. Setting clear, consistent limits for what the child may and may not do is essential. Teaching children a poison symbol such as "Mr. Yuk" or "Officer Ugg" and appropriately labeling hazardous substances may be helpful.

General Management Often a nurse may be the first person to be contacted when a child is poisoned, perhaps as a community neighbor rather than while on duty. The emergency room nurse may handle phone calls regarding an ingestion. Initial advice or treatment is critical and can reduce ultimate fatality.

Handling phone calls can be done in one of two ways — either by describing first aid step by step and instructing the parent to bring the child to the hospital or by referring the parent to a poison control center. In either case the parent may be highly anxious. The nurse must have a calming voice and give explicit directions.

There are five basic principles in the management of any poisoned child that will decrease stress and facilitate adaptation, assuming that the child is alert and stable.

1. Identify the poison. Determine what, how, when and how much the child took. Obtain any empty or full containers. Save all vomitus for analysis. Obtain blood screening tests as indicated. Time should not be wasted before treatment if determination of the ingestant is difficult.

2. Decrease absorption. Because absorption rates of substances and gastrointestinal conditions vary, there is some debate as to the extent of the time in which gastric emptying is effective. Emesis or lavage should be initiated immediately unless one of the following contraindications is present: ingestion of corrosives or hydrocarbons; central nervous system (CNS) or respiratory depression; diminished gag reflex and seizures.

The choice of emesis or lavage is a medical decision; emesis is generally favored. This can be accomplished by the administration of 15 ml of syrup of ipecac followed by a glass or two of water. Physical agitation of small children hastens the effect. The dose may be repeated in 20 to 30 minutes if one dose is ineffective; however, *additional doses are contraindicated,* since ipecac itself can be toxic. More than one or two glasses of water should not be given. With more water than this, some of the poison may be forced through the pylorus.

Causing the child to gag by stimulating the posterior pharynx or depressing the posterior tongue will also induce vomiting. Be sure that the child drinks water first and never use an unprotected finger. A blunt object such as a tongue depressor or spoon is preferred. The child should be in an inverted position with the head lower than the rest of his body if he is very young. This will prevent aspiration.

Apomorphine (.07 mg/kg) given subcutaneously is an emetic used rarely in children. In addition to inducing vomiting it causes respiratory depression, hence its antagonist, Narcan, should be readily available.

Following emesis, activated charcoal (1 to 2 tablespoons in a glass of water) may be given to bind any remaining poison, preventing further absorption. It should not be given until ipecac has been fully effective, since it will inactivate the ipecac. Toddlers may resist the unpleasant taste and consistency of the liquid.

3. Hasten elimination. Poisons already absorbed will be eliminated via the lungs, liver or kidneys. If eliminated by the kidneys, the proc-

ess can be expedited in some cases by forced diuresis and manipulation of urine pH. Diuresis must be accomplished carefully, with frequent monitoring to prevent dehydration in small children. Dialysis is sometimes indicated.

4. Carry out symptomatic management. Presenting symptoms such as coma, seizures, CNS or respiratory depression, arrhythmias or shock must be managed appropriately with supportive therapy. Maintenance of an adequate airway and oxygenation and minimizing shock are always priorities.

5. Administer an antidote. There are few true antidotes. The use of the "universal antidote" of burned toast, tea and milk of magnesia is ineffective and obsolete. When an antidote is known, it should be administered as soon as possible.

Pathophysiology and Clinical Picture Most children who are victims of poisonings present with a history of having ingested some substance; however, any child presenting in coma or with strange behavior, unexplained high fever, arrhythmias or seizures should be considered to have been possibly poisoned.[15] Such children are critically ill and care is aimed at diagnosis and giving supportive treatment. Far more often, a child presents with a history of ingesting a specific substance. Pathophysiology and symptomatology vary. A discussion of some of the more common substances follows.

Corrosives Lyes or caustics found in toilet and drain cleansers cause severe chemical burns, the degree of severity depending on the concentration of the chemical and the length of time of contact. Children may present with varying degrees of burns around the mouth and of the oral mucosa, throat and esophagus, which is not visualized. The burns may be red, swollen and oozing or more severe, with sloughing or erosion of tissue.

Alkali substances have the capability of continuing to cause damage after initial contact. Care must be taken to flood all areas with large quantities of water. Vomiting should *never* be induced in these cases, as the corrosive may cause more harm in the process. Only minimal fluid should be given orally owing to the danger of perforation. Severe burns causing perforation are accompanied by vascular collapse and shock. Subsequent healing of these lesions can produce stricture formation, particularly of the esophagus. These children should be hospitalized and treated with appropriate steroids, antibiotics and nasogastric tube feedings.

Hydrocarbons Petroleum distillates such as paint thinner, turpentine, lighter fluid, furniture polish, gasoline, kerosene and machine oil are commonly ingested substances. Ingestion can cause irritation of mucous membranes with vomiting and diarrhea and CNS depression. Aspiration occurring at the time of ingestion causes a hydrocarbon pneumonia and acute hemorrhagic necrotizing disease, usually within 24 hours. Secondary hypoxia is a major problem. Symptoms include respiratory distress, fever and tachycardia.

The odor of a petroleum distillate can be smelled on the child's breath. Emptying the stomach is a controversial issue, since to induce emesis or lavage increases the possibility of aspiration. On the other hand, to leave the hydrocarbon to be absorbed increases the likelihood of fatal systemic toxicity.

Insecticides Chlorinated hydrocarbons, such as DDT or methoxychlor, and organic phosphates such as parathion or malathion act in different ways to produce pathology. Chlorinated hydrocarbons block nerve function, causing increased salivation and vomiting, abdominal pain, tremors, CNS depression and seizures. Organic phosphates are cholinesterase inhibitors whose ingestion results in mild symptomatology such as headache, dizziness, weakness and tremor to severe symptomatology including gastrointestinal hyperactivity, respiratory distress, miosis, sweating, seizures and coma.

Treatment is supportive. The effects of organic phosphates are cumulative. Atropine and Protopam are specific antidotes for cholinesterase inhibitors.

Salicylate Aspirin is the medicine most commonly ingested by children.[19] Aspirin is found in many over-the-counter products; its presence in these products is often unknown to parents. Salicylate has various effects on the body. Of primary importance is its stimulating effect on the respiratory center in the brain, causing hyperventilation and a loss of carbon dioxide leading to respiratory alkalosis. In addition, there is a metabolic impairment leading to metabolic acidosis. Other effects include bleeding, hypokalemia and hypoglycemia or hyperglycemia. Symptoms include hyperpnea, vomiting, tinnitus, CNS derangements, hyperpyrexia and coma.

Emesis should be induced as soon as possible, because aspirin is absorbed directly from the stomach. Forced diuresis and alkalinization of the urine will hasten elimination.

Acetaminophen Poisonings with this drug are on the rise in children.[20] Acetaminophen is the active ingredient in Tylenol and other aspirin substitutes, as well as the breakdown product of phenacetin, which is found in pain relievers combined with other agents. Toxicity can cause hepatic necrosis. Symptoms include nausea, vomiting, diaphoresis and pallor. After 24 to 48 hours symptoms progress to right upper quadrant abdominal pain, decreased urine output and later to jaundice, hypoglycemia, circulatory collapse, coma, seizures and respiratory failure.

Death can occur from acute hepatic failure. Acetylcysteine (Mucomyst) is a relatively new antidote. It combines with the toxic metabolite of acetaminophen so that this can be excreted in the urine.

Vitamins with Iron Vitamins are themselves usually harmless; however, many contain iron, making them potentially lethal. Iron has a corrosive effect on gastrointestinal mucosa and can leave deposits in the liver. Symptoms occur in stages. Initially the child has gastrointestinal distress, hemorrhage, shock and coma. Symptoms subside after four to six hours and the child remains asymptomatic for 12 to 36 hours. Subsequently he can redevelop shock, hepatic failure, or later, pyloric stenosis.

There is a poor correlation between serum iron levels and clinical symptoms, and severity of toxicity is difficult to determine. Deferoxamine is used as an antidote as well as an indicator of severity. With severe overdose the urine will be pink or red following the administration of deferoxamine but will be clear in smaller overdoses.[21]

Plants Plants can cause a wide range of toxic symptoms from mild gastrointestinal distress to respiratory distress, convulsions, coma, shock and cardiotoxicity. Interested readers are referred to the article by Fosnot listed in the recommended readings.

Nursing Care The nurse may be called upon to administer first aid measures to a poisoned child. During initial contact with the poisoned child, physical care is a priority and centers on the five principles outlined earlier (p. 819). In cases of severe toxicity nursing care is a challenge. The priority is always maintaining an adequate airway, oxygenation and minimizing shock. Careful monitoring of level of consciousness and vital signs is essential. Various specimens are drawn for toxicology screening of blood, urine and gastric contents, CBC, blood sugars, electrolytes, and urinalysis; procedures are completed (gastric lavage, intubation, IV administration) and medical regimens followed. It is easy to lose sight of the child within the context of his family at such times.

Fortunately, such severe toxicity is the exception rather than the rule. Although most poisonings pose relatively little danger, the toddler and his family will be anxious and frightened. A calm, understanding attitude and a soft voice will help relieve anxiety.

Parents should be allowed and even encouraged to stay with their child and to participate in decision-making and physical care. Whenever possible, toddlers should be allowed to make simple choices and physical restraining should be kept to a minimum.

Teaching should begin immediately and be continued in the home or clinic. Instruction sheets or information booklets listing prevention, first aid and reference sources should be available in all health care settings. Repeated ingestions in a child or within a family is cause for alarm and should be referred to community health nursing services for investigation and follow-up.

Lead Poisoning

Lead poisoning can be an acute or chronic ingestion problem resulting in acute toxicity or chronic disease. Children at highest risk are of lower socioeconomic status, live in older dwellings, and are 1 to 6 years of age. Peak incidence occurs in spring and summer months.

Lead can be absorbed through the skin, lungs and gastrointestinal tract. Food, air and water all contain some lead. Pica (an appetite for unusual non-food substances) is a frequent precipitating factor in lead poisoning, with children ingesting paint chips or putty containing lead. Other sources include fruit tree spray, artist's paint and leaded gasoline.

Pathophysiology and Clinical Manifestations Acute toxicity results in gastrointestinal irritation, renal pathology and encephalopathy. Symptoms have an abrupt onset and include nausea, abdominal pain, vomiting, diarrhea, black stools, oliguria, seizures and coma.

Chronic toxicity results in degeneration of nerve and muscle cells, renal pathology, cerebral edema and bone marrow dysfunction. Symptoms appear insidiously, progressing from hyperirritability, anorexia, lethargy, intermittent GI distress, constipation and weakness to increased nervousness, ataxia, continual vomiting, impaired consciousness and encephalopathy with seizures and coma.

Diagnosis Making a diagnosis on the basis of history and presenting symptoms is difficult, since symptoms appear slowly and are similar for many conditions. A history of pica is extremely relevant. Pica may be a manifestation of iron deficiency anemia and other factors such as a diet low in calcium or a glucose-6-phosphate dehydrogenase (G6PD) deficiency. History taking and observations by the nurse will help uncover these deficiencies. Possible recent exposure to lead or lead fumes or recent change of residence should be considered.[21] The possibility that the child has played unsupervised near contaminated sources should not be overlooked.

A confirming diagnosis is made based on serial blood samples to determine accumulation of lead as well as metabolic effects. Lead flecks may appear on abdominal X-ray films or "lead lines" may be seen on long bone X-rays.

Nursing Care Acute lead poisoning is handled similarly to other poisonings. If the child is symptomatic, antidotes should be given. Chronic lead poisoning is treated on the basis of laboratory data and symptomatology. Early detection via a screening program is essential. Children with possible increased lead absorption who are asymptomatic should be assessed for exposure, and care should be aimed at removing environmental hazards. Parental involvement and education are imperative.

Children with increased lead absorption with or without symptoms will receive chelation therapy to increase excretion of lead. Edathamil disodium calcium (CaEDTA) given intramuscularly is the treatment of choice. With encephalopathy dimercaprol (BAL) may be given in addition to CaEDTA; however, BAL is contraindicated in children with G6PD deficiency.

Presenting symptoms are treated with supportive therapy. Fluid and electrolyte maintenance is important, as is continued monitoring of the child and serial blood studies. The toxic child must be observed for signs of increased intracranial pressure (changing level of consciousness, increased blood pressure, slow pulse).

During acute illness the child's and parents' fears and needs are similar to those in any poisoning. In addition, when parents are told of the possible long-term effects of lead poisoning, they need additional emotional support. Fear for their other children and guilt are expected reactions. Helping parents understand how they can help prevent further harm is far more constructive than dwelling on what has already taken place. Other stressors that could hinder the child's or family's adaptation should be identified and managed.

Prognosis is variable. Children in whom this poisoning is identified early have the best prognosis. Residual damage in other children is related to the degree of toxicity. Residual effects include brain damage, seizure disorders or hyperactivity.

CROUP

by Linda Mowad, RN, BSN

Croup refers to a pathological condition of the larynx characterized by a brassy, barking cough, a hoarse cry, inspiratory stridor and varying degrees of respiratory distress. There are a number of specific conditions that are classified within "croup syndrome," including epiglottitis, laryngitis, laryngotracheobronchitis and spasmodic laryngitis (Table 33-3). Laryngotracheobronchitis (usually referred to simply as croup) and spasmodic laryngitis (spasmodic croup) are discussed in this section. These are the most common forms of croup syndrome seen in the toddler.

Acute laryngotracheobronchitis (LTB) is most common in boys under the age of 3. It usually follows an upper respiratory infection and is most often seen in late fall or winter, during the cold season. Spasmodic laryngitis is also seen more in boys ages 1 to 3 years. It is more common in children who are anxious and excitable; a possible familial predisposition exists.[6, 21] Both forms of croup tend to recur. As the child grows, attacks tend to disappear.

Etiology

Both acute LTB and spasmodic laryngitis can be caused by a virus. Parainfluenza and influenza viruses are most common. Other organisms include the respiratory syncytial virus, measles virus and adenoviruses. Other etiological factors for spasmodic laryngitis may be allergic, psychologic or aspiration.[6, 21]

Since croup and spasmodic croup tend to recur, once a child has an attack the nurse should provide the necessary information to parents for preventing future attacks or to minimize their stressful effects. Simply being aware of the tendency of the condition to recur should alleviate some of the anxiety associated with caring for these children at home. While there are no definitive preventive measures, environmental control of temperature and humidity may be helpful. When a child has a cold the possibility of an attack should be anticipated. Air passages should be kept clear and the child adequately hydrated.

Pathophysiology and Clinical Manifestations

The symptoms associated with all forms of croup syndrome occur primarily due to inflammation with subsequent narrowing of air passages. Small children have correspondingly smaller air passages, hence even mild inflammation and edema can produce a large degree of obstruction. In addition, more than one area of the respiratory tract is usually affected.

In acute LTB the larynx, trachea and bronchi are affected. There is inflammation and edema, usually mild. It frequently follows an upper respiratory infection. Symptoms appear gradually and worsen progressively. After several days of respiratory symptoms, there is a gradually increasing brassy or barking cough, a hoarse cry, inspiratory stridor and varying degrees of respiratory distress (labored breathing; prolonged expiratory phase; expiratory stridor; suprasternal, substernal or intercostal retractions or all three). Breath sounds may be diminished and wheezes and rhonchi present. The child may have a fever, usually below 39.4° C (103° F) and may appear moderately or severely ill. Both the child and his parents will be frightened. Symptoms worsen at night.

Spasmodic laryngitis is a localized mild inflammation and spasm of the larynx. The child wakes up in the middle of the night with a sudden onset of respiratory distress and a barking cough. He has slow, labored respirations, tachycardia and cool, moist skin. Fever will be absent. Symptoms last several hours and recur for several nights, diminishing in severity. During the daytime the child is asymptomatic or has mild hoarseness.

A diagnosis of acute LTB or spasmodic laryngitis is made on the basis of history and clinical manifestations. Bacterial infection is ruled out by a culture and sensitivity testing, isolating the causative organism. These two conditions must be differentiated from more dangerous condi-

TABLE 33-3 DIFFERENTIATING CROUP SYMPTOMS

Common symptoms: Hoarseness; brassy, barking cough, inspiratory stridor, respiratory distress

Differentiating Features	Acute LTB	Spasmodic Croup	Acute Epiglottitis	Aspirated Foreign Body
Age	<3 yrs	1–4 yrs	>3 yrs	Any age
History	Gradual onset; preceded by URI	Child awakens in night with symptoms	Sudden onset; symptoms worsen over a few hours	Sudden onset of symptoms; child playing or eating; environmental hazards present, adult supervision absent
Symptoms	Fever (<40° C); mild to severe respiratory distress; worse at night	Afebrile; mild to moderate respiratory distress	Child's chin may be thrust forward; drooling; difficulty swallowing; epiglottis cherry-red; febrile (>40° C); child appears toxic	Mild to severe respiratory distress; afebrile; possibly clutching at throat
Comments	Most common	Sometimes relieved by vomiting; asymptomatic in day, symptoms recur during night	No attempt should be made to visualize child's epiglottis; child should be kept calm; emergency tracheotomy may be needed; high morbidity	Heimlich maneuver may help older child but not necessarily infants; emergency tracheotomy may be needed

tions that produce similar symptoms, such as acute epiglottitis and aspiration of a foreign body.

An aspirated foreign body lodged in the larynx or trachea can cause partial obstruction and inflammation, producing symptoms similar to croup. This diagnosis is made according to history, particularly the onset of symptoms: suddenness and time of onset, what the child was doing, presence of possible objects in the environment which could have been aspirated and absence of adult supervision. X-rays may or may not reveal the presence of an object, depending on its composition.

Acute epiglottitis usually occurs in older children (3 to 8 years), although it can occur in the toddler. It is bacterial as opposed to viral in origin. Symptoms occur suddenly over a period of hours and include a high fever (greater than 39.4° C or 103° F), hoarseness, painful swallowing and respiratory distress. The child may present with his chin thrust forward and with drooling owing to his pain when swallowing. He may be reluctant to speak or even cry. Obstruction progresses rapidly and may be complete in 6 to 12 hours, necessitating emergency tracheotomy. Diagnosis is made on the basis of history, visualization of a cherry-red epiglottis and radiological examination revealing an edematous epiglottis. If there is the slightest suspicion of epiglottitis no attempt should be made to visualize the epiglottis or otherwise stimulate the child, as such action could stimulate laryngospasm. The child should be kept calm and crying avoided. (See Chapter 42 for further discussion of epiglottitis.)

Nursing Care

Maintenance of an adequate airway is central to the care of a child with croup, whether hospitalized or cared for at home. The child must be carefully and frequently observed for signs of increasing obstruction and hypoxia. These include an increased respiratory rate, increasing pulse rate, increasing stridor, retractions, restlessness, air hunger and fatigue. Dramatic changes in the child's condition can occur quickly. Respiratory arrest from complete obstruction is a possibility. Any progression of symptoms, particularly signs of cyanosis, must be reported immediately to the physician. The giving of humidified oxygen via positive pressure (Ambu bag and mask) may force enough oxygen through the narrowing airway to maintain the child until the physician arrives. If complete obstruction does occur, insertion of a large bore needle into the trachea will provide a temporary airway; this procedure is to be followed immediately by tracheotomy. A No. 14 gauge Intercath is ideal for this procedure since the needle can be withdrawn and the catheter left in place; however, any large bore needle will do.

The use of oxygen and humidity will relieve some of the distress of croup. For acute LTB cool mist is recommended, while for spasmodic laryngitis warm mist may be better, although either can be used for both conditions. If the child is hospitalized, a croup tent provides the ideal environment. A child may be frightened and resist staying in the tent at first. Parents should be nearby and encourage the child to pretend that they are playing a game and that the tent is a house or an Indian teepee. The child's parents may have other suggestions as to how to keep him in the tent.

At home a croup tent can be improvised by placing a sheet over the top of a crib or playpen and securing it. A vaporizer (warm or cool mist) is then directed into the crib. Safety precautions must be taken so that the child is not burned or otherwise injured by the equipment. Plastic should not be used because of the possibility that the child might pull it down and smother himself. The child should be observed frequently while in a makeshift croup tent. Parents should be aware of signs of increasing obstruction and instructed to return the child to the hospital if his condition worsens.

If it is impractical to improvise a croup tent, the child can be taken into the bathroom, the door closed and the shower or tub water run to provide an environment high in humidity to relieve his distress. The child should never be left alone under these conditions.

Racemic epinephrine and 40 per cent oxygen may be administered in mist or intermittent positive pressure breathing (IPPB) to temporarily relieve symptoms. Treatments need to be repeated periodically to keep the child symptom-free.

Adequate hydration is important but can usually be achieved with oral fluids; IV's should be reserved for the dehydrated child. Oral fluids of the child's choice should be encouraged.

Vomiting is an old remedy to relieve the spasm of spastic croup and may or may not be helpful. Syrup of ipecac, 15 ml. orally followed by a glass of water, has been used to produce emesis in these children.

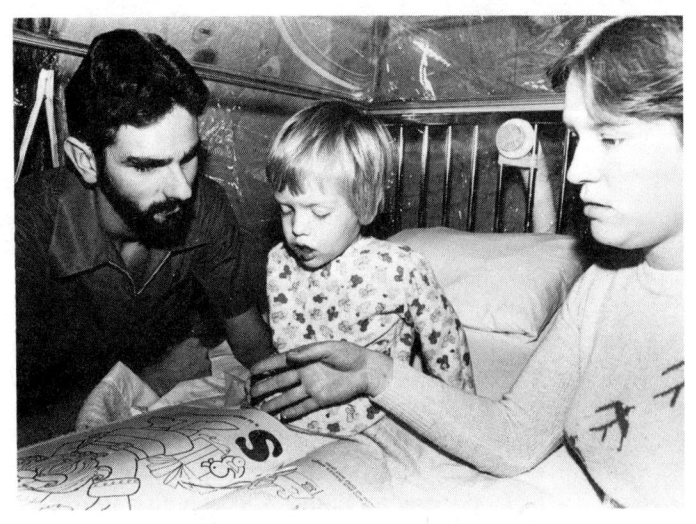

The mist tent provides an ideal environment for the child with croup; however, the tent should not hinder continued parent-child interaction.

Steroids may be given in severe croup to relieve inflammation, although their use is controversial. Antibiotics are contraindicated, since croup is a viral syndrome. Some physicians administer them to prevent secondary infection, although this practice is generally frowned upon.

A significant aspect of nursing management of croup is decreasing the child's and the family's anxiety. Croup is dramatic and frightening; respiratory distress is aggravated by anxiety. Parents should be encouraged to remain with the child, holding and comforting him. Rhythmic movements such as rocking and gentle touches will help calm the child. While in a croup tent the child should assume a position of comfort and be able to maintain physical contact with his parents. Parents should be encouraged to reach in and touch the child to reassure him and prevent feelings of isolation.

Upsetting the child should be avoided. Unnecessary procedures or extensive examinations should be deferred until the child is in less distress. Sedation is sometimes ordered, although it should be used with extreme caution as it may mask symptoms of increasingly severe hypoxia, particularly restlessness.

In order for parents to care for their child better, their own anxiety needs to be alleviated. The nurse should encourage them to verbalize their fears and anxieties. Specific instructions as to how to hold the child and measures to help relieve symptoms will help parents feel more secure in handling and caring for the child. They need to be reassured that the child will recover and to understand the course of illness and what to expect. Acute LTB lasts from several days to several weeks, sometimes with a persistent barking cough. Spasmodic laryngitis can recur for two to four consecutive nights, although the first attack is usually the worst. Both forms of croup tend to recur while the child is little. This tendency is eventually outgrown as the child and his airway grow.

Both acute LTB and spasmodic laryngitis have good prognoses. Complications from an extension of the infection occur in approximately 15 per cent of cases. Age, length and extension of illness and adequacy of management are factors that affect the outcome.

References

1. C. Archambeault-Jones, and I. Feller. Procedures for Nursing the Burned Patient. National Institute for Burn Medicine, Ann Arbor, MI, 1975
2. M. Bowden, C. Jones and I. Feller. Psycho-Social Aspects of a Severe Burn: A Review of the Literature. National Burn Institute, Ann Arbor, MI, 1979
3. P. Chinn. Child Health Maintenance: Concepts in Family-Centered Care. C. V. Mosby Co., 1979
4. A. Costello-Galligan. Using Roy's concept of adaptation to care for young children. American Journal of Maternal Child Nursing, Jan/Feb 1979, p. 24
5. A. Craft. Accidental poisoning in children. Nursing Times, 12 June 1975, p. 932
6. H. Eichenwald. Respiratory infections in children. Hospital Practice, April 1976, p. 81
7. Evaluation of Emergency Medical Services with a National Burn Registry. 1975–1978. Grant #HS-01906-01; HEW, National Center for Health Services Research, University of Michigan School of Public Health Department of Biostatistics, and National Institute for Burn Medicine
8. I. Feller and C. Archambeault. Nursing the Burned Patient. Institute for Burn Medicine, Ann Arbor, MI, 1973
9. I. Feller and K. Crane. National burn information exchange. Surgical Clinics of North America, December 1970, p. 1425
10. I. Feller et al. A Michigan burn information and triage system. Michigan Hospitals, 1977, p. 10
11. S. Gellis, and B. Kagan. Current Pediatric Therapy 9. W. B. Saunders Co., 1980
12. Isler. This technique may make tracheostomy unnecessary. RN January 1977, p. 32
13. S. Jay. Pediatric ICU — Involving parents in care. Canadian Nurse, May 1978, p. 28
14. C. Jones and M. Bowden. Nurse family interface, Burn Symposium. Symposia Specialists, Inc., Miami, FL, 1979
15. E. Keller. Poisoning in children. Postgraduate Medicine, May 1979, p. 177
16. C. Kempe et al. Current Pediatric Diagnosis and Treatment, 5th ed. Lange Medical Publications, 1978
17. D. Marlow. Textbook of Pediatric Nursing, 3rd ed. W. B. Saunders Co., 1969
18. M. McIntire. Safety packaging: a model for successful accident prevention. Pediatric Annals, Nov 1977, p. 706
19. J. Mennear. The poisoning emergency. American Journal of Nursing, May 1977, p. 842
20. H. Mofenson and J. Greensher. Controversies in prevention and treatment of poisons. Pediatric Annals, November 1977, p. 717
21. W. Nelson, ed. Textbook of Pediatrics, 11th ed. W. B. Saunders Co., 1979
22. Poisoning — an update. Clinical Pediatrics, March 1979, p. 144
23. J. Ritchie. Preparation of toddlers and pre-school children for hospital procedures. Canadian Nurse, December 1979, p. 30
24. H. Selye. The Stress of Life. McGraw-Hill Book Co., 1976
25. C. Warner. Emergency Care: Assessment and Intervention, 2nd ed. C. V. Mosby Co., 1978
26. G. Wheatley. Introduction: childhood accidents. Pediatric Annals, Nov 1977, p. 688

Additional Recommended Reading

J. Arena. Poisoning. Emergency Medicine, April 1976, p. 171

C. Artz and J. Moncrief. The Treatment of Burns. W. B. Saunders Co., 1979

L. Bailey. Mothers have needs too. Canadian Nurse, September 1978, p. 28

N. Bernstein. Emotional Care of the Facially Burned and Disfigured. Little, Brown & Co., 1976

M. Bowden and I. Feller. Family reaction to a severe burn. American Journal of Nursing, February 1973, p. 317

L. Campbell. Special behavior problems of the burned child. American Journal of Nursing, January 1976, p. 220

H. Elfert. Helping pre-school children learn to be safe. Canadian Nurse. December 1979, p. 26

H. Fosnot, Plant-ingestion poisoning from A to Z. Patient Care, 30 June 1979, p. 86

S. Frye and J. Lander. The initial management of the acutely burned child. Issues of Comprehensive Pediatric Nursing, 1976, p. 36

L. Gever. A new treatment for a new problem: acetaminophen overdose. Nursing, June 1980, p. 57

R. Goodwin. Child-resistant locks in poison control. Pediatrics, May 1978, p. 750

R. Gosselin et al. Clinical Toxicology of Commercial Products, 4th ed. Williams & Wilkins Co., 1979

C. Isler. The fine art of handling a hospitalized child. RN, March 1978, p. 41

F. Jacoby. Nursing Care of the Patient with Burns. C. V. Mosby Co., 1976

C. Jones and I. Feller. Burns — emergency care of burn victims. Journal of Emergency Medicine, March 1975, p. 13

C. Jones and I. Feller. Burns: What to do during the first crucial hours. Nursing 77, March 1977, p. 23

C. Jones and I. Feller. Proper care of the burn victim: emergent period care. Nursing 77, March 1977, p. 22

C. Jones and I. Feller. Proper care of the burn victim: acute period care. Nursing 77, March 1977, p. 72

C. Jones and I. Feller. Proper care of the burn victim: rehabilitation period care. Nursing 77, December 1977, p. 54

M. Kerr. Salicylate poisoning in children. Journal of Emergency Nursing, May/June 1979, p. 20

F. Lovejoy. Kids in crisis: priorities in poisoning. Emergency Medicine, May 1976, p. 202

A. Macy. Preventing hepatotoxicity in acetaminophen overdose. American Journal of Nursing, February 1979, p. 301

P. Rogenes and J. Maylan. Restoring fluid balance in the patient with severe burns. American Journal of Nursing December 1976, p. 1952

M. Savedra. Moving from hospital to home. American Journal of Maternal Child Nursing, Jul/Aug 1977, p. 220

J. Segal. Child and family health: Forces that shape the lives of our young. Public Health Reports, Sept/Oct 1979, p. 399

E. Smith et al. Reestablishing a child's body image. American Journal of Nursing, February 1977, p. 445

L. Talabere and P. Graves. A tool for assessing families of burned children. American Journal of Nursing, January 1976, p. 225

M. Wagner. Emergency care of the burned patient. American Journal of Nursing, November 1977, p. 1788

C. Warner, Emergency Care: Assessment and Intervention, 2nd ed. C. V. Mosby Co., 1978

M. Zitomer. Protecting children from the tragedy of burns. American Journal of Maternal Child Nursing, Mar/Apr 1977, p. 129

34 POTENTIAL STRESSES DURING TODDLER YEARS: IRREVERSIBLE ALTERATIONS IN HEALTH STATUS

by Frances White Thurber, RN, MSN

When disease of a long-term or lifelong nature compounds the normal age-centered developmental crises of the toddler, the results can be potentially devastating for both the toddler and his family. The impact of these irreversible conditions on the child and family is the subject of this chapter.

Irreversible conditions affect the child and family either for a great many years or throughout the life span, creating a state of continuous stress. Although these conditions can become life threatening, for the most part they can be adapted to by the child and the family unit, and a fairly normal life style and developmental pattern can be maintained. It is toward this end that nursing intervention is directed.

Several irreversible conditions are discussed that cause particular stress during the toddler years. Intervention to promote family adaptation is correlated throughout.

IMPACT OF IRREVERSIBLE ILLNESS: NURSE'S ROLE

The Child's Autonomy Needs

The child of this age group, according to Erikson, is striving to accomplish the maturational crisis of autonomy.[2] If the child fails to accomplish this task, he feels shame and doubts his ability to control either himself or his world.

When a long-term illness is diagnosed in a toddler, there is the potential for a major upset in this struggle for autonomy. If autonomy has been achieved, the child struggles to retain his independence. If some measure of body function control has been achieved, he continuously tries to maintain this level.

Such a diagnosis generally initiates a series of hospitalizations as well as long periods of homebound convalescence. This affects the child's abilities to master autonomy and become more independent in his functioning. Illness is a multidimensional stressor. Physically the child's abilities to master autonomy and become more independent in motor activities may be significantly reduced. Completion of daily tasks of living and engrossment in play and exploration use up most of a toddler's available energy. When his activity tolerance is reduced, caretakers are faced with the challenge of assisting their toddler to reach his maximum potential in development without compromising his physical health.

The toddler generally experiences a stage of

rapid motor development that aids and is aided by his explorative behaviors. Testing procedures or intravenous therapy may necessitate prolonged restraining measures. For this child such immobilization is intolerable and may lead to intense frustration as well as a curtailment of his autonomous strivings. The nature of the restraint at times may actually inhibit the child from utilizing previously adapted coping behaviors such as snuggling a blanket or sucking his thumb. Several studies have demonstrated that potential may exist for delay in physical, psychosocial and language skills as a result of restraint during these early formative years.[1,8]

When a child is ill, parents instinctively tend to overprotect him. If this is compounded by parental failure to perceive that this child is no longer an infant and that certain freedoms must be granted, autonomy may be further compromised. Unfortunately, the normal regressive patterns evidenced in children with chronic illness may reinforce parental overprotective behavior.

A toddler's opportunity and ability to control his life and activities is diminished when he experiences long-term illness. Therefore, those situations he can control take on new and exaggerated importance. Control of feeding is one mechanism the toddler frequently uses to assert himself. With typical negativism, he may refuse all offerings of food, merely pick at the food or decorate the floor with it. Elimination is another mechanism for asserting control in response to the restriction of illness. The child may choose to control or not to control elimination regardless of his previous mastery. His choice is strongly influenced by his parents' response to the illness as well as by his natural desire to please them.

Nursing Intervention Nursing intervention to facilitate autonomy may take many forms. Parents of a chronically ill child almost always express a need to know how their child is developing. The nurse should assess the child's developmental level using a standardized screening tool such as the Denver Developmental Screening Test (DDST) or an assessment guide such as the Washington Guide. The test should be administered at a time when the child's physical condition permits maximum cooperation. Although parents should be made aware of developmental lags so they can provide stimulation in those areas, it is essential that the nurse point out and reinforce areas of their child's normal development and emphasize how his behavior patterns have progressed.

The family should be assisted to understand their child's independence. Efforts toward self-assertion should be encouraged and maintained despite illness. This can be done by letting the toddler make small decisions, perhaps whether to take his medicine from a cup or a spoon. Unnecessary conflict should be avoided. Forcing a toddler to "give in" when it does not make a difference is counterproductive and may lead to power struggles and further frustrations. However, it is important to emphasize to parents that in spite of chronic illness, the toddler needs consistency, appropriate limits and a stable routine to order his life.

The nurse should be an effective role model of how to intervene with this child. She should provide activities and toys that will stimulate the child to explore within his limited environment. Appropriate play objects such as drums to beat and beanbags to throw provide the child with an outlet for his frustrations. Stacking and nesting toys and shape boxes into which items can be inserted especially reinforce the child's sense of accomplishment.

If energy must be conserved, caretakers may need to give assistance for task completion and provide some limits for play to avoid exhaustion. This can be accomplished without seriously hampering development if the caretaker intervenes by setting up situations that require minimal energy dissipation but meet the child's need for self-expression and independence. For example, rolling a ball back and forth on the floor can replace a game of running and chasing the ball; when dressing, a caretaker can suggest "You put on one sock while I put on the other sock."

If children must be restrained over periods of time, they should always be given an explanation for the restraint. The nurse should remove the restraint as frequently as possible to facilitate movement of extremities. Body contact, a soothing voice and perhaps a walk in the hall may ease the frustration of this child. If possible, restraints should be applied in a manner that allows the child enough freedom to touch some part of his body. This intervention is important because young children experience their body primarily through sensation.

Mealtime should be a pleasant, social experience. Optimally, no painful procedures should immediately precede or follow mealtimes. Small portions may be offered on attractive child-sized plates with child-sized utensils. A choice of nutritional snacks should be offered between but not immediately preceding meals. Praise and positive reinforcement of proper eating behavior are essential.

Parents should be made aware of the normalities of their child's behaviors as well as what responses are to be expected as the child adapts to the limitations imposed by a chronic condition.

The Child and Separation

During toddlerhood the child normally experiences intense anxiety when separated from his parents, even if only for a brief time. With the onset of irreversible disease and concomitant hospitalizations, often at great distances from home, this child is particularly vulnerable to separation anxiety. His need for safety and protection and his fears of being unable to cope necessitate their presence. If they are unavailable or their presence is limited owing to the distances involved, the child will more often move to a state of despair and then to denial. A gap may then develop between the child and his family.[7] If these hospitalizations are lengthy, the child may become a stranger in his own home. When he returns from the hospital he finds that life has gone on without him and that his siblings have established new relationships that exclude him.

Nursing Intervention Nursing interventions must be directed toward increasing the coping abilities of the child during periods of separation. This can be most effectively accomplished by decreasing the amount of separation or by minimizing its impact.

The most effective method of dealing with separation is to encourage family participation in the care of the child.[7] This is accomplished by providing live-in space or rooming-in for mothers or an alternate family caretaker. Play and recreational programs have also been instrumental in minimizing the effects of separation. Opportunities for play and diversional activities can distract the child's attention from the parents' absence.

Primary nursing is another means of assisting the child to cope with separation. This type of care provides one caretaker or team of caretakers who consistently plan and implement care; this presents an opportunity for the child to develop a close relationship with a substitute caretaker. Toddlers need one person available on a constant basis to whom they can turn for support and with whom they can establish a trusting relationship.

The impact of separation can also be minimized by maintaining as closely as possible the child's home routines. This intervention not only provides him some security in a strange environment but also aids the transition back to his own home after long or frequent hospitalizations.

Use of tape-recorded messages for playback when parents must be absent is appropriate when absences are long or frequent. In studying the responses of toddlers to tape recordings of this type, Hennessey[4] found that the children responded positively. Toddlers recognized their mother's voice and listened quietly and attentively to the recorded message. This technique, along with picture drawing and visits from siblings and grandparents, may be helpful in maintaining the child's relationship with his

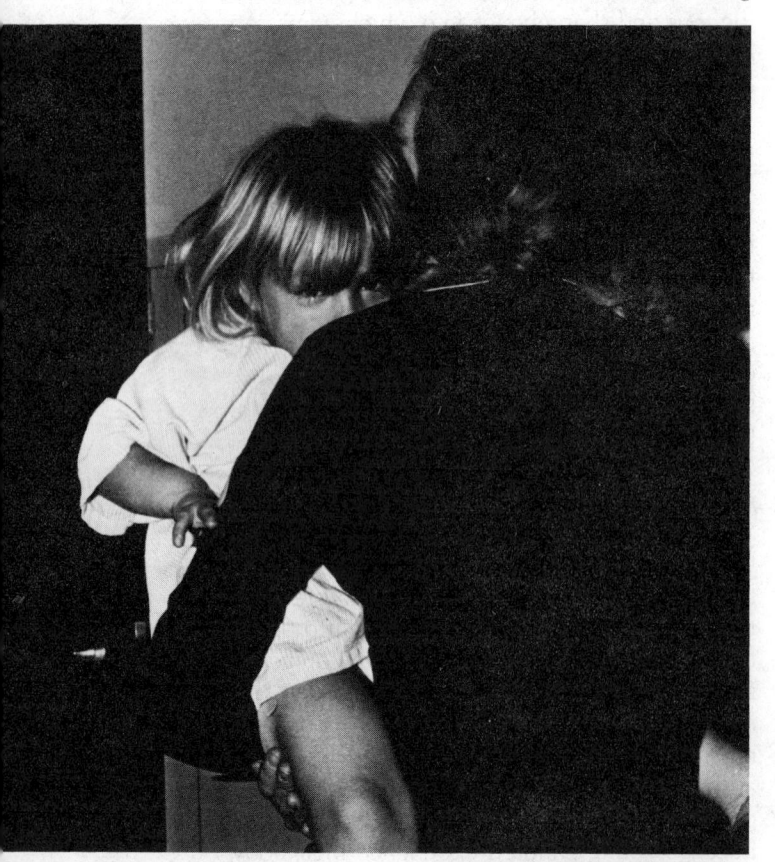

When a child must undergo frequent or prolonged hospitalization, she becomes particularly vulnerable to separation conflicts.

family during frequent or long absences from home.

Preservation of the Child's Competencies

For the toddler the development of gross motor competencies is of utmost importance. Movement through walking, climbing and exploring is the mechanism through which achievement of motor control takes place. Irreversible illness may necessitate periods of rest and limited activity. Hospitalization, at its best, imposes a more confined environment. Many disease conditions of a long-term nature impose extra limitations on a child's activities, as more rigorous safety measures often must be taken.

The chronically ill toddler may experience difficulty interacting with peers in social situations. Limitations imposed by the illness and treatment can present obstacles to the development of relationships with others outside the immediate family unit. This can lead to excessive dependency on caretakers and delays in achieving the emotional independence usually seen in young children. If the disease is particularly debilitating, the child may be frustrated that he cannot keep up with the activities of his peers.

Intellectual curiosity and cognitive development may be stifled. This can be due to the child's limited ability to explore his environment. Parents may unwittingly contribute to limits on exploration by placing too severe and restrictive constraints on the child in an attempt to protect him.

Nursing Intervention Parents should be instructed in methods to maximize the child's competencies within his limitations. Placing items and toys within the child's reach and slightly beyond easy reach will encourage explorative behavior. Exercises accomplished through creative play, which are within the child's physical capabilities, may help to restore losses in function or at least minimize further loss.

Realistic safety procedures for the child should be individualized and discussed with the family. Care should be taken to provide necessary safety without oversupervision. Home visits by nurses can be quite helpful in assisting the parents to realize where safety limits should be imposed and how to make modifications in the home environment to accomplish this.

Relationships with other persons outside the family unit should be encouraged as much as possible, especially those with peers. Parents should be prepared for the very real possibility that their child may experience frustrations if he lags behind age mates and be prepared to provide the necessary emotional support to minimize negative effects. With this kind of exposure will come the growth and competency to adapt to the lifelong limitations the condition may impose. Enrollment in an early remedial education program is essential to maximize this child's potential.

Effects on the Family

When a toddler is diagnosed as having a long-term problem it creates a family crisis that can have an enormous impact on family relationships. The family of a toddler is generally a young family, still learning how to live and cope as a unit instead of as individuals. The stress of irreversible illness at this point can either cement the marital relationship or sever it completely. In addition, this child will make increased demands on personal energy and on finances just at a time when the couple is beginning to establish some financial security.

The importance of parental time-out opportunities from the care of this child has been previously discussed. However, fulfillment of this need may be difficult. The child developmentally is reluctant to separate from his parents. He may require more care than a healthy toddler, making it difficult to secure a capable babysitter. Parents may feel acute anxiety or guilt over leaving the child to pursue their own enjoyments. Another factor is the additional cost for substitute caretakers and babysitters, at a time when the family can least afford this. Not only is the cost of sitters a problem but also their availability — many responsible sitters do not wish to take the responsibility of caring for a special child. This can be compounded by the natural resistance of a toddler to other caretakers, to necessary limitations and to essential treatment measures. Church groups and senior citizen organizations often know of people who are willing to help out in such situations. Names of specific contact persons should be provided to parents if possible.

Nursing Intervention Nurses must often intervene to help the family cope with such stresses. Community resources can be mobilized to help with the emotional and financial impact of irreversible disease. For many of these conditions, special support groups have been established whose members offer emotional support and education about the disease and suggest ways to cope with problems. These groups can also help in alleviating the babysitting problem through sharing resources and taking turns having this responsibility. In this way the financial burden can be lightened and the special care provided. Crippled Children's Services can offer financial assistance for the child's special needs.

Parents should be encouraged to share their feelings of anger and frustration. They can be helped to realize the true capabilities of their child if the positive aspects of his development are recognized along with his limitations. Knowing what to expect helps parents to prepare for what will be needed later in their child's care and to understand the needs of other family members.

Siblings should be encouraged to become involved in the care of the child, not only to share their feelings of caring but to enhance their own self-esteem. In many cases, siblings enjoy being involved in the care of this child and often assume small tasks to provide comfort or entertain.

It is imperative that the family understand its vital role in aiding the child's adaptation to the crisis of illness. Toddlers are easily influenced by the feelings of others, and it is the family's adaptation which will most affect the child's ability to cope and adjust. With the love and encouragement of his family as well as community support, the toddler with irreversible illness can adapt by learning to live within the limitations imposed by the disease. He can then realize his potential for a productive and useful future.

Three distinct disease entities — celiac disease, hemophilia and nephrotic syndrome — have particular impact during the toddler years. Their ramifications persist throughout life, necessitating continual adaptation on the part of the child and his family.

CELIAC DISEASE

Definition and Pathophysiology

Celiac disease or gluten-induced enteropathy is second only to cystic fibrosis as the most common cause of malabsorption in children. The exact incidence of the disease is unknown, as treatment is not sought for many asymptomatic children. The incidence is higher in European countries than in the United States, with estimates varying from 1:300 to 1:4000 in this country.

Peak incidence in children is between the ages of 9 and 18 months.[5] Symptoms may begin at any time after the introduction of gluten into the diet, usually at the time of cereal introduction. Affected children often have a history of digestive disturbances starting at 6 to 12 months of age.

Gluten is a form of protein contained in wheat, barley, rye and oats. The gluten itself consists of two protein fractions, glutenin and gliadin. Of these gliadin appears to be the causative agent. The exact means by which the gluten damages the mucosa of the small bowel remains obscure. However, two explanations currently exist. In the first, it is thought that an enzymatic insufficiency (dipeptidase) causes an accumulation of toxic gluten peptides. The second theory states that the gluten toxicity results from an alteration in immunologic response. The second explanation is the more preferred and is supported by the fact that any abnormalities noted in immunoglobulin level or synthesis return to normal after the preventive diet is begun. In addition, this theory is supported by the striking response to corticosteroid therapy.

Normally the intestinal mucosa is lined with tall villae whose function is the absorption of nutrients. In celiac disease sensitivity to the undigested gluten causes the villae to gradually flatten out, resulting in a reduced absorptive surface area. Digestion of fats is primarily affected, but there is also some interference in carbohydrate and vitamin absorption.

Clinical Manifestations

The resulting malabsorption leads to chronic diarrhea with large amounts of excreted fats (steatorrhea). The stools are characteristically bulky and foul smelling. Abdominal distention is present and the child appears malnourished. Due to the failure to utilize ingested calories, wasting is seen in normal areas of fat distribution, particularly the buttocks. If vitamin D absorption is impaired, bone changes occur and rickets or tetany may develop.

The disease is insidious, marked by poor weight gain and failure to grow. Two-thirds of these children are below the third percentile for weight and one-third are below the third percentile in height.[12] Anemia may also be present due to malabsorption of iron, folic acid or B_{12}, or of all three. Bleeding disorders may result from vitamin K deficiency.

Certain changes in behavior often correlate with the presence of celiac disease. These changes include irritability, lack of cooperation and eventually apathy.

The child with celiac disease may initially present as an irritable, anorexic child with chronic diarrhea, failure to thrive, a pot belly and muscle wasting. Or he may present for initial care in a state of celiac crisis. This is an acute episode of watery diarrhea and vomiting leading to severe electrolyte imbalance and dehydration, which may progress to acidosis. The crisis may be precipitated by infection, alteration in diet, or by use of anticholinergic medications, used commonly for preoperative medication.

The Nurse's Role in Making the Diagnosis

Because of the possibility of genetic transfer the nurse should be aware of significant family history when gathering assessment data. This would include information regarding family members who may have had obscure complaints of digestive problems, intermittent diarrhea or failure to thrive and gain weight. The child's dietary history should be reviewed to ascertain at what age new foods were introduced.

In evaluating the physical status of a child who is not thriving, the nurse should observe for body distribution of fat and protuberance of the abdomen. This in conjunction with frequent, foul-smelling, fatty stools that float in the toilet bowl lends credence to the diagnosis. Any failure to grow at normal pace should suggest celiac disease. The family should be told of the possibility of genetic transmission so that an informed decision may be made in regard to the advisability of having more children. It should be emphasized that although adaptation is necessary on the part of the family and child, celiac disease is usually quite well controlled by strict adherence to the dietary regimen, and that, in other respects, a normal life-style can be maintained.

Gluten-sensitive enteropathy is not difficult to diagnose. With recognition of the characteristic body changes and dispositional changes, a jejunal biopsy is usually performed.

Prior to the intestinal biopsy clotting function should be assessed. A complete blood count, platelet count, prothrombin time and partial thromboplastin time should be obtained. The nurse should know the results of clotting function tests before biopsy and should inform the physician of any abnormalities. After a six-to-eight hour fast and appropriate sedation, the biopsy is done.

Under normal conditions the procedure takes approximately 15 minutes. The characteristic histological changes in mucosa are definitive. With the child well sedated, a radiopaque polyethylene tube is passed down the alimentary canal until it lodges in the small bowel. By use of a special capsule on the tube with a small cutting edge, the specimen is taken and removed for examination. The child may resume normal feeding and activity upon awakening after the procedure. The nurse should observe the child for any signs of shock or hemorrhage from the biopsy site.

If suspected atrophy of the villae is demonstrated upon examination, this, with the presence of fecal fat, supports diagnosis. Serum proteins and immunoglobulin levels will be low owing to the protein-losing enteropathy. Radiologically, bone age may be retarded and osteoporosis and osteomalacia are often present. If the child responds favorably to a withdrawal of gluten from the diet and subsequently the condition is exacerbated in response to gluten challenge,* the diagnosis is confirmed.

Nursing responsibility during the diagnostic period is diverse. The nurse assists in collection of 72-hour stool specimens to be examined for fecal fat and coordinates collection of hematologic specimens for evaluation of anemia, protein and prothrombin levels and electrolyte imbalance. X-ray studies may be done for bone age and lower gastrointestinal function. Because of the symptomatic similarity to cystic fibrosis, a sweat test should be done. As she coordinates these procedures, the nurse should be aware of the importance of timing. If possible, tests should be scheduled so that they do not interfere with mealtimes. Honest, con-

---

*Gluten challenge means the reintroduction to the diet under controlled conditions of gluten (usually in 10 to 30 gm. daily amounts). This may be continued for two to three weeks if symptoms are absent. Patients with true celiac disease develop steatorrhea and have decreased xylose absorption.[9]

cise, simple explanations should be given to the child, without exaggeration. These explanations are best given immediately before the procedure to avoid increasing the anxiety level of the toddler. This is particularly important if his cooperation is desired in the future. The comfort and safety needs of the child should be met prior to, during and after each procedure.

The family will be a direct concern for the nurse throughout all diagnostic procedures. Because of the slow, insidious onset of the condition, the parents' ability to cope with the situation may be severely altered. Parents will be extremely worried about their child and may even question their own ability to provide adequate care. Every effort should be made to give them as much information as they are able to absorb as well as to allow time for them to express their fears and concerns.

The child with celiac disease may be irritable, anorexic, unsociable and withdrawn during the diagnostic phase and may be difficult for the parents and the nurse to deal with. The parents may be on the verge of exhaustion and occasionally need opportunities to have time out from the stress of this situation. They should also be informed that the child's irritability will quickly disappear once the diet is initiated and the intestinal tract becomes normal.

Nursing Care During the Course and Treatment of Disease

The treatment of celiac disease centers on correct dietary management. This involves the institution and maintenance of a lifetime diet free of gluten. Corn and rice as well as soybean flour may be substituted for the grain portion of the diet. Health food stores are an excellent source for many appropriate foods. Care must be taken in purchasing *all* foods, as grains are frequently used as filler or thickeners. Labels must be carefully read to avoid ingestion of grains. Foods labelled "with hydrolyzed vegetable protein" or "vegetable protein added" must be avoided. Because of the suppression of disaccharidase activity, a lactose-free diet is advocated initially to help lessen the diarrhea.

If the diet is carefully and consistently followed, a dramatic response is seen. Within the first few days the child's disposition improves; he becomes less irritable and less apathetic. A progressive improvement in muscle tone and lessening of diarrhea and decreased abdominal distention are seen.

Those seriously ill children who present in crisis may need replacement therapy with intravenous fluids, parenteral hyperalimentation and vitamin administration. A dramatic improvement has been seen in crisis when corticosteriod therapy is initiated to decrease the inflammation of the bowel. A nasogastric tube may be passed to decrease abdominal distention and should be attached to intermittent suction. When the crisis is resolved, the child returns to diet therapy for maintenance.

Prior to discharge it is imperative that parents understand what precipitates a celiac crisis. Prevention of infection should be stressed as well as maintaining the dietary regimen. If the child is to be treated by other members of the health care team, they should be made aware of his celiac status so that anticholinergic drugs will be avoided.

Within six months to one year after beginning the diet, the child with celiac disease should be within normal weight for age. Height and bone age take somewhat longer to become normal, usually two years.[12] Relapses occur whenever the child eats gluten-containing foods.

The possible correlation between celiac disease and the occurrence of intestinal lymphoma and other forms of gastrointestinal cancer is a very strong argument for remaining on a gluten-free diet for life, and should be brought to the parents' attention.

Nursing responsibility involves care during diagnosis and crisis, dietary management and instruction, facilitating the adaptation to a modified dietary life-style, as well as stimulation of appropriate emotional and developmental responses.

It is important to note that parents initially are adjusting to the potential changes in their own lives as well as feelings of guilt and may not readily absorb large amounts of information. Parents will not necessarily adjust at the same pace. Explanations may need to be detailed, and repeated and frequent feedback sessions are helpful to determine the parents' level of understanding.

Careful explanation of the role of gluten in the disease as well as a copy of the diet and recipes to bring variety to the diet should be given to the family. The family just learning of this diagnosis can contact another family with a child with celiac disease, who can share methods of coping that have worked for them. This will also provide an opportunity to ask for recipe ideas. Suggestions are helpful for making special treats for the child, such as gluten-free cookies and birthday cakes, as well as methods of making such items as pizza. Appropriate snack foods such as fruit chunks, cheese, and carrot sticks are suggested for school snacks.

A special diet is expensive and may place an added financial burden on a family. Means of rebudgeting or working out a more economical method of preparing the diet may need to be explored. Incorporating low- or no-gluten foods into the mainstream of the family diet may be beneficial, as cooking special foods for one individual is more expensive and will set the child apart.

As the child's condition improves, appropriate physical, social and intellectual activities should be initiated. This child learns early that his diet will always be a little different, and if he learns at an early age to make the correct decisions, he will adapt well throughout his life. The normalcy of his life should be stressed. It should be recognized that in essence celiac disease is a dietary problem and with correct dietary control there need be no other severe limitations.

HEMOPHILIA

Definition and Pathophysiology

Hemophilia is an alteration in the clotting mechanism and results from a deficiency in one of two different clotting factors. Factor VIII deficiency or classic hemophilia (also called hemophilia A) is the most common hereditary coagulation factor deficiency. It accounts for 80 per cent of all hereditary clotting diseases and occurs in 1:10,000 white males born in the United States.[12] It is a sex-linked recessive disorder carried by the female and transmitted to her male offspring.

The deficiency is considered severe if less than 1 per cent of the factor is present or moderate if between 1 and 5 per cent of the factor is present and the child bleeds on trauma. The condition in a child with a 5 to 50 per cent factor deficiency is considered minor, and the child may have no tendency to bleed at all except after minor surgery or dental extraction.

Christmas disease, or hemophilia B, is a factor IX deficiency and comprises 15 per cent of the cases. It also has a genetic basis and is clinically indistinguishable from hemophilia A except by factor assay.

The clotting mechanism normally functions by forming a substance called *prothrombin activator*. This may be in response to an extrinsic mechanism that begins when blood comes in contact with traumatized tissue or to an intrinsic mechanism following trauma or damage to the blood itself. The prothrombin activator then catalyzes the conversion of prothrombin into thrombin. The thrombin acts as an enzyme to convert fibrinogen into fibrin threads. Fibrin stabilizing factor acts on fibrin threads, causing meshing of red blood cells and plasma to form a clot (Fig. 34–1).

It is during the formation of prothrombin activator that the factors function. In their absence the entire mechanism is affected. The deficiency of either factor VIII or IX results in prolonged bleeding.

Clinical Manifestations and Etiology: Nurse's Role

Hemorrhage may occur in the first few days of life or following circumcision. In most cases, however, significant symptoms do not occur until the infant begins to walk. Then excessive bruising, hematoma formation and spontaneous bleeding become noticeable. Bleeding into the joint cavities, especially the knees, ankles and elbows, takes place, causing hemarthrosis. This condition produces severe pain and swelling of the joint and can lead to disability if limitation of movement becomes extreme or contracture results.

Because the etiology of hemophilia is sex-linked, the nurse should assess and identify any history of bleeding disorders within the family. It may be helpful to plot a family pedigree to discern family relationships and possible patterns of inheritance.

Nurses in the newborn nursery should be alert for circumcisions that continue to bleed. Primary-care providers should observe for signs of ecchymosis (easy bruising), subcutaneous bleeding, or swollen joints when doing well-child screening. Whenever a history of bleeding in the family is known, children should be considered at risk and carefully observed. Any siblings of an affected child should be exam-

```
                        PROTHROMBIN
                             |
Extrinsic clotting mechanism ⎫
(Tissue thromboplastin)      ⎪  Prothrombin →  ← Ca++
                             ⎬  activators
Intrinsic clotting mechanism ⎪
(Platelets, factor VIII,     ⎪
factor IX, other factors)    ⎭
                             |
                             ↓
                        THROMBIN
                             |
FIBRINOGEN ─────────────────→ FIBRIN THREADS

        Ca++ →   ← FIBRIN STABILIZING FACTOR
                   (Plasma factor XIII)

FIBRIN CLOT
```

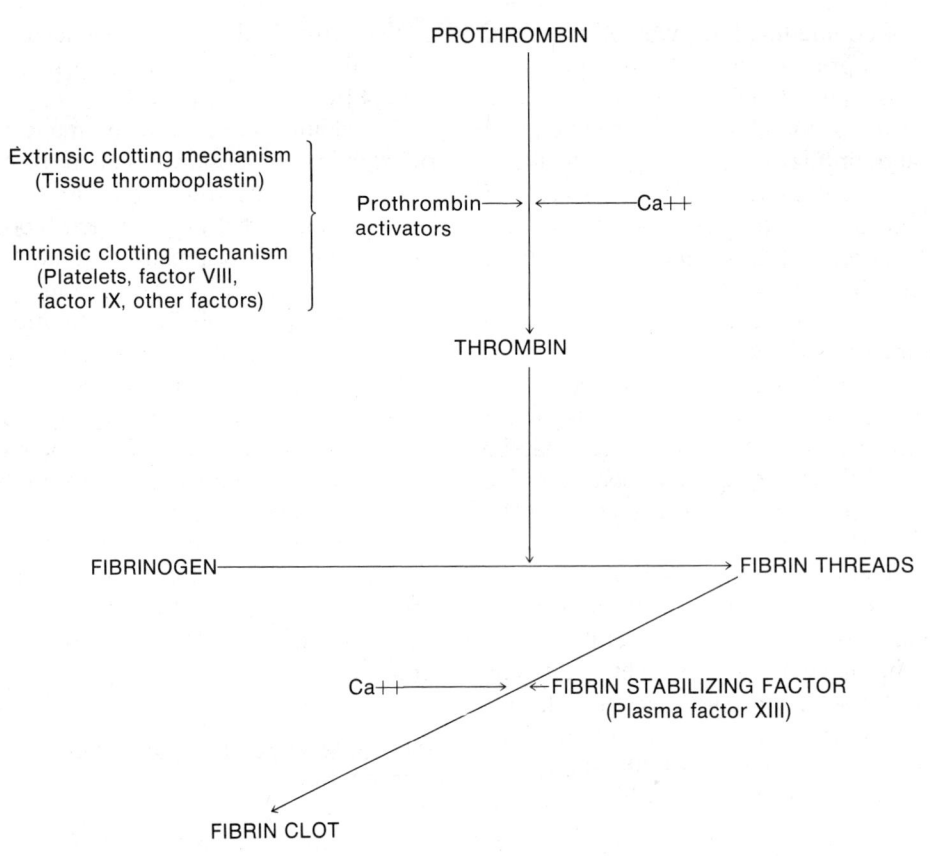

Figure 34–1. The clotting mechanism.

ined, as male siblings have a 50 per cent chance of being affected and 50 per cent of female siblings may be carriers.

Genetic counselling is appropriate if the family is considering having more children or if they need further clarification on the transmission of the condition. Although they should not be forced to have this counselling, they should realize that the option is available to them.

The Nurse's Role in Making the Diagnosis

Diagnosis of hemophilia is usually based on a history of bleeding episodes and a prolonged partial thromboplastin time. Prothrombin time and bleeding time are normal, but blood clotting time is markedly prolonged. To identify the specific factor discrepancy, factor assays must be done.

The carrier state may also be detected, as carrier females will have factor VIII levels between 30 and 70 per cent of normal but with no bleeding manifestations. The factor VIII antigen level will be approximately twice the coagulant level.

Diagnosis of hemophilia does not require physical trauma or time-consuming methodology. However, the nurse should bear in mind that in most cases the diagnosis will accompany emergency treatment for a bleeding episode. The child may be frightened and in pain. Parental anxiety levels may be extremely high in reaction to the large amount of blood loss. To allay their anxiety, the nurse should present a calm, confident and competent appearance.

Whenever this diagnosis is expected, the family will need compassion and understanding. A time and place should be set aside to allow them to express their fears and concerns as well as to hear an explanation of the implications of hemophilia. Names of local chapters of the National Hemophilia Association as well as the name of a specific person to contact may assist the parents in joining this valuable community support system.

Maternal guilt regarding the transmission of the genetic trait may also present an obstacle to adaptation. (See the Scale for Family Adaptation to Chronic Illness in Chapter 16.) Participation in parental discussion groups may help in working through these feelings. A genetic counselor may also be of assistance.

Nursing Care During the Course and Treatment of Disease

Therapy in hemophilia is directed toward three main goals: prevention of trauma, control of bleeding episodes and prevention of disability and deformity.[12] Prevention of trauma is not an easy matter, especially for children in the toddler age group. The developmental tasks of the toddler demand the freedom to explore and to test limitations.

Parents must be advised to set realistic limits for these children but not deprive them of their independence. It is more beneficial to the ultimate welfare of the child to make the environment as safe as possible. This may be accomplished by padding crib side rails, using soft chairs and purchasing only safe, unbreakable toys. All household items that can be broken or may injure should be put out of sight, or at least out of reach. Clothing should be padded, especially over points of impact such as knees. A football or hockey helmet is generally acceptable to young boys and may prevent cranial trauma. Close observation is essential at all times.

Parents should be instructed not to administer aspirin or any other medications that may affect platelet function. Prophylaxis should also include regular dental care and the maintenance of normal weight, as obesity will place added strain on damaged joints.

As the child grows older and he attends school, it is important for parents, child and school nurse to meet and plan for his special needs. Group activities with other children with hemophilia such as peer group meetings and outings or summer camp will enable the child to engage in some competitive activities and feel more in tune with others his age. The local hemophilia association is a good source of information on these activities.

When bleeding episodes do occur, replacement of the deficient factor and local control measures are the therapy of choice. Several concentrations exist for replacement of factor VIII and IX. One unit of replacement factor is defined as the amount of factor in 1 ml of fresh-pooled normal plasma. The site and severity of the bleeding will usually determine the dose of factor necessary. Whole fresh blood may be used initially if blood volume or anemia needs correction. Otherwise fresh frozen plasma or factor concentrate is transfused.

These factor concentrates, although used to treat acute episodes, are also being used prophylactically at regularly scheduled intervals to prevent hemorrhage. They are also administered prior to minor surgical procedures and dental extractions.

Local control measures are also used to control bleeding once it has begun. Topical application of adrenalin or packing the wound with fibrin foam or Gelfoam may have a hemostatic effect. Direct pressure, immobilization, elevation of the part, and application of ice packs are generally effective. In cases of severe blood loss, transfusions may be necessary.

It should be remembered that the child and family will be extremely anxious during this period of time. Keeping the child as comfortable as possible and providing explanations and reassurance will increase security and minimize anxiety.

A major responsibility in the care of the hemophiliac child is the prevention of joint damage due to repeated hemarthrosis. With appropriate pain medication, range of motion should be initiated as soon as the acute phase is resolved. Physical therapy and public health nurse referrals may be necessary if the exercise program is extended to the home. Intervention to aspirate the joint cavities or replace the joint may be needed in extreme cases.

The child should be encouraged to function at his highest level intellectually. Physical activity must be curtailed; therefore, intellectual accomplishments are more likely to fulfill his needs for self-esteem throughout his life. Parental understanding and cooperation are essential in this undertaking, especially from the father. A father generally has greater expectations for his son's athletic achievements and may even judge his masculinity on the basis of his performance.

Children with hemophilia often have repeated hospitalizations and may require extended periods of bed rest while recuperating. Adequate stimulation through play techniques as well as sensory and environmental means should be provided. The nurse should be inventive in providing a variety of quiet but stimulating activities appropriate for the age of the child. Toddlers will become particularly frustrated when physical activity is curtailed; therefore activities to dissipate energy such as hammering pegs on a pounding bench, scribbling or throwing a sponge ball can be suggested (unless wrist and elbow joints are involved).

Participation in home care programs is now available to older children and parents who are willing and able to assume this responsibility. They must be taught how to prepare, administer and monitor IVs during factor concentrate transfusions. Home care must be followed up at frequent intervals through clinic visits, telephone calls from members of the health care team, or by home visits from the team nurse or a representative of a local health agency.

Adaptation to hemophilia is not easy for the child or his family. Although family stresses initially center around guilt, this is quickly supplanted by more concrete, day-to-day worries. Hospitalization costs, medical care, and transfusion expenses place a staggering burden on the parents of this child. Insurance may help if the child is covered under a plan that includes transfusions. The replacement of large amounts of blood or frequent infusions of factor concentrate necessitate time-consuming arrangements.

A wife's employment may assist in easing the financial pressure. However, when boys are toddlers or preschoolers and are most prone to falls and accidents, it is in many cases necessary for a parent to remain home. Important decisions may have to be made regarding child care if both parents choose to work.

Family stress often alters relationships within the family. Tensions develop between father and son because of the intense dependence of the child on the mother. This may result in an overprotected child or even a rejected one. Siblings may be shown definite favor or not be given sufficient attention.

Families need long-term and continuous support from the health care team. Because discipline is difficult, parents need guidance in how to handle temper tantrums in this child. A "time-out" mode of behavior control is an acceptable disciplinary approach. Parents must be allowed to express their feelings openly, especially those of anger, hostility and guilt. Parent groups are an excellent forum for this.

Unaffected children in many cases cannot receive their fair share of their mother's attention. They are often left in the care of their father or neighbors. They may deeply resent the attention paid to their sibling.

Female siblings should be made cognizant of the 50:50 chance that they will be carriers. Feelings of inferiority, conflicts about marriage and whether or not to conceive a child are important sources of stress. Appropriate counselling is essential to alleviate the stress and help resolve these problems.

For the affected child the school experience may be unpleasant. Identification with peer groups, school loyalties, and the recognition that comes with participation in competitive and extracurricular activities may often be missed. Teachers may have problems accepting the child with hemophilia and may make him feel different from other children. This may result from a lack of understanding of the disease itself, a fear of being unable to cope with a bleeding crisis, or just as an additional burden in an already overburdened classroom. The school nurse can provide background information to teachers. She can also counsel with teachers regarding appropriate emergency care and incorporate input from teachers in establishing a realistic plan for the child's school activities.

Early counselling should be initiated in regard to a realistic vocational choice as well as in matters of sex, marriage and procreation. Sons of a hemophiliac will be free of the disease but daughters will be carriers. The provision of birth control information to the adolescent and young adult is essential.

Ultimately the child's adaptation to hemophilia is based on his perceptions of his parents' feelings, the formulation of his own positive self-image and the achievement of self-care. This adaptation can be facilitated by a positive outlook and greater availability of home care programs.

NEPHROTIC SYNDROME

Definition, Pathology and Etiology

Nephrotic syndrome is an alteration in renal function resulting from increased permeability of the glomerular basement membrane to protein. It is typically characterized by massive proteinuria, hypoproteinemia, hyperlipidemia and edema. The basement membrane of the glomerular capillary usually functions as a highly efficient barrier for serum proteins as it filters the blood circulating through it. In nephrotic syndrome, because of a defect in this membrane, massive amounts of protein are lost into the urine. The liver responds to this wastage by increasing protein synthesis. If this synthesis is insufficient, hypoproteinemia ensues.

In the normal state the serum oncotic pressure is maintained by circulating serum protein, especially albumin. As the level of serum protein diminishes, fluid leaves the intravascular space and fills the interstitial (between the cells) space. This diminishes blood volume, causing the clinical state of edema.

The decreased blood volume stimulates the adrenal gland to produce aldosterone, which increases renal tubular reabsorption of sodium and water. Normally this would correct the reduced blood volume; however, because of the lowered osmotic pressure, the fluid continues to leave the intravascular space and accumulates in the interstitial space to further compound the edema. The mechanism for the hyperlipidemia is not clearly known, but it is believed that it occurs secondarily to the hypoproteinemia.

Although pathogenesis is not clearly defined, it is thought that the kidney may be impaired as a result of an immunologic response. According to James, 80 per cent of new cases of nephrotic syndrome are classified as minimal change disease, in which the glomeruli appear essentially normal.[6] Electron microscopy reveals a change in the footing process along the outer surface of the basement membrane. This form is readily responsive to steroid therapy, with clearing of proteinuria and reversion to normal status.

Nephrotic syndrome occurs occasionally in metabolic diseases and in immune and hypersensitivity diseases such as systemic lupus erythematosus. It may follow the administration of a nephrotoxin or be associated with allergies or infections. It may also be of undetermined (idiopathic) origin.

Clinical Manifestations

A congenital form of the disease exists but it is rare. In this type the infant will usually be of low birth weight for gestational age and have proteinuria and edema. These infants fail to respond to corticosteroid or cytotoxic drug therapy, and the outcome is fatal within the first few years of life. Renal transplants have been tried on this group with limited success.

Congenital nephrotic syndrome may first be seen by the nurse who works in a newborn nursery or in a well-baby screening clinic. A baby of low birth weight for gestational age born with an extra large placenta is a child at risk. The presence of other clinical signs such as proteinuria, distended abdomen and atypical facies with wide-set cranial sutures, low-set ears and a small snub nose should alert the nurse to the possibility of nephrotic syndrome.[10] Astute observation in the delivery room for identification of infants at risk is essential.

Careful screening and developmental assessment throughout infancy will help in making the diagnosis. These children fail to gain as they should in spite of conscientious efforts to help them feed. Nursing investigation may identify other members of the family with renal disease. The congenital form is believed to be transmitted by an autosomal recessive gene. The child should be observed for an edematous abdomen, which may be indicated by an arched-back position and increases in abdominal girth measurements.

Idiopathic nephrotic syndrome is the common form seen in pediatric patients, accounting for 80 per cent of the cases. Although it may occur at any age, it usually occurs between the ages of 1 and 6 with the peak incidence between 2 and 3 years of age. Incidence approximates 2 per 100,000 population per year in North America, and the condition is seen more frequently in males.[6]

Children with the idiopathic form of nephrotic syndrome will usually present with insidious edema that has developed over a period of several weeks. Parents may report that the child has periorbital edema upon arising, which diminishes throughout the day. They may also indicate that it is difficult to find clothes and shoes that fit properly and that ankle and pedal edema seem to develop in the later hours of the day. Volume and frequency of urination are decreased and the urine is foamy and dark in color. Hematuria is uncommon. The edema is more prevalent where subcutaneous tissues are loose, such as around the eyes, neck and genitalia.

Respiratory difficulty may be present if ascites produces sufficient pressure on the diaphragm. With the increase in edema, the child becomes anorexic and lethargic. It is essential for the nurse to interview carefully and document the pattern of the edema, any prior infection and the child's pattern of development. Changes in behavior and eating patterns can also be valuable clues. It is important to note that the blood pressure in most cases will be normal.

The Nurse's Role in Making the Diagnosis

In making the diagnosis it will be necessary for the nurse to draw or assist with the drawing of blood specimens as well as to collect and examine repeated urine specimens. She must understand the fear that the child has of undergoing repeated assaults on his body. A simple explanation of what is going to take place should be given immediately before the procedure. Blood can be difficult to draw from the edematous child, as veins are more difficult to find. Rest periods may be indicated if efforts must be repeated. If the child is placed in a supine position for blood collections he should be closely watched for respiratory difficulty. After the specimen is obtained a Band-Aid is applied, and the child is consoled by the nurse and one or both parents.

Urine specimens must be screened frequently for the presence of proteins. Because of the decreased urinary output this may be difficult. The child who is toilet trained should be regularly encouraged to void in an appropriate container. If a urine collection bag is necessary, careful skin care is particularly important because of the presence of edema.

Renal biopsy may be done to examine glomerular tissue. However, usually a trial test of prednisone is given to assess response to corticosteroids. If the response is favorable steroid treatment usually is continued and the biopsy is deferred. If renal biopsy is done, the child must be prepared for a surgical procedure with appropriate play techniques and simple explanations. Parents will also need to be assured that the procedure is necessary and will require an explanation of its methodology.

Parents will be concerned with wanting to know about nephrosis, its cause and what they could have done to keep their child from getting it. The nurse should be available to answer these questions and participate with other team members in the explanation given to parents about the long-term course of the disease.

Nursing Care During the Course and Treatment of Disease

Treatment with pharmacological agents should be initiated as soon as possible. Bed rest may be instituted to bring about a mild spontaneous diuresis, but generally ambulation is encouraged. The male child may find comfort in a scrotal support during periods of ambulation.

The diet should be high in protein, with the elimination of highly salted foods. Care must be taken not to severely restrict salt because this may make food unpalatable just at a time when an increase in intake is desired. Occasionally diuretics are ordered. Fluids are usually not restricted unless the child is severely hypertensive.

Corticosteroids will usually induce remission in children with idiopathic nephrotic syndrome. A daily dose of 2 mg/kg of prednisone is given. Remission is usually induced in 6 to 14 days and is indicated by an abrupt diuresis and the absence of urinary protein. Care must be taken to observe the child for side effects of the steroids. An increase in weight and appetite, an elevation of blood pressure, obesity, moon facies, and striae may occur. Serious infections may be masked. Growth in height may be decreased. As soon as feasible, steroids are gradually tapered and only reinstituted in cases of relapse.

Patients who fail to respond to prednisone after four weeks of therapy are considered steroid resistant and are treated with cyclophosphamide (Cytoxan) in combination with the steroid. This has proven effective in reducing the incidence of relapse. The severe side effect of leukopenia will drastically increase susceptibility to infection. Hair loss can be a distressing problem to children who are already experiencing body image concerns because of the edema. Cystitis may occur and sterility has been associated with long-term use of this drug.

Nursing care for the child with nephrotic syndrome centers primarily around care of the child and family during the acute phase and preparation of the family for assuming care in the home setting.

Edema about the eyes may interfere with sensory perception and comfort. The use of eye irrigations or ophthalmic creams may be indicated. Allowing the child to sleep with his head elevated on a pillow may prevent the eyes from swelling closed and eliminate the fear associated with this.

Careful attention and meticulous cleansing of touching skin surfaces is essential; skin creases should be padded with a soft material. Supporting edematous areas with pillows may provide a measure of comfort. The child should be turned, positioned and massaged frequently. A bed cradle may be helpful in lifting bed covers off the child's skin and allowing air to flow.

As the edema diminishes the child's malnourished appearance will become visible. Getting the child to eat becomes a challenge. The nurse should make meals as attractive as possible. Smaller portions offered more frequently are often tolerated better by this child. Using a small glass with a small amount of fluid will assist in gaining the child's cooperation. The child should be weighed on a daily basis to monitor the edema and diuresis.

Body image is just beginning to emerge in the toddler and he evidences concern when parts of his body are no longer visible to him. Boys need reassurance that their penis is still there even if edema conceals it from their view. Opportunities should be provided for the child and his family to express their fears and concerns about the rapid changes in body size.

Safety must be constantly monitored, as changes in body size will alter the child's ability to move and maintain position. Bed side rails are usually necessary, and are absolutely essential with the younger child. Parents should be made particularly aware of the need for safety as they prepare to take the child home.

The child's resistance to all infections is lowered and compromised by his drug therapy. Antibiotics may be prescribed for an acute infection. The nurse should be aware that the child should not receive immunizations until he is free of proteinuria and off steroids for one year.[10] Whether hospitalized or at home, this child should be protected from exposure to other children with infections; otherwise, normal relationships with children and adults should be encouraged.

Care of the family centers around support and education. The protracted course of the disease with remissions, relapses and occasional admissions to the hospital places severe stress on the family. Although outpatient treatment is usually practical for children with moderate edema, parents must be instructed as to what indicates need for prompt medical attention and of the importance of complying with a regimen of regular office or clinic visits. Parents will also need instruction regarding the testing of urine for protein. Practice sessions should be initiated as soon as their level of readiness is deemed appropriate.

Dietary instruction should be coordinated and supplemented with feedback and question sessions. Parents should realize that the toddler's appetite will vary and may need to be stimulated. Recipes that are appetizing and that fit within the budget may be helpful. Positive reinforcement of the child's appropriate behavior may be beneficial, with appropriate rewards for eating properly. Contracting for certain behaviors may work with the child of 2½ or older. A wide variety of nutritional snacks may be offered from which the child can be allowed to choose. Patience and a positive attitude on the part of the caretaker must persist.

Skin care should be explained and opportunities given for parents to demonstrate their proficiency. Explanation should be given for the use of mild soap and cornstarch, particularly at skin folds, to prevent excoriation.

It must be remembered that although parents may understand the nature of the disease, its effect on their life style and their finances may only become clear as they live and cope with the problems. Discussion of available financial resources may facilitate early acquisition of assistance and more positive adaptation on the part of the family.

An awareness that nephrosis and the accompanying medication therapy may cause irritability and mood swings as well as physical changes should be communicated to the family. The importance of periodic rest and quiet activities should be emphasized. Parental participation in care during hospitalization should be encouraged as much as possible to maintain family ties.

As the child becomes more active, appropriate play sessions will help to distract him and enhance his normal developmental pattern. He needs this opportunity to play out his hospital experiences to facilitate mastery of the situation.

The child, his parents and siblings should be aware that the alteration in physical appearance may elicit stares and teasing from playmates and peers. If hair loss is probable, arrangements may be made for a wig. Because the child may be small for his age, people may tend to talk down to him. Parents should be aware of the child's need for self-esteem and treat him age-appropriately.

The entire manner in which a child copes with chronic renal disease depends on developmental level, internal resources and relationships with his family. The nurse should be continually assessing the family for indications of alterations in these relationships. Early referral for counselling or quiet talks in which parents can air their concerns may be beneficial.

Relationships with siblings are frequently disturbed. Siblings are resentful of the time and attention that the ill child receives and may feel neglected and unloved. Older siblings may have to take on more responsibility and experience deprivations due to the financial strains. On the other hand, the ill child may feel jealous of his siblings' liberal diet and normal peer relationships. Siblings need to be able to discuss these feelings. In some cases sibling counselling may be helpful.

Travis identifies common elements with psychosocial implications in the care of the child with renal disease.[11] These are pain, intrusive procedures, growth retardation, dependence, body image distortions, diet restriction, interruption in school or peer relationships, anxiety, heavy costs, time burdens and disrupted relationships for the family. These demands make adaptation very difficult, but with the proper support and education the family can surmount this disease.

The prognosis of children with nephrotic syndrome is generally quite good. Although relapses are common, most children respond to treatment. For children with lesions other than minimal change disease the outlook is less optimistic, with progression to renal failure necessitating dialysis and transplantation.

References

1. E. L. Dowd et al. Releasing the hospitalized child from restraints. American Journal of Maternal and Child Nursing, Nov/Dec 1977, p. 370
2. E. H. Erikson. Childhood and Society. W. W. Norton and Co., 1963
3. C. M. Fagin. Pediatric rooming-in: its meaning for the nurse. Nursing Clinics of North America, March 1966, p. 83
4. J. A. Hennessey. Hospitalized toddlers' responses to mothers' tape recordings during brief separations. Maternal-Child Nursing Journal, Summer 1976, p. 69
5. R. A. Hockelman et al. Principles of Pediatrics: Health Care of the Young. McGraw-Hill Book Co., 1978
6. J. A. James. Renal Disease in Childhood. C.V. Mosby Co., 1976
7. J. Robertson. Young Children in Hospitals. Basic Books, Inc., 1958
8. M. S. Sibinga and C. J. Friedman. Restraint and speech. Pediatrics, July 1971, p 116
9. A. Silverman et al. Pediatric Clinical Gastroenterology. C.V. Mosby Co., 1971
10. S. Steele. Nursing Care of the Child with Long Term Illness. Appleton-Century-Crofts, 1977
11. G. Travis. Chronic Illness in Children: Its Impact on Child and Family. Stanford University Press, 1976
12. V. Vaughn et al. Nelson Textbook of Pediatrics. W. B. Saunders Co., 1979

Additional Recommended Reading

S. W. Arneson and J. L. Triplett. How children cope with disfiguring changes in their appearance. American Journal of Maternal and Child Nursing, Nov/Dec 1978, p. 366

M. Boutaugh and P. C. Patterson. Summer camp for hemophiliacs. American Journal of Nursing, August 1977, p. 1288

M. N. Coddington. A mother's struggle to cope with her child's deteriorating illness. Maternal-Child Nursing Journal, Spring 1976, p. 39

D. Cornfeld. Nephrosis in childhood. Hospital Medicine, March 1978, p. 98

C. M. Edelmann, Jr. Pediatric Kidney Disease, Vol. II. Little, Brown and Co., 1978

E. Farrell and B. S. Kiernan. A positive approach to nutrition for hospitalized children. American Journal of Maternal and Child Nursing, Mar/Apr 1977, p. 113

J. H. Fergusson. Late psychologic effects of a serious illness in childhood. Nursing Clinics of North America, March 1976, p. 83

A. C. Galligan. Using Roy's concept of adaptation to care for young children. American Journal Of Maternal and Child Nursing, Jan/Feb 1979, p. 24

G. E. R. Garrett. The celiac child. Nursing Times, November 1977, p. 1708

L. J. Guhlow and J. Kolb. Pediatric IVs. RN., March 1979, p. 40

A. Hetrick et al. Nutrition in renal disease when the patient is a child. American Journal of Nursing, December 1979, p. 2152

M. W. Hilgartner. Managing the child with hemophilia. Pediatric Annals, June 1979, p. 68

M. Johnson and M. Salazar. Preadmission program for rehospitalized children. American Journal of Nursing, August 1979, p. 1421

L. Kunzman. Some factors influencing a young child's mastery of hospitalization. Nursing Clinics of North America, March 1972, p. 13

S. A. Lawrence and R. M. Lawrence. A model of adaptation to the stress of chronic illness. Nursing Forum, No. 1 1979, p. 33

J. Lazerson. Prophylactic infusion therapy in hemophilia. Hospital Practice, May 1979, p. 49

M. McCreery. Diet: first-line defense against celiac disease. RN., February 1976, p. 50

B. McNicholl et al. Variability of gluten intolerance in treated childhood coeliac disease. Gut, February 1979, p. 126

D. R. Miller et al. Smith's Blood Diseases of Infancy and Childhood. C.V. Mosby Co., 1978

S. T. Sahin. A new nursing perspective on the family with a special needs child. Nursing Forum, No. 4 1978, p. 357

C. H. Smitherman. Parents of hospitalized children have needs, too. American Journal of Nursing, August 1979, p. 1423

B. Snell and C. McClellan. Whetting hospitalized preschoolers' appetites. American Journal of Nursing, March 1976, p. 413

W. S. Yancy. Approaches to emotional management of the child with a chronic illness. Clinical Pediatrics, February 1972, p. 64

POTENTIAL STRESSES DURING TODDLER YEARS: LIFE-THREATENING ALTERATIONS IN HEALTH STATUS

by Anita Spietz, RN, MSN

THE TODDLER WITH LIFE-THREATENING ILLNESS

The toddler is egocentric, believing the world revolves around him. Because of this he is unable to differentiate himself from the world or distinguish living from nonliving or separate fact from fantasy; all these differentiations must be made to comprehend the concept of death. He can recognize physical death, but since he cannot distinguish it from life, death is considered a temporary, reversible phenomenon. Informed of someone's death, the toddler continues to talk of the person from his frame of reference of life and temporary death. Thus his conversation may at one time reflect that the person is in "heaven" and at another time imply that the person is still present or living. The concept of death as the permanent cessation of life, a universal and inevitable phenomenon, is not possible due to his preconceptual stage of thought. Although the toddler is capable of symbolic thought, he is not able to think in abstract forms nor does he possess a sense of time or space. As a result, the concept of death as understood by adults is not comprehended or thought about in children this age.

The way in which preverbal children view death is not fully understood. It is suggested that children under 3 experiment with contrasting states of being and nonbeing beginning with such games as peek-a-boo (in which the child alternates periods of terror and delight), the disappearance and return of toys (from which the phrase "all gone" is derived) and periods of sleep and wakefulness (with a marked increase in nightmares and fears of dark during toddlerhood). All of these "games" speak to the beginning awareness of absence and may support beginning ideas about death.

Explaining Death to Toddlers

There are few guidelines available to parents about how to discuss death with their dying toddler. The nurse has an obligation, however, to help parents become aware of those guidelines that do exist. Parents should be encouraged to begin by evaluating their own feelings about death. This introspection helps them to know and understand their own feelings and fears before dealing with their toddler's concept and emotions. The parents can use the opportunity to explore death with their toddler and his siblings through natural events such as the death of a bug, a pet or a grandparent. Such discussions draw out the child's questions. Having books read to him that discuss death or include death experiences may be another alternative for children this age. Not only does this provide information to the child on the subject of death but it also encourages discussion between parent and child.

Many factors such as personal beliefs, religious convictions, cultural background and comfort with the topic will influence the 'parents' response to the dying child and to his questions. When the child is dying the ultimate decision of what to tell the child must be left up to the parents. However, helping parents to recognize the importance of openness and honesty with this age group is an important nursing intervention. Toddlers are adept at sensing inconsistencies between verbal and nonverbal messages. Fabricating stories or attempting to conceal real feelings arouses considerable anxiety in toddlers and poses a real threat to the child's sense of security. Parents should also be helped to realize that children of all ages need to mourn and express their feelings in ways similar to those of adults.

The Toddler's Response to Life-Threatening Illness

The course of life-threatening illness is incongruent with all a toddler is striving developmentally to achieve — autonomy, self-control, order. As life-threatening illness progresses to its termination, the toddler typically experiences discomfort, anxiety over the separation he senses is coming (or may already be experiencing if his care is mismanaged), and fear because of the losses in control he experiences when his routines are continually disturbed and new situations are regularly introduced. His response during the early stages of his illness is usually regression, as is typical of any toddler who is taken from his familiar routines and surroundings. As his condition worsens, the toddler's fears intensify and he will likely react with aggressive acting-out behaviors or by passively withdrawing. He and his family manifest the emotions and behaviors of anticipatory grief.

Pain and Discomfort Since the toddler cannot comprehend the seriousness of his illness, his reactions are primarily in response to pain, intrusive procedures and the discomforts of actual or perceived separation. He is forced to contend not only with the procedures any ill toddler is exposed to but also with many additional diagnostic and treatment regimens of a more extreme nature that often are accompanied by "monstrous" equipment and infliction of sometimes excruciating pain. Therefore, those interventions appropriate to any hospitalized toddler are particularly important to the comfort and security of the dying toddler. Above all else, he needs his parents' presence during the experiences.

Separation Anxiety In spite of the toddler's striving for independence, he still depends on his parents for security and love. Separation from his mother (or other significant caregiver) is the dying toddler's most acute concern. Although all toddlers need their mothers during illness, the dying toddler needs her desperately in order to cope. The toddler can sense that all is not well with him and, since he equates separation or absence with death, it is apparent that the toddler is able to respond to loss long before he is able to understand death. Recognizing this, the nurse should encourage and support the mother so she can provide her toddler's care and mothering, thus postponing the separation that is inevitable with his death. The child may become totally disorganized and may panic if his care is left to unfamiliar persons. If involving the mother or a significant other in the child's care is not possible, a minimum of people should be assigned to care for the toddler while attempts are being made to draw the mother and family into the child's care.

Although the toddler's verbal abilities are not well established, he has an immense ability to sense what others are feeling and may become overtly disturbed when he sees anger, anxiety or sadness displayed by parents or family members. If the parents are upset, he becomes upset; if they are depressed and withdrawn he reacts likewise. Therefore it is critical for the nurse to help parents work through their feelings so they have the emotional reserves to care for their child and adjust to the fact that he is dying, while at the same time providing as normal a relationship with him as possible.

Breaches of Routine Unless maintaining routine is built into the plan of care, the toddler's final days can become chaotic and may lack any semblance of routine, from which he derives comfort and security. The dying toddler does not like to be treated in ways outside of usual routine and his fears become greater if he sees different routines or patterns of behavior in those around him. Dying children, especially toddlers, react most positively when routines and rituals of their daily lives are maintained. A primary goal of nursing care is to prevent maladaptation. Providing parents with an overview of behaviors representative of the healthy, trustful, autonomous responses in the toddler may aid in helping them establish priorities in providing care. It is important to periodically re-emphasize the needs of the toddler for routines, schedules, discipline and limit setting. The toddler who is allowed to have his way will become frustrated, angry and more demanding unless limits are firmly established.

The typical problems parents face with their dying toddler include difficulties in eating, sleeping, elimination, separation and independence. Providing routines in these activities of daily living as close as possible to ones he is accustomed to offers the toddler a sense of control that may otherwise be lost in the strange hospital environment. In order to carry this out effectively the nurse can interview the parents for information regarding the child's habits, routines and preferences, incorporating this information, when possible, into his plan of care. Familiar toys, clothes, and interactions that parallel his home life also help the toddler maintain his sense of autonomy.

Loss of Control As his life draws to an end, the child may experience a loss of control. Any restriction placed on the toddler's activity is met with physical resistance. The toddler's sense of autonomy may be maintained if the nurse can allow him mobility and independence, even if this means altering hospital routines. This may include such things as examining or treating the child in an upright position, since toddlers react strongly to being held in a supine position, or providing a physical environment that is conducive to the toddler's motor skills.

Working with the terminally ill toddler is both difficult and challenging for the nurse. Providing care that takes into account his concept of death, his stage of development and the quality of his family attachments will help the toddler pass through this most difficult stage of life.

The toddler speaks primarily in symbolic language (his meaning is known only to himself), his messages being more accurately conveyed through his actions. To determine how much the toddler understands about his illness, the nurse should encourage experiences for play that when observed provide insight into the child's understanding of his illness. Engagement in play therapy helps the toddler play through his fantasies and anxieties, thereby giving him an opportunity for self-expression and a means to work through his impending separation.

ALTERED HEALTH STATES

Rhabdomyosarcoma

These are highly malignant soft tissue tumors, generally of three types: embryonal, alveolar or pleomorphic. They are generally found in the urogenital tract, head and neck, limbs and trunk, and the abdomen. Metastasis is rapid and early in the course of the disease, often to the regional lymph nodes, bone marrow or nasopharynx. This tumor can occur at any age in childhood but usually occurs at less than 4 years of age.[3]

Rhabdomyosarcoma presents with superficial swelling of an extremity, urinary retention, a watery or bloody stained vaginal discharge, or tenderness and swelling of the scrotum. Epistaxis or blood-stained purulent discharge from the nose or ear, strabismus or proptosis, or generalized irritability may also occur. Weight loss, anorexia and fatigue are typical.

The use of surgery in combination with radiotherapy and chemotherapy has proved to be the most effective in improving the 5-year survival rate. Prognosis is improved the younger the child is at the time of diagnosis. The most "favorable" site in terms of prognostic indicators is the orbit; the least favorable is the abdomen.[3]

Retinoblastoma

Retinoblastomas are congenital malignant growths composed of embryonal retinal cells.

They are the most common orbital tumor of the eye in infancy and childhood. Retinoblastomas occur equally in males and females at a rate of approximately 1 in 20,000 births.[2] Although the growth may be present at birth, the average age at the time of diagnosis is 17 months, with the majority diagnosed before age 3 and rarely after age 6.

Etiology Although the mechanism of transmission is not fully understood, retinoblastomas are thought to be a result of both somatic mutations (which occur in general body cells) and germinal mutations (which occur in germ cells or gametes). Somatic mutations are not hereditary. They result in unilateral involvement and account for the majority of all retinoblastomas. Germinal mutations, on the other hand, are inherited and transmitted by the autosomal dominant mode of inheritance with incomplete penetrance. (The parent has the trait but not the disease.) The majority of germinal mutations are bilateral, with about a third resulting in unilateral involvement. If the child's parent has unilateral involvement, there is an 8 to 25 per cent risk of the child having retinoblastoma, increasing to 50 per cent when the parent has bilateral involvement. If the parents are healthy and have one child with the tumor, other children they may have may be affected with tumors. Because the incidence is high with a family history, it is extremely important for the siblings of the affected child to have a thorough examination, and that the parents be informed of the risk in subsequent children.

Clinical Manifestations and Diagnosis The tumor arises as one or more white nodules on the retina and grows at variable rates, eventually causing retinal detachment or formation of a mass on the posterior portion of the eye. The tumor cells may spread by way of the optic nerve into the subarachnoid space, producing central nervous system symptoms and death, or into the choroid and lymphatics with probable metastasis to the bone.

The most common presenting sign of retinoblastoma is the white reflex of the pupil noted most frequently by parents, and known as the "cat's eye reflex" (Fig. 35–1). A white spot on the retina during ophthalmoscopic examination is diagnostic of this tumor mass. It is extremely important to acknowledge the parents' reports in such cases. If parents mention to the nurse the appearance of any abnormality, she should attempt to elicit the reflex and refer the toddler to a specialist for confirmation.

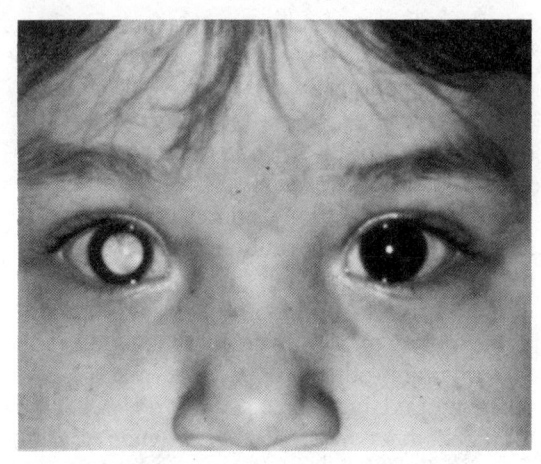

Figure 35–1 The "cat's eye reflex" of retinoblastoma. (From G. Peyman et al. Principles and Practice of Ophthalmology, W. B. Saunders Co., 1980, p. 1150.)

If the tumor is small and located on the posterior portion of the eye, the initial sign may be strabismus. Whenever strabismus is observed, a thorough ophthalmic examination is required to rule out this tumor. Loss of vision and redness or pain with or without glaucoma may be observed by the practitioner or reported by the parent. The child may complain about pain or the parent may note changes in behavior indicative of decreased vision (bumping into objects, poor coordination). Because young children do not always complain of loss of vision and the defects may not be apparent on surface appraisal, the practitioner needs to carefully check the eyes for abnormal protrusions of the eyeball, atrophy or venous congestion. A depression of the eyeball on the side where the tumor exists is often observable, or the tumor may be palpated when the eyes are closed. Eye testing may reveal reduced acuity of vision.

Diagnosis is suspected when the size of the optic canals is increased and calcification of the eye is present on radiographic studies. Calcification occurs in approximately 75 per cent of cases. Additional tests used to support the diagnosis and establish desirable treatment include carotid angiography, which localizes the process and determines the degree of malignancy, and ultrasonography, which differentiates tumor growth from normal tissue, localizes the growth and detects extensions of the tumor into the surrounding orbit and optic nerve.[1]

Treatment and Prognosis The size of the tumor and its shape and location generally dictate the type of treatment indicated. Radiation is often effective in reducing the small, localized tumors of unilateral retinoblastoma, thereby preserving vision. Other treatment options for small localized tumors include the use of cobalt plaque applicators (actual implantation of a cobalt applicator on the sclera to aid in delivering radiation to tumor), light coagulation (laser beam that destroys blood vessels to the tumor), and cryotherapy (destruction of blood vessels to tumor by freezing the tumor). In advanced cases with unilateral involvement, removal of the affected eye (enucleation) reduces the likelihood of metastasis by approximately 50 per cent. In bilateral cases, the eye with the more advanced tumor is removed and the other eye is treated with radiation or chemotherapy. In those instances in which both lesions are very advanced, both eyes are removed. Since metastasis is likely along the optic nerve pathway, a long optic nerve stump is removed with the eye to discourage or prevent metastasis. The size of the tumor at the time of removal determines the chance of survival.

If the tumor growth has metastasized, chemotherapy may be used in conjunction with radiation. Most often, regardless of treatment used, all vision is gradually lost because of the eventual metastasis or in the case of unilateral retinoblastoma, there is recurrence in the other eye. Early diagnosis is important. The stage of the disease at the time of diagnosis is most significant in determining outcome. If the tumor is detected at an early stage and adequate treatment is carried out, the prognosis is good. Once the tumor has metastasized out of the eye into the orbit, the chance of survival is minimal.

Nursing Management The care of the child with retinoblastoma and his family will depend on the stage of growth at time of diagnosis, the treatment required and whether the inheritance factor is involved.

The parents' ability to accept the diagnosis and treatment will vary according to the stage at which the tumor is detected. If diagnosed early, when treatment may be curative, parents' fear and anxiety is reduced in a short period of time. In instances in which detection occurs late in the disease process and the prognosis is poor, parents experience shock and overwhelming disbelief at the diagnosis. If a family has a history of this disease, additional feelings of guilt may evolve. The nurse must consider all these factors in devising a plan of care with the family.

When radiation is employed, the child and his parents need preparation for what is to happen and what will be expected of them. The radiation procedure requires that the child be immobile with his head held in perfect alignment. As a result the young child is heavily sedated prior to treatment. Parents need a realistic, clear explanation of the purpose of the therapy as well as the need for sedation. Depending on the size of the tumor and the amount of radiation received, the child may not demonstrate side effects until the second to fourth day. General malaise may be the first side effect. Comforting and supportive measures on the part of the parents should be encouraged by the nurse when any untoward effects of radiation are observed.

If surgery is the recommended treatment, giving consent means that parents must make an especially difficult decision at a time when they are still emotionally distressed by the diagnosis. The nurse needs to recognize the overwhelming feelings the parents are experiencing and encourage them to talk. Although they realize that the prognosis is poor if the surgery is not carried out, they may also be fearful of the disfigurement, the pain involved, or the resentment the child may have for them later on for having made the decision they did.

Once the decision has been made, the parents need preparation for their toddler's appearance following surgery. The child will have an eye patch in place that will be changed regularly by the ophthalmologist. His face may be edematous and fittings for a prosthesis do not take place until the edema subsides. Generally within three weeks the facial appearance returns to normal. It may be important to explain to the parents that the surgery will not result in a cavity in the skull; the area will appear quite normal because a sphere will be surgically implanted to maintain the shape of the eyeball. This should be repeated to them after surgery and before the child is seen. Preparation of the toddler for surgery includes determining what the child knows and understands about his illness or hospitalization and clarifying any misinterpretations. Preparing for the postoperative phase includes talking to him in terms appropriate to his development about the patch over his eye and the restraints that will be on his arms to help him remember to keep his hands away from his eyes. The nurse will reassure him that she or his parents will be with him as much as possible, and that his eyes are the only part of his body that will be operated on. Providing an opportunity for him to ask questions and engaging him in play with a doll whose eyes he can patch can help him adapt to the experience of surgery.[4] Parents need to be encouraged to participate in the teaching to provide additional support to the toddler.

Following surgery parents need to be informed of their role in quieting and comforting the child who may be physically resisting the use of restraints. Sedating the toddler may be necessary. Young children are generally encouraged to resume normal activities as soon as possible; however, it is important to remember that regression is common among this age group and is acceptable behavior. Unless complications arise, such as infection, hemorrhage or prolonged edema, the child is provided a prothesis within three weeks of surgery. Teaching the parents and child how to care for the prosthesis is critical. Techniques for insertion, removal and cleaning need to be incorporated.

Once the diagnosis has been made it is also imperative that the risk of retinoblastoma in subsequent children be discussed and genetic counselling obtained. It is also critical for the other children in the family to be examined as early as possible.

References

1. B. Conway. Pediatric Neurologic Nursing. C. V. Mosby Co., 1977
2. R. Ellsworth. Retinoblastoma. Center for Birth Defects Information Service (National Foundation March of Dimes), No. 1.1, 1978
3. P. Jones and P. Campbell, eds. Tumors of Infancy and Childhood. Blackwell Scientific Publication, 1976
4. M. Petrillo and S. Sanger. Emotional Care of Hospitalized Children. J. B. Lippincott Co., 1972

Additional Recommended Reading

The Toddler and Death

M. Atkin. Counseling Families. Nursing Mirror, 7 April 1977, p. 62
G. Calkin. Are hospitalized toddlers adapting to the experience as well as we think? Maternal and Child Nursing, Jan/Feb 1979, p. 18
H. Feifel. New Meanings of Death. McGraw-Hill Book Co., 1977
E. Grollman. Explaining death to children. Journal of School Health, June 1977, p. 336
J. Koch. When children meet death. Psychology Today, August 1977, p. 64
P. Kossoff. Telling children about death. American Baby, February 1978, p. 44
H. Schiff. The Bereaved Parent. Crown Publishers, 1977
B. Schoenberg et al. Anticipatory Grief. Columbia University Press, 1974
B. Sheer. Help for parents in a difficult job — broaching the subject of death. Maternal and Child Nursing, Sept/Oct 1977, p. 320
J. Smith. Spending time with the hospitalized child. Maternal and Child Nursing, May/June 1976, p. 164
K. Stephens. A toddler's separation anxiety. American Journal of Nursing, September 1973, p. 1553
R. Toch. Management of the child with a fatal disease. Clinical Pediatrics, July 1974, p. 419
E. Waechter. Children's awareness of fatal illness. American Journal of Nursing, June 1971, p. 1168
A. Wolff. Helping Your Child To Understand Death. The Child Study Press, 1973

Cancer in the Toddler

M. A. Bedford. Management of retinoblastoma. Modern Problems in Ophthalmology, Vol. 18 1977, p. 101
J. Benoliel and J. McCorkle. A holistic approach to terminal illness. Cancer Nursing, April 1978, p. 143
J. Francois. Conservative treatment of retinoblastoma. Modern Problems in Ophthalmology, Vol. 18 1977, p. 113
W. Höpping and G. Schmitt. The treatment of retintoblastoma. Modern Problems in Ophthalmology, Vol. 18 1977, p. 106
R. Jenson and R. Miller. Retinoblastoma: epidemiologic characteristics. New England Journal of Medicine, 5 August 1971, p. 307
J. Martinson. Facilitating home care for children dying of cancer. Cancer Nursing, February 1978, p. 41
J. Michelson et al. Fetal antigens in retinoblastoma. January 1976, p. 62
A. Reese. Tumors of the Eye. Harper and Row, 1976
J. Short. Nursing care study: enucleation of the eye. Nursing Times, 2 February 1978, p. 184

THE HOSPITALIZED TODDLER

36

by Mabel Hunsberger, BSN, MNS

Separation from parents is the single most important stressor for the young child who is hospitalized. A child between the ages of 6 months and 4 years is more vulnerable to psychological upset as a result of hospitalization than at any other age.[17] Not only is a toddler threatened by the separation from his parents, but he is removed from almost everything that is basic to his security. He must give up his crib, his favorite chair, his own plate, cup, fork and spoon in exchange for an unfamiliar hospital environment. His fear and loneliness are further complicated by his being subjected to hurtful procedures, and in most cases he does not feel well. It is only the presence and loving care of his parents or another significant person in his life that gives him a chance for even minimal psychological comfort. Having the security provided by his blanket, a teddy bear or a thread-bare cloth may bring temporary cessation of tears, but the security that the presence of his parents gives him cannot be equaled. The nurse intervenes to ease the toddler's upset and to facilitate optimal physical and psychological health of the toddler and his family by: (1) reducing the stress of hospitalization for parents, the toddler, and siblings; (2) providing opportunities for normal growth and development; (3) providing safe and developmentally appropriate nursing care; and (4) preparing the child and family for discharge.

REDUCING STRESS OF HOSPITALIZATION: NURSE'S ROLE

The nurse can assist the toddler and his family to cope with the stress of hospitalization by intervening in various ways. Areas in which the nurse can provide assistance are preparing the child and family for hospitalization, encouraging and supporting care by parents and providing explanations and suggestions to assist parents to cope with their stressed toddler.

Preparation for Hospitalization

Most of the techniques that are used to prepare preschoolers and school-age children for hospitalization are not effective for a toddler. In a review of the literature Goslin points out that positive research findings pertinent to the preparation of children for hospitalization consistently carry qualifying statements that some children, particularly the younger ones, do not seem to benefit from preparation.[7]

A toddler must be prepared for hospitalization within the confines of his mental ability. He

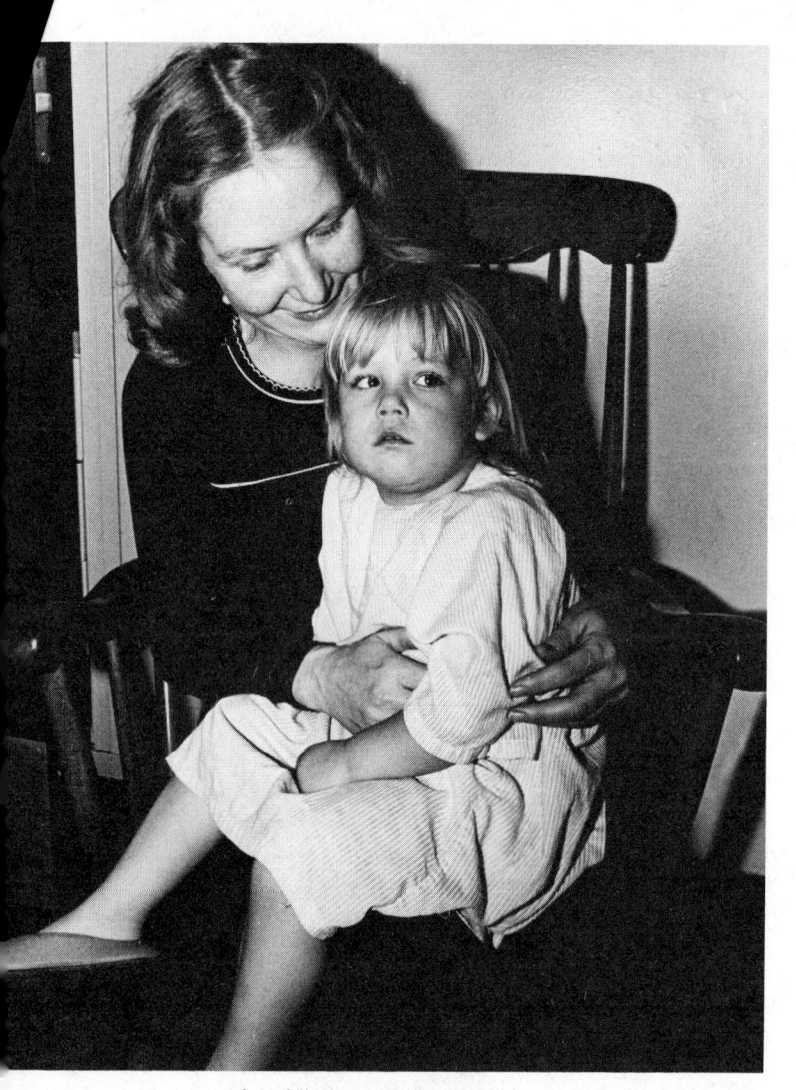

A toddler's stress is diminished by the presence of a parent whose anxiety has been reduced. A rocking chair is a soothing addition to a child's hospital room, both for the child and parent.

does not have a concept of time or causality to understand an explanation of something that is to happen in the future, nor will he understand the cause of his illness or the reason for hospitalization. Stress of the toddler is most effectively reduced by the presence of a parent whose own anxiety has been reduced.

An important role of the nurse who cares for a hospitalized toddler is to prepare the parents for the hospitalization of their child. To prepare parents the nurse should help them understand the child's illness and the reason for hospitalization; she should explain the events of hospital admission and give them some guidelines that can be used to prepare their toddler and his siblings for the hospital experience.

A common unrecommended approach used by parents when a young child must be hospitalized is to protect him from the trauma of being told that he must go to the hospital. The child is told on the morning of hospitalization that he is going to the library, to the store, to the park, or for some other pleasurable experience. The nurse must intervene to prevent parents from taking this approach. It is appropriate to tell a toddler about the hospitalization the morning of admission, but the explanation should be simple and truthful, with descriptions of a few of the nonthreatening events that will occur.[15] For example, he can be told about the environment, and about the nurses, doctors, and other children he will meet. It is appropriate to tell some toddlers two or three days before admission, but the explanation should not include descriptions of threatening procedures. A toddler can also benefit from the parents reading to him from books about hospitalization and from playing with a nurse or doctor kit a few days before admission.

Older siblings should be prepared with greater detail about the toddler's hospitalization, including explanations of who will be at home to care for them and who will be spending time at the hospital, and how much time will be spent there. If a parent will be rooming-in, this should be explained. It is important that family members not speak about the toddler's upcoming hospitalization in his presence before he has been told. A toddler understands a great deal of what he hears and can sense that something to do with him is about to happen, but he cannot express how much he understands or how he feels. Preschoolers and school-age children cannot be trusted to avoid discussion in the toddler's presence; therefore the parents should be encouraged to tell all their children at the same time.

Care by Parents

The nurse who admits the toddler to the hospital must from the moment of contact communicate a feeling of acceptance of the parents and tell them how important their presence is during their toddler's hospitalization. Whether the parents room-in or visit sporadically, the nurse's priority is to maximize the quality of the parent-child relationship. The more effective the nurse is at putting parents at ease, the greater is the toddler's security. Parental presence assists a toddler to withstand pain and stress. A toddler has no formalized concept of pain, but he experiences as terrifying an unfamiliar environment without his mother.[19] Although a toddler does not verbally communicate pain, his discomfort is expressed in aggressive physical behavior and through other nonverbal communication.[6]

Parent involvement in the care of the toddler should be encouraged and supported by the nurse. Care by parents results in better physical care; the parent-child relationship is maintained, and the parent provides ego support to the child.[11] A toddler needs each of these benefits. Most toddlers require a great deal of physical care including bathing, dressing, changing of diapers, and supervision or assistance in elimination and at mealtime. A toddler's developing autonomy is frequently manifested by resistive or dawdling behaviors during his daily physical care. He feels more secure if his parents continue to provide this care and take the time required to accomplish these tasks in the usual manner. A toddler becomes attached to those who daily meet his needs; if the parents can continue in this role the parent-child relationship can more easily be maintained. Likewise, when the toddler is subjected to frightening procedures, it is the parent who can best offer comfort.

When parents are able to room-in with their hospitalized toddler the nurse does not remove herself from the scene because "there is nothing to do." She continues to bear responsibility for the care of the toddler, assisting with daily care and providing the specialized care pertaining to the child's illness. The more complex responsibility of the nurse, however, is that of assessing the coping level of the family and intervening to maximize the comfort of each person. There are times when parents feel exhausted or frustrated by the demands of caring for their sick toddler. The nurse should be particularly sensitive to the needs of a toddler's parents, realizing that even the care of a well toddler in his own environment is a demanding job. When a toddler is hospitalized parents need assistance with their efforts to provide his day-to-day care. They need the opportunity to leave for periods of time, and they need to have contact with a nurse who makes them feel at ease to express the frustrations they are experiencing. The nurse needs considerable interaction with the toddler and his parents to assess whether the stress of caring for the toddler is too overwhelming. When it is, she can help the family identify ways in which they can be assisted to cope with the stress of the hospital experience.

Parents need ongoing explanations and support regarding their child's illness and treatments; they also need assistance in the management of behaviors that are common to the toddler when he is hospitalized.

Parents may have difficulty setting limits in their usual way because they cannot bear to oppose the child's wishes while he is ill. The nurse should provide an opportunity for parents to express the conflict they are experiencing and assure them that the security that the setting of limits affords a toddler is particularly important now that he is in a threatening environment. The nurse can also point out that if parents can continue to provide the limit setting in their usual manner there will be fewer problems of readjustment for their toddler when he returns home.[8]

Another area of conflict is the resistive behaviors that are normal for toddlers. When he feels threatened with losing control over what happens to him, a toddler may become even more resistive, with the result that parents become exhausted and frustrated. The regressive behaviors such as thumbsucking, soiling (by a previously potty-trained toddler) or the whining, baby cry of a toddler may be disturbing and embarrassing to parents. Parents may even feel that they are the cause of such behaviors and may begin to isolate themselves emotionally from their toddler, even though they are physically present. The nurse's responsibility then is not only to encourage parents to be there but to help them cope effectively with their toddler's reactions to hospitalization.

Parents are not always able to room-in with their hospitalized toddler. In spite of the available research that supports the positive effects of the presence of parents, many institutions still have limited visiting policies. Any nurse who works with young hospitalized children has a responsibility to act to bring about the goal of 24-hour visitation by parents, especially for children between 6 months and 4 years of age. When parent-child separation is inevitable because of family circumstances, the nurse must strive to work out a plan with parents that will be most beneficial to the family as a unit. Some families may need assistance to re-evaluate their circumstances and search for alternatives that will increase their availability to the toddler. The nurse cannot assume that there are no alternatives, nor can she disregard the needs of the entire family.

When parents can visit for only short periods and such visits are infrequent, the nurse must make a special effort to reduce the stress this produces for parents. Parents who are unable to visit when a young child is hospitalized often feel extremely guilty and need the acceptance and understanding of a sensitive nurse. It is especially important that the nurse does not compound their guilt by thoughtless, judgmental remarks. The nurse can suggest ways to keep the parent-child relationship intact, such as telephoning the nurse to receive a report on their toddler; for some older toddlers it is helpful if they can speak to their parents on the telephone. The nurse can also suggest that parents leave an important personal item (keys, eye glass holder, scarf) and a family photograph for the toddler. A tape recording of a parent reading a familiar story has been reported as another successful technique to help the toddler recall the image of a parent.[9]

When these parents do come to visit their toddler, the nurse should be available to provide information about the child's condition and to discuss any behaviors they find disturbing. Parents particularly need assistance with and clarification of the typical behaviors that a toddler manifests when he is separated from his parents. These behaviors are described in the discussion that follows.

Support of a Stressed Toddler

The response of a toddler to a stress situation does not necessarily have to be one of severe anxiety and long-term adverse effects. Those aspects that are the most stress-producing can be carefully managed to minimize the threat posed by a hospital experience. A toddler's security is particularly threatened by (1) being separated from his parents or other significant person, (2) being in an unfamiliar environment and having his routines and rituals disrupted and (3) feeling a loss of control and having his autonomy threatened by procedures that are painful and necessitate restraints. The nurse and family must cooperatively plan to minimize the adverse effects of these inevitable situational crises and maximize the positive experiences that can be derived from hospitalization. This presents a unique challenge to the nurse who cares for hospitalized toddlers.

Separation Anxiety The toddler is in a stage of development when his attachment to his mother is "fiercely possessive, selfish, and intolerant of frustration."[17] He does not understand why he must be separated from his parents, nor does his developmental level provide him with adequate coping mechanisms to withstand separation. There are many variables that affect the way a toddler experiences separation. The quality of the existing parent-child relationship, previous experiences with separation, the personality of the child and the type of substitute caretaking are important variables that have an impact upon the toddler's coping ability.

Robertson[17] observed institutionalized children and identified stages that a young child passes through when separated from his mother. These stages of protest, despair and denial (detachment) as described by Robertson provide useful information for the nurse who attempts to intervene when children are separated for even short periods from their parents. However, each child is unique in his response to separation, so these phases serve only as a general guide to the kinds of behavior that can be expected.

During the initial phase, *protest,* a toddler will cry desperately in an effort to summon the usual response of his parent. He violently protests the departure of his parents by screaming and clinging to them as they try to place him in the crib. During this phase parents experience ambivalence about visiting when they see their toddler pleading for them to stay. The nurse can intervene by staying with the child when the parents leave; she must, however, realize that it is not uncommon for the toddler to reject the attention of the nurse during this period. It is least traumatic for the child and the parent if the parent says goodbye and then leaves. When parents return several times in desperation to comfort their toddler, his protest is enhanced and the parents' anxiety is increased. The child should be told the truth by his parents about their leaving even though he protests; parents often need help from the nurse to understand

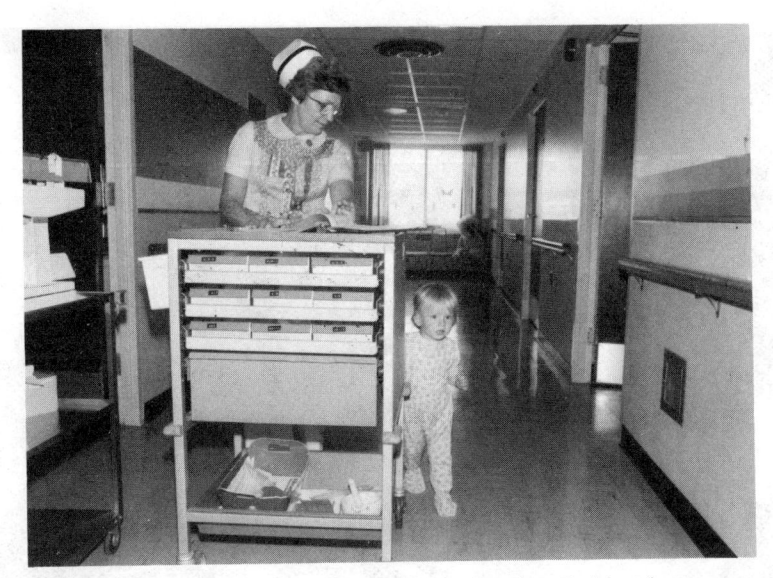

Frequent contacts can be facilitated by allowing the toddler to be close to his primary nurse as she completes her tasks.

the importance of not resorting to telling their child they are "just going for a cup of coffee." Recognizing these behaviors as a normal, healthy response, the nurse explains this to parents lest the parents feel that their visiting is causing greater trauma than staying away would cause. In spite of the trauma that this scene produces for both nurse and parent, the nurse must clearly communicate to the parent that it is essential to their child's welfare that they not curtail their visits.

The second phase is one of *despair* in which the toddler experiences a continuing conscious need of his mother. Despair or an increasing hopelessness results when the act of protest fails to bring his parents back. His despair can be recognized by his withdrawal from events and people in the environment. He rarely resists anything that is done to him and seldom cries during this stage. Apathy and depression exist, but the compliant behavior is easily mistaken as a sign of adaptation to the hospital experience. It is during this phase that the nurse must guard against misinterpreting the child's behavior when parents visit. A toddler is likely to cry intensely or have a temper tantrum when parents visit and the nurse who does not understand the nature of the toddler's anxiety concludes that the child is "better" when the parents do not visit. The young child particularly lacks a sense and understanding of time; therefore, in Robertson's words, "daily visiting touches only the fringe of his need."[17]

The third phase, *denial,* can result when a young child must stay for an extended period in the hospital and is cared for by a variety of nurses. In this child there is a return of interest in the environment with an appearance of having adapted; in actuality the external appearance is the result of a repression of feelings for his mother. The toddler no longer seems upset when parents come and go and he forms superficial relationships with many staff members, but he avoids closeness with any one person. Typically he becomes the ward favorite because he seems to be happy and responds to everyone; what he desperately needs is a trusting relationship with one individual.

A close relationship with a primary nurse is comforting when parents cannot visit regularly.

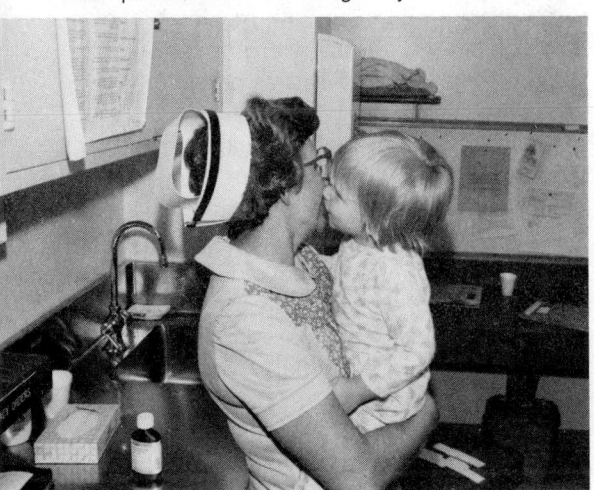

THE HOSPITALIZED TODDLER 853

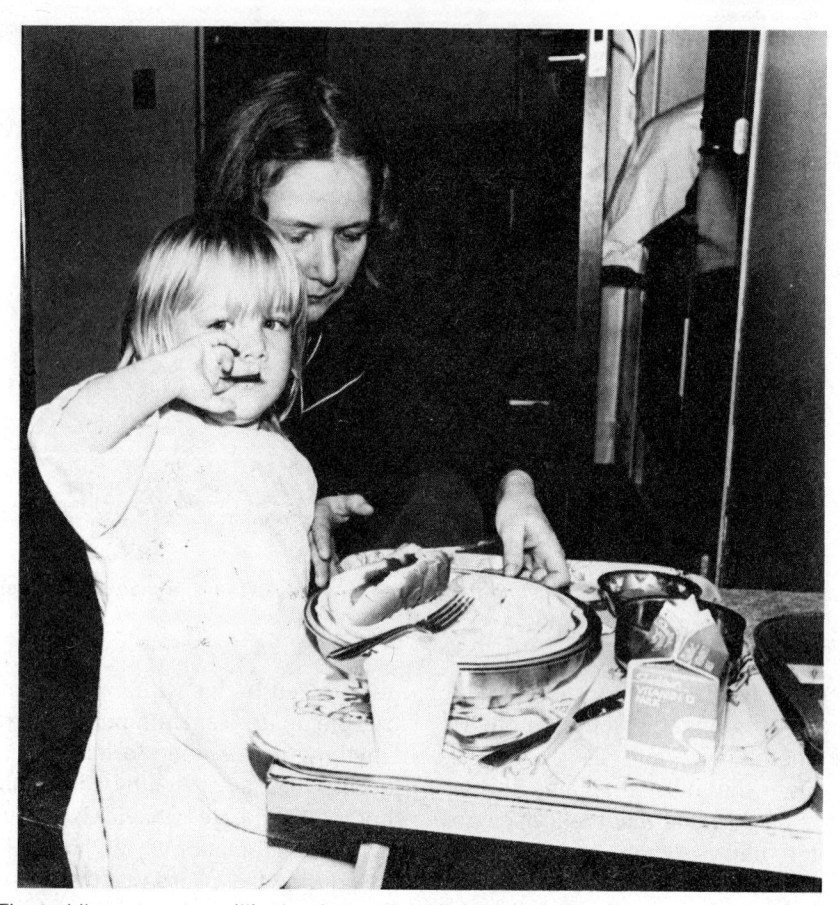

The toddler eats more willingly when served familiar foods in the presence of a parent.

To accomplish the goal of forming a trusting relationship with this child, one nurse should take the responsibility for planning his care so that some constancy of routine can be established. The primary nurse who plans his care should also care for him whenever she is on duty. The primary nurse should attempt to have frequent interactions with the toddler throughout the day. To a toddler several hours are an eternity; therefore, frequent contacts for shorter periods are more meaningful than only one or two contacts in an eight-hour period. The coming and going of the primary nurse during the day also gives the toddler practice in dealing with separation and increases his trust that the nurse will return. Additional special methods of ongoing contact should be used. It may be feasible for a toddler to follow the nurse around the unit, sit on her lap as she charts, or sit close by in a wagon or stroller as she performs other duties.

When the reasons for the parents' absence are not clear, the nurse has a responsibility to explore the family situation. The nurse can easily become engrossed with her own relationship with the toddler and disregard the reality that the relationship with parents must be maintained. The ultimate goal of the nurse is to encourage the presence of the parents so that the parent-child relationship can be maintained. When parents cannot be there the nurse should attempt to develop a trusting relationship with the child but with maximal involvement of parents through telephone calls and encouraging as many visits as possible.

Maintaining Routines and Rituals A toddler's security is dependent on doing things in the same way in the same environment. It is not feasible to retain every aspect of a toddler's routine, but the nurse can avoid serious disruption of the toddler's security by adapting his care to coincide with his established routine whenever possible. Rituals associated with mealtime and bedtime are particularly significant to the toddler. The toddler benefits from being offered foods with which he is familiar, served on his own tableware if he has this at home. The toddler is often more likely to eat for his parents than for the nurse or other strangers. Likewise, the toddler settles into sleep better if his bedtime routine at home is exactly followed during his hospitalization. Data collected about the child's routines and rituals should be incorporated into the care plan and be available to every nurse who cares for him. Even though parents are usually present, the nurse should be familiar with the child's most important routines. Bedtime rituals are particularly important to toddlers, and when parents cannot be present the nurse should provide the usual forms of security for the toddler.

Preparation for Procedures A toddler's limited cognitive ability makes him particularly likely to arrive at strange conclusions regarding painful procedures. Prugh and colleagues reported that young children reacted to threatening procedures as if they were hostile attacks and viewed them as punishment.[16] Toddlers may react to the intrusion of procedures by wildly kicking, screaming, hitting and trying to flee. They particularly respond to the visible aspects of a procedure such as needles, hemostats, tourniquets and any other strange pieces of equipment. It is not advisable to show a toddler large, frightening pieces of equipment because he will not understand their use and will be terrified by their appearance.

It is more effective to talk to the toddler about what will happen and then immediately proceed. Even though a toddler does not comprehend the content of an explanation, he can sense the feeling of caring and protection in the tone of voice, facial gestures and physical contact. It is most beneficial if the parent can be present and repeat the explanation to the toddler. The nurse can also provide an opportunity for the toddler to act out the procedure on a doll or favorite toy animal. Once the toddler is approached in performing the procedure, precision and skillful technique by the nurse are the most needed qualities. Hesitancy and pondering cause the toddler's anxiety to mount and give him the opportunity to fantasize an even greater intrusion than is about to occur.

During the actual procedure the nurse should understand that a toddler cannot be expected to cooperate and lie still. He is experiencing extreme anxiety and makes every attempt to resist the intrusion. The nurse should gently but firmly restrain the toddler and explain that she will help him to hold still. Reasons for the procedure will not be understood by a child under 3 years of age, but statements of warning such as "This will hurt" are understood by some toddlers.[2] A statement of warning that it will hurt should be followed immediately with a statement of comfort such as "It won't hurt long," or "Mommy is here to help you." Distraction by playing music, singing to the toddler, or reading a favorite story can also be helpful. The use of rhythm and imagery tends to increase the effectiveness of distractions from pain. As means of distraction, McCaffery describes the use of rhythmic breathing and pretending to be a train; these can be used to distract the attention from his pain in a child as young as 18 months.[13]

The involvement of parents whenever a toddler must undergo a procedure is another important part of relieving stress for him. Parents need to learn about the procedure before it is done even if they do not plan to be present. Such a discussion should not be carried out in the presence of the toddler since he will understand some things and misinterpret others. Also, the reaction of parents to the explanation may be alarm or concern, and the toddler is particularly sensitive to the general mood of conversations even though he does not understand their content.

Parents should be given the option to stay or leave when a painful procedure must be done. Some parents cannot cope with seeing their toddler being hurt and the nurse has a responsibility to support the parent in that decision. If a parent is made to feel that he or she *must* be present, the distress of the parent is likely to be communicated to the toddler and consequently compound his anxiety. Providing the toddler with his securities such as a blanket, teddy bear or other special objects is essential during such procedures.

Immediately before and following procedures the toddler should be cuddled and spoken to softly so that he does not interpret the procedure as a form of rejection. Even if the toddler kicked and screamed he should be praised for his efforts to cooperate or for this tolerance and he should be cuddled. Prugh[16] reported that children under 4 at times evidenced guilt after having lost control during a procedure. This was manifested by a period of time during which the child tried to control his unacceptable impulses

TABLE 36-1 TODDLER DEVELOPMENTAL NEEDS AND SUPPORTIVE NURSING INTERVENTIONS

Need	Nursing Intervention
Physical Physical freedom to explore and develop muscle skill within a safe environment.	1. Collect data to determine the type of explorative activities in which the toddler usually engages. 2. Provide small manipulative toys (boxes with lids, stack toys, nesting toys, large beads, large puzzles, equipment to color, paint and scribble). 3. Provide a crib with an enclosed see-through top when a child attempts to explore by reaching for dangerous objects or crawling out of his crib. 4. Permit supervised activities in a playroom where he can explore new toys and the unfamiliar environment. 5. Allow him to explore in his room under supervision.
Engage in large muscle activity within safe limits.	1. Collect data regarding degree of mobility attained. 2. Provide for supervised out-of-bed activities consistent with patterns at home to the degree that the child's condition permits. 3. Keep floors free from small objects. 4. Enforce the child's wearing of shoes or non-skid slippers while out of bed. 5. Provide large muscle toys (rocking horse, soft ball, indoor slide, push and pull toys).

Begin development of self-care in activities of daily living.	1. Collect data to determine level of self-care attained (eating, elimination, dressing, hygiene, bedtime care).
	 2. Provide opportunities for participation in self-care activities
	   a. Eating–Provide high chair or small table and chair, bib, and usual types of food; allow child to feed self in usual manner.
	   b. Elimination–Provide a potty chair or diapers according to usual elimination patterns. Reinforce routine as established prehospitalization.
	   c. Dressing–Permit child to assist with those activities he is capable of doing.
	   d. Hygiene–Allow child to participate in handwashing, brushing teeth, manipulating own wash cloth in tub.
	   e. Bedtime care–Allow child to participate in the bedtime story, and preparation for bed according to home routines.

Table continued on opposite page

TABLE 36-1 TODDLER DEVELOPMENTAL NEEDS AND SUPPORTIVE NURSING INTERVENTIONS *(Continued)*

Need	Nursing Intervention
Intellectual Opportunity to learn via sensorimotor and express self through imitation and pretending.	1. Provide toys that encourage exploration and manipulation. 2. For older toddler provide toys and equipment that can be used to re-enact hospital experience.
To engage in conversation with adults and children to enhance language development; to hear proper language and be encouraged to express self through language.	1. Collect data to identify extent of child's vocabulary, especially elicit data regarding key phrases and words pertaining to daily activities. 2. Allow child to complete sentences; avoid speaking for the child. 3. Reinforce words child has mastered and introduce new words. 4. Encourage group activities (play and eating) to encourage use of language between children.
To be given explanations about procedures. (The toddler can understand more than he can say.)	1. Avoid speaking about the child without explanations to him as well. 2. Explain procedures before doing them.
Emotional and Social Develop sense of autonomy.	1. Allow child to do things by himself pertaining to his own care. 2. Give child control over some of his own life: allow choices, restrain as little as possible, and praise him for completed tasks. 3. Give explanations when restraints are necessary.
Learn to separate from parent(s).	1. Encourage care by parents. 2. Assist family in coping with behaviors in response to hospitalization and separation. 3. Encourage parents to visit often even though child resists their leaving. 4. Provide primary nurse when parents cannot be present. 5. Keep image of parent in child's mind with a picture, personal belongings or a tape recording.
Learn to adapt socially.	1. Reinforce those socially acceptable behaviors mastered by the child before hospitalization (eating, elimination, play). 2. Provide play opportunities with other children.
Maintenance of usual routines and rituals for sense of security.	1. Gather data to determine important rituals and routines especially regarding bedtime (provide security objects and maintain routine re reading story, hugging, use of night light and other rituals). 2. Gather information regarding preferences in foods, toys, routines regarding daily hygiene, elimination and dressing. 3. Maintain as many home routines as possible.

and would verbally make reference to how "good" he was. The nurse should carefully assess those children whose treatment requires repeated traumatic procedures and involve the parents and health team in a search for ways to reduce the adverse effects and maximize the child's comfort.

ENHANCING NORMAL GROWTH AND DEVELOPMENT

Normal growth and development needs of the toddler can be met during hospitalization if the nurse works closely with the parents to provide individualized care. The child's physical, intellectual and emotional and social needs must be considered when planning nursing interventions (Table 36–1). Two central themes that dominate the development of a toddler are that he is becoming autonomous and that he develops through play.

A toddler who feels secure shows increasingly more autonomous behaviors. Hospitalization disrupts his familiar life of people, places and things so that he feels threatened, insecure and even punished. As he feels less secure, the spirit of "Me do it" wanes. Furthermore, hospitals are run on schedules that often do not allow for the extra time it takes to permit a toddler to do his own zipper, take off his own socks and shoes, and brush his own teeth at his own pace. Toddlers dawdle to increase their sense of control, wanting to do things in their own time in their own way. When this right is taken away, development is interrupted.

The nurse who understands the importance of these behaviors will incoporate interventions into the care plan to support the toddler's developing autonomy. Those tasks that the toddler has accomplished should be performed by him whenever possible, even though it takes him longer to do them. The toddler can also learn to perform new tasks while hospitalized, but major tasks such as becoming toilet trained, giving up a pacifier, or being weaned from a nighttime bottle should not be attempted during this time of stress.

His developing sense of autonomy is hampered frequently when he must be firmly held during procedures or by the restraint of extremities for intravenous fluids. Although it is often necessary to restrain the toddler for a procedure, the nurse should try to gain his cooperation before resorting to the use of restraint. The toddler who is restrained for an IV should be removed from restraints periodically. During this time he should have an opportunity to get out of his room, and under supervision he may even be taken to the playroom.

Need for Play

A child's intellectual and emotional and social development must be supported by play activities within the hospital. Toys can be brought to the child's bed or a small table in the child's room can provide an ideal play area. Some hospitals have designed enclosed outdoor play areas that permit activities to exercise large muscles. If he is confined to bed, it is especially important to provide for the toddler's need to explore, to be independent and to make discoveries through manipulation. Providing the opportunity to color, paint and manipulate toys that stack or come apart is appropriate for a toddler. Large puzzles, books with cardboard pages that the toddler can turn himself, and large beads to put on a heavy string are activities that a toddler enjoys. Toys that allow the child to dissipate energy, such as a pounding board with a hammer, a soft ball that can be thrown and thick crayons that can be used to scribble vigorously, can relieve a toddler of some of the frustration he feels because of limited physical exercise.

As a toddler approaches 3 years of age, therapeutic play becomes an increasingly effec-

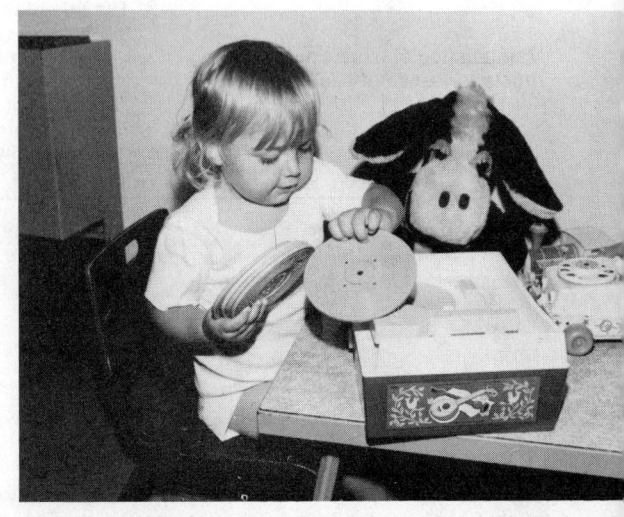

Play within the hospital is an integral part of a toddler's recovery.

tive way for him to regain some control over the hospital experiences; he can be the doer while a doll is the recipient of a procedure. Whenever possible, the nurse should let the toddler pretend to do to a doll or stuffed animal what will be done to him. This technique is effective for simple procedures such as brushing teeth, taking vital signs and even drinking milk and eating vegetables.

KEEPING THE TODDLER SAFE

Safety is a priority in the care of toddlers. Toddlers are quick, inquisitive and do not foresee danger; thus they are prone to accidents, whether at home or in the hospital. Every aspect of care has a safety component to consider. Toddlers are prone to injury during procedures and medication administration; the child can pull out the tubes of an IV because he does not understand the purpose of what is being done to him. Important responsibilities of the nurse are to maintain environmental safety and to administer medications by adapting the technique to the developmental level of the toddler.

Environmental Safety

The usual precautions that are necessary to keep a well toddler safe should be taken in planning the safety of a hospitalized toddler. (See Chapter 30 for normal growth and development of the toddler.) In addition, the nurse and parents need to be aware of the dangers posed by a hospital environment (high cribs, unfamiliar stairways and slippery floors, and medications, needles and glass). The trend toward increased freedom and mobility of children in hospitals to foster normal growth and development carries with it an increased likelihood for accidents to occur.

When toddlers are up and about on a smooth hospital floor falls are inevitable, but special precautions can be taken to reduce the number and severity of accidents. The floor should not be highly polished but should be kept clean and free of small objects that could be swallowed, or sharp objects that could be picked up by a toddler. The toddler should not be allowed to run in socks or in bare feet; in socks he is sure to slip and fall and in bare feet he may fall or step on dangerous objects — commonly, broken glass. Feet should be protected with shoes or slippers that have non-skid soles. Toddlers who are free to be out of bed must be supervised because they disappear quickly and may fall down an unfamiliar stairwell or get on an elevator.

Falls from cribs are an even greater threat in the hospital than at home. Hospital cribs are high and the floors rarely have rugs or carpet to cushion the fall. Because of the serious damage that can result from a high fall, the standards of care pertaining to cribs must reflect extreme caution. Use of an enclosed see-through crib top can prevent falls by toddlers who attempt to crawl out of their cribs. These cribs allow the toddler to stand up and be free to walk around in a safe area. The nurse should not hesitate to make the decision to use an enclosed (bubble top) crib whenever there is even the slightest indication that a toddler may climb out of the crib. Parents can provide important information regarding the toddler's usual behavior, but the nurse should also make her own assessment by observing the toddler in his crib. Even though a toddler has never crawled out of his crib at home he may do so in the hospital because of his prolonged confinement to the crib. The nurse should re-evaluate the toddler as he recuperates; he is more likely to crawl out when he is feeling better and is more familiar with the environment.

The nurse should establish safe habits while working with a toddler in a crib; nurses must observe each other and other health team members for any breach of safe practice. When the siderail is down the nurse must keep one hand on the toddler whenever her back is even slightly turned for a fraction of a second; this is a rule never to be broken. Putting the siderail halfway up and turning to get things from the bedside stand and walking away momentarily are unsafe practices. Even if a toddler is restrained it is not safe to leave a siderail down because, given sufficient time, the toddler can get out of the most complicated restraints. Parents will need explanations of these dangers and standards of care. If they leave a siderail down and walk away from the crib the nurse must take the responsibility to ensure the safety of the child by reminding parents of the rules of safety and asking them to comply.

Another aspect of care that differs in the hospital from that in the home is the use of high

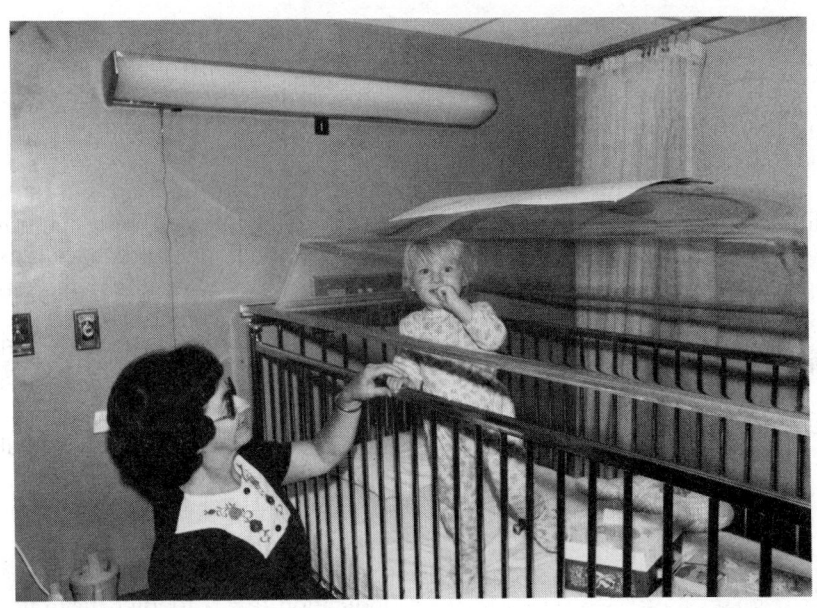

An enclosed see-through crib keeps the toddler safe from falls but free to move. Note the large poster lying across the top of the crib to provide an interesting view for the toddler while lying in his crib.

chairs. At home the toddler is likely to be at the table with his family when he is in a high chair, and it is less likely that he will stand up and fall out of the chair. However, within the hospital the nurse who is feeding a toddler may be momentarily called away, leaving the toddler alone in a high chair. It is preferable to not leave a toddler in a high chair unattended even though he is restrained. However, if a nurse must leave, the toddler must be securely restrained and the high chair should be moved into a position in which the child cannot reach a wall or furniture. If the highchair has wheels they must be locked. These precautions prevent the toddler from reaching a sturdy object and pulling on it until the chair tips and falls, a feat which the toddler is very capable of performing. If the restraining strap in a high chair is broken or missing a jacket restraint can be used or other forms of restraint can be improvised. However, even if all these precautions have been taken, the nurse should return in a few minutes.

Toddlers on the go in a hospital unit are also more prone to ingestion and foreign body aspiration. The emphasis on the use of toys and play materials within the hospital adds another area of responsibility for the nurse. Toys must be inspected for small, removable parts. Bedside stands, cupboard tops and the nurses' station are all accessible to the toddler. Diapers, safe toys and books can be stored in a toddler's room but pins, ointments, thermometers, medications, scissors, solutions, and unattended purses cannot. Discarded medications and needles or other small or sharp objects must not be thrown into wastebaskets, from which they will be retrieved by a busy, searching toddler. Medication carts can never be left unattended if unlocked. When the cart is unattended it should be stored in a medication or treatment room in which children are not allowed. The variety of colors of liquid medications used in pediatrics is particularly intriguing to the toddler.

Food, liquids and medications are sources of potential aspiration. Toddlers generally eat table foods and drink from a cup, but their level of skill varies according to age and from one child to another. The nurse should be familiar with a child's particular level of development and avoid giving foods that are too coarse or hard for him to eat safely. Popcorn, nuts, hard candy and corn are foods that are not easily managed by some toddlers. Toddlers should not be allowed to run with food in their mouth and they should be in a sitting position to take liquids and medications. They should never be allowed to be mobile with a Popsicle, or candy on a stick.

Electrical sockets are potential sources of danger to a toddler, whether at home or in a hospital. The hospital environment is particularly hazardous in this regard. Most commonly, the head of the crib is placed against the wall and the toddler can reach the plugs and sockets that are at approximately crib top level. Thus the toddler stands up, reaches over the rail and pulls on plugs, or he may insert something into an open socket. Sometimes it is possible to move the crib and lock the wheels so that the toddler cannot reach the sockets; otherwise, when a toddler insists on playing with the sockets it is necessary to use an enclosed crib top so that he cannot reach out of the crib.

Administering Medications

Children from 1 to 3 years of age resist taking medications more frequently and more intensely. A struggling toddler not only increase the to resist verbally and, most noticeably, physically. A struggling toddler not only increases the chances for an injury, but the psychological effect of tightly restraining a toddler day after day for frequent medications can seriously threaten his security and his developing sense of autonomy as he daily succumbs to the physical coercion.

To reduce likelihood of psychological upset the nurse should first try to gain the cooperation of the toddler, encourage the presence of parents and use physical gestures to console the toddler. It is particularly important for the nurse to consult parents regarding the best method and approach to use in giving medication to their child. When hints are given by parents and they are effective, the nurse should communicate this to other nurses by making a note on the medication sheet and nursing Kardex. This is particularly important for toddlers, whose security is dependent on their rituals and routines. Allowing a toddler to pretend he is giving medication to a doll or stuffed animal is an effective way to gain his cooperation.

Oral Medications A spoon, a medicine cup or a medication syringe is used to give oral liquid medication to a toddler. The usual hospital procedure is to use a medicine cup or a syringe; however, the nurse should explore whether a spoon would be more effective. When the medicine cup is used the toddler frequently prefers to hold the cup and resists taking the medication if he is not allowed to do so. In some cases the toddler wants his parents to hold the cup. The nurse should remain with the toddler until all the medication is swallowed.

When using a syringe caution must be taken to avoid squirting the entire contents of the syringe into the toddler's mouth at one time. The syringe should be placed to one side and toward the back of the toddler's mouth. The plunger is then pushed, injecting the portion of the medicine that the toddler is capable of swallowing at one time. (A 5 cc syringe of medication would require approximately two to three squirts.)

Oral medications can also be given in tablet form. Chewable tablets can usually be given to a toddler by the time he is 2 years of age. The nurse should stay with the child until the medication is chewed and swallowed. Tablets that need to be crushed can be mixed in water or flavored syrups. If the taste is extremely bitter it may be disguised more effectively in a nonessential food such as ice cream or a small amount of fruit jelly. Regardless of how medications are given, the nurse must approach the child with recognition of the developmental tasks and behaviors that will affect oral administration of medications (see Medication Guide).

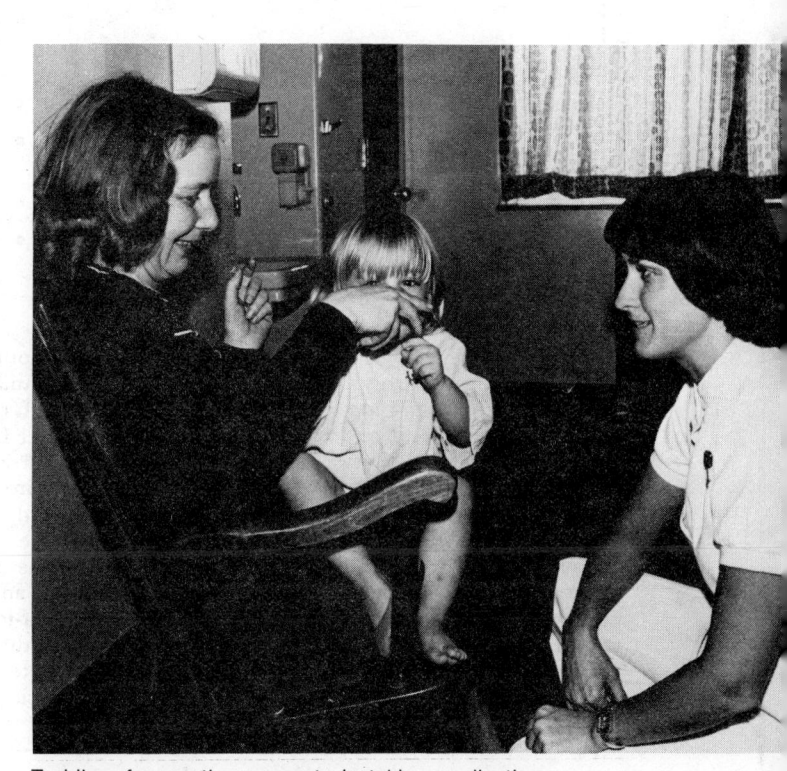

Toddlers frequently cooperate in taking medications in a supportive environment. (Notice that the nurse gets down to the toddler's eye level.)

PEDIATRIC MEDICATION GUIDELINES—12 TO 18 MONTHS

	Developmental Tasks and Behaviors	Nursing Implications
MOTOR	• Advances from standing with support to independent walking.	• Have the child choose a position for taking medication or hold him to provide control and comfort. Forcing the child to take medicine when he is lying down takes away his sense of independence and will frequently result in very resistive behavior.
FEEDING	• Begins independent self-feeding, but is still messy. • Develops voluntary tongue and lip control. • Spits deliberately.	• Home feeding habits should be considered. • Spits out disagreeable tastes effectively. Disguise crushed tablets and contents of capsules in a *small* amount of familiar solid. Be prepared to refeed.
INTERACTIVE	Autonomy versus Shame and Doubt • Indicates needs and wants by pointing. • Speaks 4 to 6 words. Uses individual jargon. • Responds to familiar commands. • Responds to and participates in the routines of daily living. • Exhibits notable independence, resistance, self-assertiveness, and ambivalence. Begins to have temper tantrums.	 • Find out what words child uses for drinking, swallowing, and how oral medicines have been given at home. • Let child explore an empty medication cup. He will likely be more cooperative if familiar items are used. • When possible, involve the parents. They are familiar and trusted persons, which is an important factor during an unfamiliar experience. • Tell parents and staff the approach used for medication. Report its effectiveness. • Allow the child as much freedom as possible. • Allow the child to assert himself by choosing a drink to wash down the medicine. • Use games to gain cooperation. • Tell the child what you expect and then follow through. A consistent, firm approach is essential.

EXAMPLE: Eighteen-month-old Simon has been in the hospital 4 days with severe gastroenteritis. He has had nothing orally and has received intravenous (IV) fluids for volume replacement and ampicillin therapy. This morning his IV was discontinued and oral ampicillin started. At shift report the day nurse states he does not take his oral medication well. She reports that she gave the suspension via syringe.

Recognizing that Simon has had experience with a variety of syringes in the last few days, the evening nurse elects to try a different approach. From talking with Simon's mother she knows Simon is used to an assisted self-feeding routine—he has his own fork and spoon and his mother supplements his efforts with another spoon. Also, he enjoys apple juice and can manage a cup fairly well by himself.

Using this "at home" activity and Simon's need to feel familiar with an object to decrease his fear, the nurse allows him to play with a medication cup, drink juice from it, and watch his mother handle and use it. Later she measures the ampicillin into one now-familiar cup and apple juice into another. She allows Simon to hold the juice cup. Simon's sip of ampicillin, given by the nurse, is alternated with a self-fed sip of apple juice. He took the ampicillin without resistance. At night shift report the nurse notes this approach was effective. She encountered no resistive behavior.

PEDIATRIC MEDICATION GUIDELINES—18 TO 30 MONTHS

	Developmental Tasks and Behaviors	Nursing Implications
MOTOR	• Walks, climbs into chair (18 mos.). Advances to running without falling (24 mos.). • Advances to obtaining and throwing small objects.	• Child is able to run away and kick. • Child may throw materials placed within his reach. Never leave medications sitting on the bedside stand.
FEEDING	• Generally feeds self. Advances to proficiency with minimal spilling. • Second molars erupted (20-30 mos.). Exhibits increased rotary chewing; manages solid food particles. • Controls mouth and jaw proficiently.	• Allow child opportunity to drink liquids from a medicine cup by himself. • Permits greater flexibility in choosing form of medication. • Child is effective in spitting out unwanted medications and in clamping mouth tightly closed in resistance.
INTERACTIVE	Autonomy versus Shame and Doubt • Has some sense of time, but no words for time (18 mos.). Then responds to "just a minute" (21 mos.). Advances to understanding, "Play after you drink this." (24 mos.). • Carries out 2 to 3 directions given one at a time. • Shows ability to respond to and participate in routines of daily living. • Helps put things away; carries breakable objects. • Exhibits independence, resistance, self-assertiveness, and ambivalence. • Throws temper tantrums frequently. • Shows pride in accomplished skills. • Does not know right from wrong. • Shows conflict between holding on and letting go.	• Tell the child getting medicine that any bad taste will only last "a minute." • Learn child's level of time awareness from nursing history. • Give simplified directions: "Open your mouth, drink, and then swallow." • Include child in establishing medicine-taking routine. • Use a firm, consistent approach. Resistive behaviors are at a peak. • Give immediate, positive tactile and verbal response to cooperative taking of medicine. Ignore resistive behavior. • Give choices when possible: "Do you want to sit in the chair or on my lap to take your medicine?"

EXAMPLE: Barbara, 28 months, has bronchitis and was admitted to the hospital 3 days ago. She has been receiving ampicillin 250 mg by mouth every six hours. Usually a delightful, playful child, she has been labeled a "brat" when it comes time to take her medicine. Nurses have emptied capsules, placed the contents in chocolate syrup, and spoon-fed her with the result of most of the mixture ending up on the nurse. Suspension form has also been tried ineffectively.

Referring to the nursing history for possible help with this child, the nurse discovers that Barbara's favorite food is now candy. Since she has demonstrated proficiency in chewing solid food and candy, the nurse suspects she might take her ampicillin as a chewable tablet. The nurse also feels that involving Barbara in the ritual of medication time might be helpful. At the next medicine time the nurse allows Barbara to pick out two 125 mg tablets herself from a medication cup. Barbara then chews and swallows them. Next she throws the now empty cup into the wastebasket. The nurse gives Barbara a chaser of choice and praises her for her help. Barbara is now a "successful helper" in taking medications.

PEDIATRIC MEDICATION GUIDELINES—2½ to 3½ YEARS

	Developmental Tasks and Behaviors	Nursing Implications
MOTOR	• Continues to develop proficiency. Basic skills have all been initiated.	• Child may be quite adept in resistive behavior.
FEEDING	• Becoming more proficient in skills. Eating likes and dislikes are definite but changeable. • May be influenced by others' reactions in responding to new food experiences.	• Medication tastes can be disguised with variable effectiveness. • A calm, positive approach is needed to gain a cooperative response from the child; quick tense approach is likely to produce similar behavior in the child.
INTERACTIVE	Initiative versus Guilt • Gives full name. • Is ritualistic. • Has little understanding of past, present, or future. • Shows concrete thinking, egocentricity. • Exhibits early aggressiveness; coercive, manipulative behavior. • Has many fantasies. • May be frightened by his "power."	• Begin asking for verbal identification of patient before giving medications. • Communicate administration methods. • Use concrete and immediate rewards. • Tolerates frustration poorly. Child's initial response to reason appears positive, but without consistent effect. • Prolonged bargaining is frustrating and frightening to the child because no one is in control of the situation. • Give a choice when possible. Do not give a choice if the child does not have one. • Begin giving simple, honest explanations of why the medication is given (not because the child was bad). • Child's sense of security is dependent upon the nurses' consistent expectations of his behavior.

EXAMPLE: Roger, 3 years old, has otitis media and ampicillin 200 mg is ordered by mouth every 6 hours. He is to get the first dose in the clinic and then treatment is to be continued at home. His mother seems reluctant to agree that he really needs the medication. Finally she says she just cannot face what she knows will be trouble because he is at "that stage" when he won't do anything he is told.

The nurse pours the ampicillin into a cup. Roger is seated on his mother's lap. The nurse says, "Roger, your ears have been hurting. This medicine will help stop the hurting. I have the medicine in a little cup for you to drink. It tastes funny, but I don't think it tastes too bad. You can hold the cup and do it yourself; your mother and I will watch." She hands Roger the cup and watches while he follows through. "Good, it's done in one big swallow. Would you like some apple juice or some water now?" the nurse asks.

When they come back in 10 days, Roger's mother reports changing from juice to gum to ice pops to lemon drops after the medication, but that the medicine all went down.

Nose, Ear and Eye Drops Nose drops are administered by placing the toddler's head over a pillow on the parent's or nurse's lap. Being placed over the edge of the bed is frightening to a toddler and should be avoided. It is necessary to have the head positioned lower than the body because the toddler cannot cooperate by sniffing the medication into the affected nasal passages. The lowered position is frightening to the toddler but the idea can be introduced through playful manipulation before the time that the medication must be given. The head must be lower than the body to allow the drops to penetrate the swollen nasal passages by gravity flow.

Ear drops are most easily administered if a toddler is held on the parent's lap. A toddler resists lying flat on his back, but he can be held in a side-lying position while the nurse pulls down and back on the pinna of the ear and gives the prescribed medication. If the nurse does not have the assistance of a parent, the toddler can be firmly held in the nurse's lap or positioned on his side on the bed. Both the nurse's hands are free to administer the medication, but the toddler's movement is restricted by the nurse's arms. The toddler should remain in position for a minute after ear drops have been instilled.

Placing cotton in the ears after administration of ear drops has some disadvantages in toddlers. The toddler may remove the cotton and put it in his mouth or he may push it into his ears farther than is recommended. If cotton is used it should be placed gently and loosely so that in the event of ear discharge, secretions are not trapped in the ear.

Eye drops and eye ointments are instilled with the toddler being held in a flat position on someone's lap or on a flat surface. The toddler often resists when anyone comes near his face; he may strongly resist administration of eye medication by flailing his arms, kicking, screaming and squeezing his eyes closed. The nurse is most successful if she can move quickly once the toddler is told what will happen. If the toddler begins to strongly resist it is extremely difficult for one person to accomplish the task; therefore it is advisable to stop immediately and summon assistance from another nurse. It is difficult to give eye medication safely to a resisting toddler and the nurse should not hesitate to ask for assistance.

Rectal Medications Administration of rectal medication may be strongly resisted by a toddler who is not accustomed to having his temperature taken rectally. A toddler's response to rectal medication may also be affected by his particular experience with toilet training. Since the toddler is just becoming aware of body sensations related to defecation he may try to expel the suppository. The suppository must be inserted past the rectal sphincter and the buttocks gently pressed together for several minutes. The suppository is not likely to dissolve for 5 to 10 minutes, but the toddler generally does not tolerate having pressure applied to his buttocks for that length of time. The toddler who is resisting by crying and kicking is more likely to expel the suppository than if he is asked to rest in his crib after it is inserted and briefly held in place. It is also helpful if a parent can hold the toddler in a side-lying position on her lap for several minutes after the suppository has been inserted. The nurse should ask the parent to check the diaper carefully on the next changing to be sure the suppository has not been expelled. The nurse should also return in 15 minutes to check the diaper.

Intramuscular Medication The technique for administration of intramuscular medication for a toddler is similar to that for any child. The ventrogluteal site and the anteriolateral thigh (vastus lateralis muscle) are the most appropriate sites for the toddler. An appropriate-sized needle is chosen according to the amount of subcutaneous tissue that is present. For an intramuscular injection the needle must be long enough to pass through the fatty layer and into the muscle. In most children between the ages of 1 to 3 years a one inch needle is adequate, but in a young toddler who still has chubby thighs a longer needle may be necessary. For most types of medication a 23 gauge needle is appropriate.

The approach to a toddler and his family when giving an intramuscular injection must take into account previous experience with injections, the parent-child relationship, and the child's developmental level. The parents should be told about the medication before the nurse enters the room. This explanation should be given when the toddler is not present, and at that time the nurse should also explain any side effects and the purpose of giving the medication. The parents should also be asked whether or not they wish to stay with their toddler and if they wish to stay, the nurse should explain to them how they can help.

Once the parent(s) have been prepared and the medication is ready the nurse should proceed to the room with the medication but keep the needle out of the child's view (e.g., inside the medication cart). The nurse can then prepare the child by briefly telling him what will happen, using terms that he best understands such as "shot" or "needle." Once the explanation has been given and the toddler has been given the opportunity to experiment in play as applicable, the medication should be administered without further delay. A toddler can best be restrained if the nurse gently leans across his torso so that his arms are free to move but blocked from the injection area. For many toddlers it is essential to have another nurse assist with the injection. The legs can then be restrained by one person and the other person can give the injection. After the procedure the toddler is cuddled and praised for his cooperation. (See Appendix VII for further instruction about injections and injection sites.)

PREPARATION FOR DISCHARGE

The nurse's goal is to discharge the toddler and his family in optimal physical and psychological health. Nursing interventions to reduce the stress of hospitalization, to maintain normal growth and development and to provide safe, developmentally appropriate nursing care have been described. With appropriate interventions in these areas during hospitalization the transition from hospital to home is eased. Upset after leaving the hospital is most common during the toddler years. The nurse must make every effort to reduce the likelihood of its occurrence.

During hospitalization the nurse should be in communication with the family regarding the effects that hospitalization is having on their toddler. The nurse should also discuss with the parents how they are handling the care of siblings in the home. If there has been ongoing communication during hospitalization pertaining to expected behavioral changes in their toddler and siblings, the nurse who discharges the family need only review with them the most common behaviors that the toddler and siblings are likely to manifest when the toddler returns home.

The reactions of siblings when a hospitalized child returns home is dependent on their age and is highly individual, but the family can generally expect that when the toddler returns home older siblings may resent the loss of attention from parents because of the toddler's special needs. The toddler returning home may show regressive behaviors in developmental tasks and show clinging and whining behaviors, and may have some sleep disturbances. Frequently it is the most recently achieved task that is lost first.[19] Parents need to be aware of the possibility of these behaviors occurring; they should be counseled to give their toddler additional emotional support by allowing him to be more dependent for a time and gradually weaning him back to his usual more independent behavior. They also need to be reminded that older siblings will resent this additional attention and that for a time an older child who was not hospitalized may manifest additional attention-getting behaviors.

It is important that nurses and parents do not have a preconceived idea that the toddler will regress and become more dependent because of a hospital experience. With careful interventions to reduce stress and enhance normal growth and development the toddler can mature and benefit from a hospital experience. The nurse and family must make every effort to capitalize on the unique resiliency of the toddler.

References

1. E. I. Barowsky. Young children's perceptions and reactions to hospitalization. In Psychosocial Aspects of Pediatric Care. E. Gellert, Grune and Stratton, 1978
2. P. Blos. Children think about illness: their concepts and beliefs. In Psychosocial Aspects of Pediatric Care, E. Gellert, Grune and Stratton, 1978
3. J. D. Calkin. Assessing small children: Are hospitalized toddlers adapting to the experience as well as we think? American Journal of Maternal Child Nursing, Jan/Feb 1978, p. 18
4. L. O. Eckhardt and D. G. Prugh. Preparing children psychologically for painful medical and surgical procedures. In Psychosocial Aspects of Pediatric Care. E. Gellert, Grune and Stratton, 1978
5. S. Everson. Sibling Counseling. American Journal of Nursing, April 1977, p. 644
6. J. H. Gildia and T. R. Quirk. Assessing the pain experience in children. Nursing Clinics of North America, December 1977, p. 631
7. E. R. Goslin. Hospitalization as a life crisis for the preschool child: A critical review. Journal of Community Health, Summer 1978, p. 321
8. C. Hardgrove and A. Rutledge. Parenting during hospitalization. American Journal of Nursing, May 1975, p. 836
9. J. A. Hennessey. Hospitalized toddlers' responses to

mothers' tape recordings during brief separations. Maternal-Child Nursing Journal, Summer 1976, p. 69
10. N. J. Kerr. The effect of hospitalization on the developmental tasks of childhood. Nursing Forum, Vol. 18, No. 2, 1979, p. 108
11. E. A. Mason. Hospital and family cooperating to reduce psychological trauma. Community Mental Health Journal, Vol. 14, No. 2, 1978, p. 153
12. M. M. McBride. Assessing children with pain. Pediatric Nursing, Jul/Aug 1977, p. 7
13. M. McCaffery. Pain relief for the child. Pediatric Nursing, Jul/Aug 1977, p. 11
14. E. A. R. Ormond and C. Caulfield. A practical guide to giving oral medications to young children. American Journal of Maternal Child Nursing, Sept/Oct 1976, p. 320
15. M. Petrillo and S. Sanger. Emotional Care of Hospitalized Children, 2nd ed. J. B. Lippincott Co., 1980
16. D. G. Prugh et al. A study of the emotional reactions of children and families to hospitalization and illness. American Journal of Orthopsychiatry, January 1953, p. 70
17. J. Robertson. Young Children in Hospital, 2nd ed. Tavistock Publications (London), 1970
18. D. Vernon et al. Changes in children's behavior after hospitalization. American Journal of Disease in Children, June 1966, p. 581
19. A. L. Wilkinson. Behavioral disturbance following short-term hospitalization. Comprehensive Pediatric Nursing, July 1978, p. 12

Additional Recommended Reading

C. Berner. Assessing the child's ability to cope with the stresses of hospitalization. In P. Brandt et al., (eds). Current Practice in Pediatric Nursing. C. V. Mosby Co., 1976

A. C. Galligan. Using Roy's concept of adaptation to care for young children. American Journal of Maternal Child Nursing, Jan/Feb 1979, p. 24

C. Isler. The fine art of handling a hospitalized child. RN, March 1978, p. 41

NURSING CARE PLAN FOR THE TODDLER WITH CIRCULATORY ALTERATION by Joyce Piazza

Nursing Diagnosis	Expected Outcome	Nursing Intervention	Rationale
Altered circulation due to congenital heart disease.	Short term: Child's circulatory status will be assessed; significant signs and symptoms of congenital heart disease will be recognized and appropriately treated. Long term: Parents will know signs and symptoms of congenital heart disease, when to notify physician of significant symptoms and participate in plans for follow-up care.	Dx: 1. Check vital signs as ordered, noting significant changes in heart rate and rhythm and in blood pressure reading. 2. Observe respiratory status. 3. Note presence and quality of peripheral pulses. 4. Check skin temperature of child's extremities. 5. Observe color of skin, nailbeds and mucous membranes. 6. Observe activity tolerance. 7. Note hydration of child and indicate if child appears dehydrated or edematous. 8. Watch for neurological changes. Rx: 1. Organize care to provide rest periods. 2. Encourage parents to engage their toddler in quiet activity. 3. Explain treatments and assessment of vital signs to child and parents.	1. Vital signs are checked to insure stability. Significant changes can indicate cardiac decompensation. 2. Depending on the cardiac defect, pulmonary circulation can be increased or decreased, causing respiratory symptoms. 3–4. Peripheral pulses, skin temperature and color are checked to determine adequacy of circulation to extremities. 5. Changes in color may indicate condition improving or getting worse. Depending on the cardiac defect, the child will be cyanotic or acyanotic. Those defects causing right-to left shunting in the heart cause cyanosis. 6. Activity tolerance is observed because child is less able to tolerate activity as cardiac condition worsens and less oxygen is circulating in the blood. 7. Fluid overload can be caused by cardiac failure. Dehydration can occur when child is receiving diuretics to treat heart failure. 8. If the child is polycythemic, as often occurs with cyanosis, he may experience neurological changes. With polycythemia the blood is viscous and sluggish; thrombus formation may occur and lead to a cerebral vascular accident (CVA). 1. Rest reduces oxygen requirements by reducing metabolic activity. 2–3. Parents being present and prepared for procedures reduces anxiety level of child and parents. Energy is conserved when the child and parents remain comfortable and calm.

		Patient/Parent Education: 1. Use a diagram to explain to parents the altered circulatory condition. 2. Make parents aware of signs and symptoms of altered circulatory status due to congenital heart disease. 3. Keep parents informed of any significant changes in their child's condition. 4. Discuss with them plans for follow-up care of their child.	1–4. Explanation (verbal and by diagram) of the altered circulatory status helps parents understand necessary treatment. Informing parents of expected signs and symptoms and the meaning of any changes in child's condition prepares them to care for child at home.
Potential for development of congestive heart failure.	Short term: Child will be observed for signs and symptoms of heart failure and managed appropriately to prevent or correct it. Long term: Parents will be aware of signs and symptoms of heart failure and of measures to take to prevent and alleviate it.	Dx: 1. Monitor pulse rate. 2. Monitor respiratory rate and listen to breath sounds. Determine if child is experiencing shortness of breath, dyspnea, or orthopnea, or having retractions. 3. Monitor intake and output; weigh child daily. 4. Measure specific gravity of urine. 5. Observe for presence and location of edema.	1. An increased cardiac rate (tachycardia) is a compensatory mechanism of the heart to increase its output. As heart failure increases, stroke volume may decrease, resulting in impaired systemic perfusion. 2. Respiratory status should be assessed because heart failure leads to pulmonary congestion. As fluid moves from the vascular space to the interstitium or alveoli of the lungs, wheezing or rales may be heard. 3. Measurement of intake and output and daily weighing are used to determine if medical treatment child is receiving is effective. As cardiac function improves, there is less retention of sodium and water and a decrease in weight is noted. 4. Specify gravity measurements are used to assess cardiac function. With reduced cardiac function renal blood flow diminishes. As a result, urinary output is reduced and specific gravity is high. (Urine is concentrated.) 5. Heart failure can lead to retention of body fluids, causing edema. As systemic venous blood pressure increases fluid collects in the interstitial spaces. *Table continued on following page*

NURSING CARE PLAN FOR THE TODDLER WITH CIRCULATORY ALTERATION (Continued)

Nursing Diagnosis	Expected Outcome	Nursing Intervention	Rationale
		Rx:	
		1. Position child to facilitate easier breathing by elevating head of bed or propping on pillows.	1. Child will breathe more efficiently when sitting upright—lungs are not compressed by pressure of abdominal organs against the diaphragm as when child is lying flat in bed. In the upright position venous return to heart and lungs is reduced, thereby diminishing pulmonary congestion.
		2. Provide a restful atmosphere. Arrange for nap periods during day and handle child minimally.	2. Rest decreases workload of heart because it reduces body's requirements for oxygen and blood.
		3. Administer oxygen as ordered.	3. Oxygen is given because child is not getting enough oxygen to the tissues when the heart is in failure.
		4. Give sedative drugs as ordered.	4. Sedative drugs assist child to rest, especially when hypoxic.
		5. Administer digoxin and diuretics if ordered. Check electrolyte laboratory reports (potassium in particular) and observe for side effects and toxicity of drugs.	5. Digoxin increases cardiac output by increasing force of contraction. Diuretics increase urinary output: Use of diuretics can lead to hypokalemia. A state of hypokalemia sensitizes the myocardium to cardiotonics (digitalis, digitoxin, digoxin).
		6. Restrict fluids as ordered.	6. Fluids are restricted because child is usually in fluid overload. Excess fluid increases workload of the heart.
		Parent Education:	
		1. Make parents aware of signs and symptoms of congestive heart failure.	1–3. Since the toddler has limited verbal ability, parents need to be taught how to assess his condition and manage his care.
		2. Teach them measures to make child more comfortable and alleviate distress.	
		3. Explain to them the need for fluid restriction and medications.	

FAMILIES WITH TODDLERS

Need for surgical intervention.	Immediate: Child and parents will be given adequate preparation for surgery. Short term: Child's circulatory stability will be maintained postop, and appropriate measures will be taken to prevent or treat complications. Long term: Child will recover from cardiac surgery and return to as normal a lifestyle as possible.	Preop: Dx: 1. Determine whether child knows surgery will be done. 2. Assess parents' understanding of surgical procedure and postop care. 3. Assess how parents feel about their child having surgery. Rx: Carry out preop routines as ordered (bath, NPO, preop meds, etc.). Patient Education: 1. Do preop teaching as appropriate for child's age. 2. Tell toddler about surgery close to the time it is to be done and give a simple explanation. Assure the child that his parents will be with him afterward. Postop: Dx: 1. Monitor vital signs as ordered. 2. Assess respiratory status by observing respiratory effort and listening to breath sounds. 3. Monitor intake and output. 4. Weigh child daily.	1–3. Often cardiac surgery involves a high risk for the child, which causes parents extreme worry. Providing them with information about the operation and postop care can help to ease fears and anxieties. 1–2. Telling toddler too far in advance may cause him unnecessary anxiety, because he does not have a concept of time. Toddlers need to be told things in simple terms because detailed explanations are not understood and may produce fear. 1. Vital signs may change after surgery because of stress put on the heart from the procedure. If changes are noted early, complications can be prevented or detected in time to take effective action. 2. Changes in breath sounds and respiratory effort may occur after cardiac surgery if child develops atelectasis or pneumonia (potential respiratory complications). 3. Accurate intake measurement is needed to make sure the child is receiving necessary fluids but not exceeding fluid restriction. Output is measured to determine if renal function has been affected by altered cardiac status. *Comparison of output with intake* warns of fluid retention. 4. Child is weighed to determine whether or not he is retaining fluids postop, as increase in weight usually indicates this. *Table continued on following page*

THE HOSPITALIZED TODDLER   871

NURSING CARE PLAN FOR THE TODDLER WITH CIRCULATORY ALTERATION (Continued)

Nursing Diagnosis	Expected Outcome	Nursing Intervention	Rationale
		5. Check incision site.	5. This is done to see if there is any bleeding from incision, or if any signs of inflammation are present. Coagulation abnormalities can cause postoperative bleeding. Wound infection is also a potential complication.
		6. Note color of skin, nailbeds and mucous membranes.	6. Changes in color may indicate improvement or worsening of child's condition. Oxygen saturation affects color. As oxygen saturation drops, cyanosis may become noticeable.
		7. Check peripheral pulses and warmth of extremities.	7. Palpable peripheral pulses and warm extremities indicate good cardiac output and peripheral circulation.
		Rx: 1. Turn child who is on bed rest. Allow child to increase activity as tolerated (up in chair; up in wheelchair; walking). Chest therapy prn.	1. Child should be turned and activity gradually increased to prevent alterations in respiratory status resulting from immobility.
		2. Lift child by placing one hand under buttocks and the other hand behind the back for support.	2. This method for lifting keeps strain off of incision.
		3. Restrict intravenous and oral fluids as ordered and gradually increase diet.	3. Fluids are often restricted to prevent fluid overload. Initially postop, only half maintenance fluids are given because child may tend to retain fluids.
		4. Administer medications as ordered.	
Increased risk of infection.	Immediate: Infectious process will be prevented, or detected early so that treatment can begin immediately. Long term: Child will be protected from infection through prophylactic measures. Child will be observed for early signs of infection.	Dx: 1. Observe for early signs of infection (redness, swelling, elevated temperature, respiratory symptoms, etc. 2. Assess parents' knowledge of subacute bacterial endocarditis (SBE) prophylaxis and ability to recognize early signs of infection. Rx: 1. Administer antibiotics as ordered whenever child has an infection, or prophylactically before surgical or dental procedures.	1–2. Infection can be detected early when caretaker is aware of signs of beginning of the infectious process. The earlier the infection is treated, the less damage is likely to occur to the heart. 1. Whenever there is a chance that bacteria may enter the bloodstream, antibiotics should be given because of the possibility of the child developing SBE.

	2. Treat any open cuts or sores as ordered. 3. Observe aseptic technique in all aspects of care, including care of catheters, chest tubes, and pacing wires. Parent Education: 1. Instruct parents regarding the need for SBE prophylaxis, good body hygiene, and avoidance of any possible sources of infection. 2. Inform parents of signs of infection, and necessity of having them treated as early as possible. 3. Give instructions to parents on how to administer antibiotics if prescribed.	2–3. The numerous catheters are potential portals of entry for bacteria. 1–3. Prevention of infection and early treatment of infections is necessary to prevent cardiac invasion by bacteria. Particularly serious are infections of intracardiac prostheses.
Potential anxiety related to separation from parents and feelings of strangeness and hurt.	Short term: Child's and parents' feelings of anxiety during hospitalization will be recognized and appropriate measures will be taken. Long term: Child will gradually return to prehospitalization behaviors and level of independent functioning as appropriate for his age. Parents will be able to cope with anxiety and can effectively care for the child.	Dx: 1. On admission to hospital, assess child's level of independence. 2. Determine if child is showing signs of regression during hospital stay. 3. Review with parents how child separates from them, and what measures they normally use or may suggest to comfort the child at time of separation. 4. Determine what parents' feelings are about their child's hospitalization in regards to having to be separated from their child, and to the treatment the child is or will be receiving. 5. Observe how child reacts to new surroundings in the hospital or to painful procedures that are carried out or both. Rx: 1. Comfort and reassure parents that child's cardiac condition is not their fault, and they need not feel guilty when they have other obligations and have to leave child.	1. Data are collected to use to evaluate effect of hospital experience. 2. Toddlers will often show regressive behavior because of their anxiety when separated from parents. 3. Similar measures can be used in the hospital if the parents tell the nurse how they comfort the child. 4. Parents often feel guilty about having to leave their child, or when the child must undergo painful treatment. 5. Unfamiliar surroundings and procedures that may cause him pain can be frightening and traumatic for a toddler because he does not understand why he is taken away from home and parents and undergoes hurtful procedures. 1. Children often sense their parents' attitudes, fears and anxieties. Helping parents to deal with their feeling will help the child.

Table continued on following page

THE HOSPITALIZED TODDLER 873

NURSING CARE PLAN FOR THE TODDLER WITH CIRCULATORY ALTERATION (Continued)

Nursing Diagnosis	Expected Outcome	Nursing Intervention	Rationale
		2. Comfort and support child when parents have to leave or when painful or frightening procedures are carried out.	2. If child feels protected his fears and anxieties will be temporary and he will be able to return to normal behavior.
		3. Provide child with familiar toys, family photos, during the absence of the parents.	3. Since a toddler cannot understand verbal assurances that his parents will return or pain will go away, providing him with familiar objects may help to ease anxiety.
		4. Allow child to express himself through play.	4. Through play the toddler can translate his feelings and act out his aggressions.
		5. Allow child to follow daily routines established at home whenever this is possible.	5. Allowing child to follow routines or rituals he is familiar with provides him with a sense of security. With routines the child feels more in control of things.
		6. Try to assign consistent personnel to care for child.	6. When a child is cared for by a staff that are familiar to him, he will experience less anxiety. He usually trusts those persons who have earned his confidence in a continued relationship.
		Parent Education:	
		1. Encourage parents to visit frequently or to room in whenever possible.	1. Parents' presence helps the toddler most in adapting to hospitalization. He feels safest when they are nearby.
		2. Explain to parents how familiar objects or comfort measures will help to ease the child's anxiety about hospitalization.	2. Incorporating familiar objects and measures used by parents into the care of the child will help him feel more secure in dealing with the strange and often frightening environment of the hospital.

Potential delayed development due to physiological limits and psychosocial limits imposed by parents.	Child will be able to function at level of development appropriate for his age within the limits imposed by his cardiac defect. Parents will be able to identify normal developmental milestones for the child, and the effect the cardiac defect has on their child's development.	Dx: 1. Determine the child's present level of development by doing DDST or other developmental screening tests. 2. Assess if cardiac defect is having any effect on child's activity tolerance. 3. Determine parents' knowledge of skills a child of toddler age should have. 4. Determine whether parents are allowing child to experience normal activities for his age, or if they are imposing unnecessary limits on his activities. Rx: 1. Provide the child with activities to stimulate the development of both motor and cognitive skills. Parent Education: 1. Provide parents with information about developmental milestones for a toddler. 2. Explain to them the need to allow age-appropriate activities and to encourage child to become independent and function with the realistic limits imposed by his cardiac defect.	1. Developmental screening tests give a good indication of whether the child is functioning at an age-appropriate level. 2. Certain cardiac defects, especially those which produce cyanosis, can cause child to become easily fatigued and unable to tolerate increased activity. This leads to delays in motor development. 3. Parents should be aware of age-appropriate skills so they can determine if their child is delayed in development. If so, they can provide necessary stimulation to encourage child's development. 4. Parents of children with heart defects tend to be overprotective, and often impose more restrictions on their child than are necessary. Restrictions can hinder the child's development. 1. Most children with heart defects have the potential to develop normally and should be given the opportunities to do so. Children will usually restrict themselves if they feel they are being overtaxed. 1-2. If parents do not allow toddler to experience age-appropriate activities, he cannot satisfy his need to explore and to develop a positive self-image. If they do everything for him, rather than encourage him to do things for himself, this is likely to discourage language development.

THE HOSPITALIZED TODDLER

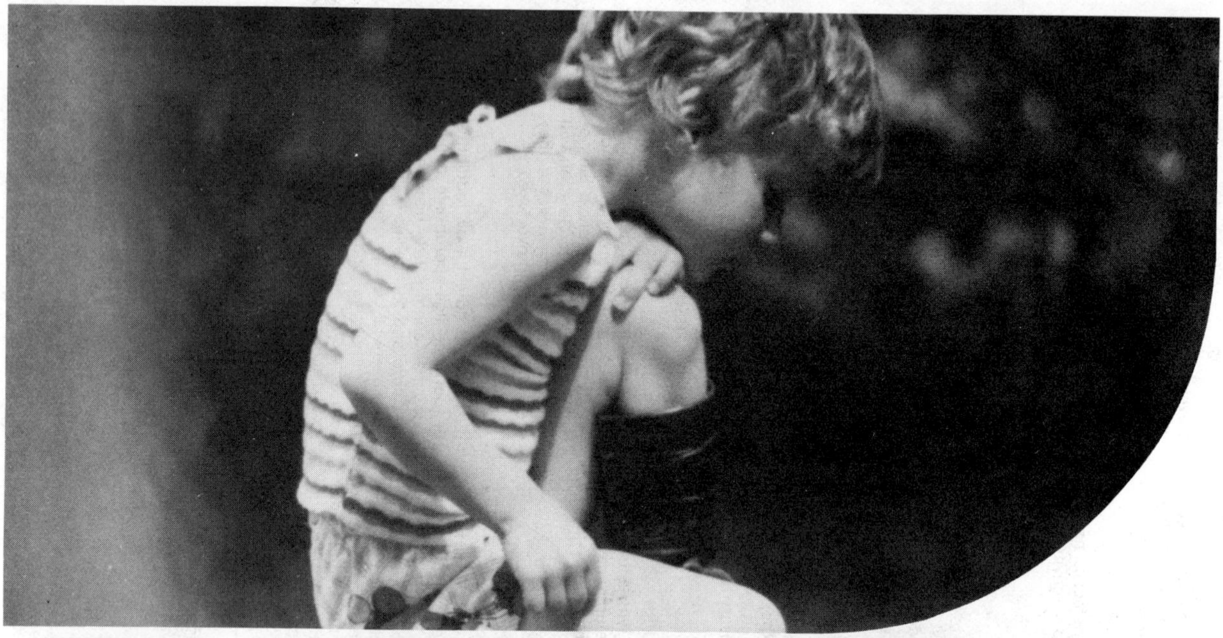

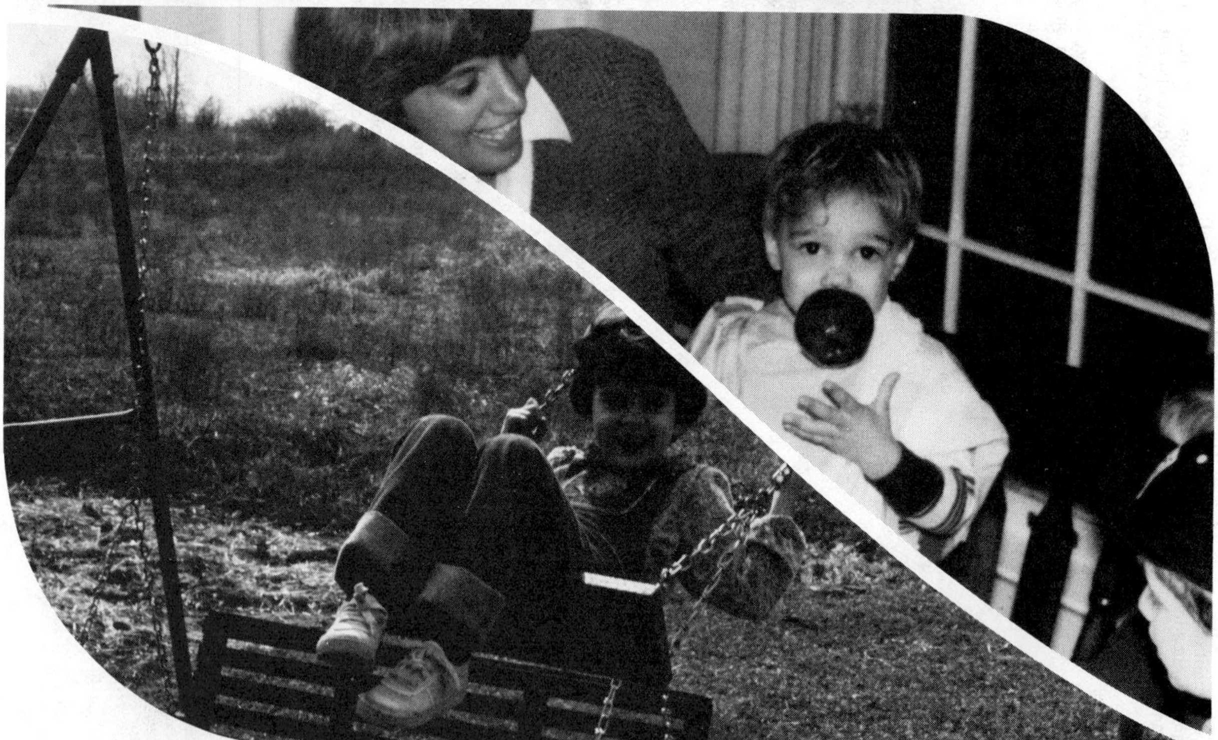

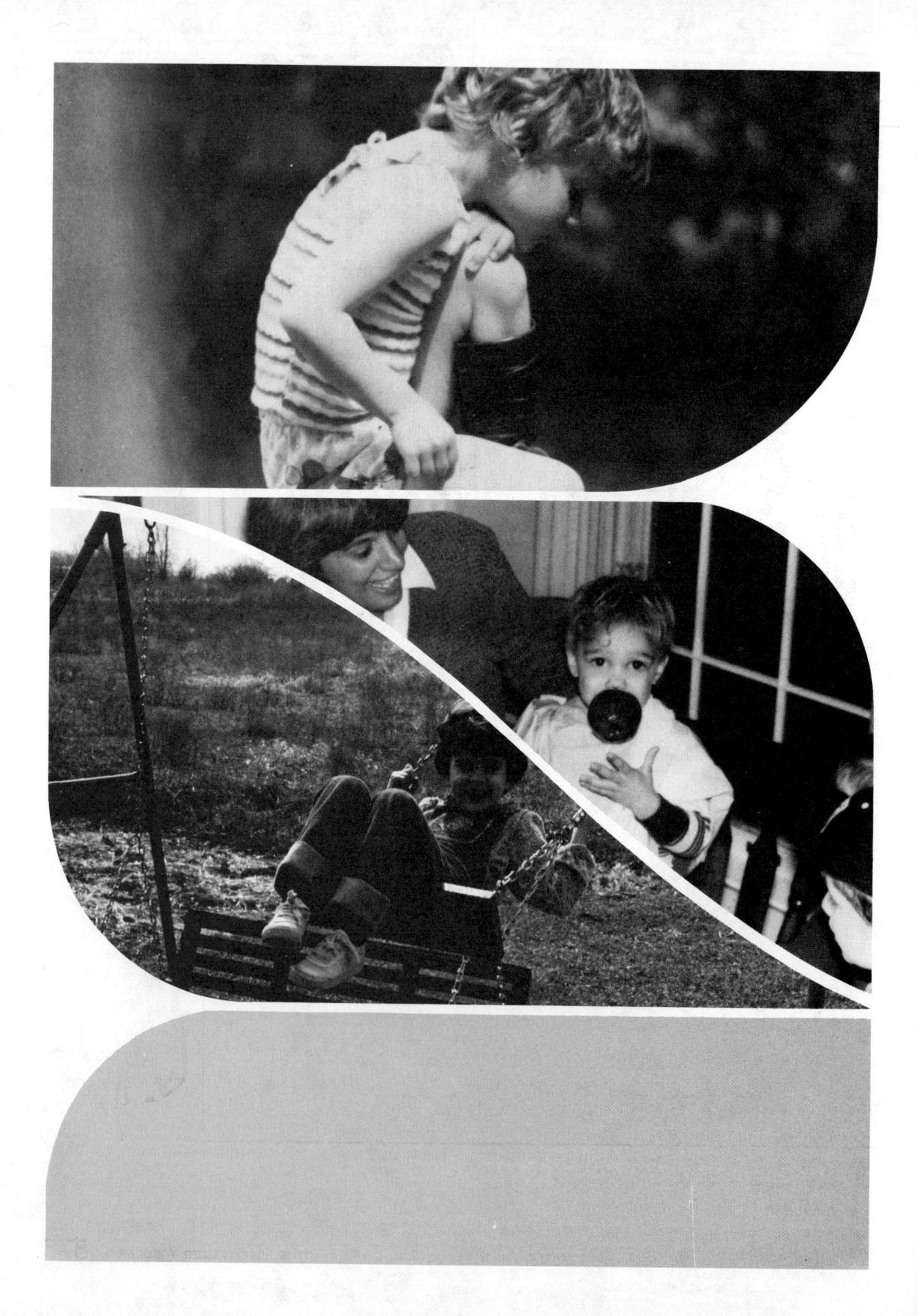

PART 6

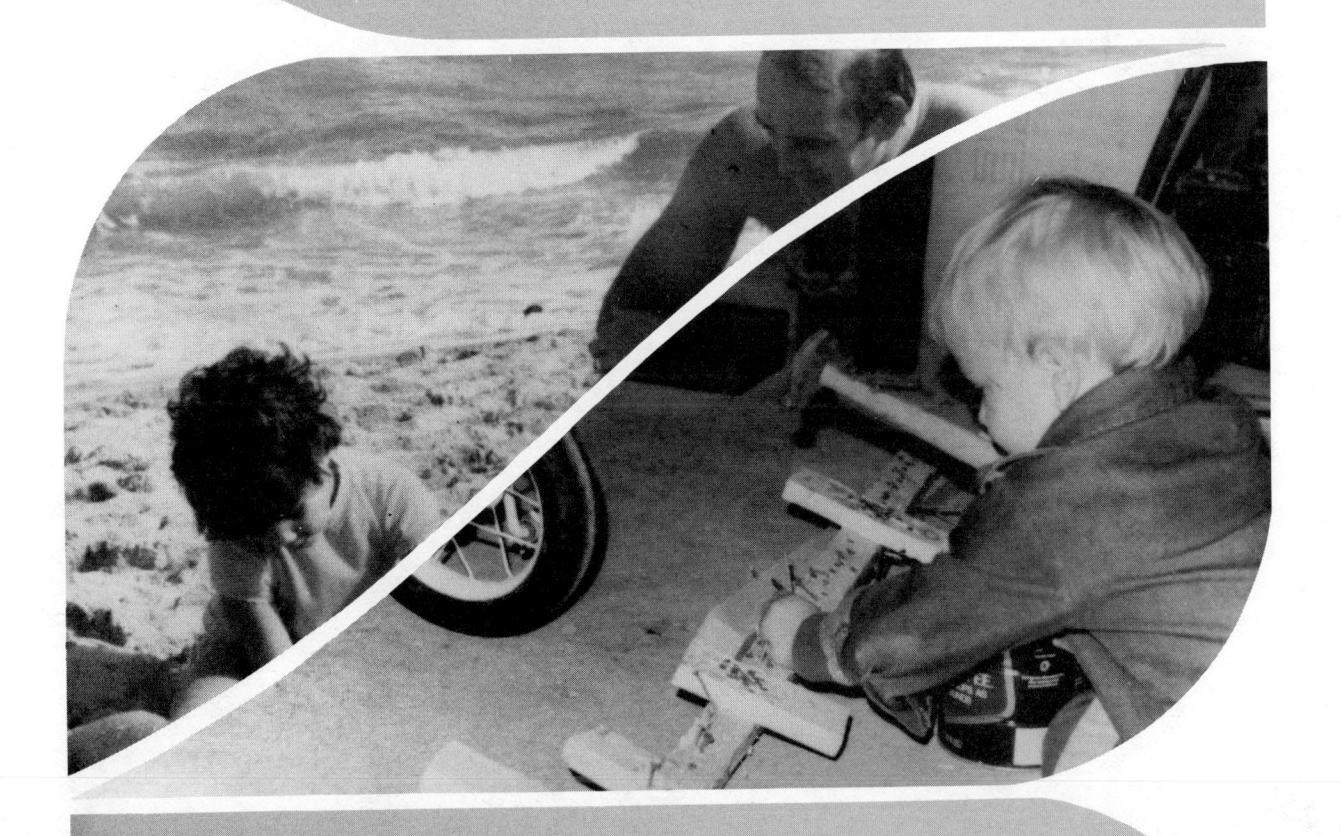

FAMILIES WITH PRESCHOOLERS

GROWTH AND DEVELOPMENT NEEDS OF THE FAMILY WITH A PRESCHOOLER: MAINTAINING WELLNESS

37

by Kathleen King, RN, MSN, PNP

The world of the preschool child is rapidly expanding both within and beyond the confines of the family unit. All family members are changing cognitively, physically, emotionally and socially, and those changes affect every family member's functioning. New relationships are forming within the family structure as parents and siblings relate to a preschool child. The nurse needs an awareness of these family interrelationships to effectively give guidance to families with a preschooler.

The family with a preschooler is confronted with the tasks of (1) allocating resources to meet the needs of a more active family; (2) maintaining satisfying communication that recognizes the preschooler's contribution; (3) establishing realistic expectations and responsibilities of family members including the preschooler and (4) cultivating relationships with relatives and the world beyond the nuclear family. These tasks are interrelated and accomplished simultaneously within the family unit. They are achieved by building upon previously established patterns of family living.

RESOURCE ALLOCATION

Preschool children, through their initiative, are becoming active members of their existing world. The dramatic increase in the use of language and affect prompts family members to respect and accept the role of the preschooler in the family. He is more individualistic, noisily demonstrating definite ideas about subjects, and expressing his needs and wants. His rapidly expanding interest in drawing, coloring, painting, cutting and pasting necessitates more supplies and space. Although it may appear that these supplies constitute a minimal strain on the family budget, when coupled with other financial requirements, they may indeed be a strain.

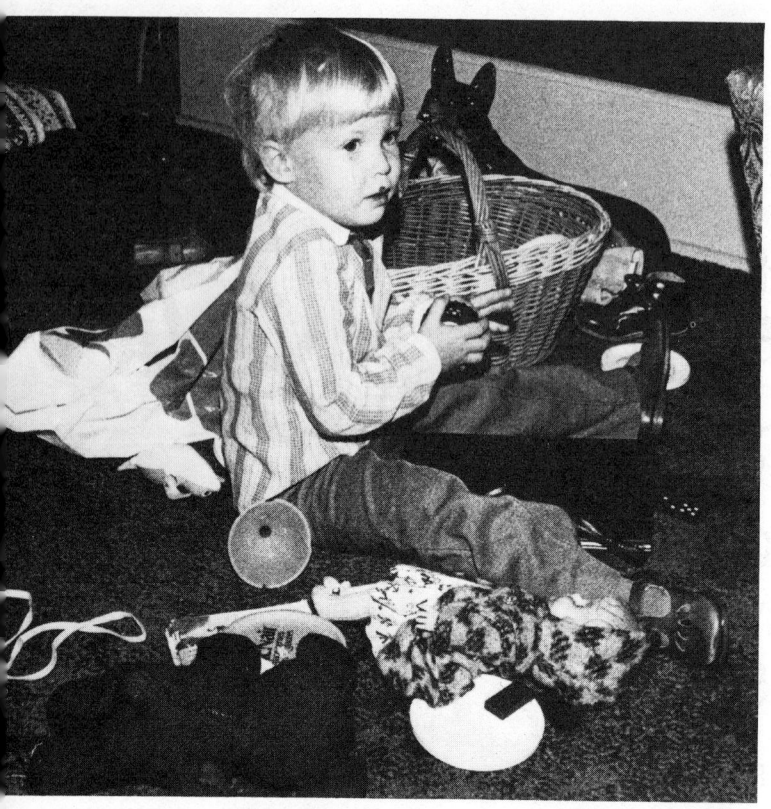

Household materials and homemade toys make imaginative play items.

The need for larger play equipment to enhance large muscle development and the need for added space to house toys, crafts and projects of the preschooler are a concern to his parents. The child needs a larger bed; additional bedrooms and a larger dining table may be needed as he grows and matures. For families on a strict budget these requirements demand reallocation of funds as well as innovative methods of using household materials to make play equipment (making paste and modeling dough; saving partially used paper for the preschooler to draw or paint on; saving safe, empty containers to utilize as building blocks or imaginative play items). Some families resolve these extra financial demands through the mother's return to work or the father's taking on an extra job.

Preschool years are active years in which accidents are not uncommon, thereby increasing financial demands on the already strained family budget. Stressing the importance of safety measures to minimize the probability of accidents is a nursing priority. Teaching these families how to determine when medical care is needed and teaching basic first aid measures to eliminate frequent emergency room visits may significantly decrease the medical costs of many families.

The preschooler comes into contact with many individuals beyond the nuclear family, being exposed to upper respiratory infections and communicable diseases. Health maintenance costs for families with a preschooler may be increased because of these frequent illnesses. Some of the expenses incurred (throat cultures, medications) may be included in insurance plans for the family. A nurse can increase the family's awareness of insurance coverage to which they are entitled.

COMMUNICATION

Parents of a preschooler may find a need to recharge their relationship after the intense years of parenting an infant and toddler. Changes are brought to the family as the child becomes increasingly independent, as he entertains himself more and plays with siblings and friends. With his increased attention span he will watch television, enjoy a sitter and read books. All this allows many parents increased leisure. This additional leisure time can be used to maintain or rebuild common interests, as well as for family activities.

Spouses should be encouraged to have private conversations that are not child related, and that stimulate and satisfy mutual intellectual needs, interests and goals. Regularly scheduled and impromptu times alone, inside or outside the home, help parents maintain themselves as individuals and as a couple, in addition to being parents. Weekend seminars, camps and classes are available to parents seeking to re-establish their own unique relationship, which may have been submerged during the years of dealing with an infant. These seminars focus on communication and dialogue to positively stimulate a couple's relationship.[3]

The preschool child's questioning can disrupt family unity and test parental patience. When a child first begins the "why" questions parents view it as a challenge to respond appropriately. However, as the "why" questions increase in frequency, often with no logical progression, parents can become frustrated with this behavior, even though the majority of parents realize the child is learning about the world through his torrent of questions. Because of the child's cognition level, he may be unable to assimilate an answer given by the parent and may require repeated explanations for the same question. This cycle of events frustrates busy, tired, overworked parents!

The preschooler's curiosity is far reaching and includes questions about sex ("Where did I come from?"), death ("Where is heaven?" "What happens to people when they die?"), and about common, everyday events. It is often the questions about sex that cause parents to be uncomfortable. Communication and attitudinal patterns within the individual family dictate how parents respond to these questions. The responses range from openness to refusal to discuss sex, or to the giving of erroneous answers to a child's probing questions.

By addressing the topic of sex-related questions and the constant "whys" with parents during well-child visits, the nurse can encourage parents to think about their responses to the inevitable questions before they occur. The nurse should encourage parents to use honest, simple, clear and open communication with their child, using correct terminology for body parts, to meet the child's immediate need. Many books are available to assist parents in formulating age-appropriate answers. The nurse should be familiar with books locally attainable and suggest use of these to parents.

Siblings will relate differently to the preschooler than they did to the toddler, and parents need to accept this relationship change as a natural, developmentally healthy event. Older siblings may now see the child who has become a preschooler as a nuisance — no longer a plaything but an individual with his own desires and needs. Verbal battles and physical aggression between siblings are not uncommon as the preschooler is increasingly capable of self-preservation. Parents need to be alert to problems of physical abuse and dominance by the older sibling so that the fragile self-concept of the preschooler is not damaged.

Jealousy between siblings may cause behavioral acting out by the preschooler or sibling. Each child needs time alone with each parent to enhance his individual identity and security as well as decrease the feelings of jealousy toward siblings or parents. Family unit play, special times for each child to discuss pertinent matters with parents or all family members, and quiet times for children to pursue individual interests may also help the family to respect each member.

The preschooler may begin to imitate the sex roles personified within the family structure. It is also during the preschool years that the child is developmentally coping with feelings of intense affection toward the parent of the opposite sex and rivalry with the parent of his own sex. This oedipal phase (oedipal or electra complex) (see discussion in Chapter 11) may cause feelings of rejection and frustration for the unsuspecting parent. Nurses can help parents understand the developmental struggle with which the child is coping, relieving undue parental stress caused by the competitive preschooler.

Parents may need some assistance in managing oedipal behaviors of their preschooler. Reinforcing with parents the need to set limits on the preschooler's affectional demands with adult sexual connotations is helpful. This, coupled with the preschooler's observations of displays of affection between his parents, aids him in resolving the feelings of the oedipal phase.

It is often during the preschool years that a couple contemplates family expansion. The nurse can facilitate the parents' discussion of having another child by helping them identify the pros and cons of this. If another child is introduced into the family's life, the preschooler will need to share his parents with a sibling — not an easy task for a child! Parents will need to reallocate their time and roles to accommodate

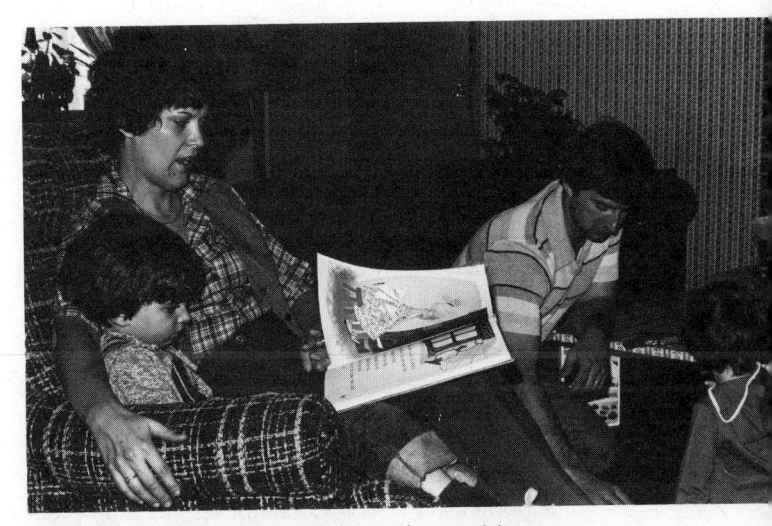

Each child needs time alone with each parent to enhance his individual identity and security. Mother and one daughter explore a picture book while father and another daughter play a quiet game.

GROWTH AND DEVELOPMENT NEEDS OF THE FAMILY WITH A PRESCHOOLER: MAINTAINING WELLNESS

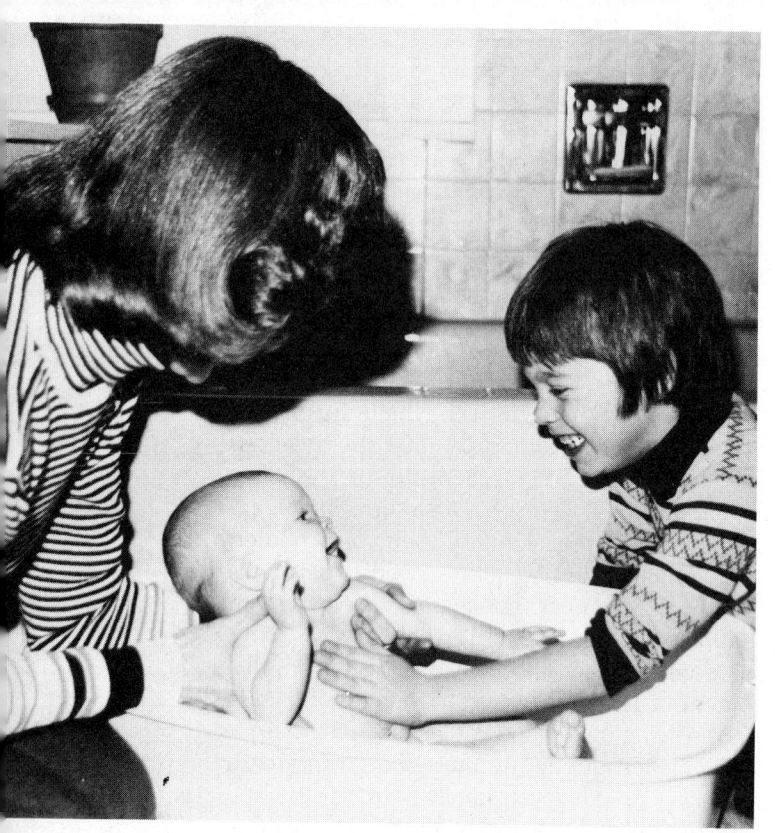

Contributing to infant care allows the preschooler to work through his feelings and adjust positively to being a sibling. (Photograph by David Trainor.)

another child without neglecting their other child(ren)'s needs. If another child is wanted, parents can ease the preschooler's adjustment to being a sibling by including him in the care of the infant, permitting him to make small decisions (selecting between two outfits for the baby to wear), and allowing him to safely act out his aggressive feelings about the infant.

REALISTIC EXPECTATIONS AND RESPONSIBILITIES OF FAMILY MEMBERS

As the preschooler develops, his increased capabilities change his behavior as well as the expectations for his behavior held by his parents, peers, siblings and relatives. The preschooler may enjoy "helping" to complete household activities such as sweeping, dusting and outside chores. Nurses should encourage parents to allow and plan for the preschooler to participate and become the active family member he or she desires or is able to be. This activity will help the child see himself as a useful family member.

Parents need an awareness of age-appropriate expectations for the child. For example, the 5-year-old child could realistically be responsible for dressing himself and tidying his room, whereas the 3-year-old may not be able to perform these tasks in their entirety. Role prescriptions may change from month to month and setbacks in behaviors are not uncommon. The use of rewards (stars pasted on a clearly designed daily worksheet or additional privileges) may be suggested to parents who have difficulty maintaining the preschooler as a contributing family member with increasing responsibilities.

Parents are also changing their role prescriptions to encompass the duties and responsibilities that correlate with expanding family needs as related to active play, crafts, reading time, formal learning activities, quiet individual times and family group activities. The constant supervision of children's activities is mentally and physically exhausting to parents. In many families with a preschooler, both parents are active in planning and supervising their child(ren)'s routine tasks. This joint parenting process allows children to see parents as a team and also frees one parent to complete household tasks, rest or pursue individual interests while the other is helping the preschooler perform activities of daily living and diversional or craft projects. Tension between spouses may accompany role changes within the family if these changes have not been anticipated or clearly delineated. Tension may be evidenced by frequent verbal or physical abuse or emotional isolation between spouses. Nurses can help parents by anticipating these possible role changes and helping parents to identify their unique response to these changes.

Parents may find themselves in a continual dilemma as their preschool child develops initiative and self-confidence. Parents do not want to stifle the initiative that both they and their preschooler enjoy, yet specific limits need to be applied to the aggressive tendencies of the preschooler. Even though the preschooler's cognition remains preoperational (lack of ability to make appropriate generalizations or to reason deductively), his cause-and-effect reasoning is advancing so that parents can utilize natural consequences of inappropriate actions as a disciplinary approach with their preschooler. The parenting approach can also consider the preschooler's developing ability to put off immediate need gratification to more fully enjoy a future event. For example, the preschooler who demands to finger paint immediately will agree to do this later when his mother explains that the child's friend is arriving later that day with paints and then he will have a better selection of equipment.

There is a change in the kind of questions preschoolers ask and in the type of information and support they need. The nurse should be familiar with available books, magazines and community-based parenting classes, as well as with techniques and theories of parenting, so that she can responsibly answer parents' questions. When working with parents a nurse needs to have sensitivity to possible individual parenting problems as well as to have the ability to give anticipatory guidance of developmental disciplinary needs. It is important that the nurse stress the individuality of each child and that proposed book methods of handling problems with the preschooler be tailored to fit the individual needs of the child.

The child's use of mass media and television is an increased responsibility for parents as, on the average, the western world's preschooler views 33 hours of television per week.[7] Preschool children are very impressionable and, with an increasing attention span are enthralled with television. Violence (physical and emotional), the sedentary nature of viewing television, noncommunication between parents and children during viewing, and the potential behavioral modeling of television characters are all factors parents should consider as the preschooler views television. The nurse can encourage parents to use television as a learning tool and only minimally as a "babysitter." Television can aid preschoolers in developing social behavior by providing competent models who relate to persons with kindness and respect. Several programs of this nature (*Mr. Rogers' Neighborhood, Sesame Street* and *Captain Kangaroo*) are available in most areas.

Parents can identify programs suitable for their preschooler's viewing by reviewing written accounts of materials to be presented before actual viewing time. Parents who watch programs with their child are in an excellent position to further the child's learning by evaluating the program as all are viewing ("Molly is really kind to Mary" or "I don't like how they treat each other").[5] Critical evaluation can help the preschooler because he has not yet separated fantasy from reality.

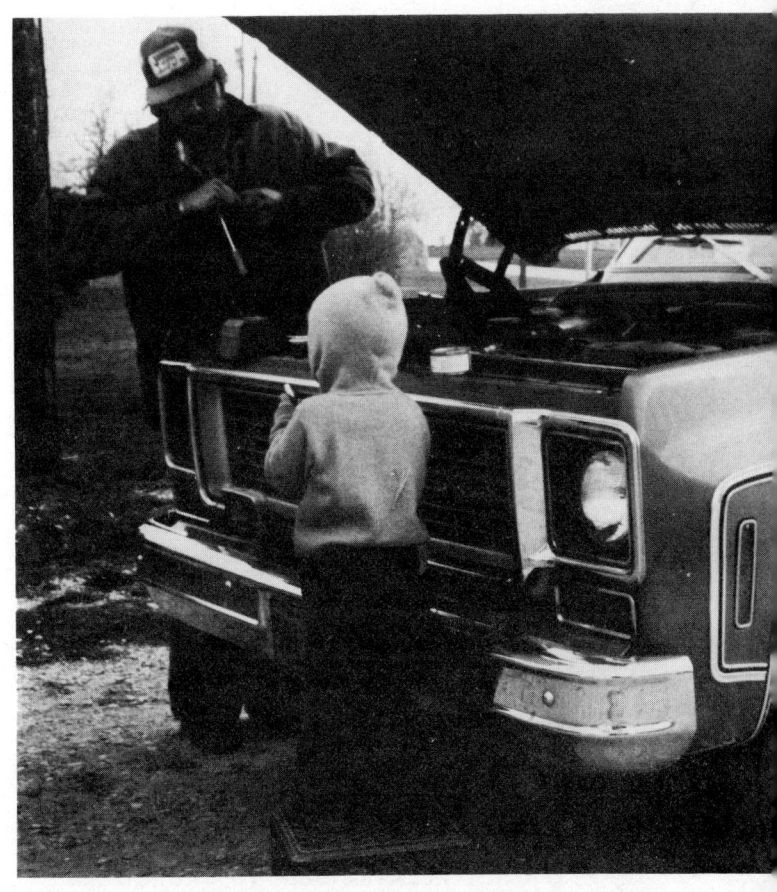

Joint parenting facilitates the need for each child to have time alone with each parent on a regular basis.

In the modern world television has, in many families, replaced valuable family group events. Unfortunately, television preempts family times of playing simple word games or card games, group games, table games, or working side by side. Such family interaction is enjoyable for the preschooler and helps advance his cognitive and social skills as well as cement family relationships.

Encouraging parents to utilize as teaching tools the many educational children's magazines (*Ranger Rick's Nature Magazine, Humpty Dumpty* or *World*) can greatly expand the preschooler's learning about the world, as well as provide an opportunity for intense interaction, learning and enjoyment among all family members through reading and discussion.

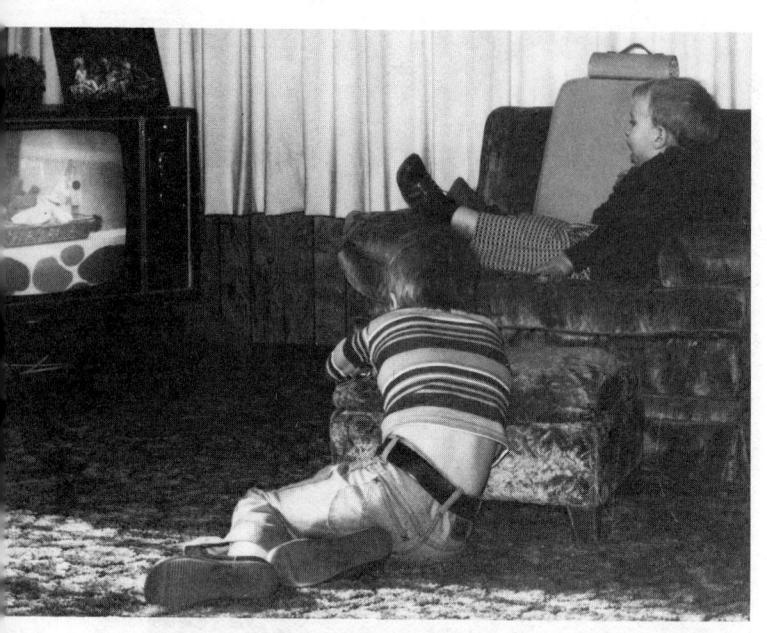

Some television programs can aid in the preschooler's development. However, it is up to parents to discriminate between good and bad programs. Television should not be used as a "baby sitter" or a substitute for human interaction and active play.

FAMILY RELATIONSHIP TO THE WORLD BEYOND THE NUCLEAR FAMILY

The nuclear family provides security and companionship as well as a safe, nonthreatening environment for the testing of the preschooler's inquisitive ideas and mannerisms. However, with increasing language and motor skills, the child is now becoming interested in his peers and other adults. Relatives of the preschool child fulfill various roles for the child, depending upon the physical distance between family and relatives. Grandparents, cousins and other relatives represent roles such as censor, educator (they show the preschooler different viewpoints on subjects), authority figure, babysitter and playmate to the child and the family.[2] By cultivating fuller relationships with relatives, the parents and the child can utilize relatives as resource persons to enhance their understanding of the family heritage and values. Also, the couple can add to their parenting skills by learning through the experience of relatives.

Cooperative play by the preschooler and his peers allows the preschooler to develop friendships and playmates beyond family members.

The community, with its increasing provision of classes for children in group play, gymnastics, crafts, religious activities and music appreciation, adds greater dimensions to the preschooler's world. Parents should begin to carefully scrutinize behaviors exhibited as a result of their preschooler's exposure to influences outside the home. Community activities also afford the entire family the opportunity to travel and attend events together (zoo, children's theatre and sports events).

Socialization with other families is changing. The preschooler can now entertain himself or play with peers for longer periods of time without direct supervision, thereby allowing parents' socializing to be more relaxed and enjoyable. In addition, parents may be more relaxed in visiting friends because the home being visited need not be as childproof as during toddlerhood. Nurses should encourage families to interact with relatives and friends, as these interactions may renew and positively influence learning for both the preschooler and his parents.

Day care arrangements or nursery schools or both are utilized by many parents as they return to the work world or seek socialization experiences for their preschooler. The nurse can facilitate day care selection by helping parents discover alternatives available in their community for the care of their child(ren). Then parents can more intelligently select the option that best meets the family's needs. Relatives and neighbors currently account for most of the informal child care arrangements in the United States.[6] However, with greater distances between nuclear and extended families, the use of grandparents or relatives as caretakers becomes increasingly difficult and other arrangements are necessary. Other day care alternatives available to the family are day care homes, day care centers and day nurseries, nursery schools, kindergarten or play schools.

Day Care Homes

The family day care home is a setting in which the child's immediate needs are attended to satisfactorily (nutrition, safety, supervised play, nap time). In this setting there are generally no activities related to long-term plans to enhance the child's individual development. Care is given for one to six children from infancy to school age. Day care homes can be of three general types: (1) several children in a care-

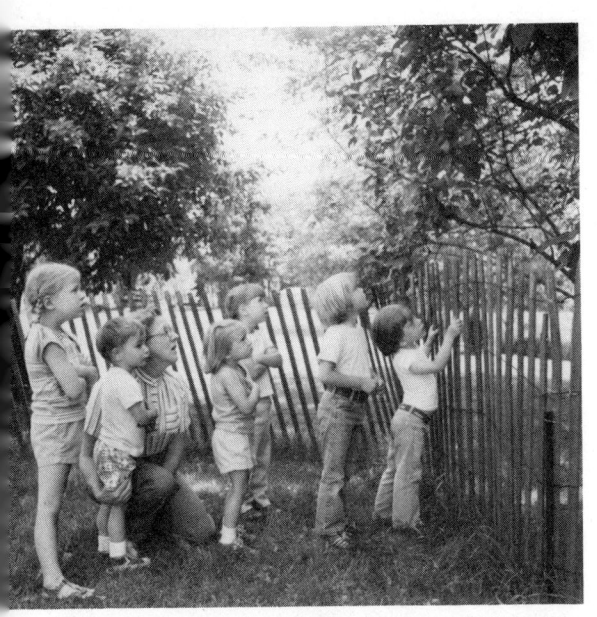

The day care center program has planned activities that are structured to stimulate the child cognitively as well as caring for physical and emotional needs. Day care homes are a popular choice of formal day care for preschoolers; these children learn about nature in the back yard.

taker's home (with or without the presence of caretaker's own children), (2) a non-family member caretaker in the family's residence and (3) a care situation in which the children (sometimes including caretaker's own children) are cared for by more than one caregiver. Day care homes are a popular choice of formal day care for preschoolers in the United States. These homes are usually located relatively close to the family's residence or to the place of employment of one parent.

Day care homes are not required to be licensed in many states. Some states do offer licensing standards for day care homes to assure safe, appropriate care. Licensing implies some of the following: proper adherence to health code for the day care residence (plumbing, heating); sufficient living space for the number of children cared for; and physical and mental stability of the caretaker. Limits are also set on the number of children a home may care for at one time. Home day care provides the opportunity for children to be in a home setting for the hours in a day they are not with their parent(s).

Day Care Center

Day care center programs are generally located in their own facility and provide daily care for children from 2 or 3 to 6 years of age. Over 50 per cent of day care centers are business enterprises, run for profit, providing mostly for physical needs of the children.[8] However, the long-term goal of the day care center includes careful attention to planning and structured environments for learning to provide for the physical, social, cognitive and emotional needs of the children who attend. The day care plan includes physical care of children, supervised play activities, rest periods, health supervision and crafts. If a parent is available during the day hours when the preschooler attends day care, the parent may be included in center activities.

The staff is generally composed of trained caretakers. Public centers administered by a unit of the state or local government and some voluntary centers administered by social agencies, settlements or churches may receive federal monies for operation. This subsidization permits parents to pay in accordance to their income level, thereby attempting to assure a worthwhile program for each child regardless of the parent's income.

Although the quality of day care varies, each state has established minimum standards for day care centers. These standards pertain to staff qualifications, physical facility requirements, code requirements, standards for child health, records and reports, nutrition, and insurance and special provisions for handicapped children.[9] Each state has its own definition of what constitutes a day care center.

Nursery School

The nursery school operates from two to five days a week for either two or two and a half hours a day as morning or afternoon sessions. Groups can be composed of children of the same age or different ages (as 3- to 5-year-olds). Various types of nursery schools exist: guided observation schools (laboratory to study growth and development, often associated with colleges and universities); cooperative nursery schools (parents are utilized as teacher-helpers, thereby decreasing tuition costs as well as including parents in their preschooler's learning world); schools with full-time teachers and no daily solicitation of parent help (private schools such as Montessori schools); child de-

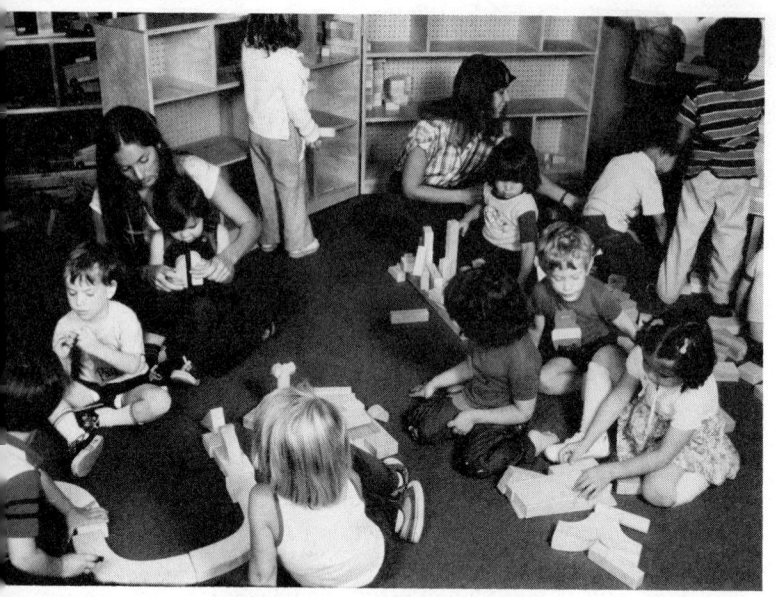

Under the supervision of skilled, competent caregivers, the preschooler has opportunities for socialization and self-expression. Note how blocks are used to develop motor skills (manipulating the blocks), social skills (working together to construct towers) and intellectual skills (identifying and matching shapes). Thus three important skills areas are practiced in what seems at first glance only to be play. (Photograph by Brian Leatart.)

velopment centers (governmental Head Start program for disadvantaged children); and schools for exceptional children.[4] Nursery schools can be nonprofit or profit enterprises, but all exist to enrich the world of the preschooler.

The nursery school will afford the preschooler socialization opportunities as well as enhance his learning about the physical environment. Free self-expression through various means allows the preschooler to develop a positive self-concept and encourages his cognitive growth. A good nursery school should afford parents the opportunity to participate in some aspect(s) of the program.[4]

Child-directed as well as teacher-directed activities are a part of the nursery school plan. Opportunities to expand language and visual acuity and develop fine and large motor coordination and to participate in school readiness activities (familiarization with numbers and letters and identification of like objects) may be a part of the curriculum. Educational models and learning objectives vary, depending upon the population served and teacher orientation.*

Play Schools

Local play schools or neighborhood play sessions are child care alternatives that many parents find helpful for occasional child care. Voluntary organizations (churches or groups of neighborhood mothers) may provide play sessions. These sessions are short-term with no planned curriculum other than babysitting, as the population served varies daily. These alternatives are used most often by the family that has a parent in the home full-time.

Kindergarten

Kindergarten for the 5-year-old is a structured learning environment available to most preschool children through local public school systems. Private facilities are available to parents who can afford the cost of a private enterprise. It is generally a half-day experience, five days a week, utilized to provide a gradual transition from home to school. Kindergarten affords an opportunity for children to develop positive attitudes toward school and to complete learning of alphabet, numbers and application of letter sounds and combinations to form words, as well as to develop abilities to think, discover, reason and concentrate on one activity for a period of time. A professional teacher is responsible for teaching the classes. Emphasis is placed upon total growth and development of the individual child as well as group experiences, thus making entrance into formal learning activities of lower elementary grades an easier transition for the child.

As the parents and child prepare for the kindergarten experience, the nurse can offer them assistance in planning and preparation. The child should know his name, father's and mother's name, address and age, and should be able to play cooperatively, dress himself, complete his own elimination and follow safety principles (can cross street safely on own). For children who have not attended nursery school or day care centers, nurses should encourage parents to have their child spend a day away

---

*An excellent discussion of various types of early childhood programs is found in The Preschool in Action, 2nd ed., M. C. Day and R. K. Parkers, eds. Allyn and Bacon, Inc., 1977.

from home occasionally to initiate the separation process imminent with school.

Day Care Evaluation

Table 37-1 identifies factors that nurses should encourage parents to identify when contemplating any type of day care for their preschooler.[4] Parents need to enumerate their exact needs as they search for a satisfactory day care alternative. For the child about to enter day care, nurses should encourage hearing and vision screening, a complete physical and developmental assessment and updated immunizations. Most centers for child care require completion of health forms and examinations prior to acceptance of the child.

Families may use a combination of day care types. Parents need encouragement to regularly evaluate child care arrangements and select alternatives if the present arrangement is detrimental to the child or family. Nursing priorities are to help parents identify the value of preparing the child in advance for day care, to help the parent and child adjust to school (separating from each other) and to help parents provide a continuity between the experiences their child encounters during day care and life at home.

TABLE 37-1 GUIDELINES FOR PARENTS SELECTING A DAY CARE FACILITY FOR THEIR PRESCHOOLER

1. Purpose(s) of the program
   Is the focus to foster development of the child?
2. Program structure
   Are there organized, continuous experiences suited to the children attending? What are the cultural expectations? Are these expectations realistic in relation to and supportive of the preschooler's developmental tasks?
3. Personnel
   Is the ratio of children to caretaker teacher realistic for the ages and needs of the children attending? Are the teachers professionally competent? Are the personnel and the facility certified? Do aides supplement the child-to-teacher ratio? What training and qualifications do they have? What is the general emotional climate?
4. Facilities
   Is the facility easily accessible to home or employment? Is the space (indoors and outdoors) adequate for the needs of active preschoolers? Are appropriate materials and equipment provided? Are the fees and manner of payment manageable?
5. Health and safety
   Are nutritious meals and snacks provided and in sufficient quantity? Are health records kept on employees and children? What are the entry requirements regarding health status? Does the facility have an established plan for ill children? Is the health status of children identified daily? Is adequate provision made for first aid and emergency care? Is there adherence to public health codes?
6. Special services
   Are special services provided for parents? For children with special needs? Are there financial adjustments to fees? What does the facility expect from the parents?

References

1. E. Duvall. Marriage and Family Development. J. B. Lippincott Co., 1977
2. E. Hurlock. Child Growth and Development. McGraw-Hill Book Co., 1978
3. W. Kephart. The Family, Society and the Individual. Houghton Mifflin Co., 1977
4. S. Leeper et al. Good Schools for Young Children. Macmillan, Inc., 1974
5. S. O'Bryant and C. Corder-Bolz. Tackling "the tube" with family teamwork. Children Today, May/June 1978, p. 21
6. R. Rapoport and R. Rapoport. Working Couples. Harper and Row, 1978
7. E. Rubenstein, G. Comstock and J. Murray, eds. Television and Social Behavior. Report to the Surgeon General's Scientific Advisory Committee on Television and Social Behavior, U.S. Department of Health, Education, and Welfare, 1972
8. M. Steinfels. Who's Minding the Children? Simon and Schuster, 1973
9. U.S. Department of Health, Education and Welfare, Office of Child Development. Abstracts of State Day Care and Licensing Requirements Part 2: Day Care Centers. U.S. Government Printing Office, 1971
10. E. Widmer. The Critical Years: Early Childhood Education at the Crossroads. International Textbook Co., 1970

Additional Recommended Reading

S. Fraiberg. Every Child's Birthright: In Defense of Mothering. Basic Books, Inc., 1977

S. Freud. (Translated by A. A. Brill) Three Contributions To The Theory of Sex. Nervous and Mental Disease Publishing Co., 1918

A. Friedman and D. Friedman. Parenting: a developmental process. Pediatric Annals, September 1977, p. 564

J. Gibson. Growing Up: A Study of Children. Addison-Wesley Publishing Co., Inc., 1978

H. Katsura and G. Millor. The difficult child in day care — a nursing challenge. The American Journal of Maternal and Child Nursing, May/June 1978, p. 166

E. Kittrell. Children and television: the electronic fix. Children Today, May/June 1978, p. 20

P. Mussen and N. Eisenberg-Berg. Roots of Caring, Sharing and Helping: The Development of Prosocial Behavior in Children. W. H. Freeman & Co., 1977

P. Payne. Day care and its impact on parenting. Nursing Clinics of North America, September 1977, p. 525

P. Pizzo. Counseling parents about day care. Pediatric Annals, September 1977, p. 593

D. Singer and J. Singer. Family television viewing habits and the spontaneous play of preschool children. American Journal of Orthopsychiatry, July 1976, p. 496

M. Sussman. The family today. Children Today, Mar/Apr 1978, p. 32

38 POTENTIAL STRESSES IN FAMILIES WITH PRESCHOOLERS

by Kathleen King, RN, MSN, PNP

Multiple sources of stress encountered by the family with a preschooler require flexible adaptive abilities of family members. Specific sources of stress include the mother's return to the work world, independence-assertion behavior, masturbation and sexual exploration by the preschooler, and incestuous behavior within the family. The family's adaptation patterns coincide with its immediate and long-term priority needs and the coping mechanisms of each individual within the family. The child who is a preschooler can be a contributing family member and facilitate the family adaptive process because of his increased ability to cooperate during certain family crises.

Dual-Career Families

In 1975, approximately 51 per cent of mothers with preschool children were employed full time outside the home.[3] The motive for working is most often *financial necessity* — money is needed to maintain or upgrade the family's standard of living. Meeting unanticipated medical expenses, inflationary costs of housing and food, and extra expenses of a preschooler (see Chapter 37), as well as family desires (music lessons, attendance at entertainment and sports events) necessitates larger incomes for families. Personal fulfillment of goals, career opportunities or a sincere enjoyment of the challenge of the work world may influence the decision for outside employment. Part-time work by one spouse to supplement full-time employment of the other spouse, full-time work by both spouses, and part-time work by both spouses are options available to dual-career families.

Many working couples find that role changes occur within the family when the mother returns to work after having been at home full time. The husband may react by covert or open expressions of resentment or jealousy of his spouse's position change in the family. The husband's resentment of his wife's earning potential or his loss of total control of the family's finances (if this has been the pattern while the mother was at home full time) may cause animosity.

Society has traditionally characterized a distinct division of labor for husband and wife — the mother is responsible for children and house duties and the father is total breadwinner. For a husband reared with this traditional concept of being breadwinner, his wife's new status may cause feelings of self-doubt. Pressure from his peers may also account for the father's ambivalence about the mother's working, thereby altering role expectations at home.

Conversely, the mother's employment outside the home may be gratefully anticipated by the father. He may be happy to be relieved of total responsibility for their financial security. The probability that he will become more intimately involved with day-to-day parenting of their preschooler and siblings, share household chores, as well as perhaps have more freedom to develop his own desires and goals apart from his work world, may add positive dimensions of joy and contentment to the spouse and family relationship. The mother's employment may necessitate increased interdependent roles within the family, as well as open up communication between spouses, cement the fathering role in childrearing and cause a greater sharing of the responsibilities for childrearing.

The mother's attitude toward working is an excellent indicator of her children's attitudes and behaviors about her return to the work world.[5] Mothers may feel guilty or resent the need to work.[5,9] These guilt feelings may be projected to their children and spouse or turned inward as evidenced by fear, anger, depression, withdrawal or low self-esteem. Through the mother's cultural and familial patterning, she may intrinsically feel that a competent mother is one who remains at home with her child(ren). This concept may be reinforced by her spouse. These conflicting feelings may initiate the use of behaviors of overcompensation (leniency in limit-setting for the preschooler), projection ("I would not need to work if my husband earned a higher salary") and rationalization ("I'd be getting away from home somehow, anyway").[9] The preschooler can usually sense these guilt feelings his mother has and may utilize the overcompensation or projection behaviors to his advantage.

Another anxiety mothers exhibit when returning to the work world is related to "letting go" of the child. While the mother is employed outside the home, she is not aware of all the happenings involving her preschooler on a moment-by-moment basis. To those mothers who feel a need to control events within their preschooler's life space, such a situation can cause stress.

In many families the woman finds she remains the primary child caretaker and housekeeper in addition to being employed outside the home.[10] Thus, the mother must cope with the stresses of inequitable division of household tasks, less time to attend to family needs, her own separation anxiety and her child's and physical and mental exhaustion from her job. Adaptation to these sources of stress (expressed or implicit) may create family tensions.

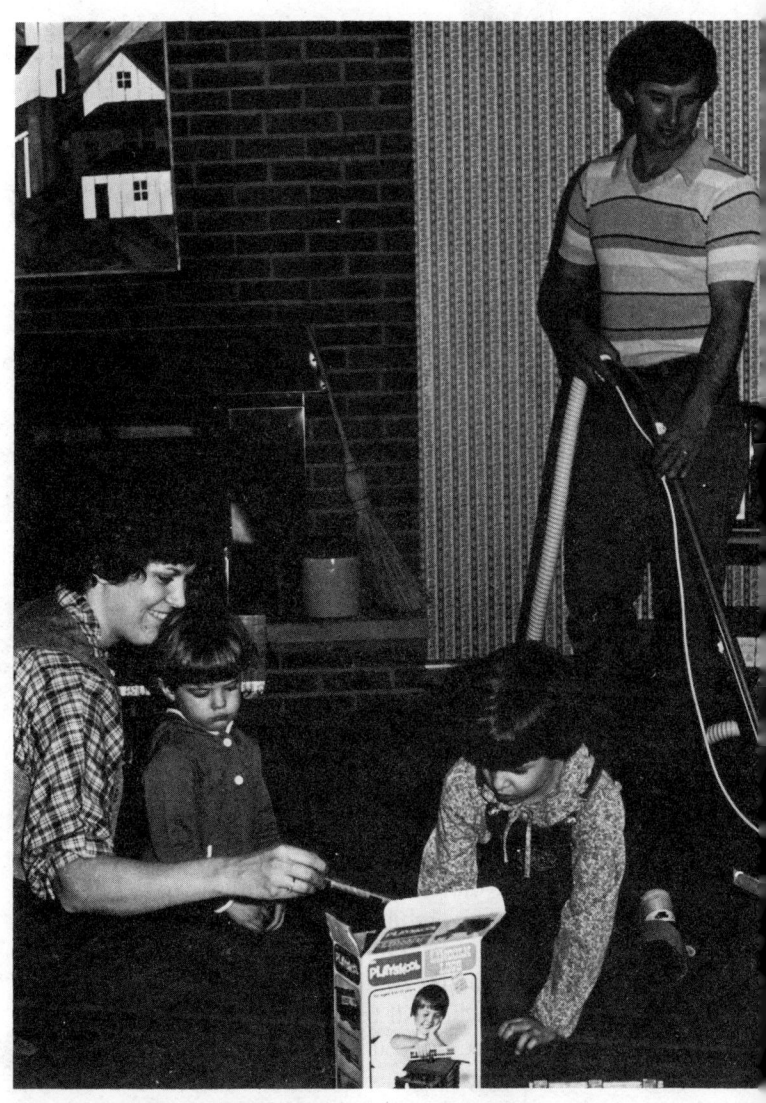

In dual-career families, shared responsibility for household chores as well as childrearing activities can add positive dimensions of joy and contentment to family relationships.

The presence of preschoolers in the family seems to contribute to lower job satisfaction for both spouses, with the mother being the most dissatisfied.[16] This dissatisfaction may occur from societal pressures for the mother to be at home, inequality in family task prescriptions or logistical problems in establishing child care. Interestingly, some mothers find it difficult to accept help for housework from their spouse or children (even though they may want and need the help) because of a need to maintain their own standards for household and child care.[10] A mother with these feelings may either attempt to complete all household tasks to maintain her standards or become frustrated with having to settle for tasks being completed by other family members and not necessarily exactly as she would prefer.

If the mother portrays a sense of pride and fulfillment in employment and discusses this fulfillment, along with any career and home anxieties, the child and family seem able to be positive and accepting of the mother's needs. Through increased self-esteem, assertiveness learning and positive reinforcement from their support systems (spouse, family, relatives, nurse) mothers are seeing themselves as complete persons in the dual roles of mother and employee.

The working mother generally delegates more responsibility, possibly giving the child a greater opportunity for creative activities. Working mothers also make a more direct effort to spend or allot time exclusively for each child, thus participating in more planned activities with their children.[2,4,5]

As the nurse works with mothers who are employed outside the home or planning to return to employment, she should explore whether attention has been given to discussion by spouses of specific role expectations to avoid implicit assumptions by one or both of them; careful planning of work schedules to allow for family times together; planning for handling of routine and nonroutine responsibilities (who will transport child to day care, what will be done if child is ill, who will deal with emergency care for children); maintaining family integrity in mornings as the mother and father prepare themselves and their child(ren) for departure; and keeping communication channels open for all family members. Dual-career families need emotional support to maintain a life style that does not yet meet with society's full approval.

The preschooler who is a member of a dual-career family can be encouraged to help his parents in tasks to accommodate daily living patterns for the family. This helps the preschooler develop skills and feelings of self-worth. It also helps to distribute family tasks. The probability of providing an equalitarian parental role model for children exists in the dual-career family, thus providing the preschooler with enriching experiences with both mother and father.[7,8]

The initial separation process for preschoolers and their working mothers can be traumatic for both of them. If the mother is confident that her decision to work is a good one, if the child is cared for in a quality day care environment, and if the mother can avoid long absences from the preschooler at times other than employment hours, the child will probably not develop undesirable long-term behaviors as a result of having a working mother.[2-4,6] If the separation process is handled in a positive, reassuring, knowledgeable manner, taking into consideration the growth and developmental level of the child, the preschooler learns that his mother will return. The nurse can help parents by teaching about the need for a gradual separation process. She can warn them to expect acting-out behaviors upon their return to get the child at the day care facility, and to reassure and express love to the preschooler during this separation process.

Masturbation

Sexual exploration is characteristic of normal growth and development of children. The preschool child discovers the pleasurable sensations accompanying self-manipulation of the genital organs. Masturbation during the preschool years is a common behavior. It is when masturbation becomes excessive or compulsive or when it is a source of anxiety to the parents because of their own level of sexual understanding or adjustment that masturbation becomes a stress in the family. Many parents' value systems include the belief that masturbation should not be allowed. When parents have concerns about their child's masturbation or when they nonverbally express anxiety (such as embarrassedly pulling away a child's hand if the child scratches himself in the genital area), the following points can be emphasized by the nurse:

1. The preschooler's body exploration is a normal growth and developmental activity.
2. Masturbation will not cause any organic disease.
3. The parents' reaction to masturbation will affect their child's feelings about his or her own body and possibly the child's future sexual adjustment.
4. As the preschooler develops more interests and activities, masturbation decreases in importance, becoming just one among many activities.

TABLE 38-1 INDICATORS OF POSSIBLE INCEST WITH PRESCHOOLERS*

Physical	Emotional-Social
1. Venereal disease	1. Extreme anxiety
2. Vaginal discharge in girls	2. Excessive fear of males
3. Urethral discharge in boys	3. Phobias; excessive fear of touch
4. Physical abuse, body mutilation	4. Expressing need to "wipe self out"
5. Difficult defecation	5. Parent reports molestation by stranger
6. Vague abdominal symptoms	6. Inappropriate sex expressions
7. Enuresis	7. Compulsive masturbation
	8. Excessive curiosity about sexual matters

*Adapted in part from workshop on Incest, conducted by N. R. Larson-Carlson, Family Sexual Abuse Treatment Program Director, University of Minnesota Medical School, Minneapolis. Sponsored by University of Michigan Continuing Education Department, November 7, 1978.

Chapter 40 discusses interventions when masturbation becomes excessive, to the exclusion of other interests and activities.

Incest

The incidence of incestuous relationships within families with preschoolers is receiving more attention as many states require reporting of sexual abuse in their child abuse statutes. Incest for families is defined according to the family's value system. For our purposes, incest will be defined as a sexual relationship between individuals too closely related to marry.[15]

Sexual exploration among siblings is characteristic of normal growth and development of children. As children's curiosity increases they test their questions by mutual looking and touching. Sexual exploration between friends at the preschool level is common, although it creates much anxiety among parents when it is discovered. By anticipating this curiosity ("If you have questions about your body or another person's body come to me and we'll find the answers to your questions"), some experimentation may be circumvented. However, children will test the accuracy of parents' answers with siblings and friends. These exploratory sessions are transient in nature and do not have lasting psychological effects on the preschooler or his sibling.[13] If parents discover sexual experimentation (suspected when preschoolers play doctor in privacy or whisper behind locked doors), limiting the behavior by redirecting activities or establishing rules about where such activity can occur is appropriate. This parental attitude does not make the child feel guilty about his curiosity, yet limits his behavior and helps him maintain a healthy attitude toward sex and his body.

Psychological damage for the preschooler involved in an incestuous relationship with a sibling may occur if the sibling is considerably older than the preschooler or if the relationship occurs over an extended period of time to the exclusion of peer socialization for the preschooler.

Incest between parent and preschooler has roots that have an emotionally significant impact upon the preschooler and the involved parent. These relationships stem from parents who have an inability to check their own impulses and are unable to discriminate their role in the parent-child relationship.[14] Patterns of general family confusion, chaotic communication, spouse misunderstandings and frustrated sexual relationship, and poorly structured family time predominate in families harboring incestuous relationships.[12, 13, 15]

Children enjoy and seek loving contact with their family members because they want to be special. The preschooler may enter into a sexual relationship with a parent to please the parent as well as feel good himself. This incestuous relationship is sincerely sought as warmth by the preschooler, but at the parental level it is a distorted search for caring and love.[12] This warmth, of course, is related to a gentle sexual relationship with a parent and is not associated with a physically mutilating child-parent relationship. Incest can occur with the preschooler in the form of sexual intercourse, oral sex, mutual masturbation or a combination of these.

Incest seems to be the least harmful psychologically for the young preschooler as compared to children in later developmental stages, as the preschooler does not yet perceive the relationship as exploitive or improper. The preschooler has not yet developed a strong conscience that has incorporated society's norms. As the child learns of society's expectations, feelings of guilt, fear and anger emerge, thereby causing individual and family stress.[13]

Table 38–1 indicates symptoms the preschooler could exhibit that should alert the nurse to suspect incest or sexual abuse of the child. The preschooler's physical and emotional health should be carefully assessed and evaluated and an immediate plan of action should be formulated for the welfare of both the child and the family. Specific behaviors (fear, disgust) exhibited by the nurse will negatively influence parents' attitudes toward seeking professional help. The nurse may express concern for the family to develop mature, stable relationships through professional guidance. Referral of the family for counselling and concomitant follow-up is a nursing priority.

The Aggressive Preschooler

Aggression in and of itself is not an undesirable behavior; it can be a positive force that helps the preschooler become an indivdual and become self-assertive. It is the overly aggressive preschooler who can be disruptive to family unity and cause parents anxiety as they try to cope with outbursts of anger. The aggressive preschooler may be inconsolable when angry, repeatedly causing discord among playmates. He may be unable to positively relate to babysitters or child care workers, and exhibit inappropriate language and physical aggression toward his parents and siblings. His aggression may cause peers and significant adults to avoid interacting with him, causing isolation from those individuals most significant to his development. Parents can become very distraught about disciplinary management of their aggressive child. Parents may react to the child by ignoring him so they will not have to deal with the behavior, may acquiesce to the child's wants and wishes to avoid further conflict, or may try to set limits and work consistently with the child.

It is important for the nurse to recognize such a situation within a family and to empathically assist parents to pursue alternate ways to meet their needs as a couple, those of their preschooler and those of the entire family. Reassurance of and discussion with parents is often a boost to their self-esteem as parents. Reminding them that any feelings the child expresses are neither good nor bad, but just feelings, may help parents realize that the overly aggressive child who freely expresses anger is not a bad child per se. He is angry and his angry feelings need to be channeled into appropriate outlets. Basically, four options are available to parents in attempting to meet the needs of this child: (1) permitting certain behaviors (fully accepting certain behaviors of the child and not trying to change them), (2) interfering with the behavior (attempting to change it), (3) tolerating some behaviors (not fully accepting the behavior, but allowing it to occur for the time being) and (4) anticipatory planning (avoiding behavior by prior planning).[11]

Certain strategies that may be helpful for the frustrated parent include: rewarding by giving approval to the child for acceptable behavior, helping the child to verbalize feelings rather than use physical aggression, showing affection (including touch), utilizing humor in discussion of the undesirable behavior or precipitating incident, setting consistent limits on behavior and following through with them and being an appropriate role model by using encouragement.[1, 11]

Such responses can help parents begin to concentrate on actions that may assist their overly aggressive child to express feelings with appropriate, socially acceptable behaviors.

References

1. L. Anderson. The aggressive child. Children Today, Jan/Feb 1978, p. 11
2. M. Bane. Here to Stay: American Families in the 20th Century. Basic Books, Inc., 1976
3. J. Curtis. Working Mothers. Simon and Schuster, 1976
4. L. Hoffman and F. Nye. Working Mothers. Jossley-Bass, 1974
5. L. Hoffman and F. Nye. The Employed Mother in America. Rand McNally and Co., 1963
6. M. Howell. Employed mothers and their families — I. Pediatrics, August 1973, p. 252
7. M. Howell. Effects of maternal employment on the child — II. Pediatrics, September 1973, p. 327
8. G. Howigan. The Effects of Working Mothers on Children. Center for the Study of Public Policy, 1973.
9. J. Lancaster. Coping mechanisms for the working mother. American Journal of Nursing. August 1975, p. 1322
10. R. Rapoport and R. Rapoport, eds. Working Couples. Harper and Row, 1978
11. F. Redl and D. Wineman. The Aggressive Child. Free Press, 1963
12. A. Rosenfield et al. Incest and sexual abuse of children. Journal of the American Academy of Child Psychiatry, Spring 1977, p. 327

13. R. Sarles. Incest. Pediatric Clinics of North America, August 1975, p. 633
14. R. Summit and J. Kryso. Sexual abuse of children: a clinical spectrum. American Journal of Orthopsychiatry, April 1978, p. 237
15. The Random House Dictionary of the English Language, rev. ed., s.v. "Incest" (1969).
16. L. Troll. Early and Middle Adulthood. Brooks-Cole Publishing Co., 1975.

Additional Recommended Reading

R. Brant and V. Tisza. The sexually misused child. American Journal of Orthopsychiatry, January 1977, p. 80

S. Colvin. A preschooler's expression of aggression in fantasy. Maternal and Child Nursing Journal, Summer 1978, p. 99

E. Duvall, Marriage and Family Development. J. B. Lippincott Co., 1977

A. Emlen and E. Watson. Matchmaking in Neighborhood Day Care. Continuing Education Publications, 1971

S. Fraiberg. The Magic Years. Charles Scribner's Sons, 1959

S. Fraiberg. Every Child's Birthright: In Defense of Mothering. Basic Books, Inc., 1977

J. Gibson. Growing Up: A Study of Children. Addison-Wesley Publishing Co., Inc., 1978

W. Homan. Child Sense. Basic Books, Inc., 1977

L. Howe, ed. The Future of the Family. Simon and Schuster, 1972

E. Hurlock. Child Growth and Development. McGraw-Hill Book Co., 1978

H. Katsura and G. Millor. The difficult child in day care — a nursing challenge. The American Journal of Maternal Child Nursing, May/June 1978, p. 166

S. Levitan and K. Alderman. Child Care and ABC's Too. The Johns Hopkins University Press, 1975

M. Steinfels. Who's Minding the Children? Simon and Schuster, 1973.

39 GROWTH AND DEVELOPMENT OF THE PRESCHOOLER: MAINTAINING WELLNESS

by Barbara Miller, RN, PNA, MA

The child from 3 to 5 years is very active, progressing rapidly in motor abilities, cognitive function and in language development. The constant practice of these abilities and skills brings amazing changes in his personality development. He becomes an individual. Some preschoolers are boisterous, outgoing, active, curious and exploring constantly, while others are quiet, shy, passive and withdrawing. One child is aggressive, while another appears totally nonaggressive. Each child develops his own "self"; some become leaders and others are content to be followers.

During this period the child develops a sense of initiative through increasing goal-directed activities, such as competition with others. The preschooler must overcome the sense of guilt that he feels for real or imagined transgressions to develop this sense of initiative. This process helps the child to develop a conscience or superego and associated standards of moral conduct. The preschooler copies or adopts his parents' moral values as he identifies with the parent. He wants to be similar to the extent that he will punish himself if he feels that he has done something his parent would not find acceptable. Another form of identification for the preschooler is sex-typing, or adoption of behavior identified with the child's sex. Much sex-typing is culturally decided, with strong parental pressure attached.

By the age of 3, the child is ready for cooperative play. He will play with others and take turns. By 4 years of age, the child will play with others for longer periods of time than he did at 3, enjoying "dressing-up" and dramatic forms of play that fit into his fantasy world. As developmental tasks are achieved, the preschooler progresses from the toddler stage of dependency to become the 5-year-old, who is independent and ready to go to school alone.

Nurses should provide information on the achievement of developmental tasks when giving guidance to parents of preschoolers. When working with the preschooler, the nurse should spend time playing with and talking specifically with the child to gain the child's cooperation and trust, especially before attempting any procedures. A preschooler is usually more cooperative than a toddler during health care and when his mother is allowed to remain close, separation anxiety is minimal.

PHYSICAL COMPETENCY

The preschooler becomes increasingly more aware of his physical competence during the years from 3 through 5. He is conscious of the skills of his peers and those of the older children he is exposed to and becomes frustrated when he is unable to accomplish the same tasks. A refinement of gross motor skills and a progressive mastery of fine motor abilities evolves during this period. Having discovered himself as a separate person by the end of his toddler years, his performance now directly affects his developing self-esteem. Assessment guidelines that characterize the preschooler's physical development are presented with emphasis on the nurse's role in helping parents stimulate their preschooler's physical competency.

Height and Weight

The preschooler's growth continues to be slow and steady as in the toddler years. On the average the preschooler grows about 2 to 3 inches a year and gains 4 to 5 pounds a year. The child's weight at 1 year of age is doubled by the end of the preschool period.

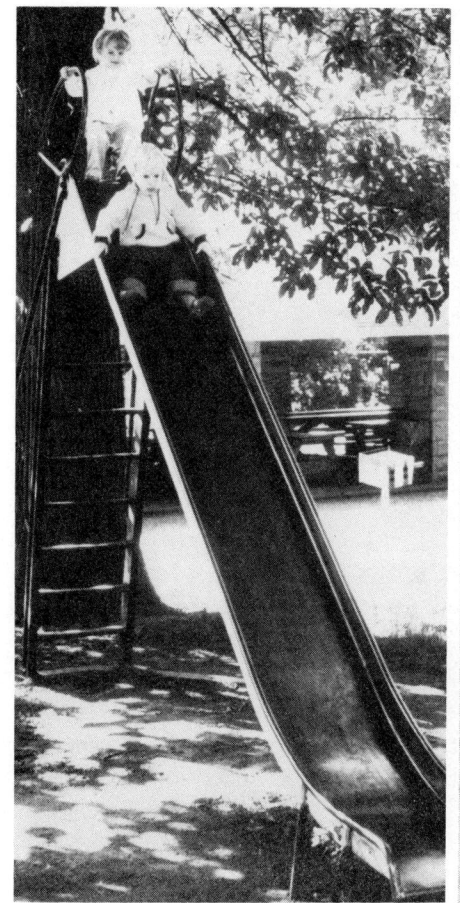

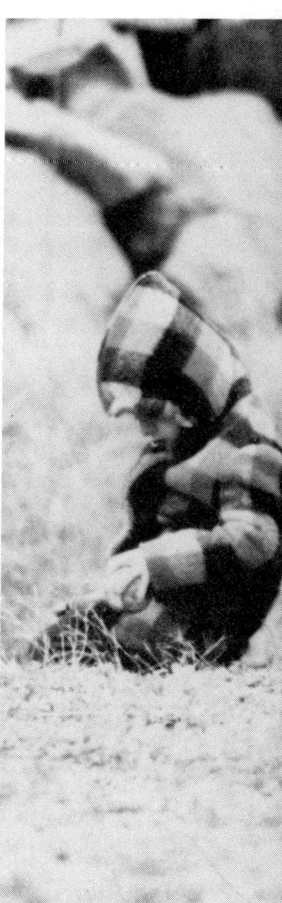

The preschooler becomes an individual. One is outgoing and active (left) while another prefers to look at the world in his own quiet way (right).

Anticipatory Guidance: Height and Weight

Once the height and weight have been taken and plotted on a graph, it is important to discuss the significance of these findings with the parent. It is easy to point out graphically to parents where their child stands, and problem areas are obvious. Many times parents do not recognize obesity unless they can see evidence of it on paper. It is important to discuss diet and activity, as well as expected weight gains in the coming year. This record will help parents to see if they are overfeeding or underfeeding their child; however it is not always the quantity of food a child eats that affects his growth but also the quality of food intake. Parents should be reassured that wide variance exists in size and stature among preschoolers.

General Appearance and Skeletal Growth

The general appearance of the preschooler is tall and thin as compared to the toddler. He looks sturdy, yet graceful and agile. The baby fat of infancy becomes muscle tissue so that his posture is erect.

At age 3, head circumference for boys ranges from 47.9 cm to 52.7 cm with the 50th percentile at 50.4 cm, while the range for girls is 46.8 cm to 52.0 cm with the 50th percentile at 49.3 cm. Head circumference is not usually measured after 3 years of age.

While observing the child standing, the distance between the medial malleoli should be noted, and if the distance is more than 2 cm with the knees touching, the condition of genu valgum (knock-knee) is present. This is a normal condition in the child from 3 to 5 years old. Also, while the child is standing, the foot should be examined for arches. Many 3-year-olds will have the appearance of flat feet due to the fat

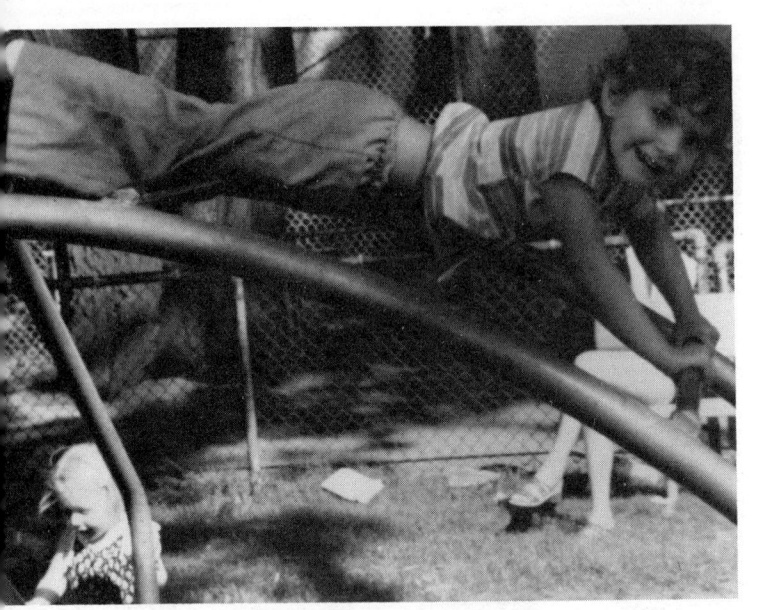

The preschooler looks sturdy, yet she is graceful and agile. (Photograph by Dan Bruggeman.)

pad that is normally present under the medial arch until the child has walked for a couple of years. Flat feet in even the 4- and 5-year-old child is not a problem unless it is causing some specific symptoms.

One of the best methods of evaluating the structure and function of the foot is to look at the child's shoe. Lateral wear on the heel and sole of the shoe indicates a well-functioning foot. Fair function is seen with even wearing of the heel and sole, and poor functioning is evident when the sole has become worn on the medial aspects.[1]

Anticipatory Guidance: General Appearance and Skeletal Growth Parents should be informed of the normal changes that will occur in their preschooler's appearance. Information and reassurance that the knock-kneed, flat-footed characteristics of their child are normal at this age can save parents the needless expense of corrective shoes. If extreme variations in these normal preschool skeletal features exist, the nurse should refer the child for further evaluation.

Parents should also be cautioned against lifting their preschooler off the ground by one hand or wrist or yanking on the child's upper extremities, usually done in an effort to hurry him or lift him over an obstacle. Such movements can cause a disorder referred to as "uncles' elbow," or "nursemaid's elbow." In this disorder the child may complain of pain in the elbow or wrist or, when the shoulder is involved, may refuse to use the arm.

Dentition

All of the primary teeth have usually erupted by the end of the toddler years and permanent teeth do not erupt before the early school-age years in most children. (See Chapter 13 for normal tooth eruption.) Toothbrushing should be a regular activity, and the child who is not drinking fluoridated water should receive an oral fluoride supplement for healthy development of the permanent teeth buds in the gums.

Preservation of the primary teeth during the preschool years is important to maintain proper spacing for the permanent teeth, to prevent decay in forming permanent tooth buds and for chewing.

Anticipatory Guidance: Dentition The first visit to the dentist should be made by 3 years of age, preferably before any dental work needs to be done. A cooperative dentist will let the child look around the office, ride up and down in the dental chair and become familiar with the instruments. After this initial visit, preschoolers should visit the dentist every six months, and at any time the parent notices any problem.

Toothbrushing, preferably after every meal but at least twice a day, should be encouraged. Because children this age enjoy imitating, it is good for them to observe adults brushing. Parents should monitor the child's toothbrushing and should assist the child in brushing at least once a day. Using dental floss to clean between the teeth is encouraged by most dentists, but usually the procedure must be completed by the parent, since a great deal of manual dexterity is required.

The practice of not seeking treatment for caries in primary teeth because "the teeth will fall out anyway" must be discouraged by nurses. Loss of a primary tooth before it is ready may cause the other primary teeth to shift over, crowding the permanent tooth when it erupts. Decay from the primary tooth can invade the permanent tooth while still in the gum.

A diet that is low in sweets and high in nutritious food should be stressed. Natural snacks should be offered, such as fresh fruit, raw

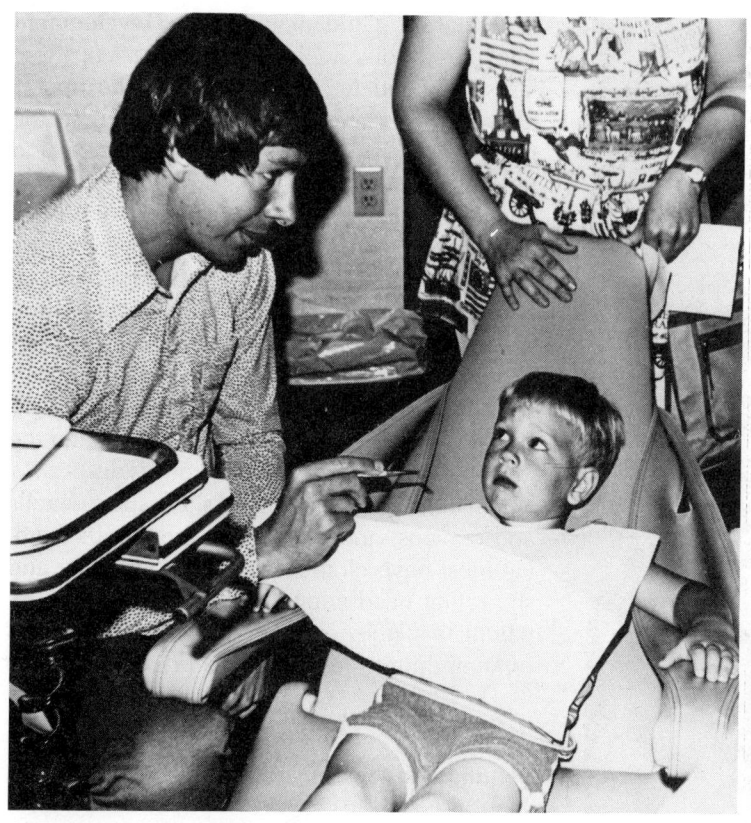

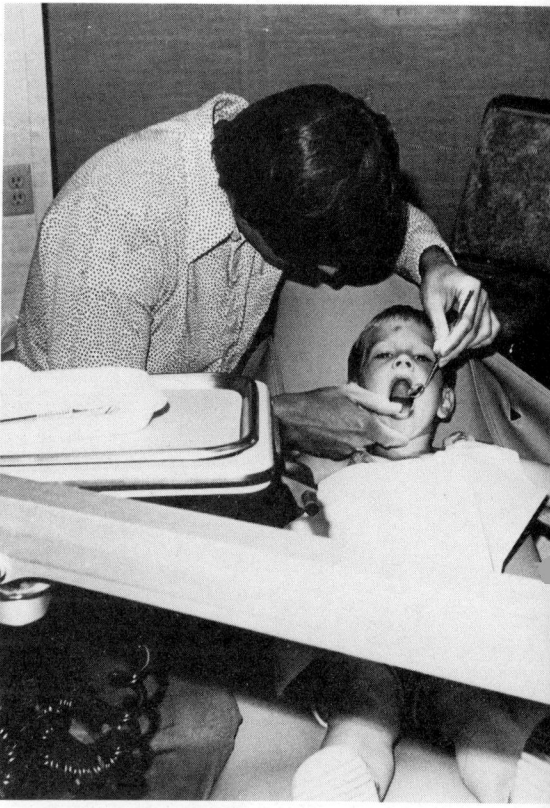

A cooperative dentist takes time to get acquainted with the preschooler and to allow him time to become familiar with the chair, the equipment and environment. Doing so usually gains the preschooler's cooperation.

vegetables, cheese and popcorn. When a child chews gum it should be sugar-free.

Motor Development

By the time a child reaches 3 years of age, his gross motor skills have reached considerable maturation due to nerve myelinization (development of an insulating myelin sheath around the nerve fibers) and the separating of nerve fibers as the central nervous system matures. Additionally, by the age of 3 the brain has grown to approximately 80 per cent of its adult size. This allows the child a greater coordination and enables him to do such things as run, go up and down stairs easily, jump up and down, jump over objects and throw a ball with some accuracy. He is able to pedal a tricycle and balance on one foot for brief periods of time. He can undress himself and, with some assistance, dress himself. He can do some simple buttoning on the front of his clothing.

By the age of 4 years, he can run easily, hop on one foot and sometimes skip clumsily. He can balance on one foot for up to 10 seconds, heel-toe walk forward, climb steps without holding on to a rail, and his movements are more graceful and rhythmic. He sits well balanced even while reaching forward and twisting and he is able to touch his nose with his finger when asked. He can generally dress without supervision, buttons well and can tell the front from the back of his clothes.

By the age of 5 years, the preschooler has developed the skill to run well, with speed and agility to play games with others. His coordination increases as his brain has increased to nearly 90 per cent of its adult size. He can balance on his toes and begin to dance with rhythm, roller skate, hop and skip, jump rope and climb on a jungle gym. He can dress without supervision and tie his own shoelaces.

In developing finer movements involving the use of the hands and fingers, the preschooler acquires increasingly more complicated skills. Mastery of these fine motor skills requires perceptual maturation as evidenced by progression in the development of eye-hand coordination.

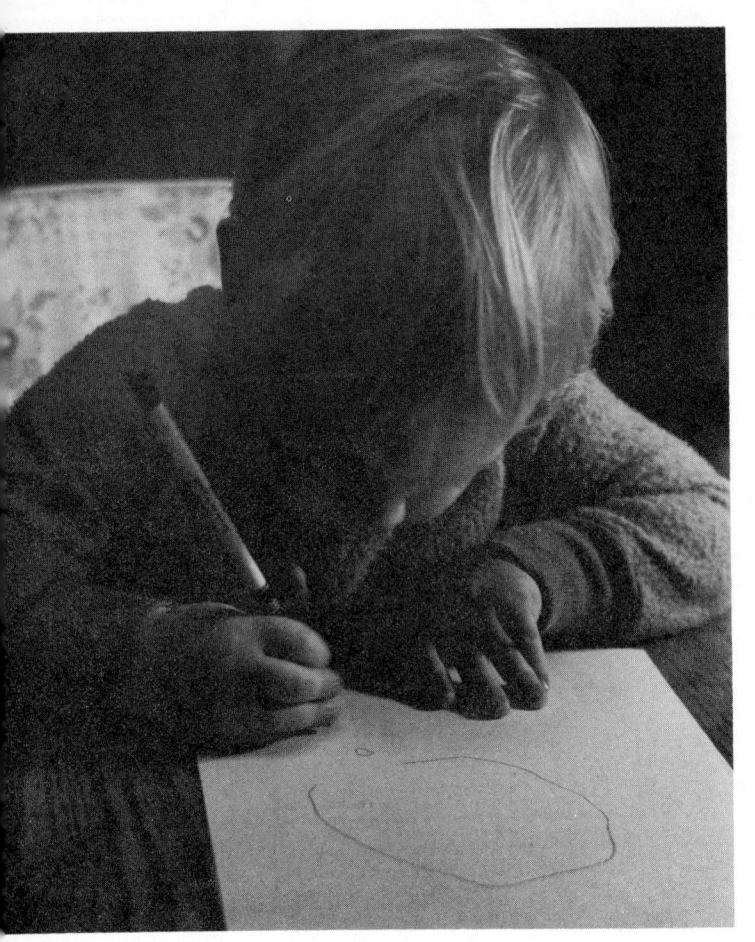

Practice produces progressive refinement of the preschooler's fine motor skills.

The 3-year-old is able to put large beads on a string, to copy a circle, to stack eight blocks on top of each other, to draw a vertical line beside another vertical line, and to cut with scissors.

By the age of 4, the child is able to cut out pictures. He can copy a cross and can imitate a square if it is demonstrated. He can draw a man with three parts and can build a bridge with blocks.

By 5 years of age, a child can draw a square without assistance; he can draw a six-part man and other recognizable objects and can hit a nail with a hammer. Again, the preschooler will not learn these skills if he has no opportunity to practice and receives no encouragement. The development of skills is not necessarily a function of chronological age, but a progressive refinement of previously learned skills.

Anticipatory Guidance: Motor Development

The preschooler will learn to do all of these tasks provided he has been given the opportunity. Nurses should explore with parents the need for the child to have some freedom and independence as he learns from his curiosity and exploration. However, safety is of utmost importance, since accidents constitute the most common cause of death in the preschooler. Safety rules must be clear-cut, consistent and simply explained to the preschooler. The child should be given praise as a reinforcement for safe behavior. Frequent punishment and constant threats will eventually be ignored, and the child becomes resentful and rebellious.

The child must have access to paper, pencils and crayons, and be encouraged to use them. He must have clothes that need buttoning and shoes that need tying to learn those skills. The parent that does everything for his child does not help him to learn and mature.

Hearing and Vision

Sensory function is highly developed by the time a child becomes a preschooler. Since a child at this age who has a visual problem is unaware of it and because amblyopia (lazy eye) becomes an irreversible condition usually by the age of 6, preschool vision screening is essential.

Vision screening is done for the preschool child with the use of the E chart, which is similar to the standard Snellen chart, with the exception that E's are used to replace the alphabet. Most preschoolers have 20/30 vision, which means that they are slightly myopic or nearsighted. This is normal until around age 8, when the vision is 20/20.

Preschool hearing testing should be done at the same time that preschool vision testing is done. Because the development of speech is dependent on the child's ability to hear, the nonhearing child is generally diagnosed before the preschool period. Occasionally a child of this age who has been treated for retardation will be found to have severe hearing loss.

Testing should be done with an audiometer, which tests pure tones in each ear separately. This is a fairly expensive piece of equipment, so it will not be found in most physician's offices. Most school systems have at least one audiometer for testing, and these can usually be used for preschool screening. On other occasions when preschool children are seen, hearing can be evaluated by a whisper. This is a very rudimentary method and is even less accurate with the young preschooler.

Other methods of hearing screening, the Weber and Rinne tests, are done with a tuning fork.

There are two types of hearing loss seen in children. One is *conduction loss,* in which there is an interference with the transmission of sound. The most common cause of conduction loss is frequent or untreated ear infections (otitis media). Temporary conduction loss occurs with upper respiratory infections. Both upper respiratory infections and otitis media are very common problems in the preschool child. The other type of hearing loss is *perceptive loss,* in which there is damage to the eighth cranial nerve. This is sometimes called nerve deafness. It is seen in children who have had serious illnesses such as meningitis; in previous years it occurred with the more commonly seen contagious diseases such as measles and mumps. Some drugs, called ototoxic drugs, are capable of causing perceptive deafness. It has been suggested that the noises from incubators and intensive newborn nurseries may contribute to perceptive deafness.

An otoscopic examination is an important part of each health appraisal during the preschool years. Preschoolers are particularly prone to upper respiratory infections and secondary ear infections. After a few ear infections the child's tympanic membrane may become stretched or perforated so that he no longer expresses discomfort when infections do occur; therefore the condition of the internal ear should be monitored regularly. Also, the preschooler's ear canal has now taken a more adult slant so that the ear is now pulled up and back during otoscopic evaluation (see illustration in Chapter 13). It is important that the child does not move during the otoscopic examination, but most preschoolers do not have to be restrained. One method that works well with this age child is to have the child cover the opposite ear with his palm, "so that the light does not shine through." He becomes so engrossed in "keeping the light in" that he will not move.

Anticipatory Guidance: Vision and Hearing Although the Snellen E test for visual acuity can identify many visual problems while they are still treatable, parents should be informed that this test in no way replaces an ophthalmologic examination. This examination should be conducted at each health appraisal or whenever the parents notice any behaviors in their preschooler that suggest visual problems (frequent eye rubbing or squinting).

There are organized preschool vision screening programs that parents should be encouraged to utilize. These programs, however, do not reach anywhere near all the children in this age group who need to be screened. Nurses can help to make these programs available in areas where they do not exist, and to make parents aware of those programs that do exist. Home test kits are also available to parents, especially those who live in areas where this screening does not exist, to do the vision screening at home. These kits can be obtained from the National Society for the Prevention of Blindness.*

It is important that eye safety be taught to preschoolers and their parents. Most eye injuries are preventable and they can cause blindness. Usually they are caused when children throw small objects at their siblings or friends. Children should be taught to use silverware for eating, not as weapons, and preschoolers should never play with knives, darts or sticks. At this age they should be well supervised during play activities. Toys should be inspected and those with small parts that are removable and can become dangerous weapons should not be allowed.

Parents should be instructed to promptly report any behaviors suggestive of hearing loss in their preschooler, such as playing alone despite the availability of peers for cooperative play, delays in speech development, or lack of response to repeated requests made in normal voice tones.

Bowel and Bladder Control

The preschooler will have bowel control and daytime bladder control, as these skills are usually learned during the toddler period. Some young preschoolers may have accidents if they become absorbed in play and need to be reminded to take time to go to the bathroom. Nighttime bladder control is usually accom-

---

*National Society for the Prevention of Blindness, Inc., 16 East 40th Street, New York, NY 10000.

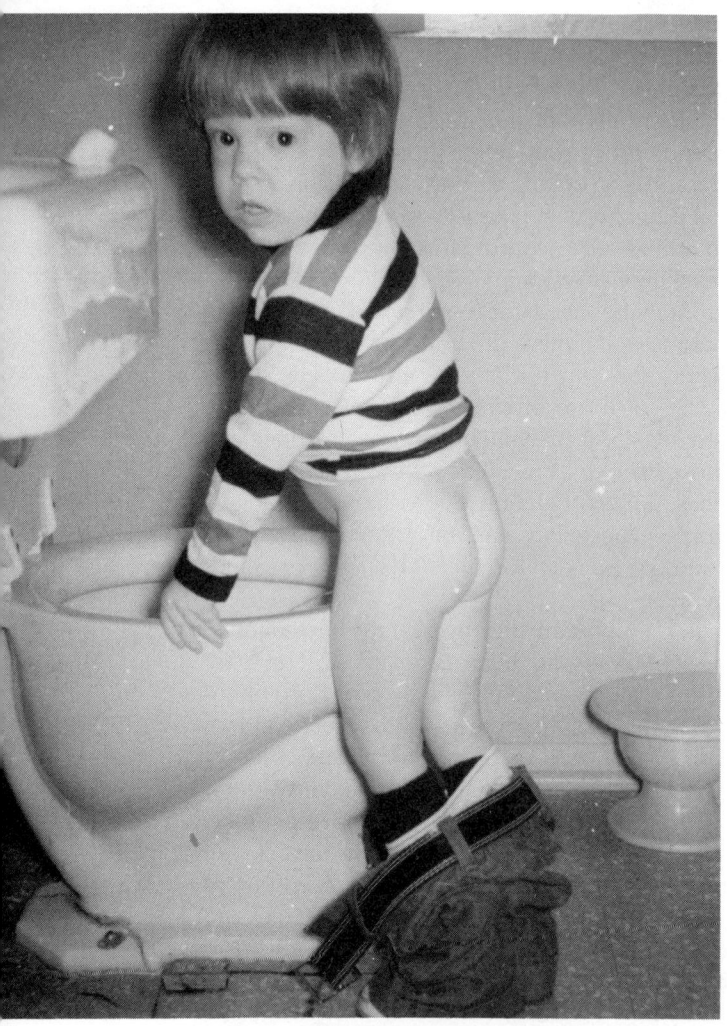

By 4 years of age the preschooler may be independent in using the toilet. (Photograph by David Trainor.)

plished between 3 and 4 years of age. By 4 years of age the child can usually manage his own clothing at elimination, and by 5 is completely responsible for the entire process.

The average urinary output in a 24-hour period for the preschooler is 500 to 780 ml. The 5-year-old voids about four to six times a day while awake, and generally sleeps through the night without getting up to void.

Anticipatory Guidance: Bowel and Bladder Control The nurse should help parents to understand that occasional bowel or bladder accidents or both are to be expected during the preschool years and that punishment will not alter this fact. The child is old enough to take responsibility for cleaning himself up and changing his clothing at such times with only minimal parental assistance. The preschooler should be reassured that his parent understands it was an accident.

The preschooler's ability to manage his own toilet activities should be permitted and reinforced by his parent(s). If the child requests privacy during these activities his request should be granted. However, the parent(s) should be nearby so that, if the child needs assistance, the parent is immediately aware of it and can come to the child's aid. Periodic reminders and checks on the child's use of hygienic measures during elimination, especially the girl's use of front-to-back wiping, is appropriate during the preschool period.

Nutritional Requirements

Nutrition for the preschool child includes the same basic four groups of food needed by adults. The child's growth remains stable through the preschool years. The child's curiosity about what is going on around him persists, so he may have little interest in eating.

Calories from proteins and carbohydrates are essential for muscle growth in the preschooler. The child in the 3- to 5-year-old range requires from 90 to 100 Kcal/kg of body weight per day. Water, an essential element for life, comprises approximately 70 per cent of the child's body weight. The principal source of water in the diet is fluids, although many fruits and vegetables that children eat contain up to 90 per cent water. The average daily requirement of water for the child of 3 to 5 is 100 to 125 ml per kg (1½ to 2 oz per pound) of body weight. Protein requirements for the preschool age child are 2 to 3 gm per kg (0.9 to 1.35 gm per pound) of body weight. The minimal fat requirement for children is unknown; however, it is felt that at least 35 per cent of the total caloric intake for preschoolers should be in the form of fats. See Appendix 5 for vitamin and mineral requirements during the preschool years.

INTELLECTUAL COMPETENCY

Intelligence

Generally intelligence is measured by a test to determine IQ. The most common test of intelligence in the United States is the Stanford-Binet, which in reality measures what the child has already learned. This test includes a variety of verbal and performance items. For example, at the 4-year-old level of the Stanford-Binet, the child is asked to name pictures that illustrate a variety of common objects, to name objects from memory, to discriminate between such forms as circles, squares and triangles, and to define such words as bat and ball. In addition, the test on this level includes repeating a ten-word sentence and counting four objects. The test is scored in terms of mental age, as a ratio of mental age over chronological age multiplied by 100. For example, a child who is 4 years and no months old who scores a mental age of 4 years and no months would have an IQ of 100.

Another common intelligence test used with preschool age children is the Wechsler Preschool-Primary Scale of Intelligence (WPPSI), which has a verbal scale and a performance scale. There are subtests within each scale and each subtest is scored in terms of the mean for the age group. The IQ is derived from the total scores on all subtests. There is a high correlation between IQs derived from the Stanford-Binet and from the WPPSI, even though there are differences in the test items given and the methods of computation.

Generally the 3-year-old child has an attention span of 10 to 15 minutes and has a beginning comprehension of the past and the future, but is primarily concerned with today. He knows his own age and can understand simple directions. He is an imaginative child, can organize his thoughts and can be bargained with.

By the age of 4, the child's attention span has increased to 20 minutes, and he has developed a concept of time. He knows what day of the week it is, how old he is, when his next birthday is, and that birthdays and holidays are particular time units and are related to parties. He can count to five and understands the concepts of one, two, etc.

The child at 5 has become less imaginative than at 4, and is interested in detail and the definition of words. He can be reasoned with logically, has become more practical and sensible and has some understanding of money. He is beginning to understand the meaning of being related to another person. His attention span is now 30 minutes, his memory is good, and he has a good sense of time, including months, years and weeks. In addition, the child should be able to solve some small problems without assistance, to start and complete activities of interest and to play without continuous supervision.

Anticipatory Guidance: Intelligence Developing the skills that are evidence of intelligence is essential to the child's enjoyment and learning in the school environment. Parents should be encouraged to help their child achieve these skills by exposing him to the concepts of time, money and memory tasks. Much of that exposure can be achieved merely by encouraging and assisting the preschooler to become independent. He should be allowed to participate in his self-care, and he should have some items that are his alone.

Language Development

"Where does the sun go at night? Why can't I go outdoors? Where did baby Susie come from? Why is it wrong? Why can't I see grandma? Why? What? Where? When? How?" This is the language of the preschooler. This is his method to learn, to get information and to gain attention, and for social experience and understanding. Response from others to these questions is essential for the child to relate to others and to problem solve. Without response, the preschooler will attempt to find refuge in a fantasy world and neglect the verbal communication that is necessary for the period of growth from infancy to school age.

At 3 years of age the child has a vocabulary of about 900 words, and is using plurals. He uses language more fluently than previously, and

The preschooler needs answers to his questions. (Photograph by Dave Trainor.)

TABLE 39-1 APPROXIMATE AGES FOR THE MASTERY OF VOWELS AND CONSONANTS

Age in Years	Sounds Usually Mastered
3–4	Most vowel sounds and p, b, m, h, w.
4–5	K, g, f, d, m, (ng) as in sing, (ya) as in yellow.
5–6	F, v, sh, l, th, s, z, r, ch, (jah) as in jar.

sings simple songs. He can make up a phrase and repeat it, not seeming to care whether anyone is listening. He talks to himself or to imaginary playmates.

By 4 years his vocabulary has increased to 1500 words, and the preschooler understands prepositions. He uses "I," talks in sentences, asks many questions and wants detailed explanations. He exaggerates, tattles and tells family problems outside the home. He is starting to know one or more colors if he has been exposed to them.

By 5 the preschooler has a vocabulary of 2100 words and uses language correctly with meaningful sentences. He talks constantly, asks questions (about the meaning of words and how things work), and can tell a story accurately, sometimes adding a little fantasy to make it "better." He can sing fairly well, count to 10 and knows some colors, again depending on exposure.

During the preschool years the child gradually masters vowel and consonant sounds. Table 39–1 shows ages at which the various sounds are usually mastered. Nonfluency typifies the preschooler's language. Probably because of his incomplete mastery of sounds, his speech lacks the smoothness and rhythm of fluent speech. Egocentric speech typical of the toddler and early preschooler yields more to social speech by the end of the preschool stage as the child learns how to both listen and initiate conversation, is able to both ask and answer questions and to offer as well as understand commands, requests or threats.

Anticipatory Guidance: Language Development The nurse is often approached by parents about the speech of their preschooler. Parents get particularly concerned when their child mispronounces sounds or hesitates in his speech. Parents should be encouraged not to expect or demand perfection in their preschooler's speech. The child should not be criticized or forced to repeat correctly mispronounced sounds or words, as such measures only serve to create speech disturbances when none originally existed. What parents can do to help their preschooler master correct pronunciation is to model the proper pronunciation of sounds in their own speech, giving special clarity to the particular sounds that the preschooler is learning at the time (see Table 39–1). Bringing to the child's attention the sounds that are present in his environment (engines running, wind blowing) and talking with him about what makes the sounds helps him learn to listen to sound and to understand what he hears.

Self-talk (talking about what you are doing) and parallel talk (talking about what the child is doing) gives the child words to think with and to describe all sorts of activities and feelings. *Sesame Street*, *Romper Room* and *Captain Kangaroo* are television programs that use the technique of self-talk. Encouraging parents to watch these with their children may help them expand their communication skills with their preschoolers.

The nurse, parents and others who interact with the preschooler should listen to the child's contributions to conversation even if he cannot be understood. This makes him feel that what is said and how it is said is important, thereby encouraging his language development.

Obscene or curse words should be ignored. The more attention that is given to this type of language, the more it is reinforced.

In addition to adults' responding to the child's attempts at communication, language is developed from their reading to the child and making reading materials available. Stories should be simple at first and colorfully illustrated to interest the child. Content should fit into the child's world of fantasy and reality, such as animals that talk as well as inanimate objects that act like humans.

Cognitive Development

The preschooler falls into Piaget's stage of preoperational thought. During this stage, the child will treat objects as symbolic of things other than what they are. For example, a block of wood becomes a car and the child will move it around like a car, making a noise as it travels. In addition, this child cannot accept another's point of view; he cannot imagine that the way he sees something might not be the way another might see it. Piaget calls this egocentrism. A preschooler feels that his experiences are universal, and the world revolves around him. This becomes obvious in his speech, in which everything is centered on himself.

The preschooler has not yet learned that a certain quantity remains constant in spite of transformation of shape. If you give this child two sets of five identical coins and count for or with him the number of coins in each set, so that he knows there are five in each, then lay them out in two rows, spreading one row out farther so that it is longer, the preschooler will tell you that there are more coins in the longer row than in the shorter row. The same thing will be observed when pouring a specific amount of water from a short fat glass into a tall thin glass; the child will tell you that there is more water in the tall thin glass because it appears higher.

Another aspect of the preoperational stage is the inability of the child to classify or sort objects in any order. For example, if the child is given a group of small toys consisting of people, animals and houses and he is asked to give you all the toys that are like the horse, he might give you all of the animals, a person and a house. He seems not to understand the difference.

Of particular importance for nurses to remember is the *centering characteristic*; that is, the centering of attention on one feature and blocking out all others. For example, when the preschooler comes to the doctor for an immunization, all he knows is the pain of the shot; he cannot comprehend the advantage for him or the need.

The preschooler is unable to comprehend that moving objects are not all alive (animism and realism); thus large pieces of equipment used in the hospital, such as the x-ray machine, EKG machine, or oxygen or mist tents are viewed as frightening and capable of attack. Health care personnel can help a preschooler understand what is going to happen to him, and what it means. Many hospitals have tours, either for children going in for surgery or for area children such as preschoolers, to acquaint them with the hospital, and some of its equipment.

Anticipatory Guidance: Cognitive Development Much of the preschooler's mastery of cognitive tasks arises from his own discoveries during play investigation. Parents can help their child learn to classify objects through verbalization of object groups that are present in the child's activities of daily living. For example, while selecting the shirt the preschooler is going to wear, the parent might say, "These are all shirts. Which do you want to wear: the blue shirt that buttons, the red shirt that zips, the green shirt that goes over your head or the brown shirt that snaps?"

Parents may need assistance to associate the fears of their preschooler as a natural developmental phenomenon created by the animism and realism that is a part of his cognitive processes at this time. When parents can anticipate that objects or experiences may create fear in their preschooler because of these cognitive processes, they can prepare their child through books about the object or experience, by gradually exposing the child to the situation through pretend play opportunities and by being present and supportive during the experience.

EMOTIONAL-SOCIAL COMPETENCY

As the preschooler's environment broadens and his interests expand, he becomes more of a social being. At 3 years of age he is friendly but still self-centered; by 4 he is not as pleasant and has become noisy; at 5 he is becoming more sociable. He becomes a companion rather than someone to care for, and can be a pleasure to be around. His imagination assists him in learning about others. He learns to get along with both children and adults, and behaves in a more grown-up manner. In his play he imitates those adults around him, mimics their conversations and manner of speaking, and loves to pretend by "dressing up" in their old clothes.

The Developing Person

Initiative and Self-Esteem The preschooler is, according to Erikson, in the stage of initiative versus guilt, which is the third stage of develop-

has unwarranted guilt feelings over obvious or secret wrongs.

Other evidences of the initiative stage include some aggressive behavior, exaggerating and making up stories, and tattling. His imaginary friend may be used to take the blame for undesirable actions. By the age of 5 he is more responsible and less rebellious. He is more truthful and cooperative, and is making progress toward Erikson's fourth stage of development.

The preschooler's developing identity gives him a sense of belonging, which provides security and gives him a sense of competence. A sense of competence, in turn, motivates the child to perform those tasks that develop his initiative. From a very early age, parents must provide safety and security in meeting the needs of the infant to start this foundation. Parents must provide both verbal and physical love that tell the child he is worthwhile, thereby contributing to his sense of worth and self-esteem. During the preschool years, the child judges his own self-worth on the basis of this competence with things, his competence with parents and other adults and his competence with peers. If he has not developed a sense of belonging and self-worth, he will be hindered in his ability to move out into the bigger world of school and community.

Anticipatory Guidance: Developing Initiative Adults, especially parents, should use praise and affection, rather than scolding and threatening, in their relationships with preschoolers. The use of physical punishment and verbal threatening as a means of controlling children this age produces a child who is anxious and fearful about the loss of parental love. Parents should refrain from comparing their preschooler with siblings or other preschoolers. Children develop at different rates, and comparing makes it difficult for the preschooler to develop a sense of competence and self-worth. Parents that are warm and accepting of their preschooler, although not necessarily always of his behavior, will help him to develop a high level of initiative.

Nurses should be observant of the interactions of the family. A home visit is especially helpful to observe the family in its normal surroundings and usual activities. By becoming more observant and listening carefully to what is not being said as well as what is being said, the nurse can see what warmth, affection and control a parent provides, and frequently what problems a child may have and why.

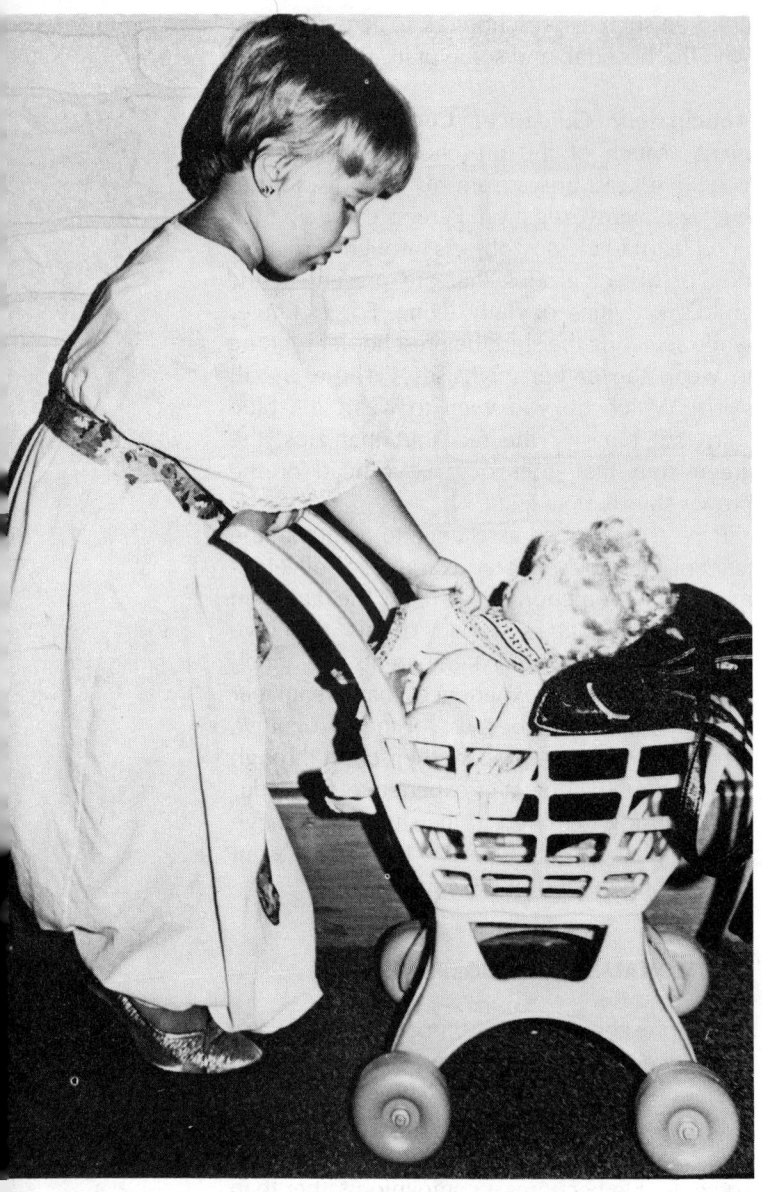

The preschooler loves to pretend by "dressing up."

ment. The main object of this stage is for the child to develop a sense of initiative instead of a sense of guilt. The vigorous preschool child is intent on *doing* and *learning,* which is observed in his endless questions, exploration (physical and mental) and his constant, intense noise. Guilt is a major hazard because much of what he would like to do is either forbidden or he is physically or mentally unable to do it. Guilt also occurs when those he wishes to please are not pleased, or when he himself is not happy with what he has done. Because the preschooler has a rigid conscience, he frequently

Developing Sexual Identity During the initiative stage the preschooler develops a great deal of sexual curiosity. As a toddler he became aware of his sex (gender identity) and the behaviors expected because of his sex (sex typing). He now exhibits and investigates his genitals as a part of his developing body image and shows curiosity about the sexual development of his friends and family (expanding gender identity to include body structure and capacities). It is not uncommon to observe a little boy pulling up a little girl's skirt, or suggesting that she take her clothes off. He is trying to learn and understand the difference between boys and girls. When a girl this age observes that the boy has a penis and she does not, she worries about what has happened to hers, and the boy has the same concerns, plus he now worries about what could happen to his.

His developing sexual curiosity and an awareness of how he differs from others makes the preschooler's sense of self more definite. He is learning about his body, what it looks like and what it can do, and all of this helps him to form his own sexual identity. Preschoolers are influenced by our culture, which tends to sex-type them. Many parents have definite ideas of how boys should behave, such as "fighting back" and not crying when unhappy, whereas girls are punished for "fighting back," but tears are acceptable. Parents may also buy toys that help endorse those cultural sex-type expectations (guns or war games for boys and dolls for girls). Boys are pressured to develop characteristics of their fathers, and girls model themselves after their mothers. By the late preschool age, the child identifies himself and others by the correct sex.

The early preschool period is a time of confused sexual relationships. The boy is thought to be jealous and competitive of his father, wishing to possess his mother solely (Oedipus complex). During this time, he brings her gifts, is protective of her, and attempts to compete with his father for his mother's love. Similarly, the "Electra complex" is seen in girls during the early preschool years and is characterized by the child becoming coy and seductive toward her father and jealous toward her mother. During this time the child watches the same-sex parent closely and imitates their behaviors in an attempt to replace them in the opposite-sex parent's eyes. By late preschool age the child begins to realize that such a sexual relationship is not possible, and he becomes involved in other activities.

It is important for the preschooler to learn the correct names and basic functions of his body parts. The child will have many questions about sex, especially where babies come from, and "Why doesn't Susie have a penis?" It is important to give accurate information, such as, "Girls are made different from boys. When a girl grows up, she can get married and if she wants, she can have a baby." Boys should be told that they are born with a penis and it is not going to go away — boys are made different from girls. If the boy has been told about girls having babies when they get married, he should be told that boys have a part in "growing" babies as a part of being the husband, so that he does not feel left out of this process.

Anticipatory Guidance: Sexual Identity Sexual exploration or sex play in the preschool child is fairly common. The preschooler learns by exploration; he should not be punished for attempting to satisfy his curiosity. Obviously sex

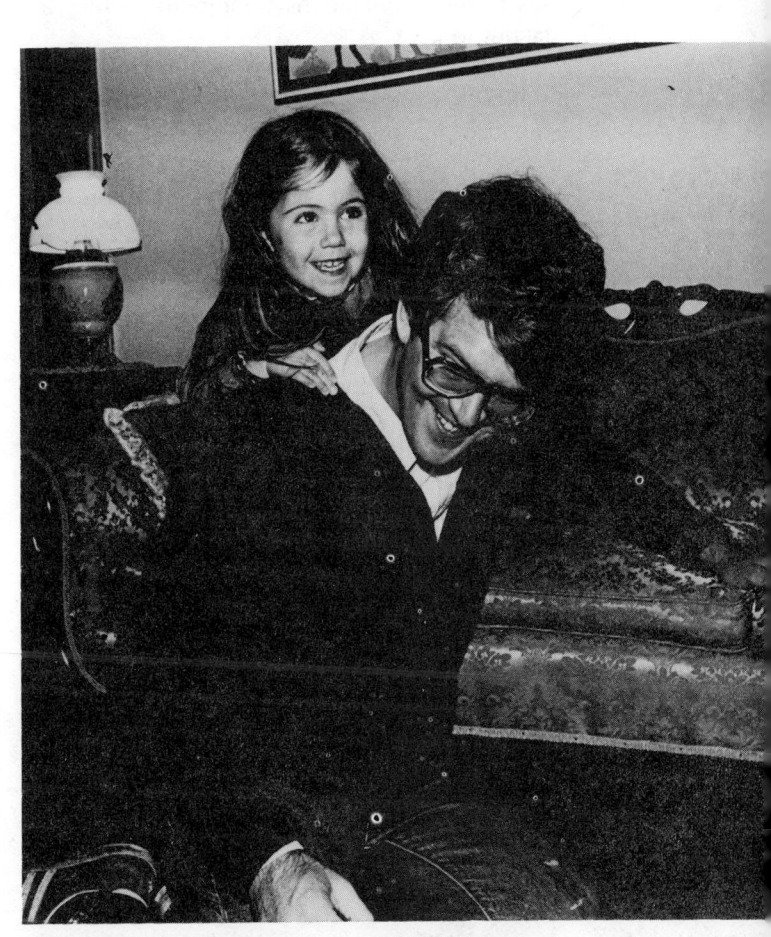

The preschooler competes for a position of closeness with the opposite-sex parent.

play is not encouraged, and limits may be enforced regarding when or where sex organ manipulation may occur, but the child should not be made to feel guilty about this very natural response to his inquisitiveness and developing sexual identity. If the child feels shame or guilt, this could affect his adult sexual functioning. The more emphasis that is placed on this behavior, the more actively curious the child will become. For the most part, once the child learns what he wants to know, genital manipulation diminishes significantly. Because many parents are disturbed by this behavior or do not feel confident about how to handle it, the nurse should always include discussion of it in the anticipatory guidance she offers.

To decrease the amount of sex-typing in the family, it is important for children to observe parents doing things together, such as housework and yardwork. Parents can provide a variety of toys, and encourage their child to play with any toy that interests him, regardless of the sex-typing connotations traditional culture attaches to it.

The child in a single parent family needs substitute experiences with a relative or family friend of the opposite sex to provide the relationship of a missing parent. In some two parent families, one parent is too busy, not interested, or out of town a great deal, and the same need is present and can be filled by an interested relative, neighbor or family friend.

Parents must be prepared to understand their children's feelings of love and hate during the time of the Oedipus and Electra complexes. The child needs to know that his parent is not going to retaliate when told "I hate you," and that he will continue to be loved. The opposite-sex parent also needs to show love, yet protect the child from sexual stimulation or rejection.

Developing a Conscience (Superego) Conscience, or superego, development is the acquisition of moral beliefs. Conscience begins developing during the preschool years as the child learns what behavior is acceptable to his parents. When the child's behavior is not acceptable, he feels guilty. The moral behavior he develops is adopted from that of his parents, as they are the ones judging him. The preschooler, during the process of identification, strives to become similar to his parents, especially the parent of the same sex. He therefore closely imitates all behaviors of that parent that he observes. During these preschool years, rules are absolute, passed by parents who are "perfect," and things are totally right or totally wrong, with the parent always right. Parents and nurses should realize the preschooler believes that sickness, accidents, and hospitalization are punishment for some real or imagined transgression.

In addition to learning right from wrong by imitating his parents, the preschooler also becomes indoctrinated into the behaviors or practices evidenced by his parents related to their religious and ethnic affiliation by imitating. Although the preschooler cannot yet discern the reasons for behaviors such as prayer or attendance at religious services, he eagerly participates in these practices as a part of his identification with his parents.

Likewise, the preschooler cannot comprehend the rationale that makes some behaviors acceptable and others unacceptable. Nevertheless, to facilitate his cognitive development he needs opportunities to question or disagree, even if he does not comprehend.

Anticipatory Guidance: Developing Conscience Many parents do not recognize the significant impact they have on their preschooler's developing moral, religious and ethical attitudes. Parents need to be aware of the role model they provide for their child. The attitude of parents and their relationships with each other as well as with their children all affect the conscience development of the preschool child. The nurse can assist parents to identify what values and attitudes they want to instill in their child and then help them to recognize their behaviors or practices that either foster or hinder their preschooler's acquisition of those values and attitudes. The nurse may encourage parents to actively and regularly participate in religious or ethnic activities that will provide their preschooler with the role models he needs, if they identify these as important in their child's development.

Parents also may require assistance to understand that their child is not ready to adopt acceptable behaviors or avoid inappropriate behaviors only from discussions or explanations of why these behaviors are correct or not correct.

Becoming Social

Rest and Sleep Routines The preschooler seems to have an endless supply of energy, and may be on the go continually. Parents need to be aware of this and initiate rest periods or periods of quiet activity, such as reading. The 3-year-old needs from 10 to 14 hours of sleep daily. He may still nap during the day, or at least rest quietly for one to two hours. By 5 years of age, the sleep requirement is down to 9 to 13 hours and the child seldom naps. Ritualistic bedtime routines continue during the preschool years and can be used as a means to postpone bedtime.

All preschoolers have a fear of the dark, and this fear is exaggerated when they are exposed to ghost stories, scary television programs or very active play before bedtime. In addition, the child this age has a vivid imagination, and at night when it is dark, stuffed animals, designs on wallpaper, rustling leaves and blowing branches become frightening objects. Many preschoolers have dreams and nightmares that waken them during the night.

Anticipatory Guidance: Rest and Sleep Routines Parents may need guidance in the management of sleep behaviors common to preschoolers. The preschooler's wish to postpone bedtime can be dealt with in various ways. Usually taking a favorite toy or blanket to bed, with a story and prayers of a specified time limit, and a consistent, regular routine encourages a readiness for bed. The endless "drink of water" and "go to the bathroom" tactics can be minimized by incorporating these two activities into the bedtime routine. Solutions to bedtime fears include monitoring TV, keeping play quiet before bedtime, removing objects that can appear scary at night and leaving a night light on. When terrifying nightmares awaken a preschooler he needs reassurance that he is safe, and that the dream was not reality. The technique of an understanding parent sitting with him and placing a light for him to see that it is safe is much preferable to that of taking the child into the parent's bed, which can easily become a habit very difficult to break. When these measures do not effectively manage the sleep disturbances or fears, additional evaluation and counselling is appropriate. (See Chapter 41 for further discussion.)

School Readiness The child's world starts with only his mother and himself, and gradually expands to include his father and siblings. After the third year, relatives and neighborhood children, then nursery school and eventually school and larger social circles become part of his world. With this expanding social circle he learns to share people with other people, starting with his mother and father.

The preschooler's attention span is increasing and his memory is improving, which allows for longer periods of play and a decrease in the anxiety of separation from home and parent. His curiosity persists, and he becomes ready to explore the outside world. When the child first expands his social circle beyond his parents, it usually is with one other child to the obvious exclusion of all others. Each positive experience encourages the child to expand this circle to larger and larger groups. The child becomes eager to make friends, quickly learning that sharing brings approval of adults and more playmates. The ability to cooperate with others is not learned overnight but takes much time and assistance from adults, parents and preschool teachers. When a child feels secure in the love of an adult, he finds it much easier to share with others.

The preschool child has increased cognitive and coping capacities as well as more communication skill, initiative and independence as compared with the younger child, and responds less violently to separations. Much of this response is based on previous experience and developmental readiness. The child must have developed sufficient ego strength and the emotional freedom necessary to transfer his dependence from his parent to other responsible adults.

The preschooler should not be put into a school situation until he is able to separate easily from the parent. This is accomplished by his having experienced periods of brief separation in the past, so that the child trusts the parent and knows he is not being abandoned. He should have reached the age in which he can play cooperatively with other children. Nothing is accomplished by putting a child in a preschool or nursery school when he is still in the stages of parallel play. This child should remain in the home with a babysitter if it is necessary for parents to work during the day. If the preschooler has had opportunities to play with other children in the family or neighborhood, he is usually ready for a preschool program by 4 years of age and some will benefit from a part-time program at 3. The child who has no contact with other children will usually benefit from a part-time program of nursery school, just to allow him to develop outside interests that are not available at home and to develop relationships with peers.

Anticipatory Guidance: School Readiness
Parents should see themselves as educators and should share activities with their children that provide learning opportunities to prepare them for school. Nature walks, with discussions of what is seen, and visits to community buildings, post offices, city halls or fire stations all help the child expand his knowledge. If available, art galleries and museums are good places to explore, as are zoos and parks. The city child gains insights from a visit to the farm, while the farm child needs exposure to the city. A ride on a train, a bus and a taxi are all valuable learning experiences, and ones that parents can share. Parents can also participate in their child's learning by playing simple games, putting puzzles together, making cookies or pudding, and sharing other simple forms of cooking with him. Providing paper, finger paints, paste, crayons and blunt scissors allows the preschooler to be imaginative and create his own art work. Reading to the preschooler is probably one of the most valuable experiences he receives, although this activity ideally should begin in infancy. Music and musical games are other opportunities for learning that the preschooler and his parents can mutually enjoy.

Educational television can also contribute to the preschooler's readiness for school. Parents should limit TV viewing and monitor programs seen. Physical activity is far more important than TV viewing.

Attending Sunday school and summer vacation bible school provide opportunities for children to learn to play and work with peers, particularly for the preschooler who is not in a nursery school program. In the nursery school, preschool and Sunday school setting, the child is provided with planned activities that ready him for the school experience. These same activities can be planned in the home, but valuable interaction with peers may be missing in the home. The day care center provides interaction with peers but usually without planned school readiness activities. Parents should be aware of the differences in preschool and day care services and plan for their child's needs accordingly.

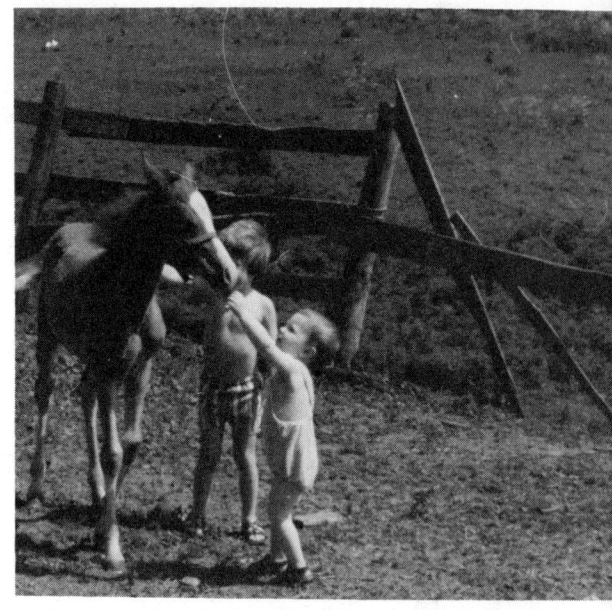

The preschool child seeks experiences that expand his world beyond home. These city children are enjoying a visit to a farm. (Photograph by Dave Trainor.)

When a day care or preschool program is chosen, parents should explain to the child what the preschool program is and why it is necessary that he spend some time there each day. Adequate preparation will help the preschooler to avoid feeling abandoned or rejected. School should be discussed at home, and a visit made to the preschool to see what it looks like and to meet the teacher. Friends or siblings already attending school can offer positive input to the preschool child. Parents should have confidence in the preschool and convey that feeling to their child. Ideally, a parent should attend school with the child at the beginning, staying for shorter periods each day, until the child feels secure. If possible, a parent should take the child each day and assure him of his or her return at the end of the day, rather than having someone do this whom the child does not know well.

HEALTH MAINTENANCE

Nutrition

Mealtime for the preschooler should be a happy time within a warm atmosphere. This should be regular and planned to include all family members present at the time. A planned quiet period for the preschooler and siblings may be

TABLE 39-2 BASIC FOUR FOOD GROUPS: PORTIONS AND NUMBER OF SERVINGS PER DAY FOR PRESCHOOLERS

Food Group/Portion Size*		Number of Portions
Milk and Milk Equivalent		4
(Requirements/day: 16–24 oz milk)		
Milk	1/2–3/4 cup	
Cheese	3/4–1 oz	
Cottage cheese	3/4 cup	
Yogurt	1/2 cup	
Ice cream	3/4 cup	
Meat and Meat Equivalent		2
(Requirements/day: 2–4 oz)		
Meat	1–2 oz	
Egg	1 (limit to 3–4/week)	
Frankfurter	1–2	
Lunch meat	1–2 slices	
Tuna	1/4–1/2 cup	
Peanut butter	2 tbsp.	
Dried peas or beans	1/2–1 cup cooked	
Vegetables and Fruits		4–5
Vegetables	1/4–1/2 cup	
Cooked		
Raw	Dark green, deep yellow—3/week	
Fruit	1/4–1/2 cup	
Canned		
Raw	Citrus: 1/day	
Fruit Juice	4 oz	
Bread and Cereal		4
Bread	1/2–1 slice	
Whole grain/enriched		
Cereal		
Cooked	1/4–1/2 cup	
Dry	1/2–1 cup	
Noodles, rice,	1/2 cup	
Macaroni, etc.		
Crackers	8–2 inch	

*Portions represent the average amount of food a preschooler might eat. Amounts actually eaten vary considerably from day to day.

necessary before the mealtime. Conversation should include the preschooler.

This is a time for the child to learn socialization skills, mealtime behavior, language skills and family rituals. Table manners at this age are best learned from observation and should not be stressed. Parents should not expect better table manners from the child than they use. Mealtime spills should be accepted, cleaned up and forgotten.

Because the preschooler continues to grow at a slowed rate, he has a small appetite. Serving small portions with seconds allowed, or allowing the child to serve himself, is preferable to serving more food than the child can eat. It is normal for the child to want more food on some days than on others (this occurs in adults), but some parents tend to think that children should always eat a specific amount of food a day.

All preschoolers still enjoy finger foods; these should be offered in some form at mealtime.

By the age of 4, most children can use a fork and can spread with a knife. Many 5-year-olds are able to cut their meat with a knife. The natural flavors of food should not be covered with seasoning, so that the child learns to accept the true flavor. All foods should be served in small amounts so the child can handle it easily. As the child learns colors, he becomes more aware of food colors, and will prefer brightly colored foods to dull ones. Table 39–2 describes the average portions and number of servings for preschoolers per day.

Assisting in food preparation also makes eating interesting for the child, and there are many helpful things the preschooler can do in the kitchen to help. He can help plan a menu and assist during grocery shopping, set the table and help wash the dishes. Some parents feel that it is too time-consuming to allow the child to help or to teach him about food preparation, but if they will take the extra time, they will be rewarded by their child's new interest in food. Letting the child plant vegetable seeds in a garden in the spring and watch the vegetables mature and then pick them, will increase his interest in eating vegetables.

Attitudes about foods and eating habits formed during early childhood will last throughout life. It is important to introduce the child to new and different foods so he can learn more about the world around him. A variety of foods increases the child's ability to select and accept those foods that contribute to a well-balanced diet. New foods should be introduced gradually, and include a variety of tastes, colors and consistencies. It is very important that foods introduced to the preschooler be accepted by adults in the home, and eaten by them at mealtimes. Most preschoolers will try new foods due to their initiative but will refuse them if other family members make disparaging remarks about the food.

Between-meal snacks should be planned at appropriate intervals and should consist of juice, fresh fruits or raw vegetables, cheese, peanut butter on crackers and other similar foods. Sweet foods should be offered infrequently, as they tend to contribute to dental caries, malnutrition and obesity. Snack time should be supervised. Snacks should not be given just before mealtimes.

If the child is growing in accordance with height and weight charts for his age and is happy and healthy, plays well and has healthy teeth, his parents should be advised that his "not eating a thing" is probably the normal decrease in diet for his age. It is important for the nurse to go over proper diet with the mother and explain the role of junk food in decreasing appetite. If the diet seems adequate, it usually is not necessary for the child to be taking supplemental vitamins.

Play

Imaginary play is a predominant form of preschool play activity. He plays house from what he observes at home and, if there are older siblings in the home, he plays school. As a toddler he played alone (parallel play), even if side by side with another toddler. This play time was spent learning to use fingers and manipulate objects. The preschooler is more coordinated and is experienced with manipulation, so these activities take up much less time.

The young preschooler starts to play with at least one other preschooler (cooperative play). He still remains somewhat selfish but is more interested in what is going on around him. By the age of 4 the child has a longer attention span and plays with groups of children. Much of this play is noisy, aggressive and dramatic. When the child reaches 5 he can play simple games with other children and can share. All preschoolers like quiet times involving such activities as coloring, pasting, cutting and being read to. They also like noisy, boisterous activities, active games, riding tricycles, playing with cars and trucks, and playing with water, mud, snow, leaves and other outdoor activities. The preschooler enjoys getting wet and getting dirty and he frequently is.

Parent(s) should provide play materials that are sturdy and simple. Many household articles make good play materials, and they need not be expensive. Play should provide physical activity through the use of balls, blocks, wagons, tricycles, swings and safe climbing materials. Creative play should be encouraged with sheets of paper, crayons, finger paints, clay, scissors,

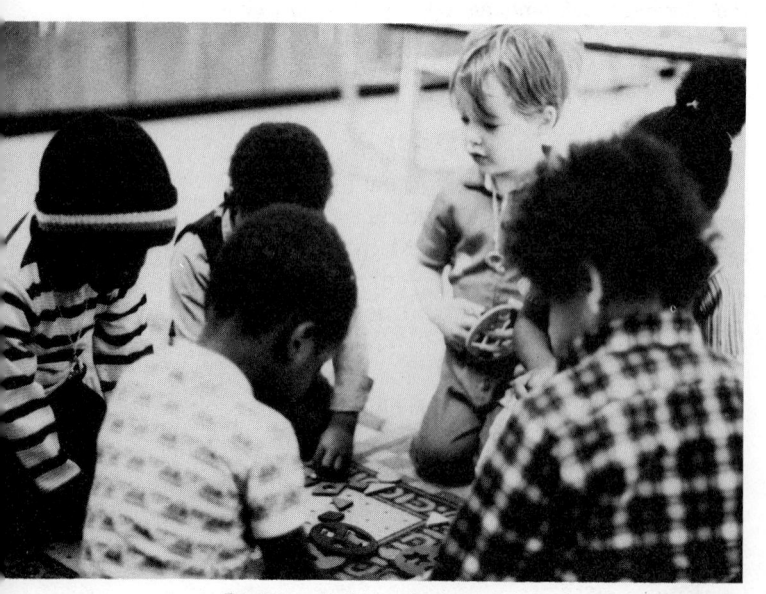

By 5 years of age, the preschooler is able to interact with peers in simple games.

boxes, cloth and yarn scraps. Dramatic play can be stimulated by providing dolls, cars and dress-up clothes. Quiet play can be encouraged with books, records and puzzles. Parents should provide opportunity, equipment, space and safety for the child during play but should avoid attempting to structure the child's play.

Safety

The preschooler is old enough to start learning about safety. His desire to imitate and his sense of initiative assist in his ability to learn safety measures. Parents should take advantage of this readiness and teach the rationale for safety rules. For example, the preschooler can comprehend why it is dangerous to cross the sreet. He is old enough to learn to look both ways before crossing streets, and to cross busy streets only with a green light if available, or with an adult.

Car accidents are still a leading cause of injury to preschoolers, and parents need to explain the rationale for use of car seats and seat belts. If the child observes the parents using seat belts consistently, he will be more likely to comply. When the child is too short to see out of the car window, use of a car seat brings less resistance than restraint by a seat belt.

The nurse should counsel parents to never leave a child in a car alone, even for a few minutes. A preschooler can very quickly set a car into motion while imitating the parent driving. The child could also climb out of the car and be injured by other cars, or get lost. Although it takes longer to unbuckle the child and take him into the store for a moment, the safety of the child is ensured. The preschooler is not mature enough to be left alone at home, responsible for himself or siblings.

An area in which preschoolers sometimes get into trouble is while playing outside and hiding from others. His poor judgment and lack of experience may lead the preschooler into dangerous hiding places, such as under cars or in abandoned refrigerators and freezers. Abandoned buildings are also favorite playing places but are unsafe and children should be cautioned about entering these. He should be taught to refuse to talk to strangers in cars, to refuse rides and to refuse gifts. The preschooler should also know his own name, address and phone number, and how to approach a policeman for help.

The preschooler's drive to imitate adult roles can lead him into dangerous play if he is not supervised and taught the safe limits of his experimentation with materials usually used by adults. Because of his curiosity and quick movement, it is wisest to keep him away from areas in which power tools or equipment are being used, sucn as lawnmowers and saws. The preschooler should be taught to use sharp objects such as a paring knife with extreme caution and never without supervision by an adult. Power tools should be stored out of his reach. If a gun is kept in the house, it should be stored unloaded with the bullets stored in a separate area, both preferably locked.

Preschoolers are intrigued by matches and fire, and they soon develop the dexterity to ignite them. Matches are best kept stored in a tight container and out of reach. The older preschooler may be allowed to accompany a parent to the incinerator and permitted to help burn trash. This measure often helps reduce the child's interest in matches. In addition, it offers an opportunity for the parent to teach the child about fire and the safety precautions needed around fire.

During the preschool years a child's play and daily activities are less supervised than in earlier years. Parents need to be cautioned to provide adequate supervision of a preschooler to prevent falls and serious accidents during play and activities of daily living. For example, a pre-

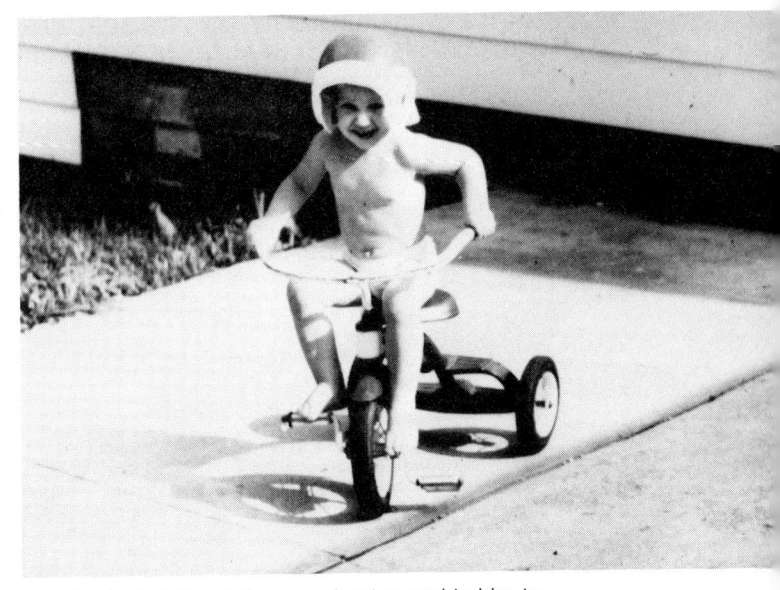

The physical skills of the preschooler enable him to enjoy a tricycle.

TABLE 39-3 SUMMARY OF PRE-SCHOOLER GROWTH AND DEVELOPMENT AND HEALTH MAINTENANCE

Age (Years)	Physical Competency	Intellectual Competency	Emotional-Social Competency	Nutrition

General 3–5	Gains 4-1/2 kg (10 lbs)
	Grows 15 cm (6 in)
	20 teeth present
	Nutritional requirements:
	  Energy: 1250–1600 cal/day
	  Fluid: 100 ml/kg/day
	  Protein: 30 gm/day
	  Iron: 10 mg/day
		Becomes aware of self and others
		Vocabulary increases from 900–2100 words
		Piaget's preoperational/intuitive period
			Freud's phallic stage
			Oedipus complex-boy
			Electra complex-girl
			Erikson's Initiative vs. Guilt
				Carbohydrate intake approximately 40–50% of calories
				Good food sources of essential vitamins and minerals
				Regular tooth brushing
				Parents are seen as examples; if Daddy won't eat it, child won't

3	Runs, stops suddenly Walks backwards Climbs steps Jumps: broad jump Pedals tricycle Undresses self Unbuttons front buttons Feeds self well	Knows own sex Desires to please Sense of humor Language—900 words Follows simple direction Uses plurals Names figure in picture Uses adjectives/adverbs	Shifts between reality and imagination Bedtime rituals Negativism decreases Animism and realism: anything that moves is alive	1250 cal/day Due to increased sex identity and imitation, copies parents at table and will eat what they eat Different colors and shapes of foods can increase interest
4	Runs well, skips Hops on one foot Heel-toe walks Up and down steps without holding Jumps well Dresses and undresses Buttons well, needs help with zippers, bows Brushes teeth Bathes self Draws with some form and meaning	More aware of others Uses alibis to excuse behavior Bossy Language—1500 words Talks in sentences Knows nursery rhymes Counts to 5 Highly imaginative Name calling	Focuses on present Egocentrism/unable to see the viewpoint of others, unable to understand another's inability to see his viewpoint Does not comprehend anticipatory explanation Sexual curiosity Oedipus complex Electra complex	Good nutrition 1400 cal/day Nutritious between-meal snacks essential Emphasis on quality not quantity of food eaten Mealtime should be enjoyable, not for criticism As dexterity improves neatness increases
5	Runs skillfully Jumps 3–4 steps Jumps rope, hops, skips Begins dance Roller skates Dresses without assist Ties shoelaces Hits nail on head with hammer Draws man–6 parts Prints first name	Aware of cultural differences Knows name and address More independent More sensible/less imaginative Copies triangle, draws rectangle Knows four or more colors Language—2100 words, meaningful sentences Understands kinship Counts to 10	Continues in egocentrism Fantasy and daydreams Resolution of Oedipus/Electra complex, girls identify with mother, boys with father. Body image and body boundary especially important in illness Shows tension in nail-biting, nose-picking, whining, snuffling	Good nutrition 1600 cal/day Encourage regular tooth brushing Encourage quiet time before meals Can learn to cut own meat Frequent illnesses from increased exposure increases nutritional needs

schooler's engrossment in play, especially imaginative play, interferes with his perception of danger. Upstairs windows should have sturdy screens or guards or both to prevent a serious fall by a preschooler, who may be engaged in "flying superman" play. A preschooler also must be closely supervised when playing around water to avoid accidental drowning. Although many preschoolers are afraid of water, they may slip and fall into the water accidentally. A preschooler's independence in daily activities should be supported by providing special safety devices (adhesive strips in the tub).

Immunizations

The need to prevent communicable diseases is essential in all children. Basic immunizations should have been completed by the preschool age. Prior to beginning school DPT and polio booster shots are given, usually at the time of the preschool examination, which is between 4½ and 5 years of age. These boosters of DPT and Polio protect the child for the next ten years. Tuberculin testing should be done at the preschool visit.

TABLE 39-3 SUMMARY OF PRE-SCHOOLER GROWTH AND DEVELOPMENT AND HEALTH MAINTENANCE (Continued)

Play	Safety	Immunization
Reading books is important at all ages Balance highly physical activities with quiet times Quiet rest period takes the place of nap time Provide sturdy play materials	Never leave alone in bath or swimming pool Keep poisons in locked cupboard; learn what household things are poisonous Use car seats and seatbelts Never leave child alone in car Remove doors from abandoned freezers and refrigerators	Basic immunization should be completed by 2 years Booster due at 4½–5 years
Participants in simple games Cooperates, takes turns Plays with group Uses scissors, paper Likes crayons, coloring books Enjoys being read to and "reading" Plays "dress-up" and "house" Likes fire engines	Teach safety habits early Let water out of bathtub; don't stand in tub Caution against climbing in unsafe areas, onto or under cars, unsafe buildings, drainage pipes Insist on seatbelts worn at all times in cars	
Longer attention span with group activities "Dress-up" with more dramatic play Draws, pounds, paints Likes to make paper chains, sewing cards Scrapbooks Likes being read to, records and rhythmic play "Helps" adults	Teach to stay out of streets, alleys Continually teach safety; child understands Teach how to handle scissors Teach what are poisons and why to avoid Never allow child to stand in moving car	TB skin test if going to preschool
Plays with trucks, cars Plays with guns, soldiers Likes simple games with letters or numbers Much gross motor activity: water, mud, snow, leaves, rocks Matching picture games	Teach child how to cross streets safely Teach child to not speak to strangers or to get into cars of strangers Insist on seatbelts Teach child to swim	Booster DPT, OPV TB skin test before school entrance

Reference

1. Physical Examination of the School Age Child: The Musculoskeletal System. Filmstrip Made by Undergraduate Dietetic Program and the Department of Nursing, California State University at Los Angeles and distributed by Trainex Corporation.

Additional Recommended Reading

M. Alexander and M. Brown. Pediatric History Taking and Physical Diagnosis for Nurses. McGraw-Hill Book Co., 1979.

U. Bronfenbrenner and M. Mahoney. Influences on Human Development. The Dryden Press, 1975

A. Chapman. Management of Emotional Problems of Children and Adolescents. J. B. Lippincott Co., 1974

M. Erickson. Assessment and Management of Developmental Changes in Children. C.V. Mosby Co., 1976

J. Malinowski. Answering a child's questions about sex and a new baby. American Journal of Nursing, November 1979, p. 1965

R. Murray and J. Zentner. Nursing Assessment and Health Promotion through the Life Span. Prentice-Hall Inc., 1975

P. Mussen et al. Child Development and Personality. Harper and Row, 1974

A. Pillitteri. Nursing Care of the Growing Family. Little, Brown & Co., 1977

P. Pipes. Nutrition in Infancy and Childhood. C.V. Mosby Co., 1977

40 POTENTIAL STRESSES DURING PRESCHOOL YEARS: MANAGING BEHAVIOR

by Jo Joyce Tackett, BSN, MPHN

Preschool misconduct is usually only temporary. It is evidence of the child's struggle to adapt to his developmental changes and the changing expectations significant others have of him. Occasionally the typical misbehavior of the preschool years becomes disturbed, most often because the child is inaccurately interpreting environmental cues (parental in particular), because the expectations made of him are unrealistic or because his temporary misbehaving has received reactions from significant others that perpetuate rather than discourage repetition of the behavior.

DIFFICULTY LEARNING AND RESPECTING OWNERSHIP RIGHTS

One characteristic of the preschooler is his creative ability to redefine reality to suit his personal needs. Although he is usually reasonable and dependable, the preschooler will alter facts or change rules, particularly in stressful situations, to save face or gratify personal desires. To do this without feeling guilt, he reshapes reality so that the object of his desire comes to be perceived as really belonging to him, or he pretends to the extent of convincing himself that he can *borrow* an object with long-term intent without being in the wrong.[1]

If limits are consistently and calmly placed on these "borrowing" behaviors and the child is helped to see how the real owner feels when his possession is taken, such misconduct will soon disappear. Parents find it easier to remain calm about these episodes if they are aware that their preschooler has not developed the cognitive skills needed to grasp the concepts of cheating, lying or stealing. This helps them to understand that the "borrowing" behavior is not plotted, intentional misconduct.

Disturbed Psychodynamics and Etiology

When behavior that ignores others' rights to ownership persists over time or develops a pattern of frequency that is excessive, a problem exists that merits parental or professional intervention or both. Persistent or excessive "borrowing" behavior is most often prompted by underlying feelings of frustration. The child may be reacting to a lack of limits that makes him feel unprotected. He discovers that if he ignores rules of ownership his parents will at least stipulate a limit on that behavior. (Even overpermissive parents will usually not tolerate disrespect for ownership and will set limits when the behavior causes them personal embarrassment or pressure from outside sources.) Such behavior may also represent a child's plea for attention; even negative attention or a hysterical parental response is better than none at all.[1]

Sometimes the behavior is actually a symptom of great disorganization in the child's life experiences that has caused him to prefer a fantasy world that is more pleasant than his real world. Because play is a part of the preschooler's world — real or fantasy — assuming ownership of others' things easily becomes a part of the behavior of the child who prefers fantasy.[1] Frequently, the preschooler is imitating the adults in his environment who have not conveyed a respect for the child's own ownership needs.[7] For example, a parent or sibling who keeps before the child the fact that the clothes he is wearing or the toys he is playing with are or were his brother's deprives the child of knowing a sense of ownership. A child cannot be expected to respect ownership if he has not experienced ownership and thereby learned what it is. Likewise, the parent who insists on the preschooler sharing everything he has is diminishing the child's sense of ownership and control over what is his.[7]

Sharing can be promoted without compromising ownership if the preschooler is allowed to put away prized toys or possessions when siblings or visitors with whom he is expected to share are around. But the child who is continually deprived of ownership experiences will "borrow" relentlessly, in search of something he will be allowed to claim as his own.[1,2,7] Very rarely is "borrowing" at the preschool stage due to the fact that the child comes from an economically impoverished home — a sense of ownership does not require wealth. One possession that is solely one's own is all that is required to gain a sense of ownership.

Disregard for ownership is an aspect of some preschoolers' behavior that is learned and maintained through social reinforcement (usually from parents), not because of some inherent flaw in the child himself.[2]

Management

Correction of this problem is directed toward the cause. The first step in intervening, therefore, is to get a history of the behavior: when it occurs, how often and how long it has been occurring, what story or reason the child gives for taking the object and whether a pattern exists in his reasoning. Information should be obtained on how the parents have handled the behavior up to now and why they are seeking help now (if they in fact have identified the problem and sought help). Whether the parents role-model ownership and respect the child's ownership needs, how much time is spent with the child usually and how much in the couple of days just prior to each episode should be ascertained. Questions regarding how much time the child spends fantasizing each day and if the child seems to be off in his own world much of the time need to be answered. The history should also document if any unusual stresses occur in the family around the time that the misbehavior occurs and the parenting style used with this child. This kind of data can help establish that a problem does in fact exist and the parents are not just overreacting to normal preschooler behavior that is temporary. This information can also facilitate identification of the cause.

If the parenting style is overpermissive, leaving the child without limits, the nurse's task will involve helping the parents establish parenting practices that are less extreme, providing the child with the guidelines for living that he seeks. The parents may simply need information to redirect their parenting, which the nurse can provide; or they may need counselling to develop confidence and comfortableness in setting and enforcing limits for their child. The nurse may be competent to do this, or she may refer the couple to an appropriate resource.

When parental response to "borrowing" behavior is hysterical, the nurse can help the parents learn that other options exist to manage the misbehavior. Often information about what is realistic to expect of a preschooler and that he has not developed a concept of stealing or lying that would make his behavior intentional is all parents need to help them respond more calmly.

When the child's disturbed behavior is being

motivated by a hunger for attention, the nurse must help the parents evaluate the time they spend with their child in terms of both quantity and quality. This process assists parents to recognize the deficits that exist. They are then able to cooperate with the nurse in planning time and activity with the child that meets his attention needs without overcompromising their life style.

If family disorganization is prompting the behavior, a long-term multidisciplinary effort is usually required to help the family become more functional, offering pleasurable experiences for the child so he need not rely on fantasy for emotional survival.

Inadequate modelling of ownership by the parents that deprives the child of ownership experiences can also be tactfully pointed out by the nurse. Using the history as a teaching aid, she can review with the parents those patterns in their own behavior that discourage the child's mastery of ownership rights. Sometimes this knowledge, coupled with information about how a child learns to respect ownership, is enough to motivate parents to change their behavior. However, if these behaviors have deep-seated emotional stimuli, counselling and a behavior modification program for the parent(s) may be necessary.

The child is not without responsibility in changing his behavior, however. A program of behavior change for the child can be instituted simultaneously with the intervention to identify and remedy the underlying cause. The following measures constitute this program and should be carried out consistently.

When the behavior occurs, the parent should:[1,7]

1. Make the child aware that you noticed his behavior.
2. Tell him how you feel about the behavior.
3. Find out his reason for the behavior or account of the situation.
4. Help the child identify whether his story is real or fantasized.
5. Insist (physically guide him if necessary) that he return the object (immediately if possible) and apologize to the owner of the object for the hurt and sorrow caused.

Reinforce the child's behavior any time he displays respect for ownership and provide the child with generous role models (parents, siblings, friends) who receive reinforcement of behaviors displaying respect for ownership regularly in his presence.[2]

STUTTERING

Behavioral disturbances in the preschool years sometimes present in the form of language difficulties, typically stammering or stuttering. Stammering is the result of involuntary pauses in the formation of words, while stuttering results from the involuntary repetition of the sounds of speech.[5]

Normal and Disturbed Psychodynamics Most children engage in stuttering or stammering behavior at some point during the years they are formulating language skills, most commonly during late toddlerhood or the early preschool years. This behavior is a natural manifestation of the child's concentrated effort to master communication skills and, at best, should be ignored. It is most likely to occur on occasions when the child is tired or experiencing extreme anxiety, or being exposed to overstimulation from his environment.[4]

These natural, temporary speech disturbances become a problem when they become persistent or cause the child extreme distress. What happens is that during the child's normal stage of stuttering or stammering some experience or some person (often a parent) draws the child's attention to his speaking. The primary basis for these disturbed speech behaviors is the result of demands on the child to impose conscious control over the involuntary act of forming words.[4,5] Thus a natural behavior is molded, ever so unintentionally, into a behavioral disturbance because of the constant pressures to impose consciousness on an unconscious act by phrases like "Try to say it over again carefully," "Say it this way," and "Think about what you are saying!" Once conscious effort is demanded, the stuttering or stammering becomes established.

Children with "keyed-up personalities" who demand more than ordinary amounts of sleep, rest and play and who are easily overstimulated or upset are especially at risk to persist in these speech mannerisms if they are brought to the child's attention. Parents who are critical of their child's speech efforts are also more likely to be critical of his efforts in other performance areas, making the child more emotionally insecure and more susceptible to development of these speech mannerisms.

Clinical Manifestations These speech mannerisms are almost always recognized first by the parents or other lay adults. If at the inception of stuttering or stammering it is dealt with by ignoring it and making sure others in the child's environment do too (a point to be made when the nurse offers anticipatory guidance), it will most likely resolve itself in a few months. If it continues for several months, despite its being ignored, parents should be urged to seek professional evaluation and not rely on hearsay approaches that usually only serve to enhance the behavior.

Management Established speech mannerisms are treated most effectively by specially prepared professionals (speech therapists). However, the nurse can complement the therapists' interventions by offering parents the following guidance recommended by the Speech Rehabilitation Institute* to help diminish the behavior:[4]

1. Avoid all urges to correct the child's speech, to force him to repeat words, or to force him to talk. (This does not mean he cannot be *encouraged* to talk.)
2. Always speak slowly, simply and calmly to the child.
3. Build the child's general emotional health with praise, affection, opportunities to excel, commendation for small gains in task mastery.
4. Keep the home climate calm to avoid overstimulation or increased anxiety levels.
5. Enforce adequate periods of rest and sleep and provide opportunity for uninterrupted free play.

SLEEP DISORDERS

Sleep problems, particularly nightmares, night terror and sleepwalking, peak during the preschool years.[9] Dreams are an essential part of sleep and average five or more in number nightly.[4] The preschooler confuses waking and dreaming experiences easily, and his dreams are extremely vivid and real to him; thus a dream may frighten this child whether it is pleasant or scary, simply because it looms so real. The fright is heightened by the fact that the preschooler's dreams usually focus on him as the active participant or central figure rather than as a passive observer.[4]

At this age a child's dream life is influenced by his immediate environment and living conditions. Nightmares are particularly common in children with a history of separation from their primary caretakers and home for three to four weeks or more.[4] Dreams are more likely to be negative during periods of poor health or family stress; however, personality is the greatest single influence on the nature of the child's dreams.[4] The neurotic or slow-to-warm child is most likely to have predominately nightmarish dreams. The difficult or hostile child is most likely to have aggressive, terrorizing dream themes.

A negative-theme dream life is also more likely in children who display exaggerated fear of the dark. Most preschoolers express some fear of the dark, but those exposed to significant others (parents, siblings, peers) who show apprehension for the dark, those for whom darkness has been used as a punishment, and those for whom death has been equated with sleep are most at risk to develop phobic fears of the dark.[4, 6, 9] The fear of darkness expressed by a child is best acknowledged as real to him and should be combined with a program of positive reinforcement and weaning from the fear. Two weaning programs that have been successful with preschoolers are described in the box.[4]

Disturbed Psychodynamics and Clinical Manifestations Normal sleep disturbances in preschoolers are basically temporary and show theme variance. A negative theme that is recurrent and exists over time is symptomatic of some underlying emotional disturbance that needs intervention. Fortunately, children express their feelings simply and clearly in their dream life, seldom with the distortion of symbolism typical of adult dreams.[4] Therefore the problem is usually identifiable within the child's description of the dream.

Night terrors differ from nightmares in pathology. Table 40–1 describes the characteristics of these dream patterns and of sleepwalking and how each is most effectively handled.

Management to Eliminate Sleep Disorders

The most definitive action to be taken in alleviating nightmares is to identify the underlying cause and eliminate it.[4] This requires an evalua-

---

*The Speech Rehabilitation Institute, 61 Irving Place, New York, NY, 10003 can be a valuable resource for information and support to parents of children with speech problems.

MANAGING PHOBIC FEAR OF THE DARK

Program 1 Leave a lamp on in the child's room on the floor near his bed. Move it gradually farther from the bed and eventually out of the room. How quickly this can be done will vary with the child. (The average is to move farther away every two to three nights.) If the lamp is moved and the child reacts negatively, move it back to its former position a few more nights, then try again. Once the lamp is out of the room a few nights, turn it off after the child is asleep. Then, a few nights later, try not turning it on at all. If the child tolerates that for several nights, he has been weaned from his fear and the lamp can be removed completely. If the child regresses during illness or other upset, go to his room and comfort him but without holding him or turning on the light and he will overcome his fear.

Program 2 Place the child in bed with the room light on, but turn it off once he is asleep, keeping the door of his room open and a hall light on. During the daytime teach the child how to turn his own light on if he awakens and wants it on if he does not already know how. Once he knows how, tell him he is a big boy and can be responsible to turn the light on himself when he wants it on at night and enforce that expectation. Each time he turns the light on, turn it back off after he is asleep. The child will eventually tire of getting up to turn on the light and will just go back to sleep.

---

tion of the child's reactions to various situations coupled with consideration of the content of the nightmares (remember children do not dream symbolically). Parents may need assistance with this process or they may require a psychological expert's input.

Intervention to diminish night terrors is less easily accomplished. Since central nervous system immaturity is a primary factor, terrors cannot be completely eliminated until the central nervous system gains more maturity. Actions can be taken to eliminate environmental or psychological stresses that may be intensifying or increasing the frequency of the night terrors. This is done in the same manner as for nightmares, although professional assistance to decipher the dream may be needed, since the child often recalls only a single image from the dream.

Steps can also be taken by parents to help the child approach bedtime in a positive frame of mind. The following activities have proved successful in enhancing the interventions described in the previous two paragraphs.[4, 5, 9]

1. Use the hour before bedtime as a cooling-down period by participating with the child in some quiet, mutually enjoyable activity such as reading a mild, happy bedtime story or talking through the day's pleasant events.
2. Help the child establish some before-bed rituals that help indoctrinate him emotionally for bed, such as a warm bath, brushing his teeth, putting his dolls or cars or teddy bear to bed, hugs from family members. Then put him to bed.
3. Distinguish between bedtime and sleep time. Allow quiet play in bed until sleep overcomes the child.
4. Teach the child where the hands on the clock are when it is bedtime so that the clock becomes a "neutral" teller of bedtime, making a game of bedtime rather than a battle of wills.
5. Do not make the child feel isolated at bedtime. Allow comforts such as a light on, the door open, soft music to make the child feel he is not alone. Also reassure the child that you are nearby throughout the night and that he will awaken safe and sound in the morning. Some parents even remind the child of some pleasant event he can look forward to the next day.

Whatever the child's sleep problem is and regardless of its frequency, parents should be cautioned by the nurse not to over-react to the child's behavior or the child will learn to use the sleep disturbance to manipulate them.

EXCESSIVE MASTURBATION

During the preschool years there is a natural, developmentally associated increased interest by the child in his genitals. All children masturbate to some degree and it is estimated that 75 per cent of preschool children do so on a fairly regular basis.[4, 5] Boys are four times more likely

TABLE 40-1 CHARACTERISTICS OF NIGHTMARES, NIGHT TERRORS[4-9]

Sleep Disturbance	Description	Behaviors Manifested	Management During Behavior
Nightmares	Psychological motivation. Anxiety expressed, worked through in negative theme. Occurs during active sleep. If child awakens, can recall all or most of dream; no recall if not awakened.	Moves around restlessly in bed, may whimper or cry but not hysterically. May or may not wake. Face may show facial grimace or expression of fear.	Do not overreact. If child crys, parent who wishes to respond to it should satisfy self that nothing is wrong (not caught in blankets, not fallen out of bed, no fever), then leave without waking child. If child awakens, give reassurance that it was only a dream and he can safely go back to sleep. Then leave; making a fuss over the child only reinforces the behavior.
Night terrors	Physiological motivation: result of immature CNS function; psychological factors determine theme. Occurs during deep sleep. Child can usually only recall a single frightening image, if anything; usually repetitive.	Sits up in bed, screaming, or assumes bizarre crouching posture; pulse and respirations increase, pupils dilated. Senses doom, intensely anxious and agitated. Appears to be staring at something in front of him with his eyes wide open. Disoriented. Does not recognize persons who respond to his distress but will gradually respond to a soothing voice.	Although the child does not recognize the adult who responds to his shrieks, reassurance and cuddling do eventually calm the child, allowing him to return to sleep.
Sleepwalking	Family trait. Lasts 1/2 to several minutes. No recall. Child's eyes are open; not awake.	Wanders around room or house. Unconscious of environment although eyes are open. Movements are rigid and repetitive. Answers in monosyllables if spoken to. Will return to bed on own.	Do not attempt to wake child but protect him from injury. Keep doors to basement, outdoors, other areas of potential danger locked. Allow child's own return to bed. If guided back to bed before ready he will usually get up again anyway.

to masturbate than girls, probably because their genitals are more accessible.[4]

Despite their knowledge of the normalcy of masturbation, most parents (especially mothers) experience anxiety over their child's display of this activity, yet the majority, fortunately, do not interfere to stop the child's behavior.[4]

Disturbed Psychodynamics and Etiology Masturbation does not usually become excessive or disturbing in the preschooler unless parents or other caretakers over-react to it or take punitive action when it occurs.[4, 5, 8] The parents' reactions impose guilt on the child that, if it persists, can penetrate other aspects of the child's sexuality and interpersonal relationships.[8] The child's emotional-social psyche is especially at risk for damage if his parents perpetuate the myth that masturbation leads to physical deterioration, impotency or lunacy.[5] Parental overanxiety creates the compulsiveness; this, and the need for the solace of inward consolation that the activity provides the child, are the unhealthy aspects of masturbation.

Excessive or compulsive masturbation sometimes is performed as a source of solace to a child who feels emotionally isolated and deprived or who is poorly adjusted in several aspects of his development. This child tends to show a preference for masturbation behavior over other enjoyable activities; the masturbation is a symptom of the child's general disorientation toward life.[4, 5] The masturbatory behavior really becomes a plea for attention and limit-setting rather than a form of inquisitiveness and pleasure that is the natural motivation for masturbation in preschoolers.[3]

Management

This first step in organizing a plan of intervention is to gather a history regarding the masturbation behavior: when it began, how frequently it occurs, circumstances surrounding its occurrence, where it occurs, parental response to the behavior, general state of parent-child relationship. Then the nurse can do a physical appraisal to rule out vaginitis (also common in preschoolers) or penile irritation. If vaginitis or penile irritation exists, treatment should be instituted to correct these conditions.

If no physiological cause can be identified, management involves steps to modify the parents' responses to the behavior and to place limits on where or when the child may involve himself in the activity.[4, 5, 8]

Education or counselling or both are needed to help the parents learn to ignore the behavior or to casually distract the child by involving him in some enjoyable interaction or activity outside himself.

Limits on where and when the activity may occur should also be established with the child. He should be informed that people do not accept the behavior being carried out publicly, using the same tone of voice that one would use to discourage spitting or nosepicking. He should then be told where the activity may be done, such as only when he is alone or only in his own room. These limits should then be calmly and consistently enforced. Punishment should never be used to enforce these limits, however.

If the child has already suffered some emotional impairment, professional psychological intervention should be initiated to reverse those feelings as early as possible.

References

1. J. Costello, Dean Erikson Institute for Early Education. Tall tales and mistaken ownership. Parents, March 1979, p. 88
2. D. Doland and K. Adelberg. The learning of social behavior. In Social Learning of Childhood by D. Gelfand. Brooks/Cole Publishing Co., 1969
3. S. Fraiberg. The Major Years. Charles Scribner's Sons, 1968
4. M. Herbert. Problems of Childhood. Pam Brooks Ltd., 1975
5. W. Homan. Child Sense. Basic Books, 1977
6. M. Jones. A laboratory study of fear; the case of Peter. In Social Learning of Childhood by D. Gelfand. Brooks/Cole Publishing Co., 1969
7. P. McDonald. Helping children learn moral values. Home Life, January 1977, p. 50
8. L. Salk. What Every Child Would Like His Parents to Know. Warner Paperback Library, 1973
9. R. Winter. The Fragile Bond. Macmillan, Inc., 1976

41

POTENTIAL STRESSES DURING PRESCHOOL YEARS: TEMPORARY ALTERATIONS IN HEALTH STATUS

by Jo Joyce Tackett, BSN, MPHN, and Barbara Miller, BSN, PNA, MA

Temporary illness does not usually disturb the preschooler too much, since he is treated at home by his own caretakers. The interruption in his usual activities is generally brief. During the acute phase of his illness, the preschooler feels too ill to care that he cannot play or carry out usual daily routines. His convalescence is another matter, however. If recuperative confinement lasts more than a day or two, the preschooler quickly becomes bored and aggravated because of the isolation from his playmates and the limitations placed on his usual actively rambunctious play.

The preschooler may also feel confused because his initiative is temporarily stifled by the limitations imposed by the illness itself, by his caretakers, or by his own spontaneous developmental regression that is a natural consequence of his illness. He needs frequent reassurances that his illness did not come about because he did or thought something wrong or bad. Simple physiological explanations, using terms the preschooler understands, should be offered for the illness and the symptoms he is experiencing. He should be allowed to make small decisions regarding his care when a choice exists. The preschooler is usually cooperative with treatment measures if he is given simple explanations of how they will help him and what he may do to assist or carry out the treatment. Such opportunities help him maintain some sense of initiative during illness.

During the acute phase of temporary illness, the preschooler will need frequent contact with his caretakers and soothing reassurances that he will soon feel better. The preschooler will continue to need regular contact with his caretakers during his convalescence as a reassurance that he has not been forgotten. He will also need frequent changes in activities to prevent boredom, which precipitates crankiness, uncooperativeness and an escalation in demands. Chapter 16 discusses several viable activities appropriate to the convalescing pre-

TABLE 41-1 CHILDHOOD COMMUNICABLE DISEASES SPREAD BY AIRBORNE DROPLETS[1-3, 5, 6]

Airborne oronasopharyngeal droplets are expressed during speaking, sneezing or coughing, or are present on freshly contaminated fomites. Virus may also be present in blood, urine or feces. Respiratory isolation and careful handwashing are required to control spread.

Disease (Agent)	Diagnostic Features	Incubation (Days)	Communicability Period	Clinical Manifestations *Prodromal Symptoms*
Rubella (myxovirus). Also called 3-day measles and German measles	Characteristic rash. Specific lymphadenopathy involving postauricular, postcervical, occipital nodes.	14–21	7 days before rash until 4 days after it disappears.	Tender, enlarged lymph nodes in post-auricular, postcervical, occipital areas (often only symptom in preschooler). Low-grade fever, anorexia, mild conjunctivitis; coryza. Slight pharyngitis.
Rubeola (paramyxovirus). Also called measles, hard measles, red measles, and regular measles.	History of URI symptoms and conjunctivitis 3–5 days before rash. Koplik spots. Characteristic rash.	10–20	5 days before until 5 days after rash appears.	Cold-like symptoms: conjunctivitis, photophobia, nasal congestion, hacky cough. Steadily increasing fever over 3–5 days. Koplik spots (white spots circumscribed in red like grains of sand in mouth opposite lower molars, then spreading to buccal mucosa) fade in 12–18 hr.
Erythema infectiosum (possibly virus). Also called fifth disease.	Flushed face of otherwise asymptomatic child; rash recurrence at intervals.	7–28	Unknown.	None.

schooler. Television does not entertain the preschooler for long and should be reserved for times when the caretaker must have a brief uninterrupted period rather than as a long-term babysitter.

Parents who have received adequate explanation of the temporary illness and verbal and written instruction in care required usually adapt easily to the situation. Their main complaint is often related to sleep loss due to need to administer medications and other treatments round-the-clock and the child's symptom-related inability to sleep. Additional reassurance is provided if the nurse maintains daily contact with the parents (home visit or phone call as indicated by the child's condition and the parents' competency and confidence in their ability to provide treatment and monitor symptoms), at least during the acute phase.

CHILDHOOD COMMUNICABLE DISEASES

The preschooler and the early school-age child are particularly vulnerable to childhood communicable diseases. It is at this time that they generally have less resistance to infectious organisms and at the same time are increasingly exposed to these organisms as they increase their social contacts beyond home. Another group of children at special risk to the childhood communicable diseases is made up of those with malignancy, those on immunosuppressive drug therapy, or those who have an

TABLE 41-1 CHILDHOOD COMMUNICABLE DISEASES SPREAD BY AIRBORNE DROPLETS[1-3, 5, 6] (Continued)

Clinical Manifestations Acute Phase Symptoms	Treatment	Complications	Prevention
Rash: Begins on face and hairline and as it clears moves to trunk, then extremities. Also pinpoint rose-red spots on soft palate. Lasts 3 days. Rosy red, dry, maculopapular character. Diffuse configuration. Systemic signs: Occasionally persistence of prodromal symptoms.	Self-limiting, mild disease. Quiet activity. Aspirin for fever or headache.	Can cross placental barrier in pregnancy causing congenital rubella with 50% chance of malformation during 1st trimester.	Vaccine after 12–15 mo of age. Isolate from pregnant females. Permanent immunity from vaccine or disease.
Rash: Begins at hairline and moves to neck, ears, face, then to trunk and then to upper and lower extremities. Lasts 10 to 15 days. Dark red, dry, discrete, maculopapular character; turns brown and scaly after 5–6 days. Fever: Peaks (40.5° C, 105° F) 2–3 days after rash starts, then subsides as rash spreads. Prodromal symptoms diminish as fever lowers. Other systemic signs: Preschoolers may have associated vomiting, diarrhea or otitis media.	Spontaneous recovery, acute disease. Bed rest until 2 days after fever subsides, then quiet activity. Isolate from persons with bacterial infections. Antipyretics, sponge baths, increased fluids for fever. Room humidification and antitussive for cough. Dimly lit room or sunglasses for photophobia. Cleanse eyes to remove crusts; keep child occupied to discourage eye rubbing.	Viral or bacterial encephalitis; bacterial-caused otitis media or bronchopneumonia.	Vaccine after 15 mo of age. Permanent immunity from vaccine or disease.
Stage 1 Rash: Bright red cheeks (slapped-cheek appearance) with circumoral pallor. Fades in 1–4 days. Stage 2 Rash: Red, symmetrical, maculopapular character. Begins 1 day after stage 1 rash disappears. Starts on trunk, then extremities and buttocks. Lasts 2–40 days. Stage 3 Rash: Periodic recurrence, especially with exercise, temperature extremes, emotional upset, or skin irritation. Fades from center in a lacy appearance.	Self-limiting, mild disease. No treatment or isolation necessary; continue usual activities. Parents may need help in explaining disease to school personnel.	Rare: arthritis, anemia, pneumonitis, encephalitis.	None. No permanent immunity.

immunological disorder. These children have greater susceptibility either because their disease keeps them from being immunized or because the disease or drug therapy reduces or alters their body's resistance to the infectious organisms. They are much more likely to develop serious complications or die from these diseases, which in other children are usually mild and self-limiting. Therefore, the nurse, especially the school nurse, has a responsibility to keep families of children at special risk informed of outbreaks in the community and to emphasize to parents the importance of trying to avoid exposing their child to these diseases.

The incidence of communicable disease in the United States has dropped significantly with use of immunization. Likewise, serious complications and mortality have decreased thanks to antibiotics and antitoxins.

The Nurse's Role

Nurses play a major role in the prevention and identification of childhood communicable diseases. A nurse must have a thorough knowledge of each disease syndrome and its treatment (Tables 41–1 — 41–3) and perform history taking and physical assessment efficiently to carry out this role effectively.

Prevention The primary means of preventing most of the childhood communicable diseases is through immunization. The nurse can be actively involved in carrying out an immunization program in any pediatric work setting;

Text continued on page 930.

TABLE 41-2 CHILDHOOD COMMUNICABLE DISEASES SPREAD BY DIRECT CONTACT AS WELL AS BY AIRBORNE DROPLETS[1-3, 5, 6]

Disease (Agent)	Diagnostic Features	Incubation (Days)	Communicability Period	Clinical Manifestations *Prodromal Symptoms*
Chickenpox *(Herpesvirus varicellae)*. Also called varicella.	Characteristic lesions of rash.	10–21	1 day before lesions until 6 days after first vesicles form.	24 hours before rash. Fever, anorexia, malaise.
Herpes zoster *(Herpesvirus hominis*–like the chickenpox virus). Also called shingles.	Location of characteristic rash; unilateral involvement. Characteristic prodromal symptoms.	4–24	Same as for chickenpox. (Person with chickenpox may give shingles to someone with partial immunity; someone with shingles may give chickenpox to child who has never had the disease.)	Pain and itching along ganglion lines for 1–5 days before lesions erupt. Pain is burning, stabbing, worse at night and with movement. Previously has had varicella at some time in past but immunity has waned or is only partial.
Mumps (myxovirus). Also called parotitis.	Characteristic swelling.	14–26	2 days before swelling until 9 days after swelling occurs.	Occurs 1–2 days before swelling. Headache; fever, often high; anorexia and vomiting; malaise.

TABLE 41-2 CHILDHOOD COMMUNICABLE DISEASES SPREAD BY DIRECT CONTACT AS WELL AS BY AIRBORNE DROPLETS[1-3,5,6]

Clinical Manifestations Acute Phase Symptoms	Treatment	Complications	Prevention
Rash: Begins on chest, spreading to entire trunk, scalp and face. Few or no lesions on extremities. Mucous membranes affected. Severity varies from mild with a few lesions to severe with hundreds. Successive crops of lesions in varying stages of formation. Crops stop appearing after 5 days. Begin as maculopapular, intact lesions on a red base, become vesicular, then rupture, forming crusts. Lesions 2–3 mm in diameter. Lasts about 2 wk. Not communicable after crusts form. Pruritic. Palatal white ulcers make swallowing painful. Systemic signs: Fever that ranges from low to 105° F according to severity of rash. Malaise.	Spontaneous recovery, acute disease. Bed rest until fever gone. Then quiet activity until all lesions crust. Once rash has entirely scabbed, may return to usual activities. Antipyretic, cool sponge bath without soap, light clothing, fluids for fever. Soft diet tolerated best if mouth lesions present. Antipruritic, antihistamine; cool, light, loose fitting clothing; keep child occupied for pruritus. Sedative if severe itching at night. Keep nails short or hands mittened; pat moistened cornstarch on lesions; antiseptic bath 2 times daily; child and caretaker wash hands often; change clothes and linen daily to prevent secondary infection. Topical or systemic antibiotic for secondary infection.	Secondary infection from scratching (cellulitis, pneumonia). Encephalitis. Reye's syndrome.	None. Permanent immunity from the disease if full-blown case. Passive immunity with IM immune serum globulin (ISG) or zoster immune globulin (ZIG) within 3 days after exposure to children at high risk for complication or fatality. Isolation of high-risk children from known cases.
Rash: Located along the ganglion of peripheral nerve roots, most commonly in the thoracic area. Always unilateral eruption that does not cross midline.	Aspirin for pain. Same as for chickenpox.	Rare. Encephalitis, secondary bacterial infection.	Same as for chickenpox.
Unilateral or bilateral swelling of parotid glands (lymphocyte infiltration of glands with cell necrosis and blockage of duct openings) and/or other salivary glands. 2/3 of cases symptomatic; 1/3 are asymptomatic. Swelling peaks by 3rd day, returns to normal by 10th day. Chewing, sour liquids or foods aggravate the earache-like pain.	Self-limiting. Liquid or soft bland diet to minimize pain. Bed rest until temperature normal, then quiet activity until swelling gone. Aspirin, warm or cold compresses for pain of swelling.	Orchitis sterility. Meningoencephalitis. Auditory nerve neuritis→ deafness. Pancreatitis.	Vaccine after 12 mo of age. Permanent oophoritis immunity with vaccine or disease, whether symptomatic or not.

Table continued on the following page.

TABLE 41-2 CHILDHOOD COMMUNICABLE DISEASES SPREAD BY DIRECT CONTACT AS WELL AS BY AIRBORNE DROPLETS[1-3,5,6] *(Continued)*

Disease (Agent)	Diagnostic Features	Incubation (Days)	Communicability Period	Clinical Manifestations *Prodromal Symptoms*
Pertussis (Bordetella pertussis bacillus). Also called whooping cough.	WBC shows progressive leukocytosis. Characteristic cough. Nasal culture positive for organism.	5-10	Throughout all stages of disease; greatest during catarrhal stage.	Catarrhal Stage: Lasts 1-2 weeks. URI-like symptoms of headache, rhinorrhea, low-grade fever, irritating cough and sneezing; anorexia.

TABLE 41-2 CHILDHOOD COMMUNICABLE DISEASES SPREAD BY DIRECT CONTACT AS WELL AS BY AIRBORNE DROPLETS[1-3,5,6] *(Continued)*

Clinical Manifestations *Acute Phase Symptoms*	Treatment	Complications	Prevention
Paroxysmal stage: Lasts 4–6 weeks. Cough worsens, developing to spasms and ends with prolonged inspiration (crow sound), a "whoop." Often followed by vomiting of large amounts of thick, stringy mucus. Child appears to be strangling during paroxysm. Paroxysms initially occur several times an hour, decreasing to 3–4 a day over time.	Hospitalization recommended in most cases. Humidification; increase liquids, suctioning to reduce mucus and keep airway patent. Small, frequent feedings; usually tolerated best if offered just after a vomiting episode to maintain hydration. IV therapy may become necessary. Minimal physical exertion, cool room temperature with good ventilation, O_2 therapy. Intubation if necessary to maintain oxygenation. Quiet environment. Seizure precautions. Avoid temperature extremes, smoke, dust. Antibiotic (erythromycin favored) to render organism noncommunicable; does not decrease paroxysmal stage. Respiratory isolation. Parental and child support: (1) In hospital—rooming in to maintain child's emotional needs, parent/child bond; teach care. Talk calmly to child during cough spasms. Age-appropriate explanations of disease and care to child and parents.	Atelectasis, dehydration, pneumonia, convulsions, hernias, otitis media, hearing loss.	Vaccine (series of 3 begun at 2 mo with boosters at 18 mo and 5 yr.) Permanent immunity with immunization or disease.
Convalescent stage: Lasts weeks or months. Any intercurrent respiratory infections may result in return of paroxysmal cough and vomiting. Gradual decrease in cough, vomiting stops, appetite returns, improved strength.	(2) At home (mild or convalescing cases)—daily contact with nurse via phone or home visit as indicated. Thorough instruction (verbal and written) regarding care of child: 1. Room humidification; keep room free of smoke, dust, temperature extremes. 2. Encourage tepid fluids; small frequent feedings after vomiting. 3. Quiet environment; seizure precautions. 4. Respiratory isolation. 5. Stay with child during paroxysms; watch for respiratory distress; stay calm; suction if equipment available. 6. Administer antibiotic therapy exactly as prescribed. Arrange for competent source of relief on regular, daily basis so caretakers can obtain rest without interruption or worry about the child. Educate regarding secondary infection and complication signs to watch for and report (see next column).		

Table continued on the following page.

TABLE 41-2 CHILDHOOD COMMUNICABLE DISEASES SPREAD BY DIRECT CONTACT AS WELL AS BY AIRBORNE DROPLETS[1-3, 5, 6] *(Continued)*

Disease (Agent)	Diagnostic Features	Incubation (Days)	Communicability Period	Clinical Manifestations *Prodromal Symptoms*
Diphtheria (Corynebacterium diphtheria)	Progressive growth of oronasal membranes. Positive culture of organism in 24 hr. (Swab under membrane or rub firmly over membrane and incubate immediately).	2–5	Until patient or carrier no longer harbors organism (identified by 3 consecutively negative cultures).	Low-grade fever, headache, malaise, mild pharyngitis.
Scarlet fever (group A beta hemolytic streptococcus) Also called scarlatina and septic sore throat.	Recent strep infection. Positive throat culture. Characteristic strawberry tongue.	1–3	10 days or course of illness.	Abrupt high fever, abdominal pain, vomiting. Headache, chill, malaise.

FAMILIES WITH PRESCHOOLERS

TABLE 41-2 CHILDHOOD COMMUNICABLE DISEASES SPREAD BY DIRECT CONTACT AS WELL AS BY AIRBORNE DROPLETS[1-3, 5, 6] *(Continued)*

Clinical Manifestations Acute Phase Symptoms	Treatment	Complications	Prevention
Severe swelling of throat and mouth. Tough, leathery, gray pseudomembrane forms on tonsils and may extend to nasal passages and larynx. If the membrane is removed, bleeding occurs and the membrane re-forms. Hoarseness, dysphagia, brassy cough, fever. Enlarged cervical lymph nodes. Airway occlusion from swelling and membrane sloughing makes breathing difficult. Nasal secretions become serosanguineous and cause excoriation of upper lip.	Hospitalization recommended. Antitoxin (IM for mild cases, IV for severe cases) to destroy toxins (first check for sensitivity with intradermal or conjunctival injection). Antibiotic helps kill toxins and prevents secondary infection. Liquid or soft diet high in calories offered in small frequent feedings. Analgesics and ice collar for headache and sore throat. Lubricant to protect lips from excoriation. Observe closely for signs of respiratory distress or obstruction; tracheostomy tray at bedside in event of obstruction. Humidification and O_2 therapy if indicated. Intake and output monitored for hydration and renal function. Bed rest for a minimum of 2 wk to prevent myocarditis. Daily evaluation of heart for signs of myocarditis. Antipyretics if fever stays up.	Respiratory obstruction. Neuritis (bilateral and self-limiting in 10 days. Renal damage (decreased output and proteinuria). Myocarditis (low BP, arrhythmia, ECG changes, rales, abdominal pain).	Toxoid (series of 3 shots begun at 2 mo with boosters at 18 mo, 5 yr and every 10 yr thereafter). No permanent immunity; immunity must be maintained through boosters. Antitoxin given to carriers.
Rash: Begins on neck, axillary folds and chest, groin, then moves to trunk and extremities. Not on face but facial flushing present. Lasts 5 days; not always present. Diffuse, dry, fine, punctate, red papules (resemble goose flesh) that blanch on pressure. Desquamates as it resolves. Dusky red, enlarged, exudate-covered tonsils; pharynx red and swollen, sore throat and dysphagia. Tongue white and furry (white strawberry tongue) first 2-3 days, then peels off and by fourth day papillae become prominent and red (red strawberry tongue); circumoral pallor.	Will subside spontaneously but complications are frequent if left untreated. Antibiotic to kill toxin—10 day course; ensure caretaker reliability in giving properly and for full course. Bed rest until fever resolves, then quiet activity during convalescence. Cool mist humidification, analgesics, liquid or soft diet for sore throat. Instruction to observe for and report any signs of complication; daily contact via phone or home visit. Motivate antibiotic compliance and monitoring for complications. Instruct in careful cleaning of clothing, linens, dishes to prevent spread.	Pneumonia, suppurative otitis media, peritonsillar abscess, rheumatic fever, acute glomerulonephritis, cervical adenitis.	Reportable to health department. Permanent immunity with disease.

TABLE 41-3 CHILDHOOD COMMUNICABLE DISEASES SPREAD BY DIRECT CONTACT WITH INFECTIOUS LESIONS, EXUDATE, OR FOMITES[1-3, 5, 6]

Disease (Agent)	Diagnostic Features	Incubation (Days)	Communicability Period	Clinical Manifestations *Prodromal Symptoms*
Impetigo (Group A beta hemolytic streptococci; occasionally staphylococci or pneumococci). Also called pyoderma and impetigo contagiosa.	Positive vesicle culture. Characteristic lesion.	2–10	Throughout infection; highly contagious, spreads rapidly.	Skin breakage or insect bite. May be none.
Cellulitis (Group A beta hemolytic streptococcus or staphylococcus).	Positive culture. Characteristic symptoms.		Throughout infection.	Previous infection, frequently impetigo.

community health nurses and school nurses are in a position to do so on a community-wide basis. Primary prevention also requires that the nurse help identify and obtain treatment for children who are experiencing infections or diseases that often precede communicable disease (e.g., strep throat). Identification and immunization of unimmunized family and social contacts who have been exposed to active communicable disease is another preventive action for which the nurse is responsible.

Another aspect of prevention is the use of control measures to prevent or minimize the spread of the disease. Control measures include appropriate isolation and early identification and treatment of existing disease.

Most children with communicable disease are treated at home; therefore, the nurse's role becomes one of instructing the family members in proper techniques of isolation and handwashing. A home visit is often the best approach to help the family identify how they can realistically confine the ill child and handle the discarding or cleaning of contaminated articles (Fig. 41–1). For example, isolation by confinement to his room may not be realistic if a child must share the room or even a bed with other family members or the entire family. Proper handwashing should be stressed, demonstrated and, if indicated, a return demonstration given to ensure that family members can comply with this basic preventive technique. Family members are more likely to carry out handwashing, hygiene, isolation and other preventive practices if they are given reasonable explanations for these procedures. The nurse should make sure parents know how many days isolation must be enforced, since parents may otherwise unnecessarily isolate the child until a rash is gone. If antibiotic therapy is needed, the nurse must ensure that the child's caretakers know the specifics of how and when to administer the antibiotic. The nurse must also determine the family's reliability in seeing that the antibiotic is given properly and for the full course. If reliability is questionable, the nurse may need to arrange for community nurse supervision or recommend hospitalization.

Specific treatment that must be supervised by the nurse if the child is hospitalized or that must be taught to family members if the child is treated at home is described in Tables 41–1 through 41–3.

Identification The nurse is often the one who first recognizes signs of communicable disease

TABLE 41-3 CHILDHOOD COMMUNICABLE DISEASES SPREAD BY DIRECT CONTACT WITH INFECTIOUS LESIONS, EXUDATE, OR FOMITES[1-3, 5, 6] *(Continued)*

Clinical Manifestations Acute Phase, Symptoms	Treatment	Complications	Prevention
Intact, erythematous papules fill with WBC's and a vesicle or pustule forms. Eventually vesicle ruptures and forms a honey-colored crust. Pruritus. Usually located around mouth and nose, occasionally the extremities, with a rapid peripheral spread. Groups of lesions form circles and arcs. Regional lymphadenitis.	Topical (few lesions, less than 50¢ piece in size) or oral (several lesions, lesions larger than 50¢ piece) antibiotic for 10 days. (Experimental data support a single injection of Benzathine Pen G as the most effective treatment.)[2] Given to promote lesion healing, decrease recurrence or spread, decrease risk of AGN. Crusts removed by soaking, then lesion scrubbed gently and thoroughly with soap at least 3 times daily. Keep child occupied to reduce scratching; mittens if necessary. Instruct in single usage of linens by the child and not exchanging with other family members.	Cellulitis or erysipelas, acute glomerulonephritis (AGN), bacteremia.	None. Maintain adequate hygiene and nutrition and thoroughly cleanse skin breaks and insect bites to reduce susceptibility. Inspect family members for contacts and treat those infected.
Involved skin and deeper subcutaneous tissues inflamed—swollen, red, firm, hot to touch. Streaking of extremity from lymphangitis. Regional lymph node enlargement and tenderness. Fever and malaise.	Bed rest. Immobilization of affected area. Oral or parenteral penicillin. Warm soaks to relieve pain.	Bacteremia, septicemia. May be fatal in neonate.	None. Culture all family members regardless of absence of symptoms and treat those with positive cultures.

or to whom parents and teachers bring their concern if they suspect symptoms. Therefore, she must become skilled in recognizing and describing various rashes and in associating them with other symptoms to identify the correct disease so that appropriate treatment can be initiated.

The nurse's evaluation should begin with a history of any known exposure by the child to any communicable disease in the past month and a history of the communicable diseases that the child is already known to have had. This information, in addition to a knowledge of the child's immunization status, aids in diagnosing the particular disease syndrome. Any systemic or prodromal symptoms experienced within the past week should also be considered and documented. The rash or lesions are most accurately examined with a magnifying glass and good lighting. A note should be made of where the rash is on the body (distribution), including where it began and how it spread. Characteristics (morphology) of the rash should be noted, including the size, color, shape, configuration and type of lesion. The stage of involution of the rash as well as any secondary changes (crusts, scaling, excoriation) should be documented.

The nurse should maintain a high index of suspicion of the possibility of communicable disease any time a preschool or early school-age child develops minor complaints (low-grade fever, anorexia, malaise, sore throat) or a rash. History and assessment findings are then useful in confirming that suspicion.

RABIES

Rabies is a disease of the central nervous system that is transmitted to man in the saliva of infected wild animals such as squirrels, skunks and bats, as well as domestic cats and dogs. Preschool children are more frequently bitten by cats and dogs. They are losing their fear of animals and think of even wild animals as potential pets but do not yet understand that certain animals can transmit serious disease. The incidence of rabies is steadily increasing in the United States.

Rabies is caused by a neurotropic virus, which travels from the peripheral nerves to the central nervous system. The disease has three stages. The first is the *prodromal*, which lasts about two to four days and is characterized by numbness, tingling and burning at the area of the bite. This is followed by fever, headache,

POTENTIAL STRESSES DURING PRESCHOOL YEARS: TEMPORARY ALTERATIONS IN HEALTH STATUS

> **ISOLATION PROCEDURES DURING COMMUNICABLE DISEASE***
>
> **Respiratory Isolation** (for childhood diseases spread by airborne droplets)
>
> > *Separate room* or screened-off area; door kept closed.
> > *Mask* worn by all persons entering room who are susceptible to the disease. (A tissue may be substituted for a mask at home but should be used only once and discarded properly.)
> > *Hands* must be washed thoroughly with soap upon entering and leaving the room.
> > *Articles* contaminated with secretions must be disinfected.†
> > *Susceptible persons* should be excluded from patient area.
> > *Clean room* by vacuuming or damp dusting daily.
>
> **Secretions and Exudate Precautions** (for childhood disease spread by direct contact with the lesions or contaminated fomites)
>
> > *Hands* must be washed thoroughly with soap before and after contact with patient or objects patient has handled.
> > *Articles* should be disposed of in sealed bag or disinfected† before reused.
> > *Susceptible persons* should avoid contact with the patient or articles he handles if possible.
>
> **Strict Isolation** (any child with undiagnosed rash or lesions (exanthema) is placed in strict isolation until diagnosis is made)
>
> > *Separate room;* door kept closed.
> > *Gown, mask, gloves* worn by all persons entering room.
> > *Hands* washed thoroughly with soap upon entering and leaving room.
> > *Articles* are discarded or disinfected† and sterilized; sealed in bag and placed in another sealable clean bag at door to remove articles or trash from room.
>
> ---
>
> *See discussion on preparation of children for isolation in Chapter 16.
> †Disinfection may be achieved through chemicals (chlorine), ultraviolet light (sunlight), or heat (boiling, baking, clothes dryer, dishwasher).

nausea, sore throat and irritability or restlessness. Increased salivation, diaphoresis and sensitivity to bright lights and noises are also evidenced during this stage.

The next stage is the *excitement* stage. The child becomes increasingly excitable and apprehensive; muscle twitching and generalized convulsions occur. Throat spasms occur when the child tries to eat or drink and even when he hears the sound of running water. The name *hydrophobia* (morbid fear of water) comes from this symptom. There is also spasm of the respiratory muscles and, at times, continuous tonic convulsions. The temperature frequently is around 39.5° to 40.5° C (103° to 105° F). This stage lasts one to three days, and many patients die during it. If the child survives he goes into the third stage, called the *paralytic,* or *terminal,* stage. There is increasing paralysis and coma and then death. Only one documented case of a person surviving rabies has been reported, and that child was treated vigorously for each symptom before the symptom developed.[7]

In dogs the incubation period is three to eight weeks, while in man it is two to six weeks but may be as long as two years. A rabid animal does not usually behave like a healthy animal; it staggers and runs blindly and is more aggressive. It may drool and hide after biting another animal or a human, since rabid animals seek seclusion for death. A rabid animal can transmit the disease by licking abraded skin or mucosa. If the animal doing the biting has been properly immunized against rabies, it will probably not transmit the rabies virus even if it was bitten by a rabid animal.

There are no complications in rabies. It is currently a uniformly fatal disease.

Prevention of the disease is of major importance. Most communities have ordinances requiring immunization of pets. Leash laws should be enforced and all stray dogs and cats should be picked up for confinement or destruction. Children should be taught early to treat pets kindly and to avoid stray or sick animals, whether tame or wild. Programs should be instituted to control wildlife population during rabies epidemics. When a child is bitten by *any animal,* tame or wild, or licked by *any unimmunized or wild animal,* the site should be washed immediately and flushed with copious amounts of soap and water, followed by an application of 40 to 70 per cent alcohol, Zephiran or iodine.[9] The child should then be evaluated by a physician to determine what, if

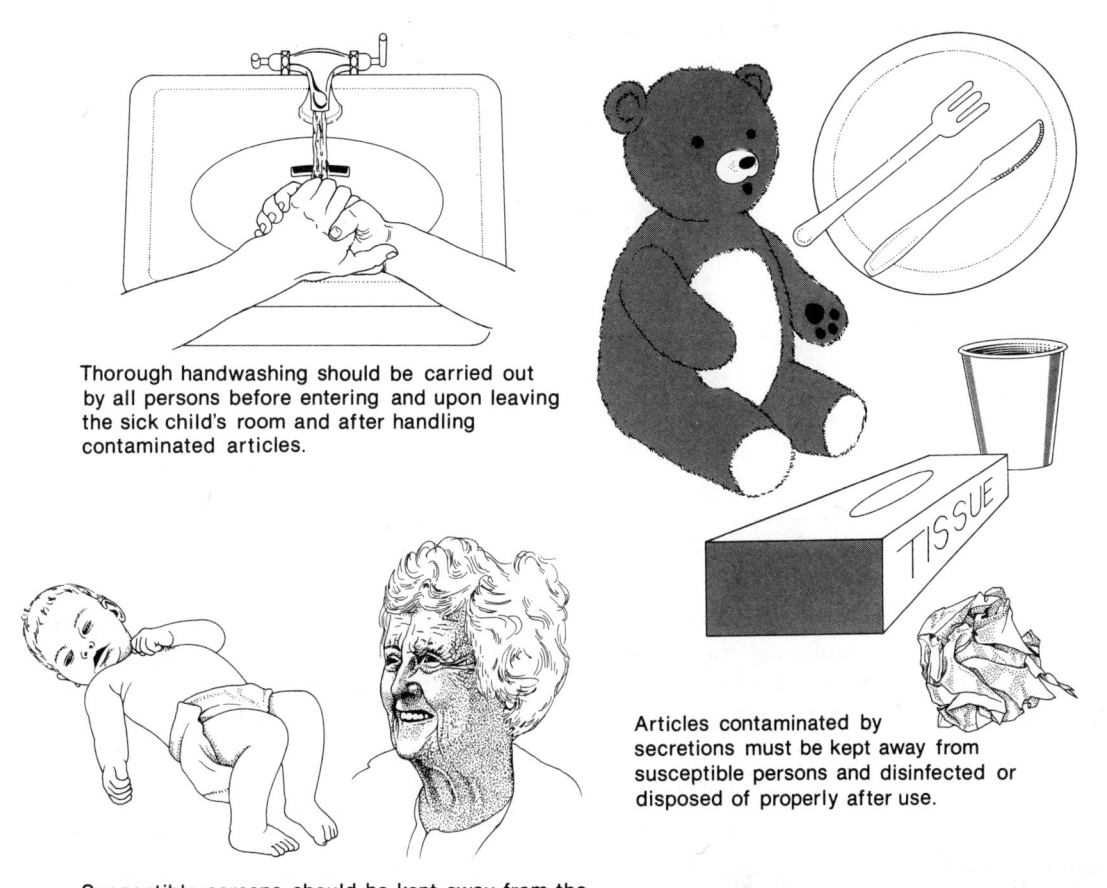

Figure 41-1 Basic precautions in the home to prevent the spread of communicable disease.

- Thorough handwashing should be carried out by all persons before entering and upon leaving the sick child's room and after handling contaminated articles.
- Articles contaminated by secretions must be kept away from susceptible persons and disinfected or disposed of properly after use.
- Susceptible persons should be kept away from the patient's area.

any, prophylactic treatment should be initiated. The wound should be cleaned again in the doctor's office. Suturing, if necessary, should not be done immediately, since it is believed that closing the wound may cause the virus to spread.[9]

History taking is very important, especially if the child was alone at the time of the bite. The child is asked to describe the animal, since he might not know what the animal was. Keeping a picture book of animals available for the small child to pick out the kind that bit him can be helpful.

The child is asked to describe what he was doing when the animal bit him. Unprovoked attacks are more likely to be from rabid animals. Many children provoke animals such as cats and dogs, without realizing it, while hugging the animal or helping it to eat. A bite from a familiar animal that is healthy does not usually produce rabies; however, the parent should be sure of the animal's immunization status and the animal should be confined for 10 days to be observed for signs of rabies. If the animal is unknown, all efforts should be made to locate it. If it cannot be located or if the animal is a bat, regardless of the bat's condition, rabies treatment should be insituted. If the animal is wild, it should be killed. When the animal has been killed or found dead, the head should be packed in ice and sent to the state Department of Public Health or to a competent veterinarian for examination. Any time a domestic animal that has been confined develops symptoms of rabies, it should also be killed and the head sent for examination.

Rabies treatment utilizes a rabies vaccine in conjunction with rabies serum (Table 41-4). The vaccine allows the child to develop his own

POTENTIAL STRESSES DURING PRESCHOOL YEARS: TEMPORARY ALTERATIONS IN HEALTH STATUS

TABLE 41-4 RECOMMENDED PROPHYLACTIC THERAPY FOR RABIES*

Nature of Exposure	Status of Biting Animal	Recommended Treatment
Single bite, minor wound or lick of broken skin (legs, arms, trunk).	a. Suspected as rabid. Unprovoked bite in endemic area. Domestic animal.	Start vaccine. Stop treatment if animal remains healthy after 5 days.
	b. Rabid animal. Animal unavailable for observation. Wild animal.	Serum and vaccine; given in 14 daily injections. Booster shots 10 and 20 days after series.
Multiple bites, major wounds (face, head, neck or finger); licks of mucosa.	Suspect or rabid animal. Unprovoked bite in endemic area. Animal unavailable for observation. Wild animal.	Serum and vaccine; given in 21 daily injections or 2 daily injections for 7 days, then one daily for 7 more days. Booster shots 10 and 20 days after primary series.

*As defined by the World Health Association Expert Committee on Rabies, U.S.P.H.S.

active immunity. The injections are very painful and often produce uncomfortable side effects including pruritus, pain and tenderness at the injection site. Occasionally the injections cause low-grade fever, confusion or shock. Epinephrine should always be on hand when injections are given for use in counteracting shock. The subcutaneous injections are usually given in rotation in the abdomen, the lower back and the lateral aspect of the thigh. Researchers are currently investigating the use of interferon as a viable rabies treatment.[7]

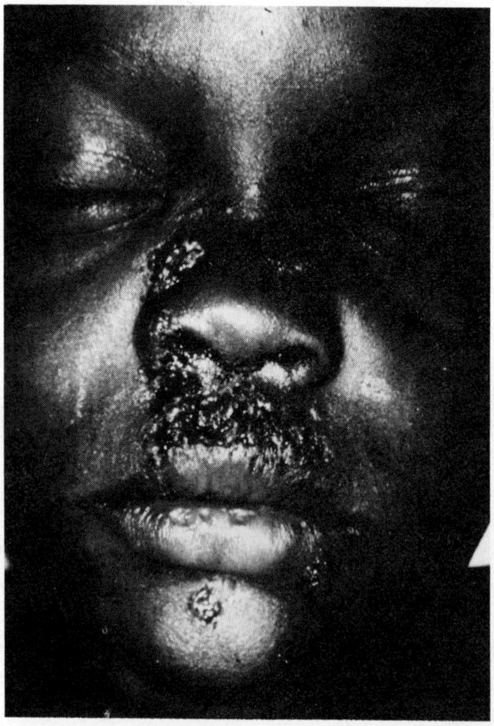

Passive immunity is provided with a hyperimmune antirabies serum that is injected in and around the wound within the first 24 hours after the bite. Sensitivity must be evaluated, since horse serum is used. Human rabies immune globulin is being researched and is being used in persons sensitive to the horse serum.[7]

The child and his parents will need substantial psychological support and preparation to cope with the long and painful treatment as well as the gravity of the situation. Instruction should be given regarding the side effects and their relief. Reassurance should be offered as to the satisfactory results obtained by prophylactic antirabies treatment in preventing this dreaded disease.

PEDICULOSIS CAPITIS (HEAD LICE)

Approximately three million cases of head lice are diagnosed annually in the United States alone. Females are affected twice as often as males, despite the trend for males to wear long hair. Pediculosis is 20 times more prevalent in whites than in other racial groups, presumably because of the difference in the makeup of the hair shaft.[8] The peak incidence is in preschool and early school-age youngsters, with a steady decline after that age until about sixth grade, when the incidence again rises somewhat.

The bloodsucking louse lives its entire life (nit

Figure 41-2 The characteristic distribution of impetigo is about the nose and chin. (From M. Green and R. J. Haggerty, Ambulatory Pediatrics, 2nd ed. W. B. Saunders Co., 1977.)

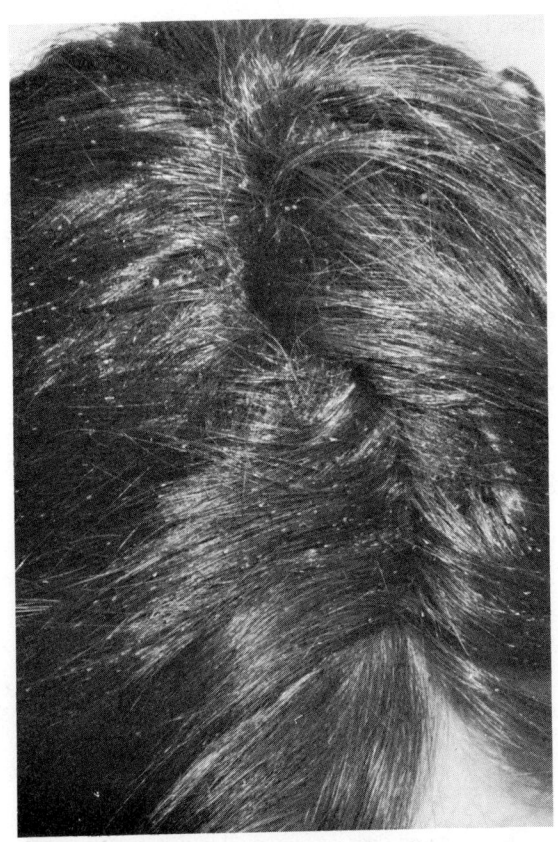

Figure 41–3 Nits on scalp hair. (From A. Domonkos, Andrews' Diseases of the Skin. W. B. Saunders Co., 1971.)

or egg to nymph to adult louse) on the head of the child it infests. The eggs, called *nits,* attach to the hair shaft by a cement-like substance and hatch within a week (Fig. 41-3). The hatched nymph matures into a mature louse in another week to 10 days and punctures the scalp with its hook-like claws to suck blood. It remains attached until it is dislodged or dies (about one month).

A child is infested either by direct contact or from fomites (comb, headgear, play wigs, clothing). Human head lice do not jump from head to head unless there is direct contact, nor are they transferred from one person to another in the breeze.[4] The nits are not communicable; only the hatched louse is. These insects avoid light or perspiration.

A week after the child is bitten, he develops an allergic response evidenced by a mild fever, malaise, intense scalp itching and enlarged cervical and occipital nodes. After a prolonged exposure, the body's sensitivity is diminished and the child becomes oblivious to the bites, i.e., asymptomatic. Occasionally a child will develop focal alopecia due to the allergic response. The nits can be seen as silvery or grayish-white, smooth and glistening specks resembling dandruff but securely attached to the hair shaft near the scalp. (Prominent locations are behind the ears and the nape of the neck.) The adult louse can be seen as a minute black speck that moves and jumps on the scalp and hair. The child's scratching during the period of allergic reactivity may result in secondary infections.

Diagnosis is made by identification of the nits and lice using a magnifying glass and strong direct lighting or a Wood's lamp. Microscopic examination differentiates the head louse from the body louse or from aphids, which can carry other diseases. Examination of the scalp is done by parting the hair in several places (especially in the region behind the ears and nape of the neck) with two applicator sticks, moving systematically from side to side and front to back. The magnifying glass or Wood's lamp is then used to inspect the exposed scalp and hair for nits and lice.

Treatment is both preventive and corrective. Preventively, children should be taught not to exchange combs, brushes, headgear or clothing with other children. Keeping hair short and clean may also help prevent infestation. At home and in settings in which a group of children are gathered, individually assigned hooks or lockers for wraps and possessions help decrease the incidence and spread of the louse. (The adult louse may survive one to two days away from the scalp.) Children found to be infested should be confined at home until 24 hours after treatment is complete to minimize spread to others. It is generally recommended that all family members be treated simultaneously; often louse infestation is so widespread that entire classrooms or schools of children are encouraged to undergo treatment. (The treatment may actually be carried out at school with parental approval.)

Corrective treatment involves three activities: (1) using medicated shampoo, (2) disinfecting fomites and (3) examination of contacts. Nonprescription (RID [includes a fine-tooth comb]; Triple X) or prescription shampoo with a pyrethrin or benzene derivative may be used and should be applied exactly according to directions. The child prone to eczema may have an allergic response to the shampoo. The shampooing must be done vigorously to be effec-

POTENTIAL STRESSES DURING PRESCHOOL YEARS: TEMPORARY ALTERATIONS IN HEALTH STATUS

tive. After the shampoo, the hair is combed (teasing backward) with a fine-tooth comb, preferably outdoors, to remove any remaining nits. All the nits must be removed. Sometimes dipping the comb in vinegar helps to loosen tightly attached nits. Itching may continue for three or four days after the insecticide shampoo, but if pruritus lasts longer than this, it is evidence of more nits and lice requiring retreatment.

All contactable items should be laundered in hot water and dried in sunlight or a clothes dryer (20 minutes on high) or ironed. Non-launderable items may be soaked in 2 per cent Lysol or one of the pediculocidal shampoos for an hour or heated in water (65° C) for 5 to 10 minutes.

All the child's contacts should be examined and treated if necessary. Family members must be treated simultaneously with the child to prevent immediate reinfestation.

Panic and anger are typical responses of parents and school officials when pediculosis is discovered. The nurse or school nurse often receives the brunt of their reaction and must learn to accept this response syndrome without taking it personally. Preventive education as well as education as to the cause, transfer and treatment of this disease prior to any major occurrence may help allay some of these negative reactions. When a diagnosis is made, feelings of guilt, shame and uncleanliness are usually provoked in the child or his caretakers or both. Constant reassurance offered by the nurse that the child is not unclean because he contracted head lice and that parents cannot be responsible if their child uses other children's possessions or comes in close contact with other children during play often produces better cooperation and reduces parental aggressive responses. School or community funds may be required to make treatment possible for children of low-income families who cannot afford the costs involved in treatment. Involvement of community health nurses may be necessary if a family's cooperation is questionable or if infestation is widespread in the community.

HORDEOLUM (STYE)

A stye is the result of an acute infection of the glands on the margin of the eyelid that produces a small abscess. There will be pain and redness, localized on the lid margin, with preauricular lymph node enlargement. The lid around the area may become tender and swollen. Superficial abscesses come to a head and rupture spontaneously with complete healing without treatment. If the abscess does not come to a head (point) on its own within one to two days, treatment consists of localizing the abscess by applying hot, wet compresses for 20 to 30 minutes four to six times a day followed by application of a topical antibiotic or sulfa ointment. If the condition does not improve, a culture and sensitivity test may be necessary to find an effective medication. Preschoolers who have repeated styes should have their vision checked, because while a stye has nothing to do with vision problems, the child with a refractive error does a lot of rubbing, and this can contribute to the development of styes. If styes tend to occur in crops, underlying staphylococcal infection usually exists, requiring both local and systemic antibiotic treatment. Rarely, incision and drainage of the abscess may be required.

References

1. A. Benenson, ed. Communicable Diseases in Man. American Public Health Association, 1975
2. S. Cohen and M. Ziai. Viral infections. In Pediatrics by M. Ziai ed., Little, Brown & Co., 1975
3. Communicable disease control in the school. Bulletin C17, Michigan Department of Public Health, June 1978
4. V. Harlin et al. Pediculosis. Its transmission and treatment in the schools. Journal of School Health, June 1977, p. 346
5. J. Hughes. Synopsis of Pediatrics. C. V. Mosby Co., 1979
6. J. Parrish. Dermatology and Skin Care. McGraw-Hill Book Co., 1975
7. E. Vella. Research in rabies. Nursing Times, 17 March 1977, p. 37
8. L. Welsh. Pediculosis at summer camp. American Journal of Nursing, June 1979, p. 1073
9. WHO Expert Committee on Rabies. Sixth report: local treatment of wounds involving possible exposure to rabies. In Communicable Disease Control Public Health Notes by United States Public Health Service, August 1973

Additional Recommended Reading

S. Cohen and G. Glass. Skin rashes in infants and children. American Journal of Nursing, June 1978, p. 1041

R. O. Grady and T. Dolan. Whooping cough in infancy. American Journal of Nursing, Jan. 1976, p. 114

P. Koblenzer. Common bacterial infections of the skin in children. Pediatric Clinics of North America, May 1978, p. 321

J. Leaning. Post-exposure treatment of rabies. Nursing Times, 17 March 1977, p. 377

A. Rice. Common skin infections in school children. American Journal of Nursing, Nov. 1973, p. 1905

N. Welsh. Recent insights into the childhood "social diseases" — gonorrhea, scabies, pediculosis, pinworms. Clinical Pediatrics, April 1978, p. 320

42

POTENTIAL STRESSES DURING PRESCHOOL YEARS: REVERSIBLE ALTERATIONS IN HEALTH STATUS

REACTIONS OF THE PRESCHOOLER AND FAMILY TO REVERSIBLE ILLNESS

by Mabel Hunsberger, BSN, MSN

A preschooler is talkative, energetic and playful. His cognitive ability is still limited (preoperational). Thus he continues to view the world egocentrically; he thinks in concrete terms and his reasoning is transductive (from one particular to another particular). His development affects the type of illness to which he is vulnerable and has an impact on his psychological response to illness.

A preschooler is more vulnerable to certain illnesses because of increased exposure to organisms as he encounters the world beyond home in day care, nursery school or kindergarten. Increased independence in self-care may make the preschooler more vulnerable to specific problems, such as urinary tract infections. Surgical interventions during this period may be required to correct gradually developing problems or for the correction of problems identified at some earlier time. Illnesses discussed in this chapter require varying lengths of time for correction or resolution, but they are not likely to have long-term effects. The nurse who cares for a preschooler with a reversible illness must be knowledgeable about the specific illness and also have some understanding of a preschooler's perception of and behavioral responses to illness. Furthermore, the nurse should be sensitive to the nature of the stress experienced by the child's family. Each child and family have unique needs during illness. The following discussion includes general reactions that the nurse should be prepared to encounter while caring for a preschooler who is ill.

A PRESCHOOLER'S PERCEPTION OF ILLNESS

When an illness is reversible, those who care for a preschooler are comforted by the knowledge that the existing problem will be corrected. The preschooler, however, does not understand the source of his illness, how long he will be ill, nor the source of the cure. Reversible illness for a preschooler can thus cause considerable stress that an adult can overlook if he fails to understand the preschooler's viewpoint. Bibace and Walsh[1] have developed useful categories to describe a child's perception of illness. They tested children from 3 to 13 years of age by using 12 "how" and "why" questions regarding illness. The categories, in sequence, according to stages of cognitive development are as follows: (1) phenomenism and contagion (preoperational); (2) contamination and internalization (concrete operational) and (3) physiological and psychophysiological (formal operational). A preschooler is in the preoperational stage and perceives illness primarily through *phenominism* and *contagion*.

Phenominism The phenomena that are identified by children as the cause of illness are usually sensory (sight or sound) but are "spatially remote and inappropriate."[1] The relationships between the phenomena and the illness cannot be explained; the causal link is one of magic or merely that the illness and the phenomena occur at the same time. For example, in response to a question about how someone got a certain illness, a preschooler might reply "from the sun" or "from the wind." A 4-year-old's explanation of illness as quoted by Bibace and Walsh follows:

> Do you remember anyone who was sick? "Yup, my brother." What was wrong? "He goed to the hospital." How did he get sick? "The wind, and he went to the doctor." How did the wind make him sick? "The wind. . . ." How did he get better? "Then he came home."

This example reflects the preschooler's centering on a concrete, single phenomenon of his own experience and without any specification of the causal link.

Contagion The child defines illness in terms of external persons, objects or events, but the source is *near to* the ill person, or the causative event occurred *before* the illness. A child who perceives illness in this way still cannot explain the causal link; illness is explained merely in terms of spatial or temporal proximity. The child sees himself as a victim of illness, but his vulnerability is more restricted. An example of a 4-year-old's explanation quoted from Bibace and Walsh follows:

> What is a heart attack? "A heart attack is falling down." Why do people get heart attacks? "You went on the bus and then you came home." How does going on the bus give someone a heart attack? "Cuz it does."

The connection between the source of illness (or cure) and the actual illness is not explained; however, compared to phenomenism the identified source is closer to the person and generally more appropriate.[1]

A preschooler's perception of illness and its cure has implications for those who care for him. He needs special help to understand that something he did is not the cause of his illness. The source of the cure is usually perceived as a person or object in close proximity or as an event occurring after the illness. The components of treatment do not necessarily fall within these definitions of " a cure." Thus a preschooler may not necessarily cooperate in a specified treatment regimen.

To help the preschooler understand his illness the nurse can make the objects and equipment related to his treatment part of his immediate environment. Handling equipment and using it in imaginative play can be encouraged to help a preschooler cope with the events surrounding his illness.

A PRESCHOOLER'S RESPONSE TO ILLNESS

A preschooler has mastered many social skills and is becoming increasingly able to tolerate separation from his parents. However, his caretakers must recognize that during illness he may demonstrate behaviors that are not consistent with his usual pattern.

Mattsson and Weisberg[4] described reactions by preschoolers during minor illnesses for which they were not hospitalized. During the acute phase of illness all children showed behavioral changes. Two distinct patterns emerged regarding their relationship with their mother in particular. Reaction I (primarily in 2-year-olds) was characterized by a clinging, whiny dependence with extreme irritability and intolerance of frustration. Reaction II (in those over 3 years of age) was characterized by a diminished interest in physical and verbal contact with a withdrawal into a "self-contained, undemanding state." These children appeared at times to be "more independent than usual" and "easy to manage."[4] The self-contained behavior may suggest a withdrawal of interest in the environment by the child, and an increased focus on his body and its needs during illness.[4]

During the convalescent phase, as the previous state of health is re-established, a change in behavior may be demonstrated. Mattsson and Weisberg noted in all children, regardless of age, an increased irritability and episodes of anger of one to five days' duration during convalescence.[4] Thus, at the time when a preschooler is expected to behave as usual because he is getting better, he may actually become more irritable and difficult to handle.

If a preschooler is hospitalized or subjected to a variety of unfamiliar procedures during an illness, additional stresses are imposed upon him. He is fearful of abandonment, punishment and bodily injury. To reduce the severity of responses to reversible illness with or without hospitalization his caretakers must give special attention to alleviating those fears associated with the illness. It has been suggested that especially preschool-age children in intensive care situations should be touched by staff members at times other than when procedures are being carried out on them; preschoolers are receptive to touch and can be soothed and calmed by it.[2] The use of a low tone of voice when explaining procedures is another suggested technique that helps frightened preschoolers gain self-control; the child has to quiet down to hear what is being said.[3] (See Chapter 45 for further discussion of the preschooler who is hospitalized.)

RESPONSE OF PARENTS AND SIBLINGS

A reversible illness may occur as an emergency or it may develop over a period of time. Regardless of the type of illness, parents are put under considerable stress by the behavorial change in their child that results and the increased demands on time necessary to provide the required physical care. An increased demand for attention by the preschooler can also be a cause of jealousy of siblings. Older siblings can be made to feel important and less in competition if they assist with tasks involved in the care of the preschooler rather than merely doing an increased share of usual household tasks.

When a preschooler demonstrates a self-contained, nondemanding type of behavior, parents and siblings can assist him by sitting quietly nearby. Activities introduced should be consistent with the mood of the preschooler. A stable, accepting environment helps a preschooler to feel secure even though he is ill.

When specific interventions are required parents need assistance in preparing the child for the prescribed treatment. Fears can be reduced by preparing preschoolers through play pertaining to the treatment, reading about it and verbal explanations. Siblings can participate in these activities to increase their own awareness of the ill child's problem.

The parents and siblings should be prepared for typical reactions during the convalescent phase. It is when a preschooler begins to feel more energtic that a period of more demanding behavior and irritability may emerge. Parents and siblings must direct this energy into appropriate activities, otherwise this behavior can become a source of conflict among and annoyance to all family members. The usual forms of discipline should be maintained throughout the course of illness.

Those who care for a preschooler need to be patient and gentle. He does not understand how he became ill nor that the illness will pass; his concern is what will happen today, and if it will hurt.

References

1. R. Bibace and M. E. Walsh. Developmental stages in children's conceptions of illness. In Health Psychology — A Handbook, G. C. Stone et al., eds., Jassey-Bass Publishers, 1979
2. R. M. Carty. Observed behaviors of preschoolers to intensive care. Pediatric Nursing, Jul/Aug 1970, p. 21
3. K. F. Gaffney. The preschooler in the emergency department. Journal of Emergency Nursing, December 1976, p. 15
4. A. Mattsson and I. Weisberg. Behavioral reactions to minor illness in preschool children. Pediatrics, October 1970, p. 604

RESPIRATORY CONDITIONS AND RELATED PROBLEMS

by Mabel Hunsberger, BSN, MSN

During the preschool years a child is particularly vulnerable to respiratory problems because of the increased exposure to organisms at child care centers, nursery school and kindergarten. Early recognition and proper management can prevent long-term consequences or a life-threatening condition. The nurse plays an important role in early intervention through the questions she asks, advice she gives to parents (especially over the phone), and care of the child during an acute illness.

PHARYNGOTONSILLITIS

Pharyngotonsillitis is an inflammation of the structures in the pharynx, including the tonsils. (Tonsillitis occurs in all cases of pharyngitis[13]). Pharyngotosonsillitis occurs at all ages but has a peak incidence during the late preschool and early school-age years. This is the time when a child is exposed to more infections outside the home. A natural hypertrophy of lymphoid tissue also develops at this time, shown in enlarged tonsils and adenoids.

The two most common causes of pharyngotonsillitis are viruses and Group A beta-hemolytic streptococci (referred to as strep throat). About 80 per cent of cases are caused by a virus and 20 per cent or less are bacterial in origin. In children less than 3 years of age the bacterium *Hemophilus influenzae* is common; streptococcal pharyngitis is rare before 2 years of age.

Viral and streptococcal pharyngitis cannot be reliably differentiated by clinical manifestations. Some characteristics of each are summarized in Table 42–1, but even these overlap considerably. Streptococcal pharyngotonsillitis thus can not be reliably diagnosed without a throat culture.

Management Viral pharyngitis is treated symptomatically, whereas streptococcal infections require antibiotics to prevent complications (especially rheumatic fever and glomerulonephritis). In viral pharyngotonsillitis aspirin generally brings about a prompt reduction in fever, whereas in streptococcal infections fever usually persists. On the other hand, antimicrobial therapy (penicillin) is so effective in streptococcal pharyngotonsillitis that fever does not usually persist longer than 24 hours after initiation of therapy.

The method of administering antibiotics varies. It is generally safe to wait for the results of the throat culture before instituting therapy.[5, 10] An exception to this is a patient with a history of acute rheumatic fever; in this case treatment should begin at the onset of pharyngitis.[10] Penicillin is the drug of choice. It can be administered orally for 10 days or by one intramuscular injection. The advantage of intramuscular injection is that the problem of lack of compliance is eliminated; however, it is a painful mode of treatment. Unless streptococcal disease has been confirmed, it is unreasonable to subject a child to this therapy when he may not need it.[5] If compliance is a problem and streptococcal infection is confirmed, one dose of benzathine penicillin is given intramuscularly to ensure adequate penicillin levels for a 10-day period. If the child is allergic to penicillin the drug of choice is erythromycin for 10 days.

The nurse has an important role in obtaining a complete health history with particular attention to the history of the illness. The nurse should also gather sufficient data to make a recommendation regarding the mode of therapy (oral or intramuscular) that would be most appropriate for the particular family.

If the child is to receive a 10-day course of antibiotics, the nurse must emphasize the importance of continuing the medication even though the child feels well and is free of symptoms. If intramuscular penicillin is to be administered, both the child and parents must be forewarned of the pain associated with the injection. Local measures can be suggested to provide relief at home, including warm baths and use of a heating pad or a warm water bottle;

TABLE 42-1 CHARACTERISTICS OF BACTERIAL AND VIRAL PHARYNGOTONSILLITIS*

	Streptococcal Pharyngotonsillitis		Viral Pharyngotonsillitis
	<2 Years of Age	>2 Years of Age	Any Age
Onset	Gradual or sudden	Sudden	Gradual
Presenting signs	Nasopharyngitis	Abdominal pain, vomiting, headache	Sore throat (often preceded by malaise and anorexia)
Fever	Slight to moderate (rarely, 102°F), often irregular	Usually high (103–104°F), but may be moderate	Slight to moderate, sometimes high (reduced by aspirin)
Tonsillar involvement	Little or none	May have any or all of following: follicular exudation, erythema of tonsils and pillars, petechnial mottling of soft palate, lymphadenopathy; or mild-to-moderate tonsillar or pharyngeal inflammation	Similar to streptococcal, although petechial mottling is less common and erythema is often less
Clinical complaints	Anorexia, runny nose, listlessness, failure to thrive, vomiting	Sore throat	Sore throat, hoarseness, cough, rhinitis, conjunctivitis
Lab results	Leukocytosis	Leukocytosis	Leukocyte count normal to high

From H. F. Eichenwald. Respiratory Infections in Children. Hospital Practice, April 1976, p. 83.
*In many children there is considerable overlap in symptomatology of viral and streptococcal disease.

parents should be cautioned to never apply a heating pad without constant attendance.

Additional symptomatic measures for sore throat include cool bland liquids, aspirin or Tylenol, warm compresses to the neck, and warm normal saline gargles (if the child is able to gargle). Parents should be counselled not to force the child to eat and to avoid liquids and foods that are irritating to the throat, especially citrus and spicy foods. The nurse should also advise the family to report similar symptoms in other family members. Recurrent streptococcal pharyngotonsillitis within the family is an indication for all family members to have cultures done.

Viral pharyngotonsillitis is usually self-limiting, requiring only symptomatic treatment. Streptococcal pharyngotonsillitis if adequately treated generally results in complete recovery. Both nonsuppurative (rheumatic fever and glomerulonephritis) and suppurative (peritonsillar abscess, otitis media, mastoiditis, cervical adenitis, meningitis, osteomyelitis, pneumonia) complications usually can be prevented with prompt treatment. Recurrent pharyngotonsillitis is no longer a universally accepted indication for a tonsillectomy.[2]

DISEASED TONSILS AND ADENOIDS

In its common usage the word tonsils refers to the two faucial tonsils (palatine) on either side of the opening of the oral cavity into the pharynx (see Fig. 13-15, Chapter 13). Adenoids (pharyngeal tonsils) are located in the midline of the posterior wall of the nasopharynx. Tonsils and adenoids, along with other lymphoid tissue, trap infection from the upper respiratory tract; tonsils also have the capacity to produce antibodies and have an important function in immunity. The size of lymphoid tissue increases to that of an adult when the child is around 6 years of age, almost doubles by age 10, then gradually shrinks to normal adult size by age 20.[8] During early childhood lymphoid tissue (including tonsils and adenoids) responds to infection by becoming larger.[6]

Indications for removal of tonsils and adenoids is a subject of much controversy. Although the nurse may not play a primary role in the decision regarding removal of tonsils and adenoids, an awareness of the nature of the controversy is helpful in her discussions with the family. It is important for the nurse to have a clear understanding of the explanation that has been given to the family by the physician regarding the need for tonsillectomy and adenoidectomy ("T & A").

Although T & A is the most frequently performed operation in children requiring anesthesia in the United States, controversy about its benefits continues. The ultimate evaluation of T & A is made by weighing the potential benefits it can provide against potential risks.[7] Some physicians still perform T & A to treat recurrent sore throats, while others recommend that it be done only in rare circumstances. Indications for the operation have not been agreed upon, but certain conditions exist in which most physicians would agree that a tonsillectomy, adenoidectomy or both is required. These are: (1) alveolar hypoventilation or cor pulmonale, (2) dysphagia, (3) sensorineural or conductive hearing loss, (4) chronic mastoiditis, (5) cholesteatoma and (6) malignancy.[7] It is also generally agreed that adenoidectomy may be indicated alone* in children under 4 years of age and that tonsillectomy is preferably deferred until after 5 years of age.

Management Once the decision has been made that removal of tonsils and adenoids is necessary, the nurse's attention should be focused on preparing the child and family for the surgical experience and providing optimal postoperative nursing care to prevent complications. Frequently the child is admitted to the hospital the evening before surgery, although some authorities recommend that the child sleep at home the night before surgery and be admitted the morning of surgery.[12] The child should be prepared for hospitalization and various procedures according to his age. (See chapters on hospitalization for specific age-related preparation.)

The nurse should perform a complete health assessment on admission, including a careful evaluation of the child's respiratory status. T & A should not be performed until several weeks after an upper respiratory infection has cleared. An elevated temperature should be reported to the surgeon. The child and the family should be assessed to identify allergies, a history of bleeding tendency, or a family history of cholinesterase deficiency.[12] In addition to these factors a submucous cleft palate (soft palate with little or no muscle) is a contraindication for adenoidectomy. It may be recognized by hypernasal speech, a history of frequent otitis media, a bifid uvula, and a palpable V-shaped notch in the posterior edge of the hard palate.[7,12]

Preoperatively the child and his parents should be prepared for what the child will experience before and following surgery. Many hospitals have special programs to prepare a child for surgery, including a film or slide-tape, a prehospitalization tour, and a play program that provides an opportunity for the child to manipulate equipment and supplies that he will see during the preoperative and postoperative experience.

Physical preparation of the child should also be explained to the child and family. Usually the child will have prothrombin time (PT) and partial thromboplastin time (PTT) tested in addition to routine admission laboratory tests of hemoglobin, hematocrit and urinalysis. Foods and liquids are withheld for eight hours before the operation to prevent vomiting with aspiration. Preoperative medication includes an injection of atropine or scopalamine to inhibit secretions and Nembutal, Demerol, or Vistaril for sedation (if needed).[3]

Special attention should also be given to the child's actual understanding of the procedure. A young child may fear "being cut" and does not understand that his operation will be done through the mouth and that an incision is not made through the neck. The child and the parents should be prepared for the child's sore throat after surgery, including explanations of what will be done for it.

Anesthesia may be given by endotracheal intubation or inhalation. The majority of tonsillectomies in children can be performed safely without intubation if the airway is safeguarded.[3] Adenoidectomy by curettage is usually performed first, followed by the tonsillectomy. The tonsils are removed by surgical dissection, with the lower pole of the tonsil being severed by scissors or a snare. Tonsillectomy and adenoidectomy may also be done separately or in conjunction with myringotomy and tube insertion. Bleeding should be controlled before the child leaves the operating room.

Postoperatively the bed is kept in a flat position, and the child is placed in a side-lying or abdominal position with the upper knee flexed. This permits the tongue and jaw to come forward and secretions and vomitus to drain from the mouth, preventing aspiration. Vital signs are checked every 15 minutes beginning immediately after the child returns from the recovery room; the nurse should watch for tachycardia, which indicates bleeding. Additionally, the child should be checked for pallor and excessive swallowing. (Swallowing indicates that blood is trickling down the child's throat.) The child's face is often flushed because of the atropine that was given preoperatively. Codeine

---

*Removal of both tonsils and adenoids in very young children may stimulate hyperplasia of other lymphoid tissue in the oropharynx.[3]

or acetaminophen are used for pain as needed, but this is seldom severe after the second postoperative day. An ice collar wrapped in a soft material and applied to comfortably fit the contour of the child's neck provides some relief of pain. Once the child is fully awake and vital signs are stable, fluids are given cautiously. Small amounts of cold liquids should be given until the danger of vomiting has passed. The most easily tolerated form of intake is a Popsicle or ice chips. The child should be observed for excessive swallowing, pallor and any change in vital signs throughout the night.

Most children can be discharged the day after surgery. Parents should be advised against giving their child hot, coarse or spicy foods for five to seven days; swimming is generally discouraged until the follow-up visit in 10 to 14 days, and any signs of bleeding should be promptly reported to the physician. A late hemorrhage (5 to 10 days after surgery) is associated with infection of the upper respiratory tract. Thus it is advisable during the recovery period to limit exposure to other children who are known to have colds. The hemorrhage occurs when the tissue (eschar) that normally forms over the raw surfaces separates prematurely in the presence of infection; parents should be aware of this but should not be made to feel that it is likely to happen. Analgesics may be necessary for the first few days after surgery for throat pain and referred pain to the ears, but pain should not persist beyond the first week.

STREPTOCOCCAL PNEUMONIA

With the availability of antibiotic therapy pneumonia has become a rare complication of Group A beta-hemolytic streptococcal infection. In the preantibiotic era it accounted for up to 25 per cent of all bacterial pneumonia and resulted in a high mortality rate.[11] Streptococcal pneumonia* most commonly occurs in children 5 to 6 years of age through young adulthood.[11] It is most frequently associated with rubeola, varicella, and scarlet fever.[14]

Most children experience a mild illness (slight fever, myalgia, sore throat) of only a few days followed by an abrupt onset of high fever, chills, pleuritic chest pain, cough, respiratory distress, and occasionally hemoptysis. X-ray findings are variable, resembling those in viral infection (interstitial pneumonia) or the purulent pneumonia seen in staphylococcal infections. (See Chapter 24 for further discussion of the various types of pneumonia.) Pleural effusion suggests a probable bacterial pneumonia; a pleural tap is required for identification of the organism and initiation of appropriate antibiotic therapy.

Management Treatment varies with the clinical findings and degree of illness. If the effusion is small, repeated plural taps may be sufficient; if the fluid contains pus (empyema), closed-chest tube drainage is necessary.[4] In some instances intubation for mechanical respiratory assistance is indicated. Large doses of intravenous or intramuscular penicillin G are usually required. The usual supportive care for a child with pneumonia includes giving oxygen and intravenous fluids and providing chest physical therapy. It is recommended that a child with dyspnea receive oxygen even though cyanosis is not apparent.[4] Intravenous fluids are administered if the child is poorly hydrated and for intravenous antibiotic administration.

The treatment phase includes numerous procedures that are painful and frightening to the preschooler, and cause parents worry. They need assistance from the health team to cope with their fears.

The most common complication is empyema. Early and vigorous chest drainage is used to prevent development of pulmonary complications later (see procedures in Chapter 17.) Acute rheumatic fever is not reported to follow streptococcal pneumonia; however, pericarditis has been reported in 1 to 10 per cent of patients with streptococcal pneumonia.[11]

EPIGLOTTITIS (SUPRAGLOTTITIS)

Epiglottitis is an acute infection of the epiglottis with a potentially fatal outcome. The epiglottis is swollen, cherry-red in appearance, and surrounded by copious secretions. The infection occurs most commonly in children between 3 to 8 years of age and is almost always caused by *H. influenzae* (Type B).

Symptoms of mild upper respiratory infection may or may not precede the sudden onset of the classic symptoms of epiglottitis. Over a period of several hours the child develops high fever,

---

*Streptococcal pneumonia in this chapter is used to describe pneumonia caused by Group A beta-hemolytic streptococcus. Pneumonia caused by Group B streptococcus, seen in neonates, is discussed in Chapter 24.

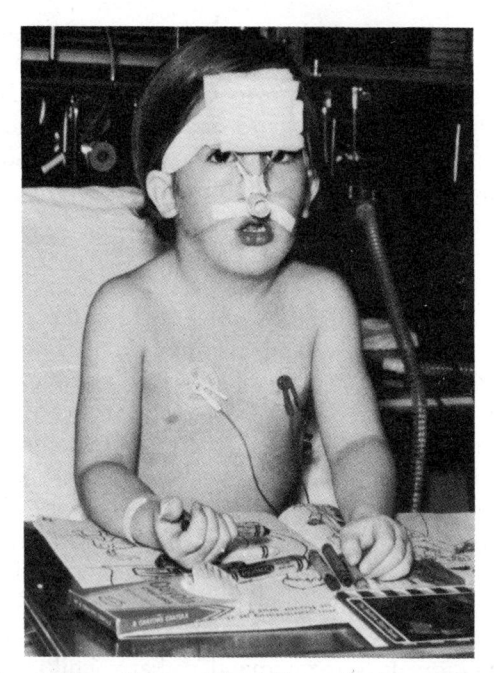

Figure 42-1 Young child with intubation treatment for supraglottitis. Nasotracheal tubes are well tolerated by most children. (From G. Barker. Current Management of Croup and Epiglottitis. Pediatric Clinics of North America, August 1979, p. 576.)

severe sore throat with dysphagia, and rapidly progresses to a state of severe respiratory distress with some inspiratory stridor, a prominent respiratory snore, and retractions. The general appearance of the child is suggestive of the diagnosis. Typically he leans forward with chin thrust forward, his mouth open with drooling that occurs because swallowing is too painful. The condition may worsen rapidly, with complete obstruction occurring within 6 to 12 hours from the time of onset.

A tentative diagnosis is based on the history and clinical presentation. Treatment is immediately instituted when there is clinical evidence that the child has epiglottitis. Under no circumstances should a throat swab be attempted before an airway is established.[1] Placing the child in a recumbent position or using a tongue depressor may produce instant obstruction and is avoided until the child is moved to a facility in which skilled personnel have appropriate equipment to establish an airway. Although x-rays of the neck may show a swollen epiglottis, they are not done without personnel in attendance who are capable of establishing an airway.

Management The nurse has an important role in the early management of these children. To avoid the catastrophe of bringing on obstruction of the airway, all team members must recognize the symptoms of epiglottitis. The nurse's ability to remain calm can reduce the child's and parent's anxiety during the emergency phase. The nurse should not leave the child unattended even momentarily until an artificial airway is established. The child is allowed to assume a position of comfort and is not asked to lie down. He is left undisturbed: no procedures are done that would cause crying or excitement. The immediate intervention is establishment of an artificial airway.

Although most authorities agree that it is unsafe not to establish an artificial airway, the preferred method of intervention is not universally agreed upon. Until the early 1960s tracheostomy was generally the accepted method of treatment, but because of the associated morbidity, mortality and length of hospital stay, alternative methods have been investigated. Nasotracheal intubation has now become the preferred method and is usually well tolerated, but its acceptance varies and some controversy continues. To maintain a nasotracheal tube a highly skilled staff must be available 24 hours a day to provide emergency care in the event of accidental extubation. Thus, in some centers in which such a staff is not available, tracheotomy is the recommended technique.[1]

Appropriate antibiotic therapy is also initiated immediately. With increasing reports of infections from ampicillin-resistant *H. influenzae*, the recommended treatment is now combined therapy using chloramphenicol (100 mg/kg/24 hrs) and ampicillin (200 to 400 mg/kg/24 hrs) intravenously. When results of antibiotic sensitivity testing are obtained, the specific effective antibiotic is continued and the other one discontinued.

The child with an artificial airway requires respiratory care, including direct humidification of the airway, physical therapy, tracheal suctioning and constant observation for signs of respiratory difficulty (increased pulse and respiration, retractions, restlessness, cyanosis). Mist can be delivered through a hood or a mist tent, whichever is most comfortable for the child. An intravenous line is required to deliver the antibiotics and maintenance fluids. These children are usually not dehydrated because they have been well until just before the rapid onset of symptoms. Accidental extubation must be prevented by applying appropriate restraints when the child is unattended; elbow restraints are usually sufficient.

A nasotracheal tube is usually kept in place 24 to 36 hours. After extubation the child is observed in the intensive care unit in a mist tent for 24 hours, then transferred to a pediatric unit. One or two days later he is discharged on antibiotics. Epiglottitis seldom recurs, but the frightening experience is not easily forgotten by the child or the family.[1]

HENOCH-SCHONLEIN PURPURA

Henoch-Schonlein purpura is a systemic disease of the vessels characterized by a purpuric skin eruption. Purpura is the term for any hemorrhagic disease characterized by extravasation of blood into the skin, mucous membranes and visceral tissues.) A generalized vascular disorder, Henoch-Schonlein purpura involves the arterioles and capillaries. The characteristic hemorrhagic rash occurs in association with gastrointestinal symptoms, joint manifestations, and, in older children, renal disease. The incidence seems to be increasing and is most common in children between 2 and 8 years of age with a 2:1 ratio of male to female.[9]

The etiology is unknown, but reports have implicated a hypersensitive response to infections (especially upper respiratory), food and drug allergies, or insect bites. The significance of a preceding streptococcal infection is uncertain.[15] Although this problem is little understood, we do know that the immune system deviates in such a way that allergens attack the surface of some cells and alter them so that the cells of the small vessels themselves produce allergens. In this way the child literally becomes allergic to his own tissues; his capillaries become fragile and permeable.

Clinical manifestations vary, depending on the parts of the body affected by vasculitis. Variable degrees of malaise, low-grade fever and anorexia may be associated with the illness. The three most common symptoms are skin eruption, joint pain and abdominal pain. These occur individually, simultaneously or sequentially.

A characteristic skin eruption is at first like that of urticaria, then progresses to a red maculopapular rash that become hemorrhagic. The rash typically shows various stages of discolorations, as is typical of any bruised area. The distribution of the rash usually involves the buttocks, extensor surfaces of the arms and legs, and lower part of the trunk but may extend to other parts of the body. Colicky abdominal pain, nausea and vomiting and occult blood in the feces are caused by the edematous and hemorrhagic intestinal wall. Occasionally perforation or intussusception (telescoping of the bowel) occurs as a complication. Joints may be puffy, warm, painful and tender, but usually are not affected for more than a few days.

Renal involvement, potentially the most serious manifestation, tends to occur early in the course of illness and is most typical in older children. While most children have no long-term effects following the acute phase, some develop chronic renal disease.

The diagnosis is made primarily on the basis of the clinical findings. The platelet count and coagulation studies are usually normal. If there is renal involvement, urinary findings include hematuria, proteinuria and casts.

Management Treatment is generally symptomatic. Contact with any identified allergen is avoided and any accompanying upper respiratory infection is treated. Corticosteroids may be beneficial if symptoms are severe, especially when there is gastrointestinal or joint involvement. Corticosteroids are thought to reduce the likelihood of an intussusception and generally provide some symptomatic relief, but they do not seem to influence the incidence of renal involvement nor alter the course of the rash.

Nursing care centers on the problem of immobility caused by the arthritic symptoms. Fine and gross motor activities are hindered. Particular attention must be given to providing quiet activities at the bedside for a preschooler who must stay in bed. The appearance of a hemorrhagic rash is upsetting to a preschooler and the discomfort of associated abdominal and joint involvement has the potential to result in whining and demanding behavior.

The child who is toilet trained may regress when occult blood, which acts as a cathartic appears in the stool. Lassitude, fatigue and abdominal cramping may cause delay in motor tasks and frustration of the preschooler's efforts at achieving these. Immunosuppressives enhance the child's susceptibility to infection; therefore peer interaction during this time may need to be reduced.

Prognosis is favorable, with complete recovery occurring in most children. However, a strong tendency for recurrence exists.

References

1. G. A. Baker. Current management of croup and epiglottitis. Pediatric Clinics of North America, August 1979, p. 565
2. T. S. Carden. Tonsillectomy — trials and tribulations. (Report on the National Institutes of Health Consensus Conference on indications for tonsillectomy and adenoidectomy.) Journal of the American Medical Association, 27 October 1978, p. 1961
3. F. I. Catlin. Otolaryngologic disorders. In Pediatric Surgery, 3rd ed., Vol. I. M. M. Ravitch et al., eds, Year Book Medical Publishers, 1929
4. H. F. Eichenwald. Pneumonia infections in children. Hospital Practice, May 1976, p. 89
5. H. F. Eichenwald. Respiratory infections in children. Hospital Practice, April 1976, p. 81
6. L. D. Frenkel and J. A. Bellanti. Development and function of the lymphoid tissue. In Children Are Different, T. R. Johnson et al., eds, Ross Laboratories, 1978
7. R. A. Hoekelman. Tonsillectomy and adenoidectomy. In Principles of Pediatrics, R. A. Hoekelman et al., eds., McGraw-Hill Book Co., 1978
8. R. A. Hoekelman. The pediatric physical examinaton. In A Guide to Physical Examination, B. Bates, ed. J. B. Lippincott Co., 1979
9. J. Hughes. Synopsis of Pediatrics. C. V. Mosby Co., 1979
10. E. B. Levin. Upper respiratory tract. In Principles of Pediatrics, R. A. Hokelman et al., eds., McGraw-Hill Book Co., 1978
11. R. A. Molteni. Group A beta-Hemolytic streptococcal pneumonia. American Journal of Diseases of Childhood, December 1977, p. 1366
12. R. L. Perkin. Tonsillectomy and adenoidectomy. Primary Care, December 1978, p. 697
13. R. J. Ruben. Nose, paranasal sinuses, and pharynx. In Pediatrics, 16th ed., A. M. Rudolph, ed. Appleton-Century-Crofts, 1977
14. W. H. Tooley and H. H. Lipow. Diseases causing reduction of the parenchyma. In Pediatrics, 16th ed., A. M. Rudolph, ed., Appleton-Century-Crofts, 1977
15. L. W. Wannamaker. Rheumatic diseases of childhood. In Nelson Textbook of Pediatrics, V. Vaughn et al., eds. W. B. Saunders Co., 1979

Additional Recommended Reading

E. H. Beachey et al. A strep vaccine: How close? Hospital Practice, November 1979, p. 49
J. K. Lewis et al. A protocol for management of acute epiglottitis. Clinical Pediatrics, June 1978, p. 494
R. T. Rowe and R. T. Stone. Streptococcal pharyngitis. Clinical Pediatrics, October 1977, p. 933
W. Shaikh et al. A systematic review of the literature on evaluative studies of tonsillectomy and adenoidectomy. Pediatrics, March 1976, p. 401
R. Wang. Streptococcal sore throat. American Journal of Nursing, November 1977, p. 1797

UROGENITAL PROBLEMS

by Evan J. Kass, MD
and Mabel Hunsberger, BSN, MSN

Preschoolers have a great deal of curiosity about the genital area. When procedures and examinations must be done that involve this area, a preschooler needs repeated explanations and opportunities to act out his fears in therapeutic play. Preschoolers are particularly adept at fantasizing events to be more threatening and intrusive than they really are. Castration and mutilation fantasies are common during the preschool years; therefore, one must clearly explain what will happen during a procedure or operation. Words should be chosen carefully because descriptions can easily become frightening if words such as "cut" and "bleed" are used indiscriminately.

A preschooler is likely to think that discomfort and pain experienced during procedures or postoperatively is a punishment for something he has done. At this age many children normally engage in masturbation and out of curiosity explore each other's genitals; thus he may interpret the surgery as punishment for these activities. The nurse can help by carefully explaining to the child why the procedures are necessary and allowing him to verbalize his fears and anxieties. Minimizing parental separation before and after surgery can help the child through this trying period.

Use of body outline drawings can be helpful to determine the child's understanding of his own body and what will be done to it. Catheterization is particularly anxiety-producing and requires that parents and the health team elicit the child's fantasies and correct misconceptions. Drawings or dolls can be used to describe procedures and the location of tubes and bandages that will be used after surgery. A preschooler can be given the opportunity to play with a doll and attach tubes and bandages as part of preoperative preparation.

The nurse should also be sensitive to the

special needs of parents whose child has a genitourinary problem. It may be difficult for parents to explain upcoming procedures to the child because they are uncomfortable in a discussion with the child that pertains to genitalia. The nurse can assist parents by encouraging them to express their feelings and discuss any fears or concerns they may have. When the genitourinary condition is one that is familial or genetic, it is often difficult for parents to talk about the problem with their child because of the guilt feelings they hold. This has particular significance for the child with a genitourinary condition because of the parents' worry about the reproductive implications of the problem. Even when the prognosis is good, the nurse should not underestimate the worry and concern that parents have about their child's genitourinary problem.

Another problem that arises for the preschooler is that he has only recently developed control over his own bodily functions and now he will either have pain when he urinates or he will no longer have control over urination because he has a catheter. The child and parents need reassurance that the previous level of control over elimination will again be achieved. Parents particularly need to be able to express their frustrations when a toilet-trained preschooler temporarily regresses. They should be advised to avoid using a punitive approach to regain their child's cooperation in toilet training.

CRYPTORCHIDISM

The testes develop on the posterior wall of the abdomen and at about the eighth month of gestation descend through the inguinal canal into the scrotum. A *cryptorchid testis* is one that has not completely descended; it may be located intra-abdominally, in the inguinal canal, at the external ring, or high in the scrotum. An *ectopic testis* is one that has deviated from the normal path of descent after emerging from the inguinal canal. It may be located in the perineum, over the pubic bone or in the femoral region. The management of both cryptorchid and ectopic testes is the same.

The incidence of undescended testes varies directly with the gestational age and weight of the fetus; that is, the smaller and more premature the infant the greater the likelihood for an undescended testis to be present. The testes cannot be felt in the scrotum in as many as 30 per cent of premature infants, while in term infants the incidence is 2 to 3 per cent. Spontaneous descent of the testes may occur during the first 6 to 12 months after birth, so that the incidence of "true cryptorchidism" is only 0.7 per cent.[13]

The etiology of this condition is unknown; however, several theories are prevalent. The first is that the testes is inherently an abnormal organ and failure of descent reflects this disordered embryological state. The second theory points to lack of sufficient gonadotropic stimulation (particularly applicable to bilateral cryptorchidism) as the cause, and the third theory cites mechanical obstruction to descent caused by fibrous bands, a short spermatic cord or an ectopic location (commonly noted in unilateral undescended testes).[2, 3, 11]

Nurse's Role in Identification Accurate documentation of the position of both testes immediately after birth and during well-baby check-ups is essential. Before the child reaches 6 months of age the scrotal contents are easily examined and the cremasteric reflex (the reflex retraction that draws the testes into the upper part of the scrotum or inguinal canal in response to cold, pain, fear and touch) is absent or rudimentary. After 6 months of age in babies, and in older boys, the cremasteric reflex becomes quite active and may simulate the empty scrotum of cryptorchidism in up to 50 per cent of boys (retractile testes). A reassuring attitude and thorough explanation of what the child may expect will facilitate the examination. If examination of the inguinal and scrotal regions in the erect and supine positions suggests an undescended testis, it is often helpful to repeat the examination with the child seated and the knees drawn up to the chest in order to diminish the cremasteric reflex. Early documentation of a testis in its normal scrotal position (4 cm below the pubic tubercle) eliminates confusion in later years. The nurse's role is to do a thorough genital examination and document her findings. Whenever the nurse is unable to palpate a testis in the scrotum she should bring it to the attention of a physician for further examination. If upon repeated examination by a physician a testis is not palpable in its normal position by the time the child reaches 1 year of age, the diagnosis of cryptorchidism can be made and appropriate management instituted.

When cryptorchidism is suspected, the child should be referred by 1 year of age to a surgeon skilled in pediatric urologic procedures.

Management Hormonal stimulation (human chorionic gonadotropin) is beneficial in children with bilateral undescended testes but is only occasionally helpful in unilateral cases. Surgical placement of the testes in the scrotum (orchidopexy) is required for most children with cryptorchidism. Most authorities recommend surgery before age 5[10]; however, evidence demonstrating structural changes in the undescended testes of these boys by one year of age would suggest that orchidopexy should be performed before age 2.[2]

To perform an orchidopexy, a small transverse incision is made in the lower abdominal skin fold and the testes and spermatic cord are freed from surrounding tissues. A hernia sac is present in up to 90 per cent of cases but is not usually detectable preoperatively, and only occasionally is it symptomatic. After an adequate length of spermatic cord is obtained, an incision is made through the skin of the lower portion of the scrotum, a pouch created, and the testis is pulled down into the pouch and then sutured to the inner wall of the scrotum. Subcutaneous sutures that do not require removal are used to close the skin incisions. The child may be discharged on the afternoon of surgery or the following morning and may resume normal activities as tolerated. Tub bathing is usually withheld for several days; however, showers are permitted.

The potential for fertility and the long-term risk of testicular malignancy should be discussed with the patient and his parents. Although the physician plays the primary role in this discussion, the nurse should have sufficient knowledge to participate effectively in counselling these families. It is important for the nurse to be present when the physician discusses these issues with the family so that she is aware of specific information that has been given by the physician. The nurse is then prepared to be supportive of the family as they deal with the effects of this information.

Specific information given to a family will vary; however, there are some facts that will assist the nurse in understanding the approach to management of cryptorchidism. Spermatogenesis is significantly impaired in undescended testes. Although orchidopexy improves the situation, the fertility rate among these patients, even when only one testis is undescended, is reduced in comparison to that of unaffected men. Additionally, the risk of developing a testicular tumor in the undescended testis is increased 20 to 50 times (normally 2 to 3 per 100,000 males) and also, to a certain extent, in its normally descended mate.[6]

The nurse, working together with other members of the health care team, can play a central role in the management of these children. Early examination and documentation of the position of the testes by the nurse may obviate a false diagnosis later in life, thus eliminating needless anxiety, costly examinations and unnecessary testing. Discussions with the patient and his family on the importance of long-term follow-up for development of tumor and for evaluation of fertility are essential. Additionally, instructing the patient in the method and importance of self-examination of the testes to check for tumor is critical because of the length of time between surgery for undescended testes at 1 to 5 years of age, and the possible development of a tumor at about 30 to 50 years of age.

HYPOSPADIAS

Hypospadias is a congenital defect in which the urethra terminates proximally and ventrally to its normally expected location, more common in males. A ventral curvature of the penis (chordee) is usually present and is caused by tough fibrous bands extending ventrally behind the urethra and reaching the glans, or adhesions between the urethra and overlying skin, or both. Hypospadias is usually classified according to the position of the urethral opening as glandular (opening at the base of the glans penis), coronal (junction of glans and penis), penile (between the glans and scrotum), penoscrotal (at the junction of the penis and scrotum), or perineal (severe hypospadias with other anomalies of the genitals). The condition occurs with an incidence of approximately 5 per 1000 births of males, and some evidence exists to suggest that a genetic factor may sometimes be important.

Nurse's Role in Identification and Diagnosis The nurse can assist in the identification of hypospadias by taking a thorough history and performing a genital examination on all newborns. Mild degrees of hypospadias may be missed on casual examination. A detailed examination is essential because if any degree of hypospadias is present circumcision should not be performed without urological consultation. Urinary incontinence is not usually manifested, since the urethral abnormality in this condition occurs distal to the urinary sphincter.

The most common associated anomaly is cryptorchidism, and should hypospadias occur with one or both testes not palpable (ambiguous genitalia) an extensive investigation to determine the appropriate assignment of sex is indicated. When ambiguous genitalia are present, assignment of gender may be delayed for several days while tests (chromosome analysis, excretory urograms and cystoscopy, or even laparotomy) are performed. The family needs the help and support of the entire health team in order to cope with their anxiety and stress during this period. The nurse can be particularly helpful to the family in dealing appropriately with inquiries of relatives and friends.

Hypospadias as an isolated anomaly or as part of a more complex syndrome may be difficult for the family to understand and accept. The nurse with other health team members can help the family understand the condition, its long-term implications and methods of management.

Management The goal of surgical management is to normalize the appearance and function of the penis. To achieve this, the fibrous bands and skin adhesions causing the ventral curvature must be completely released, and then a urethral tube must be created to allow the urethra to terminate in its expected location. The surgery may be performed in two stages separated by an interval of 6 to 12 months or all at once, depending on the degree of abnormality present and the preference of the surgeon. There are numerous types of hypospadias, and no one method of repair is universally accepted.

No special physical preparation is required for hypospadias surgery. Psychological preparation varies according to the age of the child. Surgery may be performed at almost any time but usually is done when the child is between 1 and 4 years of age. The preschooler will not necessarily verbalize his fears, nor will he completely understand what is happening to him. However, an attempt must be made to prepare him so that his fears may be diminished as much as possible. From the beginning the child should not be made to feel abnormal or different. He can be told that the opening on his penis will be moved to a position from which he can urinate more easily; telling the child that surgery will make his penis "look better" suggests that he does not presently appear normal. Preoperatively the child can be given a simple explanation about the dressing and the catheter that will be in place postoperatively. The family should be made aware of the hospitalization procedures as well as what they may reasonably expect during the preoperative and postoperative periods.

Following the operation a pressure dressing is often used to reduce bleeding and tissue swelling. The tip of the penis should be checked frequently to be sure that it is pink and viable. The dressing is usually changed by the surgeon and should not be removed unless this has been ordered. A catheter is usually placed suprapubically, perineally or transurethrally into the bladder to allow the urine to bypass the operative site. The catheter is securely taped in place to ensure free drainage and to avoid inadvertent dislodgement. Premature catheter removal or obstruction to urine flow may produce significant complications; therefore the nurse should see that the tape is secure and that urine flow is adequate. In a young child who is unattended by a parent it may be necessary to apply wrist restraints in the immediate postoperative period. Early ambulation is encouraged, often the same day as surgery.

After catheter removal (usually by the fifth to tenth postoperative day), urinary infection, dysuria, hematuria or frequency are not uncommon. A child who has not completed toilet training may regress following surgery, but this problem corrects itself promptly. Loss of bowel control may be a particular problem in the immediate postoperative period. The nurse should prepare the parents for this possibility and tell the child how to signal for help to go to the bathroom. The parents and child should also be told about the postoperative urinary symptoms of dysuria, hematuria and frequency. Parents can be particularly helpful in encouraging the child to urinate even though it is initially painful. Placing the child in a tub of warm water can be suggested if dysuria is a particular problem.

POTENTIAL STRESSES DURING PRESCHOOL YEARS: REVERSIBLE ALTERATIONS IN HEALTH STATUS

Most health care personnel have little concept of the potential complications of hypospadias repair. When counselling parents the nurse should emphasize that a successful result cannot be guaranteed with only one or two operations. She should be aware that the commonest reported complication is a urethrocutaneous fistula, in which a part of the newly formed urethra fails to heal properly, allowing an opening to persist between the urethra and the skin. Surgical correction is required if the opening does not close spontaneously.

URINARY TRACT INFECTION

Urinary tract infection is a common problem in childhood, ranking second only to respiratory tract infections. Approximately 1 per cent of neonates will have a documented episode of urinary bacteria, with incidence predominately in males at this age. After this time urinary infection is more frequently encountered in females.

Bacteria gain access to the urinary tract either via the blood stream (hematogenous), which is common in neonates, or via the urethra, which is common in females. However, in order for the bacteria to cause an infection, some other predisposing factor must be present. Therefore, a urinary tract infection should not be viewed as an isolated event but rather as a marker of some underlying problem of the urinary tract. Congenital anomalies of the urinary tract, neurogenic bladder dysfunction, and calculous disease may be the underlying problem. Since many infections seem to cluster around the time of toilet training, some investigators have suggested that the so-called persistent infantile bladder, common at this age, may be a cause of infection.[7] In this condition the child's bladder automatically contracts in an attempt to expel urine whenever a certain bladder volume is reached. Children cannot suppress this involuntary bladder contraction. Since they do not want to wet themselves, they attempt to prevent voiding by voluntarily constricting the sphincter muscles or squatting on their heels to compress the urethra between the pubis and the heel of the foot (the "curtsy maneuver"). These children typically complain of urinary frequency, urgency, urge incontinence ("urge syndrome") and will always wait until the last moment to run to the bathroom. In older children, particularly females, infrequent bladder emptying may be a cause of frequent urinary infections.

Nurse's Role in Prevention The nurse should attempt to determine if any of the conditions predisposing to infection exist and then assist the child and family to learn basic principles of prevention. All children should be encouraged to empty their bladders frequently (every 3 to 4 hours) as a basic principle of good health. Cleansing from front to back is another basic practice in good hygiene that all female children should be taught. Encouraging large fluid intake is beneficial during an acute urinary infection or in children with calculous disease; however, extra fluid intake by healthy children has not been shown to prevent urinary infections.

Other factors thought to increase the incidence of these infections are long tub baths, use of bubble bath substances, tight clothing, poor hygiene and bowel problems. Scientific evidence in support of these theories is sparse; however, if a direct causal relationship exists in a particular individual, it is reasonable to suggest eliminating that factor.

Identification and Clinical Manifestations: Nurse's Role Urinary tract infections are important not only because of the associated patient morbidity during the acute episode but also because of the renal damage that may occur. Renal scarring is found in up to 25 per cent of children after their first urinary tract infection and in a higher proportion of those with recurrent infections.[14] Urinary infection is directly associated with 18 per cent of the end-stage renal failure in children.[12] The challenge in childhood urinary tract infection is to detect the infection early and then to identify those patients at risk of developing renal damage.

The first step in detecting a urinary tract infection is the nurse's recognition of the symptoms associated with urinary infection. In older children specific symptoms localized to the urinary tract are commonly seen. Dysuria, frequency, urgency and enuresis are common complaints in children, and are readily localized to the urinary tract. However, one should note that unexplained fevers, flank or abdominal pain, anorexia and lethargy may also arise from urinary infection. The identification of urinary tract infections is particularly difficult in infants and young children because typical symptoms are usually absent. The infant may fail to gain weight or to eat properly or have jaundice, unexplained fever, colic, abdominal distention, vomiting, diarrhea, or blood on the diapers.

Urinary infections in many children are misdiagnosed because the diagnosis was not even considered; therefore it is prudent to perform a urine culture whenever possible in every ill child, especially if there is any history of the symptoms just mentioned.[8] The nurse must remember that a urinary tract infection may exist at any age in the absence of typical symptoms and a high index of suspicion must be maintained by all members of the child's health team.

Diagnosis The diagnosis is indicated by significant numbers of pathogenic bacteria in the urine of an individual with typical clinical manifestations of a urinary tract infection. However, one must always consider how the specimen was collected, because bacterial contamination in a "clean catch" urine specimen is particularly common, whereas in a catheterized or suprapubic specimen contamination is unusual.

Urine cultures are obtained in order to (1) identify the offending organism, (2) determine the bacterial sensitivity to the various antibiotics and (3) confirm the presence of urinary infection. The finding of 100,000 bacterial colonies per millimeter upon culture of a clean voided specimen is required to diagnose a urinary tract infection because of the possibility of external bacterial contamination. However, if the urine is collected by suprapubic aspiration or catheterization, any bacterial growth may be significant. No method of collection is 100 per cent accurate on a single examination. False-positive urine cultures are a common problem and expose the child to the unnecessary risk of antimicrobial therapy as well as possible future tests to determine the etiology of the infections. The single most important responsibility of the nurse in facilitating diagnosis is in correctly collecting and transporting the urine specimen. Cleansing the child properly, obtaining a fresh specimen and delivering it promptly to the laboratory are nursing priorities. (See Chapter 17 for discussion on collection of urine specimens.) If there is any doubt about the accuracy of results in the clean-voided specimen, suprapubic aspiration or catheterization is performed. (A normal urinalysis or culture never requires instrumentation for confirmation.)

The importance of the physical examination in children with urinary tract infection should not be underestimated. The abdomen should be examined for masses or tenderness (hydronephrosis, distended bladder), the spinal regions should be examined and palpated (spina bifida), and if possible the urinary stream should be observed. Parents may be asked to observe and keep a record of the child's voiding habits. Pertinent observations to be made are frequency of urination, caliber and force of the urinary stream, whether the child strains to urinate, whether the stream is interrupted, or whether there is any sign of discomfort during voiding.

Once the diagnosis of a urinary tract infection has been established, the next task is to identify those children who are in danger of developing renal damage. An excretory urogram (also called intravenous pyelogram [IVP]) and a voiding cystourethrogram (VCUG) should be performed following the first documented urinary infection in all children under 5 years of age, in all boys of every age and in any age child after all febrile urinary infections. A high probability of congenital anomaly of the urinary tract exists in these children.

The excretory urogram requires an intravenous injection of the contrast medium, which is excreted by the kidney and concentrated in the collecting tubules so that the calyces, renal pelvis, ureters and bladder may be visualized. Anatomical abnormalities such as hydronephrosis, renal scarring, or parenchymal loss, or calculi can be identified. A VCUG requires that the child be catheterized and the bladder filled with contrast material. The child then is asked to void, and x-rays are taken during this time. This test is necessary to identify vesicoureteral reflux. With this condition contrast medium will back up from the bladder into the ureter and sometimes into the kidney itself on one or both sides; normally reflux does not occur. In boys reflux may indicate urethral obstruction caused by stricture or posterior urethral valves.

The nurse should be familiar with the testing procedures and their purpose so she can assist in preparing the child and the family. Many children will be frightened by the dark room and unfamiliar people performing the tests and are unable to cooperate fully with the testing. The family should be aware that the child may experience some voiding discomfort following catheterization and may even have some blood in the urine.

Management The management of a urinary tract infection is predicated upon achieving the following goals: (1) eradication of the infection, (2) identification and correction of factors predisposing to infection and (3) prevention of recurrences. The specific treatment program varies with the type and severity of the infection; infections are described as (1) acute and uncomplicated, (2) recurrent or persistent, and (3) complicated.

Acute Uncomplicated Infection This type of urinary tract infection typically occurs in a school-age girl and is characterized by lower urinary tract symptoms (dysuria, frequency, and so forth) without symptoms of possible renal involvement (fever, flank pain). The most common offending organism is E. coli (80 per cent) and usually sulfisoxazole (Gantrisin) or ampicillin is used for treatment. Following completion of the 7- to 10-day course of antibiotics a urine sample should be checked to ensure eradication of the infection. An IVP or VCUG is not routinely performed in girls over 5 years of age with an uncomplicated urinary tract infection, but if two or three such infections are documented, investigation is warranted. However, just one uncomplicated urinary infection in a male or in a child under 5 years of age requires that an investigation be undertaken.

Persistent or Recurrent Infection A recurrent urinary infection is one that occurs after a previous episode has been successfully treated (a second new infection). In a persistent infection, the initial infection has not been completely eradicated. It is usually difficult to distinguish between these two entities, unless there is adequate documentation (negative urine culture) that the initial infection has cleared. The infection may be symptomatic but frequently is not. Since many of these infections involve organisms other than E. coli, the antibiotic should be selected on the basis of culture and sensitivity studies, whenever possible. For a recurrent urinary tract infection generally a 10- to 14-day course of antibiotic therapy is adequate; however, persistent infection or frequent recurrences may necessitate the use of antimicrobials for as long as 6 months. Children with vesicoureteral reflux managed nonoperatively are routinely given low-dose antimicrobials (a single daily dose of a urinary antibiotic) for one or more years.

Complicated Infections Complicated urinary infections are those in which there may be involvement of the kidney itself, or those with associated structural abnormalities of the urinary tract. Febrile infections, infections in children under 5 years of age or in males of any age should be considered to be in this category. An investigation of the urinary tract (IVP, VCUG) is mandatory and should be performed following the first urinary infection. Since Proteus, Klebsiella, Pseudomonas and Entercocci are the organisms that are often involved in the infection, a sample of urine should be routinely sent for culture and sensitivity studies if a complicated infection is suspected. Children with febrile infections may require hospitalization and treatment with combinations of parenteral antibiotics to control the infection; however, most of the children can be treated safely as outpatients. Adequate follow-up is essential to ensure that the infection has been controlled and to protect against possible recurrences.

The nurse can contribute to the effectiveness of the treatment regimen as well as the follow-up program by gaining the confidence and cooperation of the child and the family. All health team members should emphasize that the antibiotics must be taken as directed even though symptoms have subsided. Follow-up is essential because recurrences have been reported in 30 to 50 per cent of uncomplicated infections in young girls and may be even more common following complicated infections. The nurse and physician must work closely with the family to gain their compliance with the follow-up program. Generally in an uncomplicated infection the child should be seen shortly after the completion of antibiotic therapy and then every three to six months thereafter for two years. In children with structural abnormalities of the urinary tract or vesicoureteral reflux, it may be necessary to perform urine cultures every one to three months for several years. In these children, home or office screening tests for urinary bacteria may be informative.

VESICOURETERAL REFLUX

Vesicoureteral reflux is the regurgitation of urine from the bladder back into the ureter or upper urinary collecting system. Reflux does not normally occur in children regardless of age or sex because the ureter, after passing through the bladder musculature, courses underneath the bladder mucosa before opening into the bladder lumen. The length of this submucosal segment of ureter functions as a valve to prevent the urine from re-entering the upper collecting system during voiding or bladder filling. Reflux occurs when the valve mechanism is congenitally incompetent (primary reflux) or when a normal valvular mechanism is damaged by chronic infection or bladder outlet obstruction (secondary reflux).

Vesicoureteral reflux is important because it allows bacteria from the bladder (where most urinary infections originate) to reach the kidney where renal infection (pyelonephritis) and damage may occur. (This condition is referred to in the literature as chronic atrophic pyelonephritis, interstitial nephritis, or more recently as reflux nephropathy.) Vesicoureteral reflux is found in one third of children with urinary infections[4] and, conversely, 95 per cent of children with vesicoureteral reflux will develop urinary infection. The most common radiographic abnormality found in children with urinary infections is vesicoureteral reflux.

Diagnosis Vesicoureteral reflux is best demonstrated by the catheterized voiding cystourethrogram (VCUG). For this test a catheter is inserted into the child's bladder and the residual urine is drained. Radiographic constrast medium is dripped into the bladder until it is full, and then the child is asked to void. The entire procedure is monitored by cinefluoroscopy, and if contrast medium is seen at any stage, either in the ureter or kidney, reflux is said to be present. The amount of reflux seen during the radiographic study is classified as slight, moderate or gross, depending on the extent of the filling and dilatation of the upper urinary tract (renal pelvis and ureter). The VCUG may be performed on the same day as the excretory urogram, but to avoid confusion, should always be done first.

Management Once vesicoureteral reflux is documented, the physician must attempt to exclude any factors that might possibly predispose to the development of vesicoureteral reflux or prevent its disappearance (bladder outlet obstruction, neurogenic bladder dysfunction, and so forth). Following the initial assessment most children with vesicoureteral reflux are placed on prophylactic doses of nitrofurantoin or sulfamethoxazole-trimethoprim in an attempt to prevent urinary infection. It is thought that if urinary infection can be controlled no renal damage will occur and with time the reflux will disappear spontaneously. However, the children must take their antimicrobial medication every day, often for several years, and during this time close and continuous follow-up is mandatory to exclude breakthrough infections. If adequate compliance and follow-up is not possible, antireflux surgery should be considered.

Most of the children who eventually undergo antireflux surgery are initially managed medically[9]; only rarely is surgery required on an urgent basis. The most common reasons for surgery are: (1) failure of the medical program to prevent infection, (2) progressive renal damage, (3) renal growth arrest and (4) persistent severe reflux. Usually by the time that surgery becomes necessary the child as well as the family has been exposed to several members of the health care team on multiple occasions and should have a reasonable understanding of the disease process, as well as the reasons for surgery. The nurse should attempt to determine the family's level of understanding and either build on it or correct it appropriately. The nurse should ascertain from the urologist what has already been explained to the family and which of the several types of antireflux operations will be used so that there are no conflicting statements.

The surgical treatment of vesicoureteral reflux is called reimplantation of the ureters or ureteroneocystostomy (Fig. 42–2). In this procedure a transverse suprapubic incision is made in the skin fold, the bladder is exposed and the ureter is mobilized for a length of 6 to 7 cm. The ureter is then repositioned in a new submucosal tunnel of adequate length and sutured in place. Many surgeons place tubes up the ureters in order to divert the urine while healing takes place. These tubes are brought out through the bladder and skin, and are usually left in place for four to seven days. In addition, a urethral catheter or suprapubic tube is utilized to drain the bladder. Special attention should be given to preventing accidental dislodgement or blockage of these tubes, and output should be accurately recorded from each tube. If a bilateral

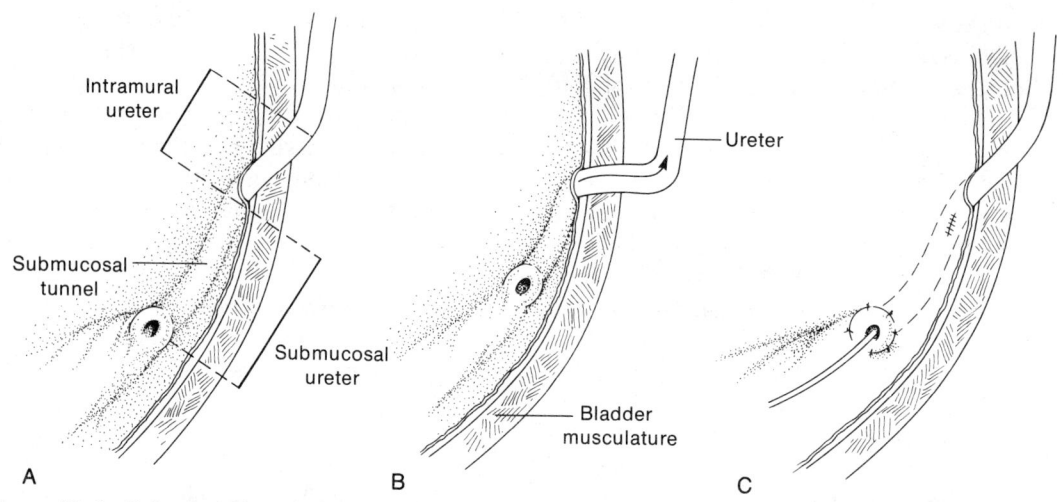

Figure 42-2 Reimplantation of ureters. A, the ureter enters the bladder at an oblique angle to form a normal ureterovesical junction. Normally as pressure in the bladder rises, the angled position of the ureter causes a temporary closing off of the lumen, preventing urine backflow (reflux). B, in vesicoureteral reflux the ureter enters the bladder at an acute angle and the submucosal tunnel is shortened. As pressure in the bladder rises, urine is directed up the ureter (reflux). C, reimplantation of the ureter is done to correct the ureterovesical angle and lengthen the submucosal tunnel to prevent reflux.

reimplantation has been performed, the ureteral catheters will drain nearly all the urine output and the bladder catheter will have minimal drainage. The child should be advised that urination will not be possible until all tubes are removed (usually 5 to 10 days). Bladder discomfort or spasms are common and are often perceived by the patient as the urge to urinate. He or she should be reassured that medication is available to relieve the spasms and that following removal of the catheters the symptoms will resolve. The child may walk while the tube is in place as long as proper assistance is provided to prevent premature removal. Bathing is not permitted until all tube and sutures have been removed.

Following release from the hospital the child's activities are usually limited for several weeks and antibiotics are continued for three to six months.

Follow-up radiographic studies are performed three to six months following surgery and then every 12 to 18 months for several years to confirm that the surgery has been successful and to exclude complications.

The surgery should be successful 95 to 98 per cent of the time. The most common complications are persistent reflux and obstruction at the ureterovesicular junction.

References

1. B. Belman and L. King. Urethra. In Clinical Pediatric Urology, P. Kelalis et al., eds. W. B. Saunders Co., 1976
2. F. Hadziselimovic et al. Surgical correction of cryptorchidism at 2 years. Journal of Pediatric Surgery, February 1975
3. F. Hadziselimovic and B. Herzog. The meaning of the Leydig cell in relation to the etiology of cryptorchidism. Journal of Pediatric Surgery, February 1976
4. W. Heale. Age of presentation and pathogenesis of reflux nephropathy. In Reflux Nephropathy. J. Hodson and P. Kincaid-Smith, eds. Mason Publishing, USA, 1979
5. W. Hecker and H. Hienz. Cryptorchidism and fertility. Journal of Pediatric Surgery, vol. 2, p. 513, 1967
6. S. Krabbe et al. High incidence of undetected neoplasia in maldescended testes. Lancet 1, 12 May 1979
7. J. Lapides and A. Diokno. Persistence of the infant bladder as a cause of urinary infection in girls. Transactions of the American Association of Genitourinary Surgeons, vol. 61, p. 51, 1976
8. A. Margileth. Urinary tract bacterial infections. Pediatric Clinics of North America, November 1976
9. C. Normand and J. Smellie. Vesicouretric reflux: the case for conservative management. In Reflux Nephropathy. J. Hodson and P. Kincaid-Smith, eds. Mason Publishing, USA, 1979
10. L. Pinch et al. Cryptorchidism: a pediatric review. Urologic Clinics of North America, vol. 1, p. 573, 1979
11. R. Prentiss et al. Undescended testes. Journal of Urology, May 1960
12. Proceedings of the European Dialysis and Transplant Association, 1977
13. C. Scorer. The descent of the testis. Archives of Disease of Childhood, December 1964
14. J. Smellie et al. Clinical and radiological features of urinary infection in childhood. British Medical Journal, vol. 2, p. 1221, 1974

POTENTIAL STRESSES DURING THE PRESCHOOL YEARS: IRREVERSIBLE ALTERATIONS IN HEALTH STATUS

by Mary Lou Frey, BSN, MSN
Mabel Hunsberger, BSN, MSN,
Jo Joyce Tackett, BSN, MPHN

The impact of irreversible conditions on preschool children and their families depends on the nature of the problem and the extent to which the disability imposes on the child and on family relationships. These conditions alter every aspect of development but especially affect the social development of the child and alter the needs of his family. How family members, particularly parents, respond to this crisis significantly affects the child's own response.

FAMILY REACTIONS

The reactions of the family to the diagnosis of an irreversible illness in the preschool period are somewhat different from those that occur when the initial diagnosis is made at birth. The family has experienced the child as normal and healthy and has invested time and energy into his healthy development. When they learn the diagnosis, these parents experience an acute sense of loss because they must alter expectations and hopes for the child's potential. Fear that the rewards and anticipated pleasure of childrearing will be lost results in depression in some families. Acute denial of the diagnosis may cause the parents to shop around for a medical expert who will state that the condition is only temporary or that the diagnosis is inaccurate. Closely associated is parental disbelief of the diagnosis, particularly if the obvious signs of illness have subsided.

Many parents, on the other hand, express a feeling of relief at learning the diagnosis, particularly if they have suspected a problem for some time and have experienced delay in confirmation of their suspicions. The diagnosis aids them in knowing what they are confronting; this helps them mobilize their resources to cope. However, overacceptance of the diagnosis may indicate unrealistic expectations that the prognosis will be favorable.

Once the diagnosis and prognosis have been accepted, family members attempt to achieve a balance between their own developmental tasks and the special needs of the child. Achieving this balance requires that parents take on new roles and make psychological adaptations because of the child's prolonged dependency needs.

During preschool years a child usually masters self-care skills that free parents to pursue their own activities. The child with irreversible illness may not master these self-care skills; therefore, the parents may be restricted in the pursuit of personal interests because of the care demands imposed by the child's handicap. These restrictions may cause resentment, leading to feelings of guilt. To compensate for their guilt, parents may become overprotective of the handicapped child. Some parents consciously or unconsciously reject the child, criticizing him for causing them inconvenience. They may neglect his care or they may inadvertently place the burden of responsibility for his care upon siblings.

At a time when most families can give progressively less time to the care of their preschooler, the family of a preschooler with irreversible illness is faced with a situation which makes ongoing demands on its time and other resources. Most working parents with a healthy preschooler can increase their financial stability by devoting more time and energy to their jobs as the child becomes gradually more independent. When the preschooler has irreversible illness, the parents have access to fewer persons who can or are willing to provide the care their child needs. So there is less opportunity for a family to increase its income during these years.

A deterioration of the marital relationship may occur as one spouse becomes engrossed in the care of the child while the other is absent from home, channeling more energy into a job, either to maintain financial stability or as a means of dealing with the situation. When one parent assumes total responsibility for the child's daily needs, a sense of isolation and separation from the child is experienced by the other.

The child's need for early remedial education, coupled with the prolonged dependency that results from his handicap, presents a separation conflict for the parents. The fewer the number of separation experiences the child has had because of his care demands, the greater is the parents' anxiety that the child cannot function without them. Overprotective parents who have not provided their preschooler with opportunities to develop self-sufficiency within the limitations of this handicap have an even greater problem separating from the child.

Siblings may resent the special attention received by the affected child or the added responsibilities given to them to maintain household routines or both. A sibling may manifest these feelings by withdrawing from the child or by making him a recipient of the sibling's feeling of frustration.

CHILD'S REACTIONS

The attitudes of others, especially his parents, largely determine how the preschooler with a disability perceives himself and his functional potential. The preschooler's inquisitive nature precipitates many questions about his illness, the limitations it imposes and any treatments used. However, it is also a developmental reality that the preschooler will probably interpret the answers as a punishment for real or imagined actions, misbehavior or bad thoughts. His inability to comprehend cause and effect relationships may lead him to blame himself or his parents for his limitations. The preschool child is also developing a new awareness of the body's capabilities. He needs positive family and social interaction to help him obtain a realistic picture of his assets and liabilities.

Most preschool children can function with the limitations posed by their disability if they can find a different route to accomplish tasks of development according to their capacity and are helped to identify with and accept their limitations. A lack of assistance and training to master developmental tasks despite limitations may lead to cranky, irritable, unpleasant, whining or demanding behavior. This can cause parents to feel guilty, resentful or inadequate. When the handicapped preschooler is allowed and encouraged to accept and adapt to his limitations, he develops the determination to try and the persistence to succeed. The success he achieves, along with the acceptance he feels from others in his environment, produces a sense of self-worth and confidence that he is capable and functional despite his limitations.

If he does not perceive himself as worthwhile and capable, the preschooler's developmental potential is compromised. A certain amount of dependency and protection is usually necessary for safety in the care of the child with a disability, but when family members become indulgent and overprotective, the child feels worthless and insecure and loses the initiative or confidence to master developmental skills. His insecurity may be evidenced by overly dependent behavior, persistent thumb-sucking, self-stimulating motor activities, shyness and withdrawal, or refusal to try new tasks.

Other factors besides parental overprotectiveness may interfere with the child's development of self-worth and confidence. Parents and other well-meaning adults may promote a sense of failure in the preschooler because of their own fears that the child cannot overcome his difficulties. They may attempt to insulate the child from peer insults, exploratory play and preschool education, anticipating that these experiences will cause him trauma. They may also communicate lower expectations for the child because of his disability. Such actions jeopardize the child's intellectual development and promote social isolation, making it difficult for him to initiate and maintain friendships or learn to handle his limitations without loss of self-esteem.

Extensive constraints may also be placed on the child's emotional development by his parents and others. Unrealistic pressure to achieve tasks beyond the child's present abilities or denial that the limitation exists force the child to invest considerable energy in trying to hide or ignore his disability. A child may be unable to succeed because of his limitation or undue pressure on him or exaggeration of his limitation by parents and peers. If his parents react to his failure with anger and frustration, he may feel incompetent and worthless. Limited physical mobility or sensory deprivation or both imposed by the disability decrease the child's exploration of his environment and diminish his opportunities to release pent-up energy and emotions.

When he feels unaccepted as he is by his family and community, the preschooler tends to have a more difficult time handling normal developmental tasks and is more likely to have developmental delays. Fearing abandonment, he may use his symptoms to gain attention or to attempt to ensure his parents' continued presence.

Dealing with chronic illness may be an especially difficult task for the preschool child as he begins to realize that he is different from his peers, especially if the defect is visible. Invisible problems such as asthma cause the child to be confused as to why limitations are imposed. His cognitive development is such that it is difficult for him to understand his disability or how the discomfort or limitations of some therapeutic regimen can be helpful to him in the future.

NURSING INTERVENTIONS

The parents need assistance to foster the developmental potential and independence of their child. Irreversible illness imposes stresses that make even the healthiest family vulnerable. The vulnerability to disintegration of the family unit as a result of a chronic illness is related to the ability of family members to modify their respective roles and redefine their personal goals and expectations to achieve equilibrium.

The nurse must recognize that the family's equilibrium depends on the nature of the child's needs, the type of disability, the family's perception of the child's limitations and achievements, and their knowledge of and capacity to maximize his developmental potential. To help family members maintain or achieve a balance between their own needs and the needs of their handicapped preschooler, the nurse must begin by helping the members identify those needs unique to their own situation. The nurse should explore with the parents ways to meet most effectively their own need to re-establish or develop their interests and career pursuits. The preschooler needs to develop social skills and increase his ability to separate; therefore, the nurse can support the family's and preschooler's development by integrating other forms of care into the life style of this family. For example, brief periods of substitute caretaking, remedial education, and visiting a grandparent for a weekend fosters a preschooler's normal development and gives parents the opportunity to pursue their own interests. The nurse's responsibility lies not only in assisting the parents to find these resources but also to help them resolve the conflict that may arise because they cannot without some guilt transfer the responsibility of care to another while pursuing their own personal goals.

The development of the handicapped preschooler is further enhanced if the nurse can support parents in child care approaches that will foster maximum independence of the child in activities of daily living. This is another area that has the potential to create conflict for parents. The nurse can help them deal with the struggle to foster independence in their preschooler in a way that is congruent with their particular style of parenting. The nurse can provide them with information about the growth and developmental needs of their preschooler and help them identify ways to expand their own capacity to stand by supportively while their child struggles to accomplish a task. Praising a child, giving him time to complete a task, and removing obvious obstacles are forms of supportive intervention.

These parents generally need reassurance that independence expressed through self-care is an integral part of their child's development. A preschooler is at an age when parents must adapt to the process of "their baby" becoming an independent school-age child. For parents with a handicapped child, this process is complicated by the child's additional dependency needs. Parents may gain considerable support from other parents with similar problems and particularly benefit by becoming involved in the child's remedial education program. In this setting they can observe child care approaches that facilitate maximum development while gaining reassurance that their own style of parenting is appropriate.

Parents often require assistance to adapt play activities to the child's capacities. For example, a child prohibited from gross motor activities because of a physical disability can enjoy vicarious locomotion through action stories to which he can add the locomotion sounds, such as "panting" when the boy in the story is running fast and "blowing" when the swing goes up toward the sky. The child who cannot pull a wagon or ride a tricycle may enjoy the sensations and imaginative opportunities of an exploratory walk or wheelchair ride. Art and music can also be satisfying substitutes for more active play.

The nurse has an important role in easing the burden of these families. Facilitating the family's access to available resources, particularly crippled children's services, can provide the continuing financial, emotional, and moral support these families need.

The siblings of a preschooler with an irreversible illness also require the attention of the nurse. When there is an older sibling, the nurse can provide the opportunity for the sibling to express feelings without the presence of parents. This gives an opportunity to express feelings of frustration as well as tell about positive experiences the child has with his handicapped sibling. When a sibling resents the time and attention given to the handicapped child, the nurse can intervene to help the sibling see that the amount of attention given is a result of the handicapped child's special needs and not because the parents prefer the handicapped child.

The nurse can assist the total functioning of the family by examining with parents and siblings their feelings about the physical care the preschooler requires. The nurse can work with parents and siblings to arrive mutually at an appropriate amount of responsibility for the preschooler's siblings. The nurse can help facilitate family decision-making; this promotes a favorable environment for siblings and parents of a handicapped preschooler. It is within this healthy functioning family that a handicapped preschooler can best learn to adapt.

POLIOMYELITIS

Poliomyelitis is an acute febrile contagious disease, caused by a virus, that may affect the central nervous system, resulting in damage to the motor neurons. Most frequently it is a mild nonspecific illness or the infection remains asymptomatic; only a small percentage of persons develop flaccid paralysis.[2]

Incidence, Epidemiology and Pathogenesis

The incidence of poliomyelitis (also called polio or infantile paralysis) has been extremely low since the advent of mass immunization programs, beginning with the Salk vaccine in 1957 and continuing today with the Sabin trivalent oral polio vaccine. Recently there have been a few outbreaks in some areas of the United States in children who were not immunized for reli-

TABLE 43-1 TYPES OF RESPONSE TO POLIO VIRUS INFECTION

Frequency	Response	Manifestations
1	Asymptomatic	Infection is not clinically apparent, but the virus may be isolated from throat and feces.
2	Abortive	Mild illness. Fever, headache, sore throat, nausea, vomiting, anorexia and malaise in various combinations, lasting a few days. In some instances there is a recurrence, which then takes on characteristics of nonparalytic poliomyelitis.
3	Nonparalytic poliomyelitis	May present as the initial form of illness or as the second phase of the abortive type (see above). CNS symptoms similar to those in aseptic meningitis, including pain and stiffness in the neck, legs, and back.
4	Paralytic poliomyelitis	Presents a few days after recovery from abortive type or may begin with nonparalytic manifestations.
	(a) Spinal form	Affects muscles supplied by the motor neurons in the spinal cord. Paralysis is associated with the signs and symptoms of the nonparalytic poliomyelitis. Distribution of paralysis is characteristically asymmetrical and scattered. It may affect all limbs, a few muscles of one or more limbs or only parts of muscles. Muscle pain, hyperesthesia and tremors usually precede paralysis. Initially deep tendon reflexes are exaggerated; they decrease or become absent as paralysis develops.[3] Although paralysis involving the extremities is most apparent, there may be involvement of the diaphragm or intercostal muscle, suggested by use of auxiliary muscles and asymmetrical chest expansion during respirations.
	(b) Bulbar form	Respiratory and circulatory centers in the medulla are affected, resulting in shallow, irregular breathing and a rapid, weak, thready pulse. Medullary nuclei of the cranial nerves may also be damaged. Manifestations may include weakness of face and neck muscles, inability to swallow normally, excessive salivation, nasal voice, and speech impairment.
	(c) Bulbospinal form	A combination of spinal and bulbar.
	(d) Encephalitic form	Clinical manifestations are those of encephalitis (drowsiness, disorientation, irritability) in conjunction with muscular paralysis.

gious reasons.[1] Poliomyelitis usually appears during the summer and early fall, occurring endemically and epidemically.

The disease is caused by one of the three polioviruses (Type 1, Type 2, Type 3). Of the three, Type 1 is the most frequent cause of paralytic poliomyelitis.

The virus spreads from pharynx to oropharynx, but in areas of poor sanitation the fecal-oropharyngeal route predominates.[2] After exposure the virus is present in the oropharynx for about a week; however, the major site of viral multiplication is the alimentary tract.

If the virus invades the central nervous system, injury to the neurons may be extensive enough to cause paralysis. The anterior horn cells of the spinal cord are affected in many paralytic patients; this is the spinal form of paralysis. Involvement of the brain stem (bulbar form), especially the medulla, is a more life-threatening form of central nervous system involvement. This bulbar form of paralysis occurs less frequently, however.[3]

The clinical manifestations range from nonspecific minor illness to rapidly progressing paralysis and death. There are four possible responses as a result of infection with poliovirus. Table 43-1 describes these in order of frequency.

Nurse's Role in Prevention

The nurse can fulfill an essential role in prevention of poliomyelitis through her efforts at determining that all children are adequately immunized. (The immunization schedule recommended by the American Academy of Pediatrics is found in Chapter 13, Table 13-2.)

Some concern has been expressed in recent

years that children have been improperly immunized as a result of poor techniques, particularly in large immunization centers. The nurse involved in immunization can help by being sure that vaccine is stored properly and administered carefully. All Sabin vaccine should remain frozen until the vial is opened. It should not be stored on the shelves of refrigerator doors, because temperature fluctuations may make the vaccine ineffective. The multidose vial should never be refrozen; remaining portions should be used according to manufacturer's instructions.

Poliomyelitis immunization is contraindicated for children with an immune deficiency or for those receiving corticosteroid therapy. No immunization should be given when a child has a fever. Children with malignancy are exempted from routine immunizations, as are those allergic to eggs, chicken or neomycin.

Another aspect of prevention that the nurse should teach is to avoid unnecessary exposure to high concentrations of the poliovirus. Isolation with enteric precautions of anyone exposed to the virus should be observed according to the local public health regulations. An infected child should not return to school until the virus is no longer present in his secretions.

Maintaining the body's resistance is an important preventive measure. An adequate diet and a balance between rest and activity are health practices to be encouraged. Routine immunizations other than poliovirus during a polio outbreak should be avoided. Also, if a tonsillectomy is performed when the virus is present in the pharynx, bulbar poliomyelitis may result.[4] Tonsillar or oronasal surgery should be avoided when diagnosed polio exists in the community.

Although outbreaks are rare today, when polio is suspected in a community, nurses can play a vital role in prompt epidemiological assessment and follow-up. It is essential that the nurse determine the immunization status of children who have symptoms suggestive of polio, particularly during summer or fall. In an epidemiological approach an investigation is made of environmental factors such as water supply, food storage and sanitation conditions and life style practices or community beliefs that might promote transfer of the virus. A family health history is taken to discover family beliefs about immunization and health care, to identify onset of symptoms in other family members, and to clarify the children's immunization status.

Nursing Management

During the early stages of polio the child is isolated and enteric precautions are observed until the child no longer represents a source of infection. During the febrile stage of illness, the child should be watched for acute respiratory distress, and bed rest is indicated. The child should lie on a firm mattress, and his body should be in proper alignment. When his position is changed, he should be rolled gently, with joints supported. Care must be taken to avoid pulling on tender muscles, which have a tendency to undergo painful spasms when stimulated. The sensory nerves are intact in all flaccid or spastic muscles. Warm, moist packs help reduce pain and spasm. Passive range of motion exercise of joints helps to prevent contractures and maintains muscle tone.

When a child has the type of poliomyelitis that affects the muscles of respiration, a respirator is used to maintain adequate ventilation. A tracheostomy is sometimes necessary to maintain a patent airway. Swallowing difficulties require the use of tube feedings or hyperalimentation to provide adequate nutrition.

The nurse can help maintain the child's intellectual competency by providing adequate sensory stimulation while he is being maintained on a respirator or is in isolation. Quiet activities such as reading stories or playing games that allow tactile stimulation are entertaining but not physically exhausting. Some form of communication needs to be established by which a child can make his needs known without language (e.g., a set of picture cards of objects and activities, such as a drink, voiding, play, that the child can use to indicate needs). Maintaining the child's social and emotional development is important, as in hospitalization for any reason (see Chapter 45 on the hospitalized preschooler).

During the convalescent stages, the child needs passive exercising of all affected and unaffected muscle groups, gradually progressing to active exercise of involved muscle groups through play.

The child who has been paralyzed by an acute case of polio can often be restored to useful muscular activity through proper treatment. In some cases reconstructive surgery and heel cord lengthening on the affected limb is valuable. Orthopedic devices such as braces, supports and special shoes may be used. Parents who are unable to afford proper treatment can find aid through a local branch of the National Foundation for the March of Dimes (800 Second Avenue, New York, NY 10017) or through services of the local public welfare or public health departments.

A child with residual paralysis who needs to use braces for mobility will require long-term nursing care and support. Exercises of the arms should begin early to build strength. Parents and the child will need to learn to care for and apply braces safely. Long-leg braces must be checked for pressure areas on stress points. Braces must be kept properly padded and their fit must be re-evaluated during growth spurts. The child with braces must be encouraged to take part in normal activities with other children. Participation in a nursery school or play group should be encouraged. The child can be helped to deal with an altered body image through verbalization, therapeutic play, and handling of the braces. The child's sense of self can be aided through emphasis by parents and health care workers on what the child can do, not what he cannot do.

Children with bulbar involvement seldom have residual paralysis. They are, however, more susceptible to upper respiratory infection than other children. Children with spinal involvement are apt to have residual paralysis if major neurons are affected. Proper bracing will decrease the risk of thoracic and lumbar scoliosis.

VISUAL PROBLEMS

Various eye conditions can cause vision problems if not identified and treated early. Five per cent of all preschool children have visual problems; 68 per cent are refractive errors, 15 per cent are caused by strabismus, 15 per cent are the result of amblyopia, and 2 per cent are traceable to other causes.[25] Refractive errors and strabismus account for the majority of preschoolers' vision problems. While prevention of these conditions is not possible because they are primarily hereditary, early identification and treatment can prevent serious loss of vision. The nurse should have a part in screening for visual problems in children. During the preschool years refractive errors and strabismus and resulting amblyopia are prevalent, and the consequences when these go unrecognized and untreated are always serious.[25]

Visually impaired (partially sighted and blind) children are usually identified before the preschool years. The nurse can aid in recognizing these conditions early so that effective treatment programs can be instituted to prevent developmental delays and lifelong maladaptive functioning. While some of these children may show developmental delays, it cannot be assumed that the more limited a child's vision is, the greater the developmental delay. Furthermore, depending on how successfully a child can learn through his remaining vision and his other senses, his development may not be delayed at all.[3]

In addition to her part in early identification of eye problems, the nurse can provide anticipatory guidance to parents on the child's development and, in the event of problems, can supply information on available resources.

Early Identification of Visual Problems

Early detection of visual problems is accomplished only through a screening program that begins when a child is born. Specific vision screening tests requiring special equipment that can be used for infants are discussed in other publications.[13] A simple approach for nurses to use is assessment of the development of vision (Table 43–2). Assessment of vision as part of well-child examinations involves various techniques listed in Table 43–3. Components of an eye examination and a description of screening techniques are included in Chapter 13.

In addition to assessing vision during health examinations, the nurse should teach families to detect a visual problem in their child. The Home Eye Test for Preschoolers is available from the National Society for the Prevention of Blindness.*

Refractive Errors

In vision, light rays enter the lens and are brought to a single point of focus on the retina.

---
*79 Madison Ave., New York, NY 10016.

TABLE 43-2 ASSESSMENT OF VISION DEVELOPMENT

Birth to 2 weeks	Eyes blink in response to bright light. Doll's eye reflex because child is unable to integrate head and eye movements. (When examiner rotates infant's head to one side, eyes lag behind). Transitory fixation develops at a distance of approximately 3 feet.
1–2 months	Regards parent's face and watches intently. Follows large moving objects in range of 90° (45° from midline) but glances are minimal for moving stimuli beyond 2 feet.
3–4 months	Visual following at 6–12 inches from face with a combination of head and eye movements through an 180° arc. Convergence on near objects now developed. Doll's eye reflex disappears. Watches own hands and feet. Fixates immediately on a 1-inch cube brought within 1–2 feet of the eye.
6–7 months	Ciliary muscle function begins and accommodation-convergence reflex developing. Eyes move together (binocular vision established). Crossing is abnormal and indicates strabismus. Hand-eye coordination is developing. Child reaches for anything seen and adjusts own position to see objects.
10 months	Pats at mirror image. Sees tiny objects and reaches for them using fingers and thumb. Follows and watches activities within 10–12 feet. Visual acuity 20/200.
12 months	Drops toys and watches them fall. Recognizes familiar people at 20 feet or more in the distance. Visual acuity 20/100.
18 months	A keen interest in pictures. Fixes eyes on small dangling toy at 10 feet. Points to familiar objects. Convergence well established.
2 years	Accommodates well. Recognizes fine details in pictures.
3 years	Attention span is fair. Fixation on small pictures or toys approaches 50 seconds. Matches letters HOVT in STYCAR test at 10 feet. Visual acuity ±20/40.*
4 years	Visual acuity ±20/30*
5 years	Visual acuity ±20/30*
6–7 years	Visual acuity 20/20*

*From B. Bates. A Guide to Physical Assessment. J. B. Lippincott Co., 1979. T. Johnson et al. Children Are Different: Developmental Physiology, 2nd ed., Ross Laboratories, 1978. S. Stangler et al. Screening Growth and Development of Preschool Children: A Guide for Test Selection. McGraw-Hill Book Co., 1980.

When the bending of the rays (refraction) and the length of the eyeball are uncoordinated, the image does not fall on a single point on the retina. Reduced acuity and discomfort related to the use of the eye are the two major symptoms of refractive errors.[14] While a child may not say that he has trouble seeing, symptoms such as rubbing of the eyes, tearing, red-rimmed eyelids and squinting should make one suspicious of a refractive error.

The work of the eye — bringing the image into clear focus — involves accommodation and convergence. Accommodation is the focusing mechanism of the eyes that allows a person to see clearly at all distances. As the ciliary muscle contracts, the curvature of the lens and its refractive strength are increased. Convergence of the eyes occurs simultaneously with accommodation in a fixed ratio. Convergence is an increasing inward movement of the eyeballs as an object is brought from a position of distance to closeness. The closer the object is brought to the child's face the greater the degree of convergence. This reflex facilitates focusing of the image at the same position on the retina of each eye, resulting in binocular vision, or fusion of the images. As the object is brought closer to the child's face, in addition to convergence, constriction of the pupils occurs.

Measurement of visual acuity is a screening test that can be done easily and quickly to identify refractive errors. The preschool years are an important time to detect these errors to help the child avoid problems in school. The nurse should understand that the eyeball grows as the child grows and that during this time refraction may change significantly. The three

TABLE 43-3 TECHNIQUES OF VISION ASSESSMENT*

Age	Techniques
Newborn	External inspection of eye (check for infection, trauma, and congenital anomalies). Check for blink response to bright light. Check for presence of red reflex and pupillary response to light. Do Hirschberg test for detection of strabismus. Check for nystagmus† with optokinetic drum‡ to establish the presence of vision.
6 months	External inspection of eye as for newborn. (A deviation or anomaly may now be apparent that was not noted in the newborn.) Test for strabismus: Use cover-uncover test or alternate cover test; Hirschberg test; check whether both eyes follow a light from side to side equally well. Observe for nystagmus. (Congenital nystagmus is present at birth but is not commonly detected before the age of 2–3 months.) Assess visual development. (See Table 43–2.) Perform ophthalmoscopic examination.
3–5 years	External inspection of eyes as during infancy. Test for Strabismus as described for 6 months of age. Behavior of child: <ul><li>Frequently rubs eyes</li><li>Brings eyes close to objects</li><li>Frequently squints or frowns in order to see</li><li>Tilts head; shuts or covers one eye</li><li>Complains of itchiness, burning, or a "dusty" feeling in eyes</li><li>Cannot see well (chalkboard, a toy, an object across the room)</li><li>Has abnormal sensitivity to light</li><li>Has more than usual difficulty adapting to low levels of illumination</li></ul> Visual acuity tested with Snellen E symbol. (Of particular importance is identification of unequal vision caused by amblyopia) Check for color blindness. Refer a 3-year-old with visual acuity of 20/50 or less and 4- or 5-year-old with 20/40 or less. (All children should be rescreened on another day before referral. Other tests of visual acuity for preschooler: STYCAR (letter matching test) Allen picture cards
School-age	Techniques for detection of visual problems is similar to that described for 3–5 year olds with the exception that as the letters of the alphabet are learned it is recommended that the standard Snellen alphabet chart is used.

*Adapted from "About Children's Eyes" Available from National Association for Visually Handicapped, 305 East 24th Street, New York, NY 10010. S. Stangler et al. Screening Growth and Development of Preschool Children: A Guide for Test Selection. McGraw-Hill, 1980. E. Hatfield. Methods and standards for screening preschool children. The Sightsaving Review, Summer 1979.

†Nystagmus is a rhythmic oscillation of the eyes that normally occurs on lateral gaze.

‡An optokinetic drum is a striped cylinder that when twirled within the baby's range of vision normally elicits nystagmus if vision is present.

---

types of refractive errors that are most common in children are hyperopia, myopia, and astigmatism. Hyperopia increases until around 6 to 7 years of age, after which it decreases gradually until adulthood; myopia usually begins around the teen years and gradually increases until adulthood.[17]

Hyperopia In hyperopia (farsightedness) there is insufficient refractive power, resulting in poor vision at any distance because the image falls behind the retina. Increased accommodative effort brings the focus of the image forward onto the retina. Children have the ability to accommodate to attain good visual acuity; however, if the hyperopia is great, correction with convex lenses may be required. The constant accommodative effort required for close work may cause eyestrain and eventually strabismus and amblyopia, to be discussed later.

Myopia In myopia (nearsightedness) there is an excessive amount of refractive power resulting in light rays coming to a point of focus in front of the retina. The only symptom of myopia is blurred vision for distance. Eyestrain and headaches are not associated with myopia. A child with myopia may be able to read without accommodative effort, because near vision requires greater refractive strength than distant vision.[14] If, however, myopia is severe, the child may have to hold the print close to see it clearly.

Concave lenses readily correct the vision of a myopic child, but the problem may become more severe during the early school years. The child may need new glasses every year or two. On the other hand, congenital myopia tends to resolve gradually with age, with a visual acuity of 20/40 by adolescence.[17] These children may or may not need corrective lenses, depending on the severity of the problem.

Astigmatism In astigmatism the curvature of the cornea is not equal in all directions. The result is that light rays are not focused symmetrically; therefore, the image is blurred and distorted. Eyestrain results from the accommodative effort that is made to bring the image into focus. The problem cannot be compensated for by accommodation on the part of the child; it must be corrected with lenses that compensate for the abnormal curvature of the cornea. Astigmatism may coexist with myopia or hyperopia.

Strabismus (Squint)

Strabismus is a condition in which there is a lack of coordination of the eye muscles. The eyes do not work together, resulting in a crossed-eye appearance. The condition occurs in about 2 per cent of all children. The normal infant may at times appear to have strabismus because of incomplete coordination between the two eyes. This results in transient ocular deviations. However, by 3 months of age the child's eyes should be focusing together.[17] Some children appear to have strabismus because of certain facial features; this is called pseudostrabismus (Fig. 43-1). The features that give a false impression of strabismus are prominent epicanthal folds and a broad, flat nasal bridge.

About 50 per cent of all children with strabismus have a positive family history for the condition; therefore, any child in a family with a history of strabismus should be followed closely. Also, the siblings of a child with strabismus should be examined frequently for this defect. The most common cause of strabismus is imbalance of the muscle alignment of the eyes, but other etiologic factors such as brain tumor, infection, retinoblastoma, myasthenia gravis, and cataracts should be considered. Whenever there is any suspicion that a child has strabismus, he must be referred for further examination.

Any type of misalignment should be of concern, and any child who does not see well with each eye should be suspected of having a serious condition.[8] Early recognition and treatment are essential to prevent amblyopia. Amblyopia develops when vision is suppressed in the eye that deviates. Without correction permanent visual loss may occur in the deviated eye.

There are two major kinds of strabismus: nonparalytic (noncomitant) and paralytic (comitant). Nonparalytic strabismus is the most common type in children. The child has difficulty seeing at close range and is likely to squint. Accommodative strabismus is a special type of nonparalytic strabismus that usually develops between 2 and 4 years of age. It has two forms: convergent and divergent. This type of strabismus develops because of a refractive error. Most children normally have a degree of hyperopia (farsightedness) until about 7 years of age. In the presence of hyperopia, accommodative effort is required to attain good vision. With accommodation there is normally an accompanying convergence reflex; a fine balance is needed between the accommodative effort and the simultaneous convergence. In the hyperopic child strabismus can result when the amount of accommodation required for clear

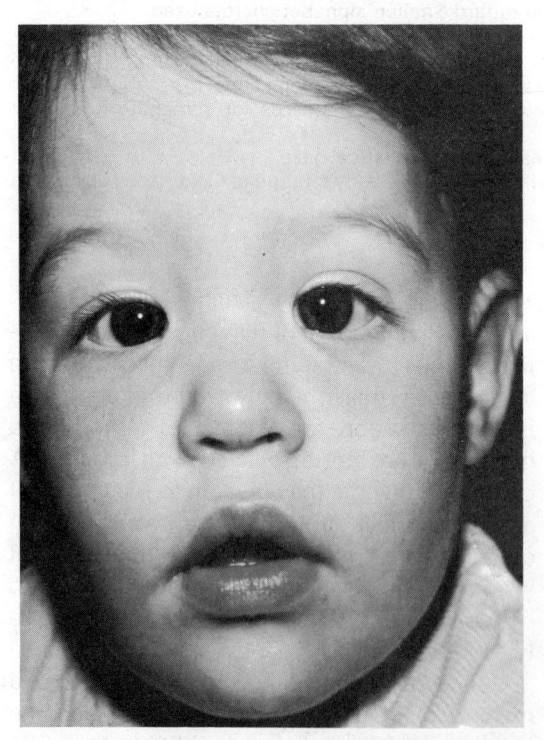

Figure 43-1 Pseudostrabismus. (From H. Scheie and D. Albert. Textbook of Ophthalmology. W. B. Saunders Co., 1977, p. 337.)

vision results in excessive convergence (crossed eyes).[22] Conversely, external deviation (divergence) occurs in myopia; this is less common but may be present at birth.

The various terms used to describe strabismus are as follows:

Words ending in:
- tropia–an active, observable misalignment
- phoria–a latent tendency to misalignment (strabismus becomes evident only during fatigue, illness or stress)

Monocular–one eye is used to fixate and the other deviates. The deviating eye is prone to the development of amblyopia.

Alternating–each eye is alternately used for fixation; vision develops more or less the same in both eyes.

Convergent (esotropia)–eye turns toward the midline (Fig. 43–2).

Divergent (exotropia)–eye turns away from midline.

Nonparalytic (noncomitant)–all muscles function but not in unison; deviation is the same in all directions of gaze.

Paralytic–caused by a weakness or paralysis of one or more of the extraocular muscles; eye appears crossed when turned in the direction of the affected muscle.

In paralytic strabismus the child may complain of headache and demonstrate lack of coordination in fine or gross movements. Double vision, or diplopia, is evident by the child's response. He may close one eye or tilt his head in order to avoid seeing a double image.

Strabismus may be obvious, or it may occur only when the child is ill or tired. Screening tests for strabismus include the cover test and Hirschberg test described in Chapter 13.

Management The goal of treatment is for the child to attain the best possible vision in each eye and, if possible, equal vision. The ultimate goal is attainment of binocular vision with stereopsis (depth perception). However, in many affected patients this cannot be achieved.[17] The type of treatment varies with the age of the child and type of strabismus. Patching of the good eye is a common method of treatment. This is done to encourage the child to use the deviating eye. In some instances, for example in the case of accommodative strabismus, the wearing of glasses may correct the deviation.

In very young children anticholinesterase drugs (miotics) such as echothiophate iodide (Phospholine Iodide) and isoflurophate (DFP) are used to correct accommodative esotropia. Inhibition of cholinesterase affects the normally fixed relationship between accommodation and convergence. Anticholinesterase causes the ciliary muscle to respond to only a minimal accommodative innervation. Consequently, as accommodative innervation is decreased, convergence is also lessened, resulting in correction of the strabismus. However, many children require surgery on the extraocular muscles to correct the misalignment of the eyes. An adjunct to glasses, patching, medications and surgery is the use of eye exercises (orthopics). Eye exercises should be prescribed by an ophthalmologist; they are useful only in selected cases.

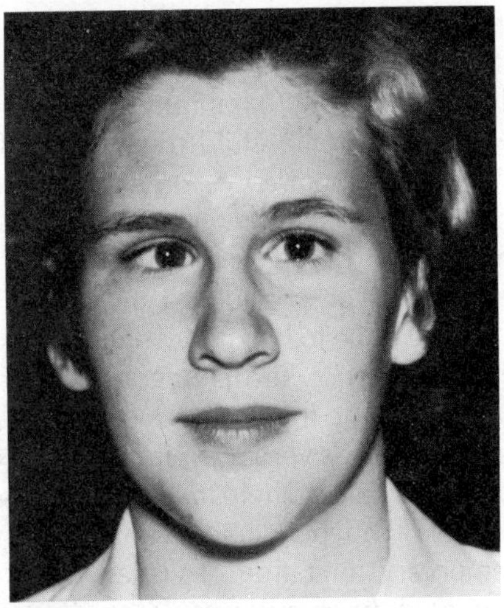

In the management of strabismus, the nurse can help the family carry out the required treatment and ensure that the child has regular eye examinations. Of particular importance is that any child who requires eye patches should be closely followed for decreased vision in the patched eye as a result of the occlusion. In very young children amblyopia can develop in the patched eye in less than two weeks.[22]

A frequently encountered problem is the young child's refusal to keep on an eye patch. When patching is required, a pair of clear glasses with a patch occluding the one eye may be more acceptable to a young child. If the condition permits, intermittent patching may be necessary during the first few days. When patching is required postoperatively the child should be introduced to this sensation before surgery by playing games that require having the eyes

Figure 43–2 Accommodative esotropia, uncorrected. (From H. Scheie and D. Albert. Textbook of Ophthalmology. W. B. Saunders Co., 1977, p. 337.)

covered. Arm restraints should also be made available for preoperative experimentation with a doll or favorite stuffed animal.

Postoperatively the child must be treated as any child with impaired vision. If both eyes are patched he must be treated as a blind child; that is, things are placed within easy reach, the environment is described and the child is told what will be done to him and what he is likely to feel before a procedure is begun. The child is allowed to handle things to discover their properties but he needs verbal explanations of color. The primary goal is to help the child maintain his usual level of independence even though he has the temporary limitation of visual impairment. The surgery is brief and usually the child can be discharged the day after.[9]

During the course of management the nurse is a resource person to the family. The negative effects of strabismus on the child's self-image and personality development can be minimized if attention is given to this potential problem early, beginning at the time of diagnosis. It is disappointing to the child and his family when the operation fails to correct the misalignment. It should be explained early that repeated operations may be necessary.

Ongoing communication with the family regarding any difficulty encountered in carrying out the treatment program is an important contribution of the nurse. The child and his family should be encouraged to express their thoughts and feelings about the operation and required treatment. The nurse should understand that when the operation is repeated it offers the same likelihood of success as did the original operation.[8] She should avoid misleading the family into assuming that successful correction will be achieved.

The nurse should decide if referral of the family to a public health nurse or public agency is needed to meet demands of long-term care. If the child is in school, the treatment plan should be explained to the school nurse and limitations on the child's school activities should be discussed.

Amblyopia

Amblyopia (lazy eye) is reduction or loss of vision in an eye that is normal on ophthalmoscopic examination.[22] A commonly accepted diagnostic sign of amblyopia is that visual acuity in the normal eye is at least two Snellen lines better than the acuity in the affected eye. There are various types of amblyopia: strabismic amblyopia, amblyopia ex anopsia and anisometropic amblyopia.

Strabismic amblyopia is the loss of vision in the deviating eye of a child with strabismus. Visual loss occurs because there is an attempt to suppress the double vision experienced by the child with strabismus. The vision in the suppressed eye fails to develop, resulting in loss of vision ranging from a minimal decrease in acuity to severely impaired vision.

Early detection and treatment of strabismus is essential to prevent strabismic amblyopia. Usually by the age of 6 years the brain has developed suppression to a degree that will not readily respond to treatment, and by 8 or 9 years of age reversal of the impairment is considered virtually impossible.[22]

Amblyopia ex anopsia refers to visual loss from disuse owing to some type of occlusion. This type of amblyopia can be caused by ptosis (drooping of the upper eyelid), cataracts and occlusion therapy for strabismic amblyopia.

Amblyopia can also result from dissimilar refractive errors in the two eyes. Hyperopia (farsightedness) is a normal condition until around 6 to 7 years of age. This condition normally requires an accommodative effort by the child to correct the refractive error. When the two eyes are not equally hyperopic, fusion may be impossible because of the differences in the images. The less hyperopic eye may then become the preferred eye because less accommodation is required. Consequently, the other eye (the more hyperopic one) becomes lazy or amblyopic. This is known as *anisometropic amblyopia*. This type of amblyopia can be prevented if discovered and treated early. Glasses are necessary to correct the refractive error and prevent the development of anisometropic amblyopia.

In addition to using glasses to correct any refractive error, patching of the good eye is the basis for treating amblyopia. The patch is usually worn during the waking hours, but some authorities even recommend that the child wear the patch 24 hours a day. Careful follow-up is essential to prevent amblyopia of the eye that is being patched. Patching may be required for as long as a year, followed by a period of time during which intermittent patching must be continued. The child and his family need reinforcement from the health team for their efforts in complying with the long-term therapy of keeping a young child's eye patched. With early identification and adequate therapy irreversible loss of vision can be prevented.

Visual Impairment

The term visual impairment includes a highly heterogeneous group of conditions. Some people with visual impairment are able to distinguish between light and dark or have good sight for distance but not for peripheral vision (tunnel vision), while others are totally blind. Visual impairment is classified according to physiological measurements (visual acuity) as well as functional ability.[3, 18]

Partial sight Physiological measurement: Children with partial sight have vision that cannot be corrected beyond 20/70 in either eye or have a limited field of vision (the widest diameter of visual field subtending an angle of no greater than 140 degrees).

Functional ability: Vision is considered partial when visual loss interferes with learning processes but still permits the use of print as a chief method of learning.

Blindness Physiological measurement: Children with corrected vision in the better eye of not more than 20/200 or a limitation in the visual field (widest diameter of vision subtending an angle of no more than 20 degrees) are considered blind.

Functional ability: A child is considered blind when other senses (hearing and touch) are relied upon as the chief means of task performance and learning.

The term *visual handicap* is usually used to describe the condition in those children with visual impairment who, even after maximum correction, are limited in their ability to learn through the visual channel.[3] Most blind children have some remaining (residual) vision that they should be encouraged to use. *Residual vision* is a term used to describe the vision of a child who cannot read print of any size but whose vision is more than only light perception.[18] Any degree of vision that a child has should be used because the eyes, particularly those of young children, benefit from use.[3]

Detection and Prevention of Visual Impairment Genetic and unknown causes are responsible for the majority of cases of congenital blindness in children. A family history of a genetic disease associated with visual loss is significant information that may lead to the early detection of visual impairment in an infant. Also, genetic counselling is an important aspect of prevention of blindness when known genetic diseases that cause blindness are identified in a family history. Prenatal screening for maternal infections that cause blindness (rubella, syphilis) and adequate prenatal care to prevent prematurity are preventive approaches in which the nurse may have responsibility.

Postnatally in preventive actions the nurse's duties include prophylactic instillation of silver nitrate to prevent blindness from gonorrheal conjunctivitis and prevention of retrolental fibroplasia by maintaining oxygen levels for prematures at a concentration not above 40 per cent. Periodic screening is essential for the early detection of congenital blindness and visual problems that could lead to blindness. If vision problems are detected, the nurse can provide close supervision of corrective measures to ensure that glasses or eye patches are worn. The nurse can also aid in early detection of tumors, infections and diseases such as diabetes and rheumatoid arthritis that can lead to blindness by taking a thorough history and performing a careful eye examination on all well-child visits. The nurse should ensure that all children receive adequate immunizations against childhood illnesses and provide safety counselling to prevent accidental eye injury. Sharp objects, fireworks, chemicals, power tools and sunlight are potential sources of danger to a child's eyes.

Clinical manifestations of specific conditions causing loss of vision (cataracts, glaucoma, retinoblastoma) are discussed elsewhere in the test. Included in this section is a discussion of the impact of visual impairment on the child and his family. Visually impaired children have the same needs as other children, but they are met through alternative means. These children need stimulation from their environment and the opportunity to get information and responses from the people around them. These children cannot get information and responses through sight; therefore, experiences must be adapted to support their physical, intellectual and emotional and social development.

Partial Sight

The dilemma of the partially sighted is best described in the words of a partially sighted child: "It is very hard when you are not really blind or sighted because you are just hanging in the middle."[18] Partially sighted children's conditions are often misdiagnosed or remain undiagnosed. Their eyes may look normal, and it is only when the child's development seems to be slow that parents may suspect something is wrong. The behavior and responses of these children are often misinterpreted. For example, when first enrolled in preschool, a partially sighted child may be viewed as clumsy or immature or as a slow learner or a behavior problem because he appears uncooperative and inattentive.

Areas in which a partially sighted child needs special help and understanding are related to communication, mobility, spatial perception and visual fatigue. The partially sighted child is often unsure of how to respond verbally to others. The intent of people's communication is often conveyed through facial expression and gestures. Because a partially sighted child's perception is distorted, he may be confused as to how to respond. Additional verbal explanations may be required to clarify the exact meaning and intent during conversation.

Mobility and spatial perception are also affected when a child has partial sight. Many of these children walk later and more hesitantly than sighted children. Their depth perception and concept of the body in space may not be developed sufficiently, resulting in clumsiness, falls and accidents.

Visual fatigue is particularly noticed when a partially sighted child begins school. Teachers, nurses and parents must recognize that behavior problems may develop because of visual fatigue. As a child's eyes tire he may become inattentive and irritable. Diagnosis and assessment of the child's vision by an ophthalmologist is essential in order to plan an educational program that best meets his needs.

Once the child's visual capacities have been established, management of the visual disability follows. This includes increasing the retinal image by magnification, increasing the sharpness of the image or using other senses (auditory or tactile) to compensate for vision loss.[26] A particularly well-accepted visual aid device for preschoolers 4 and 5 years of age is a hand-held prism telescope of six times and eight times magnification; its use is thought to possibly improve self-sufficiency and mobility later in life.[26] Other low-vision aid devices are available through low-vision aid centers. (See list of services at the end of this chapter.) However, low-vision aid facilities in the United States are primarily located in cities and are fewer in number than service organizations for the blind.[21]

In the past there has been some concern that straining the eyes might result in further loss of vision. Consequently, use of books in Braille was recommended as the major source of learning so that sight would be "saved." Now that it has been determined that using the eyes does not weaken vision, partially sighted children are reading large-print materials, in addition to using a variety of supplemental aids including talking books, tapes and cassettes, magnifiers, telescopes, and closed-circuit television enlarging devices.

The problems of the partially sighted are different from those of the blind. Many of the social and economic rehabilitative services available to the "legally blind" are not available to the partially sighted. The most important aspect of adjustment for the partially sighted child is learning to utilize his residual vision fully.[21] With adequate services and devices to supplement his vision, a partially sighted child has a chance to participate in his world and reach his maximum potential.

Blindness

Each blind child has individual needs as does any child; however, a child who is robbed of one of his most crucial senses has the special need to learn alternate ways of relating to his environment. Every area of his development is affected by a child's inability to see. The following discussion describes the impact of blindness and appropriate interventions in the areas of (1) developing human attachment, (2) motor development and mobility, (3) language cognition and learning, (4) play and socialization, (5) independence and self-concept and (6) perception of space and body image.

The *development of human attachment* is basic to a child's growth and serves as the foundation for the parent-child relationship. When a child is blind, the usual facial interplay that is used to express mutual pleasure between the infant and parents must be replaced by an alternate method of communication. The pattern of smiling and the factors that elicit it are different in a blind infant. For the sighted infant the visual stimulus of the human face elicits an automatic smile at 2 to 2½ months of age with a high degree of regularity for which there is no equivalence in the blind baby.[12] In a study of seven infants Fraiberg[11, 12] noted that from the second month on blind babies smiled in response to a familiar voice or sound and increasingly demonstrated a pattern of selective smiling in favor of the mother's voice. However, the smile was not automatic and even the mother's voice did not elicit it regularly. To help parents of a blind baby, the nurse should understand the importance that the smile has in development of a mutually satisfying relationship between parent and infant. Parents can be encouraged to hold their blind infant and talk, coo and sing to him and play lap games with him to help him learn to know them and to elicit smiles.

Even when parents and blind infants develop a maximally satisfying relationship, the smile of the blind infant differs from that of the sighted child. Blind babies have a "muted smile" and do not have expressive facial signs that depict various emotions. The absence of these signs may be read as "no affect" and are cause for parents and others to comment that "he looks depressed" or "nothing interests him."[12] The process of developing a satisfying exchange of signals between parents and their blind infant must be recognized by the nurse as a potentially frustrating experience for parents. The nurse has an important responsibility to help parents and blind infants communicate and to provide parents an opportunity to express feelings about the development of their relationship with the infant.

Motor development and mobility for a blind infant is another area that requires special intervention from parents. In the sighted child, motor development is enhanced by the child's interest in moving toward the things he can see. While auditory experiences in a blind child must replace visual experiences, an important phenomenon regarding a child's response to sound must be recognized. The sighted child reaches for and attains an object at the age of 24 to 28 weeks[9] because he can see it. However, whether blind or sighted, an infant does not reach for an object he *hears* until the last quarter of the first year. Activities of reaching and grasping for and crawling toward an object have a primary role in motor development, but the blind child is dependent on auditory stimulation for self-initiated mobility. Consequently this movement does not occur in the blind child until much later than it does for a sighted child because the sighted child moves toward the object he sees. Therefore, the immediate environment of the blind child must provide interesting sounding objects and varied tactile experiences that the child's hands will encounter while randomly moving. These early experiences with objects provide the blind infant with the necessary stimulation to progress toward a sense of self and object differentiation.

Various stimuli can be used to lure the infant to begin to move out into the space around him. Without specific intervention this infant's hands may encounter only each other or the mouth. If mouth and hand activities become fixed at this immature level, these infants are reported to show signs of impending autism.[1]

Blind babies have been reported to sit and support themselves on their hands and knees at the same time as sighted children, but these activities were not followed by creeping as they were in sighted infants.[11] Independent walking for the blind child is hampered because he lacks the visual model to imitate. A blind baby was described by Adelson and Fraiberg to walk "painstakingly at first, one step at a time, feeling his way repeatedly as he gained familiarity with his old world in a new position."[2] The median age for independent walking in blind children reported in their research is 19.25 months, 7 months later than sighted children. If the blind baby is given early experience with the interesting possibilities in the space around him and is lured into that space by the familiar voices of his parents and by interesting sounds, he will achieve the developmental task of independent walking, although at a later time than will a sighted child.

Achievement of independent walking is encumbered with fears on the part of the child as well as the parents. The child needs repeated practice to propel himself into an experience that provides new sensation; at times he may reach an impasse, when he seems to retreat from his experimentation with walking. Parents, on the other hand, fear that a delay in walking may mean that their child is mentally retarded.[10] Parents need to be prepared for these delays and may need constant encouragement to provide opportunities that will help their blind child learn the skills of mobility.

As the blind child becomes mobile parents are faced with a new dilemma — they fear that he will be injured while engaging in normal active play. During the active preschool years all children need special instructions about dangers, but they should not be prohibited from engaging in normal activities of swinging, biking, sliding and other playground activities.

Specific activities must be taught to a blind child because he cannot learn by imitation. For example, a child's legs and arms may have to be physically manipulated to show him how to skip, hop or bounce a ball. He can learn how to use play equipment such as a slide and monkey bars by feeling another child's body move or by having someone move his body through the motions.[3] While a blind child is taught the motions of these physical activities he must also be taught the rules and limitations that will keep him safe.

Successful mobility is one of the most important skills that a blind person acquires. Early intervention can determine to a large degree how independent a blind person will be in later life.[18] As a child enters school specific mobility skills can be taught by trained instructors. Blind children are taught to listen for the echo of their breath to tell them when they are about to bump into large objects. Cane technique and guide dogs are invaluable aids to independent movement. Guide dogs are not usually used until the teen years.[18]

Blindness has a profound impact on the child's abilities in *language cognition and learning*. Vocalizations and first words occur during the first year of life at about the same time in a blind child and a sighted child.[18] After this stage, however, language development in a blind child is often delayed, but the degree of visual impairment has not been shown to correlate positively with speech and language difficulties; this indicates that blindness alone is not the decisive factor.[18]

The family and environment of the blind child greatly influences his cognitive and language development. This child must be talked to and the verbalizations should be associated with concrete experiences to enable the child to understand words and concepts. The child needs to handle toys and variously shaped objects while their characteristics are being described to him.

The blind child must accept verbal descriptions by the sighted of many objects and phenomena that he cannot touch (moon, fire). Therefore he has an incomplete concept of whatever is being described. The ability to describe visual concepts verbally while having only partial or inaccurate understanding is called *verbalism*. Teaching a blind child from infancy with as many concrete experiences as possible helps the child develop concepts and is an important intervention to promote later academic learning.

School programs for the visually impaired are varied, ranging from residential schools for the blind to public school programs in which the blind are integrated. Both types of programs require special equipment and devices for the blind student. Academic achievement of blind children who have access to appropriate educational opportunities does not differ from that of sighted children.[6]

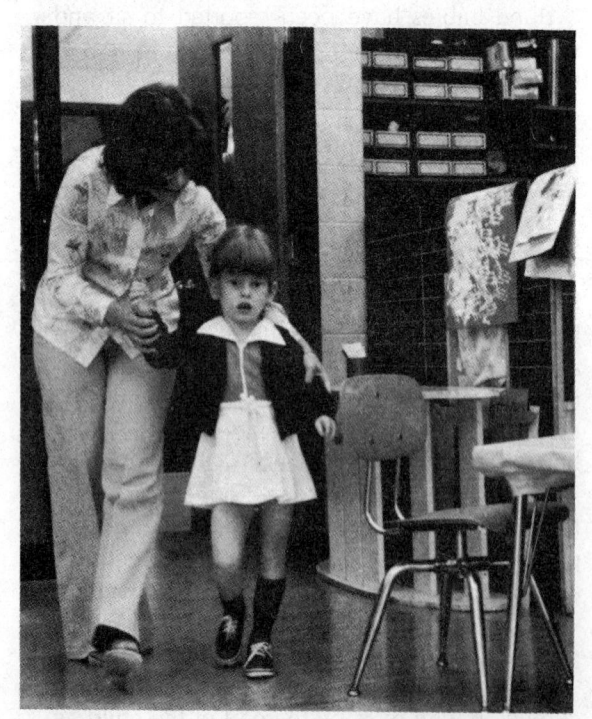

"And now we're coming to the worktable, where Barry is sitting." (From L. Alonso et al. Mainstreaming Preschoolers: Children with Visual Handicaps. DHEW Publication No. (OHDS) 78-3112. U.S. Gov't. Printing Office, p. 39.)

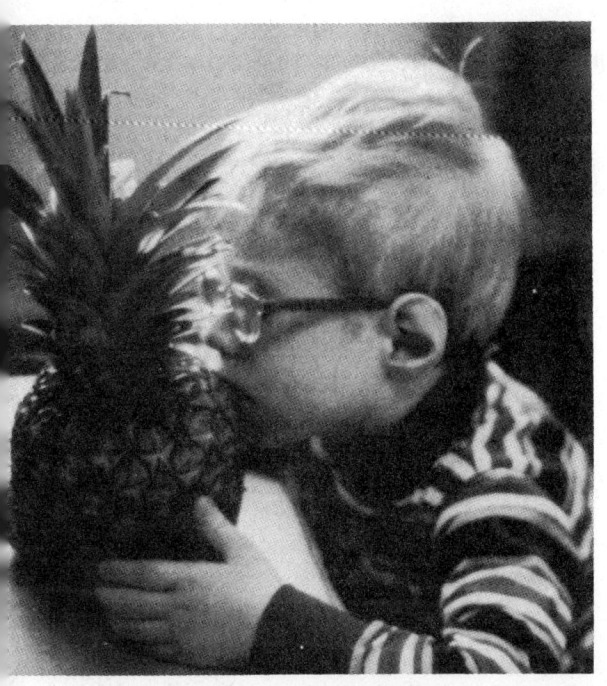

Blind children need the experience of feeling objects. (From L. Alonso et al. Mainstreaming Preschoolers: Children with Visual Handicaps. DHEW Publication No. (OHDS) 78-3112. U.S. Gov't. Printing Office, p. 67.)

Technological advances are making the printed word more accessible to blind children, but many blind scholars believe that Braille will continue to be a primary method of reading and writing for the blind.[18] Electronic reading devices in which letters are produced in tactile form are also available. Machines that actually speak the words, talking calculators and tape recordings (with a device that can increase or slow the speed of the recording) can aid the blind student.[18] In addition to educational materials the blind student may need special help in physical education and sex education, and in music, drama and art.

A blind child's *play and social skills* are profoundly affected by his visual impairment. As he becomes mobile, the active play of young children presents new problems to the blind child. In the area of physical activity his ability to learn games through imitation is limited and his ability to compete with peers is diminished. He cannot follow a rolling ball because he cannot see it. Furthermore, because he cannot imitate his peers in actions and behavior, he is unable to gain a sense of being like them.

Blind children need extra help from teachers, other children and family members during play and socialization experiences. During the preschool years when a child learns to relate to other children, the blind child be told about the activity and his body must be moved through the activity before he can understand the nature of it. Visually impaired children benefit from physical contact when being helped to accomplish a task as an alternative to being able to learn by imitation.

The choice of play materials for the blind child is based on the guideline that if a child cannot see materials well enough to learn the intended concepts or skills, substitute tactile or auditory material must be provided to teach these things.[18] When playing with a blind child, one must talk more than normally about the objects and the activity so that he will gain an accurate idea of what constitutes his environment. A wide range of textures should be available to the child, and their appearance described. During play a blind child is assisted to distinguish various sounds and the direction from which the sounds are coming. The more sensory experiences a blind child has in play, the more opportunity he has to take in information to foster his normal growth and development.

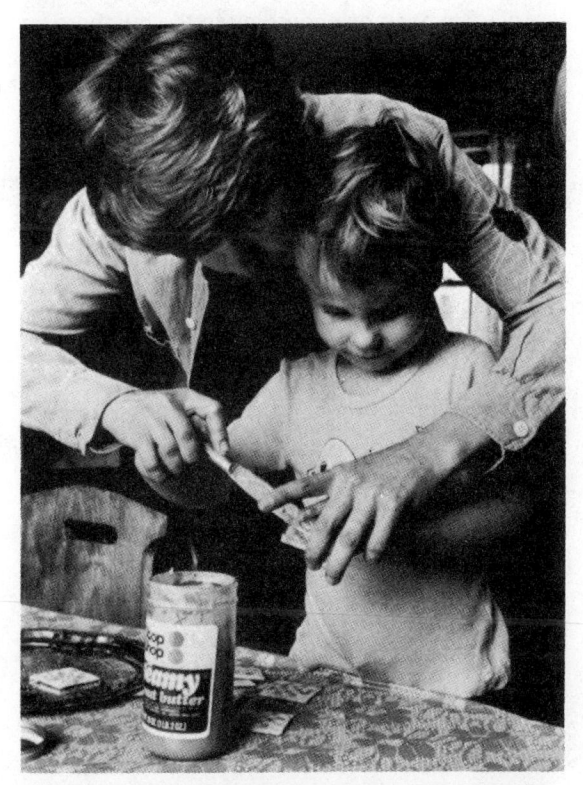

Visually handicapped children often learn best by being "moved" through an activity. (From L. Alonso et al. Mainstreaming Preschoolers: Children with Visual Handicaps. DHEW Publication No. (OHDS) 78-3112. U.S. Gov't. Printing Office, p. 48.)

POTENTIAL STRESSES DURING THE PRESCHOOL YEARS: IRREVERSIBLE ALTERATIONS IN HEALTH STATUS

PRACTICAL HINTS TO USE IN FOSTERING INDEPENDENCE IN A BLIND CHILD

Orientation and Mobility
- To move along a wall, hold arm nearest wall slightly out to the side and forward.
- Hand is in a loosely curved position with the back of the fingers touching the wall to locate openings or obstacles.
- Fingers are curved slightly inward to prevent injury at places such as door frames.
- Explain where you are going when leading a child so that he feels secure.
- Verbally describe arrangement of desks and furniture so that he can become independent more quickly.

Mealtime and Snacks
- Use real dishes — plastic or paper dishes tip and spill easily.
- A dish with a rim and some depth makes it easier for a child to use a scooping maneuver.
- Securing the dish to the table surface eliminates accidental tipping and spilling.
- Placing food in a circle and explaining its position according to the numbers on the clock is useful for children who can tell time.
- Glasses or cups should have a wide base.
- Permit children to pour their own liquids when developmentally able to do so. (Child can grip glass with one hand and place index finger slightly below the rim of the glass to feel when the glass is full.) See photograph on next page.
- By sitting behind a child in helping him learn to use a spoon, one can assist him with more natural feeding movements.
- In some cases the help of an occupational therapist should be suggested if a child has difficulty in swallowing, chewing or biting.

Dressing
- Start with undressing (outerwear, then loose clothing such as T-shirts and sweaters).
- Break tasks down into small steps, explaining each step while the child's hand is over yours as the task is performed.
- Praise the child as each step is learned.
- Tags and special identifying marks on clothes are needed to help a child choose his own outfits.

Toilet Training
- A child must be instructed verbally in a step-by-step approach, including where the potty is, how it looks, and its purpose.

From Mainstreaming Preschoolers: Children with Visual Handicaps. DHEW Publication No. (OHDS) 78–3112. U.S. Gov't. Printing Office, 1978.

The nurse can help parents provide their infant with a stimulating environment involving a variety of sounds and textural toys. During preschool years play and socialization is enhanced if the blind child is assisted in participating in normal activities of his age group, with appropriate guidance in keeping him safe while furthering his independence.

Self-stimulating mannerisms such as body rocking, eye poking, head rolling, thumb sucking and other eye, hand and head movements have been noted in blind children. These are called stereotyped behaviors. These repetitive motor activities vary in frequency, complexity and intensity. A direct positive correlation with the degree of visual impairment and the frequency of the behaviors has been reported.[18] Furthermore, these activities seem to intensify with boredom as well as under excessive stimulation. It has been suggested that self-stimulating behaviors may be done to overstimulate the labyrinth of the inner ear in an effort to compensate for loss of orientation.[24] Although the cause of these behaviors is not fully understood, early intervention to provide the opportunity of mobility, exploration and manipulation of objects is recommended to help the child substitute for them.[18]

Achieving *independence in the activities of daily living* is important for the development of a positive self-concept in all children. The blind child is particularly at risk of losing the opportunity to do things for himself because he needs special help and additional time to learn self-care skills. Being treated as a capable person by teachers, friends and family members is crucial for the child to develop the initiative that will motivate him to try to do things for himself. The nurse can aid parents by providing them with

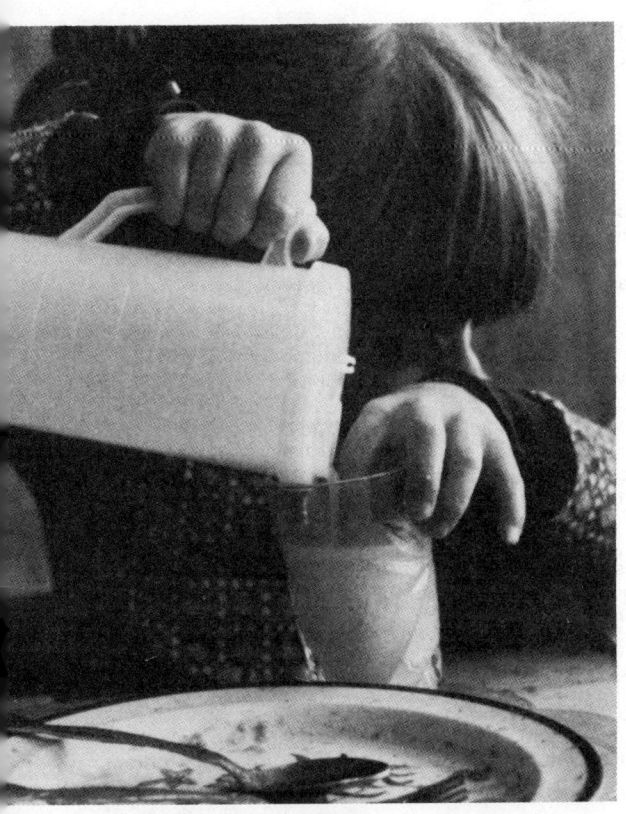

A blind child becomes independent by doing. (From L. Alonso et al. Mainstreaming Preschoolers: Children with Visual Handicaps. DHEW Publication No. (OHDS) 78-3112. U.S. Gov't. Printing Office, p. 59.)

hints that they can use to help foster independence.

The blind child develops a *body image* through tactile experiences and, once language becomes meaningful, through verbal communication and feedback. His ways of taking in information are inferior to those of the sighted child; consequently, the formation of body image is delayed.[23] Certain activities are thought to aid a child's ability to organize space in relation to his own body. For example, bending down, reaching out, and climbing under and over an object assists a blind child in developing an idea of where his body fits in relation to the larger space outside it.[4]

A problem of blind children that has been identified as indicating a deficit in body image is the "floppy" posture that some blind children tend to assume. Based on the verbal responses of blind children on tests of body image, Cratty[7] has identified four stages through which children pass in developing a body image. These are:

Phase I. Awareness of body parts, body planes and simple movements.

Phase II. Left-right discrimination.
Phase III. Body object relationships; identification of portions of the limbs.
Phase IV. Identification of body parts and body movements of another person.

Body image training as described by Cratty is organized around these four phases.

Development of body image is a central aspect of education of the blind. It cannot be left to chance that a child makes the connection of how his body relates to space. A thorough, systematic effort must be made by the sighted to help the blind child learn the dimensions of himself and his world.

HEARING IMPAIRMENT

Hearing impairment may be profound, significantly handicapping a child, or be so mild that it goes undetected for years. Both the volume (measured in decibels[dB]) and pitch (measured in Hertz [Hz]) of a sound determine whether it is audible to the human ear.

Levels of hearing impairment in decibels used to describe severity of hearing loss vary in the literature; however, it is generally agreed that persons with hearing levels exceeding 90 dB are termed "deaf."[4] For educational purposes, however, a *deaf* person is one whose hearing is disabled to a level (usually 70 dB or greater) at which speech through the ear alone, with or without a hearing aid, cannot be understood; a *hard-of-hearing* person is one whose hearing is disabled to a level (usually 35 to 69 dB) that makes it difficult to understand speech through the ear alone, with or without a hearing aid.[19] The hard-of-hearing person has sufficient residual hearing to understand speech with the use of a hearing aid, although it is difficult.

In contrast, for the deaf person vision is the primary mode of language acquisition and communication. The probable handicap that results from the various hearing levels in decibels is summarized in Table 43–4. It should be noted that the ranges differ for children and adults. It is felt that even slight hearing impairment may interfere with a child's normal development of speech and language and educational progress.[30]

The summary as provided in this table is at best only a general guide. It does not take into account important variables that the nurse

TABLE 43-4 DEGREE OF HANDICAP AND EDUCATIONAL NEED ACCORDING TO HEARING LEVELS

Hearing Level in Decibels (dB) and Degree of Hearing Loss		Effect of Hearing Loss and Educational Needs
Children	*Adults*	
Normal		Although this is considered normal hearing, those children in upper limits of this range may be affected. They may show poor language development, have problems in listening, and have reduced ability to hear information needed for academic achievement.
0–20	0–26	
Mild loss		Faint and distant speech is heard with difficulty. Child may benefit from a hearing aid and needs special seating and lighting in classroom; may need speechreading instruction.
27–35	27–40	
Moderate loss		Understands conversational speech at a distance of 3–5 feet if in face-to-face position. May be limited in vocabulary and exhibit some incorrect speech. Child in the classroom will benefit from special seating and a hearing aid; may need speechreading instruction.
36–55	41–55	
Moderately severe loss		Conversation must be loud to be understood. Child has great difficulty participating in classroom discussions. Needs special seating, hearing aid, speechreading instruction, and may need special classes for the hearing impaired to develop speech and language skills.
56–70	56–70	
Severe loss		May hear loud voices at a distance of one foot from the ear. May be able to distinguish vowels but not consonants. May be able to identify environmental noises. Speech and language is defective. Child requires full-time special education hearing aid, and program to develop language and speech.
71–90	71–90	
Profound		May hear some loud sounds but does so through recognizing vibration rather than tones. Does not rely on hearing as a primary channel for communication. Child requires full-time program with continuous appraisal of needs in regard to communication techniques.
91 or more	91 or more	

From S. R. Stangler et al. Screening Growth and Development: A Guide for Test Selection. McGraw-Hill Book Co. 1980, p. 126; F. N. Martin. *Pediatric Audiology*. Prentice-Hall, 1978, p. 38.

should always consider when assessing the impact of a hearing impairment. These factors are (1) cause and onset of the hearing loss, (2) type of hearing impairment (see later discussion on types of hearing losses), (3) presence of other impairments (physical, intellectual, emotional) and (4) interactions and relationships within the family.[30]

It is important for nurses to realize that a high percentage of children are affected by hearing loss yet it is often a subtle, undetected deficit that can seriously affect the child's development.

By 2 years of age, 1:25 children (4 per cent) will have mild to moderate hearing losses secondary to ear disease; in school-age children 7 to 8 per cent have some degree of hearing loss. Severe hearing loss is present in 1:1000 infants and 1:50 neonates discharged from intensive care nurseries.

Early detection of hearing impairment, regardless of degree, is paramount. By 3 years of age approximately 80 per cent of language growth is thought to have taken place.[12] Deafness during early childhood, occurring before the acquisition of a functional language base, seriously affects a child in all areas of development. Furthermore, mild hearing loss significantly reduces vocabulary growth, articulation skills, the ability to communicate through spoken language, the use of grammar and syntax and auditory memory skills.[14]

Regular hearing screening therefore becomes a critical feature of health assessment to prevent unnecessary sequelae to hearing deficits. An understanding of the causes and types of hearing impairment provides an important base for the nurse to carry out this responsibility.

Causes and Types of Hearing Impairment

Hearing loss may vary from mild to profound as outlined in Table 43-4. The higher the number

TABLE 43–5 ETIOLOGY OF DEAFNESS IN CHILDREN*

I. **Congenital Deafness**
   A. Genetic
      1. Deafness appearing alone due to defects in fetal development (aplasia)
      2. Deafness associated with other conditions (e.g. Waardenburg's syndrome, albinism, hyperpigmentation, visual handicaps
      3. Chromosomal abnormalities
         Trisomy 13–15
         Trisomy 18
   B. Nongenetic (prenatal and perinatal factors)
      1. Infection (maternal rubella, cytomegalovirus (CMU), toxoplasmosis, herpes simplex, congenital syphilis
      2. Ototoxic drugs (maternal ingestion of streptomycin, chloroquine, quinine, thalidomide, and possibly excessive use of salicylates)
      3. Metabolic disorders (toxemia, diabetes)
      4. Rh incompatibility
      5. Radiation (first trimester)
      6. Anoxia and birth trauma
      7. Low birth weight

II. **Adventitious Deafness**
   A. Genetic (Delayed onset)
      1. Deafness occurring alone (ostosclerosis)
      2. Deafness occurring with other conditions (Alport's syndrome, Hurler's disease, Paget's disease, von Recklinghausen's disease, sickle cell anemia)
   B. Nongenetic (Acquired)
      1. Infection (measles, mumps, chickenpox, influenza, serous otitis media, meningitis, gentamicin)
      2. Ototoxic drugs (kanamycin, streptomycin, gentamicin)
      3. Neoplastic disorders
      4. Trauma (direct injury via skull fracture or head injury or damage resulting from high noise level)
      5. Metabolic disorders (hypothyroidism)

*From F. Bess. *Childhood Deafness*. Grune & Stratton, 1977. D. Mouney. Differential diagnosis of hearing loss in children. *Pediatric Annals*, January 1980. R. Carrel. Epidemiology of Hearing Loss. In S. E. Gerber: Audiometry in Infancy, Grune & Stratton, 1977.

ABOUT DECIBELS AND HERTZ

Disorders in hearing mean that persons so affected are unable to perceive or translate the sound waves that other people hear.

Sounds are "heard" by means of vibrations, or waves, that travel from the place where the sound originates to the hearer's ear. Different sounds have different cycles, or wave patterns. A wave pattern that completes itself in one second (that is, frequency of one cycle per second) is called a Hertz (Hz), after the German physicist Heinrich Rudolf Hertz (1857–1894). The lower the pitch of a sound, the fewer cycles per second; the higher the pitch, the greater the number of cycles.

The decibel (one-tenth of a bel) takes its name from Alexander Graham Bell, whose interest in deafness led him to the invention of the telephone. Zero decibel is the least perceptible sound an average normal human being can hear (in the decibel scale, zero is not the absence of sound but rather, the threshold at which sound can first be perceived). The decibel scale used in measuring hearing ranges from 0 to 110; above that range, at 140 dB, sound produces pain.

From L. Bergstrom. Causes of severe hearing loss in early childhood. Pediatric Annals, January 1980, p. 25.

---

in decibels the greater the hearing loss. Hearing losses are also described according to time of appearance, cause and pathology involved.

Terms used to differentiate the causes of hearing loss are used inconsistently in the literature. In this discussion *congenital* is used to describe a hearing loss present at birth, whether of genetic or nongenetic origin. *Adventitious* hearing loss refers to a loss that develops after birth and may be due to genetic or nongenetic factors. Genetic-induced disorders that do not result in a hearing impairment until later in life (adventitious) are classified as having a *delayed onset* (e.g., Alport's syndrome), while deafness resulting after birth from nongenetic causes is termed *acquired*.[24] A summary of genetic and nongenetic causes of both congenital and adventitious hearing loss is outlined in Table 43–5. Of all cases of congenital deafness 50 per cent are inherited, whereas in adventitious hearing loss environmental factors are of major significance. The nurse's familiarity with the causes of hearing impairment can help her suggest preventive measures and provides a base for taking a pertinent health history.

Types of hearing impairment are categorized as central, peripheral and functional (nonorganic). *Central disorders* are those within the central nervous system, specifically along the pathway from the brain stem to and including the cortex. *Peripheral impairment* results from lesions outside the central nervous system involving any part of the auditory system from the external ear to the point at which the auditory portion of the eighth cranial nerve synapses within the brain stem.[20] *Functional or nonorganic* hearing impairment is a psychological rather than a physiological disorder in which "hearing loss" is a defense mechanism to cope with stressful situations. Of these three types central and peripheral are the most prevalent.

Central Disorders

Central hearing impairment involves brain damage that results in the inability to process information. Processing refers to reception, analysis and integration of auditory material within the central nervous system. The child is unable to interpret the auditory stimulus he receives and exhibits complex problems in speech and communication. The inability to express ideas, either spoken or written, is called *expressive aphasia; receptive aphasia* is difficulty in comprehending what one hears or reads.[20]

Children with central impairment are easily distracted, have a short attention span, and have reading difficulty when instructed by phonics.[4] This type of impairment is associated with a history of maternal rubella, diabetes, preeclampsia, prematurity and Rh incompatibility. Also, infections (meningitis and encephalitis), trauma, prolonged asphyxia and brain tumors, cysts and abscesses are among the numerous causes of central impairment.[4,6] The problem is not identifiable by hearing screening tests; therefore, a careful history and observations of behavior and speech are important methods of detection. Careful psychological and educational testing is required because children with auditory imperception (inability to understand the meaning of what is heard) resemble the emotionally disturbed.[4]

Peripheral Losses

Peripheral losses may be either *conductive* or *sensorineural*. If both conductive and sensorineural losses are present, it is referred to as a mixed loss. These classifications are based on location of the defect.

Conductive hearing impairment accounts for most hearing loss in children. There is a dysfunction of the outer (pinna and external auditory canal) or middle (tympanic membrane, Eustachian tube, or ossicles) ear that interferes with sound transmission (air conduction). The inner ear is not affected; therefore, bone conduction is normal and there is no nerve damage. Consequently, a person hears himself adequately via bone conduction and tends to speak quietly. The speech of others is understood provided he can hear what is said. Conductive hearing losses usually are the same for all frequencies, but high frequency may be heard better. Hearing levels fluctuate in the child with conductive hearing loss and are usually mild to moderate losses. The child with conductive hearing loss displays a recognizable syndrome of behaviors that include fluctuating attentiveness to his environment, poor language skills and mild behavior problems.[4]

The transmission of sound is reduced or absent when inner or middle ear pathology obstructs air conduction. Obstruction of the outer ear by cerumen or in some instances a foreign object can cause significant hearing loss. It is important for the nurse to stress that parents should not use cotton-tipped swabs or a sharp probe to clear the external canal. When a swab is used, cerumen readily gets pushed deeper into the canal and it may become impacted against the eardrum. Using a probe may cause injury to the external canal or eardrum, resulting in infection. The ear canals may also be occluded because of a defect in development. A missing canal can be constructed or an occluded canal can be corrected by surgery. Most frequently, extensive plastic surgery is required because the eardrum and bones of the middle ear are missing entirely.[20] Other causes of external ear obstructions are growths, swimmer's ear, and trauma.

The most common cause of conductive hearing loss in children is serous otitis media, an infection and inflammation of the middle ear that results in blockage of the Eustachian tube and a retracted eardrum. (See Chapter 23 for a discussion of serous otitis media.) Serous otitis media does not necessarily cause pain and the hearing loss rarely exceeds a level of 30 dB; thus the hearing loss may go undetected. Nursing interventions directed at preventing complications and the recurrence of serous otitis media can reduce the potential for hearing loss to occur. Even though decongestants and antihistamines are prescribed, these children require follow-up to repeat the otoscopic examination and assess hearing. Furthermore, when a child has had one occurrence of serous otitis media, parents should be advised to give the medications prescribed for serous otitis at the first sign of an upper respiratory infection as a preventive measure against recurrence.[11] An additional preventive measure to teach the child is how to blow his nose properly. Pressing lightly on the nostrils with fingers without pinching prevents mucus from being forced into the orifice of the Eustachian tube.

Other middle ear conditions that may produce conductive hearing loss are acute and chronic suppurative otitis media, tumors and myringitis bullosa (a viral infection of the outer layer of the eardrum resulting in blistering). Screening and auditory tests to detect conductive hearing loss are described later in this section.

Sensorineural hearing losses are the result of pathology in the inner ear (semicircular canals and cochlea) or along the nerve pathway (auditory nerve) from the inner ear to the brain stem. This loss results in acoustic distortion (difficulty in discriminating speech) and a reduced sensitivity to sound. There is typically better hearing ability for the lower frequencies than for high frequencies. There is an inability to understand what is said because many consonants are high frequency sounds and cannot be heard; thus word confusion results. Also, with a sensorineural loss one's own voice is not heard because of the deficit in bone conduction. (We hear our own voices partly through the mechanism of bone conduction.[20]) Consequently, with this type of hearing loss one speaks in what others perceive as an excessively loud voice.

Most of the babies who have impaired hearing at birth (congenital) have sensorineural impairment. However, this type of impairment may manifest itself at any time in life (adventitious). Whether congenital or adventitious the cause of the hearing loss may be genetic or nongenetic. The nongenetic factors that adversely affect prenatal and perinatal conditions (see Table 43-5) should be the focus of preventive prenatal and perinatal care. Acquired sensorineural hearing impairment can be prevented by careful management of infections in children, anticipatory guidance to prevent injury and immunizations against childhood illnesses.

Screening and Detection

The nurse plays an important part in early identification of hearing impairment. The nurse's focus on thorough history taking, behavioral observations of the child and attentiveness to parents' concerns increases the likelihood that she will detect an existing impairment. Also, her contact with families in child health settings gives her an opportunity to teach parents the normal responses to sound and language development to be expected.

Hearing screening is a nursing responsibility; therefore, an understanding of the various screening techniques is necessary. Hearing impairments can be identified through high-risk registers and various screening techniques appropriate for the age of the child (Table 43-6). While it is now possible to detect hearing loss in infancy, most children with severely handicapping hearing deficits are not identified until they are between 2.2 and 2.9 years of age.[14] An exception is children of deaf parents.

Detection in the Newborn Period The Joint Committee on Newborn Hearing* in 1973 recommended use of a high-risk register. This is a system to identify the largest number of hearing-impaired infants with the smallest number of questions; otherwise testing is not economically feasible.[9] According to the recommended criterion, a newborn is at risk for hearing impairment if one or more of the following conditions are present:

1. Family history of hereditary childhood hearing impairment.
2. Rubella or other nonbacterial intrauterine fetal infection (e.g., cytomegalovirus infection, herpes infection).
3. Defects of ear, nose, or throat, including malformed, low set or absent pinnae; cleft lip or palate (including submucous cleft); any residual abnormality of the otorhinolaryngeal system.
4. Birth weight less than 1500 gm.
5. Bilirubin level greater than 20 mg/100 ml serum.[13, 16]

Four additional important high-risk factors are multiple apneic spells in the nursery, exchange transfusions, neonatal meningitis and a five-minute Apgar score of 5 or less.[3]

---

*This committee had representatives from the American Academy of Pediatrics, The American Academy of Ophthalmology and Otolaryngology, and The American Speech and Hearing Association.

TABLE 43-6 PURPOSE AND TECHNIQUES FOR HEARING SCREENING ACCORDING TO AGE*

Age	Purpose	Technique
Newborn	Identify all hearing losses	1. High-risk register 2. Behavioral responses 3. Crib-O-Gram testing 4. Brain stem evoked response
Birth to 3 yrs	1. Identify severe hearing losses that might develop after birth 2. Detect ear conditions that may cause mild hearing losses	1. Follow-up of high risk children 2. Auditory orientation behavior 3. Assessment of speech and language 4. Tympanometry† (impedance testing) 5. Parents' impression of child's hearing and take concerns seriously

3 to 5 yrs	1. Detect conductive losses due to otitis media
	2. Detect sensorineural losses that might have developed
		1. Audiometry
		  (a) Pure-tone screening
		  (b) Non-pure tone screening
		2. Assessment of speech and language
		3. Tympanometry (impedance testing)
		4. Parents' impression of child's hearing and take concerns seriously

School age and Older	1. Maintain educationally adequate hearing 2. Detect ear disease	1. Pure-tone audiometry every 2 years 2. Tympanometry (impedance testing) 3. Parents' and teachers' concerns regarding child's hearing taken seriously 4. Tuning fork

*At each age the ear should be examined with an otoscope.
†For infants under seven months of age tympanometry is of limited validity.
From M. Downs. Early identification of hearing loss. In N. Lass et al. (ed.). Speech, Language, and Hearing. W. B. Saunders, in press. D. Cunningham. Hearing Loss. In R. Hockelman et al. (ed.) McGraw-Hill Book Co. 1978.

High-risk factors are identified by reviewing the medical record, asking parents to complete a questionnaire and by examination of the newborn.

It is recommended that all newborns be assessed and those at risk be referred for audiologic evaluation during the first two months of life. Even those infants who appear normal should be referred and followed. The nurse can assist in every aspect of this process and particularly in developing a system of adequate follow-up.

Screening by Behavioral Testing Screening by observing behavioral responses to sound stimuli is recommended to supplement the high-risk register.[8] While the infant is asleep with eyes closed and no body movement a stimulus of 90 dB is used to arouse the infant. The acceptable response is "a generalized body movement involving more than one limb and accompanied by some form of eye movement."[17] This test is not accepted as a single method of screening but is useful as a supplement to the high-risk register. While neonatal audiometers are available for precise testing, the nurse should not disregard the value of testing newborns with a bell. The bell is rung approximately four inches from the ear and should elicit an eyeblink. An eyeblink is the most common and reliably observed response to sound in neonates.[9,13] In addition to the high-risk register and behavioral testing, other techniques such as the Crib-O-Gram and brain stem–evoked response screening are described in the literature.[9, 13, 20]

Birth to Three Years of Age Once an infant has been identified as high risk, it is essential that he be examined regularly to identify hearing loss that may develop at some time after birth. It is recommended that these children have an audiological evaluation every three months through the first year.[3] The nurse can assist parents by helping them understand that although hearing tests are normal, their child is more vulnerable to hearing loss because of the presence of a high-risk factor or factors.

The nurse has an important role in screening and detection of hearing problems during all well-child visits. Assessment of hearing development should include an otoscopic examination, assessment of the infant's response to noisemakers (auditory orientation behavior) and an assessment of speech and language development.

The otoscopic examination, including pneumatic otoscopy (described in Chapter 13), uses important techniques for identification of past and present middle ear pathology. These tests must be done by skilled professionals to ensure that hearing losses are prevented. When otoscopy is performed in conjunction with tympanometry, ear problems can be detected even earlier. It can be used at any age but is of limited validity in infants under 7 months.[25]

Tympanometry (impedance testing) is an objective measurement of the compliance or mobility of the tympanic membrane in response to air pressure changes in the external auditory canal. Maximum compliance occurs when pressures on either side of the membrane are equal. Even mild disease of the tympanic membrane or middle ear influences the degree of compliance, making this test particularly useful to detect ear pathology *before* it has caused a hearing impairment.

Tympanometry is an efficient, reliable technique that is recommended to be used as a supplement to otoscopic examination and audiometric hearing tests.[22]

Three to Five Years At this age screening and detection consists of all of the techniques described for newborn to 3 years of age. In addition, audiometric screening must be done to detect any sensorineural loss that may have developed. For this age, pure tone testing using play conditioning techniques is appropriate for the young preschooler; for the 5-year-old the standard pure tone screening is appropriate.

Non-pure tone screening is another technique that can be used to test preschoolers. The child is shown a board of pictures while words are spoken to him through earphones. The child is asked to point to the appropriate picture. The first word is spoken at 51 dB and each subsequent word is presented at 4 dB less than the previous one until the 15 dB level is attained.[8] When this test is given, differences in language development and word exposure must be taken

---

TYMPANOMETRY

1. A tympanometer is an automatic instrument with a probe inserted into the ear canal. (An air-tight cavity is formed between the tip of the probe and the eardrum.)
2. A pure tone (usually 220 Hz) is then administered through the tip of the probe.
3. During the test ear canal pressure in the airtight cavity is varied automatically by the tympanometer ($\pm$ 200 mmH$_2$O).
4. As ear canal pressures vary, compliance of the eardrum changes. (Compliance decreases whenever pressures on the two sides of the eardrum are not equal.)
5. As the ear canal pressures are varied, the sound (220 Hz) is reflected back into the airtight cavity whenever the eardrum is not free to vibrate. (It vibrates best [is most compliant] when pressure against the two sides of the eardrum are equal.)
6. When pressures on the two sides of the eardrum are not equal and sound is reflected, the probe tip measures the intensity of the reflected sound in the ear canal. Thus, the compliance of the ear is evaluated by measuring the reflected sound in the airtight portion of the ear canal.
7. For a normal ear the greatest compliance is attained at 0 pressure.
8. If ear pathology is present, maximum compliance may be attained at positive or negative pressures. The amount of pressure required (whether positive or negative) to produce maximum compliance is the middle ear pressure.

into consideration. It is more appropriate for most 4- and 5-year-olds than it is for 3-year-olds.

School Age The most common method of screening hearing in school-age children is pure-tone audiometry. While the more recent development of impedance audiometry is more effective to detect ear pathology, pure-tone audiometry continues to be the predominant method for screening school-age children. The nurse's responsibility is to maximize its effectiveness by administering the test under optimal conditions. Three important criteria should be met in giving the test: (1) the environment* should be quiet to avoid false-positives; (2) the audiometer should be maintained* in proper working condition and (3) personnel conducting the test should be properly trained.[31]

The school nurse should supervise the hearing screening program, recognizing its limitations to discover hearing loss and ear pathology in its early stages. Pure-tone audiometry must always be supplemented with serious attention given to the observations and concerns of teachers and parents regarding the hearing of the child. The purpose of pure-tone audiometry is to *identify* hearing loss greater than a certain level, whereas impedance audiometry is used to discover the presence of otopathology. This is an important distinction that is not always made in discussions of auditory screening procedures.[31] Despite the advantages of impedance audiometry it is unlikely to be used in the place of pure-tone screening; therefore, the nurse's responsibility is to upgrade the conditions under which pure-tone audiometry is administered.

A school-age child can cooperate in being assessed by the tuning fork test, in addition to otoscopy, speech and language assessment, impedance audiometry and pure-tone audiometry. (See Chapter 13 for description of the Weber and Rinne tests.)

At all well-child visits the nurse should inspect the ears and examine the ear with an otoscope. Additionally, the nurse should assess the child for behavioral indications of hearing losses both by direct observation and asking for pertinent information given by parents. Physical and behavioral findings which may be indicative of a hearing loss are summarized in Table 43-7.

Management: Nurse's Role

Usually parents are the first to notice that something is wrong with their baby's hearing. It is at this point that correct management begins. On the average a full year elapses between the first suspicion and the actual confirmation that a child has a severely handicapping hearing deficit; a child with a mild to moderate hearing loss is often 3 years of age before any concerns are raised and over 4 years old before the hearing loss is confirmed.[15] This presents a serious challenge to all health professionals who care for children and especially to nurses, who are often the first to hear the concerns of parents during the process of taking a developmental history. Nurses thus can make a significant impact on the current problem of delayed intervention by taking concerns of parents seriously and making a referral for audiological evaluation.

The impact that a hearing impairment has on a child is largely affected by how his parents can accept and adapt to the impairment. Therefore, the initial focus of the nurse should be to help parents adjust to the child's handicap. Not only do parents feel disappointed about the baby's deficit, but from birth the communication interplay is altered when a baby has a hearing impairment. Parents should be encouraged to interact verbally with their child while in direct line of vision to permit the child to respond to the stimulation of facial expressions.

Parent involvement is central to the habilitation program beginning from the moment of diagnosis. They need to learn how the hearing impairment affects normal growth and development and about techniques available to maximize their child's potential. While the nurse may not be primarily responsible for counselling the parents regarding amplification, communication techniques and educational methods, she should know of the available alternatives. The nurse acts as a resource to the family to discuss any aspect of the habilitation of their child.

Impact of Hearing Impairment on a Preschooler The nurse can prepare parents for the various behaviors of their child and devel-

---

*American National Standards Institute (ANSI) Specifications 53.1 (1960) and 53.6 (1969) describe criteria for background noise and maintenance, respectively.

TABLE 43-7 BEHAVIORAL INDICES AND PHYSICAL FINDINGS ASSOCIATED WITH HEARING LOSS

A. Behavioral indices
  I. Orientation responses
   - Responds more to movement than to sound
   - Turns head and body to sound as if dependent on one ear
   - Responds to spoken sounds only when speaker's face and lips are visible
   - Responds more to changes in facial expression than to words
   - Fails to follow verbal directions
   - Lacks motor or facial response to spoken word
  II. Vocalizations and sound production
   - Monotone voice quality and inflection patterns; loud voice
   - Loss of or lack of normal babbling by 7 months of age; loss of previously acquired speech a primary indicator
   - Only parts of words vocalized; mispronounces or omits certain words
   - Bangs head or stomps foot to elicit vibratory sensation
   - Uses same sound to express pleasure, annoyance or need
  III. Visual attention
   - Attends closely to facial expression and eyes of the speaker for intent of words
   - Points and uses gestures rather than words to express desires after 15 months of age
   - Displays marked imitativeness in play
   - Is distracted by gestures and movement when in groups
  IV. Emotional and social behavior
   - Is shy, timid and withdrawn in group play
   - Lacks appropriate noises in play with dolls, animals, trucks; no preference for noisy toys
   - Displays intense preoccupation with things rather than people
   - Has puzzled, unhappy, inquiring and sometimes confused facial expression in group play
   - Is disobedient
   - Has short attention span, hyperactivity and unusual fatigue
   - Uses tantrums to call attention to self or needs in routine situations
   - Is irritable at not making himself understood
   - Appears to daydream or be oblivious to others
   - Displays unpredictable behavioral outbursts

B. Physical findings

I.	White forelock in hair line of forehead	Streak of gray or white hair; indicative of genetic defect (Waardenburg's syndrome) with hearing loss component
II.	Heterochromia	A difference of color in portion of same iris: indicative of genetic defect (Waardenburg's syndrome) that has hearing loss component
III.	Very bushy eyebrows that almost meet at the nasal bridge	Indicative of congenital defect that has hearing loss component
IV.	Impacted cerumen in external canal	Leads to a temporary conductive loss
V.	Otitis externa	Inflammation of external ear (may result from furuncle or allergy to cleaning solutions used for hearing aid)
VI.	Abnormal tympanic membrane	Retraction, bulging, air fluid levels, perforation, scarring all contribute to conductive loss; fluid in ear can lead to labyrinthitis, mastoid disease or cholesteatoma; labyrinthitis can lead to permanent damage to the hairs in the organ of Corti
VII.	Hypertrophied adenoids	Enlargement of adenoid tissue in posterior nasopharynx; may cause mild conductive loss

opmental consequences of having a hearing impairment. While a hearing preschooler is highly verbal and readily shares experiences even with strangers, the hearing impaired preschooler may be limited in social skills. With the loss of adequate expressive language there is a tendency to withdraw from social situations. Strangers and peers may not understand the speech of the hearing-impaired child and he in turn cannot understand them. The ability to hear enables a child to identify the emotional intent of the words spoken. A hearing child learns what is expected of him from contextual cues and sounds perceived in the environment.

Large groups present a particular problem to the hearing-impaired child because he hears only parts of the conversation and does not learn the rules of games well. His response may be inappropriate to the situation, resulting in teasing by his playmates who quickly dissociate him from the activity.

A hearing-impaired child tends to be more active in exploring the environment than a hearing child. He wants to see and touch everything and desires to touch faces to feel the vibrations of speech. Some people may find this type of behavior intrusive and intolerable. Also loud, unintelligible speech at the wrong time or in the wrong place may embarrass family members. Parents who cannot accept these behaviors may impose social isolation on the whole family or choose the alternative of planning activities whereby the child and one parent are always excluded in family activity. A sense of family unity may never evolve. Furthermore, older siblings may not bring friends home because they fear rejection of the family by their friends.

The child who has learned to accept his limitation and has made some progress in his developmental skills will have limited emotional problems. Temper tantrums and extremes of destructive behavior and handflapping in response to frustration are often limited in duration. The child may have some difficulty, however, in delaying gratification of needs at times or may become impulsive. His negative behavior cannot be rewarded with attention from friends and family and with the supplying of his every need. This response to negative behavior encourages a repetition of the behavior and loss of self-esteem. Eventually the child will take on a dependency role and give up trying. His major drive toward self-reliance may never succeed and his ability to solve problems will be greatly handicapped.

The preschool child is developing a social conscience about what is improper and what is acceptable behavior. Parents must set consistent and firm limits on the child and learn to expect reasonable obedience so he can learn socially acceptable behavior. Parents may tend to avoid discipline for the hearing-impaired child because they fear that he will not understand why the limitation was set. Mild, consistent disapproval with a stern "no" and facial expression of displeasure will enhance his understanding of what pleases his parents and will free him to initiate more social contact.[5] The nurse can help parents determine the normal behavior problems of the preschool period and methods to cope with them. Parents can be encouraged to balance punishment with love and acceptance, which will decrease the feelings of rejection on the part of the child. The child needs to be reassured that both parents love and accept him.

Methods of Communication

The controversy over the best method of communication is confusing to parents and to professionals. The goal of educators of the hearing impaired in the United States is to assist a child to develop the ability to "speak and understand the spoken word to the highest degree possible."[19] No present-day educators advocate only the use of the manual (sign language and fingerspelling) technique.[19] Four basic methods of communication are used in the United States: the oral method, the auditory method, the Rochester method, and total communication.

Oral Method This method has been predominant until recently. It focuses on the use of residual hearing with amplification and speechreading (lipreading). Proponents of this method believe that it is important for the deaf to be taught to talk and understand speech so that they can communicate in the hearing world of people. Gestures and signs are viewed as an interference to the development of speech. While speech and speechreading is the goal for the hearing impaired, some do not have sufficient residual hearing to distinguish sounds and words that look alike on the lips.

Auditory Method This approach is also called the unisensory or acoupedic method. In this method speechreading is not taught but rather children are taught listening skills and are expected to rely primarily on their hearing ability. This method requires early detection, powerful hearing aids and extensive parent participation.

Rochester Method This method combines the oral method (speechreading and residual hearing) with fingerspelling. Reading and writing are emphasized.

Total Communication In this approach all techniques of communication are used, including sign language, cued speech, fingerspelling, speechreading, tactile stimulation, and amplification. There is an increasing movement for the use of this method with very young children. This support may be the result of (1) evidence that deaf children with deaf parents are more successful academically than those with hearing parents, (2) the increased acceptance of sign language, (3) dissatisfaction with traditional methods with the profoundly deaf and (4) strong support from deaf adults who were trained by a rigid oral method.[19]

The nurse can explain to parents that no single method is preferred for all hearing-impaired children, but rather with the guidance of professionals the method is individualized for each child.

The child's type and degree of hearing loss and age of onset are important variables that an audiologist must consider when determining the type of communication technique most suitable for each child. The effect of hearing loss and resultant educational needs are summarized in Table 43-4.

Hearing aids are used to amplify the volume of environmental sounds only. They are helpful when one has good residual hearing. For some children, the sound becomes so grossly distorted when the volume is increased that it may create a barrier to receptive abilities. Knowing the range of sound volume loss as noted on diagnostic audiograms gives the nurse insight into determining the appropriate volume setting that is useful to the child. Consistent wearing of the aid is particularly important for a child who is just learning to adjust to wearing it. Testing and changing of the batteries will increase the effectiveness of the aid and the child's social competence. Auditory feedback (a disturbing screech that emanates from the earpiece) occurs when the volume is too high or the ear mold is improperly fitted. The child and family know how to alleviate this problem; however, the child may not hear the feedback, therefore others have to draw his attention to it.

THE SENSORY-IMPAIRED CHILD IN THE HOSPITAL

The sensory-impaired child is particularly dependent on his family at a time of stress. Despite any attempts to prepare a sensory-impaired child for what to expect in the hospital, new people and a strange environment are a threat

---

COMMUNICATION TECHNIQUES FOR A CHILD WITH A HEARING IMPAIRMENT

Hearing Aids include (1) a microphone that picks up sound waves and changes them into electricity, (2) a battery-powered amplifier to increase the strength of the signal coming from the microphone and (3) a receiver to change the amplified signals back to sound waves. Hearing aid selection with young children requires considerable time devoted to repeated evaluation and trial periods with loaned hearing aids. The various types available include an aid that fits directly in the ear, an ear-level aid that fits behind the ear, a body aid that can be worn in a pocket or attached to clothing and an aid that is built into the frame of glasses. Hearing aids are binaural (on each ear) or monoaural (on one ear). Binaural aids are more expensive but provide a more natural production of sound. Hearing aids are being fitted in infancy (on children as young as two months of age) and are considered important to effect early stimulation of residual hearing.[14]

Auditory training is the process of teaching a child how to listen to spoken language. The emphasis is on listening to natural language, not to separate speech sounds such as vowels and consonants.[13]

Speechreading (also called lipreading) is a concentration on visual clues to decipher the content of the spoken word by watching the lips, tongue and jaw. Speechreading is difficult because many English sounds require similar formation of the lips. A child's ability to speechread is improved if adequate lighting falls on speaker's face and if natural speaking is used with normal articulation and complete sentences.

Sign language is a manual form of communication in which an entire concept is communicated by the position, configuration and movement of the hands.

Fingerspelling is the spelling of a word letter by letter. Letters are represented by hand configurations.

Cued speech is the use of eight hand configurations and four hand placements supplementing natural speech. The hands are placed around the chin, cheek and neck to give clues to assist in speechreading.

Speech training is the process of teaching a deaf child to speak intelligibly. A child is taught how to regulate his voice and articulate correctly.

to his security. The stress of hospitalization is best tolerated if parents can be present to assist in orienting the child to the environment and participate in preparing him for the various hospital events. Nurses are most helpful if they work with the family to learn the child's special daily care routines and how he can best relate to others. While this is important for all hospitalized children, it is exceptionally so for a sensory-impaired child, who uses alternate methods of relating to his environment.

While rooming in by parents is encouraged and beneficial, the nurse should not expect parents to assume full responsibility for the interpretation and explanation of procedures to the child. The nurse should become increasingly adept at communicating effectively with a sensory-impaired child so that parents will feel comfortable in leaving for short periods of time. Also, if parents are to take an extensive part in the care of their child, the nurse must in turn be prepared to spend adequate time with parents to prepare them for this task. Parents have difficulty knowing what is expected of them regarding the routines and procedures of a hospital and need assistance to understand how they can participate.

Special routines of home must be maintained to provide maximum comfort to a sensory-impaired child. The nurse is responsible for collecting specific data on admission regarding special care needs of a sensory-impaired child such as hearing aids, lenses, self-care skills, and mobility techniques. Also, the level of the impairment and its effect on independent functioning must be ascertained. From this information a care plan must be developed and used by all nurses caring for the child. It is distressing to the child and parents to have to orient each "new" nurse to the child's individual needs.

The nurse who gives nursing care to a sensory-impaired child should make the necessary adaptations that will permit the child to maintain his usual method of communication and foster normal growth and development. Independence in self-care skills such as self-feeding, dressing, bathing and mobility should be maintained and encouraged, even though for a sensory-impaired child this may require additional patience and time on the nurse's part.

When a procedure is performed, the nurse must carefully assess the implications it may have for the child. For example, the wearing of a mask will cut off an important means of communication for the deaf child and restraint of the hands and arms interferes with one of a blind child's primary methods of taking in his environment. Play with other children should be encouraged to prevent the child from feeling isolated. The help of parents should be elicited to provide a play situation that is suitable to the child's abilities and is similar to his usual environment for play.

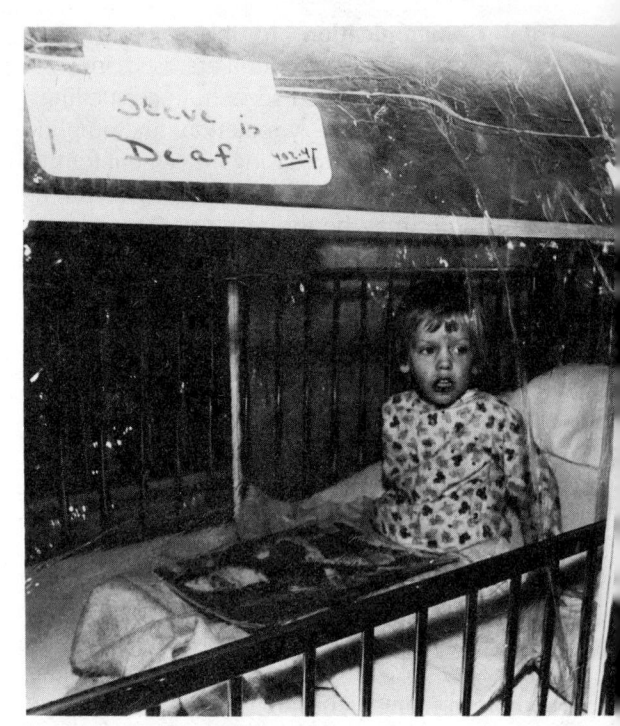

Despite any attempts to prepare a sensory-impaired child for hospitalization, a strange environment poses a serious threat to his security.

BRONCHIAL ASTHMA

Asthma is a chronic obstructive disorder of the tracheobronchial tree that evidences itself in periodic paroxysmal respiratory distress. The degree of obstruction prompting the dyspneic spells varies and may resolve spontaneously, although medical intervention is often required to reverse the asthmatic attack.

This disease usually begins in childhood, typically during the preschool years, and is more prevalent in males. Asthma persists into adulthood about 50 per cent of the time; those children who outgrow the asthma usually develop other allergies in adulthood.

Asthma is found most often in children with

inherited allergenic constitution and is, in children, most often a response to allergenic inhalants. It is believed that these children have an extraordinary sensitivity to acetylcholine and other immune response chemical mediators. Szentivanyi proposes that an imbalance of the autonomic nervous system is responsible for this hypersensitivity in that it does not respond to effectively counter the physiologic effects of these chemical mediators.[6] A genetic predisposition is undoubtedly involved, but the mode of inheritance is unclear.

Extrinsic and intrinsic asthma are the two major forms of the disease.[2] In *extrinsic asthma* the child responds allergically to external factors such as pollens, molds, animal danders, lint and dust, insecticides and other irritant odors such as smoke, smog or perfume. Less frequently the allergen is food or drugs. In *intrinsic asthma* the precipitating factor is primarily infection in the respiratory tract, usually viral in origin.

A child may react with severe symptoms to an allergenic substance at certain times and be relatively free of symptoms when exposed to the substance at other times. This is because symptom severity depends on the concentration of the allergen to which the child is exposed. For example, a child allergic to pollens will have no symptoms when the pollen count is low but will have coryzal symptoms (sneezing, rhinitis) when the count is moderate and have coryzal and asthmatic symptoms when the count is very high. The amount of the substance needed to cause symptoms in an individual is called his *allergic threshold*. Most allergic children are reactive to more than one substance. An exposure to an accumulation of substances even in low counts can cause symptoms. For example, a child can be symptom free when around a dog except in pollen season. This cumulative effect changes the allergic threshold. The higher the child's threshold, the more exposure to allergens is tolerated.

The frequency and severity of asthmatic attack may also be greatly influenced by aggravating factors such as weather changes, consumption of beverages or foods of extreme temperatures, fatigue or vigorous exercise, nonsteroidal anti-inflammatory drugs (especially aspirin), endocrinal changes such as occur during physiological or psychological distress or with puberty, and intense or persistent emotional tension (excitement, fright, unresolved parent-child conflicts). Since the factors may precipitate or perpetuate attacks, nursing attention should be directed toward helping the family control these factors or to modify their reactions to them. Education of the family must emphasize that these factors merely aggravate the asthma, they do not *cause* it.

Pathophysiology and Clinical Manifestations

Whether an asthmatic attack is allergenically or infectiously initiated, the body responds with three physiologic alterations that produce the asthmatic symptoms. In response to the allergen(s) or infectious organisms (1) the bronchial mucosa becomes edematous (smooth muscle hyperplasia); (2) thick tenacious mucus is produced in abundance (mucosal hypersecretion), causing mucus plugs that partially or completely occlude the airways; and (3) hyperactivity and hypertrophy of the bronchial smooth muscles occurs (bronchospasm). Frequently the asthmatic also has sinusitis, nasal polyps or concurrent chronic bronchitis that further compromise oxygenation. The mouth breathing of the asthmatic further thickens secretions; this further aggravates obstruction. If these physiological responses are not reversed early, air becomes trapped in the alveoli, causing air hunger and resultant hyperventilation of these tissues. The blocked inspiratory air and poor oxygen-carbon dioxide exchange ($\downarrow PaO_2$, $\downarrow PaCO_2$) lead progressively to hypoxia and acidosis. The fright and the vagal stimulation created by air hunger further aggravate the bronchospasm, increasing the severity of symptoms even more. If obstruction, acidosis and fatigue persist ($\uparrow PaCO_2$), respiratory failure and cardiac arrhythmias ensue, leading potentially to arrest and irreversible brain damage or even death.

An asthma attack may develop gradually or begin abruptly. Typically the attack starts while the child is at rest, primarily at night. Early manifestations of an impending attack are complaints by the child of chest congestion or tightness, exercise intolerance evidenced by early onset of fatigue and shortness of breath and increased sputum production, usually accompanied by a productive, paroxysmal cough. Vomiting may occur in the preschooler because of his tendency to swallow coughed-up mucus

TABLE 43-8 TYPICAL PATTERNS OF ASTHMA*

Classification	Definition
Mild	Less than six mild attacks per year *and* asymptomatic between attacks, *and* no functional impairment between attacks *and* no medication used between attacks
Moderate to moderately severe	Up to eight severe attacks per year *and* mild to moderate symptoms between attacks *and* mild to moderate functional impairment between attacks *and* on continuous medication
Severe	More than eight severe attacks per year while on continuous medication *and* moderate to severe functional impairment between attacks, steroid dependent, *or* at least 2 episodes of status asthmaticus per year

Continuous medication is defined as medication used on more than 25% of the days in the past year.
Functional impairment is defined as:
Normal functional activity—on par with peers
Minimal functional impairment—1 or 2 disability days/quarter
Moderate functional impairment—1 or 2 disability days/month
Severe functional impairment—1 or more disability days/week
A *disability day* is defined as a day on which a person stays in bed most of the day for asthma or a school day loss.

*From D. Pearlman and C. Bierman, Asthma (bronchial asthma, reactive airways disorder). In Allergic Diseases of Infancy, Childhood and Adolescence. C. Bierman and D. Pearlman, W. B. Saunders Co., 1980, p. 587.

rather than expectorate it. Wheezing often is absent at this stage.

These signs indicate the need to initiate home management measures promptly; therefore, the child and parents must be taught to recognize and respond to these early signs of attack. Without intervention these symptoms may resolve, but typically they continue over hours or days with progressive development of acute respiratory distress, expiratory wheezing and hypoxemia. If these symptoms persist for more than two hours and are unresponsive to the acute management regimen, *status asthmaticus* (unresolved bronchospasm, inspiratory wheezing and potential respiratory acidosis) develops. Termination of the attack usually is heralded by pronounced coughing with expectoration of thick sputum containing pearls of thick mucus surrounded by thin secretions and is immediately followed by a sensation of relief of air hunger and bronchospasm. Pearlman and Bierman[6] have classified the three typical patterns of asthma which may be manifested by asthmatic children (Table 43-8). In the mild case the pathophysiologic obstruction is completely reversible; in the moderate case the obstruction is only occasionally completely reversible. In most moderate and severe cases the obstruction persists to some degree, causing chronic alveolar hyperinflation and decreased pulmonary flow with or without hypoxemia. In these cases the likelihood is that the child will develop chronic obstructive pulmonary disease later in life despite proper long-term management of the asthma.

The preschool child with poorly controlled or severe asthma will have minimal endurance and energy expenditure for gross motor play activities, restless sleep patterns, and decreased interest in the environment because of slowed thinking processes as a result of high histamine levels. His peer contact will be less because he always has a cold; there will be few invitations for group play because of his socially objectionable symptoms (facial grimacing, throat clearing, sniffling, runny nose). The child may have developed a self-concept of being slow and not as bright as other children. He may also have intermittent learning disabilities secondary to sensory alterations (transient hearing loss, fatigue, restlessness) stemming from his chronic asthma symptoms.

These characteristics of children with chronic

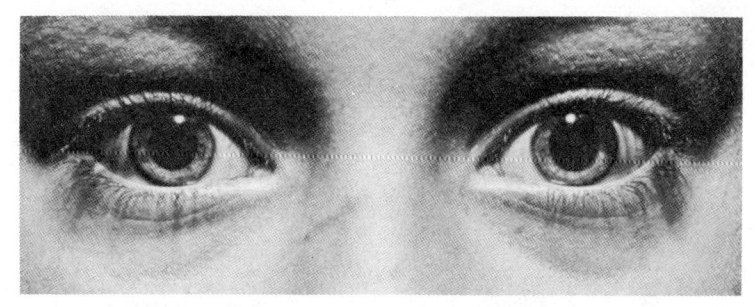

Figure 43-3 Allergic shiners. (From M. Marks. Stigmata of Respiratory Tract Allergies. Upjohn, 1977, p. 12.)

allergic disorders such as asthma are little understood and often go unrecognized. They are misinterpreted as a response to emotional disturbance when they are, in fact, a cluster of symptoms called the *tension-fatigue syndrome*. Rowe characterizes this syndrome by fatigue, even upon arising; lassitude and depression; inability to think or concentrate; general irritability and restlessness; frequent crying; musculoskeletal complaints, especially headache; and a battery of mannerisms typical of the particular allergic disorder (e.g., allergic salute in allergic rhinitis).[7] This syndrome and the associated mannerisms, often interpreted by parents or teachers as deliberate and disruptive, should be recognized by the nurse as a manifestation of allergic disease.

Eye signs of chronic allergy include allergic shiners (discoloration below the eyes) (Fig. 43-3), muddy and boggy conjunctivae, marginal upper eyelid eczema and long silky eyelashes. Nasal signs are transverse nasal crease and allergic salute (Fig. 43-4). A gaping, open-mouthed expression, gingival hyperplasia, asymptomatic pharyngeal hyperemia, geographic tongue (bald patches of oval, round or snakelike shapes) (Fig. 43-5) and elevated, pearly margins on the tongue represent oral signs. Chest signs are barrel chest, pigeon breast, and prominent lump in the upper back (see Chapter 13 for figures).[3]

Diagnosis

The nurse has a primary role in assisting in the early diagnosis of allergenic substances, re-

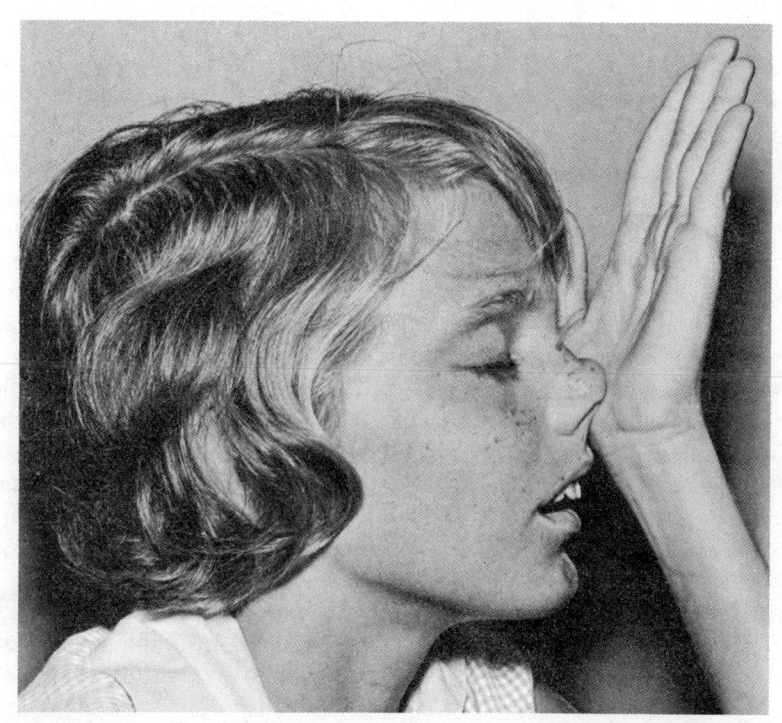

Figure 43-4 Allergic salute. (From M. Marks. Stigmata of Respiratory Tract Allergies. Upjohn, 1977, p. 1.)

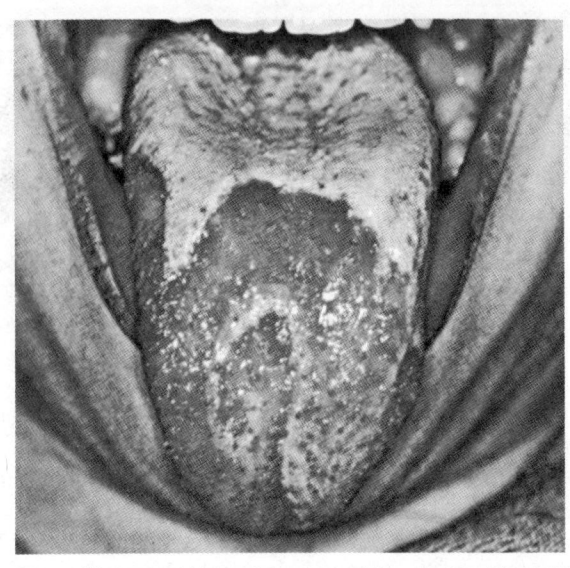

Figure 43-5 Geographic tongue. (From M. Marks. Stigmata of Respiratory Tract Allergies. Upjohn, 1977, p. 28.)

ferral to an allergy specialist and support and education of the family during long-term management of and adaptation to this problem.

Because of features in the history and physical examination that asthmatic children usually share in common, diagnosis often is possible from these alone. The history usually includes recurrent bouts of bronchitis, pneumonia, persistent coughing with colds or perhaps merely a chronic chest rattle throughout infancy and early childhood. Symptoms during these episodes historically have showed improvement after treatment with epinephrine or adrenergic drugs. Symptoms were also typically more severe at night or during early morning hours, with noticeable improvement through the daytime.

Episodes of coughing spells or coughing spells accompanied by expiratory wheezing are often reported and occur more frequently over time. These episodes typically cleared after five to seven days, usually spontaneously. Observant parents or the child may even be able to identify factors that precipitate these episodes. The preschooler's input to the history should be solicited, because he often can identify factors that parents have overlooked or misunderstood from the child's behavior.

Documentation of any known allergies should also be made as well as any family history of asthma.

Physical appraisal should include evaluation of growth over time. Growth retardation may be a consequence of chronic hypoxemia; control of the asthma usually results in a growth spurt. Blood pressure should be recorded as a baseline for comparison after drug therapy for asthma has been initiated. (Steroids and adrenergic agents may cause elevations.) Respirations should be evaluated for rate, prolonged expiration, dyspnea, retractions or nasal flaring and use of accessory muscles (shoulders rise). Skin color and capillary return of the nailbeds should be documented. A round shoulder posture indicates alveolar hyperinflation. If hyperinflation is marked, the liver will be pushed downward and palpable. The heart, too, will be displaced downward, shifting the location of cardiac maximal impact (PMI). The lungs should be auscultated for unequal breath sounds, rhonchi that clear with coughing and for presence of overt wheeze or latent wheeze produced with forced expiration. The preschooler can be stimulated to force expiration by asking him to blow a feather or a whistle with the ball removed. Cardiac rate and rhythm should be carefully assessed, because asthma drug therapy can alter cardiac function. Assessment should be done for concomitant aggravating factors such as otitis media, the swollen turbinates and gray boggy nasal mucosa of sinusitis, and healed or active eczematous skin lesions.

Table 43-9 summarizes the usual laboratory tests used in the differential diagnosis and ongoing evaluation of asthma. If the history, physical examination, and laboratory tests suggest any inhalant allergen or the results are vague, skin

TABLE 43-9 LABORATORY TESTS IN ASTHMA*

Test	Possible Abnormalities in Asthma	Comments
Complete blood count	Leukocytosis (occasionally)	Induced by infection, epinephrine administration, "stress" (?)
	Eosinophilia (frequently)	Varies with medication, time of day, adrenal function; not necessarily related to "allergy." (Often higher in "intrinsic" than "extrinsic" asthma.)
Sputum Exam White or "clear" and small yellow plugs	Eosinophils	In both "intrinsic" and "extrinsic" asthma.
	Charcot-Leyden crystals	Derived from eosinophils.
	Creola bodies	Clusters of epithelial cells.
	Curschmann's spirals	Threads of glycoprotein.
Nasal smear	Eosinophils	Suggests concomitant nasal allergy in children.
	Lymphocytes, PMN's, macrophages	Replace eosinophils in URIs.
	PMN's with ingested bacteria	Bacterial rhinitis or sinusitis
Serum tests	IgG, IgA, IgM	Often normal. May be abnormal—various patterns seen.
	IgE	Sometimes elevated in "allergic" asthma. Often normal.
	Aspergillus-precipitating antibody	Suggestive, not diagnostic of bronchopulmonary aspergillosis.
Sweat test	Normal in asthma Perform to rule out cystic fibrosis	Cystic fibrosis and asthma can coexist.
Chest x-ray	Hyperinflation, infiltrates, pneumomediastinum, pneumothorax Rule out tuberculosis	Indicated once in all children with asthma. Indicated on hospitalization for asthma.
Lung function tests	↓ FEV_1, ↓ FVC, ↓ $FEF_{25-75\%}$, ↓ PEFR; $FEV_1/FVC<75\%$	Useful for following course of disease, response to treatment.
Response to bronchodilators	>15% improvement FEV_1; PEFR	Safest diagnostic test for asthma.
Exercise tests	Decreased lung function after 6 minutes of exercise PEFR and FEV_1 >15% ↓ $FEF_{25-75\%}$ >25% ↓	Useful to diagnose asthma in children. Often abnormal when resting lung function is normal.
Methacholine inhalation test (Mecholyl test)	20% fall in lung function with dose tolerated by "normal" subjects.	Should be performed only by specialists.
Antigen inhalation test	20% fall in lung function immediately after challenge; may cause delayed response 6–8 hrs. later	Potentially dangerous; specialist only.
Allergy skin tests	Identifies allergic factors which *might* be causative factors.	Test only likely factors—selected by history.
RAST	Same significance as skin tests	More expensive than skin tests.

*From D. Pearlman and C. Bierman, Asthma (bronchial asthma, reactive airways disorder). In Allergic Diseases of Infancy, Childhood and Adolescence. C. Bierman and D. Pearlman, W. B. Saunders Co., 1980, p. 587.

ALLERGY SKIN TESTING

Skin tests involve the use of extracts from numerous common antigens. The antigens are injected onto the cutaneous layer of skin by a scratch or prick method.* If no cutaneous response occurs, an intradermal method of injection is used.† Which antigen extracts are tested is determined by the child's age, geographical and environmental exposure, and history and physical examination findings. The extracts are injected in rows, an inch apart, and in a specific pattern. The usual test sites are the arms and back. The forearm is most desirable since it is more accessible to a tourniquet should an extreme allergic response occur to one of the antigen extracts. If a child is dermatographic (mere touch causes skin erythema), normal saline may be used as a control.

The testing may be done at one visit or over a period of several visits, depending on the number and type of antigen extracts to be used. This testing may be done on any child over 6 months of age.[1] No antihistamines should be given the child for 24 hours before testing.

Preparation of the preschooler for the skin tests includes explanation of the itching and swelling of the extremity, the appearance of the polka dots around the testing areas and methods he can use to hold still during the prolonged testing period. This procedure is uncomfortable for the child and every effort should be made to support and comfort him by having a parent present to touch and soothe him, by providing pleasant distractions such as stories, picture books, music boxes, puppets or other age-appropriate diversions and by the presence of adults who are calm but empathetic to his distress. A child should *never* be left alone during the testing procedure or in the interval after when reactions may occur. Within 10 to 30 minutes after exposure reactions will occur at the site of any antigens to which the child is allergic. A positive reaction is evidenced by erythema and wheal formation at the site. Once a reaction occurs, the area should be immediately wiped off to prevent further reaction. These reactive manifestations may persist for 8 to 12 hours. Any delayed reactions (within 24 to 48 hours later) should be reported. The testers should monitor the child closely for any systemic reactions during the testing procedure. All the extracts should be removed after the testing (approximately 30 minutes). Since false positives and negatives can occur, skin testing results should be interpreted in conjunction with the history, physical examination and laboratory findings.

---

*The scratch method involves scratching the epidermis and applying one drop of extract over the scratch. The prick method involves placing one drop of extract on the skin, then pricking the skin where the extract was dropped.
†Intradermal method involves injecting .02 ml of 1:500 or 1:1000 strength extract by holding the skin taut and inserting the needle, bevel up, laterally between the outer skin layers, then rotating the bevel downward and injecting the extract.

---

testing may be done to make diagnosis more certain or to ascertain initial desired concentrations of antigens in immunotherapy.

Long-Term Managment

Asthma management is aimed at reducing allergen exposure through environmental and dietary (if applicable) modification and elevating allergen thresholds through medication and hyposensitization (if indicated). Long-term management of the preschool asthmatic child and his family begins with education. The parents and the child need information about adequate control of symptoms by proper administration of drugs, avoidance of contact with known allergenic factors, therapeutic breathing exercises to enhance the child's physical competency, prevention of infection, reduction of precipitating factors, psychotherapy in cases of extreme parent-child conflict and guidance for parents in management of the child's developmental tasks and needs. Parent groups led by qualified professionals help in solving day-to-day health and childrearing problems and emotional concerns. Table 43–10 summarizes the basic long-term management for the three classifications of asthma. Compliance to the management regimen by the child and parents is critical to the ultimate goal of preventing disability and minimizing physical and psychological side effects. Immunotherapy is sometimes given in inhalant-stimulated asthma particularly

TABLE 43-10 LONG-TERM MANAGEMENT OF ASTHMA*

Mild	Moderately Severe	Severe
1. No medication between attacks.	1. Around the clock administration (usually tid or qid) of oral theophylline and/or oral or aerosol adrenergic drug. Cromolyn sodium (qid) is given to children unresponsive to theophylline or adrenergics.	1. Treatment as for moderately severe type. Corticosteroid therapy administered at 2-week intervals in an attempt to reduce frequency and severity of acute episodes. Full corticosteroid therapy given during acute episodes, surgery, trauma or acute illness.
2. Oral theophylline or oral adrenergic drug, administered promptly when early signs of impending attack appear.	2. Oral corticosteroids daily, administered before 8:00 a.m. and gradually tapered off over 5 to 7 days for episodes of impending attack.	

Administration in all three types as applicable:
1. Antibiotics prescribed on evidence of bacterial or mycoplasma infection. Instruction should be given to stop the antibiotic if symptoms worsen and notify the doctor because some antibiotics are themselves allergenic.
2. Cromolyn sodium (inhaled dry powder) may be prescribed for seasonal inhalant-initiated asthma or for exercise-induced asthma (inhaled before exercise). *Not* to be used during acute attacks or status asthmaticus.
3. Aerosol adrenergics may be prescribed for use 20 minutes before exercise if exercise precipitates attacks. These are usually reserved for older children who can understand proper use since aerosol use can be abused.
4. Those with mild asthma who develop attacks when excited or nervous (e.g. holidays, special events) may have medication prescribed to be administered the day before and the day of the event.
5. Breathing exercises and short-interval mildly exertive sports or games are encouraged to help relax bronchioles, improve ventilation and strengthen respiratory muscles.
6. Antihistamines and expectorants may be prescribed to help reduce irritation from associated allergic rhinitis or during bouts of respiratory infection. Many doctors instruct parents to administer asthma medications to the person with mild asthma at the first sign of infection.

*From D. Hudgel and L. Madsen. Acute and chronic asthma: a guide to intervention. American Journal of Nursing, October 1980, p. 1791. D. Pearlman and C. Bierman. Asthma (bronchial asthma, reactive airways disorder). In Allergic Diseases of Infancy, Childhood and Adolescence. C. Bierman and D. Pearlman, W. B. Saunders Co., 1980.

IMMUNOTHERAPY IN ASTHMA

Immunotherapy or desensitization (allergy shots) is sometimes used when an antigen cannot be removed from the environment and exposure to it cannot be controlled in those who experience relatively severe reactions. This method of management is fairly effective with some antigens (many inhalants) and of debatable or no value in others (most ingestants, injectants, and some contactants).

Immunotherapy involves injecting small amounts of antigen extract in increasing strengths until tolerance is achieved.[1] The strength that accomplished tolerance becomes the maintenance dosage. The injections are received one or two times weekly until the maintenance dose is discovered. (This may take two months to a year.) Then the maintenance dose is administered on a regular basis at two- to eight-week intervals.[1] The immunotherapy may be given preseasonally (before the time of year when the antigen is present in quantity), co-seasonally (during the peak time the antigen is present), or perennially (throughout the whole year), which is the most common approach. The goal of this therapy is desensitization by development of hyposensitivity to the antigen. The series of regularly injected antigen stimulates development of IgG antibodies (see Chapter 23 for a discussion of allergic pathology), which block histamine release on mast cells or combine with the allergen to render it harmless.

The extract is specially titrated for the specific child and must be stored upright in a refrigerator. Before withdrawing the desired amount for injection (use a tuberculin syringe), rotate the container, then withdraw the extract from the vial without injecting air. The dose is administered subcutaneously in the lower triceps or deltoid. The site should be rotated each time, with documentation kept of the site, dosage, and any reactions. Emergency equipment should always be immediately available in case of systemic reaction. If a dose causes a systemic response or creates local erythema or edema the size of a nickel, or larger, the next dose should not be given until an allergist is consulted. The nurse should observe the child continuously the first 20 minutes after injection, and parents should watch for any reaction in the following 24 hours. Local reactions can be treated with cold compresses and oral antihistamines.

---

when the specific inhalants are ones that cannot be eliminated from the environment or their elimination would require drastic life style changes.

Children disposed to allergy need careful attention given to maintaining their general health at optimal levels with balanced nutrition, adequate rest and a relatively routine, calm home and school environment. Consultation with the child's allergist is indicated to determine which immunizations (the culture media for some vaccines is highly allergenic to some persons) may be safely given. Exposure to known illness or infection at school or in the home should be avoided as much as possible. Environmental factors known to precipitate or aggravate asthmatic attacks should be eliminated or avoided when possible (see Chapter 23 for a discussion of home allergy-proofing) but not to the extent of inhibiting experiences valuable to the child's normal growth and development or to the degree that constant family discord is created. For those children on round-the-clock medications, the schedule should be as convenient as possible. Ideally the schedule avoids school hours; when medication is necessary at school, arrangements should be made for the child to take the medication privately, without attention being drawn to this.

The nurse has major responsibility for ensuring that the child and his parents have thorough, accurate information about asthma and its management. Parents' understanding of the disease helps immensely to prevent overprotection of the child or neglect of his condition. The child should be provided with adequate information as he grows and develops so that he can increasingly take personal responsibility for his own medical and environmental management. The dangers of attempting to manage asthma with unprescribed over-the-counter drugs advertised to relieve allergic symptoms should be emphasized often. Parents should be cautioned that even under the most careful management occasional asthmatic attacks may occur and should be reassured that these attacks are not evidence of parental failure.

Management of Acute Attack

Prompt, effective treatment of an acute asthmatic attack, initiated when early signs of developing obstruction become apparent, significantly reduces the need for or length of hospitalization. When symptoms appear, prescribed home treatment should be promptly given. This treatment usually includes administering an oral bronchodilator and use of an adrenergic aerosol with a pressurized hand nebulizer. If these measures do not give relief, the child should be taken immediately to an emergency room for further treatment.

The emergency room nurse should use a calm and confident approach in managing the child in acute asthmatic distress. This measure alone aids significantly in reducing the child's and parents' anxiety.

The child should be encouraged to assume a position of comfort. (Usually Fowler's or semi-Fowler's position is preferred, but no specific position should be forced.) Oxygen (4-8 L/min.) should be administered by nasal prongs. (A mask may be used but many children resist this.) The child should be evaluated quickly for signs of hypoxemia (headache, fatigue, confusion, dizziness) or impending respiratory failure (drowsiness, diaphoresis, muscle twitching, normal or elevated $PaCO_2$). A quick data base should be collected as a basis to determine emergency interventions. The nurse should record what medications the child receives regularly as well as any given earlier in this attack, any known allergies and the onset of this episode. Lung auscultation should be done to evaluate airflow. In severe bronchoconstriction, no wheezing will be audible or it will occur with inspiration — a sign of impending respiratory failure. In less severe episodes, wheezing is heard on expiration. Wheezing that clears with change of position or coughing is due to upper airway mucus plugging and congestion. Subcutaneous epinephrine or another bronchodilator is prescribed and may be repeated two or three times at 10- 15-minute intervals. An IV (5 per cent dextrose in saline) is then started (18 gauge needle; well secured to withstand the child's coughing and restlessness) for fluid and electrolyte maintenance* and for the administration of aminophylline in case epinephrine is unsuccessful. If response was poor to initial subcutaneous adrenergic drugs, oral or IV corticosteroid therapy may be initiated early in an acute attack to help reduce inflammation. The importance of beginning this early is based on the fact that six or more hours are required for the drug to take effect and the drug may prevent or reverse status asthmaticus.[4, 6]

---

*Urine specific gravities help to establish hydration needs. Serum electrolytes should be used to determine the need for potassium replacement.

An IVAC should be used to ensure effective titration levels of the intravenous drug in the blood. Aminophylline* is initially given in a loading dose, then a maintenance dosage is achieved by continuous infusion. Theophylline blood levels should be determined before the maintenance dosage is begun; the goal is to maintain theophylline blood levels at 10 to 20 $\mu g/ml$. Additional doses of subcutaneous or inhaled adrenergic drugs may be given to control bronchospasm.

This therapy is continued until the patient has stopped wheezing and spiromatic pulmonary function is stable. If after one hour there is no deterioration, the child may be sent home; however, if there is deterioration or pulmonary clearing is incomplete, hospitalization for further evaluation is in order. Expectorants may be given to help bring up secretions but require adequate hydration to be effective. If infection exists (this may be verified by a sputum culture or chest x-ray), an antibiotic will be prescribed.

During emergency care questions to the child should be minimal and limited to those that can be answered yes of no. The child's parents should be permitted to stay with him to offer reassurance and comfort. Likewise, any security item the child has brought along should remain with him as additional emotional support. Once the attack has diminished so that the child can swallow fluids without gasping, small but frequent drinks of lukewarm liquid should be offered to help liquefy and bring up secretions.

Management of Status Asthmaticus

Status asthmaticus is a severe acute asthmatic attack that persists beyond two hours despite bronchodilator therapy and in which respiratory metabolism is imbalanced.[5] (Bronchial obstruction from a foreign object may cause similar symptoms and should be ruled out by history of onset and chest x-ray.)

The treatment as described for an acute asthmatic attack is continued in status asthmaticus. However, the child is hospitalized and huge

---

*Whenever aminophylline is given the child should be hooked to a cardiac monitor and respirations evaluated frequently. The drug can alter cardiopulmonary function.

doses of intravenous corticosteroids are given. Blood gases, respiratory status and level of consciousness are closely monitored to identify early signs of progressive hypoxemia and acidosis. If the child becomes acidotic, sodium bicarbonate is given promptly to reverse the acidosis. Sedatives and tranquilizers are avoided despite the child's restlessness because these drugs further compromise respirations. If alveolar hypoventilation (normal or elevated $PaCO_2$) persists despite the sodium bicarbonate, the child should be intubated and a volume-cycled ventilator applied to ensure adequate alveolar ventilation and possibly prevent respiratory or cardiac arrest.

As the attack diminishes oral drugs and fluids are given and, if tolerated, the IV is discontinued. Chest physical therapy (postural drainage, breathing exercises) is used to help remove all remaining secretions. Steroid therapy is gradually discontinued over a period of two to seven days. Most children can be discharged from the hospital in two to three days after the attack has resolved.

Family Management

Stress for the asthmatic child and parent at home usually involves fears of an attack that could happen when help and appropriate remedial treatment are not available immediately. The parents may fear sending the child to a day care center, leaving him with a babysitter and taking vacations very far from the local doctor or hospital. This leads to restrictions on family activity and overprotectiveness of the child with limitations to his initiative and cognitive growth. The family can learn to deal with this by learning to give epinephrine injections, and the child, after age 5, can be taught to use and carry an inhalator with him, if it is prescribed, for use in emergency situations only. With proper allergenic control, the symptoms will lessen and restrictions can be minimized.

The family's sleep cycle is often interrupted because many asthma attacks occur during the night. Occasional interruptions cause little long-term family distress, but frequent sleep disruptions can create fatigue and irritability. Giving medications just before bedtime with sufficient fluid intake may help to decrease the severity of symptoms. Loss of nighttime bladder control often accompanies the paroxysmal coughing, but episodes will decrease once allergen tolerance is achieved.

Conflicts over dependency-independency needs often occur in families of children with asthma. Sibling jealousy over preferential treatment given to the child or restrictions on freedom imposed on the entire family may lead to suppressed anger. Suppressed anger on the part of parents about life style changes can cause conflicts that are stress-producing. Persons with suppressed anger because of restrictions on the family will need to express this anger in an appropriate manner. Interventions such as financial aid, finding a babysitter qualified to care for the child in an emergency and avoidance of precipitants that stimulate attacks may help diminish family stress. The angry preschool child may benefit by using toys such as modeling clay and pounding tables to express his feelings in an acceptable way. Incorporation of the preschooler in family activity and giving him some responsibility with expectations that he will be able to meet it helps to reduce these conflicts. Equal imposition of house rules on all children helps to decrease sibling jealousy.

Many children with asthma will state that if their demands are not met they will start to wheeze and promptly do so. Physical punishment is discouraged but limits can be set on the child's behavior by using denial of a favorite activity for a reasonable amount of time. The child who picks his form of punishment and follows through on it until he gains control of himself will enhance his self-reliance and self-control. The parent must be cautioned not to make threats that cannot be enforced. The child, as he grows, needs frequent assurance from health personnel and from his parents that, although everyone involved sometimes feels frustration because of the allergy, the child himself should not feel guilt. He did not cause the allergy and it is, in fact, something beyond anyone's control. Parents may need to be cautioned against using their child's allergy as a conversation topic. (Children react to overheard conversations about themselves long before they master language.) Some parents may need counselling if they persistently use the child's allergy as a convenient excuse for his misbehavior.

If conflicts and anxieties in the family perpetuate the child's asthmatic episodes or the child

TABLE 43-11 SYMPTOMS OF CHRONIC ALLERGIC RHINITIS

Allergic shiners	Dark circles noted around the eyes from chronic nasal and sinus congestion
Allergic salute	Upward brushing of the nose tip to allay pruritus and open nasal passages; a white crease across bridge of nose may be present
Allergic gaping	Open mouth breathing, particularly during times of rest; often accompanied by a high, V-shaped palate and aseptic red throat
Geographic tongue	Shiny, bald patches with elevated pearl borders on the edge or tip of the tongue; usually associated with food allergies, but not always.
Transient hearing loss with immobile or scarred tympanic membrane	Results from chronic serous otitis media associated with persistent (allergic) rhinitis and blockage of the eustachian tube
Abnormal nasal mucosa	Pale and swollen with gray, boggy nasal turbinates
Pepper seed conjunctiva	Conjunctiva appear to be covered with pale, hardened vesicles, with or without reddened eyes; associated most frequently with hay fever.
Hypernasal voice	Vowels are heard to be muffled during episodes of seasonal rhinitis

frequently uses his asthma behavior to express and meet his emotional needs, psychiatric counselling should be sought. Parents need help in developing in their child an increasing responsibility for self-care and promoting the goal of raising the child as normally as possible. Parental attitudes of overprotection, lenient discipline, rejection or neglect negatively affect personality development. Parental love and attention when the child is well will help to minimize the use of wheezing to gain attention.

STINGING INSECT ALLERGY

The normal reaction to an insect sting is a localized reaction consisting of pain, swelling and erythema. In sensitive children the reaction does not remain localized to the area of the sting: a distant area of the body may be affected with hives, nasal or eye allergies, wheezing. The child may collapse and faint. In allergic persons, the next sting could cause death in 10 to 15 minutes. Parents are instructed to carry an allergy center insect sting kit in the car and to have one available at school and at home. The school nurse should be made aware of the child's allergic history, and the parents and nurse together can educate teachers about the need for immediate action in case of a sting. Chewable antihistamines are often carried by older preschoolers. Precautions also need to be taken to avoid stings, such as wearing neutral-colored clothing; avoiding use of scented soaps and perfumes; using insect repellent on hair, clothing and exposed extremities; staying away from commonly infested areas such as barns, fruit trees, woods or attics; and avoidance of walking barefoot.

RHINITIS

Chronic Allergic Rhinitis

Chronic allergic rhinitis is an inflammatory reaction of the nasal, conjunctival, and bronchial mucosa associated with inhalant allergy to house dust and molds in the winter months and ragweed pollens in the summer. Table 43–11 summarizes characteristic symptoms of the child with chronic rhinitis.

Diagnosis of the causative factors of chronic allergic rhinitis involves a series of skin testing procedures by the scratch, prick or intradermal methods. A particularly helpful adjunct to diagnosis is a symptom diary. The parent is instructed to prepare a daily log of symptoms according to organ system, time of day, level of child's activity, season, weather, foods consumed and geographic location. This provides good data upon which to judge the potency of the allergens suspected.

Nursing care focuses on assisting the family to maintain environmental control, support during hyposensitization, and understanding of the behavioral components of allergy. The major goal is to eliminate exposure to offending allergens or to reduce the concentration of the allergen in the environment. Many allergists believe that *poor parental understanding of environmental control is one of the most frequently encountered factors identified in poor response to hyposensitization therapy*.

Seasonal Allergic Rhinitis

Seasonal allergic rhinitis (hay fever), an inhalant allergy, involves an inflammatory symptom complex of the nasal mucosa characterized by uncontrolled bouts of sneezing, rhinorrhea, nasal congestion, conjunctivitis and pharyngitis. It is differentiated from the common cold by the presence of eosinophilia in nasal smear. The antigen or antigens are identified by skin testing.

Treatment involves avoidance of the allergen when possible. Symptomatic treatment consists of antihistamines coupled with ephedrine nose drops at bedtime. In a third to half of children with seasonal hayfever, the condition progresses to asthma. If environmental control and symptomatic treatment are ineffective, hyposensitization is necessary.

References

Introduction

1. C. Fostel. Chronic illness and handicapping conditions. In P. Brandt et al. (eds). Current Practice in Pediatric Nursing, C. V. Mosby Co., 1978
2. B. Holaday. Parenting the Chronically Ill Child. In P. Brandt et al. Current Practice in Pediatric Nursing, C. V. Mosby Co., 1978
3. J. V. Lavigne and M. Ryan. Psychologic adjustment of siblings of children with chronic illness. Pediatrics, April 1979, p. 616
4. S. Steele. Nursing Care of the Child with Long-term Illness. 2nd ed. Appleton-Century-Crofts, 1977
5. G. Travis. Chronic Illness in Children, Its Impact on the Child and Family. Stanford University Press, 1976

Poliomyelitis

1. R. Hoekelman et al. (eds.). Principles of Pediatrics. McGraw-Hill Book Co., 1978
2. D. Horstmann. Poliomyelitis. In Pediatrics, 16th ed., A. M. Rudolph, ed., Appleton-Century-Crofts, 1977
3. J. Hughes. Synopsis of pediatrics, 5th ed. C. V. Mosby Co., 1980

Visual Problems

1. E. Adelson and S. Fraiberg. Mouth and hand in the early development of blind infants. In Third Symposium on Oral Sensation and Perception. J. F. Bosma, Charles C Thomas, 1972
2. E. Adelson and S. Fraiberg. Gross motor development in infants blind from birth. Child Development, March 1974, p. 114
3. L. Alonso et al. Mainstreaming preschoolers: Children with Visual Handicaps. U. S. Department of Health, Education and Welfare Publication No. (OHDS) 78-31112, 1978
4. N. Barraga. Utilization of Sensory-Perceptual Abilities in the Visually Handicapped Child in School. B. Lowenfeld, ed., The John Day Co., 1973
5. R. Bischoff. Early childhood development of the visually handicapped. Issues in Comprehensive Pediatric Nursing, October 1979, p. 36
6. P. Chinn. Child Health Maintenance. C. V. Mosby Co., 1979
7. B. J. Cratty. Movement and Spatial Awareness in Blind Children and Youth. Charles C Thomas, 1971
8. S. Feman and R. Reinecke. Handbook of Pediatric Ophthalmology. Grune & Stratton, 1978
9. S. Fraiberg et al. The role of sound in the search behavior of a blind infant. The Psychoanalytic Study of the Child, Vol. XXI, 1966, p. 327
10. S. Fraiberg et al. An educational program for blind infants. Journal of Special Education, Summer 1969, p. 121
11. S. Fraiberg. Intervention in infancy: a program for blind infants. Journal of the American Academy of Child Psychiatry, July 1971, p. 381
12. S. Fraiberg. Blind infants and their mothers: an examination of the sign system. In The Effect of the Infant on its Caregiver, M. Lewis and I. Rosenblum, eds., John Wiley and Sons, Inc., 1974
13. J. Gwiazda et al. New methods for testing infant vision. The Sightsaving Review, Summer 1979, p. 61
14. W. Havener. Synopsis of Ophthalmology, 5th ed. C. V. Mosby Co., 1979
15. E. Hatfield. Methods and standards for screening preschool children. The Sightsaving Review, Summer 1979, p. 71
16. D. Hiles. Strabismus. American Journal of Nursing, April 1974, p. 1082
17. J. Hughes. Synopsis of Pediatrics, 5th ed. C. V. Mosby Co., 1980
18. J. Jan et al. Visual Impairment in Children and Adolescents. Grune & Stratton, 1977
19. B. Lowenfeld, ed. The Visually Handicapped Child in School. The John Day Co., 1973
20. R. Pagon. The role of genetic counseling in the prevention of blindness. The Sightsaving Review, Winter 1979-80, p. 157
21. Problems of the Partially Seeing, National Association for Visually Handicapped, 1980
22. H. Scheie and D. Albert. Textbook of Ophthalmology, 9th ed. W. B. Saunders Co., 1977
23. G. Scholl. Understanding and meeting developmental needs. In The Visually Handicapped Child in School, B. Lowenfeld, ed., The John Day Co., 1973
24. I. Siegel and T. Murphy. Postural Determinants in the Blind: Final Report. U. S. Educational Resources Information Center, ERIC Document FD 048 714, August 1970
25. S. Stangler et al. Screening Growth and Development of Preschool Children: A Guide for Test Selection. McGraw-Hill Book Co., 1980
26. A. Tongue. Low vision examination in children with visual impairment. Journal of Pediatric Ophthalmology and Strabismus, May/June 1980, p. 175

Hearing Impairment

1. L. Bergstrom. Causes of reversed hearing loss in early childhood. Pediatric Annals, January 1980, p. 13/23
2. P. Brookhouser. Early recognition of childhood hearing impairment. Ear, Nose and Throat Journal, July 1979, p. 10
3. D. Cunningham. Auditory screening. In Principles of Pediatrics. R. Hoekelman et al., eds., McGraw-Hill Book Co., 1978
4. D. Cunningham. Hearing loss. In Principles of Pediatrics. R. Hoekelman et al., eds., McGraw Hill Book Co., 1978
5. D. Dale. Deaf Children at Home and at School. University of London Press, Ltd., Warwick Press, 1968
6. H. Davis and S. R. Silverman. Hearing and Deafness. Holt, Rinehart and Winston, 1978
7. J. DiBartolomeo and S. Gerber. Pathology of hearing loss In Audiometry in Infancy. S. Gerber, Grune & Stratton, 1977

8. M. Downs. Early identification of hearing loss. In Speech, Language, and Hearing. N. Lass et al., eds., W. B. Saunders Co., 1981
9. S. Gerber and G. Mencher, eds. Early Diagnosis of Hearing Loss. Grune & Stratton, 1978
10. B. Jaffe, ed. Hearing Loss in Children. University Park Press, 1977
11. J. Kass and M. Beebe. Serious Otitis Media. Nurse Practitioner, Mar/Apr 1979, p. 25
12. E. Lenneberg. Biological Foundation of Language. John Wiley & Sons, 1967
13. F. Martin. Pediatric Audiology. Prentice-Hall, Inc., 1978
14. W. McFarland et al. An automated hearing screening technique for newborns. Journal of Speech and Hearing Disorders, November 1980, p. 495
15. W. McFarland and F. Simmons. The importance of early intervention with severe childhood deafness. Pediatric Annals, January 1980, p. 16
16. D. Meyer and U. Wolfe. Use of high-risk register in newborn hearing screening. Journal of Speech and Hearing Disorders, November 1975, p. 493
17. G. Mencher, ed. Early Identification of Hearing Loss, Karger, 1976.
18. G. Mencher. Screening the newborn infant for hearing loss: a complete identification program. In Childhood Deafness, F. Bess, ed., Grune & Stratton, 1977
19. D. Moores. Educating the Deaf Psychology, Principles, and Practices. Houghton Mifflin Co, 1978
20. H. Newby. Audiology, 4th ed. Prentice-Hall, Inc., 1979
21. Northern and M. Downs. Hearing in children. Williams and Wilkins, 1974
22. J. L. Northern et al. Tympanometry: a technique for identifying ear disease in children. Pediatric Nursing, Mar/Apr 1975, p. 32
23. J. S. Palfrey et al. Selective hearing screening for young children. Clinical Pediatrics, July 1980, p. 473
24. M. Paparella. Differential diagnosis of childhood deafness. In Childhood Deafness. F. Bess, ed. Grune & Stratton, 1977
25. J. Paradise et al. Tympanometric detection of middle ear effusion in infants and young children. Pediatrics, August 1976, p. 198.
26. R. M. Poland et al. Methods for detecting hearing impairment in infancy. Pediatric Annals, January 1980, p. 32
27. E. H. Rosenblum. Fundamentals of Hearing for Health Professionals. Little Brown & Co., 1979.
28. M. Rubin. Meeting the needs of hearing-impaired infants. Pediatric Annals, January 1980, p. 46
29. F. Simmons. Identification of hearing loss in infants and young children. Otolaryngologic Clinics of North America, February 1978, p. 19
30. R. Sweitzer. Audiologic evaluation of the infant and young child. In Hearing Loss in Children: A Comprehensive Text. B. Jaffe, ed., University Park Press, 1977, p. 101
31. S. Vargo. Auditory screening in the schools — Failure or success? Journal of School Health, January 1980, p. 32

Asthma

1. S. Bridgewater et al. Allergies in Children: recognition. American Journal of Nursing, April 1978, p. 613
2. S. Cahill. The asthmatic patient: a practical perspective. Journal of Emergency Nursing, Sept/Oct 1980, p. 14
3. R. Carty. Some facts about allergy. Pediatric Nursing, Mar/Apr 1977, p. 7
4. D. Hudgel and L. Madsen. Acute and chronic asthma: a guide to intervention. American Journal of Nursing, October 1980, p. 1791
5. S. Lulla and R. Newcomb. Emergency management of asthma in children. Journal of Pediatrics, September 1980, p. 346
6. D. Pearlman and C. Bierman. Asthma (bronchial asthma, reactive airways disorder). In Allergic Diseases of Infancy, Childhood and Adolescence. C. Bierman and D. Pearlman, W. B. Saunders Co., 1980
7. A. Rowe. Food Allergy: Its Manifestations and Control and the Elimination Diets. Charles C Thomas, 1972

Additional Recommended Reading

The Sensory Impaired Child

N. Erber. Speech perception by profoundly hearing-impaired children. Journal of Speech and Hearing Disorders, August 1979, p. 255

P. Hixson. Recognizing delayed language development in children with hidden hearing impairment. Pediatric Annals, January 1980, p. 28

B. Lovelace. The blind child in the hospital. AORN Journal, February 1980, p. 256

N. Matlein. The audiologic examination of young children at risk. Ear, Nose and Throat Journal, July 1979, p. 29

D. W. Naiman and J. Schein. For Parents of Deaf Children. National Association of the Deaf, 1978.

R. T. Sataloff. Pediatric hearing loss. Pediatric Nursing, Sept/Oct 1980, p. 16

J. Semple. Hearing-Impaired Preschool Child: A Book for Parents. Charles C Thomas, 1970

A. Shayse. Helping parents in the developmental rearing of a blind child. Maternal-Child Nursing Journal, Spring 1972, p. 55

M. Smith and P. Cloonan. Meeting the special needs of the hearing-impaired child. Issues in Comprehensive Pediatric Nursing, October 1979, p. 22

J. C. Wisner. Causal factors, identification and management of hearing impairment in early childhood. Issues in Comprehensive Pediatric Nursing, Jan/Feb 1978, p. 25

V. Varma. Stresses in Children. University of London Press, 1973

Asthma

V. Bates. Emergency management of status asthmaticus. Journal of Emergency Nursing, Sept/Oct 1980, p. 9

M. Bergner and C. Hutelmyer. Teaching kids how to live with their allergies. Nursing 76, August 1976, p. 11

J. Dewey. Ambulatory nursing: 18 ways to live with asthma. Nursing 75, May 1975, p. 48

B. Dyer. Asthmatic kids — independence. One giant step. Pediatric Nursing, Mar/Apr 1977, p. 16

E. Hawkins-Walsh and C. Pettrone. Drugs used in the treatment of pediatric allergy and asthma. Pediatric Nursing, Mar/Apr 1977, p. 12

J. Hughes. Synopsis of Pediatrics. C. V. Mosby Co., 1979

S. Kim et al. Temperament of asthmatic children. Journal of Pediatrics, September 1980, p. 483

J. Souhrada and J. Buckley. Pulmonary function testing in asthmatic children. Pediatric Clinics of North America, May 1976, p. 249

Resources for the Visually Impaired

Organizations

American Association of University
Affiliated Programs
Suite 406
2033 M Street
Washington, DC 20036

   Provides diagnostic, treatment, educational and consultant services.

American Foundation for the Blind
15 West 16th Street
New York, NY 10011

   Publishes The Journal of Visual Impairment and Blindness.

Association for the Education of the Visually Handicapped
919 Walnut Street
Philadelphia, PA 19107

   Publishes Education of the Visually Handicapped.

Council for Exceptional Children
1920 Association Drive
Reston, VA 22091

National Association for the Visually Handicapped
305 East 24th Street
New York, NY 10010

National Society for the Prevention of Blindness, Inc.
79 Madison Avenue
New York, NY 10016

Resources for Materials and Catalogues

American Printing House for the Blind, Inc.
1839 Frankfort Avenue
Louisville, KY 40200

Catalog of large-type materials, 1979
National Association for Visually Handicapped
3201 Balboa Street
San Francisco, CA 94121

Library of Congress
Division for the Blind
and Physically Handicapped
Reference Department
Washington, DC 20542

   Provides for library service to individuals who are unable to read standard print.

Catalog of Optical Aids, Optical Aid Service
New York Association for the Blind
111 East 59th Street
New York, NY 10022

Vision Center
1393 North High Street
Columbus, OH 43201

Touch Inc.
P.O. Box 1711,
Albany, NY 12201

Resources for the Hearing Impaired

Organizations

Alexander Graham Bell Association for the Deaf, Inc.
3417 Volta Place, N.W.
Washington, DC 20007

Conference of Executives of American Schools for the Deaf
5034 Wisconsin Avenue, N.W.
Washington, DC 20016

Council of Organizations Serving the Deaf
4201 Connecticut Avenue, N.W.
Suite 210
Washington, DC 20008

International Parents Organization
Alexander Graham Bell Association for the Deaf
3417 Volta Place, N.W.
Washington, DC 20007

National Association of the Deaf
814 Thayer Avenue
Silver Spring, MD 20910

National Association of Parents of the Deaf
814 Thayer Avenue
Silver Spring, MD 20910

The American Speech and Hearing Association
9030 Old Georgetown Road
Bethesda, MD 20014

The National Association of Hearing and Speech Action
Suite #201, 814 Thayer Avenue
Silver Spring, MD 20910

POTENTIAL STRESSES DURING THE PRESCHOOL YEARS: LIFE-THREATENING ALTERATIONS IN HEALTH STATUS

by Mary Waskerwitz, BSN, PNP, and Ruth M. Heyn, MD

Most people think of cancer as a disease of the elderly. Cancer, however, is the leading cause of death from disease in children over 1 year of age. The Third National Cancer Survey, which was conducted from 1969 to 1971, reported that the most common malignancies in children in the United States were, in order, leukemia, brain tumors, lymphomas (including Hodgkin's disease), neuroblastoma, Wilms' tumor, soft tissue sarcomas (including rhabdomyosarcoma), bone tumors (Ewing's sarcoma and osteogenic sarcoma), and retinoblastoma.[5] From a review of 834 patients with these diagnoses who were treated at the University of Michigan from 1962 to 1978, the percentage distribution of children according to age group is presented in Figure 44–1. These statistics also demonstrate that a majority of the patients (575) first presented with their disease as preschoolers or school-age children.

The age distribution pattern presented in Figure 44–1 shows that the diagnoses of leukemia, Wilms' tumor and neuroblastoma are common to preschoolers. These diseases and the impact of cancer on the preschooler and his family are reviewed in this chapter.

LEUKEMIA

Leukemia is the most common type of childhood cancer. Although leukemia may have its onset at any age, its peak incidence is between the ages of 3 and 4. Leukemia is a proliferation of abnormal white blood cells in the body. Death comes from secondary complications resulting from the presence in vital tissues of these abnormal cells *(blasts)*. To understand why children with leukemia die and how the leukemic cells affect the body, it is important to have a basic understanding of the origin and function of normal blood cells.

Normal Blood Components

Whole blood is composed of plasma and cells. *Plasma* is the fluid portion of the blood. The solid, or cellular, portion is composed of red cells, white cells and platelets circulating in the plasma. Red cells carry oxygen to the body tissues from the lungs. Oxygen provides tissues with a vital ingredient of all cell metabolism. *Hemoglobin* is the oxygen-carrying protein of red blood cells, which imparts a pink or red appearance to the skin, lips and nails. Normal hemoglobin from the age of 2 to 5 is about 12 to 13 gm/dl. *Platelets* are the tiny cells that promote clotting and prevent bleeding. A normal platelet count is 200,000 to 400,000. The white blood cells form the body's defense against infection. Normal total white blood count is 5000 to 10,000. The three major types of white blood cells are *granulocytes, lymphocytes* and

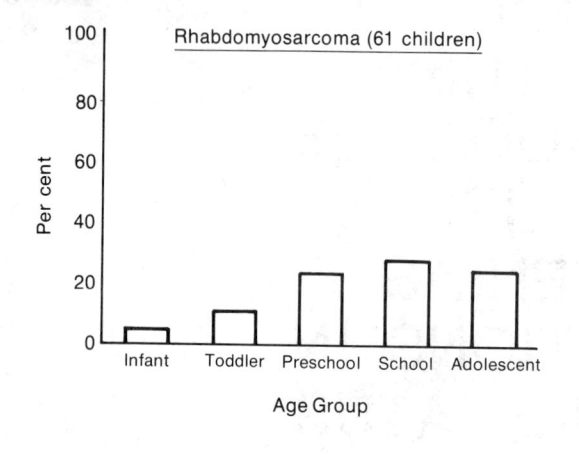

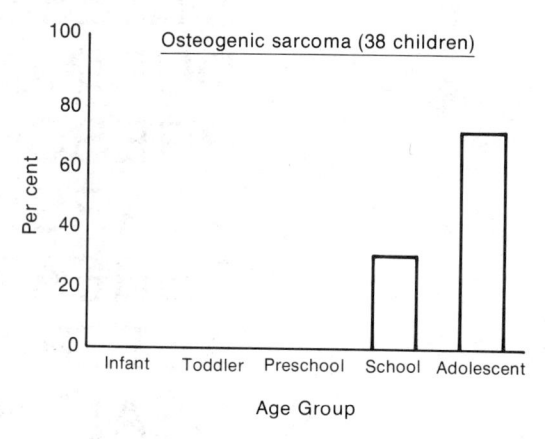

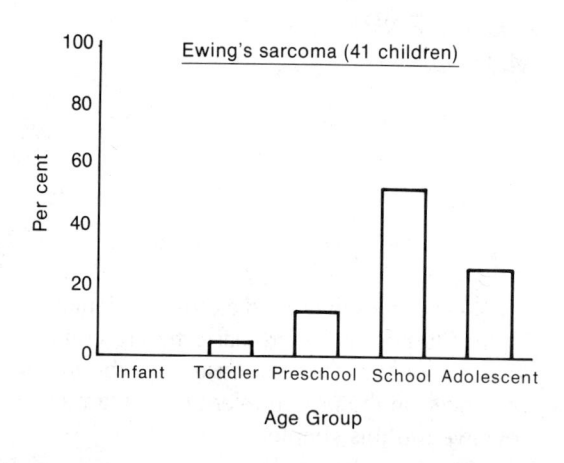

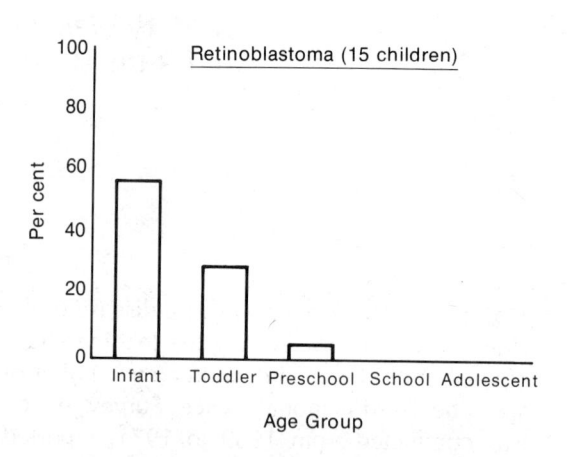

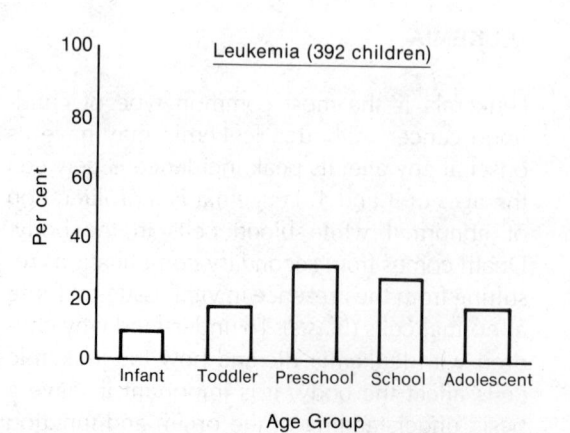

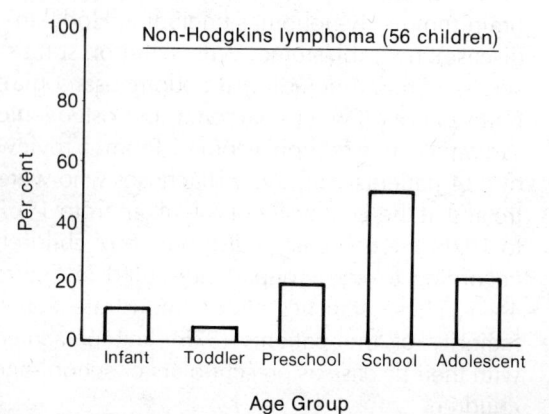

Figure 44-1 *See legend on opposite page*

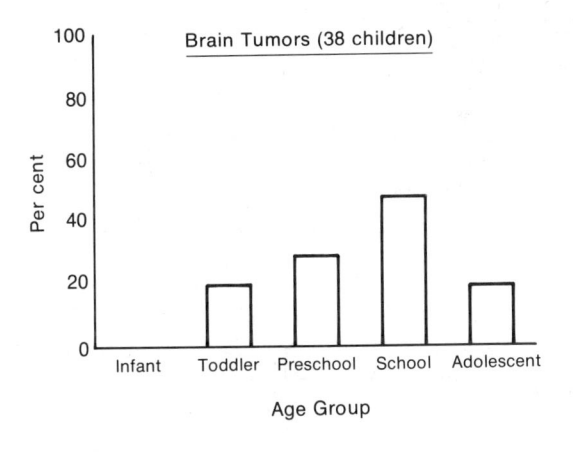

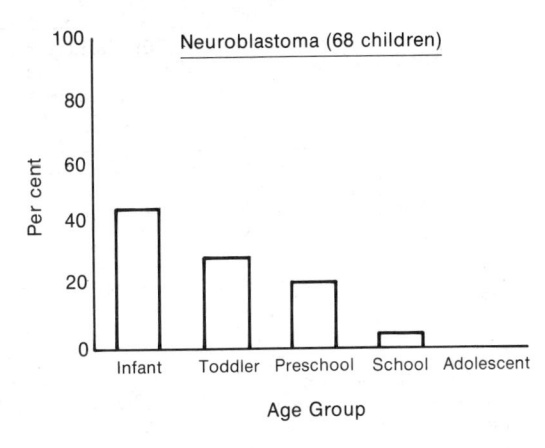

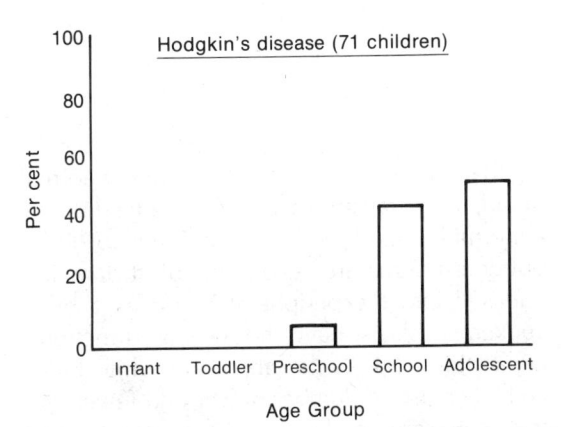

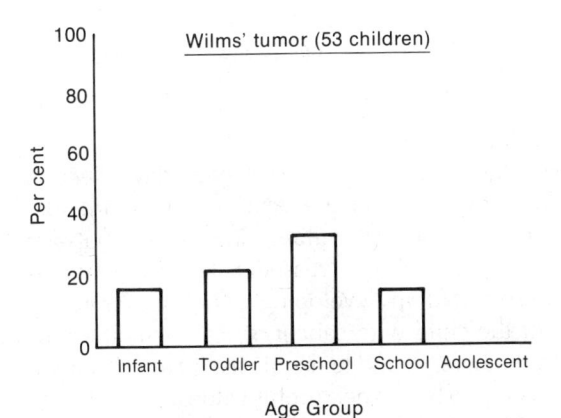

Figure 44-1. Distribution of cancer by age at diagnosis. Distribution in percentages of 834 children treated at the University of Michigan from 1962 to 1978 by age at diagnosis, using age distribution defined by this textbook.

monocytes. In addition, there are three major types of granulocytes: *neutrophils, eosinophils* and *basophils.*

While caring for children with malignant disease it is important to know about white blood cells and their specific functions. Table 44-1 summarizes the kinds of white blood cells, the proportion of these cells in the normal white blood count (WBC) and their major function. When a differential count is done, the percentage of each type of white cell is reported.

Words used to describe the most mature neutrophils are *segmented (segs), polymorphonuclear (polys), bands,* and stab cells *(stabs).* The absolute neutrophil count (ANC) is the total (or absolute) number of neutrophils in the blood. ANC is found by multiplying the percentage of neutrophils (segs and bands) in the differential by the total white count. Thus if the WBC is 8000 and the differential lists 40 per cent segmented forms, the ANC is 40 per cent of 8000 to 3200/mm³. Since neutrophils are very important in protecting against infection, the ANC is a guideline of the body's ability to fight

TABLE 44-1 CATEGORIES OF WHITE BLOOD CELLS AND THEIR FUNCTIONS

White Cell Type	Per Cent in Normal WBC	Function
Granulocytes Neutrophils	55	Ingest and digest bacteria during bacterial infection
Eosinophils	4	Summon antigen-antibody response in allergic reactions
Basophils	1	Specific action unknown
Lymphocytes	30	Effect cellular and humoral immunity; produce specific antibodies against viruses, bacteria, and other proteins
Monocytes	10	Act as phagocytes in bacterial infections and are an integral part of normal immune response via their relationship to lymphocyte function

POTENTIAL STRESSES DURING THE PRESCHOOL YEARS: LIFE-THREATENING ALTERATIONS IN HEALTH STATUS

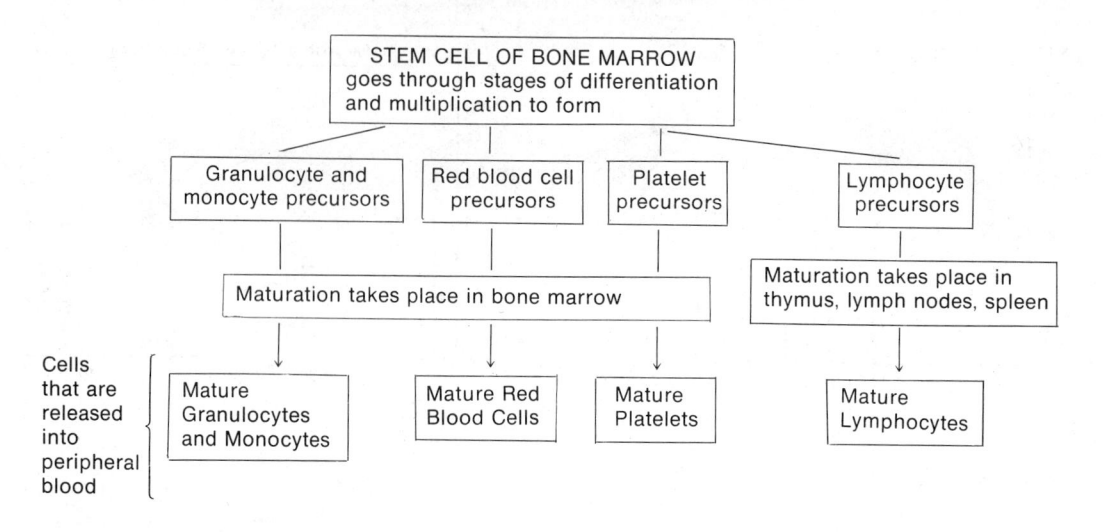

Figure 44-2 A schema of blood-cell production in the body.

bacterial invasion. Serious bacterial infection may occur when the ANC is less than 500. Knowing normal values and those that are associated with increased risk of infection is very helpful in developing guidelines for caring for the child with cancer, since chemotherapy, radiotherapy, and leukemia itself are often associated with low neutrophil values.

Blood cells are produced in the *bone marrow*, the soft material located in the cavities of bones. All blood cells arise from a common cell called the *stem cell*. Under genetic control, stem cells in the marrow differentiate to form red blood cells, white blood cells and platelets. Once a cell has differentiated into the parent cell of a red cell, a granulocytic white cell or a platelet, it continues to undergo division while maturing into a functional cell ready to work for the body. In the normal state the bone marrow releases only these mature, functional cells into the peripheral blood. Lymphocytes arise from the stem cell, but as soon as the commitment to this cell takes place, further maturation occurs in the thymus, lymph nodes and spleen. The exact site of monocytic maturation is unknown. Figure 44-2 illustrates the process of blood cell production.

Leukemia and the Blood

With the information that leukemia is a proliferation of abnormal white blood cells, and relating that information to knowledge of the normal blood, two statements can be made: (1) The abnormal white blood cell continues to divide but does not mature beyond the blast state. It is released into the peripheral blood as a blast. Leukemic blasts have no normal functional capabilities. (2) As the abnormal white blood cells increase in number, fewer and fewer normal cells are made, so that at the time of diagnosis the percentage of abnormal cells in the marrow is usually 80 to 100 per cent of the cells present. The lack of normal cells accounts for the symptoms seen in leukemia and, in large part, accounts for death from the disease.

Etiology

The etiology of leukemia is unknown. It is known that a few cases of leukemia in adults have been linked to exposure to environmental factors such as radiation or chemicals. The role of inheritance in the development of leukemia is demonstrated by the enhanced incidence of leukemia in identical twins. If an identical twin has leukemia, his twin has a 1 in 4 chance of developing leukemia. In contrast, the risk of a single child developing leukemia is 1 in 25,000.

Several genetically determined diseases have also been associated with an increased incidence of leukemia. Children with Down's syndrome, Fanconi's hypoplastic anemia, agammaglobulinemia, ataxia, telangiectasia, and Bloom's syndrome have shown a high incidence of leukemia.[5] Several of these defects are associated with immune deficiencies. Although the Ebstein-Barr (EB) virus has been associated with Burkitt's lymphoma and nasopharyngeal carcinoma, no other specific virus is known to be causally related to the development of leukemia or other malignancies. Research seeking an answer to the etiology of leukemia continues, with the investigation of carcinogens, viruses, genetics and other potential etiologic factors.

Types of Leukemia

There are several different types of leukemia, classified on the basis of the course of disease and the morphology of the cells. Each type carries its own prognosis and characteristics, making it important to know what kind of leukemia each child has.

Most childhood leukemia has an acute course (97 per cent) as opposed to a chronic one. Acute leukemia has a short history of symptoms and, without treatment, a rapidly declining course to death in three to six months. Leukemia in adults is more often chronic. Chronic leukemias have a more gradual onset and a course extending over two or more years. Chronic granulocytic leukemia is rarely seen in children, whereas chronic lymphocytic leukemia is never seen in them.[5]

The morphology of the white blood cells involved in the disease also varies. The most common childhood leukemia (80 to 85 per cent) is acute lymphocytic leukemia (ALL), which results from malignant change of the lymphocyte or its precursors and is acute in onset. Less common in childhood is acute granulocytic leukemia (AGL) and acute monocytic leukemia. Because the cells in the granulocytic and monocytic types vary so much, these conditions are often referred to as acute nonlymphocytic leukemias to cover the several types of cell morphology.

Clinical Manifestations

Recalling that leukemic blasts replace normal cells in the bone marrow, it is obvious that the child may present with decreased numbers of mature granulocytes, red blood cells and platelets. The child may have fever or obvious infection due to decreased numbers of normal white blood cells. A decrease in red blood cells and hemoglobin causes weakness, malaise and pallor. Decreased platelets may be associated with increased bruising, petechiae, or bleeding from the nose and gums. The spleen, liver, lymph nodes, thymus and kidney may become enlarged owing to an infiltration of these tissues with blast cells. Bone pain is a common symptom and is due to infiltrates in the cortex of bone or the subperiosteal area.

Making the Diagnosis

Leukemia is suspected when a child presents with the symptoms just described. If a complete blood count (CBC) is taken, the decreased numbers of normal red blood cells, white blood cells and platelets will be evident. This condition is known as *pancytopenia*. Leukemic blasts may be seen in the blood smear. The definitive diagnosis is made after examining a sample of bone marrow. To obtain a bone marrow specimen in the child, an area of accessible marrow, usually the anterior or posterior iliac crest or vertebral spine, is treated with local anesthesia. A small skin wheal and a small amount of anesthesia in the periosteum is necessary. A heavy, wide-gauge needle with a stylet is inserted into the center of bone and the marrow is aspirated with a syringe. To the naked eye bone marrow looks like blood, but when put onto slides and studied under a microscope it has characteristic histological features. Normal marrow contains less than 5 per cent very young cells *(hemocytoblasts)*. If the cells in the bone marrow specimen include more than 5 per cent blasts with leukemic morphology, the diagnosis of leukemia is made. Most leukemic patients at diagnosis will have about 90 per cent blasts in their bone marrow.

The Course of Disease and Treatment

Remission is the term used to describe an absence of leukemic cells in the marrow following treatment. A *relapse* is the reappearance of leukemic cells in a marrow that has been in remission. Once relapse has occurred remission can again be achieved, but this tends to be more difficult and the remission is less lasting with each successive relapse. Thus the major aim of initial treatment is to achieve a primary remission that lasts without relapse.

Treatment is divided into three phases. *Induction* is the term used for the initial treatment period that induces or brings about remission. Induction treatment is the most intensive and potentially the most life-threatening because the child is at high risk for bleeding and infection until his marrow is rid of blasts and again repopulates with normal cells. In addition, the treatment complications of kidney dysfunction and immunosuppression contribute to other potential problems. Induction treatment is usually given over a period of one month. The second phase of treatment includes *therapy for the central nervous system,* since this is an area in which the concentration of chemotherapeutic agents is poor. A combination of x-ray therapy to the brain and chemotherapy injected into the lumbar area of the spine is ordinarily used. The third phase is called *maintenance treatment* and provides therapy that will maintain the remission. Maintenance treatment is usually given for two to five years.

Chemotherapy

Treatment of leukemia involves the use of drugs that interfere with the production of leukemic cells. Use of these drugs, which include a variety of compounds, is known as *chemotherapy*. Most chemotherapeutic agents affect cells in the process of dividing to make new cells. Since many leukemic and tumor cells are dividing rapidly, their division and growth will be interfered with to a great extent, but many normal cells will also be affected to some degree. Chemotherapy drugs are most often used in combinations to complement and potentiate their interference with dividing cells.

Chemotherapeutic agents can be classified according to activity exerted on the tumor cells. Alkylating agents are compounds that interfere with the structure and function of DNA, combining chemically with DNA so the cell becomes damaged. Alkaloids disorganize the mitotic spindle to arrest cell division. Antimetabolites are substances similar to natural body substances that act falsely to incorporate into DNA. Synthetic hormones alter normal hormonal balance in patients to modify the growth of cancers arising from tissues that are particularly susceptible to hormonal influence, preventing effective cell proliferation. Antibiotics are chemicals produced by living bacteria that interfere with cell metabolism. Enzymes can inhibit certain cell metabolites and prevent protein synthesis.

Vincristine, prednisone, and L-asparaginase are drugs that are most often used in induction treatment of ALL. Vincristine, prednisone, 6-mercaptopurine, methotrexate, cytosine arabinoside, doxorubicin, and cyclophosphamide are drugs that can be used during maintenance. About 10 per cent of leukemia deaths are due to drug toxicity, so it is important for the nurse to be familiar with their toxicities. Table 44-2 summarizes the most commonly used agents, their generic and brand names, their classification and their major side effects.

All chemotherapeutic agents are immunosuppressive (they suppress the normal function of lymphocytes in the immune system) so patients must not receive live virus immunizations while on treatment and they must be cautioned to avoid exposure to common viral contagious diseases. If an immunosuppressed child contracts one of these diseases or receives one of these immunizations, he could develop a serious form of that particular disease because of his inability to mount a proper antibody response to the virus.

Central Nervous System Leukemia

Normal spinal fluid contains less than 5/mm^3 white blood cells and these are usually lymphocytes or monocytes. Leukemic cells probably get into the nervous system via disruption of meningeal capillaries when the peripheral blood contains blasts. The blast cells can remain in nongrowth phases for variable periods of time before increasing in number to the point of causing symptoms. Symptoms of central nervous system (CNS) leukemia are those of increased intracranial pressure and include headache and vomiting. Other manifestations include cranial nerve palsies, seizures and other neurological symptoms.

Drugs given orally and intravenously do not cross the blood-brain barrier to a very great extent so that treatment must consist of applying therapy directly into the CNS. This is done by injecting a limited number of chemotherapeutic agents directly into the spinal fluid via lumbar puncture (intrathecal) or giving radiation therapy directly to the skull and spine. Only three agents can be introduced into spinal fluid.

TABLE 44-2 DRUGS COMMONLY USED IN THE TREATMENT OF ACUTE LYMPHOCYTIC LEUKEMIA

Agent Generic Name	Brand Name	Category	Toxicity
cyclophosphamide	Cytoxan	Alkylating agent	Bone marrow depression, hemorrhagic cystitis, nausea and vomiting, alopecia
cytosine arabinoside	Cytosar	Antimetabolite	Bone marrow depression, nausea and vomiting
doxorubicin	Adriamycin	Antibiotic	Bone marrow depression, cellulitis with extravasation, red urine, heart damage, alopecia, nausea and vomiting
L-asparaginase	Elspar	Enzyme	Diabetes, pancreatitis, local reaction to injection, allergic or anaphylactic reaction
Mercaptopurine	6-Mercaptopurine	Antimetabolite	Bone marrow depression
methotrexate		Antimetabolite	Bone marrow depression, mouth sores, diarrhea, liver damage, kidney damage, increased sensitivity to sun, skin rashes
prednisone		Hormone	Increased salt and water retention, increased appetite, weight gain, glucose intolerance
vincristine	Oncovin	Alkaloid	Abdominal, leg, or jaw pain, numbness and tingling of fingers and toes, constipation, alopecia, cellulitis with extravasation

Methotrexate has been used most, but cytosine arabinoside and hydrocortisone succinate can also be given. The same drugs can also be used in combination intrathecally.

Because statistics show that at some time 60 per cent of children with leukemia will develop CNS leukemia, treatment for CNS involvement is now given as a part of initial therapy so that any cells present will be eradicated at the same time that the marrow and other tissues are cleared of blasts.[1] Most investigators have referred to such treatment as "prophylactic," since it is given when children are asymptomatic. It is successful, however, because it treats the undetected cells before there are enough to cause symptoms. Currently about 10 per cent of children still develop CNS leukemia in spite of such "prophylaxis."[3] Because of the toxicity to the marrow resulting from spinal irradiation and the lack of adequate drug concentration in the brain when drugs are given in the lumbar area, most investigators use a combination of cranial irradiation and five or six doses of intrathecal methotrexate.

CNS leukemia can occur without bone marrow relapse. However, when marrow release occurs, the CNS may again be seeded with leukemic cells.

Testicular Leukemia

The male testis is the second most common site of extramedullary* relapse. The sign of testicular leukemia is a firm, enlarged testis. This complication may occur without marrow relapse, but is often a predictor of future marrow change. It is most apt to occur in those males who have high white counts at the time of diagnosis. Treatment includes testicular radiation and systemic reinduction therapy. The development of testicular leukemia carries an unfavorable prognosis. Because testicular relapse has been a problem after therapy is stopped, biopsies of the testes are being done before chemotherapy is stopped to make sure no leukemic cells are present in the testes.

Prognosis

The outlook for a child with leukemia depends on many prognostic variables. The histologic type separates two major categories of disease.

*Extramedullary refers to leukemic cells present outside of the bone marrow.

With proper treatment a child with acute lymphocytic leukemia (ALL) has a 96 per cent chance of obtaining an initial remission and greater than 50 per cent chance of surviving five years or more. By contrast, a child with acute nonlymphocytic leukemia has a 70 per cent chance of obtaining an initial remission, but the length of that remission is usually only 9 to 12 months.[3] Acute nonlymphocytic leukemias are less responsive to available chemotherapeutic agents even when more aggressive therapy is used. For many children a survival of five years may even mean they are cured.

Studies of ALL involving large numbers of children have identified prognostic factors that indicate how children with leukemia will fare with their disease. Children who at diagnosis are 3 to 7 years of age and have total white blood counts of less than 10,000 have a 90 per cent chance of being alive five years after diagnosis and are called "good risk." Children with high white blood counts (greater than 50,000) at diagnosis have an unfavorable prognosis and only 40 to 45 per cent are alive at five years. Children who are less than 3 years or more than 7 years but have white blood counts less than 50,000 fall in between and are considered "average risk."[4]

It is important to note the continually improving prognosis for children with leukemia. In 1948 the first drug was successfully used to treat leukemia. Before that time each child who developed leukemia died. Today the outlook for children with leukemia is changing favorably as improved treatment plans are developed.

Caring for the Child with Leukemia

Special care for the child with leukemia should include emotional support for the child and his family, provision of maximal physical comfort, and management of problems that relate to low blood values and to drug side effects. Initial supportive care depends on the blood counts at diagnosis and the complications present. Nurses caring for children with leukemia should be aware of the child's current hematologic status. Such knowledge is necessary for the nurse to remain alert for the many potential problems that may arise when counts are low or abnormal. Nurses should also be familiar with each child's specific treatment plan, especially the drugs the child is receiving. Also, the nurse will likely be a main source of emotional support for the child and his family. (Discussion on the family's needs and the support the nurse can offer is included later in this chapter.) It is the nurse who has the skill and is present 24 hours a day to respond to the fears and agony that a child and family experience during the course of illness and treatment of leukemia.

Children with very low hemoglobins (anemia) must be observed for increasing fatigue, increasing heart rate, increasing respiratory rate and irritability. Red blood cell transfusions can be given to correct the anemia. Children with low neutrophil counts (ANC less than 1000) must be observed for fever or other signs of infection. If a patient with a very low neutrophil count develops infection, he will acquire antibiotics or white blood cell transfusions to help fight the infection. Children with low platelet counts (less than 100,000) must be careful to avoid traumatic injury. Epistaxis and gum bleeding are common in children with very low platelet counts. The child may require platelet transfusions to control bleeding.

Parents must be taught to understand the blood counts and must know the special care required for each low value. Appendix VIII describes the special care of a child undergoing chemotherapy and radiotherapy. The nurse is responsible to provide this care while the child is hospitalized and to teach parents the skills required for them to deliver this care when the child is home.

The goal of treatment is to achieve and maintain a remission. The doses of chemotherapy used are derived by experience and calculated by the patient's body weight or surface area. These doses may not always be tolerated; therefore, close surveillance is necessary. Drug doses are decreased when defined toxicity occurs. A child in remission maintenance usually has a normal blood count and at these times is not at additional risk for bleeding. However, even with a normal white blood count he is always at some risk for infection because of the immunosuppressive effect of the majority of the chemotherapeutic agents used. These agents decrease the functional capabilities of normal lymphocytes.

NEUROBLASTOMA

Neuroblastoma is the second most common childhood solid tumor.[2] It is a malignant neoplasm that develops in cells of neural crest origin that give rise to the adrenal gland and the sympathetic nervous system. The etiology of neuroblastoma is unknown.

The majority of children with neuroblastoma are under 5 years of age, with a peak incidence at 2 years.[2] The sites of the primary tumor (site of origin) in the body vary. Over one-half of the primary tumors occur in the abdomen. Most of these are in the adrenal gland. About one-eighth of the primaries arise in sympathetic ganglia in the chest area. Neuroblastoma commonly metastasizes (spreads beyond the primary site) to bones (especially skull, femur and humerus), bone marrow, liver and lymph nodes. Infants less than 1 year of age tend to have either localized tumors or, if they have metastases, these are usually in areas that can be readily treated. Metastases to lungs are rare. Two-thirds of patients have metastases at diagnosis.

Clinical Manifestation and Diagnosis

Children who present with neuroblastoma may look and feel very sick. The chief signs and symptoms include an abdominal mass, fever, irritability, pain that relates to bone metastases, and orbital ecchymosis or proptosis (displacement of the eyeball causing it to protrude) from skull metastases. Neurological symptoms from spinal cord compression by the tumor can occur at times.

Diagnostic studies focus on the principal sites of primary or metastatic disease. Physical examination may reveal a palpable, firm mass in the abdomen. Tumor at other sites such as in the chest may be impossible to detect on physical examination. The tumor cells secrete increased amounts of catecholamines or other tyrosine metabolites, which are excreted in the urine. Twenty-four hour urine collections for catecholamines are imperative, since they provide an excellent means of following tumor presence.

Collecting complete and accurate urine samples can be difficult in a child who is not toilet-trained and usually requires the use of immobilization devices and secure urine bags. The nurse should be particularly sensitive to the stress that immobilization causes for the child and family. Special effort should be made to provide quiet diversional activities for the child during this period. Certain foods (such as those containing high amounts of vanilla or caffeine) and medicines may create falsely elevated levels of catecholamines in urine collections. For this reason the nurse should obtain a list of these foods and drugs from the catecholamine laboratory and provide it for parents of patients collecting urines. The urine is kept in bottles that contain a special preservative acid. Ninety-five per cent of all neuroblastoma patients will have elevated catecholamines.

Specific x-rays are done to define the primary and specific metastases, if present. Chest x-ray, abdominal x-ray, intravenous pyelogram (IVP), and inferior venacavagram (IVC) may show a mass that often contains flecks of calcium. Small calcified deposits occur when areas of tumor undergo necrosis, or cell death, and become calcified. Skeletal x-rays may show lytic lesions in bones. Bone scan and liver scan may detect subtle disease in the liver and bones. Bone marrow aspiration and biopsy are performed to check for infiltrates of tumor clumps in the bone marrow. As many as half of all patients have disease that has spread to the bone marrow. Bone marrow disease may be reflected in the blood count, but the most common finding is anemia, which is not dependent on tumor involvement in the marrow. The diagnosis of neuroblastoma depends on tissue histology. This must be made from a biopsy of the primary or metastatic tissue.

Staging

The extent of disease is described in a staging system. Stage I is the classification of a localized primary tumor that has been completely resected. Stage II disease extends beyond the primary tumor but does not cross the midline of the body and is grossly resectable. Disease classified as Stage III is localized but extends beyond the midline. Stage IV involves distant metastases. Stage IV-S is a special classification that is made primarily in infants whose metastatic disease is limited to liver, bone marrow or skin.

Treatment

Treatment varies with extent of disease. Disease at Stages I and II is treated with surgical removal of the primary tumor. Stages III and IV are frequently too extensive for complete or safe surgical removal of the primary tumor. When residual tumor is present, radiation therapy may be used for Stages II and III. Radiation therapy is practical in Stage IV disease only when chemotherapy has controlled metastatic sites. Chemotherapy may be used for disease classified as Stages II and III (when surgery is incomplete) and in Stage IV. No drug regimen or combination has been found that results in more than 60 to 70 per cent initial remission rate in Stage IV neuroblastoma. Cyclophosphamide, vincristine, dimethyltriazenoimidazole carboxamide (DTIC) and doxorubicin are drugs that are presently used in various combinations and schedules.

Prognosis

The prognosis for children with neuroblastoma depends on the age of the child at diagnosis and the stage of disease. Children who are very young at the time of diagnosis have the best prognosis. Infants under a year of age usually have either localized or have Stage IV-S disease. Children with Stage I tumors have almost a 100 per cent survival while those with Stages II, III, and IV-S have a 50 to 80 per cent survival. Children with Stage IV disease have a dismal prognosis; survival in this group is between 15 and 25 per cent.[2] Preschoolers with neuroblastoma tend to have disease classified as Stage IV.

Although children with localized neuroblastoma do fairly well, those whose disease is in Stage III or IV may have a devastating course and fatal outcome. Children who die with widespread neuroblastoma have often had severe pain and growth of tumor masses in multiple sites. The terminal stages of this disease are very difficult for a family to accept, since the child's body can be grossly disfigured by the disease. When a child with neuroblastoma is dying, he and his family are very dependent on the nursing staff for much of their support and comfort.

WILMS' TUMOR

Wilms' tumor is a malignant neoplasm of the kidney that most often affects young children. The median age of incidence is 3½ years.[6]

Clinical Manifestations

The child with Wilms' tumor most often is a well child in whom an abdominal mass has been seen or felt. Sometimes parents are the first to notice increasing abdominal girth when belts or waistbands become suddenly tight. Less common presenting signs and symptoms are abdominal pain, malaise, anorexia, fever, gross hematuria and hypertension.

The initial workup for these patients is designed to define the renal mass and search for areas of metastases. Wilms' tumor may metastasize to lung, liver or bone. Intravenous pyelogram and inferior venacavagram delineate the area of the tumor involvement in the kidney and, very importantly, show the status of the other kidney. About 5 to 10 per cent of Wilms' tumors are bilateral at initial diagnosis. Chest x-ray and a complete skeletal survey are done to evaluate renal, hepatic and hematological function. Studies done include BUN, creatinine, liver function tests, CBC and coagulation studies.

Tumor Classification

The National Wilms' Tumor Study, which was organized in 1969, has provided excellent data for staging and prognosis in this tumor. Wilms' tumor is classified, using the term *group*, according to extent of disease. Tumor classified as Group I is confined to the kidney and can be completely resected by nephrectomy. Group II tumor extends beyond the kidney but can be completely removed at the time of nephrectomy. Group III represents regional spread of disease beyond the kidney with residual nonblood-borne disease in the abdomen following surgery. Group IV represents blood-borne spread of disease to lung, liver, bone or distant lymph nodes. Group V Wilms' tumor involves both kidneys.

More important than staging is the histology of Wilms' tumor. Children with tumors that show a defined degree of anaplasia or are sarcomatous in pattern make up the majority of those succumbing to this disease. Those with "favorable" histology have an excellent prognosis.

Treatment

The treatment for Wilms' tumor includes all modalities of cancer treatment, namely, surgery, radiation therapy and chemotherapy. Surgery is performed as soon as the diagnosis is suggested by physical examination and x-rays. A nephrectomy is performed, with removal of all regional lymph nodes and any regional tumor that can be resected. Radiation therapy and chemotherapy are begun immediately after the operation. Radiation is used for the tumor bed for microscopic residual disease or for the entire abdomen in patients whose disease has spread beyond the kidney itself. Use of chemotherapy depends on the initial staging and is given for up to 15 months. The drugs that are commonly used today for Wilms' tumor include actinomycin D, vincristine and doxorubicin. Metastases are treated with radiation therapy, chemotherapy and at times, surgery.

Prognosis

When patients are adequately treated, the long-term survival in Wilms' tumor is about 90 per cent. The patients who do the best are the youngest children in Groups I and II with favorable tumor histology.

Since the outlook for children with Wilms' tumor is good, a greater concern is the quality of their survival. These children have only one kidney so they must be followed closely for urinary tract infections; these must be treated to maintain good kidney function.

SUPPORTING THE CHILD AND FAMILY DURING DIAGNOSIS

When cancer is diagnosed in a preschool child, the parents may already have suspected the child's symptoms and condition could represent such an illness. Nonetheless, when the diagnosis of cancer is actually made by the physician, the parents are immediately terrified that the child will die. The nurse should be present when the parents are told the diagnosis. As the physician tells the parents that their child has cancer, they may become instantly withdrawn. They often fail to recall any of the details of initial conversations with the physicians and nurses. The nurse should take an active role in helping parents to deal with the reality of the diagnosis by participating in the frequent explanations of the disease and its treatment that are required of the health team in the ensuing days.

After the initial shock, the parents will have numerous questions. Each question must be addressed and answered with gentle honesty. The parents are depressed about the possibility of their child's death. They may feel guilty about not having sought medical attention sooner. They are angry that this is happening to them and their child. They are still in a state of shock and disbelief. The parents probably do not know any individuals on the medical-nursing team well at this point, so they may not be ready to share these feelings. The health team must be there, however, ready to offer support when the parents are ready to be more open.

The initial hospitalization of a child with cancer may be the parents' first experience with hospitals and complicated treatments. Even the simplest procedures must be explained to the child and the parents. The nurse must therefore keep abreast with the diagnostic plan so that she can prepare the child and the parents for each step. The nurse can help the child and family develop trust and feel more secure during this frightening period if she uses her skills and knowledge effectively to communicate an attitude of caring and to give accurate information about the illness and treatments. These nursing functions can relieve some of the overwhelming stress that the child and family experience at this time.

At diagnosis the preschooler does not feel well. He may be irritable, but he is not especially worried because he has felt sick before and has always gotten better. The preschooler does begin to worry as soon as he can sense uneasiness, anxiety and sadness in his parents. His inability to separate reality from unreality calls for an honest explanation of what is happening. As soon as the parents can calmly speak with the child, he must be told something about why he is in the hospital and why things that hurt are being done to him. Obviously a preschooler does not need and will not benefit from a detailed description of his disease. He should be told the name of his disease to avoid embarrassment or fears later when he is out in public and exposed to persons who may freely use the diagnostic term. He will probably be satisfied with the information that this is an illness that requires special care from special doctors and nurses. He should know that at times some of the special treatments may hurt him a little bit for a while, but that all treatments will eventually make him feel better and will help him to get better. It is very important for the parents to tell the child that they will be with him and that they love him very much.

The entire family unit immediately centers all

EXPERIENCE OF A FAMILY WHOSE PRESCHOOLER HAS CANCER

Janie Fox was a normal 3-year-old. She was a delight to her parents as they watched her protect her baby brother and laugh and play with her friends. She seemed to be progressing and developing even more quickly than her 7-year-old sister did. At times during the family's recent vacation Janie's parents were overwhelmed at the beauty and solidity of their young family unit. Their hopes and dreams for their children were limitless.

As early as one month before Janie's symptoms began, her mother had thought she looked a little pale. Since Janie had always been a healthy child, she dismissed this as a product of her own imagination. To reassure herself the following week, however, she phoned her pediatrician, who told her that many children seem to be excessively pale as a summer tan wanes. The doctor and nurse discussed Janie's diet and told her mother that more iron-containing foods might be helpful. The next three weeks passed reasonably uneventfully. There was no question, however, that Janie had not been "her usual self" over a two-day period after this. She seemed to tire more easily.

The next morning Janie did not get out of bed and was irritable. She said that her legs hurt her. In looking at her legs her mother noticed that Janie felt warm and that her legs had several large bruises that she had not noticed previously. Janie's temperature was 101.8°F. After giving her some aspirin for the fever, Janie's mother called her pediatrician and made an appointment for the same day.

Dr. Richard entered the room, having been warned by his nurse that Janie looked quite ill. Instead of the bright active child who usually chattered incessantly, he saw a pale withdrawn little girl who had numerous bruises and scattered petechiae on her face. She had very prominent lymph nodes on physician examination; the doctor did not express his alarm when he easily palpated her spleen. He told her mother that a blood count was needed to search for a cause of Janie's illness. He ordered a CBC with differential and platelet count.

Later in the day Dr. Richard returned to the examining room. To Janie's mother, he looked more troubled than she could ever recall in numerous visits spanning seven years and three children. "Mrs. Fox," he began hesitantly, "I've examined the results of the blood test and am afraid that Janie is quite ill. I would like you to take her immediately to Children's Hospital to be seen by their specialists." An alarmed Mrs. Fox asked, "What's the matter?" Dr. Richard hesitated and then replied, "She is anemic and has an elevated white blood count. She may have a problem with her bone marrow. She should be evaluated by the experts in blood diseases."

The ride of one hour to the hospital seemed to last for an eternity. What concerned Mrs. Fox most was Dr. Richard's serious tone; she had conveyed this impression to her husband on the phone. Mr. Fox had been able to leave work and join his wife on this grim drive. "What is a disease of the blood?" he asked his wife. To himself he wondered if kids could get cancer, and if so, whether his daughter had it.

Dr. Richard had phoned ahead to the hematology clinic. His message to one of the hematologists read: "Noted pallor, fever, purpura, petechiae, splenomegaly and lymphadenopathy; CBC showed a hemoglobin of 4.8 gm/dl, WBC 27,500 with 85 per cent atypical-appearing lymphocytes. Please evaluate for possibility of leukemia."

Janie arrived at the hospital in the afternoon. Shortly after her arrival someone poked the tip of her finger and gave her a Band-Aid. The nurse who initially assessed Janie was pleasant and reassuring to Janie's parents. Shortly thereafter they looked up as a relatively young doctor entered. "Mr. and Mrs. Fox," he said, "I am Dr. Davids. I will be taking care of Janie. It appears that she is quite ill. Her blood count is abnormal. I am not certain what Dr. Richard might have told you, but from her blood count it appears that your daughter has leukemia. We will need to do some special tests to confirm the diagnosis and then begin to try to make her better immediately. We will talk to you again about what tests we will do and what they show."

Mrs. Fox heard but did not really absorb Dr. Davids' words about more blood tests and some test that involved taking blood from the hip. All she heard over and over in her mind was leukemia. Yesterday her daughter was a normal child who was playing with her little brother. Today she had cancer....

its emotional energies on the child with cancer. It is easy for the mother and the father to overlook the need for sharing their anxiety and comforting each other. As soon as the child's condition is stable, they will probably need to be told to get away from the hospital for a while just to be alone together. They may need reassurance from the nurse that she will take special care of their child in their absence. Likewise, it is easy for parents to forget about the needs of the siblings at home.

The brothers and sisters are most likely scared about what is happening at the hospital. As soon as is possible, the siblings must receive an age-appropriate explanation of the child's diagnosis. They need to be reassured about their own health. For a while the parents may not have much time to spend with the siblings, so it is particulary important for them to know and feel the love of their parents. A warm, comfortable home environment is crucial at this time when parents cannot be at home. If possible, a familiar relative or friend should be in the home with the siblings. They should be encouraged to visit their brother or sister in the hospital to allay their fears of the unknown about the child, his illness or the hospital. These children are often frightened and the parents should talk with them about their fears and the seriousness of the diagnosis.

The parents may wish to have the physician or nurse describe the illness for them to relatives and friends who are important to them. This may relieve some of the burden on the parents, who may also feel responsible for supporting the anxieties and reactions of these other people.

REACTION OF CHILD AND FAMILY TO TREATMENT

Treatment will begin almost immediately. To the child this comes to mean "pokes and pains." The child will soon learn to associate white coats with painful experiences. He may cry at the mere sight of someone in white. A consistently kind and pleasant attitude from doctors and nurses will lead the child to trust in special individuals who have been caring for him.

Most children's hospitals have rooming-in programs for parents, and parents are encouraged to participate in treatments, usually as hand-holders. To the preschooler all these treatments may represent permanent damage to his body's integrity. Procedures must be explained briefly before they are performed. Even though the child and family have been told about the procedure by their physician, the nurse should again give a brief explanation. This provides an opportunity for them to ask questions that they have thought about since the initial explanation.

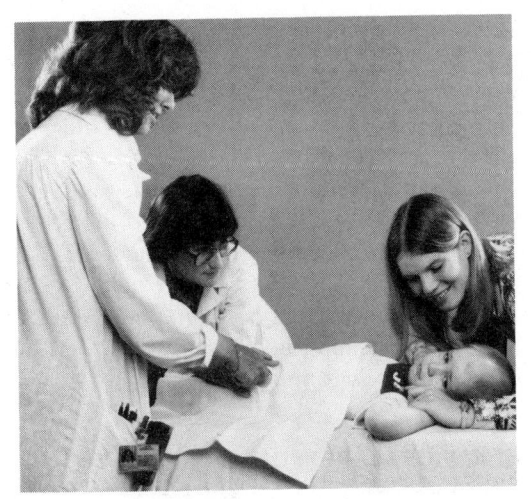

Preschoolers must feel comfortable and safe before a threatening procedure is done. A parent's presence during this bone marrow procedure helps the child endure it.

A preschooler must feel comfortable and safe before a threatening procedure is done. A parent's presence in the treatment room can provide that feeling of safety. A preschooler may squirm and fight a procedure even after an explanation of it has been given. Thus the kindest thing to do is to quietly and calmly speak to the child, handle him gently and get the procedure done quickly. The nurse can be particularly effective by talking to the child and offering encouragement to help him endure the procedure. While these painful procedures must be done as part of the treatment, perhaps some fun can be associated with the painful ordeal, such as picking a trinket from a toy box after each visit to the treatment room.

Some of the chemotherapy drugs are given in pill form. This may be the child's first experience with taking pills. Parents will need support and tips* from the nurse on getting the preschooler to swallow pills.

---

*A common method is to crush the pill and mix it with a nonessential food such as jelly, ice cream, or a sweet fruit syrup. Coating the pill with chocolate coating purchased at Dairy Queen may also help some children tolerate the taste of these drugs.

POTENTIAL STRESSES DURING THE PRESCHOOL YEARS: LIFE-THREATENING ALTERATIONS IN HEALTH STATUS

Preschoolers normally are "picky eaters," and the child at diagnosis often does not feel well enough to eat. Parents and grandparents may think that a child cannot get well unless he eats. They need to be reassured that the child will be able to tolerate not eating food for a while, and he should not be forced to eat.

The most bothersome drug side effect to parents may be hair loss. They must be reassured that most preschoolers are not ashamed of their hair loss and often cannot even be bothered to wear wigs and hats.

BEHAVIORAL RESPONSES OF THE PRESCHOOLER

When a child of any age becomes ill, regressive behavior is natural. The preschooler may now ask for his bottle or pacifier. He may want to be carried instead of walk. His vocabulary may revert to "baby talk." These behaviors may worry the parents. They fear that the child may never be "his old self" again. It is reassuring to tell parents that regression is natural and that it is asking a great deal of a 3-year-old to expect him to understand and accept this seemingly awful treatment and change of environment. The nurse must emphasize that the child's behavior will return to normal as his disease improves and as he develops trust in the situation. He needs consistency and guidance of his parents, who should not baby him but should treat him as a normal child his age.

It is natural to want to overprotect the child who is ill and may die. However, overprotection will lead only to regression and failure to grow emotionally. As soon as the family can settle down after the diagnosis of cancer is made, it is important for the nurse to help them provide for the normal growth and development needs of their preschooler. The child is just beginning to experience some independence away from his parents. He is eager to move, think and use his hands. Usually within the hospital setting there exists an opportunity to develop these skills via the hospital play program. The child should be allowed to re-enter socialization through play with peers. Also, the preschooler with cancer still needs consistency and limit-setting. It might be emotionally difficult to discipline the child with cancer, but the nurse should counsel the parents to help them understand the importance of continuing the childrearing practices that foster normal growth and development. The parents will need encouragement and assistance from the nurse to work through specific discipline issues.

HOME CARE

When the preschooler is well enough for discharge, the parents become the primary caregivers. The nurse plays a primary role in preparing parents for this responsibility from the first day of hospital admission. To care for their child at home, parents must understand the disease, its treatment and its possible complications. They must be comfortable and confident in their ability to care for their child. There is a great deal of new information for them to remember. The nurse can provide a written explanation of the disease as a ready reference for parents to use at home. Sometimes it is hard to give specific guidelines for home care, but general hints in writing are helpful. The nurse should help to design calendars of the treatment plan for parents to follow. They should have phone numbers for 24-hour medical assistance, and they should be encouraged to call if any specific questions arise. Most children with cancer will be receiving chemotherapy. The nurse should provide lists of these drugs in writing, with their possible side effects. Most chemotherapy drugs will cause low blood counts. Parents are helped to understand the different levels of blood counts so that when the child is home they can plan his activities according to any specific limitations dictated by these test results. Many parents like to keep diaries of what has been happening to the child between clinic visits. These help them to feel more comfortable as historians on the child's interim medical condition.

When the child is home, getting back into the normal family routine is very important. The child with cancer will need special medical treatment, hospitalization and frequent clinic visits, but this must not totally disrupt family life or fulfillment of the needs of each family member. Sibling rivalries can arise out of jealousy for the sick child's special treatment. Parents and friends must remember the needs of all children in the family. Each member needs special attention and loving from the others. It can be easy for the mother engrossed in caring for the child with cancer to forget this. The father may feel "left out" because he must be at work and cannot even be present at many clinic visits. The nurse should assess how the family is coping with these typical stresses and suggest that they make the clinic visits a family affair whenever possible.

Clinic visits need not mean only pain and treatment to the preschooler. The presence of a play therapist and toys in the clinic can add some fun to the day. Maybe a stop at the hamburger shop after each visit would be something to look forward to. The nurse can also suggest that the parents bring the child to visit the hospital or clinic sometimes just for fun, when no treatment must be given. With careful, thoughtful nursing interventions, the atmosphere may gradually be viewed as more comfortable and friendly.

Preschoolers like to pretend. A good way to get preschoolers to understand and accept treatments is with doctor or nurse play. Nurses can give the children some supplies from the clinic, and through play they will soon be acting out each bone marrow, spinal tap, and injection with their playmates, siblings, dolls and stuffed animals at home.

The preschooler with cancer will usually have no special restrictions on normal activity when he is at home. When blood counts warrant keeping a child in the house with quiet activity, the parents will be informed of these temporary restrictions. Depending on his diagnosis, the odds may be in the child's favor that he will live, so it is up to his parents to provide him with a normal, happy environment in which to grow.

THE NURSE'S ROLE IN SUPPORTING PARENTS

As time goes by the parents will become more relaxed, but they still will be aware each day that their child has cancer. Years ago if children had cancer, they would almost surely die. Now there is great variability in prognosis, depending on the diagnosis and stage of disease. Statistics can be offered parents, but they are difficult to apply to an individual child. The fact that much time has elapsed following the initial diagnosis does not mean that the child no longer has cancer nor that the parents can cease to be concerned about his dying of cancer. The nurse has a major responsibility to help parents through this difficult time; fears and feelings of anger and despair will need to be expressed. Parents need the opportunity to tell another caring person how it feels to be threatened by a loss of the joys that the child brings. The nurse can offer a tremendous support by being available when the family needs her for that purpose. She should also help the family to find additional resources. In many cities support groups have been formed of parents of children with cancer; these are excellent sources of information and emotional sharing. There are also national organizations for parents of children with cancer which the nurse should tell the family about.

Having a child with cancer can be a tremendous financial burden to the family. Even if the family has good medical insurance, there are still many nonmedical expenses such as transportation to the clinic, meals at the hospital, and babysitters for siblings while parents are tending to the child with cancer. Parents must be aware of all available resources in their area, such as state resources for aid to chronically ill children, the American Cancer Society and various leukemia foundations.

THE CHILD WHO DIES

Despite improving statistics for children with cancer, some children will die. When it becomes obvious that a preschooler has reached a terminal state, he will sense a change in the mood of his family. He will have many scary feelings about what is happening. He may have many questions. To a preschooler death is reversible, and he may have beautiful fantasies about what happens at death. The nurse should help parents to understand their preschooler's views of the situation. Parents should be encouraged to answer questions honestly. Preschoolers may not be able to put their feelings into words. Behavior and drawings often reveal feelings. The child needs to express his inner feelings in some way. He needs reassurance. He needs to know that his parents will always be there. Parents must know that all medical means will be used to prevent undue pain and suffering for their child.

Most parents will know when the child's fight for survival has become futile. They may never before have experienced the death of a loved one. They may have many questions in their minds about what the actual event of death is like. A staff member who is close to the family

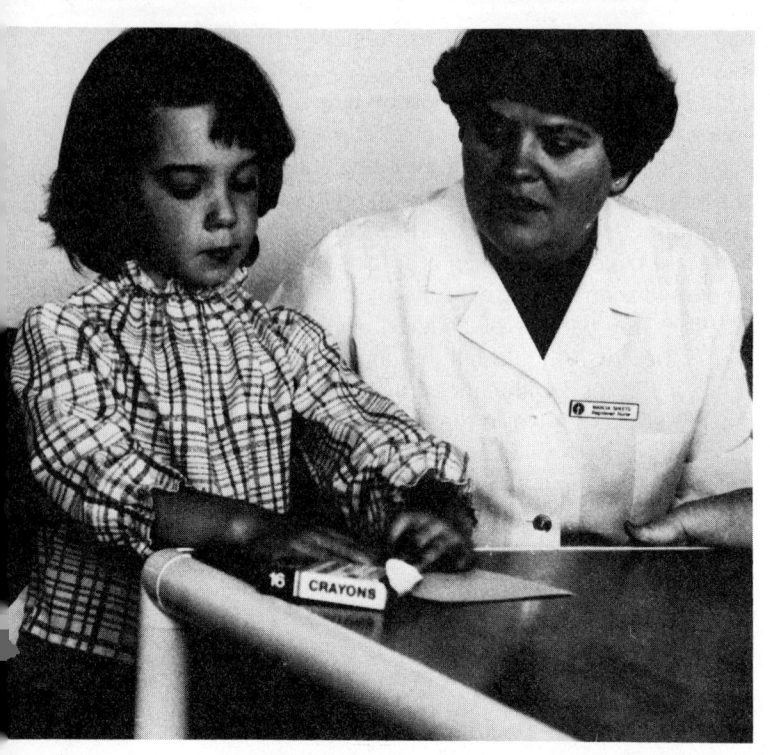

Drawings are often the best medium for the preschooler to describe her inner feelings about death and dying. (Photograph by Cynthia Stewart.)

should talk about these things with the parents. It is not morbid to talk about funeral arrangements before the child dies, so that at the time of death parents will be spared some of the agonizing chores. This concrete discussion of death will often initiate mourning, which may reduce despair at the time of death. Parents need one or two special staff members now to support them more than at any previous time.

There is an increasing trend for parents to want to have the child to die at home, where he is most comfortable. This possibility should be explored with parents. If they do wish the child to be at home, the nurse or other special staff member should prepare them for any emergency that may arise. They should have 24-hour support available to them by phone. They should be prepared for common preterminal events such as changes of consciousness, alteration of respirations, loss of bowel or bladder continence and emesis.

During this terminal stage the needs of other family members must not be forgotten. Siblings need every opportunity to release their emotions and express their fears. Contact with their dying brother or sister should be maintained as long as communication is possible to allay regrets about not having said last words or last goodbyes. A brother or sister may feel responsible for the sibling's death because of an old argument or fight. These concerns must be addressed even when they are not expressed openly by the siblings. The dying child will look and feel very sick, so the amount of time that the children spend with him is a personal decision for the parents to make. It is up to the professional team members to be aware of all these family needs and to help the parents to be aware of them.

It is emotionally very difficult for a nurse to face death in any patient. The death of a preschooler can be particularly hard for a nurse to understand and accept. She must be aware of her own ideas about life and death before she can relate to her patients and their families. Sometimes it is hard for the nurse to become involved with a child whom she knows will die. If the nurse can know that she helped a short life to be a more comfortable one, she will be rewarded inwardly and embraced outwardly for her care by the grateful parents of the child.

The family that has come to rely on the persons in the cancer center cannot be forgotten once the patient has died. A social worker or community health nurse can help families get through these difficult times. The child may be dead, but he will never be forgotten. He will be a part of his parents' and siblings' everyday life forever. Many parents realize the bond of friendship that has grown between them and the health team during the child's illness. As a sign of this friendship, parents should be urged to come back to see the team members at any time. It is rewarding to know that a large number of parents return to visit frequently, and some have been willing to talk with other parents and continue to be active in parent groups.

References

1. M. Donaldson and H. Seydel, eds. Trends in Childhood Cancer. John Wiley & Sons, 1976
2. A. Evans et al. Diagnosis and treatment of neuroblastoma. Pediatric Clinics of North America, October 1976, p. 161
3. A. Mauer et al. Current progress in the treatment of the child with cancer. Journal of Pediatrics, October 1977, p. 531
4. D. Miller. Prognostic factors in childhood leukemia. Journal of Pediatrics, October 1975, p. 672
5. W. Sutow et al., eds. Clinical Pediatric Oncology. C. V. Mosby Co., 1977

Additional Recommended Reading

L. Baker. You and Leukemia. W. B. Saunders Co., 1978

H. Bloom et al., eds. Cancer in Children: Clinical Management. Springer-Verlag, 1975

G. J. D'Angio et al. The treatment of Wilms' Tumor. Cancer, August 1976, p. 633

W. Easson. The family of the dying child. Pediatric Clinics of North America, November 1972, p. 1157

G. Foley and A. McCarthy. The child with leukemia: the disease and its treatment. American Journal of Nursing, July 1976, p. 1109

T. Greene, ed. Cancer in children. Nursing Clinics of North America, March 1976, p. 11

P. Groncy and J. Finkelstein. Neuroblastoma. Pediatric Annals, July 1978, p. 73

G. Hammond et al. The team approach to the management of pediatric cancer. Cancer, January 1978, p. 29

L. Helson. Neuroblastoma: early diagnosis, a key to successful treatment. Pediatric Annals, May 1974, p. 46

M. Pearse. The child with cancer: impact on the family. Journal of School Health, March 1977, p. 174

P. Pendergrass. What is Wilms' Tumor? A Parent's Guide, Division of Hematology/Oncology, The Children's Orthopedic Hospital and Medical Center, Seattle, 1977

D. Powers. Wilms' tumor, recent advances and unsolved problems. Pediatric Annals, May 1964, p. 55

S. Schiefelbein. Children and cancer, new hope for survival. Saturday Review, 14 April 1979. p. 11

J. Simone. Childhood leukemia: the changing prognosis. Hospital Practice, July 1974, p. 59.

45 THE HOSPITALIZED PRESCHOOLER

by Jo Joyce Tackett, BSN, MPHN

The preschool years are fairly stable for the child and thus for his family. He has mastered most body functions and self-care skills; he is increasingly sociable and cooperative with peers, siblings and adults; and he has mastered language enough to express most of his needs in nonstressful circumstances. The preschooler has come to recognize his own body as an intact whole with much potential, as well as with limits. He now spends his time initiating activities, mostly through play and incessant questions, that will satisfy his keen curiosity and prepare him for the larger world of school.

To understand the impact hospitalization has on the active, inquisitive preschooler, the nurse must know where the child is in his development and what developmental tasks he is presently attempting to accomplish. This knowledge guides her approach to the child and her identification of his age-specific needs during the hospital experience. A three-year study conducted by Johnston and her associates revealed that both young and older children and adolescents react to hospitalization according to (1) their perceptions of the experience, which are directly influenced by their developmental level, (2) their parents' understanding of the reason for the hospitalization as expressed in their behavior and in their explanations to the child, and (3) the preparation the child had for hospitalization and/or the number of previous hospitalizations the child has had and the memories and fear he retains from those previous experiences.[8] Nursing actions should be geared toward understanding the child's perceptions by observing his behaviors, especially during play, and noting his questions; misconceptions, common at the preschool age, should be confronted and corrected. The nurse should also learn the parents' perceptions of the hospitalization and take action to meet their needs so that they can be more relaxed and confident and more able to help the preschooler during the stressful hospital experience. This action is especially important when a preschooler or younger child is hospitalized because he relies more on his parents' attitudes and explanations than those of the nurse or other strangers providing care. Nursing action also should be taken to provide the child with adequate preadmission or readmission preparation whenever possible, to reduce his distorted memories or fears associated with the unknown or created by fantasy, which is at its height during preschool years.

IMPACT OF HOSPITALIZATION ON THE PRESCHOOLER'S NEEDS

Hospitalization, even when action is taken to prepare the child and support his development during the confinement, is highly likely to be anxiety-producing for the preschooler.[7, 9] The experience can hinder his initiative-seeking behaviors, threaten his newly established concept of an intact body that he controls, and jeopardize the progress he was making in separating from his parents without conflict.

Physically, the preschooler has successfully achieved control of most body functions, allowing him a fair amount of self-control in most activities of daily living. The stress of hospitalization usually leads to some degree of regression in this mastery as the preschooler attempts to cope.[13] This regression is frustrating and confusing to him. Having just mastered self-care, he finds it threatening to relinquish it. The preschooler greatly fears the loss of control over these daily routines. He needs help to regain self-control so that he does not experience shame and further regression (Table 45-1 contains nursing interventions specific to this age group). When he is not receiving adequate assistance, the preschooler lets the nurse and his parents know either by becoming inactive, uncooperative and withdrawn or by becoming hyperactive, overaggressive and displaying pseudo-independence. (In pseudo-independence, he refuses comforting or assistance and acts as though he does not care if the parent is there or not.[3,7]) Which way he responds is mostly determined by individual temperament and the type of responses he has learned to expect from caretakers through these behaviors. The withdrawal or aggression is usually expressed in relation to the very activities toward which he feels a loss of control (eating, elimination, sleeping).[8,13]

Intellectually the preschooler is still egocentric. Perhaps the greatest difficulty hospitalization creates for him lies in the guilt and shame he experiences that stem from his egocentric belief that being in the hospital is a punishment for something he did or thought.[1,2,7,9] His thinking is intuitive and magical, creating for him a rich fantasy life. During hospitalization, the distortion of perception that arises out of his egocentric and magical thoughts works against him. He constructs unfathomable fantasies and fears out of the strange hospital "Land of Oz." The preschooler has usually mastered basic language skills under normal circumstances but may still have difficulty verbalizing his needs and feelings during stress. With help, the preschooler can avoid or master unrealistic fears during hospitalizations and can progress in his ability to verbally communicate his needs effectively, even under stress (see Table 45-1).

Emotionally and socially the preschooler is taking initiative to gain some control over his environment and increase his independence. He needs limits set for him so that his active imagination and adventurousness do not harm him. He continues to rely on rituals and routines in the activities of daily living to preserve his sense of trust and security during this period in his development. Although he now separates from his parents more easily, with only initial conflict over the separation, he will still resist separation during illness and other periods of stress.[12] The preschooler is in an oedipal phase of development, during which he prefers the opposite-sex parent and will, toward the end of this stage, focus his flirtations on nonparent,

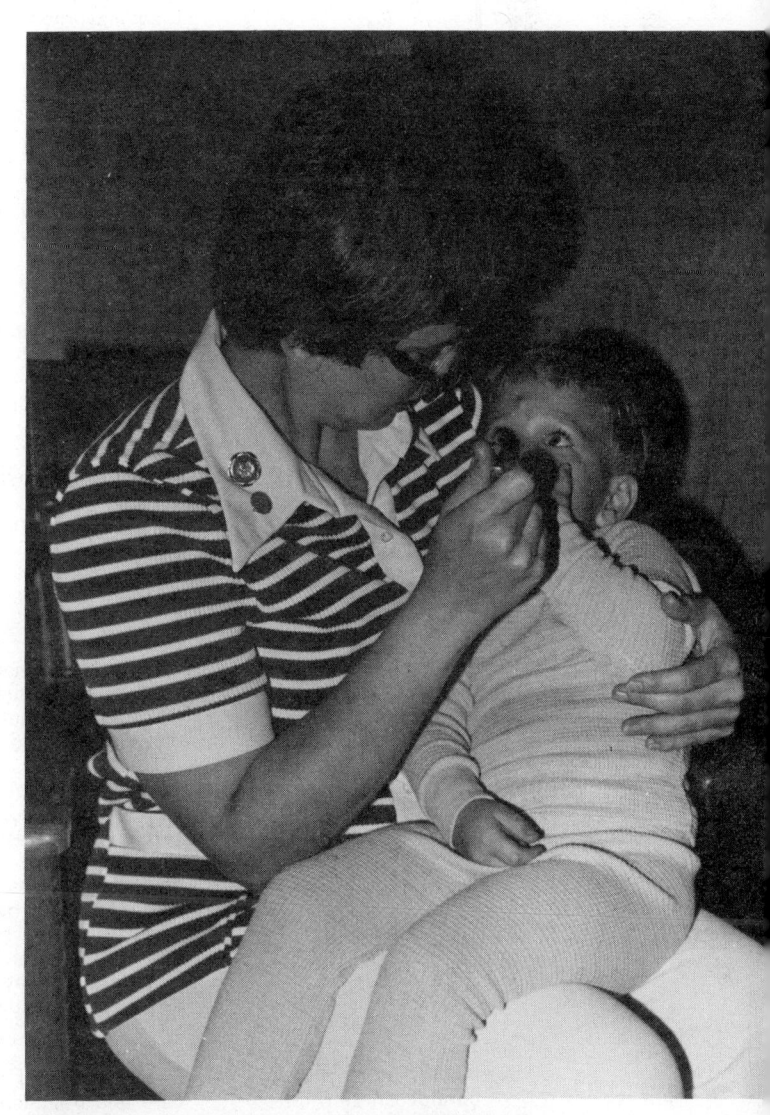

Withdrawal or aggression may be expressed by the hospitalized preschooler in relation to the activities toward which he feels a loss of control.

TABLE 45-1 PRESCHOOLER DEVELOPMENTAL NEEDS AND SUPPORTIVE NURSING INTERVENTIONS

Need	Nursing Intervention
I. *Physical* A. Maintain control of body functions.	1. Learn during admission interview the level of control child usually has at home and any patterns that exist for eating, elimination, sleep, and words used for each. 2. Develop care plan to allow for these patterns as much as possible. 3. Reassure when accidents in elimination occur; do not reprimand or punish. 4. Praise successes in self-control. 5. Provide age-appropriate motor stimulation.
B. Continue development of self-care in activities of daily living.	1. Learn during admission interview the self-care tasks child performs at home 2. Develop care plan to allow for continued self-care when possible; provide some opportunities for decisions on care, especially in aspects of care in which child's condition or treatment prohibits self-care. 3. Allow for usual eating practices: provide foods child is used to, finger foods, favorite foods and eating utensils from home; allow family members to eat with child if isolated or to feed if child must be fed; allow eating at child-sized table with hospitalized peers if not isolated; follow child's usual rituals, such as prayer before eating. 4. Allow for usual elimination practices: provide potty chair (from home if preferred) or regular toilet as child is accustomed to; if mobility is restricted, offer to assist child to toilet or bedpan at usual eliminating times. Keep call bell near so child may get *prompt* assistance at other times. (Preschoolers still have difficulty "holding off" eliminatory processes.) Stay with child or provide privacy as child is accustomed. 5. Allow for usual rest and sleep practices: allow night light if child is used to one or requests one; provide quiet, uninterrupted period during child's usual nap or rest time if nap still taken; allow usual sleep time attire to be worn; if not contraindicated, allow usual sleep position and amount of cover and pillows used at home; bring any special sleep items (blanket, pacifier, toy) from home. 6. Permit child to dress at least partially in own clothing during daytime.
II. *Intellectual* A. Egocentric thinking: protect from sense of guilt.	1. Reassure repeatedly that no one is to blame for his condition or hospitalization. 2. Reassure that only necessary treatments will be done and they will not be done without telling him first. 3. Provide activities (play, arts and crafts, stories) that stimulate intellectual development.
B. Preoperational cognition yields intuitive, magical thoughts: protect from fears created by active imagination.	1. Explain all procedures, especially describing what he can expect to experience through his senses, before doing them. 2. Provide for dramatic and therapeutic play; make available safe procedural equipment and dolls during education sessions, in play room, at bedside. 3. Do not talk about the child in front of him unless he is included in the conversation.
C. Developing expressive language.	1. Encourage his questions and ask questions to learn his fears, fantasies and misperceptions (correct these when possible) as well as giving him experience expressing himself verbally during stress. 2. Encourage child to tell stories about his drawings or to tell you a "story" about procedures or other experiences he has in the hospital. These also reveal fears and fantasies as well as helping him master self-expression. 3. Teach him new words related to simple anatomy and physiology, his disease or treatment, and hospital equipment and personnel. This helps him learn to relate intelligently in health consumer–provider interactions as well as expanding his vocabulary.
III. *Emotional-Social* A. Initiative to master control of his environment, develop independence.	1. Encourage child to participate in self-care and hygiene and in medical care and treatments. (The preschooler is able to be cooperative if given adequate instruction and permission to participate.) 2. Meticulously observe safety precautions. 3. Promptly take action to remove offensive smells and preserve orderliness. The preschooler, as a result of having mastered toilet functions, is keenly aware of smells and disorder and is upset by them. 4. Permit and encourage child's own decision-making regarding care and treatments when actual choices do exist.

Table continued on opposite page

TABLE 45–1 PRESCHOOLER DEVELOPMENTAL NEEDS AND SUPPORTIVE NURSING INTERVENTIONS *(Continued)*

Need	Nursing Intervention
	5. Praise any evidences of competence in all areas of development (self-care, learning new words, helping with a treatment, cooperation during stressful procedures). 6. Solicit and respect child's suggestions regarding care, room environment changes, toys in room, etc.
B. Limit setting.	1. Enforce safety rules; give simple explanations for rules (child must be in crib or bed with rails up even if he is used to big bed without rails at home). 2. Clearly and appropriately define his limits on activity due to illness (isolation from other children while disease is communicable). Since child's concept of time is undeveloped, give him some idea of how long the limitation will be by associating it with concrete things he is familiar with ("You can go to the playroom Saturday. That is the day that cartoons are on TV all morning." or "You can drink water and other drinks again when *Nurse's name* comes to care for you this afternoon"). 3. Learn during admission interview if there are any home rules parents want continued during hospitalization (only certain TV shows may be watched or TV is allowed only so many hours a day, teeth are to be brushed after each meal, limited beverages are allowed after suppertime) and enforce those not in conflict with treatment regimen. Explain to parents reasons that any cannot be enforced.
C. Rituals offer security.	1. Find out child's usual routines and rituals during admission interview, carry these out by integrating them into the care plan as much as possible. 2. Encourage parents or other family members acquainted with the rituals to be present and help child carry out mealtime, bedtime, other significant rituals. 3. Ask parents to bring from home those objects related to child's rituals or other security items or both.
D. Learning to separate without conflict.	1. Provide for a primary nurse for each shift. 2. Permit and encourage unlimited parental visits and participation in planning and giving care. 3. Allow parents to remain and comfort child, if desired during treatments or procedures parents cannot or do not wish to do; primary nurse present as parent surrogate during parental absences to stay with and comfort child. In addition to the emotional comfort parents provide, research shows their presence contributes to earlier recovery and fewer complications.[8] 4. Let parents do as many of the "caretaking" tasks as possible. 5. Ask parents to bring in familiar toys, family photos, personal belongings that can be left with child as reminders of them during their absence. 6. During care make up pleasant stories about home activities including names of family members in the stories or encourage child to tell stories about home and family activities. 7. Provide opportunities for child to become acquainted with other children and parents who may "fill in" as sources of comfort during parental and sibling separations. 8. Help parents identify ways to keep child in contact with siblings or peers who cannot visit (phone calls, tape recordings, notes, pictures).
E. Resolve oedipal conflict; minimize associated intrusive, mutilative and pain fears.	1. Give thorough explanations and continued reassurance about what will happen to the child's body as a result of a treatment or procedure; it is especially important to reassure of continued presence and intactness of genitals when these body parts are involved. 2. Handle genitalia as little as possible and use gentleness when handling is necessary. Some children respond better if their hand is used with the nurse's in handling the genitalia. 3. Avoid use of intrusive procedures or treatments whenever possible (preschooler copes with axillary or oral thermometer better than rectal). 4. Observe for silent attachment (oedipal attachment) to staff member(s) as evidenced by flirtations, admiring expressions, preferences for that individual(s), coyness. Ensure that the child receives warm, positive responses from favored adult(s) that help resolve oedipal feelings through healthy identification and nurturance of self-confidence. 5. Help parents understand ambivalence regarding each parent that is part of oedipal struggle as expressed by variations in response to them (love and hate, compliance and defiance, clinging and independent rejection). These responses fluctuate more during hospitalization when the child suspects parental punishment, too.

opposite-sex adults whom he admires and who treat him warmly. Exhibitionism and genital inquisitiveness is associated with the oedipal phase, accompanied by some sexual fantasies and fears that arise from the preschooler's great imagination. Very little stimulus is generally required from the child's environment to set off his imagination.

Hospitalization tends to pose the greatest threat to the preschooler's emotional and social development.[1, 7] He feels a demise of the control he had been gaining over his environment. Particularly if he is immobilized or isolated, he may lose the initiative to try to satisfy his curiosities. Unless nursing personnel carefully plan for preservation of the routines and rituals that the child is accustomed to at home, he is left without the security they afford him. His hospitalization is stressful, so separation from the family becomes a source of emotional turmoil, especially if he has experienced few or no separations lasting for many hours or overnight in the past. He tends to perceive the separations as punishment by his parents and fears abandonment. His oedipal crisis causes him to fear body mutilation, pain and invasion of body orifices; this is possibly the preschooler's greatest fear during hospitalization.[7, 9, 11] Appropriate parental and nursing interventions can eliminate many potential emotional and social anxieties of the hospitalized preschooler through adequate communication and careful planning to preserve familiar routines (see Table 45–1). Also, parents can bring to the hospital objects with which the child is familiar.

NURSING ACTIONS TO MINIMIZE DEVELOPMENTAL TRAUMA DURING HOSPITALIZATION

The nurse needs to give continuous attention to all aspects of the preschooler's development — physical, intellectual and emotional and social — but the emphasis will vary with the phase of hospitalization. Hospitalization can be divided into four phases: preadmission, admission, treatment phase and discharge.

Preadmission or Pre-readmission Phase

Ideally the preschooler should have an opportunity to learn about and see inside the hospital while he is well or at least before he is admitted. Hospitals in many communities have organized programs and tours designed to orient children to the hospital and its environment. Many well-written books and good records are available that parents, nursery school teachers and office or clinic nurses might use. With these, the preschooler may be exposed to common hospital sites and to routines, personnel and procedures (see the bibliography at the end of the section on hospitalization in Chapter 16). Some good film strips about the hospital experience are available from local libraries or the Association for the Care of Children in Hospitals.* Some hospitals have also organized pre-readmission programs to help the child being rehospitalized to overcome any distorted memories or fantasies left over from previous hospitalization.

The preschooler may enjoy meeting the nurses he will see or who will care for him in the hospital sometime during a tour or preadmission visit to the pediatric unit. He may also be receptive to having some time to play in the hospital play area during this visit. These experiences allow him to become familiar with the

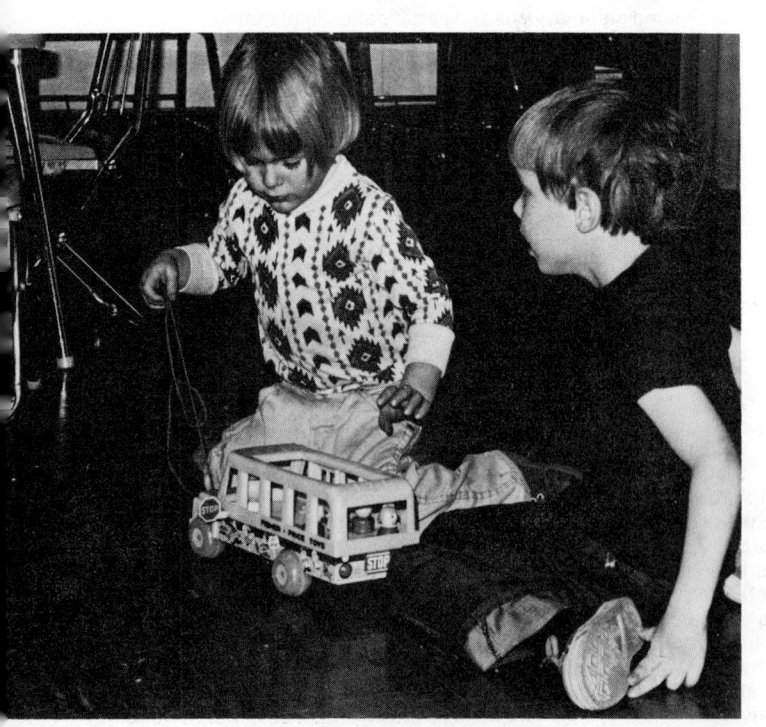

The preschooler enjoys having some time to play in the hospital play area during his preadmission tour and visit.

*ACCH has headquarters at 3615 Wisconsin Ave., Washington, DC 20016.

setting during a period when he is not under the stress of being admitted. Some hospitals also arrange for the primary nurse assigned to a child who is scheduled for admission to make a home visit before the admission. During this visit the nurse can answer the child's questions and those of his parents, as well as use books or other visual aids to expose the child to hospital routines.[5]

Admission Phase

If there is no preadmission history available at admission, a history or interview should be done during admission to learn the child's usual level of functioning in terms of body control and self-care, his usual routines, and the rituals that are associated with activities of daily living at home. Particular attention should be given to the child's eating patterns and food preferences, toilet habits and words used to described elimination, and usual rest and exercise patterns. The child's reactions to toilet accidents should be documented, and how these are viewed and handled by the parents at home. Security items and items associated with rituals should be identified by the parents.[7]

If he is able, the preschooler should be allowed and encouraged to participate in the interview as a beginning toward participation in his treatment. Such participation gives him some sense of control and independence that is so important to him developmentally. He should be given a tour of the unit if he has not had a preadmission tour. After he has been

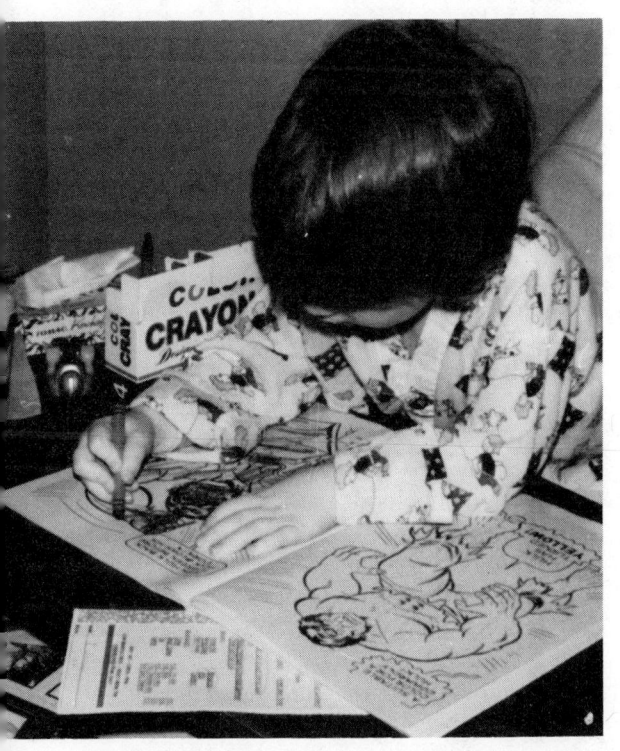

Once the preschooler has "settled in" on admission he may find release from anxiety in play in his room or in the pediatric unit play area. (Photograph by David Trainor.)

A MODEL PRE-READMISSION HOSPITAL PROGRAM

Johnston and Salazar[8] described a pre-readmission program for children of various ages in a California hospital in which research on the program was collected. This research supports the program as a model that other hospitals can use to develop similar programs.

As part of the hospital program, the child and family are assigned a volunteer ombudsman who accompanies them through the diagnostic departments during the diagnostic clinic visit that precedes hospital admission, explaining procedures as they are done. The family then participates in a group session (usually composed of several families together) to express their concerns and ask questions to which they are given concrete, honest answers. They also watch an 18-minute videotape that is designed to produce feelings and awaken memories of previous hospital experiences. The nurse watches the reactions of various family members during the videotape; immediately following viewing, they discuss the adaptations in routine hospital encounters that can be made to meet the needs of the particular child and family. During this discussion information is exchanged regarding separation, the roles of parents and siblings in the hospital environment, home care and other relevant topics. The nurse who viewed the tape with the families and led the group discussion is responsible for seeing that the staff of the pediatric unit is informed of the adaptive changes before the child is admitted so that the changes can be incorporated immediately into the child's care plan.

Following the group session the child is examined by the doctor or nurse practitioner and a history is collected. The child returns in three days for hospital admission. Research in this setting has proved that this pre-readmission process takes an average of 1½ hours as compared to 3 or 4 hours when families are left on their own.

introduced to his roommate and primary nurse, the preschooler enjoys helping arrange his bedside space with his mementos from home as a part of "settling in." If the preschooler is well enough, he may also find release from anxiety through play in his room or the unit play area. By allowing the child these considerations, the nurse can significantly facilitate his beginning adaptation to the strange hospital environment. If possible, admission diagnostic procedures should be done on an outpatient basis before the day of admission or if that is not possible, the procedures are ideally postponed until several hours or a day after admission.[7,8]

Treatment Phase

Although the child continues adapting to the hospital environment, which was his main task during the admission phase, his major task during the treatment phase is to cope with the treatment procedures and unfamiliar individuals and equipment that are required to manage his illness. Two activities toward which the nurse and parents contribute are most relevant to the preschooler's success in coping with this phase of hospitalization.[1,9] They are (1) educating the child about what to expect during the procedures and about the people and equipment involved and (2) providing materials and opportunities for dramatic and therapeutic play so that the child can work through his fears and fantasies.

Education The preschooler needs teaching about his disease, including simple anatomy and physiology, and about the procedures and treatments used to diagnose or correct it. Also, any misconceptions that occur during the hospital experience should be clarified.

The preschooler responds best when the information he needs during his hospital encounter is given by his primary nurses.[7] After discussing with the physician the medical information he wants shared with the child and family,* the nurse should question the parents on what their understanding is of the disease, procedure or other subject being taught and inquire what they have explained to the child and how the explanation was given. The nurse can clarify any misunderstandings the parents have and provide additional information as needed. This knowledge guides the nurse's decisions about where to begin with the child. Studies show that if parents are cooperative and supportive, the preschooler benefits from their presence during teaching sessions.[7,9] They can be encouraged to participate in providing explanations because they usually know best the words their child is used to and at what level he comprehends.

Neutral words should be used in explanations to avoid stimulating the child's imagination or producing mutilation fears. For example, in describing a surgery the nurse should say "make an opening" instead of "cut" and "the bandage may look pinkish and wet" rather than "there may be blood on the bandage." The preschooler is very interested in what his body looks like and what the names are for various parts. He is able to comprehend simple anatomy and physiology if visual aids such as body outlines, pictures or organ models are used. Body outlines are particularly appealing to the preschooler because he is familiar with the

Body outlines as teaching aids are particularly appealing to the preschooler and provide insight for the nurse into the child's understanding of his body and disease process.

---

*Some hospitals have teaching protocols for various diseases and procedures that have been jointly approved by nursing service, medical staff and hospital administration.

concept of the flat body from his storybooks and his own crude "people" drawings. The material to be taught should be covered in two or three sessions to avoid overwhelming him with information. The preschooler's attention span is usually only 20 to 30 minutes and he loses interest in a topic if it is dealt with too many times.

Before starting a session the nurse should find out what the child already knows and understands about the topic(s) to be discussed. Beginning with questions such as "How did you know you had to come to the hospital?" or "What did your parents tell you about (topic)?" reveals the child's knowledge base, his fantasies that may need correcting, the areas in which he needs reassurance, and information that should be emphasized. Denial of knowledge should not be taken at face value in the preschooler. He may deny knowledge because he thinks the disease will go away or the procedure will not take place if he denies its existence or knowing anything about it.

A story approach might be used with the denying child to obtain his contributions and questions. An example might be a story about a child in the hospital who knows he is sick or that a procedure is to be done but is afraid to ask questions because he wishes it would go away or would not happen and how much better he feels when he finally asks questions. Sometimes just saying "If I were you I'd sure want to know all about (topic)," stimulates the child to talk.

Questions should be answered honestly and briefly. (The nurse must learn to hear the preschooler's actual question and answer it only; he does not want an elaborate speech.) Repetition of information may be necessary before the preschooler fully understands explanations. His lack of understanding is communicated verbally through questions and nonverbally through uncooperativeness and defiance.

When teaching is done about a procedure, the timing of the instruction is important. The child should have adequate time to work through the explanations but not enough time to let his imagination get carried away with fantasies. If the preschooler is verbal and appears to be adapting adequately to his environment, explanations can be given the day before a procedure is to take place. The early preschooler who is not as adept at verbalizing his feelings and questions and any preschooler who is having trouble adjusting to hospitalization should be given an explanation shortly before

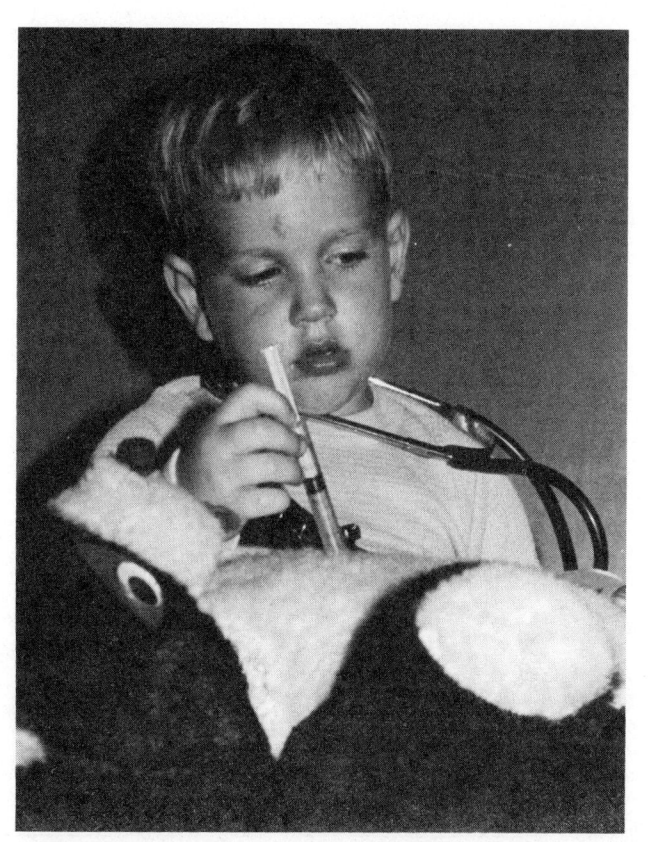

The preschooler needs some time for therapeutic play with equipment and dolls before and after a procedure.

the procedure. The child is given permission to object to the procedure (it is ok to cry or yell) but is also given an understanding that he has no choice as to whether the procedure will be done or not. The use of body outlines, dolls and other visual aids facilitates the child's comprehension of explanations and encourages his questions. Preferably, time is allowed for some therapeutic play with the equipment and a doll or the nurse both before and after the procedure.

Two procedures that almost every hospitalized preschooler is confronted with are taking medications orally and receiving injections. If consideration is not given to the preschooler's developmental level, these procedures can be traumatic or, at the very least, a source of battles of the will. The accompanying illustration provides guidelines useful in preventing defiant behavior during medication administration to the preschooler. Injections are a source of fear to the preschooler because of the pain and intrusion of his body that he anticipates. Needle

PEDIATRIC MEDICATION GUIDELINES—3½ TO 6 YEARS

	Developmental Tasks and Behaviors	Nursing Implicatons
MOTOR	• Develops proficiency of coordination. Can identify the parts of a complete movement or task.	• Child can attempt and master pill taking.
FEEDING	• Exhibits olfactory, gustatory, and kinesthetic refinement.	• Disguising tastes is generally less effective than it is at younger ages. Child can distinguish medicine tastes and smells.
	• Begins to lose temporary teeth (5 yrs.).	• Loose teeth may need to be considered when selecting form of medication.
INTERACTIVE	Initiative versus Guilt • Makes decisions.	• Child should be active in making decisions which affect him.
	• Sense of time allows enjoyment of delayed gratification. • Is able to tolerate frustration. • Seeks companionship. • Shows pride in accomplishments.	• Rewards which are not immediately received and social interaction can be used as effective motivators. Child is able to understand the purpose of medications in simple terms.
	• Has ability to follow directions and remember several instructions for a period of minutes to hours.	• Teaching can have long-term benefits.
	• Exhibits developing conscience. Needs limits set to help control his frightening sense of "power."	• Prolonged reasoning or arguing may frighten the child; a simple command by a trusted adult may be more effective.
	• Exhibits genital interest, general mutilation fears.	• Explain the relationship between cause, illness, and treatment. Use simple terms.
	• Illness often seen as punishment.	• Give control when possible—child needs to make choices.
	• Shows changeable response to parents.	• Child may be more cooperative in medicine taking for the nurse than for the parent.

EXAMPLE: Orlando, a 4-year-old with repeated pneumonia secondary to cystic fibrosis, has been treated repeatedly with ampicillin. The nurse remembers that previously the suspension form was used with no resistance. But with this admission Orlando has been refusing the familiar suspension.

After watching him swallow whole jelly beans during an afternoon playtime, the evening nurse tries giving him ampicillin capsules at bedtime. She explains the pills are medicine like the pink liquid but that the shells they have stop the medicine from tasting so bad. She points out that they are the same size as the jelly beans he took while playing. Other things she tells him include how he can place the capsules far back in his mouth and swallow water to help "wash" the pills down to his stomach. By bedtime the next day, medication refusal is no longer a nursing problem.

Medication guide. Reprinted by permission, Ormond and Caulfield. American Journal Maternal Child Nursing, Sept/Oct 1976, p. 325.

---

play can help him work out some of this fear. In addition, the needle and syringe should not be flaunted or referred to in front of the preschooler nor hidden when the nurse comes to give the injection.[2]

Once the preschooler knows he is to receive an injection, it should be given promptly. The preschooler is usually more receptive when the injection is given by a nurse with whom he is familiar and who has spent time with him when procedures were not involved. Although this age child can often cooperate to lie still during the injection if his fears have not been given time to escalate, it is safer to have a second adult nearby to help restrain the child if necessary. Holding the child's arms in a restraining position in case it is needed, the second adult can preserve the child's sense of self-control by simply saying "Let me help you hold still." Putting a decorated Band-Aid over the site is comforting to the preschooler and helps reassure him that his body is still intact (now all his blood cannot get out).

The vastus lateralis and ventrogluteal muscles are equally acceptable sites for intramuscular injection in the preschooler, as is the posterior gluteal muscle if the child is well developed.[2] Some preschoolers rebel against use of the vastus lateralis; in this case the other two sites should be given preference. (Appendix VI describes the proper techniques for administering these injections.) Especially when the posterior gluteal muscle site is used with the preschooler, reassurance should be given that the shot is not a punishment, as children this age usually associate any assault to their "bottom" as punishment. A simple explanation of what the shot will do (make you stop hurting) usually is adequate to dispel the child's feelings of being punished. The most important point for the nurse to remember is that injections are more stressful to the preschooler (due to mutilation fears, concern about body intactness, punishment perception) than to children in any other age group. Therefore, prompt administration and immediate postinjection support is mandatory. Provision of a toy or involvement in an activity that permits release of frustration and aggression after the shot is also therapeutic.[2]

Play Play is the major activity of the waking hours in a preschooler's life. It is a natural avenue for self-expression, the medium through which he masters his developmental tasks, and the major resource for learning about his world. It is only logical, then, that play is therapeutic in relieving his stress during hospitalization. Play for the hospitalized preschooler not only promotes his development, it also provides an important outlet for aggressive or hostile feelings, allowing him to work through his fears and fantasies that are multiplied during hospital experiences. It also helps him master reality.

Unlike other forms of play, therapeutic or dramatic play is not intended to be diversional or recreational. Its purpose is to allow the child to overcome his anxieties, at least to the degree that he can cope with the events in his environment. During nondirective therapeutic play, the preschooler is in control, subjecting others (a doll, stuffed animal, parent or nurse volunteer) to the very event he fears as he experiments with various ways of reacting to it. In the process he acquaints himself with the tools (the toys in this form of play), procedures, and the roles of patient and "procedure-doer" that he believes to be part of the event creating stress. During therapeutic play, the nurse has an opportunity to gain insights into the child's perceptions, feelings and needs related to the event(s) the child is enacting.

Other forms of play may also be used to gain insight into the preschooler's perspective while emotional release is provided to the child. Role-playing (the child becomes nurse or doctor and the nurse, parent, volunteer or doll becomes the patient) is one such form. Role-playing is an effective means of gaining the preschooler's cooperation.[1,4]

Puppet play is a universal way to communi-

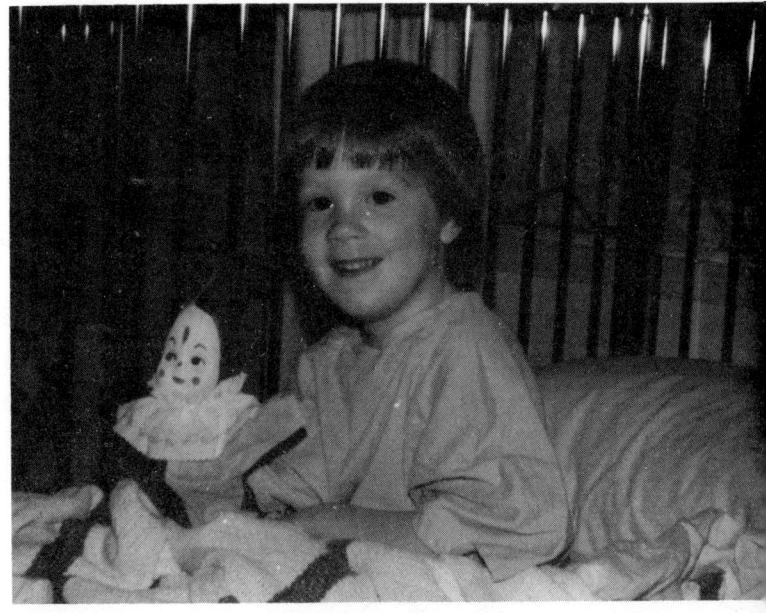

Puppet play is a universal way to communicate with and gain insight about the preschooler. (Photograph by David Trainor.)

cate with and gain insights about preschoolers. Puppets are usually successful in drawing out even the most slow-to-warm child at this age. Puppets may be dressed to represent hospital personnel, parents and siblings, animals or popular TV characters. The puppet seems to free the preschooler to express ideas, feelings and fears he would not share in direct conversation.

The preschooler also finds release in creative play materials (fingerpaints, water, crayons) and "aggression toys" (bean bags, pounding boards, balls, clay). Items for therapeutic, puppet, creative and aggressive play should be available to the hospitalized preschooler in a play area and in his room. Free access to these items allows the child to select the means of release he prefers at whatever time he prefers. (See Chapter 12 for further discussion of play and play theory).

Discharge Phase

The main objective during this phase is to identify any misconceptions the child has about his hospital experiences and correct them. The child should be encouraged to talk (a puppet is often helpful in initiating conversation) about various experiences he has had while hospitalized so that memory distortions can be identified.[2] If photographs have been taken during the hospitalization they will provide the child with reminders of the actual experience, thereby helping him to recall it realistically and to distinguish between what he imagined and what really happened. The preschooler should also be allowed to take safe, disposable equipment home with him so he can continue to work through his feelings in therapeutic play.[1]

The nurse should encourage parents to keep the hospitalization experience open to discussion with their preschooler so that he has opportunities to reaffirm what really happened. Parents should also be informed that the preschooler needs continued reassurances that he was not responsible for the illness or hospitalization for weeks or months after these events are over. The preschooler and his family should be invited to return for visits to the unit after discharge. Such visits help correct memory distortions and decrease anxiety in the event the child needs future hospitalization.

NEEDS OF THE PRESCHOOLER'S FAMILY

The preschooler's stress at being hospitalized is often accentuated to the extent that anxiety is exhibited by his parents. Therefore, incorporating the parents' needs into the child's plan of care is functional in aiding the child's own adjustment to hospitalization. Chapter 16 discusses the general impact hospitalization has on parents and siblings when a family member is hospitalized.

The preschooler's parents also have some unique needs. The biggest problem of hospitalized preschoolers' parents is the tendency to forget how independent their preschooler has become and to treat him in ways he perceives as "babyish" or demeaning to his independent self-concept. Such parental behavior encourages and reinforces regressive behavior in the ill preschooler.[9] Frustrated by his regression, the preschooler then becomes noncompliant and ambivalent toward the parents, reinforcing their sense of guilt and helplessness. Without intervention, an unhealthy cycle is put into action.

The nurse, through anticipatory guidance regarding the behaviors and needs of hospitalized preschoolers and through role modelling, can help parents preserve their preschooler's independence during his hospitalization. Involving parents actively in planning care communicates that they are important to their preschooler and that they know him best.[6] They can be helped to feel capable and useful by participating in the supervising of their child's self-care and assisting in or doing those tasks the child is unable to handle himself. The most valuable contribution parents probably make to their preschooler's hospital adjustment is their participation in the child's preparation for procedures. To children at the preschool age, parents are still essential interpreters and translators of the language of the outside world; therefore their involvement in their child's education is just as important as their presence and their ability to provide comfort during hospitalization encounters.

Working together from a developmental perspective, parents, primary nurse and the child himself can prevent or minimize many of the potential fears and fantasies to which he is vulnerable during hospitalization.

References

1. A. Azarnoff. Mediating the trauma of serious illness and hospitalization in childhood. Children Today, Jul/Aug 1974, p. 12
2. P. Brandt et al. Injections in children. American Journal of Nursing, August 1972, p. 1402
3. J. Calkin. Assessing small children: are hospitalized toddlers adapting to the experience as well as we think? American Journal Maternal Child Nursing, Jan/Feb 1979, p. 18
4. J. Conlin. Role playing with Paddy. Nursing '80, May 1980, p. 136
5. C. Crawford and M. Palm. Can I take my teddy bear? American Journal of Nursing, February 1973, p. 286
6. K. Frieberg. How parents react when their child is hospitalized. American Journal of Nursing, July 1972, p. 1270
7. A. Galligan. Using Roy's concept of adaptation to care for young children. American Journal Maternal Child Nursing, Jan/Feb 1979, p. 24
8. M. Johnston and M. Salazar. Preadmission program for rehospitalized children. American Journal of Nursing, August 1979, p. 1420
9. E. Oremland et al. The Effects of Hospitalization on Children. Charles C Thomas, 1973
10. E. Ormond and C. Caulfield. A practical guide to giving oral medications to young children. American Journal Maternal Child Nursing, Sept/Oct 1976, p. 320
11. M. Petrillo and S. Sanger. Emotional Care of Hospitalized Children. J. B. Lippincott Co., 1980
12. M. Smart and R. Smart. Preschool children: Development and Relationships, 2nd ed. Macmillan Inc., 1978
13. K. Tekely et al. Regressive behavior in a hospitalized preschool child. Maternal Child Nursing Journal, Fall 1978, p. 185

Additional Recommended Reading

P. Cormier. Indentification of typologies derived from children's behaviors in the hospital as predictors of psychiatric upset. Journal of Psychiatric Nursing, June 1979, p. 28

F. Erickson. Play Interviews For Your Year-Old Hospitalized Children. Child Development Publ., 1978

J. Haliburton. Valuable helps for frightened children. Dimensions in Health Services, May 1979, p. 39

C. Hardgrove and A. Rulledge. Parenting during hospitalization. American Journal of Nursing, May 1975, p. 836

N. Kerr. The effect of hospitalization on developmental tasks of childhood. Nursing Forum, No. 2 1979, p. 108

P. Patterson. Chospitology — the art and science of rendering hospitalization as benign an experience as possible for a child. Dimensions in Health Services, May 1979, p. 12

S. Port. Trends in pediatric hospitals. Dimensions in Health Services, May 1979, p. 51

C. Smitherman. Parents of hospitalized children have needs, too. American Journal of Nursing, August 1979, p. 1423

B. Snell and C. Mclellan. Whetting hospitalized preschoolers' appetites. American Journal of Nursing, March 1976, p. 412

G. Terry. A 5 year old boy's aggressive and compensatory behavior in response to immobilization. Maternal Child Nursing Journal, Spring 1979, p. 29

NURSING CARE PLAN FOR THE PRESCHOOLER WITH A URINARY ALTERATION
by Margaret Alderman

Nursing Diagnosis (Problem)	Expected Outcome	Nursing Interventions	Rationale
Alteration in excretory or regulatory function Decreased or absent urine output due to: • altered urine production • dehydration • obstruction • retention • decreased renal blood flow or Increased urine output due to: • altered urine production • fluid overload • metabolic disorders	The child's fluid balance will be maintained.	Dx: 1. Strictly measured intake and output. 2. Daily weighings. 3. Observe for pain or discomfort on urination. Pain is manifested in the preschooler by irritability, facial expression, muscular tenseness and restlessness or change in vital signs. 4. Palpate bladder every 3–4 hours. 5. Record vital signs and blood pressure.	Dx: 1. Measurements of intake and output show the balance between the amount of fluid presented to the body and its ability to process it. Potential fluid overload or dehydration can be identified. 2. Daily weighings reveal sudden fluid shifts (gain or loss) that reflect the ability of the kidney to excrete fluid. 3. Pain on urination may be due to infection, stones, bleeding, tumors or bladder spasms. The preschooler is not able to specifically localize pain. His concept of pain is so vague that he may not be able to state his need for pain relief. Nor is he able to understand that a painful procedure (shot) will alleviate pain, so he is medicated as indicated rather than offered the choice of receiving a pain "shot." 4. Palpating bladder helps the nurse intervene before serious bladder distention can cause kidney damage. 5. Vital signs and blood pressure indicate the body's ability to perfuse the kidney.

		6. Record specific gravity, pH, blood, ketones, sugar on each void.	6. Specific gravity, pH, blood, ketones and sugar indicate the kidney's ability to concentrate fluid, filter substances.
		7. Check the patient for hydration status.	7. Decreased urine output may be related to dehydration. Increased output may be related to fluid overload.
		Rx:	Rx:
		1. Force or restrict fluids as ordered.	1. Depending on cause of decreased output, fluids may need to be increased (dehydration, inadequate blood flow) to present more fluid to kidney or may need to be restricted to prevent overload that kidney cannot handle.
	The child will not experience urinary obstruction or retention.	2. Empty bladder completely and regularly by natural or artificial means as ordered.	2. Complete bladder emptying prevents reflux, infection and discomfort. Preschoolers who have only recently gained urinary continence feel pride in maintaining control. With increased urinary output it may be more difficult to do this without assistance.
		3. Administer drugs as ordered.	
Potential urinary tract infection (UTI) due to: • reflux • stasis • obstruction • retention • contaminated catheters	The child will be free of urinary tract infections (UTI).	Dx: 1. Record color, clarity and odor of urine.	Dx: 1. Urinary infections cause urine to look dark and cloudy and have a foul smell.
		2. Obtain culture specimens as ordered.	2. Identifying the causative organism is prerequisite to treating infection.
		3. Record intake and output.	3. A pattern of frequent output of small amounts of urine indicates UTI. Intake is recorded to ensure that adequate fluids are provided to promote "flushing" of kidneys and prevent urinary stasis.

Care Plan continued on following page

NURSING CARE PLAN FOR THE PRESCHOOLER WITH A URINARY ALTERATION *(Continued)*

Nursing Diagnosis (Problem)	Expected Outcome	Nursing Interventions	Rationale
		Rx: 1. Administer medications as ordered. 2. Force fluids as ordered. 3. Empty bladder completely by natural or artificial means as ordered. 4. Provide increased dietary acids.	Rx: 2. Adequate intake must be maintained to "flush" kidneys and assist excretion of cells, casts and sediment produced by infection. 3. Urine provides a good culture medium for bacteria, and residuals left in the bladder support infection. 4. Acids are excreted by kidney, producing a urine pH that restricts and inhibits bacterial growth.
	Child will be able to discuss and demonstrate proper toilet hygiene and elimination practices.	Child/Parent Education: (for Problem 1 and 2) 1. Instruct child and significant other in toilet hygiene (washing hands before and after eliminating and wiping from front to back). Reinforce instruction regularly. 2. Explain the importance of responding promptly to the urge to void and of taking time to empty the bladder completely at each void.	Child/Parent Education 1. Proper toilet hygiene reduces likelihood of causing or spreading genitourinary infection. The preschooler has developmental ability to manage this task but becomes preoccupied easily with other activities. 2. Preschooler has cognitive ability to comprehend simple cause-and-effect relationships, can understand that hygiene reduces the likelihood of urinary retention, stasis or infection.

1030 FAMILIES WITH PRESCHOOLERS

Inability of kidney to regulate body electrolytes or to excrete waste products or medications.

The child's electrolyte and acid-base balance will be maintained.

Dx:
1. Evaluate serum electrolyte studies, blood urea nitrogen (BUN), uric acid and creatinine levels.

2. Observe child for sign of
   - acidosis (depression of CNS with altered level of consciousness)
   - alkalosis (stimulation of CNS causing overexcitability, nervousness, tetany, convulsions, tingling sensations)
   - electrolyte imbalance (disorientation, confusion, muscular rigidity or flaccidity, cardiac changes depending on the specific electrolyte in imbalance).

3. Observe all kidney patients for toxic drug reactions or further impaired kidney function.

4. Measure urinary pH on each void.

Rx:
1. Carefully administer or restrict intake of electrolytes as ordered.

2. Protect a disoriented patient from injury.

Dx:
1. Kidney regulates body's balance of sodium, potassium, bicarbonate, magnesium and calcium. Kidney excretes urea, uric acid and creatinine to control blood levels of waste products.

2. The kidney is a major body organ for maintenance of acid-base balance through its regulation of body electrolytes and excretion of metabolic wastes. Electrolyte disturbances may cause clinical changes before lab results return.

3. Because kidney receives 25% of cardiac output and is the obligatory excretory route for most drugs, these patients are at high risk for drug toxicity or additional drug damage to kidney itself.

4. Kidney maintains acid-base balance by excretion of bicarbonate, hydrogen ions and acid end products of metabolism.

Rx:
1.

2. A common sign of electrolytes or acid-base disturbance is disorientation or agitation.

Care Plan continued on following page

THE HOSPITALIZED PRESCHOOLER 1031

NURSING CARE PLAN FOR THE PRESCHOOLER WITH A URINARY ALTERATION (Continued)

Nursing Diagnosis (Problem)	Expected Outcome	Nursing Interventions	Rationale
		3. Provide renal diet as ordered: • low protein • carbohydrate and fat calories • vitamin supplements	3. Due to inability of kidney to handle waste products of protein metabolism, dietary protein may be restricted. Low-protein diets provide inadequate supplies of vitamins. Adequate nonprotein calories are necessary to prevent endogenous protein metabolism. An exception is nephrotic syndrome in which a generous protein intake is desirable.
		4. Work with parents to identify patterns of intake best suited to child.	4. Each child has his own patterns of drinking and eating. If these natural rhythm needs for order and consistency can be met within the dietary limitations, maximal satisfaction can be provided.
	The child will have maximum opportunity to receive gratification at meals despite dietary restrictions.	5. Give small frequent feedings if possible.	5. Stomach capacity of the preschooler is limited, as is his ability to delay gratification; therefore small frequent feedings may better meet his needs.
		6. Provide socialization during mealtimes.	6. The preschooler is moving from parallel play into cooperative play and is learning to relate to others outside his immediate family. Meeting the need to socialize may increase gratification of restricted meals.

	7. Provide maximum skin care.	7. Due to build-up of waste products in the skin, it becomes itchy. Restricted diets (especially protein) increase skin fragility and the chances of pressure sores, infections and breakdown.
Parent can describe the dietary needs of their child with renal dysfunction and can write meal plans that reflect this knowledge.	Child/Parent Education: 1. Instruct parents in dietary needs of child on a renal diet, including ways to vary diet and keep extra expense minimal without compromising it. • dietitian referral • referral to resource for financial assistance	Child/Parent Education: 1. Parents are responsible for maintaining their preschooler on the renal diet for as long as necessary. Diet must be varied since clinical state and therefore dietary needs differ with the stage of renal disease. These diets require careful preparation and can be expensive.
Parent can state the symptoms of acid-base or electrolyte imbalance.	2. Inform parents of symptoms and pathophysiology of acidosis, alkalosis or electrolyte imbalance. Stress significance of sharing this information with the preschooler's other caretakers.	2. Parents must recognize kidney dysfunction in their preschooler and seek intervention. Since the preschooler's world is expanding to include other caretakers, that responsibility also extends to them.
Complications of Renal Dysfunction Long-term: Potential hypertension, anemia or alteration of vitamin D metabolism.		
The child's blood pressure will be maintained within safe limits. The child will be free of anemia. Bone growth will be maintained.	Dx: 1. Monitor blood pressure regularly.	Dx: 1. It is believed that pressure sensors in the kidney or chemical receptors in the body stimulate production of renin when blood flow to kidney is reduced. Renin sets off a chain reaction that increases blood pressure and blood flow to kidney by increasing sodium reabsorption, water retention and plasma volume expansion.

Care Plan continued on following page

THE HOSPITALIZED PRESCHOOLER

NURSING CARE PLAN FOR THE PRESCHOOLER WITH A URINARY ALTERATION (Continued)

Nursing Diagnosis (Problem)	Expected Outcome	Nursing Interventions	Rationale
		2. Regularly monitor: • Blood studies (Hgb, Hct, total solid protein) • Urine for blood and protein • Pulse and respirations	2. Bone marrow suppression may occur due to a deficiency in or absence of production of erythropoietin by the failing kidney. Renal failure further increases the potential for anemia because of an increased tendency to bleed (due to impaired platelet function). Dietary restriction of protein further increases the risk of anemia. Severe anemia produces tachycardia and tachypnea.
		3. Regularly monitor serum blood for calcium levels.	3. When kidney function is altered vitamin D production is decreased, causing less calcium absorption from the gut. Lowered calcium and ineffective action of vitamin D prevent adequate bone mineralization.
		Rx: 1. Administer drugs and regulate diet as indicated on the basis of kidney function.	
		2. Provide adequate rest or activity as indicated by kidney function.	2. An increased metabolic rate places increased demands on already compromised kidney(s).
	Parent will name potential complications of kidney impairment and (1) identify diagnostic methods	Child/Parent Education: 1. Explain to parents and child the reason for each diagnostic and preventive measure.	Child/Parent Education: 1. If parents understand reason for diagnostic and preventive measures, cooperation in diagnosis and compliance in treatment is fostered.

1034 FAMILIES WITH PRESCHOOLERS

	for early recognition of complications, (2) identify preventive measures.	
Interference in motor, intellectual and emotional and social development.	Parent will state how interventions can be adapted to developmental level of child.	2. Teach parents to prepare child for tests, procedures or surgery in developmentally appropriate ways (use simple language and line drawings or dolls to demonstrate to child). 2. Parents act as "interpreters" and "translators" for the preschool child. Their participation in child's preparation (if possible) will facilitate his understanding. Preschoolers like to learn the names of different parts of the body, especially the genitalia. Use of dolls help child to visualize the body's outside appearance and to understand through play the equipment and procedures to be used in his treatment.
	The preschooler will have opportunities for development consistent with physical condition and developmental age.	Dx: 1. Identify what the child knows about his problems. 2. Take a history from parents to identify sexual attitudes to determine specifically how parents are dealing with their preschooler's interest in exploration of genitalia. Dx: 1. The preschooler may misunderstand what is happening to him because of limited ability to conceptualize. He is dominated by his perceptions of things. He will always come to some conclusions about what is happening but his limited ability to distinguish fantasy and dreams from reality may cause erroneous beliefs. (The child who must have repeated catheterizations for residual urine may imagine the catheter is a snake that will bite him.) 2. A preschooler has increased sexual curiosity. Although the genitalia may not be affected in a specific urinary problem, the preschooler understands the body in a limited way and does not separate urinary

Care Plan continued on following page

THE HOSPITALIZED PRESCHOOLER 1035

NURSING CARE PLAN FOR THE PRESCHOOLER WITH A URINARY ALTERATION (Continued)

Nursing Diagnosis (Problem)	Expected Outcome	Nursing Interventions	Rationale
			from genital problems. The parents' reactions to their child's sexual curiosity will determine how the preschooler normally expresses this curiosity and has implications for the nurse's approach with the family and the child.
		Rx:	Rx:
		1. Allow genital play and exploration within limits of physical needs and parents' values, recognizing that the need for this behavior may be increased.	1. Normal fears of castration and mutilation are compounded when urinary problems exist. The child will attempt to reassure himself through exploration of his own body. Interference with this normal process may generate feelings of being bad or that something is wrong with his body.
		2. Provide activities that challenge the child and are within his activity restrictions but that do not overextend his capabilities.	2. For the preschooler learning is done through play. Children this age may repeat an activity until they master it and then totally reject that activity for another more complex one. The preschooler is capable of learning manual or fine motor skills. These are more difficult, but are easier to provide for the child with restricted activity. If too complex a challenge is given, frustration can be increased rather than relieved.

3. Allow for aggressive release in play and for crying and expression of verbal anger during procedures or treatment. Opportunities for therapeutic play through dolls and puppets should be provided.

Child/Parent Education:
1. Explain the relationship between urinary problems and the preschooler's temporary alteration in bladder or bowel control.

Parents demonstrate acceptance of child's regression in bowel or bladder function associated with urinary problems.

3. The child who cannot explore his environment has decreased learning experiences and physical outlets for anger and aggression. The preschooler can control some of his actions if his needs are channeled into nondestructive activities within his therapeutic restrictions. Fears regarding intrusive procedures can be expressed in therapeutic play. Activity involved in this play also provides an outlet for aggressive behavior.

Child/Parent Education:
1. Loss of elimination control may be physiologically associated with the disease process or a psychological response to altered routine and increased focus on elimination.

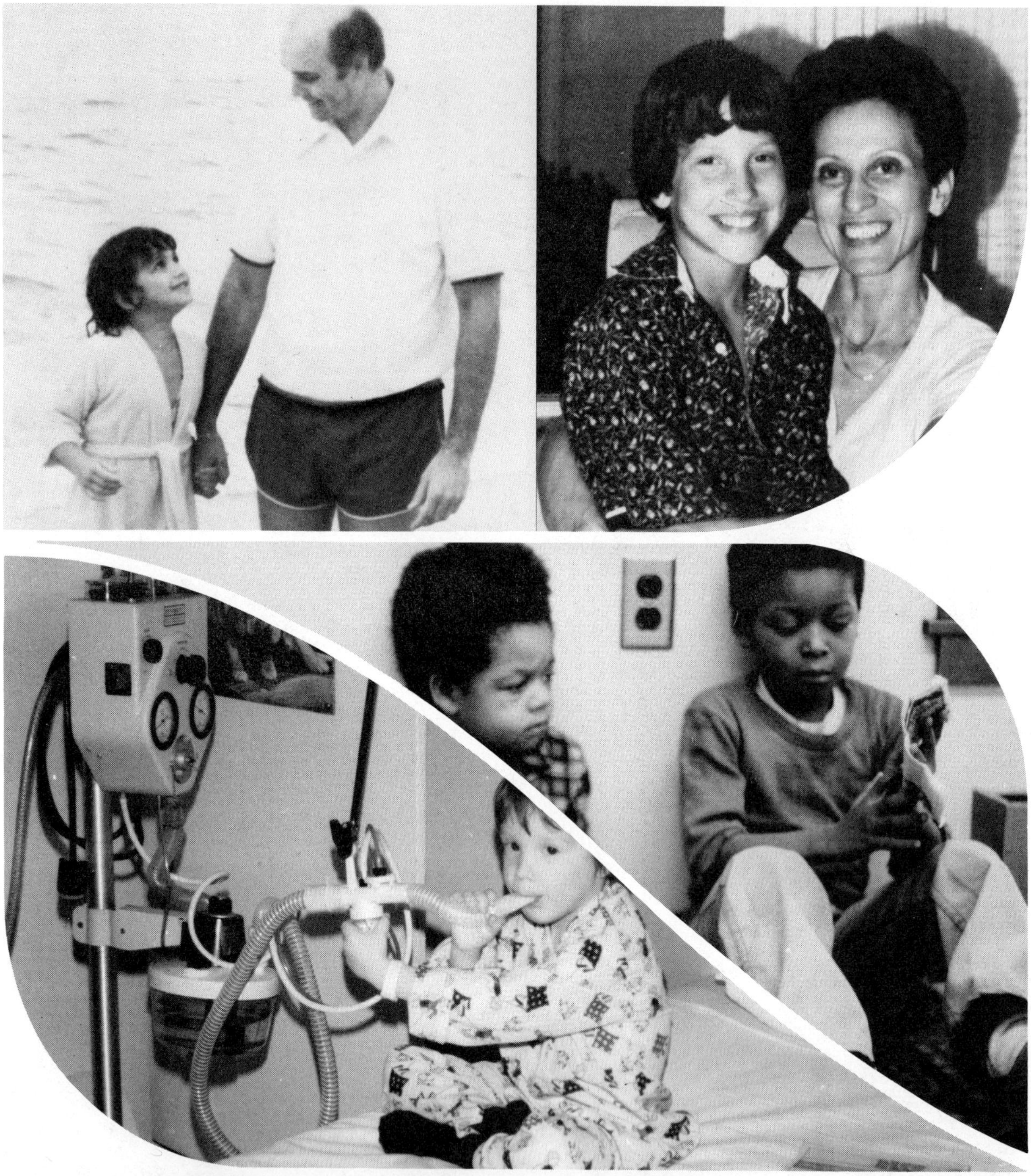

PART 7

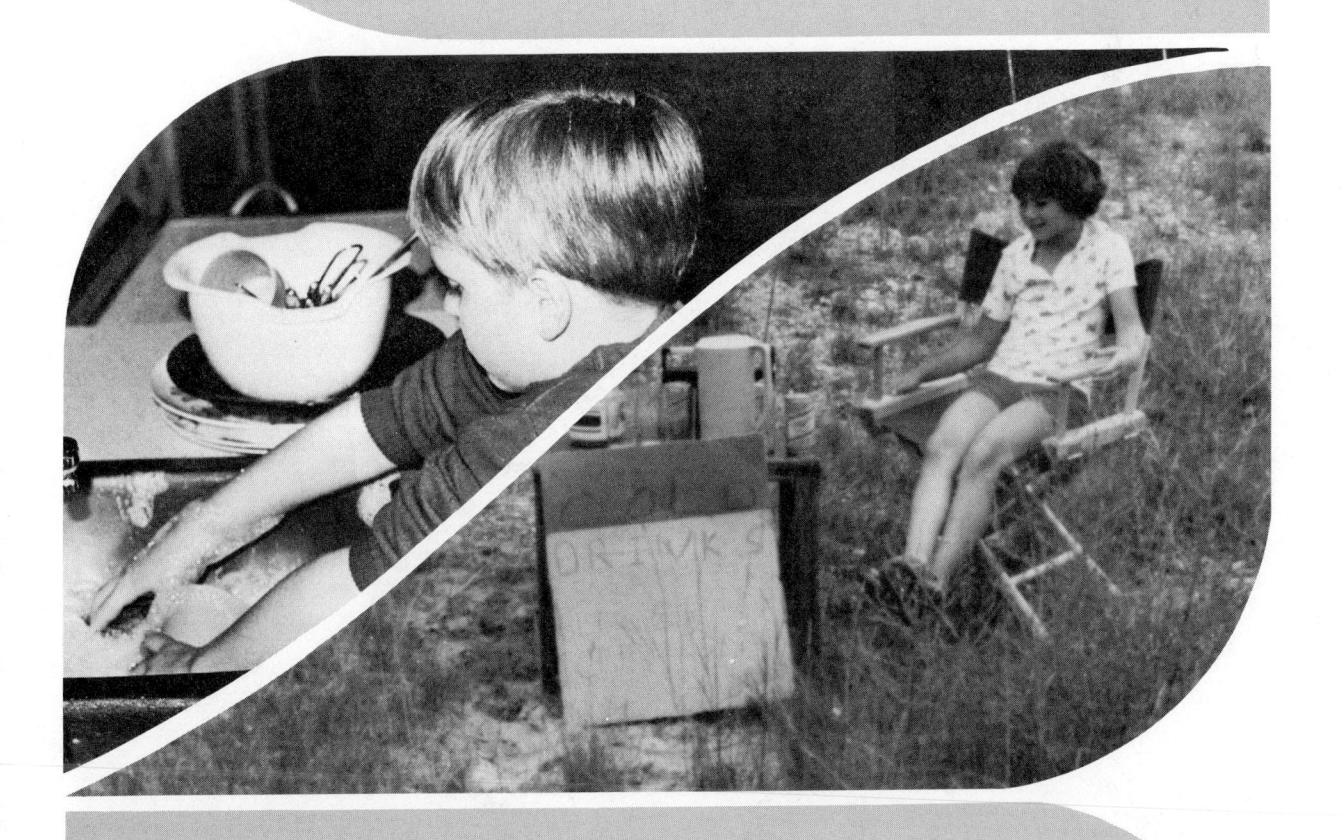

FAMILIES
WITH
SCHOOL-AGE
CHILDREN

GROWTH AND DEVELOPMENT NEEDS OF THE FAMILY WITH SCHOOL-AGE CHILDREN: MAINTAINING WELLNESS

by Evelyn McElroy, RN, PhD,
and Jo Joyce Tackett, BSN, MPHN

The United States contains 48.5 million school-age children between the ages of 6 and 12. Second only to the family, the school is the major socializing agency available for transmitting values as well as knowledge to children.

This chapter describes common needs of families with school-age children, presents the developmental tasks of families with children in the age group from 6 to 12 years, and considers methods of adapting to life changes encountered. Available support systems are discussed. Interventions aimed at promoting the well-being of the child and family are described.

As individual family members move from one life stage to the next, family life is marked by changing relationships, with family functions at one stage superseded by responsibilities of the next. The willingness of parents to accommodate to changes in their growing children as well as to progress in their relationship with each other determines the degree and quality of the family unit's functioning.

The family with school-age children is confronted with three major areas of change that constitute the family's developmental tasks. These are: (1) adapting to the child's expanding world as he moves into school and the world of teachers and peers, (2) expanding family communications and activities to recognize the school-ager's readiness for independent thinking and greater responsibility both within and outside the family unit and (3) maintaining financial solvency as family costs escalate to meet the needs of school and extracurricular activities.

ADAPTING TO THE EXPANDING WORLD OF SCHOOL

One changing characteristic of all school-age children and their families is the need to adjust to a world no longer totally controlled by parents and the home environment. Beginning school is an event that creates anxiety in some

> Carrie Hearn began first grade last Monday. Carrie was fortunate in having had the experience of attending nursery school in her neighborhood. There she had developed some friendships that could be continued as her preschool playmates also entered elementary school. In addition, Carrie's mother had accompanied her to school and had ensured that she arrived at the appropriate room, was introduced to her teacher, and became involved with another little girl who lived in the same block. Three factors helped Carrie meet the new challenge of beginning first grade: having past experiences in a school setting, encountering a new situation with the support of her mother and locating an old friend.

children; this situation can be mitigated by anticipating potential sources of difficulty. An example of a successful adaptation to first grade is shown in the boxed material above.

As the child begins school the family must deal with the new parameters presented by school and peers (Table 46–1). The child may for the first time experience being labeled (e.g., "Fatso," "Skinny," "the kid from Becker Street") and prejudice. With exposure to differing moral attitudes and beliefs, the child and his parents must now contend with the incongruities between family beliefs and expectations and those of peers at school. In addition, the child who by now is beginning to handle sibling rivalry is faced with the new situation of peer rivalry as he competes with other children for the teacher's attention and approval.

As the child begins absorbing the values of the peer group and school, conflict often arises. Home becomes a testing ground for new ideas and behaviors — parents are sometimes nonjudiciously compared with teachers and cooperative preschool darlings can become relentlessly sassy school-age teases. The inevitable consequence of this, even in the best-adjusted families, is some degree of conflict, particularly between parent and child; between home and school; or between home and peer groups, especially with the older school-age child. Some parents perceive the decrease in control over their child's life as threatening; they sense a progressive impotence as parents. They may respond with alarm or anger directed toward the child or the school (usually the teacher). Sometimes parents over-react as their child expresses new ideas or imitates peer behaviors, trying them on for fit. Parents may impose overly strict rules or punishment in response to the experimentation. Other parents give up, refusing to set any limits at all on these experimental ideas and behaviors. Many parents, however, find comfort from sharing concerns and frustrations (not to mention the humor created by some of their children's experimental antics) with parents in similar situations. These parents, although they sometimes feel like packing their bags and running away or hiding out for a day, usually set realistic limits on their children's experimental activities, pray a lot and wait out this phase in their children's development.

As the child approaches and settles into school, teachers and peers become especially significant to him and can represent valuable support systems in his school adjustment. Caplan describes support for the child as occurring when:

Other people are interested in him in a personalized way. They speak his language. They tell him what is expected of him and guide him in what to do. They watch what he does and judge his performance. They let him know how well he has done. They reward him for success and punish or support and comfort him if he fails. Above all, they are sensitive to his personal needs, which they deem worthy of respect and satisfaction.[2]

Such support may be of an enduring or short-term nature. Characteristic functions of support systems are helping to mobilize a person's psychological resources, sharing his tasks, and providing him with extra supplies of materials, tools, skills, and cognitive guidance to improve his handling of his situation.[2]

The extent to which teachers possess the attributes of support systems allows them to function as facilitators in the child's attempt to adapt successfully to school. By making expectations clear, guiding his efforts, judging his products and rewarding in success or comforting in failure, a teacher can influence a child's sense of industry. According to Erikson, good teachers "know how to alternate play and work, games and study. They know how to recognize special efforts, how to encourage special gifts."[6]

In regard to enhancing a child's motivation to achieve and master particular knowledge or skills or develop talents, the teacher can be a vital supporter. According to Jerome Kagan, the motive for mastery has as its foundation three goals: "the desire to match behavior to a standard, the desire to predict the environment and the wish to define the self."[8] The first goal becomes realized as the child continually acquires new ideas about the world. The child tries to simulate many phenomena by putting into practice some of the ideas he has learned, such as taking apart a miniature motor similar to repairs of real cars performed by a parent. The teacher can guide the child in his efforts to meet standards by helping him define certain strategies and persuading him that he possesses intellectual talents that, if used, can lead to success. For the second goal, in his attempt to predict outcomes the child strives to master unknown situations. The school-ager tries to predict what will happen in school, how well he will do on a test or how many hits he will get in the afternoon baseball game. In the learning environment, a teacher can promote successful guessing by providing basic general knowledge and encouraging children to apply their understanding to various phenomena. For the third goal, in terms of the child's attempt to define himself, the teacher can play an important role in making each child aware of his or her special areas of competence. She can construct work groups in which each child has one area of relatively superior skill, whether it be in music, art, or physical coordination, or reading, writing, and arithmetic. This process also helps build an expectancy of success and permits the child to define himself as a person with certain skills.[8]

In a similar fashion, the teacher can play an important part in preventing development of feelings of inferiority in the child. Besides structuring the learning situation so a child can experience relative success, the teacher can contribute toward the maturing of positive feelings toward self and others. Barbara Biber applied mental health principles in the school setting. Her premise assumed that "self-feeling (self-concept) in childhood is, to a large degree, an introjection of the opinions and attitudes of important adult figures."[1] The implications of this for teachers go beyond merely providing a warm and accepting climate. Teachers must have knowledge of childhood developmental processes in psychodynamic terms. Maturity in children must not be equated wholly with reasonableness — there must be an appreciation for the creative potential inherent in fantasy,

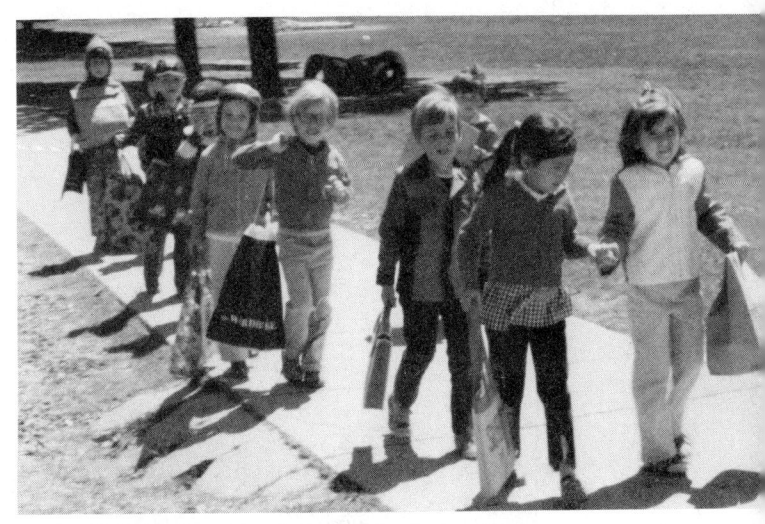

As the child begins school, the family deals with the new parameters of school and peers.

and actions should be based on the expectation that growth will be gradual, wavering, regressive and uneven. Of the teacher, Biber says "Recognizing conflict as inevitable in the growth process, she is not surprised by children's fears, weaknesses, guilt, anxiety. She is able to help children feel comfortable in having their troubles, doubts, and shame known to her with the confidence that they will not be discounted."[1]

Erikson indicated that "the development of a sense of inferiority, the feeling that one will never be 'any good,' is a danger which can be minimized by a teacher who knows how to emphasize what a child can do and who recognizes a psychiatric problem when she sees one."[6] By being sensitive to a child's personal needs and deeming them worthy of respect and satisfaction, the teacher can be a source of emotional support merely by listening to and understanding problems, even if they are outside the scope of solution within the school. Thus by guiding the child's attempts to achieve and providing the cognitive skills to master situations, the teacher can enhance the attainment of a sense of industry. Likewise, by treating the child as an individual in his own right and recognizing variations in the growth process, a teacher can be instrumental in preventing feelings of inferiority. Both of these qualities are important attributes of people in support systems.

Peers can also become important members of

TABLE 46–1 TASKS OF CHILDREN, PARENTS, TEACHERS AND NURSES IN FACILITATING SCHOOL ADJUSTMENT[10]

Statement of Adjustment	Child's Tasks	Parents' and Teacher's Role in Facilitating Task Achievement	Nurse's Role in Assisting Parents, Teachers, Child
Diffusion into larger world (5 or 6–8 yr).	1. Must adapt to differences in teacher's and parents' disciplinary approach and behavioral expectations.	1. Parents and teacher should communicate their respective expectations for the child to identify extreme differences and to work out compromises that permit him to meet expectations of each and so that parents and teachers can mutually reinforce their expectations.	1. School nurse can help organize parent-teacher interaction (e.g., preschool roundups; parent-teacher-nurse conferences) or mediate in conflicts. a. During preschool roundup or school physical, learn what child's and parents' expectations for school are.
	2. Must compete with peers for teacher's attention and approval as teacher replaces parent for large portion of day.	2. Teachers should avoid obvious favoritism in classroom, give individual attention and praise to each child, avoid comparisons of achievement.	2. School nurse can offer guidance to teachers and intervene in unhealthy child-teacher relationships. a. During preschool registration or school physical, evaluate parent-child relationship for problems as these often carry over to teacher-child relationships.
	3. Must learn to handle blatant, hurtful honesty and downright rudeness of peers without damage to self-concept.	3. Peer activities and behaviors need close adult supervision.	3. Nurse in well-child facilities or schools can provide this guidance to parents and teachers.
	4. Needs to test out new ideas and behaviors in security of home environment.	4. Parents need to recognize developmental function of "trying on" ideas and behaviors incongruent with family's but set reasonable limits on how much and what type of "trying on" is to be allowed.	4. Nurse in well-child facilities or schools may offer this anticipatory guidance.
Disorganization created by disparities between home and school or peers (8–10 yr).	1. Must learn to concentrate on cognitive achievements as he settles into school life.	1. Parents and teachers need open communication about cognitive tasks that are being focused on at any one time and skills the child finds difficult so that both parties can support his mastery of those skills.	1. School nurse observations in classroom will help identify children having difficulty with this task. Investigation of state of health, sensory organ function, and neurological, physical and emotional function should follow to determine source of problem in achieving task.

1044 FAMILIES WITH SCHOOL-AGE CHILDREN

	2. Must learn to integrate peer values in a manner that does not deny family values and to transfer family values into larger world in socially acceptable ways.	2. Parents and teachers must understand that just as a child falls as he learns to walk so will he fall as he learns to think. These falls during school age are typically boasting, teasing, fighting, lying, cheating, sassing and whining.	2. School nurses should regularly monitor playground and classroom activities to identify extricated children and then set the task force (parents, teachers, nurses, other pertinent school or health personnel) in motion to uncover source of problem and offer help.
		3. Teachers and parents need to develop the art of overlooking minor falls and feel comfortable seeking help for more serious or persistent falls. Children left alone with their peer group often overcome problems with peer assistance rather than adult intervention.	3. Well-child facility and school nurse should evaluate child's behavior patterns and self-concept at each contact to pick up clues that all is not well in his emotional and social relationships. Nurse in clinic or school should offer parental/teacher anticipatory guidance regarding handling of behavior problems.
Disposition of compromise between home and larger world (10–12 yr).	1. Must take increasing responsibility for initiating and carrying out own learning activities at school and home; find internal satisfaction in performance.	1. Family and teacher must acknowledge child's ability to manage responsibility and allocate responsibilities in which child can take pride and feel success.	1. Nurse in any setting in contact with parents and teachers may offer this anticipatory guidance. Nurse may role model of such interactions in her dealings with child.
	2. Must take interest in organized school and peer activities to be accepted as a group member.	2. Parents need to see developmental advantage of child's involvement in organized activities and plan with child how he can get to these, financially handle the expenses involved and still manage home and school responsibilities. Teachers should understand the need for such involvement and appropriate homework reasonably.	2. Same as 1 above. Nurse may help family learn about community activities available to children this age and of financial assistance available through schools, community clubs, churches.
	3. Must become capable of maintaining appropriate personal conduct (control impulses, resist temptation) with little or no adult supervision.	3. Child should be given increasing opportunity to go to school, religious and peer functions unattended by parents and be praised for reports of good conduct. Digression from appropriate conduct should be dealt with in accordance with the seriousness of digression. Parents need to communicate faith in child's ability to handle himself adequately.	3. Same as 1 above.

GROWTH AND DEVELOPMENT NEEDS OF THE FAMILY
WITH SCHOOL-AGE CHILDREN:
MAINTAINING WELLNESS

the child's support system. An extra feature of these "supporters" is that there is a greater likelihood for enduring relationships in light of the fact that a child normally progresses through his school years with the same peers, in contrast to the yearly exposure to different teachers. In terms of the child's need to develop a sense of industry, to feel good about his products and to compete with others for recognition, his peer group watches what he does, judges his performance and lets him know how well he has done. Typically this latter process is conveyed through inclusion or exclusion from group activities. Essentially, a child looks to his peers to measure his own skills and worth. According to Maier, "A sense of accomplishment for having done well, being the strongest, best, wittiest, or fastest are the successes toward which he strives. The child wards off failure at almost any price."[11] Thus the child looks to others for an appraisal of his skills and develops pride in his abilities according to how peers evaluate him.

A specific factor that enhances the indentification of peers as "significant others" is their ability to share the tasks of a child. This occurs between younger groups of peers as well as older groups. Between the ages of 6 and 8, activities are organized around playful games. There is little formality or organization; groups collect by chance and consist of whomever shows up on the sidewalk or street corner at a particular time. The children may have little other association with each other, yet there is a mutual participation in fun activities. As children grow older, particularly around age 10 or 11, peer groups become more organized around common interests and planned events. There may be nature clubs, fan clubs or secret societies with special rules, and plans may be made in advance, such as going to the movies, building a fort or having a picnic. In addition, chumships develop between children, usually of the same sex, and best friends become inseparable. They attend activities together as well as share intimate thoughts, feelings, hopes, fears and doubts. Some chumships may be brief, but subsequent intense and exclusive relationships between one child and another usually develop within a short time.

A study by James Youniss demonstrated that peers share tasks with one another and are sensitive to one another's personal needs.[13] The intent of the study was to examine how children establish and maintain their social relationships. Specifically, Youniss focused on the concept of affirmation as it pertained to communication among children. The first phase of the study consisted of asking children ranging in age from 6 to 12 to tell short stories about affirmation in which they indicated that they liked someone, described that they were friends and described that they showed kindness to someone. In the second phase, Youniss presented to the subjects a series of stories about friendship initiatives. In one story a child asked another to play. In another story one child was depicted as being new (and lonely) at school, and another child asked him to play. In the final story, one child did not feel like playing but offered to play anyway because another child made the request. With each of these stories the subjects were asked: (1) to decide which child was kind, (2) to tell why they thought the child was kind and (3) if the character in the story was depicted as unkind, to project what he should have done to be considered kind.

The results of the study indicated that for the first part of the investigation, children in the youngest group, the six-year-olds, usually told stories about sharing material goods and playing with one another. Children in the middle group, 9 years of age, generally constructed stories about playing; and children in the oldest group, the 12-year-olds, frequently told stories about one child assisting another. This latter finding reflected a gradual movement of children toward an identification of affirmation (liking) with offering assistance. In contrast to the younger children, who demonstrated liking by doing something "with" another child, the older children equated liking with doing something "for" another child.

Likewise, the results of the second phase indicated a progression toward demonstrating kindness by meeting a specific need on the part of the recipient. The younger children often told stories of sharing toys or food with another child or generally just playing with him. The children in the middle age group emphasized more of an "inviting" another child to play, rather than simply engaging in playful activities. Finally, the older children demonstrated a more sophisticated notion of sharing feelings and thoughts with a friend and offering psychological comfort to an unhappy person. There was more evidence of displaying kindness in relation to someone's specific need, such as helping someone with school work or consoling someone whose dog had died.

Each of these results points to the specific features of peer group relationships in terms of their uniqueness as support systems. Encouraging school children to share in tasks offers the additional qualities of mutual understanding and emotional support that can lead to expression of feelings and meaningful friendships, thereby decreasing the likelihood of a child feeling isolated and inferior.[5]

Role of the Nurse in Facilitating Adjustment

The possible implications are numerous for the nurse in the school setting to facilitate the child's adjustment within the framework of the support systems afforded by teachers, peers and family. Through direct personal interactions with a key individual, the teacher, the nurse may not only be able to clarify a particular crisis situation but also may provide support for the supporter. Both tasks may be needed in view of the fact that the quality of any teacher-student relationship is partly determined by factors that each party brings to the relationship. Some authors have referred to teachers as "substitute mothers."[12] Not only is the child's first teacher usually a woman, but she typically also performs nurturing functions such as praising "good" behavior and punishing "bad," and providing emotional support when needed. As a result, the behaviors and attitudes that a child has developed in relation to his mother are frequently transferred to the teacher. According to Mussen and colleagues, "If the child views his mother as nurturant and accepting, he is likely to approach the teacher with the same positive attitude. If, on the other hand, the child has hostile feelings toward a rejecting mother and has generally behaved aggressively toward her, he may transfer these responses to the teacher."[12] These distortions may cause strain on the teacher-student relationship, particularly if a great deal of ambivalence or conflict exists between the child and the mother that can become intensified during states of crisis for the child. Similarly, the teacher may experience periods of stress in her own life that affect her relationships with students. When a particular child experiences stress at the same time that a teacher is dealing with her own troubles, the result may be a displacement of the teacher's problems onto the child. The child may become labeled as a "problem child" instead of a "child with problems."[2] By intervening directly through personal interaction with the teacher, the nurse, by remaining aware of the teacher's defense mechanisms, can provide within their framework an objective opinion as to methods of handling the situation. Such intervention could relieve the tension between the child and the teacher without placing blame on either person and, more importantly, would provide support for the supporter.

The nurse may be in a more advantageous position than the teacher to deal with crisis situations, since school performance is associated with teachers' evaluations.[3] In any family the child's learning problems may impinge on the goals and aspirations of the parents. A child may be perceived as a psychological extension of the parents, the bearer of their genetic traits and the product of their childrearing efforts. If the child fails in school the parents may see themselves as failures. Feelings of guilt, doubt and anxiety may turn into anger, which is projected onto the school. Principals, teachers, learning disabilities specialists and remedial instructors may not be able to obtain the trust and confidence of the parents because these educators are often the conveyers of bad news regarding the child's achievements. In situations such as these, the nurse may be more successful in engaging the family in counselling and may be more effective herself in any therapy efforts. Thus, such actions may relieve some of the tension between school personnel and individual children and indirectly provide support for the supporters.

In terms of intervening in the peer support system, the nurse can be instrumental in facilitating the availability of supporters. By working directly with individual children, suggestions can be given as to how to improve their skills at making friends, thereby increasing the number of other children they can turn to for support.

The nurse solicits the family's support by offering them anticipatory guidance that will help them to "let go" of their child without feeling they have lost him to the larger world of school and community. This guidance is readily offered during preschool roundup conferences as a component of interaction during the child's physical examination for school and can be ongoing as a part of parent-teacher-nurse sessions at parent-teacher organization meetings or scheduled conferences.

In summary, factors that seem to foster school adjustment are a positive regard for a child's individuality by parents, teachers and peers; a willingness among these support groups to respond appropriately as he signals needs; an atmosphere within the family and school that is conducive to growth; and the availability of effective support systems. By assessing the family unit and classroom routinely for psychosocial dysfunctions, the nurse can identify "stressors" and develop appropriate methods of intervention.

Table 46–1 summarizes the major challenges of the school-age child, his parents and teachers to achieve adequate school adjustment. Nursing actions to facilitate the child's and family's adjustment are also listed.

EXPANDING FAMILY COMMUNICATION AND ACTIVITIES

Expanding communication and activities during the school-age years involve two interwoven processes: the process of letting go by parents and the process of taking on progressively more independence and responsibility by the school child. These two processes are accomplished in the milieu of family group activities or projects as well as activities the child participates in away from home and without parental supervision.

Letting Go

Letting their child go is one of the hardest tasks parents must undertake. It begins during the school-age years as the child leaves home for school and culminates in late adolescence or early adulthood when the child leaves to make a home of his own. A mother summarized "letting go" by saying, "It takes a closed mouth, a loving heart and an open door."[14]

Letting go requires that parents free their child to make increasingly more of his own decisions, learn from his own choices and experiences and take progressively more responsibilty for himself and his actions. Letting go also involves allowing the child to experience hurt and humiliation when his choices were unwise, to feel the exuberance of having done something "all by himself," and to know the satisfaction that comes from working with others because he chooses to. Parents grant this freedom by keeping their mouths closed and hands at their sides when they are tempted to give the child advice, assist him in tasks or baby him. Giving in to these temptations only alienates the child and impairs his development of independence and responsibility.

Along with this spirit of allowing the child his freedom, parents need to communicate faith in his competence and resilience. The child who knows that his parents believe in him and are proud of him has fewer failures and bounces back quicker when he does fail. The child who experiences belittling of his ideas and efforts and whose parents communicate doubt in his abilities usually complies with their expectations for failure.

Keeping an open door requires giving the child room to make his mistakes and offering support or comfort while he recuperates from the lapses in self-confidence and self-esteem that his mistakes or failures create. Actual assistance or advice is offered only at the child's provocation. The nurse cannot make parents let go of their school-ager but she can help them understand the need for and benefits of such action to the developing child. Putting parents in touch with other parents who are now or have in the recent past gone through this stage with their children is often supportive, especially for parents who are resisting "letting go."

Ensuring that the child is being assimilated into groups that conform to family and community expectations can be comforting to parents as they cope with the gradual loss of their child's attention. This can be augmented by encouraging the establishment of contacts with other families who possess similar values and by reinforcing socialization experiences that help the child make the emotional shift from family to peers to the larger society. Parental participation in the child's activities should continue but will take different forms than it did earlier. For example, instead of playing baseball with Johnny, who now prefers to be with his peers, the father may provide transportation for the team, be a volunteer at the neighborhood recreation center where Johnny and his friends defend their title, or be a proud spectator.

Parents may need to be encouraged to invite their school-age child to participate in family projects and outings that are appropriate to his interests, talents and developmental level. His freedom to become involved in or help organize family activities and his parents' respect for his contribution to this cooperative endeavor can reinforce the school child's self-worth, self-esteem and convey feelings of belonging that could provide a positive frame of reference for addressing group activities outside the family. The nurse should encourage parents to speak of the unique contributions made by their children. In this manner individual differences that contribute to identity formation will be encouraged. It is important to recognize that in addition to involvement in family activities, children need to be given separate time with parents. The nurse involved in counselling parents should bring this to their attention.

Progression in Independence and Responsibility

The school-age child is ready for increased independence and responsibility both at home and away. Even the early school-age child is capable of caring for his room, making his bed and helping with household tasks such as meal preparation and clean-up, vacuuming and dusting, and garden work. By age 8 most schoolagers are responsible enough to run short-distance errands alone, take full charge of pet care, help wash the car and entertain younger siblings, and to do other moderately demanding jobs. By 10 years, the child is usually interested in a paper route, lawn task or other after-school and summer jobs to supplement his allowance. He can also help with household repairs and prepare simple meals alone. By this age he also wants to go some places alone with peers such as the movies or a ball game or to school activities. Most grade schoolers can handle themselves adequately in public (often manifesting better behavior than they display at home) and the opportunity to go alone to public activities with peers builds their self-confidence to meet new situations.[7]

Parents can also draw upon community organizations to provide opportunities to develop their school-age child's independence. Obtaining his own library card is an event that frequently is important to a child in this age group. As a result of such an extension outside the home, other activities may evolve. For example, the children may attend a puppet show while parents use the free time to peruse new books or do some shopping until the show is over. Other children may choose to become involved in organizations such as church groups or boy or girl scouts and by late school age to become involved in volunteer organizations and participate in boy-and-girl activities such as "mixers."

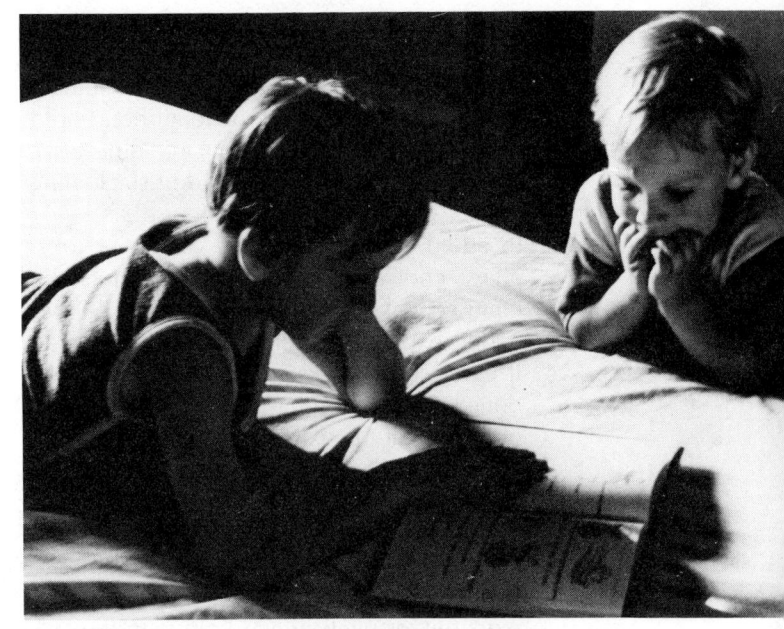

By middle school age, the child is responsible enough to run errands alone, take charge of pets or entertain younger siblings.

School-age children also need areas in the home that provide privacy to take advantage of opportunities to become involved in personal activities separate from those of other family members. The sanctity of places to keep diaries and special mementoes needs to be respected. Rules that safeguard the person's right to privacy need to be developed and clearly communicated to family members. Parents should use consistency in dealing with violations of these rules. As children approach adolescence the need for even more privacy must be anticipated.

The nurse's role in fostering progressive independence and responsibility in the school-age child lies primarily in the provision of information, support and guidance to parents as they attempt to lessen their control over the child. Directives to parents for yielding independence and greater responsibility to their children as provided by Foster[7] can be useful for the nurse's anticipatory guidance. Foster's recommendations are:
1. Praise the child's independent efforts at re-

sponsibility; do not criticize or condemn poor results.
2. Do not label tasks as being male or female responsbilities; instead, rotate all household jobs to lessen the monotony of some tasks and to diminish the likelihood of slackening quality in the job done.
3. In addition to providing a variety of jobs, allow choices in duties; this permits the child to make maximum use of his abilities and to explore different interests.
4. If carelessness creeps into work heretofore done well, either rotate tasks or increase the challenge of the existing task.
5. When a child shirks his task, letting him suffer the natural outcome is usually the most effective management. However, flexibility in demands is needed. If the child has other demands on his time such as homework, either pitch in and help with the task or temporarily take it over.
6. Check work performance while the child is still around; do not tolerate slipshod work or redo it for the child as long as it is a task within his capabilities to do well.

Such anticipatory guidance from the nurse may serve to prevent unnecessary family conflict. To provide opportunities for the child to master competencies expected for his developmental stage yet to reasonably restrict him from situations that are beyond his coping ability requires a balance not easily obtained. To allow children to make mistakes and to learn from them is often difficult for parents. Group discussions with other parents who have successfully coped with similar situations may be a useful modality for the nurse to suggest.

MAINTAINING FINANCIAL SOLVENCY

Families with school-age children are expected to continue to provide for the physical safety and economic needs of their members and to obtain enough goods, services and resources to survive. Because of heightened financial and social pressures as the child enters school and participates in extracurricular activities, and the increased time available as he attends school for longer periods of time, mothers who did not work outside the home previously may begin employment. In addition, both fathers and mothers may "moonlight," work overtime, or seek promotion to positions of greater responsibility and stress. The demands of employment will require some shifting of roles and responsibilities of some or all family members.

A major concern of the nurse should be that the shifting of responsibilities does not place undue responsibility on the school-age child so that he is not free to pursue play, outside activities or school tasks. Another concern is that he not be given responsibilities or independence beyond his capabilities or level of maturity. (See Chapter 47 for discussion of the "latchkey" schoolchild.)

Studies have shown that the attitude toward working of the working parent (especially the working mother) influences the children's emotional adjustment.[9] If parents want to work and if they like their jobs and provide adequate substitute caretakers while they are at work, their working has been shown to have no adverse effect on the child. Consequently, assessing parental (especially maternal) attitudes toward work may be useful to nurses in identifying families at potential risk for psychosocial problems.

The nurse may provide assistance to families to help them to assign fairly responsibilities among family members, to set family priorities and to simplify household demands whenever possible. The nurse may also help the family find reliable substitute caretakers during the parents' work hours.

References

1. B. Biber. Integration of mental health principles in the school setting. In Prevention of Mental Disorders in Children, G. Caplan, (ed.), Basic Books, Inc., 1961
2. G. Caplan. Support Systems and Community Mental Health. Behavioral Publications, 1974
3. C. Connolly. Counseling parents of school-aged children with special needs. Journal of School Health, February 1978
4. M. Dess. Lessons in letting go. Home Life, December 1976, p. 36
5. W. Damon. The Social World of the Child. Jossey-Bass, Inc., Publishers, 1977
6. E. Erikson. Identity, Youth, and Crisis. W. W. Norton and Company, Inc., 1968
7. C. Foster. Developing Responsibility In Children. Science Research Associates, 1976
8. J. Kagan. Understanding Children — Behavior, Motives and Thought. Harcourt-Brace-Jovanovich, Inc., 1971
9. K. Keating. Are working mothers attempting too much? Better Homes and Gardens, October 1978, p. 22
10. J. Laige. The school-aged child and his family. In Family Health Care: Developmental and Situational Crises, by D. Hymovich and M. Barnard, McGraw-Hill Book Co., 1973.

11. H. Maier. Three Theories of Child Development. Harper and Row, 1969
12. P. Mussen et al. Child Development and Personality, 4th edition. Harper and Rowe, 1974
13. J. Youniss. Catholic University of America, 1976

Additional Recommended Reading

C. Caplan and Killilea, eds. Support Systems and Mutual Help. Grune and Stratton, 1976
E. Erikson. Youth and the life cycle. Children, Mar/Apr 1960, p. 43
B. Farber. Family Organization and Interactions. Chandler Publishing Co., 1964
C. Feldman and N. Krigsman. When I have a sixth grader. Children Today, Jul/Aug 1977, p. 2
J. Langer. Theories of Development. Holt, Rinehart and Winston, 1969
S. Oden and S. Asher. Coaching children in social skills for friendship making. Child Development, June, 1977, p. 495.
F. Roberts. The little backseat driver. Parents, November 1978, p. 106
I. Weiner and D. Elkind. Child Development: A Core Approach. John Wiley and Sons, Inc., 1972

47 POTENTIAL STRESSES IN FAMILIES WITH SCHOOL-AGE CHILDREN

by Evelyn McElroy, RN, PhD,
and Jo Joyce Tackett, BSN, MPHN

Potential stresses of families with school-age children depend on many factors, including the behavioral style or temperament of the children, parental perception of the youth and expectations for their behavior, the marital relationship, effectiveness of family support systems, and circumstantial factors such as financial pressures, illnesses and myriad events affecting the family. These factors influence how the family deals with "stress" and must be considered when evaluating a child's response to school, since the effects of family discord are often acted out by the youth in the school setting.

In families with school age children the most commonly encountered stresses are those associated with separation and the dangers inherent in releasing the youth to the world outside home. All parents experience some degree of stress upon "letting go" of their youngster to the school system, which requires day-long separations of parent and child. Likewise, the broader social exposure that school creates forces families to cope with attitudes of prejudice and potential threats to the child's safety during his hours away from home.

This chapter considers some of the psychosocial dilemmas of families with school-age children who are at greater risk for distress during this period. Disruptions or distortions in the normal process of parent-child separation during school-age years often are symptoms of earlier problems in these relationships (overdependency, overprotection, unreasonable developmental expectations, psychosexual conflicts) that have persisted or increased because of the child's required attendance and participation in school or his developmental maturation. Other stress factors may have occurred more recently within the family that adversely affect separation, such as divorce, illness or death of a parent, the main caretaker's working outside the home, or a geographical move with the subsequent loss of friends and change of school. Such factors, whether their effects are long-term or temporary, may upset the family balance and produce dysfunctional behavior among its members. Often the conflict within the family is projected onto one member, who becomes a "scapegoat" or who produces symptoms indicative of emotional disturbance. If the family conflicts are displaced to the school-age child, school difficulties, peer problems and maladaptive affectional relationships frequently are found.

The school nurse frequently is a member of the interdisciplinary team that develops a treatment plan for the school-age child who is having problems; assessment of family interaction is often the nurse's task. Observations gained from family interactions provide the nurse with information about strong and weak character traits of members, the problems they face and their methods of coping with issues.

A family interview, preferably in the home, is essential to the nurse in gaining an understanding of problems of school-age children and in planning with families how to manage these problems. In addition to specific verbal information collected during the interview, equally important is observation of the family members' behavior during the interview itself. For example, the nurse can observe and note the father's sitting back and leaving it to the mother to tell the story and to discipline the child, the child's willingness to stay put during the recitation of his problems, and his increasing restlessness and distracting activity as the nurse draws the mother's attention away from him and to more neutral ground. From such observations can be developed a working hypothesis that the child's apparently "problem" behavior at least works for him in that through it he keeps his mother's attention. An appropriate intervention might be to applaud the mother's obvious extra effort in trying to deal with the child, and to engage the father in helping the mother to back off and become less involved in the child's behavior.

No behavior occurs in isolation and no intervention is aimed at one family member alone. The nurse's energies are directed toward observing the family system in action and abstracting from that observation the repetitive patterns of interactions among family members that support the problem behavior. With this information the interdisciplinary team can establish strategies to help the family members manage their stress in a way that does not precipitate problem behavior in their school-age child.

INAPPROPRIATE SCHOOL ASSIMILATION

A major task of parents with school-age children is "letting go." When parents have extreme anxiety about letting go of their child and freeing him for the new experiences that school and peer activities afford, his response is typically maladaptive. Two syndromes that arise out of acute separation anxiety between the school-age child and his caretakers(s) are school phobia and speech phobia (elective mutism). Although both of these syndromes may be precipitated by circumstantial factors such as those described earlier, a neurotic parent-child relationship is usually the primary underlying factor. Characteristically one parent (usually the mother) has overinvested in the child for several years as a means of fulfilling his or her own emotional needs that are unsatisfactorily met in adult (spouse) relationships. The child, stifled from normal emotional development as a result of overprotection and overindulgence, adopts the syndrome to control the domineering parent to avoid separation from that parent. (See Chapter 29 for a detailed discussion of overprotective, domineering parenting.) School phobia is discussed in Chapter 49.

Elective Mutism

In elective mutism, or speech phobia, the child refuses to speak or speaks selectively only to certain people or in certain situations. The lack of speech has no organic basis yet persists over months or years and is perceived by the child as a means of punishing the people who have offended him.[10] This silence and social isolation and withdrawal bring about a negative relationship with teacher and peers that interferes with academic achievement. The secondary effects of elective mutism are often more crippling than the silence itself.

Etiologically, studies have shown the existence of a neurotic relationship between mother and child in which the mother fosters overdependence in the child and the child responds by becoming mute to control the mother. This response of the child carries over into his other relationships, especially those with persons in a similar role as the mother such as the classroom teacher. This neurotic behavior of the child may be potentiated by the child's or other family members' predisposition to shyness, defects in speech articulation, thought disorders and extreme sensitivity to others' behavior toward them.[7,10] A number of children with elective mutism have also had in common a history of mouth injury or trauma at the time when the child was learning speech.[5,10] The incidence is significantly greater in girls.

Diagnostic findings are consistently similar among electively mute children. Typically the

TABLE 47-1 A SAMPLE APPROACH TO MODIFYING THE ACADEMIC PROGRAM TO CORRECT MUTISM[7, 8, 10]

Goal	Interventions
Help the child develop a satisfying social relationship.	1. Designate one person, preferably female, to work with child and mother. Person may be school nurse, speech therapist, social worker, etc. • With mother: Teach communication skills and techniques for dealing with mute child. Help her develop ways to achieve satisfying adult relationships to meet her emotional needs. Teach alternative parenting methods. • With child: Teach appropriate social responses through role modelling and reinforcement techniques. Establish rapport and trust, build child's general self-esteem.
Require audible responses in interactions with the one person.	1. Demand speech in interactions between the child and this one person. Begin by reinforcing nod responses; then require sounds. Progress to vocalization of single words and eventually sentences. 2. Ignore mute responses or other forms or nonverbal communication. 3. Reinforce all audible responses.
Generalize speech behavior to all school interactions.	1. Bring teacher into interactions with child and the one person with whom child has used speech. Instruct teacher to use same methods to elicit speech. Gradually increase length of interactions between child and teacher while steadily decreasing time other person is present. 2. Select one confident child from classroom to relate with child and role-model appropriate social responses. Reinforce mute child's outgoing responses. 3. Let mute child choose another child to add to play group each day until group is 5 or 6 in number. Continue reinforcing outgoing responses and speech (if it occurs). 4. Tape record mute child reading while alone or with the person who has established rapport. 5. Include mute child with group (from No. 3 above) for reading; play tape recording of mute child reading to the group. Continue reading group activity with this group until child reads within the group. Reward child's participation and verbalization. 6. Take child to classroom for reading group. Reward verbalization. 7. Include child in half-day then day-long classroom activities and insist on verbalization; reinforce this. 8. Include child in recess activities and set up situations requiring verbal exchange with other teachers, school personnel and children from other classes. Instruct adults in school environment to insist on and reinforce verbalization and to ignore nonverbal communication.

physical and neurological examination shows no defects and average or above-average intellectual and learning ability. The child has no satisfactory relationships and is lacking in social drive. An unresolved symbiotic relationship with the mother persists in which the mother is overly anxious about and overly protective of the child. Before the muteness, which usually commences in late infancy or toddlerhood, the child's speech development was normal. When the child abandons his muteness, verbalization and language development are very nearly age-appropriate despite the lengthy period of silence. Family responses show obvious reinforcement of the muteness, and the child receives the communication after a time that his muteness is expected.

While a few electively mute children resume talking spontaneously, most require treatment to overcome their problem. The earlier after onset that intervention is initiated, the more rapid is the progress toward resolving the problem. Unless severe intellectual limitations or thought disorders exist, prognosis is typically good for recovery. Treatment involves: (1) psychological counselling for the mother, (2) modification of the school curriculum as necessary to insist on verbalization (Table 47-1), and (3) refusal by all persons relating to the child in the treatment program to permit silence. Initiated early, this program of treatment is usually short-term.

PREJUDICE

Once a child reaches school age, his parents can no longer cushion or protect him from the prejudice of others that may exist because of the child's size, beliefs, color, ethnic background, family social status or neighborhood of family residence. Parents can take measures, however, to help their child build self-confidence and the ability to relate tolerantly to those who are prejudiced against him or her.[3] With these qualities the child can deal with this byproduct of life in a diverse society without severe loss of self-esteem or detriment to emotional or social development. Children also need direct, honest answers when they question why they or someone else is different. They need regular reassurance that because they are different does not mean they are "bad" or less worthy than their peers.

In dealing with a situation in which there is prejudice against a child, parents can make use of available literature and music and provide for the child's and family's participation in ethnic, religious or social events to help answer the child's questions and to provide him with a sense of belonging and reassurance about his difference.

When the child is confronted with others' prejudice against himself, he will react in a fashion similar to the way his parents have responded in the past. Therefore parents should develop skill in handling prejudice in a positive way. There is no one best way to confront prejudice against oneself, but using a calm, forceful approach is probably most effective.[3]

Children sense their parents' prejudices and imitate those same prejudices in their peer group. By school age, the best approach of a person trying to help the child overcome his prejudices toward others is to discuss frankly these prejudices with him, encouraging him to formulate his own ideas and opinions rather than bearing the burden of a parent's preconceived ideas. Ideally, of course, the parent also works to overcome that prejudice.

Parents can expose children positively to all kinds of people. Family friendships and social interactions with families of diverse backgrounds help the child develop an early appreciation for the richness that people's differences can lend to living. Such a child will not adopt prejudiced ideas that arise from knowing nothing about other cultures or life styles.

Children need to learn that no one need tolerate discrimination and that legal assistance in dealing with and protection against discrimination do exist in the United States.

Parents may need help to realize that prejudice is learned and that parents are the primary teachers. If parents provide opportunity for exposure to the diverse cultures of America and keep communication lines open on this subject, they will be helping their child to grow up with a clearer view of the world and a self-confidence that allows tolerance of others' ignorance.

THE LATCH-KEY CHILD

A potential source of conflict in families with school-age children centers on the different expectations held by parents and children in regard to freedom, privileges and responsibilities. That conflict is usually increased when only one parent is available to the family or when both parents must be away from home several hours a day on a regular basis.

The parents of over 30 per cent of children growing up in this decade eventually will be divorced. Another 5 to 10 per cent will be living with a single parent because of annulment of the marriage, separation of the parents or death of a parent.[1] In addition, in well over half of American families, the main caretaker also works outside the home.

These statistics indicate that in many families adults are away from the home more than in previous decades; this results in less supervision and more household responsibility for millions of children. Children who are given responsibilities beyond the usual age-appropriate norms and who are expected to perform in a manner beyond their developmental level are frequently referred to as "latch-key" children. These children are frequently expected to come home after school, clean the house, do laundry, care for the younger children and possibly even prepare dinner. The children frequently are not permitted to "waste time" in activities considered by the parents to be unimportant. Consequently, these children may not participate in school activities; they may not have friends or appear to enjoy life. The excessive demands made on them by their parents frequently result in a passive attitude toward life. It is also possible that the anxiety transmitted to the children by the parents may be manifested in psychophysiological symptoms resulting in excessive absences from school. The nurse must assess the child for symptoms of depression, which include an apathetic approach to life, loss of appetite, failure to gain weight or grow adequately and sleep disturbances.

The nurse's initial approach to a suspected "latch-key" child may be to conduct a family interview. By the time they encounter a nurse the parents may have a sense of incompetence and failure, and may exhibit anxiety about how their competence as parents will be viewed by professionals. In fact, under the stress of the moment, many parents who have successfully raised older children and have been quite competent in dealing with all the transitional and developmental issues involved forget their own history of success. The nurse can ease this anxiety in a few moments of interviewing, often through no more than a question like, "What did you do that worked so well with your older children?" With such phrasing the situation can be normalized, and the parents can recall their past success and see themselves as competent to deal with the present situation. This is essential, because the nurse operates on the assumption that family members do have the competence to deal with their current problem, and that they are not currently utilizing their strengths because of the constraints of the overwhelming life situation in which they find themselves. When there are no older children, parents can be asked to identify previous stressful situations in raising this child with which they successfully coped.

It follows from the nurse's belief in the capabilities inherent in the family that the counselling role for her excludes trying to solve the family's problems herself — giving advice and instructions about what to do. The task is to create an environment in which the responsibility struggle can be acted out in the session, and in which family members can experience success in solving their problems.

In the case of the "latch-key" child, the nurse may suggest that the husband and wife or single parent simplify home life and relieve the child of some responsibilities. The husband may be encouraged to assist the mother to back off from overzealous housecleaning or meal preparation. They may need to identify the household and child care tasks that could be shared more equitably between them. The nurse will not, however, tell the husband how to help his wife or tell the couple how to split home tasks, for the experts on that issue are the two people involved.

Likewise, a single parent may need encouragement to list activities that could be eliminated from a busy schedule and to plan options that could reduce time spent in commuting to and from work. The parent might think of affordable resources to help manage household chores and thus free up time to be spent with the children or to reduce the children's inappropriate home responsibilities.

A couple may be instructed to use the session to discuss the kinds of things that the husband can say or do to interrupt his wife when she is overworking and signals she can use to let him know she needs his help. The goal of these interventions is to provide the child with enough freedom to risk trying new experiences that could lead to greater independence without placing excessively unrealistic demands on him. Some professionals have had success in reducing the discrepancy between parental viewpoints and realistic responsibility for children of various ages by holding "parenting" groups in which parents assemble, discuss problems, and learn about themselves and others. Anticipatory guidance for parents as the child grows regarding the amount of responsibility that is realistic developmentally in relation to the child's developmental needs can help prevent the problem of latch-key children.

SEXUAL ASSAULT

The exact incidence of sexual abuse in school-age children is not known, but of those cases reported nearly 90 per cent are girls 10 to 11 years old.[9] Sexual assault to preadolescent children differs from rape in that the child-victim is not old enough to give consent legally and vaginal intercourse occurs in relatively few cases (less than 5 per cent) in this age group. Both of these conditions are essential to the legal definition of rape. Sexual assault is defined legally as the manual, oral or genital contact by an offender with the genitalia of the victim.[2] The child may participate willingly or unwillingly; either way it is assault.

Statistics from reported cases reveal that 97 per cent of sexual assaults are carried out by men from all social strata, the median age of the men being 31 years. One-fourth to one-third of offenders are strangers to the child; the incidents are usually one-time assaults.[9] The remainder of offenses are committed by someone with whom the child is acquainted and typically involve a series of assaults over an extended period of time.[4] Incest (sexual assault or rape between family members) is discussed in Chapter 38.

Sexual assault is typically reported by a parent or other caretaker, a family friend or the teacher to whom the child has confided the incident or who has witnessed the offense. In the classroom, children who have been assaulted frequently appear tired, have circles under their eyes, and are not as spontaneous as their peers. Bruises are sometimes apparent if physical force accompanied the assault. Other findings that may suggest sexual assault are suspicious physical findings such as blood in the child's undergarments, dried semen on the genitalia and thighs, itching or scratching the genitals, pelvic inflammatory disease and oral or anal lesions. Any venereal disease diagnosed in the school-age child should arouse suspicion of sexual assault or rape.

When sexual assault has been witnessed or is reported, three phases of assessment are required: an interview with the child, a separate interview with the parents and an examination of the child. Before her involvement in the assessment, the nurse should be aware of the legal implications involved in sexual assault within the state and of available support resources within the community.

Interview with the Child

The initial goal of the nurse who will interview a child suspected of being sexually abused is to respond to the child's immediate reactions. This response may vary from mild fear to panic to a complete lack of concern or guilt. The child's age, relationship to the offender, the degree of physical trauma and the family's reaction to the event are primary determinants of the child's response. The young child (under 9 years) responds more to the behavior than to the event itself because she does not have a concept of the sexual nature of the event. The older and more mature school-age child who does associate sexual meaning to the event is more apt to respond with panic and guilt. The more familiar the child is with the offender and the more threats the child has received to keep silent, the more fear and guilt the child can be expected to express. If physical trauma has been associated with the event, the child's reaction is also more severe. If the offender was gentle and caring, the child is often not disturbed until she observes the family's anxious reactions. Children whose families react with grief, anger or repulsion, or who punish the child or lament a sense of personal guilt greatly increase the trauma to the child. Those who react calmly in the child's presence and communicate continued love and acceptance of the child cause less trauma.

The interview with the child can help determine the extent of physical examination needed and the child's perception of the event. It can provide a description of the offender (if the interview is a part of the legal investigation); the child's level of coping with the situation can also be assessed. The child should be interviewed alone if she is verbal. If parents are to be present, they should be interviewed first and informed of how their response will affect the child.

The child is encouraged to talk about the event(s) using an open-ended approach such as, "Tell me what happened the time X was with you" or by asking the child to draw a picture of "what happened" and attempt to describe the incident from the picture.[4] The picture is not intended for psychological analysis but rather as therapy and to encourage conversation. Information should be documented in the child's words to avoid misinterpretations. Some children may need to act out the event (child as the offender and interviewer as the child or use of puppets or dolls to represent the two persons) in order to describe it. Table 47–2 identifies other specific details the interview should elicit.

Interview with the Parent(s)

Four types of parental reaction are typically associated with a child's sexual assault. Some parents deny the suspected or reported assault, insisting that the child is lying. Others threaten the child to try to make the child keep silent. These are more common reactions when the assailant is a family member or someone the family knows well.

Many parents feel intense guilt because they think that they did not adequately protect or

TABLE 47-2 ASSESSMENT OF POSSIBLE SEXUAL ASSAULT[4,9]

I. Child interview/parent interview
   A. Areas of physical injury or manipulation
   B. Date, time and type of sexual contact
   C. Whether child examined by an adult; if so, adult's findings
   D. Whether child has urinated, bathed, had a douche or been cleaned in any way since the assault
   E. If the child has begun menses; if so, date of last period, whether child has been taking oral contraceptives
   F. Known allergy to penicillin

II. The Physical examination
   A. External – check for:
     1. Any redness, bruising, raised areas or marks on labia majora
     2. Any swelling of labia minora, obscuring hymen or urethra
     3. Absence of scarring or recent rupture of hymen
     4. Vaginal bleeding
     5. Any lacerations, swelling or abradement of anus, urethra
   B. Internal – check for:
     1. Any redness, lacerations, lesions of vaginal canal
     2. Any evidence of bleeding
   C. Other findings; taking of specimens
     1. Loose hairs on child's underpants or genitalia; sample of child's own pubic hair, if present, for comparison
     2. Cotton pad wiping of thighs, buttocks, genitalia for later testing of semen secretions
     3. Swab of vagina (anus and mouth if applicable) for semen; saliva specimen for secretor status
     4. Blood sample for blood type and group
     5. Gonococcal smear swabbed from assault site
     6. Pregnancy test, if applicable

---

supervise their child and respond by overprotecting or rejecting the child. Some parents manage to remain calm, accepting the fact that the event has occurred and utilizing their energy to support the child. All parents experience a sense of anger toward the offender; some also feel anger toward the child for "allowing" the assault.[4]

Parents are interviewed to determine their reaction to the event, their legal intentions and how they will cope at home, and to assess their understanding of their child's needs during this time. Instruction regarding the child's needs and how they can help to meet these can be provided. The nurse can also inform them of available legal and community supports. If a parent expresses little concern or interest, an immediate referral to an official body such as a department of children's services (or a comparable community service) should be initiated.[4,6]

The Physical Examination

If vaginal penetration has not occurred, a complete pelvic examination is unnecessary. The assessment (Table 47-2) involves a visual inspection of genitalia, anus and mouth, collection of a specimen for venereal disease testing, and if dried secretions are evident, a specimen for semen evaluation. General examination of the body for any physical injury is also conducted. If intercourse did occur, a speculum examination of the vagina should be conducted under analgesia or anesthesia to rule out any internal injuries. If the child has begun menses, testing for pregnancy is also done.

Both the parents and the child should be prepared for the examination. Explanation should include that the child will be examined for any trauma, and reassurance should be offered that the pelvic examination (if applicable) will be done under analgesia or anesthesia by a physician. Consent forms will need to be signed by legal caretakers for the pelvic examination, for collection of evidence and for release of information to the police. If a parent will be supportive and is willing and if the child agrees, he or she should be with the child during the examination. Otherwise a nurse should remain with the child to offer support and be ready to repeat explanations of procedures. The child should be told what the examiner will do and why, and the sensations that will be felt during each procedure should be described. Showing the child the swab for the venereal disease tests and letting her touch it usually helps diminish her anxiety.

The child should be allowed to remove her own clothing if able. Otherwise a parent should remove it. Many school-age children respond best when a drape or sheet is not used; this allows them to see better what is happening and feel less secrecy about their genitals.[4]

The child should be asked if she would like to have a "special" person or object, such as a doll, present. During times of stress security objects can be comforting.

Intervention

After physical assessment all wounds are cleaned and dressed. Warm baths may be prescribed to relieve pain and decrease swelling. Instruction is given for the child or parents to observe for any bleeding or discharge and report this immediately. Prophylactic tetanus booster for the child with wounds and a single dose of polycillin for children who have had penile entry into any orifice is administered.[4]

Psychological intervention is essential to help the child and the family resolve their feelings about the event so that normal family living can resume as quickly as possible. In addition to explaining all procedures and the results obtained to parents, the nurse should warn them that the findings may not prove or disprove sexual assault. They will also need reassurance that most children successfully cope with the emotional and physical aspects of the situation without residual effects as long as the situation is dealt with calmly. Parents may need information about the child abuse laws of their state (the nurse should be familiar with these) and how other authorities will be involved.

Both the child and the parents are encouraged to talk about their feelings regarding the experience with one another or another trusted adult or health professional, but are discouraged from discussion with friends, schoolmates or work associates, who have a harder time understanding the situation. If the child previously has been left alone for any length of time during the day, parents should arrange for another female to be with her while they are away until some time has passed after the event. Most children do not require long-term medical care, although the nurse may maintain daily phone contact for a week. Then she may have periodic follow-up contact for several months to determine if counselling is needed or desired and how the family is adjusting. She may also need to support the family through legal proceedings.

References

1. ADM facts heard at family conference. ADAMHA News, 13 June 1980, p. 3
2. J. Breen. The molested young female. Evaluation and therapy of alleged rape. Pediatric Clinics of North America, August 1972, p. 718
3. K. Brown. How parents can best fight prejudice. Family Circle, 13 December 1977, p. S2
4. L. Gorline and M. Ray. Examining and caring for the child who has been sexually assaulted. American Journal of Maternal Child Nursing, Mar/Apr 1979, p. 110
5. M. Herbert. Problems of Childhood. Pan Books, 1975
6. K. Lehman. The sexually abused child. Nursing 77, May 1977, p. 68
7. G. Reed. Elective mutism in children: a reappraisal. British Journal of Child Psychology and Psychiatry, April 1963, p. 99
8. E. Rosenbaum and M. Kellman. Treatment of a selectively mute third-grade child. Journal of School Psychology, January 1973, p.26
9. R. Sullivan et al. Child Molestation. Academy of Family Practitioners, March 1979, p. 127
10. H. Wright, Jr. A clinical study of children who refuse to talk in school. Journal of the American Academy of Child Psychiatry, April 1968, p.603

Additional Recommended Reading

I. Berlin. Advocacy for Child Mental Health. Brunner/Mazel, 1975
M. Burgdorff. Legal rights of children, implications for nurses. In Symposium on Child Psychiatric Nursing, E. McElroy, ed. Nursing Clinics of North America, September 1979, p. 405
A. Burgess and L. Holmstrom. Sexual trauma of children and adolescents. Nursing Clinics of North America, September 1975, p. 551
U. Capraro. Gynecologic examination in children and adolescents. Pediatric Clinics of North America, August 1972, p. 511
R. Colligan et al. Contingency management in the classroom treatment of long-term elective mutism: a case report. Journal of School Psychology, January 1977, p. 9
R. Gittelman. School phobic children. Today's Education, Nov/Dec 1976, p. 41
K. Keating. Are working mothers attempting too much? Better Homes and Gardens, October 1978
E. Kelly, Jr. School phobia: a review of theory and treatment. Psychology in the Schools, January 1973, p. 33
W. Kennedy. School phobia: rapid treatment of fifty cases. Journal of Abnormal Psychology, April 1965, p. 285
E. Parker et al. Social casework with elementary school children who do not talk in school. Social Work, May 1960, p. 64
B. Schmitt. School phobia — the great imitator: a pediatrician's viewpoint. Pediatrics, March 1971, p. 433
L. Schultz. Rape Victimology. Charles C Thomas, 1975

48 GROWTH AND DEVELOPMENT OF THE SCHOOL-AGE CHILD: MAINTAINING WELLNESS

by Elaine C. Smith, RN, PhD

The school-age period, 6 to 12 years, is characterized by slow but steady physical growth, refinement of neuromuscular skills, and rapid expansion of cognitive and social skills. It is a time for "doing" and mastering the ever-expanding world of things and people. During this period the foundations are laid for future adult roles in the world of work, recreation and social interaction.

Statistically, the school-age child has the lowest rates of mortality and serious morbidity of any age group.* In a health interview survey conducted in the United States, 95 per cent of this age group was reported to be in good or excellent physical health.[11]

The primary goal for the nurse in working with this age group is to promote optimal competencies within the child and to assist the child and parents to appreciate the importance of and the interrelationship between physical, intellectual, emotional and social competencies.

---

*1975 death rate per 100,000 population: Under 1 year = 1641.0; 1 to 4 years = 70.8; 5 to 9 years = 35.7; 10 to 14 years = 35.7; 15 to 19 years = 101.5.[12]

PHYSICAL DEVELOPMENT

To assess the physical competency of a school-age child, the nurse must be aware that each child has a unique growth pattern. Although the most obvious measures of physical growth are increases in height and weight, other indicators of normal development, such as neuromuscular ability, sensory organ development, tooth eruption and other measures, are included in a complete assessment of physical competency.

Body Proportions: General Appearance

Height and Weight During the early school-age period the child's progress in height and weight is relatively slow and steady at approximately 5.5 cm (2 in) per year for height and 2.5 kg (5.5 lbs) per year for weight.

Boys are an average of an inch taller and two pounds heavier than girls in the early school-age period. (The average weight in early school-age years is 40 to 50 pounds and the average height is 44 to 48 inches.) The yearly increment in height and weight is comparable for boys and girls through age 9, when it begins increasing more rapidly for girls than for boys. By age 12 girls are an inch taller than boys and two pounds heavier. This preadolescent growth spurt for girls, beginning between 10 and 12 years, is an initial sign of pubertal maturation. Boys typically have to wait another two years for the acceleration in growth; that is, between 12 and 14 years.

Although a slow and steady growth pattern applies to school-age children as a population group, a given child may not follow it precisely. Growth charts (Chapter 13) provide for individualization of the assessment in that increases in height and weight are plotted sequentially from year to year. Growth is not constant. Periods of acceleration occur at different times in any group of children, with the overall pattern evening out over time. Often children experience an acceleration in height during the spring and in weight during the fall of the year.

As with other assessment tools, growth charts are effective only if plotted and interpreted correctly. Marked deviations from the growth chart curve require further evaluation. Moderate deviations may be the result of individual growth patterns and may need further follow-up if they persist. Untoward deviations in height or weight are more frequently the result of illnesses than their precursor. Consequently, these measures have limited value as a screening device for early identification of health problems.

Anticipatory Guidance: Height and Weight
Because school-age children may not receive annual health assessments, the school physical examination for the first grade is an opportune time for the nurse to discuss expectations about increases in height and weight with children and parents. With the advent of regular school attendance the child is faced, usually for the first time, with large numbers of children his age. Comparisons of self to others are inevitable. Children and parents should be helped to understand that genetic endowment, nutrition and exercise are major determinants of increases in height and weight in the *healthy* child.

The height and weight chart should be reviewed with the child and parents. Parents can be taught how to weigh and measure the child accurately so that together they can plot the child's growth between health assessment visits. The child's birthday is an opportune time for plotting height and weight. With this activity,

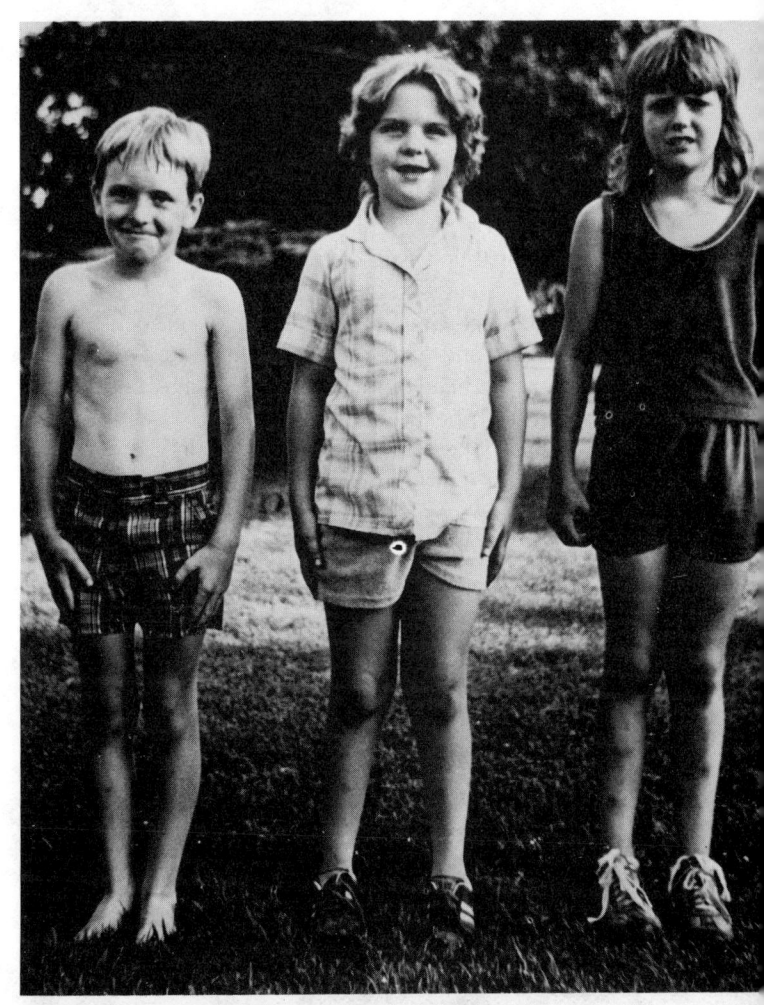

These three nine year olds exemplify the typical variations in size of children the same age during the school years.

the child can attain a sense of accomplishment through knowing his exact growth over time and learn a valuable lesson about the usefulness of self-comparison as a yardstick for progress. The natural tendency is to compare self to others, and the child this age needs to learn the value of comparison of his own progress over time.

Body Composition Body composition, as measured by the percentage of body weight attributed to organ weight, muscle mass, body fat and extracellular fluid, changes little during the school-age period. Body fat remains at approximately 15 per cent of total body weight in the school-age child. Muscle mass and extracellular fluid increase by 1 to 2 per cent at this age, while organ weight decreases by 1 to 2 per cent. Until the adolescent growth spurt, body composition for boys and girls is comparable.

The lymphatic tissues such as tonsils and adenoids grow rapidly during the school-age period, with growth reaching a peak toward the end of the period. Thereafter, involution of lymphatic tissue occurs.

Skeletal Growth The rate of growth of the trunk and extremities continues to exceed that of the head during the school-age period. Although head circumference increases little, remodeling of facial bones occurs. The frontal sinuses, present in rudimentary form from birth, become visible by x-ray during the early school years, and the other sinuses enlarge. Because of facial bone remodeling, the eustachian tube gradually assumes a more downward, forward and inward direction than previously.

By age 10 or 11 years, the distance from the crown of the head to the symphysis pubis is approximately equal to the distance from the symphysis to the sole of the foot, and remains so thereafter. Because of these variations in the rate of growth between the head, trunk and extremities, the center of gravity of the body with erect posture moves from a point just below the umbilicus at age 5 to below the crest of the ilium by 13 years. Improved balance of the older school-age child is attributed to this lower center of gravity.

The overall bodily appearance of school-age children also changes — they tend to look thinner than preschool children and adolescents. As skeletal growth progresses, the "rounded" shoulders, slight lordosis and prominent abdomen of the early school years gradually give way by the end of the period to a more erect posture.

Anticipatory Guidance: Body Composition and Skeletal Growth Knowledge about body composition and skeletal growth can provide the nurse with a base for guiding parents and children in dealing with selected health problems that might occur during this age period. If enlarged tonsils and adenoids or susceptibility to ear infections are of concern, simple explanations about the growth patterns of lymphoid tissue and the direction in which the eustachian tube lies are helpful. Understanding that normal growth can alleviate selected health problems can be especially helpful to the child. The awareness that no relative increase in body fat is expected until the adolescent growth spurt can alert parent and child to a potential problem with obesity if the child starts to "fill out."

Adults (parents or teachers) may become unduly concerned about the posture of an early school-age child, when, in actuality, normal growth will alleviate the "rounded" shoulders, lordosis and prominent abdomen of that age group. Posture should be considered satisfactory if a straight line can be visualized to pass from the front of the ear through the shoulder and the greater trochanter to the anterior part of the longitudinal arch of the foot (Fig. 48–1). Seeing that the child has regular physical activity and regular changes in position when sedentary is more effective in promoting good posture than exhortations to stand straight. A healthy,

Note the changes in posture from preschool to school age and to adolescence.

rested child typically assumes a balanced, comfortable posture.

Excessive exercise to develop a specific skill that places undue strain on a bone or joint should be avoided. Because the bones are still ossifying, they cannot tolerate pressure and muscle pull as well as mature bones can. In addition, growth of bone, muscle, tendon and support tissues may not be synchronous, especially during the preadolescent growth spurt. For these reasons, children are more prone to injury from excessive exercise than adults. Caution also needs to be exercised in carrying heavy loads. Heavy loads, such as books or a pack of newspapers, should be shifted periodically.

Motor Development

The word that best describes the neuromuscular development of the school-age period is *refinement*. The basic mechanisms involved in neuromuscular skills already have been acquired; however, they are rudimentary. The school-age period is the time for refinement and expansion of those skills.

Gross Motor Skills Physical activity seems to be a natural and strong impulse for the school-age child. The child seems driven to "be doing" something with his hands, feet and body. During the early school years before refinement of motor control, physical activity seems somewhat aimless, as can be observed in the restlessness of the first grader. By the time the child is ready to embark into adolescence, this physical activity is more controlled and directed toward specific goals such as those found in sports.

The six basic gross motor skills that are refined during this age period are running, jumping, sequencing foot movements, balancing, throwing and catching. Steady improvement in all six basic motor skills is seen in the school-age child if he is given the opportunity to practice them.

Most children practice these skills during play and delight in the experience as well as in their accomplishments in skill development. The games of childhood, which seem to pass from generation to generation, provide experience in the basic gross motor skills. Examples include running in tag, hide-and-seek and red rover; jumping, sequencing foot movements and balancing in skipping, jumprope, hopscotch, bicycling, skating, skate boarding, scrimmaging

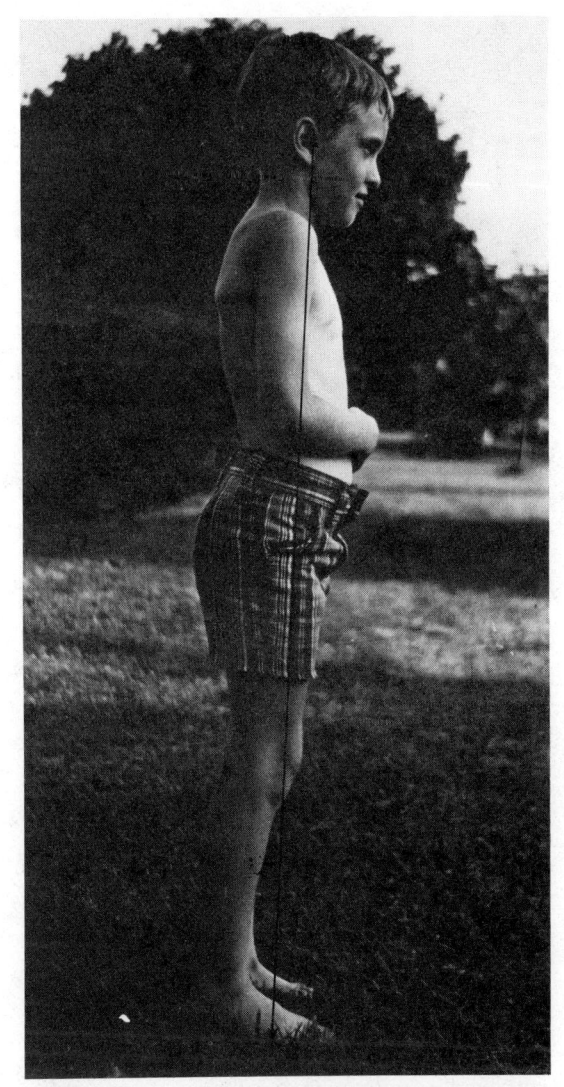

Figure 48-1 A straight line that passes from the front of the ear through the shoulder and the greater trochanter to the anterior part of the longitudinal arch of the foot indicates satisfactory posture during the school-age period.

and tug of war; and throwing and catching in many games. In most games of school-age children coordination of the basic skills is required and complex movements evolve.

Even in physical activities other than play the school-age child seems intent on testing out what can be accomplished with his body. While he is engaged in a motor activity such as walking down the street, a puddle is to walk in, to see how big a splash or how small a ripple can be made. An ice-covered sidewalk is to see how far one can slide on two feet without falling. This child explores the world with and through his body.

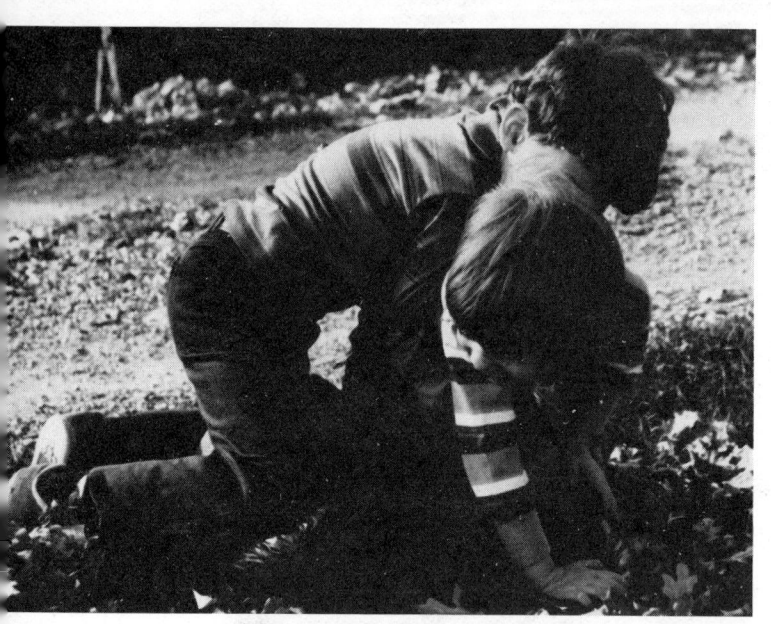

Scrimmaging provides experience in gross motor skills. (Photograph by Dave Trainor.)

Play of a child changes over time in keeping with the development of motor skills. The 6-year-old has boundless energy and rudimentary skills. Consequently, play is active, somewhat disorganized and requires rather simple skills such as running, jumping, throwing, skipping. The 7-year-old seems more cautious, quiet and intent on acquiring skills such as sequencing foot movements, balancing on a bicycle, throwing and catching. The 8-year-old has greater smoothness in movements and becomes more involved in group activities than previously. The 9-year-old works intently on and takes great pride in demonstrating motor skills and strength. Competitive team sports are of interest, and disparity between the skills of individuals becomes more apparent than previously. During the 10th through 12th year muscular control and skills in all gross motor areas are established. Just as the school-age period was ushered in on a child who experienced a great need for physical activity, it ends on the same note. The 11- to 12-year-old is energetic, although sporadically, and very active physically. Because of the preadolescent growth spurt this increased physical activity may appear more clumsy than a year or so earlier.

Fine Motor Skills Although the fine motor skills lag behind gross motor skills, they progress approximately at the same rate. Six-year-olds can cut with scissors and can paste, can button and zipper their clothes, and can copy a triangle, draw a man with 12 details and use a pencil for printing. However, skill in these activities tends to be uneven in development, and they may be performed clumsily. The 7-year-old ties his shoes, copies a diamond and draws a man with 16 details. At 8 years, cursive writing begins, and at 9 eye-hand coordination is well developed, and the child can manipulate objects skillfully enough to benefit from hand crafts.

The reaction time or speed in performing fine motor skills, such as tapping, turning small objects and removing and placing pegs, increases rapidly from 6 to 9 or 10 years, after which the rate of improvement gradually slows. Accuracy of movement improves markedly from 5 to 9 years and then less rapidly to adolescence. Girls tend to have better dexterity of hands and fingers than boys and tend to perform fine motor skills at a greater speed and more accurately than boys.[15]

Anticipatory Guidance: Gross and Fine Motor Skills The healthy school-age child will pursue gross and fine motor activities if provided with the opportunity. Parents should be encouraged to provide these opportunities for a variety of reasons. The benefits of physical activity are numerous, including the promotion of bone growth, enhancement of learning and the promotion of fitness and a physically active life style.

Although the genes determine the basic growth and shape of long bones, environmental factors are influential also. The complex development of cartilage, established embryologically, into mature adult bones entails growth in length and width, changes in bone density and maintenance of shape and integrity. Although the exact mechanisms are not clear, intermittent energetic compression of the entire cartilage, aided by gravity, weight-bearing, and muscle contractions, is indispensable in keeping children's bones growing at the required rate.[2] Bone density also is influenced by physical activity, with inactivity resulting in deossification. Activity has even more influence on bone density than nutrition does. Only extreme deficiency of calcium and vitamin D will cause deossification, while it is often found on x-ray after only a few weeks of inactivity.

Periods of physical activity also enhance aca-

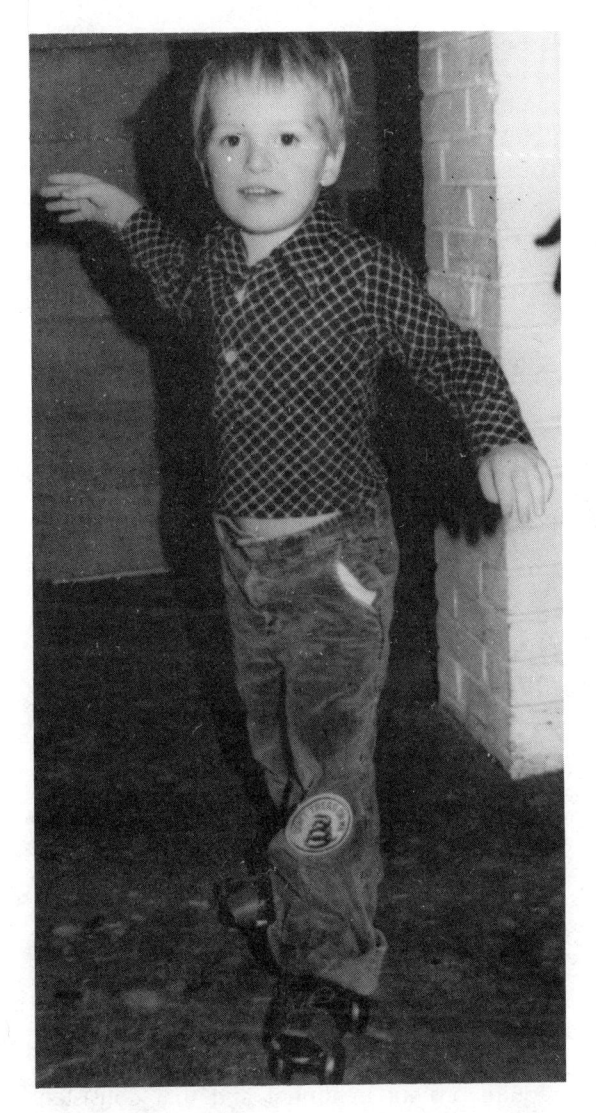

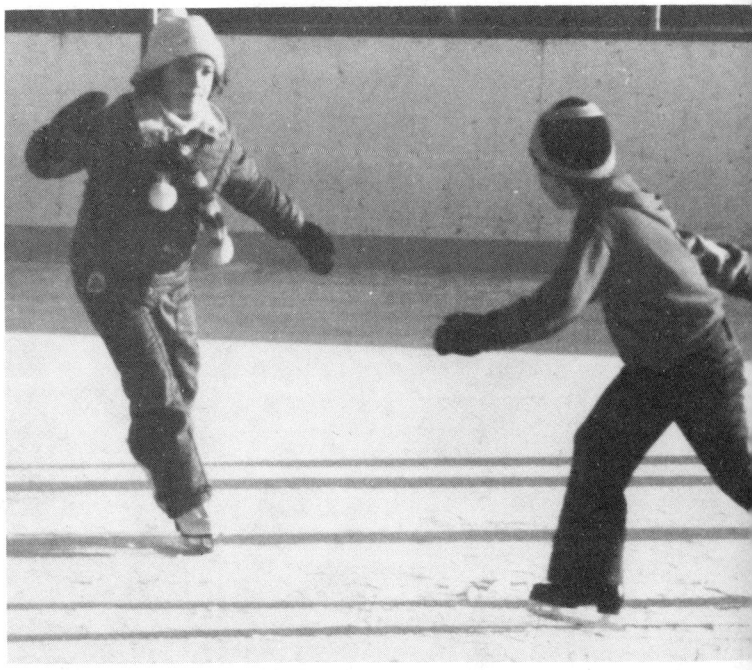

The 6-year-old (left), although energetic, has only rudimentary motor skills, while the 11-year-old (top) has established control of motor skills that makes him look organized and graceful.

demic learning. Schools have long recognized this phenomenon and have provided recess periods for gross motor activity. Research also has demonstrated the positive influence of such motor activity on learning. One of the largest and most notable studies showed that in a school in which classroom time was decreased by one-third and that time was devoted to physical education, children performed better academically than their counterparts whose school maintained the regular schedule. Even though the time of instruction was decreased by a third, the children did as well or better on scholastic tests than their counterparts.[1]

Physical fitness is almost synonymous with physical activity. A physically fit child who finds pleasure in gross motor activity usually carries this fitness and pleasure into adulthood. Childhood provides a unique opportunity for promoting healthful exercise habits, because of the child's propensity for delighting in gross motor activity.

The opportunities parents provide for gross and fine motor activities need not be elaborate nor expensive. A great deal of gross physical activity can take place in a relatively small space. Walking or jogging can be a family affair. Advantage can be taken of community programs and parks.

For fine motor activities, paper, pencils, crayons, water colors, scissors, string, beads, empty food cartons and so forth can be implements for creative activities.

The child should be encouraged to pursue physical activities. Limits may need to be set on television viewing if it interferes with more positive pursuits. Increased competency in skills

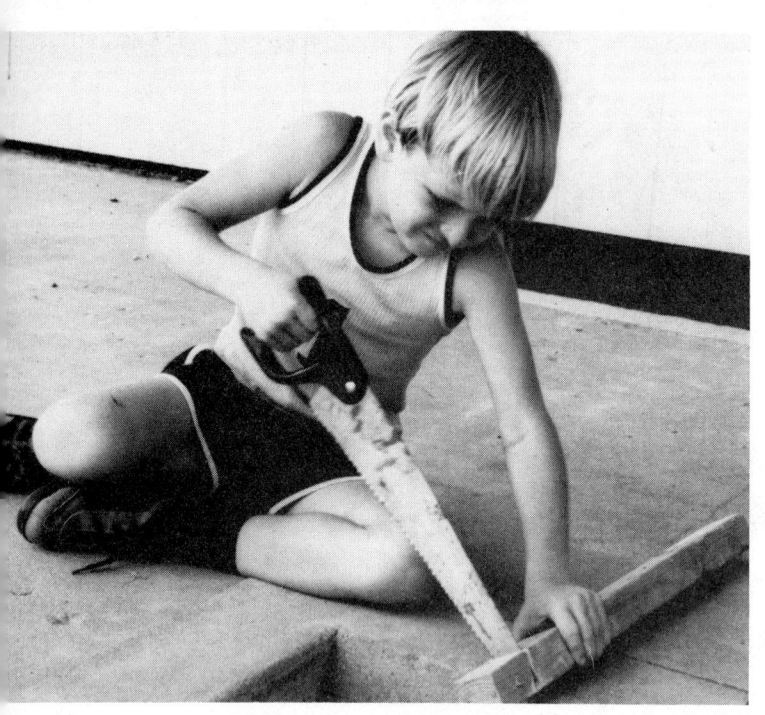

The 9-year-old has coordination of eye and hand that allows him to manipulate objects and benefit from a variety of projects and crafts.

should be rewarded by praise that is deserved, but not exaggerated.

Sensory Organ Development

A major thrust of the school-age period is exploration of the world. Normal development of the senses, especially those of sight and hearing, are crucial to this exploration. Therefore, the competency of the sense organs is vital to the child's overall development. No assessment of the school-age child is complete without a careful examination of the eyes and ears.

Nearly 75 per cent of ocular development is completed during the first three years of life. The final growth phase, affecting only the posterior segment of the eye, proceeds at a very slight and steady pace until approximately 15 years. The crystalline lens is the only component of the eye that continues to grow throughout life. Its growth, associated with alterations in its shape, pliability and refractive index, has important implications for visual acuity.

The normal hyperopia of the young child gradually diminishes during the early school-age period owing to the growth of the posterior segment of the eye globe. If the eye axis grows to be longer than average, myopia results. This refractive error, which tends to manifest itself between 8 and 10 years of age, usually increases until ocular and body growth are completed.

The ear and the sense of hearing are well developed by school age. Overall mild hearing losses (not exceeding 25 decibels) usually do not produce communication problems for the school-age child. (Chpater 43 discusses hearing losses and visual losses in detail.)

Anticipatory Guidance: Sensory Organs Parents need to be aware of the symptoms of visual problems and should be encouraged to follow through to have them corrected. If corrective lenses are prescribed, every effort should be made to help the child look upon them in positive terms and to encourage him to wear them as directed.

Eyestrain should be avoided for the general well-being of the child. Causes of eyestrain include using poor lighting (either too little or glare) and poor posture while reading, reading too-small print, reading in a moving vehicle, doing close work or watching television or films for prolonged periods without rest or change of focus. The child should be taught how to rest the eyes by simply changing the gaze from near to distant vision (and vice versa) for a few minutes. To prevent hearing problems, parents need to be aware that middle ear infections require prompt treatment and that consistent follow-up and hearing tests are indicated for recurrent otitis media. Immunizations also should be encouraged as primary prevention for complications of the communicable diseases that may cause nerve (perceptive) hearing losses.

The parents and child should be informed that trying to remove wax from the ear canal with a hairpin or similar implement probably will only impact the wax more firmly against the tympanic membrane and may even damage the membrane.

Eye-Hand Coordination

The development of eye-hand coordination is related to development of gross and fine motor skills. By age 9 years, the child works well with both hands concurrently on large and small motor tasks but shows preference for either the right or left hand.

Lateral preference for using left or right hand, foot and eye is established during the school-age period. Preference is determined by asking the child to perform a task such as throwing a ball or writing for the hand, kicking a ball for the foot, and looking at a distant object through a short paper tube for the eye. Children of early school-age tend to show mixed preferences, but by the end of the period most children have established preferences for all three body parts. In the establishment of laterality, foot preference seems stronger than hand preference, while eye preference seems the weakest and the last established.[3]

Ability to discriminate left from right on their own bodies is achieved about two years before hand preference is established. Almost all children can make this discrimination on their own body by age 7, and all can by 11. Discrimination of left and right on others follows self-discrimination.[5] The perceptual ability to imitate the movements of another person standing facing the child, however, presents a more difficult task, and the skill may not be acquired until adolescence.

Anticipatory Guidance: Eye-Hand Coordination The child should be encouraged to participate in activities that promote eye-hand coordination. The lateralization for hand, foot and eye preference is a natural process that gradually evolves over time. Parents and teachers should not pressure a child to use either right or left hand, foot or eye. The physical activities that promote the development and refinement of gross and fine motor skills are the same activities that promote eye-hand coordination and lateralization.

Teeth

One of the most obvious developmental milestones to occur during the school-age period is the loss of all 20 primary teeth and their "replacement" by 30 of the 32 permanent teeth. The last two permanent teeth to erupt, the third molars (wisdom teeth), lag behind the other teeth by an average of eight or more years, not erupting until the twenties. All further discussion of tooth development excludes these third molars.

The eruption or appearance of a tooth is only one aspect of tooth development, albeit the most obvious. A review of the total process of tooth development is important to an accurate assessment of the school-age child.

For each of the 52 teeth (20 primary and 32 permanent), development of the tooth matrix and its calcification proceeds in the same orderly manner from crown to roots. The time lag between the start of the calcification until eruption of each permanent tooth is six to nine years, depending on the particular tooth. Full development of the root structure takes another two to four years. Calcification of the first molar, the first permanent tooth to erupt at age 6, begins in utero; all permanent teeth start calcification by age 3 years and all are completely calcified by about 8. The first teeth to complete root development are the central incisors at 8½ to 11 years, while the last to complete root development are the second molars at 15 to 16½ years.

Because of the length of time between the initiation of calcification and the actual emergence of a tooth, its soundness at eruption is not as dependent on current health and nutritional status as it is dependent on previous health status. If local trauma, severe nutritional deficiency, severe infection and high temperature or ingestion of tetracycline at an early age has disrupted normal tooth development, the tooth appears with hypocalcified opaque white areas or dark yellow discolored areas.

Although severe and prolonged undernutrition may delay eruption of the teeth, tooth development is largely impervious to environmental factors. Genetic factors are the major sources of differences between individuals in tooth development and eruption. For example, siblings tend to resemble each other more in the timing of eruption than do nonrelated individuals. Tooth development in females is slightly ahead of males, as is that of United States blacks as compared with whites.

Because teeth and bones are of different embryological origins, there is little correlation between height or onset of puberty with tooth development. Tooth development, therefore, seems relatively independent of other body systems.[8] (See Chapter 13.)

The normal sequence of the emergence of permanent teeth and shedding of primary (deciduous) teeth are important to proper occlusion; that is, the alignment of the chewing surface of the maxillary (upper) teeth to the mandibular (lower) teeth when the jaws are closed. Symmetry is evident in the eruption of teeth on the right and left sides of the jaw, but slight asymmetry is evident for the maxillary and mandibular teeth.

Anticipatory Guidance: Teeth Preventive care is essential between the beginning of calcification and the eruption of the teeth. The child should become increasingly involved in explanations about preventive practices and in assuming responsibility for his own dental health during the school-age period.

The 6- to 8-year-old does not usually possess the required fine motor skill to be totally responsible for flossing the teeth but should be able to do a fairly adequate job of brushing them. Nor does this age child have the cognitive skills to appreciate the rationale behind the preventive measures for increasing the resistance of the teeth and reducing bacterial activity and amount of fermentable carbohydrates in the mouth. Neither is the child of this age future oriented enough to appreciate preventive practices. However, the child is still very dependent on adults and looks to parents and teachers for guidance. Good dental health practices can be instituted and will be followed at this age because they are the "thing do do" or the "rules." Teachers can be very influential and effective during this period in promoting good dental health practices.

From the age of 9 on, the child has the fine motor and cognitive skills and is future oriented enough not only to assume total responsibility for dental health practices but also to understand simple explanations and appreciate the rationale for preventive dental health practices.

Premature loss of primary teeth due to dental caries or accident can be prevented. Parents need to be aware of the importance of the primary teeth. Dental hygiene and regular visits to the dentist should be instituted during the preschool period so as to prevent the premature loss of these teeth to decay.

Sleep and Rest

At the beginning of the school-age period the child usually averages 11 to 12 hours sleep per night. The amount of sleep per night gradually diminishes to an average of 9 to 10 per night at age 12. A healthy child ordinarily seeks the amount of sleep required to meet health needs.

If a preschool child has developed the habit of retiring for sleep at a late hour and sleeping late in the morning, difficulties can be anticipated with the start of regular school attendance. Parents can be advised that this difficulty can be resolved by making the retirement hour earlier and earlier over a period of several months before the start of school.

To promote sleep, a period of quiet activity just prior to bedtime is advised. An exciting or stimulating television program is not included in the category of quiet activity. Overstimulation, either physical, mental or emotional, can have an adverse effect on the restful sleep that is the norm for the school-age child.

If a child who usually sleeps well experiences sleep problems without apparent reason, he may be upset or worried about some aspect of school or home life. This cue should be followed up with the child and efforts made to alleviate the problem.

Elimination Skills

Most healthy school-age children experience no difficulties with elimination skills. Bowel and bladder control are usually well established. However, when a child is under undue stress temporary lapses are not unusual. For discussion of problems with bowel and bladder control see Chapter 49.

Nutrition

As has been noted previously, the school-age years are characterized as a period of relatively slow and steady growth. The exception is the preadolescent growth spurt at about 10 to 12 years for girls and 12 to 14 years for boys.

Until the adolescent growth spurt, the nutritional needs of the child are relatively stable, with the need slightly increased for quantity (to accommodate the increases in height and weight) rather than quality. The adolescent growth spurt is accompanied by an increase in appetite and total caloric needs, with the budding adolescent being noted for having an insatiable appetite.

Proportionately, however, in calculating the daily needs for calories, protein, and water per

TABLE 48–1 NATIONAL NUTRITION SURVEY MEAN INTAKE COMPARED TO RECOMMENDATION FOR AGES 6 THROUGH 11 YEARS

Nutrients	Intake*	Recommendations†
Calories	2060	2360
Protein	76 gm	36 gm
Calcium	1073 mg	900 mg
Iron	10 mg	12 mg
Vitamin A	4088 IU	3500 IU
Vitamin C	75 mg	40 mg

*First Health and Nutrition Survey, 1971–72.[10]
†Based on recommended daily dietary allowances, Food and Nutrition Board, National Academy of Sciences–National Research Council, revised 1974.

kilogram of body weight, a slight and steady decrease in requirements is seen. Calorie requirements decrease from approximately 90 per kg (41 per pound) at age 6 years to 70 per kg (32 per pound) at age 12 years; protein from approximately 3 gm/kg to 2 gm/kg; and water from 100 ml/kg (1½ ounces per pound) to 75 ml/kg (¾ ounce per pound).[17] In a well-balanced diet for this age, as well as for other ages, the approximate distribution of calories is 15 per cent protein; 35 per cent for fat and 50 per cent for carbohydrates.[17]

Just as the school-age period is noted for being probably the healthiest of any age period, it also is one with relatively few nutritional problems. The results of the biochemical tests included in the federally sponsored nutrition survey in 1971–72 indicated that fewer school-age children had nutritional deficiencies than those in age groups that precede or succeed this age. In the age group of 6 to 11 years inclusive, less than 5 per cent had low values for hematocrit, serum iron, serum protein or serum vitamin A. Ten to 15 per cent of the age group had low values of transferrin saturation, which is a measure for binding and transport of iron. Approximately 16 per cent of white children below the poverty level were deficient, while approximately 10 per cent of the white children above the poverty level and blacks at both levels were deficient in transferrin saturation.[10]

Table 48–1 compares the survey findings for mean intake of selected nutrients with the recommended intake for the school-age group. This comparison indicates that the school-age children in this probability sample had a slight deficit in iron and total calories. They exceeded the recommendations in all other nutrients, especially in protein and vitamin C. Although the deficits were not severe, they could be assumed to lead to deficiencies if prolonged.

Deficits in total calories especially are problematic. Even when the total sample was divided into groups by race and economic level, the white above-poverty level group averaged only 2118 calories rather than 2360 as recommended. The black below-poverty level group only averaged 1690 calories, a marked deficit. A marked deficit in calcium and iron also was evident in this latter group. The survey would seem to indicate that as a population group the school-age child seems relatively well nourished, with the possible exception of iron and total calories. However, segments of this population group may experience severe deficiencies.

Information about eating habits as well as kind and amount of food eaten is essential to the total evaluation of nutritional status. Snacks are common for school-age children and often consist of empty-calorie foods that can interfere with proper nutrition.

Various forms of interviews are used to assess nutritional status (see Chapter 13). From the interviews, an assessment can be made of a child's diet. The results should be compared to the recommended food intake and average size of servings for a child of that age (see Appendix V for recommendations). This comparison should disclose possible deficiencies that will need to be included in anticipatory guidance.

The sufficiency of the food intake cannot be assessed adequately or altered appropriately without considering the family's cultural background, financial status and food preferences. The community cultural and socioeconomic status, along with food availability within the community, also affect the amount and kinds of foods that the family and child can obtain.

In anticipatory guidance these factors must be taken into consideration, as must community resources available.

The concern of the federal government for the nutritional status of its youth has long been evident. The first legislation of significance to the school-age group was the National School Lunch Act of 1946, which supports and promotes nutritious school lunches at reasonable cost or free to those who cannot afford it. In 1966 a similar program to support and promote school breakfasts was initiated. By 1975, 80 per cent of the public and nonprofit private schools in the nation participated in the school lunch program.[7]

Anticipatory Guidance: Nutrition As a child enters school and moves from the confines of the home and its immediate environment, other influences become increasingly important to the child's health practices. These influences can be both positive and negative. Ideally, the teacher, the school nurse and perhaps peers will have a positive influence on health practices, including eating habits.

Health education is an important and integral part of a school curriculum. As late as 1978, the American Academy of Pediatrics reaffirmed its support for health education in the schools. Although school nurses can contribute directly to the health education program by teaching selected content, a more effective role is to serve as a consultant and resource person for teachers. Health education, to be truly effective, must be a consistent and integral part of daily classroom instruction — something no school nurse could possibly accomplish or schedule.

Education in nutrition and in dental health overlaps and therefore instruction is combined for these. An example is the fact that nutritious snacks also promote dental health. Suggestions about anticipatory guidance for dental health discussed previously apply equally to nutrition education.

In health education about nutrition, cultural factors play a greater role than in most other topics of health education. Children need to learn that a great variety of foods, taken in proper quantities, will meet their daily requirements in nutrition. Respect for their own cultural heritage and for that of others can be an indirect benefit of well-planned nutrition education.

Because school-age children do not have control over meal preparation at home, nutrition education should extend into the community so as to include the parents. School-age children do have control, however, over intake at meals and need to have sufficient knowledge to select appropriate types and quantities of available foods. Breakfast and snack intake needs special emphasis, because it is often deficient in quantity or quality.

Obesity may be a problem in the school-age population as well as other populations. In addition to eating excessively, the obese child often does not exercise as much as the average-weight child. A vicious circle may ensue; the more obese the child, the more difficult it is for him to keep up with the other children in physical activity, and the more he resorts to eating as consolation. Motivating the child to reduce may be difficult. Often having the child keep a daily diary of everything eaten will provide the basis for an individualized regimen of diet and exercise.

INTELLECTUAL AND LANGUAGE DEVELOPMENT

Although physical development during the school-age period is characterized as slow and steady, cognitive development is characterized as rapid and expanding. It is as though physical development in general is held somewhat in abeyance so that all the child's energies can be directed toward cognitive development. That is not to say that physical development ceases; it continues unabated and contributes much to cognitive development. Neurological development, including refinement of the corpus callosum of the brain at age 7 or 8, promotes the expansion of cognitive competency.

Intelligence

Intelligence is generally considered to be the ability to learn or acquire and retain knowledge. Included is the ability to learn from experience and to apply previously learned knowledge to a new situation. Intelligence is assessed by various tests. The Stanford-Binet test is widely used and is established as one of the most reliable intelligence tests. The Wechsler Intelligence Scale for Children is used widely also.

Results of intelligence tests must be interpret-

The American Academy of Pediatrics believes that it is necessary to reaffirm its support for the concept of school health education, from kindergarten through grade 12, for all schoolchildren in the United States.

A basic concept of pediatrics is prevention, and health education is a basic element in the delivery of comprehensive health care. The public is continually bombarded by the media about the high cost of medical care and the overutilization and incorrect use of medical facilities. The media also writes about the problems of increasing promiscuity and illegitimacy; the money wasted on quackery; practices that are detrimental to the health of people in the United States; and the lag in the dissemination of new health information and facts to the public. The Committee on School Health believes that community health education programs, of which school health education programs from kindergarten through grade 12 are an integral part, are one of the most viable methods to help alleviate these and similar problems. Therefore, the Committee on School Health makes the following recommendations and urges action for them at state and local levels.

1. Health education is a basic education subject, and it should be taught as such. Health education is compatible with other traditional subjects and can enhance the contribution that other basic subjects make to general life experience, understanding, and skills.

2. Planned, integrated programs of comprehensive health education should be required for students from kindergarten through grade 12. Instruction should be given by teachers qualified to teach health education. The health curriculum should be planned and be appropriate for the age and maturity of the children at each grade level. A comprehensive health education program should include the following subjects: courses that yield an understanding of basic biology, physiology, and genetics; accident prevention; venereal disease; alcoholism; mental health; parenting; sex education; drug abuse; environmental and consumer health; and preventive medicine.

3. The health education program should help teach students to use the facts and the concepts discussed for healthful living and for making knowledgeable decisions to solve personal, family, and community health problems.

4. Financial support must be assured for health education programs because proper funding is critical in developing effective programs. Local boards of education and state and federal government bodies dealing with education must be convinced to continue or increase their portion of funding for health education programs. Funding should also be sought from corporations, foundations, and private and governmental agencies that have specific interests (such as heart, cancer, alcoholism, or mental health). The most effective way to provide education about these specific subjects is to incorporate them into a well-planned, comprehensive health education curriculum.

5. Comprehensive health education programs in elementary and secondary schools should be directed by qualified health educators functioning in consultation and cooperation with school personnel, parents, students, physicians, and health agencies in the community.

6. Health education should be a part of every elementary and secondary teachers' training program. Professional preparation programs in health education should be developed in the schools of education. These schools should set high standards and have requirements as exacting as those requirements for other fields of instruction. All teachers should be required to complete courses in health science.

7. School districts, other public agencies, the medical community, and private agencies should intensify their health education programs for adults as part of a coordinated community health education effort.

COMMITTEE ON SCHOOL HEALTH

Donald E. Cook, M.D., *Chairman;* Conrad L. Andringa, M.D.; Karl W. Hess, M.D.; Leonard L. Kishner, M.D.; Samuel R. Leavitt, M.D.; Stanley F. Novak, M.D.; Kenneth D. Rogers, M.D.; J. Ward Stackpole, M.D.; Casper Wiggins, M.D.

Statement of the Committee on School Health of the American Academy of Pediatrics. Published in *Pediatrics*, 1 July 1978, p. 117. (Copyright American Academy of Pediatrics, 1978.)

---

ed with caution, especially the results of group testing, the usual testing method. These tests are encumbered by the problem common to any paper or pencil test — their results depend on the motivation to do well on the test and the well-being of the child at the time the test is given. Reading skill, practice on specific skills involved in the test, as well as luck in guessing correct answers, affect results; the tests may not be not truly reflective of mental ability.

Since the late 1960s, intelligence tests have been the subject of controversy, primarily because of misuse of test results to "label" and track children educationally. Blacks, Hispanics and other children not exposed to white mainstream middle class experiences are at a disadvantage in taking the tests. Much effort is being devoted currently to development of tests that will not discriminate against underprivileged or culturally deprived children.[13]

Anticipatory Guidance: Intelligence Intelligence tests of whatever variety should be considered only as screening tools to be used to help the child reach full potential. IQ can and does change. If used appropriately, the tests can help the parent and the child recognize the child's strengths and weaknesses and set realistic goals and expectations for the child.

The sense of competency in one's own ability is important to the school-age child. Whatever his mental ability, a child needs to be appreciated for what he can do competently. Comparison of the child's own accomplishments and competency over time helps him to see his own progress and to acquire self-esteem.

Parents can promote intellectual competency by stimulating the child's desire for achievement and by offering a variety of experiences that foster mental development. The values the family holds about intellectual pursuits profoundly affect a child's achievement orientation, as well as the experiences to which he is exposed. Certainly a child who is exposed to books and magazines in the home and sees parents reading with interest will have an orientation to achievement and intellectual pursuits different from that of a child who is exposed to neither situation.

Cognitive Development

During the school-age period, the child's thought processes undergo dramatic shifts. According to Piaget, at the beginning of the school-age period these thought processes are characterized as intuitive thought; they move into concrete operations at about 7 or 8 years of age and from there into formal operations at about 11 or 12 years.

The Intuitive Stage With intuitive thought (6 to 7 years), thinking is based on immediate, unanalyzed relations between any particular environmental phenomenon and the child's own viewpoint. For example, to this child anything that moves is alive. Conversations tend to be monologues because the child thinks others think as he does and can even read his mind.

The child may recognize two or more characteristics of something in the environment but focuses his attention or thought on only one characteristic at a time. He cannot consider wholes and parts at the same time; attention is focused either on the whole or a part but not on both simultaneously.

These characteristics of intuitive thought lead the child to make gross misinterpretations of phenomena. They do not provide the cognitive tools for organizing the world of people, places and things into systems. Those cognitive tools are provided through "operations" — first, concrete operations for dealing with people, places and things that can be experienced through the senses, and then formal operations for dealing with abstracts and for playing with ideas.

The Concrete Operations Stage During the stage of *concrete operations* (8 to 10 years), the child steps outside his own thought processes and realizes that his way of thinking is not the only way. Real conversation and sharing of information become possible. Gradually, the egocentric and fluctuating rules for games and behavior give way to democratically derived rules for games and reasonable expectations for behavior.

The child can now decenter, or take into consideration more than one characteristic or attribute of an object or environmental phenomenon at the same time. He can consider the various parts of a whole while maintaining the concept of the whole. Other important characteristics of the child's thought processes are that he can retrace the steps he took mentally in arriving at a conclusion. He also realizes that there may be more than one way of arriving at the same conclusion.

When the child enters the stage of concrete operations, all characteristics of the stage are not necessarily available to him in all situations. For example, the child discovers the conservation of substance at 7 or 8 years by realizing that changes in shape do not change the quantity of such substances as clay. However, he does not discover the conservation of weight until he is about 9 or 10 years old and does not discover the conservation of volume until about 11 or 12 (measured by displacement of water when an object is immersed).

Concrete operations not only have a powerful influence on the acquisition of knowledge for the school-age child but also profoundly affect his emotional and social life. Illustrative of the changes seen in the emotional and social life of the child during this coordination of concrete operations are the child's concepts about causality and chance, moral feelings and judgments, use of rules for games, and perceptions of reality.

Prior to age 8 or 9 years, the child's concept of chance is lacking. Everything has a reason — often based on immediate, unanalyzed relations between environmental events. For example, falling down and skinning a knee may be attributed to disobeying Mother an hour or so earlier. Not only does everything have a reason, but because of the young child's egocentric thought patterns, the reason often centers on self. For example, the child may think a parent has become ill because the child angrily wished it so. With the realization at age 8 or 9 years of the concept of chance, life becomes much more benevolent for the child than previously.

In a similar manner, the changes in moral feelings and judgment make life more benevolent during the period of concrete operations than during the intuitive stage. For the 6- or 7-year-old, the many rules of behavior are immutable. Rules are based on what adults direct and are taken literally. The child is likely to judge an act in a unidirectional way as absolutely right or absolutely wrong. He is likely to consider that an act is bad if it elicits punishment, and he tends to be very harsh in the punishment he would prescribe for another child who has broken a rule.

As concrete operations become available to the child, the absolutes become tempered by the realization that the same act may be viewed in many different ways by different individuals. The intentions that prompted an act now are taken into consideration. Through interaction and cooperative endeavors with peers, the child develops respect for them and for himself and realizes that rules evolve through mutual consent and the democratic process of consensus. Rules are no longer absolute and immutable but can be changed by either mutual consent or extenuating circumstances. Punishment the child would recommend now becomes less harsh, more specific for the infraction, and is no longer considered absolutely necessary. Moral judgments are increasingly more independent of adults as the solidarity between peer groups of children grows and a morality based on cooperation develops.

Rules used for playing games also undergo the same type of change as do moral feelings.

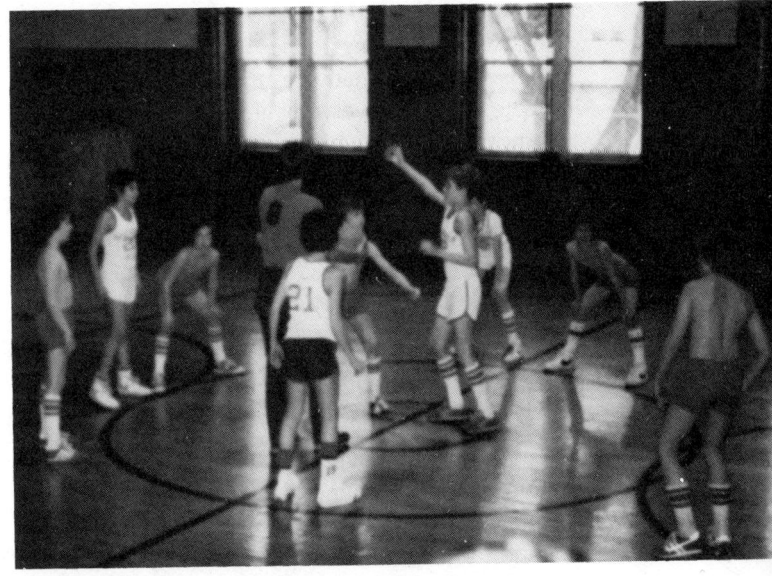

As the school-age child achieves the stage of concrete operations, play becomes more cooperative and team play involving rules becomes a popular activity. (Photograph by Charles William Jameson.)

As the child moves away from egocentric thinking and appreciates the viewpoints of others, he becomes increasingly capable of cooperative play and team play involving rules. This play is in contrast to that of the early school-age child, who likes to play games with rules but exhibits only a partial understanding of them and thinks the child with whom he is playing understands the rules in the same way he does. In actuality, the age-mate may have a completely different understanding of the rules. The young child plays the game as he understands it, without real concern for what others are doing. In the game nobody loses and everybody wins because the purpose of the game is to have fun in a group activity.

After age 7 or 8 years, games are characterized by increasing structure, with common observance of rules and mutual surveillance to make sure all players observe the rules. The spirit of the game is honest competition, with some players winning and others losing according to the rules. True communication, cooperative play and mutual respect are now possible. After age 10 or 11 years, handicaps are even added to games when appropriate, for to win over a less-skilled opponent is no win at all.

From ages 8 or 9, the behavior of the child also evidences an increased perceptive ability, with attendant self-criticism of activities such as drawing. Drawings consequently seem less creative and imaginative as the child tries to replicate reality. In everyday life, the age of 9 years is known as the age of erasures, in which the child demonstrates increased dissatisfaction with his efforts if his drawing does not appear realistic.

During the stage of concrete operations (8–10 years) the child works hard to discover how the world of people, places and things, which he can experience through his senses, functions. A major deficiency, however, is the child's inability to work with abstractions, hypotheses and propositions removed from the concrete and present observation; that is, to play with ideas. This deficiency is removed at age 11 or 12 years as the child moves into adolescence and the stage of formal operations.

Anticipatory Guidance: Cognitive Development During the intuitive stage parents and teachers may utilize a variety of "think games" to nurture the child's development of concrete operations. (For example, several cups of different colors and progressive sizes may be used to help the child learn ranking and arrangement of objects by common characteristics; a variety of objects or pictures may be used to help the child learn to compare, contrast and classify items that are alike and different in some way.) Similarly, games can be used with the older child to help him master temporal and numerical concepts.

Parents should be encouraged to have patience and allow their school-age child to do some of his own problem-solving. They may need to be reminded that trial and error is a valuable part of learning problem-solving. Parents should not expect the school-age child to handle more than one big problem at a time, and they should be cautioned to expect some fluctuation in the school-ager's skill at problem mastery.

Play continues to be a necessary main activity if the school-age child is to progress cognitively. Through play, group games and peer interaction the child learns the cognitive concepts necessary to cooperation, compromise, persuasion and productivity. Parents may need help from the nurse to understand this valuable function of play to their child.

Language Development

As might be expected from the profound changes in cognitive development, language development progresses rapidly during the school-age period.

An assessment of the progress in language development includes examination of the three interactive components of language itself: *phonics*, or speech sound, *syntax*, or grammar, and *semantics*, or meaning in language forms such as words and sentences. The assessment is not complete, however, without looking at the personal and social uses of language for the child.

Speech usually is fluent and the voice well-modulated in the 6-year-old. Also, *articulation*, or phonically correct speech, is usually good, with the possible exceptions of thr, shr, sk, sh, ch, s, j and z sounds. By 7 or 8 years, however, these sounds should be pronounced correctly.[14, 15] Articulation difficulties may result from physical problems such as cleft palate, hearing losses, or true cultural factors. Apparent speech defects may be a consequence of the child imitating the speech patterns of the home or neighborhood environment.

Syntax, or grammar, is usually correct by 6 years of age and the child can form five or six word sentences. Semantically, the 6-year-old has 2,500 to 3,000 words in his vocabulary, can carry out commands involving three to four actions, and comprehends "if," "because" and "why."[14]

Research indicates that a basic qualitative change in both syntactic and semantic development takes place at around 7 years of age when concrete operations begin to be established.[15] Complex and compound sentences are used increasingly after that age. Nuances of word meaning, whether standing alone or included in a sentence, are comprehended increasingly. In addition to increasing his vocabulary, the child learns new meaning and more subtle connotations for old words. Whereas younger school-age children typically define words by offering descriptions of the thing signified or examples of its functions, the older school-age child tends to employ explanations or synonyms. At the end of the school-age period, word meanings increasingly approximate those of adults.

Illustrative of the expansion in mental processes involved in language are the typical questions the child asks during the school-age period. As children advance in age, their questions become less global (Why?) and more specific (What? Where? Who? Which?) and, finally more definitive (How?).

The language of the school-age child has a distinctive quality, with unique personal and social functions. This language is a part of the culture of childhood — the behavior pattern of humor, rituals and games that are passed down from one generation to another of children without adult intervention or input. An adult can teach a child how to play checkers, but only children teach other children the rhymes, chants and rituals of childhood. Some of these chants and games can be traced back in time to the middle ages and beyond. This remarkable durability indicates the effectiveness of language in helping the school-age child meet his abiding need to master and control his expanding world and to acquire a social identity with peers.

The countless chants and magic-making words of the school-age child provide a sense of control in a sometimes frightening and bewildering world. Chants accompany many ancient games such as London bridge, ring-around-a-rosy, jumprope and ball bouncing. Some are saved for special occasions: "Ladybug, ladybug fly away home" "It's raining, it's pouring, the old man is snoring" "Star light, star bright, first star I see tonight." The words tend to have a magical quality for the school-age child, as well as being fun to say.

Humor is also expressed through language. The verbal humor of the early school-age child is usually expressed in riddles. Riddles can provide the child with a sense of authority or power. So much of what adults say is incomprehensible or difficult to understand; a riddle can create for a child a situation in which he is the authority with the answer. Likewise, jokes, which become more common around ages 8 or 9, often tend to disparage adults, and thus release tensions the child may experience about his inadequacy in knowledge and power in relation to adults.

Social identity with peers is promoted also through the use of chants, rituals and humor. But social solidarity with peers to the exclusion of adults and other groups of children is attained primarily through the secret language so prevalent with peer groups after the ages of 8 or 9 years. Secret language provides the child with a sense of belonging to a particular group and a sense of power that comes with knowing something adults and other peer groups do not know. If the code of the language is broken by adults or others, the secret language is merely changed to provide another exclusive language. Nicknames are another manifestation of group solidarity. To be given a nickname by the "in" group means one really belongs. Even to be given an offensive nickname means recognition.

Language during the school-age period is the vehicle for expanding knowledge as well as personal and social growth of children.

Anticipatory Guidance: Language Development As with other aspects of development, the child needs to be provided with opportunities to exercise and expand his language skills. Exposure to pronunciation and usage of society's mainstream and to reading should be provided.

Currently, some controversy exists about encouraging use in the classroom of minority ethnic languages such as "Black English," which supposedly helps the minority child develop a positive identity. The arguments for and against such a policy are too numerous to recount here. Awareness of the controversy, however, is pertinent to the anticipatory guidance given to parents and children. The ultimate decision about language usage in the home is theirs.

Parents can facilitate their school-age child's language development in the expression of feelings and thoughts by encouraging discussion of their child's ideas, plans and reactions regularly. Likewise, parents can be urged to express their own feelings, observations and ideas to their school-age child so that he learns the appropriate words to describe his own feelings and thoughts. Such discussion opportunities not only help him develop his vocabulary and learn correct grammar (provided proper grammar is used by his parents), but such activity helps to keep communication lines open between parent and child as he approaches adolescence.

Anticipatory guidance about the personal and social uses of childhood language helps parents conjure up at least hazy memories of the chants, rituals and secret languages they used as children, facilitating their acceptance of these language forms as a part of growing up.

EMOTIONAL AND SOCIAL DEVELOPMENT

The major thrust of emotional and social development in the school-age period is the introduction of the child into society, primarily the society of peers, and his evolvement as a competent doer and member of that society. This emotional and social development is related to and runs parallel with physical and intellectual development and language development. Separating them is somewhat artificial but provides for a more coherent picture of development than considering all three facets together. Included in the discussion of emotional and social development are temperament, emotions, culture, and the developing person.

Temperament

Because of their awareness of the individual differences between children that could not be accounted for by developmental theories, health professionals who deal with children have welcomed the work of Thomas and Chess on temperamental styles.[16] Although innate characteristics of temperament seem to be relatively stable, their expressions may vary over time, being influenced by environmental and intrinsic developmental factors. Therefore, an understanding of the nine major categories of temperament provides a means of seeing how the individual child approaches learning tasks and how he interacts with peers and adults. These factors involved in temperament are activity level, approachability, adaptability, intensity of reaction, threshold for stimulus, mood, distractibility, attention span and persistence.

A child's innate *activity level* is not likely to present problems in the child's adjustment to school if it is of an average or low level. However, a high activity level may make it difficult for the child to settle down to sedentary activities in the classroom. Opportunities for regular motor activity are important, especially for the child with a high activity level, as is patience on the part of the teacher and parent.

The child who has a personality characterized by high *approachability* responds well to new situations, people, places and learning demands, and usually is a joy for a teacher. On the other hand, the child who initially withdraws from new situations and is "slow to warm" may be misjudged by teachers and adults as being slow mentally or noncooperative. This child needs extra time or repeated exposures to new materials to function optimally and to maintain a sense of dignity and self-worth.

The quality of high *adaptability* helps to counteract the effects of high withdrawal in new situations. With extra time or repeated exposures, the child with high withdrawal and high adaptability will function well in new learning situations. However, if the child has high withdrawal and low adaptability, new learning situations will create great difficulty for both the child and the teacher. Much patience and individualized attention is needed to prevent failure in academic achievement for this type of child. Early successes in overcoming difficulties with new learning situations will help to motivate the child to persist despite high withdrawal and low adaptability in subsequent new situations.

With many children, one can judge their interest, moods, likes and dislikes with great accuracy merely by observing their reactions to situations or people. These are children with moderate to high *intensity of reaction*. However, for those with a mild intensity of reaction, simple observations of their responses will not give an accurate evaluation. For these children, the teacher or other adult must be alert for more subtle cues to accurately assess their reactions and to respond to them appropriately.

Children vary greatly in their ability to discern visual, auditory, or tactile stimuli. The hypersensitive child with a low *threshold for stimuli* may be distracted easily in a classroom situation, while the child with a high threshold may be oblivious to the small stimuli. The child with a low threshold is likely to pick up small nuances in voice and behavior that go unnoticed by the child with a high threshold. Consequently, the child with a high threshold may need more detailed instructions to carry out a task than the child with a low threshold.

The quality of *mood* also varies among children. The good-natured child with a typically positive mood is likely to be treated more positively than the ill-natured child with a negative mood. Responses to both types of children are likely to reinforce their prevailing quality of mood. The child with negative mood may feel "picked on" and find confirmation for his feeling that a negative response is appropriate for the predominantly negative world in which he lives.

A child who is highly *distractible* may be aware of extraneous visual and auditory stimuli in the environment, while the child with low distractibility will be able to concentrate on the task at hand with only peripheral awareness of the extraneous stimuli. The latter child usually has the advantage in the classroom situation. However, in the social situation the child who is highly distractible often has capacities for social sensitivity, empathy and constructive behavior that are lost to the child with low distractibility.

Attention span and *persistence* are the last two of the nine temperament characteristics. In the classroom situation long attention span and marked persistence are assets, while short attention span and low persistence are usually liabilities. However, unusually long attention span and marked persistence can lead to stubborn insistence on completing a task even if another activity is called for.

These temperamental qualities tend to occur in clusters, to form what Thomas and Chess call "easy," "slow-to-warm" and "difficult" children, each having special vulnerabilities that can be offset.[6]

Anticipatory Guidance: Temperament Awareness of the temperamental styles of a given child helps the teacher, parent and nurse to adapt their responses to the child to best meet his needs. What works with one child will not work with another of a different temperament. A "canned" preoperative teaching program may be ideal for one child but may alienate another who has a different temperament style.

The reactions of children to illness, injury and hospitalization will vary according to temperament characteristics. The nurse must assess the temperament characteristics of the child if nursing care is to be optimal.

Easy children tend to be a joy to all and usually adapt well to the demands for socialization and school life and in health care situations. The key to optimal response for slow-to-warm children is that they be given time to adapt at their own pace. Patience is required in working with these children. If pressured, their reactions tend to be exaggerated. Difficult children are most vulnerable to the demands of socialization, that is, the demands for altering spontaneous responses and patterns to conform to the social rules of living with family, schoolmates and peers. However, once these children do learn the rules, they function easily, consistently and energetically. The greatest risk period for them is the long adaptation period, and much patience and encouragement is called for in helping them adapt. The transition from home to school is a crucial period in their school life. See Chapters 3 and 9 for further discussion of temperament and management of temperament types.

Emotions

Emotions contribute to total personality patterns and enrich life if properly used. By age 6, the major emotions of anger and aggression, fear and worry, jealousy, and love and affection are fairly well established. During the school-age period, emotional expression becomes more organized and controlled. The major movement is from primarily *physical* expression to *verbal* expression of emotion.[18] The intensity of emotional expression, of course, depends on the temperamental characteristics of the child.

The major task for the maturing child is to control and express emotions in a manner acceptable to the society in which the child lives. An acceptable expression, however, varies with the subcultural groups within that society. Some subcultural groups are more demonstrative in emotional expression than others. What may be acceptable at home may not be acceptable at school or with a peer group. Consequently, the child must learn not only to control the expression of emotion but also to learn acceptable ways for expression in different environments. Usually, if the home is a safe haven in which the child can count on abiding love, emotions can be expressed more openly there than in other environments.

A major mental health goal in the school-age period is for the child to accept his emotions and to learn to express them in socially acceptable ways. Anticipatory guidance for the parents and child is directed toward this goal. The discussion of the major emotions that follows includes essential considerations to include in anticipatory guidance.

Anger is a common emotion of childhood. The usual cause for anger is that the child finds himself in a situation in which he is not able to do what he wants to do. The situation may be one in which the child is restrained or inhibited by adults or peers who enforce limits or behavior, by circumstances such as stormy weather, by objects such as a defective tool, or by the child's own lack of skill. Any of these situations may precipitate an outburst of anger. Physical states such as hunger or fatigue may cause an otherwise benign situation to be anger-provoking. Also, if expressions of anger are rewarded by the child being given his own way, or if parents are overly concerned about expressions of anger, the child may use it inordinately.[18]

Two periods during childhood are especially anger-provoking for the school-age child. One of these periods is during the transition from home to school, when skills are rudimentary and when many new situations are experienced that thwart the child's desires. The other period is at about 8 or 9, when children tend to tease and criticize each other excessively. During both these periods parents need to be patient and understanding and help the child work out his concerns.

As the child becomes better able to control motor skills, to use words more glibly and to understand rules for behavior, life becomes more reasonable and the child is able to bring anger under control. Verbal rather than physical expressions of anger increase with age. The self-centered anger of the school-age years gives way increasingly at the end of the period to anger triggered by injustices to others or social conditions. However, such anger is more typical of the adolescent than of the school-age child. Such anger can be and is used constructively as the energizing force for social action.

As verbal expressions of anger become more available to the child, so do more covert or devious methods of expression, such as sassing, sulkiness, sneering, belittling, plotting, arguing or scapegoating.

Probably the best way to help a child to learn to use anger as a constructive force is to help him verbalize the anger, to examine honestly the circumstances that triggered the anger, and to figure out how those circumstances can be changed, or if they cannot be changed, what can be done about them. Providing models of acceptable expressions of anger is also important. As with adults, physical activity can take the edge off the child's anger. Also, role playing, either through puppetry or doll play, can help a child work through angry and aggressive feelings and to master them.

Aggressive behavior usually is a result of anger but is different from simple expressions of anger. It often involves intentional injury to an animal or human or destruction of an inanimate object. Behavior such as hitting another person is fairly common in the young school-age child. However, from age 10 years on, when aggressive tendencies are better controlled, it occurs rarely. Aggression tends to be better tolerated by society in boys than it is in girls. The same methods for helping a child control anger apply to controlling aggression.

As the world of the school-age child expands, so do his worries and fears. Although fears and worries are learned, they are not necessarily related to actual experiences.

During the early school years, fears and worries tend to be related to family and school. Children worry about such things as parental illness or death, not being liked, getting into trouble and getting hurt, and about being harmed by supernatural beings or monsters, wild animals, or the dark. With age, children's fears and worries become more generalized in many respects, as well as more personalized

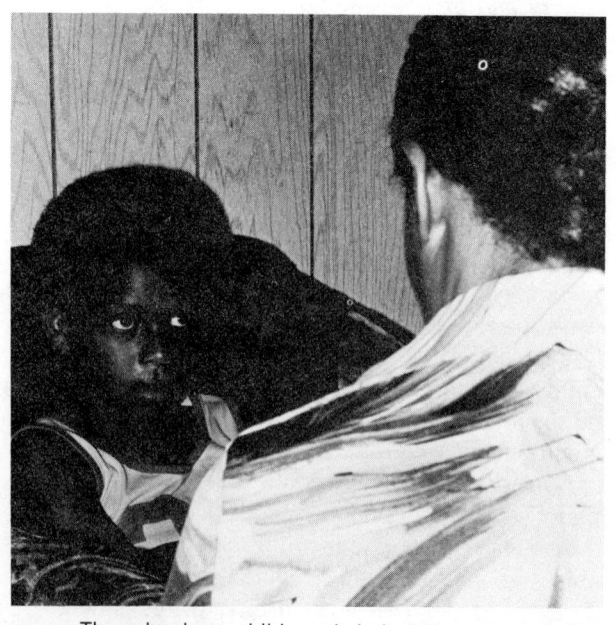

The school-age child needs help to learn to verbalize his anger and to examine the circumstances that triggered the anger so he can learn to use his anger constructively.

and realistic than previously. They increasingly worry about self and possible failures and about scoldings or embarrassment related to specific situations. Mass media opens the door to more generalized fears such as those involving cancer, air pollution, cigarette smoke and war. Fear of such supernatural beings as monsters is abandoned around age 10. Consequently, horror stories and films may be fun or therapeutic for the child 10 or older, while they are very frightening for the younger child.

Fear or worry can be of value if it is not excessive. It warns children of danger and can motivate learning or healthful behavior. Excessive fear, however, can narrow a child's field of experience and damage self-concept. A positive self-concept is a powerful deterrent to excessive fears and worries. Frank discussion of fears and worries, successful experiences in overcoming specific fears, and role models who display mastery over fears can help a child master his own fears and worries.

Episodes of *jealousy* are virtually unavoidable in childhood. An older sibling is often jealous of a younger one because of special privileges and the attention of parents, while the younger sibling is jealous of the older for similar reasons. The perspectives are different, but the supposed reasons are the same. Jealousy stems from insecurity in a relationship and is often accompanied by feelings of anger or inferiority. Its frequency of occurrence decreases with age. As the child matures in cognitive development and moral judgments and his concepts of rules become more mature, he is better able to ward off feelings of jealousy. A positive self-concept and time spent by parents with each child also deter feelings of jealousy.

The need for *love* and *affection* seems to be an innate, basic human need the fulfillment of which is essential for normal development. Just as a child needs to be loved, he needs to love himself and others.

The average school-age child will be able to accept and to give love, but the expressions of love and affection are less overt than with the younger child. The young school-age child is usually reluctant to kiss and hug a parent in public, while the child 10 years and older will avoid such a display with vehemence. This does not mean the school-age child loves the parent less, only that love and affection are expressed in more covert ways, such as just being near parents or trying to please them. Likewise, the parent expresses love and affection by showing

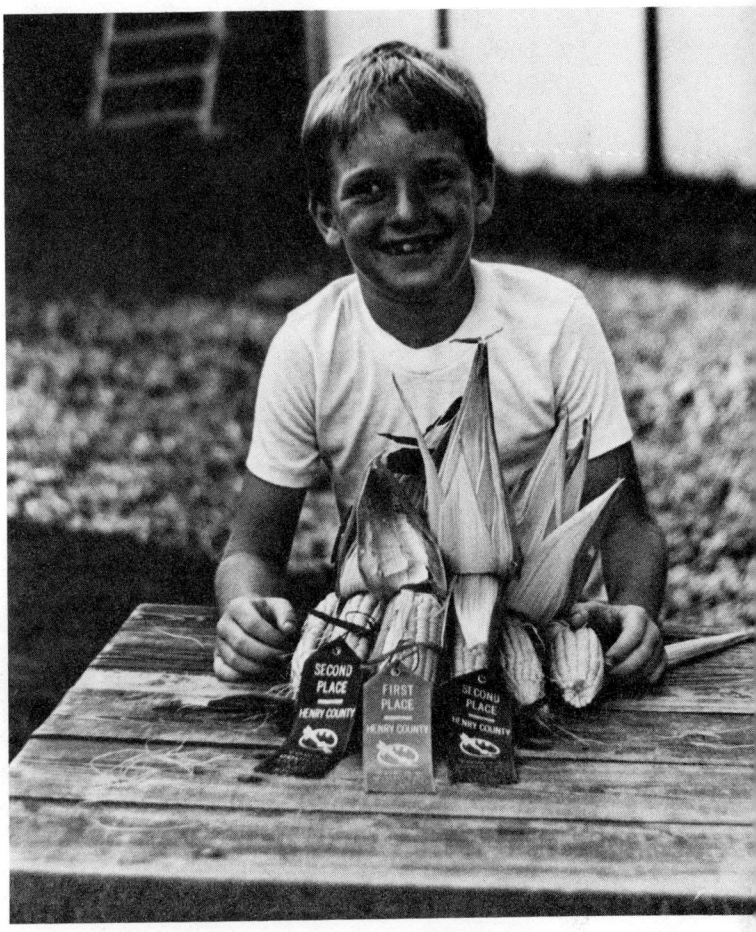

The school-age child builds self-esteem through his accomplishments and evidences of competency.

genuine interest in the child and what he is doing. With peers, expressions of affection are shown by the desire to be with them and to share experiences with them.

Joy, or *happiness,* is allied closely to love. Joy can be experienced by sharing an experience with a loved one. Joy is experienced also in circumstances that promote self-love or self-esteem, such as completing a difficult task. In this age period when the triumph of the sense of industry over the sense of inferiority is a major developmental achievement, joy is found in accomplishments and the sense of competency.

The child develops his basic *emotional pattern* during the school-age period. Basic character formation takes place during these years. Character traits are stabilized, as are the fundamental ways for dealing with people and things. With proper guidance and models for the child to emulate, the pattern will be healthy and carry him through successful adolescence and adulthood. All emotions have a purpose if used wisely. Anger that is just can lead to social concern and reform. Fear and worry can be motivators for positive action and cautions for avoiding negative action. Jealousy can promote empathy and identity. Affection and joy give meaning to life.

Culture

A major change in a child's life occurs with the onset of the school-age years — the child is introduced into society and the extrafamilial culture. This is a fundamental social change for the child. Greater and greater demands are placed on him. At the same time, he is treated in a less personal way than previously. His individuality is lost in the large group structure of which he becomes a part.

During the school-age years, the basic values of the culture are inculcated. In every society, even the most primitive, these are the years when the knowledge, laws and customs of the civilization are passed on. They are crucial years both for the society and for the child. Basically, the child brings with him to this stage the culture of his family and his ever-expanding cognitive skills, thirst for knowledge and urgent sense of industry or need to master the world. The child is ripe for absorbing cultural values.

Although the child is ready for it, this inculcation of culture may be somewhat traumatic, especially if the cultural values of the family differ from those of society at large or from the school or peer group. The child must learn to reconcile the differing values in a way that makes sense to him and that he can live with.

Fortunately, this process of inculcation of culture and reconciliation of differing values is not thrust on the child all at once. The process is slow and gradual. It proceeds primarily through the peer group, which becomes a major force in the life of the school-age child at about 8 or 9.

Prior to age 8 or 9 years, children of both sexes socialize informally. The group composition more or less depends on who is available and is interested in the same activity. At about 8 or 9 years, a marked change appears in the social groupings, with a cleavage occurring between sexes, and a pattern of strong affiliation and loyalty evolving for a particular group or gang of the same sex. The group or gang provides the support system for the child to emancipate himself from adult rules and to declare independence from them. Secret languages or codes and odd mannerisms of behavior and dress are developed to further this independence. The group almost takes on the form of a secret society with formal rites. The child becomes somewhat of an immigrant whose host culture is the subculture of childhood and whose parents live in a hopelessly old-fashioned foreign culture. The child no longer overtly looks to the parents and adults for rules of conduct and behavior. Covertly, however, the child is still very dependent on the parents for guidance and maintains the essence of their value system. It is through group membership, however, that mutual respect and cooperation evolve that Piaget considers essential to the moral development of the child.

Toward the end of the school-age period, the lore of belonging to a secret society abates, and groups and gangs are more likely to be organized around particular kinds of activities and functions. At this time, too, the child's activities are focused around a best friend of the same sex with whom all areas of life can be discussed. Together they may belong to more than one group, depending on their interests. These in-

At about 8 or 9 years strong affiliation for a particular group or gang of the same sex emerges. (Photograph by Dan R. Bruggeman.)

terest groups do not require the fierce loyalty and solidarity of the previous group structure.

The structure of childhood social groups progresses roughly through three stages — from a global or undifferentiated group of children to a highly differentiated group with an exaggerated structure to an articulated functional unit. As the child progresses through these stages, he is socialized into the peer culture. At the next developmental stage, adolescence, socialization is to the social culture of the community at large.

The cultural values inculcated through the peer group are a mixture of the family cultural values of each of the group members and the values promulgated by the schools and religious groups to which the children belong and the mass media to which the children are exposed. The children actively "try on" differing approaches, insofar as cognitive processes allow.

Conflicts may arise between the family's cultural values and those that the child is exposed to in the peer group. A family may be very prejudiced against a particular racial or ethnic group, and the peer group may not be, or vice versa. The peer group might think that experimenting with smoking or drugs is the thing to do, while the family is opposed to such activity. In such situations, the child must resolve the conflict by choosing one viewpoint or the other. Family influence, however, is still very strong with the school-age child. If open lines of communication have been the family pattern, the child will look to the family for guidance in resolving cultural conflicts.

The Developing Person

The major thrust in psychosocial development in the school-age period is the establishment of the ego quality of *industry versus inferiority* — Erikson's fourth stage. As Erikson stated:

One might say that personality at the first stage crystallizes around the conviction "I am what I am given," and that of the second, "I am what I will." The third can be characterized by "I am what I can imagine I will be." We must now approach the fourth: "I am what I learn." The child now wants to be shown how to get busy with something and how to be busy with others.[9]

Erikson described what he meant by the term *sense of industry:*

Children become dissatisfied and disgruntled without a sense of being useful, without a sense of being able to make things and make them well and even perfectly: this is what I call the sense of industry.[9]

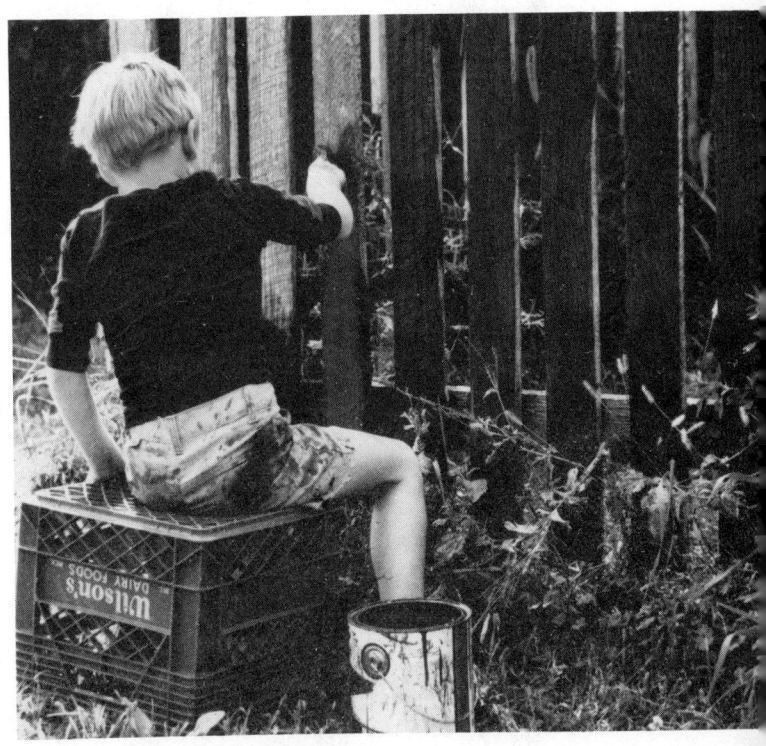

The school-age child is industrious.

The child becomes involved in production of things, work completion, division of labor, equality of opportunity, and positive identification with those who *know* things and know how to *do* things.

As is clear from Erikson's words, the ego quality of industry versus inferiority has both personal and social implications. On the personal level, the focus is on the competency of the individual, especially in physical and cognitive skills. Previous discussion of these skills demonstrates the progress the normal child makes in these areas. The child's psychic energies are directed toward the acquisition and perfection of these skills. "Industrious" is an apt description of the school-age child.

The danger of this stage is that the child will find his physical and cognitive skills wanting and will develop a sense of inadequacy and inferiority rather than industry and competence. Few children, however, are incapable of developing competence in some area of activity. Likewise, few will be capable of developing competence in all areas of activity.

A sense of inferiority in some areas of activity is inevitable for the vast majority of children. As

Erikson points out, the "versus" in the stage designations does not mean that the negative component is not present; it means only that for successful completion of the stage, the positive component must outweigh the negative component in the equation. The school-age child, therefore, needs to recognize his limitations and to accept them without a diminution of self-esteem. Not everyone has artistic talent, but just because an individual does not have artistic talent does not mean the individual is less of a person than one who has this talent. The same holds true of any type of activity. Successful completion of this stage, then, means that the child comes to recognize his abilities as well as his liabilities and with that recognition develops a sense of competence, pride and self-esteem for what he can do. Competition among individuals is very much a part of this stage. Through competition with peers, the child gains recognition of personal assets and liabilities.

The social implication of the stage of industry versus inferiority means primarily that the child becomes a productive member of a social group of peers in preparation for becoming a productive member of society as an adult. The development of cooperative and collaborative working relationships based on mutual respect is the major social goal of this stage of development. Again, competition is very much a part of this process, but with respect to social goals, it is group or team competition rather than individual competition. The child learns to respect the abilities of others and to take pride in the accomplishment attained through group activities. He learns that the strengths and weaknesses of individuals, including his own, can be counterbalanced in group activities. And, perhaps the hardest lesson of all, the child learns that the accomplishments of others do not diminish his own.

This major achievement of a personal and social identity as an industrious and competent individual and group member occurs rather slowly over the entire span of the school-age period. The characteristic behaviors of the child at each age from 6 to 12 years illustrate this gradual progression.

The 6-year-old is noted for almost constant activity; the whole body seems to be involved in almost anything and everything he does. Throwing a ball involves the entire body; telling a story involves gesturing with the arms and face. Much spontaneous dramatization is evident during this sixth year. The child tends to be restless and indecisive and needs activities that require use of the large muscles. Group activities are entered with enthusiasm, but the child is not yet ready for cooperative play, often leaving a game if he does not get his way or if he is distracted by something else. Behavior is often explosive, with temper tantrums reaching a peak at this age. Rudeness is common, especially at home and at play. The conscious or moral judgment is strict, literal and unreliable. Cheating is frequent but against the child's conscience. The child may behave very differently at home and at school. This is not an easy age for either child or parent. Probably the most endearing characteristics are the child's eagerness to learn and to "help" adults by performing tasks for them. Adults, parents and teacher, are very important to the child, and direct imitation of their mannerisms is frequent. Parental affection, patience and praise are extremely important to the child throughout this difficult year.

The 7-year-old is full of vitality and energy but is more cautious in exercising it in play than the 6-year-old. The child also is cautious, self-critical and anxious to do things correctly in the activities that he undertakes. He is talkative and starts to use words to express anger rather than physical means. He enjoys songs, rhythms, fairy tales, myths, nature stories, comics, television and movies. A rudimentary understanding of time and money values is evident. He assumes responsibility better than the 6-year-old, and is very concerned about what is right and wrong even though he may take things that do not belong to him. He is sensitive to the feelings and attitudes of both peers and adults, wanting them to like him. A spontaneous awareness of and sensitivity about sex makes him modest and concerned about self-exposure. He becomes concerned about fairness but has difficulty in accepting criticism or blame. He is especially dependent on the approval of adults and needs a warm, encouraging, friendly relationship with adults.

The 8-year-old is eager to do things and does them with more smoothness and poise than previously. Group activity takes on increasing importance and the child seeks it out actively, disliking to be alone. Segregation by sexes is obvious, and the child chooses a best friend of the same sex. However, these friendships tend to be unstable, and the child may have several best friends in sequence during the year. Play outdoors may be vigorous but the child also seeks quiet activities, and dramatic play is very popular. Collections of miscellaneous objects are common and are treasured. The child is eager to learn and usually enjoys school. Areas of interest expand beyond the immediate environment. Time concepts are expanding, and the child tries to relate himself to the past and present. He can recognize the difference between real or historic characters and fictitious ones in movies or on television. The 8-year-old is beginning to understand and accept other people more than previously, recognizing individual differences. He begins to see himself in relation to others and has a beginning capacity for self-evaluation. Conscience is less rigid than previously, and he begins to resent parental authority, looking more to the group for support. Behavior is likely to be better away from home. Although the child moves increasingly to the peer group for support, he continues to need much praise and encouragement from adults.

The 9-year-old is fairly responsible, reasonable and dependable. Individual differences in abilities and skills between children become more distinct and clear both to adults and to the children themselves. The same-sex groups or gangs of childhood are all important. Conformity within the group is accentuated and the group may leave out a child who is different in any way. New forms of independence from adults are attained through the peer group. The parents are reappraised to a more realistic level. The former image of the parent as all powerful and all knowing is devalued down to a more human level, and new authorities are set up against parents. Hero worship becomes prominent. The child has an increased attention span and the capacity to plan and complete a fairly complex project with little or no help from adults. Interests expand rapidly. He is interested less in fairy tales and fantasy and more in his community and country and in other countries and people. The scope of interest includes babies, and both sexes enjoy interacting with babies and small children. As part of their interest in learning about the world around them, they are interested in learning about the origin of babies and how they grow. The 9-year-old is self-sufficient, self-critical, and somewhat of a perfectionist. He has a strong sense of fairness and right and wrong and is mature enough to accept blame for wrongdoing. However, he does not like to be talked down to. The child needs the support of parents and adults in his efforts to become more self-sufficient personally and to become a productive member of the peer group.

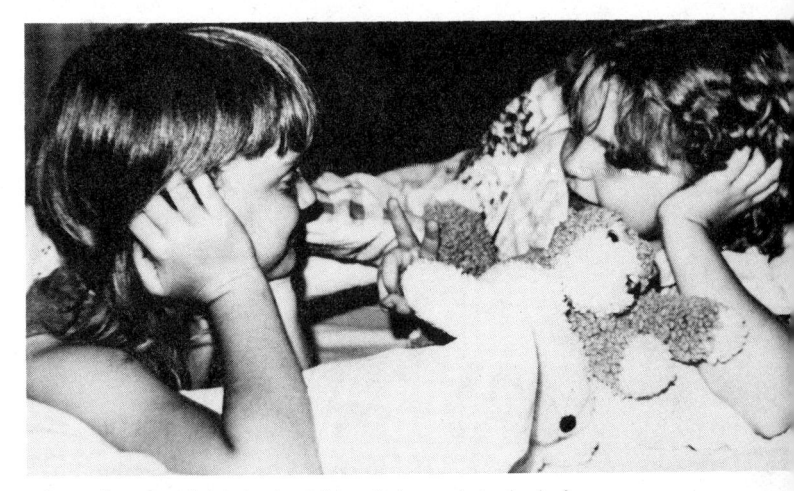

Spending the night at a best friend's home is typical of the school-age period.

The most obvious change at 10 years is the differences between the sexes. Girls often start sexual maturation and are more poised and socially mature than boys, who start puberty approximately two years later. The solidarity of the sexes, however, is still very evident. Team

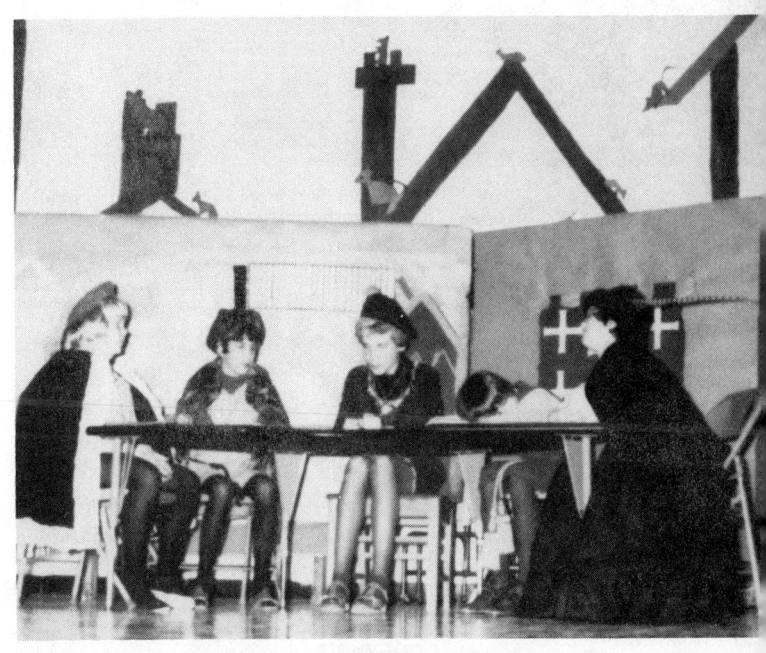

The middle school-age child enjoys acting and dramatic play.

Children continue to reappraise parents and become self-conscious of them and about them. Some children develop a "foundling" fantasy in which these ordinary people could not possibly be his parents, and he fantasizes that his parents are some glamorous figures. However, the child is still very dependent on the love of parents and implicitly accepts certain standards of the family.

Differences between the sexes are even more apparent in 11- and 12-year-olds, because of differences in timing of onset of puberty. However, many behaviors are characteristic of both sexes. The sex cleavage is often intensified, and frequent expressions of resentment and disgust toward the opposite sex are common. Girls are the first to break down the cleavage by becoming "boy crazy." Sexual concerns are often discussed secretly with a best friend or a cohesive peer group. An increase in curiosity and

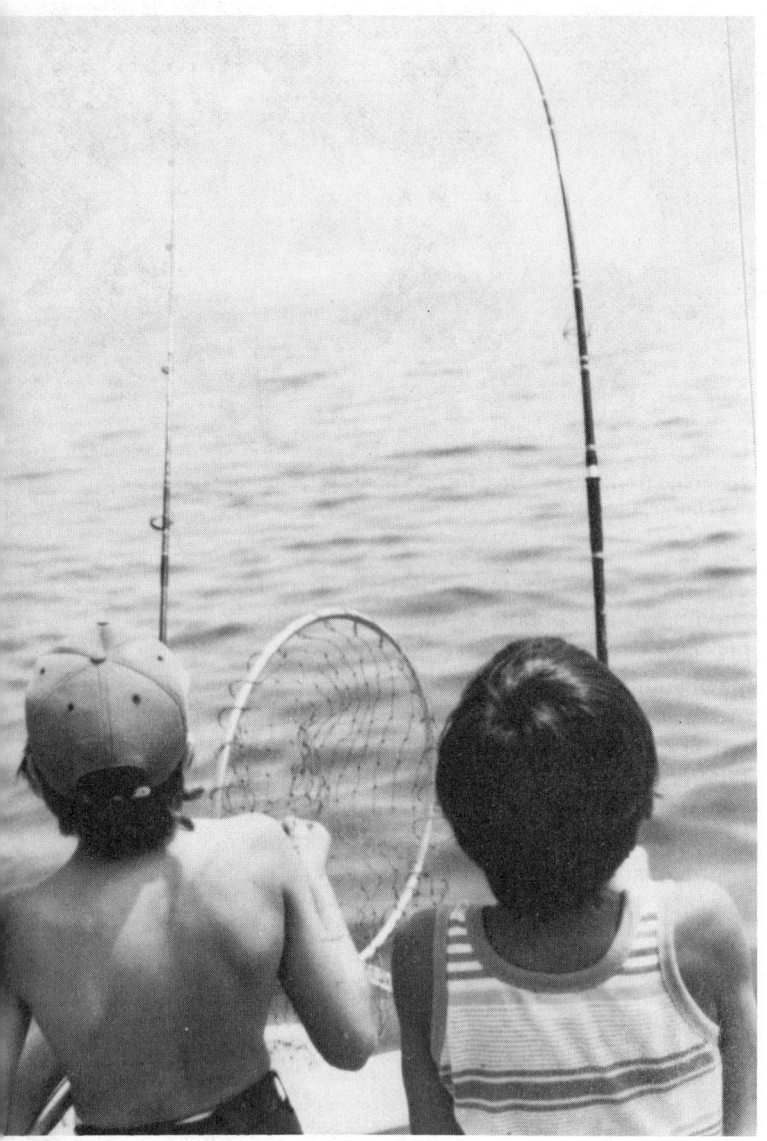

Toward the end of the school-age period, collections give way to lifelong hobbies. (Photograph by Charles William Jameson.)

sports and cooperative activities are prominent, and the child readily submits to the rules of the game. A stable and lasting friendship with someone of the same sex is formed, and a separation through a move to a distant new home by either child may be very traumatic for both. Collections are no longer miscellaneous but very distinct and organized and may lead to a lifelong hobby. Hero worship continues. Interests in the world of people, places and things continue to expand, and a strong moral sense of good and bad is expressed about many of them.

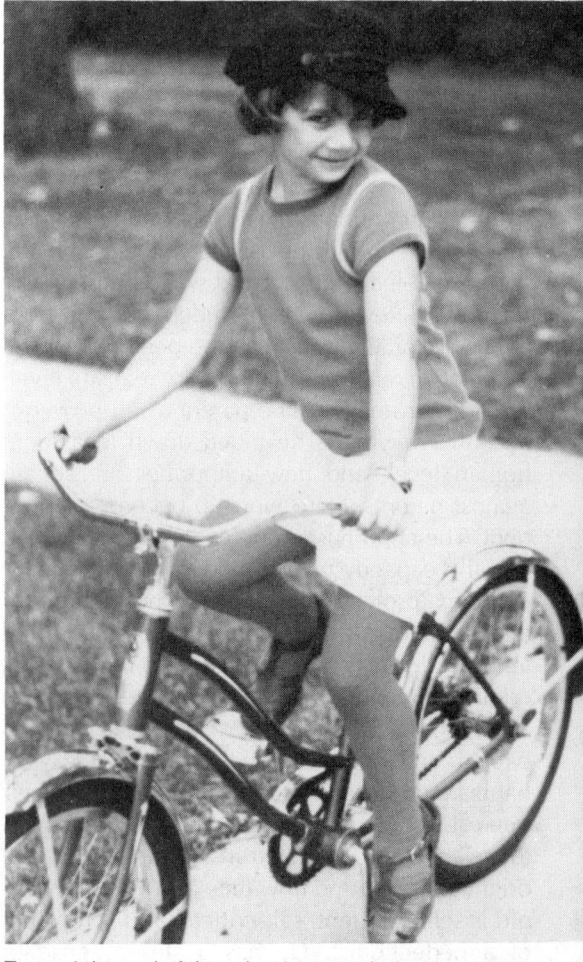

Toward the end of the school-age period, although the sex cleavage is often intensified, girls become flirtatious and boys begin to tease. (Photograph by Dan R. Bruggeman.)

physical and intellectual activity in both sexes is seen. Tension outlets of nail biting and foot twirling may appear, as may compulsive behavior, fears, and aches and pains of unknown and benign origin. The relationship with the family may be ambivalent and oscillating, with the child wanting to be independent, especially of the mother. The child is secretive and demands and needs privacy. Increased unruliness, sloppiness and dirtiness are often evident. Parents are often astonished to hear how well these same children behave in other settings. Membership in groups and clubs that are organized around a specific function are of increasing importance. Team games and sports are very popular. As with the other ages of the school-age period, 11- and 12-year-olds need parents' support in this difficult transitional period. Their need for privacy needs to be respected, as does their need for peer activities.

This overview of the behavioral characteristics of the child as he progresses through the school-age period illustrates the tremendous progress the child makes in personal and social competency. They are not easy years for either the child or parents. The parents' understanding of the typical behavior of the child, however, will help them provide the support the child needs to progress in his long struggle for a sense of industry and competency as opposed to inferiority and inadequacy.

HEALTH MAINTENANCE

The school-age period is a relatively healthy one for children. In 1975, the death rate per 100,000 estimated population of children 5 through 14 years was 35.7.[12] By far, the leading cause of death is accidents, including both motor vehicle and other accidents. This fact indicates that safety education is of primary importance in health maintenance efforts for this age group.

Acute illnesses, especially respiratory illnesses, are fairly common with this age group. Over half the acute illnesses reported are due to respiratory conditions. The average number of days of restricted activity for illness per child in the 6 through 16 age group is approximately 10, with approximately 5 school days lost due to illness.[11] Although acute illnesses are to be expected as a normal part of life, this information about the incidence of acute conditions indicates that prevention of respiratory conditions should be included in health promotion efforts for this age group.

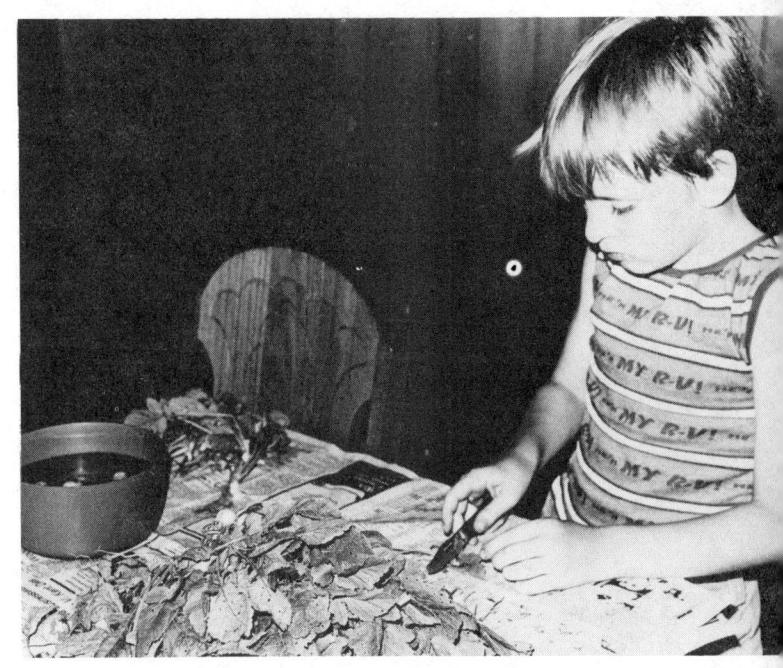

By 9 years the child can assume responsibility for assisting with meal preparation and clean-up.

The following concerns need to be included in a health promotion program: nutrition, play, safety, immunizations, sex education and value clarification.

Nutrition

Proper nutrition, discussed previously, is essential for the health and well-being of children. A properly nourished child is less susceptible to acute illnesses and is better able to develop the physical, intellectual, emotional and social competencies so important to this age group.

One problem area in nutrition for this age group is that children may become too busy and involved to eat properly. Children like structure and rituals, and adults can use this to the advantage of both themselves and their children. Regularity of meal and snack times gives children the structure they need around which to plan activities.

Mealtimes also should be pleasant occasions to look forward to and to provide opportunities for social interaction with the family. The 6 or 7 year old may find it difficult to sit through a meal and may need to be excused early. By 9 years, the child's table manners are good and he can also assume responsibilities for assisting

TABLE 48-2 COMPETENCY DEVELOPMENT OF THE SCHOOL-AGE CHILD

Age (Years)	Physical Competency	Intellectual Competency	Emotional-Social Competency
General: 6–12	Gains an average of 2.5–3.2 kg/year (5½–7 lbs./year). Overall height gains of 5.5 cm (2 inches) per year; growth occurs in spurts and is mainly in trunk and extremities. Loses deciduous teeth; most of permanent teeth erupt. Progressively more coordinated in both gross and fine motor skills. Caloric needs increase with growth spurts.	Masters concrete operations. Moves from egocentrism; learns he is not always right. Learns grammar and expression of emotions and thoughts. Vocabulary increases to 3000 words or more; handles complex sentences.	Central crisis: industry vs. inferiority; wants to do and make things. Progressive sex education needed. Wants to be like friends; competition important. Fears body mutilation, alterations in body image; earlier phobias may recur, nightmares; fears death. Nervous habits common.
6–7	Vision reaches adult level of 20/20. Gross motor skill exceeds fine motor coordination. Balance and rhythm are good—runs, skips, jumps, climbs, gallops. Throws and catches ball. Dresses self with little or no help.	Vocabulary of 2500 words. Learning to read and print; beginning concrete concepts of numbers, general classification of items. Knows concepts of right and left; morning, afternoon and evening; coinage. Intuitive thought process. Verbally aggressive, bossy, opinionated, argumentative. Likes simple games with basic rules.	Boisterous, outgoing, and a know-it-all, whiney; parents should sidestep power struggles, offer choices. Becomes quiet and reflective during 7th year; very sensitive. Can use telephone. Likes to make things: starts many, finishes few. Give some responsibility for household duties.
8–10	Myopia may appear. Secondary sex characteristics begin in girls. Hand-eye coordination and fine motor skills well established. Movements are graceful, coordinated. Cares for own physical needs completely. Constantly on move; plays and works hard; enforce balance in rest and activity.	Learning correct grammar and to express feelings in words. Likes books he can read by himself; will read funny papers, scan newspaper. Enjoys making detailed drawings. Mastering classification, seriation, spatial and temporal, numerical concepts. Uses language as a tool; likes riddles, jokes, chants, word games. Rules guiding force in life now. Very interested in how things work, what and how weather, seasons, etc., are made.	Strong preference for same-sex peers; antagonizes opposite-sex peers. Self-assured and pragmatic at home; questions parental values and ideas. Has a strong sense of humor. Enjoys clubs, group projects, outings, large groups, camp. Modesty about own body increases over time; sex conscious. Works diligently to perfect skills he does best. Happy, cooperative, relaxed and casual in relationships. Increasingly courteous and well-mannered with adults. Gang stage at a peak; secret codes and rituals prevail. Responds better to suggestion than dictatorial approach.
11–12	Vital signs approximate adult norms. Growth spurt for girls; inequalities between sex is increasingly noticeable; boys greater physical strength. Eruption of permanent teeth complete except for third molars. Secondary sex characteristics begin in boys. Menstruation may begin.	Able to think about social problems and prejudices; sees others' points of view. Enjoys reading mysteries, love stories. Begins playing with abstract ideas. Interested in whys of health measures and understands human reproduction. Very moralistic; religious commitment often made during this time.	Intense team loyalty; boys begin teasing girls and girls flirt with boys for attention; best friend period. Wants unreasonable independence. Rebellious about routines; wide mood swings; needs some times daily for privacy. Very critical of own work. Hero worship prevails. "Facts of life" chats with friends prevail; masturbation increases. Appears under constant tension.

with meal preparation and clean-up. The younger child can help, too, but may be somewhat erratic in his ability to carry through on assigned tasks. Tasks for the younger child need to be simple, such as putting the napkins on the table or clearing away his dishes. Undue pressure on skilled performance should not be applied so that the child can acquire a sense of competence and pride in contributing to family welfare.

Play

It has often been said that play is the work of children. When consideration is given to what play does for the development of physical, cognitive and social competence, this might even be considered an understatement.

Play is of vital importance to the acquisition of the ego quality of industry versus inferiority. Children acquire physical competence and skills through play involving gross and fine motor activity. Active involvement in play promotes cognitive development, and through

TABLE 48-2 COMPETENCY DEVELOPMENT OF THE SCHOOL-AGE CHILD *(Continued)*

Nutrition	Play	Safety	Immunizations
Fluctuations in appetite due to uneven growth pattern and tendency to get involved in activities. Tendency to neglect breakfast due to rush of getting to school. Though school lunch is provided in most schools, child does not always eat it.	Plays in groups, mostly of same sex; "gang" activities predominate. Books for all ages. Bicycles a must. Sports equipment. Cards, board and table games. Most of play is active games requiring little or no equipment.	Enforce continued use of safety belts during car travel. Bicycle safety must be taught and enforced. Teach safety related to hobbies, handicrafts, mechanical equipment.	
Preschool food dislikes persist. Tendency for deficiencies in iron, vitamin A and riboflavin. 100 ml/kg of water per day. 3 gm/kg protein daily.	Still enjoys dolls, cars and trucks. Plays well alone but enjoys small groups of both sexes; begins to prefer same sex peer during 7th year. Ready to learn how to ride a bicycle. Prefers imaginary, dramatic play with real costumes. Begins collecting for quantity, not quality. Enjoys active games such as hide-and-seek, tag, jumprope, roller skating, kickball. Ready for lessons in dancing, gymnastics, music. Restrict TV time to 1–2 hours/day.	Teach and reinforce traffic safety. Still needs adult supervision of play. Teach to avoid strangers, never take anything from strangers. Teach cold prevention and reinforce continued practice of other health habits. Restrict bicycle use to home ground; no traffic areas; teach bicycle safety. Teach and set examples re harmful use of drugs, alcohol, smoking.	TOPV and DPT boosters if not received at age 5.
Needs about 2100 calories/day; nutritious snacks. Tends to be too busy to bother to eat. Tendency for deficiencies in calcium, iron and thiamine. Problem of obesity may begin now. Good table manners. Able to help with food preparation.	Likes hiking, sports. Enjoys cooking, woodworking, crafts. Enjoys cards and table games. Likes radio and records. Begins qualitative collecting now. Continue restriction on TV time.	Stress safety with firearms, Keep them out of reach and allow use only with adult supervision. Know who the child's friends are; parents should still have some control over friend selection. Teach water safety; swimming should be supervised by an adult.	TD vaccine if series not previously received.
Male needs 2500 calories per day; female needs 2250 (70 cal./kg/day). 75 ml./kg. of water per day. 2 gm/kg protein daily.	Enjoys projects and working with hands. Likes to do errands and jobs to earn money. Very involved in sports, dancing, talking on phone. Enjoys all aspects of acting and drama.	Continue monitoring friends; Stress bicycle safety on streets and in traffic.	

playful experiments on the environment, the child discovers much new knowledge and many new cognitive skills. Some parents may need assistance in the continued need of this age child for ample playtime. Socialization to the peer group is acquired primarily through the play of children. Peer group and team activities are important to the school-age child's developing peer identity, not just during the school year but also during summer months. Parents may need information about community facilities, programs and camps that provide opportunities for play experiences. A childhood without ample opportunities for play is no childhood at all. The value of play cannot be overestimated in the promotion of a healthy childhood.

Safety

Safety education is of primary importance in health maintenance efforts for the school-age group. Accidents are by far the leading cause of death. Because motor vehicle accidents account for nearly half the deaths due to accidents, automobile safety should be stressed. Children like rituals, and one ritual that should be automatic is buckling up the seat belt. Children can learn also the rules of the road, and included in the rules is proper behavior in the automobile so that the driver is not distracted from the primary task of driving the car.

Although motor vehicle accidents are a major cause of death, over half of the accidents of this age group occur inside the house or on adjacent property.[12] Home safety measures therefore also assume major importance. Boys are twice as likely to have accidents as girls. According to one study, the most common commercial products involved in these accidents were bicycles, glass, swings, skateboards and nails.

Caution in play and other activities needs to be stressed to the child. However, caution should not be overly stressed because excessive caution or fear can inhibit normal development. A certain number of skinned knees and bruises seems inevitable in the normally developing child.

Children need to be taught the proper use of tools, toys and implements. If skateboards must be used, proper protective gear should be worn. The child can be challenged to figure out proper safety precautions to use in various activities and with various implements. If this exercise becomes habitual, the child will carry it through into adulthood.

Immunizations

If the child is up to date in immunizations and has received a dose of DPT (diphtheria, tetanus toxoids combined with pertussis vaccine) and TOPV (trivalent oral poliovirus vaccine) as recommended during the fourth to sixth year, no further immunizations are required until adolescence. Any child who does not receive his DPT vaccine by age 7 will receive a Td instead, since pertussis vaccine is not given beyond this age. Tetanus toxoid is administered as a booster promptly after any injury that involves a compound fracture, gunshot or other penetrating wound and for any wound not easily cleaned or debrided. When the child has had no previous tetanus immunization or if he is not seen the day of the injury, tetanus antitoxin or human tetanus immune globulin is given and tetanus toxoid immunizations are begun (given at a different site) at the same time.

Common Concerns

Two major concerns pertaining to the child that need to be faced by parents during the school-age period are sex education and drug education. The older school-age child urgently needs to acquire factual knowledge and values about both. The younger school-age child needs to have his questions answered in terms appropriate to his cognitive development, but the older child needs more specific information and clarification of values.

The older school-age child can assimilate factual knowledge about menstruation, nocturnal emissions and reproduction if he or she has a repertoire of information about the anatomy and physiology of the human body. If sex education is given in isolation, the assimilation of it is problematical. If given in isolation it also gives undue emphasis to sexual function as the only bodily function of importance. If presented in context with a study of the wonderful human body, it becomes a natural process to be respected as are all other natural processes of the body. If given in this context, certainly the 11-year-old can assimilate the information, and the 9-year-old can handle introductory information.[4]

Because sex education is so value laden, parents need to take an active part in it. Although factual information may be given in school, parents need to be aware of what is taught and in what context, so that they can respond to the child's questions appropriately and provide value clarification. Otherwise, questions will be answered and values clarified within the peer group only and this situation is often one of "the blind leading the blind."

With the increasing availability of drugs to younger children, children need to be made aware of the harmful effects of drugs. Rather than scare tactics, emphasis is more effectively placed on how drugs hinder the ability to accomplish all the feats so important to the age group.

Table 48-2 summarizes the competencies of the school-age child which serve as a basis for all anticipatory guidance.

References

1. D. Bailey. The growing child and the need for physical activity. In School-Age Children, Development and Relationships, 2nd ed. M. S. Smart and R. C. Smart. Macmillan Inc., 1978
2. D. Bailey et al. The influence of exercise, physical

activity and athletic performance on the dynamics of human growth. In Human Growth, Vol. 2: Postnatal Growth, F. Falkner and J. M. Tanner. eds. Plenum, 1978
3. L. Belmont and H. Birch. Lateral dominance and right-left awareness in normal children. Child Development, June 1963, p. 257
4. A. Bernstein and P. Cowan. Children's concepts of how people get babies. In School-Age Children, Development and Relationships, 2nd ed. M. S. Smart and R. C. Smart. Macmillan Inc., 1978
5. D. Boone and T. Prescott. Development of left-right discrimination in normal children. Perceptual and Motor Skills, February 1968, p. 267
6. S. Chess. Temperament and learning ability of school children. American Journal of Public Health, December 1968, p. 2231
7. M. Chow et al. Handbook of Pediatric Primary Care. John Wiley & Sons, 1979
8. A. Demirjian. Dentition. In Human Growth, Vol. 2: Postnatal Growth, F. Falkner and J. M. Tanner, eds. Plenum, 1978
9. E. H. Erikson. Identity and the life cycle: Selected papers. Psychological Issues Monograph, January 1967
10. Health status of children: A review of surveys 1963–1972. U.S. Department of Health, Education, and Welfare, Publication No. (HSA) 78–5744, 1978
11. Health United States–1975. U.S. Department of Health, Education, and Welfare, Publication No. (HRA) 76–1232, 1976
12. Health United States–1978. U.S. Department of Health, Education, and Welfare, Publication No. (PHS) 78–1232, 1978
13. L. Laosa. Nonbiased assessment of children's abilities: historical antecedents and current issues. In Psychological and Educational Assessment of Minority Children, T. Oakland, ed. Brunner/Mazel, 1977
14. G. Lowrey. Growth and Development of Children, 7th ed. Yearbook Medical Publishers, 1978
15. M. Smart and R. Smart. School-Age Children — Development and Relationships, 2nd ed. Macmillan Inc., 1978
16. A. Thomas and S. Chess. Temperament and Development. Brunner/Mazel, 1977
17. V. Vaughn and R. McKay, eds. Nelson Textbook of Pediatrics, 11th ed. W. B. Saunders Co., 1979
18. J. Williams and M. Stith. Middle Childhood — Behavior and Development. Macmillan Inc., 1974

Additional Recommended Reading

E. Anthony. The child's discovery of his body. Physical Therapy, October 1968, p. 1103

S. Arieti. The Intrapsychic Self. Basic Books, 1967

D. Ausubel and E. Sullivan. Theory and Problems of Child Development, 2nd ed. Grune and Stratton, 1970

J. Boettcher and K. Boettcher. Sex education for fifth and sixth graders and their parents. American Journal Maternal Child Nursing, Jul/Aug, 1975, p. 218

E. Erikson. Childhood and Society, 2nd ed. W. W. Norton, 1963

S. Fomon. Nutritional disorders of children — prevention, screening, and followup. U.S. Department of Health, Education, and Welfare, Publication No. (HSA) 77–5104, reprinted 1977

S. Garn. Body size and its implications. In Review of Child Development Research, L. W. Hoffman and M. L. Hoffman, eds. Vol. 2, Russell Sage, 1966

A. Gesell and R. Ilg. The Child From Five to Ten. Harper and Row, 1977

R. Gardner. Understanding Children. Jason Aronson, 1974

M. Green and R. Haggerty. Ambulatory Pediatrics. W. B. Saunders Co., 1968

I. Graller. The best school nurse program in America. Parents, November 1978, p. 86

M. Holliday. Body composition and energy needs during growth. In Human Growth, Vol. 2: Postnatal Growth. F. Falkner and J. M. Tanner, eds. Plenum, 1978

N. Larreck. Do you have TV interference? Today's Education, Nov/Dec 1978, p. 39

A. Nizel. Preventing dental caries: The nutritional factors. Pediatric Clinics of North America, February 1977, p. 141

F. Ohler. Oral Health Behavior: acquisition and maintenance. The Journal of School Health, November 1976, p. 522

R. Pantell et al. Taking Care of Your Child — A Parents' Guide to Medical Care. Addison-Wesley, 1977

G. Pearson. Nutrition in the middle years of childhood. American Journal of Maternal Child Nursing, Nov/Dec 1977, p. 378

J. Piaget. The Psychology of Intelligence. Littlefield, Adams, 1966

I. Shorr and C. Neuman. Office assessment of nutritional status. Pediatric Clinics of North America, February 1977, p. 253

M. Siemon. Mental health in school-aged children. American Journal Maternal Child Nursing, Jul/Aug 1978, p. 211

E. Smith. Are you really communicating? American Journal of Nursing, December 1977, p. 1966

L. Stone and J. Church. Childhood and Adolescence. Random House, 1965

W. Vinacke. Concept formation in children of school ages. In The Child, A Book of Readings, J. M. Seidman, ed. Holt, Rinehart and Winston, 1960, pp. 294–302

49 POTENTIAL STRESSES DURING SCHOOL-AGE YEARS: MANAGING BEHAVIOR

by Mary Sue Jack, RN, MS

Four common problems that affect school-age children are discussed in this chapter: enuresis, encopresis, school phobias, and antisocial behavior. The nurse in the primary care setting who works with children affected with these should remember three points:

1. *The seriousness and the intensity of these behaviors vary from child to child.* For example, a child who does not want to go to school on a particular day because of fear of a test that day cannot be considered in the same manner as a child who absolutely cannot go to school at all; yet both of these children have a form of *school refusal,* or *phobia.* The first child's reaction to school is mild and normal, whereas the second child and his family should have some form of therapy. The importance of recognizing the degree with which each child is affected by these problems is seen when one plans management for a child and the child's family. Individual differences must be assessed and planned for accordingly.

2. *It is important to recognize that each of the issues discussed has multiple causes.* In this chapter consideration is given to some of the possible causes of each problem; however, the list is by no means exhaustive. During each situation in which the practitioner is called upon to work with this child and his family, the many possible causes of the conditions must be carefully considered. A complete and thorough history is the best tool; the child, the parents and siblings should be included. The practitioner may want to gather data from people other than the immediate family. When the child enters school, a whole new group of people becomes important. Peers and teachers have a great influence on the child's behavior. By using these persons in collecting data, the nurse will have a wider, truer picture of the child and can more accurately assess reasons for behavior. Knowing that there are many factors contributing to a child's problem will allow the nurse to use resources more skillfully.

3. *Preventing these problems is the best approach.* The nurse can begin anticipatory guidance in relevant areas such as discipline, toilet training and school attendance long before

problems involving these occur in the child's life. The nurse's knowledge of growth and development can be used to help parents watch for and manage potential problem situations. The nurse, as a primary care provider, can alert parents to clues which signify that trouble may be developing in a particular area. Most of the behaviors of school-age children have been developing for a significant amount of time. Early identification and counselling for prevention is the most effective management of the issues.

ENURESIS

Enuresis is defined as the involuntary passage of urine by a child over the age of 5 years. It can occur during the day (diurnal enuresis), during the night (nocturnal enuresis) or at both times. A child who has never been totally continent is said to have *primary enuresis*. A child with *secondary enuresis* has experienced a period of dryness of at least three to six months after toilet training was completed.

Anywhere from 15 to 26 per cent of all children are enuretic.[2] According to research data, enuresis occurs more frequently in boys. It is seen more in children of lower socioeconomic classes. Children in large families more frequently have enuresis. There are also data supporting a familial tendency toward enuresis: 32 per cent of fathers of enuretic children were bed wetters; 20 per cent of the mothers of bed wetters were enuretic as children.[2] In a study of children raised in a kibbutz, 44 per cent of siblings of bed wetters were also bed wetters, even though they were raised by separate nurses.[2]

Etiology

There are several theories regarding the etiology of enuresis. All or part of each one might be operating in a given child. It is important for the nurse to be aware of the possible causes of enuresis in order to offer the optimal management of the problem.

The first cause that must be considered is an organic defect. There may be a physical problem or disease process present in the child. Dribbling urine may be a manifestation of an infection, diabetes or epilepsy.[12] There may be an anatomical abnormality of the urinary tract. Some investigators have reported enuresis in children with a history of food allergies.[3] In performing the physical examination it is important to rule out all of these possible organic causes.

There may be a psychological cause for a child's enuresis. Some practitioners believe that the child is using enuresis to "get back" at the parents for some "unfairness." The child may be reacting to too-strict control or to unrealistically high expectations the parents have for his behavior and performance. Or "getting even" with the parent may be for a reason unknown to the child, parent or nurse. Parental response to the enuresis may perpetuate this problem. Use of shaming or punishment techniques gives the child further reason for "getting even." In children with secondary enuresis having a psychological component, a threatening event or anxiety-producing situation has usually occurred, such as the birth of a sibling or threatened school failure that precipitates the bed wetting.[12]

There is good support for the theory that enuresis is caused by a developmental or maturational delay in the child. Studies have shown that the child with enuresis has a smaller functional bladder capacity than a nonenuretic child.[12] This means some children are not physically ready for full control of urinary function at the time considered "average." They do not have adequate bladder size or sphincter control to last an entire night without voiding. Support for this theory is seen in the fact that enuresis spontaneously disappears in many children as they get older.

Some children have only diurnal enuresis; environmental stresses are most prevalent in these cases. Some causative factors in this situation may be: (1) nervous tension in a given situation such as school, (2) shyness on the part of the child in asking his teacher in front of classmates to leave the room to urinate or (3) reluctance of some children, particularly girls, to use unfamiliar toilets.[2]

Management

The management of a child with enuresis begins with a careful history. It serves not only as the principal tool with which to collect data but also offers the opportunity for the nurse to establish a caring relationship with the child and parents. This history should be obtained in a comfortable environment, with the information being given by the parents and the child. The nurse should maintain a calm, nonjudgmental attitude, supporting the strengths of the parents. Many times parents simply need to vent their feelings regarding the enuresis and to sort out the approaches they have attempted and the results of their attempts. The nurse should emphasize the fact that this family sought help as a positive step toward eliminating the enuresis. The history-taking session itself can be an important intervention in the management of enuresis.

In many instances, the enuresis has been present for months or years. Therefore it is important to know why the family sought assistance *at this particular time*. It may be that the enuresis had not been viewed as a problem by the parents until friends or relatives began saying that the child is "not normal." Or perhaps the enuresis has become a social problem for the child. "Sleeping over" at a friend's house is a popular activity, and the child fears the humiliation of wetting the friend's bed. Many practitioners think that enuresis should not be treated until it limits the normal activities of the child. It is believed that since so many children spontaneously stop enuresis, putting them through the regimen required to manage the problem might be more traumatic than wetting the bed.

The family history contributes to the management of enuresis. Determining that one or both parents was enuretic can help allay some of the child's concerns about the future, particularly in the area of marriage. Knowing that a parent had the same problem and was able to overcome it helps the child deal with this problem. A family history of urinary tract problems may give direction for defining the etiology of this child's enuresis, suggesting that enuresis might be a symptom of an organic problem.

The past medical history of the child should be reviewed. A history of urinary tract infections may contribute to the cause of this child's enuresis. The prenatal history should be reviewed for any possible neurological complications in the child prenatally or during birth that might contribute to incontinence. The allergic history of the child and family helps rule out allergies as the cause of enuresis. Developmental milestones should be discussed in order to assess the child's progress.

Elimination patterns of this child must be elicited in the history. Toilet training methods used should be discussed. Sometimes too early and too rigid toilet training can contribute to a child's enuresis.

Methods used by parent and child for handling enuresis are significant. Enuresis is an emotional issue and the nurse needs to know the attitudes and feelings of all involved. Knowledge of past attempts to deal with the problem gives important insight into management issues. Shaming and punishing the child the next morning are of no value; in fact, these approaches are harmful. They compound the child's existing feelings of inadequacy and "differentness." All attempts made at controlling the enuresis should be discussed, including the child's response to each attempt and the degree of success achieved with each effort.

The history should include the number of bed-wetting episodes per week, the approximate amount of urine passed (at night and during the day), and the frequency with which the child urinates during the day. These facts give a clue to whether the child's functional bladder capacity is small. Some practitioners feel that the enuretic child sleeps more deeply than the normal child; depth of sleep can be assessed by inquiring about the difficulty with which the child is aroused from sleep. It is important to know if the enuretic episodes are becoming more or less frequent and whether they can be related to any stressful event in the child's life. It should be determined if the child has ever been continent, and if so, for how long.

Data collection should include a general physical examination, with special attention to the genitourinary function. Color, stream and odor of the urine should be assessed. Frequency, dribbling, dysuria or hesitancy in beginning urination should be noted to rule out organic causes. The neurological system should be reviewed with parents and child for any abnormal behavior or activity. Height and weight should be noted. Blood pressure should be checked for evidence of renal disease. The abdomen should be palpated for masses or tenderness. External genitalia should be examined for any gross abnormalities. Observations as to cleanliness and hygiene should be made. Any signs of allergic manifestations may be noted.

Laboratory testing should include a check of specific gravity and checks for glucose, protein and blood. If the index of suspicion from the history is high for urinary tract infection, a urine culture should be done.

Treatment

Enuresis is a highly treatable condition.[14] In planning a management program, it is important to have the cooperation of the child and the parents. Otherwise, success with management of enuresis is unlikely. During the history and physical, the nurse has the opportunity to assess the child's and parents' motivation to overcome the enuresis. The child can assume a large role in affecting cure, but parental support and reinforcement is essential. Similarly, if the parents seem eager to work on the problem and the child is apathetic, positive results will not be forthcoming. This must be a joint venture.

Many health care providers will not start a program with children of 5 or 6 years due to the high incidence of spontaneous resolution of the enuresis.[5] With older children there are several interventions that can be tried. If a small functional bladder capacity is diagnosed, efforts to enlarge the bladder may be attempted. These include having the child drink a large amount of fluids during the day and wait to urinate until discomfort is felt at least once each day. Restriction of fluids after dinner (or after 6 p.m.) may yield positive results. The child should void just before bedtime. There is some controversy as to the effectiveness of having parents wake the child to urinate when they retire. Some think this "lifting" is beneficial, since nocturnal urine production is highest in the early hours of sleep.[14] Others believe that it contributes to enuresis since the child does not really wake up at this time — thus "lifting" teaches the child to urinate in his sleep.[8]

Some physicians prescribe medication for children with enuresis. Imipramine is the drug of choice. The exact mechanism of this drug is not agreed upon by practitioners. Some think that it acts to increase bladder capacity. It may act as an antidepressant in emotionally disturbed children so they stop wetting the bed. It may act as a stimulant so the child does not sleep as deeply and can wake up to urinate.[6] It does not stop enuresis in some children, and the long-term result with its use is not significantly better than in those cases that spontaneously resolve. And it is not without danger to the child; neurological side effects and overdoses are potential problems. Gualtieri believes that imipramine should be used only in those cases in which more conventional methods have not been successful.[6]

Another method of treating children with enuresis involves use of a mechanical device, installed on the child's bed. An alarm goes off if the child begins to wet the bed, thus waking the child so he can finish urination in the toilet. In principle, this should condition the child to wake up when urination begins. These devices have varying degrees of success. Their strength seems to be with older children; however, the relapse rate is quite high (35 to 79 per cent).[3] Success depends on several variables: (1) proper functioning and installation of the device, (2) placing of the child so that he sleeps directly on top of the device so the urine touches the sensing mechanism, (3) the child waking up and (4) the child not disconnecting the apparatus. Rashes on the buttocks are a complication of this treatment.[3]

Whichever plan of treatment is chosen by the nurse, parents and child, the method of reinforcement is critical. None of the plans will work if the child does not receive positive reinforcement from parents for dry nights. Some families put gold stars on a chart for dry nights. Special activities can be used as positive reinforcers. The reward must be meaningful to the child and must be consistently given.

As with many childhood disorders, prevention is part of the key to enuresis. Early in the life of each child some consideration should be given to appropriate toilet training methods. This topic should be discussed with parents by the nurse long before the child is ready to be toilet trained. Knowledge of the cues or developmental milestones that indicate a child's readiness for toilet training will reduce the likelihood of too-early toilet training attempts.

Another factor to be considered is the provision of a warm, convenient place for the child to urinate. If the child must go down a long, dark hallway to the bathroom, he will not be as likely to get up in the middle of the night to void. A warm bathroom with a night light is much more conducive to nighttime use.

ENCOPRESIS

The most widely accepted definition of encopresis is dysfunction in which a child regularly passes formed or semi-formed stool in locations other than the toilet. In most cases this is associated with chronic stool retention. A few have incontinence without clear evidence of withholding.[7] Encopresis is further differentiated into *primary encopresis,* in which bowel control has never been achieved, and *secondary encopresis,* in which the child has been continent of stool for a period of months.[10] Fecal soiling may occur during the day as well as at night. It frequently accompanies a time of stress in the child's life.

Seven per cent of children are constipated and 7 per cent of these experience fecal soiling.[2] Encopresis is seen more frequently in boys than in girls.[4] It is seen in children from disrupted families more frequently than in children with intact families.

Etiology

Etiologic factors in encopresis do not seem well-defined at this time. This condition is like so many others in childhood — causes are many and components of each theory may be involved for any given child. The role of the nurse is to identify the causal factors in each child's situation so as to more effectively plan a management program. For this reason, the nurse needs to be acquainted with the various popular etiologic theories.

Encopresis may have a psychological basis arising from a variety of possible factors. For some reason the child learns, at a very early age in some cases, to withhold stool. It could be in response to improper toilet training. Toilet training might have been started too early or coercive tactics might have been used. Having a bowel movement may be uncomfortable to the child because of a fear of the toilet or of being left alone in the bathroom. Some deep-seated emotional problem is usually present with encopresis.

Some data indicate that there may be a genetic cause or predisposition to encopresis. It is believed that children with encopresis absorb more water from the fecal mass as it passes through the colon, thus making the mass more difficult to expel.[15] This theory might explain why constipation is present in these children from infancy.

There may be an organic basis for encopresis. A neurological problem or anatomic abnormality might cause fecal soiling and constipation. The child may have internal or external anal lesions that cause pain during the passage of stool.

Clinical Manifestations and Diagnosis

When a child has reached schoolage, bowel patterns are no longer obvious to the parents. Therefore, parents are not aware that the child is constipated. But parents are aware when fecal soiling occurs. The initial obvious conclusion of the parent is that the child has diarrhea. This complaint of diarrhea is sometimes the reason why health care is sought by a family. Other symptoms that may or may not be present are abdominal pain, lethargy, poor appetite and large, painful stools.[10] Many parents approach the health professional not because of diarrhea or constipation concerns but because of the frustration and embarrassment the soiling causes and the ambivalent feelings it is creating in them and the child's peers toward the child.

The diagnosing of encopresis and constipation begins with a careful, thorough history. This history should assess the child's daily habits and the psychosocial milieu of the family. Information about family dynamics is necessary to identify causative factors and to plan successful interventions. Parenting methods should be assessed. The primary person responsible for the care of the child should be identified — the mother or father, a sibling or a babysitter — because of the important role the primary caregiver has in the management of this condition. While obtaining the history, the nurse should observe the child's interactions with the parents in order to assess the health of the parent-child relationship.

The dietary history should be explored. Junk food, whole milk and limited fluids contribute to constipation, as do irregular eating times. Developmental milestones may be significant. The age at which bowel continence was achieved (if ever) is important.

A history of toilet training should be obtained. Inconsistent or coercive means to induce bowel control have been shown to contribute to the development of encopresis.

A description of elimination patterns is a necessary part of the history. Past medical history can be helpful; a long-standing problem with diarrhea or constipation might be significant. What the nurse means by diarrhea and constipation should be made clear to the parents. Amount and frequency of stools should be noted. If constipation has been present, the nurse will want to determine how this constipation has been treated and with what results. The issue of fecal soiling should be discussed, giving attention to how it has been treated at home and with what results. Some practitioners believe that parents who actively intervene when their child soils are reinforcing the encopretic activity because the child finds pleasure in the intervention. The touch of the parent in giving an enema or cleaning the perineum after soiling is enjoyable to the child and thus reinforces encopretic behavior.

Physical examination should be conducted, with special attention paid to neurological aspects. By eliciting a normal anal "wink" (response to a pin prick to anus), one can assess the neurological status of the anus. The abdomen may be mildly distended. Upon palpation, fecal material distending the colon may be felt. Bowel sounds may be normal or slightly diminished. Usually fecal material can be seen around the anus and in the underwear.[4]

Management

Once the diagnosis of encopresis has been confirmed by history and physical examination, the parents, child and nurse can set up a management program. Simple and specific explanation of the problem is the first step. This is particularly important, since this child most likely presented with diarrhea. The first goal of the program is to clear the impaction if it exists. These children usually have a large amount of stool distending the lower colon. Enemas are given on varying schedules until the impaction is removed. Depending on the regimen, this will take approximately 24 to 48 hours. It may be done at home or in the hospital depending on the family and the protocol being used.

Next an oral laxative is started, along with the establishment of a program of regular elimination patterns. The child is expected to sit on the toilet for a specific amount of time at regular times during the day. There should be proper foot support for the child — the feet should be at an angle whereby pushing can be comfortably done. A diet high in residue and low in milk is started. Fluids are encouraged. Children this age often respond well to the regimen when it is explained to them as though they were "in training" like an athlete, only the regimen they will follow is to improve the condition of the bowel (to return its elasticity and normal tone).

The parents and other family members will be affected by this treatment program. It may mean a diet change if they ordinarily do not eat a high-fiber diet. All members should be told to help enforce the toilet program of the child, but shame or ridicule from them will threaten a successful outcome. All family members (including siblings) should be involved in the management of encopresis.

As regular bowel habits are attained, dosage of oral laxative is gradually tapered. In most programs, a normal bowel pattern without oral laxatives is established within three to six months. Failures in management of encopresis are most often due to noncompliance. Giving an aura of hope to these children and involving families in the management are ways in which the nurse can motivate compliance.

Family therapy may be warranted in some cases. Knowing the family dynamics and community resources can aid the nurse in deciding whether to refer the family for counselling.

Prevention is the key to encopresis. The nurse working with families with young children should always carefully review elimination patterns with parents. Anticipatory guidance should be given regarding toilet training. Parents should wait until the child demonstrates readiness; his natural inclination to imitate adult behavior is an advantage. His readiness is indicated by his discomfort at having a stool in the diaper and interest in the toilet and the fact that there is some regularity to his bowel patterns. When bowel training is begun it should be in a warm room where adequate foot support for pushing is provided. If he desires, the child should be allowed privacy at this time. The nutrition of the child should be examined; junk food and irregular eating habits should be avoided. The child should be encouraged to exercise often. (See discussion of toilet training in Chapters 29 and 30.)

SCHOOL PHOBIA

The child with school phobia presents a challenging management problem to primary caregivers and school authorities. This child and his family need much support and guidance to achieve the child's comfortable return to school and interaction with peers.

Children suffering from severe school phobia are so immobilized by this that they cannot attend school. Hysterical, frantic behavior will be manifested when any attempt is made to urge this child to go to school. Different from the truant who does not want to go to school, the child with school phobia truly wishes to attend school but simply cannot force himself or herself to go when the hour arrives.

To understand school phobia more clearly, it is helpful to think of its severity as plotted on a continuum. At one end is the child with minor somatic complaints on school days when there is a test or presentation that is dreaded — a fairly normal reaction. At the other end of the continuum is the child whose anxiety is absolutely immobilizing. These are the children who become hysterical on the morning of a school day. Each child reacts to his school phobia with different degrees of intensity. This is of particular significance as the management of the child is considered.

Incidence and Etiology

There have been few studies in which the incidence of children with school phobia has been reported. Although it can occur at any age from 5 to adolescence, its peak incidence is at about 11 years of age. It occurs with equal frequency in boys and girls.[9] The children affected are of average or above average intelligence.[9] The number of children with this condition being seen by primary care providers is increasing, perhaps due to the fact that in the past these children were referred to truant officers. In terms of prognosis, younger children (under 11 years) have a more favorable outcome with therapy than do adolescents.

There are two theories as to the etiology of school phobia. However, when working with school phobic children, the nurse should realize that the etiologic factors for each child may be a combination of both or part of these theories; very seldom does the phobia have a single etiology.

The first theory that is held by some psychiatrists is that school phobia is basically a form of *separation anxiety*.[13] The child is not so much afraid of what will happen at school as of what will happen at home while he is attending school. This child is extremely fearful of leaving the home environment. In most studies, the mother is the parent the child feels closest to and is most fearful of leaving. These studies also show that the parent (usually the mother) fosters feelings of dependency in this child. In fact, while the mother verbally encourages the child to attend school, she holds the child's hand very tightly. This oversimplification is used to illustrate an extremely complex relationship between child and mother. Intellectually the mother realizes that her child must attend school; however, her dependency on this child is so great that actually having the child separate from her is extremely difficult. Phrases such as "I don't know what I'll do when you're gone," subtly reinforce the child's dependent state. It is felt that the mother has hidden hostilities toward herself for having to depend on a child and toward the child for being so dependent. The marital relationship often is not a healthy one. The father has characteristically withdrawn from the situation, thus offering no or minimal support to the mother. In attempting to repress these unacceptable hostilities, the mother becomes overprotective of this child so that the child will not recognize these "non-motherly" feelings. And as her overprotection increases, the child becomes more dependent on her and more reluctant to leave her to participate in normal activities such as school. This theory might be useful in explaining why some children have dreaded school since the beginning of their school experience, but it cannot clearly explain why a child with previous good school attendance develops a school phobia.

There is a second theory that is used to explain why a child with normal patterns of school attendance suddenly refuses to go. Leventhal believes that children with school phobia have an unrealistic view of their abilities.[9] They overvalue themselves — think themselves capable of feats beyond their talents. For instance, they see themselves as popular, well-liked and competent. When their peers and teachers in school do not support this view, they feel threatened and humiliated. Their self-image is damaged, perhaps to the point that they will refuse to attend school. For these children school becomes a difficult task because they feel constantly threatened. At home they receive family input that reinforces their too-high opinion of themselves, while at school they feel insecure and uncomfortable. This theory would explain why a child with good school attendance initially later starts finding excuses to miss school and, finally, refuses to attend at all.

In both of these theories there is an identifiable precipitating event that motivates the child's ultimate reaction to school. Events such as the birth of a sibling or unhappy experiences at school threaten the child so severely that refusal to attend school results. Children who separate with difficulty as well as those with unrealistic perceptions of their abilities have likely been slightly irregular in their school attendance. When the precipitating event occurs, school attendance becomes noticeably irregular or the child may cease to attend school completely.

A phobia has been defined as "severe and excessive fear aroused by a particular object or situation and characterized by an extreme desire to avoid the object."[1] In considering causes for a child's refusal of school, one must remember that it could be an acquired fear. There may be an object, person or situation in the school setting that arouses the child's fear to the point that refusal to attend occurs. Another child might be bullying this child. A particular class may be distasteful or difficult. Or the object of fear might not be readily identified either by the child or the family.

The source of a child's school phobia is not always obvious. Each one of the factors discussed might be influencing a given child. A child with an unrealistically high self-image may have an overprotecting, dependent mother, or there may be a frightening or humiliating situation that must be routinely faced at school by a child with a falsely positive self-image.

Clinical Manifestations and Diagnosis

School phobia presents in the form of somatic complaints; symptoms are varied. They reflect the severity of school phobia. Abdominal pain, headaches and general malaise are the most common symptoms; others are nausea and vomiting, anorexia, muscle aches and occasionally a low-grade fever. The child most commonly does not complain of fear of school. As the symptomatology is so varied and nonspecific in this phobia, the primary care provider is challenged to determine the underlying issue. If a mother brings the child to the physician or nurse with the complaint of "frequent abdominal pain," an in-depth history is essential in recognizing that the primary issue is that the child does not want to go to school.

Diagnosing the school phobic child's problem begins with a careful, thorough history. Clarification of statements and open-ended questions are of inestimable value. A specific area on which to concentrate is the past medical history. How much illness has this child had? How frequently did illness keep the child out of school? On careful questioning, it is often seen that the school attendance of this child has been sporadic and that somatic complaints have often been the reason. It is not until the parents and child start adding up these absences that they realize their frequency.

Another pattern that may be apparent when discussing the child's past medical history is the timing of symptoms. Symptoms displayed by children with school phobia are rarely seen during holidays, summer vacation or weekends. The symptoms are most prominent Sunday evenings or on a school morning and virtually disappear by afternoon. When obtaining a history from a school-age child, the nurse always should ask the child directly about school, being alert for the attitude displayed. Information from the child regarding friends and activities at school should be obtained. One reason to explore the child's feelings about school is to assess for factors causing the child's fear.

Because theories support that there is a precipitating event in the life of a child with school phobia, the nurse should pay special attention to recent life events. Occurrences such as birth of a new sibling or recent death or absence of a parent or other family member could precipitate an acute episode of school phobia. Dealing with these situations may eliminate the school phobia.

During the initial interview and history, the nurse should pay particular attention to the nonverbal communication taking place. How do the mother and child react to one another? Is the mother dominating the conversation to the point that the child is unable to speak? If this is happening, separating the mother and child and interviewing each alone might be effective. If the father is present, an assessment should be made regarding his role in the family situation and interaction. If the father is not present, an attempt should be made to interview him at another time. Since school phobia is so intimately related to family dynamics it is important, when obtaining the history, to have as many family members contributing as possible. When planning interventions for treatment, including all family members from the start helps ensure their commitment to participation in the management.

As was stated earlier, these children rarely present with "school phobia." They generally appear with a minor physical complaint such as a recurrent headache or stomachache. For this reason it is important for the practitioner to perform a complete physical examination, with particular attention given to the systems involved in the "chief complaint."[13] The physical is done to reassure the child and the parents that the child is physically well and to rule out an organic basis for the complaint. Simple tests such as throat cultures or urinalysis are sometimes performed, depending on the reason for seeking health care. Hearing and vision screening are especially important in this child. School problems are often manifestations of difficulties in hearing and vision.

Management

After the history and physical, the nurse assesses the severity of the problem for the child and parents. The nurse should evaluate parental anxieties related to the child's blatant unhappiness, their desire to eliminate his dread of school, and their concern over how the absences will affect his school work and over their legal responsibility to ensure his school attendance. It is at this point that the decision is made as to whether this child and family should be referred to a qualified therapist such as a psychiatrist or mental health nurse. These families tend to have multiple issues facing them and long-term therapy is often the only way to manage the problems. The literature regarding school phobia generally recommends referral to a mental health provider.

The major goal of management with these children is to get them back in school as rapidly as possible. Staying home from school deprives the child of the experiences needed to mature normally. The longer this child is allowed to stay out of school, the more difficult it will be for him to eventually return.

As plans are being formulated for the return to school, school authorities should be included, as their input is vital for the success of the program. The feasibility of the plan will depend on school facilities and the cooperation of teachers, counselors and administrators. Planning for return to school must be made cooperatively with the individual child and family. If the plan does not include all these, the chances of success are diminished. The plan could be for the child's return to school for two hours every day for a week in the counselor's office and then a gradual return to the classroom (desensitization technique), or an immediate return to the classroom.

Two fundamental considerations must be considered by the nurse in facilitating the plan: the fact that (1) school attendance is mandatory by law and (2) whether the child is capable of resuming a place in the community of peers.

Family therapy is often helpful in a given situation with school phobia. The decision whether or not to refer the family must be made by the primary care provider.

Close follow-up of these families is important as they attempt to alter long-standing patterns of behavior, because they will need much support and guidance. The parents may have many anxieties regarding the child and his relationship to school. Parental needs are important in the management of this issue and should be assessed by the nurse. The nurse is often in a position to be supportive and to help the family deal with issues that arise along the way.

As is the case in so many issues that arise in childhood, the best approach to school phobia is prevention. Early in the life of a child, the nurse can assess the separation patterns that are present. Anticipatory guidance and support to parents who have difficulty separating from their infant can prevent major separation problems from occurring later in the child's life. As the nurse works with young families, she can assess parenting skills and communication patterns. During the preschool examination, time should be spent with the family discussing school and the feelings the parents and child have about attending school.

ANTISOCIAL BEHAVIOR

Disturbing behaviors are sometimes manifested by school-age children that are contrary to societal norms. The testing of right and wrong through stealing, lying and cheating is sometimes seen in school-age children as they develop their moral code. Working through these temptations helps a child develop a conscience, if the situation is properly managed. School-age children are exploring their environment in earnest. Rules and regulations learned from parents are now being tested in their expanding world. Parents may not know about some of their child's growth and development stresses; when antisocial behavior suddenly manifests itself in their previously well-behaved child, they find this extremely disturbing and frustrating. They may seek assistance from the nurse in managing this behavior.

While this antisocial behavior is disturbing, parents should be encouraged to continue to discipline the child according to past and existing patterns in order to facilitate his quick passage through this stage. Parental expectations of the child should remain constant. When faced with disciplining a child who has stolen an object, a parent may be overwhelmed with the enormity of the issue and be unable to act effectively. One mother who discovered her school-age boy had obtained 30 dollars dishonestly did not know how to discipline him, so she did nothing until three weeks later when she sought help from her health care provider. It is important to point out that, until this situation arose, this particular mother felt confident about her parenting skills. But her beliefs about cheating were so strong that when she saw her son behaving dishonestly, her feelings prevented her from acting and caused her to have some self-doubts regarding her parenting skills. This reaction in a parent is not uncommon.

School-age children are beginning to observe and judge the behavior of significant others in their lives. They are now aware when parents or other adults do not always behave in the honest way they are expected to behave. Ignoring parking tickets, speeding and other such common behavior among adults is confusing to the child who has been constantly admonished to be truthful and honest. In light of these confusing messages from the adult world, the child experiments with some of these issues while attempting to form a superego.

Cheating is commonly seen in the early school-age years. At age 5 or 6, the child may not have a clear understanding of the rules of a game or activity. The child may have an extremely competitive spirit to the extent that cheating at a particular game is more tolerable than losing.[16] The developing superego coupled with an inability to fully understand rules often results in cheating behavior. It is usually of a benign, innocent nature and as the child matures will disappear. If cheating should persist and influence school or social performance, the parent or school authorities may seek help for the child.

Lying

A lie is a deliberate falsification with the intent to deceive.[2] In judging a statement to be a lie, it should be remembered that children, particularly under the age of 6 to 7 years, have a very active fantasy world. Through their fantasies, they are learning about the real world and how they fit into it. In the early school years the child often has difficulty differentiating between fantasies and reality. Sometimes the child will speak his fantasies; the adult may not recognize this and label it a lie without giving thought to the child's developmental level. However, the child is not deliberately telling a falsehood with the intent to deceive. It is therefore difficult to say that a child under the age of 6 or 7 years tells "lies."

Most children at one time or another tell a lie; it is a normal part of the exploration of childhood. It is when the lies become excessive or destructive that intervention is necessary.

Bakwin and Bakwin differentiate types of lies. The most commonly occurring lies are:[2]

1. Fantastic lies. These are the lies that come from the child's fantasy world. They are useful in helping the child learn about the real world.
2. Imitative lies. Adults are apt to embellish stories to a certain degree; the child imitates this behavior.
3. Lies of exaggeration and attention-seeking. These lies are told by the child to peers and adults for self-enhancement. These lies serve the purpose of compensating for real or imagined incompetencies or to build up wavering self-esteem.
4. Lies of convention. These are the "white lies" that are told generally in order to prevent hurt to others.
5. Defensive lies. These lies are told usually to escape punishment. They may also be told in an attempt to measure up to unrealistic expectations that have been set by someone else.

Stealing

A certain amount of stealing is normal in the early school years. These children are curious about everything around them. They love to collect things and are particularly attracted to brightly colored, interesting objects. The school-age child is developing a superego. Although he is learning right from wrong and "mine" from "his," these concepts are not fully internalized. Therefore, temptations are not always resisted — if a child sees something he wants, he sometimes takes it. This limited idea of property sense is somewhat understandable in light of adult role-modeling. Parents going through each other's belongings and through their children's belongings add confusion to the child's sense of ownership.

Stealing is a particularly disturbing problem to parents. The nurse may be asked for advice by parents. Bakwin and Bakwin list four causes of stealing:[2]

1. A lack of sense of property rights. Some parents do not allow their children any privacy either in time or possessions. They do not role-model for the child any concept of ownership. Thus the child does not learn to differentiate between what does and does not belong to him. Certain needs of children that can be met by parents are conducive to the prevention of stealing: (1) a child needs privacy; (2) a child needs some possessions that are his alone, especially clothes or toys; (3) a child must be taught early to respect the property of others.
2. Bribery. School-age children steal in order to have the means by which to obtain the favor of classmates and peers.
3. Desire to possess. One characteristic of the school-age child is a desire to collect. If he is not supplied with the means (allowance or pocket money) of purchasing additions, he may steal items to augment the collection.
4. Revengeful stealing. The child may steal to "get back" at parents for some unfair disciplinary measure or too-high expectations.

Identifying and Managing Antisocial Behavior

The issues of stealing, cheating and lying are emotional ones; children and families attempting to deal with these problems are frustrated, anxious and frequently feel guilty. The nurse must maintain a calm, nonjudgmental attitude and accept this family to effectively work with it. The practitioner's own feelings about the issues must be examined. A beginning therapeutic relationship should be established during the initial history-taking session.

It is important to be aware of family dynamics and communication patterns. Such observations may provide a major clue to the reasons the child is acting in an antisocial manner. The nurse should assess the type of restrictions and expectations the parents have of the child. Activities and interests of the child should be explored. Discipline measures and the granting of allowances should be discussed.

The nurse must realize that the child's behavior affects all family members. The parents may feel inadequate in preventing undesirable behavior in the child; other siblings may feel embarrassed by his behavior. Communication patterns may be disrupted because of the child's behavior. Recognizing the family members' needs surrounding this child's behavior helps the nurse identify desirable interventions.

Lying The practitioner must determine if the child is in fact lying, or if the child is merely sharing a fantasy world with parents who are mislabelling the statements as lies. If it is determined that the child is deliberately lying, the motivation behind the lies becomes paramount.

When the reason for a child's lies has been determined, proper therapy can be initiated. Depending upon the experience and attitude of the nurse, the child and parents may be referred to a mental health worker. Excessive lying is often symptomatic of deeper family pathology and is appropriately referred by the nurse, who will want to follow the child's progress by communicating with the mental health counselor.

If the nurse chooses to manage this issue, a problem-solving session with parents and child might facilitate successful resolution. Helping the family look at communication among its members, motivation behind the child's lies, and some possible interventions may be the best approach to overcome the problem. Frequently parents will identify behaviors that might have caused the child to lie. Working with the parents and child may improve the health of relationships within the family. Sup-

NURSING ACTIONS: FACILITATING MANAGEMENT OF SCHOOL-AGE BEHAVIOR PROBLEMS

Enuresis

Provide parents and child with accurate information on prevalence, etiology, and familial tendency.

Assure that organic causes are investigated and ruled out.

Obtain a complete history, including possible psychological causes and current stresses the child is experiencing.

Establish communication with child and parents; cooperation and understanding of all members in household is needed in management.

Encourage parents to provide positive reinforcement as child develops control.

Discourage shaming and punishment as methods of management.

Encopresis

Obtain a complete history, including dietary habits, toilet training experiences, and family interactions.

Clear impaction if necessary.

Institute program of regular daily elimination habits.

Provide guidance to family regarding importance of high-fiber diet, fluid consumption and adequate exercise.

Refer family for counseling if there is evidence of significant family dysfunction (see Chapter 5).

School phobia

Be aware that a child with school phobia often appears with minor physical complaints — stomachache or recurrent headaches.

Ensure that complete physical examination is carried out; school problems may involve hearing or vision difficulties.

Differentiate, with involvement of child and family, between normal mild fear or dislike of school and severe disabling anxiety.

Be open minded in listening to the child's complaints about school. Children may fear *real problems* — abusive teachers, street crime, school bullies or gangs, a vicious dog.

Serve as advocate for the child with school authorities or parents if needed; a nurse may be the only person aware of problems contributing to school phobia.

Antisocial behavior

Recognize that a nurse cannot impose her values on child or family.

Help parents realize that some antisocial behavior is "value testing" by a child and is a normal part of maturation.

Give parents guidance on what may be reasons for child's lying: fantasies, imitative lies, exaggeration and attention-seeking, and desire to avoid punishment.[2]

Give parents guidance on what may be reasons for child's stealing; lack of sense of property rights, bribery, desire for possessions or revenge.[2]

---

porting the parents as they begin intervening to eliminate the child's lying may be the nurse's primary role.

Prevention of a child's lying is the first defense. In giving anticipatory guidance to parents, discipline should always be discussed. Parents' feelings and attitudes about disciplining their children should be elicited. Too-strict discipline measures seem to promote lying in some children. The nurse may tactfully suggest to parents that their expectations of their child's behavior are high and unrealistic. If expectations are realistic, a child will not be forced into telling lies.

Stealing To intervene effectively with school-age children who steal, the nurse must determine the reason(s) for the stealing. The reason is not likely to be discovered until a mutually trusting relationship is established between the nurse, the child and the parents. Family dynamics may have to be explored, depending upon the cause that is identified. This complex issue may be resolved optimally by referring the child and family to a mental health clinic. Depending upon the severity and the outcome of the stealing episodes, legal authorities may be included in the management of this problem.

The nurse may choose to work with this family regarding the issue of stealing. Suggestions from the parents as to how comfortable they are in handling this problem and the intervention options that are acceptable to them should be considered first. To prevent further episodes of stealing, the parents should be encouraged to handle the situation matter-of-factly, allowing the child to see how upset they are. By clearly demonstrating to the child that stealing is unacceptable behavior and will not be tolerated, further stealing may be prevented.

Parents can also help their child stop stealing by removing tempting items. Loose change should be out of sight. Pens and pencils should be in drawers, except for the items that belong to the child. By removing "stealable" items, the parents can reduce the internal conflict experienced by a child who steals. Wanting the object while knowing it is not one's own is frustrating for the child. Helping to prevent stealing and administering consistent discipline if it occurs are two interventions that may alleviate the behavior.

References

1. S. Ambron. Child Development. Rinehart Press/Holt, Rinehart & Winston, 1975
2. H. Bakwin and R. Bakwin. Behavior Disorders in Children. W. B. Saunders Co., 1972
3. M. Cohen. Enuresis. Pediatric Clinics of North America, August 1975, p. 545
4. J. Fitzgerald. Encopresis. In Ambulatory Pediatrics by M. Green and R. J. Haggerty, eds. W. B. Saunders Co., 1977
5. M. Green, Enuresis. In Ambulatory Pediatrics by M. Green and R. J. Haggerty, eds., W. B. Saunders Co., 1977
6. C. Gualtieri. Imipramine and Children: A review and some speculations about the mechanism of drug action. Diseases of the Nervous System, May 1977, p. 368
7. R. Hoekelman et al. Principles of Pediatrics: Health Care of the Young. McGraw-Hill Book Co., 1978
8. W. Homan. Child Sense. Basic Books, 1977
9. T. Leventhal and M. Sills. Self-image in school phobia. American Journal of Orthopsychiatry, Vol. 34, 1964, p. 685
10. M. Levine. Children with encopresis: a descriptive analysis. Pediatrics, September 1975, p. 412
11. M. Levine and H. Baksu. Children with encopresis: a study of treatment outcome. Pediatrics, December 1976, p. 845
12. J. McKendry and D. Stewart. Enuresis. Pediatric Clinics of North America, November 1974, p. 1019
13. P. Nadar et al. School phobia. Pediatric Clinics of North America, August 1975, p. 605
14. D. Shaffer. Nocturnal enuresis. Nursing Times, 22 April 1976, p. 616
15. D. Sieber. Encopresis: a discussion of etiology and management. Clinical Pediatrics, April 1969, p. 225
16. F. Ug and L. Ames. Child Behavior. Harper & Brothers, 1955

Additional Recommended Reading

E. Christopherson and M. Rapoff. Eneuresis treatment. Issues in Comprehensive Pediatric Nursing, Mar/Apr 1978, p. 34

T. Kenny and R. Clemmens. Behavioral Pediatrics and Child Development. Williams and Wilkins, 1975

E. Lessers et al. Steps in the return to school of children with school phobia. American Journal of Psychiatry, March 1973, p. 265

POTENTIAL STRESSES DURING SCHOOL-AGE YEARS: TEMPORARY ALTERATIONS IN HEALTH STATUS

by Anne E. Hartson, RN, MA

Temporary alterations in health can have several ramifications for the school-age child and for parents, siblings, peers, teachers and the school nurse.

Family functioning is disrupted in several ways. Medical bills or hospitalization or both can add a temporary financial burden. Usual routines may need to be altered to allow for doctor appointments, visits to the hospital and compliance with treatment regimens. Anxiety, guilt and fear may affect interactions of family members.

The school-age child with a temporary alteration will be affected in areas of cognitive, emotional and social and physical development. Learning experiences in school may be interrupted by doctor appointments or hospitalization. The child may experience frustration or anger because of his need to depend on parents and other adults at a time when he is seeking control over his life. Interactions with siblings may be affected by jealousy because of extra attention given to him. Peer contacts may be limited, particularly if hospitalization is required. A temporary change in the child's physical appearance may cause him worry and thus interfere with his developing self-concept. The school-age child spends a great deal of time engaged in physical activities at home and school. Having to curtail these may put additional stress on him.

The nurse has an important role in helping the child, parents and siblings cope with these alterations by providing support, preparing them for treatment procedures, teaching about the condition and offering anticipatory guidance on preventive measures. Resolution of the child's problem and restoring family functioning is the primary goal.

CUTANEOUS PROBLEMS

Scabies

Scabies is an infectious skin condition frequently seen in school-age children, causing a vesicular or papulovesicular eruption. An epidemic of scabies has existed worldwide since 1964;

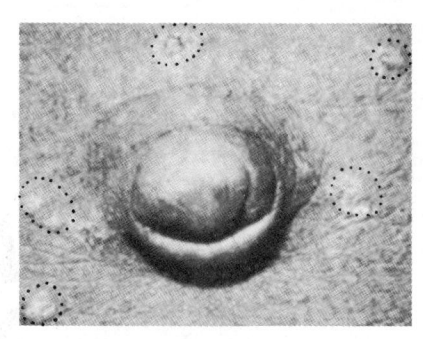

Figure 50–1 Papular and eczematous lesions of the abdomen are usually present in a "spokelike" periumbilical arrangement in classic scabies. (From M. Orkin. Scabies in Children. Pediatric Clinics of North America, May 1978, p. 373.)

scabies has been pandemic in the United States since 1974.[8] There are several forms of scabies. The most common "classic scabies" is transmitted by direct contact with a person infested with the *Acarus scabies (Sarcoptes scabiei)*, or itch mite.

The adult female itch mite, approximately the size of a grain of sugar, digs into the superficial stratum corneum of the epidermis and forms a burrow, leaving debris and feces. Each day for approximately a month burrowing continues a few millimeters and the female mite lays two to three eggs. The adult mite then dies and the eggs mature to an adult form in 10 days. The skin of the infested person reacts in an allergic fashion and small vesicles and papules form.

Identification of scabies is difficult and often it is misdiagnosed in children. Although it is often classified as a "social disease," it occurs in all socioeconomic levels, and cleanliness is not a protection.[7] Children who bathe regularly will remove many of the mites, and the burrows may be impossible to detect. The nurse may use an ink pen to trace the burrows to the vesicle (mite hill) in an attempt to visualize the lesion. Because scabies is transmitted by direct contact, it is imperative that all family members be treated for scabies regardless of the presence of lesions. It is not necessary to treat fomites,* because the mite will survive only two to three days away from human skin.

Children infested with the itch mite will first experience nocturnal itching. Pruritus is increased with the warmth of the bed and occurs only after sensitization to the mite and debris, usually a month after infestation. Scabetic lesions will usually be present on the sides or webs of the digits of hands and feet, extensor surface of the elbows, anterior axillary skin folds, glans penis, scrotum and abdomen (Fig. 50–1). The nurse will recognize initial lesions as small erythematous, excoriated papules. These may appear eczematous if the child has had pruritus and scratching resulted.

The diagnosis of scabies must be made microscopically by identification of the mite from skin scrapings. It is imperative that the nurse provide factual information regarding the transmission of the mite in an attempt to alleviate guilt feelings of the parents and child. Notification of local health authorities is not required with individual cases, and parents will be relieved to know that confidentiality will be maintained. Examination by a physician is imperative for appropriate treatment.

Gamma benzene hexachloride (GBH) is the usual treatment for scabies.[5] Sulfur and Crotamiton are recommended for infants and young children because of the possibility of central nervous system toxicity with GBH.[8] The infected child and all family members should initially bathe, towel dry and then apply the scabicide from the neck down, being especially careful to apply between the fingers and toes and in the genital area.[7] Bathing should be repeated 12 hours after application of the scabicide. One application is usually sufficient, although some physicians may recommend a second treatment in one week.[8] Clothing in direct contact with the skin should be washed in hot water and dried. Underclothes and bed linens should be changed with each bath.

Treatment is usually very effective if instructions are followed correctly. Many parents will want to overtreat their child, and it is imperative that instructions be provided verbally and in writing.

Allowing the child an opportunity to ventilate feelings and providing basic information about the disease and treatment will be a major role for the nurse. School-age children with scabies may feel ashamed or guilty. An understanding of the condition will help the child cope and maintain a positive self-image.

Tinea Pedis

Tinea pedis (dermatophytosis), more commonly known as athlete's foot, is a fungal disease.

---
*Fomites are inanimate objects such as combs or clothing that serve to transfer infectious organisms from one person to another.

Fungal infections develop when a person has an altered homeostasis, providing a conducive environment for the organism. Conditions that promote pathogenic fungal growth include immunosuppression and hyperhydrosis. Although tinea pedis is not frequent in the young school-age child, its incidence increases near puberty.

Trichophyton rubrum, T. mentagrophytes and *E. floccosum* are the usual causative organisms. The appearance of tinea pedis can range from an acute inflammatory vesiculobullous eruption to a dull erythema and scaling (Fig. 50–2). An acute episode initially involves the intertriginous area of the fourth and fifth toes and extends to the plantar surface of the foot. Skin maceration, scaling, vesicles and fissures result. The absence of vesiculation and the presence of moccasin-like scaling occurs in chronic tinea pedis and is usually limited to a small area between the toes.

Prevention of tinea pedis is virtually impossible, because the organisms are present on most people. However, proper foot hygiene is an important health consideration for all school-age children. Instruction should include the importance of daily bathing and careful drying between all toes. Many children now wear nonventilated shoes, which provide an excellent growth medium for fungus, especially during the summer months when their feet are warm and moist. Nurses should encourage older children to go barefoot when appropriate or to wear sandals, which allow the feet to stay dry. Early treatment of a fungus-infected toenail may prevent an episode of tinea pedis and complications from secondary infections.

Children complaining of itchy feet with signs of scaling and or vesicle formation should be referred to a physician for diagnosis and treatment. Diagnosis can usually be made clinically; however, tissue scrapings examined under a Wood's lamp will confirm suspicions.[16] Some children experience discomfort and burning from the vesicles. A child unable to walk probably has a secondary infection in conjunction with acute tinea pedis.

Treatment for acute tinea pedis is somewhat involved, and parents will need specific written instructions. Systemic treatment is with oral griseofulvin and a broad-spectrum antibiotic. Parents and child need to be shown how to apply wet compresses to the foot for 20 minutes four times a day. Local treatment of the vesicles with wet compresses is continued until the blisters heal, and then topical antifungal agents are used. The child with tinea pedis should be instructed to wear cotton socks and to alternate between pairs of shoes to allow complete drying. Parents and siblings need to be informed that the skin condition is not contagious; however, the exchange of socks and bath towels should be prohibited. If the child is not in acute distress, arrangements should be made to allow him to continue with school. The child with a severe case of acute tinea pedis may feel some resentment at having to temporarily curtail ambulatory activities, particularly physical education or athletics that stimulate foot perspiration, or because he cannot walk. The school nurse should discuss the child's condition with his teacher so that the child's discomfort and lack of participation in some activities will be understood. The teacher responsible for gym classes should be informed so that attention is given to proper hygiene.

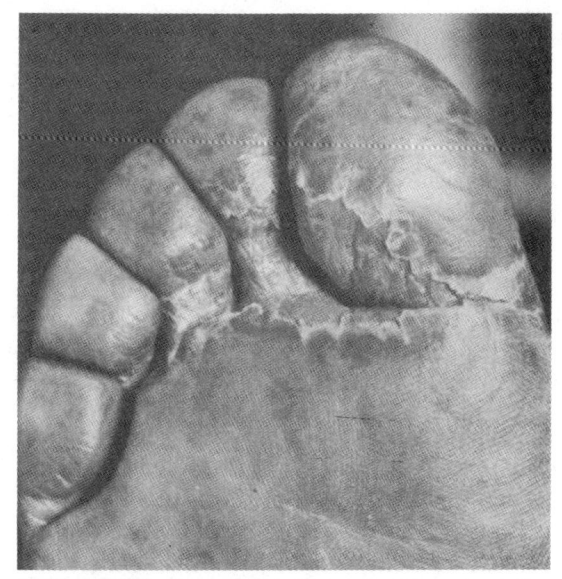

Figure 50–2 Tinea pedis. (From A. Domonkos. Andrews' Diseases of the Skin, 6th ed. W. B. Saunders Co., 1971.)

Chronic tinea pedis may be treated with nonprescription topical antifungal medications such as Tinactin or Whitfield's ointment. Application of the ointment must be continued for three to four weeks after healing has occurred.

Furuncles

Furuncles, or boils, may occur at any age. In children they are most commonly seen in staphylococcal carriers and those with chronic nutrition problems, immune deficiency states and other debilitating diseases.[4] A furuncle is an acute localized perifollicular staphylococcal abscess of the skin and subcutaneous tissue that undergoes necrosis and suppuration.[4]

Development of a furuncle results from obstruction of a sebaceous gland or ingrowth of a hair follicle. A small pustule enlarges around the hair follicle, becoming firm, red and tender. The lesion becomes fluctuant and will eventually drain purulent material, allowing healing to occur in one to two weeks.

Nurses working with children identified as "at risk" should facilitate early treatment by teaching the signs and symptoms of furuncles. When teaching good skin care to children, they should include a description of furuncles, and children should be cautioned against "picking" at infected hairs. Recurring furuncles may require checking family members for staphylococcal carriers. Furuncles occur only in areas of hair follicles — most commonly the neck, buttocks, extremities, perineum, axillae and face. The child may initially experience itching but usually will ignore the pustule until it enlarges and causes pain. Malaise and an elevated temperature (38.3 to 38.9° C or 101 to 102° F) are other presenting symptoms. Diagnosis is made by isolation of the *S. aureus* from the purulent drainage. Referral to a physician is warranted if the child is experiencing intense pain and the lesion does not drain spontaneously. Occasionally systemic treatment with a synthetic penicillin is necessary.

Nursing care for home management of a boil includes careful instruction on good handwashing, avoiding hand contact with the pustule and disposal of drainage in a closed container. The application of warm, moist compresses may alleviate some of the child's discomfort. Children with draining lesions may attend school if bandages are used to cover the area. Clean, dry gauze is placed over the area but may need to be changed while the child is in school. The nurse can help in changing the bandage and evaluating if further treatment is necessary. This is also an opportunity for the nurse to demonstrate proper handwashing and disposal of the soiled dressing. She should also assess the child's discomfort. If pain is severe or the child is self-conscious about the bandage, attendance at school should not be mandatory. The school nurse should contact the child's teacher and arrange for make-up work to be done at home. Children with furuncles will benefit from knowing that the skin infection is only temporary and there will be no residual scarring.

Carbuncles

Carbuncles represent a more severe and extensive skin infection than furuncles. The incidence of carbuncles is greater in males and is seen most often in children with diabetes, hypogammaglobulinemia, and other resistance-lowering diseases.[5]

The perifollicular abscess affects adjacent hair follicles and drains through multiple openings in the skin; thus carbuncles are often described as multiple furuncles. Sites for abscess development are similar to those described for furuncles. The simple pustule develops slowly, enlarges to the size of an egg or an orange, and causes extensive pain. When carbuncles drain, the entire center lesion may slough off a large amount of necrotic material, leaving a large ulcerated area. The ulcer will granulate in several weeks, but a scar is usually present.

Recurrence of carbuncles is common, and children prone to development of this skin condition should avoid skin irritation from constrictive clothing.

School-age children will experience general malaise, fever, chills and complain of severe pain. The nurse will easily recognize a carbuncle from its large size, red color and tenderness. Any child presenting with this skin condition should be referred to the physician for diagnosis and immediate treatment.

Management usually includes systemic antibiotics, rest and warm, moist compresses. Analgesics may be needed if the pain is severe. Occasionally excision of the carbuncle is necessary to promote drainage. The nurse should prepare the child and parents for the excision in these ways: (1) describe the procedure and equipment to be used, (2) describe possible pain the child may feel and (3) discuss how the child wants to deal with treatment, as whether to have parents present. Adequate preparation for treatment enhances the child's coping abilities and promotes parental support.

The physician has a responsibility to inform the child and parents that a residual scar may be present after healing has occurred. Nurses can be helpful in allowing children an opportunity to express concerns over scar formation; however, with the exception of facial lesions, most children adapt well.

TRAUMA

Epistaxis

Nosebleed, or epistaxis, occurs twice as often in children as adults.[11] Anterior epistaxis is visible because the blood flows down and out through the nostril. Posterior bleeding is less common and more difficult to assess because the blood flow is down the back of the throat and children often swallow the drainage.

Most episodes of epistaxis arise in the anterior inferior part of the nasal septum called Kiesselbach's plexus.[11] Causes of epistaxis include the following: (1) major trauma (fractures), (2) nose picking resulting in irritation of the superficial blood vessels, (3) chronic upper respiratory infections that produce inflammation and ulceration of the mucosa and (4) bleeding disorders.

Prevention of trauma is a primary goal for all nurses. Health teaching for children and parents should include a discussion on proper nose blowing, and provisions for adequate humidity in the atmosphere when upper respiratory infections occur.

Nosebleeds are often frightening, and the nurse must calm the child while trying to control the bleeding. The child should be encouraged to sit quietly with his head tilted forward* while the nares are compressed for five to 10 minutes. Ice may also be applied during compression of the nares. Eighty per cent of nosebleeds will stop spontaneously when clotting occurs.[11] If bleeding continues, a piece of cotton should be inserted into the nostril and the child transported to the physician. The physician will insert cotton with a few drops of epinephrine for five minutes to control the bleeding and keep the child in the office until the bleeding has stopped. Then the doctor will remove the cotton. An explanation of the treatment prior to the procedure will usually allay the child's fears and gain his cooperation. Persistent bleeding may require the use of a silver nitrate stick, which is applied to the superficial vessels. Another form of treatment is the use of electrocautery. If cauterization is needed, it is important to forewarn the child of the burning odor and sound. Nasal packing (gauze wad inserted to fill nostril, creating direct pressure to the bleeding vessel) is used only when bleeding is profuse and persistent, usually in hemorrhagic diseases. Petroleum jelly is applied to the nares to prevent crusting of blood or irritation. This measure also alleviates the tendency of the child to pick at crusted areas.

Because epistaxis episodes are usually short-term, most children and parents will need only immediate support. Parents should be cautioned that if excessive amounts of blood are swallowed, the child will probably have some dark, tarry stools. However, after the bleeding is controlled the nurse should direct her attention to teaching preventive measures to the child and parents.

Frostbite

Frostbite, or tissue freezing, results from extreme exposure to cold. Environmental conditions, including low temperatures, high humidity and high wind velocity, will increase the rate of heat loss from the body. Children are a high-risk population because most do not comprehend early warning signs of exposure.

Cold causes arteriolar vasoconstriction, resulting in a decreased blood flow and interference with oxygen transport; tissue anoxia is the end result. With tissue freezing, the particles form in the extracellular spaces and draw water from surrounding cells. Cell dehydration and the destruction of intracellular structures results.

School nurses working in cold climates can play an important role in the prevention of frostbite. The education of parents, children and teachers on appropriate outdoor clothing for insulation is essential. Several layers of light clothing, including cotton or cotton-lined underclothes, shirt and pants of woven fabric, a sweater and a down coat or parka, are the best protection. Children playing outdoors should be instructed to wear two pairs of socks (cotton and wool), a hood or hat and mittens or gloves. Young school-age children should not be allowed to play outside in extremely low temperatures. Older children should be instructed to warm themselves when hands or feet begin to sting.

Blanching of the skin and a stinging sensation

---

*This is done to prevent blood from trickling into the pharynx.

are the initial signs of impending frostbite. Numbness will follow and the exposed area will appear white or mottled, feel cold and hard and be without sensation. Deep frostbite will cause the tissue to blister. The nurse must quickly assess the appearance of the frostbite and institute appropriate first aid measures to prevent further tissue damage. Any child with white or mottled skin after cold exposure should be referred for medical evaluation and further treatment. During school times, treatment for mild frostbite can be managed by the school nurse.

The child should be in a warm place and the affected part can be rewarmed gradually by blowing hot breath on the part or holding warm hands firmly on the area.[14] For deeper frostbite it is essential that the part be rapidly rewarmed; slow thawing causes further tissue damage because some refreezing of tissue occurs.[18] If the child is close to medical facilities he should be transported immediately, keeping the part frozen. In isolated areas, rapid rewarming in a water bath (90 to 106° F) should be done prior to transport.[13] It is imperative to avoid refreezing the affected area during transport. Children with severe frostbite will need to be hospitalized and receive long-term treatment similar to that for the burn victim.

Support for the child with mild frostbite should include a discussion as to why it is essential to rewarm the affected part. Stinging sensations may be frightening to children, and it is important for the nurse to explain the normalcy of these sensations. Parents may feel guilty over allowing their child to play outside; therefore it is important to allow them to ventilate feelings and then to focus on preventive measures. Siblings should also be included in a discussion of prevention and appropriate first aid measures.

Bicycle Accidents

Bicycle riding is a favorite activity for many children and adolescents. Unfortunately, the number of bicycle-related injuries and deaths has increased. Injuries involving bicycles lead the U.S. Consumer Product Safety Commission's list of product-related injuries.[15] In 1977, 1100 deaths resulted from bike accidents; 540 deaths occurred in the 5 to 14 year age group. Bike injuries constitute a large percentage of pediatric outpatient and hospital admissions.

These injuries vary from mild abrasions, contusions and lacerations requiring minimal first aid to multiple injuries of the head, trunk and limbs. The seriousness of the injury is determined by the type of accident. Collisions with automobiles account for a high percentage of deaths from craniocerebral trauma.[15] Simple falls are associated with a high risk for trunk injuries caused by the impact against the handle bars. Improperly worn shoulder bags can become wedged in the front wheel and the child thrown head first over the bicycle, causing facial injuries.

Establishment of an open airway is the first priority for the emergency room nurse treating a bicycle accident victim. Further assessment will include an evaluation of the child's cardiovascular and neurological status. Addressing the child by name, speaking in a calm voice and providing an explanation of who you are and what you are doing will decrease the child's anxiety and gain his cooperation.

After an initial assessment it is necessary to obtain a history of the injury from the child or parents; when, where and what occurred. The parents should be allowed to remain with the child during treatment or rejoin the child as soon as possible after treatment. Most parents experience tremendous guilt feelings when their child is injured. Listening and encouraging verbalization will help parents deal with these feelings. Parents will have many questions about the treatment and the severity of the injuries sustained that the physician or nurse or both should answer. The extent of the child's injury will determine the prognosis. If the child is hospitalized, he, his parents and siblings will experience the stress caused by an unexpected crisis.

Studies have shown that many school-age children are ignorant of traffic signs and terms. A bicycle safety education program similar to the driver training programs should be conducted by all elementary schools. Parents can also get information on bicycle safety to discuss with their child from their local motor vehicle and license registration bureau.

Head Injuries

About 200,000 children a year are admitted to U.S. hospitals for observation and treatment following a head injury.[16] Accidental falls, bicycle, and motor vehicle accidents are the major cause of head injuries in children.[12]

Head injuries result from a physical change of the head in relation to its environment. During a fall, a child's head is in constant motion and is stopped abruptly when it hits the ground. This is the acceleration-deceleration phenomenon common in head trauma. The sudden deceleration causes the child's brain to move inside the cranium, with resulting injury to tissue and blood vessels.

Most head injuries are minor and do not cause loss of consciousness. The child will be examined by the physician and sent home with specific instructions for the parents. The child may vomit and appear pale, apathetic or irritable. Any child who does not regain consciousness within a few minutes after an injury or who shows progressive loss of consciousness will need immediate medical attention.

If the nurse is present at the accident scene, she should establish an airway and quickly assess the child's neurologic status. The child should not be moved until an emergency vehicle is available to transport him. Parents need to be contacted immediately to obtain permission for emergency treatment.

Concussion Concussion frequently occurs in children who have experienced more than minimal head trauma. The injury involves reversible neuronal damage that precipitates an immediate, transient altered consciousness (drowsy, lethargic or unconscious) that may last minutes or hours, followed by prompt recovery without immediate sequelae. The loss of consciousness is related to a disruption in brain stem activity. Upon arousal the child is pale or flushed, may be diaphoretic and usually complains of headache and may vomit for up to 48 hours. The child also experiences a memory loss of the facts about the accident.

Because a concussion is caused by a hard blow to the head, it is imperative to closely assess the child for signs of intracranial hemorrhage or fractures. A hematocrit (Hct) should be done to determine any decrease suggestive of internal bleeding intracranially or elsewhere. Skull x-rays are done if fracture is suspected. The nurse should monitor speech ability, pupil size, limb movements and muscle strength, and state of consciousness at 15- to 30-minute intervals.

If the injury occurs away from home, notification of parents is essential. When phoning the parents, the nurse should describe how the child is feeling and what occurred, and that a medical examination is needed to rule out possible cranial injury.

Home or hospital management depends upon the severity of signs and the parents'

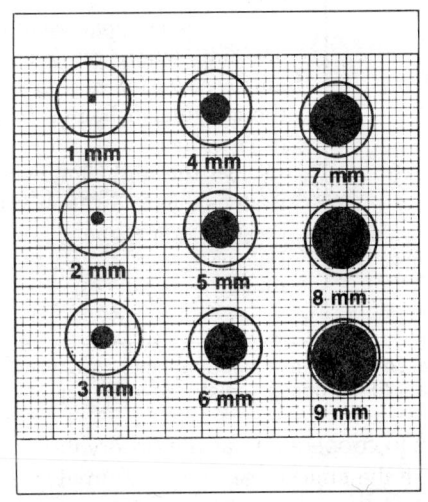

> **SPECIFIC RECORDING OF PUPIL SIZE**
>
> Pupil size is a significant evaluation factor in every neurological check. Yet, documentation of pupil size is often very subjective and vague, lacking a systematic terminology or method of documentation. Terms such as moderate, dilated, or pinpoint have many different meanings to different individuals.
>
> Marshall and her colleagues have established a method of estimating and recording pupil size more accurately, which helps maintain consistency from one neurological check to the next. This method utilizes EKG paper onto which various possible pupil sizes have been charted. A pinpoint pupil equals 1 mm (size of one small square on EKG paper). A moderately dilated pupil is 5 mm (size of a large square on EKG paper). A fully dilated pupil is 8 to 9 mm. The nurse can then refer to this chart to establish the dilation in millimeters at each neurological check.
>
> We propose that an EKG strip become part of the neurological checklist. Pupil size would then be filled in at each neurological check, providing a flow sheet of the patient's pupil size from which comparisons can be made as to improvement or deterioration of neurological status as related to pupil size.
>
> Reprinted from Tips and Timesavers, September issue of Nursing 78, Frances Marshall, author. Copyright © 1978 Intermed Communications, Inc.

> ## INSTRUCTIONS TO PARENTS—
> ## CARE OF THE CHILD WITH A HEAD INJURY
>
> Although your child has been thoroughly examined for evidence of head injury, and the examining physician has determined that it is safe for your child to return home, certain signs of trouble may appear within the next 48 hours. During this time, please observe your child carefully and telephone your doctor should any of the signs listed below develop. *Be sure that you review all these signs with the examining physician to be sure you understand them before you leave the hospital.*
>
> 1. *Excessive drowsiness.* Your child may well be exhausted by the ordeal experienced after a head injury. However, you should be able to rouse the child easily, as you would normally from a deep sleep. If not, notify your doctor.
>
> 2. *Persistent vomiting.* In most cases, children will vomit one or two times following a severe head injury. Should the vomiting recur more than once or twice, or should it begin again hours after it has ceased, notify your doctor.
>
> 3. *Eye problems.* If one pupil appears to be larger than the other, or if your child complains of seeing double or if the eyes fail to move together appropriately, notify your doctor.
>
> 4. *Unsteady gait or movement.* If your child does not use either arm or leg as well as previously or is unsteady while walking, notify your doctor.
>
> 5. *Speech difficulty.* If your child's speech becomes slurred, or the child is apparently unable to talk, notify your doctor.
>
> 6. *Headache.* If severe headache occurs, particularly if it increases in severity and is not relieved by aspirin, notify your doctor.
>
> 7. *Convulsions.* Should a convulsion occur, place the child on one side, where he or she cannot fall, and be sure that there is ample room for him or her to breathe. Stay with the child until the convulsion begins to subside and notify your doctor *as soon as possible.*
>
> On the night following the head injury or during any nap, it is advisable to awaken your child every 3 hours to look for any of these danger signs.
>
> Doctor: _____
> Phone: _____

Figure 50–3 Form of instructions to parents caring for a head-injured child. (From R. Reece and J. Chamberlain, Manual of Emergency Pediatrics. W. B. Saunders, 1974, p. 690.)

ability to cooperate in astute observation of the child. If the child rouses with minimal stimulus and shows no signs of hemorrhage, increased intracranial pressure or neurological sequelae he may be observed at home; otherwise hospitalization for 24 to 48 hours is indicated. Whichever place the child is observed, he should be aroused at regular intervals to determine pupil size, limb strength, speech ability and level of consciousness. He should not receive sedatives, although he may receive analgesics for headache or antipyretics for fever. Many emergency rooms provide a printed form of instructions for parents similar to the one in Figure 50–3. This information on what to observe should be provided for the parents, both verbally and in writing, before the child is released. As level of consciousness improves, the child should be reoriented as to where he is and what happened and then confined to quiet activity. Full recovery usually occurs in 24 to 48 hours, at which time the child may return to school.

Contusions Contusions result from severe head trauma, causing bruising or laceration of brain tissue with associated local edema at the site of the blow (coup) or opposite the site (contracoup).[16] This child shows signs of shock, develops progressive alteration in consciousness over a period of hours, and may be convulsive or ataxic. A child with a contusion may be confused, irritable or amnesic. Careful observation for flow of cerebrospinal fluid* or blood or both from the nose should be done; these signs indicate basilar skull fracture.

Diagnostic neuroradiological studies, including x-rays, computerized tomography (CAT scans) and cerebral angiography are done to determine amount and location of injuries. The CAT scan is most commonly used because of its safeness and reliability. Providing the child's parents with specific information on the diagnostic tests will help allay their anxiety.

In the absence of signs of increased intracranial pressure (papilledema or pupil changes), a lumbar puncture may be done to decrease the severity of headaches or improve the state of consciousness. Sedatives are avoided but Valium or Dilantin may be administered for agitation or seizures. Antipyretics are indicated for fever. Attention must also be given to maintaining an adequate airway in patients with impaired cardiorespiratory function. If the child's condition deteriorates and the coma deepens, surgical intervention to relieve increased intracranial pressure may be necessary. Other treatment includes the use of steroids (dexamethasone) and osmotic diuretics to reduce cerebral edema.

Prognosis for the child with a contusion depends on the severity of tissue damage. Less than 10 per cent of all head injuries result in neurological impairments.[3] However, the child will be hospitalized. The family will need ongoing support during hospitalization and after discharge, since these children may exhibit disruptive behavior changes when under stress.

Epidural Hematoma Epidural hematomas result most often from a tear in the middle meningeal artery with a sudden accumulation of blood, which presses on the underlying cerebral tissues. Concussions, contusions or fractures may cause the hemorrhage between the skull and dura. Without surgical intervention the hematoma causes increased intracranial pressure and the mortality rate is 100 per cent.[2] This hematoma is more common in the school-age years than at any other age.

Any child who awakens from a concussion, is alert and then loses consciousness with signs of increasing intracranial pressure should be examined immediately for a possible epidural hemorrhage. Diagnosis is made with skull x-rays, echoencephalography and cerebral angiography, if time permits. These measures also help to localize the hematoma prior to surgery. Immediate surgical intervention is mandatory when signs of focal weakness, unilateral pupil dilatation and respiratory distress appear. The prognosis depends on the duration of the child's unconsciousness and on the preoperative status.

Although head injuries in children are very common and often relatively benign, it must be stressed that head trauma can cause permanent neurological sequelae (convulsive, neuromotor, learning or behavioral) or even death. It is estimated that about 20 per cent of children with more than minor head trauma develop such sequelae.

Sports Injuries

Children's involvement with sports may vary from competitive contact sports such as football, basketball or wrestling to noncontact and recreational sports such as swimming, tennis, running and archery. All forms of sports have an important role in the child's physical, emotional, social and mental development. Physical development is enhanced by improving the child's strength, stamina and fine and gross motor skills. Sports provide an opportunity to learn lifelong recreation activities. Interactions with other children and adults help expand the child's social environment. Sports also serve as an acceptable outlet for release of aggression and frustration.

The incidence of sports injuries in children is difficult to ascertain. Experts feel that banning all children from contact sports in an attempt to prevent injuries is futile. Many children are seriously injured during nonsupervised "roughhousing" activities. The majority of injuries

---

*Cerebrospinal fluid must be differentiated from nasal mucus. This is easily determined with pH paper tape (pH of CSF is 7.4; nasal mucus 6.6) or Dextrostix (CSF is positive for glucose; nasal mucus is negative).

suffered in organized sports are relatively minor abrasions, lacerations, contusions and strains. However, because school-age children are entering a rapid growth period and have an immature musculoskeletal system, they are prone to serious injury. Soft tissue injuries can range from severe sprains with a complete tear in the ligament to a partial or complete rupture of the tendon. Fractures and dislocations are possible with any sport, and adequate treatment must be provided to prevent permanent disability.

Other potential problems include nutrition and heat stress. Children actively involved in competitive sports need guidance on the importance of eating balanced meals regularly and high carbohydrate, light meals just before competition. Young athletes often waste a great deal of money on unnecessary vitamins and protein supplements in an attempt to increase physical strength.

There is always a danger of heat exhaustion or heat stroke when exercising in hot weather. Girls are especially sensitive because their body temperature must rise two to three degrees higher than is necessary in boys before perspiration and body cooling occurs. Precautions should be taken by providing frequent rest periods and water or other liquids.

Prevention of sports injuries begins with a complete physical examination, including x-rays and laboratory work. X-rays are needed to detect any skeletal abnormality such as scoliosis that would contraindicate contact sports. It may be necessary to help the child choose an acceptable alternate activity when a chronic health problem such as epilepsy or asthma is present. However, if the child's condition is controlled with medication and the activity is supervised by an adult there is usually no problem with sports participation. Other preventive measures include proper conditioning, protective equipment that is fitted to each child, appropriate facilities and immediate access to emergency medical care.

Finally, before the child begins participating in any competitive sport, the following questions should be raised and the issues discussed: (1) Is the child participating because he wants to or as a result of parental pressure? (2) How is the child or parent going to feel if he does not make the team or the team loses? (3) Are both the parent and child ready to make the time commitment necessary? (4) Are both aware of the possibility of an injury?

Sports should be an enjoyable part of a child's life and with appropriate guidance the child can be helped to select a sport appropriate to his optimal development with minimal risk of injury.

LEGG-CALVÉ-PERTHES DISEASE

Legg-Calvé-Perthes disease, coxa plana, osteochondritis, and Perthes' disease are all synonyms for a condition of the femoral head caused by a vascular disturbance that produces an ischemic necrosis. The condition is four times more common in boys than girls, with the usual onset at 4 to 8 years of age.[9] Specific etiology is unknown.

The disease process is self-limiting in about 36 months and has three stages: (1) aseptic necrosis (x-rays show opacity of the epiphysis [condensation]); (2) revascularization (the epiphysis is mottled and fragmented [fragmentation]); and (3) reossification with gradual reformation of the femoral head (regeneration).

The nurse's early identification of affected children will aid in treatment, although it will not necessarily ensure a better prognosis. The disease process has usually reached the second stage before signs and symptoms become apparent. The child may be limping on the affected leg. He has pain in the groin that may be referred to the thigh or knee. Pain increases with activity and decreases with rest. Inspection of the affected leg may show atrophy of the buttock or thigh muscles and a decrease in range of motion. The child will initially be admitted to the hospital and placed on bed rest. If pain continues after several weeks with limited range of motion, a definitive x-ray diagnosis can be made.

The goal of treatment for Perthes' disease is to prevent deformity of the femoral head from the stress of weight bearing.[9] Treatment plans include methods to prevent subluxation and extrusion by keeping the femoral head inside the acetabulum. Complete bed rest with Buck's traction for one to two years used to be the treatment of choice.[10] This method obviously put an inordinate amount of stress on the child and his family. Physicians now recommend a period of bed rest and traction in abduction until maximum range of motion is obtained.[9] Then the child is fitted with a nonweight bearing brace device or a harness (Fort harness),

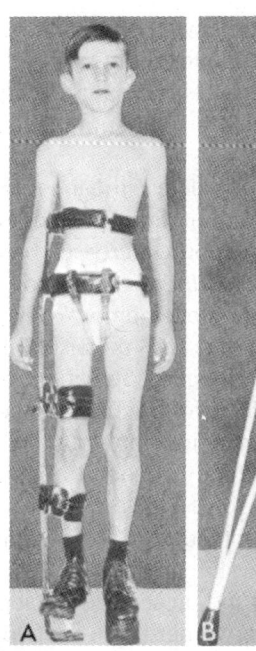

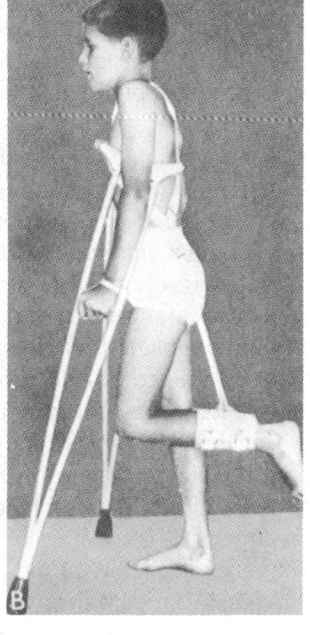

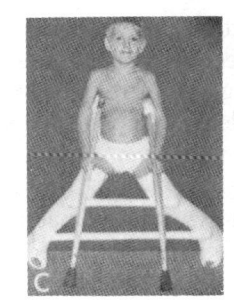

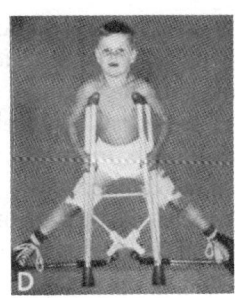

Figure 50-4 *A*, weight-relieving brace (Taylor) for Legg-Perthes' disease. This method is being replaced by more effective techniques. *B*, sling and crutches (Snyder) for Legg-Perthes' disease. *C*, abduction plaster casts (Petrie) for Legg-Perthes' disease. *D*, abduction brace (Bobechko). (From R. Salter. Textbook of Disorders and Injuries of the Musculoskeletal System. Williams and Wilkins, 1970, p. 277).

which prevents weight bearing on the affected side (Fig. 50-4). The child must use crutches, but his mobility is greatly increased. Some physicians do not believe that weight bearing is detrimental as long as the femoral head remains in the acetabulum; they suggest use of bilateral long leg casts with an abduction bar.[10] Atrophy of the extremity is prevented with nonweight bearing exercises. Surgery is sometimes used for reconstruction of the femoral head but seldom yields much success.

Confinement to a hospital bed can be extremely stressful to an active youngster. Attempts should be made to provide the child with a variety of toys and games that can be played in bed. The nurse should assist the child in maintaining contact with siblings and peers during hospitalization via phone calls or visits, if permitted.

Even though Perthes' disease is self-limiting, management of the child at home and school can present a challenge. The removal of bikes, skates and similar toys will alleviate parental worry and diminish frustration for the child. Making the home environment safe may include removal of loose rugs and rearrangement of furniture to allow for the larger spaces required to ambulate with the braced crutches. The nurse can be of assistance by encouraging the child to continue his school work during hospitalization and at home. She can also prepare the child's teacher and classmates before the child's return to school. It is important to the child's development for him to continue with normal activities even with this temporary handicap.

Siblings may resent the extra attention and special treatment that is given to their brother or sister. Warning parents of this possibility may help prevent the situation or at least help them understand it. It is difficult for parents to continue routine home activities, but most will be willing to try in an effort to maintain an environment that best meets the needs of their child.

Prognosis for Perthes' disease depends entirely on the severity of the femoral involvement and the age at onset. Generally the younger the age of onset, the better the prognosis.

PRECOCIOUS PUBERTY

True precocious puberty is arbitrarily defined as the onset of puberty before age 8 in girls and age 9 in boys. Approximately 1 to 3 per cent of girls will experience precocious puberty; boys are affected less often. The cause of onset is idiopathic in 80 per cent of girls and 50 per cent of boys.[6]

The exact mechanism that inhibits gonadotropin secretion before puberty is not known. However, at puberty central nervous system maturation allows a reduction in hypothalmic sensitivity to the negative feedback effect of sex steroids, and the pituitary gland increases FSH and LH secretions. The release of gonadal sex hormones also increases, and secondary sex characteristics appear.

Precocious puberty triggers the premature maturation of the hypothalmic-pituitary mechanism that brings on puberty. Girls will experience development of the breasts, vagina, uterus and external genitalia and the onset of menstruation. Pubic and axillary hair growth will result from adrenal androgens. In boys precocious puberty is evident by an enlargement of the penis and testes and the presence of spermatogenesis.

Early breast development, the presence of pubic hair or the onset of menstruation are usually the first signs observed by the nurse. Any boy or girl in elementary school experiencing a rapid increase in height and weight should be further assessed by the school nurse. If signs of pubertal development are present, the child should be referred to a physician, preferably an endocrinologist, since, although precocious puberty is sometimes idiopathic, it can also be associated with a variety of potentially serious disorders. The parents should be consulted before the referral to discuss the nurse's observations and to provide an explanation of possible diagnostic procedures. Parents should be encouraged to provide the child with a simple rationale for the examination, based on the child's developmental level and sexual awareness. The nurse's matter-of-fact approach will help parents avoid over-reacting to the situation.

Diagnostic procedures can be extensive and lengthy. The parents and child will need continued support throughout the procedures. An initial history, including the onset of secondary sex characteristics and familial history of adolescent development, is important. Physical examination will include the genitalia, and sedation may be needed in girls for a pelvic examination. Young children often have fears concerning their genitalia, so an understandable explanation to the child before the examination is of paramount importance. Skeletal x-rays to determine bone age are necessary, because bone age is greater than one would expect from linear growth charts. Blood tests for serum gonadotropin levels will be performed. A 24-hour urine test for 17-ketosteroids is needed. Tests to rule out cerebral abnormality include an electroencephalogram and pneumoencephalography.

The physician must also determine the rate of sexual development, and if it is progressive. Girls may be referred with only increased breast development (*premature thelarche*) and no other signs of pubertal development. Precocious appearance of pubic and axillary hair is termed *premature adrenarche*. Specific treatment is limited to close follow-up for these incomplete types of precocious puberty.

The treatment for sexual precocity depends on an accurate diagnosis. If a CNS, adrenal or gonadal tumor is present, surgery is necessary. Treatment for idiopathic precocious puberty is not very satisfactory at the present time. Depo-Provera 150 mg IM every other week for two to four years until the child reaches 8 years of age will decrease breast size and stop menstruation.[6] However, use of long-term steroids results in side effects that may be more detrimental to the child than the condition warrants. There is no treatment available to stop the accelerated bone growth, and approximately 50 per cent of girls will reach adult height at five feet.[6]

Psychological support must be a primary part of the treatment plan. It is important that the child and parents understand that the condition is harmless, even though the symptoms will continue. All efforts must be made to prevent emotional trauma in the child by emphasizing that the changes are "early" and not "abnormal." Children will not have precocious intellectual or social development even though their appearance would suggest otherwise. The school nurse can work with school personnel to prevent difficulties that can arise from peer interactions, especially in physical education classes. If menstruation is inevitable, the nurse should help parents prepare the child for this. Some parents may be concerned about a possible pregnancy, and contraception may be warranted.

Siblings must be included in the management plan in an attempt to alleviate fears they may experience. The nurse is an excellent person to offer an explanation of the condition and to encourage siblings to treat their brother or sister as they normally would.

Children with precocious puberty will cope well with this condition if they are given adequate support during the prepubertal years.

Usually by 10 to 14 years of age the child's peers will be developing secondary sex characteristics and the trauma will have passed. Reproductive capabilities are not affected by the condition.

References

1. Accident facts. National Safety Council, Chicago, 1978
2. S. Carter and A. Gold. Neurology of Infancy and Childhood. Appleton-Century-Crofts, 1974
3. B. L. Conway. Pediatric Neurologic Nursing. C. V. Mosby Co., 1977
4. D. J. Demis et al., eds. Furuncles and Carbuncles. In Clinical Dermatology, Harper & Row, 1979
5. M. Domonkas and N. Anthony. Andrew's Diseases of the Skin, Clinical Dermatology. W. B. Saunders Co., 1971
6. S. Emans et al. Pediatric and Adolescent Gynecology. Little, Brown & Co., 1977
7. M. Green and R. Haggerty. Ambulatory Pediatrics II, Personal Health Care of Children in the Office. W. B. Saunders Co., 1979
8. P. Jacobs. Fungal infections in childhood. Pediatric Clinics of North America, May 1978, p. 357
9. E. Kamhi. Legg-Calvé-Perthes disease. Postgraduate Medicine, October 1976, p. 125
10. C. Larson and M. Gould. Orthopedic Nursing. C. V. Mosby Co., 1978
11. R. Lingeman. Epistaxis. American Family Physician, December 1976, p. 79
12. J. Mealey and C. Thomas. Pediatric Head Injuries. Charles C Thomas, 1968
13. W. Mills. Out in the cold. Emergency Medicine, January 1976, p. 134
14. D. Pascoe and M. Grossman. Quick Reference to Pediatric Emergencies. J. B. Lippincott Co., 1973
15. J. Paulson. Accidents. In Pediatrics Update Reviews for Physicians, A. J. Moss, ed., Elsevier, 1979
16. V. Vaughan et al. Nelson Textbook of Pediatrics. W. B. Saunders Co., 1979

Additional Recommended Reading

American Academy of Pediatrics. Competitive athletics for children of Elementary School Age. Pediatrics, October 1968, p. 703

P. Barelli. The management of epistaxis in children. Otolaryngologic Clinics of North America, February 1977, p. 91

T. DeLapp. Taking the bite out of frostbite and other cold weather injuries. American Journal of Nursing, January 1980, p. 56

F. Glickman. Dermatology in General Medicine. PSG Publishing Co., Inc., 1979

M. Korting et al. Diseases of the Skin in Children and Adolescents. W. B. Saunders Co., 1979

M. Low. Sports and the young athlete. Journal of School Health, October 1969, p. 514

F. Nezamis. The child with a head injury. Issues in Comprehensive Pediatric Nursing, Jul/Aug 1977, p. 30

J. Parks. Endocrine disorders of childhood. Hospital Practice, October 1977, p. 93

M. Sayers. Pediatric trauma. In Craniocerebral Trauma, R. Touloukian, ed., John Wiley and Sons, 1978

W. Sinton. Preventing athletic injuries in children. Consultant, June 1978, p. 49

D. Styne and S. Kaplan. Normal and abnormal puberty in the female. Pediatric Clinics of North America, February 1979, p. 123

N. Welch. Recent insights into the childhood social diseases — gonorrhea, scabies, pediculosis and pinworms. Clinical Pediatrics, April 1978, p. 318

J. Winter et al. Normal and abnormal pubertal development. Clinical Obstetrics and Gynecology, March 1978, p. 67

G. D. Zuidema et al., eds. The Management of Trauma. W. B. Saunders Co., 1979

51 POTENTIAL STRESSES DURING THE SCHOOL-AGE YEARS: REVERSIBLE ALTERATIONS IN HEALTH STATUS

by Anne E. Hartson, RN, MA

The school-age child who experiences reversible illness, especially if the illness requires a period of hospitalization, finds the disruption to his normal activities at home and school frustrating emotionally and socially. He is confronted with separation from peers who are increasingly important to his self-image and security, and, if hospitalization occurs, the separation extends to his parents and siblings, who are still important sources of support in the school-age child's daily living. At a time developmentally when children prefer to be very active physically and intellectually, reversible illness forces temporary limitations and confinement.

The school-age child's psychosocial task of industry is also compromised briefly by reversible illness. With restrictions on what he can make, his industrious energy may be stifled unless alert, understanding and creative parents and nurses provide him with optional means of releasing this energy.

Parents can usually handle stress posed by the illness itself if they are given adequate information about the illness and its treatment and the usually favorable prognosis. A greater source of stress for them is often related to their child's reactions to his illness as expressed through increased aggression and uncooperativeness or by regression in development. The nurse may help alleviate parental anxiety associated with the child's behavior by reassuring them that his responses are typical and by enlisting their aid in minimizing his frustrations that precipitate these behaviors.

Whether the child is treated in the hospital or at home (convalescence is usually at home in reversible illness), provision should be made for him to maintain daily contact with his peers through their visits, phone calls and notes. The same provision should be made for daily contact with the child's siblings. Parental visitation (during the hospital phase) and active participation in treatment should be encouraged and supported. A teacher should visit the child, whether at home or in the hospital, after the acute phase of the illness to help him stay abreast of his class and to keep him intellectually active.

The child should be kept informed about his disease and the progress of his recovery. The school-age child is very curious about his body, what happens to it during illness and how it goes about recovering from illness. The nurse should take advantage of this natural curiosity to educate the child not only about his disease but about health in general.

The nurse should make herself available on a daily basis to answer this child's questions and listen to his worries and feelings, encouraging verbalization as an avenue to release frustration and aggression. Toys that allow release of aggressive feelings should be provided; these should be chosen according to the physical limitations imposed by the disease. Therapeutic play provided by the nurse, teacher or play therapist offers the child another opportunity to gain some sense of control and release aggressions. The child's anxieties are also lessened if he is provided with regular daily opportunities to make decisions relative to his care. Decision options should not be offered, however, in situations in which there is no option. These actions by the nurse and parents can help the school-age child adapt to his reversible illness in a way that facilitates rather than hinders his recovery.

REVERSIBLE INFLAMMATORY PROCESSES

Acute Glomerulonephritis

Acute glomerulonephritis is a term used to describe several specific renal disease entities. The most common type in childhood is poststreptococcal glomerulonephritis. The peak age of occurrence of acute glomerulonephritis is at 5 years and usually affects boys twice as often as girls. A streptococcal infection of the throat or skin usually precedes this immune-complex disease by two to three weeks.

The incidence of acute glomerulonephritis associated with streptococcal pharyngeal infections peaks during the winter and spring months. Development of this disease following cutaneous streptococcal infections is common in hot climates during the summer months, when insect bites and abrasions increase. Not all children with Group A beta-hemolytic streptococcal pharyngeal or cutaneous infections will develop acute glomerulonephritis, because only specific nephritogenic strains will affect the glomeruli. Prevention is possible for approximately 50 per cent of children with streptococcal pharyngitis if early antistreptococcal treatment is initiated.[6] Appropriate treatment of insect bites and abrasions may inhibit the development of cutaneous streptococcal infections and thus decrease the risk of this disease. Streptococcal infections are easily spread in overcrowded areas in which hygiene is poor and poverty is rampant. When a child contracts acute glomerulonephritis, family members should have throat cultures, and those with positive results should receive penicillin.

Pathophysiology and Clinical Manifestations Antibodies form against the streptococcus antigen, producing a precipitate that is entrapped in the middle glomerular membrane, and an inflammation of the glomeruli ensues.[8] A large number of white blood cells collect in the glomeruli, and endothelial cells along the glomerular membrane proliferate to fill the glomeruli and capsule. Many of the glomeruli that are not blocked will develop a greater membrane permeability, allowing large amounts of protein to leak into the glomerular filtrate. If the membrane ruptures, red blood cells can also pass into the glomerular filtrate and in very severe cases the glomeruli may be permanently damaged. The effect of the pathological changes is a decrease in the glomerular filtration rate. Sodium and water retention cause edema and hypertension, which are probably due to decreased glomerular filtration rather than an increase in renin secretion.[6, 11]

The signs and symptoms of acute glomerulonephritis are acute in onset and will usually be present 10 days after a pharyngeal infection and approximately three weeks after a cutaneous infection. A decrease in volume of urine and a dark cola-beverage color of urine may be first signs of acute glomerulonephritis. The child usually does not appear very ill; however, a slight puffiness of the face, usually around the eyes, may be noticed (Fig. 51–1). The child will probably be frightened by the change in his urine and call attention to it. When questioned,

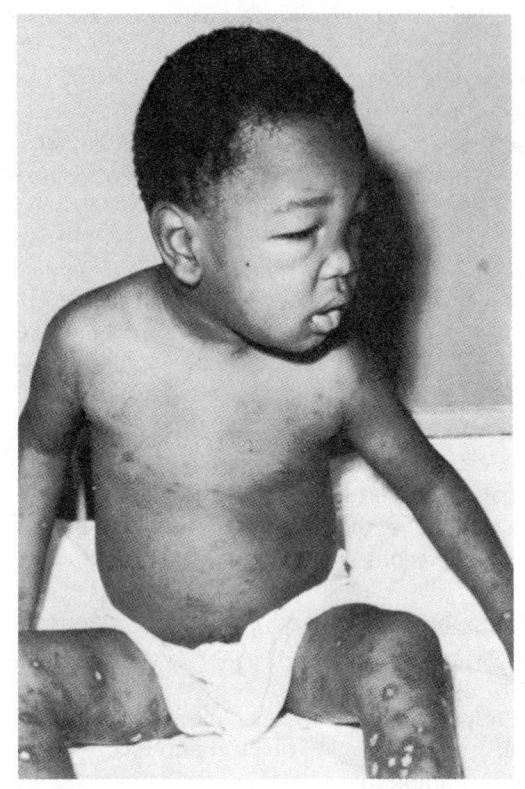

Figure 51-1 Acute glomerulonephritis. Note periorbital edema, prominent abdomen, healing impetiginous lesions on the legs. (From James, J. A.: Renal Disease in Childhood, ed. 3, St. Louis, 1976, the C. V. Mosby Co.)

he may complain of mild abdominal or flank pain.

When a child presents with these symptoms the nurse should first obtain a history of recent skin or throat infections. The nurse's assessment will also include checking for periorbital edema, enlarged cervical lymph nodes, tonsillar exudate, healing pyodermas (pustular skin lesions), decreased urine output, lethargy, and the presence of mild to moderate hypertension (120–180/80–120 mm Hg). Some children have more striking symptoms, including signs of cardiac overload or seizure activity precipitated by acute hypertension.

Regardless of the presentation of symptoms, any child with unexplained dark-colored urine will need to be examined immediately for a diagnosis.

A definite diagnosis of acute glomerulonephritis is made from laboratory results and a positive culture for Group A *beta-hemolytic streptococci*. The urinalysis will usually show an increased specific gravity (>1.020), 3 to 4+ protein, and the presence of red blood cell casts. The BUN and creatinine will be elevated in 50 per cent of cases due to the impaired glomerular filtration. Other laboratory results include the presence of an increased antistreptolycin O (ASO) titer, a decrease in serum complement activity, mild leukocytosis, increased erythrocytic sedimentation (Sed) rate and a mild anemia (Hgb 10 to 11 mg/dl). The child with cardiac symptoms should have a chest x-ray to rule out cardiac enlargement and pulmonary vascular congestion. An electrocardiogram is warranted because changes that show on the ECG may result from hyperkalemia. Renal biopsy is rarely needed for diagnosis.

Renal disease has an ominous sound to parents. It is important to establish an accurate diagnosis quickly in order to alleviate anxiety. The course of acute glomerulonephritis is short, approximately three weeks, and most parents will handle this stress period well if given information on the disease and its treatment by a supportive nurse. Providing the child with an age-appropriate explanation of the disease is important to gain cooperation and decrease anxiety. A 7-year-old will benefit from being shown a simple picture of the kidneys on a body outline, with an explanation that "the kidneys are sick but will get better." Laboratory procedures can be very frightening and painful to any child, and preparation before the procedure is needed. Providing the child with a doll on which to practice "drawing blood" is an excellent method to allow expression of anger resulting from painful procedures.

Hospitalization is required for treatment of acute glomerulonephritis unless the symptoms are extremely mild and the child is not hypertensive. For home management the parent will need to be taught how to check the child's blood pressure and urine. These procedures are done daily so that if the child develops hypertension or oliguria, he can be hospitalized for closer supervision and treatment. The hospitalized child will feel ill during the acute edematous phase, which lasts one to two weeks. Bed rest is required during the hypertensive and edematous phase and play activities should be provided as the child's condition improves. Although hospitalization for the child with acute glomerulonephritis is only temporary, siblings should be encouraged to visit.

Drug treatment for hypertension, usually reserpine and hydralazine, will be needed if diastolic pressure is 100 mm Hg. Because encephalopathy is a complication of hypertension, close monitoring of blood pressure and observation for signs of headache, dizziness, vomiting and seizures are important. Edema and oliguria are monitored through daily weighing and recording of intake and output. Management of intake and output is achieved by restricting fluid intake to equal insensible water loss, use of diuretics (furosemide), a sodium-restricted diet (low to no added salt), and potassium restriction until urine output is more than 200 to 300 cc/day. If cardiac failure occurs, digitalis therapy will also be necessary.

Diuresis of approximately 3 liters/day will occur after the initial edematous phase. The child's urine will begin to clear and his blood pressure will decrease. Bed rest can be discontinued at this time if there is no edema and the child's weight and blood pressure are stable for 24 hours. The child is discharged two to three days after the diuresis if gross hematuria is absent and the BUN is less than 30 mg/dl.[11] The importance of keeping follow-up appointments should be discussed with parents.

Once discharged, the child can be up and about but should continue to engage only in quiet play. Avoiding strenuous play for several months may be necessary until the urine is clear of red blood cells.[11] The child usually returns to school in 7 to 10 days. The school nurse should be informed of any activity limitations so that teachers can be provided with instructions and explanations of the disease and its management. Prophylactic penicillin is sometimes prescribed to prevent intercurrent infections during the convalescent period, although the recurrence rate is low. Prognosis for complete recovery is excellent, with only 5 per cent of children developing chronic glomerulonephritis.

The progression of chronic glomerulonephritis is variable, and most children will have few problems with the disease. However, if the disease progresses to the final stages, the end result is renal failure because glomeruli are replaced with fibrous tissue and no longer function.[8] Hemodialysis or renal transplantation or both will then be needed.

Rheumatic Fever

Rheumatic fever is a collagen disease involving the heart, joints, central nervous system, skin and connective tissue. The incidence of rheumatic fever has decreased in the United States, but approximately 0.3 per cent of American children acquire the disease annually.[18] The disease is most prevalent in the school-age child of 6 to 8 from the lower socioeconomic group. It is still the leading form of acquired heart disease in children and the most common serious preventable disease of childhood.[5]

Although rheumatic fever is usually preceded by a Group A beta-hemolytic streptococcal infection, not all children with pharyngeal streptococcal infections develop the disease. It has been theorized that rheumatogenic streptococci (present in certain strains of streptococcus) cause an autoimmune or allergic reaction.[18] Efforts are being made to develop a streptococcal vaccine. The streptococci release proteins, and antibodies form to react with different tissues in the body.

The development of Aschoff bodies (a type of inflammatory lesion) in the heart muscle, connective tissue and other muscles causes endothelial proliferation and eventually necrosis.[14] Cardiac valve injury, the most serious complication, occurs when Aschoff bodies develop on the heart valves. Damage results when these large hemorrhagic, fibrinous lesions grow along the inflamed edges of valves, most commonly the mitral valve. Scarring occurs and eventually stenosis, months or years later.

Clinical Manifestations Because pharyngeal streptococcal infections usually precede the development of rheumatic fever by two weeks, it is important to institute treatment with penicillin early. Any well child complaining of a sore throat should have a culture done to rule out streptococcal infection. Unfortunately two-thirds of children with streptococcal pharyngitis never have this infection treated by a physician.[18] Nurses working with low socioeconomic families should be especially aware of the necessity of obtaining throat cultures on children. All nurses working with this population should know that rheumatic fever is most frequent during winter and spring, tends to occur in families, has a high recurrence rate, and is best prevented by early diagnosis and treatment of pharyngeal strep infections.

The onset of rheumatic fever is often insidious; the child may merely appear tired and apathetic. Figure 51-2 illustrates the body's involvement in rheumatic symptoms. One of

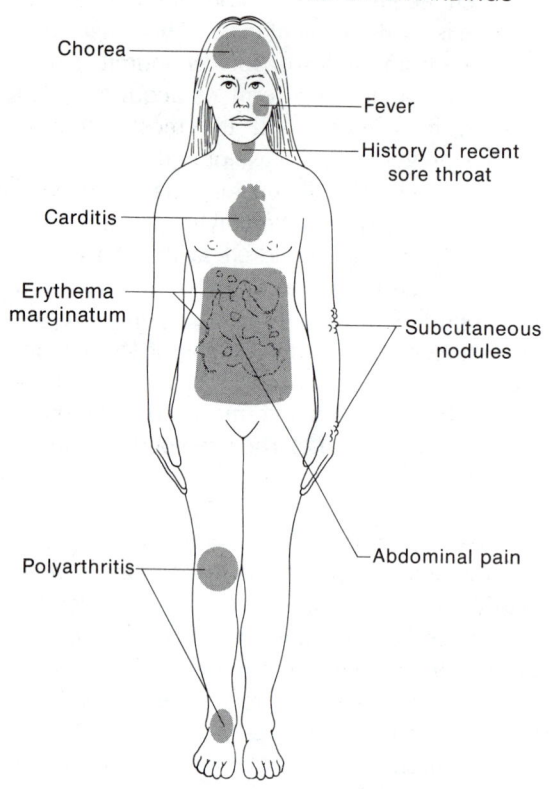

Figure 51-2 Manifestations of rheumatic fever.

the first symptoms the child complains of may be joint tenderness, with the area appearing swollen, red and warm. Arthritic symptoms will usually first develop in the knee and ankle joints and then migrate to the wrists, elbows and hips. The child may complain of joint tenderness for a few days to several weeks. Signs of carditis, including tachycardia, cardiomegaly and murmurs, will be seen in approximately 40 per cent of children with the first attack.[24] Other symptoms of rheumatic fever may include Sydenham's chorea (see discussion later in this chapter), erythema marginatum, subcutaneous nodules and epistaxis. Erythema marginatum manifests as a nonpruritic rash with pink macules appearing on protected parts of the body. Firm, nontender subcutaneous nodules on the joints and scalp occur when the disease is well established. Epistaxis is seen in only 10 per cent of children with rheumatic fever.[24]

Nurses working with school-age children must be alert to the initial symptoms. Joint pains should not be dismissed as "growing pains." Growing pains can be differentiated from rheumatic joint pain because the pains from growth are relieved or disappear during rest or sleep, whereas rheumatic joint pain is not relieved. History and physical assessment findings may further differentiate the two types of pain.

Nurse's Role in Management Hospitalization of the child is usually required if rheumatic fever is suspected. The nurse should explain to the child that he must be hospitalized so that tests can be performed to find out why he is not feeling well. Further explanations of specific diagnostic procedures will be needed for both the child and the parents.

A definitive diagnosis must be made so the child may avoid unnecessary psychological stress and long-term drug therapy. The revised Jones Criteria (Table 51-1) is commonly used for diagnostic purposes. The presence of two major or one major and two minor criteria plus a history of a preceding streptococcal infection usually indicates rheumatic fever.

The treatment goal is to reduce stress on the heart and relieve joint pains. Once the diagnosis is established, antibiotics are given to destroy any remaining Group A beta-hemolytic streptococci. Penicillin is the drug of choice, with erythromycin for penicillin-allergic children.

Aspirin is the most commonly used anti-inflammatory agent for arthritic symptoms and mild carditis. Because it may be needed for several months, especially after steroids are discontinued, monitoring for salicylate toxicity and bleeding tendencies is imperative. If the carditis is extensive and the child has signs of congestive heart failure, digoxin, diuretics and

TABLE 51-1 JONES CRITERIA (REVISED) FOR GUIDANCE IN THE DIAGNOSIS OF RHEUMATIC FEVER

Major Manifestations
    Carditis
    Polyarthritis
    Chorea
    Erythema marginatum
    Subcutaneous nodules

Minor Manifestations
Clinical
    Previous rheumatic fever or rheumatic heart disease
    Arthralgia
    Fever
Laboratory
    Acute phase reactions
    Erythrocyte sedimentation rate, C-reactive protein leukocytosis
    Prolonged PR interval

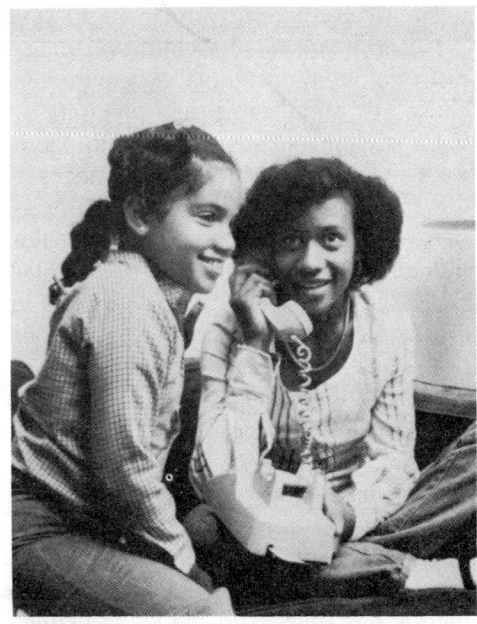

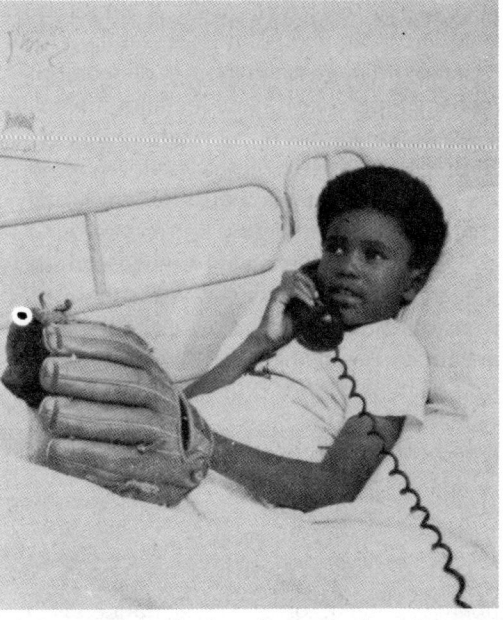

Telephone calls to or from siblings or visits with them help to reduce the boredom of bed confinement while helping the ill child to maintain a sense of family intactness. (From Help for the Family's Neglected "Other" Child. Copyright 1979, American Journal of Nursing Company. Reproduced with permission from MCN, the American Journal of Maternal Child Nursing, Sept./Oct., Vol. 4, No. 5.)

steroids may be given. Steroids often cause mood swings, and it is essential that parents, siblings and the child be aware of the source of this emotional lability. Steroid therapy may be continued for four to six weeks, and the child may develop manifestations of Cushing's disease.

The child will need complete bed rest during the acute period to prevent carditis or its complications. Physicians vary in their opinions on the enforcement of strict bed rest and may allow minimal activity if the child experiences great anxiety about being kept in bed. The range of required bed rest varies from 7 to 10 days if no heart disease is present. Three weeks to three months may be required if carditis occurs. Bed rest is discontinued when the inflammation, the sedimentation rate and the enlargement of the heart decrease.

The child confined to bed is subject to boredom, anxiety and dependency on parents and adults for meeting his needs. The nurse can minimize stress in several ways. If the child is interested, she can provide age-appropriate reading material on rheumatic fever. Most school-age children will comprehend a simple explanation of the disease and its effect on the body. Activities to decrease boredom may include allowing sibling visitations, telephone calls to siblings and peers, television, radio, table games and reading. Any child confined to bed is going to need someone to serve as a sounding board for release of anger, fear and frustration. Ideally, during hospitalization the child can be assigned a primary nurse in order to facilitate the trust relationship needed to help the child work through these feelings. The child needs encouragement to be an active participant in his treatment by making decisions about meals and daily routines.

After the acute stage (usually a week to 10 days) the child is placed on a regimen of benzathine penicillin G given intramuscularly every four weeks to prevent recurrence of the infection. This prophylactic drug therapy must be continued throughout childhood and may be prescribed for the rest of the child's life. Oral penicillin may be taken only if the child and parents are very reliable; this route does not have a high compliance rate.

The child who misses several weeks or months of school may have a difficult time keeping up with his class. Completing homework gives the child a sense of normalcy and accomplishment; therefore, the child should be encouraged to continue school work as soon as the acute stage has passed. At this time the child may begin a limited activity program with provisions for rest throughout the day.

The child's prognosis is good if antibiotic treatment is continued. This is essential, for there is a tenfold increase in the risk of developing another streptococcal infection after the first attack of rheumatic fever.[5] In approximately one-third to one-fourth of the children with carditis, the cardiac status will improve during the acute stage or in the following 10-year time period. Heart disease is still the most serious complication of rheumatic fever, although deaths are rare after the first attack. The child with rheumatic heart disease is susceptible to subacute bacterial endocarditis. Good oral hygiene practices and antibiotic treatment before dental and other surgical procedures help to reduce that susceptibility.

Sydenham's Chorea

Sydenham's chorea, or St. Vitus dance, is a manifestation of juvenile rheumatism. It will often precede, follow or present itself with other signs of rheumatic fever, although chorea and carditis seldom occur together. Prepubescent girls are affected two to three times more often than boys. The rapid, involuntary muscle movements are caused by a diffuse meningoencephalitis that affects the cerebral hemispheres, basal ganglia, and pia arachnoid.

The child may appear clumsy and may tend to drop things. Teachers may report problems with inattention, emotional lability, and a decrease in clarity of speech and handwriting in a child with no previous problem. The nurse, upon examining the child, may note a hyperextension of the fingers and wrists when the hands are outstretched. A weak grip and intermittent muscular contractions or twitching may be noted. These signs may develop suddenly or over several weeks.

Diagnosis is usually made by clinical signs of frequent, purposeless bilateral movements of the trunk, face and extremities. An elevated sedimentation rate is present in 50 per cent of patients. The cerebral spinal fluid is normal.

A thorough explanation of the condition and reassurance that it is transient will help parents cope with this disturbing disease. Some children become extremely irritable and exhibit inappropriate laughter or crying. Movements may also be very violent. Parents need constant reassurance that the disease will run its course without causing residual damage to the child.

Nursing care for the child will include bed rest in a quiet, unstimulating environment, because any stimulation may precipitate the involuntary movements. A bed with padded rails for the child's protection may be necessary until the movements cease. A high calorie diet is needed to provide the additional calories required for the child's increased muscular activity. Frequent small meals can be used to avoid the fatigue of eating a large meal. The child may be so weak or tire so easily that assistance with feeding may be necessary. Sedatives may be given to control the chorea and allow the child to rest.

The nurse needs to understand the effect of this disease on the child and family in order to provide consistent, supportive care. This disease results in a variety of complex interactions within the family. The school-age child's need to be independent now presents a challenge to the family because of the danger imposed by the child's inability to control his own movements. Simple tasks such as pouring hot water, carrying something breakable or using a sharp knife become unsafe. The child's inability to complete a task well thwarts the development of self-esteem. The dilemma of not being able to accomplish even simple tasks results in outbursts of irritable, demanding behavior. The child needs calmness, patience and continued expression of affection from those who interact with him daily. Those who love and care for him in turn need a periodic break from this care to gain new perspective.

The nurse has two roles in supporting the child and family: first, to provide a quieting effect on the child herself, and second, to teach family and others about the child's needs and how to make necessary changes in his environment. She can suggest that family members simplify daily tasks of living, provide periods of rest and lessen demands made on the child. Siblings can help by adapting their own life to the needs of the school-ager, but they need to be able to continue their usual activity as much as possible to minimize the development of anger toward the child.

The course of the disease may continue for approximately 10 weeks, with neurological signs subsiding completely upon recovery. The prognosis for the child to return to normal activities is good, although some instances of psychiatric disturbances have been reported in long-term follow-up studies.[24]

Appendicitis

Acute appendicitis is the most common surgical emergency in children and, although the mortality rate has steadily declined, this condition is still the cause of many preventable deaths. The disease tends to occur slightly more often in boys.

The appendix is located at the end of the cecum and has no apparent function. Etiology of the disease is an obstruction of the appendiceal lumen, usually by a fecalith (hardened feces). Secondary obstruction may result from inflammatory changes of blood-borne or enteric infections or from pinworms, stenosis or kinking. The obstruction causes inflammatory changes in the mucosal wall, which becomes edematous and filled with leukocytes. This distention causes the blood supply to be compromised. Gangrene and perforation result. Perforation of the appendix allows bacteria to escape and produces a generalized peritonitis or a localized abscess (confined by the adjoining omentum).

Clinical Manifestations and Diagnosis Appendicitis has an acute onset. It is not uncommon for the child with appendicitis to appear in the school nurse's office complaining of severe abdominal pain. Many children will not be comfortable standing upright and will attempt to lessen discomfort by bending over and guarding the abdomen with their hands. It is difficult to assess the location of pain because the child is fearful of anyone touching his abdomen. However, the nurse can ask the child to show her "where it hurts" and avoid palpation. The presence of vomiting, low-grade fever and periumbilical or right lower quadrant pain (at McBurney's point) should alert the nurse to seek immediate medical assistance for the child. Pain elicits a fear response; therefore during the examination the nurse calmly explains what she is doing and that parents will be contacted. She should tell the child why it is necessary to see a physician.

Because appendicitis is an emergency, there is little time available to prepare the child adequately for the diagnostic work-up. If at all possible, parents should be encouraged to stay with the child. Letting the parents know that the nurse is aware of their concern and will answer their questions helps them cope with their anxiety.

The physician will need to palpate the abdomen to assess for rigidity and tenderness. Adequate preparation will decrease the child's tendency to tense his abdominal muscles. If the inflammation is located in the pelvic area the abdominal examination may be negative. A rectal examination is mandatory but uncomfortable, and should be done last. School-age children are modest and it is important to explain the necessity for rectal examination and to provide privacy. Rectal tenderness may indicate a local abscess or perforation.

Diagnostic tests will include blood studies, urinalysis and x-rays of the chest and abdomen. A leukocytic count of 14,000 to 16,000 cells per mm and pus cells present in the urine are significant. X-rays will aid in excluding the possibility of pneumonia and may show the presence of a fecalith. The physician must also rule out other possible causes of acute abdominal pain, including severe constipation, urinary tract infection and acute gastroenteritis.

Management Perforation occurs frequently in children, so when a diagnosis is made the child is scheduled for an emergency appendectomy. Contraindications to immediate surgery include the presence of a high fever, dehydration or sepsis, all of which must be controlled before the child is anesthetized.

If perforation did not occur and there was no abscess, the child usually remains in the hospital for a three- to four-day period. Nursing care includes monitoring the IV and vital signs, assessing the incision at dressing changes, encouraging ambulation, deep breathing and coughing, and observing for signs of abscess formation (increased pain, restlessness, irritability and a decrease in ambulation). The child will experience pain from the incision, and pain medication should be offered. Many children hesitate to ask for medication because they are afraid of a "shot." The nurse should obtain an order for oral medication to be given as soon as the child can tolerate liquids, usually 24 hours after surgery.

The child with an abscess or perforated appendix will return from surgery to his room with an IV, a Penrose drain in the incision, and a nasogastric tube. The child will be given parenteral antibiotics for the period of hospitalization, usually 10 days. The child is acutely ill and needs intensive nursing care during the immediate postoperative period.

Recovery for the child without peritonitis is rapid, and he may return to school a week or two after surgery. Strenuous exercise should be curtailed for several weeks. School personnel will need to know of these restrictions in order to ensure the child's compliance.

Guillain-Barré Syndrome

Guillain-Barré syndrome, also known as infectious neuronitis or acute polyneuritis, is a disease of the peripheral or cranial nerves or both causing varying degrees of motor and sensory disturbances. Although relatively uncommon, it may affect children of both sexes between the ages of 4 and 10, as well as adolescents.

Peripheral and cranial nerve fibers undergo degenerative changes from an inflammatory process. Another pathological change of the fibers is a segmental demyelinization of unknown etiology, although some authorities believe the myelin is attacked by sensitized lymphocytes.[17] The disease tends to occur after bacterial or viral infections and is associated with influenza, diphtheria, scarlet fever, mumps, rubeola, rubella, typhoid fever and respiratory infections in over half of reported cases. The nurse's role in prevention consists of encouraging parents to complete and maintain their children's immunizations, and teaching hygiene measures for handwashing, nose blowing and coughing to help control the spread of infection.

Clinical Manifestations and Diagnosis Signs and symptoms may occur several days after an infection. The child may hesitate to walk or run because his legs "feel funny." Peripheral neuritis usually starts bilaterally in the legs with weakness and numbness that extends up to the arms and hands. The progressive paralysis usually peaks at 7 to 10 days, with 50 per cent of children affected showing some improvement by the second week. However, the recovery period is lengthy, varying from 2 to 18 months. Deep tendon reflexes will be decreased or absent and the child may complain of muscle tenderness or cramping pains upon examination. Assessment of paresthesia (altered sensation of the limbs) is very important but may be difficult in the young child. The child's vague complaints should be taken seriously.

Cranial nerve involvement is usually not evident initially, although the seventh and eleventh cranial nerves may be affected as the disease progresses. Ten to twenty per cent of affected persons will have sufficient involvement of the abdominal and thoracic muscles to cause respiratory insufficiency.[17] Any child experiencing sensory disturbance in his limbs or having difficulty talking or swallowing or all of these symptoms needs immediate medical attention.

Admission to the hospital is required for diagnosis and treatment. The physician will need to rule out the presence of viral and infectious diseases, especially those altering muscle function such as poliomyelitis. It is extremely stressful for parents and siblings to observe a child with signs of paralysis. Helplessness at not being able to do anything and guilt that help may not have been sought early enough are paramount, and the nurse will need to reassure all family members that everything possible is being done to help the child. Having someone to answer questions, explain procedures and listen to concerns is therapeutic for the family.

A lumbar puncture is required to assess the cerebral spinal fluid for an increase in protein and cell count; both are present in Guillain-Barré syndrome. This test is usually frightening to the parents and child. The nurse should thoroughly explain the procedure, including why it is necessary, what it feels like, how long it takes, and what position the child needs to assume during the procedure. If parents do not feel comfortable staying with the child during a lumbar puncture, the nurse should assure them that she will be present to comfort the child and hold him in position.

Although an electroencephalogram (EEG) is a painless procedure, preparation of the child is needed to alleviate fear and ensure cooperation. Findings may show denervation and decreased nerve conduction velocity.

Clinical signs of a symmetrical ascending paralysis and the positive findings from the lumbar puncture and the EEG are diagnostic of Guillain-Barré syndrome. As soon as the diagnosis is made the parents and child should be given an explanation of the disease and treatment.

The Nurse's Role in Management Nursing care during the acute stage is supportive and consists of promoting the child's comfort, preventing deformity and assessing respiratory status. Irritability, restlessness and pain from nerve root involvement may be present. An indwelling catheter for urinary retention or incontinence may be needed. Maintaining adequate nutrition and hydration is important, and parenteral fluids are needed to prevent aspiration if there is involvement of the ninth or tenth cranial nerve. Respiratory paralysis will necessitate transfer to the intensive care unit, for the child will require a tracheostomy and possibly use of a ventilator. Corticosteroids, when given early in the disease process, may hasten recovery.

Prevention of contractures is a primary need during the entire disease process, and physical therapy with passive range of motion to all extremities is needed at least every four hours. Repositioning the child every one to two hours will help prevent deformity and skin breakdown.

Care during recovery will involve several health professionals. The occupational therapist and the physical therapist will help the child recover muscle strength and motor abilities. Bracing or splinting may be needed for the child with residual muscle weakness. The activity or play therapist has an important role in providing the child with appropriate energy-releasing activities. Immobilized children often express a wide range of behaviors, including withdrawal, aggression, noncompliance and loneliness. The nurse who understands this will be able to accept some aggressiveness and noncooperation. However, providing the child with outlets for his aggression and frustration through therapeutic play, physical exercise within the limits of the disease, and verbalization of feelings can minimize the behaviors and facilitate healthy coping.

The long recovery period can be emotionally and financially draining for the entire family, and a medical social work referral is useful. Discharge planning should include a community health nurse referral to assist with home management and arrangements for a homebound teacher to help the child with school work. Prognosis is good, with 95 per cent of these children having complete recovery.

Osteomyelitis

Osteomyelitis is a rapidly developing bloodborne bacterial infection of the bone and its marrow.[19] The metaphyseal area of the long bones in the legs and arms is affected. The disease commonly occurs in school-age children, with boys affected four times more than girls.[19]

Osteomyelitis is a localization of infectious organisms that enter the blood from primary sources such as skin or respiratory infections. *Staphylococcus aureus* is the causative organism 80 to 90 per cent of the time. Inflammation with hyperemia and edema begins in the spongy tissue and marrow of the metaphyseal region of the bone. This causes an increase in intraosseous pressure and local pain, because the bone is unable to expand. Pus forms and interferes with circulation. Eventually there is thrombosis, leading to necrosis and bone death. The area of dead bone separates, forming a separate area called a sequestrum. The infection spreads via the bloodstream, causing septicemia. It also spreads laterally under the periosteum, causing abscess formation. If the epiphyseal plates remain intact there is no direct spread of the infection; however, the presence of septicemia may allow an infection to develop in another bone.

Primary prevention includes eliminating factors that lower one's resistance to infection. Adequate nutrition, rest and maintenance of skin integrity are important in avoiding infections. Health education programs should teach children how to stay healthy as well as teach basic first aid for skin cuts and abrasions. Appropriate treatment of all skin lesions and infections is essential in the prevention of osteomyelitis.

Clinical Manifestations and Diagnosis A sudden fever and local tenderness and pain are the first signs of osteomyelitis. The child hesitates or refuses to use the involved limb because of severe pain. Upon examination the nurse may see evidence of a cutaneous infection or injury. Early treatment is imperative and any child with the symptoms described should receive immediate medical attention. School nurses should suspect osteomyelitis in any child with musculoskeletal complaints and pain. Diagnosis involves the following: (1) obtaining a careful history of recent infections or local injuries or both; (2) clinical signs of fever, severe pain and swelling at the end of a long bone; and (3) an elevated sedimentation rate, leukocytosis and a positive blood culture.

Bone x-rays are not diagnostic, because bone destruction will not be evident until 10 days after the onset.[9, 19] The diagnosis may precipitate parental feelings of guilt for not having prevented the infection, and the nurse should be supportive in allowing the parents to verbalize these feelings. Taking time to explain the infection and the treatment regimen will help allay some anxiety.

Signs of septicemia are usually apparent 24 hours after the onset of fever. The child is acutely ill and needs bed rest with analgesics. Blood cultures are drawn immediately and parenteral antibiotic therapy begun. The usual course of treatment lasts three to four weeks. A nutritious, high calorie diet facilitates bone healing.

The child's pain is intense and he will be afraid for anyone to touch him or the bed. Before the child is moved for any reason, an explanation is given of what will be done and how the painful area will be protected. It is usually necessary to use two people, one to support the joints above and below the affected area, and one to move the child's body. Splints or traction is sometimes used to immobilize the extremity and promote comfort.

If the child shows no signs of improvement within 24 hours, surgery is done to decrease pressure and allow drainage of the pus. After bone surgery, it is imperative that aseptic technique be observed during dressing changes.

Because the child with osteomyelitis must be hospitalized for several weeks, the nurse must know the effects of hospitalization on the school-age child (see Chapter 54). The major problems confronting the child with osteomyelitis are immobility and pain. Immobility limits the child's ability to control his environment. The nurse should allow the child to make decisions about daily routines. Maintaining contact with siblings and peers is important for the child's socialization. School work should be continued after the acute phase. Parents should be encouraged to visit frequently and bring favorite books or toys to alleviate feelings of loneliness and separation. Engaging the child in therapeutic play or body drawings allows him to work through feelings about painful procedures. The nurse must be attuned to both verbal and nonverbal expressions of pain and give pain medication as needed.

Both the parents and child will need thorough instructions on activity restrictions after discharge. It is necessary to avoid falls and jerky movements; therefore the child will need to continue with quiet play activities until the physician recommends otherwise. Siblings usually are happy to have their brother or sister home again with the hope that their lives may regain some normalcy. However, the child will not be able to share in household responsibilities for some time, and siblings may resent this. Therefore, they should be included in the discharge planning discussion and helped to view the situation realistically.

The prognosis for complete recovery is good if effective antibiotic treatment was initiated early. However, the possibility of chronic osteomyelitis exists and the child will need to be monitored closely by his physician. Fortunately, mortality rates from septicemia have decreased with antibiotic therapy.

FRACTURES

Falls on playgrounds, pedestrian and bike accidents, and casualties of participation in sports all contribute to the high incidence of fractures in school-age children. A fracture is defined as a break in the continuity of bone. The fracture can be either complete, in which the bone and periosteum separate completely, or incomplete

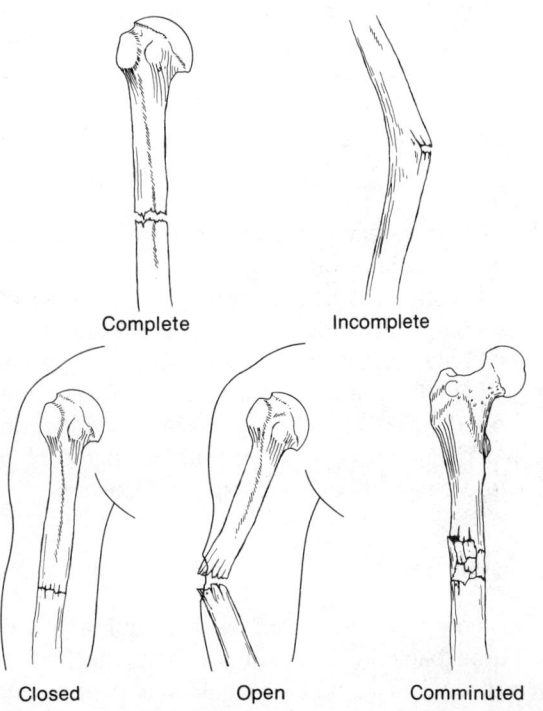

Figure 51-3 Types of fractures.

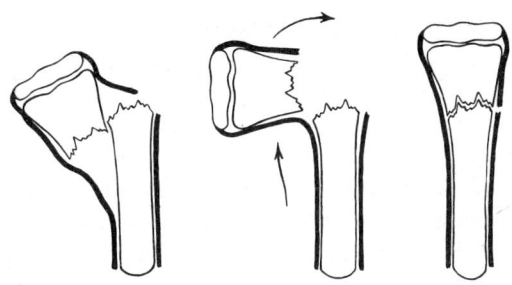

Figure 51-4 The periosteal hinge. Left, a fracture with an intact periosteum on one side. The other drawings illustrate the manner in which this should be used to reduce the fracture, using the hinge to prevent overcorrection of the deformity. (From R. Salter. Textbook of Disorders and Injuries of the Musculoskeletal System. Williams and Wilkins, 1970.)

(greenstick), in which the bone bends or splits but does not break completely. In addition, fractures are classified as either closed (simple) or open (compound). In an open fracture, there is a wound in the skin that communicates with the bone. The bone may or may not protrude through the skin surface. A comminuted fracture consists of three or more bone fragments and an impacted fracture is one in which one part of the bone is jammed into another.

Physiology and Pathophysiology A child's skeletal physiology is distinctly different from an adult's. Types of fractures, treatment and management vary in several ways. First, greenstick fractures are the common type in children because their bones are more porous and flexible. A child has greater osteogenic activity than an adult and bones heal more rapidly. Children also have a very thick periosteum, which is often used as a hinge to facilitate closed reductions (a form of fracture treatment) (Fig. 51-4).[19] Finally, the chance for deformity is decreased because remodeling* or epiphyseal plate growth will often correct the malunion.

When a bone is fractured there is hemorrhage at the site and a clot forms between the two ends of tissue. A few days after the injury a large number of chondroblasts and osteoblasts are present at the injured area. Immobilization of the bone is important so that cartilage and calcified matrix can start callus formation (bony tissue that forms at the fracture). Calcification of the callus continues until the fracture is completely united. Total healing is evident when the callus is replaced by mature bone, usually in several weeks or months.[17]

Fractures of the clavicle, elbow, radius, ulna and femoral shaft are the most common injuries in children. School-age children spend a great deal of time in activities that develop their musculoskeletal abilities. Their need to investigate and their lack of inhibition often lead to risk-taking. It is impossible to protect a child from all injuries; however, every child should learn safety rules at home and school.

Nurse's Role in Prevention, Assessment and Management Nurses can help prevent childhood fractures by discussing with parents the importance of keeping stairways free of toys, avoiding use of loose throw rugs, and encouraging adult supervision on playgrounds. School nurses may be involved in promoting bicycle safety programs, fostering the use of safety patrol crossing guards, and discouraging contact sports for school-age children.

Emergency Care Any injured child should be thoroughly assessed by the nurse before being moved. Establishing an open airway is the first priority and tilting of the head or artificial respiration may be needed. Bleeding must be controlled and this may necessitate applying direct pressure proximal to the fracture. Compound fractures should be covered with a sterile dressing to help prevent infection. Pain and local hemorrhage from the fracture may cause shock; pallor, tachycardia and hypotension are early signs of shock. The child should be kept lying still and covered for warmth. Back or neck injuries are always a possibility, and the child should never be moved until it is determined that no injury exists. Before the child is examined for fractures, he should be offered an explanation of what will be done. Talking to them usually helps children to relax; the child can be asked to give an account of what happened.

Pain that increases upon movement of the affected limb is the most obvious symptom. Other signs include swelling over the fracture site, ecchymosis, decreased mobility of the affected limb and deformity. (Deformity may be minimal with greenstick fractures.) In some children the thick periosteum will stabilize the fracture enough to allow weight bearing or limited use, so movement does not immediately rule out a fracture. The area distal to the fracture may feel cool, appear discolored and have a decreased or

---

*Remodeling is the buildup of new bone or callus after a fracture that results in a reshaping of the bone to its typical straight appearance.

absent pulse. These are signs of vascular impairment and indicate the need for careful splinting and immediate medical attention.

Splinting is necessary to support the joints above and below the site and to prevent further extension of the fracture and damage to vessels and tissues. The extremity must be immobilized before moving the victim. Commercially available standard splints consist of a padded board that is bandaged to the extremity; an air splint is zipped over the extremity and inflated by blowing air into the intake valve. In emergencies, improvised splints made with magazines, newspapers, boards, pillows or the victim's own body can be utilized. Pillow splints can be used for fractures of the foot, ankle, tibia or knee. For elbow or forearm fractures, instruct the child to cradle the arm close to his body or use a sling. (The reader may refer to the *American Red Cross First Aid Manual* for specifics on splinting.)

When immobilization is completed the child should be taken to the emergency department for treatment. Emergency rooms are noisy, frightening, and completely foreign to most children, and the parents or nurse should stay with the child for support. A history of the accident is important but often difficult or impossible to obtain from an apprehensive child. The nurse on duty should try to obtain a description of what happened from the person who transported the child. X-rays of the involved part are needed before treatment. The extremity should remain splinted during x-raying. In children it is difficult to diagnose trauma to unossified bone and an x-ray of the opposing limb is used for comparison. An undisplaced epiphyseal plate injury will not be evident on the x-ray; therefore, the physician should carefully assess the area for tenderness before eliminating the possibility of a fracture. Blood and urine tests will be needed if the child is in shock or has multiple injuries.

Casting Hospitalization is needed for treatment of open fractures and those requiring traction. However, almost all fractures of long bones can be treated with closed reduction, a process of realigning bone fragments, and cast application to hold the bones in place during healing. Before the fracture is reduced (treated), a sedative is given to promote relaxation of the muscles and decrease the child's anxiety. X-rays are retaken after the reduction.

The nurse has an important role in preparing the child for cast application. If time permits, the nurse can demonstrate the procedure on a doll or show the child a picture with the type of cast to be used. Plaster of paris casts are most commonly used, although lightweight fiberglass is now being utilized. The nurse may assist the physician by supporting the limb and explaining the casting process to the child.

Nursing Care of a Child with a Cast

Nursing care of a child who has recently had a cast applied must involve two components: (1) care to assure drying of the cast and adequate circulation to the limb and (2) instructions to the family for preventing complications such as breakdown or injury to the skin of the extremity.

After application of a cast, about 24 hours are needed for drying. During this time the child's position should be changed every 30 to 60 minutes to assure that the cast dries completely on all surfaces. The cast should be uncovered during this time.

Elevating the affected limb with pillows immediately after the cast is applied will help to prevent swelling. Circulation distal to the cast should be checked frequently. As indications of adequate circulation, the digits should be warm to touch and pink, and have normal sensation and immediate capillary refill after blanching. Any change in these parameters may indicate a compromise of circulation and should be reported. If a cast is applied after surgery or over an open wound, draining material may appear on the cast. In order to monitor the amount of drainage, it is helpful to draw a circle around the area with a pen and write the time and date on the cast. Any concerns about the amount of drainage should be discussed with the physician.

To prevent skin breakdown around the cast several steps may be taken:
1. Inspect the skin at the cast edges for any redness every day.
2. "Petal" the cast. (This is done by cutting two-inch pieces of tape with one rounded edge. These pieces of tape are placed around the cast edges.)
3. Massage with lotion around the cast edges to increase circulation and prevent breakdown.
4. Wash the skin around the cast with alcohol to toughen the skin.

Care of the cast at home involves protecting it

from damage and observing it to detect possible complications. The following points should be reviewed with parents before the child is discharged:

1. The cast must be kept dry; it can be protected with a plastic bag during bathing. A sponge bath may be easier than a tub bath.
2. Soiled areas of the cast can be cleaned with a damp cloth and cleanser. Expose the area after cleaning to dry it completely.
3. Do not allow the child to poke pencils or other objects under the cast, because this may damage the skin. If the area under the cast itches, a hair dryer can be used to blow cool air under the cast. Be sure the hair dryer is set on "cool."
4. Development of any foul smell from the cast or areas of drainage should be reported immediately. This may indicate an infection.
5. Other possible danger signs that should be reported include complaints of numbness in the digits distal to the cast, a dusky appearance of the extremity, the extremity feeling cold to touch or looking swollen, and the child reporting pain after the initial 24- to 48-hour period in the cast.

Discharge instructions should be provided verbally and in writing to the child and parents. Instructions should include a warning to watch for signs of circulatory impairment. Any complaints of numbness, tingling, pain or inability to move warrant an examination by the physician. The child should not experience pain once the cast is applied. Most children adapt very well to limitations on their activity resulting from the cast. Discharge instructions to the child should include:

1. Do not bang or hit your cast.
2. Do not let your cast get wet.
3. Do not put anything inside your cast.
4. Do not scratch underneath your cast.
5. *Tell your parents or another adult if your arm or leg hurts, feels numb, tingles or looks different.*

Children will need repeat x-rays during the healing process, usually in three to four days and then weekly until the cast is removed. The child should be prepared before cast removal. After the cast is off, the child and family should be told to use skin lotion or allow the excess dry skin to come off when bathing. Full function of the limb is usually regained by allowing the child to participate in all usual activities except contact sports.

The child's overall reaction to a nonhospitalized fracture will depend on his age, prior experience with injury, support given during the treatment, and the effect of the fracture on his usual activities. A very active child will resent not being able to go swimming, play ball or ride a bicycle. Although children's fractures heal quickly, the time may seem incredibly long for the child, and the nurse should encourage the child to express these feelings. She should provide positive reinforcement to the child who takes good care of his cast and, if possible, allow the child an opportunity to view his x-rays during the healing process. Most children are very interested in learning about their bodies and now is an excellent time to teach about the relationship of nutrition to healing.

Traction Traction is used when fractures require more immobilization than cast application can provide. The pulling force of traction will initially decrease muscle spasms and fatigue the muscle, aiding in reducing the fracture. With traction, skeletal muscles act as a splint for the fracture to allow alignment and reduction to be maintained. The main disadvantage of traction is the necessity of hospitalization and prolonged bed rest.

Equipment used varies according to the orthopedist, the age of the child and the type of fracture. However, all children require a bed with an overhead frame for attachment of the traction apparatus and a firm mattress or the use of bed boards to prevent flexion contractures. Traction may be *fixed* with the apparatus attached at the foot of the bed or *balanced* with a series of pulleys and weights. An overhead trapeze may be allowed and should be utilized whenever possible to aid in providing nursing care.

Nurses working with traction will need to remember several basic principles. *Continuous* traction is used for reduction and immobilization. Some types of traction, applied with non-

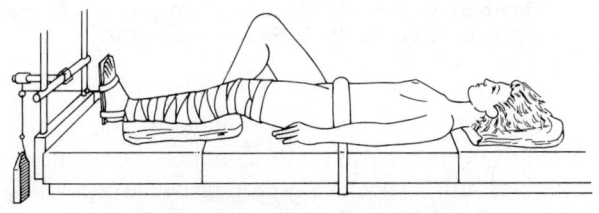

Figure 51–5 Buck's extension.

POTENTIAL STRESSES DURING THE SCHOOL-AGE YEARS: REVERSIBLE ALTERATIONS IN HEALTH STATUS

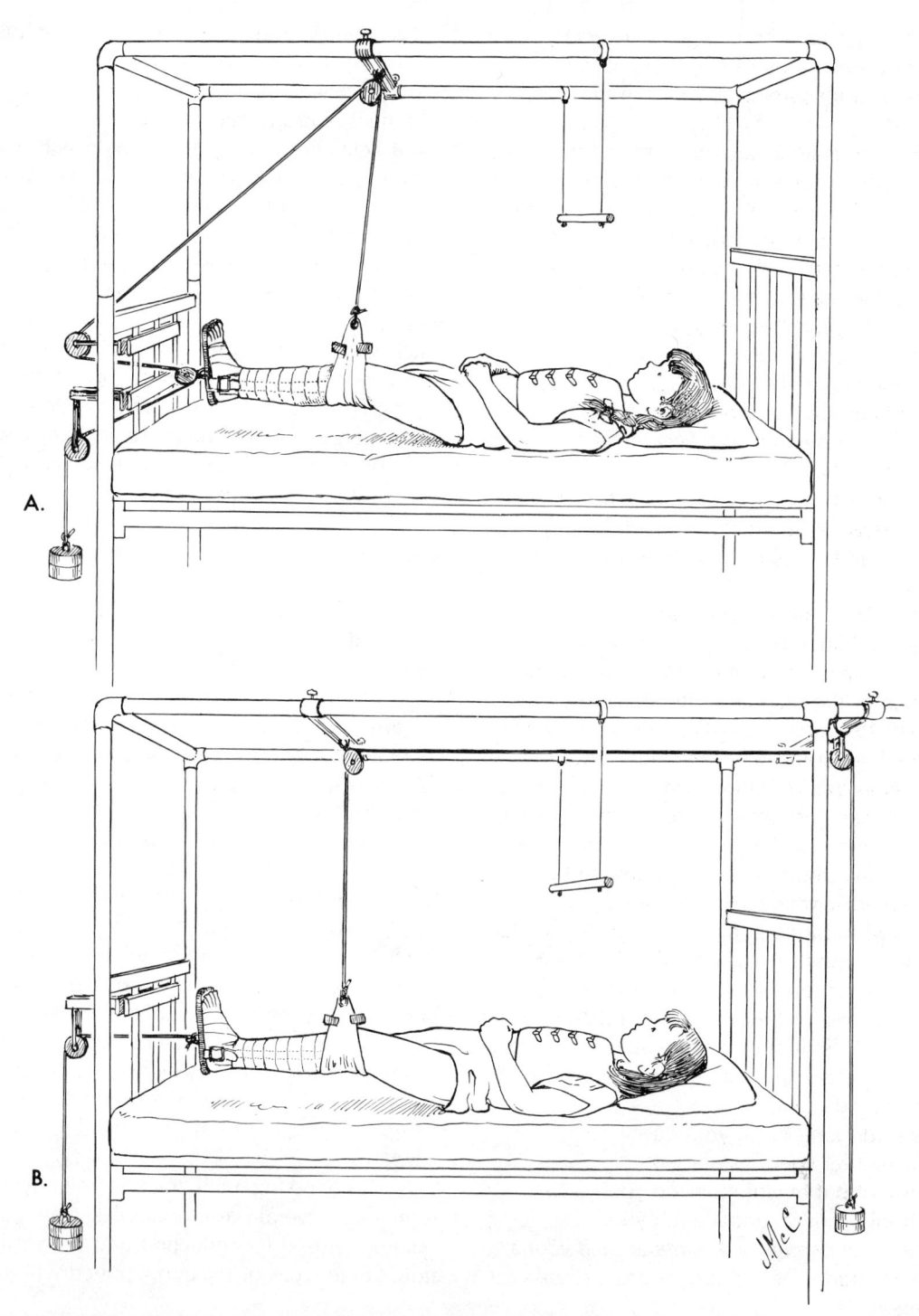

Figure 51-6 Russell skin traction (A) and split Russell Traction (B). (Drawing modified from M. Tachdjian. Pediatric Orthopedics, W. B. Saunders Co., 1972.)

adhesive strips, may be *intermittent*. The nurse must never interrupt or discontinue the traction unless this is specifically ordered by the orthopedist. Careful observation of the traction apparatus should include checking the following: (1) weights should be the correct ordered amount and should hang free, (2) ropes should be in good condition and (3) ropes should be in the center of the pulley and hang free from the bed to avoid friction. Specific orders regarding the child's position are given by the physician to ensure the

1130 FAMILIES WITH SCHOOL-AGE CHILDREN

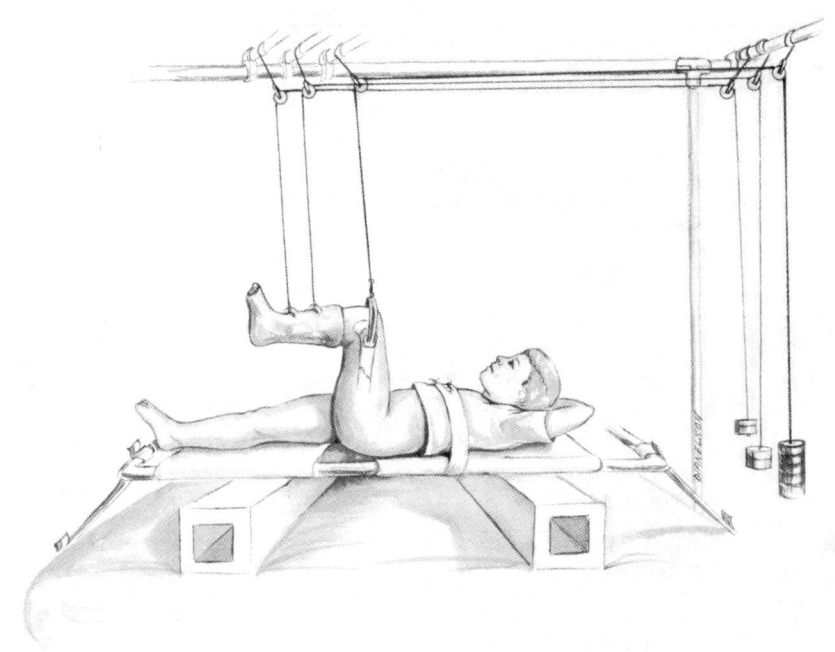

Figure 51–7 Ninety-ninety skeletal traction with wire through the distal femur. (From J. Tachdjian. Pediatric Orthopedics, W. B. Saunders Co., 1972.)

correct body alignment necessary to facilitate the traction pull.

Types of traction include skin, skeletal and manual. *Skin traction* is applied directly to the skin with adhesive or nonadhesive strips, bandages or slings. *Skeletal traction* provides a stronger pull and is applied directly to the skeleton via the Steinmann pin or Kirschner wire inserted through a bone. The application of Crutchfield tongs for cervical traction is also a form of skeletal traction. *Manual traction* is provided when a person's hands maintain pull on the fracture during cast or traction application.

Lower Extremity Traction *Buck's extension,* a type of skin traction, is used for fractures of the femur, hip and knee contractures, and conditions requiring immobilization of the lower extremity. The traction pull is obtained by applying straps (unilateral or bilateral) to the child's extended leg(s) and connecting these to weights at the foot of the bed (Fig. 51–5). An elastic bandage is wrapped around the straps with care to avoid putting pressure on the peroneal nerve. Buck's extension provides only a slight pull and is usually only a temporary form of traction. Countertraction (pull in the opposite direction) is provided by the child's body; therefore it is essential that he not slip down in bed. The child is usually positioned supine or prone.

Russell's traction is often used for femoral shaft fractures. A sling provides support to the knee and skin traction is applied to the lower extremity (Fig. 51–6). The traction pull is in two directions, from the knee sling (vertical pull) and from the spreader or footplate (longitudinal pull), which is connected to the leg straps. The child is in the supine position with countertraction provided by raising the foot of the bed. Nursing care must include keeping the sling wrinkle-free to avoid skin irritation and to reduce pressure on the popliteal area.

If a stronger pull is needed for reduction of a femoral fracture, *90–90 traction* (hip and knee flexed at a 90-degree angle) is used. A wire or pin is inserted through the distal femur to provide skeletal traction and a short leg boot provides suspension of the lower leg (Fig. 51–7). It is essential to assess the pin or wire carefully for signs of infection and proper placement; a loose pin must be readjusted by the orthopedist. Some physicians will specifically order the pin site to be cleansed with an antisepetic solution. Corks or gauze is used to cover the ends of the pins to prevent injury.

Balanced suspension is often used in conjunction with other traction devices for older children and adolescents. Support of the hip and knee is provided by a metal ring (a Thomas splint) and the Pearson attachment (Fig. 51–8). The leg is

POTENTIAL STRESSES DURING THE SCHOOL-AGE YEARS: REVERSIBLE ALTERATIONS IN HEALTH STATUS

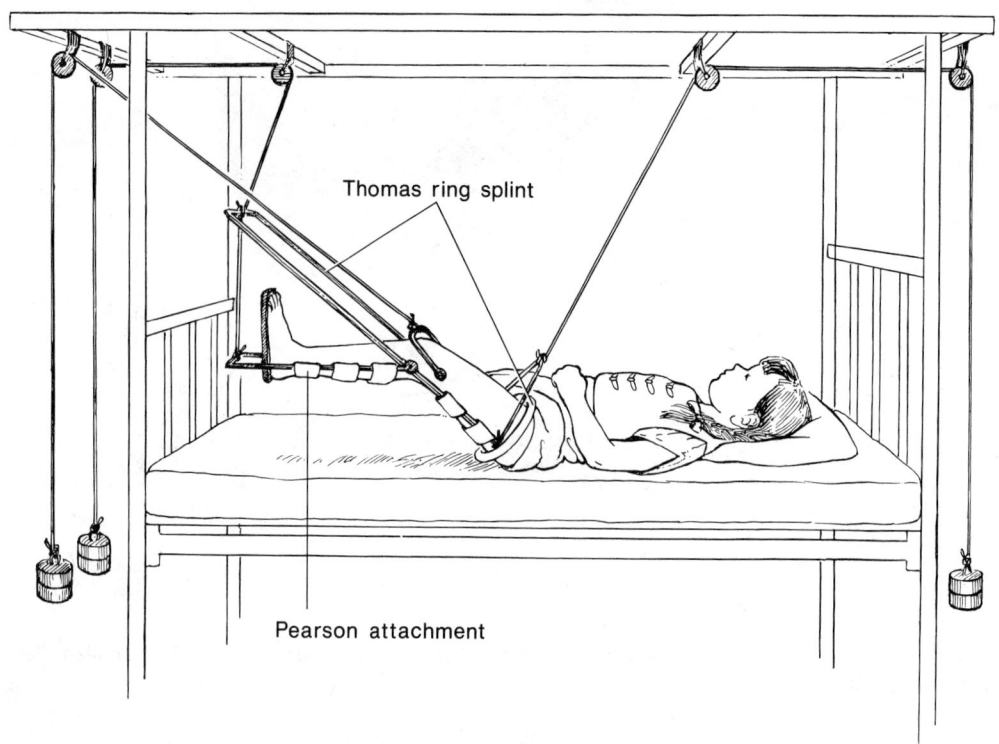

Figure 51-8 Suspension traction with wire through the distal femur with Thomas splint and Pearson attachment. (Drawing modified from M. Tachdjian. Pediatric Orthopedics, W. B. Saunders Co., 1972.)

supported by heavy canvas, which covers the Pearson attachment and Thomas splint. As the child moves, the suspension apparatus adjusts without disturbing the traction pull. This allows the child greater movement and is helpful in long-term treatment.

Bryant's traction is a form of skin traction used to treat a fractured femur in children under 2 or children who weigh less than 14 kg (30 pounds). It is not used on heavier children because the extra body weight poses a danger of impairing circulation.

Both the child's legs are suspended above him at a 90-degree angle of flexion from the hips with pulleys and weights (Fig. 51-9). The child's buttocks are slightly raised off the bed from the countertraction created by his own weight. The child's legs are attached to the pulleys by a footplate. The footplate is attached to the foot soles by adhesive strips that are secured to the legs with elastic bandages; these bandages extend from the foot to the groin. Room is left between the plate and feet for toe and foot movement to prevent contractures. Both legs are always suspended, even if just one is involved.

The child is placed on a sheepskin to minimize pressure points. Often he is placed on a Bradford frame and jacket-restrained to prevent turning or twisting out of alignment. This child is also monitored closely for Volkmann's syndrome* because the nature of this traction and the body position maintained increase the risk of this complication.

Upper Extremity Traction *Sidearm* or *Dunlop's traction* is used for supracondylar fractures of the elbow. The upper arm is abducted and the forearm is placed in a 90-degree angle from the plane of the child. Pull is obtained in two directions: one in line with the upper arm (longitudinal) and the other in line with the lower arm (perpendicular to the upper arm). Dunlop traction is obtained by using either skin or skeletal attachment, depending on the amount of pull required. When skin traction is used, traction straps are placed on the upper arm and lower arm. When a greater pull is needed a

---

*Volkmann's syndrome (Volkmann's ischemic contracture) is a condition in which contractures of the fingers and wrist or knee result from ischemia of the muscles of the forearm or lower leg produced by arterial insufficiency. The insufficiency is a consequence of spasm or arterial occlusion that leads to anoxia then muscle necrosis and contractures if allowed to progress.

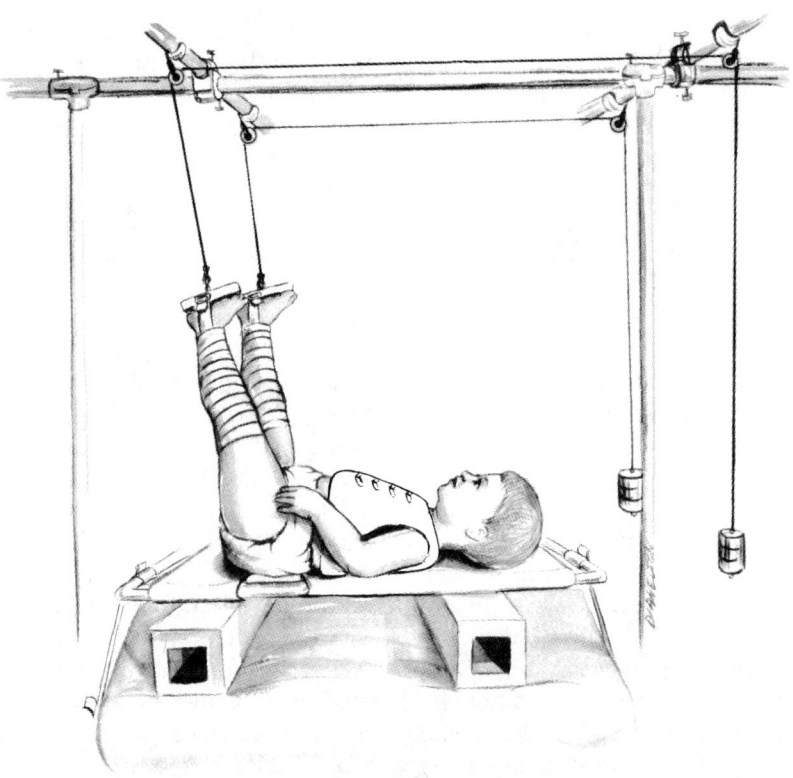

Figure 51-9 Bryant's direct overhead traction. (From M. Tachdjian. Pediatric Orthopedics, W. B. Saunders Co., 1972.)

skeletal wire or pin is placed through the condyles of the humerus to allow for an additional pull to the upper arm; skin traction is used for the lower arm. Countertraction is provided by placing the bed of the affected side on shock blocks.

Neurovascular assessment is critical to detect early signs of Volkmann's syndrome. Critical signs requiring immediate action to prevent the ischemia include: (1) severe increase in pain, (2) inability to palpate peripheral pulses, (3) extremity cyanosis, (4) loss of sensation and (5) loss of function.

Cervical Traction Cervical traction is used for cervical injuries and muscle spasms. This traction maintains the head in a neutral position by the weights attached to the soft or hard head halter. The head of the bed is elevated 15 to 20 degrees and a pelvic sling is applied so that body weight serves as a countertraction.

Nursing Care During Traction

The child in traction requires skilled and creative nursing care if physical and emotional health is to be maintained. Immobilized children are subject to muscle atrophy and deformities. Exercise of all extremities is essential for the child to maintain range of motion and muscular strength. A foot board or foot plate is used with lower extremity traction devices to prevent foot drop. Neurovascular assessment (checking the extremity for numbness, tingling, cold, pallor, pain, loss of sensation or movement) is a vital nursing function and should be continued for the duration of traction.

Skin care is often difficult with children in traction. Pressure areas, especially over bony prominences, develop quickly and the nurse must assume responsibility for assessing the child's entire body. Use of sheepskin does not eliminate the need for massage of the sacral area and scapulae. Use of skin oils or powders should be avoided because they tend to cake and irritate the skin. The use of two folded sheets, one for the top and one for the bottom of the bed, will facilitate care by making linen changes and movement easier. Fracture pans will make elimination easier for the child and nurse.

Immobility tends to decrease the child's appetite; poor nutritional status hampers bone

POTENTIAL STRESSES DURING THE SCHOOL-AGE YEARS: REVERSIBLE ALTERATIONS IN HEALTH STATUS

healing. Most children will quickly adapt to eating in the traction position when provided with foods they like. An increased fluid intake will help prevent renal calculi and constipation.

Hypostatic pneumonia can be a complication of prolonged bed rest. The child can be encouraged to breathe deeply by using colored water blow bottles or balloons. The child's position should be changed whenever possible.

Younger school-age children will need a restraint (jacket or belt) when placed in the traction device. The restraint should be applied from the onset of traction so that the child does not view this as a punishment for movement but rather as a part of the traction apparatus. All children should be given an age-appropriate explanation of the device and shown a picture before the traction is applied. The child should also be told the signs to report, what he may and may not do in terms of movement, and how he can help in his care. This may help allay some anxiety, but nurses should expect the child to experience an adjustment reaction to being placed in traction.

Immobilized children may become angry, irritable, apathetic or depressed. The nurse can help the child learn to cope with his inability to move in several ways. First, the child in traction should not be isolated; he needs a roommate. Whenever possible, the child should be transported to the playroom for a change of environment and for group activities. Recognizing the child's inability to see progress, the nurse should keep him informed of x-ray findings. The child's bed can be decorated with photographs, cards, mobiles to supply visual stimuli and emotional support. Enlisting the aid of activity therapists, occupational therapists, and hospital teachers is helpful in providing a regular schedule of activities. Parent and sibling and peer visits should be allowed and encouraged as frequently as the child can tolerate.

CHILDHOOD OBESITY

Childhood obesity is a major nutritional problem for all health professionals because approximately 12 to 30 per cent of children are affected.[10] Although the potential for serious physical and emotional health problems is great, the incidence continues to increase in large part because of inadequate prevention or treatment. Humphrey's study found an incidence of 12.8 per cent obesity in elementary school children.[10]

There is much confusion about the terms overweight and obesity. The overweight child simply weighs more than the average child of the same age and height. Obesity is defined as being "overfat," having an excess percentage of body fat and not just an excess number of pounds.[26] The label of obesity is applied when a caliper measurement of skinfold thickness shows body composition to be greater than 20 per cent fat. Body weight can be used as a reliable obesity measure only when age, height, sex and body build are also considered.

Many factors (genetic, environmental, social, psychological and nutritional) have been related to the etiology of obesity. Unfortunately, except for an identifiable endogenous cause in endocrine or metabolic disturbances, there is no simple causal explanation. One theory states that cellular composition is a factor in the development of obesity.[1] According to this theory, everyone has different adipose cellular composition, with some having an excess number of adipose cells (hyperplastic) and others having a normal number of overfilled adipose cells (hypertrophic). It has been hypothesized that when the obese person with hyperplastic cells loses weight, the cells decrease in size but not in number. A state of imbalance then exists in the body, and it strives to regain its equilibrium by returning to the obese state.[3] If this hypothesis were proved to be true, the prognosis for treatment would be very poor; however, insufficient data are available.

Environmental influences are significant in the development of obesity. The Ten State Nutritional Survey found that children of obese parents were three times as likely to be obese as children of lean parents.[22] Other studies have shown a high percentage of obesity in only children, children suffering the death of a parent, children of lower socioeconomic status, and those born to mothers over 35 years of age.[7]

Family attitudes toward food have a definite effect on eating habits. Some families tend to use food as a reward, as a form of entertainment or as a solace to appease family members' disappointment or stress. These practices tend to produce their effects as early as infancy (see section on infant obesity in Chapter 24).

Attitudes that give rise to the practices are likely to result in habitual overemphasis on and overindulgence in food, substantially increasing the risk for obesity. Children's attitudes toward foods are also influenced by television advertisements promoting "junk foods." Modern living has prompted the use of more pre-prepared convenience foods high in sugar and sodium; this also contributes to the rise in obesity statistics.

All the circumstances discussed contribute to an excess caloric intake; however, this excess alone is not enough to cause obesity. Most authorities believe that the problem is an ingestion of calories beyond caloric expenditure. Obese children do not necessarily eat more but do tend to be less active than nonobese children, thus promoting fat storage.[3, 25]

The Nurse's Role in Assessment and Prevention

Being knowledgeable of the etiological factors of obesity is helpful in identifying children at risk. However, primary prevention beginning in infancy should be the nurse's goal, for obese infants tend to become obese children. Pediatric nurses working in clinic or well-child centers should obtain explicit nutrition histories in an attempt to help caregivers avoid overfeeding. Nutrition teaching should include a list of nutritional snacks and discussion of appropriate serving sizes for children of different ages and the relationship of activity to caloric needs. (Nutrition needs are discussed in each age-specific growth and development chapter.) The value of lowfat and nonfat milk should be emphasized. A part of the child's health maintenance visits should include use of growth charts and standardized skinfold measurements to detect growth patterns. Calipers (see Chapter 13) are used to measure the thickness of the pinched skin and the underlying subcutaneous tissue, which gives a good picture of the total body fat.

Careful observation of growth patterns should alert the nurse to early signs of a weight problem. Obese children, in addition to weighing more than their peers, also grow more rapidly in height. Puberty tends to come early with fusion of the epiphyses, causing adult height to be below average. The nurse has a major responsibility to discuss the problem with the parent tactfully and recommend a medical referral for a complete physical examination to eliminate an organic cause. Some health professionals may not understand the problems of obesity. The nurse should contact the physician directly to discuss her concerns and promote continuity of care. Obese children know they are fat, but they and their families may not understand the need for a medical referral. It is essential to explain fully the rationale for a diagnostic evaluation to gain the child's cooperation.

For the physical examination, a history of the child's growth pattern, familial growth patterns, present and past eating habits, and physical activities is obtained. Using the format of "what happens on a typical day" is helpful in eliciting the detailed information needed. Parents and siblings need to be included in the diagnostic process, because the problem involves the entire family. Other tests include anthropometric measurements and a battery of psychological tests, useful in evaluating the child's emotional state.

The child, parents and siblings will need some time after the diagnostic visit to decide if the problem warrants treatment. Mowery feels that the *family* must "recognize the need for weight control and want to implement a plan of change" for such a program to be successful.[15] The nurse should be available to answer questions concerning the diagnosis and possible treatment, and she should respect the child and family's final decision.

The Nurse's Role in Management

A lot of time and money is spent in treating obesity, with minimal long-term success. For success it is important that a team approach be utilized with the family. The health professionals should be skilled in working with children with problems of obesity.

Drugs (appetite depressants) and intestinal bypass surgery should not be used in treating children. Attempts to limit the child's caloric intake by using only a calorie-restricted diet are not effective, because with this device alone the child's eating habits and activity patterns are not changed. The goal is to develop healthy lifelong nutritional practices.

The most effective approach is a combination of diet control and behavior modification — weight loss with a change in eating behavior.[2, 7, 23, 25] The first step of the program will involve collecting baseline data on the child's caloric intake, eating habits, and daily activities. The child should be started on a low calorie, nutritious diet that provides the necessary calories for growth rather than on a diet that severely restricts calories. Such a diet may impair development or cause health problems. Caloric requirements should be based on the child's age, height and activity level. Realistic goals, which make allowance for indulgence in birthday treats at school and low calorie afternoon snacks, are needed if the weight-reduction program is to be successful. The long-term goal of behavior modification is to bring about improvement in the child's self-esteem and body image through a loss of weight. Therefore, obtainable short-term goals of desirable eating habits, rewarded immediately, are important in continuing to motivate the child and his family. A contract outlining the program (developed jointly by the child and health professionals) should be signed by the entire team.

Although behavior management programs are effective if followed carefully, many families are not able to follow through with the necessary record-keeping and ongoing team appointments. Failure tends to perpetuate the view that "nothing will work," and further treatment may never be sought.

School nurses can assist by helping the child develop a record-keeping system at school. Ongoing encouragement and reinforcement for success are very important to the child. Nurses can also hold group sessions with obese children. Obese children tend to have very negative feelings about themselves, and providing a safe environment where feelings can be shared with peers is extremely important in helping the child build his self-esteem. Obese schoolmates can help in fostering weight loss by setting up a "buddy system" to offer support at night and on weekends.

The prognosis for the obese child who fails to lose weight is grim. Although the obese adult does not necessarily have a higher mortality rate, authorities document that heart disease, hypertension, kidney disorders and diabetes all correlate with childhood obesity.[3, 12, 21, 25, 26] Severe psychological damage may occur in the child who has been ridiculed by his peers and isolated from them. The obese child tends to remain obese as an adult and will continue to be discriminated against when trying to enter college and when seeking employment.[25]

DENTAL PROBLEMS

The Need for Orthodontia

Dental orthodontia is a specialized area in dentistry in which malocclusions are treated. *Malocclusion* is a term used to describe the condition when the teeth of the upper and lower dental arches are not in proper alignment. If a severe malocclusion is present, the child may experience speech dysfluency, mastication problems, facial deformities, and eventual loss of teeth in adulthood. Significant psychological problems often occur in the child with an untreated malocclusion.[20] Peer or sibling rejection will perpetuate the child's poor body image.

Malocclusions are skeletal deformities of the mandible and maxilla, usually genetically caused.[20] Skeletal facial development may predispose an individual to malocclusion: bone size of jaw may not correspond to tooth size, the mandible may deviate posteriorly or may be hypertrophic or the face may be asymmetrical. The child with premature loss or prolonged retention of primary teeth and tooth loss that interferes with the normal chewing position may also develop a bite problem. Nurses are often asked by concerned parents if their child's teeth will be damaged by thumb or finger sucking. Experts agree that there is no permanent damage if the sucking stops before the permanent anterior teeth erupt. The school-age child is more likely to have a malocclusion when the oral habit continues during the mixed dentition period.*

Early recognition of malocclusion will allow intervention at the appropriate time and prevent the psychological and dentition problems that commonly follow. Although nurses are not experts on occlusions, assessment of the overall dentition should be a part of every child's health maintenance visits. Many children do not routinely have dental care, and the nurse is often the person who first recognizes a potential problem. A very common malocclusion is an anterior open bite caused from digital sucking during the mixed dentition period. To check for this the nurse should have the child clench his

---

*Mixed dentition period refers to the overlap in time during which the child has both primary and permanent teeth.

teeth and determine if the anterior maxillary incisors contact the lower teeth. If there is no contact there may be a problem of occlusion. The presence of jumbled, crossed, or missing teeth should also alert the nurse to the possibility of an occlusion problem.

Convincing parents that a pedodontic or orthodontic referral is needed may be difficult, especially if the parent has not formerly recognized the problem or is not a firm believer in the necessity of dental care. An explanation of eventual long-term problems should be provided. Orthodontic treatment is expensive and many families cannot afford to receive treatment. Nurses may be able to help the family obtain financial help from community service groups or refer the child to a dental college that may provide treatment for a reduced fee.

Diagnosis should be done by an orthodontist specializing in orthodontics or children's dentistry (pedodontist). Cephalograms (skull x-rays) will be needed to establish the extent of the problem.

The child's acceptance of the need for treatment will depend on his prior experience with dentists and his present awareness of the problem. Children need a thorough explanation of the problem, including why treatment is necessary, although the child who has been teased about his teeth will usually readily accept treatment.

Orthodontic treatment improves the child's occlusion and thus his facial appearance. The type of treatment depends on the age of the child and the type of problem. Use of appliances, fixed or removable, is the usual treatment for school-age children.

Removable acrylic appliances require a great deal of cooperation from the child, since he is responsible for wearing the device and may see the dentist only every six months. With fixed appliances, the child will be seen every two to three weeks. Headgear that provides cervical traction may be used to reduce the treatment time and aid in a more permanent occlusion correction.[16]

Appliances require conscientious oral hygiene measures. Proper brushing after meals is necessary to prevent the development of caries beneath the appliance. School nurses can be helpful in encouraging the child to follow through on brushing and reinforce a nutritious diet. The child will also need verbal support that the treatment is effective. Pointing out the changes on x-rays and taking periodic photographs help tangibly to reinforce the progress being made.

The child with a disturbed body image may feel worthless. School nurses should intervene early to help the child identify his positive attributes. It may be necessary to refer the child to a counselor or school psychologist for ongoing therapy. Involving the child's teacher is important so that consistent positive reinforcement can be provided at school.

Dental Caries

Although malocclusion, which affects approximately one-third of the school-age population, constitutes a dental problem of importance, by far the most important and prevalent dental problem is caries, affecting approximately 98 per cent of the population.[30] In addition, these two dental problems are interactive, with a major cause of tooth loss being decay from dental caries. This holds true for both premature loss of primary teeth and for loss of the permanent teeth. Dental caries thus constitutes a problem of major significance.

The widely accepted explanation for the formation of dental caries is that the tooth enamel and dentin are decalcified by acidogenic (acid-forming) microorganisms, which are maintained in the mouth by fermentable carbohydrates. The microorganisms most commonly involved are lactobacilli and aciduric streptococci, and the fermentable carbohydrates most commonly involved are sugars. The tooth surfaces most susceptible to attack are located where the fermentable carbohydrates and bacteria are prone to accumulate; that is, the contact areas between the teeth and grooves or fissures on the chewing surface of teeth. This accumulation takes the form of plaque, a sticky transparent coating that becomes firmly attached to the tooth surface.

This explanation for dental caries leads to a three-pronged approach to a prevention program: (1) increase the resistance of the tooth to acids, (2) reduce activity of microorganisms, and (3) reduce the amount of fermentable carbohydrates in the mouth.[29]

The ingestion or topical application of fluorides increases the resistance of tooth enamel to acids. For maximum benefit ingestion should be consistent throughout tooth development, which takes place throughout childhood. Fluorides are provided in most communities via the water supply system at a concentration of one part per million. In communities in which fluorides are not provided, the ingestion of a daily supplement of sodium fluoride with vitamins is available. Topical application of stannous fluoride is available through the dentist and through tooth dentifrices.

Bacterial activity can be reduced by proper oral hygiene. Teeth should be brushed after each meal if possible. Brushing before bedtime is especially important, because the acid-producing activity of bacteria normally increases in the environment of the mouth during sleep. If brushing is not possible after eating, the mouth should be rinsed with water. To cleanse between the teeth where bacteria and plaque are likely to accumulate, dental floss should be used at least once a day.

Repair of cavities and restoration of deep developmental grooves and fissures in the teeth also reduce bacterial activity. Semiannual visits to the dentist are recommended so that early repair and restoration are accomplished before extensive damage is done to the tooth. The role of reducing the amount of fermentable carbohydrates in the mouth in preventing dental caries cannot be overstated.

Canker Sores

A canker sore is a small, painful crater-like ulcer on the mucus membranes of the oral cavity, appearing singly or in groups. These ulcerations occur most often in the 10- to 20-year-old.[13]

There is no known cause of canker sores, although two theories are currently accepted.[13] The first states that ulcers result from hypersensitivity to the "L" form of *Streptococcus sanguis*, an organism commonly found in the mouth; the second is that an autoimmune reaction of the oral epithelium may also cause ulcer formation.

There is no specific treatment and the ulcers will heal spontaneously within a week or two. Some people are more prone to develop the ulcers. Most school-age children will call their parents' attention to a canker sore. Treatment with topical tetracycline may decrease the pain and shorten the course.[13]

References

1. H. Barnes and R. Berger. An approach to the obese adolescent. Medical Clinics of North America, November 1975, p. 1507
2. K. Brownell and A. Stunkard. Behavioral treatment of obesity in children. American Journal of Diseases of Children, April 1978, p. 403
3. T. Coates and C. Thoresen. Treating obesity in children and adolescents: a review. American Journal of Public Health, February 1978, p. 143
4. B. Conway. Pediatric Neurologic Nursing. C. V. Mosby Co., 1977
5. C. DeAngelis. Pediatric Primary Care. Little, Brown and Co., 1979
6. K. Drummond. Acute glomerulonephritis. In Nelson Textbook of Pediatrics. V. Vaughan et al., eds. W. B. Saunders Co., 1979
7. M. Golden. An approach to the management of obesity in childhood. Pediatric Clinics of North America, February 1979, p. 187
8. A. Guyton. Textbook of Medical Physiology. W. B. Saunders Co., 1976
9. M. Hammerschlag. Osteomyelitis. In Manual of Emergency Pediatrics, R. Reece, ed. W. B. Saunders Co., 1978
10. P. Humphrey. Height/weight disproportion in elementary school children. Journal of School Health, January 1979, p. 25
11. J. James et al. Renal Disease in Childhood. C. V. Mosby Co., 1976
12. R. Laur et al. Coronary heart disease risk factors in school children: the muscatine study. Journal of Pediatrics, May 1975, p. 697
13. R. McDonald and D. Avery. Dentistry for the Child and Adolescent. C. V. Mosby Co., 1978
14. R. Mitchell. Disease in Infancy and Childhood. Churchill Livingstone, 1973
15. B. Mowery. Family oriented approach to childhood obesity. Pediatric Nursing, Mar/Apr 1980, p. 40
16. F. Orr. Headgear. In Minor Tooth Movement in the Growing Child, M. Cohen, W. B. Saunders Company, 1977
17. S. Robbins and M. Angell. Basic Pathology. W. B. Saunders Co., 1976
18. K. Roberts. Manual of Clinical Problems in Pediatrics. Little Brown and Co., 1979
19. R. Salter. Textbook of Disorders and Injuries of the Musculoskeletal System. Williams and Wilkins Co., 1970
20. J. Salzmann. Practice of Orthodontics. J. B. Lippincott Co., 1966
21. A. Stunkard and M. Mendelson. Obesity and the body image: I. Characteristics of disturbances in the body image of some obese persons. American Journal of Psychiatry, April 1967, p. 1296
22. United States Department of Health, Education, and Welfare. Ten state nutritional survey. (DHEW) Publication No. HSM 73-8704. Washington, D.C.: Government Printing Office, 1972
23. R. Wang and J. Watson. Contracting for weight reduction — making the sacrifices worthwhile. The American Journal of Maternal Child Nursing, Jan/Feb 1978, p. 46
24. L. Wannamaker. Rheumatic fever. In Nelson Textbook of Pediatrics, 11th ed. V. Vaughan et al., eds., W. B. Saunders Co., 1979
25. W. Weil, Jr. Current controversies in childhood obesity. The Journal of Pediatrics, August 1975, p. 175
26. R. Werner. Weight reduction and weight control strategies for obese individuals: a case for behavior modification. The Journal of School Health, December 1976, p. 602

Additional Recommended Reading

E. Bovill and M. Chapman. Skeletal injuries. In Quick Reference to Pediatric Emergencies, D. Pascoe and M. Grossman, eds., J. B. Lippincott Co., 1973

H. Brashear and R. Raney. Shand's Handbook of Orthopedic Surgery. C. V. Mosby Co., 1978

P. Bray. Neurology in Pediatrics. Year Book Medical Publishers, Inc., 1969

P. Canwright and M. Campbell. Nursing care of the child and his family in the emergency department. Pediatric Nursing, Jul/Aug 1977, p. 43

J. Chamberlain and N. Feins. Appendicitis, acute. In Manual of Emergency Pediatrics, R. Reece, ed., W. B. Saunders Co., 1978

M. Chapman and E. Bovill. Osteomyelitis. In Quick Reference to Pediatric Emergencies, D. Pascoe and M. Grossman, eds., J. B. Lippincott Co., 1973

H. Chernoff and M. Kreidberg. Rheumatic fever. In Manual of Emergency Pediatrics, R. Reece, ed. W. B. Saunders Co., 1978

R. Copeland. Obesity in school children. Nursing Times, 11 January, 1979, p. 18

R. Crow and J. Fawcett. Child obesity — obesity in infancy. Nursing Times, 11 January 1979

C. Donahoo and J. Dimon, III. Orthopedic Nursing. Little, Brown and Co., 1977

J. Farrell. Illustrated Guide of Orthopedic Nursing. J. B. Lippincott Co., 1977

M. Gellin. Digital sucking and tongue thrusting in children. Dental Clinics of North America, 1979, p. 187

R. Gottleib. Acute glomerulonephritis. In Manual of Emergency Pediatrics, R. Reece, ed. W. B. Saunders Co., 1978

A. Hetrick et al. Nutrition in renal failure: when the patient is a child. American Journal of Nursing, December 1979, p. 2150

E. Kaplan. Acute rheumatic fever. Pediatric Clinics of North America, November 1979, p. 817

R. Klima et al. Body image, self-concept, and the orthodontic patient. American Journal of Orthodontics, May 1979, p. 507

P. Kryschyshen and D. Fischer. External fixation for complicated fractures. American Journal of Nursing, February 1980, p. 256

C. Larson and M. Gould. Orthopedic Nursing. C. V. Mosby Co., 1978

C. Lewis. Body image and obesity. Journal of Psychiatric Nursing, January 1978, p. 22

G. Lloyd-Roberts. Orthopaedics in Infancy and Childhood. Appleton-Century-Crofts, 1971

B. McDonald and P. McEnery. Glomerulonephritis in children. Pediatric Clinics of North America, November 1976

A. Nizel. Preventing dental caries: the nutritional factors. Pediatric Clinics of North America, February 1977, p. 141

J. Ogden. Injury to the immature skeleton. In Pediatric Trauma, R. Touloukian, ed. John Wiley & Sons, 1978

M. Rang and R. Willis. Fractures and sprains. Pediatric Clinics of North America, November 1977, p. 749

N. Rowe. Childhood obesity: growth charts vs. calipers. Pediatric Nursing, Mar/Apr 1980, p. 24

J. Schaller. Arthritis and infections of bones and joints in children. Pediatric Clinics of North America, November 1977, p. 775

P. Schoenecker and J. Ginsburg. Injuries of the lower extremities. In The Management of Trauma, G. Zuidema et al., eds. W. B. Saunders Co., 1979

B. Schwaninger and N. Vickers-Schwaninger. Developing an effective oral hygiene program for the orthondontic patient: review, rationale and recommendations. American Journal of Orthodontics, April 1979, p. 447

C. Seltzer and J. Mayer. Greater reliability of the triceps skin fold over the subscapular skin fold as an index of obesity. American Journal of Clinical Nutrition, September 1967, p. 950

R. Singh. Orthopedic emergencies. In Immediate Care of the Skin and Injured Child, S. Dube and S. Pierog, eds. C. V. Mosby Co., 1978

J. Vipperman and P. Rager. Childhood coping: how nurses can help. Pediatric Nursing, Mar/Apr 1980, p. 11

M. Winick. Childhood Obesity. John Wiley & Sons, 1975

G. Wright and D. Kennedy. Space control in the primary and mixed dentitions. Dental Clinics of North America, October 1978, p. 579

52 POTENTIAL STRESSES DURING SCHOOL-AGE YEARS: IRREVERSIBLE ALTERATIONS IN THE SCHOOL-AGE CHILD'S HEALTH STATUS

INTRODUCTION

by Jo Joyce Tackett, BSN, MPHN

The school-age child with irreversible illness is faced with potential conflict in achieving several of his developmental tasks. Four tasks that pose particular problems are: (1) attaining or retaining satisfying peer relationships, (2) adjusting or adapting to school, (3) becoming progressively more independent in functioning and decision-making and (4) fulfilling a sense of industry, as defined by Erikson.

During the school-age years peers become an increasingly important source of support, self-esteem building and identity development. The irreversibly ill child may find his peers less than supportive, especially if his illness prohibits him from participating in many of the peer group's activities. Some children cope with this by developing "loner" types of hobbies and investing their energies in being studious academic achievers. For other children, the price of not being a part of the peer group is too great, so they forfeit their treatment regimen to do what they must in order to be a part of the group. Still other children learn ways to gain peer recognition without compromising their treatment regimen. Which approach an individual child uses to cope with this dilemma is strongly influenced by the amount of parental support the child has received from the beginning of his illness and the image the child has of himself ("special," normal with limits, handicapped, a "freak" or outsider) as shaped by family attitudes and behaviors toward him. Another influential factor is how much help the child's peers have had in understanding the child's disease and the adult models (parents, teachers, school nurse) that they have observed interacting with the child.

School often brings conflict for the irreversibly ill child. Limitations imposed by the illness or by the periodic interruptions to school attendance for treatments or hospitalization may make mastery of basic educational foundations difficult. The child may have to be sent away from his familiar neighborhood and friends to a school that can meet his special learning needs.* With school entry the child may realize for the first time that he is different from his peers, especially when the disease and symptoms can be felt but not seen. His disease, besides potentially or actually compromising his independence and ability to compete, may cause him to be excluded from peer activities, subjected to ruthless statements and judgments by his peers, or even treated with withdrawal by other children and parents who fear that the illness may somehow be contagious.†

The school nurse or community health nurse usually provides much of the necessary intervention when the irreversibly ill child is able to attend school and resume the activities of daily living. It is essential, therefore, that the nurse (and teacher) know the status of the child's disease (mild or severe; in remission or relapse). The nurse provides the principal, teacher and other involved school personnel with information and instruction regarding the disease and its management (especially when it affects the child's school functioning or when treatment must be provided during school hours). The nurse may also prepare the child's peers for his return to school.

A positive approach that avoids needless restrictions, keeps the child at as near normal activity as possible, and that provides substitute activities when limitations are necessary should be emphasized. Effort should be made to keep the child involved with his healthy peers and included in their activities. Since there is a greater incidence of "school phobia" in children with irreversible disease, the nurse should be alert to early signs of this behavior, such as frequent, unjustifiable complaints to the school nurse or frequent unexplained (or flimsily explained) absences. The nurse, teacher and parents should encourage and if necessary insist on daily school attendance. Parents may need substantial encouragement and support from the nurse while they convince their child to attend school. The school nurse is also responsible to see that a homebound teacher is arranged for when needed.

To protect the child from additional disease or complications, the school nurse may need to remind parents to keep up their child's childhood immunizations (unless contraindicated by the disease) and to tell parents of any infectious outbreaks for which their child may be at special risk. A cooperative endeavor between home and school can help eliminate or minimize the conflicts a child with irreversible illness would otherwise experience at school.

The school-age child should be becoming progressively more independent of adults in his activities of daily living and in decision-making during the school years. The irreversibly ill school child may have limitations that hinder his independence development in one or more areas of living, thereby frustrating his need to become independent. Sometimes the limitation is not within himself but is imposed from outside by parents, teachers, peers or other segments of society that disallow him progressive independence in function or thinking. The nurse should regularly assess the child's social environment for evidence of unnecessary restrictions for which the illness is merely used as an excuse. Additional education or professional counselling may be needed to help the child or the restricting individuals in his environment or both see the extent of the child's limits to independent function in a more realistic manner.

The school-age child's psychosocial task is to be industrious — to investigate, create and do. The school child with physical or mental limitations that interfere with being productive needs extra support. He needs recognition for what he accomplishes and also for his *effort*, for *trying*. He should be presented with achievable challenges and rewarded when he masters them.

Care should be taken not to underchallenge

---

*Every school corporation is now required by law to provide services to meet the needs of all children in the populace they serve; however, not every school in the corporation must be so equipped. Thus the child may have to be bussed to the school in the corporation that can best accommodate his needs. That school may not be the one his neighborhood friends attend.

†L. Robbins and N. Kacen. How should the teacher view the chronically ill pupil? Today's Education, May 1971.

this child, however. The expectation that he at least should try should be communicated and enforced by parents, teachers and other significant persons in his life. It takes a great deal of patience and willpower to stand by and let this child do for himself and to let him experience failure and recover to try again, rather than doing things for him. The nurse can be an important figure in encouraging, teaching and modelling this behavior for others in the child's daily life.

Parents are also affected in special ways when their irreversibly ill child is of school age. The sorrow that parents experience when they have to accept that their child has an irreversible illness often increases when the child enters school. The more atypical the child is in appearance or function and the more his ability to function in school activities is compromised, the greater that sorrow is likely to be.

Parents now may have to decide on the setting in which their irreversibly ill child will receive his school experience — in a regular school program, a special education program, and institutional setting — and how they will absorb the extra costs any special schooling or ancillary services may create.

The hardest part of releasing their child to school for some parents is the necessity involved of freeing the child to become more responsible for himself and to develop self-care skills required to carry out aspects of his treatment regimen in their absence.

For these and many reasons unique to the child and his family, parents need the support of other families who are in or have been in similar circumstances. If parents have not already been introduced to a parent support group, the nurse should arrange for this by the time the irreversibly ill child reaches school age. Sometimes parents who have heretofore not felt a need for such involvement or who have been reluctant to join such a group are now ready for such exposure and support. The health team supervising the child's long-term care should be especially alert to conflict related to school entry and school continuation. Prophylactically, extra support and contact should be provided by the team during this time of potential crisis. Pulling together as a team, the child's family, the health providers and school personnel can help to make the irreversibly ill child's school years as happy, productive and memorable as they are for any other child.

OSTEOGENESIS IMPERFECTA

by Frances Bontrager Greaser, RN, MSN Ed

Incidence and Pathophysiology Both types of this disorder, congenital osteogenesis imperfecta and osteogenesis imperfecta tarda, are rare. In both types, the pathology lies in the immature development of osseous tissue, with the first type apparent at birth and the second apparent after the first year of life. It is an autosomal hereditary disorder involving the connective tissue. Since there is defective osteoblast formation, immature bone structure results. This is a systemic disease in which the mesenchyme and some of its derivatives such as the sclera, bones and ligaments are defective, resulting in inadequate cellular formation. The condition is considered an inborn error of metabolism.

In congenital osteogenesis imperfecta, fractures may be incurred during the birth process, or evidence of intrauterine fracture may be present. Because of the defective periosteal bone formation, the shafts of the long bones have reduced cortical thickness. The infant may be born with a deformed spine because of intrauterine fractures. Those children who survive may suffer fractures from any slight trauma and may never learn to walk because of frequent falls. The limbs may have angulations, and there may be growth retardation because of epiphyseal trauma. The child may also develop kyphosis or scoliosis if the vertebral bones are involved.

Osteogenesis imperfecta tarda is transmitted as a dominant hereditary trait. Frequently, more than one family member may have the condition. It usually develops after the first year of life and is not as severe as the congenital type. There may be fewer fractures after puberty. It is very difficult to make a clear distinction between the two.

Clinical Manifestations In both types the symptoms are the same. Because of the disturbed formation of periosteal bone, the cortex is thin and immature. The mesenchyme is halted in its development of connective tissue, and the sclera appears blue and thin. The skin has a transparent look, giving the child a delicate and fragile appearance. These children are usually short, owing to frequent fractures. Because of the involvement of the osseous labyrinth, there may be auditory disfunction. Cataracts also occur frequently. The child bruises easily, and a tendency for frequent epistaxis may be present. There may be immature and deformed dentition. The child will frequently experience pain at the fracture site, with resultant redness, heat and swelling.

Nursing Care The most beneficial intervention that can be made is to assist the child and his family to accept the condition. The child will undoubtedly have repeated hospitalizations and be in traction frequently. Both the hospitalizations and the restricted physical activity can cause anger and resentment. Immobilization is a threat to the child's need for independence and the frequent disruption of schooling and limited social activity can cause feelings of inadequacy and bring about withdrawal and personality changes.

The family needs the support of a caring nurse who can give anticipatory guidance into areas in which the child can function independently and still be alert to the need for protection from trauma. If the child enjoys physical competitive sports, he may need to accept a more sedentary role of being umpire or scorekeeper. These children frequently find satisfaction in spectator sports or enjoy reading or studying.

The nurse must be alert to the possibility of hearing loss, frequent dental caries or loss of fillings. The family should be taught the principles of good cast care and emergency splinting, and the signs and symptoms of fractures and how to transport a child with a fracture. If the child is inactive, constipation may be a problem.

As the nurse listens to the child's physical history and the family history, she may assist in restructuring the child's life to attempt to avoid fractures. There is no effective treatment for the condition other than adequate nutrition and good physical and orthopedic care. Oral administration of magnesium oxide appears to decrease the number of fractures and lessen the degree of constipation.[37]

The first tendency of the family is to overprotect the child, but this can cause emotional crippling. The child and the family can be helped to see that most people are handicapped in some way. Since the child's physical skills are limited, he should be encouraged to develop leadership skills that will allow him to continue to be a part of a peer group. Hobbies should be encouraged. He must have as much involvement as possible with his peer group. The condition should be explained to his friends and they should be encouraged to accept him for what he can contribute.

The child will undoubtedly be absent from school frequently. The teacher should keep in close communication with the child. If possible, his academic work should be continued in the hospital or home if he is immobilized. If the parents have not arranged for this, the nurse should initiate a contact through the parents. Children who cannot achieve physically often achieve academically.

The quality of the family values and the members' relationships with each other are evidenced in the child's acceptance of his handicap. Sibling competitiveness should be discouraged and the child allowed to develop his own personhood despite the handicap. A broken personality could be a greater handicap than the actual disease. Family members should be exposed to genetic counselling.

MINIMAL BRAIN DYSFUNCTION: LEARNING DISABILITIES

by Frances Bontrager Greaser, RN, MSN Ed

Minimal brain dysfunction (MBD) is not a reportable pathology, and its symptomatology and definitions vary. There is no standard criterion to aid in diagnosis. Minimal brain dysfunction is a medical term for a group of learning or behavioral disorders. Educators refer to affected children as "learning disabled." Unofficial estimates indicate that between 3 and 15 per cent of school-age children have some form of minimal brain dysfunction. Boys are affected more frequently than girls.[37]

A broad definition would include all children who exhibit a disorder in one or more of the basic psychological processes involved in understanding or using a spoken or written language. This may be manifested in a disorder of listening, thinking, talking, reading, writing or spelling. It includes conditions referred to as *perceptual handicaps* and to *brain injury, hyperactivity, dyslexia*. It does not include problems primarily caused by retardation, hearing or motor impairments, emotional disturbances or cultural disadvantage.

Pathophysiology Children with minimal brain dysfunction are of normal or above-average intelligence and do not show any major pathology. While some have learning disabilities, others may have motor coordination disability and others may have speech or auditory perceptual problems. A child may have a combination of motor and sensory problems. These children are recognized as having some "soft signs" that are found in approximately 50 per cent of those affected.[25] These signs include clumsiness, short attention span, mild speech impairment, impulsiveness, awkwardness, talkativeness, destructiveness, distractability, hyperactivity and social immaturity. Very few children have all these characteristics, but the diagnosis is suspected when a child exhibits a variety of these. Some of these traits are usually present in children under 6, but when present beyond ages 7 or 8, they may indicate abnormality. A child performing within a six-month grade level* is usually not considered learning disabled. Many learning disabled children do poorly in tasks demanding verbal or auditory skills. Minimal brain dysfunction is the single most important cause of school underachievement in school-age children.[25]

When the brain is damaged, its complex function is disrupted and messages are not transmitted. This disruption makes it difficult for the child to interact in the usual way. The extent of disruption depends on the area affected and the extent of damage. There is also a complicated interaction between the physical defect and the child's psychological and social environment.

Etiology The cause is unknown. It is important that the diagnosis be made and special attention provided early because of potential psychological damage that might be done to the child. Diagnosis is made through neurological and psychological testing and observation. The developmental history of the child is very important. This should be given by the family if possible in the security of the home and not by observations made when the child is under stress in the physician's office or is undergoing extensive testing.

It is believed that certain parts of the brain of the child with minimal brain dysfunction mature more slowly than others. This would explain why a child who is easily distracted or is unable to remember basic concepts can gain a longer attention span or improved memory in later years. Infection and injuries may also contribute to the cause. Chronic lead poisoning has been considered a cause of a minor degree of perceptual and cognitive impairment and motor incoordination.

Clinical Manifestations There are over 100 varieties of learning disabilities.[25] Many children are disabled in more than one area. Categories most often referred to are perceptual or

---

*A child performing at a level within 6 months of the normal grade level.

motor handicaps, learning disabilities, neurological learning disorders, conceptual handicaps, hyperkinetic syndrome, cerebral dysfunction, and dyslexia. Most become apparent in the preschool or primary grade years. However, many children are not helped and are given a "social promotion" to the next grade and finish school without being able to read. Many children are difficult to discipline, since they do not readily learn from past experience. These children also have difficulty understanding or following instructions. For example, children with visual perceptual disabilities may not understand what they see. They may be unable to trace or draw a circle or square or copy these from a blackboard. Children with auditory perceptual disabilities may not understand a series of instructions; as a child who may not be able to carry out three consecutive directions such as "Go to your room, turn on the light, hang up your clothes."

Although children are not hospitalized because of minimal brain damage, the symptoms can be recognized by an alert nurse. Early referral is of prime importance in assisting the child. Parents frequently recognize symptoms but are told the child will outgrow the condition. This is unfair, since the child needs special help immediately to prevent further disability. Many children with learning disabilities are receiving help earlier today because teachers in day care and preschool programs recognize the symptoms and initiate therapy. Parents are usually relieved to know that someone else has also recognized some of the "soft signs" and that help is available.

Children with minimal brain dysfunction require special attention, but this should never be given at the expense of siblings. The child with specific problems must be helped to learn to cope in his environment despite his handicap and should not be allowed to use this handicap as a reason for requesting special favors. Nor should he be excused from certain experiences because of his lowered competencies in academic skills. Nurses can encourage parents to involve the child's siblings by explaining honestly that the child has a special problem and that everyone will be required to help him. This can minimize sibling competitiveness and aid in family cooperation.

Children younger than the child with minimal brain dysfunction may develop at a faster rate, and the child may be threatened and embarrassed by a normal younger sibling. All children should be praised for their accomplishments and allowed to grow at their own rate. The child should not be compared with his siblings, nor should there be a sense of competition. The child should never receive the impression that he is not loved as much as his siblings. Nurses should be supportive to parents and help them in giving each child the individual attention he needs. Every family member is involved in building a wholesome, nonthreatening, noncompetitive, affirmative relationship.

Management Management for any of the specific conditions in minimal brain dysfunction must be provided by a team. Unless this is done, the child can become confused and his symptoms can increase. Team members should include the family, a physician, a psychologist, a teacher, a nurse and a specialist in the discipline in which the child needs help. Various screenings must be done for auditory and visual acuity. Along with the developmental history, serological studies, including those for lead intoxication, should be done.

Regardless of specific diagnostic conditions, there are some general guidelines to be observed. The nurse or social worker can assist the family in implementing them:

1. There must be consistency. Parents need to agree in the approach to child care. A definite time schedule for eating, sleeping, schoolwork and play should be planned by the family and followed consistently. Siblings and parents must evaluate their feelings, for the child readily becomes aware of any tensions he is causing.
2. Keep frustrations at a minimum. The frustration level can be increased as the child learns to function more maturely.
3. Reward the child for work well done. Verbal praise is reward enough. Minimize defeats and build on strengths. Encourage positive self-concept.
4. Assign simple tasks with simple directions. Show what is to be done, rather than relying on verbal commands. Give only one direction at a time.
5. Special school therapy should be continued at home. Simple motor skills can be learned through play and repetition.

One of the nurse's greatest contributions is to assist the family in using community resources.

The Association for Children with Learning Disabilities (ACLD) is a parent group in which strength and support is found through exchange of concerns and ideas.

Some children need to attend special classes for learning disabilities until they are able to adapt to a more complex and confusing environment. The child, however, should be included in regular classes to the degree that he can tolerate. It is very important that he not be singled out from his peers as being different. Peers should be given a simple explanation of a learning disability so they can more readily accept the child.

The earlier an insult to the brain area is discovered, the greater the possibility of correction through remedial education. Earlier discovery in the preschool years will diminish problems in school. Many children's symptoms decrease after they reach puberty.

Hyperactivity

Incidence and Etiology Diagnosis is difficult; it is based on history and on psychological and neurological evaluation. The condition occurs more frequently in boys than in girls. It is the most common minimal brain dysfunction condition.

Hyperactivity is a behavior disorder caused by dysfunction in some area of the brain. The dysfunction causes neurologically based, non-goal–directed activity in inappropriate amounts.

Factors in the child's history, such as prematurity or low birth weight, perinatal anoxia, head injury with unconsciousness, prolonged febrile seizures or meningitis, may predispose a child toward hyperactivity or other learning disabilities. History is important but not adequate for diagnosis. Definite etiology can remain obscure, but it appears to involve a delay in the maturation of cerebral inhibitory function. The effect of dietary factors continues to be researched and is a controversial issue.

Clinical Manifestations The child manifests little impulse control, has a short attention span, is easily distracted, is very active and has immature control of small muscles. The symptoms can be noted during infancy and the preschool years; they reach a peak during middle school years and gradually diminish during adolescence. Some individuals, however, continue to have symptoms of emotional maladjustment in adulthood. The term learning disability is not interchangeable with "emotional disturbance."

Nursing Care The hyperactive child's behavior can be very irritating and disruptive to others. The child's behavior must be identified as either neurologically based activity or as undisciplined behavior. Help for the child must be initiated immediately; it involves placing the child in a structured environment with a minimum of external stimuli. The child should be in a special education class with a teacher qualified in learning disabilities. The diagnostic team continues to evaluate the academic and social development of the child as he matures and gives guidance as he progresses.

The attitude of the child's family is important, since the child's destructive activity may have caused open hostility in siblings. They may suffer embarrassment and resentment at the antisocial behavior of this family member, and thus limit their own social involvement. Parents may repress feelings of inadequacy or guilt and may need counselling. Tension and stress in the home may increase the anxiety of the child, who frequently is under pressure to achieve. This increases his anxiety and triggers more unacceptable behavior.

The observant nurse watches for cues and is supportive to the family in their most difficult responsibility of caring for this child. If the child must be hospitalized for any condition, his anxiety will be heightened. The hospitalized hyperactive child should have continuity of care from the same nurses and a quiet, relaxing environment in which caregivers' answers and explanations will lessen his anxiety. This child functions best in a structured, controlled environment. The term slow learner, underachiever, hyperactive or any such label should never be used within the child's hearing, since these often place psychological limits on the child's interest in achieving.

The nurse should encourage the family to allow the child to relax at home without emphasizing academic skills. Frustrations should be minimized until the child is better able to adapt to the environment. The nurse must be aware of the expense and embarrassment caused by the child's impulsive behavior and refrain from being judgmental of the parents.

Behavior modification, or *operant conditioning,* is considered by some to be bribing the child or creating the expectation of a reward for each task well done. It is, however, wise to consider giving simple rewards for attainable goals, gradually increasing the complexity of the task and lengthening the time span. A series of short "contractual" assignments with an immediate reward encourages the child toward achievement. Most hyperkinetic children have low self-esteem, and verbal praise is rewarding enough. Food should not be used as a reward.

The child's behavior should be reinforced with praise when the task is done well and inappropriate behavior or responses should be ignored. The child will do best academically in a structured, closed classroom setting in which he learns through repetition and reinforcement. The development of keen auditory, tactile, visual and verbal skills should be stressed.

The use of medication for behavior control remains in dispute. Medication is usually prescribed only when attempts at modifying environment and approach have not produced a change in behavior. Medication may reduce distractibility and impulsivity and improve the attention span, but it does not produce learning. It is, however, effective in allowing the child brief moments of control in which he can concentrate. A firm, consistent environment and an awareness of the family's needs is undoubtedly as therapeutic as reliance on drugs.

Most frequently used drugs are the amphetamines, such as amphetamine sulfate (Benzedrine), dextroamphetamine sulfate (Dexedrine) and methyl phenidate (Ritalin). These drugs stimulate the release of norepinephrine and thus produce a calming effect. All medications should be prescribed in small doses and gradually increased until the desired effect is reached. It is extremely important that the family be in close communication with the doctor and school during the time medication is administered. The doctor must be kept informed of any unusual activity or change in behavior. The family should also be advised of the side effects, which are loss of appetite, blurred vision and sleeplessness. In some cases, there has been growth retardation that could have been caused by interference with the release of growth hormone.[11] The medication regimen must be closely supervised and discontinued as soon as the child can cope with his environment. In most cases, the medication is not given over weekends or during the summer when the child is not in an academic setting.

Prognosis The prognosis for a child who is hyperactive depends upon the age when therapy was initiated and the external guidance he receives from family members, his teacher and other significant persons in his life. If the child develops self-confidence, he will be able to achieve and become a self-sufficient adult. Parents should insist that the school provide remedial educational services for their child. This is the child's right. The medical or diagnostic team may need to be supportive to the family in communities in which academic facilities have not yet been established.

The nurse in the school or hospital setting can support the teacher in emphasizing the importance of individualized, noncompetitive care. Because of his maturational and developmental lag, the child needs guidance from a patient, kind, significant person who will encourage him through repetition in a relaxed atmosphere. The child can develop school phobia if too much pressure is placed on learning. The feeling of incompetence may also contribute to immaturity in self-help skills.

Dyslexia

Reading disorders are a major cause of school failure. About 15 per cent of children beginning school each year have dysfunctions in reading skills.[2] The term *dyslexia* is loosely used to describe the child who is two or more grades below his peers in reading level. Of this group, approximately 2 to 3 per cent have either primary or developmental dyslexia.[1] Children with this pathology should be differentiated from those with reading difficulties primarily due to lack of exposure to learning opportunities. Developmental dyslexia is more frequently found in boys than in girls. There is no known single cause of the condition.

Pathophysiology and Clinical Manifestations It appears that *primary dyslexia* is usually familial. It may be due to weakness of one or several learning processes or immaturity of a certain part of the brain. *Developmental dyslexia* results from cerebral dysfunction and is evidenced in specific learning disorders of reading,

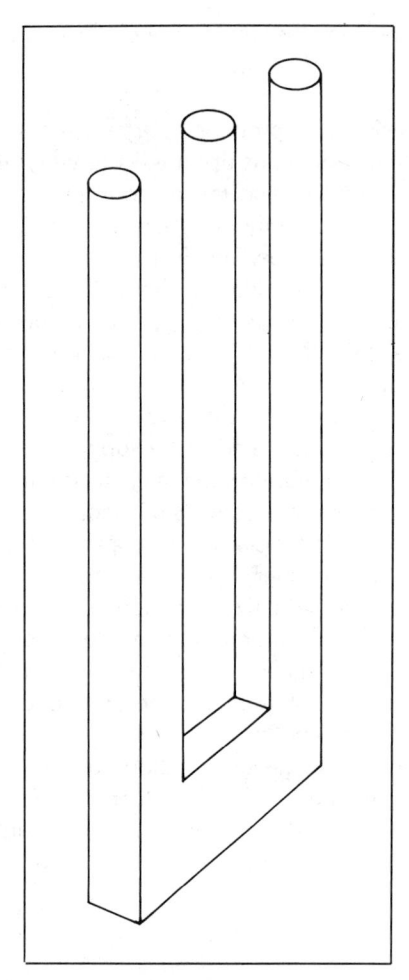

Figure 52-1 This drawing causes a perceptual dysfunction similar to that encountered by the dyslexic child in everyday activity.

spelling and writing. The child can hear and understand statements but cannot read them. There seems to be a blockage or misconnection in the transmission of the written word from the eye to the higher brain centers in which the messages are integrated and relayed to the appropriate sensory area. The child with dyslexia may be unable to distinguish between similar-appearing letters, such as b and d. Letters may appear upside down or reversed. He may read "on" for "no" or "was" for "saw." Letters are frequently seen in mirror image.

Diagnosis and Nursing Care The diagnosis is made through a battery of tests, including appropriate psychological evaluations. The dyslexic child is usually of average or above average intelligence. Since this is not a condition that warrants hospitalization, the nurse in that setting may have limited exposure to dyslexia. However, as a community health person, the nurse must be aware of the symptoms and further preventive intervention. Early recognition is the key to diminishing this problem. The child needs the assistance of a reading specialist. Individualized program planning in a structured setting with limited stimuli should be provided. If therapy is initiated early, the child can attain the same reading level as his peers within a few years. If the problem is not recognized until the child is in the third or fourth grade, the response will be less favorable.

The nurse who does vision screening using a Snellen or an E chart can aid in the detection of visual perceptual problems. If a problem is suspected, the family should be informed and a referral made for a differential diagnosis by an ophthalmologist.

Arriving at a definite diagnosis will relieve family tension, since family members will have been aware of a problem and may have suspected retardation or emotional disturbance. Since children with dyslexia are usually of average intelligence, they frequently act out their frustrations by adopting an "I don't care" attitude or by using physical strength to show competencies lacking in other areas. Very sensitive children may develop feelings of inferiority and may regress in other areas. Early detection and treatment can help prevent secondary emotional scarring.

The child should receive special help in remedial reading but should participate equally with his peers in other activities. There should be no discrimination because of lack of skill in one specific area. If his peers understand his specific need, they can more readily accept the child as one of the group. The family should be encouraged not to emphasize reading excellence but to reinforce the teacher's structure and allow the child to excel in other areas until he gains competence in reading. The family and the school must constantly maintain open communication and help the child avoid feelings of inadequacy or being different.

The child should be taught through repetition and reinforcement. Letters that are confusing to him can be taught by using various forms of sensory stimulation such as letting him "feel" the letter that has been cut from sandpaper, wood, soft textured material or paper. Letters may be color-coded or traced in sand. Each letter should be mastered well before the next letter is taught. Various types of classroom learning machines to enhance reading skills are also available.

The nurse should help the family determine how it can maintain a relaxed and pleasant environment. A local parent group will be ready to share strengths and concerns. Suggestions for enhancing learning at home include those measures discussed in the section on minimal brain dysfunction, as well as the following:

1. Provide informal learning exposure. Reading to the child will enlarge his vocabulary and create interest in the printed page. Use clocks, road maps and calendars. Teach him to recognize safety words such as "stop," "danger" and "poison." Reinforce lessons of "left" and "right" through play.
2. Improve coordination through the use of basketball hoops, and playing "catch." Buy hand-eye games such as jacks or pick-up-sticks. Many games teach a child to count and involve use of small muscles.
3. Break down complicated tasks into small steps. Be sure the child is comfortable with each step before he attempts the next. Reward with praise. Do not scold or show impatience if he does not grasp the concept the first time.
4. Assure the child that he is loved and is an important family member.

DEVELOPMENTAL DISABILITIES

by Frances Bontrager Greaser, RN, MSN Ed

Definition The President's Committee on Developmental Disabilities defines the term as a handicapping condition originating in the developmental period (before age 18) that is attributable to *mental retardation, epilepsy, cerebral palsy,* or *autism.* A developmental disability is one that constitutes a substantial handicap to a person's ability to function in society and that can be expected to continue indefinitely.

Historical Overview Deviations from "normal" have always been confusing and threatening to a misunderstanding society. Historically, records indicate that some American Indian tribes killed any child born with a handicap. An African tribe warded off evil spirits through use of the disabled. The Sudanese believed that handicapped people were a curse and left them to die. The ancient Hebrews saw the disabled as sinners or disability as a result of sin. Some Nordics considered handicapped people gods. During the Middle Ages, they were believed possessed by the devil and were burned as witches.

In the Renaissance, a new concept emerged and these individuals were considered unfortunate and were hospitalized. Much later they were institutionalized and kept from society.

The studies of Aristotle and Galen, who had special concerns about epilepsy and imbecility, have been the basis for further study. However, even in today's scientific age there are those who consider the impaired as cursed or demon-possessed. Many countries still have no special educational facilities for the disabled. The disabled in most parts of the world are still labeled, isolated and denied opportunities for further development.

There is a tendency for people to become frightened or uncomfortable with anyone who is "different." We are conditioned to expect the routine. Society as a whole continues to be surprised by the accomplishments of the visually impaired and continues to stare at twisted bodies in wheelchairs and ignores the retarded. Those who deviate from the norm have been stereotyped and given an inferior place in society.

It is also common to view the impaired as objects of pity — this is debasing and debilitating for them. The child with an impairment is first of all a person and wants to be recognized as such. It is only in a competitive society that people are forced into certain molds and expectations. In spite of this, a child must be freed to be his own person and to express himself in his unique way.

POTENTIAL STRESSES DURING SCHOOL-AGE YEARS: IRREVERSIBLE ALTERATIONS IN THE SCHOOL-AGE CHILD'S HEALTH STATUS

MENTAL RETARDATION

Incidence Approximately 3 per cent of the population is in the moderately to profoundly retarded range.[23, 27] Mild mental retardation appears to be more prevalent among the socially disadvantaged. According to the President's Committee on Mental Retardation, approximately 85 to 90 per cent of cases of mild retardation that do not show identifiable organic or physical cause are associated with conditions arising from the environment.[27]

The American Association for Mental Deficiencies has defined mental retardation as a subaverage general intellectual functioning that originates during the developmental period and is associated with adaptive behavior.[2] The definition is specifically developmental in its approach, and with differentiation from impairment following damage in adulthood. The retarded child is classified according to the developmental tasks that are appropriate for his age. Mental retardation should not be confused with mental illness or emotional disturbance. Three levels of mental retardation are usually identified.

1. Mildly retarded; educable. Such a person may be hard to identify and is often physically normal. In school, mildly retarded individuals are able to learn academic skills up to approximately sixth grade level, and as adults often acquire vocational and social skills necessary for independent living. The majority of mentally retarded individuals are mildly retarded.
2. Moderately retarded; trainable. A person whose intellectual functioning is such that academic achievement is significantly impaired but who can learn self-care, social and some vocational skills.
3. Profoundly or severely retarded. A person who, with special training, may be capable of a significant degree of self-care but will need supervision throughout life. Many are incapable of any self-care skills.

Etiology Over 250 causes of mental retardation have been identified.[27] Most causes fall into four groups of etiological factors, but some are difficult to differentiate. These etiological classifications involve genetic, neonatal and perinatal, infancy and childhood, and social-cultural-familial factors (Table 52–1).

TABLE 52–1 FOUR TYPES OF FACTORS INVOLVED IN CAUSING MENTAL RETARDATION

1. **Genetic Factors***
   Phenylketonuria
   Cerebral lipoidosis
   Galactosemia
   Hypoparathyroidism
   Hypoglycemia
   Gargoylism
   Kernicterus (Rh factor)
2. **Neonatal and Perinatal Factors**
   Inadequate prenatal care
   Premature birth
   Use of drugs during pregnancy
   Anoxia during or after delivery
   Birth injury
   Dehydration
   Maternal factors
     Rubella in first trimester
     Malnutrition
     Toxemia
3. **Factors Operative in Infancy and Childhood**
   Infectious diseases
   Accidents
   Ingestion of intoxicants
   Asphyxia
4. **Social-cultural-familial Factors**
   Emotional rejection
   Nutritional deficiency

*Due to an alteration of the normal genetic information stored in the DNA molecules.

Nursing Care The nurse will note that some of the causative factors can be avoided. Teaching aspects of prevention cannot be overemphasized, because prevention is the most important tool in combating retardation. Nurses should always stress the need for immunization against rubella, encourage health care during pregnancy and recommend giving human immune globulin to prevent Rh hemolytic disease. They should be sure that all infants are appropriately screened for phenylketonuria. The nurse must know the community resources available and be able to follow through on referrals from the diagnostic team. If the etiology warrants it, nurses should encourage all siblings or intellectually impaired children to have genetic counselling.

There are many variables that condition family life, but problems are intensified when one member is disabled. The moment the disability is diagnosed, the emotional tone of the family changes. Parents, in their earnest effort to cope, and because they themselves frequently know so little, often give siblings an unhealthy view of the diagnosis. It is during this period of extreme crisis and stress that the health care team must be supportive in stimulating acceptance and

> **NURSING CARE OF THE INTELLECTUALLY IMPAIRED CHILD**
>
> A. Restoration and maintenance of physical competency
>   1. Care is based on keen observation and providing a climate of acceptance and confidence. The care plan is developed with the family and should include as much normalcy as possible. The care is specific to the medical problem and the child's mental and physical competencies.
>   2. The nurse should cultivate astute observational skills and follow through appropriately on observations.
>   3. Know cues of discomfort.
> B. Restoration and maintenance of intellectual competency
>   1. Auditory stimulation: provide records, radio, television, music, story telling. Be available personally. Speak directly to the child. Ask him questions that can be answered with a "yes" or "no" if he is nonverbal. Observe his eyes for response.
>   2. Visual stimulation: provide colorful play objects, pictures.
>   3. Tactile stimulation: Provide a variety of play activities involving textures.
>   4. Explain all procedures in simple terms. Repeat them each time the procedure is done.
> C. Restoration and maintenance of emotional and social competency
>   1. Arrange for continuity of care to be provided by a significant person.
>   2. Encourage and reinforce socially acceptable behavior.
>   3. Encourage positive family and peer interaction.
>   4. Provide favorite toys to give security.
>   5. Provide structure in settings as near to normal as possible.

hope. The impaired child has a right to family acceptance.

The hospitalized child with mental retardation should be treated for the condition for which he is admitted, but his special needs must be recognized. His care is adapted to his specific need, with a comprehensive and individualized plan geared to his developmental level. This plan should allow for his self-expression, independence and progress at a slow rate.

A significant person should be permitted to stay with the hospitalized child to reassure him that there will be continuity of care. The care plan should have family input on the child's specific likes and dislikes, fears, favorite activities, and any other information on the child and his rituals of daily living that will make hospitalization easier for him. If the child does not communicate verbally, the nurse should be aware of expressions or symbols that are important.

The child with severe mental retardation along with physical handicaps presents complex problems that require a team of experts familiar with the condition. The child with severe brain damage may have vision and hearing deficits that may not have been discovered because the child has no way of knowing that his vision or hearing is impaired. The alert nurse will observe for any symptoms of sensory deficit.

Mentally retarded children are unable to do abstract thinking. Most can comprehend simple explanations, but concrete examples must be given. For example, instead of the nurse saying that she will return after a while, she should show him where the hand on the clock will be when she will return.

Most retarded children enjoy music. A record player and some of the child's favorite records will help ease hospital anxiety. The child should have his favorite toys with him. Toys or games that give immediate reward ("busy boxes," in which something happens when you pull a string or open a drawer) will stimulate motor activity and develop observational skills.

If the child must have surgery, a family member, school nurse or familiar person should stay with him. Procedures should be simply explained. If the child is to have a tonsillectomy, a simple "The doctor is going to fix your throat so it won't hurt as much later," might be adequate. The nurse must always be honest.

Role playing and looking at pictures of doctors in their surgical attire is therapeutic. The child could be given a mask or surgical cap to play with before surgery. If the child has a fracture, a similar cast could be applied to a doll. This can be taken off to show him that the cast is not permanent.

The physical needs of the mentally retarded

POTENTIAL STRESSES DURING SCHOOL-AGE YEARS: IRREVERSIBLE ALTERATIONS IN THE SCHOOL-AGE CHILD'S HEALTH STATUS

child are basically no different from the physical needs of all people. Their body systems, for the most part, function normally, but mental and motor response are restricted. Since all body systems are interdependent, any system might be directly or indirectly affected. It is the nurse's responsibility to observe verbal and nonverbal clues and know how to interpret them.

Medical information should be interpreted by the nurse to the family. She will need to be comfortable in the role of consultant and confidante. She will frequently be asked questions produced by deep hurt and despair. Listening and observing are more important than pious words.

Mental retardation can never be an isolated diagnosis — it affects every family member. Parents and siblings need special help in understanding the pathology and their relationship with the involved child. Parents need to be especially concerned that they do not neglect other family members because of the time a brain-damaged child demands.

The child should be included in as many family activities as is feasible. Favorite picture books, picture card games, and activities that provide an immediate response will help entertain the child while travelling. Food as a reward or pacifier should be kept at a minimum. The child who is well accepted as a family member is not catered to but expected to take his turn in activities. This is part of the maturation process.

Professionals should encourage parents to develop interests outside the home so that no one person is responsible for providing constant care. Guilt feelings can cause overprotection. Siblings should not be expected to forfeit their social activities and relationships for the impaired child. Although qualified babysitters are difficult to find, the family needs time away from the impaired child when internal pressures become too intense. Many communities have facilities for respite care that provide families a brief reprieve. Camps for the handicapped benefit the child and the family. Unless the family has internal strengths it is at risk for dissention.

Introducing one family to another that has a brain-damaged child of similar ability can help both find support. Many families of retarded children become involved in local groups that provide the community with an understanding of the handicapped. The National Association of Retarded Citizens was started by a parent group. Membership in Youth NARC is open to all interested young people between the ages of 13 and 25. There are more than six hundred local Youth Association for the Retarded units throughout the country.

Siblings play an important part in the child's development. When there is a healthy acceptance of the diagnosis, the child will be involved in family activities and will not be excluded from the sibling's circle of friends. The child will feel acceptance and love and will enjoy the richness of a full life. Siblings, however, need to be prepared for the onslaughts of a cruel, uninformed world that continues to tease and deride those who are disabled. Siblings have a unique role in altering public attitudes by example and education.

The nurse must remain sensitive to the daily hurts of the family and not become calloused in her attitude. She must be aware that each family situation and child is unique and, although the family must develop its own way of adapting to changes in many life patterns, the professional team stands by supporting, caring and guiding.

The family sets the tone of acceptance for the community. If the family demonstrates care and concern for the child, the community will more likely respond with the same acceptance.

The nurse and the family involved in the care of children who are mentally impaired should remember some basic facts:
1. Retarded children have the same fundamental physical and emotional needs as all children.
2. Each child needs food, clothing and shelter.
3. Each child needs acceptance and recognition of personal worth.
4. Each child needs love.
5. Each child needs the experience of accomplishment paced at his level.

The extent of these needs may vary, but every child has the same basic rights as does each of us.

The nurse is an important member of the diagnostic team. Her observational skills in noting gross and fine motor movements, visual and auditory acuity, and emotional responses are important in diagnosis. Although psychological testing is required in the evaluation of the child's mental status, the final evaluation should

> **GUIDELINES FOR GENERAL ASPECTS OF CARE OF THE MENTALLY RETARDED CHILD**
>
> 1. Learn from the family what the child can do. Encourage self-care.
> 2. Recognize the emotional problems and defense mechanisms of the family.
> 3. Build a climate of confidence. Be honest and prove yourself trustworthy.
> 4. Do not give the family unrealistic assurance, but encourage hope.
> 5. Stimulate auditory, visual, and tactile sensation for the child.
> 6. Provide structure.
> 7. Talk to the child frequently. Explain procedures simply.
> 8. Focus on what the child can do. Praise him for what he does well.
> 9. Ignore negative behavior. If the child screams for attention, ignore the screaming, but come as soon as he is quiet. Praise him for the length of time he can wait quietly without screaming.
> 10. Set goals and limitations. Let the child know the expectations.
> 11. Expose the child to normal experiences.
> 12. Encourage new explorations.
> 13. Make situations as normal as possible. Convey confidence.
> 14. Make appropriate referrals and follow-through.
> 15. Allow some stress and challenge and small failures. Allow the dignity of risk and the freedom to fail but give assurance that the child is accepted whether he succeeds or fails.
> 16. Do not compare the child to others of similar diagnosis.
> 17. Allow competition at the child's level in play and sports, but discourage threatening competitive situations beyond the child's abilities.
> 18. Be consistent! Never make threats or promises you do not intend to follow through.
> 19. Encourage independence. Never perform a task the child can learn to perform himself. Assist him but gradually diminish your assistance until the child performs independently.
> 20. The "three R's" of mental retardation are *Repetition*, *Routine*, and *Relaxation*.

due to lack of external stimuli. In this case, with exposure to positive experiences, some degree of maturation and learning will take place.

Children should be encouraged to use all their abilities. Emphasis should be placed on the child's capabilities. Parents should be asked to tell what the child does well rather than what he cannot do. The adage "Build on the weakness of his strength" is frequently cited. In this process, the strengths of the child are reinforced, and gradually the unwholesome behavior is diminished. If the child has learned to tie his shoelaces, this process might be enhanced by learning to tie other ribbons, thus developing improved finger dexterity. If he has learned to feed himself, encourage him to pour liquids from pitcher to glass or to pour sand from one bottle to another. This will improve eye-hand coordination. The process should be initiated at the point at which a child performs well. The child will want adult and peer approval, and if he receives affirmation for what he does well but no response for inappropriate behavior, he will quickly perform appropriately for approval. The inappropriate behavior will usually diminish. As the child gains competence and confidence, the negatives will lessen.

Since nurses are in leadership positions and have many opportunities for changing attitudes, they need to examine their own emotions of fear, discomfort, anger or desire for escape when they are exposed to people with impairments. The child will quickly sense the attitude behind the all-important interactions with the nurse. There can be no therapeutic relationship if the child does not feel acceptance. Children are quick to recognize the emptiness of care given in a sense of duty. The nurse giving care will see a person of potential within an imprisoning shell that needs to be broken.

Helping the Family Teach the Retarded Child If the child is intellectually able to make basic decisions, he must learn to accept responsibility for his own safety. Siblings should not be held responsible or punished for actions performed by a brain-damaged child. The child must be taught to accept responsibility for his own actions, with the same guidance his siblings received. The task and discipline should commensurate with his developmental level.

One of the frustrations of the family is fre-

be made by a team, with special attention given to adaptive behavior in the child's family environment. Intelligence testing, without considering adaptive behavior, often labels a child and limits expectations. His cognitive lag may be

POTENTIAL STRESSES DURING SCHOOL-AGE YEARS: IRREVERSIBLE ALTERATIONS IN THE SCHOOL-AGE CHILD'S HEALTH STATUS

quently found in the need for guidance in sexual matters. The nurse should be prepared to assist the family to establish some guidelines. The child has undoubtedly already absorbed the verbal and nonverbal cues of the family's attitude about each member's sexuality. The child's questions about sex should be answered honestly, factually and simply. If the child has the awareness and curiosity to ask, he deserves the courtesy of an appropriate answer. Parents may need to initiate a discussion if the child does not ask. The level of comprehension (and explanation) depends upon the degree of mental impairment, but the basic approach to sex education is the same.

The school-age child is faced with physical changes, and the boy may be frightened if nocturnal emissions and penile erections are not explained. A girl should certainly have received anticipatory guidance about menstruation. Children need to know that, just as it is not socially acceptable to urinate in public, so is masturbation done in private, but parents should not make the child feel guilty. The child's sexuality is part of him, and an open acceptance of it frees the child to develop a better self-image. The manner in which sexual matters are discussed may be more meaningful than the verbal message.

Parents are frequently concerned with communication skills they can develop with their handicapped child. Many impaired children have speech pathologies and should be receiving speech therapy. The following suggestions will be helpful for reinforcement at home. Parents should be reminded that facial expression and voice tone are more important than words spoken. The method of communication depends upon the degree of mental impairment.

1. Don't do the child's talking for him. Let him try to express himself verbally as well as he can. Take time to listen.
2. Let him be an active part of family conversation, even if he is only able to contribute an occasional "yes" or "no."
3. If the child is nonverbal, teach him cues for a yes or no response, such as looking down for no and smiling for yes. Ask questions that require only a yes or no answer.
4. Plan a scheduled 15 minutes each day for speech correction if necessary. This should be the only time the child's speech is corrected. Don't nag. Praise him when he speaks properly.
5. Speak frequently to the child, using vivid explanations (the noisy, green truck; the red book; the soft, white blanket).
6. Do not accept gestures or pointing. Name the object and encourage the child to repeat the name. If he has the ability to speak, insist that he say the word before the object he wants is given. For example, insist that the child say the word "milk" and do not accept pointings or gruntings. If he makes a reasonable effort, give the milk but continue to work on quality.
7. Provide many auditory experiences by reading simple stories or playing suitable records. Allow the child to sing along or respond to rhythm.
8. Praise his successful speech. Whenever he makes an effort toward a new word, reward him immediately with a verbal response.
9. Use short, simple sentences and repeat words frequently.
10. Never refrain from talking to a retarded child because you do not know what to say. Speak to him as you would to any other child, and pick cues from his response, and include him in group conversation.

Before a child can learn to speak, he must know how to chew, suck, blow and swallow. Speech can be reinforced at home by correlating the retarded child's self-feeding skills with the speech program. Teaching an impaired child self-care skills requires much time, patience and repetition, but the results are gratifying in terms of the family's satisfaction and the child's self-esteem. The child usually wants to become independent, and patterns must be established early before dependency habits become established. As he learns one skill, he develops more confidence in conquering the next.

If the child is severely brain damaged, developing self-feeding skills may be problematic, but in most cases the following suggestions that the nurse can make to the parent will be helpful. Have the child sit in a comfortable position with feet on a firm surface. With your hand over the child's dominant hand, assist him in bringing the spoon from the dish to his lips. There are various wrist movements involved in getting food from a dish to a spoon and then to the mouth. This procedure will need to be repeated for many sessions and may take months. Gradually move your hand from his hand to his wrist, and eventually you will be assisting by only a guiding touch on the elbow. Do not be concerned about spillage but encourage neatness. The same procedure can be applied to holding a cup of milk. Begin with food the child enjoys, such as applesauce. Gradually add new textures and flavors, but reward him with his favorite food. Encourage finger foods. Be sure that food is placed in the back of the child's mouth and not just on the tip of the tongue. Peanut butter on the upper or lower gums or between the gums and cheeks encourages tongue manipulation and mandibular movement that is necessary for both speech and chewing.

Helpful hints for teaching dressing skills include:

1. If the child is learning to tie his shoe, let him practice on an adult shoe. The child can slip his foot into the shoe and can play "pretend adult" games while learning.
2. Sew large buttons and enlarge the buttonholes on an adult blouse or shirt. The child can then lift the apparel and watch what he is doing.
3. Name tags on the neck bands of coats, slip-on sweaters and tops teach the child his name and identify the front and back of garments.
4. If the child has trouble getting his coat on, have him put the coat on the table, with the lining side up and the collar toward him. The child faces the coat, puts an arm in each sleeve and then raises his arms over his head. This procedure is also used for slipover sweaters and tee shirts. The neck label will identify the front and back.
5. To teach a child to put on his socks, put the sock in position over his toes and let him pull it over his heel and ankle.

Toilet training for a brain-damaged child cannot be hurried. It is important that it be done at a point at which both child and mother are relaxed and ready. A routine must be established and carried out in a calm, comfortable way, with the mother explaining all actions to the child. As she takes the child to the bathroom, she says, "Here we go to the bathroom" and "Down go Jenny's pants" as she puts her hand over the child's hands and "Up goes Jenny" as the child is placed on a comfortable stool with foot support. An adult should stay with the child so that someone is there to give immediate reward when the child performs appropriately. To be effective, the reward must be something the child particularly enjoys. If there is no result in five minutes, wipe the child and calmly remove him. Again, put your hands over the child's hands as you both pull the pants back into position.

Establish a pattern for bowel movements by noting on a calendar the time of elimination over a two-week span. Take him a few minutes before the average time and repeat the procedure. Watch the child's face and listen for particular sounds. Dress him in clothes that are simple to remove. If the child cries, discontinue and try a few weeks later when he may be more ready.

According to Erikson, the school-age child should have developed a sense of trust, autonomy and initiative and is now engrossed in developing a sense of industry. These developmental stages are equally important for the intellectually impaired child, but the developmental levels are delayed. The child will perform according to realistic expectations; however, if he is pushed beyond his ability, there will be withdrawal and regression. Intellectually impaired children need a supportive, nurturing environment in which they are allowed to develop at their individual level.

The Retarded Child in the Community The most frequent time of recognizing mental retardation is at birth, age 3, and age 6. The child should receive therapy and be enrolled in a stimulating program as soon as the diagnosis is made. Because of the proliferation of preschool programs and day care centers, astute teachers are recognizing symptoms and making early referrals. Early intervention and stimulation results in greater intellectual awareness. Most states have mandatory education programs for retarded children that provide for bus transportation and an educational experience.

As the child progresses and has adequate preparation, he should be integrated into regular classes with his peers, or "mainstreamed." This allows for normal social activities and new experiences with peers. Segregating groups of people from the mainstream of society is seen as dehumanizing. Mainstreaming gives all children an equal opportunity to participate in community and school activities. However, the teacher needs special orientation to the child and must keep open communication with the family. There is grave danger that with mainstreaming, the child will no longer receive

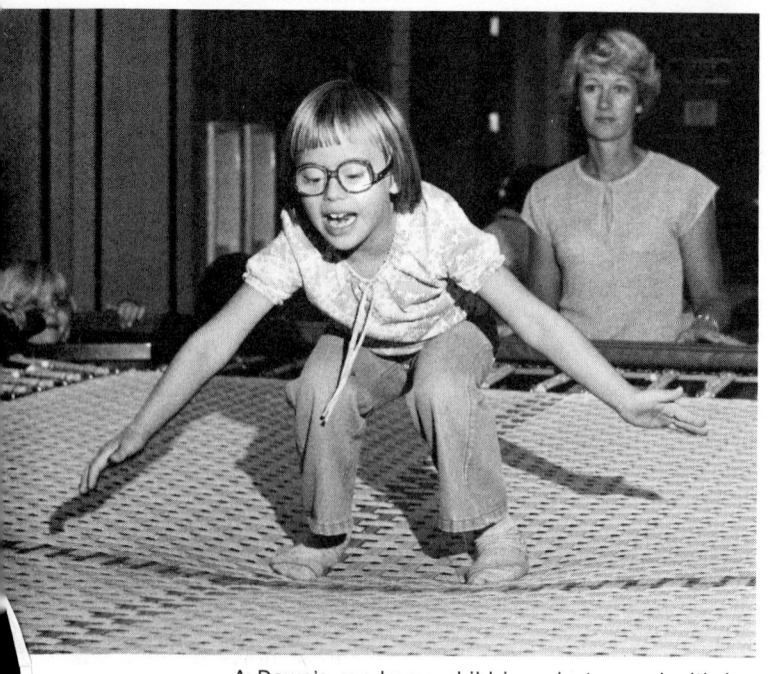

A Down's syndrome child is mainstreamed with her peers for a class in motor skills. (Photograph by Howard Zehr; Joint Schools Special Education Program of Elkhart County, Indiana.)

individualized help and may regress academically.

The process of "normalization," first developed in Sweden, makes available to every retarded person opportunities and conditions of everyday life as close as possible to the norm and patterns of other people. It implies as normal a routine of life as possible. This means the child with an impairment will be integrated into as many normal experiences as he is capable of participating in his condition.

Within the past few decades, great strides have been made in creating community awareness of the needs of brain-damaged children. Consequently, they are more readily accepted. There will undoubtedly always be retarded children, but if today's medical and nursing personnel will focus on preventive measures, a greater percentage of children previously labelled retarded will be able to enjoy a richer and healthier physical and emotional environment.

Microcephaly

Microcephaly is a rare condition characterized by a small skull and severe mental retardation. Primary microcephaly is caused by arrested brain growth in utero. The brain is not formed to the usual size, resulting in diminished skull growth. Secondary microcephaly occurs after injury and is accompanied by neurological manifestations.

The *primary* congenital pathology is an embryological defect and may be caused by an autosomal recessive disorder or a chromosomal abnormality. Other suspected causes are maternal rubella in the first trimester, toxoplasmosis and maternal exposure to repeated x-rays. *Secondary* microcephaly is caused by an insult to the nervous system during the latter part of the third trimester, or perinatally or postnatally, after which the brain stops growing normally. Etiological factors include anoxia, traumatic delivery, neonatal infections and metabolic disorders. The secondary type is first recognized by symptoms of neurological impairment.

There is no increased intracranial pressure in primary microcephaly because the brain has stopped growing. The criterion for microcephaly is a head circumference of 33 cm or less in a 6-month-old baby and 43 cm or less in an adult. The head must be disproportionately small in comparison to the rest of the body.

Primary microcephaly can be recognized in a child at birth: the skull is small and conical. Face and ears are normal but the child has a receding forehead and the back of the head is flattened. Physical growth is delayed and many children have spinal curvatures and vision defects. In the secondary (acquired) type, the symptoms of microcephaly depend on the age of the child when the trauma occurred. The degree of mental retardation is dependent upon the degree of injury.

A supportive health team can be most helpful when the family faces this crisis. The parents and any siblings of the affected child will endure deep grief. Although the infant may have an attractive face, the absence of a well-formed skull gives him an abnormal appearance. There are no words or actions more helpful than the quiet, assuring presence of a professional person who indicates that she cares.

Since no medication or specific therapy exists at present for the child with microcephaly, treatment is symptomatic. The parents and siblings will need continued support in acceptance and care of this child. The degree of mental retardation depends on brain formation, although most children are severely retarded.

The local community typically adopts the attitude of the family members, and if they show a wholesome acceptance of the child regardless of the degree of handicap, the community will share this.

There continues to be much study and evaluation of this pathology. The best treatment is prevention, and with proper immunizations, prenatal care and avoidance of infections in infancy, the pathology can be diminished. Siblings should have genetic counselling. The care described in the preceding section on mental retardation is applicable to the child with microcephaly.

Down's Syndrome

Down's syndrome affects both sexes equally. It occurs approximately once in each seven hundred live births[32] and is chiefly found in whites.[25] The trisomy 21 type occurs more often in children of women over the age of 35. As maternal age increases, the incidence increases. Down's syndrome is a consequence of faulty cell division, which results in an infant of reduced intellectual functioning.

Pathophysiology and Etiology Down's syndrome is based on a chromosomal aberration; instead of the normal 46 chromosomes, each cell has 47 (with the exception of translocation). Although there are many types of chromosomal deviations, there are three which are most common: In trisomy 21 (G) there is a failure of the two chromosomes of pair 21 to separate during gametogenesis, thus producing an abnormal ovum. The cause of the aberration is unknown. It is rarely familial. In *translocation*, the deviation occurs when extra chromosome 21 material attaches itself to another chromosome in group D (13/15) or group G (21/22). The chromosome count in these individuals is still 46, but there is an extra amount of chromosomal material. This aberration is rare; it can be inherited and is not related to maternal age. In *mosaicism*, cells of different chromosome counts are present in the same individual. Some skin cells may show 46 chromosomes, while liver or blood cells may show 47. This type is also rare and is not related to maternal age or heredity. Trisomy 21 is the most common.[8]

Exact cause of the chromosomal aberrations is unknown, although Down's syndrome is more common in infants of mothers who are older. Various theories have been suggested but not proved. Paternal age makes no difference.

In most cases there is little relationship between the type of chromosomal deviation and the degree of mental deficiency. However, in a study of the development of individuals with mosaicism and trisomy 21 Down's syndrome, determined through chromosomal analysis, it was shown that the mosaicism group demonstrated significantly higher intellectual potential, better verbal facility and fewer visual perceptual difficulties than the trisomy 21 group.[8]

Clinical Manifestations There are over 50 confirmed physical characteristics of Down's syndrome.[36] Not all signs appear in all cases. Some of the most common are:
1. "Flattened affect" characterized by a flattened, broad nose and protruding tongue
2. Absent Moro reflex
3. Muscle hypotonia and short stature
4. Dysplastic ear
5. Flat nasal bridge and small nose
6. Excess skin at back of neck causing a broad, short appearance
7. Slanted eyelids producing the Mongolian effect caused by inner epicanthic folds
8. Hyperflexible joints
9. Brushfield spots on the iris with short, sparse eyelashes
10. Simian crease on the palm of the hand
11. Usually short and stubby fingers

Not all of these may be present at birth, but if the diagnosis is questionable, chromosomal analysis, or *karyotyping*, should be done. Some signs are seen at a later date. The extra chromosome seems to have resulted in an unfinished child. Along with the external sign, some Down's children have cardiac involvement such as atrial or ventricular septal defect and patent ductus arteriosus. Some are prone to respiratory and eye infections. There appears to be a higher incidence of leukemia among them. Some, on autopsy, have been discovered to have fatty liver deposits and undersized thyroid glands.

Diagnosis and Nursing Care This pathology is readily diagnosed at birth because of some of the obvious signs. There are undoubtedly few other diagnoses that cause as much grief, confusion and loneliness in parents as this one, ending their happy anticipation of a "normal," healthy baby. How the diagnosis is presented to the family is crucial, an event the family will always remember. This is a highly sensitive and emotional time; parents' acceptance of the child and the diagnosis cannot be rushed, for time is the only healer of the hurt. Parents have anticipated a child they do not have; they are mourning this normal child and they feel guilty about their confused emotions. They should be assured that these are typical reactions and that no one is to blame for their child's anomaly. The nurse may be the most supportive person to stand by, listen, and help them formulate the questions they must ask.

Acceptance of the child varies with the value orientation of the family. Parents who value academic excellence may have a great deal of difficulty accepting a child with limited intellectual potential. There is a wide range of intellectual ability among children with Down's syndrome. Although some are seriously affected mentally, others function at a relatively high level. Down's syndrome children cannot be classified in one category, although similar signs and symptoms may be present. Most children, however, continue to function at half their chronological age up to the age of 12. They never seem to catch up with peers.

Because of recent governmental assistance in special education, it is now mandatory that education be provided for all children with handicaps. Most communities have access to special educational facilities. The infant with Down's syndrome is in some ways more fortunate than one with a hidden diagnosis, since therapy can soon be initiated. Infant stimulation increases awareness and alertness. Some who have had early intervention are now participating in regular elementary classrooms with continued special assistance.

In years past, there was little help or support for the families and their child, and institutionalization was frequently recommended. With the academic opportunities of today, parents are encouraged to keep the child in the home setting, in which he can be socially and academically stimulated. One of the most important comforts the nurse can give is to assure parents that help is available. If possible, a relationship with another family with a child of similar diagnosis and ability should be established. Many communities have a "parents of mongoloids" group in which concerns and strengths are shared. The nurse must know the community resources available.

Down's syndrome children of school age usually have delayed psychomotor development. Speech is commonly delayed; the child may need speech therapy. In the classroom psychomotor activities are incorporated into the school day; children can learn much through play activity. Some children learn to read on a low level, but they cannot do abstract thinking. Although few achieve an IQ above 75, society has yet to learn what can be accomplished if the child is treated as a worthwhile member and given unlimited opportunities and exposures.

Siblings of Down's syndrome children are frequently embarrassed because of this child; older siblings have questions about heredity and wonder whether they too will produce a Down's child. They fear social ostracism because of the affected family member. Karotyping should be done on siblings of the retarded for genetic counselling. Fetal cells obtained by amniocentesis as early as the eighth week of pregnancy may be cultured in vitro and the information made available.

The Down's syndrome child is a social person and enjoys contact with people. As the nurse helps the family members toward acceptance, they will become aware of the contribution the child can make to the family and the community. The Down's child should be among peers, since he learns much through imitation. He should be exposed to as many normal experiences as possible and should not be deprived of opportunities to learn and grow.

These individuals are commonly happy, frank and honest people and have many lessons in values to teach us. As society learns to accept people for what they are, and not for competitive or intellectual performance, the retarded person can be enjoyed and accepted. When a Down's child is hospitalized with any medical problem, discipline and structure should be enforced, and no concessions made "because he is retarded." The child soon learns who he can manipulate. He should be treated respectfully.

Because of modern science, these children are expected to live a normal life span. Previously they usually died of respiratory illness or cardiac pathology while fairly young. Many communities now have group homes for retarded persons where they are under adult supervision and can enjoy semi-independent normal living.

CEREBRAL PALSY

There are an estimated 25,000 babies born with cerebral palsy in the United States annually. Although exact statistics are unavailable, sources estimate there are 1.5 to 5 per thousand live births.[37] Cerebral palsy involves a difficulty in controlling the voluntary muscles due to damage to some area of the brain. It is a collective term that indicates paralysis of the pyramidal motor system, which consists of the motor cortex, cerebellum and basal ganglia. It occurs before birth or during the early years of life. Damage is permanent and is not progressive. Children with cerebral palsy may have normal or superior intelligence, although damage to the cognitive area of the brain is frequent. It is a general term that indicates a pathology but does not indicate the area of damage; therefore the term actually indicates a symptom rather than a diagnosis.

Each individual inherits two brain areas with the same potential. The tendency to be left or right-brained is inherited. Constant usage establishes a pattern. Functions such as chewing, walking and feeding become automatic with usage, but for a cerebral palsied child they must be learned through lengthy repetition. Since one area of the brain has been damaged, the child must develop patterns through the receptors of another brain area.

Pathophysiology A wide range of neuromuscular disability and many types of cerebral palsy exist, depending upon the brain area involved. Five major types are: (1) athetoid, (2) spastic, (3) ataxic, (4) rigidity, and (5) mixed. The child with the *athetoid* (dyskinetic) type has damage to the basal ganglia. This is recognizable by uncontrolled and involuntary movements. Since there is damage to the basal ganglia that controls involuntary movement, any stimulus causes a sudden jerking. This frequently increases in intensity during emotional stress. The incidence of accompanying hearing loss is high.

The child with *spastic* cerebral palsy has damage to the cortex, which is one of the most common types of cerebral palsy. These children are recognizable by their very tense muscles. There is total contraction to stimulus, and when the child is startled, hyperirritability of muscle tone is apparent. The child must make a conscious effort to relax. A tight heel cord causes him to have a talipes equines (walk on toes) walk. Convulsions are more common in these children. They may have strabismus and usually have more difficulty in speech and oral musculature control.

The *ataxic* is a less common type, and the affected child has damage to the cerebellum that controls equilibrium — he appears to walk as if in a drunken stupor. Both position and touch are affected. Children with ataxia frequently have ocular problems. They must be helped to develop a freedom from falling.

The next two most common are *rigidity* and *mixed*. The child with rigidity has resistance in both flexor and extensor muscles and is in a constant state of tension. It is not unusual for a child to have more than one type of cerebral palsy (mixed).

Etiology Over half of the children with cerebral palsy received damage to the motor area of the brain during the prenatal period. Some of the causes are listed in Table 52–2.

Clinical Manifestations and Nursing Care
Early symptoms in the newborn are absence of normal reflexes, irritability, feeding problems, poor motor development and poor muscle tone. Nurses who recognize these symptoms should report them to the physician so that early diagnosis and treatment can be initiated. Physical or occupational therapy and infant stimulation should be begun as soon as the family has had time to consider the problem objectively. The degree of pathology will vary, but the thera-

TABLE 52–2 CAUSES OF CEREBRAL PALSY

Faulty development in utero
  Rh factor
  Rubella in first trimester
  ABO incompatability
Complications at birth
  Combination of prematurity and precipitate delivery
  Anorexia (lack of oxygen in blood)
  Toxemia from maternal medication overdose
  Asphyxia from cord around the neck
  Trauma during delivery
Postnatal period
  Infections (encephalitis, meningitis)
  Trauma
  Poisonings
  Cerebral vascular accidents

POTENTIAL STRESSES DURING SCHOOL-AGE YEARS: IRREVERSIBLE ALTERATIONS IN THE SCHOOL-AGE CHILD'S HEALTH STATUS

peutic aim is to help the child develop skills in speech, arm coordination for feeding and self-care, walking and learning ability.

Many children with cerebral palsy have multiple handicaps. The most common are speech and hearing impairment, mental retardation, oculomotor impairment and convulsive disorder. Assistance should be available through interdisciplinary teams consisting of a speech and hearing therapist, a pediatrician, a nurse, a social worker, an occupational and/or physical therapist, a neurologist and a family member(s). The long-term aims of management involve developing the child's abilities to the extent possible and preventing eventual deformities or complications.

Although medications such as levodopa have given relief for some athetoid children and peripheral nerve blocks have decreased symptoms in a few spastic children, the most promising specific treatment for cerebral palsy is the surgical implantation of a cerebellar pacemaker. Its exact action has not been physiologically explained, but its success in improving functioning relatively quickly has been impressive.[5]

Nursing care needs to be highly individualized for the age of the child and the degree of pathological involvement. Most cerebral palsied children are highly motivated toward independence. Because muscle tension increases caloric catabolism, they are given a high caloric diet. If possible, the child should be taught early to develop independent feeding skills. Proper positioning in a fitted chair with sturdy foot support is very important. An adequate fluid intake is necessary. Since many of these children wear braces, the nurse must be alert to good skin care and must be especially observant if the child is nonverbal. Drugs as relaxants or to control seizures are given, and the nurse must observe for symptoms or side effects.

One of the most important aspects of quality nursing care is the emotional support given the child and the family. The interdisciplinary team must aid the family through the periods of grief and adjustment and allow them to accept the child and see him in perspective — a family member who must learn to use all the abilities he has. The family must be aware that the pathology cannot be cured but, with therapy, new patterns frequently can be established.

If the child has had only minimal exposure to learning or is limited in his ability to respond, his IQ needs to be compared with his adaptive ability. The child should be exposed to new experiences and given opportunities for learning. Educational opportunities, including transportation to classes, are now the right of the handicapped. If feasible, the child should attend a regular class with peers. If needed, speech therapy or physical therapy should be provided as part of his school experience. The child should not be singled out as being "different."

The United Cerebral Palsy Agency was started as a group of parents. Parents and siblings should become aware of the national and community support systems available to them. Summer camps for handicapped children or Special Olympics can help the child see that he is not alone in his particular handicap, and he can gain strength from healthy relationships.

Because of heroic measures now being performed in neonatology nurseries, more children are being salvaged. Predictably, this has led to an increase in the number of children with handi-

The importance of properly fitting braces is emphasized during a conference of the teacher, the school nurse and the mother of a child with cerebral palsy. (Photograph by Howard Zehr; Joint Schools Special Education Program of Elkhart County, Indiana.)

capping conditions. However, more research is also being done and attempts are being made to prevent many neonatal pathologies. Communities should be aware of the needs of children with handicapping conditions. The prognosis of the child with cerebral palsy depends on all factors relating to his condition and the attitude of the child, his family and the community.

EPILEPSY

Epilepsy is fairly common, occurring in approximately 3 per cent of all children.[5] Initial symptoms are most frequently noted in one of three periods: the first two years of life, at 5 to 7 years, and at the onset of puberty. Infantile convulsions are not to be confused with epilepsy. The term *epilepsy* refers to a group of neurological conditions characterized by abnormal electrical-chemical discharges in the brain. The discharges are manifested in various forms of physical activity called *seizures*.

Pathophysiology Normally, each cell receives impulses from other cells. Cells react only if the impulse is strong enough. Normal neurons have thresholds strong enough to withstand daily pressures, but injury to these areas may result in seizure activity. *Organic epilepsy* is defined as recurrent seizures due to demonstrable brain damage, often caused by birth injuries or cerebral infections. *Idiopathic*, or *acquired*, *seizure* designates activity that has developed without any identifiable cause. A seizure is a transitory disturbance in consciousness of motor, sensory, or autonomic function that is due to uncontrolled electrical discharges in the brain. It manifests itself by lack of consciousness and abnormal muscle tone. A seizure is not a disease but rather a symptom.

Grand Mal Seizure These seizures appear to begin in the reticular formation of the brain stem. The child has loss of consciousness and falls to the floor. Eyes become dilated, glassy and expressionless. The shape of the mouth may become distorted; this gives the child a grotesque facial appearance. The arms become rigid and flexed. Legs are motionless. The body becomes tense and the jaws clamp shut. Thoracic and abdominal muscles contract and the child becomes cyanotic owing to the rigid musculature that hinders breathing. The autonomic nervous system is stimulated and the child begins to salivate. This phase usually lasts less than a minute, then the child enters the *clonic phase* and the entire body begins to jerk. After a short time, the child appears to relax but cannot be easily aroused. During this period the child may urinate or defecate involuntarily. Convulsions in children are not commonly preceded by an aura, although older children have been known to have headaches before having a seizure. The alert adult may notice a pattern of eye movements, staring, or giggling that might predictably be followed by a seizure. This is not an age-specific symptom.

Petit Mal Seizure These seizures are due to uncontrolled electrical discharges in the brain. A transitory disturbance in consciousness occurs, during which the child may stop activity and stare into space, exhibit rapid eye blinking, or have a brief loss of consciousness. Sometimes there is uncontrolled tongue movement. Petit mal epilepsy almost always starts in childhood after the age of 3 and frequently stops at puberty. There is little change in behavior during the seizure activity, and the seizure may not be noted by others in the child's immediate vicinity. Some affected children can initiate this seizure by hyperventilating.

Myoclonic Seizures This form is characterized by sudden, brief muscular contractions. There may be slight jerking of an extremity that occurs repeatedly or only one time. *Infantile myoclonus* (massive spasms) is common in children under 3, while *akinetic myoclonus* is common in children 3 to 12 years of age.

Akinetic Seizure A sudden loss of muscle tone and position control occurs. The child may fall, but he cannot protect himself during the fall because of loss of reflex control. Seizures usually appear before age 15 and the condition is hereditary.

Focal Motor Seizure There are also many types of focal (restricted to one area) motor seizure activity without generalized activity. These are not age specific and usually have an organic origin. One focal seizure, the *Jacksonian* seizure, begins with localized activity in an extremity, and as the electrical impulses spread to the cortical areas, the clonic seizure activity spreads to various body parts and may become generalized. *Abdominal* epilepsy is a rare condition in which some children experience recurrent episodes or abdominal pain without any convulsive activity. It begins with a sudden onset of pain in the mid or upper abdomen and lasts only a few minutes. The pain is intermittent and reappears at intervals of a few days or a week. During this time, the child is usually nauseated and may be disoriented but remains conscious. After the attack, the child falls asleep and feels well upon awakening. *Psychomotor* (temporal lobe) seizures range from brief losses of consciousness to lengthy periods of purposeless activity. They are usually preceded by an aura of abdominal disturbance, headache, or visual and auditory sensations. Activity after the seizure is characterized by postictal sleepiness and amnesia regarding events that occurred during the seizure. This type seizure comprises a third of all seizures but is more common during late childhood and adulthood.

Clinical Manifestations and Nursing Care Two types of seizure activity are noted. *Tonus* refers to muscle tone — the body becomes rigid. There is loss of consciousness, eyes become fixed, the head is held back in slight opisthotonus, arms are flexed, hands are clenched and extremities stiffen. Twitching, or *clonus,* begins at a focal point and may become generalized. Spasms involve the respiratory muscles and breathing becomes irregular. The child may become cyanotic and is unable to swallow saliva. His pulse becomes weak.

Nursing care is focused on the physical and mental attitude of the child and his family. Today's child with epilepsy is more fortunate than such children even 50 years ago, since there is now a healthier attitude toward this problem. With more information available to the public, some of traditional stigma attached to the disease is lessening. The school-age child with epilepsy has a complex problem, since he has a strong need for peer approval and acceptance. Physical changes and stress may trigger a seizure and he may resent having to take medication, or he may not want his peers to know about his condition for fear of rejection.

Nursing care of an epileptic child hospitalized for his disease must be given objectively, with an adequate understanding of the disease and its treatment. Since the first exposure to a seizure is a frightening experience, the nurse should seek opportunities to view films or to observe a child having a seizure before she cares for such a child. Seizure activity is bizarre and the nurse must be comfortable with her own feelings about it. Total acceptance of the person and his disease is helpful in controlling the symptoms.

Not all children who have seizures are hospitalized; it is only for further diagnostic evaluations and control of lengthy seizure activity that hospitalization is required. Diagnostic tests include skull x-rays, brain scans, pneumoencephalograms and electroencephalograms. Electroencephalograms record the cyclic changes in the brain and help localize involved areas. Interpreting electroencephalograms in children is much more difficult than in adults because of the wide ranges of normality in children. This study is informative but is not a substitute for further types of diagnostic evaluation. It is imperative that the nurse explain procedures to the child and the significant person with him. Intense anxiety can cause seizure activity. Coloring books and cartoons are available to help inform the child about various diagnostic tests as well as the disease itself. The child should be allowed to express his feelings through conversation or drawings. Questions must be answered simply and honestly. Assure the child that many people with epilepsy are able to lead nearly normal, productive, happy lives.

The care of the child with epilepsy must be consistent at the hospital and at home. Care must be structured by the team; epilepsy cannot be cured, but most seizure activity can be controlled by medicine. Various medications are effective for different types of epilepsy. The nurse must understand the function of the medication and its side effects and must be sure to record any suggestive symptoms. Medication must be given regularly.

Some drugs have the potential for creating an adverse effect on the hematopoietic system, liver and kidneys. This may become manifest through symptoms such as fever, sore throat, enlarged lymph nodes, epistaxis and petechiae. It is the nurse's responsibility to know the medication and be alert to the action of the drug and its possible toxic effects. Table 52–3 shows some of the more commonly used drugs. This information must be shared with the family.

Anticipatory guidance must be given in the child's adjustment to an irreversible pathology. Understanding the family life style will give the nurse some cues concerning the amount of

TABLE 52-3 MOST COMMONLY USED DRUGS IN THE TREATMENT OF EPILEPSY

Drug	Type of Seizure	Side Effects	Comments
Phenobarbital	Grand mal Petit mal	Drowsiness, irritability, hyperactivity	Safe. Has a very pungent taste. Most useful in combination with other drugs. May cause personality changes.
Dilantin	Petit mal Jacksonian Myoclonic Other focal seizures Psychomotor	Causes gingival hyperplasia, nystagmus, rash, anorexia, nausea and vomiting, thrombocytopenia, leukopenia	Generally effective and safe. Regular massaging of gums lessens hyperplasia. Used in combination with phenobarbital. Periodic blood count.
Valium	Myoclonic Jacksonian	Lethargy, ataxia	Also useful in generalized status epilepticus.
Zarontin	Psychomotor Petit mal	Nausea and vomiting, rash, lethargy	Give with food. Have monthly blood count.
Tridione	Petit mal	Rash, photophobia, nausea, irritability, aplastic anemia	Have monthly blood count and Hgb.

reinforcement they will need in acceptance and care. They will also need to know the possible side effects of treatment medications used. Exercise for the child should be encouraged, since seizures are less likely to happen when the brain is active. Encourage the family to allow the child to engage in competitive sports and to minimize their comments on his epilepsy. If the disease is accepted matter-of-factly and explained in terms peers will understand, the child will more likely be accepted and social stigma can be avoided.

Siblings are a vital part of the team. Their social life should not be affected because there is epilepsy in the family. They play a vital role in helping the affected child find acceptance in school. After the child is diagnosed as being epileptic, the school nurse or teacher should prepare the students for the child's return by explaining the pathology of epilepsy. This will greatly lessen the child's anxiety. The school-age child is especially at risk for absenteeism if seizures are not controlled. This can hinder academic achievement. Many epileptic children are also mentally retarded, but the majority are of average intelligence.

A staff conference at school, including the physical educator, can be a means to define the child's needs. The staff should know the type of medication the child is taking and any side effects. There is a tendency for school personnel to either pamper the child or restrict activities unduly. If the child has akinetic seizures, a helmet might be needed when the child is engaged in physical activity, since this type of seizure is difficult to control. The helmet should be removed during sedentary activity. The child should not be further damaged psychologically by being labelled as "different." Encourage the family to provide a Medic-Alert* identification bracelet for the child to wear at all times.

An acceptance of this condition by parents can never be hurried. The nurse should allow the parents to stand away and watch the activity of the child during a seizure with someone else helping him. Explain what is happening, and encourage calmness and confidence. Involve the family in the plan of care during a seizure. Assure them that the most important intervention is to prevent the child from injuring himself and to maintain a patent airway. Nothing can be done to stop the seizure. No attempt should be made to hold the child or resist seizure activity. If the child is in bed, the side rails or crib sides should be padded. Clothing should be loosened and toys that could injure or suffocate the child removed. If possible, have the child lie on a side to aid breathing. Do not attempt to put anything in the child's mouth. If seizures are extreme, a suction machine or oxygen may be necessary. If the child is at home and seizures are extreme, he should be brought to the hospital by ambulance. After the seizure, accurate reporting should include the activity of the child

---

*Medic-Alert bracelets are available at drug stores, jewelers or the Medic-Alert Foundation, Turlock, CA 95380.

POTENTIAL STRESSES DURING SCHOOL-AGE YEARS: IRREVERSIBLE ALTERATIONS IN THE SCHOOL-AGE CHILD'S HEALTH STATUS

> **NURSING CARE OF A CHILD WITH EPILEPSY**
>
> Care is always focused on the child and not the disease, and is based on his emotional and physical needs.
>
> A. Maintenance and Restoration of Physical Competency
>   1. Know the action of specific medications and be alert to toxic reactions.
>   2. Physical stress (including hyperexia) can trigger seizure. Guard against avoidable events that could stimulate seizure activity.
>   3. Give a high caloric diet to compensate for catabolism during seizure activity.
>   4. Encourage physical and mental activity.
>   5. Encourage daily elimination.
>   6. Teach good oral care including gum massage to discourage overgrowth of gum tissue.
>   7. Teach the importance of taking medication routinely.
>
> B. Maintenance and restoration of intellectual competency
>   1. Encourage the child to develop one area of expertise.
>   2. Encourage continuation of academic achievement in the hospital setting.
>   3. Encourage questions about diagnosis. Give simple information on epilepsy that the child can understand and provide picture books for him to keep.
>
> C. Maintenance and restoration of emotional and social competency
>   1. Encourage continued healthy relationship with peers.
>   2. Build a healthy self-image. Reinforce abilities.
>   3. Contact the school to initiate an awareness of epilepsy and a welcoming of the child when he returns to school.
>   4. Encourage siblings in their understanding and acceptance of the pathology.

before the seizure, length of seizure in minutes, the part(s) of the body involved, site where contracture or twitching began, type of movement, posture of body and any incontinence before or after seizure activity.

The manner and attitude of the family is very important to the child. If a seizure is handled calmly, the child will have less fear. After a seizure (or convulsion) is over, the child is frequently confused and embarrassed. Assure him that all is well. Care is directed toward the child and not the seizure.

Prognosis If the child is properly medicated, seizures can be controlled in over 50 per cent of cases. In an additional 30 per cent, seizure activity can be reduced so that persons with epilepsy can lead normal, productive lives.

One major effort toward prevention is better postnatal care. Because of modern medical skills and technology, many high-risk infants are saved, but at the expense of some form of irreversible damage. They may have epilepsy as a secondary effect. Since there is a hereditary element in some forms of epilepsy, genetic counselling is recommended for their siblings.

The Epilepsy Foundation of America has a bibliography of literature available. Most states have an epilepsy foundation, and many communities have local chapters. Parents and families can gain strength through contacts with other parents. The foundation makes medication available at a reduced rate. Speakers are available for school or community groups. It also provides individual and group counselling.

AUTISM

Autism is a rare condition in which a child has severe problems in communication and behavior and an inability to relate to people in a normal manner. It seems to occur more frequently in males. It can be suspected as early as a few weeks or months after birth, or not until 2 or 3 years of age.

Psychodynamics and Clinical Manifestations The autistic child fails to develop normal social relationships. The child demonstrates ritualistic and compulsive behavior; change in routines or surroundings may provoke tantrum-like rages. The child is detached, withdrawn, and unresponsive. He appears to have disturbance of perception, speech and language and sometimes mobility as well as inability to relate. This child does not react to either verbal commands or sounds. He may not show a response to very loud, sudden noises. He shows no reaction to new persons or objects in his environment and may walk into objects as if he does not see them. There is lack of response to tactile or painful stimuli. He seldom makes eye contact. Speech and language may be delayed, and echolalia (repetition of sounds) is common. The child frequently flicks, twirls, or spins toy objects rather than playing with them appropriately. There is little peer interaction and infrequent or delayed social smile. The child is disinterested in people and surroundings but has an unusual interest in inanimate objects. He is unable to perform two tasks simultaneously. Vision appears to be more peripheral than central. Frequently, the head is held to the side, and the child walks on the ball of his foot, frequently and habitually flapping his hands.

Etiology and Nursing Care Little is known about possible causative factors or conditions preceding or accompanying autism. It is considered by some to be "a physical disease of the brain."[28] It appears to be biogenic rather than psychogenic in origin. There is some evidence that severe perinatal distress and autism are related. The disturbance in perception is likely due to an undefined neuropathophysiological process.[28] The child has impaired ability to use sensory input.

To establish the diagnosis, the child must have shown symptoms of specific disturbance of developmental rate, perception, relatedness and language before the age of 3. The pathology may be idiopathic or be in conjunction with other diseases affecting the central nervous system.

A primary person should give care and attempt to help the child become person-oriented rather than object-oriented. The child and his family need the help of educators skilled in the care of autistic children. The family undoubtedly will need special support, since there will be feelings of inadequacy, guilt and low self-esteem. If there is no mutual agreement on discipline, there may be parental distance and family breakdown. Siblings become embittered or angry, and family members suffer fatigue and frustration. Mothers especially suffer from psychotic trauma because of the 24 hour responsibility of a disruptive child. The whole family will benefit from counselling and a relationship with an understanding and sympathetic significant person(s). Respite from care should be available periodically.

Dr. Leo Kanner in 1943 described a group of children as having "autistic disturbances of affective contact."[26] There has been much study and research since then, but the problem continues to be mystifying. This child is bewildering to parents, and it is difficult to get a developmental history because of periodic changes in symptoms. His head banging and similar bizarre behavior may lead to self-mutilation. The autistic child is not usually admitted to the hospital for the condition, although he may be admitted for a diagnostic evaluation. There is as yet no medication or treatment that alters its course. Previously, these children were institutionalized and did not have access to a stimulating environment or a warm, symbiotic relationship with a caring person.

The most effective management of an autistic child is a structured educational program and the environment of a special classroom. This should be begun as soon as the symptoms are recognized. Behavior modification is used in an attempt to change the child's autistic symptoms. Positive reinforcement in the form of food, affection or activity (feed the gerbils, water play) should be given immediately when the child responds appropriately. Accurate and detailed recording is necessary to note change in behavior. In a group setting, adverse conditioning such as a sharp "NO, Timmy!" or insisting that he sit on a chair removed from the group may eventually be effective. Any momentary awareness must immediately be rewarded to help draw the child from his world of fantasy and introversion into the world of reality.

Ideally, there should be an initial conference in the home to observe the child in the family setting. The attitudes of siblings and parents can best be evaluated in a nonthreatening setting. All family members can contribute to a discussion of the child's habits, routines, favorite objects and preferred foods. If there are specific things that frighten the child, this should also be noted. The family should continue to be in close communication with the teacher to establish continuity of care and provide a consistent home environment.

With the assistance of a warm, caring teacher, the child will receive guidance in impulse control, gross and fine motor coordination, language development, as well as academic and social training. The diagnostic team evaluates the child's intellectual abilities as well as any physical contributing factors. Deafness and developmental aphasia must be ruled out. Intelligence of these children usually is in the functionally retarded range.

Consistent and structured care from a limited number of receptive people can allow the child to develop at his own speed in an individualized academic setting. Despite the intensive, individualized treatment that many children are receiving, thus far approximately two-thirds of autistic children remain autistic all their lives.[28]

The National Society for Autistic Citizens is dedicated to the education, welfare and treatment of all children with severe disorders of communication and behavior. This is an active organization with annual national meetings and continued lobbying for the rights of autistic people.

DIABETES

by Sandra Merkel, BS, MSN,
Lisa Parker, BS, MSN, and
Anne Karr, BS, MSN

DIABETES INSIPIDUS

Diabetes insipidus is a disorder of water metabolism caused by a deficiency of antidiuretic hormone or by an inability of the kidney to respond to the hormone. Antidiuretic hormone (ADH) is synthesized in the nuclei of the hypothalamus. Granules containing ADH are transported down axons that terminate in the posterior pituitary. These granules are stored and then released in response to physiological stimuli: increased plasma osmolality, decreased blood volume and a fall in blood pressure. ADH then acts on the convoluted tubules of the kidney to increase the reabsorption of water.

Central diabetes insipidus, which is a deficiency of ADH, may be primary or secondary, depending on the presence or absence of underlying disease. In one-third of children affected, a specific cause cannot be found; their disease is called *idiopathic*.[30] The familial form is very rare. The major cause of diabetes insipidus is a lesion of the posterior pituitary resulting from a tumor or a head injury or operative damage. *Nephrogenic* diabetes insipidus is a rare renal tubule disorder in which the tubules do not respond to ADH. It is transmitted as a sex-linked characteristic primarily affecting males. Nephrogenic diabetes inspidus appears shortly after birth.

Clinical Manifestations All forms of diabetes insipidus are characterized by polyuria, nocturia, polydipsia, low urine osmolality and hypernatremia. Irritability relieved by water but not by milk is a sign of diabetes insipidus in an infant. Growth failure, fever of unknown origin and rapid loss of weight with dehydration are common in the affected infant. In the older child enuresis may be the first sign. Children with diabetes insipidus do not perspire and thus skin is dry and pale. Dehydration is not common in older children because they are able to get water. The excessive thirst that these children have is not life threatening, but it does interfere with play, learning and sleep. The urinary output of a child with diabetes insipidus can be between 4 to 10 liters a day. Frequent trips to the water fountain and bathroom may disrupt the classroom, and children with diabetes insipidus may be unduly punished by teachers or ridiculed by classmates ignorant of their condition.

Diagnosis The nurse's role in the detection of diabetes insipidus is to be alert to the signs and symptoms and to follow up on parental concerns about the child's excessive thirst or fluids consumed. Parameters that should be assessed pertaining to urine are output, specific gravity and the presence of glucose. Children with neoplasms, with head lesions from trauma, or neurosurgery need to be monitored closely for acquired diabetes insipidus. Fluid intake, output and specific gravity need to be determined at least two to three times a day. Sometimes the signs of diabetes insipidus disappear as cerebral edema decreases, but if they return or persist, this should be reported to the physician.

In addition to assessment, the nurse takes an active role in the diagnostic tests by preparing

NURSING CARE IN DIABETES INSIPIDUS

A. Maintenance and restoration of physical competency
   1. Observe for symptoms of dehydration.
   2. Evaluate laboratory results for electrolyte imbalance.
   3. Provide water at all times within reach.
   4. Guard against pyrexia or infections.
   5. Record and describe stool and elimination patterns.
   6. Encourage activity.
   7. Encourage good nutrition in pleasant surroundings.
B. Maintenance and restoration of intellectual competency
   1. Encourage questions. Explain pathology and need for medication and water.
   2. Encourage normal experiences.
   3. Notify school and encourage academic routine.
   4. Provide for privacy.
C. Maintenance and Restoration of Emotional-Social Competency
   1. Include the family in plan of care. Encourage questions and discussion.
   2. Encourage interaction with peers.
   3. Contact school nurse or teacher for student understanding of diagnosis.
   4. Encourage normalization activities.
   5. Encourage genetic counselling.

the child and family, monitoring psychological changes and supervising restrictions. A water deprivation test is administered as the first part of the diagnostic process. This test needs to be fully explained to the child and parents. Being deprived of water will be difficult for the young child to understand, and the parents may find it hard to listen to constant requests for water. Surveillance may be required to prevent any surreptitious water intake. Seven hours of no water for a child with diabetes insipidus usually results in a depletion of extracellular fluid, a rise in plasma osmolality and weight loss.[16] The urine remains colorless, with a specific gravity unchanged between 1.001 to 1.005.

Parameters including weight, specific gravity and temperature need to be measured and recorded accurately. The danger of a water deprivation test is severe dehydration. Usually the fluid is prohibited only until weight loss is 3 to 5 per cent. A compulsive water drinker without the disease will concentrate urine during this test and will not usually have severe weight loss.

After the deprivation test, responsiveness to ADH is determined. Patients with central diabetes insipidus will respond by concentrating urine while those with nephrogenic diabetes insipidus will not respond. Skull x-rays and other neurological studies are ordered to determine presence of lesions or injuries.

Management Once the specific diagnosis is determined, treatment is prescribed. The nurse then needs to implement an educational plan that meets the goal of home or self-management. As with any diagnosis of a chronic illness, the parents may first react with shock or denial. They may feel responsible for the illness either because of genetic transmission or injury to the child, or they may believe that they should have sought medical help sooner. The school-age child may see the illness as a punishment, or he may be unduly expectant that his problems of frequent urination will be solved. Initially, the nurse provides an opportunity for the family members to discuss their fears and feelings and assures them that the child can be helped by treatment.

To be able to manage diabetes insipidus at home, the parents need education concerning the disease process, signs and symptoms to monitor, the importance of keeping accurate records, administration of medication and when to seek medical attention. The teaching plan should include not only specifics about the treatment but also items that will assist the family in adjusting to a chronic illness and knowing how to plan for age-appropriate independence for the child.

The control of nephrogenic diabetes insipidus may be difficult. Chlorothiazide is given to lower the glomerular filtration rate and increase absorption of fluids. These children need water at frequent intervals and in sufficient amounts to prevent dehydration and fever. Sometimes a low protein and low salt diet is prescribed to decrease urine obligatory water loss.

The central form of diabetes insipidus is

POTENTIAL STRESSES DURING SCHOOL-AGE YEARS: IRREVERSIBLE ALTERATIONS IN THE SCHOOL-AGE CHILD'S HEALTH STATUS

treated by replacing the antidiuretic hormone with vasopressin. The administration of lypressin, a nasal spray of aqueous vasopressin, is painless but it needs to be repeated every two to six hours. A cotton ball inserted in the nose at bed time may provide longer relief. Nasal mucosa irritations from allergies and upper respiratory infections will interfere with absorption. Pitressin tannate in oil is effective for 48 to 72 hours but needs to be administered intramuscularly. Intramuscular injections are inconvenient and painful and parents may find it difficult to adhere to the plan.

In preparing the medication, warming the vial and shaking for nearly 7 minutes will resuspend the pitressin in the oil. If the parents do not prepare the pitressin adequately, an inaccurate dose is given and relief is not obtained for as long a time. A new synthetic vasopressin analogue, desmopressin (DDAVP), is available as an aqueous solution for intranasal administration. The duration of this drug's action is 8 to 20 hours and has permitted longer relief with a convenient administration method. Desmopressin is administered through a flexible catheter that is filled with the medication and then blown into the nose. This method can be used with infants and children who cannot sniff by using an air-filled syringe.[18]

In preparation for home management of diabetes insipidus, the nurse develops a teaching plan that includes information about disease process, measurement of urine output and specific gravity, medication, signs and symptoms of problems and how to record data. Accurate records of the amount of medication and concentration of the urine allow the parents to determine the effectiveness of medication.[24] The parents and the child need to be educated, and as the child matures, responsibility for self-care is gradually given to him. The child should wear identification tags to prevent mismanagement when he has problems and the parents are not in attendance. The school needs to be informed so that the child has unrestricted use of the bathroom and can have water when he needs it. Friends and school are an important part of the school-age child's life. The nurse can assist the family in discussing feelings and making plans for increasing independence and self-management so that the child can participate in activities with his peers.

DIABETES MELLITUS

Diabetes mellitus is a metabolic disorder caused by an absolute or relative lack of the pancreatic hormone insulin. Without insulin, normal body functions are inhibited, creating aberrations in metabolism of fat, protein, and carbohydrates. Diabetes can occur as a primary disease of unknown cause or as a secondary disease resulting from a pancreatic disorder or hormonal problems. Primary diabetes has two classifications: Type I, insulin dependent diabetes and Type II, noninsulin dependent diabetes. Type II, which accounts for 90 per cent of the diabetic population, comes on gradually and usually occurs later in life. These people usually produce insulin, but their bodies cannot use it efficiently. Insulin dependent diabetes can occur at any age but usually develops during childhood or puberty. It results from a total lack of insulin, and the symptoms occur quickly. The insulin dependent child must receive prompt treatment to prevent ketoacidotic coma. Because they rely on exogenous insulin, these patients are often more labile and prone to such problems as ketoacidosis, hyperglycemia and hypoglycemia.

The cause of *insulin dependent* (juvenile onset) diabetes mellitus is not known. There is some genetic component to diabetes, but the risk of transmission is not as great as once thought. Some statistics suggest that a child of a diabetic parent has a greater chance of developing diabetes before the age of 10. There is some belief that specific environmental factors such as infectious agents are often important in triggering the onset.

Pathophysiology Insulin is the primary hormone for regulating the level of glucose in the blood. It is secreted by the beta cells of the pancreas, which function as sensors of blood glucose levels. A negative feedback system exists whereby incremental amounts of carbohydrate stimulate the secretion of proportionate amounts of insulin. In fat cells, insulin promotes the uptake of glucose and the storage of triglycerides. In muscle cells, insulin increases the transport of glucose and amino acids into the cell. In liver cells, insulin enhances conversion of glucose into glycogen and also inhibits the release of glucose from the liver. In addition, insulin enhances protein synthesis throughout the body.[15]

> ### NURSING CARE IN DIABETES MELLITUS
>
> A. Prevention, restoration and maintenance of physical competency
>   1. Recommend a diet low in carbohydrates.
>   2. Inform the child and family that insulin should be administered according to need.
>   3. Allow adequate calories to maintain growth and development.
>   4. Encourage health habits: good dental care, frequent bathing, careful nail clipping. Encourage foot care, guarding against foot infection.
>   5. Encourage exercise to decrease blood sugar.
>   6. Encourage routine vision examinations to detect early eye changes or vision problems in the diabetic child.
>   7. Observe for symptoms of insulin shock or acidosis.
>   8. Interpret lab reports to the child and his family.
>   9. Encourage the child to have some form of sugar with him constantly. (Commercially prepared glucose is available.)
>
> B. Prevention, restoration and maintenance of intellectual competency (The child under 6 is unable to understand the reason for injections or diet control; at 6 to 12 he is curious, wants to learn, and needs peer contact and approval.)
>   1. Answer questions openly. Encourage questions.
>   2. Allow child to function as independently as feasible.
>   3. Teach child and family the principles of body metabolics and need for ancillary insulin.
>
> C. Prevention, restoration and maintenance of emotional and social competency (Diagnosis can cause identity crisis.)
>   1. Encourage peer contact through visits, phone calls, tapes, etc.
>   2. Encourage open discussion of diagnosis.
>   3. Introduce the child to another child with diabetes.

In insulin dependency states, glucose is not readily available for energy, triggering the conversion of stored substances into glucose. The fat cell attempts to provide fuel by mobilizing fat stores. The liberated triglycerides yield free fatty acids, which are then converted to ketoacids by the liver. In muscle cells, lack of insulin activates their glycogen stores. Insulin is not necessary for the transport of glucose into the liver. However, when insulin release is suppressed, glycogenolysis and gluconeogenesis occur so that glucose can be fed into the system. In the diabetic, the conversion of glycogen to glucose creates an abnormally high blood glucose level. When the amount of glucose exceeds the renal threshold, *glycosuria* develops. In addition, the excreted glucose acts as an osmotic diuretic, causing large quantities of water and salts to be lost. Dehydration with severe sodium, bicarbonate and potassium depletion occurs.

Ketoacids (produced by the liver from the breakdown of fat) accumulate in the blood and are likewise excreted by the kidneys. The accumulation of ketoacids and concomitant excretion of bicarbonate cause a fall in plasma pH and metabolic acidosis. In addition, the acidosis and osmotic diuresis also cause a decrease in total body potassium.

Treatment with insulin, water and electrolytes reverses the catabolic state created by insulin deficiency; blood glucose levels fall, fat breakdown stops, ketones are no longer produced, pH and serum bicarbonate levels rise and potassium balance is reestablished.

Diagnosis and Management The diagnosis of insulin dependent or juvenile diabetes is usually straightforward. Classic symptoms of polyuria, polyphagia, polydipsia and weight loss are prominent and occur in at least three-fourths of all cases.[29] Fasting blood glucose levels are also elevated and glycosuria is evident. Hospitalization is usually indicated once symptoms are present, as metabolic changes can lead rapidly to diabetic ketoacidosis. Insulin therapy should be instituted and is dependent on the severity of child's condition. The severity can be divided into three stages, with specific clinical manifestations and management for each.

Diabetic Ketoacidosis (DKA) Diabetic ketoacidosis is the most acute stage and includes dehydration and electrolyte imbalance. Kussmaul respirations and CNS depression may also be present. A child in this condition needs emergency treatment. If untreated, DKA can

TABLE 52-4 ABNORMAL LAB VALUES IN UNTREATED DIABETIC KETOACIDOSIS (DKA)

Laboratory Findings	Abnormal Value
Serum glucose ↑	300 mg/dl often > 500 mg/dl
Glycosuria present	>2% often >5%
Ketones present in blood and urine	
Plasma bicarbonate ↓	10 mEq/l or less
Serum pH ↓	<7.3 often <7.1
Serum potassium ↑ or ↓ (Total body potassium ↓)	
Serum sodium ↓	<130 mEq/l
BUN ↑	Possibly > 20 mg/dl
WBC ↑	Often 15,000/mm³
Red cells, white cells and casts ↑ in urine	

lead to coma, vascular collapse and death. Abnormal lab values that may be observed are summarized in Table 52-4.

Treatment with large doses of regular insulin (2 units/kg of body weight) is indicated for children in DKA.[14] The amount per kilogram varies with the mode of administration. A continuous infusion of intravenous regular insulin is the preferred method of treatment because hypotension from dehydration may make subcutaneous perfusion poor.[9] Additional small doses of regular insulin can be given subcutaneously or IM. Fluid and electrolyte therapy is the same as for any dehydrated acidotic child. Glucose is administered when the blood level comes down to 300 mg/100 ml because total body glucose is low and insulin treatment will deplete these stores. Hypoglycemia should be prevented by careful monitoring of glucose levels in blood and urine.

The child in DKA is in critical condition and needs constant observation. To prevent development of a bolus of insulin, IV insulin should be administered with the use of a regulating pump device such as an IVAC. However, the use of a device of this kind does not preclude nursing responsibility to frequently count the number of drops per minute that are being delivered. When insulin is administered through plastic tubing there is an initial binding of a small amount of insulin with the plastic. This occurs on the initial dose; subsequent doses administered through the tubing are not affected. Vital signs should be taken frequently with special attention given to pulse rate. The pulse will become fast and pounding as epinephrine is released in response to hypoglycemia.[14] Blood glucose determinations can be made at the bedside with the use of Chemstrips. Accurate intake and output should be recorded with testing of glucose and ketones of each voided specimen. Any emesis and the concentration of urine are important to note. Large amounts of potassium are administered IV to replenish losses from tissue breakdown and excretion. Insulin therapy assists in driving potassium back into the cells and may result in hypokalemia with the possibility of arrhythmias and cardiac arrest.[13]

The child in this condition is often unconscious or disoriented but is occasionally alert and oriented. It is important to keep him informed what is happening to him, with simple explanations of his treatment procedures and the personnel and equipment involved. Basic comfort measures are an integral part of this child's nursing care.

Diabetic Ketosis The ketotic child has hyperglycemia, glycosuria, ketones in blood and urine, and possibly dehydration. However, serum pH is normal and there is no evidence of CNS depression. Treatment with regular insulin is indicated, 0.5 unit/kg of body weight being the usual initial dose.[14] Subsequent doses (0.25 to 0.5 unit/kilogram) are given to the ketotic child every four to six hours. When the child's condition is stabilized, the usual regimen of one or two insulin injections a day can be instituted.

The role of the nurse in caring for a child in this metabolic state is similar for that of the child in DKA: insulin therapy, vital signs, recording fluid intake and testing urine for glucose and ketones. However, this child is encouraged to eat and drink plenty of fluids. In addition, the child can be assisted in learning and performing parts of his care (e.g., urine fractionals). As the child begins to feel better, a more structured eductional program should be started.

Hyperglycemia In this state, abnormal amounts of glucose may be found in the blood and urine, but ketones are not present. Insulin requirements are usually 0.25 to 0.5 units/kg of body weight as an initial dose given in four equal doses.[14] The child may continue on his usual diabetic diet. The child is not "sick"; therefore, nursing care for the child with hyperglycemia focuses on activities of daily living. The child is encouraged to be up and about, exercise and take an active part in the educational program and ward activities.

Reaction of the Child and Family The diagnosis of diabetes can put an enormous strain on the family. It is imperative that the care of the child with insulin-dependent diabetes also include psychological and emotional support for the child and his family. In order for the family and child to learn about diabetes, they must be given time to adjust mentally to the diagnosis. Initially the parents may react with shock, disbelief and feelings of guilt. It is important to answer questions honestly, dispel old wives' tales, and to encourage the family and child to express their feelings and fears. The family needs to know that although the condition is not curable, treatment and a productive life are possible.

It is not unusual for parents to feel that it is their fault that the child got sick. Anger, fear, resentment and denial are normal reactions. Parents have to come to grips with their feelings before they can learn about the disease. Parents who do not adjust to the diagnosis may find it difficult to accept their child. They will grieve for the healthy child who formerly existed but who is now lost to them and may become overinvolved in activities such as work to avoid the child. Shame and embarrassment may lead to less involvement with friends or blaming the child for their own failures.[35]

The school-age child with diabetes often feels that he is being punished for some act. A child at this age may still have difficulty separating fact from fantasy. Frequently all he really understands about his disease is the pain and physical symptoms he feels. Play therapy can be a useful adjunct to help him work through his feelings and fears. The child wants to be like all other children, but the diabetes does make him different. There are injections to be taken, a routine to follow and he cannot always eat the refreshments at parties. The child must come to realize that diabetes is not in itself a barrier to a happy life. The child can still participate in most activities. Learning new routines will take time, and self-management is not always easy. The nurse, through education and emotional support, assists the family to accept the diagnosis and adjust to the changes.

Goals of Treatment The goals in treatment of the school-age child with diabetes are (1) metabolic control, (2) self-care through education and (3) normal growth and development with participation in age-appropriate activities. Strategies for meeting these goals should be individualized for each patient. These are long-term goals and need not be realized by the end of the hospitalization. This is an important point for both the family and health care professional to acknowledge. The amount and nature of information the child and family must assimilate can be frightening. They need time to understand the information and absorb its meaning for them.

Successful management of the school-age diabetic requires a comprehensive approach, incorporating several health care disciplines. Studies show that patients who are treated from the onset of diabetes by a multidisciplinary team adjust better to the requirements of treatment than those treated initially by a conventional approach.[21] Each member of the team is responsible for helping to identify educational needs of the family as well as contributing in their area of expertise. The nurse identifies educational needs, works on those appropriate to her discipline, serves as a liaison between medical personnel and the patient, and organizes the physical and psychological care given to the patient and his family. Those representing other disciplines that have a place on the team include the physician, the social worker, the dietician, the physical therapist and the psychologist. It is important to remember that the family is as important on the team as each health care practitioner, and it is essential to keep the lines of communication open among all team members.

Metabolic Control The main components of the diabetes treatment plan are insulin, diet and exercise. When the child's condition is newly diagnosed, the family needs a simple explanation of the basic facts. As time progresses, families are ready for more detail and self-management techniques. After a thorough assessment an individualized education plan is formulated.

TABLE 52-5 THE HOURS OF ACTION OF DIFFERENT INSULIN PREPARATIONS

Name/Type of Insulin	Onset	Peak	Duration
Short acting			
Regular	½–1°	2–4°	6–8°
Semilente	½–1°	2–4°	8–10°
Intermediate			
NPH	1–2°	6–8°	12–14°
Lente	1–2°	6–8°	14–16°
Long acting			
Ultralente	4–6°	8–12°	24–36°
PZI	4–6°	8–12°	36–72°

Insulin Most patients use insulin that is a beef and pork mixture. In cases of insulin resistance, allergy or religious preference, pure beef or pork insulin is available. In the past, insulin has been available in different strengths, such as U40 (40 units/cc), U80 and U100. Insulin to be used for treatment of these patients now is primarily available in U100 strength (100 u/cc). Semilente and crystalline zinc (regular) insulin are considered short-acting; lente and NPH, intermediate; and ultralente, long-acting. Table 52-5 describes the hours of action of each. Different types are often mixed in one syringe to allow for increased insulin action at various times.

Insulin that is being used daily can be stored at room temperature. Extra vials should be kept refrigerated, and freezing or exposure to heat should be avoided at all times. Insulin and syringes can be purchased at any pharmacy. In some states a prescription is not needed. Different sizes of U100 syringes are available. Most children find low-dose syringes easier to read.

Insulin is given like other subcutaneous injections. Cloudy insulins should be rolled gently between the hands to mix the insulin precipitate with the solution without creating bubbles. Air bubbles in the syringe should be removed, because they make the dose inaccurate. After the site is selected and prepared with alcohol, the skin is pinched up and the needle injected at a 90-degree angle. A 90-degree angle is recommended since insulin syringes have ⅝ inch to ½ inch needles, and this assures that the insulin is placed in the subcutaneous tissue. A short needle placed at a 45-degree angle usually propels the insulin into the intradermal region. If the needles being used are long and the patient has a great deal of fat he should be taught to inject at a 45-degree angle. Aspiration can be difficult for a child and is not required.

When mixing insulins, the rapid-acting insulin should be drawn up first. This is recommended to avoid confusion of dose at home and to decrease the incidence of rapid-acting insulin being contaminated with long-acting insulin.

Injections are given in the buttocks, the abdomen, the anterior and lateral aspect of the thighs and the lateral aspect of the arms. Young children find that keeping a record of sites with a body map is useful to avoid overuse of sites. When sites are overused, hypertrophy or localized atrophy of subcutaneous fat occurs. Avoiding hypertrophied areas usually results in gradual improvement. Monocomponent insulin, a highly purified extract, is sometimes injected directly into the atrophied areas. It is felt that this purified extract may stimulate the build-up of tissue and improve its appearance.

Diet Although dietary management is most commonly directed by a dietitian, it is important for all team members to be aware of the basic guidelines. The dietary intake should meet the following goals: (1) dietary intake must be adequate to ensure normal growth and development, (2) the diet distribution and food intake must aid in good metabolic control and (3) the diet should cause minimal changes in previous eating habits, life style or schedules.

These goals are achieved when the child follows an exchange type of meal plan as recommended by the American Diabetes Association and the American Dietetic Association. Foods are divided into groups: milk, bread, meat, vegetable, fruit and fat. Calories are distributed with approximately 50 per cent carbohydrate, 20 per cent protein and 30 per cent fat. The child usually has three meals and two to three snacks every day. Assessing the amount of food eaten before diagnosis is the best indicator of caloric need. The meal plan is then adjusted according to activity and food preferences.

Team members should continuously screen for diet problems. The child should not be separated from the rest of his family for meals, and the diet for the child with diabetes should fit the culture and life style of the family. The diet plan should be a guide to the family, not a strict regimen. Weighing and measuring are not necessary after the first few weeks. Whenever possible, the child should participate in diet planning.

Table 52–6 COMPARISON OF RESULTS USING 2-DROP CLINITEST, TESTAPE, AND KETODIASTIX

2-drop (gtt) Clinitest	0% Neg		Trace	½%	1%	2%	3%	5%
Testape	0% Neg	1/10% +	¼% ++	½% +++		2% ++++		
Ketodiastix	0% Neg	1/10% trace	¼% +	½% ++	1% +++	2% ++++		

Exercise In order to achieve adequate blood glucose control, children and parents must recognize the importance of the balance between energy expenditure (reflected by activity), energy availability (reflected by food intake), and insulin action (necessary for effective energy utilization).[33] Exercise increases energy expenditure and food requirements. After prolonged or strenuous exercise, the need for extra calories may last 24 to 38 hours.[33] Insulin seems more effective during exercise. Mobilization of insulin seems to be increased when the body part containing the injection site is exercised, causing blood insulin levels to increase more rapidly than without exercise. Glucose used rapidly after exercise replenishes glucogen stores. Extra calories should be taken before, during and after exercise to prevent hypoglycemia.

Although exercising of muscles seems to utilize glucose more efficiently and lower the blood sugar, this is true only if a sufficient amount of insulin is present. Progressive hyperglycemia can result from exercise when blood glucose levels are above 300 mg/dl and some ketosis is present.

Regular exercise at the same time daily is the most beneficial for blood glucose control. This is not always feasible for children, whose activity is often erratic. Therefore, families must be helped to understand how to maintain the balance between insulin, diet and exercise.

Urine In order to monitor the balance between insulin, diet and exercise, urine testing for glucose and ketones is recommended. However, since the urine may have been in the bladder for some time before the child voids a specimen, testing may not always correlate with blood glucose levels. For this reason urine tests should be one of many indicators evaluated when determining blood glucose levels.

There are many methods for qualitative urine testing for glucose and ketones (Table 52–6). The two-drop Clinitest method is recommended for children who tend to "spill" (excrete) large amounts of glucose. The corresponding color chart measures up to 5 per cent glucose. This is not to be confused with the five-drop Clinitest method, which uses the same reagent tablets but has a different method and color chart. The five-drop method does not measure past 2 per cent glucose. Simplified methods for qualitative readings, such as Testape and Diastix, are available but do not measure glucose past 2 per cent. Qualitative methods such as Clinistix are not recommended for measuring urine glucose. A plastic strip with a reagent area is recommended when testing urine for ketones. All urine testing supplies can be purchased at a pharmacy without a prescription.

Urine should be routinely tested for glucose before meals and at bedtime. During school, a lunchtime test can be awkward or embarrassing and is often skipped. Testing for ketones should be done when glucose tests indicate 2 per cent or greater. If the child is not feeling well, testing for glucose and ketones should be done at each voiding.

There are several ways to collect urine for testing. Testing a fresh voided specimen is most commonly recommended. Some authorities believe that a second voided (also called double-voided) specimen is more accurate. In this method the first sample is discarded and a second sample, taken 20 to 30 minutes later, is tested. However, requiring a child to urinate that frequently can often cause family stress and results in no urine testing at all; therefore the fresh voided specimen approach is recommended with children.

Testing materials can become inaccurate. To determine reliability the product should be checked to see that the expiration date shown on the label has not been exceeded, then its performance should be checked against materials that are known to give positive results. For glucose-testing materials, a sugar-containing beverage is used in place of urine. For ketone-testing materials, nail polish remover containing acetate is used. All results should be grossly positive. With any testing method used the directions should be followed exactly. All materials must be protected from excess light and moisture. They should never be refrigerated, and bottle caps should be kept tight.

All urine tests must be recorded on a chart. The records can be one indicator of blood glucose control for the family and can be reviewed at clinic visits. Quantitative urine collection is also a useful indicator of control. This is when all urine is collected over a period of time such as 6 hours or 24 hours and stored in a jug. The results describe how many grams of glucose are eliminated during a 24-hour period. Ideally, children should spill less than 10 per cent of their total caloric intake.

Education For Self-Care Although parents of young diabetic children have overall responsibility for management of care, the child can assist in his own care. Taking even small responsibility, e.g., wiping the top of the insulin vials, can increase the child's confidence and pride. When nurses promote and educate parents to expect self-care by the child, they assist in decreasing parental control. This increases independence before adolescence, when promoting of self-care is more likely to create stress between parents and children. To determine which self-care elements a child can handle, it is necessary to assess his ability to read, problem solve, count, follow directions and manipulate equipment. It is important to teach a child those skills that he can master so that he can succeed. A short list of self-care tasks may be gradually expanded until the child can manage independently. For example, a 5-year-old may find it difficult to manipulate a syringe, but he can clean the injection site. As the child develops, he can gradually assume more responsibility. Table 52–7 shows one way expectations can be set for children. When a child completes the first list, he moves on to the next.

Establishing self-care can be difficult for some children. In this case, a psychosocial assessment can help identify the reason for the difficulty. Does the family have difficulty with adjustment? Do parents promote dependency? Once the family members discuss the cause of the problem, they can often develop an approach that encourages self-care.

Behavior modification can be helpful. Simple contracts between parents and the child may encourage behavior changes. The child can also earn points for set tasks and spend them on predetermined rewards. All approaches require an agreement between both parties. Close follow-up by the nurse affords support and assistance to the family to make changes as they are needed.

Self-Management Self-management means that the family is able to alter insulin, diet and exercise independently as needed. Families must be able to analyze diabetes records and make needed adjustments. When the insulin

---

TABLE 52–7 AN EXAMPLE OF GRADUAL PROGRESSION IN SELF-CARE SKILLS

LIST 1

I, _____ , must be able to perform the following activities before going home:

- _____ State how I feel when I am hypoglycemic (low blood sugar).
- _____ State what to take for hypoglycemia (low blood sugar).
- _____ Be able to test my urine for glucose (sugar).
- _____ Be able to test my urine for ketones.
- _____ State the frequency of my urine test and how to record it.
- _____ Be able to fill out my hospital menu using diet plan.
- _____ Wear an identification tag saying I have diabetes.
- _____ State that I can participate in activities with my friends.

LIST 2

I, _____ , must be able to perform the following activities before going home/or in _____ (time):

- _____ State how to prevent hypoglycemia.
- _____ State how I feel with hyperglycemia.
- _____ State what to do about hyperglycemia.
- _____ State effects of diet, insulin and exercise on blood glucose levels.
- _____ State action, name, and strength of my insulin.
- _____ Be able to draw up and give my insulin.
- _____ State that diabetes does effect my whole family.

dose is changed, records of the past two to three days should be reviewed. The urine tests should average less than 1 per cent without frequent hypoglycemic episodes. When tests are elevated, the appropriate insulin should be increased not more than 10 per cent.

In the case of illness, parents should maintain close observation and do (or have the child do) frequent urine tests for glucose and ketones to prevent ketoacidosis. Insulin administration must always be continued during illness. The amount can be determined by appetite, exercise and urine test results. For nausea or vomiting or both the usual meal plan must be exchanged for liquids and soft foods containing carbohydrates. During any illness, forcing fluids can lessen the chances of dehydration. When vomiting and ketosis persist, hospitalization for rehydration may be necessary.

When the child requires surgery, he may receive nothing by mouth for a period of time and receive an intravenous infusion of dextrose and water. During this time regular or fast-acting insulin is given subcutaneously every four to six hours. Adjustments are made according to blood sugars.

A sliding scale whereby an arbitrary amount of insulin is given for an arbitrary amount of urine glucose should not be used. This negates the emphasis on reviewing all components of treatment — insulin, diet and exercise — before changing the insulin dose.

Maintaining Normal Growth, Development and Activity A chronic illness not only causes physical symptoms and problems for a child but requires that a family deal with the illness on a daily basis. One of the hardest things for a child and family to do is to learn how to live with a chronic illness such as diabetes. Good control is essential but overemphasis of the diabetic regimen can restrict activity and the psychological development of the child. An environment in which the parents always tell the child what to do and constantly emphasize the restrictions will not provide flexibility for the child to learn self-management. The child may respond by taking very little responsibility or by becoming angry and demanding.

Behavior problems that arise in the school-age child are often related to anxiety, pain from the injection, monitoring urines, and the diet. Parents should be encouraged to remain flexible and not always demand perfect adherence. A relaxed routine that allows an opportunity for learning will provide security and acceptance. Family counselling to deal with diabetes and its treatment may be required if the relationship between the child and parents does not allow for metabolic control and age-appropriate development.

The school-age child may find it difficult to tell friends about the diabetes, fearing he will be teased. The child may also give false information about diet, urine glucose or social interactions to avoid criticism or to get extra attention.[17] Role playing, puppets and other such methods may assist the child in learning how to confront the world without always having adult intervention.

Mothers often do most of the diabetic management for the child and can resent the father for not becoming involved. Fathers and siblings should be included in education and follow-up care. Blame for causing or transmitting the disease is less likely to occur when the whole family understands and takes responsibility for management. Although the child with diabetes is the one who is physically affected, the siblings also require consideration. Siblings may exhibit somatic distress such as fatigue, irritability or restlessness to gain attention. The nurse can discuss with

The diabetic child should be taught those skills of self-care that he is emotionally, intellectually and developmentally able to master.

POTENTIAL STRESSES DURING SCHOOL-AGE YEARS: IRREVERSIBLE ALTERATIONS IN THE SCHOOL-AGE CHILD'S HEALTH STATUS

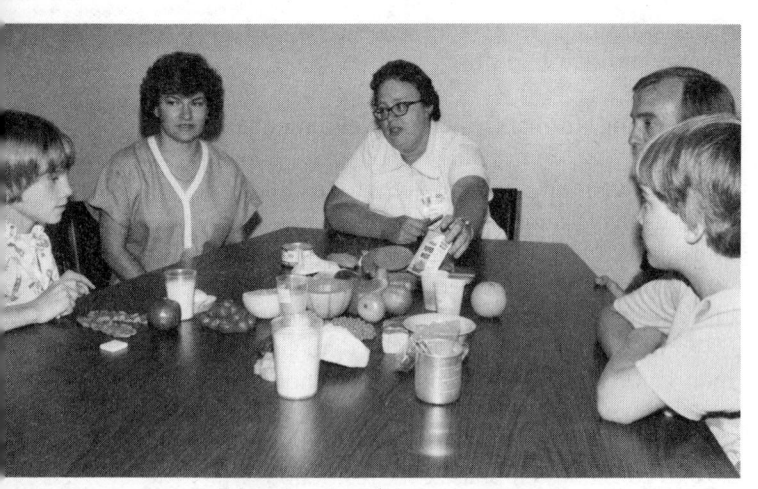

Education for diabetes management should include the whole family. Here the father and siblings as well as the mother and diabetic child learn about diet control.

the parents ways that the siblings can participate with the diabetic care. Explanations of normal sibling rivalry need to be reviewed as well as ideas given on how to reward the well sibling for his support and participation. It is appropriate for the nurse to spend time answering questions for the siblings and in assuring them that they had no part in causing the diabetes.[6]

Parents may find group discussions helpful because of the opportunity to talk with other parents of children with diabetes. The child may also enjoy seeing and talking with other children with diabetes. The American Diabetes Association (ADA) and the Juvenile Diabetes Foundation (JDF) are nonprofit organizations that sponsor activities such as workshops, group sessions and camps. The family needs to be informed of these organizations as well as other available community resources.

Living With Diabetes: Long-Term Care Only through continuous, ongoing health care can the child and his family receive supportive and preventive diabetic care. Follow-up care can be provided by an outpatient clinic, a private physician's office or a community health nurse. When a child is first diagnosed as having diabetes, he is usually scheduled for an appointment one to two weeks after discharge from the hospital, with community health nurse supervision in that interval. This gives the family time at home to experience living with diabetes. The first clinic visit must include opportunities for the family to ask questions and for the staff to review education and discuss family adjustments. Once the child and family feel comfortable with the diabetes, regular appointments may be scheduled about every three months. Even though the family is doing well, regular appointments are needed because the child is growing and family needs may change. Parameters to assess are height and weight for a determination of growth pattern, reflexes and sensation, and urine for glucose, ketones and protein. The nurse should observe the child giving insulin and testing urine and should assess his understanding of diabetes. Home records are useful in determining the family's ability to adjust the treatment plan and can be used for teaching. The nurse also must assess the child's history, dietary intake, adherence to treatment, and adjustment. Metabolic control is assessed by testing blood glucose levels, quantitative urines for glucose, and sometimes a glycosylated hemoglobin A_{Ic} (HbA_{Ic}) determination. Blood glucose levels do not give a complete picture as they indicate only one point in time, and the child's anxiety associated with drawing blood can elevate the levels. Urine tests give information about the amount of glucose excreted in one day. Studies are showing that measurement of a hemoglobin component (HbA_{Ic}) can be useful in documenting the degree of hyperglycemia during a two- to four-month span. HbA_{Ic} represents the accumulation of glucose that occurs in erythrocytes of all persons, normal or diabetic.[3] If blood glucose is high, HbA_{Ic} would be high. This determination gives information about glucose levels only during the life span of the erythrocytes.

Traveling or vacationing requires advanced planning. Insulin and meal adjustments are made when traveling in different time zones. When traveling by air, supplies and extra insulin should be carried on to the plane. Luggage can be lost or stored in varying temperatures. Airlines will usually serve a diabetic meal if notified in advance. Carrying a note from a physician or nurse may eliminate any questions at customs about insulin syringes. Extra food, sugar and supplies need to be carried in case transportation is delayed or the family is stranded or in the event that plans change. Before traveling to a foreign country with a different language, the family should learn to say or write key phrases such as "I have diabetes. I need to eat something sweet immediately."

Ketoacidosis Infection, nonadherence to management, emotional stress or inability to adjust to the disease can precipitate ketoacidosis. After the period of intensive care has passed, the nurse begins her assessment of the possible reasons that ketoacidosis developed to help prevent its recurrence. If lack of knowledge is identified, then teaching is needed throughout the period of hospitalization and a community nurse's referral may be needed for follow-up at home. Severe or chronic stress may be a factor when a child has frequent episodes of ketoacidosis. It has been suggested that the natural response to stress is the release of catecholamines, which simulates glyconeogenesis and may lead to hyperglycemia. Periodic assessments of family life and adjustment to diabetes may indicate that a child is having difficulty dealing with stressful situations. Individual or family counselling can be helpful in learning how to handle stress.

Hypoglycemia Besides understanding the etiology of low blood sugar, the child and family must know specific symptoms and how to treat hypoglycemia or insulin reaction. Most children are aware of oncoming insulin reaction. Hypoglycemia symptoms usually occur quickly and the child must either treat it himself or request help. The child should carry sugar cubes rather than candy, because children in particular may misuse candy. Teachers, bus drivers and other adults responsible for the child need to be alert for symptoms. It is advisable that fruit juice or sugar be available for emergencies. Even though some diabetic children can be manipulative, they should always be treated for symptoms of hypoglycemia. At the beginning of each school year the parents and child can meet with the appropriate personnel and review aspects of diabetes. With the family's permission, the nurse can also contact the school to provide information or suggestions.

Hypoglycemia symptoms reflect glucose deprivation in the brain. The area of the brain that has the greater oxygen consumption and need for glucose will be affected sooner by low blood glucose.[26] Table 52-8 describes the symptoms that arise from oxygen deprivation in various parts of the brain in the order in which they will be affected. The physiological response to lowering the blood sugar follows a pattern. First, the parasympathetic nervous system becomes excited and the child becomes hungry or nauseated. Then cerebral functions change, with the child yawning and being tired. As the sympathetic nervous system responds, the child may have an increase in pulse, respirations, blood pressure and sweat or may have tremors. These symptoms do not depend upon absolute blood glucose readings.

Whatever the level, if a child's circulating glucose has dropped sharply, he will need food to avoid the effects of an insulin reaction. The immediate treatment is ingestion of 10 grams of fast-acting carbohydrate. (See Table 52-9 for 10 gm carbohydrate equivalents.) After the child has responded to the fast-acting carbohydrate, a supplement of slowly digestible carbohydrate such as milk or bread should be eaten to help restore liver glycogen. If the symptoms do not disappear, the dosage of 10 grams of simple carbohydrate is repeated.

In severe cases, when a child cannot take oral glucose due to decreased consciousness, it is necessary to administer glucagon. Parents are given a prescription for the glucagon. It is stored in the refrigerator, requires mixing and needs to be checked periodically for expiration. Glucagon stimulates the glycogen-producing process within the liver. Because the effect of glucagon lasts only one hour and liver stores might be depleted, it is important that the child have some extra carbohydrate. If these measures do not work, intravenous glucose is required. For emergency use glucose products such as decorating icing in a tube can be squeezed into the mouth. The solution is absorbed through oral tissues and

TABLE 52-8 SYMPTOMS OF OXYGEN DEPRIVATION IN VARIOUS PARTS OF THE BRAIN

Areas of the Brain	Symptoms
Forebrain	Somnolence, perspiration, hypotomia, tremor
Thalamus	Restlessness, loss of consciousness, tachycardia
Midbrain	Tonic spasms, Babinski sign, inconjugate occular deviation
Hindbrain	Coma, shallow respirations, hypothermia, no pupillary reaction to light

TABLE 52-9 TEN-GRAM CARBOHYDRATE EQUIVALENTS

4 oz orange juice
2 tsp corn syrup or honey
2 tsp grape jelly
5 Lifesavers
4 animal crackers

POTENTIAL STRESSES DURING SCHOOL-AGE YEARS: IRREVERSIBLE ALTERATIONS IN THE SCHOOL-AGE CHILD'S HEALTH STATUS

swallowed by reflex. The best treatment for hypoglycemia is preventive. Mealtimes must remain regular. If a meal is delayed, a snack should be given. Frequent episodes of hypoglycemia need to be evaluated by the health team. Because changes in blood glucose cannot always be predicted, children of all ages must wear a bracelet or necklace identifying them as having diabetes. These can be purchased at drug stores, jewelers or from the Medic-Alert Foundation.*

Somogyi Effect A child who is requiring more and more insulin without a decrease in urine glucose may be exhibiting the Somogyi effect. This phenomenon is caused by an excess of insulin resulting in hypoglycemia followed by hyperglycemia and ketonuria. Unnoticed insulin reactions occur during early morning or late evening. The low blood glucose triggers a release of catecholamines, which raises the blood glucose and stimulates ketonuria. This rise in blood sugar is often treated with more insulin, when in reality less insulin is required to avoid the initial hypoglycemia reaction. The nurse needs to carefully question the child and parents for subtle symptoms of hypoglycemia such as morning headaches, night sweats and nightmares.[19]

Complications Diabetes mellitus is a chronic illness with the potential for long-term complications. In an attempt to achieve metabolic control, some patients are using Chemstrips or Dextrostix with reflectometers† at home to determine actual blood glucose. This permits them to adjust insulin based on blood glucose in addition to urine glucose.

Various infusion pumps have been tested in the attempt to develop an insulin delivery system that approximates the control of the blood glucose by the pancreas. Presently these pumps deliver a specific amount of insulin determined by individual metabolic tests. These devices are worn externally and require the person to deliver insulin manually at meals and other specific times. This device relies on patient adherence and does not seem to be any more convenient than injections are. Ongoing research involves internal closed loop devices that could be programed to deliver varied amounts of insulin through the day in response to food and exercise. This would eliminate the need for injections.

Even though there is some evidence that metabolic control will prevent or delay complications, a child should not be told that he will have no problems if he follows all the rules. Degenerative changes appear in young adults who have had diabetes for 10 to 20 years. Statistics recently compiled indicate that after 20 years of having diabetes there is a 40 to 50 per cent incidence of retinopathy and nephropathy[34]

Background retinopathy involves the small vessels of the retina which weaken and hemorrhage. Proliferative retinopathy has progressed to the surface of the retina, resulting in hemorrhages into the vitreous that can lead to blindness. Diabetic nephropathy is a thickening of the glomeruli membranes that results in kidney disease. Proteinuria, elevated blood pressure and dependent edema are indications of decreasing kidney function. The possibility of arteriosclerosis is increased in diabetic patients and can interfere with circulation in the heart, brain and extremities. Obesity, cigarette smoking, high blood pressure and elevated blood cholesterol contribute to the development of arteriosclerosis.

Peripheral neuropathy is common, resulting in tingling, decreased sensation and reflex changes. Autonomic neuropathy is less common but can result in diarrhea, incontinence, impotency and changes in heart rate and blood pressure.

Factual information about complications needs to be given to the family so that they understand the need for continued health care. Complications should not be used as a threat to improve adherence to the treatment plan. A balance between insulin, diet, and exercise provides metabolic control and has the potential to delay complications. The health care team can help the child and family to achieve this goal. The family and the child need to be alert to body system changes so that they can report them to the health care team. A young child usually is not interested in details and facts about complications but he does have some fears and misconceptions or knows someone who has diabetes complications. The nurse needs to provide opportunities to discuss fears and then provide honest and factual informa-

---

*Medic-Alert Foundation, International, Turlock, CA 95380.

†A device that indicates the exact amount of blood glucose on a dip stick.

tion. If the child fears criticism from the nurse when he shares his problems and mistakes, he will be reluctant to inform the nurse about changes in his body. Diabetes does not have to be a barrier to a happy childhood, adolescence or adult life but it does take continuous care, education and support. A nurse should never promise a child a normal life with diabetes; rather she should assure him that he can be helped to live with his diabetes.

JUVENILE RHEUMATOID ARTHRITIS

by Anne Hartson, BS, MSN

Juvenile rheumatoid arthritis (JRA) is a term used to describe a group of diseases that affect the joints, connective tissue and viscera. Children can have any of three types of JRA: polyarticular (involvement of multiple joints), Still's disease (systemic JRA), and pauciarticular (involvement of one to five joints). Although this disease is sometimes reversible, more often it is chronic, persisting for many years with periods of remission and exacerbation.

JRA is characterized by chronic synovitis that may result in loss of motion in the involved joints. Joint involvement is caused by an inflammatory process whereby the synovial tissue becomes edematous and hyperemic. Swelling in the affected joints is a result of an increase in synovial fluid and thickening of tissues. The enlarged synovial tissue adheres to the articular cartilage; destruction of cartilage may occur with continued synovitis.

The etiology of JRA is not known, although bacterial and viral infections have been hypothesized.[12] Other investigators believe that a hypersensitivity reaction may be involved.[31]

Prevention of JRA is impossible, although there is a relationship between periods of stress and exacerbations of the disease.[12] The nurse can assist parents in understanding the etiology of the disease because many parents feel responsible for not having taken some action to prevent the illness.

The Differential Diagnosis

The diagnosis of JRA is difficult and the child's condition often remains undiagnosed for a long period of time. Any child presenting with joint swelling requires a complete examination immediately. Physical examination includes assessment of the joints for redness, warmth, swelling, tenderness, limited motion, muscle atrophy and contractures. Assessing for lymphadenopathy, splenomegaly and hepatomegaly is also essential, because the degree of involvement varies according to the type of JRA.

There may be ocular involvement in the pauciarticular type of JRA. If left undetected and not treated, this involvement may result in iridocyclitis and eventual blindness. An ophthalmological examination should be included during the diagnostic period.

A history of recent infections, fever, weight loss, anorexia and decreased general activity contributes to the diagnosis of JRA. Other specific diagnostic criteria are included in the discussions of the three types of JRA.

Polyarticular JRA Up to 40 per cent of children afflicted with JRA have the polyarticular type. Girls are affected twice as often as boys and the onset peaks at 1 to 2 years of age and again at 8 to 10.[20] Symmetrical large joints of the knees, wrists and ankles as well as the small finger joints will appear swollen and tender from the inflammatory process. Parents may first notice a problem when their child has difficulty getting out of bed in the morning. He may need to help to get up, or he may learn to slide out of bed. The mild to moderate pain and stiffness will dissipate as he goes about his normal activities during the day. A daily temperature elevation manifesting a low-grade fever may or may not be noted.

A nursing assessment may reveal a history of weight loss and vague complains of malaise and anorexia. Lymphadenopathy is present in approximately 40 per cent of children and a few may have splenomegaly and hepatomegaly.[20] Subcutaneous nodules may be present on the finger joints, elbows and heels.

POTENTIAL STRESSES DURING SCHOOL-AGE YEARS: IRREVERSIBLE ALTERATIONS IN THE SCHOOL-AGE CHILD'S HEALTH STATUS

Laboratory tests are not very useful in the diagnosis of JRA. Children with the polyarticular type may have a mild anemia associated with the chronic disease. Specific serologic tests for the presence of the rheumatoid factor are usually not helpful; however, a positive test may be obtained with this type.[20]

Still's Disease Systemic JRA is most common in children less than 5 years of age, with boys affected slightly more frequently than girls.[10] The child feels very ill during the acute stage but, excepting for the fever, is generally well. The acute onset begins with daily temperature spikes of 102° or above followed by a rapid return to normal. The child will often have a recurring rheumatoid rash with the fever (erythematous macules on the trunk, arms, face and lower extremities) for several months or years.[10, 12] Arthritic symptoms may be present at onset, and the majority of children develop arthritis within six months. These children may show signs of morning stiffness by holding their extremities partially flexed when lying or moving.

Upon examination, the child's liver and lymph nodes (axilla and groin) are enlarged. Splenomegaly may be present but is usually not extensive. Cardiac involvement, usually a mild pericarditis without dyspnea or pain, occurs in about 10 per cent of children with the systemic type of JRA. Laboratory test findings include neutrophilic leukocytosis (WBC of 15,000 to 50,000 mm^3), anemia, and an elevated erythrocyte sedimentation rate.[10]

Pauciarticular JRA Children with pauciarticular JRA usually appear well and have only mild systemic signs of a low-grade fever or malaise. This type occurs in 40 to 50 per cent of children with JRA. Onset peaks in children from 1 to 4 years of age but can occur any time from 6 months to 15 years of age.[22] Joint involvement is usually insidious, with the child experiencing pain, swelling, and decreased motion in the large weight-bearing joints. The knee is the most frequently affected, with involvement of the ankle and hip following. Hip involvement may indicate a tendency for the disease to progress to the polyarticular type.[22] Ocular involvement is most common in children with an onset at a young age (1 to 4 years) and is most typically a chronic, progressive iridocyclitis. A mild anemia and a normal or slightly elevated white blood count are commonly present.

Because the diagnosis is so dependent on the clinical signs and history, an accurate diagnosis can be made only after eliminating other inflammatory diseases and assessing for joint involvement. Feelings of anger, frustration, and guilt on the part of the parents may persist during the long diagnostic period. Most parents are not acquainted with arthritis in children and will envision a permanent deformity or disability. Others may be angry with their physician or feel guilty for not having sought medical attention earlier.

Nurse's Role During Course of Treatment

Nurses can help parents cope with their child's disease by giving repeated thorough explanations of the disease and being available to talk about specific concerns. The child will also need an explanation of why his joints are swollen and difficult to move. School-age children may feel that the illness is a punishment for a wrongdoing. These feelings must be explored and dealt with, for the child is usually faced with an irreversible disease. Helping the child adjust to the diagnosis is an ongoing process that is enhanced by involvement of school personnel.

Hospitalization is necessary during the acute stage and exacerbations of the disease. The goal of treatment is to return the child to his normal activity as soon as possible by maintaining joint function. This necessitates a team approach that actively involves the child and his parents.

Salicylates are the most effective medication used in controlling the inflammatory process. ASA given every six hours will maintain therapeutic blood levels (a blood salicylate level of 20 to 30 mg). To prevent gastric disturbances, enteric-coated salicylates should be used or the medication should be given with food. Maintaining the child on long-term salicylate therapy necessitates close monitoring for signs of toxicity. Parents and child should be instructed to observe for respiratory difficulty, unusual drowsiness or CNS disturbances.

If no relief is obtained after a trial period of six weeks, other drugs, including ibuprofen (Motrin) and indomethacin, may be used. Gold salts are occasionally used in treating children with JRA. Although gold therapy has been effective, it requires a great deal of patient cooperation. The injections are given weekly or biweekly with extensive laboratory tests required before each treatment to check for toxicity.[12, 31]

Use of corticosteroids is controversial because, although a marked improvement is obtained, the side effects of long-term usage are very serious. Steroids are appropriate for the child with systemic JRA who fails to respond to other drugs, is acutely ill with cardiac problems, or has iridocyclitis.[12, 31] Steroids should be discontinued as soon as possible.

Physical therapy is a major aspect of the child's treatment. Even the acutely ill child will need ongoing therapy to maintain joint range of motion (ROM). Treatments may include whirlpool baths, active and passive ROM exercises, and paraffin soaks or moist heat applications to the involved joints. These help in maintaining joint motion and muscle strength. Encouraging the child to assist in self-care activities such as bathing, tooth brushing, or hair combing is an easy method of actively exercising the upper extremities and promoting independence. Table games, television viewing or reading may be effective distractors for the uncooperative child during exercise periods.

It is imperative that proper body alignment be maintained at all times; otherwise, the child with arthritic pain will assume the position he finds most comfortable, that is, flexion. A firm mattress and sandbags to hold the hips in a neutral position will aid in preventing hip and knee joint flexion. Children with cervical spine involvement should use only a very flat pillow to prevent a permanent forward position of the head.

Various splints may be needed during the course of the disease to decrease inflammation, contractures and ankylosis. Types of splints include: (1) *resting* splints that immobilize the inflamed joints, (2) *functional* splints that immobilize only the affected joint and allow distal movement, and (3) *corrective* splints that are used only after the acute stage if joints are deformed.[7]

Before discharge a home visit should be made to assess modifications needed to promote the child's independence at home. An elevated toilet seat, clothing that is easily fastened, and a wheelchair shower will allow the child to resume some normal activities without help.

Direct contact with the school nurse and the child's teacher should be included in discharge planning. School desk modifications may be needed and arrangements should be made for daily exercises at school. Classmates should be prepared with an explanation of the disease and the importance of including the child in as many activities as possible. Most children in remission can participate in all activities except contact sports; swimming is especially beneficial.

Irreversible illnesses are expensive in terms of time and money. Repeated hospitalizations, drug therapy, special equipment and the exercise regimen place much stress on the entire family. The social worker or community health nurse may be able to obtain adaptive equipment (wheelchair, braces) from state Crippled Children's Services or the National Easter Seal Society For Crippled Children and Adults.

Parents will need ongoing counselling with the nurse or social worker to avoid overprotecting the child and neglecting other children. Siblings should be included in the discharge planning and ongoing counselling, for they must also learn to cope with a disruption in their lives.

Most arthritic children will benefit from contact with other children with the disease. This is an especially effective method of helping the child learn to deal with body image changes, pain and recurrent interruptions in activity. Continuous counselling may be necessary, and this should be provided by someone with whom the child has developed a good relationship.

To promote a healthy adjustment to the disease, the child must be treated as normally as possible; otherwise, he will feel different and handicapped. If the child is old enough, he should be given some responsibility for taking medications and following through with the exercises. This will promote his cooperation and independence, both of which are very necessary for this long-term condition.

The prognosis for JRA varies, depending on the type and on the degree of functional disability. Children with Still's disease may develop chronic polyarthritis and disability; however, the prognosis is usually good. The course of polyarticular JRA varies and the child may have no exacerbations; 30 per cent will still have the disease 15 years after the onset. Children with pauciarticular JRA usually have no disability, although the disease has many periods of remission and exacerbation. This type may progress to polyarticular JRA. Each of the types has the potential for joint deformity and growth disturbances, thus it is essential to continue medication and exercises until the physician discontinues treatment. It may be necessary to have reconstructive surgery for severe joint deformities. Ongoing slit eye examination are essential to detect iridocyclitis, which may develop years after the onset. Mortality rates are low and usually result from infections during long-term steroid therapy.[12]

References

1. M. Brenton. Mainstreaming. Today's Education, Mar/Apr 1976
2. H. Bruen. The dyslexic child. Pediatric Annals, February 1977. p. 129
3. R. Cole. The significance of hemoglobin A$_{1c}$ in diabetes mellitus. Upjohn, 1978
4. Conversion to U100. Diabetes Forecast, Jan/Feb 1979, p. 27
5. B. Conway. Pediatric Neurologic Nursing. C. V. Mosby Co., 1977.
6. M. Croft. Help for the family's neglected other children, American Journal of Maternal Child Nursing, Sept/Oct 1979, p. 297
7. W. Donavan. Physical measures in the treatment of JRA. In Juvenile Rheumatoid Arthritis, J. Miller, III. PSG Publishing Co., Inc., 1969
8. Fisher, Koch and Donnell. Comparison of mental development in individuals with mosaicism and Trisomy 21 Down's syndrome, Pediatrics, November 1976
9. S. Genuth. Constant intravenous insulin infusion in diabetic ketoacidosis. Journal of the American Medical Association, 19 March 1973, p. 1348
10. L. Gorin. Stills' disease: systemic juvenile rheumatoid arthritis. In Juvenile Rheumatoid Arthritis, J Miller III, PSG Publishing Co., Inc., 1969
11. M. Gross. Growth of hyperkinetic children taking Methylphendrate, Dextroamphetamine or Imipram Neodexipramine. Pediatric Annals, September 1976
12. B. Grossman. Juvenile rheumatoid arthritis. Current Problems in Pediatrics, October 1975, p. 3
13. D. Guthrie and R. Guthrie. DKA: breaking a vicious cycle. In Managing Diabetes Properly, P. Chaney, ed. Intermed Communication, Inc., 1977
14. D. Guthrie and R. Guthrie. Nursing Management of Diabetes Mellitus. C. V. Mosby Co., 1977
15. A. Guyton. Textbook of Medical Physiology. W. B. Saunders Co., 1976
16. W. Hung et al. Pediatric Endocrinology. Medical Examination Publishing Co., 1978
17. R. Jackson and R. Guthrie. The Child with Diabetes Mellitus. Upjohn, 1975
18. M. Kasman. Evaluation of a new antidiuretic agent, desmopressin acetate (DDAUP). Journal of the American Medical Association, 20 October 1978, p. 1896
19. M. Keyes. The Somogyi phenomenon in insulin-dependent diabetics. Nursing Clinics of North America, Sept 1977, p. 439
20. D. Kredich. Polyarticular juvenile rheumatoid arthritis. In Juvenile Rheumatoid Arthritis, J. Miller III, PSG Publishing Co., Inc. 1969
21. Z. Laron et al. A multidisciplinary comprehensive ambulatory scheme for diabetes mellitus in children. Diabetes Care, Jul/Aug, 1979, p. 342
22. C. Lindsley. Pauciarticular juvenile rheumatoid arthritis. In Juvenile Rheumatoid Arthritis, J. Miller III, PSG Publishing Co., Inc., 1969
23. D. Marlow. Textbook of Pediatric Nursing. W. B. Saunders Co., 1977
24. J. McFarlane. Diabetes insipidus. Pediatric Nursing, Nov/Dec 1975, p. 6
25. M. Olson. Minimal cerebral dysfunction: the child referred for school-related problems. Pediatric Annals, Aug 1975, p. 69
26. J. Petrokas. Explaining axioms for sick days. In Managing Diabetes Properly, Intermed Communication Inc., 1977
27. President's Committee on Mental Retardation. White House Conference on Handicapped Individuals, U.S. Government Printing Office, Volume 5, 1975
28. E. Ritva. Autism: Diagnosis, Current Research and Management. Spectrum Publications, 1976
29. A. Rudolph, ed. Pediatrics. Appleton-Century-Crofts, 1977
30. W. Segar. Primary disturbance of water homeostasis. In Pediatrics, A. Rudolph, ed. Appleton-Century-Crofts, 1977
31. J. Schaller and R. Wedgewood. Rheumatic diseases. In Nelson Textbook of Pediatrics, V. Vaughan et al., W. B. Saunders Co., 1979
32. T. Shetty. Some neurologic, electrophysiologic and biologic correlates of the hyperkinetic syndrome. Pediatrics Annals, May 1973
33. J. Skyler. Diabetes and exercise: clinical implications. Diabetes Care, May/June 1979, p. 307
34. M. Sperling. Diabetes mellitus. Pediatric Clinics of North America, February 1979, p. 149
35. P. Steinhauer et al. Psychological aspects of chronic illness. Pediatric Clinics of North America, Nov 1974, p. 825
36. P. Wender. Minimal brain dysfunction in children: diagnosis and treatment. Pediatric Clinics of North America, February 1973, p. 187

Additional Recommended Reading

Assistance to States for Education of Handicapped Persons. Office of Education; Health, Education and Welfare, Pamphlet No. 250, 1977

G. Bacon et al. A Practical Approach to Pediatric Endocrinology. Yearbook Medical Publishers Inc., 1975

A. Baden. Children with arthritis: some everyday help. Nursing '73, December 1973, p. 22

C. Banion and L. Ling. The child with diabetes. Comprehensive Pediatric Nursing, September 1978, p. 21

R. Bauer and T. Kenny. Psychological management of juvenile diabetes. Pediatric Annals, June 1975, p. 72

D. Blevins. The Diabetic and Nursing Care. McGraw-Hill Book Co., 1979

A. Bloom. Diabetes Explained. Medical and Technical Publishing Co., 1975

M. Briya and R. Bolin. Epilepsy, a controllable disease. American Journal of Nursing, March 1976, p. 388

L. Buscaglia. The Disabled and Their Parents: A Counseling Challenge. Charles B. Slack, Inc., 1975

P. Chinn. Child Health Maintenance. C. V. Mosby Co., 1979

B. Collier and D. Etzwiler. Comparative study of diabetes knowledge among juvenile diabetics and their parents. Diabetes, January 1971, p. 51

E. Crosby. Childhood diabetes: the emotional adjustments of parents and child. Canadian Nurse, September 1977, p. 20

A. Damasio and R. Mauer. A neurological model for childhood autism. Archives of Neurology, December 1978, p. 777

F. Dubowski. Children with osteogenesis imperfecta. Nursing Clinics of North America, December 1976, p. 709

R. Ehrlich. Diabetes mellitus in childhood. Pediatric Clinics of North America, November 1974, p. 871

B. Forman et al. Management of juvenile diabetes mellitus: usefulness of 24-hour fractional quantitative urine glucose. Pediatrics. February 1974, p. 257

D. Guthrie. Diabetic children: preparing them to live. In Managing Diabetes Properly, Intermed Communications Inc., 1977

D. Guthrie. Exercise, diet and insulin for children with diabetes. Nursing '77, Feb. 1977, p. 48

D. Guthrie and R. Guthrie. Juvenile diabetes mellitus. Pediatric Clinics of North America, December 1973, p. 587

R. Kaufman and B. Hersher. Body image changes in teenage diabetics. Pediatrics, July 1971, p. 123

C. Kennel. Outpatient management of the juvenile diabetic. Pediatric Nursing, Nov/Dec 1976, p. 19

D. Kiser. The somogyi effect. American Journal of Nursing, February 1980, p. 236

B. Lawson. Chronic illness in the school-aged child: effects on the total family. Maternal Child Nursing, Jan/Feb 1977, p. 49

G. Lipkin and R. Cole. Effective Approaches to Patients' Behavior. Springer Publishing Co., 1973

H. Love. The Mentally Retarded Child and His Family. Charles C Thomas Publishing, 1971

J. McFarlane. The child with diabetes mellitus. Pediatric Nursing, Sept/Oct 1975, p. 6

J. Moens. Coping with diabetes insipidus. The Canadian Nurse, April 1979, p. 18

T. Pendleton and B. Grossman. Rehabilitation of children with inflammatory joint disease. American Journal of Nursing, December 1974, p. 2223

J. Petrokas. Explaining axioms for sick days. In Managing Diabetes Properly. Intermed Communication Inc., 1977

G. Prazer and M. Felice. The psychological and social effects of juvenile diabetes. Pediatric Annals, June 1975, p. 59

M. Roberts and M. Canfield. Behavior modification with a mentally retarded child. American Journal of Nursing, April 1980, p. 679

J. Scholler. Arthritis and infections of bones and joints in children. Pediatric Clinics of North America, November 1977, p. 4

D. Schumann. Insulin reactions: Fighting Fear and Fact. In Managing Diabetes Properly, P. Chaney, ed. Intermed Communications Inc., 1977

J. Simmonds. Psychiatric status of diabetic youth matched with a control group. Diabetes, October 1977, p. 921

O. Simpson and M. Smith. Lightening the load for parents of children with diabetes. Journal of Maternal Child Nursing, Sept/Oct 1979, p. 293

R. Thompson. The management of diabetes mellitus in the adolescent. Medical Clinics of North America, November 1979, p. 1349

V. Vaughan, Nelson et al. Textbook of Pediatrics, 11th ed. W. B. Saunders Co., 1979

Additional Resources and Information

Ames Division, Miles Laboratories, 1127 Myrtle St, Elkhart, Ind. Brochures and information on diabetes.

American Diabetes Association, Inc., 18 E. 48th St., New York, N.Y.

Association for Children with Learning Disabilities, 5225 Grace St., Pittsburgh, Pa.

Diabetes in the News, 3553 W. Peterson Avenue, Chicago, Ill. Free newspaper subscription.

Epilepsy Foundation of America, Washington Office, 1419 H St., N.W., Washington, D.C.

Eli Lilly and Company, Indianapolis, Ind. Information on diabetes.

National Association for Retarded Citizens, 2709 Avenue East, Arlington, Tex.

National Easter Seal Society for Crippled Children and Adults, 2023 W. Ogden Ave. Chicago, Ill.

National Epilepsy League, Inc., 203 N. Wabash Ave., Chicago, Ill.

National Society for Autistic Citizens, 169 Tampa Ave., Albany, N.Y.

President's Committee on Mental Retardation, Washington, D.C.

United Cerebral Palsy Association, 66 E. 35th St. New York, N.Y.

53 POTENTIAL STRESSES DURING SCHOOL-AGE YEARS: LIFE-THREATENING ALTERATIONS IN HEALTH STATUS

by Marcia N. Sheets, RN, MSN
and Anita L. Spietz, RN, MSN

HOW THE SCHOOL-AGE CHILD PERCEIVES DEATH

The school-age child's intellectual skills are developed by observation and by the frequent use of trial-and-error learning. He constantly and progressively reorganizes ideas. The school-age child develops and reorganizes his concept of death as he has exposure to death and as he examines dead things. The dead fly on the window sill, the dead plant, the squashed bug, the dead dog that was hit by a car in the road, the dead bird, the goldfish floating on its side at the top of a fish tank in the classroom are all stimulants for questions about death. He moves gradually from understanding death as a reversible, temporary phenomenon to one of irreversibility and permanency. While cartoons, stories and movies constantly fantasize the powers of their hero or heroine to survive life-threatening episodes, the school-age child also may have experiences with "real death." The child may experience the death of a pet or a grandparent; this may cause him to re-examine his ideas about the permanence of death.

The child in early school age may evidence a concept of death that contains components of both the "preoperational" and "concrete" phases of development. For example, to the chagrin of the mourning parents, he may expect his dead grandfather to join the family at the dinner table, while at the same time he may know that his dead pet dog will not return for *his* evening meal.

Those who have studied the school-age child's concept of death have observed that he deals with ideas about the *process* of death and dying, the *causes* of death and dying, and the *occurrence* of death.[1, 2, 6, 8, 11, 15, 20, 21]

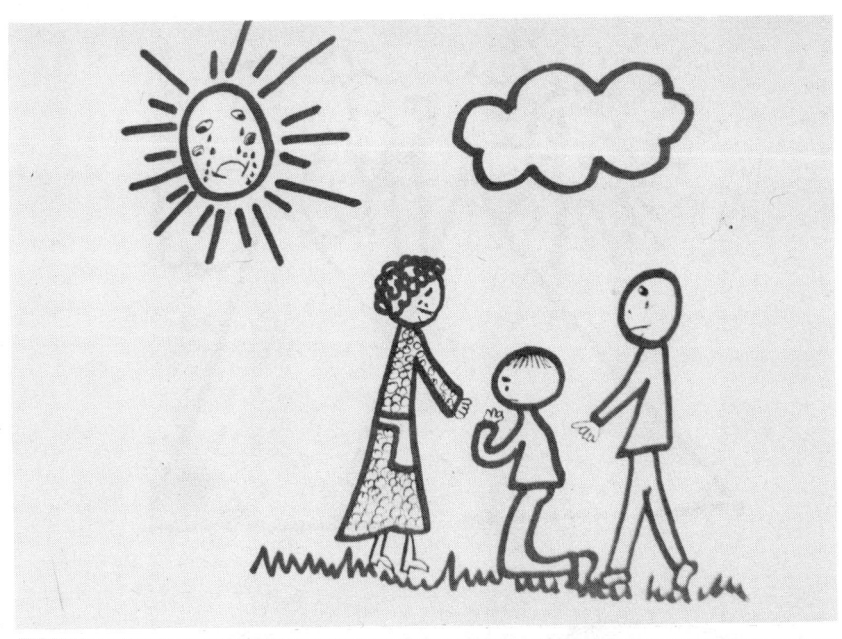

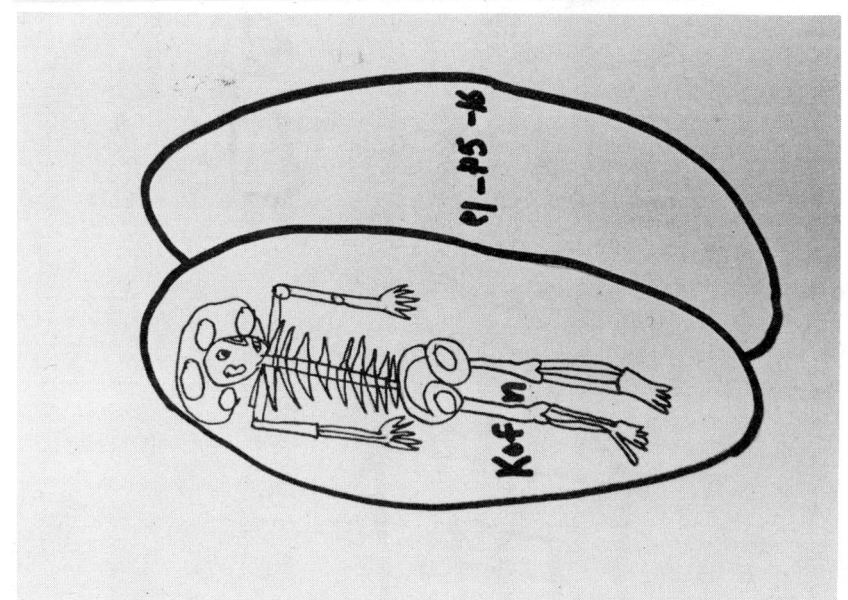

A, "A little boy dying on his front lawn—his mother and father are watching over him. They are sad. The sun is sad, too." *B,* "This is somebody dead." The school-age child is intrigued with the process of dying and with death. The two pictures illustrate a school-age child's concept of death.

Process and Occurrence of Death

The school-age child is intrigued by the process of dying and of death. He may examine dead animals, watch a dying worm, save something that has died or even dig up something that is dead to re-examine it. He draws pictures of dead people with emotions reflected in their faces. The dead person may not be able to move but he can still feel and think. Often pictures of skeletons replace pictures of the dead person. As the child matures, he begins to view death as something "seasonal" or "cyclic" in nature, a part of the natural order of the universe.

The school-age child is interested in observing "who death happens to." By this age the child has possibly been exposed to the death of a pet or to the death of a grandparent. His logical conclusion, then, is that death happens to old people and animals. He seldom thinks that death happens to children his own age or that

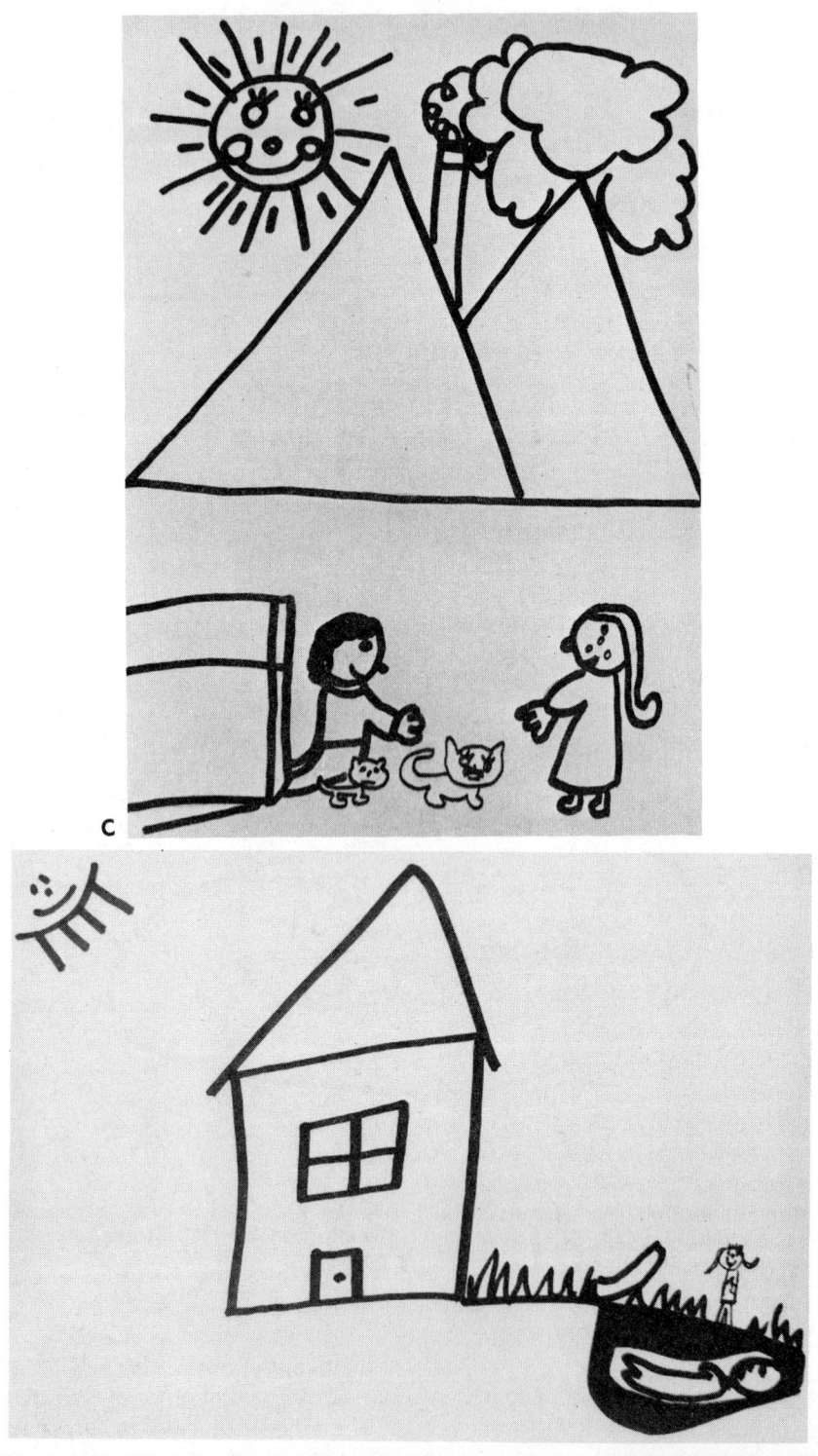

C, "This is when my kitten died. Mrs. Jones from next door came over to help the cat have her babies and I was sick that day. The baby kittens died because the mother cat had an infection in her tummy and if we didn't take her to the doctor she would have died." *D*, "The little girl was digging a hole with her shovel and she buried her grandpa and she's first praying and then she's going back to her house. She's supposed to be kneeling." The school-age child concludes from his experience that death comes to animals and old people.

death will ever come to him. As the child matures, he begins to realize that death can occur in younger people, and perhaps it does in a school-mate, friend or sibling. Gradually most school-age children realize that death is universal and that every living thing will eventually die, including his parents and himself. This may not become clear to some children, however, until adolescence.

Causes of Death

The school-age child's perception of the causes of death may include accidental death, violence, overeating or undereating, sickness or pain. Magical thinking is operative in the early school-age child, so that he may believe that he can cause someone's death just by wishing it or thinking about it. "I wish you were dead!" spoken in anger to a sibling who later develops a serious illness or is involved in a serious accident may be interpreted by the school-age child as the cause of the illness or the accident. Misbehaving, he believes, can also cause death. The young school-age child usually views death as something concrete that comes from the outside, out of the dark. Later the child begins to realize that the cause of death is internal — that the live thing or person himself dies and death does not usually attack from the outside.

Questions that may elicit perceptions of the causes of death are: "What makes animals die?" "What makes people die?"

Since magical thinking may still be operable within the child, it is important to clarify that misbehaving or wishing it does not cause illness or death.

Questions that may elicit the child's perception relative to the reversibility or permanence of death include: "Can an animal or pet who was dead ever come alive again?" "Can a person who was dead ever come alive again?" "How long does a pet stay dead?" "How long does a person stay dead?"

Although it is extremely difficult, if not impossible, for some parents to openly discuss death with a school-age child, the openness that develops around the subject will free the child and the family from the "conspiracy of silence." Ideally, death has been discussed before a child becomes ill in the same fashion that sex and birth are discussed. If talking is impossible, the child may be encouraged to draw pictures of his ideas about death. Parents and siblings can also join in this activity. Less threatening subjects

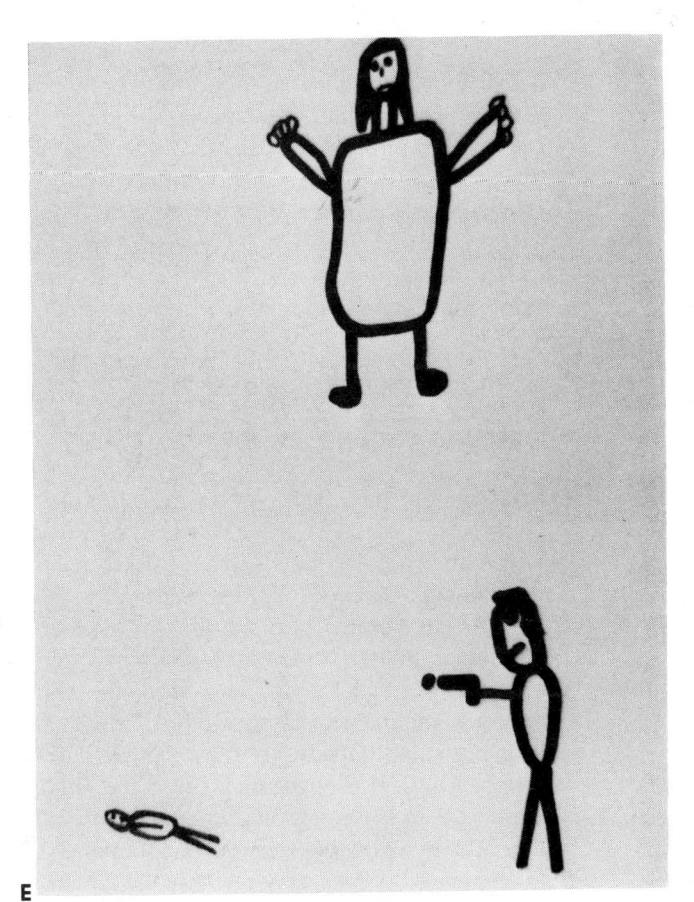

E, "This guy shot him and that's God up there." The school-age child perceives the causes of death to include accidents, violence, illness or pain.

such as a family pet may be drawn to put the family at ease.

The nurse must recognize that, unless the well-being of the child is in serious jeopardy, the parents must make the decision to discuss death with a child with life-threatening illness. They are the most effective providers of support to the child. It is through the parents that the child can be reached. Often the decision clearly becomes one of what to tell and when to tell rather than to tell or not to tell. It is quite clear, though, that "who should tell" is the parents.

The choice that most often proves harmful to the relationships within the family is maintaining the conspiracy of silence. This occurs if the family does not talk with the child at all about the reason for hospitalizations, treatments or tests. During this process the seriously ill child easily misinterprets what is happening and why it is happening and does not have the opportunity to validate his perceptions or clarify the reasons for what is happening to his body and his physical abilities. However, if the family relationship prior to the diagnosis of a terminal illness was wrought with difficulties and stresses, it is unlikely that during this highly stressful time the family will begin to communicate clearly. In fact, the added stresses may provide the stimulus for family disintegration.

SCHOOL ATTENDANCE AND THE SCHOOL-AGE CHILD WITH A LIFE-THREATENING CONDITION

An important part of the life of the school-age child is, of course, school. The change in behavior that has led to the diagnosis of a life-threatening or irreversible illness may affect the child's behavior in school and in his social and emotional milieu. Before the diagnosis of a brain tumor, for instance, the school-age child may become ataxic, may begin to demonstrate irritability and fatigue or may vomit during school. Physical changes may cause the child's classmates to tease or taunt him. The terminally ill child may be viewed by schoolmates as "contagious," which may result in social isolation and teasing.

Unless the alteration in health status is sudden or acute, the social changes that affect the child with a life-threatening disorder may lead to rejection, and school phobia may become a real problem. Parents must have input into the decision of when the ill child is ready to attend school rather than passively waiting for the physician to determine the time. Otherwise the child may lounge around home without the stimulation of school, which is so necessary to him cognitively, emotionally and socially. Being aware that children with life-threatening illness may develop a fear of attending school, the nurse can assist the family by encouraging the normal continuation of school participation regardless of periodic exacerbations of the illness. The nurse should work with the school nurse or directly with the teacher to set up appropriate standards for school attendance and other special considerations. Some children need to leave the classroom for naps or need to take medication during the school day. By careful planning, they can be assisted in meeting their special needs without noticeable school day disruption. However, some parents fear separation from their terminally ill child, causing them to unconsciously foster their child's school fears. At times counselling may help the child and family to deal with the problems associated with school attendance.

All children must learn to take care of themselves in the school environment, but the terminally ill child must learn to fend for himself while coping with physical and emotional changes. Although it is painful for both the child and the parents, the adults (parents and teachers) must, whenever possible, allow the child to work out the struggles and stresses imposed by the change in health status. If the child is not allowed to develop the skills to cope, he then interprets adult intervention as a confirmation of his feared inability to deal with difficulties or as a confirmation of his weakness and lack of control.[3]

TELLING THE CHILD ABOUT HIS TERMINAL CONDITION

The school-age child who faces life-threatening illness may begin to alter his view of death. This change is not sudden, but a gradual transition as his social, emotional and physical environment changes.

Because adults tend to protect and shelter children from knowledge of or experiences with death, the decision concerning sharing information about the diagnosis of a life-threatening disease with a child is a major task for most parents. Authorities disagree on whether or not the knowledge of having a terminal illness in fact changes the child's concept of death — does it accelerate his conceptual development, or does it only serve to increase his anxiety? Eugenia Waechter has demonstrated that children between the ages of 6 and 10 with a fatal prognosis are probably not only aware that they are dying but are also able to express that awareness verbally.[18]

Even though there is still controversy about whether to tell or not to tell the child about his disease and his prognosis, it is important for the nurse to assist the parents as they deal with this question and support them in their decision. She must actively listen to their concerns and fears and provide clarification of their child's diagnosis, treatment plan and prognosis as far as it can be determined. Whatever their decision, the nurse must encourage the parents to deal with the child as openly and honestly as possi-

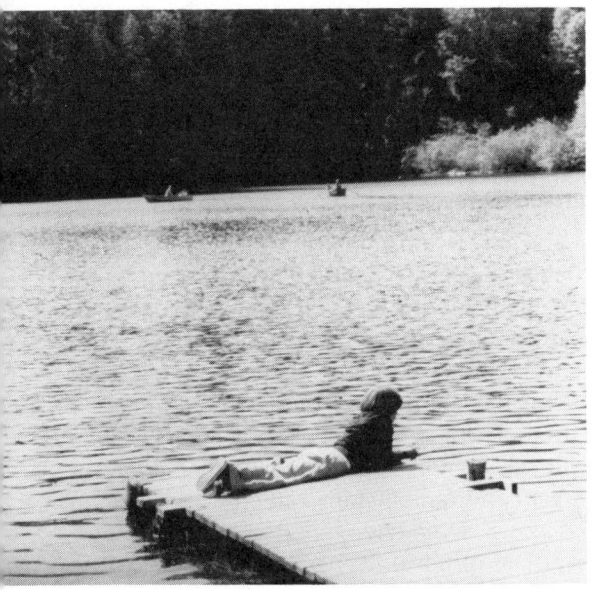

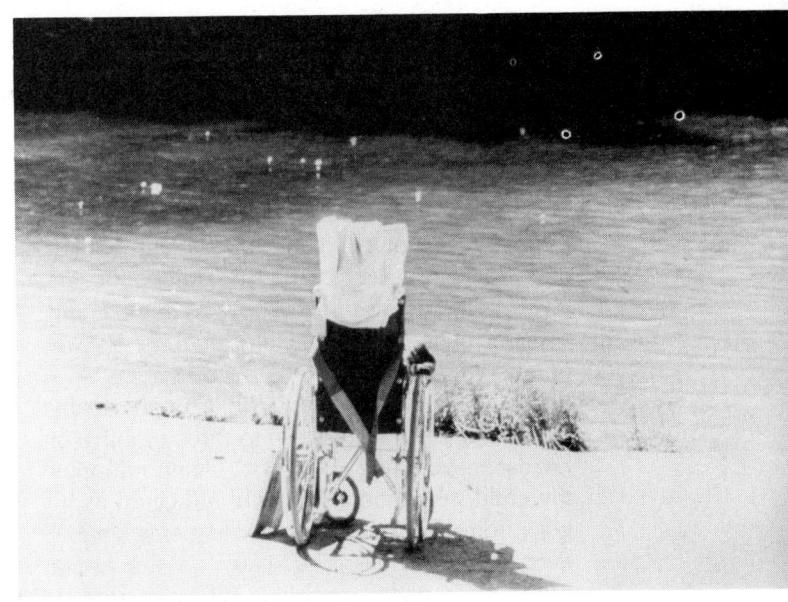

In the spring there was life. By fall it was gone. (Photographs by Cynthia Stewart.)

ble, since the child can best cope with the disease, treatment and death if the lines of communication and support are open throughout the family.

How to tell the school-age child about the diagnosis of a life-threatening disease partly depends upon the child's cognitive skills. The nurse must assess the child frequently in terms of his ability to understand those concepts necessary to comprehend death and assist the parents as they provide information to the child. The nurse or parents or both may use questions to elicit the child's understanding of various components of the concept of death. During the discussion with the child, clarification can be provided and family values/beliefs reinforced. Questions to determine previous experience with death are: "Did you ever have a pet that died?" "Did you ever know a person who died?"

At times, children's reports of previous experience with death may vary from parents' reports of the child's experience with death. Often parents assume that the child was too young to remember when a friend, family member or pet died. Some children also assume that someone is dead who has not been seen or heard from. One young school-age child, for example, was asked in a Denver Developmental Screening Test (DDST) to complete the analogy "Mother is a woman, Dad is a_____." After a few moments of thought, the child answered "soul." The mother was very shocked since the father was not in fact dead, but the parents had been separated for a year and a half. The perception could then be clarified.

Questions to determine knowledge of the process of death are: "What happens after something dies?" "Does it hurt to die?" "How do people or things die?" "What do people do after they are dead?" Misconceptions can be corrected, depending on the child's response and age. Assurances should be made that while the time before death may involve pain (and there are medicines to keep it minimal), death itself does not cause pain.

ALTERED HEALTH STATES

Intracranial Tumors

Approximately 75 per cent of all childhood malignancies (excluding leukemia) occur in the nervous system. Of these about 15 or 20 per cent are intracranial tumors. About two-thirds of these intracranial tumors are *infratentorial*,* occurring in the posterior third of the brain, and about one-third are *supratentorial*, occurring in the anterior two-thirds of the brain.[4]

---

*The tentorium is the dura mater located between the cerebrum and cerebellum supporting the occipital lobes.

Medulloblastoma

This infratentorial tumor is characteristically found in the area of the fourth ventricle. The course of the illness is rapid as the tumor spreads to the meninges of the brain and the spinal cord. Metastasis to the bone marrow and lungs may be noted if diagnosis or treatment are delayed or unsuccessful. This tumor occurs about four times as often in boys as in girls, and peak incidence occurs in children under 5 years of age.[17]

The child with a medulloblastoma usually has a short-term history (up to three months) of headache, vomiting and ataxia. Deterioration of the child's condition is usually indicated as he goes from being able to walk to being unable even to stand unassisted. Later, as the tumor grows, the child is unable to sit unassisted or even to hold up his head. Nuchal rigidity and head tilting are eventually noted. Papilledema is severe and easily recognizable.

Surgical removal of most of the tumor decreases symptomatology and re-establishes unobstructed flow of cerebral spinal fluid and subsequently decreases intracranial pressure. Although total resection of the tumor is usually not possible, this treatment is considered palliative. The use of combination therapy including total nervous system irradiation and oral or intravenous chemotherapy has resulted in a short-term response in some children. The use of intrathecal or intravenous methotrexate may result in a remission of symptoms from the tumor.[7] With aggressive combination therapy the five-year survival rate is 35 per cent and the 10-year survival rate is 25 per cent. Prognosis is poorer for younger patients.[17]

Astrocytoma

Cerebellar This infratentorial tumor is often cystic in nature and is usually located in one lobe of the cerebellum and later expands to midline, especially to the pons, the midbrain and the medulla. It does not "seed" along the cerebral spinal fluid pathway as other tumors such as medulloblastoma are apt to do. This tumor occurs slightly more frequently in girls than in boys, and the peak incidence of occurrence is usually around 8 years of age.

The child with cerebellar astrocytoma usually presents with a history (about 3 to 6 months) of morning headache, vomiting and anorexia. Ataxia of gait and incoordination of hands appear much later than do the overt signs of increased intracranial pressure. The child may gradually become irritable and lethargic, but this is usually so subtle in onset that parents may not be able to indicate just when the behavioral changes began. The child may develop a squint and complain of double vision. Ophthalmological examination reveals papilledema. An increased head circumference with separation of the sagittal suture may be noted on x-ray.

Complete surgical resection is often possible with this tumor. The combination therapy of surgery and radiotherapy often ensures a good prognosis. Some have reported a five-year survival rate of up to 90 per cent with the use of combination therapy.[4]

Brain Stem Gliomas

This infratentorial tumor is located in the brain stem and presents with severe neurological signs and symptoms before any sign of increased intracranial pressure is noted. The tumor appears to be a cauliflower-like growth on the external surface of the brain stem. It is fast growing and is usually diagnosed within two months of onset of early symptoms and signs. Peak incidence of occurrence of this tumor is in children 5 years of age. Both boys and girls are equally affected.

Neurological signs, including ocular palsies, nystagmus, ataxia, dyplopia, squint, difficulty in swallowing and talking, lack of hand coordination, weakness of limbs and facial weakness, drooling, and urinary retention are noted. Due to the difficulty with swallowing, aspiration of both food and fluids may be noted with subsequent bronchopneumonia. Progressive urinary retention usually leads to urinary tract infections. These secondary infections are usually the cause of death in these children.[5]

Surgery is useful only in diagnosis of brain stem gliomas, because the critical vital centers would be compromised by surgical excision of the tumor. Radiotherapy, although palliative, does extend the survival from a few months to a few years. Chemotherapy has not been proved useful with these tumors.

Craniopharyngioma

This is a congenital solid tumor with cystic areas located supratentorially, which is usually slow

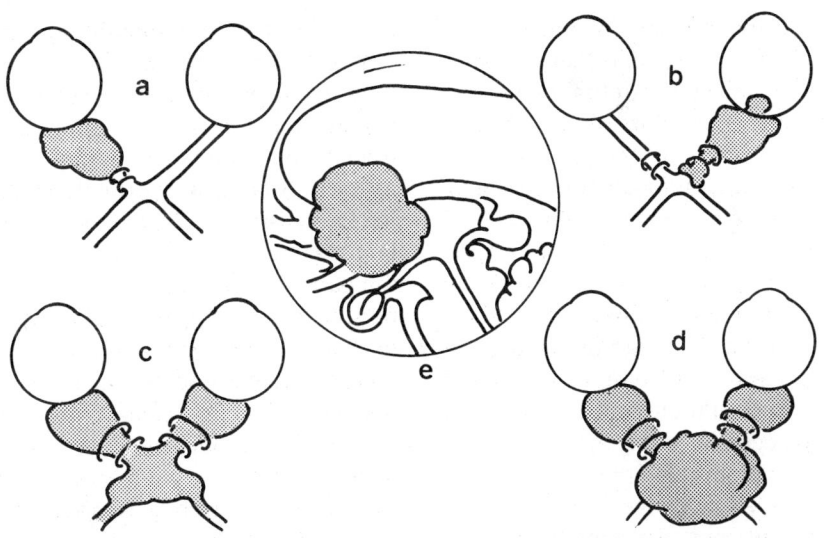

Figure 53-1 Gliomas of the optic nerve. The types shown are (a) confined to the nerve orbit, (b) extending into the globe and proximally to the chiasm, (c) diffuse involvement of both optic nerves and the chiasm, (d) further extension of tumor tissue from the major mass around the chiasm and extending into nearby cerebral substance and (e) obstructing the third ventricle. (Courtesy of P. Jones and P. Campbell, Tumors of Infancy and Childhood, Blackwell Scientific Publications, 1976, p. 264.)

growing and benign.[17] The tumor grows and extends upward and backward to involve the optic chiasm and the third ventricle, which causes obstructive hydrocephalus. The peak incidence is noted around 13 to 16 years of age.[4]

Signs and symptoms relate to the growth patterns of the tumor. Visual field deficits are noted as the tumor extends and progressively places pressure on the optic chiasm. If it is left untreated, blindness results. If the tumor extends into the third ventricle and obstructive hydrocephalus occurs, signs of increased intracranial pressure may be noted. Irritability, lack of ability to concentrate, headache, obesity and diabetes insipidus may be noted as pituitary dysfunction occurs.

Three modes of treatment are utilized: (1) total resection of the tumor, (2) subtotal resection of the tumor with the use of radiotherapy postoperatively and (3) surgical biopsy without resection and primary treatment by the use of radiotherapy. The prognosis is good with treatment, and the child can live a nearly normal life with endocrine function support, such as growth hormone, adrenocorticotrophic hormones or gonadotrophic hormones or all three.[4] According to Van Eye, "Most failures occur within three years. The outlook for children with craniopharyngioma treated in an institution with experience in either radical surgery and/or radiotherapy, together with pediatric endocrinology and general pediatric oncology support, should be excellent."[17]

Astrocytoma

Cerebral These supratentorial tumors usually have features of malignancy. An invasive solid tumor, it grows to be very large. The frontal lobe is most often involved, with extension into midline structures, basal ganglia and the thalamus. The peak incidence of the occurrence of this tumor is in early adolescence. It occurs slightly more often in boys than in girls.[5]

The child with cerebral astrocytoma usually presents with symptoms such as headache, vomiting and apathy. These are all indicators of increased intracranial pressure. Other neurological signs such as diplopia, focal seizures, ataxia and incoordination may also occur. Weakness of limbs contralaterally is sometimes noted.

Rarely is surgical resection possible. Radiation is palliative and is sometimes used in conjunction with chemotherapy. The prognosis is poor, with the average survival being about a year.[4]

Optic Path Gliomas

These benign slow-growing, supratentorial tumors are found with five different presentations: (1) confined to the nerve in one orbit, (2) extending from the optic chiasm into the eyeball, (3) diffuse involvement bilaterally of the optic nerves and the chiasm, (4) bilateral involvement of optic nerves and chiasm with extension into the adjacent cerebral tissue and (5) obstructing the entire third ventricle (Fig. 53–1).[5] Peak incidence of diagnosis is between birth and 5 years of age, although diagnosis may not be made until well into adolescence.

Neurological signs such as strabismus and nystagmus may be noted. Decreased visual acuity, diabetes insipidus, obesity and short stature may also occur. If the tumor invades the third ventricle, signs of increased intracranial pressure may exist. Proptosis (forward and downward displacement of the eyeball) is one of the earlier symptoms. In infants, failure to thrive may be noted, with general failure of growth. Café-au-lait spots are sometimes seen in patients with this tumor.

Surgical excision is sometimes possible when only one of the optic nerves is involved. The greater the involvement, the less the possibility for total resection. At times a total enucleation of the eye is recommended. Invasion of vital centers is usually the cause of death. Radiation therapy may be either curative or palliative, depending upon the extent of the invasion. If the optic chiasm is involved, radiation therapy is the only treatment of choice.

Ependymoma

This tumor originates from ependymal cells that form the lining of the spinal cord and the cavities of the brain. Therefore this tumor may be found either supratentorially or infratentorially. These tumors appear to be "embryonal tumors" and are, in fact, sometimes diagnosed at birth. This tumor occurs slightly more frequently in boys than in girls. Its peak incidence of occurrence is around 2 or 3 years of age.[4, 5]

The child with an ependymoma usually presents with a short-term history (one to three months) of vomiting, a clumsy gait and headaches. Clinical signs of papilledema, ataxia and incoordination of the hands are usually noted. The clinical presentation is very similar to that of the child with a medulloblastoma, and until surgery the tumors are not distinguishable.

It has been found that when this tumor occurs infratentorially it is benign, although it does invade the brain stem.[4] Compromised cardiorespiratory function may be noted if the onset is acute (less than one month), and the prognosis is poor. Limited range of motion of the neck may signal extended growth of the tumor.[5] If the ependymoma is located supratentorially, the frontal and parietal lobes are most generally affected. Metastasis is usually to the surrounding brain tissues.[4] These tumors may grow quite large before any signs or symptoms are noted by the parents. There may be a gradual change in personality, making the child irritable, fatigued or sluggish. The treatment is surgery, but usually complete tumor resection is not possible. Radiation of the entire central nervous system is recommended but still does not improve the five-year survival rate very substantially. The survival rate currently is about 13 to 22 per cent.[4, 5] Chemotherapy is sometimes effective and is instilled through an Ommaya reservoir. Figure 53–2 illustrates this reservoir. A description of its use follows later in this chapter.

Diagnosing Intracranial Tumors

Since many of the early symptoms of intracranial tumors are similar to those of common childhood illnesses — nausea, vomiting, headache and irritability — early diagnosis is usually difficult. Changes in behavior in school such as decreased performance and irritability or fatigue may be attributed to school phobia or some problem that the child "will outgrow." It is usually not until significant physical changes have occurred that medical assistance is sought. Ataxia, seizures, hemiparesis or cranial nerve deficits usually lead to numerous tests to determine the child's medical problem.

If a brain tumor is suspected, an entire battery of diagnostic tests must be endured by the school-age child and his parents. Such procedures may include multiple neurological examinations, computerized tomograms (CAT scans or EMI scans), cerebral angiography, skull films, ventriculography, brain scans, lumbar punctures, myelograms, electroencephalograms, bone marrow biopsies and surgical biopsies.[10]

Although the medical necessity of performing these diagnostic examinations may have been explained to the parents, the nurse must assess the parents' and child's need for further information or repeated information as the testing proceeds. During the diagnostic phase, the family is usually anxious and may be experiencing disbelief at the possibility that their child may have a brain tumor — no fate could be worse to many families. The nurse must assist the family

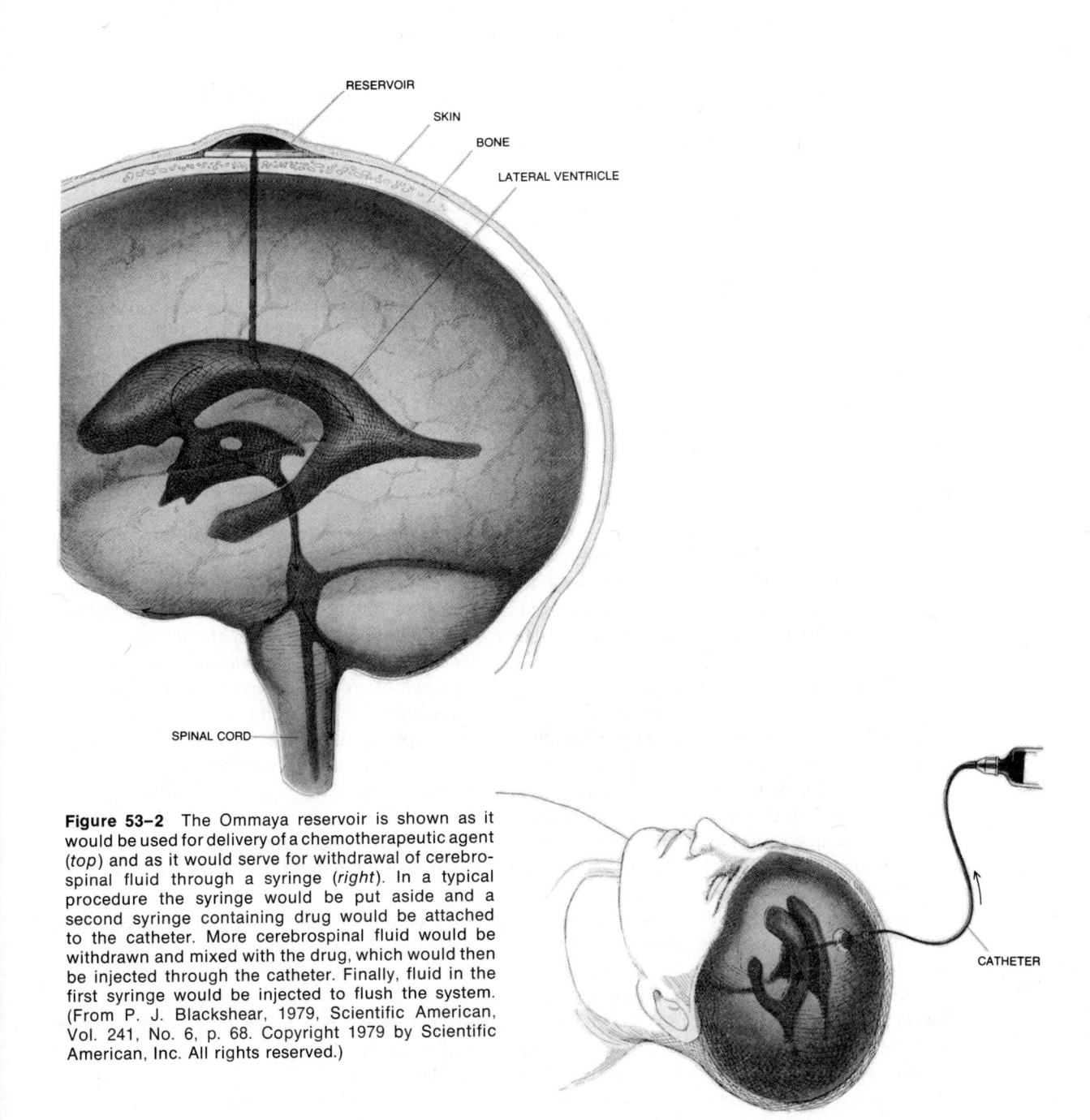

Figure 53-2 The Ommaya reservoir is shown as it would be used for delivery of a chemotherapeutic agent (*top*) and as it would serve for withdrawal of cerebrospinal fluid through a syringe (*right*). In a typical procedure the syringe would be put aside and a second syringe containing drug would be attached to the catheter. More cerebrospinal fluid would be withdrawn and mixed with the drug, which would then be injected through the catheter. Finally, fluid in the first syringe would be injected to flush the system. (From P. J. Blackshear, 1979, Scientific American, Vol. 241, No. 6, p. 68. Copyright 1979 by Scientific American, Inc. All rights reserved.)

through this phase by recognizing that even though written consent may have been obtained, "informed consent" may not in fact be operative. In other words, if the family, in their attempt to cooperate in efforts to care for their child, signed the permit for specific procedures without fully understanding the procedure or the possible complications related to it, then *informed* consent has not been given.

The nurse must continually assess the family as they cope with the many procedures and the scientific and medical jargon to which they are suddenly exposed. It is imperative that the nurse be able to provide information regarding the actual procedure to be performed, what the child can expect to feel and see during the procedure, what is expected of him, and where his parents will be. The parents should be permitted and encouraged to accompany the child to the procedure and to stay through the procedure if feasible. The nurse should provide support to the child in the absence of his parents during a procedure. Parents must not be made to feel guilty if they choose not to remain with the child during a procedure.

The school-age child needs to know the whereabouts of his parent(s) if they do not accompany him to the procedure. He also needs to know, if possible, how long the procedure will take, in terms that he can understand. For instance, if the child is still in a preoperational cognitive stage he may require an explanation such as: "After you wake up from sleeping, your mommy and daddy will be right here by your bed with you." The child in the concrete stage will be assisted by an explanation such as: "Your dad has taken your sister to school, but in an hour, after you get back from your x-rays, he will be in your room to see you."

Since several of the diagnostic procedures are done with the assistance of preoperative medications, the nurse should teach the parents and child about preoperative and postoperative routines such as the need to be "NPO," having an IV started, having dressings on after the procedure, or the need to cough and deep breathe postoperatively. The nurse should help the parents and child to understand each diagnostic procedure and their role during the testing phase. Since the diagnostic phase may be initiated very quickly, the nurse must be aware of the family's need for direct and succinct answers to questions and directions. It is important that the nurse avoid the use of jargon with the family, communicating as clearly as possible during this time of confusion, fear and shock.

Treatment of Intracranial Tumors

The treatments generally utilized to treat intracranial tumors are radiation therapy, chemotherapy or surgery or combinations of these.

Radiation Therapy Radiation therapy is most often used in combination with surgery or may be used alone as a palliative measure. There are some situations, such as with medulloblastoma, in which radiation therapy, chemotherapy and surgery are utilized together; however, surgery and radiation therapy are preferred to effect palliation or remission.

The child undergoing radiation therapy has unique needs that must be addressed in terms of nursing management. Short-term goals involve assisting the child and his family to understand what this treatment means to them. What value has been placed upon this therapy? Do they understand what radiation therapy can and cannot do? Are their expectations realistic, or are they inconsistent with what can actually be accomplished by radiation therapy?

The nurse must also assess the level of fear and anxiety associated with the treatment. The child needs information regarding his expected behavior during the therapy as well as information about possible side effects. The impact of side effects can be minimized by exposing him to symptomatic children who have adjusted well. This interaction gives the child a realistic perspective on the side effects he may experience and facilitates his questions and adaptation. Symptom management is important once side effects occur. During periods of bone marrow depression, temporary withdrawal of the child from school should be considered. See Appendix VIII for additional nursing care during radiotherapy.

Information regarding the length of treatment in terms of the entire therapy program needs to be provided and understood. A written account of the treatment regimen should be given to the parents so that expectations are based on fact and fear is reduced.

Surgical Resection Surgical resection is often used with intracranial tumors, although total resection is often not possible due to the invasiveness of some tumors such as medulloblastoma, the embryonic nature of some cells such as noted in ependymoma, and because of the close proximity of the tumor to vital centers such as in the brain stem gliomas. At times, surgery is done only for diagnostic purposes because the tumor cannot be diagnosed by clinical symptoms. Parents need to be impressed, prior to surgery, with the fact that the tumor may be inoperable and that palliation will be the most that can be achieved.

Chemotherapy Chemotherapy is somewhat limited in its usefulness for the treatment of intracranial tumors. However, this is an area of challenge to medical clinicians that may see many changes as clinical research progresses and as physicians continue to learn ways of treating intracranial tumors.

The Ommaya Reservoir is a mechanical device, a permanent reservoir and catheter, which is placed in the ventricular system or tumor to facilitate the instillation of drugs. This facilitates the process whereby water-soluble drugs reach the brain.[17] Implanted pellets or pumps are also used to provide a continuous supply of medication (Fig. 53–3). Currently it is used on a limited basis but may provide more effective chemotherapeutic effects with children with intracranial tumors. See Appendix VIII for a discussion of nursing care in radiotherapy and chemotherapy.

In some tumors, such as craniopharyngiomas and optic path gliomas, pituitary dysfunction may occur. In these situations, growth hormone, corticosteroids or gonadotrophic agents or all three may be provided to maintain nearly normal endocrine functioning in the child.

Intracranial tumors often cause seizure disorders either before diagnosis or after further invasion of the tumor. Anticonvulsive drugs are utilized to control seizure activity. Most children with the diagnosis of a brain tumor will be given anticonvulsive medication prophylactically.

Medications for relief of pain and control of nausea or vomiting or both must be provided to the child to promote comfort and decrease stress for the child and his family. Other methods of pain control may be useful. Reduction of anxiety and maintenance of a comfortable and nonstressful environment will enhance the effect of certain pain medications and modes of care. The use of soft music or not-so-soft music (as desired) may serve as a distractor and put the child at ease. Some children prefer to watch television or to have someone read to them. Some prefer to watch the activities of the rest of the family.

Tumors of Soft Tissues (Non-Hodgkin's Lymphosarcoma)

One of the malignant tumors of the reticuloendothelial system, this tumor is composed of lymphocytes derived from bone marrow cells. Sites commonly affected are the ileum, the anterior mediastinum, the neck and the nasopharynx. Although it occurs at any age, a peak incidence is evident between the ages of 5 to 10 years. The ratio of boys to girls is more than 2:1.[5] If the lymphosarcoma affects the

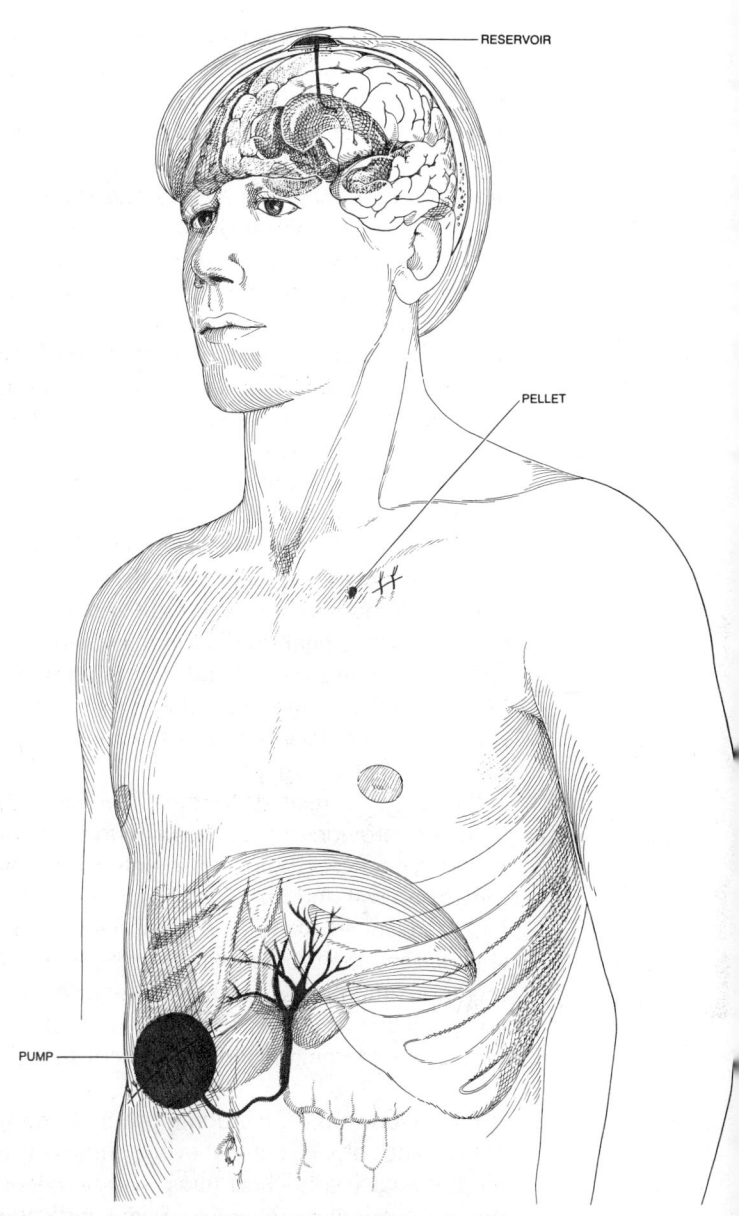

Figure 53–3 Implantable devices are shown in a hypothetical patient (hypothetical because no one person would be likely to have all three devices at once). The device under the scalp is the Ommaya reservoir, which gives access to the cerebrospinal fluid. The pellet, consisting of a concentrated drug, is implanted just under the skin. It releases drug mainly through erosion. The implanted pump has a fluorocarbon propellant that maintains a constant pressure on a supply of drug so that the pump can deliver drug at a constant rate to a vein or an artery. (From P. J. Blackshear, 1979, Scientific American, Vol. 241, No. 6, p. 67. Copyright 1979 by Scientific American, Inc. All rights reserved.)

ileum, signs of abdominal pain, a palpable mass and an intussusception with a possible obstruction may be noted. Palpable lymph nodes in the neck and other peripheral areas may exist. Anemia is common and splenomegaly may be noted.[5] The staging process utilized in determining the progression of the disease is like that used in Hodgkin's disease* although the diagnostic process may differ. Accurate staging is accomplished by physical examination, blood studies (smears with the goal of clearly identifying abnormal lymphocytes), bone marrow aspiration, chest films, bone studies and excretory urography. Lymphangiography may also be carried out along with lung tomograms and bone, brain and liver and spleen scans and perhaps abdominal ultrasound.

There is some controversy surrounding the optimal plan of treatment for the child with non-Hodgkin's lymphoma. When the disease is fairly well localized (stages I and II), chemotherapy or total body irradiation is utilized. Chemotherapy and regional irradiation may be utilized with children in stages III and IV.[16] Surgery may be indicated to remove localized diseased tissue. It is also indicated to resect areas of gastrointestinal tract obstruction.

Prognosis is related to the stage and the treatment provided. It has been found that patients receiving combined chemotherapy have longer survival and improved response. With a more advanced stage and treatment with a single agent, the prognosis is poor.[16] The use of high-dose intrathecal methotrexate with citrovorum factor rescue has been shown effective in prevention of central nervous system metastasis.

Follow-up studies, including physical examination and blood counts every three to six months with yearly chest films, will be needed once remission is achieved. Some indication exists that relapse may occur up to 10 or 15 years after remission has been achieved, although complete remission is possible.[16]

Reye's Syndrome

Reye's syndrome was first described by Reye and associates in 1963 as acute encephalopathy associated with fatty degeneration of the viscera affecting mainly the liver, brain and kidney.[13]

Incidence The actual incidence of Reye's is unknown, since reporting of cases is not required in all states. While approximately 360 cases were reported in 1977, the incidence is probably much greater, because increased awareness of the disease and improved diagnostic methods make it possible to detect the syndrome early, resulting in decreased mortality rates. Mortality rates range from 6 to 7 per cent in some states and as high as 40 per cent in others. Reye's affects children ranging from 2 months to adolescence, with peaks occurring in children 6 and 11 years of age.[19] The mortality rate is highest in children under 2 and in those who convulse.

Etiology Although several theories exist on the possible cause of Reye's, the theory most widely accepted today suggests that the condition is a reaction to the interaction between a virus and a toxin. (The viruses B-type influenza and varicella (chickenpox) in interaction with such toxins as herbicides or insecticides or both.) Annual incidence of Reye's is directly proportional to outbreaks of influenza and chickenpox. Other theories that have been proposed include defects in the Krebs' cycle* and the urea cycle,† faulty lipid metabolism and genetic metabolic predisposition to Reye's.

Clinical Manifestations The history generally reveals that the child was ill with flu-like symptoms for approximately a week, healthy for a few days and then developed repeated episodes of vomiting that lasted for two or more days, accompanied by an altered state of consciousness that progressed. Upon examination the child appears healthy, although he may be agitated, confused or combative. Signs include slight tachycardia, normal blood pressure and normal or low-grade fever. Neurologically there is no evidence of increased intracranial pressure. Pupils are generally reactive and no papilledema is evident; nuchal rigidity is absent although hyper-reflexes are characteristic. The liver is generally not palpable and there is no evidence of jaundice. Initial electroencephalogram is generally abnormal and shows a pattern unique, but not exclusive, to Reye's.[9]

---

*See Chapter 62 regarding staging of Hodgkin's disease.

*A series of enzymatic reactions occurring in most aerobic organisms, involving oxidative metabolism of acetyl units, especially during respiration, to provide cellular energy.
†A cyclic series of reactions that produce urea.

Diagnosis After other diseases that present similar signs and symptoms (such as diabetes mellitus, drug overdose, salicylism, meningitis, encephalitis or acute hepatic failure) have been ruled out, Reye's is suspected. The more promptly the diagnosis is made, the better the prognosis.

Laboratory tests used in making the diagnosis of Reye's include blood glucose levels, serum ammonia, liver function tests (SGOT, SGPT, LDH, CPK), and prothrombin time. If the laboratory report shows normal or low blood glucose levels, elevated ammonia levels (80 per cent of affected individuals have this), elevated liver function tests and increased prothrombin times, a diagnosis of Reye's is confirmed. The need for hepatic tissue to confirm the diagnosis of Reye's is controversial. A liver biopsy may be indicated when deviations from the typical clinical picture are found. Microvesicular fat droplets found on liver biopsy are diagnostic of the syndrome.[19]

Treatment Because Reye's develops quickly and progresses rapidly, treatment must be instituted immediately. The recommended first step is to begin intravenous administration of 100 per cent glucose as soon as blood samples are drawn and to place the child in a pediatric intensive care unit (ICU).[12]

Treatment will depend on the clinical stage of the disease. Lovejoy and associates have provided a framework of clinical stages of Reye's that aids in determining modes of therapy, evaluating treatment methods and comparing cases. Each stage is defined in terms of clinical features of the disease and laboratory findings. The clinical features of Reye's include:[9]

Stage I: lethargy, drowsiness, vomiting, elevation in serum liver enzymes, grade I electroencephalogram.

Stage II: disorientation, combativeness, hyperventilation, tachycardia, pupillary dilation, hyperactive reflexes, purposeful response to painful stimuli, bilateral Babinski reflex, elevation in blood ammonia and serum liver enzymes, grades II, III or IV electroencephalogram.

Stage III: coma, persistent tachycardia and hyperventilation, upper midbrain involvement (loss of ciliospinal reflex, pupillary dilation, decorticate posturing in response to painful stimuli, bilateral Babinski reflex), persistent elevation in blood ammonia and serum liver enzymes, and grades II, III or IV electroencephalogram.

Stage IV: deepening coma, further rostral-caudal progression of midbrain involvement (sluggish pupillary response to light, decerebrate rigidity and decerebrate posturing to painful stimuli, bilateral Babinski reflex), decrease in blood ammonia and serum liver enzyme activity, grade III or IV electroencephalogram.

Stage V: coma, loss of response to painful stimuli and to light, cessation of spontaneous respiration, continued improvement in blood ammonia and serum liver enzyme activity, grade V electroencephalogram.

Although it is difficult to predict whether the disease will progress to the serious form, Weeks suggests the best protocol for evaluating the disease is based on the clinical staging, correlating the staging with electroencephalographic grade.[19]

The child with Reye's is acutely ill and requires continuous care. When a child is admitted to the intensive care unit with Reye's, the nurse has many things to do in order to monitor the slightest change in his condition. These include: (1) 50 cc of blood must be drawn, (2) intravenous lines must be established and (3) Foley catheter and nasogastric tubes are inserted. If the child is in at least stage II, an intracranial pressure line is inserted in the lateral ventricle and the child is intubated and placed on a volume-controlled ventilator. The body weight of the child must be known for use as a baseline by which to measure fluid balance. Neurological appraisal needs to be made by the nurse, since the disease can progress rapidly. The neurological assessment includes hourly checking and recording of deep tendon, Babinski, and doll's eyes signs, pupillary reflexes and the child's state of consciousness and posturing.[19]

Since both clinical and pathological evidence suggest that increased intracranial pressure (ICP) is a significant factor affecting the mortality rate of patients with Reye's, treatment should initially involve reducing increased ICP by controlled ventilation, fluid restriction, use of diuretics and possibly exchange transfusions. Surgical decompression of the brain may also be necessary in some cases.

Continuous monitoring of ICP is recorded by way of a ventricle catheter placed in the lateral ventricle through a burr hole in the frontal bone, since it is impossible to determine from clinical signs alone if the child is developing increased intracranial presure. It has been the observation of Shaywitz that control of intracranial pressure is far more effective when even slight elevations are treated promptly.[14]

To keep ICP below 24 mmHg, fluids are restricted to decrease the amount of fluid to the brain. The patient is hyperventilated to maintain PCO_2 at 20 to 25 mmHg, which is also to reduce pressure. Osmotic diuretics are used to increase serum osmolality, which leads to dehydration of the brain cells and a decrease in ICP. Corticosteroids are effective in reducing pressure, although the mechanism is poorly understood. It is effective within 12 hours after administration and lasts approximately 24 hours. Mannitol is an effective agent in rapidly reducing ICP, requiring only five minutes to take effect, with the effect lasting for 90 to 150 minutes.[14] Hypothermia is an alternate method used for ICP that is not responsive to other measures. If ICP does increase, the nurse needs to first suction the patient, then bag (ventilate) to decrease PCO_2 levels until the pressure decreases, administering medication if bagging fails to hold it down. Nursing care must be designed to provide necessary physical care without elevating ICP. As a result sedation may be required before any physical routine such as percussion and care of skin and positioning.

Additional supportive therapy for the patient with Reye's includes close monitoring of fluid intake and output. Accurate recording is necessary for maintaining optimal fluid and electrolyte balance to decrease cerebral edema.

Since a constant danger in these children is hypovolemic shock, vital signs and central venous pressure need to be recorded hourly. Because many laboratory tests serve as a guide for therapy, the nurse needs to be aware of and arrange for them. These tests include analysis of serum electrolytes, hematocrit, blood urea nitrogen (BUN), glucose, serum osmolality, and blood gases.

In addition to these measures, respiratory maintenance is critical in reducing the incidence of infection. Percussion and modified postural drainage are used to prevent or treat pulmonary complications. Since the child is on a volume-controlled ventilator, inspiratory pressure, humidification and temperature of the child and ventilator should be checked frequently to promote proper maintenance and care.

Depending on the clinical stage of the disease, it may be necessary to sedate and paralyze the child, using pancuronium bromide, to maintain hyperventilation and decreased ICP for a period of 24 hours. Pancuronium bromide (Pavulon) is the paralytic agent of choice since it does not cause histamine release as does curare. If the patient tolerates this maneuver and blood gases return to normal, the sedation is stopped and the child is extubated.

Impact of Reye's Syndrome on the Family: Nurse's Role As in other instances in which there is sudden onset of illness with possible impending death, parents experience feelings of shock, disbelief, anger, denial and guilt for not having done things differently or sooner. In addition to these feelings, parents of children with Reye's often express fear because of their limited knowledge about the disease, its unpredictable nature and clinical course. Since the average duration of time from onset of vomiting to full recovery of consciousness is approximately 99 hours, with the average coma lasting 30 hours, parents need to know as much as possible about the disease to alleviate any guilt involved and to reduce their anxieties.[9]

Although the physical care of the child is demanding of the nurse's time, the needs of the family cannot be overlooked. If it is impossible for the intensive care nurse to provide the supportive care required by these families, arrangement for other personnel to do this should be made. The nurse caring for the child needs to familiarize the family with the intensive care unit (ICU), providing explanations for treatment procedures and apparatus necessary in providing therapy for their child. If the child is comatose, the nurse needs to caution the parents not to discuss his condition while in his presence, since comprehension is often possible. Counselling parents to explain events or activities to the child as though he can understand and encouraging them to touch him are constructive suggestions that may aid in diminishing the shock of seeing their child comatose.

Physical care of the child is critical during the comatose state. However, social and emotional needs of the child should not be overlooked. Weeks describes a behavioral pattern unique to Reye's children that occurs upon their awakening from a comatose state; knowing about this aids in providing care.[19] At first the children appear withdrawn and disoriented, capable of responding only to basic questions about physical needs. They cannot remember past events in the ICU and become quite anxious and upset when procedures are unexplained or if they see another person convulse or in arrest. Like all children, they are upset by separation from their parents and feel powerless in the events and decisions that are affecting their lives. The feeling of powerlessness can be observed in their lack of resistance to procedures and treatments.[19] The goal of the ICU nurse needs to be that of reorienting and restructuring the child's environment so that he comprehends procedures and is allowed the opportunity to make choices and exert control over his environment regardless of how insignificant this may seem. Parents also need to be encouraged to bring familiar things from home and spend as much time as possible with him.

Once the child is moved out of ICU (24 to 48 hours after awakening), it is important for the ICU nurse to provide the pediatric staff with information regarding the child and family's physical, social and emotional needs. Recovery is generally rapid in those who survive; however, many children with Reye's suffer chronic impairment or die. The direction and support received by the child and his family during the period of hospitalization will strongly influence their acceptance and resolution of the condition. Referral and follow-up care are crucial for parents in such circumstances.

Literature About Death

R. Bach. Jonathan Livingston Seagull. Avon Books, 1973
R. Blue. Grandma Didn't Wave Back. Franklin Watts Publishing, 1972
M. Wisi Brown. The Dead Bird. Young Scout Books, 1958
V. Cleaner and B. Cleaner. Grover. J. B. Lippincott Co, 1970
J. Fassler. My Grandpa Died Today. Behavioral Publications, 1971
E. Grollman. Explaining Death to Children. Beacon Press, 1967
A. Harris. Why Did He Die? Lerner Publishing, 1965
J. Kavannaugh. Celebrate the Sun. Nash Publishing, 1973
V. Lee. The Magic Moth. The Seabury Press, 1972
J. Little. Home from Far. Little, Brown & Co. 1965
M. Miles. Annie and the Old One. Little, Brown & Co., 1971
D. Orgel. Mulberry Music. Harper & Row, 1971
M. Rawlings. The Yearling. Charles Scribner's Sons, 1939
N. Roach. The Last Day of April. American Cancer Society, California Division, 1974
G. Rock. The House Without a Christmas Tree. Alfred A. Knopf, 1974
S. Silverstein. The Giving Tree. Harper & Row, 1964
D. Smith. A Taste of Blackberries. Thomas Y. Crowell Co., 1973
S. Stein. About Dying: An Open Family Book for Parents and Children Together. Walker Publishing, 1974
J. Viorst. The Tenth Good Thing About Barney. Atheneum Press, 1971
E. White. Charlotte's Web. Harper & Row, 1952
M. Williams. The Velveteen Rabbit. Doubleday, 1958

Other Guides to Literature on Death

C. Aradine. Books for Children about death, Pediatrics, March 1976, p. 372
Fynn. Mister God, This Is Anna. Holt, Rinehart & Winston, 1975
G. Mills. Books to help children understand death. American Journal of Nursing, February 1979

References

1. W. Easson. The Dying Child: The Management of the Child or Adolescent Who Is Dying. Charles C Thomas, 1970
2. S. Friedman. Psychological aspects of sudden unexpected death in infants and children. Pediatric Clinics of North America, February 1974, p. 103
3. J. Gyulay. The Dying Child. McGraw-Hill Book Co., 1978
4. K. Hausman. Brain tumors in children. Journal of Neurosurgical Nursing, March 1979, p. 8
5. P. Jones and P. Campbell, eds. Tumors of Infancy and Childhood. Blackwell Scientific Publications, 1976
6. G. Koocher. Why isn't the gerbil moving anymore? Discussing death in the classroom and at home. Children Today, Jan/Feb 1975, p. 17
7. P. Kornblith and R. Linggood. Cancer of the brain and central nervous system. In Cancer: A Manual for Practitioners, American Cancer Society (Massachusetts Division), 1978
8. E. Kübler-Ross. On Death and Dying. Macmillan, Inc., 1969
9. F. Lovejoy and associates. Clinical Stages in Reye Syndrome, American Journal of Diseases of Children, February 1963, p. 749
10. L. Miller. Neurological assessment: a practical approach for the critical care nurse. Journal of Neurosurgical Nursing, March 1979, p. 2
11. M. Nagy. The child's view of death. Journal of Genetic Psychology, 1948, p. 3
12. M. Prilock et al. Reye's Syndrome: early recognition is vital. Patient Care, 15 January 1978, p. 187
13. R. Reye et al. Encephalopathy and fatty degeneration of the viscera: a disease entity in childhood. Lancet, February 1963, p. 749
14. B. Shaywitz et al. Prolonged continuous monitoring of intracranial pressure in severe Reye's syndrome. Pediatrics. May 1977, p. 41
15. M. Sheets. An investigation of the school-age child's concept of death. Master's Thesis, University of Washington, 1975
16. A. Skarin et al. Malignant lymphomas. In Cancer: A Manual for Practitioners, American Cancer Society (Massachusetts Div.) 1978
17. J. Van Eye. Malignant tumors of the central nervous system. In Clinical Pediatric Oncology by W. Sutow et al. C. V. Mosby Co., 1977

18. E. Waechter. Children's awareness of fatal illness. American Journal of Nursing, June 1971, p. 1168
19. H. Weeks. What every ICU Nurse should know about Reye's Syndrome. American Journal of Maternal and Child Health, January 1976, p. 231
20. A. Wolf. Helping Your Child to Understand Death. Child Study Press, 1973
21. A. Wolff. Children Under Stress. Pelican Books, 1973

Additional Recommended Reading

The School Child and Death

M. Adams. A hospital play program: helping children with serious illness. American Journal Orthopsychiatry, July 1976, p. 416

S. Anthony. The Discovery of Death in Childhood and After. Basic Books, 1972

E. Berman. Scapegoat. University of Michigan Press, 1973.

R. Burns and S. Kaufman. Kinetic Family Drawings (K.I.D.): An Introduction to Understanding Children Through Kinetic Drawings. Brunner/Mazel Inc. 1970

J. DiLeo. Young Children and Their Drawings. Brunner/Mazel Inc. 1970

J. DiLeo. Children's Drawings As Diagnostic Aids. Brunner/Mazel Inc., 1973

J. DiLeo. Child Development: Analysis and Synthesis. Brunner/Mazel Inc., 1977

D. Fredlund. Children and death from the school setting. Journal of School Health, November 1977, p. 533

E. Hart. Death education and mental health. Journal of School Health, September 1976, p. 407

R. Kellogg. Analyzing Children's Art. Mayfield Publishing Co., 1970

G. Koocher. Talking with children about death, American Journal of Orthopsychiatry, April 1974, p. 404

I. Martinson. Home Care For the Dying Child: Professional and Family Perspectives. Appleton-Century-Crofts, 1976

I. Martinson. Home Care: A Manual for Implementation of Home Care for Children Dying of Cancer. University of Minnesota Press, 1978

A. Maurer. Maturation of concepts of life. Journal of Genetic Psychology, March 1970, p. 101

B. Mount et al. Death and dying: attitudes in a teaching hospital. Urology, December 1974, p. 741

M. Petrillo. Emotional Care of Hospitalized Children: An Environmental Approach. J. B. Lippincott Co., 1972

E. Plank. Working With Children In Hospitals. The Press of Case Western Reserve University, 1971

D. Popoff. What are your feelings about death and dying? Nursing 75, Aug/Sept 1975, Parts I, II, III

J. Spinetta et al. Anxiety in the dying child. Pediatrics, December 1973, p. 841

Brain Cancers

J. Clausen. Cancer diagnosis in children: cultural factors influencing parent/child reactions. Cancer Nursing, October 1978, p. 395

J. Menkes. Textbook of Child Neurology. Lee and Febiger, 1974

M. Meyers et al. Survival and Mortality for Children Under 15 Years of Age. American Cancer Society, 1976

F. Pilapil and K. Studva. Cancer chemotherapy: Programmed instruction in cancer care. Cancer Nursing, August 1978, p. 337

D. Smith et al. Nursing care of patients undergoing combination radiotherapy. Cancer Nursing, April 1978, p. 249

W. Fietz et al. Family sequelae after a child's death due to cancer. American Journal Psychotherapy, July 1977, p. 417

M. Walker. Treatment of brain tumors. Medical Clinics of North America, September 1977, p. 1045

Reye's Syndrome

B. Conway. Textbook of Child Neurology. C. V. Mosby Co., 1977

M. Edwards. Reye's Syndrome. Nursing Times, July 1977, p. 1039

M. Flammary and J. Holm. The child with Reye's Syndrome. Nursing 76, June 1976, p. 80c

J. Haller. Recent developments in etiology and therapy of Reye's syndrome. Clinical Neurosurgery, 1978, p. 591

J. Menkes. Textbook of Child Neurology. Lea and Febiger, 1974

S. Newman. Reye's syndrome: success of supportive care. New England Journal of Medicine, November 1978, p. 1079

S. Page et al. Reye's syndrome: an overview of nursing and medical management. Issues in Comprehensive Pediatric Nursing, May 1977, p. 41

M. Pichichero et al. Recurrent Reye's Syndrome. American Journal of Diseases of Children, November 1978, p. 1097

E. Stassi et al. Pulmonary manifestation of Reye's syndrome: a mechanism of endogenous toxicity producing acute respiratory failure. Respiratory Care, April 1978, p. 384

M. Thaler. Metabolic mechanisms in Reye's syndrome: end of a mystery. American Journal of Diseases of Children, March 1976, p. 241

54

THE HOSPITALIZED SCHOOL-AGE CHILD

by Jo Joyce Tackett, BSN, MPHN

Because of the intellectual and emotional progress he has made during preschool years, the school-age child has fewer adjustment problems during hospitalization. He is now able to tolerate parental separation. Although he is not totally free of separation anxiety, he is more reality oriented. Unreasonable fantasies and fears are fewer in number and severity, and he is eager to form relationships and have experiences outside his family and home. Handled adequately, hospitalization may be perceived by the school-age child as an adventure during which he can learn many new things and make new friends. Regressive behavior is less frequent in school-agers; if regression does occur, this child will typically display the type of fears characteristic of preschoolers: fears of mutilation, monsters and separation.[3]

The predominant fears of the hospitalized school-age child are fears of bodily injury or loss of self-control and of death.[2] To reduce these fears, the nurse can provide procedural explanations, allow the child to participate in planning and doing his own care, and give instructions and honest answers about the child's illness and prognosis. Freed of excessive anxiety with the help of the nurse, the schooler is ready to make the most of his hospitalization as a growth experience.

As with care of children at other ages, care by the nurse of a school-age child is most effective when designed around the child's developmental needs or tasks. Therefore, knowledge of school-age growth and development is imperative to construction of a realistic care plan.

IMPACT OF HOSPITALIZATION ON NEEDS: NURSING IMPLICATIONS

Physically the school-age child has achieved complete control of body functions and the physical self-care required in daily living. This independence in self-care reinforces a healthy image and builds self-confidence; therefore, allowing the ill child to perform his own tasks of daily living during the hospital experience, at least to the degree he can tolerate, is of obvious importance. School-age children are intent on developing their fine motor skills. They need to continue practicing fine motor tasks during hospitalization so that they can keep abreast of their peers. The nurse can make use of this developmental challenge by actively involving the child in the education regarding his disease and treatment and by inviting him to participate in aspects of his treatment that require fine motor function (Table 54–1).

Intellectually the school-age child is in the period of concrete operations. He bases perceptions on reality progressively more often than on fantasy. Most of the fears he retains involve situations that threaten to cause him loss of

TABLE 54-1 DEVELOPMENTAL NEEDS OF SCHOOL-AGE CHILDREN AND RELATED NURSING INTERVENTIONS

Need	Nursing Intervention
I. Physical A. Complete control of body functions and self-care.	1. Allow independent self-care to extent feasible by treatment restrictions and child's tolerance. 2. Praise for whatever self-care child does do. 3. Attempt to maintain usual routines related to body function and self-care.
B. Develop fine motor skills.	1. Provide materials for fine motor activities (pencils and crayons, scissors, Legos, computer games, hospital equipment safe for play that requires finger manipulation). 2. Encourage child to draw pictures of body and its parts during discussions of disease and treatment (see Fig. 54-1.) This gives nurse feedback as to accuracy of child's interpretation of information given. 3. Encourage child to "take notes" during patient education sessions — gives practice in fine motor dexterity required for printing or writing. 4. Teach child to participate in treatments that give practice in fine motor skills.
II. Intellectual A. Developing rational thinking, reality orientation.	1. Provide scientific descriptions of the child's disease and body responses during educational sessions or in reply to his questions. 2. Offer a rationale for each procedure before doing it and during education sessions. This knowledge helps the child to maintain self-control during procedures and to participate when feasible. 3. Provide child with rules about what he may and may not do during hospitalization, because of the disease or during a treatment. Some children enjoy writing out a list of rules to post at their bedside. 4. Determine if child perceives the hospitalization as a punishment; intervene as for preschooler if he does. 5. Provide opportunities for child to make decisions about his routine, treatments and daily care whenever choices actually exist. The middle school-age child enjoys helping to devise his care plan and seeing it written out on the Kardex or chart.
B. Mastering concepts of conservation, classification, combination skills.	1. Allow child to participate in care by helping to keep track of intake and output, writing down his vital signs, counting the seconds or adding up the minutes it takes to complete a procedure. 2. Encourage the child who can tell time to inform the nurse when it is time for a procedure or when it is time to stop the procedure (when time to take out thermometer, when time to take off wet, warm soaks, etc.). 3. Encourage scrapbook making, collections, diary keeping (according to child's interests) during hospital stay.

Table continued on opposite page

control or bodily injury.[2] He accepts that there are various points of view beyond his own. Because he can now reason out cause-and-effect relationships, he is intrigued by the scientific process and wants scientific explanations regarding his disease, the sensations he can expect during his hospitalization, and the rationale behind his treatments.[11]

Rules help the school-age child think rationally. If rules are not provided, he will construct his own rules, which are often more rigid than those an adult would supply. The early school-age child still perceives that injuries and misfortunes such as put him in the hospital are punishment for his own misdeeds; he will need the same reassurances of blamelessness that the preschooler required. As he loses his egocentric focus, the school-ager relies more on past memories and reason to make decisions; magical thinking disappears by middle school-age (8 to 10 years). The concepts of conservation, classification and combinations (time, space, numbers) are mastered during school-age years; he is then able to solve concrete problems that he can manipulate or mentally visualize. This intellect may be advantageously utilized to involve the child actively in planning and carrying out his treatment regimen (Table 54-1).

The school-age child has mastered language and is now learning to use that language to express his needs and feelings during stress

TABLE 54–1 DEVELOPMENTAL NEEDS OF SCHOOL-AGE CHILDREN AND RELATED NURSING INTERVENTIONS (Continued)

Need	Nursing Intervention
	4. Utilize these concepts in teaching sessions. 5. Provide games that require use of these concepts (card games, Monopoly, Yatzee). 6. Provide hospital school or tutor schoolwork.
C. Vocalization of feelings during stress.	1. Encourage child to verbalize feelings associated with hospitalization, disease, procedures by asking him questions ("How does it make you feel to have to miss school and be away from your friends?" or "Tell me what it is like to have to lie still for 30 minutes while those compresses are on.") 2. Schedule a few minutes each shift to be available simply to talk with the child, time not associated with any specific care or procedure. Let the child know that this is a time when he can talk about whatever he likes or ask any questions he has. Encourage parents to do the same.
III. Emotional and Social A. Latency — channel drives into socially acceptable behaviors; peer relations.	1. Do not place girls and boys in the same room. 2. Provide opportunities for the school-age child to interact with other hospitalized school-agers. 3. Determine if child has preschool residual concerns re genitalia; manage as for preschooler (see Chapter 45). 4. Help child maintain peer group contact via phone calls, letter writing, tape recordings, peer visitation, photo exchanges. (Teachers and parents are usually willing to help arrange these things.) 5. Arrange group education sessions for children with similar problems. Include discussions of how problems are similar and how they differ. Involve children in teaching each other about anatomy and physiology, disease process, treatment, under nurse supervision. 6. Treat any separation anxiety as for preschooler (see Chapter 45). 7. Encourage parents to express affection toward their hospitalized school-ager and to continue setting limits as before hospitalization.
B. Industry and associated developing self-concept.	1. Praise cooperation efforts, self-care accomplishments, participation in treatments and any other achievements. Praise honestly and often. 2. Provide opportunities for built-in successes several times daily. (Assign tasks the child is known to be able to accomplish.) 3. Provide opportunities for peer cooperation and competition. (See whether child or roommate can have largest fluid intake by noon, assuming each is to have fluids pushed, or solicit roommate's help in entertaining an immobilized child). 4. Actively involve child in his care and treatments. 5. Balance quiet and solitary activity with more active and peer activity as tolerated.

rather than using regressive or defiant behavior to communicate. Stollak's[20] research produced a communication model that effectively draws out the child's unverbalized reactions and opens up verbal communication. Stollak applied the model to children's drawings and play activities in stressful situations such as hospitalization. Using this model the nurse, parent or play therapist communicates that (1) she understands the child's needs, (2) she accepts the feelings he is expressing and (3) she can identify what she feels about the child's thoughts or actions. Table 54–2 summarizes Stollak's model. The nurse using this model helps the school-ager learn how to describe his feelings and teaches parents a new way to cope with their child's feelings and behaviors at home. If he is not given opportunity for verbal expression during his hospitalization, the school-ager will revert to the behavioral expressions characteristic of his earlier development.

Emotionally and socially the school-age child begins undertaking tasks that will lead him into healthy, productive adult relationships once the tasks are refined in adolescence. One challenge of this period (latency) is the channelling of emotional, physical and sexual drives into socially acceptable behaviors. The early school-age child (6 to 7 years) may have residual fears from preschool years regarding the genitalia. This period is one of general intolerance toward

TABLE 54-2 STOLLAK'S COMMUNICATION MODEL TO FACILITATE THE CHILD'S VERBALIZATION OF FEELINGS[20]

Feeling Adult Communicates	How Feeling Communicated	Benefit to Child
Understanding	Adult communicates directly to child that she is aware of and understands the child's need — i.e., tells the child what she thinks he is feeling and what he seems to need or want.	Adult's verbalization helps child understand his feeling and learn words to describe the feeling.
Acceptance	Adult clearly states that she accepts the child's feelings and needs but not necessarily the behavior he is using to express the need or feeling. All *feelings* should be accepted.	Maintains child's self-esteem. Reassurance in knowing he is accepted despite his feeling or need.
Identification	Adult states what she thinks and feels about the child's thoughts, feelings and actions. If action unacceptable: Exact message is given as to how the adult wants him to express his feeling right now (give 2–3 options if possible). Exact message is given as to way(s) adult would like him to express the feeling in the future.	Informs child that others also have feelings and that his feelings or actions create feelings in others. Child learns socially acceptable means to express his feelings and needs during stress.

opposite-sex peers; same-sex peers develop gangs or clubs and engage in intimate "best friend" relationships. Out of these relationships comes the learning of sex roles and the "give-and-take" prerequisite to healthy heterosexual relationships that come later in life. These factors should be considered when making room assignments and structuring activities on the hospital unit.

The hospitalized school-age child worries about whether he will retain his peer group memberships and what the group is saying and thinking about him in his absence.

To the extent that he is invested in non-family relationships, the school-age child is able to bear parental and sibling separation.[7] What he needs from parents during his school-age years is assurance that they love him and that they will provide limits to help him maintain self-control. This affection and limit-setting is increasingly important during periods of crisis such as hospitalization.

The school-ager thrives on doing things and seeing how things work. His industrious nature is tempered by a fear of failure. He tends to depend almost entirely on external evidence of his worth and is continually self-critical. At this most critical stage in his developing concept of self, the school-ager needs lots of praise, frequent built-in successes and assistance to maintain self-control.[7] Although he compares himself regularly with his peers and siblings, he cannot tolerate such comparisons to be made by parents or others. Table 54–1 describes nursing actions to meet the school-ager's emotional and social needs.

NURSING ACTIONS TO FACILITATE ADJUSTMENT TO EACH PHASE OF HOSPITALIZATION

At any age adaptation is facilitated when the unknown becomes the known. The school-age child, with his ability to reason and comprehend cause and effect, is readily instructed in what to expect during his hospitalization, provided that parents, nurses or others in his environment have made an effort to prepare him.

Preadmission Phase

As with the preschooler, books and film strips are excellent sources of information that can be reviewed to prepare the school-age child for his hospital encounter. If the school-ager reads these himself, time should be provided to discuss what he read and his reactions to it with an adult who can offer additional information and correct any misconceptions. The school-age child also benefits from a hospital tour while he is well (see discussion of hospital tours in Chapters 16 and 45).

A few creative pediatric hospital units have

even devised "pre-op parties" for children scheduled for surgery.[5] The children come to the pediatric unit for a party a couple of weeks before admission. Time is allocated for therapeutic play with hospital equipment and attire as well as other age-appropriate toys and games. After the playtime, refreshments are served, and a slide presentation showing the entire hospital routine for a surgical patient is shown by one of the pediatric nurses. The nurse who narrates the slides also encourages questions and answers any the children may have. The party lasts about an hour but saves hours of extra nursing time required by the child who is not adapting to the hospital experience because of lack of preparation and information.

Some hospital units also arrange for a home visit by the primary nurse before admission. During this visit the child is introduced to the hospital environment through storybooks or film strips and the nurse answers the child's and parents' questions to prepare them for the hospital experience.[17]

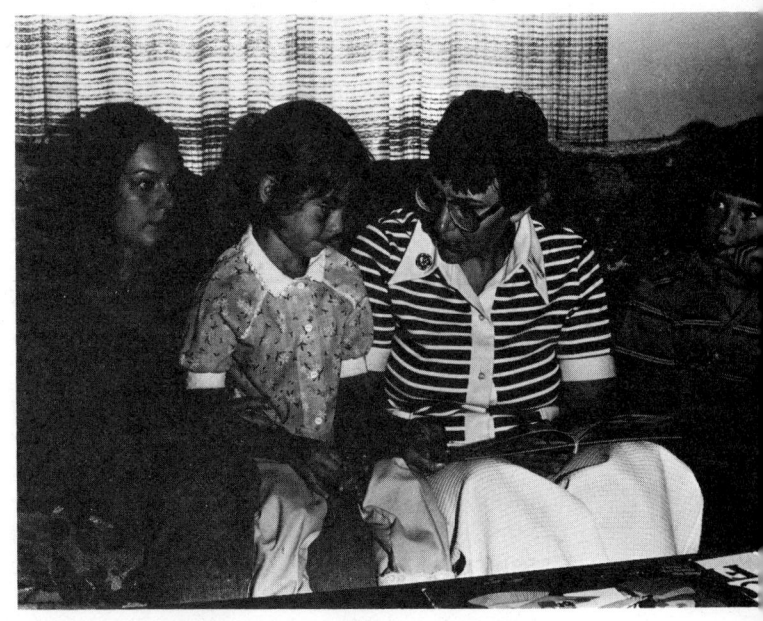

During a preadmission home visit, this nurse introduces the young patient and her family to the hospital environment through stories, and discussion of their concerns.

Admission Phase

Adams'[1] studies revealed that most children have only vague, general and usually distorted ideas about why they are being hospitalized and what will happen to them while they are in the hospital. In addition, Adams found that parents usually had an equally vague understanding of their child's hospitalization. This lack of knowledge was responsible for increasing the typical fears and anxieties associated with the child's health state and with giving over his care to strangers. Parents also worry about the impending separation and effects on their other children during this crisis. Rasmussen and Murphy's study also revealed the admission experience to be confusing to the child and his parents.[17] Their suggestion to help the child adapt and maintain control during hospitalization, starting from the moment of admission, is for the nurse to look at the pediatric unit — its activities, personnel and equipment — through the child's eyes. The nurse can then respond to the child's needs, questions and fears from his point of view.

The school-age child can and should be encouraged to contribute to his admission interview. The nurse facilitates the child's involvement by addressing her questions and conversation directly to him. Seeking his opinions reinforces his concept of self-worth, gives him a sense of control and affords the nurse an opportunity to learn his perceptions and fantasies. Once the child has contributed his information the nurse can then ask the parents to fill in any additional information and she can elicit their questions and concerns. Ideally the school-age child is interviewed separately from his parents; this is easily facilitated when the interviewing room has a play area at one end or in an area connected by an open door (allows child to see that his parent is still around). The nurse should address some questions to each parent if both are present so that each is included and has an opportunity to contribute to the interview.

The end of the interview with the child and then with the parents affords the nurse a good opportunity to talk about the purpose for hospitalization and what is likely to happen, to discuss how the child and parents will each be able to help in the plan of care, and to share any rules applicable to the child or parents during the hospital stay. (These rules should be in writing, too.) The nurse should voice her understanding that the parents know what is best for their child and that she will need them to work with her to see that his needs are met in the hospital.

If the child has not previously toured the unit he should receive a tour and be introduced to a few other children and his roommate(s). Explanations should be offered for all admission procedures and instruction given as to how the child may cooperate or participate to get procedures over quickly. The school-ager is still young enough to benefit from a primary nurse; ideally the primary nurse introduces him to others on the unit and provides the procedural explanations, staying with him during the procedure if his parents cannot. Rasmussen and Murphy also suggest that, once the child is situated in his room, he be asked if there are any objects in the room that he is unfamiliar with and introduce him to these objects and their function. The child should be encouraged to investigate and handle these objects in the nurse's presence and should be given simple, neutral but truthful answers to any questions the objects prompt.

Parents should also be encouraged to care for their child as they would at home and should be shown how things are done and where objects and facilities are found that they may need during the hospital stay. Clear guidelines should be provided regarding what parents may do themselves and what the nurse will do for them. They will also benefit from an introduction to another parent whose child is hospitalized on the unit.

Treatment Phase

Although the school-age child adapts without too much trauma to his hospital stay, there are nursing actions that will facilitate his adaptation. These include (1) preparing him for procedures and treatments through education sessions, (2) providing opportunities for expression through play and verbal exchange, and (3) allowing and encouraging the child's active participation in planning and carrying out his treatment regimen.

Education The school-age child wants explanations about his disease process and treatment plan. He needs to be provided with a rationale for each procedure before it is done; such knowledge helps him to maintain control and cooperate during the procedure. The teaching plan for this age child is like that for the preschooler (for a review see Chapter 45), but he is more enthusiastic and is able to reason, so content can be more complex. His attention span is longer, allowing him to pay attention to a topic for 30 to 45 minutes if he is actively involved in some way; he can handle slightly more content per session than can the preschooler. Expressions of questions, concerns and feelings should be encouraged and explored. Body outlines, models, games and puppets can be used to help him visualize verbal explanations and to solicit his active involvement.[10, 15, 16, 20] The boxed material summarizes what research has revealed is the typical view of the school-ager regarding the body. The nurse should determine what the school-age child's response to use of a doll is likely to be before using one for demonstrating procedures. Some school-age children enjoy dolls; others are embarrassed at the idea of "playing with" a doll.[16] Sometimes acceptance is obtained by referring to the doll as a "dummy" or "model" and by using a doll that is "grown up" (Barby and Ken dolls). Many of these children, especially those of early school age, still benefit from therapeutic play that allows handling of the equipment and doll or dummy play.[6]

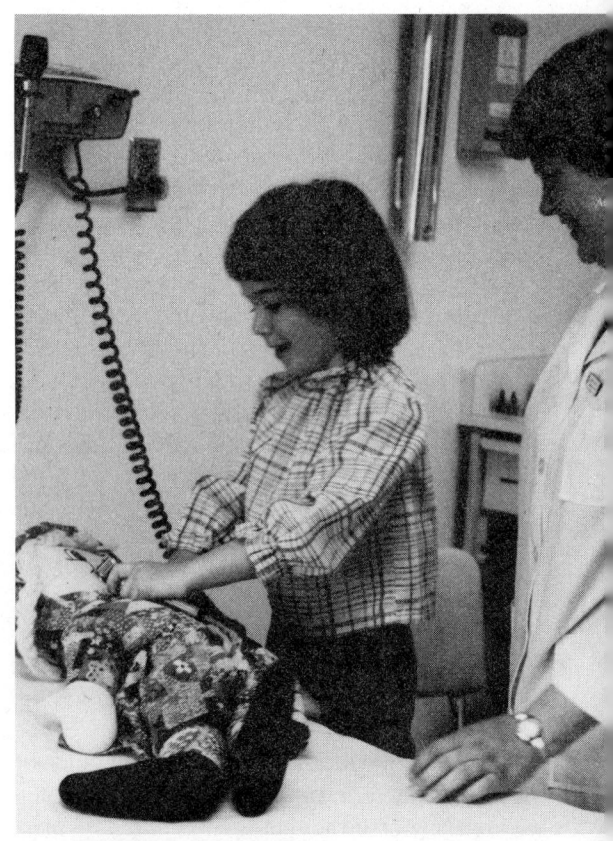

The school-age child, especially if under 9, will benefit from therapeutic play. This girl gives her doll an examination just after she herself has undergone one. (Photograph by Cynthia Stewart.)

HOW THE SCHOOL-AGER VIEWS HIS BODY

Research conducted by Nagy[14] and later by Gelbert[8] revealed how children perceive their bodies in terms of content and function at various ages. Body outlines were used along with interviews to learn what children think their bodies contain, how body contents function and where these are located. The early school-age child (6 to 7 years) tends to maintain a preschooler view of the body that centers on what is ingested and egested (Fig. 54-1). Thus, the body is perceived to be composed of food, water, urine and feces. In addition, the early school-ager also recognizes bones, brain, and eyes as body parts. The middle school-age child (8 to 10 years) concentrates more on permanent body parts, including muscles, bones, and the heart (usually drawn as a valentine shape) and blood vessels (Fig. 54-1). He also identifies eyes and a brain, which he believes is made of bone (probably associated with the skull). The middle school-ager usually locates the stomach low in the abdomen and overestimates its size. The liver is also included in his drawing. He associates the heart with breathing.

The older school-age child (11 to 12 years) identifies the same body parts as the middle school-ager (Fig. 54-1), although the location and size are usually more realistic with the exception of the stomach, which remains oversized and low. At this age the child begins to associate the relationship of the lungs and heart to breathing and circulation.

Individual children, regardless of age, may also identify organs with which they have had special experiences. For example, the child who has had frequent ear infections or a myringotomy includes the ear canals in his drawing. If pain or surgery has been associated with an organ, that organ often will be drawn in a distorted or oversized manner.

Procedural instruction can be provided a day or two in advance with a quick review just before the procedure, unless the child is immature. In this case instruction should immediately precede the procedure. The nurse should be honest and specific about what parts of the body will be involved in the procedure, since the school-age child retains fear of bodily harm.[2]

Because the school-age child is preoccupied with body function and fears body injury, he needs procedural instructions that cover what will happen, with an emphasis on the sensations that he can expect and the behaviors that are acceptable during the procedure (what he may do or not do that will help).[11, 12, 19] His developing concept of temporality makes him keenly interested in knowing the timetable of events.[12] Allowing time for the school-age child to verbalize his fears and feelings permits him to formulate a reality focus that increases his ability to cope with the procedure and the pain involved.[19] Shaefer[18] found that school-age children respond positively to group education sessions and often are supportive of each other.

Since the school-age child may be embarrassed by crying or screaming, he should be offered alternative outlets for pain or fear such as squeezing the parent's or nurse's hand, counting, engaging in diversional conversation, or clenching his teeth; if he does scream or cry he should not be shamed ("Big boys don't cry") but reassured that such expression is normal and OK. Most school-age children still prefer a parent's presence during procedures and passively seek contact with their eyes or through facial expression, but they should be offered the option of having or not having a parent present. The school-ager is able to hold still for a procedure and usually invests most of his energy in retaining self-control.[4] If he receives praise for holding still and for other evidence of cooperation or participation, the likelihood of his future cooperation is increased.

Even though the school-age child has mastered language, his behavior continues to be the best indicator of the presence and intensity of pain. This child's physical responses are those typical of an adult, including skin pallor or flushing, elevation in vital signs, pupil dilation and diaphoresis. Verbal complaints of pain are often disguised as requests for comforting or distraction or pleas for companionship.[19] The middle school-age child can rate the intensity of his pain on a scale from 1 to 10, and all school-age children can describe what helps to relieve their pain.[12] Nonverbal expressions of pain may include grimacing, fist or jaw clenching, rigidity, twisting or turning, and movement away from a painful situation. Pain intensity is

Age 3 yr 11 mo   Age 7 yr 6 mo

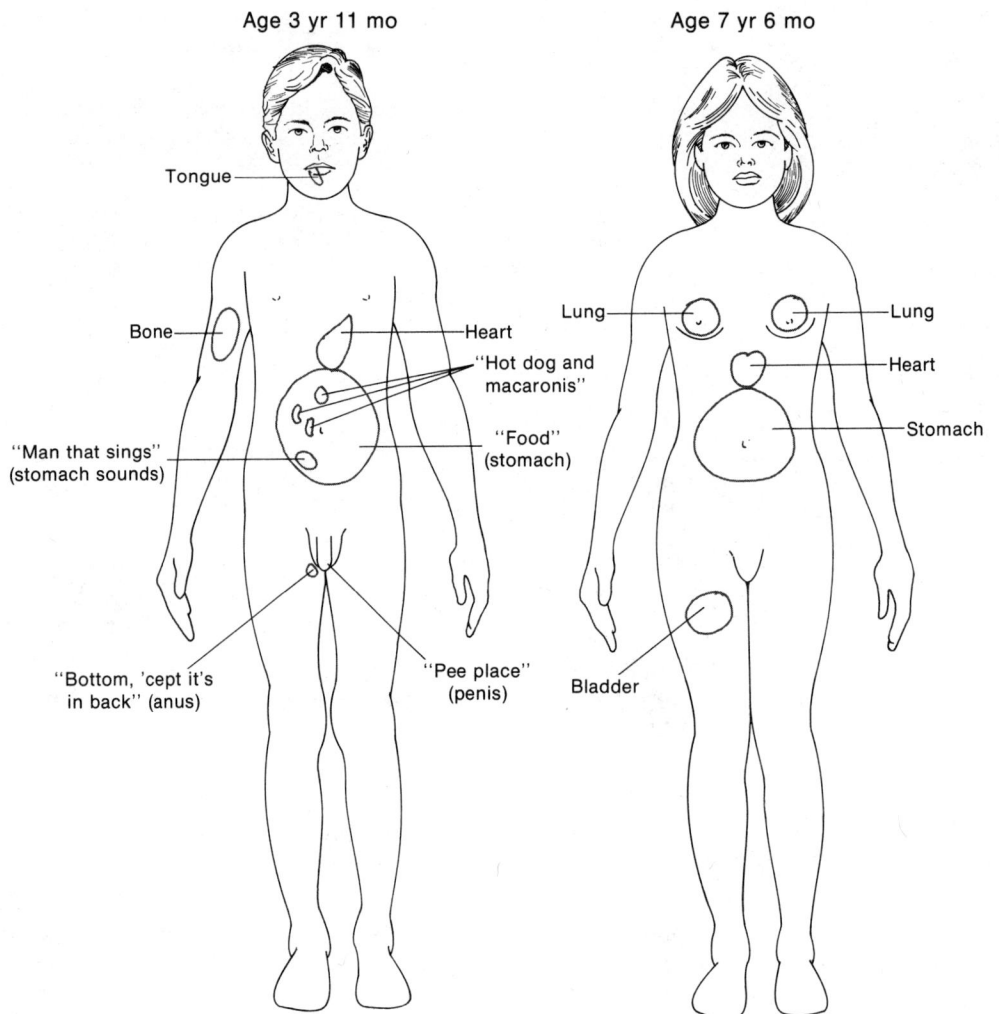

Figure 54-1 How a school-age child views his body. Examples of children's placement of body organs on a pre-drawn form.

TABLE 54-3 A COMPARISON OF PAIN PERCEPTION IN THE YOUNG SCHOOL-AGE AND OLDER SCHOOL-AGE CHILD[9, 19]

Young School Age (5–7 years)	Older School Age (8–11 or 12 years)
Fears body mutilation.	Fears body injury.
Cannot localize or describe pain.	Can define intensity of pain on scale of 1 to 10; can point to region of pain if pain is not constant.
Pain equated with punishment. Perceives infliction of pain as deliberate and mean.	Understands the reason for pain if it is explained and sees inflicted pain as necessary to improve health.
Not reassured by statements that the pain will be brief or soon be over.	Understands and is reassured by the time limits of pain (has learned temporal concept).
Determines what is painful and how to react to pain by others' reactions and by the nature of equipment involved.	Exaggerates every little scratch, tends to brag about his hurts and compare his hurts with those of his siblings and peers. He submerges his fear of pain in bravado (especially boys) or nervous behavior (more in girls). Fears being treated like a baby or succumbing to tears during pain.
Centers on one object as the source of pain.	Comprehends cause(s) of pain. Pain creates self-anger because this age child dislikes physical restrictions imposed by pain.

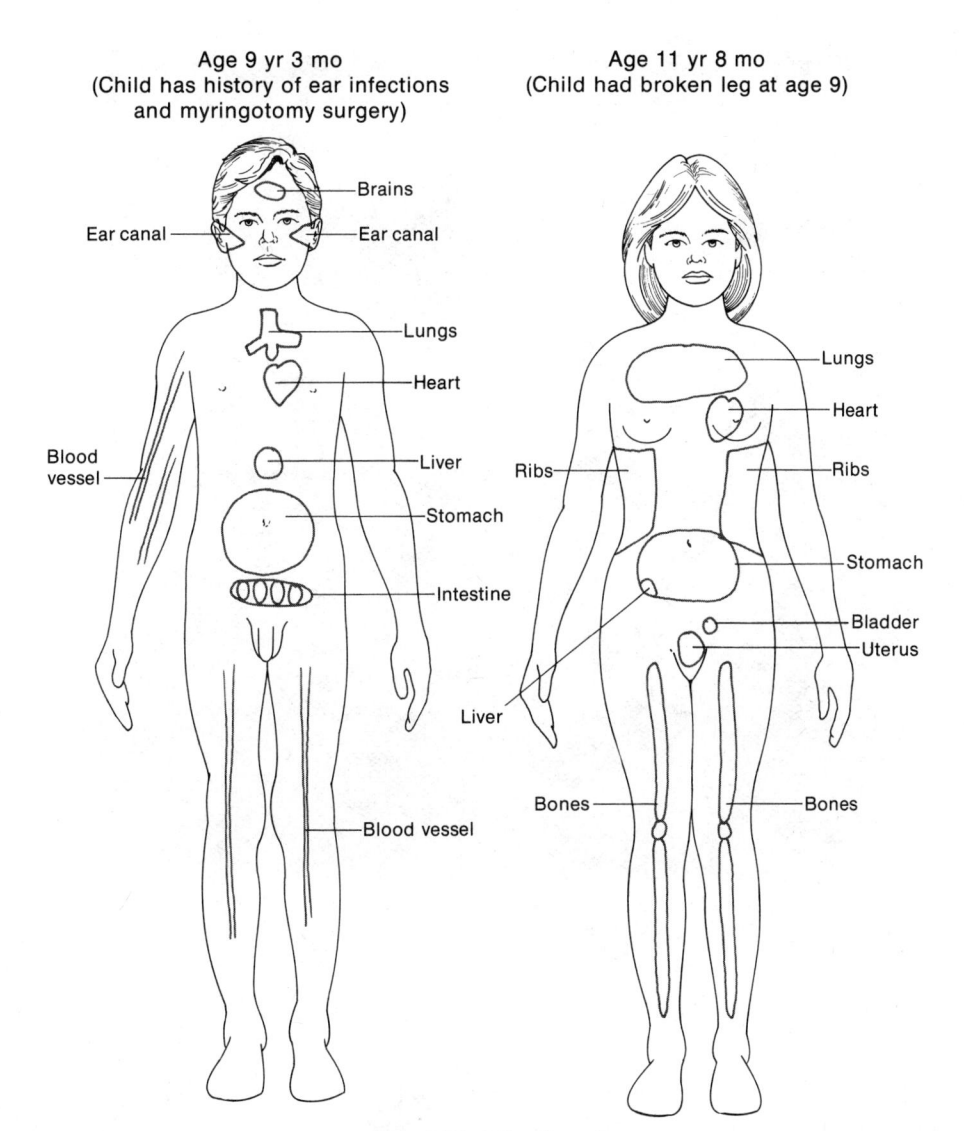

Age 9 yr 3 mo
(Child has history of ear infections and myringotomy surgery)

- Brains
- Ear canal
- Ear canal
- Lungs
- Heart
- Blood vessel
- Liver
- Stomach
- Intestine
- Blood vessel

Age 11 yr 8 mo
(Child had broken leg at age 9)

- Lungs
- Heart
- Ribs
- Ribs
- Stomach
- Bladder
- Uterus
- Liver
- Bones
- Bones

Figure 54–1 Continued

usually identified as increasing when parents leave, when the child is tired, just before an anticipated unfamiliar procedure, or during other stressful experiences.[12] As pain increases the child withdraws from interaction with his environment, becoming increasingly preoccupied with his body.[12] Table 54–3 compares what the research of Shultz[19] revealed as the characteristic perceptions of early school-age and middle school-age children to pain.

The nurse should be alert to assess signs of pain in the school-age child and help him to verbalize his pain if possible. Little research is available on the frequency and amounts of dosages of analgesics effective for children. Since the tendency is for the child to convey his pain nonverbally, pain and its effective relief are often overlooked. McCaffery[13] has investigated several nonpharmacological modes for pain relief that the nurse may readily employ with school-age children. The most obvious approach is to learn from the child and his parents what they have discovered relieves the pain and apply those techniques.

Before painful procedures the likelihood of pain should be acknowledged and discussed with the school-age child so he has time to play out his fears and diminish his fantasies regarding the pain or the procedure or both. Pain relief measures can also be taught and practiced before the painful event. Children with extremely high anxiety may be taught the relief measures without the description of the painful event ahead. Distraction that focuses the child's thoughts away from the pain is very effective in

THE HOSPITALIZED SCHOOL-AGE CHILD

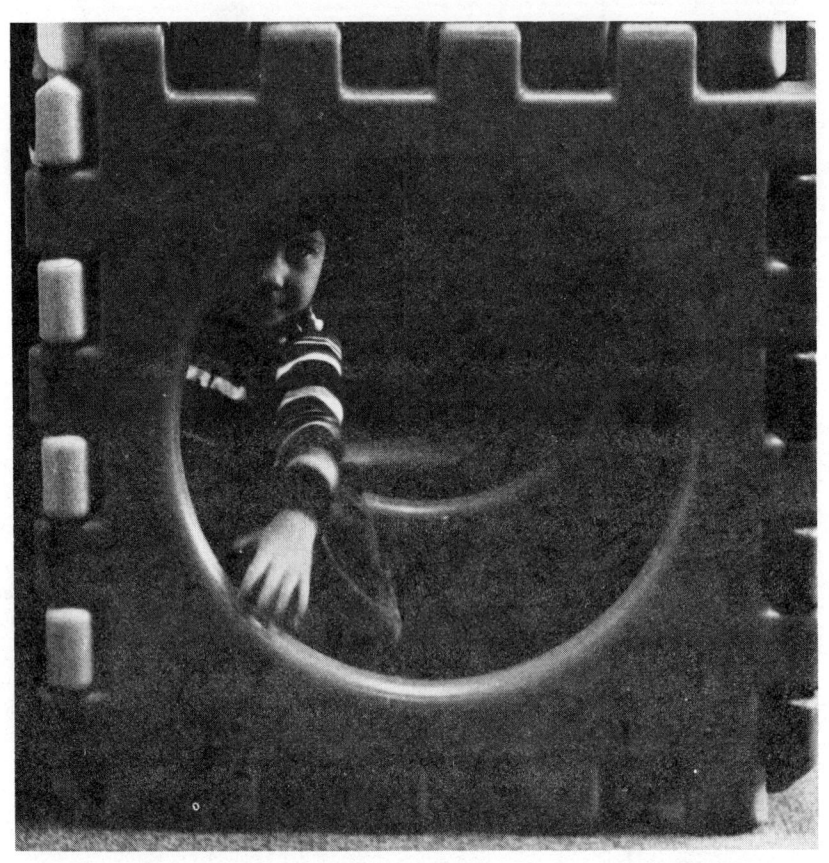

Hide-and-seek and other organized games are preferred by the school-age child over unstructured group play in the hospital play area. (Photograph by Cynthia Stewart.)

reducing pain intensity. Counting, rhymes and riddles, games such as "I'm hiding in . . . ," reading stories, or chants and blowing that employ the techniques of relaxation breathing (like that used during labor) are all distractors with appeal to the school-age child. Relaxation techniques might include music, massage or instructing the child to begin yawning or to go limp like a rag doll may also successfully relieve pain. Cutaneous stimulation (rubbing, massaging, vibrating) of moderate intensity that is rhythmic and constant decreases the transmission of pain impulses and thereby reduces pain. All these techniques may be initiated by the nurse and taught to the child so that he may use them, or parents or siblings may be instructed in how to employ these techniques with the child.

The school-age child usually handles two common procedures — taking oral medication and receiving injections — without much trauma. He generally cooperates in taking oral medicines, although younger school-age children prefer to chew pills rather than swallow them whole. If the oral medication has a bad taste when chewed or if it is in capsule form, the child may manage to take it whole if it is offered with a spoonful of ice cream or applesauce to help it slide down.

The recommended injection site for school-age children is the ventrogluteal muscle.[1] This site is easily located because of the readily palpable bony landmarks; it contains no important nerves or blood vessels and is a large muscle mass with minimal subcutaneous tissue. Use of the vastus lateralis site is frequently opposed by the school-age child, but it should be used along with the ventrogluteal and posterior gluteal sites when frequent injections or long-term intramuscular therapy is likely. The school-age child also copes better with injections when they are administered promptly and when he is given a choice as to site. (See

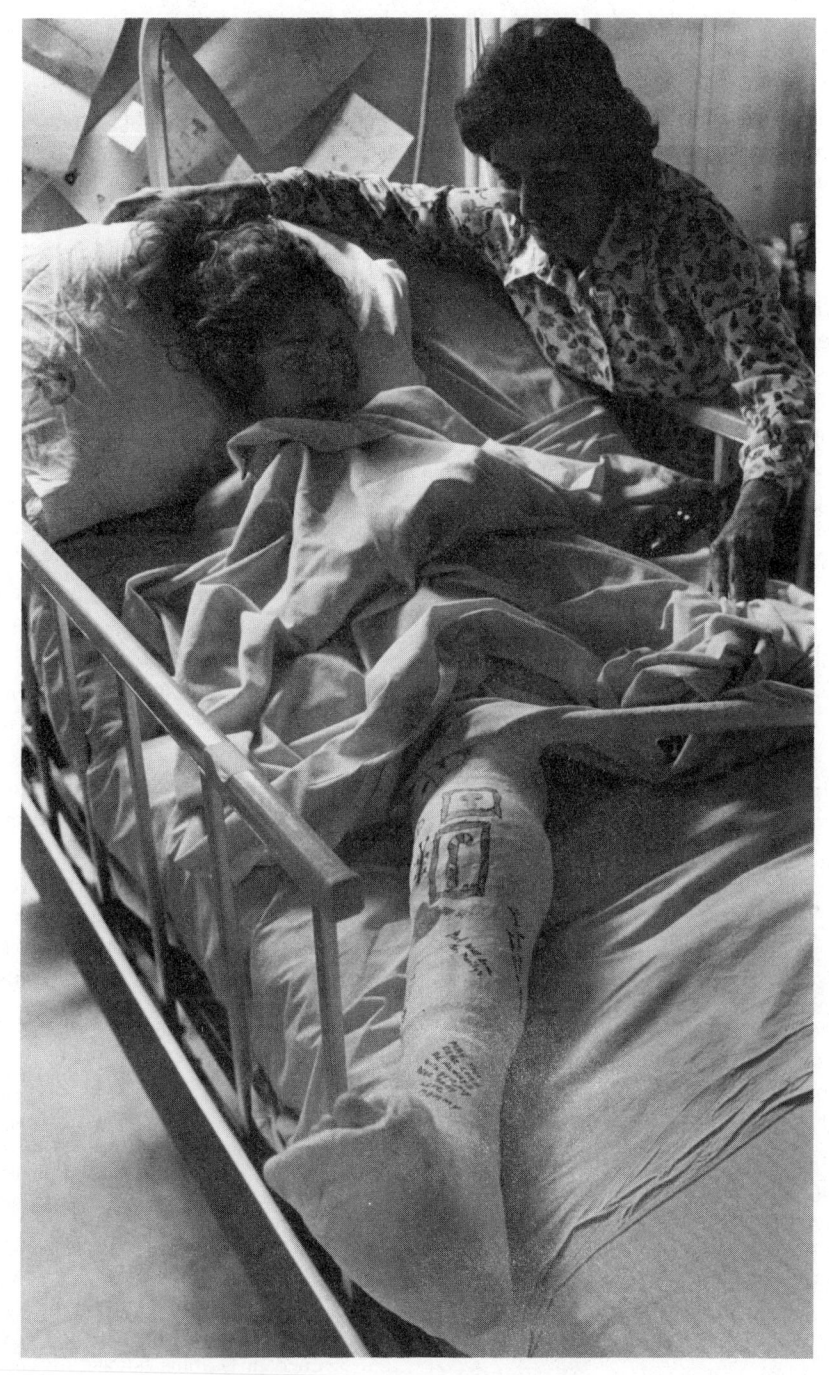

The hospitalized school-age child needs to know that her family loves her and is thinking of her.

Appendix VII for an illustration of injection techniques.)

Play Although the school-age child preserves some of the fantasy and drama in his play from his preschool days, his play has changed in several recognizable ways. He has added rules, ritualistic behaviors and language chants ("Step on a crack, break your mother's back") and team activities. The nurse or play therapist who organizes structured play activities on the school-age unit should keep these facts in mind. School-agers tend to prefer games, both active and sedentary, to unstructured group play. The school-age child also enjoys the reprieve of

THE HOSPITALIZED SCHOOL-AGE CHILD 1211

quiet and solitary activity (board games, reading books, writing stories or drawing pictures). Although he can now read books on his own, he still enjoys being read to occasionally. Therapeutic play equipment should remain available to the school-age child but should not be forced upon him.

Participation in Care The school-age child's industrious drive makes him an eager candidate to participate actively in his treatment regimen. He still finds security in a routine and willingly helps to structure what the routine will be. His understanding of time makes him capable of "helping" the nurse stay with the planned routine. Although he will require supervision, the school-age child can perform a large variety of treatments himself after adequate instruction and practice. The opportunity to actively participate in planning and doing his care bolsters the school-age child's self-concept, stimulates him intellectually and provides opportunity for refinement of motor skills. School-age children can also be invaluable in helping to teach or motivate self-care in their peers.[18]

Discharge Phase

Nursing actions for the school-age child during the discharge phase are similar to those for the preschooler (see Chapter 45). Having him write or tell a story about his hospital experience is a useful way to discover any misconceptions he has about this experience. These misconceptions should be corrected through discussion. The young school-age child is particularly interested in taking home mementos of his experience to show his peers. School-agers also appreciate the invitation to revisit the unit at any time, since they will have made some peer attachments if their hospitalization has been of any appreciable length.

NEEDS OF THE FAMILY

Even though the school-age child is moving away from his family toward peer influence, parents and siblings still remain a major influence in his life. He needs parents now who relate as adults, not pals — he needs someone he can turn to during stress and count on to set limits and control him when he cannot. These facts are evident when the school-ager is hospitalized. Although he does not need them continually present, he does need frequent assurances that his parents love him and that they are thinking about him. He will want them present during painful procedures and when he is feeling acutely ill.[16] The school-age child does not require the presence of one parent over the other as the younger child does. This fact helps parents share in the task of being with their sick child with less guilt.

Parents may need assistance to respect and permit their child's contributions to his own treatment regimen. The nurse can provide reassurance that the child's participation is welcomed by the staff and can encourage the parents' participation in the teaching process and in supervising their child in self-care.

Although the school-age child's family experiences the same needs, feelings and concerns as other families when any of their children are hospitalized (see Chapter 16 for the impact of hospitalization on families), parents whose hospitalized child is of school age usually adapt to the fact of hospitalization with less conflict than those with younger hospitalized children. This is attributable to the fact that the school-age child is more independent and can verbally express his feelings and needs; therefore parents feel less of a need to be continuously present to interpret their child's needs to hospital staff.

References

1. M. Adams. The hospital through a child's eyes. Children, February 1965, p. 102
2. E. Astin. Self-reported fears of hospitalized and nonhospitalized children aged 10 to 12. Maternal Child Nursing Journal, Spring 1977, p. 17
3. M. Ageel. Reactions of a hospitalized school-age child to separation and restricted mobility. Maternal Child Nursing Journal, Fall 1978, p. 163
4. P. Brandt et al. Injections in children. American Journal of Nursing, August 1972, p. 1402
5. S. Condon. Daytime hospital for children. American Journal of Nursing, August 1972, p. 1431
6. B. Elmassian. A practical approach to communicating with children through play. American Journal of Maternal Child Nursing, Jul/Aug 1979, p. 238
7. F. Erickson. Helping the sick child maintain behavioral control. Nursing Clinics of North America, December 1967, p. 695
8. E. Gelbert. What do I have inside me? How children view their bodies. In Psychosocial Aspects of Pediatric Care by E. Gelbert, Grune and Stratton, 1978
9. J. Gildea and T. Quirk. Assessing the pain experience in children. Nursing Clinics of North America, December 1977, p. 631
10. C. Green. Larry thought puppet-play "childish" but it helped him face his fears. Nursing 75, March 1975, p. 301

11. J. Johnson et al. Easing children's fright during health care procedures. American Journal of Maternal-Child Nursing, Jul/Aug 1976, p. 206
12. M. McBride. Assessing children with pain. Pediatric Nursing, Jul/Aug 1977, p. 7
13. M. McCaffery. Pain relief for the child. Pediatric Nursing, Jul/Aug 1977, p. 11
14. M. Nagy. Children's concepts of some bodily functions. Journal of Genetic Psychology, March 1953, p. 199
15. M. Norbeta. Caring for children with the help of puppets. American Journal of Maternal Child Nursing, Jan/Feb 1976, p. 22
16. M. Petrillo and S. Sanger. Emotional Care of Hospitalized Children. J. B. Lippincott Co., 197
17. M. Rasmussen and C. Murphy. Hospital admission through a child's eyes. Pediatric Nursing, May/June 1977, p. 43
18. S. Shaefer. Communicating with children: teaching via the play discussion group. American Journal of Nursing, December 1977, p. 1960
19. N. Shultz. How children perceive pain. Nursing Outlook, October 1971, p. 760
20. G. Stollak. What Happened Today: Stories For Parents and Children. Kendall/Hunt Publishing Co., 1973

Additional Recommended Reading

M. Audettle. The significance of regressive behavior for the hospitalized child. Maternal Child Nursing Journal, Spring 1974, p. 31

P. Azarnoff and S. Flegal. A Pediatric Play Program. Charles C Thomas, 1975

F. Erickson. When 6-12 year olds are ill. Nursing Outlook, July 1965, p. 48

D. Memalo. Body image concerns of a six year old boy. Maternal Child Nursing Journal, Fall 1978, p. 175

E. Plank. Working With Children In Hospital, 2nd ed. Year Book Medical Publishers, 1971

J. Robertson. Young Children in Hospital. Tavistock Publishing, 1970

M. Smart and R. Smart. School-Age Children: Development and Relationships, 2nd ed. McMillan, Inc. 1978

NURSING CARE PLAN FOR THE SCHOOL-AGE CHILD WITH NEUROLOGICAL ALTERATION
by Florence Nezamis

Nursing Diagnosis	Expected Outcome	Nursing Interventions	Rationale
Altered Neurological Status	1. a. Immediate: The patient's present neurological status will be maintained, attempting to prevent further damage by prompt treatment. b. Short term: The patient's neurological deficit will be diagnosed and, if possible, specific treatment given to resolve the cause. c. Long term: The patient's neurological status will be stabilized by discharge and he will achieve optimum functioning.	Dx: 1. Monitor vital signs. 2. Monitor pupillary reaction, level of consciousness, movement of extremities, occurrence of vomiting. 3. Record presence and position of headache; record seizure activity, noting frequency, duration, involved parts and apnea. Rx: 1. Maintain IV and fluid restriction. 2. Elevate head of bed 15°–30°. 3. Notify physician of any significant neurological changes or seizure activity. 4. Seizure precautions. Patient Education: 1. The child and/or significant other can state reason for frequent neurological assessment.	Dx: 1. Vital signs will change if intracranial pressure increases, causing hypertension, increasing pulse pressure, bradycardia, and irregular stertorous respirations. 2. Decreasing level of consciousness is earliest sign of increasing intracranial pressure. Generalized symptoms result from increased pressure being exerted throughout the brain, producing a widespread dysfunction of the nervous system. 3. Location of a headache and description of seizure activity gives information on location of lesion or injury. Rx: 1. Fluid overload will increase intracranial pressure — usually kept at 2/3 maintenance level. 2. Gravity may aid in draining cerebral spinal fluid (CSF) to decrease intracranial pressure. 3. Prompt notification and treatment will assist in preventing further damage. 4. This will prevent physical injury. Patient Education: 1. Knowledge that frequent assessment is necessary to determine degree of neurological stability and does not necessarily indicate that the child's status is critical puts anxiety in perspective. School-age child is usually cooperative if he is included and given reasons for interventions.

POSTOPERATIVE PERIOD (WHEN SURGICAL INTERVENTION IS INDICATED)

Dx:
1. Monitor vital signs q15" × 4, if stable q30" × 4, if stable q1° × 2, if stable q2°; q4° after 48°.
2. Neurological assessment (pupillary response, level of consciousness, movement of extremities, vomiting).
3. Check head dressing every 2 hr and record amount of drainage.
4. Observe for gastric bleeding by checking stools for occult blood.
5. Observe for CSF fluctuations within the ventriculostomy system every 2 hr.
6. Record amount and character of ventriculostomy drainage every shift.

Rx:
1. Child's head and ventriculostomy bottle should remain at level set by physician.
2. Maintain IV and fluid restrictions.
3. Give pain medication as ordered and note effectiveness.
4. Administer mannitol and/or steroids.
5. Encourage milk products as tolerated — give antacids as ordered.

Dx:
1. Increased pulse pressure, hypertension, bradycardia and irregular labored breathing results if intracranial pressure rises.
2. Increased intracranial pressure causes widespread nervous system dysfunction.
3. Clear or serous drainage denotes CSF leakage and could lead to infection if untreated.
4. Steroid therapy to reduce cerebral edema can result in gastric irritation and ulcers.
5. CSF fluctuation shows the patency of the system. If CSF does not fluctuate, the patient will begin to show signs of increased intracranial pressure.
6. Sanguinous fluid denotes bleeding within the ventricular system that may require surgical correction.

Rx:
1. If patient's head is lowered CSF will not drain; if it is raised too much CSF will be drawn out by gravity.
2. Fluid overload increases intracranial pressure. A deterioration in neurological status may occur as fluids are increased and steroids are tapered.
3. Pain can increase intracranial pressure.
4. These drugs reduce cerebral edema.
5. Milk and antacids will help decrease acidity in stomach and decrease chance of ulceration while on steroids.

Care Plan continued on following page

THE HOSPITALIZED SCHOOL-AGE CHILD 1215

NURSING CARE PLAN FOR THE SCHOOL-AGE CHILD WITH NEUROLOGICAL ALTERATION (Continued)

Nursing Diagnosis	Expected Outcome	Nursing Interventions	Rationale
		Patient Education: 1. The child or significant other can state signs and symptoms of increased ICP.	Patient Education: 1. Neurological deterioration can occur 2 weeks to 1 month after injury or postoperatively.

Interruption of emotional and social and intellectual development associated with physiologic emotional instability.	School-age child will have opportunities for developmental age that considers developmental age and personality changes.	Dx:
		1. Observe, assess and document emotional status regarding irritability, aggressiveness, or frequent fluctuations in emotions.
		
		Rx:
		1. Maintain an established daily routine that considers school-age child's physical, emotional and social and intellectual needs:
		  A. Primary nurse.
		  B. Hospital school and school work.
		  C. Peer group activities appropriate to neurological status.
		  D. Consistently scheduled time for procedures and treatments.
		2. Reassure re behavior. Diversion during procedure. Quieting environment. Sedation if too much tension. Use quieting toys and activities.
		3. Encourage parental participation in his daily routine care.
		
		Patient Education:
		1. Child and caretakers can state the reason for his change in personality.
		2. Parents can identify how to adapt behavior management during hospitalization to home and school.
			Dx:
			1. Medication may be required to control bizarre or disruptive behavior. Traumatized brain tissue, especially of frontal lobe, may result in interference in volitional control, personality and judgment.
			
			Rx:
			1. Things the school-age child can anticipate such as familiar activities and a consistent caretaker following a routine will be less threatening to him and help restore some sense of security. Peer participation, recognition and approval are becoming important to this child.
			2. Punitive measures will not change behavior since it has a physiological basis over which he has no control.
			3. The school-age child fears loss of parental affection. Their love for him must be reinforced no matter what behavior he manifests.
			
			Patient Education:
			1. Parents will be more tolerant of child's behavior if they understand it is physiologically based rather than purposeful misconduct.
			2. Though emotional lability is temporary, it may last 6 months to 1 year.

Problem	Goals	Orders
Interruption of motor development associated with paresis.	Short term: Patient's extremities will be maintained with full range of motion preventing contractures. Long term: Patient will reach optimum functioning in activities of daily living by discharge.	**Dx:** 1. Observe and record the degree of paresis every day. **Rx:** 1. Active and passive range-of-motion exercises to all extremities. 2. Assist patient in turning side to side every 2 hr. 3. Maintain adequate body alignment. 4. Back care at least every 4 hr. 5. Refer family to appropriate resources to obtain needed home care equipment. 6. Encourage child's independence in his self-care tasks as tolerated. **Patient Education:** 1. Child and/or significant other will be given information on and/or can demonstrate: the purpose of range-of-motion activities, exercise regimen, use of home care equipment. 2. Parents recognize their child's need for independence and can identify in what areas he can achieve self-care.	**Dx:** 1. Physical therapy program should be adapted every day to the child's improved or deteriorated status. **Rx:** 1. Unless muscles and other structures are stretched daily, will become atrophic and contracted. 2–4. Turning, maintaining proper body alignment and back care will provide adequate circulation to skin. This will decrease chance of skin breakdown over pressure points. 5. Social service, community health nurse or home care coordinator can assist family in obtaining necessary equipment. 6. School-age child is capable of and seeks increasing independence in self-care activities. This independence reinforces a healthy self-image and builds self-confidence. **Patient Education:** 1. This knowledge is essential to the child's participation and cooperation in his care. It increases the likelihood that he will comply with the regimen. 2. This understanding helps parents accept and encourage their child's self-care.

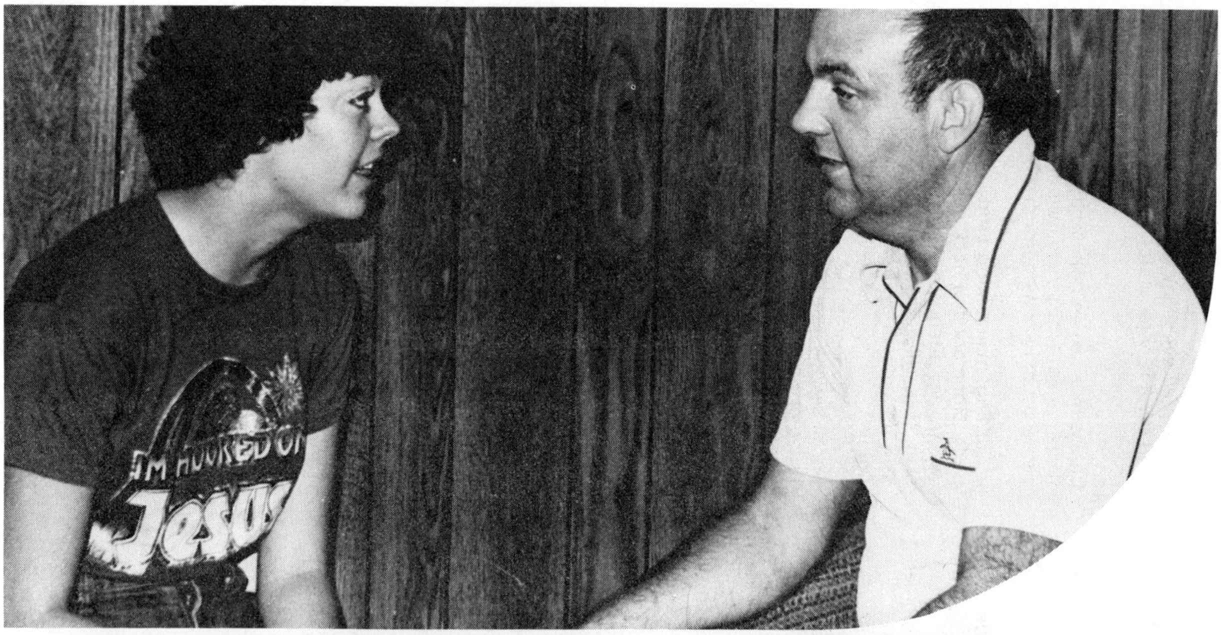
HOOKED ON

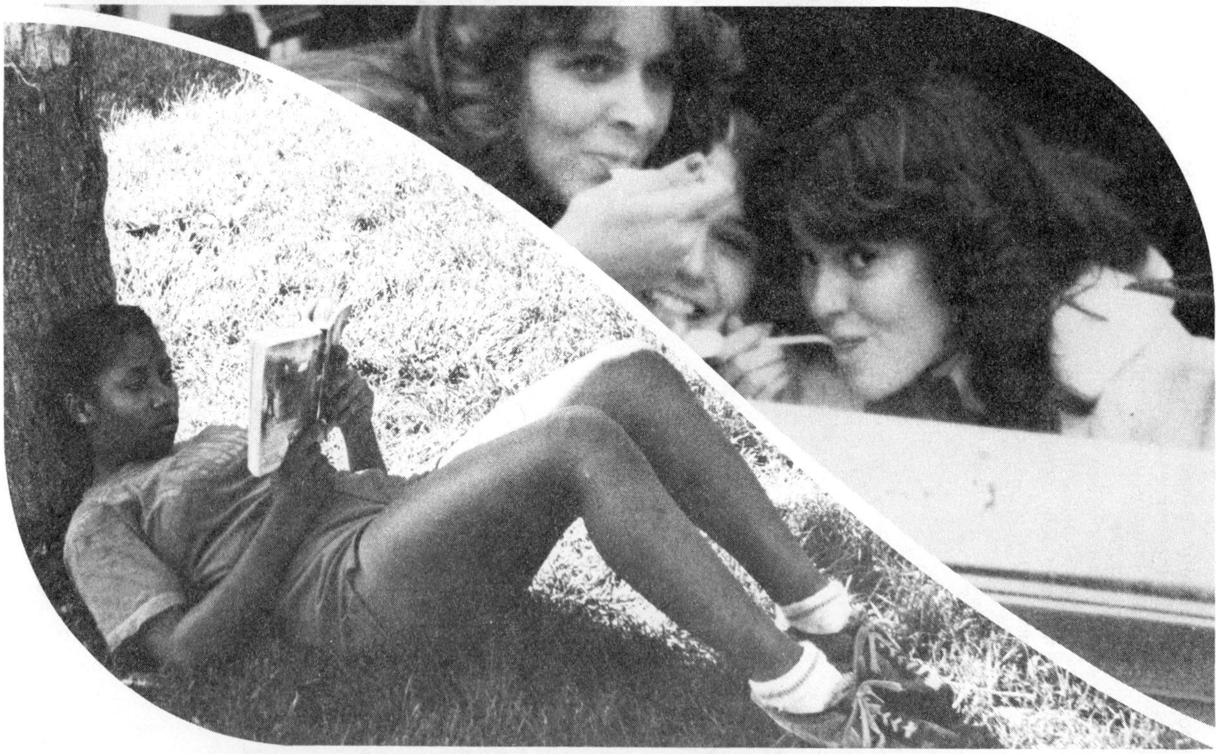

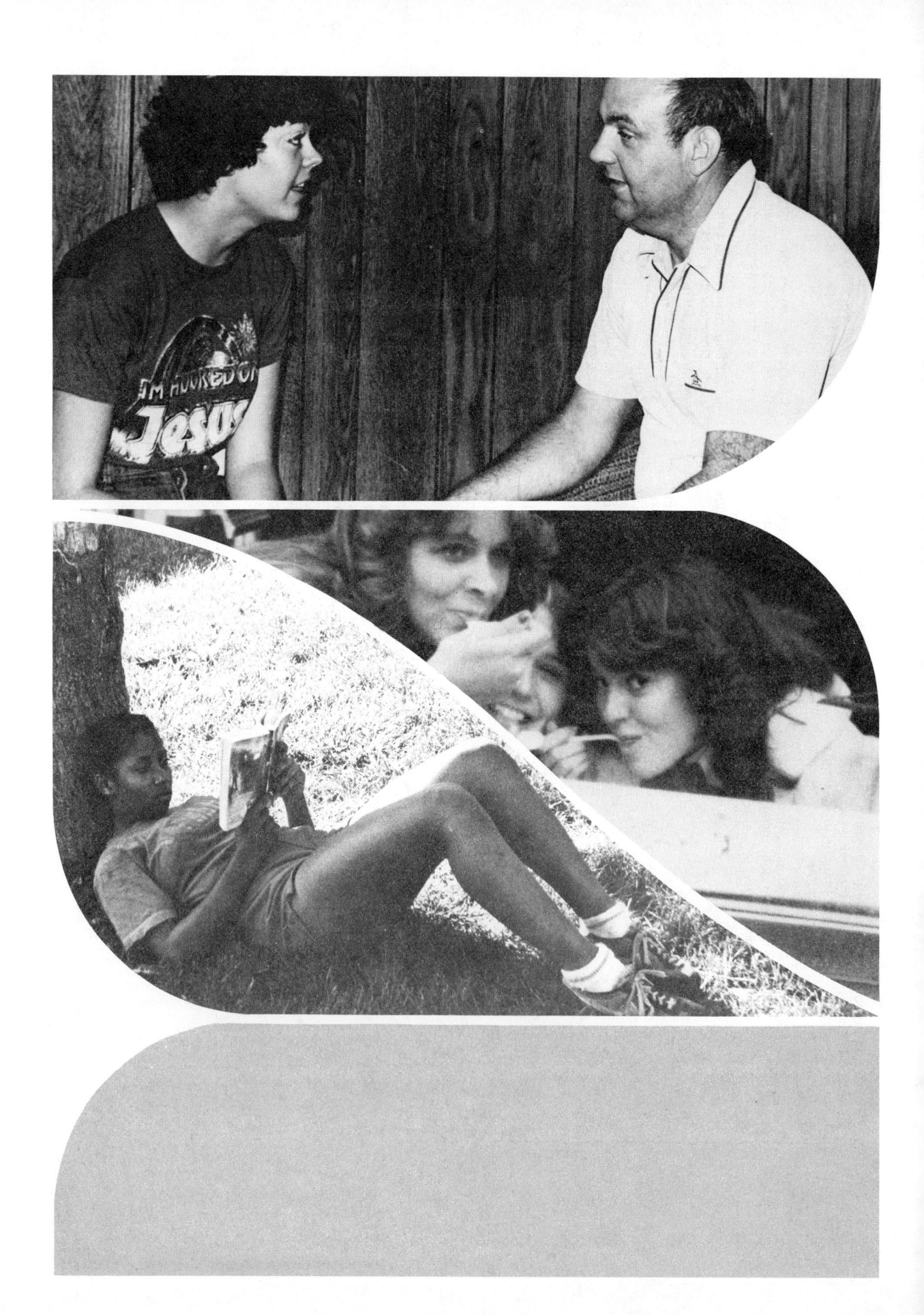

PART 8

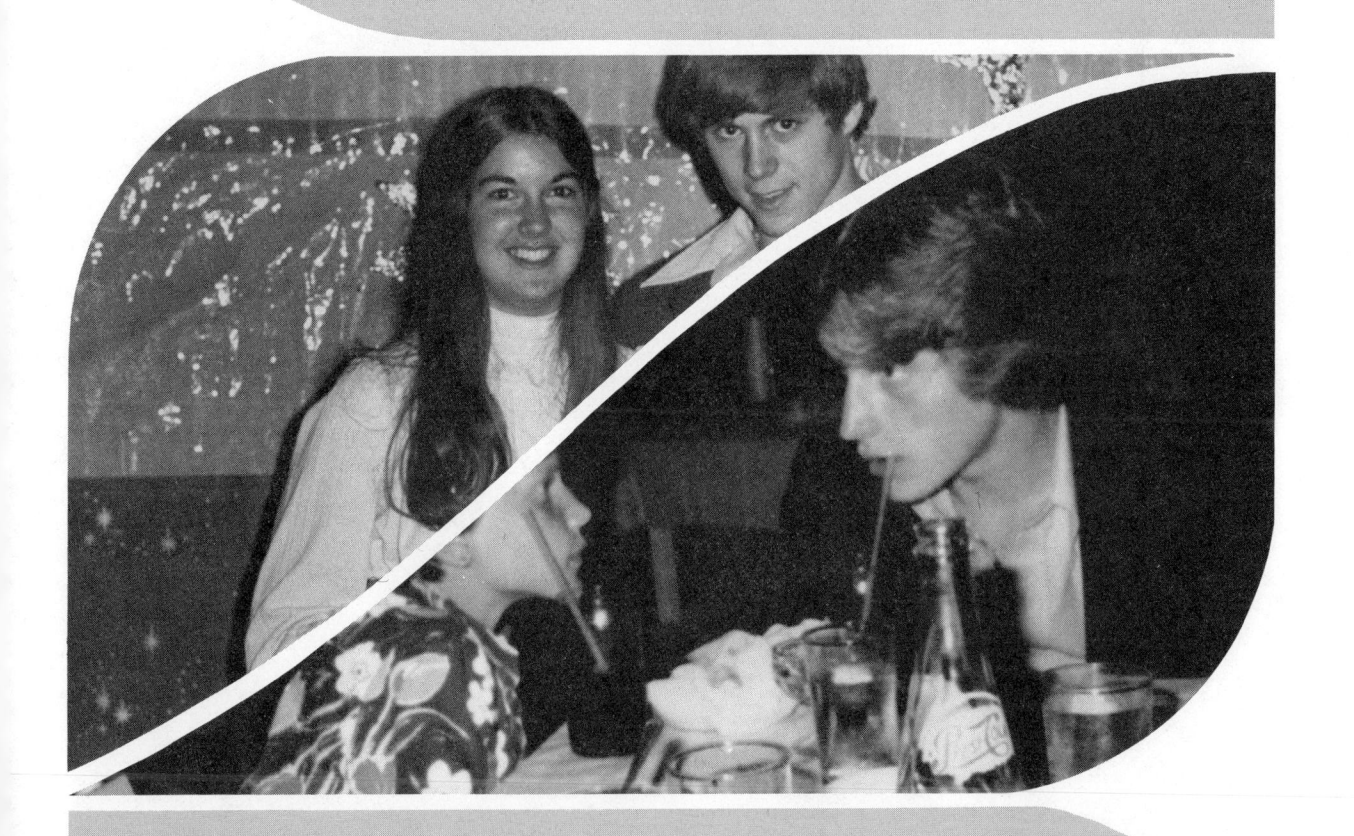

FAMILIES WITH ADOLESCENTS

55 GROWTH AND DEVELOPMENT NEEDS OF THE FAMILY WITH ADOLESCENTS: MAINTAINING WELLNESS

by Mary Arbour, RN, MSN Ed

The adolescent stage of family life begins when the oldest child is 13 and ends when that child leaves the family home to live his own life as an autonomous person.[2] The intervening years for the family may be as few as 4 or as many as 10. Should the child choose a career requiring many years of educational preparation, or if job opportunities are limited, the years of dependency may be even longer.

The adolescent experiences physical and emotional changes that occur at the same time his father and mother are undergoing maturational and menopausal changes. The stress of these developmental changes makes it challenging for the family to pass through these years quietly, unobtrusively and without some turmoil. The family has to learn a completely new repertoire of communication skills, social skills and adaptive skills. Frequently, these skills are not easily acquired. Through knowledge of life-span growth and development of the individual and an understanding of family developmental tasks, the nurse can be prepared to assist the family in its adaptation during the adolescent stage of family life.

REALLOCATION OF RESOURCES

The family developmental task of providing resources for widely differing needs of family members becomes immediately apparent in the home with an adolescent.[2]

Space The demand for increased privacy by the adolescent causes conflict between him and younger siblings. The adolescent's need for space to entertain a widening group of friends may cause conflict between the teen and his parents.

Although parents may not be able to actually increase the space available to their adolescent, they may rearrange home furnishings to include special interest areas more acceptable to him. The designation of places for conversation, listening to records and tapes, watching television and playing musical instruments will not eliminate the sounds of the adolescent in the home, but it may reduce angry feelings on the part of other family members. In some families, the location of the telephone is a critical issue. The laughter, shrieks and giggles punctuating the

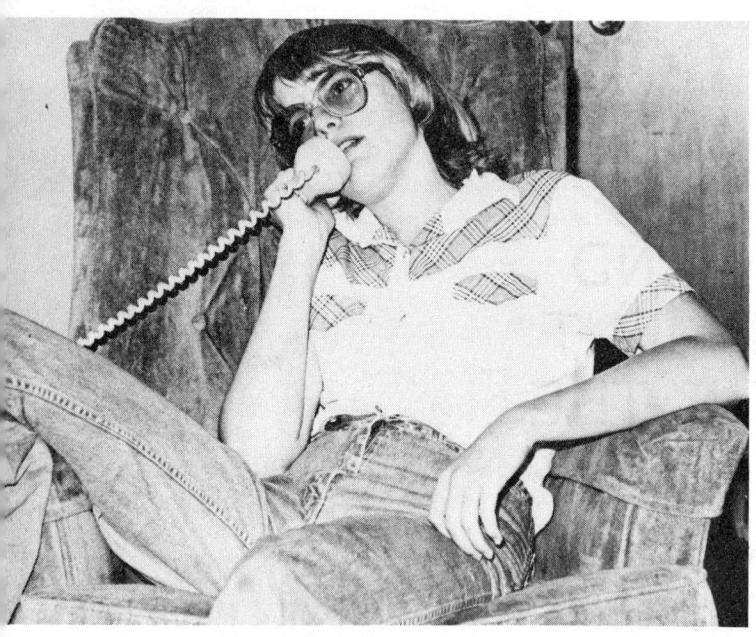

Location of the telephone becomes a critical issue during the teenage years.

teen's long telephone conversations can be a constant irritant to other family members. One family, unable to provide telephone jacks in their adolescent's rooms, solved the problem by placing the telephone in the utility room. When the firedoors were closed, privacy while telephoning was assured for all members of the family.

The adolescent's increasing social awareness and self-centered need to make a good impression on peers often results in open criticism of the home furnishings. Parents who recognize this developmental expression of the child will react by seeking the adolescent's opinions in selection or arrangement of the furniture. They will allow the youth the opportunity to organize and decorate his or her own room to satisfy adolescent tastes. Resolution of this conflict usually results in the home providing variety in decorating features, with some that appeal to the tastes and needs of each member.

Money Families with adolescents usually become acutely concerned about money.[2] Even when the family has engaged in democratic processes to manage money, during this stage a new emphasis on money becomes apparent. Parents who are future-oriented have usually anticipated the problems of ever-increasing costs in the social life of the adolescent and the rising costs of education or vocational training or both. If the adolescent has not been involved in family financial planning, he should be included now. The adolescent is responsible enough to be discreet about disclosure of family finances to adults and peers. Knowing the money needs of the family can often provide the incentive the teen needs to become increasingly independent and seek employment outside the home.

Usually, first jobs for the adolescent are near home and he can feel supported by the family. The youth experiences elation and gratification and his parents experience pride when he shows off his first money earned away from home. Parents must recognize that this money belongs to the child. Parents may make suggestions or provide guidelines as to its use, but the ultimate decision regarding the expenditure or saving of his earnings belongs to the teen. Many parents advise their children to accumulate some of their earnings for future education. Through family discussions of the allocation of money, the adolescent should be informed of those educational expenses for which he is expected to be responsible and those which he can depend upon his family to assume. Education beyond the legal requirements of the state is ideally a shared goal and a shared responsibility of all family members.

Adolescents who have participated in family financial decisions are usually supportive of parents' decisions to increase the family income. Such decisions may include extra hours

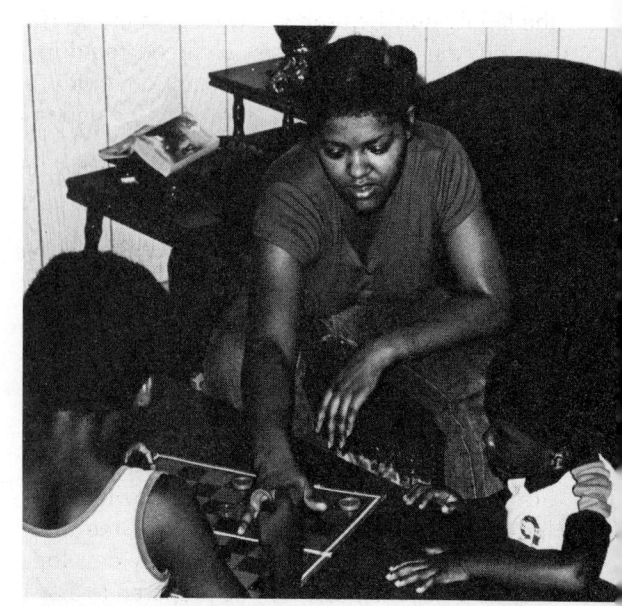

Babysitting is a common method of earning money during adolescence.

1222 FAMILIES WITH ADOLESCENTS

requires that adolescent family members intensify the work of their developmental task of sharing responsibility for family living by assuming their share in home management.[2]

In family living there are always tasks to be accomplished on a regular basis. Some tasks are routine and may be in the category of "chores," while others are creative. Some parents tend to assign the "chores" to their children and reserve the creative activities for themselves. The adolescent usually interprets this division of labor to mean that his parents do not trust him to do anything beyond routine chores.

Parents should be urged to take notice of their adolescent's contributions to family living and commend him for successful completion of assignments. Special recognition should be given for assuming additional tasks. The adolescent can also manage assigned responsibilities of a creative nature. This approach to accomplishing family activities necessary for daily living leaves a positive imprint on the child's self-esteem.[1]

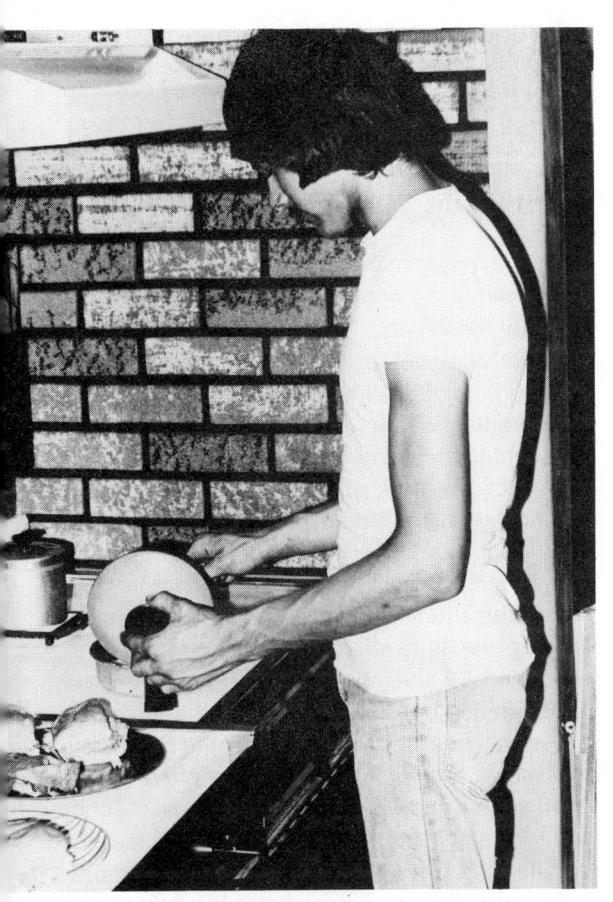

Adolescent family members can assume greater responsibility in home management. This may be a necessity if both parents are employed away from home.

of work by the father, the acceptance by the mother of a job and employment by the adolescent. If any one of these decisions is made by the family, the implementation will cause changes in roles and functions of all family members.

DIVISION OF LABOR AND RESPONSIBILITY

The nurse can assist the family to cope with the stress experienced as new roles are learned and incorporated into family functioning. Probably a decision that the mother should be employed outside the home creates the most disequilibrium in the family. The nurse may help the family to understand that tasks the mother has performed for years may now be done in less detail or shared by other family members, with different outcomes than when done by the mother. Because the outcomes are different does not necessarily mean they are unsatisfactory. The family must agree on what is expected of each member. Often the mother's employment

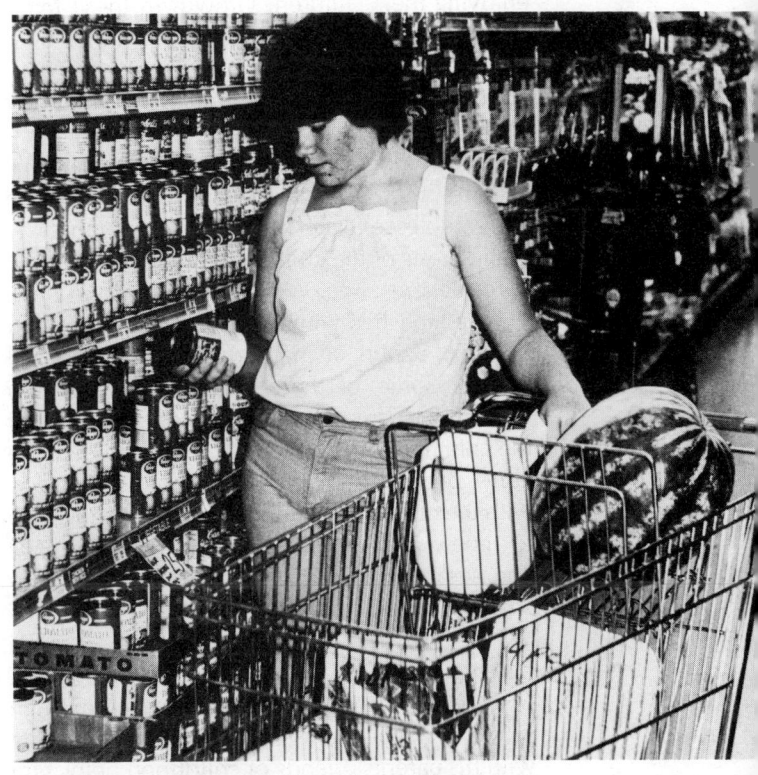

The adolescent does not like being assigned only routine chores, but she does appreciate taking responsibility that provides a challenge and an opportunity to learn useful skills.

GROWTH AND DEVELOPMENT NEEDS OF THE FAMILY WITH ADOLESCENTS: MAINTAINING WELLNESS

REFOCUSING THE SPOUSE RELATIONSHIP

In the family time span designated as the adolescent stage of family development, Duvall states that a major developmental task may be putting the marriage back in focus. Sometimes the demands of being parents are so all-consuming there is no time for self-expression by either spouse.[3] As a result the marital relationship weakens at a time when spouse cohesiveness and cooperation is essential.

The adolescent stage of family life can be an opportunity for parents to take more time to be a couple. It is not that the demands of being a parent are less at this time, but rather that they are different. The adolescent's involvement in wider social experiences, activities outside the home and dating leaves parents with more time to be alone. With this increased opportunity for self-expression, the couple can regain the initiative to be attractive to each other. Adolescents need parents who model heterosexual love as a rewarding and satisfying experience.[3]

Parents who enjoy each other usually value enjoying their children. Growth in these families is obvious. The parents take pride in their own accomplishments and those of their children. The family's security is evidenced in their ability to establish clear limits and in the positive interactions they have with each other.[29]

Some peer associations for parents of the early adolescent are frequently determined by the interests of the child rather than those of the parents themselves. Working relationships have to be established with other parents involved in the PTA, Scouts or many other youth-centered groups. Some of these relationships develop into lasting friendships. More often, however the common bond is the children, and when the child outgrows the activity, the associations with the other parents stop. Parents are now free to renew and strengthen ties with old friends and seek new relationships with persons who share common interests.

The renewal of friendships on the part of his parents is helpful to the adolescent. If he has been concerned about graduation from high school and leaving his friends, seeing and being with his parents' friends of childhood helps him to recognize some continuity in life. The adolescent may also gain a different perspective of his parents as he listens to his parents and their friends talk about the "old days," their aspirations, the times they "dropped the ball" and their successes.

MAINTAINING COMMUNICATION

An atmosphere of open communication is a fundamental component of living successfully with an adolescent. According to Duvall, there are two factors operating in the parents' ability to communicate with their adolescent: one is the parents' willingness to listen and the other is acceptance of and affection for their teen.[2]

One of the more difficult aspects of communication with the adolescent is his fluctuating emotional state. Parents may need assistance in recognizing their child's behavior as a form of communication. Sometimes parents' attempts to keep the lines of communication open are perceived by the adolescent as "picking" on him. Parents should be helped to recognize that constructive criticism is necessary to help their adolescent grow, but it should be offered with compassion and should not be an exercise in fault-finding. The most destructive effect of fault-finding on the adolescent is the lowering of his self-concept. This reduces his confidence in his ability to solve problems and in his interpersonal relationships.

An important element of communication with adolescents is that they recognize insincerity in communication. The adolescent does not accept praise from his parents in generalities. He discards as meaningless such praise as "you are very artistic." He wants his specific accomplishments recognized: "Your macramé wall-hanging is beautifully worked."

Many parents are threatened when their adolescent disagrees with them. Disagreements need not lead to destructive arguments. Parents must insist that opposing views are expressed in a respectful manner. Expressions of opinions and feelings should never be considered an invitation to argue. The parents' point of view should be presented reasonably and calmly no matter how much the child provokes the parent by pouting or unfair accusations. A good sense of humor may help turn a situation around, but humor may also be perceived by the adolescent as humiliating.

Open communication is destroyed if parents resort to humiliating their adolescent. He usually responds by being resentful. It is not uncommon for the adolescent to communicate his resentment with silence. This can be one of the most destructive techniques used in communicating. Silence on the part of the adolescent can indicate contempt, but more important is its statement of refusal to cooperate in problem solving. The adolescent's silence is usally not altered by demands of "talk to me." Silence may best be ended by the parent telling the child what his silence is communicating and confronting him with the facts.

In any discussion of communication with the adolescent it is imperative to address the importance of listening. Successful communication with the adolescent involves active listening, necessitating a real time commitment on the part of parents. Anyone who has worked or lived with an adolescent learns that he will talk about the most trivial matters for long periods before actually stating his concerns. The parent may need assistance in recognizing that the parent's interest and willingness to hear him out are being tested. (One mother stated that she usually knitted about four sweaters a year as she listened to her adolescent children. The patterns of the sweaters were always simple, freeing her to actively listen to her teen's feelings and opinions.) Anything the parent does not understand should be made clear through questioning. When parents complain that they cannot get through to their child, many times it is because they are not letting their adolescent come through to them.[4]

Family life during the adolescent stage is usually very busy with too many things to do, too many places to be at the same time and too little time for family interactions. The family may need assistance to enable them to arrange priorities in their life activities so that time is available to listen to each other. It is not enough for parents to feel love for their adolescent; they must also be able to communicate it by treating his opinions as worthy of consideration and by disciplining him in a manner that makes him

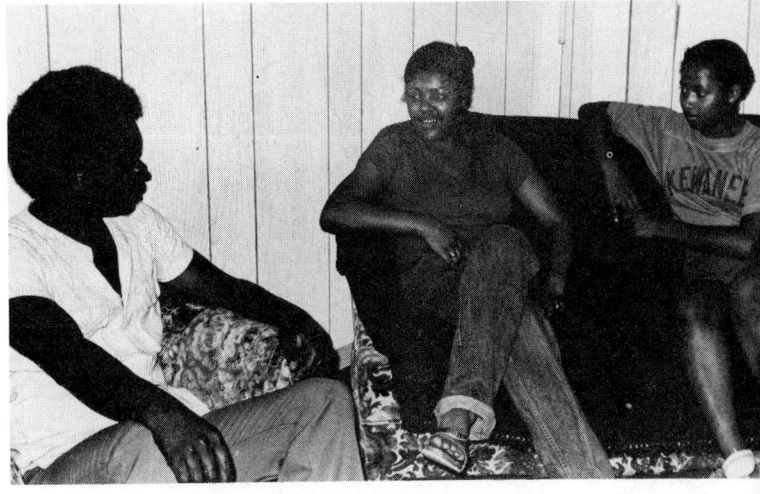

The adolescent needs parents who will listen actively and willingly to her concerns and ideas.

feel valued and enables him to become a unique person who achieves his full potential.

The nurse who works with families to assist them in their successful accomplishment of developmental tasks during the adolescent stage of family should recognize how she can contribute to healthy family living. As the intertwining tasks are anticipated and met without undue stress, the nurse needs to be aware of her role as a facilitator of the family as it grows to achieve the highest purpose of this stage: to care for the adolescent so that he matures to become responsible for his own beliefs and behavior and looks forward to success in his own family.

References

1. D. Briggs. Your Child's Self-Esteem. Doubleday & Co., Inc., 1970
2. E. Duvall. Marriage and Family Development. J. B. Lippincott Co., 1977
3. V. Satir. Peoplemaking. Science and Behavior Books, Inc., 1972
4. S. Wahlroos. Family Communication. Macmillan Inc., 1974

56 POTENTIAL STRESSES IN FAMILIES WITH ADOLESCENTS

by Mary Arbour, RN, MSN Ed

Some families with an adolescent seem to be riding a carousel, unable to reach the stop switch. The stress of the uncertainty of the ride is plainly visible. Other families do not perceive the situation of living with an adolescent as stressful. These families are able to provide for the growth and development needs of their teen and the family unit without disturbing their equilibrium.

The balanced family does not suffer stress because it does not allow the adolescent to place guilt on the family. If the family at any time loses control of the game plan, it will succumb to the stress situation. When the adolescent is concerned with his perception of how miserable and unfair his situation is, his first line of defense is an attempt to make his family, parents and siblings feel responsible for his condition. Should the parents respond with guilt feelings, they are entering into the adolescent's game and at that point the adolescent is in control. Parents may need help to recognize this behavior on the part of their adolescent and to prevent the internalization of guilt.

At no other stage of family life is it as critical for the family to recognize its value to society and for members to maintain a high sense of self-worth that cannot be dissipated by the adolescent. However, even though the family strives to meet the challenge of living with the adolescent, the intensity of the forces operating in the family may create situations that result in stress for the family. With the exception of a few segments of American society, such as the Jewish whose males go through bar mitzvah, there are no rites of passage, no age requirements to designate adulthood. Entry into the adult stage is primarily dependent on educational achievement and occupational potential. Merton describes the adolescent as one who is "poised on the edge of several groups but fully accepted by none of them."[7] This results in vacillation on the part of all family members regarding role functions and expectations for the adolescent. It contributes to the confusion of the dependence-independence struggle of the adolescent and adds to the potential for stress during adolescence.

Erikson has identified the central problem of the adolescent as one of identity and role confusion.[7] Successful resolution of the identity crisis requires both societal acceptance and role confirmation.

Role confusion may be attributed to an overprotective environment that permits the adolescent too little autonomy to develop his identity. Frequently, parents engage in activities that tend to slow down the adolescent's attempts to choose a career, to free himself from the family, to choose friends of the opposite sex and to integrate himself. The adolescent is thus required to deal with unrealistic parental restrictions along with his own insecurities about himself. This combination of forces creates rebellion in the adolescent, which is difficult for him to handle or for his parents to understand. Added to this is the adolescent's perceived helplessness and inability to understand that he is often as opposed to himself as he is to his parents.

PARENT-ADOLESCENT DIFFERENCES

Parents and adolescents are generally separated by eons of differences. If this were not true, the evolution of society would have taken light years longer. That parents will have difficulty with, take exception to and struggle through the differences is expected behavior. Adolescents and parents have different views in philosophy and about educational preparation and the value of certain habits and attitudes of the adolescent.[3] Parents need to understand that these differences should not result in reprimand or criticism of the adolescent.

The adolescent may perceive that never in his whole life has he been the brunt of so much negativism on the part of his parents. To protect himself from harsh criticism, the adolescent may isolate himself from the family. However, when the bonding between the adolescent and his parents has been constructive and nurturing, communication generally does not disintegrate.

Parents may need assistance to recognize the destructiveness of nagging and instruction in the use of actions and expressions that will continue to enhance their adolescent's self-esteem. In families in which there are strong kinship ties that are not interrupted by geographic distance, the adolescent may notice that his parents are not in conflict with his grandparents and that it is possible to develop rewarding relationships between generations. Parents who successfully handle parent-adolescent conflicts have learned to keep quiet often and allow the consequences of their adolescent's actions to silently and naturally take place.

ADOLESCENT SEXUALITY

The sexual development of the adolescent is a process that may cause anxiety and stress within the family. Few parents claim to be experts in sex education. Adolescents recognize immediately any awkwardness or hesitation on the part of their parents to discuss the subject. It is important for parents to express their feelings and admit to their concerns when discussing sexual development and attitudes toward sex with their teen. For the teen to hold positive attitudes about sex, it is essential for him to observe interactions of emotionally mature adults, to have a positive relationship with the parent of the opposite sex, and to see discipline used to foster growth and not to control family members. The adolescent who learns that sexual contact is most fulfilling when it involves caring, commitment and sensitivity to the best interest of others does not generally resort to indiscriminate sexual experimentation.[1]

The idea that sexual urges cannot be controlled is not true. The best guard against the adolescent engaging in promiscuous sexual experimentation at a time when the sex drive is high and peer pressure is excessive is for the family to promote their adolescent's self-esteem. When the adolescent believes in himself and likes himself, he is able to take a stand on moral issues. In this context the adolescent can be guided to think about the consequences of sexual activity to himself and to others. Parents may help their children to think through some difficult situations in advance and consider the consequences of their actions. Such anticipatory guidance may help the adolescent handle difficult situations and not become caught up in the situation or the intensity of emotion.

The actual incidence of sexual assault against adolescents or committed by adolescents is unknown. Sexual trauma most frequently discussed by adolescents is the "dating rape."[4] Parents need to understand some of the practices used in the socialization of the adolescent that may contribute to the problem. If an adolescent is dominated by parents and others in authority, he may use sex as a means to control. On the other hand, the adolescent who is dominated may become sexually submissive. If parents are overpermissive, the adolescent thinks only of his own needs and is totally selfish. His premise is that his sexual desire is reason enough to use his date for self-gratification.

Another aspect in the socialization of the

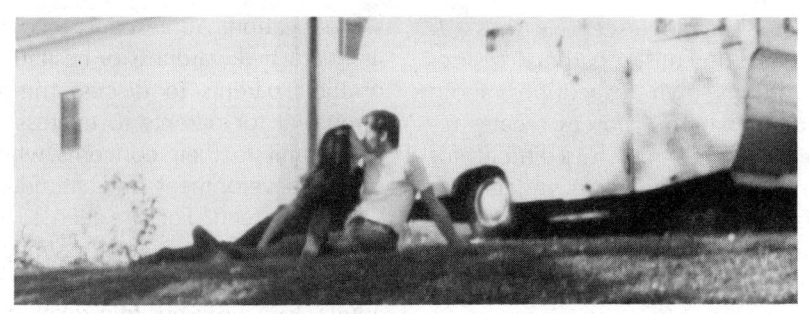

Parents can guide their adolescents to understand that sexual urges will be powerful but that expression of these urges holds corresponding responsibility to others as well as to themselves.

adolescent that influences the dating rape situation is the value parents attach to "feminine" and "masculine" behaviors. The adolescent girl is expected to be considerate, caring and nurturing. She may believe it is required of her to extend these qualities and to regard her date's sexual advances as expression of a need she should fulfill. For the adolescent boy, aggressiveness, dominance and strength are manly qualities. Since the male is generally accepted as the aggressor in the sexual relationship, it is not surprising that the adolescent boy confuses sex and aggression. For the boy involved in dating rape, it may be a means of proving his manliness and his heterosexual prowess. Submission on the part of the girl denotes femininity.

The adolescent's parents need to understand the importance of role-modeling to clarify these conflicts. Girls need to observe that the qualities of nurturing and caring are not synonymous with weakness and submission, and for boys sexual aggression and dominance of his date are not synonymous with the adult male role. Parents can be helped to guide their adolescent to understand that his sexual urges will be powerful but that sexual acts require responsibility to other persons as well as to themselves.[1]

When the victim of rape is an adolescent the emotional responses of parents are of such intensity that they may be unable to support their child. Siblings of the victim may respond in the same manner. The nurse must select those counselling strategies that will enable the family to mobilize its strengths to assure adequate immediate medical care and to plan for long-term counselling to build the family's self-esteem as a responsible, caring family.

DRUGS AND THE ADOLESCENT

The widespread and increasing use of illegal drugs by the adolescent is putting tremendous pressures on the youth and his family. The cry from the teen is a request to society to "do something about it" and from the family the cry is "What can we do about it?" Parents may need assistance to understand that group pressures on the adolescent continue to result in many offenses against himself, his peers and his family. The user of illegal drugs usually shows the personality composite of denial, ignorance about the common drugs of abuse, the need to gain control of his environment and the need to convince his peers of his power. These are danger signals the parent needs to look for in individual members of their teen's peer group.[5] In addition, adolescents who use illegal drugs are generally those who "do not belong," who have a poor record in school and who have difficulty in dealing with authority. Parents should also be aware, when observing their adolescent's friends, that those adolescents who use illegal drugs also use significantly more coffee, cola drinks, aspirin, alcoholic drinks and tobacco. Since most of these substances are classified as stimulants or drugs, the use of them by this group is not surprising.

Marijuana is the illegal drug considered least dangerous by the adolescent himself. Users and nonusers are generally expressing a more favorable attitude toward the drug. This should be cause for concern on the part of the family. The data are incomplete regarding marijuana. Parents should also recognize that there is a great deal of difference between occasional use for the purpose of experimentation and habitual use.

The response to the parents' question of what they can do about the use of illegal drugs is complex. Parents may find it helpful to join with other parents, school officials and the community in providing stabilizing influences and activities for their adolescents. Such activity may include participation in recreational programs, pursuing special interests such as sports, music or mechanics, or obtaining work experiences in which the adolescent works for money or in which he contributes services to individuals or the community voluntarily. Ensuring that the adolescent gets adequate nutrition as well as providing motivation for achievement and a respect for authority are important toward stabilizing his behavior. Fundamental to achievement of this goal is open communication without fear on the part of the adolescent or the parent of being reprimanded for expressing opinions or sharing feelings. Interestingly, adolescents who use drugs generally indicate that communication with their parents is inadequate.[2] They say that if they had a drug related problem or any other problem, they would turn to a friend rather than to their parents. Regardless of whom the adolescent chooses as a confidante, that person must communicate feelings of honesty, openness and risk-taking with the adolescent.

With the prevalent use of illegal drugs among adolescents and the resulting anxiety on the part of their families, attitudes on the use of alcohol have modified in some communities. In spite of the current controversy, the use of alcohol by adolescents under voter-determined age limits is illegal. However, parents recognize that the laws governing the legal drinking age in reality control only the places in which the adolescent may drink. The laws have not been effective in controlling whether or not the adolescent drinks. Parents' anxieties generally stem from the adolescent's response to peer pressure, which may result in abuse of alcohol and in alcohol toxicity, accidents and illegal acts. Parents now have a double-edged responsibility—to teach abstinence from alcohol because the law requires it and to teach responsible attitudes toward alcohol use. For adolescents to develop responsible attitudes toward alcohol use, parents should teach that the critical issues are how a person feels about alcohol and why he drinks.

In the past parents have taught that drinking leads to personal disaster. This concept is not supported by fact, because the majority of people who use alcohol do so without problems. The idea that teaching the serious health consequences of using alcohol will make the adolescent afraid to use alcohol is also a false hope. These and other approaches have not reduced the incidence of use of alcohol by the adolescent. (This also applies to the use of cigarettes.) The goal of teaching about alcohol use is to prevent irresponsible drinking. For some adolescents, responsible drinking may mean an occasional drink with their peers, for others it may mean the use of alcohol to celebrate certain family or religious feasts, and, for still others, it may mean abstinence from the use of alcohol.

THE ADOLESCENT'S PEER RELATIONSHIPS

Adolescence is a time when a person seeks friends to fulfill his need to be liked, to be accepted and to belong to a group.[24] The adolescent moves away from his family, and his friends become the bearers of his ideals and standards. Making friends is an important developmental task. As the adolescent becomes more and more resistive to the parent's admonitions about behavior acceptable for them, the adolescent doubles his efforts to act like and dress like his selected friends of the moment.

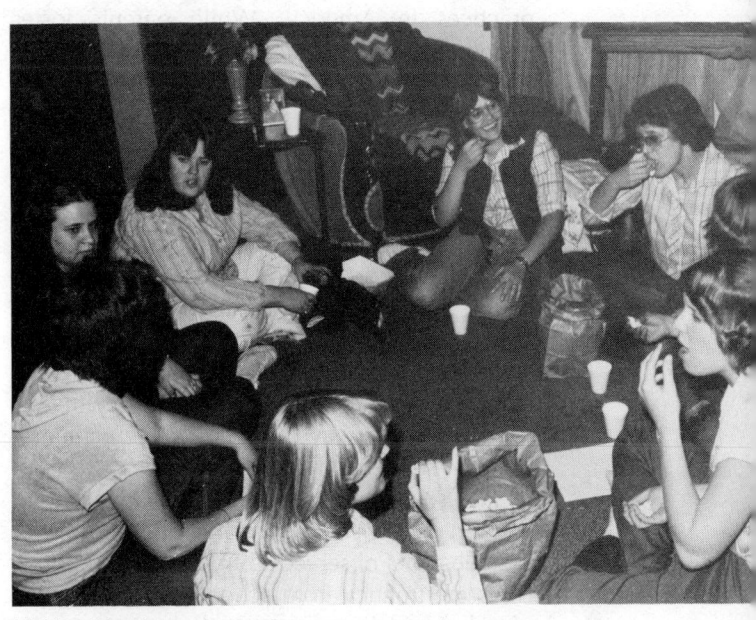

Making friends and belonging to a group are important developmental tasks of the teen. They seek friends who will fulfill their need to be liked, accepted and to "belong." Friends become the bearers of the teen's ideals and standards.

Many times the adolescent's selection of friends and his allegiance to them produces a stressful situation for the family. Parents may need help to understand that this exaggerated conformity to peer groups is a manifestation of the adolescent's process of achieving identity and independence from his parents. He desperately needs approval, and since he is moving away from dependence on his parents, he needs the support that approval from friends provides. Once parents recognize the adolescent's desire and need to make friends, their attention becomes focused on the "desirability" of the friends selected. The nurse may assist the family to understand that the adolescent needs to test a wide variety of friendships that may include those adolescents from differing cultural, social and economic backgrounds. The choice of lasting friends can be influenced by parents making themselves available to discuss family value systems, to participate in activities of interest to the child and his group, and to foster strong kinship and generational ties.

THE ALIENATED ADOLESCENT

The nurse who intervenes with families in the adolescent stage of family development should assist them to recognize a paradox in parenting practices in America. While parents foster youngsters' dependency needs during childhood, they suddenly expect a high degree of self-sufficiency as the children become adolescents and young adults. Most youth then insist that this independence is exactly what they want in their drive toward mastering the adult world, and begin seeking their peers to gratify any residual dependency needs. Others, acutely grieving the loss of maternal dependency they want desperately to regain, do not perceive the adult world as a desirable place to enter. To cope, they totally deny any feelings or needs they may have for dependency, alienating themselves from any commitments to their family, society or the world that promises no comfort or dependency gratification. Some of the behaviors observed in this group of adolescents are truancy from school or dropping out of school, delinquency, or belonging to the "rock" subculture, or all of these.[2]

A behavior that is the target of increasing concern for parents and professionals working with families is the "cult" movement in the youth culture. The danger to the youth who becomes entrapped in the cult is the mind-controlling techniques used to change his personality. It is important for the parents and the adolescent to recognize the covert activities used by leaders of cults to indoctrinate prospective members.[3] Any group the adolescent becomes involved with should be investigated early on by his parents.

Families of the alienated adolescent are frequently blamed for their adolescent's alienation. This attitude neglects to take into consideration the external forces operating to influence the older adolescent's development. These parents may need guidance to understand the circumstances in their teen's life that undermined the values and ideals of the family, and to recognize that the family cannot know the intensity of the pressures external to it that the adolescent experiences. The nurse's assistance may be required to help the family cope with their grieving for the alienated adolescent and to help identify their strengths for maintaining self-esteem.

The nurse who works with families of adolescents must be committed to developing a repertoire of nursing interventions to assist those families to adapt to each family member's individual maturational crises and family developmental situations. Some interventions are counselling, using behavior modification techniques and applying role change theory and communication theory. The nurse must be dedicated to increasing her knowledge of families and contributing through research to the growing body of knowledge of family nursing care.

References

1. D. Briggs. Your Child's Self-Esteem. Doubleday & Co., Inc., 1970
2. M. Brinkley and L. De Ridder. Comparing drug users with nonusers. NASSP Bulletin, National Association of Secondary School Principals. April 1973, p. 81
3. F. Conway and J. Siegelman. Snapping. Dell Publishing Co., Inc., 1979, p. 15
4. J. Hyde. Understanding Human Sexuality. McGraw-Hill Book Co., 1979, p. 385
5. K. Keniston, The Uncommitted: Alienated Youth in American Society. Dell Publishing Co., Inc., 1965
6. N. Kiell. The Universal Experience of Adolescence. Beacon Press, 1967
7. W. Sze. Human Life Cycle. Jason Aronson, Inc., 1975
8. R. Warner, et al. Drug abuse prevention: a behavioral approach. NASSP Bulletin: The National Association of Secondary School Principals, April 1973

Additional Recommended Reading

D. Browning and B. Boatman. Incest: children at risk. American Journal of Psychiatry, January 1977, p. 69

S. Callahan. Parenting: Principles and Politics of Parenthood. Doubleday & Co., Inc., Penguin Books, 1974

A. Chapman. Management of Emotional Problems of Children and Adolescents. J. B. Lippincott Co., 1974

R. Cloward and L. Ohlin. Delinquency and Opportunity: A Theory of Delinquent Gangs. The Free Press, 1960

M. Collins. Child Abuser. PSG Publishing Company, Inc., 1978

J. Dobson. Hide or Seek: Self-Esteem for the Child. Fleming H. Revell Company, 1974

E. Erikson. Insight and Responsibility. W. W. Norton and Co., Inc., 1964

E. Erikson. The Challenge of Youth. Doubleday and Co., Inc., Anchor Books, 1965

E. Erikson. Identity and the Life Cycle, with an Introduction by D. Rapaport. Psychological Issues, Monograph 1, vol. 1, no. 1. International Universities Press, Inc., 1959

W. Glasser. The Identity Society. Harper and Row, Perennial Library, 1975

J. Hyde. Understanding Human Sexuality. McGraw-Hill Book Co., 1979

G. Kaluger and M. Kaluger. Profiles in Human Development. C.V. Mosby Co., 1976

C. Kempe and R. Helfer. Helping the Battered Child and His Family. J. B. Lippincott Co., 1972

T. Lidz. The Person. Basic Books, Inc., 1976

R. Laing. The Politics of the Family and Other Essays. Random House, Inc., Vintage Books Edition, 1972

J. Peters. Children who are victims of sexual assault and the psychology of offenders. American Journal of Psychotherapy, March 1976

A. Schneiders. Adolescents and the Challenge of Maturity. The Bruce Publishing Co., 1965

M. Smart and R. Smart. Adolescents: Development and Relationships. Macmillan, Inc., 1978

N. Talbot, ed. Raising Children in Modern America. Little, Brown & Co., 1976

N. Woods. Human Sexuality in Health and Illness. C.V. Mosby Co., 1975

57 ADOLESCENT GROWTH AND DEVELOPMENT: MAINTAINING WELLNESS

by Janet Allen-Lia, RN, BS, MS

The term adolescence comes from the Latin word *adolescere*, meaning "grow up." Remembered by many adults as a time of turmoil, adolescence is that period between childhood and adulthood.

Adolescence is a phenomenon of industrialized, developed societies. As child labor laws were passed and education became compulsory, the process of assuming adult roles emerged as a distinguishable separate period of development, called adolescence. Conversely, in developing countries children are expected to learn adult roles early, not permitting the extended period of maturation and dependency we know as adolescence. The United States has no universal "rites of passage" into adulthood. There is no magic hour when the child turns into an adult. If it is graduation from high school, what of the drop-out? If it is living on one's own, what if the son or daughter chooses to continue to live in the parents' home? If it is parenthood, is the 12-year-old mother an adult and the 30-year-old childfree person not? There is some common agreement that the passage into adulthood covers that period of sexual maturation beginning at approximately 12 and ending around 21. (Puberty refers to the purely biological stage of sexual development during which physical changes occur that make reproduction possible. This chapter seeks to identify the normal growth and developmental needs of the adolescent (physical, intellectual, emotional and social) and how parents and professionals can help the adolescent meet these needs.

PHYSICAL GROWTH AND DEVELOPMENT

Young people mature at different rates, beginning and leaving puberty at different ages. The adolescent stage is characterized by a steady progression of physiological changes that require an adaptation of body image. Dramatic physical changes require the adolescent to adjust to his new appearance and to develop a feeling of comfort inside his maturing physical body. Furthermore, the adolescent must cope with the emotional and social pressures that accompany these physical changes. These changes may overwhelm the adolescent or they can be used as the foundation for learning adaptation mechanisms useful later in life. The understanding of young people by parents and other adults is crucial to smooth progression through adolescence.

The Growth Spurt

Adolescence is the only time after birth that the velocity of growth significantly increases. During puberty, both males and females attain the final 20 per cent of their mature height. Most of this growth occurs during a "growth spurt" that lasts two to three years. This spurt usually occurs two years earlier for females than for males. The beginning age is variable, from 9.5 to 14.5 years of age for girls and 10.5 to 16 years for boys.

During their growth spurt, boys average an eight-inch height gain, with four inches attained during the peak year (around age 14). During the growth spurt a girl's average gain is over three inches per year. At 18 more than 99 per cent of growth has occurred and only about one inch in height remains to be gained.

Growth follows a pattern, with almost every part of the body being affected. The legs usually lengthen first, causing the youth to appear lanky and awkward, then the thighs become wider. Next the shoulders broaden, followed by trunk growth. Facial bones change, particularly the mandible and maxilla. The maxilla grows forward and the ramus of the mandible lengthens.

Body Composition

Skeletal changes are dramatic during adolescence. Skeletal mass doubles, contributing significantly to weight gain in puberty.

Muscle or lean body mass and non-lean body mass (principally fat) double during puberty. In males muscles increase both in number of individual cells and in size, while in females muscles increase only in size. This probably accounts for greater male strength, but the cause is unclear. At the time of physical maturation females average twice as much body fat as males. Total body fat in males actually decreases during puberty.

The heart, lungs, liver, spleen, kidneys, pancreas, thyroid, adrenals, gonads, phallus and uterus double in size during puberty. It is also thought that the digestive tract enlarges. In contrast, the tissues of the lymphatic system (thymus, tonsils, adenoids and portions of the spleen) decrease in size. Reasons for this decrease and its relationship to antibody production remain to be investigated.

Adult visual levels were attained by 6 years of age. Adolescents have normal adult hearing, although they are sometimes accused of "selective deafness," or hearing only what they want to hear. Pulse, respirations and blood pressure values reach adult norms by 15 to 16 years of age. (See Chapter 13 for vital sign values during adolescence.)

Sexual Maturation

Sexual maturation involves the development of primary and secondary sexual characteristics. The total process is not considered complete until about 20 to 21 years of age. Primary sex characteristics involve the physical and hormonal changes necessary for reproduction. Secondary sex characteristics, while not necessary to reproduction, are the characteristics that externally differentiate male from female.

Regulation of this onset of puberty is a complicated and not fully understood process. Tropic hormones are produced in the pituitary gland but are thought to be the result of a "feedback" mechanism. The hypothalamus becomes less sensitive to negative feedback with increasing age and begins to produce releasing factors. These gonadotropic-releasing hormones then signal the pituitary to secrete gonadotropic hormones such as FSH (follicle-stimulating hormone). FSH in turn stimulates both the growth of ova in the female ovary and the growth of sperm-producing cells in the male testes. Cells in the ovary and testicle produce female and male sex hormones, respectively. Estrogen (female hormone) is produced by the ovary, and testosterone (male hormone) is produced by the testes. These hormones are responsible for development of the secondary sex characteristics. Sex hormones are also produced by the adrenal gland so that both sexes have some of both male and female hormones.

Many practitioners and investigators have observed the more or less orderly (although widely variable) progression of sexual development in both sexes. The description and labeling of these stages by Tanner[12] are generally accepted as guidelines to normal development (Tables 57–1 and 57–2; Fig. 57–1). These tables enable an examiner to determine the stage of development, to detect abnormalities and to guide the adolescent as to changes to expect next.

TABLE 57-1 CLASSIFICATION OF SEX MATURITY STAGES IN BOYS*

Stage	Pubic Hair	Penis	Testes
1	None	Preadolescent	Preadolescent
2	Scanty, long, slightly pigmented	Slight enlargement	Enlarged scrotum, pink texture altered
3	Darker, starts to curl, small amount	Longer	Larger
4	Resembles adult type, but less in quantity; coarse, curly	Larger; glans and breadth increase in size	Larger, scrotum dark
5	Adult distribution, spread to medial surface of thighs	Adult	Adult

*From V. Vaughan et al. Nelson Textbook of Pediatrics. W. B. Saunders Co., 1979.

Female secondary sexual development during puberty involves increase in size of the ovaries, uterus, vagina, labia and breasts. Body hair appears in the pubic area and under the arms; menarche occurs. The first visible signs of sexual maturity are pubic hair, breast buds or both. These developments occur in orderly fashion but do not necessarily occur together. Each aspect of development (growth, pubic hair, breast appearance) must be evaluated to determine if the young woman is developing normally. For example, it is rare for a girl to reach pubic hair stage 3 or 4 without breast development. In this case, the girl should be evaluated for the presence of hypothalamic, pituitary or gonadal dysfunction. The vast majority of girls will achieve adult breast size by age 19. There are no normal standards for breast size and no correlation exists with hormones, heredity or height. There is some correlation between weight and overall breast size. Some studies have indicated that black girls are significantly more advanced in development of secondary sex characteristics than are white girls of the same chronological age.[36]

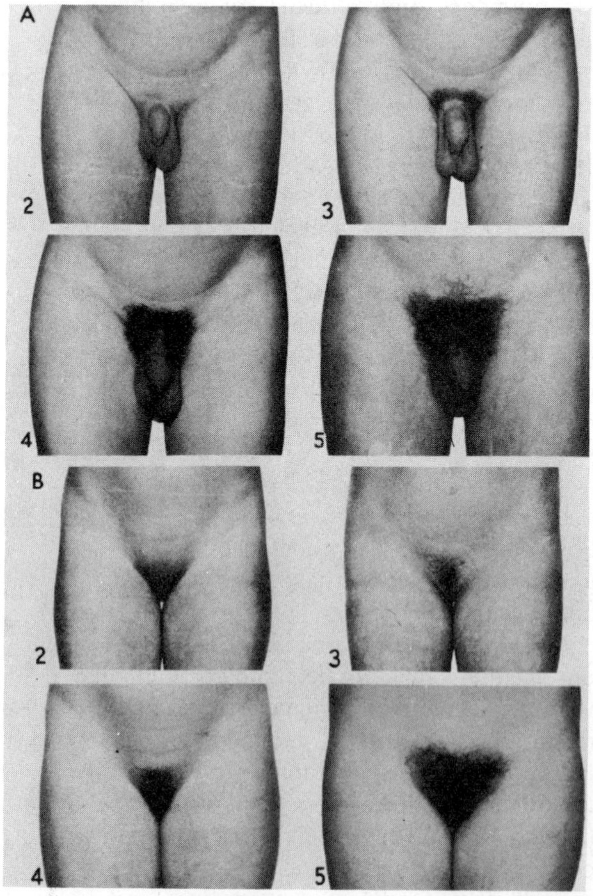

Menarche (the appearance of menstruation) has occurred earlier each generation; present-day adolescent females begin menstruating at an average age of 12 years and 3 months as compared to age 17 a hundred years ago. Reasons for these changes are unclear, but effects of environment, nutrition and better health care are most likely responsible. Menarche occurs at about the time the growth spurt slows. About 99 per cent of girls will reach menarche within five years after beginning breast development. If no evidence of puberty can be seen by age 13, a medical assessment should be done. Menarche usually occurs at stage 4 (Table 57–2).

Male secondary sexual development consists of genital growth and the appearance of pubic and body hair. The first event is usually enlargement of the testes. During puberty the testes, epididymides and prostate will increase their prepuberty size seven times. As the testes enlarge, so does the scrotum; the scrotum devel-

Figure 57–1 Sex maturity ratings of pubic hair changes in adolescent boys and girls. (Courtesy J. M. Tanner; from V. Vaughan et al. Nelson Textbook of Pediatrics. W. B. Saunders Co., 1979, p. 49.)

TABLE 57-2 CLASSIFICATION OF SEX MATURITY STAGES IN GIRLS*

Stage	Pubic Hair	Breasts
1	Preadolescent	Preadolescent
2	Sparse, lightly pigmented, straight, medial border of labia	Breast and papilla elevated as small mound; areolar diameter increased
3	Darker, beginning to curl, increased amount	Breast and areola enlarged, no contour separation
4	Coarse, curly, abundant but amount less than in adult	Areola and papilla form secondary mound
5	Adult feminine triangle, spread to medial surface of thighs	Mature; nipple projects, areola part of general breast contour

*From V. Vaughan et al. Nelson Textbook of Pediatrics. W. B. Saunders Co., 1979.

ops rugae and becomes darker in color. The next sign is growth of the penis and a few tufts of long, straight and slightly pigmented pubic hair. The genitals progress to near adult size before more pubic hair appears. The final stage of hair growth is to adult type, with hair extending to the medial thigh areas.

Ejaculation has usually occurred in boys by stage 3 and probably earlier. Spermatozoa are almost always present. Stage 4 must be reached before the full adult number of sperm are present.

The male growth spurt occurs at about the same time as penile growth and about a year after the increase in testicular size. If growth has not begun by sexual development stage 4, the boy should be evaluated for thyroid dysfunction, growth hormone adequacy or chronic disease. Generally, a boy who is short at stage 4 will continue to grow but will be shorter than average as an adult.

Males normally experience an increase in size of breast areola. About 30 per cent or more will also experience some bilateral, nontender increase in size of the breasts. Transient breast tenderness is also common. Facial and axillary hair appear at about stage 5. Breaking and deepening of the voice also occur at this stage.

Anticipatory Guidance: Physical Development

Because most adolescents do not ask questions they may have about their body changes or lack thereof, adults around them must anticipate questions. These questions can be answered in a nonthreatening, casual manner to avoid embarrassing the adolescent. Adolescents are quick to sense a "put down." Both boys and girls observe their peers, see variations in development, and compare themselves to those around them. These variations produce anxiety in those who develop slightly earlier or later than their peers.

Anticipatory Guidance for Females Menarche is a rather late occurrence in female sexual development. Therefore, when a girl who has not begun the growth spurt nor developed breast buds is anxious about not menstruating, the nurse can inform her of the order in which this development occurs and reassure her that sexual characteristics have a wide range of rate of development. Statistically, the adolescent girl should begin menstruation by age 13½ (or 5 years after breast development begins) and, if she has not, medical evaluation is indicated.

It is also normal for a young woman to experience irregularity in the amount of menstrual flow and in the spacing of periods. She can be reassured that for the first year or more her periods will be unpredictable. What is more, emotional changes affect the menstrual cycle; the teenage girl may find that her period is delayed during times of stress such as final examinations.

The school-age or prepubertal adolescent girl should be prepared for the onset of menstruation. Parents should be advised to obtain menstrual supplies for the girl long before she will need them. Their use should be explained and the girl allowed to become familiar with them. Though there is no reason to actually attempt insertion of a tampon, the girl should be allowed to keep the menstrual supplies in her room and consider them hers. Myths that baths and physical exercise should be avoided during menstruation should be dispelled. Menstruation is a normal physiological process that requires additional attention to hygiene but generally does not interrupt normal activities of the adolescent girl. If menstrual discomfort does occur, it usually does not happen until several months after menarche (after periods become ovulatory.)

When her period begins the girl's mother (or another trusted adult) should reassure her and make her feel that an important, happy event has happened. She should be helped to properly use the pad or tampon, and to insert the tampon, change it frequently and dispose of it properly.[7]

Another aspect of anticipatory guidance for a girl is self-examination of the breasts. While breast cancer is rare in teenage girls, the habit of self-examination is best learned while the girl is keenly aware of and concerned about her body. See Chapter 13 for a discussion of breast examination.

Anticipatory Guidance for Males One of the major concerns of boys is their height; most want to be tall. If a boy's growth spurt has not occurred by the time his genitals are at stage 4, he should be medically evaluated. After an examination is done, and if no abnormalities are found, the nurse should provide an opportunity for the boy to express his feelings about being short. In 85 per cent of males who are shorter than average, the cause is familial. Health professionals should concentrate on helping the boy who will not be tall to feel good about himself.

Size of penis is also a major concern for adolescent boys and adult men. If this concern exists, the boy should be reassured that penile size is not important in sexual intercourse, since only the outermost third of the female genital area is sensitive; a longer penis would not increase the female's pleasure. Information that it is impossible to estimate the size of an erect penis from its flaccid state and that, in general, there is greater enlargement of a small penis than a large one upon erection may also be reassuring.

Erections and nocturnal emissions (wet dreams) are signs of sexual development; however, these are often sources of great embarrassment for the young man. He should be reassured that they are normal and that the frequency of the unwanted erections will gradually decrease.

Uncircumcised boys need to be taught to retract the foreskin and carefully cleanse the glans, if they have not already learned to do so. Serious infections can result if this is not done. Also, the foreskin should be returned to its normal position over the glans to avoid constriction and edema of the glans.

The absence of one testicle is not a serious problem when growth and development are normal. The boy should be reassured that one testicle will not decrease his fertility, physical health or sexual functioning. Boys should be educated to seek medical help if they experience testicular pain. There are several conditions, some serious, that can occur in males, including injury, torsion of the testicle and epididymitis. In addition, young men should be taught self-examination of the testicles. The best time to examine the testes is right after a hot bath. The fingers are placed under each testis and the testicle is gently rolled between the thumb and fingers. The testes are oval, measuring about 4×3 cm. The epididymis on the back of the testicle should not be confused with an abnormal lump. Lumps should be examined immediately by a doctor, as testicular cancers detected early have an excellent prognosis.

COGNITIVE DEVELOPMENT

Anyone working closely with adolescents needs to be especially aware of the third and fourth stages in development of cognition — concrete operations and formal operations, according to Piaget's teachings (see Chapter 10). Adolescents will leave the concrete operational (third) stage of development and enter the formal operational stage at different ages. It is important to be able to identify the stage of thinking in order to have some idea of what to expect from the particular young person the nurse is dealing with as well as to know how to approach and explain things to him.

During concrete operations, logical reasoning at the concrete level is greatly increased. As a result the teenager's understanding of mathematics, people and relationships becomes clearer. An important concept that develops at this stage is *conservation*. Before this stage a child is unable to tell that a fat short glass and a tall skinny glass may hold the same volume of liquid. Children also become able to classify. For example, a concrete operational child can tell that dogs and cats are both animals and that poodles and collies are both dogs. However, the concrete operational child is unable to conceptualize values. He cannot apply past

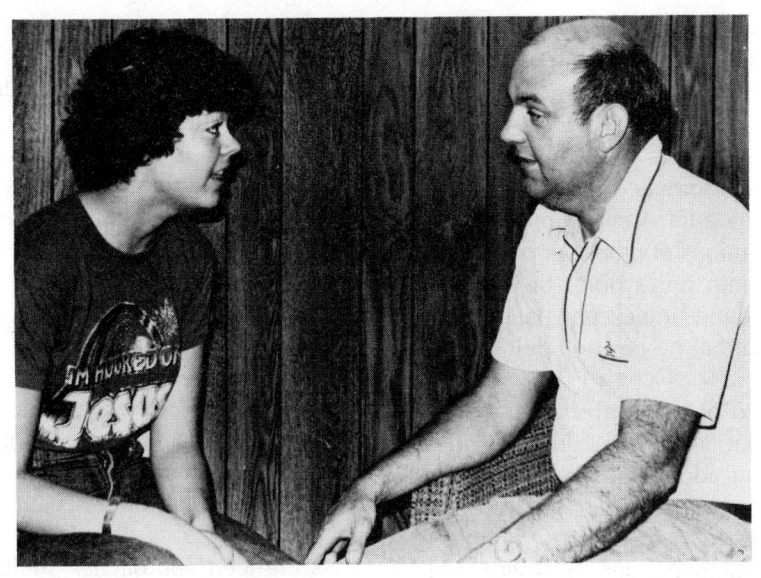

The adolescent has reached the stage of development at which she can discuss issues logically with an adult.

experiences and facts to predict probable future events. He is also unable to experiment with variables to reach a solution in a systematic way.

The formal operational (fourth) stage is the final Piagetian stage. It is only by questioning that an examiner can determine if a child has entered this stage; it is unrelated to physical development. Generally, it occurs somewhere between ages 12 and 19. Experiments have shown that some people never enter this stage of logical reasoning.

Piaget stated that formal thinking involves two major aspects: thinking about thoughts and separation of the real from the possible. At this stage children become able to use abstract logic and examine relations, classes and dimensions. They become able to construct hypotheses and, through deductive reasoning, test them logically by considering several variables. They seek scientific proof rather than relying on experience alone. They become able to vary a single factor mathematically and systematically while keeping others constant to determine cause and effect.

This change from concrete to formal thinking makes scientific appreciation and discovery possible. It enables adolescents to argue logically with adults. They are now able to examine issues and values from other people's points of view and discover their own values and ideas. Adolescents develop the ability to plan *realistically* for their own future. They can also study history with some understanding of time sequences. The boredom of school disappears when they can relate a present activity with future goals.[9]

Closely associated with cognitive functioning is the teenager's moral development. While his thinking is concrete, the adolescent displays conventional morality. He behaves in the manner that he believes or has learned will maintain or gain him approval by those in positions of authority. He has a respect for rules, because he perceives them to have been established in man's best interest. As the teenager matures into more formal thinking in late adolescence, Kohlberg* has reported that his morality changes, taking on post-conventional characteristics. (See Chapter 10 for further discussion of Kohlberg's stages of moral development.) The teen now makes behavioral decisions on the basis of internalized principles and his individual conscience. His behavior in a situation is determined by what he perceives is humanly and personally right for him.

Anticipatory Guidance: Cognitive Development

How can the foregoing knowledge help the nurse help adolescents and their parents? Before

---

*Kohlberg, L., Stages in Development of Moral Thought and Action. Holt, Rinehart and Winston, Inc., 1969.

the entry into formal operational thinking, adolescents may discuss problems with parents, but often the adolescents' arguments are critical of the parents and related to what could be or might have been. Parents' viewpoints are not easily understood or tolerated. These handicaps combined with the adolescent's limited ability to discern the emotions of other people make it important to explain one's point of view and feelings to the young adolescent patiently instead of assuming that he has an adult's ability to "pick up vibes."[6]

Being unable to perceive abstractly a situation or pattern that is not immediately evident causes many young adolescents to be criticized. If an adolescent member of a family seems repeatedly to attempt a task and is unable to complete it in a mature manner, parents need to realize that the reason may be the youth's developmental stage rather than laziness or disobedience.

Upon entering the formal operational stage young people are for the first time able to think about their values and reasoning processes. Often this new ability leads adolescents to idealism. They are able to question their own and their family's religious affiliations. It may become a major time of unrest for the teenager if he finds that he disagrees with the basic religious values he has always considered unquestionable. Some young people feel so alienated that they become part of a counterculture, a "true believer" movement, or some "radical religion." Parents and adults should openly discuss religion and values with adolescents. They should not force their point of view but offer a point of reference.

Poor school performance is a problem experienced by some adolescents and is often a problem of cognitive development that is troublesome to parents. The process of learning is complex; after a complete history and physical examination, the school is usually the best source of advice and referral for such problems. Learning disabilities can and do lead to emotional problems and often result in the child's dropping out of school and other behavioral problems. Parents need to show interest in school work, assist with homework and keep in close contact with teachers to be able to spot correctable problems.

EMOTIONAL DEVELOPMENT

According to Erikson,[3] the adolescent has the emotional task of establishing his identity or he will succumb to role confusion. The young person is now able to examine his beliefs in relation to another's point of view. People outside the home begin to exert significantly greater influence. A sampling of many different beliefs allows the teenager to try out a variety of characteristics and observe the reactions each produces and eventually to settle on an identity that is distinct but integrated and personally acceptable. If this does not happen, the young person may either remain confused about who he is or may settle on a negative identity, such as "dummy."

As the teen approaches adulthood, he must contend with establishing intimacy or being emotionally and socially isolated. At this time the young person reaches out to another and learns to share intimately. Originally Erikson associated intimacy with commitment and marriage. However, this stage applies even if permanent commitment is deferred to a later time. It involves the ability to share a meaningful relationship based on love and acceptance, and to care about others. Failing to complete this stage leads to a deep sense of isolation.

Anticipatory Guidance: Emotional Development

Adolescents tend to be concerned with themselves and view the world in terms of how it

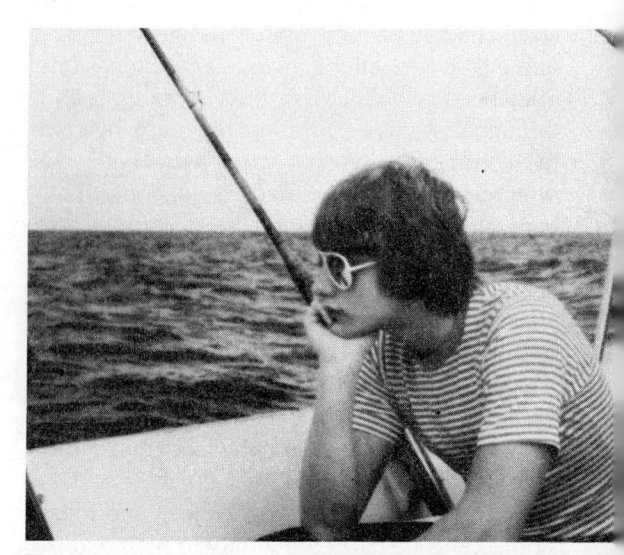

The teenager spends a great deal of time thinking about who he is as he searches for an identity that is uniquely his.

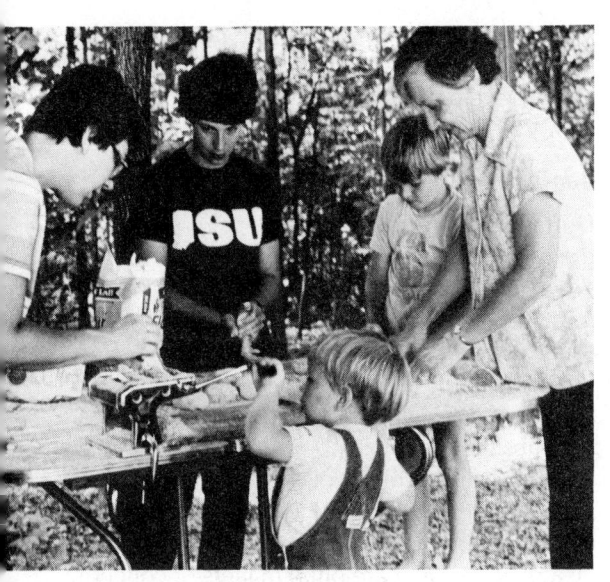

The teenager should be expected to participate in family projects and share home responsibilities without expecting monetary reimbursement.

affects them.[2] They imagine that others are watching them critically. This is one reason most early adolescents tend to enjoy being alone for periods. Their egocentrism and the fact that they usually feel powerless and vulnerable motivates defensive behavior toward their siblings and parents. Parents, with accurate information about cognitive and emotional development, play an extremely important role in guiding their teenagers through these critical stages.

Feelings of inferiority arising from incomplete resolution of stage 3 (industry versus inferiority) or from role confusion (stage 4) may lead to maladjustment that persists through life and often leads to serious consequences for society. Parents play a critical role in increasing and maintaining their adolescent's self-esteem. First, the success and self-esteem of the parents is influential in establishing self-esteem in the adolescent. Parents should pay attention to their own needs and growth. Second, parents should accept an adolescent for just *being* and let him know often that he is liked. Third, parents and teachers can emphasize positive aspects of the adolescent and not magnify negative aspects or failures. Assistance in developing his strengths builds self-confidence.

His search for identity leaves the adolescent open to many influences, which can be either constructive or detrimental both to the person and to society. Adolescents often identify intensely with charismatic figures, from political personages, religious leaders, film or music stars or professional athletes to local gang leaders. The adolescent who desperately wants "to be somebody" may, without guidance and support, settle for something which is ultimately self-destructive.

One help to developing a secure identity is investigation of vocational opportunities and the making of career plans. Parents should discuss future plans with their son or daughter. Parents cannot choose an identity for their child, however. Who or what he or she becomes must be the young person's personal choice; but parents can offer advice from their own experience when it is solicited. Open communication lines help the young person seek advice and bounce ideas off the adult without fearing ridicule or criticism.

In addition to expressions of love, both verbal and physical, adolescents need rules, guidance and discipline. The teenager needs responsibilities at home geared to his stage of development that are done as a part of meeting family goals, not for pay. Teenagers are old enough to get part-time, after-school and summer jobs and should be encouraged to do so. If possible, financial enterprises should be encouraged such as raising an animal for sale or growing vegetables to sell. The teen should also be able to manage his own checking and savings accounts and to assist in family budgeting. Every opportunity should be used to help the adolescent feel good about himself. Recognition should be given to the teenager by providing positive verbal feedback and by displays of affection and approval. Teenagers need opportunities to contribute to others. Volunteer work, running errands for an elderly neighbor, taking food to a sick friend or any other unpaid good deed will help the teenager develop a positive self-image. Organizations such as Boy and Girl Scouts and 4-H help adolescents learn and develop a sense of pride and accomplishment.

Some early signs of emotional problems can be detected by parents. Often it is not a specific behavior but rather the sudden appearance of a behavior, such as resistance to rules or avoidance of family activites, sudden change in friends or withdrawal from peers altogether, that indicates a problem is developing. Signs of depression may be conveyed by physical com-

ADOLESCENT GROWTH AND DEVELOPMENT: MAINTAINING WELLNESS

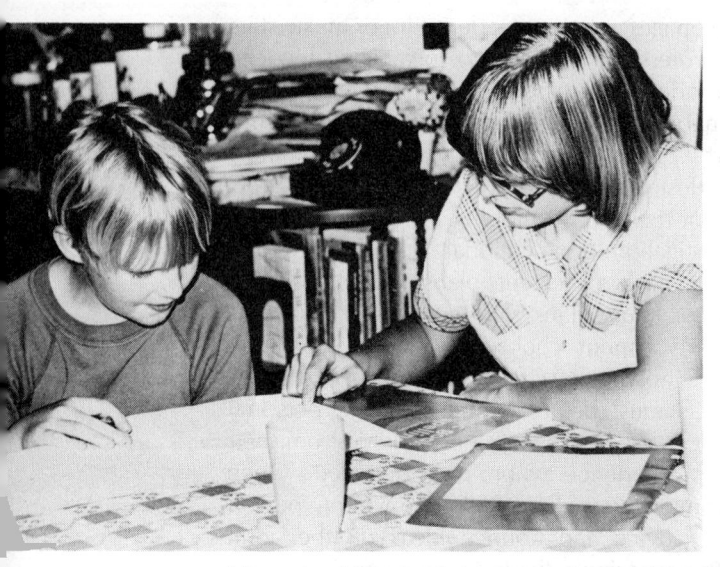

After-school tutoring is one way a teenager can earn money and build a positive self-image in the process of helping others.

plaints, headache, excess fatigue or sleeping, and poor appetite. A particularly stressful life event or series of events may trigger psychological or physical symptoms. Some of the early signs of depression are lack of interest and pleasure in life, boredom, poor concentration, diminished school performance, use of drugs or alcohol and suicidal thoughts.[7] Teens may report having difficulty in school or in making friends. The nurse should assist the adolescent and the parents to come to the realization that special help is necessary when these symptoms are present. When a referral is needed, the nurse can assist the adolescent and family in attaining such assistance.

SOCIAL DEVELOPMENT

According to Havinghurst,[5] there are nine developmental tasks of adolescents.

(1) Accepting one's body and consolidating sex role

(2) Expanding peer relationships to include both sexes

(3) Gaining emotional independence from family members

(4) Achieving economic independence

(5) Selecting and preparing for a vocation

(6) Developing adult intellectual skills and concepts

(7) Becoming socially responsible

(8) Preparing for marriage and family responsibilities and

(9) Developing realistic values in harmony with the world.

Body Acceptance and Sex Role Mastery

During adolescence the biological changes are dramatic and erratic. They begin and end at different ages for different individuals. Young adolescents usually construct an ideal body image using either admired models or fantasy. They usually closely observe older adolescents and adults to see what they may anticipate. During the transition from early to middle adolescence, a more realistic image of their body develops. At this time there may be dissatisfaction, especially if there is some physical abnormality. Height and weight are often matters of concern. By the end of middle adolescence the young person is generally comfortable with and has a realistic image of his body.[2]

By around age 3 the child had learned what sex he was, and expected behaviors because of his sex have been reinforced since his birth. By the end of his preschool years, as he resolved the impossible sexual relationship with his opposite-sex parent, he accepted and began to imitate a sex-role preference. His relationships with same-sex peers have helped to reinforce that preference and have begun shaping his sex-role identity. During early adolescence these same-sex peer relationships are intensified and take the form of gangs or cliques, which provide the opportunity to experiment with sex roles among equals and to learn some peer group expectations regarding heterosexual relationships.* By midadolescence the teenager tests out mature sex-role behaviors in direct heterosexual socialization so that by late adolescence the prominent social relationship involves one person of the other sex, with peer group identity diminishing steadily in importance.

Expanding Peer Relationships

School and the peer group divisions that the school environment affords become the teen's social "miniworld." Banned from participation in adult society and insulted by the society of childhood, teenagers are forced to shape their own subculture or group identity to preserve their sense of belonging. The Crowd (teen soci-

---

*Each clique or gang has an identifiable group of the opposite sex with whom it exchanges heterosexual feedback and interaction.

ety) and its more rigidly defined cliques and gangs (a hierarchy of classes or subgroups within the crowd; subdivision is based primarily on "popularity") compose the teen subculture to which the teenager can belong and identify while he begins the painful process of being independent from family and childhood.

In early adolescence peer group relationships are mostly with the same sex. Friendships become much more intimate than in childhood. Personal secrets that are shared with friends would never be told to an adult. Often the alliances are transient and friends are used for support. Jealousy is common. Sometimes early intimate friends remain lifelong friends. Early adolescents are curious about members of the opposite sex but are puzzled about how to approach them. Conformity in dress and opinion is important, reinforcing belonging needs. Parents are still considered ultimate authorities.

Middle adolescence is characterized by some contact with the opposite sex and less intense association with the same sex. The telephone becomes important, because it reduces the embarrassment of being observed while talking with a member of the opposite sex. Late adolescents can usually date with more self-confidence. Peer groups become less important and usually one dating partner emerges. By the end of adolescence the teen has usually developed behaviors and an identity that readies him for participation in an adult society of peers.

Emotional Independence From Family

Independence from family influence is a major developmental struggle of adolescence. As cognitive abilities reach the formal operational stage, the adolescent is able to evaluate the values of his family. Early adolescents usually use parents for role models and accept their authority. As adolescence progresses the teenager continually tests his parents and more and more freedom is demanded. By midadolescence a typical complaint is that parents give too little freedom and do not trust the adolescent. This is in conflict with parents' views: parents feel that both the freedom and trust they do offer is abused.

Parents have less and less influence in decision-making as their adolescent progresses. Teens often find another adult in whom to confide. Late adolescents find their parents easier to consult. They have found ways to satisfy their need for affection and intimacy outside

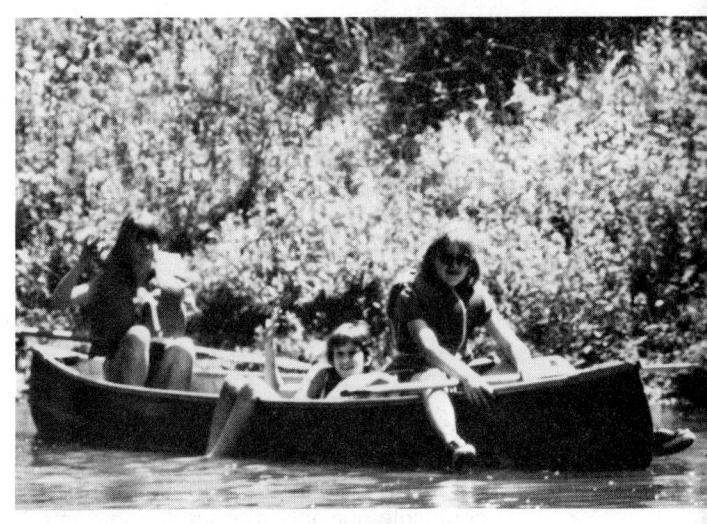

A few close friends are reserved for intimate sharing that is free of role-playing and the charades of group interaction. Often these early friendships last a lifetime.

home, to take responsiblity for the behavioral choices they make and to construct their values out of a sense of self rather than from rebellion so that they no longer perceive their parents as threats to their autonomy but as comrades in an adult world. During the interlude of adolescence parents must learn to be comfortable in addressing their children in an adult relationship. For many parents this task is not fully accomplished until their children become parents.

Economic Independence

Economic independence may or may not be related to a decision regarding life work. Adolescents become increasingly aware that dependence on parents will terminate in the near future. The early adolescent's idealistic vocational choice eventually gives way to more realistic appraisal of potential. Girls as well as boys may find the decision about life work difficult and frightening. Parents exert more influence than peers, both as role models and by persuasion. In this area, teachers also have influence on vocational choice by the kind of feedback and reinforcement they offer students about their capabilities and skills.

Developing Adult Skills

The development of adult intellectual skills and concepts is related partly to cognitive stage and partly to experience. As discussed earlier, abstract concepts such as "values" cannot be evaluated before the formal thinking stage. Parents can assist their young adult by explaining the reasons behind their own behaviors. For example, when the parent buys a new car, explanation should be offered as to why it is best to bargain, ask questions and compare before purchasing. Likewise, reasons are given for why, when seeking a job, one always dresses neatly, displays good hygiene and uses good manners.

Becoming Socially Responsible

Becoming socially responsible means being accountable not only to oneself and one's family but to the community as well. As social development takes place, more thought is given to how one's own behavior affects other people — before one acts in accordance with one's own desires. By now the teenager should understand the impact of destroying public property, causing others anguish or injury, and withholding the contribution of his own potentials to decision-making or tasks. It is necessary to be able to perform abstract thinking to understand that responsibility builds trust and facilitates the development of cooperative relationships. As a person's social responsibility is developed, he or she is also likely to become more politically active. Incorporation of a "world view" into decision making is a late task of adolescence.

Preparing for Family Responsibilities

Marriage and family responsibility follows social responsibility. At Erikson's intimacy stage, young people desire to fill the affection gap left in separation from the mother. This task is accomplished at different ages by young people. Preparing for family relationships involves more than just the capacity for intimacy. Teenagers can gain some perspective for the responsibility of family living if they are included in family budgeting and decision-making. In addition, a sense of child care responsibility is stimulated by activities such as babysitting and volunteer work in nursery schools or day care centers. Many schools now incorporate family living classes as curriculum requisites. In these classes teenagers look at the broad picture of managing a home and maintaining healthy family relationships and the ways in which society aids and hinders families in those efforts.

Anticipatory Guidance: Social Development

The role of parents is to prepare the child to successfully cope with what is in the world. Since puberty is occurring at earlier and earlier ages, children may look like adults when they are still children. Although their bodies appear mature, adolescents need the help of professionals and parents to cope with the many stresses they experience in the social realm. The nurse should encourage parents to provide information regarding the biological changes that account for the adolescent's sexual drive. Furthermore, professionals and parents have a responsibility to ensure that information that the adolescent has about sexual intercourse, reproduction and birth control is accurate (see later section on birth control).

The nurse can act as a resource person to parents to help them maintain communication with their adolescent. Parents should encourage their teenager to entertain friends at home. This communicates an acceptance of the teen's friends and gives parents an opportunity to get to know the people who are influencing their child's attitudes and behaviors. Parents should be encouraged to explain their own values and the rules they wish to maintain within their own home. When adolescents do not comply after clear explanations, parents should be supported in their decision to apply reasonable forms of punishment. (See Chapter 3 for discussion of parenting skills and styles.)

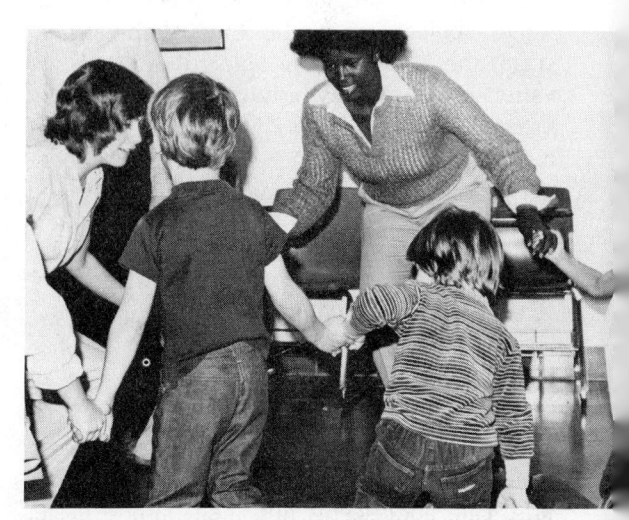

Teenagers' experiences with children help to broaden their understanding and appreciation of childrearing as a part of family life.

The boundless energy and limitless curiosity of adolescents can easily be channeled into constructive activities such as sports and hobbies. Teens should be encouraged to be creative, take outside classes (dance, music, tennis, swimming, cooking), join organizations or participate in volunteer work.

ADOLESCENT HEALTH CARE

Problems of adolescents are poorly researched. Too few studies have been done to help practitioners guide adolescents through probably the most hazardous and important time of their lives. More research is needed in the areas of the biological processes of puberty, nutritional requirements of adolescents, their intellectual development and socialization, better approaches to the delivery of adolescent health care and health education, and the effect of television, drugs and environment on adolescent physical, intellectual, and emotional-social development.

Health care is rapidly becoming specialized for adolescents. For years it was informally considered part of both pediatrics and adult health care. Certainly the needs of adolescents are similar to those of both children and adults. However, adolescents also have unique needs based more on their stage of development than on physical differences. Teenagers have often felt out of place in both pediatric and adult health care settings.

In the 1950s the special health needs of teenagers was recognized. Dr. Roswell Gallagher, a Boston internist, was a leader in this movement.[8] Several outpatient clinics were opened that centered on diseases prevalent in adolescents, such as rheumatic heart disease and diabetes. These clinics were highly successful and were followed by adolescent hospital inpatient units and an increasing number of outpatient units specifically for adolescents.

The federal government has begun to establish adolescent health care clinics. Some of these focus on specific needs such as birth control while others are comprehensive in their approach and still others are research-oriented. Other services available to adolescents include school health programs and college health services. Several cities have responded to the emergency health needs of adolescents (particularly runaways) by establishing free clinics. San Francisco's Haight-Ashbury district free clinic and Boston's mobile medical van are examples of these. Crisis hot lines have been set up in various cities and serve as effective entries for adolescents into the health care system. Other approaches include multiservice centers where medical and counselling services are available. Services for teenage parents are also becoming more common.

There are still gaps geographically and categorically in the meeting of adolescents' health care needs. One major gap is the need for services for the parents of adolescents. Discredited by adolescents and health professionals alike, parents may be an important key to prevention and treatment of many common adolescent health problems.

Conferences on adolescent health are being held and attended by representatives from many disciplines. Adolescents themselves often make significant contributions. Research, knowledge and education in the area of adolescent health are expanding.

ADOLESCENT HEALTH MAINTENANCE

Adolescents should be seen by a physician or other primary care provider at least every two years, even if no problems arise. During routine health visits the health professional should provide guidance and counselling based on the individual needs of the adolescent. The anticipatory guidance as described for physical, intellectual, emotional and social development is basic to adolescent health maintenance — as it is at any age. Special additional areas in which the health care provider working with adolescents requires knowledge are personal hygiene, dental care, nutrition, and birth control.

Personal Care

Adolescents are known both for sleeping "all the time" or chronically "burning the candle at both ends." The actual amount of sleep required by an adolescent covers a wide range. Rather than state a specific number of hours, it is wiser to advise parents to be cognizant of their adolescent's sleep patterns and symptoms of fatigue. Many other effects can result from a lack of adequate sleep, such as crankiness, accidents and frustration. If the sleep pattern changes suddenly, a call or visit to a primary care provider is in order.

A sufficient amount of exercise, sunshine, and fresh air is important to young people's emotional as well as physical health. Fresh air and change of scene can reduce tensions built up by the relative immobilization of the classroom. Adolescents, especially younger ones, often object to dressing for the weather. T-shirts in a snow storm and leather jackets in hot weather are inappropriate and parents should be encouraged to trust their knowledge of such matters. Daily bathing with special attention to genitalia is necessary in warm weather; two to four times a week is sufficient for cold weather.

Depending on when initial childhood immunizations were completed, DT and oral polio boosters as well as periodic tuberculin testing will be necessary sometime during the adolescent years.

Dental Care

Adolescent years are peak years for dental caries and yet preventive and therapeutic treatment by dental professionals is one of the most neglected needs of teenagers. Dental care is often a low financial priority of families.

Several important reasons exist for making the repair and maintenance of adolescents' teeth a priority. Adequate nutrition is nearly impossible when teeth hurt or are missing. Fresh fruit and vegetables, for example, are difficult to eat with missing, aching or decayed teeth. Appearance is extremely important to teenagers; teens with decayed teeth usually have problems with self-esteem, while healthy, white teeth help the teenager develop a positive self-concept.

A full set of permanent teeth is expected by age 13 with the exception of the wisdom teeth, which erupt by 22 to 23 years. Adequate dental maintenance includes proper brushing at least twice a day, daily flossing and a visit to the dentist every six months. An adequate supply of fluoride is needed to help prevent cavities and can be obtained from treated drinking water (1 part per million), topical application in the dentist's office or in oral fluoride tablets if the drinking supply has no fluoride. Schools may add fluoride to their drinking water in areas in which local water lacks fluoride.

Nutrition

Nutritional requirements during adolescence have yet to be adequately explored. However, teenagers are usually free to eat as they choose and must be informed of good nutrition. Often their parents are equally unaware of what constitutes good nutrition. When an abundant food supply is available, most teenagers get an adequate supply of nutrients.[2] Some problems occur, however, in impoverished families and with fad diets or weight reduction diets. For example, fresh fruits and vegetables are expensive and poor families may lack food sources of vitamins A and C and iron. Dieting teens sometimes eliminate bread and milk, thinking these foods are fattening; these foods are essential to good nutrition.

Caloric and protein requirements increase for boys from age 11 to 18. Girls have a slightly increased protein need but caloric needs decrease from age 11 to 18. The iron needed by the adolescent is almost double that needed by the adult male or the woman past menopause. Iodine is necessary for proper thyroid function and the need rises sharply during the growth spurt. Calcium required for skeletal and dental growth also increases during the growth spurt. Niacin and thiamine needs increase during adolescence in males. Most of these nutrient needs drop after adolescence. Table 57–3 describes the servings of each food group needed by adolescents.

A 24-hour nutritional assessment may be made by the nurse as for any other age. (See Chapter 13 for nutritional assessment.) Signs of nutritional problems that the nurse may watch for during routine physical examinations are summarized in Table 57–4.

Relating nutrition practices to appearance for the adolescent is an effective way for the nurse

TABLE 57–3 DAILY FOOD GUIDE FOR ADOLESCENTS

Food Group	Servings
Milk and milk products	4
Meats	3
Fruits and vegetables	4
Vitamin C source	1
Vitamin A source	1
Breads and cereals	4

TABLE 57-4 CLINICAL SIGNS INDICATIVE OF NUTRITIONAL DEFICIENCIES

General appearance	Lethargy, excessive or inadequate body fat, muscle wasting
Skin	Dryness, flakiness, scaling, roughness (follicular hyperkeratosis), pallor
Mouth	Angular fissures, redness at corners of mouth (cheilosis); redness, swelling or atrophic papillae on tongue; red, swollen or bleeding gums
Teeth	Severe caries
Eyes	Pale conjunctivae
Nails	Spoon-shaped, brittle or ridged
Hair	Dull, easily plucked

to obtain the teenager's interest in nutrition. Adolescent obesity is discussed further in Chapter 60.

Birth Control

The menstrual cycle, male and female growth and development, birth control, and facts about sexually transmitted diseases are subjects that should be discussed with all young men and women. A discussion of basic information on birth control follows. Sexually transmitted diseases are discussed in Chapter 60.

With the number of teenage (and preteen) girls who engage in sexual intercourse, it seems that there is hardly a "too young" age at which to begin teaching girls how to protect themselves from pregnancy. Although first periods after menarche begins are usually anovulatory, some girls do ovulate from the beginning. Also, since menarche is occurring earlier, today's sexually mature girls do not have the same cognitive development for decision-making that earlier generations have had.

While sexually active teenagers and pregnant teens get a lot of publicity, about half of teenage girls decide to postpone intercourse. Professionals should include in their histories questions about the teenager's decision regarding sex. It is important that the adolescent realize that a choice exists and that it is acceptable to wait.

For those teens who choose to be sexually active, the nurse has a primary role in helping them make informed decisions about birth control. Sometimes parents, in their haste to be "liberated," try to force teens into use of birth control when it is not needed. Parents and professionals must constantly be aware of their own values and keep them separate from those of their children and their clients.

Withdrawal is a method of birth control used by some teens. It is free, involves no devices and is always available. The couple have intercourse until just before ejaculation. Then the penis is removed from the vagina and the sperm is deposited at a distance from the vagina. The biggest problem with this method is its low rate of effectiveness. The reasons for this are that some sperm escape even before ejaculation and timing of withdrawal before the moment of ejaculation is very difficult to control.

The *condom,* or rubber, is another common birth control device used by teens. Condoms are relatively cheap, available without the need to visit a health care professional and allow a male to control his fertility. They prevent pregnancy by providing a barrier between the penis (sperm) and the cervix (ovum). The failure rate is fairly high unless the condom is used with foam, which increases its effectiveness to near that of the contraceptive pill. Some precautions for the young client using condoms are: (1) buy a good brand, (2) keep condoms away from heat (such as body heat from keeping them in a wallet), (3) be sure to put the condom on before the penis gets anywhere near the vagina, (4) leave a one-half inch space at the end of the condom, (5) be sure to hold on to the condom when the penis is withdrawn from the vagina and (6) if the rubber breaks or tears, insert contraceptive foam immediately. Condoms also offer some help in preventing the spread of venereal disease.

Contraceptive foam may also be used alone. The foam is placed in the vagina before intercourse by means of an applicator. The foam then blocks entry across or through the cervix and immobilizes or kills the sperm. Use with condoms greatly increases effectiveness of the foam, which also serves as a lubricant. The user must remember to: (1) shake the can 20 times before dispensing, (2) fill the applicator completely full, (3) insert the foam just before intercourse, (4) insert as far as comfortably possible so the foam will cover the cervix, (5) avoid douching for at least eight hours after intercourse and (6) wash the applicator with soap and warm water. Foam also helps prevent trichomoniasis and gonorrhea. Allergies to foam can sometimes be prevented by switching brands.

The rhythm method is another method used

by some adolescents. Unfortunately, many are grossly misinformed about this method. Its use requires knowledge, skill and motivation to be successful; however, even when used properly, it is not very effective. There are three techniques involved in natural family planning. One is the *calendar method*. This is based on the fact that ovulation usually occurs 14 days before the onset of menstruation in a regular 28-day cycle. Sperm live for two to three days and the ovum survives about 24 hours. The woman must chart her cycles for at least 8 months, then subtract 18 days from her shortest cycle and 11 days from her longest cycle; the period of time between those days is her fertile time. For example, if her longest cycle (space between first days of two periods) was 30 days and her shortest was 25 days, she should abstain between days 7 and 19 of her cycles. The second technique is *basal body method*. This involves taking a rectal temperature immediately upon waking. Immediately before ovulation the temperature drops slightly and a sharp rise is seen immediately after ovulation. After a woman feels sure of her cycle, she may resume sex three days after the rise in temperature. The third technique is the "mucus" method. This is based on body changes around the time of ovulation. Often a woman will experience pain, a sense of heaviness or other body symptoms at ovulation. The consistency of cervical mucus also changes from thick to the consistency of egg white, which can be stretched between slides or fingers at a distance of 6 cm or more. A central problem with this method is that adolescent girls have irregular menstrual cycles. It is also not a preferred method of adolescents because it requires abstinence for a period of time each month and time calculations are complicated.

The *intrauterine device* (IUD) is one of the methods for which the young woman must seek medical advice. The device is a small plastic appliance sometimes containing copper or progestin, inserted into the uterus. Its mechanism of action is not known, but conception can occur. The IUD prevents implantation of the embryo on the uterine wall, thus interrupting the sequence of pregnancy. Some conditions that contraindicate the IUD include active pelvic infection, pregnancy, abnormal Pap smear, abnormal uterine bleeding and allergy to copper (if the device contains copper 7). Some doctors will not insert IUD's into young women who have never been pregnant, because of their greater incidence of pelvic infection when using an IUD.[7A] IUD's are relatively effective in controlling pregnancy. It is somewhat easier to insert an IUD during menses, and if the device is placed at this time, a pregnancy is unlikely to exist already. Insertion is likely to cause some cramping or nausea, so it is a good idea to have someone else drive the girl home after insertion of the IUD. Precautions to warn the user about are: (1) because the IUD may fall out, the string should be checked monthly after each menses; (2) there is a chance that the IUD may perforate the uterus; (3) there is an increased chance of developing pelvic inflammatory disease and (4) IUD's can be responsible for reduction in fertility because of tubal scarring during healing of pelvic inflammatory disease. IUD users should call their doctor immediately if a period is missed or if symptoms of vaginal infection occur.

The *diaphragm* is a dome-shaped latex cup with a flexible rim that is inserted into the vagina. It must be fitted by a health professional, both for size and type. The aim is to fit the largest size comfortable, because the interior third of the vagina expands when the woman is sexually excited. The diaphragm is always used with a spermicidal cream, foam or jelly and serves to hold the spermicidal agent against the cervical os.

Effectiveness is directly correlated with proper use of the diaphragm. The diaphragm is inserted no more than two hours before intercourse by folding and inserting it, jelly side up, into the vagina, or by use of an applicator. It *must* be checked by inserting a finger into the vagina to feel for the cervix (feels like a big nose) inside the dome's rim. Subsequent intercourse must be preceded by an application of more spermicide. To remove the diaphragm, a finger is hooked on the rim and it is pulled down and out.

The wearer must be sure to leave the diaphragm in place at least six hours after the last intercourse and should not douche. The diaphragm should be washed and dried carefully, dusted with cornstarch, and kept in its case. A return visit is necessary to have the fit checked after one to two weeks of use and after a pregnancy, pelvic surgery, weight gain or loss of 10 to 20 pounds, or if any discomfort is experienced. An advantage of this method is that during menses the diaphragm holds the menstrual flow. One diaphragm should last about two years but should be checked regularly near a light for holes or tears. For the discharge that occurs after use, wearing of a tampon or mini-pad may be necessary. Diaphragms are preferred by women concerned about the effects of pills and IUD's. The diaphragm has the additional advantage of getting the woman better acquainted with her body.

Oral contraceptives, or birth control pills, are used by 10 to 15 million women in the United States. The oral contraceptives containing a combination of estrogen and progestogen suppress ovulation by inhibiting the secretion of hypothalamic gonadotropin-releasing hormone, and may also act directly on the pituitary to inhibit release of gonadotropins. The combination pill also causes development of "hostile cervical mucus," which decreases the chance of sperm penetration. Contraindications to using the pill include cardiovascular disorders, liver problems, malignancy, and pregnancy.*

The pills are taken once a day for 21 days, followed by a 7-day "off" period, before another 21-day cycle is resumed. The 28-day cycle of pills (containing 7 days of inert pills) is recommended for the adolescent because with it she simply takes a pill every morning instead of having to interrupt and resume the sequence.

To be given a prescription for oral contraceptives, a girl must have a complete physical examination, including a pap smear, hematocrit, blood pressure test and tests for syphilis and gonorrhea. The worst (life-threatening) side effects of oral contraceptives are blood clots in the legs, pelvis, lungs or brain; liver tumors and hypertension.

The nurse can be helpful in counselling the young woman in the importance of taking her pill every day. If a pill is missed, two should be taken the next day. If two or more are missed, the girl should avoid intercourse until menses occurs or use another contraceptive method in addition to completing the rest of the pill cycle. Any side effects such as spotting, nausea or weight gain should be reported to a doctor or nurse practitioner. Questions should be encouraged. The girl's nutritional requirements of vitamins C, B_6 and B_{12} and folic acid are increased by taking oral contraceptives.

Many people have suggested that giving oral contraceptives to adolescents encourages sexual activity. Shearin[11] found in his study that oral contraceptives neither increased the frequency of intercourse nor the number of partners. It is the author's experience that adolescents know when they are in danger of becoming pregnant and none have requested birth control without need.

Counselling Adolescents

When counselling adolescents about sex-related problems, the nurse may get complaints from parents. Usually the parents are angry; their anger arises from frustration and guilt that the young person has sought help from someone other than them. Parents need reassurance (without breaking confidentiality) that it is common for youngsters to do this. (Recalling with parents that they probably did not ask their own parents sex-related questions at this age may help them understand their adolescent.) It is especially important to emphasize to parents that it is to their credit that their adolescent is responsible enough to seek help independently when needed, a fact for which they can feel proud.

It cannot be emphasized too much or too often that the respecting of confidentiality is probably the most important element in obtaining a teen's trust. The nurse should encourage the teenager to discuss sexual matters with parents if possible. Included in confidentiality is the basic rule that a consultant should never leave her client's records where others can read even the name. Also, she should not give out personal information over the telephone; the caller may not be who he says he is. She should not call an adolescent's home for any reason unless she has written permission; parents get suspicious.

Legal considerations are important when treating adolescents. In some cases, there may be a conflict between the need to provide health care to minors and the objective of maintaining confidentiality. A child is considered by law to be incompetent to consent to his or her own health care. Most states consider the age of maturity to be 18. Some states have "emancipated minor" provisions in statutes whereby a minor may give consent for health services under certain circumstances. Many states have passed legislation allowing a minor

---

*There are other contraindications and the reader is referred to *Contraceptive Technology*,[4] which is published annually, for a complete discussion of all birth control methods.

to obtain contraceptive services and to be treated for sexually transmitted diseases or drug abuse without parental consent. Some states also allow provision for psychiatric treatment without consent. The nurse should be aware of the laws in her state and of the policies in the setting in which she works.

There is seldom excuse for failure to provide information to youth or to obtain the young person's consent before seeking information. Many courts have adopted a "mature minor doctrine" whereby, if the minor is judged by the health care practitioner to be capable of understanding the nature and consequences of the treatment and it is for the minor's benefit, the practitioner may give treatment. The information necessary to informed consent for birth control can be remembered by the acronym BRAIDED:[4]

*B*enefits of the method
*R*isks of the method
*A*lternatives to the method
*I*nquiries about the method are encouraged
*D*ecision to withdraw from using the methods is OK
*E*xplanation of the procedure: what to expect, what to do
*D*ocumentation of the above.

References

1. E. Anthony. The Reactions of Adults to Adolescents and Their Behavior. In The Psychology of Adolescence. A. Esman, ed. International University Press, 1975
2. W. Daniel. Adolescents For Health and Disease. C. V. Mosby Co., 1977
3. E. Erikson. Childhood and Society. W. W. Norton and Co., 1963
3a. W. Harlan et al. Secondary sex characteristics of boys 12 to 17 years of age: The U.S. Health Examination Survey. Journal of Pediatrics, June 1979, p. 293
3b. W. Harlan et al. Secondary sex characteristics of girls 12 to 17 years of age: The U.S. Health Examination Survey. Journal of Pediatrics, June 1980, p. 6
4. R. Hatcher et al. Contraceptive Technology 1978–1979. Irvington Publishers, Inc., 1978
5. R. Havinghurst. Developmental Tasks and Education. David McKay Co., Inc., 1972
6. A. Jersild et al. The Psychology of Adolescence. Macmillan Co., Inc., 1978
7. J. Meeks and C. Schwarzbeck. Understanding the Nature of Depression in Young People. Adolescent Medicine, July 1979
7a. R. T. Mercer. Perspectives on Adolescent Health Care. J. B. Lippincott Co., 1979
8. H. Miller. Approaches to Adolescent Health Care in the 1970's. DHEW publication (HSA) 76-5014, 1975
9. M. Pramik. Too short/too tall. Transitions, Vol. 2, No. 2, 1979
10. H. Sebald. Adolescence, A Social Psychological Analysis. Prentice-Hall, 1968
11. R. Shearin. Contraception for Adolescents. American Family Physician, March 1976, p. 117
12. J. Tanner. Growth at Adolescence. Charles C Thomas, 1962
13. H. Yahraes. Parents as Leaders: The Role of Control and Discipline. National Institute of Mental Health, DHEW Publication (ADM) 78-613, 1978

Additional Recommended Reading

1. J. Cassidy. Teenagers in a Family Planning Clinic. Nursing Outlook, November 1970, p. 30
2. M. Chard. An Approach to Examining the Adolescent Male. American Journal of Maternal Child Nursing, Jan/Feb 1976, p. 41
3. W. Daniel and R. Brown. Adolescent Physical Maturation. Journal of Current Adolescent Medicine, June 1979
4. Eleven Million Teenagers. Alan Guttmacher Institute, 1976
5. E. Erikson. Dimensions of a New Identity. W. W. Norton and Co., Inc., 1974
6. K. Fontaine. Human Sexuality: Facilitating Knowledge and Attitudes. *Nursing Outlook*, March 1976
7. S. Gordon and I. Dickman. Sex Education: The Parents' Role. Public Affairs Pamphlet # 546, 1978
8. J. Kagan and R. Coles, eds. 12 to 16: Early Adolescence. W. W. Norton and Co., Inc., 1972
9. F. Koestler. *Runaway Teenager*. Public Affairs Pamphlet # 552, 1977
10. J. Kosidek. Improving Health Care for Troubled Youth. American Journal of Nursing, January 1976
11. K. Reichert. Primary Care of Young Adults. Medical Examination Publishing Company, 1976
12. G. Stephens. The Creative Contraries: A Theory of Sexuality. American Journal of Nursing, January 1978
13. A. Ticky and L. Malasanos. The Physiological Role of Hormones in Puberty. American Journal of Maternal-Child Nursing, Sept/Oct 1976, p. 384
14. G. Wells. Reducing the Threat of a First Pelvic Exam. American Journal of Maternal Child Nursing, Sept/Oct 1977, p. 304

58 POTENTIAL STRESSES DURING ADOLESCENCE: MANAGING BEHAVIOR

by Linda Bond, RN, MSN

Adolescence is characterized by turbulence stemming from the new feelings within and from the awesome pressures exerted on the young person by a multitude of external sources. Limited life experiences, feelings of infallibility, and an underdeveloped sense of self are factors that lead adolescents to engage in activities that can have serious or even devastating health consequences.

Many adolescents traverse these years with only minor and temporary upsets, while others find adolescence full of problems. Resources such as a strong family support system, friendship with stable individuals, involvement in structured peer activities, and satisfactory experiences in school all contribute to a smooth transition to adulthood. Adolescents who lack support resources and who cannot cope with the stresses of this turbulent time are the ones who may resort to socially unacceptable modes of behavior.

Among the issues discussed in this chapter are delinquent behavior among adolescents; suicide; physical mistreatment, neglect, and sexual abuse of adolescents by parents or other adults; sexual stresses; the status of adolescent runaways; drug misuse; and school attendance problems. The problems confronting adolescents and their families are often part of larger social issues. Both the causes and consequences of these problems involve not only the individual family unit but also the schools and society in general. The nurse may not be in a position to provide direct interventions in all problems that she sees. Nevertheless, there are important contributions to be made by the profession. As individual issues are discussed, emphasis is placed on *the role nurses can play in casefinding efforts* to identify troubled youth or families, the *role nurses have in providing education* for both adolescents and parents, and the *nurturing role nurses have* in providing support and understanding for families and adolescents.

Certain patterns of behavior or characteristics (Table 58–1) may be diagnostic of those adolescents at high risk for adjustment problems. While no single characteristic or pattern of behavior is symptomatic, a combination of these is recognized as indicative of a potentially dangerous situation in terms of life adjustment. Not all adolescents experiencing difficulties with coping are living within a discordant family situation (Table 58–2), but the two situations certainly are related and increase the risk of maladjustment during adolescence.

TABLE 58-1 CHARACTERISTICS OF ADOLESCENTS AT RISK FOR SOCIAL PROBLEMS

Poor self-concept
Severe mood changes
School problems
Antisocial behavior
Substance abuse
Decreased verbal communication
Sleep disturbances
Prolonged grief reaction following divorce, death, or severing of a romance
Communication problems at home
"Loner"
Friends of questionable reputation
Premature "growing up"

A recent Michigan study on health and adolescence concludes that the 10- to 19-year-old age group comprise one-fifth of the population.[1] This only indicates the percentage of population in a single state but suggests that adolescents make up approximately 20 per cent of the total population in the United States. Problems associated with this age group have an impact on the total population, but probably most significant are their effects upon the individual family unit.

DELINQUENCY

As *Time Magazine* states, "People have always accused kids of getting away with murder. Now that is all too literally true."[30] Crimes and delinquent acts committed by adolescents have moved beyond the prank stage to pose a major threat to society, particularly in urban areas. Exact figures related to the number of delinquent acts committed are difficult to obtain, although the Federal Bureau of Investigation reports a staggering increase in the number of arrests for violent crimes in the period from 1967 to 1976. The most startling figures are those involving crimes in the 17 and below age group. According to this report, juveniles between the ages of 7 and 18 are the group most prone to commit crime in the nation. An increase of 98 per cent in crime was seen in this age group as compared with an increase of 65 per cent in the 18 and over age group.[31]

Delinquency is not limited to boys; more girls are becoming involved in crime. In 1975, 11 per cent of juveniles arrested for violent crimes were girls.[30]

Peer pressure or influence operates in delinquency. Delinquent acts are often the work of more than one youth or of a gang. Gangs, once glamorized in movies, are now organized and possess identifiable characteristics such as leadership and prescribed lines of authority.[28] Today gangs are composed mostly of males in their late teens. These gangs are both mobile and sophisticated in their use of hit-and-run tactics to rob and steal.

What differentiates delinquent from nondelinquent boys? Smith and Walters concluded that while both groups came from similar backgrounds, distinguishing factors in delinquent boys were (1) poor or no relationships with their fathers, (2) strong involvement with their mothers, and (3) broken homes.[28] These findings coupled with individual problems such as deviant classroom behavior, truancy, or running away present a clear picture of the potentially delinquent youth.[10] Further conclusions are drawn from a study by Cahoun. He concluded that white youths were more likely to commit delinquent acts as attention-seeking behaviors, whereas black youths committed crimes that would yield money.[6]

Delinquency is associated with all social strata, but youth from middle and upper class homes tend to be involved in less serious incidents. Delinquency among juveniles may reflect repressed desires of their parents that communicate to them a "boys will be boys" philosophy. Middle and upper class adults, especially males, protect their sons by either paying for damages incurred or overlooking the incidents. These practices, if operational, let youth involved in irresponsible, illegal and destructive acts get off essentially free. Youthful offenders released from assuming responsibility for their crimes may feel smug, but adults

TABLE 58-2 FAMILY SITUATIONS THAT JEOPARDIZE NORMAL ADOLESCENT DEVELOPMENT

Divorce
Death of one parent
Frequent family relocation
Insufficient parental guidance
Frequent absences of one parent
Drug or alcohol abuse
Step-parent
Poor relationships between family members
Mental illness
Economic deprivation
Faulty communication patterns

perpetuating this practice are interfering with their child's transition to responsible adulthood.

Youth involved in delinquent behavior expend energy that is normally directed toward meeting the developmental tasks of adolescence. Delinquency may have life-long ramifications for the individual, but these are secondary to the stress placed on the family unit at the time of each occurrence. Families escape neither the emotional consequences of nor financial responsibility for delinquency. Parents, responsible for their children until they reach the age of majority, may respond to these additional stresses by retreating from the family unit. Family discord can lead the troubled youth to further alienation from society's accepted behavior code.

The problem of delinquency has reached epidemic proportions in some areas and affects all facets of society. Efforts to stop the increasing crime rate have had varying degrees of success, but none have been entirely successful, so the problem continues.

Some urban areas have reduced the juvenile crime rate by adopting a "get tough" policy. Rehabilitation of most youth is possible. It is estimated that only 10 per cent of the youngsters who tangle with the law are incorrigible offenders.[30] Various modes of prevention, restoration and rehabilitation have been tried. The reality shock approach portrayed in the film documentary *Scared Straight,* while violent, has had success in some areas. Youthful offenders are taken to prisons, given tours, and spend time locked in the depths of the institution with inmates. The prisoners present a very realistic view of the type of life that will probably follow if the adolescents continue on their delinquent path.

If convicted and sentenced to imprisonment, adolescents face the prospect of crowded conditions. This form of punishment has not proved successful in preventing further criminal activity. There is a high cost in maintaining facilities to house youthful offenders in this manner. Group homes have been tried as an alternate to prison, but also with limited success.

Unique programs such as Outward Bound have also been tried. Groups of youth have been taken into a wilderness situation and forced to learn survival through individual and group efforts.[30] Youth involved in this program have shown positive behavior for at least the first year after participation. The most successful programs of rehabilitation are those that aim to reassert the youths' individual responsibility.[30]

The solution to the problem of juvenile delinquency lies in prevention. Families cannot be held totally responsible for the acts of individual members. Individuals at some point must assume responsibility for their own behavior.

One solution may lie in reappraisal of the family as a social institution, with appropriate reorganization to provide more structure and controls for the developing youth. A stronger emphasis on the role of the father could do much to alleviate the problem of delinquency. Fathers who develop a loving, supportive relationship with their sons can do much to guide them in positive and productive directions.[11] Role models play an important part in the way a youth develops. If the adolescent is not allowed to be involved in activities that integrate both youth and adults, an important opportunity is lost. Those activities that involve only youth tend to lack both structure and direction.

Social programs organized by groups and institutions such as churches may in part provide an answer to the problem of how to avert juvenile crime. Activities carried out under the auspices of an organization are structured and usually integrate age levels to give them meaning and purpose. Schools too can assist in preventing juvenile crimes by re-evaluating and restructuring curriculum offerings to make them more meaningful to a population representative of all youth rather than exclusively to those who are college bound. Job offerings are important to satisfy the need for money and to divert energies away from criminal acts committed to obtain money.

Nurses, *as concerned citizens,* are urged to support efforts toward prevention of juvenile delinquency according to their own political beliefs. *As professionals,* nurses have special responsibilities. The only contact between the nurse and a youth may be in an acute care setting. Although this is only a transient contact, total patient assessment is in order, including an emotional-social assessment. Signs that should alert the nurse to the need for intervention are (1) failure to accomplish developmental tasks, (2) deviant behaviors or attitudes exhibited by the youth, (3) signs of family disorganization, or all three. Interventions should begin with the youth, but including the family is critical. The nurse can apprise parents of the situation, help them understand it, and then work with them to find solutions. If the family cannot solve their problem, referrals to resource people and agencies may be the intervention of choice.

The nurse employed by a social service agency is likely to encounter the family of the delinquent youth or those families particularly vulnerable to the problems of delinquency. Nurses specially instructed in mental health concepts are valuable in agencies in which a team works to rehabilitate individuals or groups of youth.

Nurses who are sensitive to the broad range of human needs and potentials can contribute to the prevention of delinquency through family counselling and by participating in community and school activities that provide opportunities for healthful interactions with youth.

SUICIDE

Voluntarily ending one's own life, or even attempting to end one's life, has ramifications not only for the family but for all society. Trying to understand what causes a person to resort to suicide as an answer to life's problems can be a deeply frustrating experience for anyone involved, whether a health professional, friend, teacher, or family member. It is particularly incomprehensible that an adolescent should feel problems so greatly as to find suicide the only solution.

Suicide as a cause of death is second in incidence only to accidents and homicide within the adolescent population. The number of victims of suicide has increased markedly over the past two decades, with the most noticeable rise being in the 15 to 19 age groups.[9]

There is speculation that the actual numbers of deaths by suicide may be even higher than reported figures. Since suicide produces tremendous guilt feelings in the survivors, death in which suicide is not clearly evident may be attributed to natural causes or labeled accidental.[11] An example is the single-vehicle automobile accident in which a direct cause cannot be determined. These cases are sometimes labeled "autocide."

A difference exists between adolescent boys and girls regarding successful suicidal efforts. Dr. Calvin J. Frederick, Chief of Emergency Mental Health and Disaster Assistance for the National Institute of Mental Health, states that girls are more likely to attempt suicide and that this should be interpreted as a cry for help. Boys have a much higher suicide rate, up to four times that of girls. Culturally, crying out for help is not considered masculine, so boys become desperate before resorting to drastic action.[31] Another fact of importance is that with each succeeding attempt at suicide, success becomes more likely.[19]

Suicidal methods vary between the sexes. Girls are likely to use passive methods such as ingestion of pills. A wide variety of drugs are used, including those purchased "over the counter" such as tranquilizers, barbiturates, and sometimes combinations of drugs, depending upon accessibility. Boys, in contrast, resort to more quickly lethal methods such as gunshot or hanging.

Causative factors related to adolescent suicide or attempted suicide are difficult to isolate. Suicide most likely results from the compounding of several factors. The biochemical changes that occur with the onset of puberty can lead to depression. Sudden shifts in attitude or emotion in the adolescent happen without warning and for no apparent reason, leaving parents and others baffled. The task of gaining a sense of identity can lead to feelings of self-doubt and low self-esteem, particularly when the adolescent compares himself with his peers. Feelings of isolation result when the adolescent perceives that his peers have greater independence as interpreted from the social behaviors of the group. Modes of dress, interactions with the opposite sex, and independence in transportation and finance are but a few examples of social behaviors that have exaggerated importance in adolescence.

Other causative factors, both physical and social, have been cited. Minimal brain dysfunction, characterized by (1) poor academic function, (2) poor self-image and (3) feelings of hopelessness, has been identified in adolescents who attempt suicide.[25] The suicidal adolescent is often the product of a disrupted family situation.

Suicide attempts show a direct relationship to the amount of stress placed on the adolescent. Statistics reveal higher suicide rates among high school drop-outs and college students than their counterparts.[19] Other differences are noted in geographical locations. The Northern states show a higher suicide rate among black youths, whereas in the South the rate is higher among whites.[19] Although an increase in the number of suicide attempts has been noted among the 10- to 14-year-old age groups, these youths have neither the accessibility to destructive means nor the physical maturity to carry out some of the methods.[32]

Professionals who work with suicidal youths feel that suicides do not just happen but that the victims give repeated warnings. The warnings, while subtle, are multiple. Parents too often fail to recognize changes in behavior that signify an altered emotional state. Parents cope by using denial. Nurses and teachers are aware of the multiplicity of factors that influence adolescent behavior. These professionals may be the only adults with sufficient contact time to detect significant deterioration in an adolescent's behavior and outlook.

Signs of depression precede any attempts at suicide. The signs displayed by the adolescent may differ from those in the adult but nevertheless are progressive and therefore none should be discounted. Some signs are decline in school performance, disregard for personal appearance, changes in eating and sleeping patterns, increased use of drugs or alcohol, or both; threats of suicide and talk of death along with "getting affairs in order" type of behavior, including giving away prized possessions.

The impact of the suicide problem has been recognized, studied and actively attacked, but the problem continues to plague us. The American Association of Suicidologists has been established to coordinate national suicide prevention centers. The magnitude of the problem generally in the nation and particularly in urban areas has stimulated establishment of crisis intervention centers. One service offered through these agencies is a telephone hotline manned by professionals and trained volunteers. Callers are encouraged to talk through their concerns while the volunteer evaluates the immediate need of the caller. Crisis intervention techniques, along with referrals to appropriate agencies, constitute a large portion of services rendered by the telephone counselors. Telephone interventions have been successful in helping some people, but major concern still remains for individuals who have advanced to a stage of desperation beyond asking for help.

Crisis intervention techniques avert some suicides, but reduction in the numbers of deaths and attempts lies in prevention. One approach to prevention is education. Young adolescents should be involved in a comprehensive educational program. There is need to apprise them both of the scope of the suicide problem in their age group and of the progressive stages of deterioration in individuals leading to acts of desperation. Adolescent participation in prevention needs to be increased; that is, adolescents need to be granted permission through the educational process to report the indications of potential suicide in their peers. A report of this kind could save a life. Adults who have contact with adolescents need similar education so they too can recognize and report any signs of impending suicide attempts.

Rehabilitation of adolescents attempting suicide can be attempted through group therapy sessions. Nurses with appropriate training may find a satisfying role in organizing such sessions and serving as group leaders. Education and life experiences contribute to preparing nurses to help each participant to identify positive aspects of his life. Topics of mutual concern should be discussed, including suicide. Discussion of issues and exploration of alternative modes of coping can assist the troubled youth.

ABUSE OF ADOLESCENTS

Child abuse is a collective term for a variety of forms of mistreatment. Generally this social problem is addressed in young children, but information is being compiled that confirms child abuse is also a problem among the adolescent age group. Abuse within this population is in the forms of physical mistreatment, neglect and sexual abuse.

Manifestations of abuse are less dramatic in older children, but are nevertheless traumatic. Signs of physical abuse tend to be less severe due to maturation of the body and the youth's ability to flee from attack. Neglect, both physical and emotional, while potentially less devastating to the adolescent, still has long-term implications. Physically the youth can probably take care of himself, but emotionally the support and understanding of parents is still necessary for healthy development. Sexual abuse is more common than was once thought and produces long-term emotional consequences for both the youth and the family.

The crisis of adolescence produces several potentially stormy years. Although many adolescents and their parents have never read any descriptions of developmental tasks, they are acutely aware of changes occurring during adolescence. Conflict between the two age groups results as the adolescent strives to accomplish those tasks. Some parents have difficulty accepting movement of the adolescent away from the home into the world. Parental influence declines during this stage as youths place increased worth on the opinion of their peers. Most parents want their young adults to value and abide by the moral code and standards the youngsters were taught as children. In most instances, the standards for both generations coincide; but when adolescent behavior diverges from those standards, it causes grave concern to parents and can lead to conflict. Parents who have placed great confidence in their adolescents have been shocked, angered and hurt when confronted with evidence of noncompliant behavior.

Parents, too, face their own crisis in middle life. Factors such as unfulfilled ambitions, waning physical strength and declining health may contribute to the situation. Juxtapose the adolescent's striving to accomplish tasks that will move him into adulthood with parents attempting to work through their own crisis period, and a potentially volatile situation can emerge. Families not previously plagued by an abuse problem may develop one due to the many tensions that now abound.

Additional stresses that can contribute to creating a climate for abuse are social problems such as alcoholism, drug misuse and mental illness.[5] Parental emotions linked to changing relationships between themselves and their children, especially between fathers and daughters, can lead to abuse.[21] An accumulation of causative factors rather than a single incident is responsible for the problem of adolescent abuse.

All forms of abuse interfere with healthy development. Identification of abused adolescents is not easy, as they tend to live with the situation rather than report it and risk further abuse.[22] Adolescents may bear the evidence of physical abuse for long periods after the incident. Bruises are slow to fade, and if located on regularly exposed skin surfaces, can be a source of embarrassment. Turtleneck sweaters or other seasonally inappropriate attire may be a sign that the youth is trying to cover unsightly lesions.

Neglect or physical abuse of long standing produces other manifestations. Retarded physical growth can result from long-term undernutrition. Unsightly scarring or missing teeth, along with other physical signs, cause the youth to have a poor self-image and to be socially reticent.

Emotionally abused children may never be able to relate to others in a normal manner. The degree of emotional impairment is dependent on the duration of the abuse. The youth subjected to abuse throughout his life potentially has more adjustment problems than the person who is abused just for behaving as a typical adolescent.

Cognitive development may be inhibited in the abused adolescent. Several factors contribute to the delay. Absenteeism leads to poor progress in school and inability to keep pace with classmates. A hostile home environment discourages the adolescent from keeping up with homework assignments. In fact, if the adolescent has been continually belittled over the years, his motivation to succeed in school may be very limited.

Sexual abuse or incest produces few physical signs. This form of abuse may not become a problem until a family's youngsters enter the adolescent age group. Adults cite the adolescent as being seductive, thereby contributing to the situation. Adolescents, responding to new feelings within themselves, may fail to halt sexual contact; in fact, they may participate willingly. Sexual abuse occurs among both sexes, although it is more commonly reported with adolescent girls.[16] Incest occurs in immediate family combinations or with close relatives. Nonrelated adults living in a household may also be sexually involved with the adolescent.

The social stigma attached to sexual abuse and incest contributes to the lack of reporting to authorities. Noninvolved family members may be aware of a sexual abuse situation but choose to keep the secret.[22] Guilt, shame or threats of violence are other reasons that an aberrant situation goes unreported. The women's movement has been instrumental in bringing attention to the abuse problem. Women are finding the courage to defend themselves and their children by speaking out on issues previously repressed.

Recognition of abuse in the adolescent population has been slow to emerge due in part to feelings of "they get what they deserve" or "they are big enough to care for themselves." Unless abuse results in major injury to the adolescent, health care workers have little contact with that age group. Casefinding must be done by adults having regular association with adolescents, such as teachers or school nurses.

A report of suspected abuse must be initiated before interventions can be instituted. Rehabilitative efforts will rely heavily on mental health techniques and must involve the entire family. Failure of the family to resolve their conflicts, or of the abusing adult to use the services of a support group such as Parents Anonymous, is cause for removal of the adolescent from the home. Foster care homes have been used for adolescents from severely disorganized families either as a temporary measure or a permanent arrangement.

Interdisciplinary efforts have been initiated to curb child abuse. Presently, most group efforts involve treatment of the problem rather than prevention. Nurses will be actively involved in treating the abused adolescent and his family, but more important is the role that can be established to aid in prevention of abuse. Education for parenting is one significant contribution toward prevention of abuse.[18] Parents of adolescents subject to severe stress will benefit greatly from resources such as support groups. The emotional release supplied by group sessions led by the nurse can be instrumental in preventing abuse of the older child.

Nurses or other adults working with abused adolescents use resources at hand to combat the problem. In areas with limited or ineffectual resources, the national youth emergency number (toll-free; 1–800–621–4000) may provide a key to additional services.

Education for the public is a major step needed to resolve the abuse problem. Dissemination of information about causes of abuse, the cycle of abnormal childrearing, and legal responsibilities of the public to report suspected abuse are necessary prerequisites to resolving the abuse problem.

SEXUAL ACTIVITY

Body changes occurring during puberty, along with heightened feelings resulting from those changes and associated hormonal activity, may make adolescents feel strange and confused about themselves. Physiological changes, peer pressures and societal expectations of teenagers propel them toward heterosexual relationships.

Sexual experimentation is common in the adolescent years. The cultural norm in the United States, especially in traditional middle class families, is for parents to withhold sexual information, thinking that avoiding discussions regarding sex will somehow inhibit sexual experimentation. This premise has not proved to be accurate.

Early maturation, coupled with changing cultural norms for sexual behavior, has led many young people, especially girls, into heterosexual relationships early in the teen period. Immaturity and ignorance regarding sexual activity result in a stressful situation with no easy solutions. If pregnancy is the outcome of early sexual activity, many consequences await the young mother, her family and the father of the child.

Exact figures regarding numbers of youth involved in sexual activity are difficult to obtain. A major deterrent to compiling such information is parents' reluctance to let their children participate in sex-related studies. Significant conclusions have been drawn from retrospective studies such as those done by Kinsey. Teen pregnancy and increased incidence of venereal disease serve as the basis for identifying sex-related conditions as major health issues to youth. Hearings sponsored by the American Nurses Association on the health needs of youth held in 1978 revealed that health care providers repeatedly identified and dealt with sex-related problems in their practices.[3] Conclusions of a study on adolescent health needs conducted by the Michigan Department of Public Health in that same year identified four health problems, two of which were pregnancy and venereal disease. The Michigan study demonstrated higher rates of sexual activity in urban areas and an increase in the numbers of adolescents under 15 who were sexually active.[1]

The publication *11 Million Teenagers* presents statistics that show the prevalence of adolescent sexual behavior to be high.[8] This study revealed: half of the 21 million youths between 15 and 19 are sexually active; one-fifth of the 8 million 13- and 14-year-olds have had intercourse; and one million teen pregnancies occur every year in the United States, with an additional 30,000 pregnancies occurring in girls under 15 years of age. Such statistics are shocking to much of society. However, regardless of a nurse's personal values and moral feelings about adolescent sexual activity, as a health professional she must be aware that many adolescents are sexually active and that they and their families may need sexual education and counselling.

The need for intimacy, a close personal friendship, is cited by Mitchell as a compelling reason for the adolescent to become involved in a sexual relationship leading to problems.[20] Seeking out one person for a close relationship, to share innermost feelings and confidences, has strong sexual implications if that person is of the opposite sex. The feelings generated by such an intimate relationship may be interpreted as love and expressed sexually. Great pain ensues when those adolescent romances disintegrate.

In many American families, the goal of parents is to prohibit their children from sexual activity until marriage. Many parents are not comfortable discussing sexual matters with their children. Information disseminated focuses largely upon the negative aspects of sexual relations. Sexual conduct is not openly discussed. Some parents are unaware of the nonverbal lessons they supply about their own sexuality and attitude toward sex, or that these cues have been emitted and received since the child was born.

Families vary greatly in disciplinary practices and rules for members' conduct. In large families there is sometimes relaxation of the rules for younger siblings. These youngsters tend to act far more grown-up than their peers because they emulate older siblings. The loosening of controls does not mean the adolescent will be sexually active, but the opportunities are certainly greater. Conversely, an authoritarian parent who sets up strict rules for conduct may cause the adolescent to rebel. That rebellion can include forbidden sexual activity.

Deterioration of the family unit has been cited as a cause for adolescent sexual problems. Society generally has relaxed its attitude toward sex. The youth culture movement of the 1960s and '70s has exposed us to new music, dance, moral patterns and behavioral codes. Although many adults have not been in agreement with precepts of the movement, they have felt powerless to halt it. Some adults, too, have been poor role models for their adolescents, as they have found themselves confused by changes in society. Some adults have discarded traditional ideals such as marital fidelity; others still hold traditional beliefs.

Although sexual problems are not isolated within one particular socioeconomic level, a correlation does exist between orientation toward future goals and intimacy with a member of the opposite sex. In a study examining the frequency of romantic involvement among high school students, Larson and associates concluded that going steady may be a sign of insecurity as well as lower educational and occupational aspirations.[15] Life goals appear to provide the adolescent with purpose, and therefore less time and inclination to become seriously involved in a sexual relationship.

Homosexual experimentation may take place, particularly in early adolescence. Kirkendall and Rubin question whether this is a stage of development in actual homosexuality or whether such behavior arises merely out of curiosity and experimentation. Nevertheless, boys in particular may pass through a stage of sexual activity with a same-sex peer. Many theories have been postulated regarding the cause of homosexuality, but none is universally accepted. One research study suggests that teens of either sex with high levels of androgens prefer sexual activity with females, while low levels of androgens in either sex are associated with sexual preference for males.[17]

Homosexual experimentation in adolescence is not a positive prediction of sexual preference as an adult. Parents and other adults learning of homosexual activity will react according to their own level of understanding and moral code. Kappelman indicates that sexual preference falls along a continuum from exclusively homosexual to exclusively heterosexual, with individuals falling between classed as bisexual.[13] He further indicates that youth have a need to explore alternate life styles, particularly in the more open culture of the late twentieth century. As the youth moves out of adolescence into adulthood, it is likely that he will select the traditional heterosexual life style. Nurses as health professionals can help provide accurate, nonjudgmental information on this subject to adolescents and families.

Sexual experimentation of any type makes the adolescent a prime candidate for some very turbulent times. While some may experience few problems, others will have guilt feelings stemming from their awareness of violating a prescribed social code. This, in particular, can lead to isolation and severed relationships with both family and friends. Of course, pregnancy and the accompanying turmoil is a major threat to the sexually active youth. Also, the incidence of venereal disease is increasing dramatically among teens due to increasing sexual activity and numbers of partners.

Families do not escape the consequences of adolescent sexual activity, either. When confronted with evidence that their adolescent has a sex-related problem, parents' responses vary from anger to disappointment. Adolescents need room to grow and exercise their decision-making ability. Parents sometimes have difficulty determining their approach to discipline that is neither too strict nor too permissive. Parents with an open attitude that allow their youth to approach them with problems and concerns possess an important resource to avert social problems, including those of a sexual nature.

Society does not escape the impact of the adolescent sexual revolution. If this is symptomatic of the "times" and evidence of deterioration of traditional social institutions such as the family, then other facets of life must be similarly affected. Homosexuality, while no longer classified as a disease, is not a universally accepted life style. Controversy weighs heavy around the issue.

Prevention of sexual problems is not entirely possible, but education is a useful tool in assisting both adolescents and adults to make informed decisions. Adolescents deserve the right to be made aware of the options and consequences of early sexual activity. Education for parents will not only increase their awareness of present-day realities but enable them to express feelings about sex to their children in a positive manner. Parents can also be helped to feel more comfortable in discussing sexual issues with their children.

Adolescents need factual information about all aspects of sexuality. Many parents feel that all information of a sexual nature should be generated in the home. The increase in sex-related problems gives evidence that adolescents lack adequate information in spite of this. Schools, in response to the problem, have incorporated family life education into their curricula. A number of school systems have met with stiff resistance from parents, including legal action to block implementation. The situation is still far from being resolved.

In the area of sexual problems, nurses can make significant contributions because they have information on the topic and are in positions to identify potential and existing problems. Nurses can serve as resource persons, caregivers, educators, confidants, and lobbyists for the right of adolescents to have access to information that will dispel myths and misinformation presented by both adults and peers. Nurses have an obligation to stay abreast of the latest literature and research findings in the field. The scope of professional nursing practice encompasses problem identification and appropriate referrals.

RUNAWAYS

Persons leaving home without notice or just dropping out of sight are not a new phenomenon. Adolescents in increasing numbers are trying this mode of coping with life events. Estimates are that one million youth leave home in this way every year.[21] The time away for the adolescent is likely to be short, although some leave for extended periods and a few never return.

Boys are more frequently runaways than girls, although the gap is narrowing.[2] Young adolescents, 13 and 14 years old, are also succumbing to the phenomenon. The "flower child" era of the late 1960s gave rise to the current popularity and acceptability among youth of running away. All segments of society are plagued by this problem.

A number of reasons have been cited to explain why adolescents choose to drop out, to leave home, and attempt to negotiate living independently. Some reasons are strife within a family from social situations such as divorce or death of a parent, societal mobility or discipline that is either too strict or too lenient. Wolk and Brandon studied adolescent runaways and determined that these youth possess a poor self-concept, suffer from anxiety, self-doubt and defensiveness and have problems in relating to others.[83] Berry believes the increased number of runaways can be attributed to glorification of the experience by the media. He further concludes that adolescents are misled into believing that running will solve their problems rather than adding to an already complex situation.[4]

Many adolescents are unaware that it is against the law to run away. If parents or guardians want to press charges, a warrant can be issued for the runaway's arrest. Although locating a runaway may be difficult and may not be a priority among law enforcement officials, arrest can result.

Runaways tend to go one of two places when they leave home. Many choose the home of a friend, whose parents may not initially comprehend the situation. These youth ordinarily do not stay away long, usually returning home in a few days. The second destination is a large city, where one is easily lost in the crowd. Often the youth has failed to make preparations for survival so will have little money and no place to live. Once his money is gone, the youth is forced to live by his wits. To obtain money the youth may attempt to secure a regular job, but lack of qualifications will limit both his choices and his earning capacity. This plight of the runaway is recognized by drug dealers, panderers and other unsavory individuals. The jobs offered to these youth may place them in jeopardy of detection by legal authorities and subject them to other hazards of illicit activities. Lack of adequate housing and poor nutrition further complicate the youth's life. The difficulties of day-to-day survival, along with emotional turmoil, compound their feelings of desperation.

Families may be aware of deterioration in the potential runaway adolescent's life. Not all runaways come from a deplorable home situation. Parents may be totally surprised and bewildered when the adolescent is found missing. In some instances warning signals alert adults to a youth's need for help. Those signals include severe mood changes, school problems and antisocial behavior such as conflicts with police.[4] Most youth elect to communicate their need for help only once, although some will become chronic offenders, causing their parents to feel vindictive and angry each time they disappear.

In 1974, the United States Congress recognized the magnitude of the runaway problem and enacted legislation to provide funding for halfway houses, counselors and other resources. Most metropolitan areas have resources for runaways, including temporary shelter, food and counselors to help reunite families. Runaway houses have rules that the youth must call home within 24 hours after arriving, not necessarily to disclose his whereabouts but to inform his parents he is alive. Detroit Transit Alternative is an example of this type of resource. Huckleberry House in the Haight-Ashbury section of San Francisco was established early in the 1960s to lend assistance to large numbers of runaways. Travelers Aid services are located in most cities and can also be of assistance to runaways. Additional resources are available through the National Runaway Switchboard (1–800–621–4000, except Alaska and Hawaii).

Prevention rests in recognition of problems confronting the adolescent before he feels unable to cope with them and drops out. Social institutions and persons working within them may be valuable resources to assist the youth to work through problems. Helping parents to recognize problems plaguing their children may also help diminish the large number of runaways.

Nurses, particularly school nurses, can serve in a unique way with troubled adolescents. Knowledge of normal behaviors and sensitivity to alterations in the pattern of development can serve as impetus for referrals to resource persons or agencies for early intervention, counselling in particular.

DRUG MISUSE

The scope of drug misuse within the adolescent and young adult population is not easily deciphered. Drug misuse encompasses a variety of substances, including tobacco, alcohol, marijuana and "hard drugs." Substances commonly included in the category of hard drugs are the narcotics, (primarily heroin), the stimulants (cocaine* and amphetamines), and the hallucinogens (LSD, mescaline and PCP). In popular opinion, the term drug abuse is generally equated with the illegal acquisition and use of mind-altering subtances, particularly hard drugs. Fear associated with the use of illegal drugs has led some adults to view alcohol ingestion as somehow "not serious," probably because of the social acceptability of alcohol use among

---

*Cocaine is designated a narcotic under the U.S. Controlled Substances Act. It is usually considered a stimulant, however. Its effects on the body are very similar to amphetamines, although more transient.

adults.[23] However, alcohol use is actually the most widespread substance abuse problem among adolescents.

Adults serve as poor role models in the use of tobacco, alcohol and marijuana. Warnings of potential dangers to health have been ignored. The statements issued by the U.S. Surgeon General have done little to halt cigarette smoking. Making the purchase of cigarettes illegal for persons under 18 has not halted smoking among that population. The numbers of females who smoke is increasing; one can only speculate whether this is due to the new independence of females. Females have now caught up to males in the use of both alcohol and drugs.[26]

Researchers believe that people drink due to environmental factors or influences and that it is a learned behavior.[7] There are nine million alcoholics in the United States and a half million of those are in their preteen and teen years.[7] Public concern regarding alcohol and marijuana can be seen in states such as Michigan, where the legal drinking age has been changed twice in the past five years, from 21 to 18 and back to 21. The most persuasive argument in returning the age to 21 was motor vehicle accident statistics, along with concern that the 18-year-old was supplying alcohol to younger friends. Change in the legal drinking age met with strong protest from students in university communities. Several cities reacted to the student protest by enacting ordinances to levy fines against those caught breaking the law. Fines are very minimal for first-time offenders and become more stringent with succeeding convictions. Marijuana use is treated similarly, particularly in university towns.

A single cause for drug abuse is difficult to isolate. Wright has assembled a number of possible causative factors: availability of substances coupled with curiosity about the effects of a drug, family dissention and breakdown in relations between parents and their youth, need for peer acceptance and approval, boredom, poor self-image and social inequities.[34] Socioeconomic status does not provide immunity for its youth due to heavy interplay of the factors listed. Likewise, geographic location is no deterrent, although illegal hard drugs are less likely to be available in rural areas.

Adolescents casually involved with drugs may only be imitating their peer group, particularly if the social norm for the community includes cigarette smoking and parties where alcohol or marijuana use is sanctioned. The mind-altering effects resulting from use of those drugs can lead to involvement in irresponsible acts, including sexual experimentation or reckless driving, which have serious consequences. Young persons who become physically or psychologically dependent on drugs (termed *addiction*) may abandon a previous life style to concentrate major effort toward supplying their drug needs. Malnutrition, retarded growth or hepatitis are a few consequences of drug addiction. Mental burn-out or death are the ultimate disastrous outcomes of drug misuse. Emotional stress is generated from the distorted life style, guilt over drug dependence, and concentrated efforts to obtain enough money to keep up with the body's need for drugs. Alienation from family and friends, too, will have a deleterious effect on the emotional well-being of the youth.

Families are vulnerable to the ill effect of drug misuse. Use of cigarettes or alcohol by a youth may cause family disappointment. Marijuana use is also viewed by many without major alarm, most concern being due to the legal implications, unknown long-term effects on the body, and worry that use will lead to hard drug use. Parents whose children become deeply involved with illegal drugs are bewildered, disappointed, angry with the system and the suppliers, and fearful for the well-being of their child.

Society collectively does not escape the throes of adolescent drug misuse. Loss of potential human resources is most tragic. Loss resulting from thievery and other crimes is difficult to calculate.

Society's youth movement, with changing fashions, life styles and music, may be instrumental in perpetuating drug abuse. Adolescents emulate heroes both in life style and habits, including drug use as a way of coping with life. Youth lack maturity and experience to realistically evaluate the impact that drug use can have on their lives.

Programs to cure drug abusers and rehabilitate them vary in their success. Support groups such as Alcoholics Anonymous are helpful to teens involved with alcohol, providing they admit to having a problem. Drug detoxification centers have been established to help youth "beat the habit." For the person addicted to heroin, there are methadone programs in many cities to provide a controlled drug supply for the addict. Regardless of programs available, the ultimate decision rests with the adolescents. According to Johnson and Klotkowski, "For any drug abuser to choose 'no drugs' as a viable alternative in his life style, he must see himself as capable of making that choice; he must alter his devastatingly inadequate self-concept; he must realize that he has the strength and capability of handling himself in the day-to-day world without dependence on drugs."[12]

What can families do to prevent drug misuse by their children? Attention to a stable and loving environment at home is most significant. The nurturing resulting from a supportive atmosphere is of utmost importance in helping the youth develop into a self-reliant individual. Further, parents need to examine their own life style and decide if they rely heavily on substances such as alcohol or prescription drugs to help them cope with stress. Concentration on health and healthful living are habits that can be instilled in children, provided the concepts are introduced early in life.

Youth from a less fortunate family situation may have to rely heavily on society to provide nurture. Schools house children for a large portion of their growing years. Supportive teachers and school personnel, along with curricula structured to include drug education, can aid in prevention of drug misuse. Adolescents can be easily confused about the use of tobacco and alcohol because of the variety of attitudes to which they are exposed. School programs with a positive emphasis on health can aid in prevention.[23]

Nurses can be instrumental in curbing drug misuse among youth through educational programs and role modeling. Ideally they can contribute to such programs in both the planning and teaching phases, or as resource persons for drug education programs.

Challenging career opportunities are available for the nurse interested in working with drug abusers in either a hospital or rehabilitation setting. Many times admission to a substance abuse center is against the wishes of the patient, so early nursing actions will be directed toward establishing trust. The drug addict has been pictured as a manipulator who is sometimes less than truthful and who is very threatened by authority.[12] Appropriate intervention will provide inclusion of the family in the treatment program. The recovery process can be both slow and painful, without any guarantee of success.

SCHOOL ATTENDANCE

The general expectation in the United States today is for every youth to graduate from high school. Presently each state has laws making school attendance compulsory until 16 years of age. A high school diploma is a prerequisite for a majority of jobs today. The importance attached to the goal of finishing high school is supported by numbers of high school graduates; in 1962, 66 per cent of those entering high school graduated, while in 1975 the figure rose to 75 per cent.[27]

Expectations for educational achievement fluctuate with the times and economic level of the family, although formal education beyond high school has become the expected norm for many middle and upper class families. The educational level of the parents will also influence school attendance.

Deviations from the expectation of regular school attendance can be classified. Some of those categories of youth are

1. Pushouts: students forced out of the educational system by subtle pressures or indifference to their needs.[29]
2. Dropouts: students electing to leave the system before completing their education.
3. Those who have never attended school: youth who have not had the opportunity to attend because no school is available to meet a special need, or because parents have successfully avoided authorities and not enrolled their children in school.
4. Truants: youth who stay away from school without permission.

Some students do not attend school regularly because school facilities are poor or dangerous. Another reason for poor attendance is that students do not see the existing school system and the courses offered as being relevant to their lives. Schools located in ghetto areas of cities and on Indian reservations are examples. Rice describes deplorable conditions found in Indian schools as just one phase in the cold war waged to keep Indians repressed in our society.[24] For some minorities, the desegregation rulings by the United States Supreme Court have been of some help in achieving equality in education.

Schools have been given the formidable task of preparing children for life. This includes providing instruction in cognitive skills and preparing youth for earning a living and functioning in society. Cooperation of other social institutions including the family is necessary to accomplish the task.

The individual who does not regularly attend school is deprived of both the education and socialization that it offers. The youth jeopardizes his ability to compete in the employment market. The adolescent who does not attend school will likely not find a satisfying full-time job, leaving him with idle time and a lack of purpose. Consequently, his choice of activities may be poor and result in confrontation with the law. The complexities of modern technology, and resultant styles of living, make it imperative that each youth embark on adult life as well prepared as his peers.

Families can be responsible for aberrant school attendance patterns, particularly if they place little value on education. In such instances, attendance at school is not enforced, or the youth may be kept out of school to assist with maintaining the family. Families may also suffer long-term consequences if their child does not complete his education. Problems stemming from lack of an education can have a disruptive effect upon the family and, in severe cases, lead to its disintegration. Financial reverberations can be felt for a lifetime as the youth's earning potential is reduced and parents may have to supplement his income. The tradition in many families is continued feelings of responsibility even after a child reaches adulthood.

The norm for adults in the United States is that they be law-abiding citizens and financially independent. For persons who meet these two requirements, society as a whole takes a "live and let live" attitude. Educationally deprived citizens disrupt that balance. First, their contributions to the greater society will undoubtedly be minimal or nonexistent. Second, a great probability exists that they will need public assistance. Unfinished schooling and criminal activity are not directly related, but the potential for one to lead to the other exists, and if realized costs society both money and loss of human resources.

Some school systems have responded to the variety of needs of youth in their districts. Curriculum variations have been instituted, with increasingly larger blocks of vocational and technical courses included. The aim of such courses is to provide entry-level work skills for the youth not interested in continued academic pursuits. Vocational courses span two or three years and include a work component so that the youth graduating from high school can immediately find meaningful employment.

Other alterations to traditional school patterns include night school classes. The community education component of some school districts offers a wide variety of evening classes, both for adding academic credits and for enrichment. In these classes, young people can complete credit requirements for graduation. The adolescent who had personality conflicts during traditional sessions may find this alternative appealing, as many of his fellow classmates will be adults.

Success in school is greatly influenced by home environment. Parents need to realize the impact of their encouragement on a child's progress in school. Sensitivity to the strengths and the weaknesses of their child, along with knowledge of the philosophy and operations of the local school system, can help parents negotiate the system to ensure a meaningful educational experience for their child. There are times when parents underestimate the potential of their influence on their child and need the guidance of a professional to realize their importance to the nurturing of their child.

Legislation enacted to update educational content is a continued necessity. The initial step in this process is to inform legislators of problems related to school attendance. Forced school attendance is not the answer to the educational ills of today. Instead, changes are needed in programs so students will value educational achievement and want to attend school.

References

1. Adolescent Health Care Services in Michigan. Bureau of Personal Health Services, Michigan Department of Public Health, April 1978
2. L. Ambrosino. Runaways. Beacon Press, 1971
3. ANA hearings underscore youth health needs. The American Nurse, 30 November, 1978
4. J. R. Berry. Why they run. Parents' Magazine, June 1978, p. 47
5. M. Brenton. What can be done about child abuse. Today's Education, Sep/Oct 1977, p. 51
6. G. Cahoun, Jr. Ethnic comparison of juvenile offenses and socioeconomic status. Clearing House, October 1977, p. 58

7. W. Dankenbring. The teen-age alcoholic. Life and Health, April 1977, p. 26
8. 11 Million Teenagers: What Can Be Done About the Epidemic Adolescent Pregnancies in the United States. Alan Guttmacher Institute, 1976
9. Final Mortality Statistics Report, 1976. National Center for Health Statistics, U.S. Department of Health, Education and Welfare Pub. No. 78–120, 30, March 1978
10. K. C. Garrison and K. C. Garrison, Jr. Psychology of Adolescence. Prentice-Hall, 1975
11. N. A. Hart and G. C. Keidel. The suicidal adolescent. American Journal of Nursing, January 1979, p. 80
12. E. Johnson and D. Klotkowski. Turning an addicted patient on to turning drugs off. R.N., May 1978, p. 91
13. M. Kappelman. When your teenager needs you the most. Family Health, August 1977, p. 44
14. L. A. Kirkendall and I. Rubin. Sexuality and the life cycle: a broad concept of sexuality. In Focus: Human Sexuality, Annual Editions. Dushkin Publishing Group, Inc., 1977–1978, p. 142
15. D. L. Larson et al. Social factors in the frequency of romantic involvement among adolescents. Adolescence, Spring 1976, p. 7
16. R. Lempp. Psychological damage to children as a result of sexual offenses. Child Abuse and Neglect, April 1978, p. 1478
17. M. D. Margolese. Homosexuality: a new endocrine correlate. Hormones and Behavior, January 1970, p. 151
18. N. L. McKeel. Child abuse can be prevented. American Journal of Nursing, September 1978, p. 1478
19. M. S. Miller. Teen suicide. Ladies Home Journal, February 1977, p. 72
20. J. J. Mitchell. Adolescent intimacy. Adolescence, Summer 1976, p. 275
21. C. Remsberg and B. Remsberg. What happens to teen runaways. Seventeen, June 1976, p. 150
22. C. Remsberg and B. Remsberg. An American scandal: why some parents abuse teens. Seventeen, May 1977, p. 154
23. J. C. Reynolds. The drug education gap. Clearing House, September 1976, p. 10
24. F. P. Rice. The Adolescent: Development, Relationships and Culture. Allyn & Bacon, 1975
25. R. D. Rohn et al. Adolescents who attempt suicide. The Journal of Pediatrics, April 1977, p. 636
26. Sexes equal in alcohol, drug use. Science News, 30 April 1978, p. 277
27. M. S. Smart and R. C. Smart. Adolescent Development and Relationships. Macmillan, Inc., 1978
28. R. M. Smith and J. Walters. Delinquent and non-delinquent males' perceptions of their fathers. Adolescents, Spring 1978, p. 21
29. The 2.4 million children who aren't in school. U.S. News and World Report, 22 March, 1976, p. 43
30. The youth crime plague. Time, 11 July, 1977, p. 18
31. Upsurge in violent crime by youngsters: results of a study. U.S. News and World Report, 17 July, 1978, p. 55
32. D. A. Williams et al. Teenage suicide. Newsweek, 28 August, 1978, p. 74
33. S. Wolk and J. Brandon. Runaway adolescents' perceptions of parents and self. Adolescence, Summer 1977, p. 175
34. J. S. Wright. The psychology and personality of addicts. Adolescence, Fall 1977, p. 399

POTENTIAL STRESSES DURING ADOLESCENCE: TEMPORARY ALTERATIONS IN HEALTH STATUS

by Jo Joyce Tackett, BSN, MPHN

Adolescents and young adults seem to be particularly vulnerable to three categories of temporary health problems: acne, certain infectious ailments and menstrual disturbances. These are discussed in this chapter, and nursing interventions to prevent or manage the altered health states will be identified.

ACNE VULGARIS

One of the most common and most humiliating stressors of adolescence is acne vulgaris. A physiologic skin response to pubertal hormonal changes, acne vulgaris is an inflammatory disturbance involving the pilosebaceous follicles (follicle and sebaceous gland complex).

Acne is considered a disease of adolescence because of its pubertal onset and peak incidence (16- to 20-year-olds) during that stage of development. It is estimated that 90 per cent of adolescent boys and 80 per cent of adolescent girls experience acne of varying severity.[8] Although acne is self-limiting for most adolescents, it can persist well into the adult years.

Pathophysiology and Etiology

Acne usually runs a prolonged course and may manifest itself earlier in females, often preceding menarche by one to two years. The increased levels of hormones, especially androgens, in the adolescent body appear to stimulate growth of the sebaceous glands, increase gland secretions and promote more frequent follicular epithelial necrosis. These responses alter the follicle, causing a greater likelihood of occlusion of the distal hair follicle canal. This occlusion causes an accumulation of sebum, keratin, fatty acids, bacteria and dead epithelial cells within the follicle. This *noninflamed* lesion is called a *comedone;* it may be either plugged (whitehead) or open (blackhead). The comedone may resolve itself at this noninflammatory stage or, if enough debris and bacteria collects within the follicle, it will become inflamed and rupture into the dermis. *Inflamed* lesions are called *papules,* or *nodules.* An otherwise harmless bacteria, *Corynebacterium acnes,* is drawn to the sebum spilled into the dermis and hydrolyzes the sebum into fatty acids, which further irritate the dermis, causing formation of pustules and cysts. Those inflamed lesions that become cystic frequently form a scar as they resolve.

Lesion resolution, whether noninflammatory or inflammatory, can be aggravated or perpetuated by a variety of external stimuli, which include manipulation by pinching or squeezing, use of some cosmetics and preparations and creams for oily skin, and perspiration and temperature extremes. Iodides tend to increase the inflammatory process. Secondary infection with *Staphylococcus albus* frequently results from hand contact with the lesions (either resting the face on the hand or manipulating lesions), or use of hair styles in which the hair rests on the face or forehead. Severe physical or emotional stress, inadequate sleep, premenstrual hormonal changes and some medications (stimulants, steroids) can aggravate the inflammatory process of acne. There is no evidence that dietary factors (chocolate, cola beverages, greasy foods) cause acne or encourage inflammation. Some persons are, however, allergic to these substances and may have an acne-like response to the ingestion of them. Masturbation does not cause acne, but emotional pressures placed on masturbatory activities by the adolescent's significant others can encourage or perpetuate acne lesions.

There does seem to be a family predisposition for more severe acne, probably associated with an inherited tendency to have weaker follicle walls.[1] Acne lesions, although most prevalent on the face, may appear on the upper chest or upper back, where sebaceous glands are larger than hair follicles. A family tendency seems also to influence which body areas have acne involvement.

Management

Acne should never be dismissed as an inevitable fact of growing up that must simply be tolerated and ignored to the extent possible. Such attitudes on the part of parents or health professionals lead to unnecessary physical discomfort and possibly disfigurement associated with permanent scarring. Even more destructive is the injury to self-image and self-esteem as a result of the embarrassment and self-consciousness the acne causes at a time when identity development is crucial.

Seldom does treatment shorten the course of or cure acne, but reasonable management can control the severity of the inflammatory process, reduce scarring and improve appearance.

No one treatment regimen seems to adequately achieve these aims in all individuals. Self-treatment is seldom effective and may act adversely to aggravate the condition. Reasons for poor success, whether the treatment is self-prescribed or professionally prescribed, are the adolescent's tendency to be inconsistent in his compliance with the treatment, his lack of understanding of this long-term disease process that often causes him to experiment with a multitude of commercial products, and his possibly erratic emotional state. These factors define the first step needed to manage this disease.

Whatever treatment regimen is tried, health professionals intervening need to begin by educating the adolescent about the pathophysiology and etiology of acne. (Myths and fears need to be replaced with factual information.) The youth needs to understand that treatment will be lengthy and will not totally prevent or cure his acne state. He must be impressed with the importance of faithfully complying with the treatment regimen, despite a seeming lack of improvement, if successful results are to eventually occur. Understanding of these facts by parents is also important to their cooperation with and reinforcement of the plan of care. Therefore they should either be included in these initial discussions or provided the same information in a separate session before specific treatment is initiated. The nurse may also see the need during this session to increase the parents' understanding of what acne means to their teen.

These interventions by the nurse are often desirable actions to motivate the youth or his parents to follow through on her referral recommendation to a dermatologist. Once treatment is prescribed she can help interpret the therapy as specific and practical actions the adolescent can understand. She can periodically monitor the youth's compliance and help him to see the gradual improvement of his condition. (Color snapshot close-ups every three to six months give the youth visual evidence of the steady changes in his skin condition that go unnoticed under daily observation.) She can tactfully remind parents not to use nagging as a means to keep their child compliant. The nurse may also be the one who instructs the teen in the use or application of the treatment modalities. During each interaction with the youth the nurse should attempt to positively reinforce his self-image and self-confidence.

General Management General management is geared toward an appraisal of and improvement in the adolescent's general health practices. Such measures might include restructuring of routine to ensure adequate rest and sufficient exercise. Enforcing good personal hygiene, including frequent shampoos, and making changes in home, school or peer environment to reduce unnecessary emotional stresses may be appropriate. Correction of any eliminatory or menstrual irregularities may be indicated. If the youth has a food sensitivity, that food should be eliminated from his diet long enough to determine its impact on the disease. Obesity does not cause acne, but weight reduction will decrease the emotional tension obesity causes.

Management of the acne process is a widely debated issue among dermatologists and to date no one treatment protocol has gained majority consensus or demonstrated widespread success. What is apparent, however, is that the management for noninflammatory acne necessarily differs from that for inflammatory acne.

Management of Noninflammatory Lesions

Treatment of comedones is aimed at reducing the formation of noninflammatory lesions and removal of those that do form. The regimen may involve one or several of the following measures.

1. *Free the skin of external occlusion.* This measure would include conscious effort to avoid resting the face in the hands and to alter hair style to pull hair away from the face and forehead. The skin is kept clean by frequent cleansing; frequency is individually determined. Some areas such as nose, chin or forehead may need more frequent cleansing than others. The youth should use ordinary soap (not lanolin base or perfumed) or use medicated soap (such as Neutrogena, Acne-aid, Saymen). Lukewarm water should be used and a wash cloth is optional, but if used, should be used gently, not abrasively. (Some dermatologists discourage use of a wash cloth because of the unconscious tendency to use it roughly or to draw out blackheads, which stretches the follicle and weakens it.)

Astringents, although they remove surface oils, are equally ineffective and may irritate the dermis.[1] If chafing occurs, the frequency of washing should be decreased. Once the soap has been gently lathered into the skin it should be rinsed; the process should be repeated and then the skin either patted dry or permitted to air dry.

2. *Free the skin of internal occlusion.* Peeling agents may be applied topically to increase desquamation and epithelial cell turnover and to reduce the level of accumulated fatty acids, thereby reducing the accumulation of follicle debris. These preparations contain such active ingredients as keratolytic agents (sulfur, resorcinol, salicylic acid), benzoyl peroxide, or vitamin A acid. They are usually applied at bedtime, although some are contained in special cosmetic preparations for day-long action. Some drying and scaling is desirable for effectiveness, but erythema or chafing should not be induced. If these reactions occur, they indicate the need to reduce the frequency of application or dosage strength or both.[1] Individuals with dry or fair skin usually respond more rapidly and more strongly to peeling agents. Preparations with vitamin A acid will cause sun sensitivity and a tendency to burn and may enhance cancer-causing effects of the sun on the skin.[9] Benzoyl peroxide and vitamin A acid should not be combined; however, they may be used on alternate days. Ultraviolet light (sunlight or quartz sun lamps) acts as a peeling agent if exposure is limited to that amount of time required to produce mild redness within 24 hours. Time may be lengthened as tanning occurs. Sleeping during exposure should be avoided.

3. *Mechanical expression of comedones.* Mechanical removal of comedones hastens skin improvement and reduces the likelihood of developing inflammatory lesions. A comedone

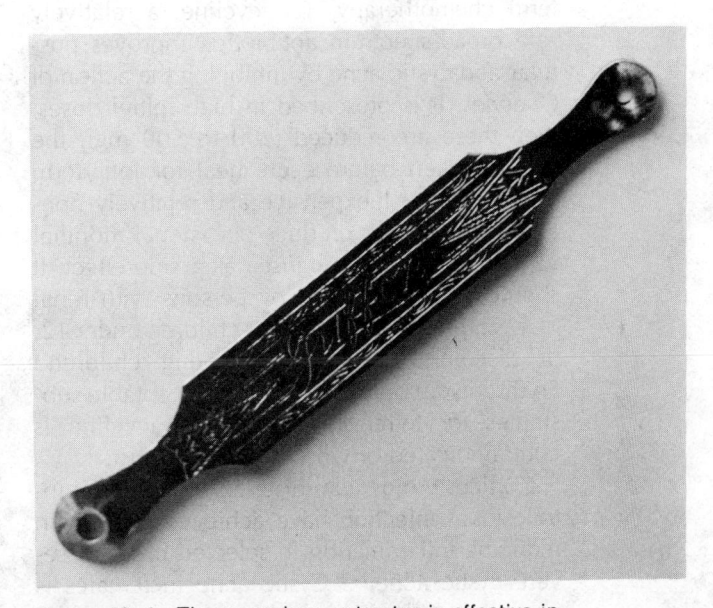

Figure 59-1 The comedone extractor is effective in nontraumatically removing blackheads.

extractor is effective in nontraumatically removing blackheads; it is used by placing the hole over the blackhead and applying direct pressure against the skin to expel the debris from the follicle. The extractor should be washed with soap and either wiped with alcohol and stored in a clean container, or stored in alcohol between uses. A few comedones can be removed daily or on some scheduled basis. Initial instruction and practice should be under the supervision of the physician or nurse in the office but the procedure can then be done at home by the teen or a capable family member. Since whiteheads are not open to the skin surface, their removal requires a slight piercing of the epidermal covering with a Bard-Parker No. 11 blade before expression with the extractor. Some dermatologists confine this procedure to their office, allowing only removal of blackheads at home.

4. *Oral administration of zinc sulfate* after meals has proved successful in reducing the occurrence of new lesions in some persons but does not currently have widespread approval.[9]

Management of Inflammatory Lesions The major aims of management of inflammatory acne are controlling infection and preventing or reducing scar formation. Treatment may involve one or more of the following therapies:

1. *Chemotherapy.* The predominant measure for treating pustulae and cystic lesions is long-term chemotherapy. Tetracycline, a relatively safe broad-spectrum antibiotic, improves pustular and cystic acne by inhibiting the action of *C. acnes.* It is prescribed in high initial doses, then these are reduced (200 to 500 mg); the drug is taken before each meal for long-term maintenance.[1] Inexpensive and relatively non-allergenic, it does produce occasional monilial vaginitis or transient nausea as a side effect. It should not be ingested by persons with renal disease, pregnant women, or children under 12. (It discolors the teeth in young children.) Erythromycin or lincomycin are acceptable substitutes for tetracycline when tetracycline is contraindicated or when sensitivity exists.[1]

Corticosteroids administered orally or by intralesional injection have achieved success in reducing inflammation in selected cases of severe cystic acne.[1,9] Cystic acne in females is improved with cyclic oral estrogens; these reduce sebum production.[3] There is usually an initial flareup of the acne the first weeks or months before noticeable improvement begins. The estrogen does carry the same risks as other hormonal preparations; therefore it should be reserved for selected severe cases in females.

2. *Acne surgery.* Minor surgery, performed to incise and drain extremely suppurative lesions, is occasionally appropriate, although it is usually reserved as a last resort if chemotherapy proves ineffective.[1]

3. *Dermabrasion.* Sometimes therapy is sought after disfigurement by scars has already developed or after therapy has not been completely successful and some scarring has occurred. It cannot be performed during active disease nor does it completely eliminate the scarred appearance, but it can render deep scars less noticeable. The procedure involves anesthetizing and freezing (hardening) the area, then abrading the skin with a high-speed rotating wire brush or steel wheel. It is reserved for the most severe forms of acne.[9]

INFECTIOUS DISEASES OF ADOLESCENCE

Although the adolescent is by and large resistant to most communicable disease, there are a few for which he seems to be a predominant host. In this section mononucleosis, influenza, tinea cruris (jock itch) and chalazion are discussed.

Infectious Mononucleosis

Infectious mononucleosis is a mildly contagious disease presumed to be viral in origin. Onset of this disease may be acute or insidious, and it is self-limiting.

The dating years (12 to 25) are the peak years for contracting this disease; this is the basis for the lay description of mononucleosis as a "kissing disease."

Etiology and Pathophysiology A herpes-like virus, the Epstein-Barr (EB) virus, is currently believed to be the causative agent in infectious mononucleosis.[9] Although the disease is occasionally epidemic, it is more often mild, and occurs only sporadically within a community. It is thought to be transmitted by direct contact with contaminated saliva of the infected individual. The incubation period varies from two to six weeks.[6]

Once the EB virus is contracted, it causes

mononuclear infiltration of the lymphatic system, producing a generalized lymphadenopathy and symptoms of an infectious process. The virus will eventually infiltrate almost every body organ in varying amounts throughout the course of the illness.

Clinical Manifestations Individuals vary in the severity with which they experience symptoms. Symptoms indicating infection usually begin with a moderate fever that gradually increases over the span of a week, although occasional patients do experience a high fever that persists longer. The fever is typically accompanied by anorexia, fatigue and a sore throat that may evolve into pharyngitis or tonsillitis.[6] About 20 per cent of infected youth experience a rash, mainly on the trunk, during the course of the fever. As the infection progresses, the youth complains of headaches and body aches. Hepatic involvement is almost always present, producing hepatomegaly and some degree of jaundice. About half of infected individuals also have splenomegaly. All these symptoms usually begin declining within a week to 10 days. However, the fatigue may linger for weeks or months, making it difficult for the youth to maintain his usual level of activity. This is probably the most frustrating element of this disease from the youth's perspective and one that his parents and the nurse must help him cope with in a realistic manner.

Diagnosis Until fairly recently it has been difficult to differentiate mononucleosis from leukemia or respiratory infections with strep throat. Lymphocytic leukocytosis is a positive finding in all three, as is an elevation of serum alkaline phosphatase. Atypical lymphocytes do not appear in peripheral blood until four to six days after the disease's onset.[6] About the same time, heterophil agglutination (Paul-Bunnell test) greater than 1:160 or rising may occur, being diagnostic if coupled with an appropriate symptomatic history.[6] However, an inexpensive test that is easily done and can identify the EB organism early has been discovered. This slide examination, called a spot test or monospot, is a rapid, highly sensitive test that specifically diagnoses infectious mononucleosis.[9]

Management No chemotherapy agent (other than interferon, which is scarce and very costly at present) has yet been found that is effective in preventing or curing infectious mononucleosis. Treatment primarily involves comfort measures to relieve symptoms. Aspirin may be given to relieve headaches and muscular aches; gargles and hot drinks ease a sore throat. Nutrition counselling that stresses the intake of a high calorie soft diet during the acute stage may be needed. Bed rest for the first couple of weeks or until fever subsides seems to be associated with earlier return to a normal activity level. Exposure to people during the first week or two of acute symptoms should be minimal to reduce the risk of secondary infection.

The young patient, used to being socially and physically active, needs reassurance that his confinement is temporary and that activity can be gradually resumed after the acute phase of the illness. The nurse may need to help the teen and his family determine a realistic schedule for returning to his usual activity level over a period of two to three months. Instruction should include an explanation that the youth should avoid receiving immunizations for about six months after resolution of the illness because cellular immune reactivity remains reduced for some time after symptoms have disappeared.

Influenza

Influenza (flu) is an acute, highly contagious infection of the respiratory tract that tends to occur in epidemic proportions (20 to 30 per cent of the population each year) during the months from September to April.[5] The elderly, young children and young adults seem to have the least resistance to the various influenza viruses and are most likely to develop complications such as pneumonia, encephalitis or acute kidney failure. Youth are probably susceptible because of their characteristic life style in which nutritious food may not be eaten and the growing body's need for sufficient rest and sound sanitary practices may be ignored. Also, those with chronic disease may resist health maintenance restrictions that control the disease but interfere with their being "one of the crowd."

Etiology and Pathophysiology Three virus groups are responsible for influenza (Table 59-1). Each of those groups also has a number of differing strains, all with the potential to cause influenza symptoms, which is why a person can

TABLE 59-1 THE INFLUENZA VIRUSES

Viral Group	Epidemic Frequency	Virulence
Virus A-1	Every 2-3 years	Causes severe body responses (symptoms)
Virus A-2 (Asian)		
Virus B	Every 3-6 years	Moderate body response
Virus C	Every year	Mild body responses; brief illness (24 hrs)

experience "the flu" numerous times. Antibodies that develop to make a person immune to the flu virus that caused his recent influenza attack will not transfer immunity to the hundreds of other strains that he may be exposed to over time.

Influenza viruses are transmitted from the nose and mouth, becoming airborne each time the infected individual opens his mouth or sneezes. They can then be inhaled by anyone nearby. Once inhaled by a susceptible individual, these viruses create a severe inflammation of the epithelium of the upper respiratory tract and bronchioles. The inflammatory response produces edema and submucosal hemorrhages of these tissues which, in turn, increase the person's vulnerability to bacterial superinfections and their associated complications. The inflamed mucosa heal within two weeks; unnecessary exposure to other pathogens should be minimized during that interval. Unfortunately, infected individuals harbor and expel the influenza virus hours to days before their symptoms become obvious.

Clinical Manifestations Once respiratory tract mucosa have become inflamed, the whole body responds with acute symptoms of sudden onset.[2,6] Initial symptoms are typically a fever that rises rapidly to high levels (more than 104° F is not uncommon), accompanied by intermittent chills, both of which subside in two or three days. Other symptoms that occur simultaneously with or several hours before the fever may include sore throat, a hacking but nonproductive cough, nasal congestion without discharge, headache with facial flushing, or conjunctival congestion. As the fever progresses, common complaints include anorexia, malaise and muscular aches, particularly of the back and extremities. These symptoms usually linger 24 to 48 hours after the fever has subsided, leaving the person temporarily disabled and prostrated. However, influenza symptoms of a C virus origin may expend themselves within 24 hours. In most individuals, symptoms of even the more severe A viruses will subside within three to seven days, although the person may continue to tire easily and feel weak for several more weeks.

Diagnosis Diagnosis is usually made on the basis of symptoms alone, particularly during epidemics. Viral throat cultures and serological complement fixation or hemagglutination tests may identify the causative organism during the peak of the infection and for a few days after symptoms have receded. A fourfold increase in viral neutralizing antibodies verifies influenza. However, these are cumbersome procedures and the patient usually recovers before the test results are known. The tests are useful, however, in identifying the virus group that is producing the epidemic.[4]

Management Treatment of influenza is aimed at controlling the organism's spread, providing comfort measures to control symptoms and preventing secondary infection.

Control of pathogen spread requires that individuals suspected of having infection be placed in respiratory isolation, whether at home or in the hospital. Exposure to others should be kept minimal and preferably should be limited to immunized persons. This is especially difficult for adolescents active socially to accept. Provision should be made for them to maintain telephone contact with their peers. They will require a variety of diversional activities (books, television, school work, hobby materials, games) that discourage boredom and depression while encouraging bed rest. Explanations should be provided of why the isolation is important as well as importance of proper disposal of Kleenex, covering of sneezes and coughs, and attention to personal hygiene to decrease the chances of bacterial superinfections.

Comfort measures and control of symptoms

involve the administration of analgesics (aspirin, Tylenol) to relieve headache and muscular discomfort. Fever can be controlled with antipyretics by encouraging drinking of fluids and by keeping the room temperature at a moderately warm to slightly cool level. High humidity and fluids also help relieve irritation in the throat and respiratory tract mucosa. Lozenges may also be soothing to the inflamed throat. The most important intervention to control symptoms and to reduce likelihood of secondary infection is bed rest for four to seven days (at least two days after the fever is gone). This is important because severity of the symptoms and incidence of bacterial superinfection is directly related to the amount of rest the patient obtains.[6]

In addition to bed rest, sound hygiene practices and minimal exposure to others as means of preventing secondary infection, antibiotics may be used prophylactically or when symptoms endure longer than four days. (Superinfection is usually suspected when symptoms last beyond this time or seem to become worse.[4]) Actions can also be taken to discourage pneumonia, the most common complication of influenza. The patient should be reminded to turn in bed or change his position frequently. He can be instructed to take several deep breaths and cough five to 10 times every hour while awake to keep all the lung fluid circulating and oxygenated.

Of course, the wisest management of influenza is preventing its occurrence. Even though acquired immunity is not yet possible, influenza vaccination with annual boosters is 70 to 90 per cent effective in preventing this disease.[2] Its usefulness in healthy children is debated, but it is more likely to be used as new, more purified forms of the vaccine are introduced. One-fourth of vaccinated individuals will experience slight erythema at the injection site.[7] Immunized children may develop a low-grade fever or feel slightly sick for several hours.[6] If a person receiving the vaccine already has a respiratory infection such as a cold, the symptoms may worsen for a couple days. Persons with egg allergy may have an allergic reaction if vaccinated. A very rare reaction (1 per 100,000 vaccinated individuals) known as Guillain-Barré syndrome has occurred in a few persons, but the majority recover without residual effects.[7]

Bed rest seems to be the key factor in preventing complication and ensuring prompt recovery in those individuals who contract influenza. Nurses and other health professionals have an obligation to inform the public of this fact and to help adolescents, with their desires to remain active socially, to comply with this intervention.

Tinea Cruris (Jock Itch)

Jock itch is a ringworm infestation of the groin that occurs primarily in pubescent males and adult men.

Two ringworm fungi (*Epidermophyton floccosum* and *Tinea rubrum*) invade the medial proximal aspects of the thighs, the crural folds and the scrotum, living off the dead keratinized skin and hair tissues of that area. Individual susceptibility is poorly understood, but poor hygiene, heat, friction, maceration in the groin area and obesity are predisposing factors.[1] Direct contact with the organism when any of these condition exists makes the young man a potential host to the fungus.

The fungal invasion is characterized by round, sharply delineated lesions, with the pubic hairs of that region broken off. These pruritic lesions vary from a scaly, red area to a painfully edematous, boggy one. Diagnosis is confirmed by presence of the fungi on direct microscopic examination of the scales.

Management involves comfort measures such as wet compresses or sitz baths to relieve the itching and swelling, irradication of the fungi with local applications of tolnaftate liquid (Tinactin) or a similar antifungal preparation, and education regarding personal hygiene and management of other predisposing factors. The youth also needs reassurance that this temporary condition in no way alters his sexuality, since any infections of the involved body region are typically perceived by young men to be somehow affiliated with venereal diseases such as syphilis or gonorrhea (there is actually no association). His parents, if they have awareness of their son's ailment, may need similar assurance and education to correct misconceptions they may hold about the disease.

Chalazion

A chalazion is caused by chronic bacterial invasion of sebaceous glands in the eyelid. Although the chalazion may begin in childhood it often does not become pronounced until adolescence, when the girl starts using eye make-up.[6] The granulomatous cyst created by the infection remains localized as a firm, nontender swelling that is covered by freely moving skin. It can be diagnosed by visual examination or, if the cyst is draining, by a culture of the exudate.

Management involves application of local heat to bring the cyst to a head and application of a topical antibiotic to eliminate the bacterial source of the infection. The teen should also be encouraged to reduce or discontinue her use of eye make-up, or if she will not avoid the make-up, to at least thoroughly remove it daily and cleanse the eyelids with a mild soap and water. If the chalazion persists despite these actions, surgical drainage of the cyst is effective.

MENSTRUAL DISTURBANCES

Severe menstrual disturbances are common to adolescence. Many teenage girls are frightened or embarrassed when their menstrual cycle does not coincide with that characteristic of their peers, yet they may experience even more anxiety about seeing a physician to have their suspected menstrual dysfunction evaluated.

Any teen undergoing a gynecological examination should be offered reassurance by the nurse that she will be present during the examination. The girl should be given information about normal menstrual function, genitourinary hygiene and desirable nutrition to maintain an adequate blood iron (Hgb) level and provided with explanations of what to expect during the examination.

Amenorrhea

Amenorrhea is a term describing a delay in the menses. *Primary amenorrhea* is a temporary delay in menarche in the girl over 17 years of age. This girl will also have delay in other pubertal characteristics if the source of her amenorrhea is delayed puberty. Amenorrhea associated with delayed puberty may be a secondary effect of hypopituitarism, adrenal hyperplasia, malnutrition, Turner's syndrome, endocrine tumors, persistent thyroid dysfunction, diabetes mellitus or other chronic disease. However, some girls with primary amenorrhea may have otherwise normal development. These girls will complain of monthly low abdominal pain and evidence normal estrogen production, but experience no menstrual flow. Possible causes are absence or congenital malformation of the female genital structures (imperforate hymen or abnormal shape or position of uterus or vagina) or an inability of the genital structures to respond to hormonal stimulation.[6] *Secondary amenorrhea* is used to describe delays between menstrual periods of 12 months or more during the two years after onset of menarche or absence of three or more periods once menarche has been established. The most common etiologies for secondary amenorrhea are emotional disturbance and pregnancy.[9]

Diagnosis Diagnostic procedures are aimed at identifying the cause of the amenorrhea, since the menstrual history alone will establish its existence. In primary amenorrhea, there is a lack of estrogen effect on vaginal smears and a normal follicle-stimulating hormone (FSH) level in the urine. These factors negate pregnancy as the cause for the estrogen absence.[6] A normal buccal chromatin pattern eliminates gonadal dysgenesis as the cause of primary amenorrhea. Physical examination or x-ray studies (vaginography) will be useful in identifying or ruling out genital malformation as the cause. A lack of virilization and a normal level of 17-ketosteroids excludes an adrenal etiology. A pregnancy test establishes whether secondary amenorrhea is due to pregnancy or to emotional distress.

Management Primary amenorrhea associated with simple delayed puberty requires no treatment. However, if the delay of menarche is causing the teenager undue emotional stress, hormonal therapy successfully initiates menses. Management of other cases of primary amenorrhea requires identifying and treating the specific causal factors (surgical correction of malformations, surgical or radiation therapy for tumors, chemotherapy to counteract adrenal or endocrine dysfunction, adequate maintenance in chronic disease processes, improved diet in malnutrition).

In secondary amenorrhea, if pregnancy is the cause, the teen must be provided with necessary information and support to make an informed decision regarding continuing or terminating the pregnancy and then referred to the appropriate agencies to help her carry out her decision. If emotional distress is the causative agent, the girl should be referred for professional counselling.

An obvious role of the nurse, regardless of the form of amenorrhea or its cause, is to provide information and explanations that will aid the girl and her parents to understand the pathophysiology involved and the management options available to them. Guidance to parents may be needed to help them recognize the need for and provide support and encouragement to their daughter until she establishes menarche.

Dysmenorrhea

Dysmenorrhea is menses associated pain or discomfort. It is common to many women, especially during adolescence. The etiology is not specifically known, nor do there seem to be any primary contributing factors other than that the female has experienced ovulation. The progesterone level just after ovulation seems to be associated with dysmenorrhea, probably because progesterone prompts uterine contractions that occur in forceful, irregular waves.[9] These intermittent contractions cause alternating constriction and dilation of the endometrial circulation, producing ischemia, edema and necrotic sloughing. Low pain tolerance may be the reason why some women experience seemingly intolerable discomfort while others describe no discomfort at all associated with this physiological process. Mental tension or anxiety experienced during this period of the menstrual cycle may serve to further increase ischemia or may leave the woman less tolerant of pain than she usually is.

Clinical Manifestations *Primary dysmenorrhea* is evidenced by complaints of cramping, abdominal pain, backache or leg ache that is intolerable or incapacitating without the presence of any pelvic pathology. *Secondary dysmenorrhea* may or may not occur in a monthly cyclic pattern. Associated with pelvic infection (endometriosis), peritonitis, systemic infection, adhesions or other pelvic disease, the secondary form of dysmenorrhea will also cause symptoms that are typical of the underlying disease process.

Diagnosis and Management Identification of dysmenorrhea and differentiating whether it is primary or secondary in nature require a careful menstrual and general health history. A thorough gynecological examination aids in ruling out pelvic abnormalities. If secondary dysmenorrhea is suspected, laboratory tests to establish an infection are indicated.

Primary dysmenorrhea management involves educating the young woman about the normal physiology of menses so that she can understand why she experiences the discomfort and relieving her of the fear of disease. A mild analgesic helps some women to carry out their normal routine during this period of their menstrual cycle. If pregnancy is not desired, estrogen therapy to prevent ovulation eliminates the pain in many young women who would otherwise experience dysmenorrhea. Numerous exercises similar to those recommended to relieve discomfort during pregnancy, such as knee-chest positioning, pelvic rocking and controlled breathing for relaxation, successfully reduce dysmenorrhea. If psychological factors are involved, professional counselling is indicated.

Adolescent girls who suffer from dysmenorrhea are often accused of using this as an excuse to avoid activities they would rather not participate in. A few do so, but for many young women dysmenorrhea is a very real, incapacitating problem. The nurse, through a careful history and astute observation, can usually differentiate the abuser from the girl actually experiencing incapacitating dysmenorrhea. Both patients, however, need guidance in learning healthy ways to cope.

Menstrual Irregularity

Irregularities in timing of periods and amount of flow are common in adolescence. The irregularity is characterized by either inconsistent intervals between periods, inconsistent length of periods, or inconsistency in the amount of flow from one period to the next. The girl's development otherwise is that of a normal adolescent. Usually this condition resolves itself by the third year after onset of menarche. Occasionally, however, irregularity persists throughout the menarche years or until completion of the first pregnancy.

A familial tendency for this disorder exists, and a careful history usually reveals a family history of similar menstrual patterns. Genitalia abnormalities should be ruled out in a thorough physical examination and, if indicated, x-rays.

Normal levels of FSH, 17-ketosteroids, and estrogen in vaginal mucosa exist in familial menstrual irregularity. Occasionally thyroid dysfunction prompts the irregularity; therefore, thyroid function tests should be performed to determine if that is the etiology.[6]

Menstrual irregularity is frustrating to the teen age girl or woman who experiences it. Unpredictability of the onset of a period encourages insecurity about herself at a time when the teen is already struggling with self-identity. Therefore, this girl needs to be reassured that many women experience this problem and that she is not a freak. She also needs information about normal physiology of menarche, including the fact that wide variation in menstrual patterns exists among women. If menstrual flow frequently tends to be excessive or prolonged, progesterone taken during the third week of her cycle over several months is effective in controlling flow. Thyroid extract is needed in situations in which thyroid dysfunction exists; this successfully manages menstrual irregularity.

Premenstrual Tension

Premenstrual tension is actually a syndrome of symptoms that many women experience a few days to a week prior to menstruation. The syndrome may include several or all of these complaints: headache, bloating of the abdomen or entire body, weight gain, lethargy or depression and breast discomfort. The etiology is unclear, but it appears to be associated in some fashion with the water and sodium retention created by progesterone production. The symptoms are relieved once menstrual flow begins.

No specific treatment has been identified, but several actions initiated by the woman herself have been found to be helpful in minimizing symptoms. These actions, taken during the third week of the menstrual cycle, include: (1) decreasing water and salt intake, (2) actively exercising for 15 minutes each day, (3) wearing a well-fitted supporting bra, (4) increasing sleep by one or two hours at night, (5) taking extra effort with hygiene and appearance to boost morale, and (6) making a daily effort to smile, laugh, and do something that brings personal pleasure or satisfaction.

References

1. S. Cohen and M. Ziai. Viral infections. In Pediatrics, M. Ziai, ed. Little, Brown & Co., 1975
2. R. Corman. The facts about flu. American Lung Association Bulletin, October 1977, p. 10
3. N. Esterly. The skin. In Pediatrics, M. Ziai, ed. Little, Brown & Company, 1975
4. J. Evans and C. Singleton. Acne: The scourge of adolescence. Issues in Comprehensive Pediatric Nursing, 1976, p. 60
5. M. Gilson. Primary amenorrhea: a simplified approach to diagnosis. American Journal of Obstetrics and Gynecology, September 1973, p. 400
6. L. Harris et al. The neck, ears and respiratory system. In Pediatrics, M. Ziai, ed. Little, Brown & Company, 1975
7. J. Hughes. Synopsis of Pediatrics. C. V. Mosby Co., 1979
8. K. Jones et al. Communicable and Noncommunicable Diseases. Canfield Press, 1970
9. J. Parrish. Dermatology and Skin Care. McGraw-Hill Book Co., 1975

Additional Recommended Reading

A. Benenson, ed. Control of Communicable Diseases in Man. American Public Health Association, 1979
W. Cunliff and J. Cotterill. The Acnes. W. B. Saunders Co., 1975
F. Shurin. Infectious Mononucleosis. Pediatric Clinics of North America, May 1979, p. 315

POTENTIAL STRESSES DURING ADOLESCENCE: REVERSIBLE ALTERATIONS IN HEALTH STATUS

by Jo Joyce Tackett, BSN, MPHN

The adolescent who develops reversible illness, especially if the illness involves an interval of hospitalization, finds the disruption to his activities at school and with peers extremely frustrating. If the illness or its management changes his appearance or limits him physically or socially, he may become embarrassed and angry.

The teenager's psychological task of developing a healthy identity makes him extremely fearful of any actual or perceived alteration to body image that reversible illness creates. This vulnerable self-concept is further compromised if his illness has a sexual component, since this is an aspect of his development to which the adolescent is extremely sensitive.

Managing the reversible illnesses to which the teen is particularly susceptible requires understanding on the part of parents and the health team of the meaning of these illnesses to the teen. The management of these health problems should be approached in a sensitive manner; the teen should be included as an active partner in both planning and implementing the treatment.

The teenager's cognitive maturity allows him to participate readily in his plan of care. He craves details and will want all the facts about his illness and the effects that the illness or treatment measures will have on his immediate health state as well as his future life style. If he is approached with honesty and respect, he can usually be relied upon to be cooperative. He will need support, however, if he is to carry out those aspects of treatment that may be contradictory to peer pressure or societal conformity. That support ideally should come from other teens who have experienced the same illness and its associated problems.

Whether the teenager is treated at home or in the hospital, provision for maintenance of peer contacts and school achievement should be ensured. If communicability of the disease prevents direct contact, peer relations can be kept up by phone, tape recordings and notes. Hospital- or homebound teens can be provided with assistance to maintain academic progress, depending on the resources and procedures of the involved school administration. While an ado-

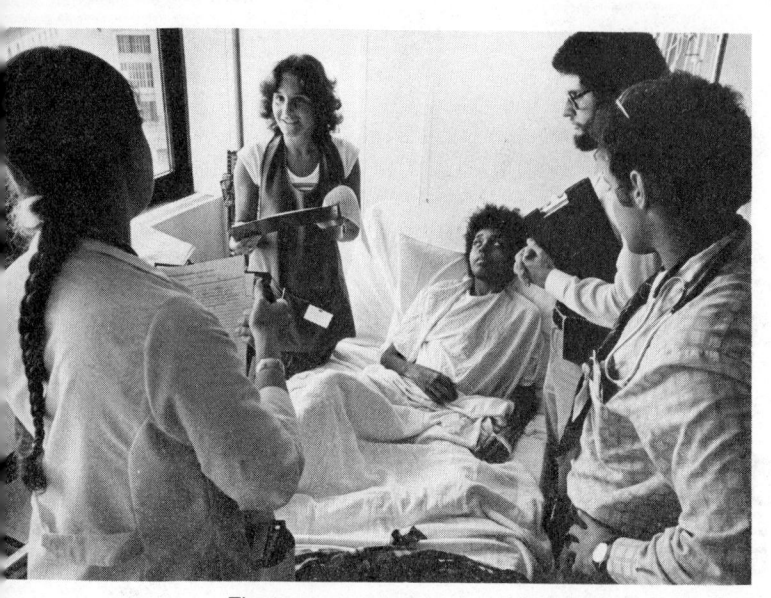

The teenager needs to be respected as a contributing member of the health team planning care. The teen who is not a respected participant experiences insult to her self-concept and is less likely to cooperate in the treatment program. (Courtesy of the Children's Hospital of Philadelphia.)

lescent is hospitalized, the nurse should make herself available some time during each day to talk with and listen to the teen so that he has an opportunity to ventilate feelings and gain a clearer perspective on concerns the illness imposes.

Such actions taken by those involved in the diagnosis and treatment of reversible illnesses during adolescence can help minimize the threats to body image and self-concept that the adolescent faces and help reinforce his developing identity as an important person worth being cared about.

SPINAL ABNORMALITIES

Spinal abnormalities such as kyphosis, lordosis and scoliosis are commonly identified and treated during the adolescent growth spurt that begins sometime between the ages of 10 and 15 years. These abnormalities are exaggerations of the natural spinal curves that may occur as a result of organic or structural vertebral changes or as a result of persistent poor posture. Kyphosis (humpback or hunchback) is an exaggerated angulation forward (convexity) of a natural vertebral curve, most commonly the thoracic curve. Exaggerated inward (concavity) spinal curvature, usually of the lumbar spine, is called lordosis (swayback). Lateral deviation of the spine, creating a side-to-side or S-shaped curvature, is scoliosis. Prior to adolescence children display developmental spinal curve exaggerations to accommodate the changes in their center of gravity. By adolescence normal adult curvature should be attained.

Kyphosis and Lordosis

Kyphosis (Fig. 60–1) may be either congenital (Scheuermann's disease) or postural. Congenital kyphosis accounts for about 5 per cent of cases and is the result of a disturbance of the epiphyses of the thoracic vertebrae. It is almost always associated with back pain, especially during effort to attain normal-appearing posture. This anomaly is not outgrown; it usually progresses, with an increase in pain and development of compensatory lordosis if aggressive treatment is not initiated. Successful treatment is usually achieved with a Milwaukee brace, although surgery is occasionally necessary.

The other 95 per cent of cases of kyphosis seen in youth are caused by habits of posture. This postural form is particularly common in the female adolescent, probably because of the round-shouldered slouch that she assumes during prepubertal and pubertal years to "hide" breast development and to make her seem less noticeably taller than her male peers, whose growth spurt comes later. An exercise program

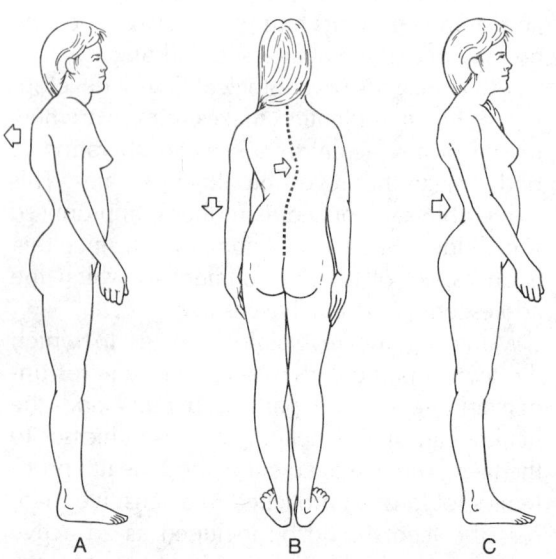

Figure 60–1 Skeletal abnormalities of adolescence. *A*, kyphosis, *B*, lordosis and *C*, scoliosis.

TABLE 60–1 CLASSIFICATION OF SCOLIOTIC DEFORMITIES

Type	Features	Etiology	Usual Management
Nonstructural	No specific vertebrae changes or rotation.	From outside spine:	
	Flexible curve, easily corrected by bending forward or toward convex side of curve.	1. Malnutrition 2. Muscle spasms from injury 3. Pain 4. Poor posture related to poor lighting, vision problem, hearing problem, negative psychological attitude, too-sedentary life style, postural carelessness, chronic fatigue.	Active and passive exercises. Correct etiological factor(s) causing curvature. If uncorrected, structural deformity will develop.
	C-shaped curve.		
Structural	Visible vertebrae, bony changes and fixed rotation toward the convexity.	Congenital malformation of vertebrae (hemivertebra, failure of segmentation of vertebra, rib fusion).	Exercise program and bracing or casting. Spinal fusion with casting or bracing and exercise program.
	Inflexible or rigid curve, not corrected by bending. Bending produces a rib hump that is the result of vertebral rotation and muscle distortion.	Neuromuscular asymmetrical muscle paralysis (neurofibromatosis, cerebral palsy, various muscle anomalies).	
	S-shaped curve results from a major curve (usually thoracic) and compensatory minor curves above and/or below the major curve.	Idiopathic with at least 70–80% suspected to be the result of dominant sex-linked inheritance (passed from father to daughter and mother to son or daughter); can skip generations (incomplete gene penetrance) and, when expressed, varies in severity (variable gene expressivity).[10, 13]	

that emphasizes proper sitting and standing, along with measures to increase the girl's self-esteem, usually bring about successful correction of postural kyphosis, although a Milwaukee brace is occasionally necessary if the kyphosis does not resolve within two to three years.

Lordosis (Fig. 60–1) is almost always a compensatory curvature associated with kyphosis or scoliosis. It is a normal compensatory curve of young children that corrects itself slightly earlier in males. Any lordosis that persists after 8 years of age should be evaluated for the underlying cause. Treatment is the same as for kyphosis.

Because of the characteristic uncooperativeness of many adolescents in doing things that they "have to do," very few will want to do the daily exercises required for spinal correction, especially if being overseen by a parent. Better success is achieved if the exercise program is supervised by a competent physical therapist who can relate to the emotional stresses of growing up. Exercises are supervised on a weekly basis initially, with the frequency decreased as the adolescent incorporates the exercises into a daily routine. The program will also be more successful if built around postural sports (weightlifting, track, dancing or swimming) that strengthen shoulder, abdominal and lumbar muscles. Success depends on the adolescent's motivation and the relationship achieved between the youth and the parent or therapist supervising the exercise program.

Scoliosis

Scoliosis is the most common skeletal deformity of adolescence, being manifested in about 15 per cent of youth between ages 10 and 21; it occurs predominantly in girls.[8] Although the deformity has usually been present before puberty or adolescence, the rapid vertebral growth that occurs during this period causes it to progress faster, making the characteristic C- or S-shaped curvature more apparent. If the deformity progresses very much, the physical changes can result in impaired cardiopulmonary function, neurological damage as a result of tethered nerves and development of an unhealthy self-image.

Scoliosis may be either nonstructural (postural; functional) or structural (Table 60–1). Structural scoliosis is further classified as congenital, idiopathic or neuromuscular, according to etiology (Table 60–2). Idiopathic scoliosis, the most common type, is more severe near puberty. It has three forms: infantile, juvenile and adolescent. This classification is based on the age of the child at diagnosis (Table 60–2). Variations in the degree of severity occur in any of the scoliotic forms.

The basic pathophysiology of scoliosis is a lateral deviation (most often a right thoracic curvature) of the spinal column from midline that may or may not involve rotation or deformity of the vertebrae (Fig. 60–1). The deviation is a consequence of weakened muscle strength from any one or a variety of genetic, environmental or physiological factors. During progression of the curvature that occurs at the growth spurt, pressure exerted on the vertebrae cause them to become wedged (Fig. 60–2). If structural changes begin occurring early, when extensive spinal growth is taking place, a more severe curvature abnormality will be created. Correctional prognosis is best when the curvature is identified and treated while it is still mild. Because idiopathic adolescent scoliosis is most prevalent, the remainder of this discussion will deal with that class of scoliosis.

Diagnosis Early identification of scoliotic curvature cannot be overemphasized, because early intervention greatly improves the prognosis and diminishes the length of time needed for treatment and the accompanying emotional trauma. The procedures to diagnose scoliosis are simple and take little time, yet several factors tend to impede early diagnosis in youth. The child between 10 and 15 (the peak ages for incidence) is usually healthy and, as a consequence, frequently does not have a yearly physical. Even when a physical is included in health maintenance for a child this age, a back examination is often overlooked or inadequately done. In addition, the vertebral changes of scoliosis often progress slowly and may go unnoticed. The adolescent, whose identity and peer group similarity is so easily threatened, may not report a deviation even when it is noticed. The majority of parents do not see their teenage daughters undressed and visualization of the bare back is necessary to observe early curve deformity.

Two fairly recent practices are currently improving early identification of scoliosis, and the nurse can actively endorse these or initiate them

TABLE 60-2 ETIOLOGICAL CLASSIFICATION OF STRUCTURAL SCOLIOSIS

Classification	Etiology and Pathophysiology	Diagnostic Features	Treatment
Congenital scoliosis	Embryologic malformation of spine during third to fifth embryonic week.	Anteroposterior and lateral x-rays verify curvature and identify anomalous vertebrae.	Early treatment essential; usually spinal fusion before preschool age to stabilize progressive curves.
	Localized or generalized deformity: hemivertebra (only half formed), failure in segmentations (vertebra segments do not fully separate) and rib fusion are typical anomalies.	Usually other congenital anomalies coexist; urinary tract anomalies most prevalent.	Complete evaluation for any other anomalies; intravenous pyelogram recommended as a minimal screening.
	Thoracic curves most common.	Secondary neurologic symptoms from long-term spinal cord tethering.	
		Secondary signs: short trunk; sacral area hair tufts; unequal leg length; cafe-au-lait markings.	
Neuromuscular (paralytic) scoliosis	Secondary to neuropathic or myopathic disease (polio, cerebral palsy, muscular dystrophy, neurofibromatosis, myelomeningocele) that results in muscle imbalance.	Presence of primary neurological or muscular disease.	Occasionally bracing stabilizes progression if no structural changes.
	Initially flexible, becoming rigid as progresses; tends to progress after skeletal growth completed:	Anteroposterior and lateral x-rays verify curvature.	Spinal fusion with Harrington rod instrumentation usually necessary if structural change present.
	Long C curve—generalized neuromuscular disease with severe muscle weakness.	Rib hump may or may not be present, depending on flexibility of curve.	
	S curve similar to idiopathic scoliosis—result of localized muscle imbalance.		
Idiopathic scoliosis	Dominant X-linked inheritance in 70–80% of cases justifies evaluation of all family members when one is diagnosed.[6]	See below for individual forms.	See below for individual forms.
	S-shaped curvature most common with vertebrae changes and rotations.		
	See below for individual forms.		

Table continued on following page

TABLE 60-2 ETIOLOGICAL CLASSIFICATION OF STRUCTURAL SCOLIOSIS *(Continued)*

Classification	Etiology and Pathophysiology	Diagnostic Features	Treatment
1. Infantile idiopathic scoliosis	Occurs in first years of life; often associated with intrauterine position. More in males, rare in U.S., common in Britain. Usually left thoracic curve.	Occurs before 4 years of age. Verification of curve with antero-posterior and lateral standing and side-bending x-rays.	50% resolve spontaneously. 50% rapidly progressive and require spinal fusion.
2. Juvenile idiopathic scoliosis	Occurs in middle childhood, usually around 6 years. Usually right thoracic curve. Sexes are equally affected.	Occurs between 4 and 10 years of age. Standing and side-bending x-rays verify curve severity.	Will not resolve spontaneously. Bracing or Orthoplast Jacket usually adequate. Spinal fusion indicated if rapidly progressive or curve is severe (55 to 60 degrees).

3. Adolescent idiopathic scoliosis	Occurs between age 10 and skeletal maturity.
	
	Most prevalent in U.S.; seven times more common in females.
	
	May or may not progress during growth spurt.
	
	Various curves possible.[11]
		Occurs after age 10.
		
		Positive screening test findings:
		  Scapular prominence
		  Rib hump
		  Shoulder asymmetry
		  Spinal curves
		  Hip asymmetry
		  Deeper creasing one side of waist
		  Torso malalignment when standing erect
		  Anterior rib and breast asymmetry
			Will not resolve spontaneously.
			
			Exercise program alone ineffective.
			
			Milwaukee brace or Orthoplast Jacket or spinal fusion with/without Harrington rod instrumentation or Dwyer instrumentation. (Cast or traction may be used preoperatively or postoperatively.)

Suggestive signs: unequal hemline, back pain, poor posture, attached earlobes, cavus (high arch) feet.

Lumbar curve (T11 to L5)
Fairly common.
Majority are left.
Seldom any compensatory curves.
Minimally deforming but does become rigid, causing arthritic pain during childbearing and old age.

Right thoracic curve (T4 to L1)
Very common.
Severe cosmetic defect and cardiopulmonary impairment if untreated.
Usually compensatory left minor curves above and below major curve.
Much vertebral change and rotation.

Double major curves
Right thoracic and left lumbar prominence most common combination.

Thoracolumbar curve (T4 to L4)
Very common.
Long curve.
Moderate cosmetic deformity.
May cause rib and flank distortions.

Cervicothoracic curve (C5 to T4)
Rare.
Usually to left.
Shoulder asymmetry only cosmetic problem.

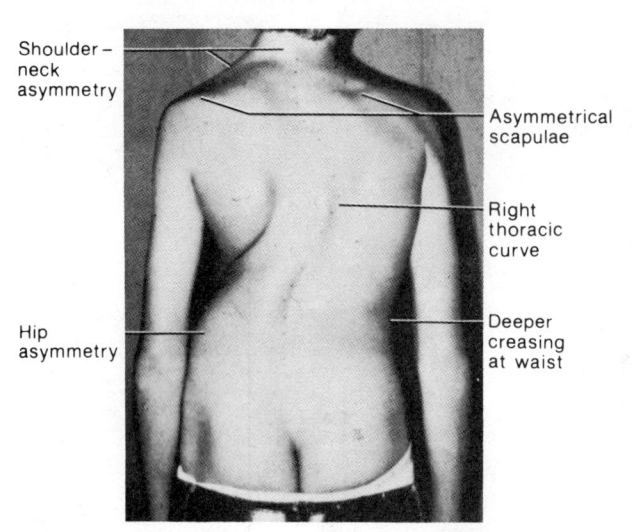

Screening of youth 9–15 promotes early detection of scoliosis. Adequate screening requires complete exposure of back, chest and hips.

Observe child from front while he is standing erect, assessing for:
- Shoulder asymmetry (shoulder elevated on convex side of scoliotic curve).
- Anterior rib asymmetry.
- Breast asymmetry (one breast may appear higher, larger or more protruding than the other).
- Hip asymmetry (one hip may protrude).

Observe youth from side and back while he is standing erect, assessing for:
- Shoulder asymmetry.
- Scapular asymmetry (scapula on convex side of curve higher).
- Rib cage asymmetry (rib cage prominent on convex side of curve).
- Waist asymmetry (waist fuller, more creased on convex side of curve).
- Hip asymmetry.
- Drop a plumb line (tape measure) from occiput to check for trunk malalignment—indicated when plumb line does not pass through gluteal fold. (If line passes through gluteal folds but curves are visible, compensation is indicated.)
- Malalignment of spinous processes. (Mark each process with a marker pen. Line formed is not straight in malalignment).

Observe youth from back while he bends over, feet together until back is parallel to floor and arms dangle freely (forward bending test), assessing for:
- Thorax asymmetry (posterior rib hump may appear on convex side of curve).
- Hip asymmetry.

Run measuring tape from anterior superior iliac spine to medial malliolar at ankle, assessing for:
- Asymmetry in leg length.

Figure 60–2 Screening procedure.

in her own community. One practice is the initiation in several states of statewide school scoliosis screening for all school-age youth as a part of the school health program. The other is the screening of all siblings in families in which a case is diagnosed. This practice has been initiated by many nurses, physicians and orthopedists as a result of the research that has revealed a genetic etiology of the condition.

Screening for scoliosis involves observing the child while he or she is walking, standing erect and bending forward. The discussion under Figure 60–2 describes the specific observations that are included in a thorough screening evaluation.

A child suspected of having scoliosis after screening should be referred for further evaluation by the nurse to the family physician or a competent orthopedist experienced in treating scoliotic deformities of adolescence. The teen and parents should be informed of the possibility of a deformity and of the importance of early intervention (ideally between 12 to 15 years of age) to possibly avoid surgery or cosmetic deformity.[10] The nurse can also inform the family that the evaluation does not involve any painful or lengthy procedures but includes a thorough history and complete physical examination and x-rays of the spine and chest. Families who hesitate to initiate diagnostic evaluation or treatment measures because of their costs may be reassured that finances from crippled children's services (as part of local social services or health departments) are available.

The nurse may be involved in collecting the history data and accompanying the teenager during the physical examination. Pertinent history includes the child's age, the age at which deformity was first noticed or suspected, and the parent's and youth's impression of the curve's progression since it was first noticed. Age at onset of sexual development, a history of dental development, rate of growth through infancy and childhood, and any subjective complaints (fatigue, pain) should also be documented for the orthopedist's evaluation. The nurse involved in initial screening or the nurse working with the orthopedist often becomes the liaison between the teen, his or her family, the orthopedist and many other team members, ensuring that follow-up of screening and diagnostic recommendations occurs.

X-rays of the anteroposterior and lateral spine are required to verify whether the curvature is structural or functional, to determine the extent of vertebral changes and rotation, and to estimate the correctability of the deformity.

Management Treatment of scoliosis is a long, drawn-out ordeal that requires a great deal of cooperation from the teen and parents to perform the treatment regimen consistently and to keep follow-up appointments, both of which are essential to successful correction of scoliotic deformity. The nurse has a critical role in motivating the family to seek medical advice and to practice treatment measures and in supporting them through the years required for correctional therapy.

Two modes of treatment have been successful in correcting scoliosis: bracing and spinal fusion. Each requires adherence to a daily exercise program if maximal success is to be achieved. This program can be supplemented by activities of interest to adolescents (swimming, weightlifting, dancing, track) that strengthen back, shoulder and abdominal muscles. It cannot be overemphasized that an exercise program alone has been shown by data from years of research to be ineffective in stopping or correcting scoliotic progression.

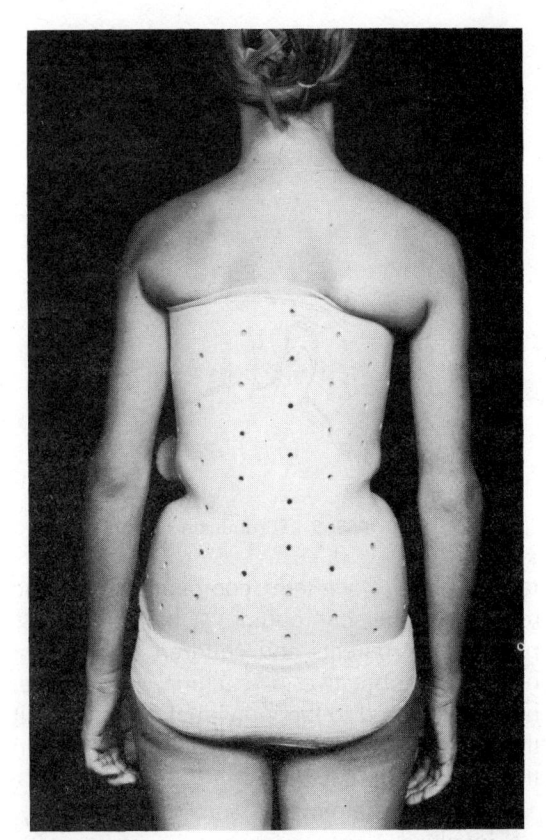

Figure 60–4 Orthoplast jacket. (From D. Hungerford. Spinal deformity in adolescence. Medical Clinics of North America, November 1975.)

Nursing Implications of Nonsurgical Management

The nonsurgical treatments employed to treat scoliosis include the Milwaukee brace, the Orthoplast jacket, and various casting and traction methods (mostly used preoperatively to improve spinal flexion or postoperatively to maintain alignment during fusional correction or at both times). Table 60–3 describes each of these methods, including when each is indicated, potential problems and general nursing care required. Figure 60–3 shows a Milwaukee brace, Figure 60–4 an Orthoplast jacket, Figure 60–5 the Turnbuckle cast, and Figure 60–6 a localizer cast.

Before the selected form of nonsurgical intervention is begun, parents and the teen need in-depth preparation to maintain correct management at home and to understand the impor-

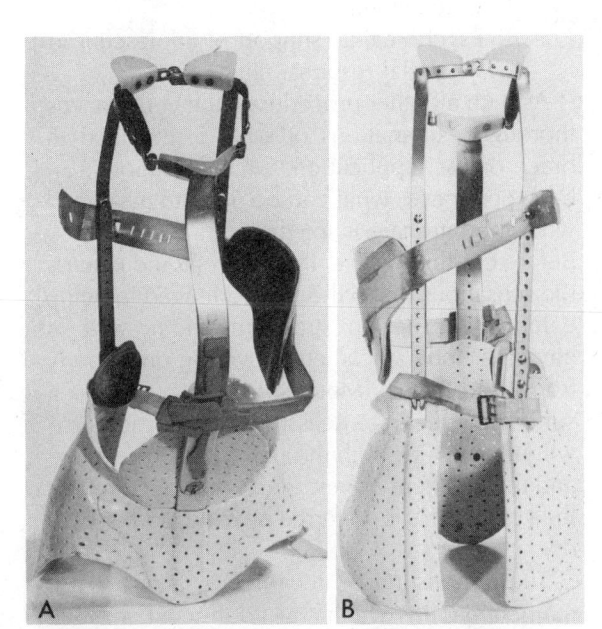

Figure 60–3 Milwaukee brace. (From M. Tachdjian. Pediatric Orthopedics. W. B. Saunders Co., 1972, p. 1210.)

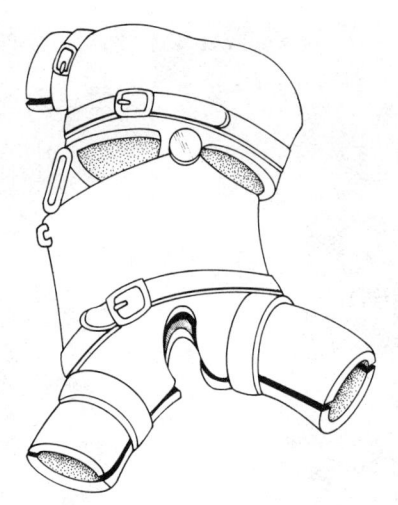

Figure 60-5 Turnbuckle cast.

tance of their long-term compliance with the regimen. Anderson* outlines a basic teaching program for parents and children in terms of behavioral objectives. Teaching, of course, must be tailored to the individual situation, but the following guidelines can help the nurse plan the topics to be covered.

1. Normal anatomy of spine; terminology involved
2. Causes of spinal deformities
3. Causal factors in specific person involved, when known

---

*B. Anderson. Carole, a girl treated with bracing. In The Patient with Scoliosis. American Journal of Nursing, September 1979, p. 1592.

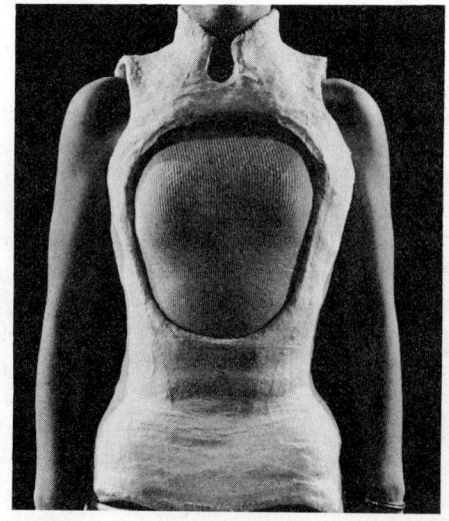

Figure 60-6 Localizer cast. (From R. Rothman and F. Simeone. The Spine. W. B. Saunders Co., 1975, p. 376.)

4. Various approaches to nonsurgical management (observation, exercise, casting, bracing, traction)
5. Reasons that specific management program was selected for person
6. Course of management program to be expected
   A. Sequence of events
   B. Anticipated outcome
   C. Frequency of check-ups
   D. Purpose of procedures during management (measurements, x-rays, sequential photography)
7. Self-care activities
   A. Application of brace (or other device)
   B. Skin care
   C. Appliance care and cleaning
   D. Clothing selection
   E. Exercise and maintenance of activities
8. Potential problems (e.g., advancement in curve, pressure sores)
   A. How to recognize
   B. How to prevent
9. Psychosocial impact of management program
   A. Self-image of adolescent undergoing treatment
   B. Peer acceptance
   C. Fears, anxieties, need for control
   D. Concerns about normal adolescent sexuality development
10. Responsibilities of parents during child's treatment program
    A. Care activities
    B. Psychological support of adolescent
    C. Financial responsibilities

As with all other procedures, the youth needs thorough explanations of what is involved in brace or cast application, what sensations can be experienced, what can be done to assist and what the rationale is for the appliance or cast. Before casting is done, the nurse should discuss the sensations that will be experienced in being balanced prone on straps in midair and of having a body stockinette covering one's body from head to toe. (Most patients complain of a suffocating feeling.) Reassurance that the nurse will be with the youth throughout the procedure and that a parent or best friend may accompany the youth if this is preferred provides some security.

These nonsurgical techniques attack three major areas in which the adolescent may be vulnerable: self-image, developing sexuality and peer acceptance. The adverse cosmetic effect of the brace or cast can be extremely threatening to the sensitive self-image of the adolescent. The child must learn how to handle the reactions and curiosity of other people and at the same time incorporate the brace or cast into his or her own self-image. The school nurse can be invaluable as a listener during the early adjustment period; a phone call or invitation to stop by the health center every few days is greatly appreciated by most teens during the anxious first days back in school. The teen and family members should be encouraged to handle public and peer curiosity with honest confrontation ("I see you are curious about my brace. Would you like me to tell you about it?")

A part of the teenage girl's self-identity is the development of a sense of femininity and sexuality. That the brace or cast hides the developing feminine figure is a source of anxiety to the adolescent. She fears that boys will find her unattractive, that the appliance will hinder breast development and that with the brace she cannot compete with her female peers in attractiveness. Reassurance should be offered that breast development is in no way diminished by the appliance. Attention and hugs received from male relatives and family friends often provide the reassurance the girl needs to retain her sense of feminine attractiveness. During evaluation examinations, the nurse should make every effort to preserve the teen's privacy, because being observed in her underwear does not hold the same meaning for the teen that being observed at the beach in a bikini does.

Nonsurgical techniques also impinge on the teen's feelings of peer acceptance. The brace or cast makes it difficult for her to wear the halters, bikinis and filmy fabrics so popular among teens and so important to "being one of the crowd." The appliance represents visible evidence that she is different from her peers at a time in her development when it is important to conform to peer norms and standards, including those of appearance.

Facing school and peer reactions the first day is one of the hardest tasks the scoliotic girl must confront. Her adjustment is eased tremendously when the school nurse has prepared the teacher or teachers and classmates ahead of time for her return. The nurse may plan with the girl to teach her peers about scoliosis and her treatment and to answer their questions on her first or second day back with the assistance and presence of the school nurse. This has been cited by many scoliotic youths as the most helpful activity in their adjustment back into school and their peer group. Teen activities such as camp or slumber parties also help to desensitize the girl to her brace or cast.

Nonsurgical techniques may also be perceived by the teen or her parents to place constraints on her independence and social life. Most teens are surprised and reassured to learn that they may participate in any activity they choose except for aggressive contact sports (sometimes horseback riding and skiing are also excluded). However, even with this knowledge the teen must still deal with the fact that the brace or cast must be worn for several years and with the problems of fatigue and overheating induced by the appliance. The nurse should help ensure that the teen has some say, whenever possible, in her treatment, and that an effort is made to show the girl at each evaluation the progress being made as a result of the treatment (compare x-rays from one time to the next or take postural photographs at each visit to compare). Reassurances about not needing surgery should not be made at any time, however, as surgery does remain a possibility.

Many braced teens have found that for study at home an adjustable drafting table relieves some of the muscle tension created by sitting and that a beanbag chair is the most comfortable for reading, resting or TV watching. Avoiding carrying heavy or bulky things and avoiding carrying anything for a long time helps reduce fatigue. Overheating is a result of having little skin surface exposed to the air and is a real problem even in cool weather. Talcum and an undershirt help absorb the moisture. Frequent application of body deodorant and a midday change of perspiration-saturated clothing helps to maintain a sense of freshness. The importance of a daily shower or bath is obvious.

As with any other health problem that persists over time, the most effective support system is contact with others who have the same problem. The nurse should be able to find or organize a scoliotic support group for the newly diagnosed scoliotic adolescent and for parents.

Parents will need reassurance to relieve the guilt feelings they experience when their child is diagnosed as having scoliosis, especially as a result of discovery of the genetic etiology of this condition. Overcoming these guilt feelings is

TABLE 60-3 NONSURGICAL MANAGEMENT OF SCOLIOSIS

Management	Indications	Related Nursing Measures
Observation Frequent measuring of curves and x-ray evaluation to monitor improvement, stabilization or progression of curves.	Mild curves of less than 20°	Emphasize that further intervention will be required if curve progresses and that cardiopulmonary compromise may occur.
Usually an exercise program also prescribed.		Emphasize that checkups every 3 months are essential to effectively monitor status of curve. Teach exercise program or refer to physical therapy for such instruction.
EXTERNAL BRACING *Milwaukee brace* A combination of straps, pads and metal struts are used to straighten the spine and hold it in position.	Curve of 20°–40° in skeletally immature spine.	Instruct and demonstrate and require return demonstration of the following:
Brace may be removed for 1 hour for personal hygiene; the brace is worn continuously otherwise.	Sometimes indicated in greater than 40° curve if patient a poor surgical risk.	• Brace application and removal (imperative to prevent skin breakdown) • Brace maintenance and cleaning • Exercises
May have daily exercises prescribed additionally.		Instruct in proper skin care: • Daily bathing • Undershirt under brace to absorb perspiration and protect skin from brace. • Tincture of benzoin, moist tea bags (tannic acid), or alcohol daubed on skin areas where brace rubs or creates pressure to toughen skin and decrease skin breakdown • Wear underpants over brace for easier toileting
The patient is gradually weaned from the brace over a 1–2 year period when spinal maturity is nearly complete.		Endorse all activity except horseback riding, driving and contact sports.
Low profile (Pasadena) brace is available, which is similar to Milwaukee brace but does not require neck ring.		Work in collaboration with school personnel and school nurse to coordinate adjustments of school program. Counselling • Frequent follow-up evaluations imperative. • Psychological adjustments to brace and altered body image

Orthoplast jacket
Plastic jacket similar to Milwaukee brace but less aesthetically distracting.

Costs considerably less than Milwaukee brace.

CASTING
Turnbuckle
Full body cast with wedges cut over convexity of curve; adjusted periodically to cause progressive, gradual curve correction.

Involves lengthy hospitalization and immobilization (See Nursing Care Plan, Chapter 63)

Localizer cast (Risser)
Full body cast that immobilizes the spine in alignment.

Same as for Milwaukee brace.

Seldom used today.
Rigid curves.

Preoperatively to stretch curve and tissues.

During surgery to maintain alignment.

Postoperatively to maintain correction until healing is progressed.

Same as for Milwaukee brace.

Teach cast care (Chapter 51).

Assure patient the cast will not alter breast development.

See care plan in Chapter 63 for comprehensive nursing care of the patient immobilized with a musculoskeletal disorder.

Same as for turnbuckle cast.

TABLE 60-4 SURGICAL MANAGEMENT OF SCOLIOSIS[16]

Management	Indications
Spinal Fusion (Arthrodesis) One-stage procedure. The paraspinal muscles are stripped from the lamina of the vertebrae to be fused. The vertebrae are fused and a bone graft (usually autogenous from one iliac crest), which is broken into matchstick pieces, is placed along one entire fusion area to promote bone formation.	Curve progression despite bracing or casting. Many paralytic and some congenital curves do this. Thoracic scoliosis with associated lordosis seldom responds to bracing. Physiological cardiopulmonary compromise. Progressive pain and fatigue despite non-surgical measures. Must be done prior to skeletal maturity for maximum correction. Lumbar scoliosis of 30 degrees with associated lordosis often causes such imbalance that surgery is indicated.
Harrington Rod Instrumentation Posterior approach by which a series of rods and hooks are implanted on the concave side of curve to apply distraction and/or on the convex side of curve to apply compression to the posterior spinal elements.	Harrington factor of 5+ (obtained by dividing number of vertebrae involved in the curve into the degree of the curve) and spinal fusion indications.
Dwyer Instrumentation Anterior approach by which spine is exposed from the front and bolts are inserted transversely through each vertebral body. The bolts are attached to a cable that is applied to the convexity of the curve. The intervertebral discs between adjacent vertebrae are removed and the vertebrae are pulled together.	Same as for Harrington procedure.

important to their ongoing participation in management of the teen's condition and to the prevention of an overprotective response. They need reassurance that they will eventually be able to look at their teen without noticing the brace or cast that causes feelings of surprise and sorrow, and that the need to protect their child from the sometimes tactless public will also pass. Whether counselling of parents takes place with the adolescent or separately, parents need to be taught as much information about intervention effectiveness as does the teen. They also need the listening ear of the nurse and an opportunity to be supported by other parents who have been through or are going through the same experience. Assistance and referral should be offered to help offset the costs of equipment and its upkeep and of follow-up evaluations, special furniture and the clothing that wears out so fast because of the appliance.

Nursing Implications of Surgical Management The most commonly used surgical management is now a one-stage spinal fusion (arthrodesis) procedure. (Table 60-4 contains a description of surgical interventions.) The procedure is done under general anesthesia and usually involves about two weeks of hospitalization, after which the teen is discharged fully ambulatory in a localizer walking cast (Risser). The cast is either applied at the end of the surgical procedure or 8 to 14 days postoperatively. It is changed at three months after surgery so that x-rays can be taken to assess early fusion and maintenance of correction. The cast is worn for another six to nine months before being removed permanently. Follow-up evaluations are necessary every three to six months for three to five more years to ensure maintenance of correction. Restriction on horseback riding, skiing and skating activities is necessary until the cast is removed; restriction on heavy-contact sports continues until follow-up is no longer necessary (three to five years).

Spinal fusion may be done alone or in conjunction with either Harrington or Dwyer instrumentation (Table 60-4). The Stryker frame is used for the patient who has Harrington instrumentation. The teen should be given an explanation of the frame and a chance to prac-

TABLE 60-5 POSTOPERATIVE ACTIVITIES AFTER SPINAL FUSION

First 24 to 48 hours
    ICU care; sometimes patient stays in ICU until cast is dry if applied during surgery.

    *Monitoring of vital signs, circulation and neurologic status of extremities every 1 to 2 hours, more often if indicated.

    *Cough and deep breathe, IPPB, or spirometer every hour for several days, frequency gradually decreased depending on pulmonary function test results.

    Catheterization if no voiding by 12 hours postop.

    IV fluids and antibiotics given; monitoring of intake and output.

    Patient kept NPO with nasogastric tube until peristalsis resumes (usually 2 to 4 days).

    Thoracotomy care given if Dwyer procedure done.

    Large frequent doses of narcotic given to relieve bone pain and muscle tension in spine.

    *Cast discomfort reported and relieved promptly.

    Patient may have assisted ventilation, especially if preop pulmonary function tests were 30% or less of expected function.

    *Meticulous skin care and hygiene practiced.

    Chest tubes, Hemovacs used to facilitate drainage from chest and graft site.

    Cardiac and central venous monitoring done.

    *Patient turned every hour (rolled pillow support to supine/side lying positions for Harrington, side to side for Dwyer); firm, flat bed.

By the 4th day
    Turning every 1–2 hours continued.

    Nasogastric tube and Foley catheter removed.

    *Diet high in protein, vitamin C, thiamine, iron and bulk; low in calories.

    Daily bowel evacuation of feces and flatus. (Suppositories, laxatives and diet may facilitate.)

    Push fluids to maintain hydration and prevent renal calculi; monitoring of intake and output continues; IV may be stopped.

    *Encourage diversional activities; prism glasses allow reading and TV watching, long tongs help adolescent feel independent in reaching bedside items.

By 8 days postop
    Sutures removed.

    X-rays taken.

    First cast or new cast applied.

    Teaching begun to family about cast care and other skills required for home care after discharge.

By 14 days postop
    Patient turns self at least every 3 to 4 hours.

    Does active and passive range of motion exercises; isotonic and isometric exercise.

    Assumes activities of daily living to extent feasible.

    Enters physical therapy.

    Has progressive ambulation; discharge when patient can walk and climb stairs independently.

*Intervention continued from time initiated throughout hospitalization.

tice manipulating it before surgery. Immobilization in bed is required after the Dwyer procedure.

In addition to preoperative teaching begun two days before surgery that prepares the youth for what to expect during and after operation, he should be given a chance before surgery to practice voiding in a supine position and to eat horizontally. Honest, open communication should be maintained between the teaching nurse and the teen throughout the preoperative period to ensure that the youth's anxieties and questions are dealt with. The youth should be informed that the surgery involves an incision from T1 to the sacrum at midline. The procedure should be described in terms the youth understands, and he or she should be told when the cast will be applied and how it is done.

Teaching regarding the postoperative period should emphasize the teen's participation in recovery. Table 60–5 outlines the typical postoperative period and can be used as a guide to prepare the teen and parents for what to expect. Psychological care during the postoperative period is extremely important. The teen will experience periods of depression and withdrawal. Diversions in which the teen's specific interests are involved are extremely helpful during this time, as are visits from peers, family and other scoliotic teens.

After discharge the family takes the responsibility of helping the teen do things he cannot do for himself. They should be provided with a resource person whom they may consult 24 hours a day. Periodic home visits from a community health nurse are supportive to the family and facilitate evaluation by the health team as to the adequacy of management and compliance at home. The school nurse should become involved in assisting the teen to adjust to return to school.

COMMUNICABLE DISEASES OF ADOLESCENCE

Adolescents are highly susceptible to two of the four leading communicable diseases in the United States: venereal disease and viral hepatitis. (Venereal disease leads and viral hepatitis ranks fourth.) The adolescent may be embarrassed to seek assistance when symptoms become apparent and hesitant to reveal contacts for epidemiological follow-up. The nurse working in settings in which these diseases are diagnosed or treated must have a sound understanding of adolescent development, a genuine interest in this age group and their needs and a nonjudgmental, tactful manner that encourages rapport.

Viral Hepatitis

There are now three etiological classifications for viral hepatitis. The first two types, hepatitis A and hepatitis B, have been recognized for some time, but hepatitis C (non-A, non-B hepatitis) is a recent research discovery.[1] Hepatitis A and hepatitis B were for a long time referred to as infectious hepatitis and serum hepatitis because of a recognized oral-fecal mode of transmission in A and parenteral mode of transmission in B. However, research has shown that both types can be transmitted parenterally and nonparenterally so that the names serum hepatitis and infectious hepatitis are no longer accepted. Hepatitis A refers to clinical disease with a short incubation period and hepatitis B to clinical disease with a long incubation period. Hepatitis C refers to clinical disease resembling hepatitis B, but in which tests do not confirm hepatitis A or B antigens. Table 60–6 summarizes the similarities and differences in characteristics of each of the hepatitis forms.

Pathophysiology and Diagnosis Infection of the liver by any of the hepatitis viruses results in patchy liver cell necrosis from viral and lymphocytic infiltration. In most cases sufficient antibodies are produced to prevent liver damage.

The allergic response stimulated by antibody formation causes the gastrointestinal, neuromuscular, dermatological and cold-like symptoms characteristic of hepatitis (Table 60–7). The decreased metabolic and synthesizing function of the liver from the infiltration makes the liver incompetent to handle fatty or fried foods and alcohol and drugs (Table 60–8) during the course of the infection. Bile blockage is a consequence of the edema of the hepatic ducts that results from the allergic response. This blockage causes accumulation of bile in the blood, feces and urine and then the skin (icteric phase) (Table 60–7). If bilirubin levels persist for too long or become too high (>15 to 20 mg/100 ml), as may occur in severe infection, the brain is affected. Pre-coma symptoms occur (Table 60–7) and, if untreated, eventually lead to coma or death.

TABLE 60-6 CHARACTERISTICS OF HEPATITIS A, HEPATITIS B AND HEPATITIS C[3, 18, 20]

Characteristic	Hepatitis A (Short-Incubation Hepatitis)	Hepatitis B (Long-Incubation Hepatitis)	Hepatitis C (Non-A, Non-B Hepatitis)
Agent	Hepatitis A virus (IH virus, HAV virus)	Hepatitis B virus (SH virus; HBV virus; HB Ag)	Unknown
Serum markers (i.e., specific elements of the virus that can be recognized in blood serum)	None	HB_sAg (Hepatitis Australian antigen or HAA; Dane particle) and anti-HB_sAg (the antibody), HB_cAg and anti-HB_cAg (the antibody), e antigen (HB_e Ag) (possibly a host antigen produced by virus infected liver cells)	None
Mode of transmission (Direct or indirect transmission possible in all 3 types)	Primarily oral route via all secretions (stool, urine, semen, tears, menses) and in contaminated food (especially shellfish), breast milk, and water. Also parenteral route via serum, blood or blood products. Virus will cross placental barrier in 3rd trimester	Primarily parenteral route via serum, blood and blood products; also by oral route as in hepatitis A. Virus will cross placental barrier in 3rd trimester	Parenteral route after multiple transfusions (15+ units) or injections from contaminated equipment. No oral route has currently been established.
Incubation period	15–60 days	60–180 days	15–160 days
Recovery time	Average 4 weeks	Average 6–12 mos	Average 6–12 mos
Carrier state	No	Yes (persistence of HB_sAg in blood for years or life)	Unknown
Seasonal variation	Greatest incidence in winter; rare in summer	None	None
Pre or post exposure prophylaxis	ISG 80–90% effective; may cause long lasting natural immunity	HBIG or ISG effective for 3–4 mos	Unknown

TABLE 60–7 CLINICAL MANIFESTATIONS OF VIRAL HEPATITIS AND NURSING MANAGEMENT[3, 19]

Phase	Symptoms	Nursing Management
Prodromal or preicteric phase (2–14 days)	Nonspecific gastrointestinal symptoms: nausea, vomiting, diarrhea, anorexia, RUQ tenderness.	1. Dramamine if nausea or vomiting is severe. 2. Small, frequent feedings of high carbohydrate, moderate protein low-fat foods; avoid fried foods; carbonated beverages usually tolerated well; avoid temperature extremes in food.
	Nonspecific neuromuscular symptoms: malaise, myalgias and arthralgias, weakness, unusual fatigability, headache.	1. Hot or cold compresses to relieve aches and pains. 2. Bed rest.
	Cold-like symptoms: coughs, coryza, pharyngitis, photophobia.	1. Darkened room to relieve photophobia. 2. Cold steam vaporizer to humidify air and relieve cough and pharyngeal irritation. 3. Patient should wear a mask if coughing or sneezing to prevent airborne spread of virus. 4. Benadryl to aid in rest and sleep if symptoms disturb sleep.
	Fever: Low grade (<102°) in type "A" to pyrexia (>102°) in types "B" and "C".	1. Cool, nondrafty room. 2. Lightweight clothing. 3. Tepid bath if pyrexia persists.
	Dermatologic symptoms: rash, hives, edema, pruritus.	1. Benadryl to relieve itching and promote rest.
	Accumulation of bilirubin in secretions from impaired liver function and blockage of bile duct occurs 4–5 days before onset of icteric phase: Clay-colored stools (bile pigments) Dark urine (bilirubinuria) Elevated serum bilirubin (>2.5 mg/100 ml) Elevated SGOT and SGPT (>2000)	1. Avoid drug ingestion (Table 60–8) especially narcotics, sedatives, birth control pills. 2. Avoid alcoholic beverages. 3. Avoid inhaling toxic fumes (cleaning fluids). 4. Watch for signs of bleeding in secretions, bruising easily, prolonged bleeding after injections or lab punctures.
	Alkaline phosphotase 2–3 times the normal value from accumulated abnormal liver products.	
	Leukopenia and lymphocytosis (2–20%).	
	Prothrombin time increased (>2–3 seconds more than control) from liver's decreased ability to absorb vitamin K or to manufacture clotting factors.	

Icteric or jaundiced phase (2–3 weeks; may not occur in mild cases)	Gastrointestinal and neuromuscular symptoms initially intensify, then gradually resolve.
	
	Temperature returns to normal. Hepatosplenomegaly and posterior cervical lymphdenopathy may develop.
	
	In moderate or severe cases:
	Serum bilirubin elevates further (5–20 mg/100 ml).
	Serum transaminase elevates (400–4000 u IU).
	
	Pre-coma symptoms (only in severe cases): Irritability, ascites, tremors of extremities, difficulty writing or drawing simple designs, sweet and musty breath odor, hepatic encephalopathy. Serum bilirubin very elevated (20 mg/100 ml).
	
	Elevated serum ammonia (impaired liver function to convert ammonia to urea).
	
	Decreased serum albumin (3.5 gm/100 ml) because liver inadequately metabolizes amino acids into protein; this increases risk of decubitus ulcers.
		1. Continue actions listed above until symptoms are resolved.
		2. Strict isolation measures. *THIS IS ESSENTIAL DURING ALL THREE PHASES UNTIL LAB TESTS REVEAL RESOLUTION OF INFECTION.*
		   a. Infected teen not allowed to handle or prepare family food.
		   b. Separate laundering of linens and clothing; dried in clothes drier or sunlight.
		   c. Separate eating utensils; disposable or washed separately in high temperature dishwasher cycle.
		   d. Avoid sexual activity, kissing or other oral contact until jaundice resolved.
		   e. Teen's toothbrush, razor, tissues kept separate from rest of family's articles.
		   f. Use of separate bathroom if possible; if not, good handwashing after elimination and washing of toilet seat after use with Lysol or similar antiseptic.
		   g. Teen's secretions should not be handled without wearing gloves.
		3. Monitor mental and neurological status at least every 8 hours in severe cases.
		4. Measure abdominal girth daily in severe cases.
		5. Careful skin care, avoidance of pressure areas, and measures to maintain adequate peripheral circulation in severe cases.
		6. Low-protein diet if pre-coma symptoms occur; low-sodium diet if ascites occurs.
		7. Corticosteroid therapy to enhance excretion of ammonia in stools.

Recovery phase (4 wks to 1 yr)	All symptoms subside except fatigability which persists; gradual slow recovery of normal activity levels.
	
	Intermittent SGOT elevations.
	
	Type B:[18]
	20% incidence of relapse.
	Occasionally carrier state develops (no antibodies were formed due to immunological incompetence) or chronic hepatitis with or without cirrhosis (antibody response inadequate to clear the infection).
	
	Rarely fulminant hepatitis with progressive liver failure that is usually fatal (excessive e antigen antibodies creating an anaphylactic response) develops.
		1. Measures to decrease teen's sense of isolation, frustration, depression:
		   a. Someone regularly available to solicit and listen to teen's feelings.
		   b. Keep phone accessible to permit contact with peers.
		   c. Teach teen reasons for restrictions on activities and complications to be avoided by his cooperation.
		   d. Arrange for homebound teacher so teen does not fall behind.
		   e. Provide opportunities for teen to have peers in home for quiet interaction until he can resume school and social activities.
		2. Monitor how teen is tolerating increases in school and social activities since he may ignore his body's response to the activity.
		   a. Help teen schedule rest periods, longer hours of sleep at night as needed.
		   b. Involve school personnel in scheduling times for teen to relax during school day.

*Best screening test for hepatitis.

TABLE 60-8 A PARTIAL LIST OF DRUGS TO AVOID IN HEPATITIS

acetaminophen (Tylenol)
chlorambucil (Leukeran)
chlordiazepoxide (Librium)
chlorothiazide (Diuril)
chlorpromazine (Thorazine)
chlorpropamide (Diabinese)
diazepam (Valium)
diphenylhydantoin (Dilantin)
estrogens
ferrous sulfate
imipramine (Tofranil)
indomethacin (Indocin)
isoniazid
meprobamate (Equanil)
methotrexate
methyldopa (Aldomet)
nicotinic acid
oral contraceptives
penicillin
phenobarbital
probenecid (Benemid)
prochlorperazine (Compazine)
propoxyphene (Darvon)
sulfonamides
tetracyclines
tolbutamide (Orinase)
trimethobenzamide (Tigan)

Diagnosis is made on the basis of a history that supports either direct contact with infected secretions or blood or indirect contact with infected fomites (shared cigarettes or eating utensils; a contaminated needle or razor in contact with broken skin; ingestion of contaminated food, and so on) as well as physical examination and laboratory findings that typify the usual clinical picture (Table 60–7). Microscopic blood evaluation (HAA study) is required to differentiate hepatitis A from hepatitis B virus. More sophisticated and expensive serologic testing (HAV test) is required if it is important to differentiate hepatitis A or C virus. (C type is present if HAA study for B antigen is negative and the HAV test for A antigen is also negative.) Determination of the amount of e antigen present in type B hepatitis may be significant prognostically. It is believed that this may be a host antigen that is directly associated with progressive liver damage after acute hepatitis B infection that progresses to chronic active or fulminant hepatitis.

Clinical Manifestations and Their Management Hepatitis B usually has an insidious onset of symptoms, with pyrexia and dermatological symptoms predominating. Hepatitis A usually has a sudden onset with gastrointestinal symptoms predominant. The symptoms are the same for any of the types (Table 60–8) but type A usually progresses from the prodromal to icteric phase in 5 to 7 days as opposed to the 2-week prodromal course in types B and C. Likewise the recovery phase is much shorter in type A, lasting an average of 4 weeks as opposed to the 6- to 12-month recovery phase in the other types. A mild case of any of the types may result in an anicteric (no jaundice) second phase. Type A hepatitis generally presents a less severe clinical picture than types B or C, and the patient is less likely to develop complications.

The typical symptoms of viral hepatitis and the reasonable management of those symptoms are described in Table 60–7. Whether hepatitis is treated at home or in the hospital depends on the severity of the disease and the amount of liver damage and whether the family is able to maintain strict isolation measures in the home environment.

Venereal Diseases and Vaginitis

The VD epidemic, primarily among teens and young adults (peak ages 15 to 24 years), has made venereal disease the number one communicable disease in our nation. Despite the discovery of penicillin to treat gonorrhea and syphilis and widespread education efforts, these two diseases and genital herpes simplex persist and increase yearly. The nurse plays a vital role in preventive education regarding venereal diseases as well as in casefinding and encouraging prompt treatment. Table 60–9 summarizes the features of these three diseases as well as the treatment currently recommended for them.

Vaginitis Trichomoniasis and candidiasis are probably the most widespread sexually transmitted diseases in the United States today and frequently appear together as vaginal infections.[12] Trichomoniasis ("trich," "TV") is a protozoan harbored asymptomatically, it is believed, in the vaginal tract in one of every five women.[14] Although men may be carriers, they are seldom symptomatic. The disease is transmitted by contact with infected perianal discharges during sexual intercourse or to an infant by passage during birth. This chronic perineal disease characteristically shows as a vaginitis producing a thin, foamy, yellowish discharge with foul odor. If the discharge is excessive, vulvar irritation is typical, with itching, burning and chafing that may extend to the anal and thigh regions. Diagnosis is made by microscopic examination of the discharge. Oral Flagyl is about 95 per cent effective in curing this disease. Use of a condom for intercourse can help prevent both spread of or reinfection by this protozoan.

Candidiasis is caused by a yeast-like fungus (Candida albicans). A normal vaginal inhabitant of 40% of women, the fungus is usually kept in check by normal vaginal flora, with flare-ups likely to occur during pregnancy, hormone therapy (use of birth control pills), antibiotic therapy or other physical or emotional stress factors that cause alteration in the pH and flora levels of the vagina. The infection may also be introduced by fecal contamination of the vagina or during intercourse with a person harboring the fungus. Candida causes intense, intolerable vulvar and vaginal itching and the abundant production of a watery discharge of a thick, white, cheesy substance. The profuse discharge may cause the pruritus to extend to the rectum and thighs and, if scratching occurs, secondary bacterial infection is likely. Diagnosis is made from either culture or microscopic examination of the vaginal discharge and treated with antifungal vaginal or oral medication. Use of a condom helps prevent both spread and reinfection.

The nurse plays a major role in helping young people understand that venereal disease and vaginitis are not the result of poor hygiene, nor a cause for shame. Teenage girls need to be taught that only two types of vaginal discharge — menstrual flow and a clear vaginal secretion at the time of sexual excitement — are normal, and that venereal diseases can be transmitted to a fetus during pregnancy or birth.

Both prevention and prompt treatment of any genitourinary symptoms are the individual's responsibility to his or her own body. Several preventive measures can be taken by the teenager who chooses to become sexually active, including (1) using a condom to reduce the likelihood of genitourinary disease and pregnancy, (2) washing the perianal region well with soap and water after sexual contact, (3) urinating after intercourse (more effective for males), and (4) being selective in sexual behavior, by avoiding contact with persons known to be infected.[14]

Although these are simple preventive measures, they are often unrealistic in terms of adolescent sexual activity. A teen's sexual activity is often sporadic, casual or unplanned — a consequence of sexual curiosity and experimentation. Thus the teen is unlikely to begin the sexual contact prepared with a condom or with thoughts about the possibility of the partner being infected. Nor are restroom facilities likely to be readily available for prompt use after sexual activity.

Nurses working with teen populations should make sure that literature about these diseases is readily available to teens and that information about recommendable clinics for the diagnosis and treatment of these communicable diseases is visibly posted (hours, locations, fees, client conditions). Most states now permit physicians to treat minors for venereal disease without parental consent.

Nurses involved in educating teens about sexuality or the sexual diseases must evaluate their own sexual attitudes. The nurse's personal sexual attitudes do not matter to the teen whom she is teaching or counselling, but her ability to be comfortable with the teen and to discuss the issues in an environment in which both nurse and teen respect each other as individuals with responsibility for their own decisions and behaviors is imperative to gaining the teen's attention and cooperation.[4] "Rap" sessions in which a group of teens and young adult leaders (nurses, for example) discuss feelings and facts about a problem and devise practical solutions have become a popular mode for educating teens about venereal disease.

A nonjudgmental approach and the assurance of confidentiality are the minimal essentials to whichever method is used to teach or counsel adolescents in sexual matters. The counselling role of the school nurse-teacher is especially worthy of attention because of the tendency of youth to trust and consult a school nurse rather than other adults in their environment. The school nurse can also be politically influential in helping identify inadequate health services for teens in the community and in arousing public support for provision of readily available and adequate health care.

ADOLESCENT OBESITY

Obesity as an adolescent health problem appears to be increasing. Adolescent obesity is almost always the result of a caloric intake that

TABLE 60-9 CHARACTERISTICS OF THE VENEREAL DISEASES[5, 7, 14, 17, 21]

Venereal Disease (Pathogen)	Transmission	Incubation	Symptoms	Diagnostic Tests	Treatment
Gonorrhea (*Neisseria gono*)	Direct contact, usually sexual; fomite contact up to 24 hrs after fomite contaminated.[21]	2–14 days (average 3–5)	*Early signs:* Copious mucopurulent discharge from phagocytosis, vaginal in female and urethral in male. Pharyngeal if oral sex. Pain and frequency of urination from urethritis. 90% of females and 10% of males are asymptomatic. *Other possible signs:* Cervicitis, salpingitis, peritonitis, PID, and abscesses of Skene's or Bartholin glands in females. Epididymitis and abscess of prostate glands in males. *Late signs:* Arthritis, endocarditis, sterility.	Culture of discharge for gonococcal growth (GC smear) positive. Visualization of discharge in infection on physical exam.	Simultaneous treatment of infected individual and all identified sexual partners with oral (probenecid) or intramuscular (procaine penicillin G, Trobicin) penicillin. The National Institute of Health is currently developing a gonorrheal vaccine. No permanent immunity.
Syphilis (*Treponema pallidum*)	Direct contact, usually sexual, during infective stage. Transfusion.	Primary stage 10–90 days (average 3 wks)	*Primary—infectious:* Chancre (painless, indurated ulcer) that heals spontaneously in 2–3 weeks. Located at site where pathogen entered.	Reactive STS (presence of spirochete in blood produces reaction to certain animal antigens); VDRL most common test. STS negative at this stage. Visualization of chancre on physical exam.	Primary/Secondary stages: 2,400,000 u benzathine pen G IM or 4,800,000 u procaine
		6–24 wks	*Secondary—very infectious:* Skin and mucous membrane rash, lymphadenitis, fever, headaches, sore throat that disappears spontaneously. Lasts few months to several years.	STS reactive; becomes nonreactive if treated now.	Pen G (half of dose in each buttock) followed by 1,200,000 u of either type pen G at 3 days and 6 days after initial dose.

1294 FAMILIES WITH ADOLESCENTS

	2–4 yrs	*Early latent* – may be infectious: No physical symptoms.	STS reactive	*Latent stages:* 3,000,000 u pen G given IM (half of dose in each buttock to be repeated at 7 and 14 days after 1st dose.)
	After 4 yrs	*Late latent* – blood infectious: No symptoms	STS reactive	VDRL repeated each month for 3 months after treatment completed to establish cure; damage done to body before treatment is not reversible.
		Late active: Gummas in skin, bones, liver, stomach. CNS involvement • 10% optic atrophy, deafness • General paresis Cardiovascular involvement in 80% cases • Aortic insufficiency or aneurysm • Endarteritis Insanity		No immunity is developed.
Genital herpes simplex (*Herpesvirus hominis* [HSV-2])	Direct contact, usually sexual.	3–7 days	*Symptomatic phase:* contagious. Minor itching or extensive rash of genital region followed by a cluster of blister-like lesions that then rupture and ulcerate; these are pruritic and painful, especially during intercourse. Painful urination, inguinal lymphadenitis and pain, fever, malaise. Symptoms disappear spontaneously after 2–6 wks. Many cases asymptomatic. *Dormant phase:* symptoms absent but reappear with emotional or physical stress during which person again is infectious; once a person is infected, virus is harbored for life, though recurrences are less severe and last about 2 wks. Cervical cancer 8 times more likely in women with HSV-2 virus.	Viral culture of lesions. Scraping and staining of ulcer tissue with Papanicolaou solution demonstrates characteristic giant cells and viral inclusion bodies. Antibody blood titer of HVH-2 21 or more days after infection.	Incurable. Treatment aimed at pain relief, fostering healing of lesions and preventing other infections. • Pain medication • Use of condom during intercourse to prevent spread of HVH-2 or infection with other pathogens. • Local application of red dye (0.1% proflavine) followed by light exposure repeated in 18 hrs. This shortens course of lesions but is controversial because of increased risk of tumor formation. Antiviral agents are being developed that may be effective against HSV-2. Cesarean section in all pregnancies if active sores exist at time of birth.

substantially exceeds the adolescent's energy needs and caloric expenditure. Usually the obesity has existed before adolescence, often since infancy. Obese adolescents are typically physically inactive; they show advanced skeletal and sexual maturation, are tall for their age, and the females experience early menarche. Emotionally this adolescent has low self-esteem, feels rejected and depressed and is socially isolated. All of these factors foster the boredom and inactivitiy that whet the appetite to eat for self-gratification and something to do. Thus a self-perpetuating cycle of eating and rejection develops. Often several family members are caught up in this cycle, indicating the need for family counselling to effectively end the cycle for the obese teen.

Weight reduction programs appeal to the obese child as he or she reaches puberty because of social pressures for peer acceptance, especially by the opposite sex. The teen is likely to try many remedies for obesity tantalizingly advertised by financially motivated persons. The problem with these remedies, besides the fact that they may jeopardize the teen's general health, is that they do not change basic eating behavior or the factors motivating that behavior. Therefore, the remedies produce a weight loss that is short-term at best and serves only to undermine the teen's fragile self-esteem and promote depression.

Motivated by the sad statistic that 80 to 85 per cent of fat teenagers remain obese into adulthood, UCLA researchers developed a program, called the Adolescent Weight Reduction Program, with a multidisciplinary approach that during its first years has had at least a 70 per cent success rate in producing substantial long-term weight loss in teens.[15] This author believes that a program such as UCLA's could readily be initiated by nurses working with obese teens (especially school nurses, who have a "captive audience" available to them). The program has three goals: (1) weight loss in teens who are 20 per cent or more over ideal weight, (2) development of sound eating and exercise habits that will be maintained into adulthood and (3) promotion of healthy psychological adjustment. Each teen entering the program goes through a physical and psychological assessment to determine the extent of obesity (anthropometry), current physical endurance or stamina (treadmill test, vital signs), current activity level (24-hour physical activity recall for a school day and weekend day), medical history (birthweight, age at onset of obesity, any chronic disease, previous weight loss efforts and outcome), family obesity or obesity-related disease, and motivation for weight loss. (This motivation is evaluated by tests of self-concept, peer adjustment, personality, and school performance and a personal interview with the teen to learn reasons for coming for help and who initiated the referral.) A 24-hour recall diet history and information about family eating patterns are also obtained to determine daily caloric intake, adequacy of nutrients and family patterns that reinforce overeating. Laboratory tests are minimal — CBC, urinalysis, VDRL and PPD skin test — to get a general picture of the teen's health status. A glucose tolerance test is included if a family history of diabetes exists, and fasting triglyceride levels are tested if cardiovascular disease exists in the family. Questionnaires filled out by the school counselor and gym teacher can be used to compare with the teen's evaluation of his school and peer adjustment and physical activity level.

Interventions in the program include a return to physical education class if the teen has not been participating, psychiatric referral if severe psychological disturbance is suggested by assessment findings, and initiation of a dietary and activity program. An initial diet of 850 calories per day is prescribed and explained by a dietitian. The diet involves an exchange system; it includes a variety of foods and can be modified to the individual teen's food likes and dislikes. A list of foods that can be eaten at will and recipes, general dieting hints and ethnic menus are also provided. The caloric intake is extended to 1000 calories per day after an initial successful loss period of at least a month.

An individual activity program is developed with the teen's participation; activities are chosen in which the teen has some interest and is most likely to participate. The school nurse may also organize group exercise sessions to help teens maintain their activity program and provide reinforcement, at least initially, until the teen incorporates exercise into his or her life style.

The teens meet weekly to have their weight checked. (At this time the dietitian answers questions, provides extra diet education and offers psychological reinforcement.) This session is followed by a coed rap session led by a psychologist. For this session the group divides according to age: those under 14 meet together, as do those over 14. Behavior modification measures can then be introduced and feelings and problems the teens are facing can be discussed. At monthly intervals the nurse reviews the individual teen's progress with him, checks skinfold measurement and blood pressure, assesses for any problems and offers encouragement.

This successful program approach is presented here as a guide from which nurses can develop their own programs to help teens conquer obesity before adulthood and find a more gratifying way of life.

References

1. J. Alter et al. Transmissible agent in non-A, non-B hepatitis. Lancet, February 1978, p. 716
2. B. Anderson. Carole, a girl treated with bracing. American Journal of Nursing, September 1979, p. 1592
3. K. Baranowski et al. Viral hepatitis. Nursing 76, May 1976, p. 31
4. M. Brown. Adolescents and VD. Nursing Outlook, February 1973, p. 99
5. R. Caplan and W. Sweeney. Advances in Obstetrics and Gynecology. Williams & Wilkins Co., 1978
6. H. Cowell et al. Genetic aspects of idiopathic scoliosis. Clinical Orthopedics, November 1972, p. 121
7. S. Golub. VD, the unconquered menace. RN, March 1970, p. 38
8. P. Hill and L. Romm. Screening for scoliosis in adolescents. American Journal of Maternal-Child Nursing, May/June 1977, p. 156
9. C. Holt de Soledo. The defect: classification and detection. American Journal of Nursing, September 1979, p. 1588
10. H. Keim. Back deformities. Pediatric Clinics of North America, November 1977, p. 871
11. H. Keim. The Adolescent Spine. Grune and Stratton, 1976
12. L. Lanson. From Woman to Woman, 2nd ed. Alfred A. Knopf, 1977
13. G. MacEven. A look at the diagnosis and management of scoliosis. Orthopedic Review, June 1974, p. 9
14. W. McNab. The "other" venereal diseases: herpes simplex, trichomoniasis and candidiasis. Journal of School Health, February 1979, p. 79
15. E. Meyer and C. Neumann. Management of the obese adolescent. Pediatric Clinics of North America, February 1977, p. 123
16. L. Micheli, et al. Surgical Management and Nursing Care of Scoliosis. American Journal of Nursing, September 1979, p. 1599
17. M. Nelson et al. New Therapy for Acute Gonorrhea: Spectinomycin IM. U.S. Public Health Service, 1974
18. A. Persich. Hepatitis B antigen: advancement in knowledge quickens (a review). American Journal of Medical Technology, June 1977, p. 568
19. A. Peterson. Acute viral hepatitis. Nurse Practitioner, Jul/Aug 1979, p. 9
20. D. Seto. Viral hepatitis. Pediatric Clinics of North America, May 1979, p. 305
21. N. Welch. Recent insights into the childhood "social diseases" — gonorrhea, scabies, pediculosis, pinworms. Clinical Pediatrics, April 1978, p. 320

Additional Recommended Reading

B. Anderson and P. D'Ambra. The adolescent patient with scoliosis: a nursing care standard. Nursing Clinics of North America, December 1976, p. 699

M. Barrett. Surviving adolescence in a back brace: Laura's experience. American Journal of Maternal Child Nursing, May/June 1977, p. 160

A. Berenson, ed. Control of Communicable Diseases in Man. American Public Health Association, 1975

D. Cantrell. Scoliosis: screening potential victims. RN, November 1976, p. 55

D. Craddock. Obesity and Its Management. Churchill-Livingstone, 1978

D. Dane et al. Virus-like particles in serum of patients with Australia-antigen associated hepatitis. Lancet, January 1970, p. 695

B. Davis and R. Stuart. Slim Chance in a Fat World: Behavioral Control of Obesity. Research Press, 1974

J. Hughes. Synopsis of Pediatrics. C. V. Mosby Co., 1979

A. Lore. Adolescents: people, not problems. American Journal of Nursing, July 1973, p. 1232

D. McElroy. Nursing care of patients with viral hepatitis. Nursing Clinics of North America, June 1977, p. 306

S. Love-Mignogna. Scoliosis. Nursing 77, May 1977, p. 50

H. Mitchell et al. Nutrition in Health and Disease. J. B. Lippincott Co., 1976

A. Nemir. The School Health Program. W. B. Saunders Co., 1975

C. Neumann, Obesity in pediatric practice. Pediatric Clinics of North America, February 1977, p. 117

N. Raynolds, Teaching parents home care after surgery for scoliosis. American Journal of Nursing, June 1974, p. 1090

E. Riseborough and J. Herndon. Scoliosis and Other Deformities of the Axial Skeleton. Little, Brown & Co., 1975

C. Sells and E. May. Scoliosis screening in public schools. American Journal of Nursing, January 1974, p. 60

B. Stone et al. The effect of an exercise program on change in curve in adolescents with minimal idiopathic scoliosis. Physical Therapy, June 1979, p. 759

Vaccines against gonorrhea. U.S. News and World Report, 10 September, 1979, p. 64

61 POTENTIAL STRESSES DURING ADOLESCENCE: IRREVERSIBLE ALTERATIONS IN HEALTH STATUS

by Kathleen Underman Boggs, RN, MSN

IMPACT OF IRREVERSIBLE ALTERATIONS ON THE ADOLESCENT

Irreversible illness is disruptive to all the developmental tasks with which the adolescent is struggling. The illness makes him at least periodically or in some facets of living continually dependent when achieving independence is critical. He is faced with a drastic blow to his self-image, just at the time when he is trying to stabilize his identity. He is forced to consider the limitations that this lifelong illness place on his vocational, educational and sexual opportunities just at a time when he had thought all the options in the world were his just for the choosing. He stands out as different from his peers during a developmental stage in which his conformity and likeness to "the crowd" is crucial to his emotional separation from his family. If the adolescent with irreversible illness is not given assistance to help him develop an attitude that he is "special but capable," his development into an adult is severely hampered.

Signs that the adolescent is not adjusting usually fall within one or more of three categories of behavior: (1) depression, (2) overdependency or (3) nonadherence to the treatment plan. His depression is the adolescent's reaction to the decreases in body function and his loss of freedom and independence. In his depression he may either blame himself (*introjection*) or his parents (*projection*) for the illness. Overdependency arises out of becoming too comfortable with the extra attention received and lessened demands placed on him due to the illness. This overdependency is often reflected through regressive behavior. (He will not do things he is capable of doing.) Nonadherence to the treatment plan is a manifestation of denial in some teens and an expression of independence in others. Obviously the consequences of any of the maladaptive behavior patterns can be severe.

The continuation of the teen's healthy personality development in the face of irreversible illness is critically influenced by his parents' acceptance of the illness and by the reactions of others significant to him. The youth needs frequent reassurances from parents, peers, teachers and the health team that he is doing a good job managing his illness. He should be treated as an adult as much as possible and given increasing responsibility for his own care as he accepts and adapts to his illness. A major emphasis of nursing is patient education. The teenager needs accurate, detailed information about his illness — what causes it, what to expect from it, what it means in terms of his educational or vocational interests, how it will affect his appearance and sexual function, how independent it will permit him to be. The "can do's" rather than the restrictions should be emphasized. Involvement in the teaching of the sick youth by another adolescent with a similar illness who is coping well gives the youth a model and peer support.

The youth's independence should be preserved as much as possible. Parents may tend to encourage dependency as part of "caring for" their sick son or daugher. They may assume more of the adolescent's physical care than is necessary or impose limits beyond those that the treatment regimen requires. The adolescent himself may fear any movement toward independence, thinking that he may be unable to survive by himself. Allowing him to make many decisions pertaining to the when's and how's of his care gives the teen a sense of control. Preparing him with the skills for self-care greatly increases his physical freedom from others. He should be provided with opportunities for living away from home for short periods once his initial adjustment to the illness has occurred. Many church or youth camps make accommodation for chronically ill youth, and there are also camps for teens who have particular irreversible conditions.

Problems may develop in the adolescent's attempts to initiate peer interactions, especially with members of the opposite sex. Chronically ill teens may have trouble gaining peer acceptance if their illness causes obvious deviations and thus threatens the normal adolescent's sense of physical adequacy. The establishment of a positive sense of self and an identity can also be affected. Since the adolescent is chronically ill, he must incorporate his illness into his identity. Factors associated with altered physical appearance, fatigue and resultant decreased academic achievement and limited participation in usual adolescent activities can contribute to diminished self-esteem. A sense of identity can also be adversely affected if the adolescent uses his illness as a means of manipulating parents, teachers and peers.

Nurses have successfully used groups to provide patient or family support. For example, adolescent support groups or informal teen activity groups have been established for hospitalized patients. Community support groups or advocacy groups have been founded in many communities and provide physical and psychological support as well as current information about treatment and research. For example, the Lupus Foundation is an extremely active, well-organized support group. Referrals can be made to other professionals or to community agencies when counselling is indicated for the patient or his family. The nurse can help the adolescent think of acceptable, appealing activities that will allow peer contact without exceeding limitations set by the physician. For example, if strenuous physical activity is limited, he may still be part of many team sports as a student manager. Within an institutional setting it is especially important to structure acceptable ways for an adolescent to express his aggressiveness, his independence and his sexuality.

During an acute exacerbation the youth may be so depleted that he desires only to be left alone. It is not uncommon for an ill adolescent to withdraw from others as a way of coping. Nurses need to differentiate therapeutic withdrawal from that caused by unhealthy coping. Self-defeating, maladaptive types of withdrawal may be prevented through structured activities and allowing the adolescent choices in controlling his daily care schedule within reasonable limits.

The teen should be encouraged to participate in clubs, activities and other social interaction with peers who have similar interests, not just with peers who have a similar disability. A regular school setting with modified activities is best for the youth's adjustment; however, his teachers need honest information about his disease and his capabilities. With this kind of exposure the teen learns to live openly with his handicap and to answer questions gracefully. He learns that he is special but capable.

DELAYED PUBERTY

Few problems cause greater potential distress to a youth than delayed puberty. As peers grow taller and develop sexually, the youth who retains his child-like appearance may experience anxiety, embarrassment or depression. Behavior changes that indicate his distress may range from nonparticipation in gym class to complete withdrawal from friends. The degree of concern expressed by parents about their child's delayed puberty varies with the degree of distress they perceive in their child and their own past experiences about the age and nature of expected physical changes.

Age is a general criterion upon which to base an investigation to determine causes for delayed puberty. A girl who reaches the age of 13½ years or the boy who passes his fourteenth birthday without displaying any sign of pubescence needs to be evaluated. The child's genetic heritage and previous growth rate need to be considered, as slower-growing children tend toward later sexual development. Developmental age, as determined by skeletal x-rays, may be a more accurate criterion on which to base investigation than chronological age. A complete medical history can be significant also, in that chronic illness tends to result in a delay in development of secondary sex characteristics in many children.

In rare cases delayed puberty is associated with some alteration in endocrine function or a chromosomal abnormality. Frohlich's syndrome is a condition characterized by a lack of genital development (*sexual infantilism*) and obesity. The youth retains a childish appearance. Other symptoms may include headaches, vomiting and loss of vision. The syndrome occurs as a result of a lesion in the area of the pituitary gland or endocrine hypofunction. Treatment involves irradiation or surgical removal of the tumor, substitution therapy for endocrine hypofunction and psychological counselling.

Turner syndrome (*gonadal dysgenesis*) is a chromosomal abnormality affecting one out of every three thousand girls. It is attributed to a lack of one of the X chromosomes (XO), resulting in a total of only 45 chromosomes in most girls with this condition instead of the normal 46. Secondary sex characteristics fail to develop and ovaries are abnormal, resulting in sterility and primary amenorrhea. Physical characteristics most commonly associated with a diagnosis of Turner syndrome include webbed, short, broad neck; low hairline at the back of the neck; high palate with small mandible; protruding, "lowset" ears; broad chest with widely spaced nipples; and short stature. These girls may have some difficulty in spatial orientation due to a deficiency in their perception; however, they usually have normal intelligence. Some of these children have associated renal or circulatory anomalies. A developmental history reveals normal growth throughout childhood with the absence of the typical growth spurts. The pubescent girl does not have breast or genital maturation. Treatment consists of administration of estrogen hormones at the time of puberty in order to promote a more feminine appearance. An increase in height may be accomplished by administering androgen hormones; however, virilization side effects can be disturbing to a girl already feeling different from her peers. No form of treatment currently yields fertility. These girls and their parents benefit immensely from supportive pyschological therapy.

ALTERED PSYCHOLOGICAL STATUS

As a young person moves from his family toward psychological and physical independence and attempts to establish a separate identity, he may stretch his coping mechanisms beyond their limits. In some individuals this leads to temporary maladaptive behaviors. In other instances such stressors trigger chronic alterations in the youth's mental health status such as profound depression or schizophrenia.

Schizophrenia

The term schizophrenia refers to psychotic behavior caused by a disintegration in mental functioning. A current definition would identify the schizophrenic as a person whose lack of integrated thought process is manifested by disturbed behavior, emotions and speech.

Many people working in the psychiatric field prefer to differentiate between adult schizophrenia and adolescent schizophrenic reaction. This differentiation is based on the premise that such a condition in an adolescent is limited to a few years and has an excellent prognosis for total recovery. Whatever its title, this behavior disturbance is relatively common in adolescents. One survey of youth found a 7 per cent incidence of schizophrenic reactions.[2]

Etiology No one factor has been identified as the cause of schizophrenia. Some theories suggest a biological-genetic-biochemical etiology.

This somatogenic viewpoint attributes schizophrenia to deficiencies in metabolic or neural functioning or to genetic factors, citing studies that report a significantly higher incidence of schizophrenia among family members, especially twins. Other theories support a psychodynamic-sociologic-developmental etiology, suggesting that disturbances in interpersonal relations are at the root of the illness. This psychogenic viewpoint supports disturbed family relationships as the causative factor. Parents, especially mothers, have been characterized as being emotionally cold to the child, keeping him at a distance or confusing him by conveying inconsistent messages and by failing to acknowledge the validity of his own feelings. Parents themselves may behave inappropriately for their age and sex, acting out their own conflicts in their relationship with the child. Most likely a multiplicity of factors can be implicated.

Clinical Manifestations Nurses and other members of the health care team may be unaware of the adolescent's need for help until he is confronted with a crisis situation and this becomes apparent. A number of factors may contribute to this lack of awareness. The youth himself may be unaware of anything but a growing sense of unhappiness. To an adolescent, asking for help is developmentally inconsistent with his inner drives for mastery and control. Until recently, seeking professional help has also carried some social stigma. Nurses and other health professionals need to incorporate assessment of mental health status as part of adolescent health screening, since youth are particularly prone to emotional disturbances.

Psychotic behavior in a youth may be obvious from early childhood, or it may be triggered by the developmental crisis of adolescence. Adolescent developmental tasks overwhelm a youth with a shaky ego and heighten his already existing fears, resulting in a loss of his sense of self. Feelings of ambivalence in his quest for independence, or hostility due to unmet dependency needs, are feared. These conflicting feelings and his poorly developed self-concept may lead to overt schizophrenic behavior characterized by delusions, hallucinations and inappropriate emotional reactions. As the level of anxiety increases, it becomes more and more difficult for the youth to distinguish between fantasy and reality. The earliest symptoms may be noted as behavioral changes or alterations in habits. For example, the neat child becomes sloppy or the casual child begins to rigidly adhere to routine. In the early stages of this illness, the youth may begin to exhibit overt signs of his struggle to maintain contact with reality by displaying rituals, phobias or obsessive-compulsive behaviors. For example, he may fear germs to the point of refusing to touch door knobs, using a tissue to open a door or washing his hands repeatedly. As his personality structure continues to disintegrate, the youth exhibits obvious schizophrenic symptoms of paranoid delusions or hallucinations. He regresses to infantile behaviors, is unable to control impulses and may have activity changes varying from apathy to aggression. Depersonalization and motor and speech disturbance become apparent.

Nursing Role in Establishing Diagnosis Diagnosis and intervention is based on an accurate data base. The nurse collects information from the parents about the history and progress of the illness. Observations of parent-youth interactions and the effectiveness of the youth's interactions with his environment are documented. Other needed information may include the extent to which the youth is able to differentiate his body from his environment; the extent of his impulsivity, regression or bizarre behavior; whether he engages in any self-mutilating or aggressive behavior; and whether he can distinguish between reality and fantasy.

Nursing Management During Schizophrenic Reaction Caring for a schizophrenic youth in a pediatric setting makes unusual demands on the nursing staff. The youth's bizarre behavior may disrupt a unit designed primarily to serve medical needs. The nurse who reacts emotionally to the disturbed youth's behavior cannot function therapeutically. For example, the nurse who gets angry and punishes the youth who hits her is responding nontherapeutically. Repeated episodes of disruptive, acting-out behavior can make members of the nursing staff feel they are losing control. Repeated attempts to help a schizophrenic youth may be rebuffed as he attempts to avoid any close interpersonal encounter. Such rejection of "helping" overtures can leave a nurse feeling helpless or inadequate. The nurse must recognize her own feelings about the disturbed youth and must recognize that the behavior is symptomatic of his illness. Group conferences with all health team members will help the nurse plan consistent, therapeutic interventions.

Treatment of adolescent schizophrenic reaction consists of controlled manipulation of the youth's external environment and alteration of his internal environment through the administration of behavior-altering drugs. The use of electroshock therapy has been discouraged by most therapists. Environment manipulation attempts to relieve some of the stress factors that have led to the youth's personality disintegration. This change may be accomplished by hospitalizing the youth on a general pediatric unit or in a residential treatment center specializing in psychiatric care. Another option is to treat the youth on an outpatient basis while working with his family to change the home environment. Emphasis is placed on helping family members recognize and change those patterns of interactions with the youth that have contributed to his illness. In either inpatient or outpatient community settings, the goal of nursing is to maintain contact with all family members and to facilitate their involvement in the overall treatment plan. The priority nursing goal is to provide an environment in which the child can safely attempt to reintegrate his personality.

In creating a therapeutic environment for the hospitalized schizophrenic youth, a major nursing task is the establishment of a stable, supportive relationship between the youth and the nurse. This relationship differs from the one he has with his therapist, which usually involves analytical attempts to explore the basis of existent fears and fantasies. The nurse's daily continuing contact with the youth allows her to design interventions that will help him substitute more useful and appropriate behaviors for those that are less than acceptable, bizarre and dysfunctional.

While regressive behavior may be tolerated at first, the nurse's goal is to foster the development of more responsible behaviors. In relating to the youth, the nurse attempts to increase his orientation to reality and to validate only his perceptions that are accurate. Realizing that some theorists believe bizarre behavior is utilized to avoid interpersonal contacts previously found to be painful and confusing, the nurse can plan interactions designed to gradually restore trust. Appropriate interactions are geared to reinforce only behaviors in which the youth is differentiating people and self from objects in the environment (maintaining eye contact, feeding or caring for himself, appropriately handling objects, relating to persons).[3] The nurse reinforces these appropriate behaviors by rewarding the youth. Initially reinforcements might consist of food or some valued object or privilege. Eventually the nurse tries to move toward social reinforcers such as a smile or motion indicating approval.[3] Nursing care might include assigning the same staff people to interact with a patient and limiting the number of other contacts. The youth might be encouraged to engage in familiar, safe hobbies, and his family can bring in some of his personal possessions to help alleviate some of his anxiety. Situations or stimuli that seem to increase the youth's anxiety level should be noted and eliminated as far as possible.

As the relationship between the youth and nurse develops, he may resist continued moves toward greater closeness. Eventually he may develop trust in the nurse, therapist and others in the hospital, and this trust will help him tolerate close relations with others. Initially it may be wise to avoid close physical contact. Touching the youth is open to misinterpretation or may even threaten him. The nurse should structure experiences that will allow the teen to repeat desired, rewardable behaviors. These types of nursing interventions can assist the youth to move toward adoption of more appropriate social behaviors.

If medications, especially tranquilizers and antidepressants, are prescribed, the nurse will have responsibilities in their administration. This may be more difficult with adolescents, who may view any drug as an attempt by adults to gain control over their behavior. Responsible nursing care includes making sure the youth has actually swallowed medication so that at a later time it will not be necessary to cope with an attempted suicide by means of hoarded drugs. Knowledge of the drugs and their associated side effects is essential. Some of the phenothiazine drugs have been reported to occasionally cause liver damage and lower blood counts. Minor irritating side effects can range from dry mouth to rashes, constipation, hypotension and changes in muscle tone or alertness.

Nursing observations of patient-parent interactions can provide insight into family dynamics. As the nurse works with family members in an attempt to get them involved in the treatment program, an important function is to give information. Visits to an inpatient facility allows opportunity to explain parts of the treatment program that may be misunderstood, such as behavior modification schedules used with the youth. Hospital or residential treatment may be combined with home visits for the weekend or brief holiday periods. In anticipation of these visits, the nurse supports the family, helping them to feel competent and comfortable with the treatment regimen, and teaches them about administering prescribed medications. Another aspect of nursing support to the family is assisting them to identify the youth's progress.

Specific nursing measures can facilitate adaptive behavior and defuse disruptive behaviors. In any treatment program it is important to avoid entering into a power struggle with a disturbed youth. Setting clearly understood limits serves to guide both the staff and the youth. The care plan should identify expectations and limits for behavior in order to provide consistent care. The success of any treatment program that sets limits on acting-out behaviors is dependent on the ability to enforce such limits. The disturbed youth is especially vulnerable to inconsistency and is frightened by feelings that things are out of control. This is true even when he seems to constantly be testing how far he can go. Various techniques for handling out-of-control behavior have been devised by treatment centers and include use of locked patient rooms, isolation rooms, or physical restraint of the youth with or without simultaneous discussion of the effects of his behavior. Rewards are offered to reinforce socially acceptable behaviors. Positive reinforcement concepts are widely used and accepted as therapeutic. Some proponents of behavior modification would include negative reinforcements (*aversive therapy*) in their treatment programs to help extinguish unacceptable behavior. Negative reinforcement ranges from isolating the youth for only a few minutes to administering an electroshock immediately following an unacceptable behavior. The latter is much more controversial, bordering as it does on punishment.

Depression

The exact incidence of depression in adolescence is unknown; however, it is a common health problem during the teenage years. Depression has also been identified in infants, manifested by poor growth and poor eating patterns. Occurrences of depression in school children have also been noted but are often masked as physical complaints such as headaches or behavioral problems such as enuresis.

Clinical Manifestations The nurse needs to differentiate between normal periods of depressed moods, which are brief and fade away, and profound depression, which persists and tends to get progressively worse. A youth with this latter type of depression behaves noticeably in an irritable, tense manner and gives indications of lowered self-esteem. In identifying depression, the nurse will note that depression in adolescents takes different forms. In some situations the depression will resemble adult depression. The youth may appear withdrawn; he may talk freely about feeling sad and lonely, rejected and depressed; or, overwhelmed by feelings of despair and hopelessness, he may express suicidal thoughts. However, more often teenagers mask signs of depression by a variety of behavioral or somatic changes. Their defense against depression may take the form of somatic complaints such as changes in eating patterns ranging from anorexia to overeating, digestive complaints such as constipation, changes in sleeping habits ranging from insomnia to persistent fatigue, or changes in productivity such as slow speech, slow thought processes or even school failure.

Behavioral changes may present in the form of destructive, disruptive, or aggressive acting-out behavior. The youth may become defiant, truant or delinquent or may repeatedly run away from home. In further attempts to deny depression, adolescents may resort to drugs, alcohol or sexual promisicuity.

Since transient, recurrent episodes of depression commonly occur throughout the adolescent years, it is important to differentiate between "normal" developmental depression and chronic depression, which persists and interferes with mastery of adolescent developmental tasks. The degree and duration of any depression should be assessed. In obtaining a history the nurse may frequently find that there has been some significant change in a close relationship. Perhaps within the family there has been a shift in relationships or a death. Sometimes there is a history of the breakup of a relationship with a girl or boy friend, an abortion, or a diagnosis of illness. These forms of loss provoke grief, anger and depression that, in the maladapted youth, lingers.

Nursing Management

Once the existence and severity of the depression is recognized, the nurse's role involves seeking appropriate referrals so that a therapeutic treatment plan can be established. The plan is ideally designed in consultation with a therapist, psychologist, psychiatrist and psychiatric nurse. A relationship should be established with the depressed adolescent in which the nurse is seen as a caring professional. Early intervention might include acknowledging how "down" the youth seems and helping him express his concerns.

The nurse also needs to recognize the adolescent's nonverbal communications or acting-out behaviors as expressions of his depression. Attempts should be made to validate these observations with him, helping him to understand that this is his way of signaling distress. As a prerequisite to any therapeutic interaction, the nurse must develop an awareness of her personal feelings and reactions to the adolescent's behavior. Another necessity is appropriate limit setting and protection of the youth from himself and of the larger community from his destructive acting-out behavior.

The family of the adolescent may need support and assistance during this time of stress. It is important to maintain contact with the family through open, honest communication. Many of the behaviors displayed in this adolescent may stem from long-existing maladaptive coping mechanisms, developed in response to family situations. The nurse needs to assess the family's expectations and demands. Family members need to become involved in the treatment plan. They need guidance in identifying causative factors within family relationships that contribute to the teenager's depression. Identification of serious family problems necessitates a referral to a family therapy program.

In every phase of nursing there are opportunities for nurses to use their anticipatory guidance skills. Sharing information about growth and development norms and age-related developmental behaviors can be of great assistance to parents. Nursing interventions that enhance parenting skills will help develop healthy parent-child relationships. Open communication maintained between parent and youth contributes substantially to the youth's mental health. Promoting trust and communication and eliminating friction between parents and children are major responsibilities of the nurse.

SYSTEMIC LUPUS ERYTHEMATOSUS

Systemic or disseminated lupus erythematosus is a long-term inflammatory disease of connective tissue, one of a group of several collagen diseases. Collagen diseases such as arthritis and lupus are referred to as autoimmune diseases. Until recently lupus was thought to be a rather rare disease of young women who became acutely ill, developed heart and kidney abnormalities, and often died. The medical community is gradually recognizing that lupus is more common and is, in fact, the second most common collagen vascular disease, led only by rheumatoid arthritis. The apparent rise in lupus occurrence may be attributed to one or all of three factors: increased awareness of the disease process, better diagnostic criteria or an actual increase in incidence. Symptoms of lupus may be vague or transitory and tend to mimic a number of other diseases. Lupus occurs seven times more often in females and is more prevalent in nonwhites. The initial diagnosis is most often made during the adolescent or young adult years.

The exact cause of lupus is obscure. It can affect any organ system or combination of organs, producing long-term disability. Typically periods of remission alternate with periods of exacerbation, called *flares*. Researchers are exploring suspected etiological factors such as altered immune reactivity, genetic predisposition and environmental trigger factors such as viruses. Many cases of lupus are known to have been precipitated by specific factors such as severe sunburn, infection or other major stress. In rarer instances, lupus-like symptoms have been noted after use of certain drugs such as penicillin and phenytoin.

Clinical Manifestations

Lupus typically presents with a skin rash; this may be a butterfly-shaped rash (Fig. 61–1) cov-

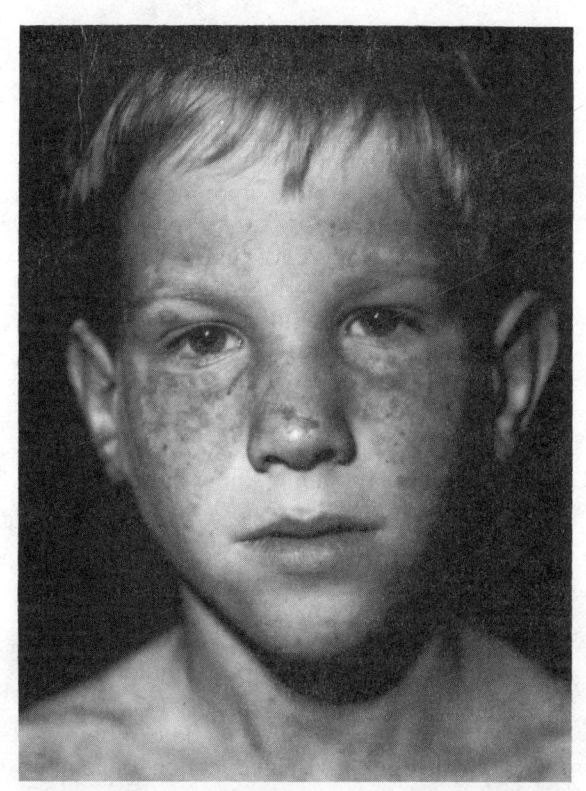

Figure 61-1 Discoid lupus erythematosus with typical butterfly distribution, atrophy and depigmentation of skin. (Courtesy of Dr. L. Schweich. From W. Kelley et al. Textbook of Rheumatology. W. B. Saunders Co., 1981.)

ering the cheeks and nose, but it can also occur in peripheral areas. It is a macular-papular type of rash and is a major symptom found in approximately 50 to 80 per cent of cases. Another frequently occurring symptom is joint inflammation and its associated pain. More than 90 per cent of all lupus patients develop arthritis-like symptoms sometime during the course of their illness. Other symptoms of lupus include low-grade fever, weight loss, fatigue, muscular weakness, anorexia, sore throat and inflammation of various organ systems. Inflammation and pain in the chest area associated with pericarditis, myocarditis or pleurisy may also be present. Lymph glands may enlarge, especially in the cervical area. Vascular changes can produce areas of ulceration or can lead to central nervous system involvement in the form of seizures, paresis or even alterations in personality. Renal involvement occurs in a significant number of persons and is one of the most serious manifestations of this disease.

Diagnosis

The period before diagnosis may be lengthy and usually involves a number of expensive visits to doctors and hospitals. Lupus symptoms are difficult to differentiate from those of other conditions. Lupus is usually diagnosed only after months of varying physical and mental complaints. Many persons who are eventually diagnosed as having lupus recall being repeatedly told that nothing was wrong, or recall being made to feel that their complaints were psychological. The months spent awaiting a diagnosis can be extremely stressful for the youth and family. Frustrating initial experiences with health professionals may create ambivalent or angry feelings in individuals who ultimately need to establish a trusting relationship with physicians and nurses. Eventually, the history and the symptoms reported by the patient, together with the laboratory data, lead to the diagnosis.

Laboratory tests done to examine components of blood or serum can detect certain abnormalities, but positive findings may not be present at all or only intermittently. Some of these findings are characteristic of a number of other diseases. For example, antinuclear antibodies (ANAs) may be found, but these are also present in juvenile rheumatoid arthritis. A positive test for ANAs indicates that the person's antibodies are reacting against his own body cells and their basic component DNA. Almost all children with lupus have positive ANA tests. A decreased serum level of complement, a serum protein, occurs in lupus. A complete blood count might show abnormally low levels of red and white cells and platelets. During an exacerbation or active phase of lupus, a special type of leukocyte may be seen in laboratory examination of blood or tissue fluid. The presence of this cell, known as the *LE cell,* is characteristic but not absolutely diagnostic for systemic lupus.

There is a skin test available that some physicians believe can help document the diagnosis of lupus, the *lupus band test.* A very small biopsy of skin is obtained from a nonrash area and stained for microscopic examination. In individuals with systemic lupus, deposits of antibodies can be visualized under the epidermis, giving the appearance of a straight line or band. The nurse should offer a simple, accurate explanation as to the purpose, techniques and minimal discomfort associated with these tests. The final diagnosis currently is based on the presence of any four of the 14 lupus symptoms designated by the American Rheumatology Association as criteria for the diagnosis of systemic lupus erythematosus. These criteria are: (1) facial erythema, (2) discoid lupus (nonsystemic lupus manifested in the form of skin eruptions), (3) Raynaud-like symptoms such as peripheral pallor and cyanosis, (4) alopecia, (5) photosensitivity, (6) oral or nasopharyngeal ulcers, (7) arthritis without any deformity, (8) presence of LE cells, (9) false-positive serology test for syphilis, (10) proteinuria, (11) cellular casts in the urine, (12) pleuritis or pericarditis, (13) psychosis or convulsions and (14) altered blood counts indicating decreased numbers of white and red blood cells and platelets.[4]

Nursing support of both the youth and the family is essential during the stressful time while diagnostic tests are being performed. Anger because of a delayed diagnosis is a fairly common reaction and may be a sign of anxiety. Recognizing this may help the professional deal with the situation by responding to the underlying cause rather than to the anger itself. It is important to recognize that many young women with lupus express their anger in the form of depression. Nursing support to the family may consist of agreeing with them (validating) that waiting is difficult and then reinforcing their persistence to seek a cause for the child's complaints.

When the diagnosis is definitely established, the nurse will need to give information about the nature and expected course of lupus. This is especially important, since lupus is not a well-publicized disease. Since much of the older literature describes the serious and fatal effects of lupus, outdated information from libraries or friends can be frightening. The informed nurse can provide current, more encouraging information about the treatment of lupus.

Management

Current treatment of lupus in its early stages emphasizes good nutrition and frequent rest periods. Analgesics may be prescribed. As the disease develops there is continued emphasis on adequate nutrition and rest. Patients are advised to reduce the amount of stress inherent to their life, a difficult challenge during adolescence. Moderate doses of corticosteroids may be prescribed to control flares. Larger doses of steroids may be needed if the disease becomes more active, particularly if kidney function is affected (lupus nephritis). If lupus nephritis does not respond to steroids, immunosuppressive drugs may be prescribed.

Since there is no cure for lupus, nursing care focuses on long-term management. Many youth with lupus need continuing encouragment to focus on the gains that will ultimately occur if they follow what may appear to be a restrictive treatment regimen. In formulating a nursing care plan, it is important to determine not only what the youth and family know but also what they want to know. In one survey of lupus patients, three prime areas of concern were identified: (1) a need for information about lupus, (2) problems with acceptance and (3) concerns about employment and acceptance by peers.[7] Information about lupus symptoms, side effects of medication, activity limitations, and techniques for dealing with fatigue can be provided by the nurse. The education of family members and friends is an important area of nursing involvement.

Since lupus is characterized by periods of remission, there will be times when the youth feels quite well and wishes to resume former activities. However, caution must be taken to prevent overexertion during intervals of remission. Overactivity may occur as an effort to deny the diagnosis. Such overexertion can lead to a worsening of symptoms. Neglecting precautions against exposure to sun or infection, as well as physical or psychological stress, can cause exacerbation.

Nurses need to promote the teen's intellectual and physical adaptation. The most important nursing role is usually not the giving of actual physical care but rather providing the necessary education of the youth and his family, including teaching him to manage his own care. Providing information about the nature of lupus may help promote an acceptance of the need for lifelong management. Knowledge about the potential destructive effects of lupus on the body, especially the kidneys, may reinforce the importance of taking prescribed medicine.

If steroids are used, the nurse informs patients about the greater risk of infection and the expected side effects. Initially, several doses of corticosteroids per day may be required to suppress the inflammatory process. Once the inflammation is controlled, the physician may reduce the amount and frequency of dosage, thereby minimizing the unpleasant side effects associated with steroid usage. Even when these side effects are within normal range from a medical standpoint, they may cause grave concern to the adolescent, who is particularly concerned with physical appearance. The long-term side effect of fat redistribution may lead to a rather husky appearance, a distressing occurrence to a maturing young woman. Other side effects such as fluid retention, weight gain and unusual hair growth may become disturbing if obvious enough to threaten self-esteem and provoke ridicule from peers. If immunosuppressive drugs are employed, the individual needs information about the increased risk of anemia or infection. Occasionally the use of antimalarial medications may be attempted in the hope of reversing the inflammatory process. The nurse needs to know that such drugs carry the potential for irreversible retinal damage.

In dealing with problems of mood changes, lack of acceptance of the illness and altered body image, nurses need to recognize that teens have tremendous difficulty coping with lupus. Not only do changes in their body image affect their developing sense of self-esteem and self-confidence, but the loss of control over the activities of their daily living is particularly stressful. Many find it difficult to cope with the activity restriction and marked fatigue that accompany lupus.

Changes in personality and behavior may be noted by the youth's family. Such changes occur not only because of physical limitations the illness imposes but develop as a result of the pathology of lupus. Previously established coping mechanisms and personality influence the way a person responds to these stresses. Teaching family members that behavioral changes result secondary to changes in the nervous system and also occur as a result of steroid medication may foster the family's acceptance of behaviors that cause stress.

Living with lupus affects a person's entire life style. Alterations occur in relationships with family and friends. The ability to plan for the future may be affected. Maturing girls may question whether they will be able to handle commitments to career, marriage and motherhood. Appropriate nursing responses create an atmosphere allowing freedom to express fears. Sharing information about those who have learned to live with lupus, leading full active lives, may encourage youth with newly diagnosed lupus. Arranging meetings with others who have successfully worked through these problems may also be helpful.

Specific nursing care to meet physical needs includes teaching and demonstrating simple range-of-motion exercises, which can assist in retaining muscle strength and joint mobility. Inflammation of joints is common but rarely results in significant residual deformity. Aspirin helps control joint pain. Stronger analgesics may be needed when more severe pain is associated with other lupus complications.

Additional teaching might include specific suggestions of ways to avoid known trigger factors. For example, since avoiding even a few minutes of direct exposure to the sun's rays is important, specific suggestions could include wearing long-sleeved shirts, broad-brimmed hats or using sun-screening lotion while outside. Parents can be advised to buy sun screen shades for automobile windows. Recommendations will vary with physicians, but many suggest avoiding immunizations and certain drugs such as penicillins, anticonvulsives such as phenytoin and antihypertensives such as Apresoline. The nurse might suggest the wearing of a Medic-Alert bracelet. Suggestions about avoiding fatigue should be based on knowledge of the youth's life style and developmental needs. The recommended requirement of 10 hours of rest or sleep per day might be best met by use of a pre-dinner nap rather than early bedtime.

Early recognition of possible life-threatening complications is essential. Appropriate teaching will ensure that the youth and parents recognize early symptoms of nephritis. The need for periodic monitoring of kidney function should be stressed.

In addition to physical and psychological stressors affecting the entire family of the lupus patient, there is a drain on the family's financial resources. A referral to social services for financial assistance and counselling might be advantageous. Financial assistance or other help might be available from private community agencies such as the Kidney Foundation or from governmental agencies such as crippled children's services. State and local support groups such as the Lupus Foundation provide psychological support and information to members. Emphasis on the things the youth can do may help him develop a way of life that will accommodate the limitations of the illness while allowing personal growth and adaptation within the family system.

TUBERCULOSIS

Tuberculosis (TB) is a long-term, communicable disease caused by a bacillus, *Mycobacterium tuberculosis*. In developed countries the morbidity and mortality rates for this disease have dramatically declined in the last 50 years. However, in many countries tuberculosis remains a leading cause of death. In the United States recent statistics from the Communicable Disease Center document approximately nine hundred new cases of TB each year in children under 4 years of age.[5] In older children and young adults reported cases average three thousand. Total reported new cases for all adults and children approximate thirty thousand per year.[5]

Children are the most vulnerable to this infection during their first three years of life and again during the two years before, during and after puberty. Many factors have contributed to decline in the incidence of TB in children. Earlier diagnosis and treatment of infected adults, who are a primary source of infection for children, has been accomplished by comprehensive public health screening programs. These programs identify and test all known contacts of people diagnosed with active tuberculosis. Another important factor in declining incidence has been the discovery and use of new, effective antituberculin drugs. Public health nurses making field visits to patients' homes have succeeded in effecting an increased compliance with drug therapy. Under current laws, food handlers and all school employees are required to receive annual TB screening tests for detection of exposure to the bacillus. Routine screening by simple skin testing of babies between the ages of 12 and 18 months has also contributed to the control of tuberculosis in children.

Etiology and Pathophysiology

The usual mode of communicability is inhalation of aerosolized sputum (cough spray) from another infected human. The spread of tuberculosis *(Mycobacterium bovis)* by drinking milk from an infected cow has almost been eliminated in the United States due to mandatory pasteurization of commercial milk.

Once a susceptible child inhales bacilli, organisms begin rapid multiplication in lung tissue, alveoli or in lymph glands draining lung areas. Following an incubation period of 2 to 10 weeks, the child will demonstrate a systemic hypersensitivity as evidenced by a positive skin test. In this test bacilli are injected immediately under the epidermis, forming a wheel. If the child has been exposed to TB and subsequently formed antibodies, a local induration will develop at the injection site. This simple skin test can be used as a screening tool to detect exposure to TB.

Most children exposed to inhaled *Mycobacterium tuberculosis* mobilize a defensive inflammatory reaction. As a part of this defensive reaction, white blood cells, especially macrophages, are deployed to attack and kill invading bacilli. As further defense, the body walls off small infected areas by the formation of tubercles. Caseous or fibrous tubercles prevent the further spread of infective organisms. Unfortunately, tuberculosis bacilli possess remarkable abilities to remain dormant in this necrotic tissue for many years. If at some later date the child's resistance is decreased, bacilli may begin to multiply, causing active disease.

The term *primary lesion*, or *focus*, denotes the original site of infection. The *primary complex* includes the primary lesion and any nearby lymph nodes that have been invaded. In many children, once the primary lesion is contained in tubercles, subsequent healing will occur through a process of calcification. Although these calcified tubercles may later be visible on x-ray, they do not indicate active disease. In older children the healed primary lesion is visualized as a scar or shadow. In both cases it is important to explain to parents the distinction between these findings and active tuberculosis. In some children the body's defense mechanisms fail to successfully control the primary lesion. After inhalation the bacilli may continue to multiply and spread by direct extension into nearby tissues. Or the bacilli may enter the blood and circulate to other sites, setting up multiple foci of infection, resulting in *miliary tuberculosis*.

In summary, following the primary lesion, possible subsequent outcomes are: (1) complete healing, (2) persistent quiescent lesions, (3) direct extension of infection at the original site,

TABLE 61-1 COMMON TUBERCULOSIS SCREENING TESTS

Test	How Administered (Use inner [volar] surface of forearm)	Read In (hr)	Negative Reaction	Doubtful Reaction	Positive Reaction (Retest with Mantoux)	Absolute Positive Reaction
Tine (OT)	A four-prong multiple puncture button containing old tuberculin is pressed into the inner forearm 2 to 4 in below bend of elbow, after site is swabbed with alcohol and allowed to dry.	48–72	0–2 mm induration	Papule 2 mm	One or more papules 2–5 mm or larger in diameter	Vesiculation*
Sclavotest (PPD)	A spring-activated multiple puncture device containing dried tuberculin purified protein derivative (PPD) solution on hidden prongs is placed on the under forearm, previously swabbed with alcohol. Gentle pressure on the device activates the prongs, which puncture skin to a preset depth. May be stored at room temperature.	48	0–2 mm induration	Approximately 2 mm induration	<2 mm induration	Vesiculation or coalescence of 2 or more puncture sites*
Mantoux (PPD)	PPD 5 tuberculin units (5 TU) in 0.1 ml solution is injected intradermally at the forearm inner surface, using a #27 needle tuberculin syringe after site has been cleansed with alcohol. A wheal is produced if the injection is intracutaneous. Keep PPD solution out of sunlight and refrigerate if possible.	48–72	5 mm	5–9 mm induration		10 mm induration

*Manufacturer suggested.

(4) spread of infection via the circulatory system to sites outside the lungs or (5) possible reactivation of the lesion at a later date should the patient become debilitated.

Identifying and Diagnosing Active Disease

The communicability of TB is increased by conditions of poverty and crowding, which foster poor hygiene. Factors such as malnutrition and fatigue can lower resistance to tuberculosis. There is a higher incidence of TB among nonwhite and Indian Americans and in large urban poverty areas that house transient peoples arriving from areas in which TB is widely disseminated.

In assessing whether a child is at risk for TB, the nurse must recognize that children are usually infected by adults with progressive cavitary lesions. These adults discharge droplets containing infective organisms into the air. Droplet residue remains in the air for long periods of time. However, prolonged contact is usually necessary before a child develops active disease.

Periodic testing of children to determine whether they have been exposed can be done by the nurse using any one of several skin tests (Table 61-1). In these tests, a small amount of specially treated tuberculin is injected intradermally. If the child has been exposed to TB, he will develop a skin reaction forming an area of induration (hard raised spots) at the site of injection. Sometimes this is accompanied by erythema. Since the nurse is responsible for administering and interpreting these skin tests she must measure, or teach the parent to measure, the width of the palpated elevated area. The presence or absence of redness should be disregarded. Reactivity to a skin test may be suppressed if the child is malnourished, under severe stress, or receiving steroids or immunosuppressive drugs. Children with doubtful readings on multiple puncture tests are retested using the Mantoux test.

Skin testing is not reliable if done within four weeks following a case of measles, or following vaccination with live virus. The American Academy of Pediatrics recommends that TB screening tests be done at one year of age and then annually or once every two years, depending upon incidence in the total community.[6] Conversion from a negative to a positive skin test is evidence that the child has been exposed to TB. It does not mean he has active disease.

If a positive skin test results from the screening, the nurse may assume the major responsibility for explaining the significance of a positive skin test to parents and to the child. At this time the nurse obtains a health history for each family member in an attempt to identify the source of the infection. All contacts are listed so that they may be screened also. The nurse provides information about further diagnostic measures and arranges for treatment. Family members need counselling as well as information. Many adults view TB not only as a serious threat to life but also as a threat to the integrity of their family unit.

Children with positive skin reactions receive chest x-rays to determine the presence and extent of active lesions. A diagnosis of active disease is documented if sputum smears show the presence of bacilli. Gastric washings to obtain swallowed sputum are sometimes done. A child may be hospitalized for this procedure; he receives nothing to eat during the night and until test completion. In the morning a nasogastric tube is inserted and stomach contents are lavaged and removed for microscopic examination. Obtaining sputum from a young child can be extremely difficult. Physicians often prefer to waive such tests rather than submit the child to a period of hospitalization, placing him on medication instead.

In some countries a BCG (bacille Calmette-Guérin) vaccination is given to produce immunity to the bacillus. This artificial immunity is effective for at least 10 years. Widespread use of BCG vaccine has not been adopted in our country, primarily because it would eliminate skin testing as an effective case finding tool.

There is a dangerous trend away from routine TB screening. Failure to implement screening programs may result in subsequent failure in diagnosing TB in its early stages. The effect will necessarily be an increase in incidence and also an increase in serious complications such as miliary TB and TB meningitis. Such complications are largely preventable with early diagnosis and treatment.

The majority of children diagnosed with tuberculosis have a noncomplicated pulmonary primary focus and are not infectious. The organisms are confined to a small area of the lung and the child has little or no coughing. However, if a child (usually a teenager) develops a cavitary lesion and is coughing up sputum containing bacilli or if the child has direct drainage from an infected site, he is a potential source of infection. Isolation precautions for all items contaminated with organisms and respiratory isolation precautions are required.

Most children will not have any symptoms and will be unaware of their tuberculosis until diagnosis. Knowing that symptoms in children are minimal, the nurse observes for low-grade fever, slight cough, history of fatigue, weight loss or anorexia. Recognizing age and risk factors can assist the nurse in case finding, but mass screening is the key to early identification.

Management

Management stresses four major interventions: (1) general supportive measures such as adequate rest, gradual resumption of activities, diet, prevention of other infection; (2) drug therapy; (3) emotional support and in some cases (4) surgery.

Rest, Activity and Diet. Ensuring that an active youth follows the treatment prescription for adequate rest can present difficulties. Fortunately, bed rest is required only when miliary TB has affected the child's weight-bearing structures. Bed rest may be desired on occasions when the child is feeling particularly ill and should be enforced during bouts of fever.

There are no restrictions on physical activities during treatment for active TB except that participation in competitive sports is discouraged. Nurses should counsel youth and parents about the need to avoid excessive fatigue, and recommend brief rest periods during the day. Sports that do not require strenuous physical activity may appeal to youth.

A nutritionally balanced diet is also part of the treatment program. Nurses cannot assume that children are receiving an adequate diet. A diet history should be obtained by collecting a 24-hour food intake diary kept by the youth. This diary can be an effective tool for both evaluation and teaching. Infected persons usually have reduced retention and utilization of nutrients; therefore, the youth's diet should be carefully planned so that what is taken in is highly nutritious and particularly rich in foods supplying protein and calcium.

Intercurrent infections encourage the spread of tuberculous processes and retard their healing. The additional stress caused by such infections seem to suppress inflammatory response

TABLE 61–2 DRUG TREATMENT OF TUBERCULOSIS

Organisms	Drug	Daily Dose (per 24 hr)	Route	Duration of Treatment (mo)	Possible Toxic Effects	Comments
Sensitive to usual drugs	Isoniazid (INH)*	10-30 mg/kg (up to 300–500 mg total) give in one or two doses	PO, IM or IV	12–18	Peripheral neuropathy, hepatotoxicity (adults)	Use the larger dose in patients in whom rapid inactivation of the drug is likely (Eskimos, Japanese, Korean) and in tuberculous meningitis; good diffusibility
	Para-aminosalicylic acid (PAS)	200-300 mg/kg (up to 12 gm), divide into two to three doses after meals	PO or IM	6–18	Gastric irritation, fever, rash, jaundice	Used as NaPAS, KPAS, CaPAS, resin, or flavored powder; give after meals
	Streptomycin (STM)	20 mg/kg (up to 1 gm), single daily dose intitially then three times weekly	IM	2–4	Ototoxicity, vestibular damage	For serious tuberculosis only; discontinue when clinical improvement is definite
	Ethambutol	15-20 mg/kg, divide into two to three doses	PO	12–18	Optic neuritis	
Resistant† to INH and/or streptomycin	Ethionamide	15-20 mg/kg (up to 1 gm) divide into two to three doses	PO	12–18	Gastric irritation, liver damage	Give after meals; diffuses well into CSF
	Rifampin (RIF)	15-20 mg/kg (up to 600 mg)	PO	12–18	Hepatotoxicity	Good diffusibility

*Pyridoxine (25-50 mg daily) is probably not necessary for children less than 11 years old.
†Additional drugs used when resistant to INH and/or streptomycin.
From *Report of the Committee on Infectious Diseases* 18th ed., 1977. American Academy of Pediatrics (Red Book), p. 291. Used with permission. Copyright American Academy of Pediatrics, 1977.

and decrease allergic responsiveness. The youth should limit his exposure to crowds and to infected persons until active disease has been controlled. This requires observant screening of family members, relatives and friends during the period of active disease.

Drug Therapy. The American Academy of Pediatrics advocates that all infants, children and adolescents with positive skin tests be treated with isoniazid (INH) for 12 to 18 months.[6] When there is evidence of active tuberculosis, such as demonstrable lesions on a chest x-ray, a combination of two antituberculosis drugs is often prescribed. Usual combinations are INH and para-aminosalicylic acid (PAS) or INH and rifampin. (See Table 61–2 for a description of the common TB drugs.) Factors to consider in choosing drugs are effectiveness, side effects, palatability and cost. Some of these drugs are much more expensive than others, although most health departments provide the medications free to residents in the geographical areas they serve.

Offering information about the side effects of medication and the importance of faithfully taking drugs each day for the entire 12 to 18 months is a crucial nursing action. Explanation of the serious consequences of failure to take medication as prescribed is an appropriate part of the education. Family members, especially parents, are sometimes upset that a child has to take medication for such a long period of time.

Other family members, especially those of the grandparents' generation, tend to remember the time when tuberculosis was greatly feared. They may have an inaccurate understanding of current treatment and prognosis, as well as incorrect opinions about diet and the amount of activity that should be permitted. If family members are to be actively involved with caring for the infected youth, they must also be given information currently available about the disease and its management.

Nurse's Role in Management Nursing functions in regard to population screening and seeking out contacts, especially for the purpose of locating the source of the infection, have already been described. Another role of the nurse is to help implement the prescribed treatment program to prevent further spread of the disease. Teaching children and their families about the disease may serve to facilitate their adaptation. The young adolescent may not be future oriented but should still be reassured that tuberculosis will not adversely affect most of the goals he will eventually have.

Nurses must be willing and able to meet the physical, intellectual and emotional-social needs of each youth. Specific care measures are determined by the extent and type of tuberculosis. The plan of care must be appropriate for the child's level of understanding and development and take into consideration his particular coping ability. Assisting a youth to assume responsibility for some of his treatment and rehabilitation goals is a nursing intervention that may ensure his cooperation.

Some youth may feel that a stigma is attached to the diagnosis and may respond by withdrawing from friends and activities. Even during the time that the initial nursing history is requested, the youth may feel constrained when asked to list all his recent contacts. He may think his friends will resent being named or being exposed to this disease. If the source of the infection turns out to be one of his friends, this can cause some friction. If the source is one of his own parents, the youth may experience some negative feelings toward that parent. Tuberculosis, like most other long-term illnesses, tends to increase or prolong dependency. This may be resented and contribute to the youth's feelings of discouragement.

Nurses can help the youth structure outlets for energy or aggressive feelings. Adolescent support groups are becoming popular. Such groups allow youth with long-term illnesses to ventilate their feelings and also provide peer support for members. Nurses need to recognize that anger is often expressed as rebellion against treatment orders or boredom and lack of interest in activities or school work. Fears about never again being completely well should be anticipated by the nurse and dealt with by frank discussion of the optimistic outcome for successful treatment of tuberculosis. Teenagers usually respond positively to visits from friends. Occasionally, however, a youth may try to avoid these contacts, fearing that his friends will be afraid of catching his TB.

Youth with active TB are frequently treated on an outpatient basis and may return to school when their sputum is negative for bacilli. Although there is some controversy about allowing youth with infective TB in school, returning them to school and their peer group as soon as is safely possible may motivate them to comply with the drug regimen. Until a return to school is feasible, specific plans to avoid disruption of intellectual achievements may include a hospital or homebound teacher.

Another stressor deserving consideration is when a youth with tuberculosis is from a family whose members are not United States citizens. These families may fear having their child's tuberculosis reported, which may result in deportation of any family members who are illegal aliens. An ethical question must be faced by nurses and medical personnel caring for families of illegal aliens. If the family thinks that medical care givers will report the tuberculosis to government officials and deportation will result, they will be reluctant to seek treatment, may not follow up with treatment, may fail to identify all their contacts, or may drop out of the community, thereby curtailing treatment efforts.

Surgery Whether surgical intervention is desirable depends upon the site, nature and extent of the active tuberculosis focus and the degree of compliance with and effectiveness of drug therapy. Vigorous antibiotic therapy is usually continued despite surgical removal of the involved organ or body tissue to help ensure subsequent healing.

With adequate treatment the incidence and complications of TB should continue to decline.

References

1. W. Anyan. Adolescent Medicine in Primary Care. John Wiley & Sons, 1978.
2. G. Godeene. Depressive and schizophrenic reactions in adolescence. In Medical Care of the Adolescent, 3rd ed., J. R. Gallagher, et al., Appleton-Century-Crofts, 1976
3. J. Huber et al. Comprehensive Psychiatric Nursing. McGraw-Hill Book Co., 1978
4. L. Miceli. Systemic lupus erythematosus: a renal review with a pediatric perspective. Journal of American Osteopathic Association, July 1979, p. 800
5. Communicable Disease Committee. MMWR: 1977 annual summary, U.S. Department of Health, Education and Welfare, Public Health Service, Vol. 26: No. 53, September 1978
6. Report of the Committee on Infectious Diseases, 18th ed. American Academy of Pediatrics (Red Book), 1977

7. J. White. The nurse who manages, the nurse who intervenes, and the nurse who cares for the patient with systemic lupus erythematosus. Michigan Lupus Foundation, December, 1978

Additional Recommended Reading

H. Barnes. The problem of delayed puberty. Medical Clinics of North America, November 1975, p. 6

P. Beeson et al. Cecil Textbook of Medicine, 15th ed. W. B. Saunders Co., 1979

H. Clarizio and G. McCoy. Behavior Disorders in Children. Thomas Y. Crowell Co., 1976

A. Copeland. Textbook of Adolescent Psychopathology and Treatment. Charles C Thomas, 1974

W. Daniel. Adolescents in Health and Disease. C. V. Mosby Co., 1977

A. Dorin. Adolescent sexuality/adolescent depression. Pediatric Nursing, Jul/Aug 1978, p. 4

J. Gallagher et al. Medical Care of the Adolescent. Appleton-Century-Crofts, 1976

K. Glaser. The treatment of depressed and suicidal adolescents. American Journal of Psychotherapy, April 1978, p. 2

A. Hofmann. Adolescents in distress. Medical Clinics of North America, November 1975, p. 6

L. Jelneck. The special needs of the adolescent with chronic illness. American Journal Maternal and Child Nursing. Jan/Feb 1977, p. 57

C. Kempe et al. Current Pediatric Diagnosis and Treatment. Lange Publications, 1978

E. Kendig. Chronic Lung Disease in Children. Hospital Practice. May 1977, p. 5

S. Leichtman and S. Friedman. Social and psychological development of adolescents and the relationship to chronic illness. Medical Clinics of North America, November 1975, p. 6

V. Lynch. Narcissistic loss and depression in late adolescence. Perspectives in Psychiatric Care, Jul/Sept 1976, p. 3

Rheumatology: systemic lupus erythematosus: take a brighter view. Patient Care, August 1976

A. Rush and A. Beck. Cognitive therapy of depression and suicide. American Journal of Psychotherapy, April 1978, p. 2

E. Sills. Juvenile rheumatoid arthritis and systemic lupus erythematosus of the adolescent. Medical Clinics of North America, November 1975, p. 6

Systemic Lupus Erythematosus: a case study. Nursing '78, September 1978, p. 28

J. Toolan. Therapy of depressed and suicidal children. American Jounral of Psychotherapy, April 1978, p. 2

62 POTENTIAL STRESSES DURING ADOLESCENCE: LIFE-THREATENING ALTERATIONS IN HEALTH STATUS

by Marcia N. Sheets, RN, MSN
and Anita L. Spietz, RN, MSN

HOW THE ADOLESCENT PERCEIVES DEATH

The adolescent has grown beyond the school-age child in his conceptualization of death. His more adept thinking processes allow him to develop a more mature concept of death. His concept of death reflects a greater comprehension of the complexities that have plagued man for centuries. He no longer views death as reversible, temporary or happening to someone other than himself. He queries the role of death within the universe and his own finiteness. He now views himself as alone in his individuality and senses his own mortality. With the advanced treatment modalities available for treating children with life-threatening illnesses, there is an increased likelihood that these children will survive to adolescence. Consequently, the nurse will sometimes need to help such an adolescent cope with impending death.

When a life-threatening illness is diagnosed during adolescence, the use of denial by the adolescent and his family during the early phases of diagnosis and treatment is not only to be expected but also to be viewed as a sign of hope. The expression of hope is healthy and needs to be fostered matter-of-factly so as to provide support for the youth undergoing severe stress. During this denial phase, an open, supportive, accepting attitude must be evidenced by the nurse, so that as the grieving process proceeds, family members will recognize her as a person with whom to discuss and explore their fears and feelings about the forthcoming death of their young adult.

If a life-threatening illness is diagnosed or if a long-standing illness worsens during adolescence, the adolescent may begin to readjust his view of death. This change is not sudden but a gradual transition as his social, emotional and physical environment changes. The overwhelming injustice of death is wrestled with by the family as well as the health team working with it. Most adults have difficulty accepting the prognosis of a terminal illness; the adolescent struggles, and has even fewer "developed" and "tried" defense mechanisms to assist in coping with death. His ability to cope is based both on his cognitive mastery and his opportunity to successfully utilize effective coping mechanisms.

The process of dying for an adolescent, whether the illness is sudden or life-long, is completely incongruous with all that he finds important—his physical attractiveness is diminished and his prowess is replaced by progressive weakness and body dysfunction. The independence and self-identity that the adolescent perceives as so important are progressively altered.

The adolescent's reaction to dying is one of extreme anger toward all with whom he has contact. He feels that everyone, including God, has failed him. He may experience guilt or depression because he cannot cope with his resentment and anger. It is much more difficult to care for the dying teenager because the angry behavior that is testimony of his need for love and care keeps everyone at a distance or forces them away completely. His family, and especially his friends, react by avoiding him or the subject of death or both. As a result the youth feels rejected by all who matter to him and he retaliates with more anger or by withdrawing.

The more mature adolescent or young adult copes more effectively with his death, usually experiencing only short-lived anger that is promptly replaced by attempts to make the most of his relationships in the time he has left. He may attempt also to accomplish at least some of his life goals in the short time that remains.

Partly because of his angry behavior and partly because of the limitations caused by the life-threatening illness and impending death, the dying adolescent's social milieu begins to change, with the development of new peer group relationships within the hospital and outpatient settings. Although a few close friends may remain part of the peer group of the dying adolescent, those who are living through life-threatening events themselves increasingly become supportive and understanding in a way that is not possible for those who are apart from that experience. Often the frequently hospitalized adolescent begins to depend upon the hospital staff as a definite part of the peer group to which he relates. There he often finds more openness, understanding and acceptance of the physical changes, emotional changes and body changes happening to him than his peers can offer.

Those involved in caring for the dying adolescent need to recognize that overt behaviors often are not an expression of his real needs and fears. He needs time and an atmosphere that will allow him to come to grips with the fact that death is happening to him.[3]

The dying adolescent needs to be treated as autonomously as possible, since he is usually struggling to remain as independent as possible during the high stress associated with his state of being. Noncompliance may be viewed as an attempt to control his own self-care or as an attempt to deny the seriousness of his condition. Patience and support must be provided during this time. Parents also may be feeling a great deal of ambiguity as they try to support the independence of the adolescent and also do "what is best for him." They may feel extreme frustration in trying to reach both these goals. Information about the disease process, treatment plans and rationale and prognosis is essential to the adolescent at this time. The realities of the situation must be made explicit to him so that informed decisions about care and self-care may be made. Some parents take on the role of decision-maker at this time. They become overprotective and actually set limits to the behavior that they consider acceptable. Many adolescents need the security that these parameters provide, while others need to be able to make their own decisions regarding the quality and length of their lives.

The adolescent may find that he sometimes needs to become dependent upon his parents again and he may be very angry, even enraged, at the injustice, asking "Why me?" and declaring "It isn't fair." The nurse can assist the adolescent and his family to accept the somewhat unpredictable behavior that expresses his anger and that is usually projected toward the staff and his parents. By identifying the normality of the behavior under the circumstances, the nurse provides support to the family unit. She can also provide opportunities for the adolescent to make decisions about his own care. She can deliberately ask for the youth's opinions, suggestions, preferences or choices and, whenever possible, these choices and preferences should be honored, thereby assisting the dying adolescent in his quest for independence and self-respect.

The death of an adolescent or young adult affects all who have come in contact with him. The youth's zest for living and his wonderment at accomplishment is unmatched by that of people in any other period of development. It is difficult to see such a life shortened by fatal illness, but it is sometimes awesome to see the courage with which he is able to approach his death.

Several of the alterations in health status that may force the adolescent to confront the reality or possibility of death are discussed in this chapter. Although there has been an awareness of the illness (such as in muscular dystrophy and cystic fibrosis) for a period of time, it is during adolescence that one's own mortality is realized and that death is comprehended in a way similar to an adult. When a life-threatening illness is diagnosed during adolescence, there may be a sense that all the growing-up years were for nothing. There is an overwhelming feeling in all those who know the young person of the unfairness of the situation. A young person whose life shows promise is suddenly limited by an alteration in body chemistry that will rob society of his potential.

ALTERED HEALTH STATES

Bone Tumors

The most frequently occurring malignant bone tumors of late childhood are Ewing's sarcoma and osteogenic sarcoma.

Ewing's Sarcoma Ewing's sarcoma is a bone tumor characterized by anaplastic cells with no connective tissue, which occurs predominantly in patients under the age of 20, with the peak incidence during the period of adolescence.[17] There is greater incidence of Ewing's sarcoma in boys than in girls.[6] It is a rare nonosseous tumor arising from bone marrow.

The site of the primary tumor could be almost any bone of the body, but about half of the tumors occur in the femur, tibia or humerus.[6] Metastasis from the primary site is to the lungs, viscera or subcutaneous tissues. At times pathological fractures occur; the site and extent of the fracture dictates the severity of the symptoms.

Osteogenic Sarcoma (Osteosarcoma) Osteogenic sarcoma is an osseous tumor of the bone that affects the mesenchyme and is seen predominantly during the time of bone growth spurts and in areas that demonstrate rapid growth, such as the distal femur, the proximal tibia and the proximal humerus. Metastasis may occur to the lung (the usual site), lymph system, viscera or subcutaneous tissues.

Due to the fact that the areas of bone growth (distal femur, proximal tibia, proximal humerus) are most often affected, it is rare to see osteogenic sarcoma before the preadolescent period of development. According to Jaffee, approximately 300 cases of osteogenic sarcoma are diagnosed each year in the United States.[6] There is a greater incidence of osteogenic sarcoma in boys than in girls.[7]

Making the Diagnosis The child with a primary tumor of the bone most often presents with a mass, which is often initially painless. Less frequently, pain precedes awareness of a mass.[17] The pain may be mild or transient, dull or aching. Referred pain may be noted if the primary lesion occurs in the hip.

While providing wellness care to the adolescent, the nurse may be involved in the early identification of a bone tumor. A nursing history may elicit information relative to the changing health status of the adolescent, particularly in the area of decreasing weight, decreasing energy levels, pain, fever, difficulty in ambulation or an awareness of a mass. The physical examination may reveal a mass in an extremity or the trunk. The youth may describe a fall or an accident that occurred several weeks before the onset of symptomatology. An immediate medical referral must be made when a bone tumor is suspected.

If a bone tumor is suspected, the adolescent must undergo a series of medical diagnostic tests. Such procedures may include a variety of radiographic examinations such as computerized tomograms (CT scans), arthrograms, bone scans by radioisotopes, and chest films. Other tests include routine hematologic studies, liver studies, and bone marrow aspiration.

The surgical biopsy is critical in the determination of the diagnosis of primary sarcoma of the bone. Prior to the biopsy, radiation therapy is employed to inactivate the tumor cells, thus reducing the possibility of "seeding" other tissues or establishing metastases by the bloodstream. The definitive diagnosis is then made by closely examining the youth's medical history, the results of the diagnostic tests and histologic examination of the bone specimen. Ideally, specialists such as a pediatrician, a diagnostic radiologist, a pediatric oncologist, a surgeon and a pathologist make the diagnosis jointly.

Although the medical necessity of performing

these diagnostic examinations may have been explained to the adolescent and his family, the nurse must assess their need for further information or repeated information as the testing proceeds. Since the shock that is probably being experienced at this time may alter the family's ability to comprehend the information presented the first time through, the nurse must continually assess the level of "informed consent" that is operative. The nurse needs to be prepared to provide exact information regarding the actual procedure to be performed, whether or not the procedure will be painful, and how the adolescent is expected to act (what he must do during the procedure, what he will be aware of, and so forth). If possible, the nurse should accompany the youth and parents to the test if the adolescent indicates a high level of anxiety about the procedure. It should never be assumed that the adolescent would not want someone with him during the procedure, although each adolescent must be individually assessed. The information provided prior to a procedure will assist the adolescent in coping before and during the procedure.

Incisional biopsy, scans, bone marrow aspirations, and arthrograms are uncommon procedures with which most youths are unfamiliar. The nurse needs to assist the adolescent to prepare for these by providing instructions and answers to questions the adolescent or the family may have. During each procedure a brief explanation of purpose before each step is done facilitates an environment of trust and maintains open communication.

The diagnostic period is a time of fear and tension, as decisions are awaited. The answers and instructions provided need to be direct and succinct — the family is probably already overloaded with jargon and scientific terminology. The nurse may effectively assist the family by being selective about the words used and the amount of information shared at this time. It is important that information not be withheld from the family in an attempt to reduce stress. Once the diagnosis is confirmed, new needs emerge. The nurse must continually assess the family's understanding of the treatment selected for their child.

Treatment The treatments generally utilized to treat the child with Ewing's sarcoma or osteogenic sarcoma are radiation therapy, chemotherapy or surgery, or a combination of these three.

Radiation therapy is generally the treatment of choice for the primary lesion of Ewing's sarcoma. The aim of this treatment is destruction of the tumor and retention of adequate function.[17] Along with the radiation therapy, multidrug chemotherapy is utilized in a series of cycles administered over one or two years. The drug regimen currently utilized for this sarcoma includes Adriamycin, Cytoxan, actinomycin D and vincristine given over 18 months.[17] (See Appendix VIII for appropriate nursing care when a child undergoes radiation therapy.)

Chemotherapy is designed to treat the cancer cells by destroying or altering the DNA or RNA component of the dividing cells. Multiple drugs are given in a series of cycles, administered over one to two years and started at the time of the primary therapy (radiation or surgery). Although several drug regimens are currently being studied, the drugs include high doses of methotrexate with leucovorin rescue, Adriamycin alone, methotrexate and Adriamycin combined with such other agents as Cytoxan, vincristine, and melphalan. (See Appendix VIII for actions of these drugs.)

Most of these regimens cause considerable toxicity that interferes with the adolescent's everyday living.[17] Many physiological and psychosocial needs already created by the primary therapy become even more pressing during this time.

An assessment of the patient's understanding of the primary treatment must be done before any chemotherapy-related teaching can begin. Due to the fact that anxiety and shock are operative during the diagnostic period and the induction or primary phase of treatment, the nurse must provide or repeat information concisely as the family is ready and able to accept it. The family should be monitored as to their understanding and subsequent consent during the course of treatment. Inappropriate use of medical terminology and jargon must be avoided. The nurse may assist the family by clarifying the terminology used.

The use of experimental drugs or treatments forces a legal issue for the nurse, youth and his family. The risks undertaken, as well as the benefits of the treatment, must clearly be described to the best of the physician's and nurse's abilities, given the most current clinical information available.

The amount of physical discomfort associated with the use of certain chemicals and treatments must clearly be described to the youth and his family before the treatment. Toxic effects and complications must be discussed as well as the means available to counteract those toxic effects or complications or both. The medications that will be available for the control of pain, nausea and vomiting need to be described. The nursing care plan, which is written and determined totally in conjunction with the entire oncology health team, the adolescent and his family, can serve as a form of contract between the nurse and the client.

Often the adolescent will come to the outpatient clinic for laboratory tests, treatment or administration of medications. The nurse needs to assess the patient and the family for their understanding of the drug regimen, side effects and toxic effects being experienced. The need for support during this time is assessed. The nurse must also consider the family's need for consultation after they have left the outpatient clinic. She must tell them how she can be reached to assist them and also how to react during a medical emergency. She can help the family to identify certain resources and back-up facilities within the community if the adolescent is having a medical complication or severe toxic side effects. Phone assessment may be done to determine if the symptom management following chemotherapy will require a return to the outpatient clinic.

Compliance in self-administration of drugs is sometimes a problem. One study has indicated that as many as 59 per cent of the adolescents studied were noncompliant.[16] Compliance can be greatly increased if a good pretreatment education program is provided.

Surgical management is another option available in the treatment of bone tumors. Depending upon the efficiency of the combination therapy of radiotherapy and chemotherapy in destroying the primary tumor cells, or depending upon the stage of the disease at the time of diagnosis, surgery may be used in treating Ewing's sarcoma. However, surgical management is indicated after a firm diagnosis of osteogenic sarcoma has been established. If the entire bone is removed, a disarticulation is performed; therefore, above-the-knee or hip disarticulation or hemipelvectomy may be the procedure utilized. A transosseous amputation is utilized if the entire bone is not removed. There is disagreement about the efficiency of this technique due to the hazard associated with seeding of adjoining tissues prior to and following the procedure.[17]

Preoperative Teaching The adolescent, who at this stage of his development is already acutely aware of his body and his body image, needs extremely sensitive care during this severely stressful time. He needs information before the surgery about what will be done to his leg or arm. He needs much reassurance that the amputated limb will be treated with respect and care. He needs to know what alternatives exist before providing consent for the procedure — a request that most adults never make!

The independent life style that he may have been striving for may seem to be disintegrating at this time. Will the boy be able to drive a car? Will any girl want to dance with him? How can the girl amputee wear a bathing suit or shorts? Who will want to engage in sexual activity with him or her now? These and other questions may or may not be answerable. The adolescent needs an accepting person to listen to his rage and his fear. The youth's behavior at this time is to be viewed by the nurse and family as an attempt to cope in the best way possible.

Specific answers regarding the care of the stump after surgery, the fitting of a prosthesis during or after surgery, and a plan for physical and occupational therapy will assist the adolescent in coping with an amputation. Specific care measures to ensure the healing of the stump must be undertaken. The fear of pain is common before a surgical amputation. The adolescent needs constant reassurance that pain relief will be provided promptly after surgery.

An explanation of what to expect after surgery is essential. The youth needs to be told that he will come back from the recovery room with a hard plaster cast on his "stump" (a new word for his leg). As Bakke notes, ". . . it is sometimes difficult at first to use the word 'stump' with these teenagers. It doesn't sound much like a functioning body part, but that is exactly what it will become after a period of physical therapy and rehabilitation."[1] The purpose of the cast is to shape the stump, reduce edema and to allow early ambulation. The cast may be held in place with shoulder straps if the youth has had an AK (above the knee) amputation. A Hemovac may be utilized for the first day to assist in the removal of the initial drainage.

"Phantom pain" should be discussed preoperatively. The adolescent needs to be reassured that a phantom sensation, a normal proprioceptive and sensory memory of the amputated limb, may exist for several months and may affect ambulation. Phantom pain can become a chronic, debilitating syndrome that may be associated with the lack of acceptance of body changes and the inability to incorporate those changes into the youth's body image. Pain may also be related to physical changes in the stump. The presence of infection, occurrence of ischemia or muscle cramping may cause burning, sharp or aching pain. The nurse must be aware of each of these possibilities relative to the youth's experience of sensations and must provide appropriate information to help him understand them.[1]

Postoperative Care A prime goal for the adolescent with an amputation is early ambulation. The earlier the return to ambulation, the earlier the youth will be able to regain his independence. The adolescent may want to keep his stump covered with blankets or pajamas and may not want to become involved with other adolescents on the ward. He may not even want to look at his leg or touch it, or he may avoid any reference to his "stump" altogether. The nurse can assist in the process of acceptance of the newly amputated limb by conveying an accepting attitude. She can assess his readiness to look or to touch as she provides routine hygienic care. She can provide privacy to the adolescent so that he will begin to explore on his own. Of significant value is the acceptance by another person important to the youth of the mutilation or the severe insult to the body that has occurred. As other members of the health team begin to inspect the stump and to assist with rehabilitative efforts, the adolescent usually begins to become more accepting of the change. The nurse can encourage the youth to assist in the positioning of the stump. He can also be taught to lie prone for a half hour three or four times a day and to keep the stump flat so as to prevent flexion contractures. The youth can also be taught to avoid abduction and external rotation.[1]

Physical therapists are often involved in assisting the adolescent to regain ambulation skills. A tilt table may be used in the first day after operation. The cast is fitted with a steel pylon (serving as an extension of the limb) to which is attached a prosthetic foot. Weight bearing is facilitated by the use of this prothesis. Parallel bars assist the youth as he begins light weight bearing. He gradually progresses to partial weight bearing and is assisted with crutches. Discharge from the hospital often occurs about 10 days after the amputation. Cast changes occur on an outpatient basis.

When the cast is removed, the Ace bandage is tightened more distally than proximally. The purpose is to assist in the shaping of the stump.[1]

The adolescent must increase his self-care skills as his rehabilitation progresses. The stump must be carefully inspected for signs of breakdown and drainage from the suture line. The youth should be informed of the signs of infection so that he can identify any breakdown early and get prompt treatment for it.

Prognosis Although definite increases in the five-year survival rates have been made through the continued research being conducted, the adolescent who is diagnosed with a bone tumor must deal with the ever-present possibility of metastasis and death. Before the advent of chemotherapy, the prognosis for a child with Ewing's sarcoma was poor, with only 5 per cent of children surviving beyond five years. Current expectations are for cure in approximately 60 to 70 per cent of treated cases.[6] The disease-free survival rates for the child with osteogenic sarcoma who has been treated with the combined modality approach appear to be greater than 50 per cent at five years.[17] This represents a major advance in the medical treatment of osteogenic sarcoma.

Hodgkin's Disease

Hodgkin's disease is a malignant lymphoma characterized by neoplastic proliferation of lymphoreticular portions of the reticuloendothelial system involving lymph nodes, bone marrow, and spleen or liver or both.

In the United States, about 5000 to 6000 new cases of Hodgkin's disease are diagnosed each year. A slightly higher incidence is noted in males than in females.[15] There also appears to be increased frequency in Jews and whites, according to Skarin.[15]

The pathophysiology of Hodgkin's disease is not clearly described to date. There are some suggestions about the etiology of the disease described in the literature. A viral cause has been postulated because virus-induced tumors have been seen in laboratory animals. Some evidence suggests that Hodgkin's disease may be associated with abnormalities in T cells with resultant impairment in cellular immunity.[15] The etiology of this disease is still under scientific investigation.

Most often the adolescent with Hodgkin's disease presents with lymphadenopathy, usually in the supraclavicular or cervical area. About half of these youth present with the disease confined to the lymph node areas above the diaphragm. The disease is progressive in that it spreads from one lymph node area to the next most contiguous lymph node group. There are occasions during which the spleen also becomes involved. Symptoms of fever, night sweats, weight loss or pruritus may be evident in the adolescent with Hodgkin's disease.

Diagnosis Diagnostic testing, including laboratory tests of C-reactive protein, erythrocyte sedimentation rate, serum fibrinogen determination, liver function studies and haptoglobin, may be done. Radiographic examination of the chest may demonstrate mediastinal adenopathy in 40 to 60 per cent of patients. Lymphangiography is useful to outline the appearance of retroperitoneal nodes; surgical biopsy of the painlessly enlarged nodes may be conducted.

The controversial "staging laparotomy" for diagnostic purposes is said to provide the only definitive diagnosis of the disease. It should not be performed haphazardly and should only be done when a significant therapeutic decision will be based on the outcome of the laparotomy. Some argue that the value of the staging laparotomy is to determine the involvement of the spleen in the disease process.[13] The staging derived from the laparotomy follows:[15]

Stage I. Disease limited to one anatomical region or to two contiguous anatomical regions on the same side of the diaphragm.

Stage II. Disease in more than two anatomic regions or in two noncontiguous regions on the same side of the diaphragm.

Stage III. Disease in lymph node regions on both sides of the diaphragm but not extending beyond involvement of lymph nodes or spleen; if spleen is involved the subscript S is used (for example, III_S).

Stage IV. Involvement of extralymphatic organs (for example, bone marrow, lung, pleura, liver, bone, skin, gastrointestinal tract); if a single extralymphatic site is involved, the subscript E is used (for example, stage II_E).[15]

All patients are subclassified A or B to indicate the absence of presence respectively of one or more of (1) unexplained weight loss of more than 10 per cent of body weight, (2) unexplained fever with temperature above 38° C and (3) night sweats.

If the decision is to perform a staging laparotomy, the nurse needs to assist the adolescent and his family to prepare for the surgical procedure. She must provide answers to questions regarding routine preoperative and postoperative care and also assist the family by being available to support and listen while they attempt to cope with their anger, shock and disbelief.

Treatment The use of radiotherapy in the treatment of Hodgkin's disease, combined with chemotherapy generally provides the most optimism in the prognosis. Treatment is administered according to the diagnostic staging determination.

Stages IA and IIA. Radiation therapy is usually provided.

Stages IB, IIB, and IIIB. Combination chemotherapy (several cycles) plus the use of nodal high-dose irradiation is usually provided.

Stage IIIA. Combination chemotherapy (several cycles) plus the use of nodal high-dose irradiation is usually provided.

Stages IVA and IVB. An aggressive combination chemotherapy is used with radiation therapy limited to extensive areas of disease in an effort to decrease the probability of recurrence in those areas.[15]

Research dealing with various clinical approaches to effective chemotherapeutics is currently ongoing in the medical community. The use of single chemotherapeutic drugs has met with limited success. Efforts are currently being directed toward the utilization of combination chemotherapy programs with the use of MOPP (nitrogen mustard [Mustargen]), vincristine (Oncovin), procarbazine, and prednisone.)[15] MOPP is given cyclically, depending upon laboratory data and levels of blood counts. The therapy is totally discounted when no clinical or radiographic evidence of disease is found. See Table

TABLE 62-1 MOPP COMBINATION CHEMOTHERAPY IN HODGKIN'S DISEASE

MOPP Drug	Route	Action	Side Effects
Nitrogen mustard (Mustargen)	IV	Forms covalent bond with DNA and RNA, interfering with their synthesis	Nausea, vomiting, bone marrow depression
Vincristine (Oncovin)	Oral, IV	Arrest mitosis in methaphase	Neurotoxicity, alopecia, bone marrow depression, constipation
Procarbazine		Probably acts like Mustargen though precise action unclear	Nausea, vomiting, flu-like symptoms, delayed myelosuppression
Prednisone	Oral	Unknown	Edema—moon facies and weight gain; hypokalemia and sodium retention; increased susceptibility to infection; gastrointestinal bleeding and easy bruising hursutism

62–1 for the actions and side effects of MOPP therapy.

Adolescents with the disease diagnosed at stages I to III have a survival rate at five years of 80 to 90 per cent with a disease-free survival of 73 per cent for patients with stage I, 69 per cent for those with stage II, and 61 per cent for those with stage III disease. The overall five-year survival rate for patients with stages III and IV treated by MOPP chemotherapy is 70 per cent at five years. At 10 years the rate of complete remission is 50 per cent. Presence of "B" symptoms decrease the survival rate for patients, but there is relapse-free survival for many of these patients.

Muscular Dystrophy

Muscular dystrophies comprise one of the most prevalent muscle diseases in childhood. They are hereditary, familial diseases characterized by gradual onset in early life, with atrophy and weakness of the proximal muscles. Although the etiology is unknown, a defect in metabolism of creatine is suspected owing to increased serum levels in affected individuals.

There are three major types of muscular dystrophy: (1) Duchenne's muscular dystrophy, (2) the facioscapulohumeral form, and (3) the limb-girdle type. The various forms of these dystrophies are presented in Table 62–2, which describes pattern of inheritance, age of onset and progressive involvement. Since Duchenne's is the most common muscle dystrophy in childhood, it is presented here in greater detail.

Duchenne's Muscular Dystrophy (Pseudohypertrophic) The most common type of muscular dystrophy in childhood is transmitted as an X-linked recessive disorder in which males are primarily affected. The onset is between 2 and 6 years with death resulting between the ages of 15 and 25 from cardiac complications or respiratory infections. It is a relatively common disease with an incidence of about 1 per 25,000.[9]

The course of the disease is gradual, with initial symptoms often overlooked. Presenting symptoms include bilateral involvement of the pelvic girdle with later progression to the shoulder girdle. Parents or playmates often notice initial signs of the disease in the young child. They may note that the child is clumsy, has a waddling gait, frequently falls, and has difficulty climbing stairs, riding a tricycle or rising to a sitting position. An early sign of pelvis weakness is the manner in which affeced children rise from the floor. The child positions himself on all fours, then extends his knees and climbs up his thighs with his hands (Gower's sign). As the disease progresses muscle atrophy is noted. In spite of the atrophy, pseudohypertrophy of the calves, thighs and upper arms results from fatty infiltration of the muscle fibers. Contractures and joint deformities are not uncommon. Walking is generally possible until approximately 12 years of age. Occasionally mental deficiency is observed in these children. Involvement of the diaphragm, myocardium and auxilliary respiratory muscles

TABLE 62-2 THE PRIMARY MYOPATHIES OF MUSCULAR DYSTROPHY

Primary Myopathies Muscular Dystrophy

Major Types	Alternate Names	Type of Inheritance	Clinical Onset	Initial Symptoms	Progression	Treatment
Pseudohypertrophic	Duchenne	Sex-linked recessive, transmitted through unaffected females. There is a 50% probability that male offspring will be afflicted, and a 50% probability that female offspring will be carriers.	Early childhood	Swayback, a waddling gait, and difficulty in rising from the floor and climbing stairs, due to pelvic girdle muscle weakness. Fat deposits replace wasting muscle tissue in the calves.	Rapid, ultimately involving all the voluntary muscles. Death usually occurs within 10–15 years of clinical onset.	None. Physical therapy may delay atrophy of disuse of healthy muscles and antibiotics control secondary illnesses, but neither halts the dystrophic process.
Facioscapulohumeral	Landouzy-Dejerine	Autosomal dominant, transmitted by either parent to children of both sexes, with a 50% probability of incidence.	Early adolescence, occasionally in the twenties.	Lack of facial mobility, difficulty in raising arms over head, forward slope of shoulders, due to initial weakness of face and shoulder girdle muscles.	Very slow, often with intervals in which the disease marks time. Average life span rarely shortened, despite considerable disability.	None. Physical therapy may delay atrophy of disuse of healthy muscles and antibiotics control secondary illnesses, but neither halts the dystrophic process.
Limb-girdle	Includes Juvenile Dystrophy of Erb	Autosomal recessive, transmitted to children of both sexes **only** when both parents carry the defective gene. 25% may then be disabled, and up to 50% carriers.	Any time from the 1st to the 3rd decade of life.	Usually weakness of the proximal muscles of both the pelvic and the shoulder girdles.	Variable, sometimes slow and sometimes fairly rapid. Disability may remain slight and some patients live to old age.	None. Physical therapy may delay atrophy of disuse of healthy muscles and antibiotics control secondary illnesses, but neither halts the dystrophic process.
Muscular dystrophy of late onset		Not known to be hereditary. Affects both sexes.	4th or 5th decade of life.	Weakness of the proximal muscles of the pelvic girdle.	Variable.	None. Physical therapy may delay atrophy of disuse of healthy muscles and antibiotics control secondary illnesses, but neither halts the dystrophic process.
Myositis						
Polymyositis		None	Any time of life.	Proximal muscle weakness not connected with any identifiable systemic disorder.	Variable, may be mild and chronic, severe and chronic, or rapidly fatal. Occasional periods of remission.	Corticosteroid therapy brings marked improvement in many cases.
Dermatomyositis		None	Any time of life.	Similar to polymyositis symptoms, with the addition of a reddish skin eruption on face and upper trunk.	Similar to polymyositis.	Corticosteroid therapy brings marked improvement in many cases.

Adapted from chart of Differential Diagnostic Characteristics of the Primary Diseases Affecting the Neuromuscular Unit. Made available through the Muscular Dystrophy Associations of America, Inc.

does not occur until the final stages of the disease.

Diagnosis Diagnosis is based on the clinical features of the disease, family history and measurement of serum enzyme levels. Both serum creatine phosphokinase (CPK) and serum glutamic-oxaloacetic transaminase (SGOT) are increased until late in the disease. Electromyography (EMG) reveals a disease of striated muscles with low voltage action potentials. Muscle biopsy is used to detect degeneration of muscle fibers and fatty infiltration.[9]

Confirming the diagnosis of muscular dystrophy is often a frightening and anxiety-producing period for parents. A young child may not understand the meaning of the diagnosis, but as he approaches adolescence he must deal with the threat of impending death.

Preparation for muscle biopsy and electromyogram varies with the age at diagnosis. The onset is usually in the preschool years; therefore, before the biopsy the child should be told that he will be asleep and that a small cut will be made and a tiny piece of muscle removed. Vital signs and drainage from the incision will need to be monitored following the procedure. In preparation for the electromyogram both parents and child need to be informed of the procedure, in which small needles are placed in the child's muscles to record contractions. For the young child needle play is appropriate; for an older child an opportunity is provided to ask questions and clear explanations must be given. Regardless of the age of the child, the nurse should plan to be present during the procedure.

Treatment Although no treatment exists for arresting the course of the disease, there are several activities that need to be carried out to maintain optimal levels of functioning. Therapy needs to be symptomatic, preventive and supportive, focusing not only on the pathophysiology of the disease but also the emotional and social needs of the child and family, which change as the child develops and the disease progresses.

Symptomatic treatment requires that the nurse assess the patient and his family for their understanding of the disease process, attitudes toward the condition and coping abilities. A priority of nursing is development of an activity-exercise program that allows for independence to promote maximum development. Through childhood to adolescence and young adulthood, active exercise aids in improving muscle strength, and passive range-of-motion exercises and physiotherapy help prevent contractures. Strenuous exercises, however, may increase muscle atrophy. If for any reason the patient is on bed rest, it is very important that range-of-motion exercises be given to maintain muscle strength.

Respiratory infections and aspiration pneumonia are fairly common in these children. Prompt treatment is required because such children are unable to cough effectively, resulting in pooling of mucus in the lungs. Postural drainage and antibiotic therapy are generally helpful.

Prevention of obesity, a common problem in the presence of muscular dystrophy, is paramount. Since obesity leads to premature loss of ambulation, nutritional status of the patient needs to be assessed. Caloric intake should be adjusted in accordance with his level of activity. A balance between rest, activity and adequate nutrition is necessary for the prevention of fatigue and obesity.

Provision of genetic counselling for the immediate and extended family is one of the primary approaches to muscular dystrophy. Simple serum enzyme levels of CPK determine carrier status.

Supportive care is the most demanding intervention in this disease. Although the family of a child or adolescent with muscular dystrophy will have many problems to deal with, the nurse can help allay fears, anxieties and misunderstandings of the disease through teaching, active listening and coordination of the patient's care.

Teaching parents and patients the importance of exercise and the danger of immobility promotes a more positive attitude toward the disease. Knowing that they have a role and can participate in therapy often provides the stimulus needed for parents to become involved in their child's care, reducing anxieties or fears. The parents' role in helping build their child's self-esteem aids immeasurably in reinforcing his attitude of cooperation in maintaining an exercise program.

In addition to teaching, assessment of the home environment for possible problems is important. Provision of equipment that may assist in therapy and assisting the family in solving everyday practical problems that arise when a child is handicapped are essential. Such help may range from aiding parents in determining the best way to alter a stairway to accommodate a wheelchair to helping them modify the patient's environment to encourage his independence. Children with muscular dystrophy encounter difficulty dressing, bathing and eating which must be modified to help the child and the adolescent gain fullest potential.

Parents should be strongly encouraged to register with the Muscular Dystrophy Association since the association has a number of services to offer patients and their families. Providing information on camp programs and parent groups will help parents lead less isolated social lives.

Dermatomyositis

Dermatomyositis is a multisystem disease producing inflammatory involvement of the muscles during the childhood years and is often difficult to differentiate from muscular dystrophy. It is characterized by low-grade fever, fatigue, red indurated skin lesions over cheekbones and nose, weakness of proximal limbs and trunk muscles, loss of reflexes, and pain. The course of the disease is variable, with muscle weakness beginning in neck, thighs and shoulder girdle and developing slowly or quickly, with varying degrees of severity. The disease has an unknown etiology, affects females more than males, and has an onset generally after two years of life. If untreated, death results in approximately 40 per cent of the cases; however, if treatment with corticosteroids is instituted within six months of the onset, pain is diminished and muscle function improves.[9] Physical therapy is used to promote muscle strength and prevent contractures.

Cystic Fibrosis

Definition and Incidence Cystic fibrosis (CF) is the most common fatal genetic disease in Caucasians. It is estimated to affect 1 in 1600 to 2000 newborns, occurring in males and females with equal frequency. Seven to 25 per cent of children with cystic fibrosis present symptoms as early as the newborn period with "meconium ileus." The remaining children may show onset as early as the first few months of life with recurrent respiratory infections that usually receive differential diagnosis. The life span of children with cystic fibrosis continues to increase. The average age of death in the 1940's was one year of age; however, with the advent of antibiotics and various modes of treatment, these children are now living to adolescence and early adulthood. Affected males generally outlive females six to one by twenty years of age.[4]

Etiology Cystic fibrosis is transmitted by the autosomal recessive mode of inheritance. Ap-

Some adolescents with irreversible alterations in health are able to participate in recreational activities with special facilities and counselling, such as this summer camp for teenagers with muscular dystrophy. (Courtesy of Muscular Dystrophy Association—National Office, New York.)

proximately one in 20 to 25 people carry the gene for this disease. Presently there is no means of detecting carrier status or the disease in utero. It can be recognized in the newborn in 80 per cent of children by screening for increased albumin content (greater than 20 mg per cent) in the stool. Although this is not a routine practice, it seems reasonable to detect such a serious condition as cystic fibrosis early, since early diagnosis and therapy appear to reduce morbidity and increase the length and quality of life.

Pathophysiology The exact cause of cystic fibrosis is unclear; however, it is generally believed to involve a generalized dysfunction of the exocrine (mucus-producing) glands with varying degrees of severity. The basic problem is thought to occur at the cellular level, reflecting an alteration in a protein, possibly an enzyme, primarily affecting epithelial tissues. The organs most commonly affected are the lungs, sweat glands, paranasal sinuses, salivary glands, pancreas, liver, intestine, reproductive tract and tear glands. Although the lungs are not exocrine glands, they are composed largely of epithelial cells.

Research with conflicting results has made it difficult to separate the primary and secondary effects of the disease. There do appear to be several functions disturbed in the affected cells, which give rise to the clinical features of the disease. These include an increased amount and viscosity of mucus, elevation of sweat electrolytes, defect in autonomic nervous system function, abnormal substances in sweat and saliva affecting the function of exocrine glands, and possibly an inability to metabolize vitamin A or lipids.

The primary factor that is responsible for the clinical manifestations of the disease is the production of increased amounts of thick mucus that causes obstructions in lungs, sinuses, pancreas, intestine and sweat glands. Instead of producing thin-flowing fluid, the glands produce a thick, tenacious mucus that causes obstruction mainly in the pancreatic ducts and bronchi. The ducts and secretory acini become dilated and the exocrine parenchyma undergoes secondary degeneration with progressive fibrosis. Because the pancreatic enzymes are unable to reach the duodenum, malabsorption results. The disturbance of this function is noted in excessive stool fat and protein content. In lung involvement, the bronchioles are obstructed first, followed by the main bronchi, resulting in chronic lung disease and progressing into emphysema due to obstructive overinflation.

Signs and Symptoms Since the two main organ systems involved in the disease are the respiratory and gastrointestinal tract, the presenting signs and symptoms generally result in complications of these systems. Symptoms of the disease are variable, differing in degree of severity; in fact, many are not readily apparent until quite late in life. The most common presenting signs are poor weight gain with excessive appetite, persistent coughing with excessive mucus, and wheezing. Additional signs are salty taste of skin, nasal polyps and bulky, foul-smelling stools.

Most children who are affected have a history of chronic pulmonary disease with onset as early as birth, but their condition is often not diagnosed for years. Initial symptoms include a dry, nonproductive cough, followed by obstruction of bronchioles resulting in secondary infection and respiratory distress. As the thick, tenacious mucus accumulates, the flow of air is impaired, with subsequent decrease in the vital capacity of the lungs and an increased residual volume causing obstruction and dilatation. As the disease progresses, the functioning alveoli are overaerated. This causes the chest to distend, resulting in the barrel-shaped chest. If ventilation is significantly impaired, clubbing of the fingers and toes and cyanosis is observed.

Pancreatic involvement is apparent in approximately 85 per cent of children with cystic fibrosis. The earliest clinical manifestation, "meconium ileus," may be apparent at birth. Signs of this are intestinal obstruction, including abdominal distention, dehydration, absence of stools and vomiting. As cystic fibrosis progresses, children have a markedly impaired ability to digest food because the pancreas is unable to secrete the enzymes. The pancreas itself shows dilation of ducts and, in later stages, diffuse fibrosis with leukocytic infiltration. Causes of malabsorption include obstruction of the pancreatic ducts and absence of the enzymes necessary for conversion of food into products that can be absorbed by the intestines. Since the enzymes (trypsin, lipase and amylase) capable of breaking down fats and proteins are absent, the child characteristically has large, loose, foul-smelling stools in normal frequency and appears undernourished (distended abdomen and thin extremities). These, coupled with the child's excessive appetite, are often the initial signs that cause parents to seek care.

Diagnosis At least two of the following four diagnostic criteria are required in order to confirm a diagnosis of cystic fibrosis: (1) a positive sweat test, (2) presence of chronic lung disease, (3) pancreative insufficiency and (4) family history of the disease.[11] The sweat test is believed to be the most reliable (98 per cent) diagnostic test and a diagnosis is rarely made without it. The sweat test involves a painless collection of sweat from the forearm of the child. To assure an accurate test, it is strongly recommended that the test be done in a medical center that performs a large number of these tests each year. Measurements of sodium and chloride levels above 60 mEq/L are considered diagnostic, levels between 45 and 60 mEq/L are considered suggestive. Children with the latter should have the test repeated. Two positive sweat tests, especially when accompanied by other symptoms, confirms the diagnosis.[14] The diagnosis in a family should alert the physician to have sweat tests performed on all siblings.

In addition to the sweat test, chest x-rays confirm chronic lung disease with emphysema. Pulmonary function studies reveal decreased vital capacity and tidal volume, increased airway resistance and decreased forced expiratory volume due to recurrent bronchial infections.[5] To determine pancreatic involvement, stool studies for trypsin and fat content are undertaken. (The stool sample must be fresh or one that was frozen immediately.) Trypsin is absent in over 80 per cent of the cases and up to 30 mg of fat may be excreted when the pancreas is affected.

Although the diagnostic tests are not traumatic, the child and parents need to have a thorough explanation of the procedure and equipment involved. In the case of the sweat test, a small electric current carrying the drug pilocarpine is placed on the forearm (thigh of infants) of the child to stimulate the sweat gland (iontophoresis). The sweat is then collected by filter paper. A simple explanation of the procedure and allowing the young child to handle the apparatus is helpful in alleviating anxieties.

There is no discomfort caused by the electrodes but the appearance of the apparatus may be frightening! Encouraging parents to be present during diagnostic procedures is supportive to the child.

Treatment Treatment for the child with cystic fibrosis is individualized and aimed at promoting an independent life as he matures and enters adolescence. Promotion of good nutrition, prevention of pulmonary infection, and a healthy psychosocial adjustment to the disease by the child and family is mandatory. A variety of treatments are used to deter the disease.

Physiotherapy plays an important role in the treatment of the patient with cystic fibrosis. It begins at the time of diagnosis, regardless of the child's age or condition. Therapy consists of postural drainage, breathing exercises, postural correction, hydrotherapy, inhalation therapy, pulmonary function testing and the support, teaching and encouragement of the family.[8]

The purpose of pulmonary therapy and breathing exercises is to maintain good pulmonary hygiene. Postural drainage is a method of draining the lungs by placing the patient in various positions. Postural drainage is carried out two to four times daily prophylactically and more often during acute infections or bed rest. Parents and patient (when appropriate for age) must be taught how to carry out postural drainage since it must be done every day. The entire procedure takes approximately one hour a day. Breathing exercises help the patient with cystic fibrosis aerate his lungs to their maximum capacity. In the young child, the exercises take on the form of a game, such as blowing soap bubbles or blowing out candles. Older children are encouraged to place their hands over the upper and lower portion of their chest to feel movement as they inhale and exhale. These exercises are carried out daily before, after or during postural drainage.

Children with a chronic chest condition frequently develop poor posture. Daily exercises that help in maintaining good posture include back extension, shoulder exercises and standing erect against a wall.[8] Another important part of therapy for the cystic child is swimming or hydrotherapy. This type of exercise helps build the muscles of respiration while encouraging good breathing habits. Children and adolescents should be encouraged to participate in sports and activities that promote good breathing habits.

tibiotic therapy only if there is an infection, others use it prophylactically. If used prophylactically, different antibiotics are given in rotation to prevent drug resistance. During acute infections, when the mucus becomes highly viscous and difficult to expectorate, mucolytic drugs are provided via inhalation to thin out bronchiole secretions. Expectorants, particularly the iodides, are most frequently used.

Diet and gastrointestinal considerations are also important in the management of CF. The underlying problem in children with cystic fibrosis is the inability of the pancreas to produce sufficient amounts of the enzymes needed to digest protein, fat and carbohydrates adequately.[12] Treatment consists of pancreatic enzyme replacement to promote growth, adequate nutrition and normal bowel movements. A tablet or powdered form of animal pancreatic enzymes is taken orally at each meal. The amount of extract will vary with the child's diet, activity level, number of bowel movements per day and type of stools. Since each enzyme unit aids in the digestion of specific amounts of protein, fat or carbohydrates, the number taken daily will vary. It is not unusual for an active teenager to require from 80 to 100 tablets a day. Since the enzymes are specific and only partially replace normal pancreatic function, a low-fat, high protein, high calorie diet may be prescribed to promote weight gain and digestion of foods. Although this is the most accepted dietary plan, many cystic fibrosis centers are promoting the elimination of all dietary restrictions. The rationale is to provide a better psychological adjustment for the children, especially for those who are at an age when peer relationships and independence are important. The suggested alternative is to increase enzymes to match intake. Experience has shown that older children are able to determine for themselves what their systems can best handle and decide what needs to be eliminated. Due to the severe fat malabsorption, supplements of lipo-soluble vitamins in water-miscible liquid are given daily in twice the recommended daily allowance. Patients are encouraged to use salt generously, since salt depletion through perspiring is a danger. During hot weather supplemental salt tablets should be given orally to prevent heat exhaustion.

Emotional adjustment to the diagnosis is often overwhelmingly difficult. The thought of

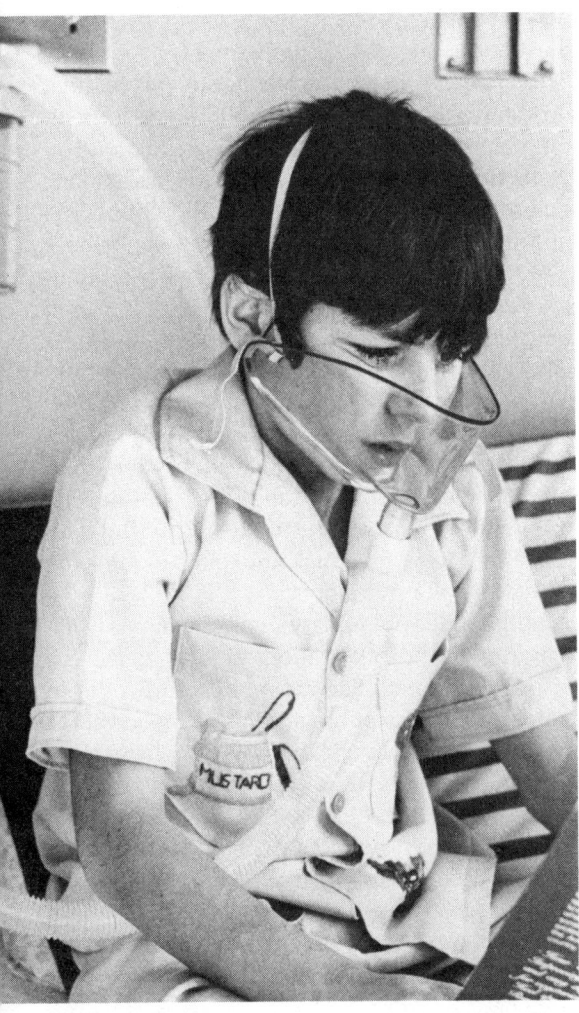

An adolescent boy with cystic fibrosis undergoes inhalation therapy. His disease is responsible for his slight build (4'7" and 62 pounds at age 15). Because of his size and breathing limitations he cannot participate in some active sports, but he attends school full time and takes part in many school and church activities. He is a responsible, active participant in his own care program, which includes daily postural drainage and medications and percussion and antibiotics during lung infections. (Courtesy Cystic Fibrosis Foundation, 6000 Executive Blvd., Suite 309, Rockville, MD 20852.)

Inhalation therapy is used to liquefy mucus and to prevent and treat infections. Prior to postural drainage, moist air is provided via inhalation to loosen bronchial secretions, aiding in their evacuation. Inhalation therapy is administered by a nebulizer or mist therapy. If given prior to postural drainage, it aids in breaking up the mucus so that the cilia can clear it from the lungs. Pulmonary function tests may be carried out routinely to provide the physician with information regarding the functioning of the lungs and therapy needed.

The use of antibiotics as a preventive measure is controversial. Many physicians prescribe ana potentially fatal illness stimulates an acute anticipatory mourning reaction in family members, including feelings of denial, avoidance, shock and disbelief, followed by information seeking. Anger is also a common manifestation of this stage, since parents see the doctor as having failed in not diagnosing the condition earlier. Often parents who have "known something was wrong" express ambivalent feelings about the diagnosis. They experience shock and guilt over learning the poor prognosis but are relieved to finally have a diagnosis for their child's chronic condition.[10]

At the time the parents are informed of the diagnosis the nurse should make every effort to be with them to clarify it and to provide support because the response and understanding of parents at this early phase can have long-lasting effects on the child's perception of himself and his illness. Parents specifically need careful explanation of the disease, information regarding the therapy involved, and additional support because they have not only been faced with the fatal outcome of the disease but also the treatment for which they must assume full responsibility. It is also necessary to recognize that the ability of many parents to take in information regarding the disease during this early stage is limited. Reiteration and provision of written material is important.

Counselling should also begin at the time of diagnosis. A common response of parents is to become overprotective, creating anxiety and poor self-image in the child. Knowing that children with cystic fibrosis are now living to adult life aids in decreasing parents' feelings of hopelessness and their inclination to avoid overprotectiveness.

Hospitalization Hospitalized children with cystic fibrosis have many special needs. Special care must be given to cleanliness of the perianal area. Frequency and characteristics of the stools are recorded to aid in enzyme replacement. The child's respiratory functioning is assessed frequently to identify lung complications.

Preparation for discharge includes teaching the parents and child how to carry out postural drainage, how to provide inhalation therapy by nebulizer and how to give enzymes at home. To teach postural drainage correctly, it is necessary to demonstrate through pictures and to have parents practice. (See Chapter 17 for illustrations of postural drainage.)

Intercurrent infection may result in frequent hospitalizations for these children. All treatments must be continued with an increase in the amount of percussion and postural drainage due to the decreased activity of the child. One of the most difficult infections to treat in these children is the *Pseudomonas aeruginosa* organism because it is sensitive only to drugs that can be given intravenously. Treatment of this infection requires 10 to 14 days of intravenous carbenicillin. Mucolytic drugs may also be necessary in liquefying mucus during these periods of acute illness. During acute illness the child may become anorexic and the special diet usually taken may be restrictive. Ensuring adequate intake is essential and may require the assistance of a nutritionist.

Additional pulmonary complications that may require hospitalization include atelectasis or pneumothorax. Such complications result in sudden shortness of breath. While the former is treated by pulmonary therapy, the latter may require insertion of a chest drain to allow pleural air to escape. Most patients with cystic fibrosis die from pulmonary complications. The clinical picture is known as cor pulmonale; in this, progressive hypoxemia strains the right ventricle causing failure and the development of congestive heart failure.[12]

Home Management Research has shown that parents who take an active part in their child's therapy show more positive acceptance and adjustment to the child's long-term, fatal illness.

Care of the sick child at home, while demanding of a parent's time and energy, may also be very satisfying. The initial stage of care following diagnosis seems to present the most problems for parents, since they are attempting to learn as much as they can about their child's disease and their responsibilities for his care. At the same time, it is not unusual for the child to rebel against changes in diet and the interference of his routines and playtimes for postural drainage.

Coordination of follow-up care for the family is crucial. Although the outpatient clinic looms significantly in the life of this child, home care is equally important. Visits by public health nurses should be made during the first weeks to assist the family in any immediate problems and to assess the environment, which may need modification for the patient. Guidelines that may assist in assessing the frequency of visits include the degree of parental anxiety with equipment, therapy and diagnosis; problems with basic management, deterioration of the child's condition; or clinic absenteeism.[2] Direct contact between the community health nurse, clinic nurse and hospital nursing staff is essential in assuring that parents are not stressed and confused by conflicting advice. Information on community services available and sources to contact for services is an integral part of home care.

References

1. K. Bakke. Nursing considerations for the adolescent osteosarcoma patient with amputation. Oncology Nursing Society Forum, October 1978, p. 14
2. M. Buchanan. Pediatric hospital and home care: easing parent's problems. Part 2. Nursing Times, 17 March 1977, p. 39
3. R. Caughill, ed. The Dying Patient: A Supportive Approach. Little, Brown & Co., 1976
4. S. Giammona. BDIS: Birth defect imformation retrieval system. RELI. 1 (National Foundation March of Dimes), Cystic Fibrosis No. 237, 1979
5. J. Jacobs. Cystic fibrosis as it affects the patient and family. Respiratory Therapy, Nov/Dec 1977, p. 52
6. N. Jaffee et al. Integrated multidisciplinary treatment for pediatric solid tumors. In Cancer: A manual for Practitioners by the American Cancer Society, Massachusetts Division 1978, p. 279
7. P. Jones and P. Campbell, eds. Tumours of Infancy and Childhood. J.B. Lippincott Co., 1976
8. B. Mallinson. Seven rules of physiotherapy, Part 3. Nursing Mirror, 24 August 1978, p. 18
9. J. Menkes. Textbook of Child Neurology. Lea and Febiger, 1974
10. C. Mikkelson et al. Cystic fibrosis: a family challenge. Children Today, Jul/Aug 1978, p. 22
11. L. Morris et al. Cystic fibrosis: making a correct and early diagnosis. Journal of Family Practice, April 1978, p. 754
12. B. Phillips. Cystic fibrosis. The challenge in research and management. Part 1. Nursing Mirror, 24 August 1978, p. 13
13. G. Sahakian. Management of Hodgkin's and non-Hodgkin's lymphomas. Medical Clinics of North America, March 1975, p. 387
14. J. Selekeman. Cystic fibrosis: what is involved in the home treatment program for children, adolescents and young adults. Pediatric Nurse Mar/Apr 1977, p. 32
15. A. Skarin et al. Malignant lymphomas. In Cancer: A Manual for Practitioners by the American Cancer Society, Massachusetts Division, 1978, p. 249
16. S. Smith et al. A reliable method for evaluating drug compliance in children with cancer. Cancer, January 1979, p. 169
17. H. Suit et al. Sarcomas of bone and soft tissue. In Cancer: A Manual for Practitioners by the American Cancer Society, Massachusetts Division, 1978, p. 239

Additional Recommended Reading

The Dying Adolescent

J. Benoliel and R. McCorkle. A holistic approach to terminal illness. Cancer Nursing. April 1978, p. 143

W. Easson. The family of the dying child. Pediatric Clinics of North America, November 1972, p. 1157
E. Erikson. Identity, Youth and Crisis. Norton Books, 1968
D. Fochtman. How adolescents live wilh leukemia. Cancer Nursing, February 1979, p. 27
S. Sontag. Illness as Metaphor. Farrar, Straus & Giroux, Inc., 1978
J. Schowalter et al. The adolescent patient's decision to die. Pediatrics, January 1973, p. 97.

Bone Tumors

M. Akahoski. High-dose methotrexate with leucovorin rescue. Cancer Nursing, August 1978, p. 319
R. Chan et al. Management and results of localized Ewing's sarcoma. Cancer, March 1979, p. 1001
P. Chang. Progress in the treatment of osteosarcoma. Medical Clinics of North America, September 1977, p. 1027
J. Clausen. Cancer diagnosis in children: cultural factors influencing parent-child reactions. Cancer Nursing, October 1978, p. 395
S. Greer. Psychological consequences of cancer. The Practitioner, February 1979, p. 173
I. Hall, ed. Medical and Pediatric Oncology. Alan R. Liss, Inc., 1978
P. Hetzel et al. Overall principles of cancer management Part IV, chemotherapy. In Cancer: A Manual for Practitioners by the American Cancer Society, Massachusetts Division, 1978
N. Jaffee. Current concepts in the management of disseminated malignant bone disease in childhood. Canadian Journal of Surgery, November 1977, p. 537
R. Jenkin. Radiation treatment of Ewing's sarcoma and osteogenic sarcoma. Canadian Journal of Surgery, November 1977, p. 530
M. Kjosness and L. Rudolph, eds. Thoughts of Young People with Cancer. Division of Hematology/Oncology of The Children's Orthopedic Hospital and Medical Center (Seattle, WA), 1978
N. Lovejoy. Preventing hair loss during adriamycin therapy. Cancer Nursing, April 1979, p. 117
M. Myers et al. Cancer incidence survival and mortality for children under 15 years of age. Professional Education Publication, American Cancer Society, 1976
C. Pratt. Management of malignant solid tumors in children. Pediatric Clinics of North America, November 1972, p. 1141
N. Schroper. Psychosocial aspects of management of the patient with cancer. Medical Clinics of North America, September 1977, p. 1147
D. Smith et al. Nursing care of patients undergoing combination chemotherapy and radiotherapy. Cancer Nursing, April 1978, p. 129

Hodgkin's Disease

V. DeVita, Jr. et al. The chemotherapy of Hodgkin's disease. Cancer, August Supplement 1978, p. 979
D. Girvan. Staging laparotomy for Hodgkin's disease in children. Canadian Journal of Surgery, September 1978, p. 409
S. Hellman et al. The place of radiation therapy in the treatment of Hodgkin's disease. Cancer, August Supplement 1978, p. 971
M. Keaveny and L. Wiley. Hodgkin's disease — the curable cancer. Nursing 75, March 1975, p. 48
S. Rosenberg et al. Combines modality therapy of Hodgkin's disease: a report of the Stanford trials. Cancer, August Supplement 1978, p. 991

D. Siveet et al. Hodgkin's disease: problems of staging. Cancer, August Supplement 1978, p. 957

R. Young. Patterns of relapse in advanced Hodgkin's disease treated with combination chemotherapy. Cancer, August Supplement 1978, p. 1001

Muscular Dystrophy and Dermatomyositis

B. Conway. Pediatric Neurologic Nursing. C. V. Mosby Co., 1977

J. Cotterill et al. Dermatomyositis after immunization. Lancet, 25 November 1978, p. 1158

T. Furakawa et al. X-linked muscular dystrophy. Annals of Neurology, November 1977, p. 414

D. Gardner-Medivin. Muscular dystrophy: can it be prevented? Nursing Times, 31 August 1978, p. 1441

L. Garibaldi et al. Clinical and therapeutic aspects of dermatomyositis in childhood. Minerva Pediatrics, 30 November 1978, p. 1793

N. Karagan et al. Early verbal disability in children with Duchenne muscular dystrophy. Developmental Medicine and Child Neurology, August 1978, p. 435

M. McGaughlin et al. The family with muscular dystrophy. Journal of Practical Nursing, August 1976, p. 14

R. McKeran. The muscular dystrophies. Nursing Times, 30 September 1978, p. 1515

N. Pickard et al. Systemic membrane deficit in the proximal muscular dystrophies. New England Journal of Medicine, 19 October 1978, p. 841

M. Roses et al. Evaluation and detection of Duchenne's and Becker's muscular dystrophy carries by manual muscle testing. Neurology, January 1977, p. 20

M. Zatz. Diagnosis, carrier detection and genetic counseling in the muscular dystrophies. Pediatric Clinics of North America, August 1978, p. 557

Cystic Fibrosis

R. Bonforte. Variability in cystic fibrosis. Journal of American Medical Association, 20 October 1978, p. 1855

I. Boyle et al. Emotional adjustment of adolescents and young adults with cystic fibrosis. Journal of Pediatrics, February 1976, p. 328

J. Duberly et al. The nurse teacher and carer for mother and child, Part 2. Nursing Mirror, 24 August 1978, p. 13

D. Garrison. Parents' understanding of genetic risk data in genetic counseling. Journal of the American Medical Association, 8 December 1978, p. 2631

S. Johnson. High-Risk Parenting. J.B. Lippincott Co., 1979

P. Liberi. Cystic fibrosis. Nursing Care, December 1977, p. 22

J. Littlewood. Neonatal screening: the present position. Midwives Chronicle, May 1977, p. 91

A. Norman. Cystic fibrosis. Nursing Times, 18 November 1976, p. 1804

M. Phinney. Review of cystic fibrosis. Comprehensive Pediatric Nursing, August 1978, p. 54

D. Quinton. Fact Sheet: For Young Adults and Adults With Cystic Fibrosis. Cystic Fibrosis Foundation, March 1975

J. Ritchie. Nursing the child undergoing limb amputation. American Journal of Maternal Child Nursing, Mar/Apr 1980, p. 114.

G. Russell. Cystic fibrosis: clinical aspects, Part 1. Nursing Times, 23 March 1978, p. 846.

G. Russell. Cystic fibrosis: genetic and social aspects. Part 2. Nursing Times, 23 March 1978, p. 846.

THE HOSPITALIZED ADOLESCENT

by Sandra Merkel, RN, MSN

Adolescence has been described as a period of transition, a period in which society has authorized a delay of adulthood. This authorization grants time for the person to integrate all the changes required to move from childhood to adulthood. Illness and hospitalization pose threats to the adolescent's accomplishment of this transition. Critical to an understanding of the impact of illness or hospitalization in this age group is a knowledge of the major issues or developmental tasks of the period.

A definition of adolescence by age is somewhat arbitrary, since adolescence can begin and end at different ages for different people. The adolescent period is characterized by profound biological and psychosocial changes. The biological changes of rapid skeletal growth and reproductive development begin sometime before the teen years (10 to 12 years old). Around the ages of 12 to 13 years the young person looks to peers and explores different adult roles in defining his personality. These movements away from home signal the beginning of psychosocial changes from childhood. The culmination of adolescence occurs at 18 to 23 years with the emergence of an independent adult. To assume the adult role the adolescent must become emancipated from his parents, define his role and answer the question "Who am I?"

EMANCIPATION

Emancipation is achieved by separating the close and dependent ties to parents. This independence and the establishment of inner controls cannot be completed without some degree of frustration, rejection and anger. As the adolescent tries out independence, opposition to the rules and ideas of parents is normal. Parents and adults are often frustrated with these attempts of independence because they no longer are able to exert the same amount of control as with a younger child. Emancipation is a gradual process that requires adults to tolerate this testing while still providing attention and limits for the adolescent.

ROLE DEFINITION

To establish a meaningful role in society the adolescent must use his mind to develop inner controls and a moral code. Not only must he stand alone in the environment, he also needs to develop meaningful relationships with the opposite sex.

The ability for abstract thinking develops at about age 12, allowing the adolescent to interpret observations and develop concepts. The adolescent enjoys acquiring new information and often engages in long discussions about the world. This intellectual ability permits the adolescent to perceive the present and future implications of illness. He can be expected to participate in decisions related to hospital treatment. The development of a sense of self-esteem encourages the achievement of sexual identity. One of the adolescent's primary concerns is physical appearance and attractiveness to the opposite sex. Threats to his body image, which is a person's way of perceiving his physical appearance, may diminish self-esteem and sexual identity. During the process of deciding upon a career or vocation the adolescent explores adult roles. Often adults other than parents are cast as idealized role models. The model is perceived as a perfect hero or heroine. Health professionals, especially if a young adolescent is hospitalized, may be seen as the perfect friend or surrogate parent.

ADOLESCENT DEVELOPMENT APPLIED DURING HOSPITALIZATION

In order to provide nursing interventions to an ill adolescent, the developmental level and physical status of the individual must be determined. A nursing assessment provides a framework for the care plan. The nursing focus can be that of merging what is known about the present physical and emotional status with the adolescent's developmental competencies and needs for future growth. A division of adolescence into three phases is beneficial in remembering the developmental issues of this period: early adolescence (12 to 14 years), middle adolescence (14 to 18) and later adolescence (18 to 21). Characteristics of these divisions are listed in Table 63–1.

When an adolescent is admitted to the hospital, the admission assessment and interview lay the foundation for his hospital experience. Subject to the nature of the illness and stability of the patient, he needs to be introduced to the hospital environment and the people around him. A tour of the unit and a brief explanation of the routine is a good way to begin to establish a relationship. The assessment and interview should be carried out in privacy in a separate room. Most adolescents express themselves better if separated from their parents. The parents can be interviewed later and then explanations of what to expect can be given to the family as a unit.

Hospital Admission Assessment

A framework or guideline for the admission assessment is useful when organizing questions and data. Three major areas to consider for the

TABLE 63-1 CHARACTERISTICS OF THREE DIVISIONS OF ADOLESCENCE

Early Adolescence (12-14 Years)
1. Puberty development is advanced.
2. Body-image issues are dealt with.
3. The individual is concerned with physical status.
4. Relationships are formed with persons of same gender and later with members of the opposite sex.
5. Long periods are spent away from home.
6. The individual is willing to be accountable to parents.

Middle Adolescence (14-18 Years)
1. Physical growth is nearly complete.
2. Independence conflicts are at a peak.
3. Group dating progresses to steady dating of one individual.
4. The individual may be attractive to the opposite sex but egocentric.
5. The peer group is the social monitor.
6. The individual rejects parental controls but depends upon them.

Later Adolescence (18-21 Years)
1. A role in the community is defined.
2. Nearly all decisions are made independently.
3. The individual requests family input but makes own decision.
4. Relationships with the opposite sex involve mutual concern and sharing.

adolescent patient are physical status, learning and thought ability, and family and social patterns.

After the adolescent is asked to describe his illness or reason for hospitalization, each of the functional body systems is assessed for problems. All body systems of an adolescent can be expected to be at optimal, or peak, performance. A thorough reproductive assessment is indicated for the adolescent in order to determine if he has undergone puberty and to assess his knowledge of reproduction and his health habits in general. Questions about sexual activity and birth control are often more easily handled when talking about social interactions and dating. Changes in body odor occur during adolescence and create special hygiene needs, so information should be collected about the condition of skin and teeth and about cleanliness practices. The assessment of learning ability is necessary to identify educational needs and plan health education. Questions about school, grades, solving problems and what is fun to learn will provide information in this area.

The social assessment includes learning about the adolescent's friendships with peers as well as family relationships. Answers to questions about hobbies, group activities, sports and people who give support and about experimentation with drugs will provide information on the degree of role definition accomplished. Questions as well as observations about parents' interaction with the adolescent will help in assessment of the adolescent's relationships with his parents. Finally, discussions about religion, occupational decisions and relationships with other adults may complete the admission assessment. The understanding conveyed by the nurse during this assessment will assist in alleviating some of the adolescent's anxiety about being in the hospital. It will also provide some understanding of how the adolescent views his illness.

IMPACT OF ILLNESS

Since adolescents are narcissistic about their bodies, any illness may be a threat to body image. The adolescent's body image will play a role in how he reacts to the illness. Disfigurement, loss of function or a change in appearance is especially difficult for the adolescent to handle. He must learn to accept and work with a new and different body. An appropriate nursing intervention when the body image is threatened is to encourage talking about the adolescent's feelings and fears regarding the changes or loss of body function (Table 63–2). From this verbalization the nurse gains understanding of what the adolescent sees as a threat and what he perceives will happen. Nursing action after this would include identifying and reinforcing the adolescent's strengths while including flexible visiting hours, availability of a telephone, and encouraging letter writing to help maintain relationships with supportive peers and siblings. When the adolescent's own peers are not available to him during hospitalization, he should be provided with options for relationships within a new peer group of other hospitalized adolescents. Teen meetings on the unit, a room structured for adolescent group activities, and group recreation or entertainment activities provide opportunities for the hospitalized adolescents on the unit to establish peer relationships and mutual support.

The age at which illness or hospitalization occurs is significant because of the wide variance in development between 12 and 21 years of age. The early adolescent is less overwhelmed by enforced dependency and allows his parents to act on his behalf. The major concern for this age group is physical appearance, function and mobility. Illness or hospitalization or both are least well tolerated by the adolescent in the middle years (14 to 18). The dependency and decreased control of life occurring as a result of hospitalization are in conflict with the drive for independence. The late adolescent usually uses the family for support and can tolerate some dependency. The main threat in the older teen is that illness poses a potential blocking of career goals and life style.

In addition to the age of onset, the nature of the illness may influence how the adolescent reacts to hospitalization and treatment. The adolescent has the mental capabilities to make distinctions between short-term illnesses and permanent changes in his body. A long-term or chronic illness, especially if disabling, may create limitations in the amount of achieved independence. The degree of conflict between a chronic illness and freedom depends upon how the adolescent has integrated the illness into his life style. When a chronic illness has begun in early childhood, special care requirements often have been incorporated into the family structure. Parents may attempt to relieve feelings of guilt or anger by providing close monitoring of the illness or by giving special attention and privileges to the child. In this case the parents create additional problems for the adolescent by promoting dependency and blocking the road to emancipation. The adolescent patient may also take advantage of his family by using the illness to secure privileges and attention.

Whether the illness is of a chronic or an acute nature, the adolescent is concerned with death. His concept of death approximates that of an adult; he perceives the irreversibility of death. The impact of dying is particularly difficult for the adolescent, for he is aware of losing everything just before or just as he achieves adult status and an answer to the question "Who am I?" He may also mourn the things he will never be able to achieve, such as the experience of attending college and of marriage and children. Because adolescents think about death, it is essential that they be told the nature of their illness. This explanation should be given by the physician in terms that the young person can understand. Prospects for treatment and expect-

TABLE 63-2 DEVELOPMENTAL ISSUES OF ADOLESCENTS AND NURSING INTERVENTIONS

Developmental Issues	Interventions
A. Physical	The nurse may provide:
1. Rapid skeletal growth	1. a. Nutritional information on diet, snacks, weight control b. Dietitian referral to assist with special dietary needs c. Health information to assist adolescent in forming health habits d. Information on hygiene measures; means of bathing
2. Puberty	2. a. Information on the reproductive system b. Answers to questions about reproductive function c. Information on preventive health maintenance, breast examination, birth control
3. Decreased tolerance to dependency, immobility and pain	3. a. Assistance to move out of bed and around the unit b. Mechanisms for expression of frustration c. Recreation activities d. Physical and occupational therapy to increase independence, muscle strength and mobility e. Permissions for temporary leaves from hospital f. Prompt administration of pain medication with thorough explanation of pain and analgesic
B. Cognitive	
4. Anxiety from fear of unknown or due to misinformation	4. a. Orientation to environment, routines and expectations b. Thorough explanation and preparation for procedures and instructions c. Use of scientific terminology d. Discharge preparation e. Public health nurse referral f. The keeping of promises
5. Interruption of schooling or change in career goals	5. a. Opportunity to complete school work b. Use of school teachers in health plans c. Reinforcement of realistic career goals
C. Emotional-social	
6. Concerns about body image and sexuality	6. a. Encouragement of verbalization of fears and concerns b. Privacy c. Utilization of youth's own belongings and clothes d. Assistance with grooming needs (e.g., hair washing, nails) e. Compliments about youth's strengths
7. Rejects adult control—strives for independence	7. a. Encouragement of self-care b. Flexible limits c. Opportunities for adolescent to participate in setting goals, planning care and choosing options d. Opportunities for appropriate decisions and control e. Psychiatrist and social worker referral
8. Needs peer contact and approval	8. a. Opportunities for friends to visit and call b. Recreation activities that stimulate adolescents to gather c. Unit meetings for adolescents d. Passes to go home or to school or social functions e. Opportunities for appropriate calls to friends
9. Needs family support	9. a. Encouragement for parents to visit and stay when adolescent needs or wants them b. Opportunities for parent meetings for parents to discuss issues and get support c. Encouragement of sibling visits d. Support to maintain family unit e. Encouragement of chaplain visits f. Encouragement of use of appropriate community resources

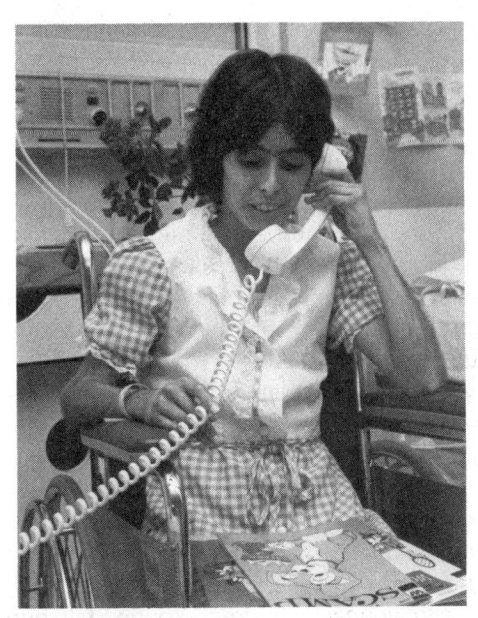

The hospitalized teen adjusts to her situation more easily if she has the means to maintain contact with her friends and family. (Courtesy of the Children's Hospital of Philadelphia.)

ed course should also be discussed. The nurse's role is to provide review, support and additional education as the adolescent needs it. The danger in not being honest or in not explaining to the adolescent is that, if left alone, he will use his fantasy thoughts in an effort to figure out what is happening.

A sudden or an acute illness can be devastating to the adolescent. Even though the illness and hospitalization may be short-term, they are restrictive, force dependency and interrupt mastery and control. The more time the adolescent is allowed for preparing and planning his absence from school and friends, the greater the degree of his acceptance of the restrictions of being hospitalized. Often the final football game or the class dance are more important than surgery. Consequently, a planned surgical procedure is often easier to accept than injuries sustained in an accident. Automobile accidents and trauma from accidents in general are frequent causes of hospitalization for the adolescent. The disfigurement, immobility and guilt, especially if a friend has died in the accident, may lead to feelings of helplessness and despair. This group of adolescents requires nursing interventions geared to their physical status, with a gradual increase in emphasis on the issues of returning to their family and friends. An adolescent in severe pain or acute physical distress wants help immediately. He does not tolerate pain or the wait for relief well. Prompt administration of analgesics and recognition of the adolescent's fear of losing control, or panic, are necessary nursing interventions.

IMPACT OF HOSPITALIZATION

No matter what the nature of the illness is, the experience of being hospitalized produces anxiety for the adolescent. Some of this anxiety can be attributed to internal factors such as thoughts about the effect of illness on the body. A large portion of anxiety can result from external factors. The adolescent has been removed from his family and friends and now is faced with a new environment in which he has little control. No longer can he lock himself in his room and play music, raid the refrigerator for a snack or talk for an hour on the telephone. Instead there are procedures and examinations that invade his privacy and body. Health professionals tell him what needs to be done; often he is not allowed to make independent decisions. Consequently the hospital environment accentuates his feelings of powerlessness and dependency. The adolescent is especially vulnerable to this loss of control. Horney explained how an anxious adolescent may cope with hospitalization, uti-

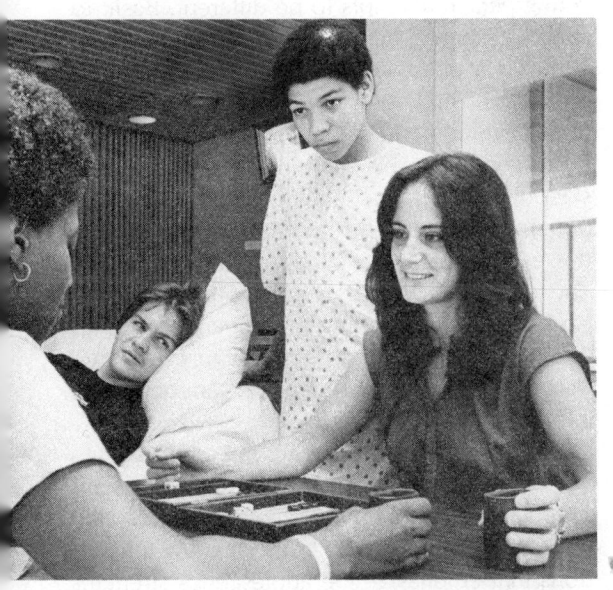

Teen activities on the hospital unit provide opportunities for establishing peer relationships and mutual support. (Courtesy of the Children's Hospital of Philadelphia.)

lizing three predominant patterns of response to other people.[1]

1. The adolescent may cope by moving toward people. In this way he accepts his helplessness and, in spite of his fears, tries to win the affection of others. By complying with the rules and treatments the adolescent does not feel isolated. He interacts and is friendly with all the patients on the unit.
2. He can also cope by moving against people. He is determined to fight and rebel. He does not trust others and wants to be strong and independent.
3. He may cope by moving away from people. He builds up a world of his own and keeps himself apart because he believes that people do not understand him.

Recognizing these response patterns may help the nurse to understand why one day an adolescent passively goes to a test while the next day he opposes all efforts of assistance. There are other reactions that relate directly to the individual adolescent's coping behaviors. Denial, projection and intellectualizing are common behaviors in the hospitalized adolescent.

Just as hospitalization is a crisis for the adolescent, it is a crisis for the parents. They have a natural concern for their son or daughter, but their ability to be supportive is influenced by their own past experiences and fears related to hospitals and illness. Parents may interpret the illness as their punishment for neglect of the child and so may feel guilty. They may see themselves as failures for not preventing the illness. Mothers may enjoy the nurturing role that is required when their adolescent is dependent, and then may find it difficult to return to the conflicts of independence that are inevitable when the adolescent is well. The adolescent may respond better to the staff nurse's requests than to the parents' requests; this may cause the parents to resent the nurse in her role as the primary caregiver. The parents and siblings may resent the time that must be spent and the changes made in normal routines that are required to provide support to the hospitalized adolescent. The amount of support available from and contact with their parents influences the amount of anxiety experienced by adolescents. Parents are often expected to be in control and supportive without any nursing intervention or assistance. The nurse should understand the role of parents, and consider and provide support for them when their adolescent requires hospitalization.

THE NURSE AND THE ADOLESCENT

At times, caring for the hospitalized adolescent and his family can be frustrating and demanding. The normal conflicts that can arise when an adolescent tests out independence, coupled with his possible nonadherence to treatment routine and hospital regulations, often cause anger and irritation among members of a nursing staff. The adolescent often uses the hospital unit as a stage, seeking attention by pranks, arguments and refusals. Just as parents lose control over their adolescent, with an adolescent the nursing staff members do not have control over bedtime, eating and waking as they do with younger children. Young staff nurses starting out in their profession may have difficulty with certain adolescents owing to overidentification with the youth. These nurses can see themselves facing death, separating from parents or being unsure about the future. One pitfall to avoid in working with youth is that of taking their side and being very critical of the parents' ability to care for and support the adolescent. This defending of the adolescent alienates parents and can make them feel inferior.

Working with adolescents and their parents requires tolerance and acceptance of unpredictable ideas and behaviors that occur when the young person attempts to be different. Basic to effective approaches with the adolescent and family is a philosophy that interactions should be based on an understanding of normal adolescent development. This normal development knowledge must be combined with an understanding of the impact of illness and hospitalization. In her relationship with the adolescent, the nurse must be honest, caring and respectful. The nurse can initiate a good relationship by explaining what is going to happen. This gives the adolescent some control because fear and misunderstanding can make anyone feel panic.

When the nurse encourages the adolescent to verbalize concerns, fears and questions, this produces an environment in which he can gain information and develop trust. Ongoing interactions that emphasize the adolescent's strengths while promoting realistic goals help him define his role and develop his identity. Arguments over nonadherence or lack of cooperation are

> I agree to do my range of motion exercises at 10:00 a.m., 2:00 p.m., and 8:00 p.m. The nurse will remind me one time.
>
> Date: _____
> Signatures: _Adolescent, Nurse_

A sample contract.

not effective or productive. The adolescent cannot answer questions such as "Why did you do that?" He does not know why, but he can explain how difficult it is to follow a treatment plan when what he really wants is freedom. Questions such as "How is it living with diabetes?" will get more information and will not result in an adult-adolescent clash. The adolescent needs to have some control over his environment. When health professionals allow him to make decisions and have some independence in treatment, the adolescent learns to be responsible. Rewards can be built into an adolescent treatment plan, by linking privileges to responsibilities.

In a hospital setting some limits are necessary. Appropriate boundaries need to be established, but they need to be flexible and communicated in an understanding manner instead of an authoritarian manner. Adolescents can be encouraged to do as much self-care as possible, but this does not decrease the nursing time they need. Thorough and scientific explanations of what is happening to them must be given. They also need to be cared for by those who are sensitive to their fears and conflicts.

Contracts often work well with adolescents because they encourage participation. A contract is an agreement between two parties that spells out expectations of each regarding a behavior or situation. A nurse and an adolescent can write out the treatment program outlining the adolescent's participation as well as the nurse's responsibilities. A contract can be as simple as an outline of things that need to be learned before going home. The adolescent agrees to learn them and the nurse and the adolescent agree upon a time when she will teach them. A contract can also be developed with specific rewards given for defined accomplishments. In drawing up a contract with an adolescent, the first step is to clarify goals. The adolescent needs to explain his goals and the things he is willing to do in meeting those goals. A sample contract is shown in the boxed text at the top of the page.

The mechanism of contracting allows the adolescent to exercise his right to choose as well as participate. This gives control to the adolescent and yet allows the nurse to set limits. One important element in a contract is that the goals or behaviors are achievable by both the adolescent and the nurse. Care must also be exercised so that compliance with a contract is seen as an accomplishment and not simply as obedience.

Discussions about school, friends and hobbies are effective approaches with the adolescent. Adolescents usually are eager to discuss numerous topics at length. These explorations and challenging conversations assist in the clarification of their values. The nurse is often seen as a person who may know some answers. Topics about reproduction may come up, and it is appropriate for the nurse to inform the adolescent that it is OK to ask questions in this area.

Just like procedures and treatments, medications need to be explained thoroughly to the adolescent. He should be told the name of a medication and reason for it being given. Alertness for side effects and knowing when to call the nurse or physician for help can be expected from the adolescent. If the adolescent understands the reasons for the medications he is more likely to participate while in the hospital and follow through at home.

An adolescent does not usually tolerate pain well; therefore, prompt administration of pain medications is required. Relief of pain and an explanation that addiction will not occur during the few days that an analgesic is needed will decrease his anxiety. Standard precautions involving medications such as taking the appropriate dose of the correct medication, using the correct method of administration and monitoring the effects of medication need to be explained to the adolescent, as with any hospitalized patient. If choices and decisions are possible, the nurse should allow the adolescent some control; if not, proper limits need to be implemented. Advance warning and preparation, especially about injections and IV's, are appreciated by the adolescent. The choice of intramuscular injection sites is similar to that for an adult, because the adolescent has adequate muscle tissue. Caution must be taken to assess the amount of tissue, especially in emaciated or small adolescents. Adolescents usually prefer the arm site if its use is possible. An injection in the thigh seems quite painful and use of the gluteus maximus is embarrassing. Establishing a rotation pattern, while giving the adolescent a choice, facilitates participation and acceptance.

In working with parents of the adolescent the nurse can serve as a model, showing and assisting the parents to help their child during dependency states and to allow freedom and control when dependency is not desirable. Parents are often intimidated by their adolescent's anger and anxiety. The nurse can explain the relationship between developmental issues and hospitalization. Parents usually do not volunteer information about problems with the family such as their own feelings of guilt and frustration, and sibling jealousy. Parents need to talk to the nurse and be given the opportunity to receive support instead of always being expected to be pillars of strength themselves.

SUMMARY

Adolescents are no longer children and yet they are not adults. Their needs are special and specific as they attempt to integrate all the changes that occur from the onset of puberty. Any interruption in the adolescent's efforts to stabilize and accomplish his developmental tasks represents additional stress upon the inherent process of obtaining independence and establishing an identity. Hospitalization places stress on the adolescent; the forced dependency of being ill is in absolute conflict with the need to be independent. The goal of health professionals who work with hospitalized adolescents is to support and assist them to return to the business of growing up and realizing the full potential of life.

References

1. B. Conway. The effects of hospitalization on adolescence. Adolescence, September 1971, p. 79
2. A. Hofman et al. The hospitalized adolescent. The Free Press, 1976

Additional Recommended Reading

A. Altshuler and A. Seidle. Teen meetings: a way to help adolescents cope with hospitalization. American Journal of Maternal Child Nursing, Nov/Dec 1977, p. 348

P. Blos. The child analyst looks at the young adolescent. In Twelve to Sixteen: Early Adolescence. W. W. Norton & Co., 1972

J. Forest. The contract and nursing practice. Nursing Papers, Summer 1975, p. 14

Guidelines for adolescent units. Developed by the Adolescent Care Study Section, Association for the Care of Children in Hospitals. Presented in Washington, D. C., June 1978

L. Jelneck. The special needs of the adolescent with chronic illness. American Journal of Maternal Child Nursing, June 1977, p. 57

E. Oremland and J. Oremland. How to care for the between-ages. Nursing 74, November 1974, p. 42

J. Schowalter and R. Lord. The hospitalized adolescent. Children, April 1971, p. 127

NURSING CARE PLAN

NURSING CARE PLAN FOR THE ADOLESCENT WITH MUSCULOSKELETAL ALTERATION

by Sandra Merkel

Nursing Diagnosis	Expected Outcome	Nursing Intervention	Rationale
Impaired mobility related to: • Congenital anomalies • Trauma • Inflammatory changes • Disease process • Disuse atrophy.	Adolescent will be independent in ambulation and activities of daily living within physical limitations with/without assistance.	Dx: 1. Observe for deformity, swelling, asymmetrical movement and posture. 2. Observe and measure joint motion and muscle strength. 3. Assess ability to carry out activities of daily living. 4. Assess ability to ambulate and move about bed. Tx: 1. Provide physical and occupational therapy referrals to assist with evaluation, provide treatment and adaptive equipment. 2. Range of motion – passive and/or active – to unaffected body parts. 3. Exercise of affected areas when ordered by physician. 4. Utilize adaptive equipment (overhead trapeze, splints, extenders) to encourage patient to improve movement. 5. Administer medication as ordered. 6. Position for comfort and prevention of complications.	Dx: 1–4. Thorough assessment is necessary to determine level of mobility and independence. Objective data provide baseline to measure changes and plan nursing care. Tx: 1. Use expertise of health team. Nurse assumes a coordinating role because of her knowledge of patient and his family. 2–3. Disuse of muscles may result in atrophy. The adolescent's participation in exercises gives him a part in his recovery. 4. Adaptive equipment facilitates self-help and mobility, important to the adolescent. 5. Medication may promote recovery of function or reduce spasm or pain that limits movement. 6. Proper positioning provides support to affected areas and relief of discomfort while preventing contractures.

Adolescent will have an opportunity to verbalize effects of impaired mobility in his life.	7. Encourage and praise ability and attempts at self-help and mobility. 8. Encourage verbalization of anger/frustration related to dependency and impaired mobility. 9. Arrange personal belongings, supplies and appropriate items within patient's reach. 10. Assist as needed with activities, hygiene, eating and mobility. 11. Maintain immobilizing equipment: traction, casts, splints and braces.	7-8. The adolescent's cognitive level and egocentric focus make him responsive to verbal reinforcement and capable of putting his feelings and needs into words. Verbalization as a psychological release stimulates problem solving. The nurse can help him identify areas in which he can retain his independence. 9-10. This provides assistance and promotes and encourages independence. 11. Malfunctioning or misfitting equipment may increase physical problems and be psychologically embarrassing; it may discourage mobility within limits of equipment.
Adolescent will state restrictions on activity and describe changes or plans that will need to be made. Adolescent will describe and understand what to expect from medical and nursing treatment plans.	Patient Education: 1. Explain and review information about musculoskeletal problem, restrictions in activity, what to expect from procedures and equipment. 2. Demonstrate to patient how to use equipment and adapt routines for self-care. If time permits before procedures that will limit mobility, allow teen to practice altered means of performing activities of daily living (eliminating or eating flat or with head down, being turned on a Stryker frame or circo electric bed).	Patient Education: 1. The adolescent can understand restrictions and his treatment process so that he will cooperate with and adhere to treatment plan. He can comprehend relationships, analyze data in a problem-solving manner, and make plans about his situation. 2. Practicing these activities gives teen some sense of mastery and independence before immobilization, thereby diminishing his frustration and giving him a more realistic idea of what the immobility will be like.

Table continued on the following page.

NURSING CARE PLAN FOR THE ADOLESCENT WITH MUSCULOSKELETAL ALTERATION (Continued)

Nursing Diagnosis	Expected Outcome	Nursing Intervention	Rationale
Potential changes in neurovascular system related to: • Casting • Surgical procedures • Traction • Extended immobility • Disease process • Injuries • Over-replacement of blood loss • Braces.	The neurovascular system will be closely monitored and changes promptly noted and reported. The adolescent will not experience further loss of sensation or function	Dx: 1. Assess color, temperature, edema, capillary refill, sensation and motion every hour for 24 hrs, then every 4–8 hrs. Assess for signs of thrombophlebitis (local pain, redness, swelling, warmth). 2. Monitor pulse, respiration and blood pressure and pulses distal to the immobilized part at least every 4 hrs. 3. Monitor intake/output as indicated; carefully regulate IV fluids. 4. Assess for unrelieved pain. 5. Assess other neurological functions: • Headaches, vision • Bowel/bladder control • Pain, spasms • Level of consciousness. Tx: 1. Position to decrease edema or compression of muscles and nerves. 2. Recommend use of anti-embolus stockings. 3. Administer anticoagulants as ordered.	Dx: 1. Close monitoring of neurovascular system is needed to determine status and diagnose muscle ischemia, thrombosis formation or neurological damage. 2. Alterations in vital signs signal cardiovascular or neurological distress. 3. Immobility and treatments may cause edema that can compromise neurovascular function. 4. Unrelieved pain and extreme pain with passive or active motion can be a sign of a compartment syndrome. 5. Neurovascular compromise and immobility may cause alteration in neurological stimulation of other body systems. Tx: 1. Elevation to decrease edema should be above level of heart. Elevation for 24–72 hrs past injury or casting is important. Do not use rubber or plastic pillows under a wet cast; they do not allow heat to disseminate. 2. Embolus formation is a risk any time there is immobilization or compromised circulation. 3. ASA is given for pain, for treatment of rheumatoid arthritis and as an anticoagulant.

		4. Administer specific medications and note side effects. 5. Change position at least every 4 hrs around the clock using all positions not contraindicated; support immobilized parts with sand bags or orthopedic pillows. 6. Apply cold or heat as ordered. 7. Encourage range of motion exercises if not contraindicated. 8. Do not massage calves of legs. Patient Education: 1. Explain purpose of close monitoring and preventive measures. 2. Instruct adolescent to notify nurse of neurovascular changes. 3. Demonstrate correct method of positioning and proper use of equipment.	5. Change of position and correct support of body parts enhances circulation and diminishes risk of embolus or pneumonia. 6. Cold application decreases blood flow and edema. Application of heat increases circulation or relieves pain or spasm. 7. Disuse of muscles may cause venous pooling and muscle atrophy. 8. Vigorous massage may dislodge blood clots in deep veins. Patient Education: 1–3. Knowing the need for close monitoring and treatment will help adolescent participate in and adhere to treatment. Encouraging him to take responsibility in his positioning and in informing staff of neurovascular changes increases his sense of self-control and independence.
Pain related to injuries; surgical procedures, casting, or disease process.	The adolescent will be comfortable.	Dx: 1. Assess type, location, severity of pain and response to analgesics or sedatives. 2. Assess for areas of pressure, compression and swelling. 3. Observe for nonverbal signs of pain (grimaces, reluctance to move). 4. Learn which pain relief measures adolescent has used in the past.	Dx: 1–3. Thorough assessment is needed to determine presence and degree of pain. Pain is influenced by subjective and psychological factors. Adolescents generally exhibit low pain tolerance, possibly associated with their egocentric focus. 4. Greater pain relief usually is achieved when adolescent participates in the process of providing it.

Table continued on the following page.

THE HOSPITALIZED ADOLESCENT 1343

NURSING CARE PLAN FOR THE ADOLESCENT WITH MUSCULOSKELETAL ALTERATION (Continued)

Nursing Diagnosis	Expected Outcome	Nursing Intervention	Rationale
		Tx:	Tx:
		1. Administer analgesics promptly.	1. Adolescent has decreased tolerance to pain.
		2. Institute treatments and procedures at least 1/2 hour after pain medication.	2. Procedures are more easily tolerated after comfort measures.
		3. Do not jar bed, traction, Stryker frame.	3. Environmental factors influence comfort; jarring can cause or intensify pain.
		4. Position and elevate to ease pain.	4. Proper positioning and prevention of edema diminish stress and tension on bones and muscles, thereby diminishing pain or spasm.
		5. Provide privacy if pain is severe.	5. The adolescent fears and becomes embarrassed by loss of control owing to pain.
		6. Provide opportunity for rest periods and adequate night sleep.	6. Adequate rest increases the ability to cope with pain and general discomfort.
		7. Utilize adequate number of staff personnel to move patient.	7. Movement without adequate support of affected area may cause discomfort or disrupt alignment of injured parts.
		8. Use adaptive equipment that may decrease pain (fracture bed pans, slings).	8. Adaptive equipment aids the teen in more independent functioning with less pain.
		9. Provide diversional activities (games, TV, hobbies, phone, music, conversation, books).	9. Activities help divert the teen's attention from his discomfort and diminish anxiety associated with potential pain.
	Parents will be able to provide support and institute measures to assist in decreasing pain.	10. Encourage patient to participate by using pain relief measures such as relaxation exercises, warm baths.	10. Participation in relief of pain allows adolescent some control.

	11. Support family members as they interact with the adolescent having pain.	11. It is difficult for parents to observe their child in pain; helping parents realize that they can be a diversion from this pain for the teen can ease their feelings.
		Patient Education:
Adolescent will be knowledgeable about treatments and will be told that pain will occur.	Patient Education: 1. Inform adolescent that pain will occur; explain cause and how long it usually lasts. 2. Instruct adolescent to notify nurse about pain. 3. Explain procedures and equipment. 4. Explain to parents about adolescent's reaction to pain and instruct them in relief measures.	1–4. Preparing the patient to expect pain and explaining relief measures decreases anxiety and increases trust and participation.
Potential skin breakdown related to extended periods of immobility and irritation/pressure from immobilizing equipment.	The adolescent's skin integrity will be maintained.	Dx: 1. Inspect skin for signs of irritation, redness or broken areas every 2–8 hrs. Note cast edges and bony prominences.	Dx: 1. Pressure areas have diminished circulation; this increases risk of skin breakdown for them and for areas in constant contact with moisture.
		2. Assess for numbness or tingling.	2. Numbness or tingling under a cast or brace may indicate pressure. If tingling stops it may indicate skin breakdown.
		3. Assess for odor from cast.	3. A musty odor from a cast indicates that secretions have penetrated into cast material; area becomes a breeding ground for infectious organisms.
		4. Monitor temperature if indicated by presence of any of the above signs.	4. Elevated temperature may indicate skin infection in areas of skin breakdown.
		Tx: 1. Provide skin care every 4 hrs and prn: • Wash thoroughly • Dry completely • Rub/massage pressure areas	Tx: 1. Alcohol and tincture of benzoin toughen skin; lotion softens skin; powder cakes, inviting microorganisms. Washing and drying well keeps skin free of

Table continued on the following page.

THE HOSPITALIZED ADOLESCENT 1345

NURSING CARE PLAN FOR THE ADOLESCENT WITH MUSCULOSKELETAL ALTERATION (Continued)

Nursing Diagnosis	Expected Outcome	Nursing Intervention	Rationale
		• Apply alcohol or tincture of benzoin to toughen, especially over bony prominences and areas resting on bed or equipment.	infectious organisms. Rubbing stimulates blood flow to muscles and skin.
		2. Position changes every 2–4 hrs.	2. Position changes allow skin to receive adequate circulation; inspection and care are more easily provided.
		3. Use padding or support equipment (heel protectors, petal cast, air mattress, all-foam pads, plastic bubble sheets; water bed)	3. Padding may help prevent pressure or rubbing on skin and nerves.
		4. Cast care (see Chap. 51).	4. Proper cast care prevents development of pressure points under cast and accumulation of secretions on skin surface of cast that encourages skin breakdown.
		5. Maintain preventive environment: dry, clean sheets, rough edges of casts, splints petalled.	5. Dry skin, bedding and clothes prevent irritation, rashes and itching.
		6. Assist with skin care of adolescent if necessary.	6–7. The adolescent prefers to maintain hygiene independently, but when limitations exist, will cooperate to have help if he realizes importance of skin maintenance and if his modesty is preserved.
		7. Recognize feelings of embarrassment related to perineal care.	
		8. Provide adequate protein and caloric intake to meet nutritional needs of healing.	8. With injury to skin and other tissues, increased amounts of protein and calories are required for the healing process.
		Patient Education:	Patient Education:
		1. Explain and demonstrate skin care, including significance of keeping skin intact.	1. Adolescent can participate in and take responsibility for skin care.
	The adolescent will be knowledgeable about self-care of skin and will know when		

Potential gastrointestinal changes related to extended immobility, superior mesenteric artery syndrome.	The adolescent will not become constipated. The adolescent's cast will be clean and dry.	2. Instruct patient to notify nurse about changes in skin or any discomfort. Dx: 1. Monitor bowel sounds every 4 hours when indicated. 2. Record frequency and character of stools every day. 3. Record frequency, type and amount of nausea/vomiting every 8 hrs. 4. Assess abdominal pain. Tx: 1. Advance diet slowly postoperatively. 2. Encourage fluids, especially fruit juices. 3. Include high fiber foods in diet. 4. Administer laxatives and stool softeners as ordered (usually if no stool in 3 days). 5. Provide privacy during elimination. 6. Protect cast, incisions, and open skin areas from stool. 7. Encourage activity and exercise as permitted. Patient Education: 1. Explain reasons why gastrointestinal status may change and importance of nursing care to maintain function.	to tell nurse or physician about problems. Dx: 1–4. Monitoring of parameters provides data to determine if changes are occurring. Tx: 1. Decreased mobility often results in alterations of gastrointestinal system (constipation, paralytic ileus). 2–3. Food, fluid and activity influence gastrointestinal function. 4. These measures assist in maintaining bowel function until mobility is increased. 5. Privacy facilitates elimination and preserves modesty. 6. Soilage of cast or contamination of incision must be prevented. 7. Activity facilitates normal bowel activity. Patient Education: 1. Understanding reasons for monitoring and treatment will encourage adolescent to participate in and adhere to care program.

Table continued on the following page.

THE HOSPITALIZED ADOLESCENT 1347

NURSING CARE PLAN FOR THE ADOLESCENT WITH MUSCULOSKELETAL ALTERATION (Continued)

Nursing Diagnosis	Expected Outcome	Nursing Intervention	Rationale
Potential urinary changes: • Incontinence • Retention • Infection • Renal stones • Renal involvement related to decreased mobility	The adolescent's excretion of urine will be maintained.	Dx: 1. Monitor intake and output. 2. Monitor urinary specific gravity. 3. Check for protein. 4. Monitor color and characteristics of urine. 5. Monitor temperature. 6. Monitor urine for culture and sensitivity if indicated. 7. Palpate bladder for distention.	Dx: 1–6. The finding of any abnormalities supports the likelihood of urinary complications; intervention can be prompt. 2 through 5 should be monitored at least every 8 hrs. 7. Bladder can be holding large amounts of urine and patient may not feel the urge to void.
	The adolescent will be independent in urinary excretion with/without assistance.	Tx: 1. Force fluids to two times the daily intake unless contraindicated. 2. Offer cranberry juice diluted in water or ginger ale tid. 3. Maintain closed drainage system of urine. 4. Assist with credé maneuver (Fig. 25–3) and intermittent self-catheterization until adolescent masters the technique. 5. Position patient with head of bed up when emptying bladder (unless contraindicated). 6. Protect cast, incision and traction equipment from urine soilage.	Tx: 1. Less mobile patients can develop urinary retention and renal calculi due to sluggish kidney function. 2. Cranberry juice increases urinary acidity thereby helping to prevent bacteruria and retarding calculi formation. 3. A closed system prevents contamination of urinary tract by infectious organisms. 4. Most teens can master these techniques if given proper instructions; they prefer independence in these tasks. 5–6. Emptying bladder in horizontal position is difficult. 6. Urine soilage of casts causes odor, softens plaster and increases possibility of skin irritations and infection.

		Patient Education: 1. Explain reasons for care associated with urination. 2. Demonstrate procedures that assist or encourage self-care. 3. Review signs and symptoms that should be brought to the attention of the nurse or physician.	Patient Education: 1–3. The adolescent is able to understand and take responsibility for self-care.
Potential respiratory distress related to musculoskeletal changes/injuries in thoracic region, extended periods of decreased mobility and surgical procedures and effects of anesthesia.	The adolescent's respiratory status will be closely monitored and changes recorded and reported. The adolescent will demonstrate how to cough, deep breathe and use incentive spirometer.	Dx: 1. Monitor temperature, pulse, respirations every 4–12 hrs. 2. Monitor breath sounds every 4 hrs when indicated. 3. Observe and record character, productivity of cough. Tx: 1. Cough and deep breathe every 4–8 hrs. 2. Use incentive spirometer every 4–8 hrs. 3. Encourage fluids to maintain hydration. 4. Turn side to side and prone to supine if not contraindicated. 5. Give medication for pain as needed. (Use IM for first 12–36 hrs after surgery.) Patient Education: 1. Explain/review reasons for preventive measures. 2. Demonstrate and then have adolescent demonstrate before procedures the expected breathing exercises.	Dx: 1–3. Decreased mobility, compression and alterations in air exchange cause respiratory embarrassment or distress. Tx: 1–2. Breathing exercises stimulate air exchange and movement. 3. Adequate hydration assists in preventing mucus from being thick; aids with coughing and removal. 4. Moving prevents secretions from stagnating and facilitates their removal. 5. Pain will influence respiratory rate and character. Patient Education: 1–2. There will be increased participation and ability to carry out techniques when expectations are explained before surgery.

Table continued on the following page.

NURSING CARE PLAN FOR THE ADOLESCENT WITH MUSCULOSKELETAL ALTERATION *(Continued)*

Nursing Diagnosis	Expected Outcome	Nursing Intervention	Rationale
Potential infections related to open wounds/fractures, surgical procedures, immobility.	Patient will be free from infection.	Dx: 1. Take temperature every 4 to 12 hrs. 2. Observe wounds, incisions, pin sites for redness, swelling, drainage. 3. Note odor or discoloration of cast. 4. Assess for pain. Tx: 1. Wash hands thoroughly before and after giving care and between procedures. 2. Wound/incision care as ordered. 3. Pain care as ordered. 4. Prevent urine/stool contamination of wounds and incisions. 5. Administer antibiotics as ordered. 6. Encourage adequate nutrition to promote healing and prevent anabolic state. Patient Education: 1. Explain purpose of plan of care. 2. Demonstrate self care and explain signs of infection to monitor for.	Dx: 1–4. The phagocytosis process in response to bacteria or foreign material is monitored by observation of these parameters. Tx: 1–4. Aseptic and clean technique is necessary to prevent osteomyelitis and other infections from bacterial contamination. 2–6. Destruction of body tissues due to infection requires healing and repair. Rest, nutrition and removal of infection is necessary for this process. Patient Education: 1–2. The adolescent has the cognitive skills to monitor for infection and the psychological need to be a participant in his care.
Potential changes in body weight related to	Fluids and foods will be provided to meet metabolic	Dx: 1. Weigh every 3–7 days.	Dx: 1–4. Loss of appetite can be expected with some decreased

1350 FAMILIES WITH ADOLESCENTS

impaired mobility, anorexia, extensive caloric intake.	needs, promote healing and maintain growth.	2. Determine caloric needs. 3. Assess daily caloric intake. 4. Determine caloric expenditures. Tx: 1. Offer choices of fluids and foods; incorporate teen's favorites. 2. Encourage adequate intake of protein, carbohydrates and fats. 3. Supplement diet with snacks. 4. Encourage family/friends to bring favorite foods and to eat with the teen. 5. If allowed and legal, offer 1–2 beers per day for anorexic patient. 6. Discourage candy and high caloric foods if weight needs to be maintained and not gained. 7. Adjust calories according to expenditure and goals. 8. Referral to dietitian. Patient Education: 1. Explain, review and reinforce information about caloric requirements during immobility and for healing.	mobility and disease processes. It can also be a sign of depression. Increased eating may result from stress or boredom. Tx: 1–4. Utilizing psychological and social factors of eating may increase appetite or willingness to eat. 5. Alcohol can stimulate appetite and provide increased calories. 6–7. These empty foods diminish appetite, decreasing intake of nutritious food. Weight gain may result because excess calories cannot be expended during immobility. 8. Dietitian should provide an appetizing, nutritious diet and should therefore be informed of teen's needs and preferences. Patient Education: 1. Adolescent is able to participate in controlling weight gain or loss.
Potential injuries due to environmental hazards, equipment malfunction or impaired mobility.	The adolescent will be free from injuries while under nurse's care.	Dx: 1. Assess institution and home environment for safety hazards.	Dx: 1–3. Equipment should be checked for proper function and safety before it is used with a patient.

Table continued on the following page.

THE HOSPITALIZED ADOLESCENT 1351

NURSING CARE PLAN FOR THE ADOLESCENT WITH MUSCULOSKELETAL ALTERATION (Continued)

Nursing Diagnosis	Expected Outcome	Nursing Intervention	Rationale
		2. Note and record any accidents or equipment failures.	
		3. Assess for injuries if accidents or equipment failures occur.	
		Tx: 1. Use safety straps when transporting patient in a wheelchair or on a stretcher.	Tx: 1–2. Patient with altered mobility may have decreased strength and altered balance; if this safety need is explained the teen can cooperate without loss of self-esteem.
		2. Use safety straps when adolescent is learning to walk with equipment or with a cast.	
		3. Utilize enough personnel when assisting patient to move or when using special equipment.	3. A patient with impaired mobility is difficult to move. Enough personnel and proper body mechanics can prevent injuries to staff and patient.
		4. Adolescent should wear sturdy, non-slip shoes.	4. Non-slip shoes decrease chance of falls.
		5. If patient is in traction, check for frayed or loose ropes, proper position and up in bed, and tight knots. Cover sharp edges.	5–6. Utilization of safety procedures will help demonstrate self-care to adolescent and prevent further injuries.
		6. Elevate head of bed slowly.	
	The adolescent will be able to describe ways to prevent accidents and injuries.	Patient Education: 1. Explain how adolescent can help maintain a safe environment.	Patient Education: 1–2. An understanding of what to expect and knowledge of how he can contribute increases the teen's cooperation and self-esteem.
		2. Explain that a cast increases weight.	
		3. Warn teen of potential for difficulties when ambulation begins: weakness, hypotension, fatigue.	3. Orthostatic hypotension may occur when patient has been on extended bed rest.

Nursing Diagnosis	Goal	Intervention	Rationale
		4. Explain ways to be safe at home: ambulating in slippery conditions; exiting house in emergency situations.	4. Understanding safety needs and planning precautions will help to prevent injuries.
Anger and frustration related to loss of control, dependent status.	The adolescent will be able to make choices within restrictions.	Dx: 1. Assess how adolescent usually expresses anger and frustration. 2. Determine the degree of independence that can be expected or permitted. 3. Assess adolescent's ideas and goals for independence.	Dx: 1–3. This information provides a basis to help the adolescent plan realistic ways to retain control and independence within limits of his situation.
	The adolescent will have an opportunity to express feelings associated with loss of control.	Tx: 1. Encourage verbalization of anger. 2. Provide opportunities to express anger (dart games, art, punching bags).	Tx: 1. If impaired mobility restricts one's usual pattern of relieving frustration, discomfort from anxiety arises. 2. The loss of control of strong feelings with temper outbursts or tears is ego-alien to most young people. It may lead to feelings of guilt and loss of self-esteem.
	The adolescent will utilize other methods than mobility to assert independence and control.	3. Allow adolescent to choose and control environment and treatments within limits (choose bath time, exercise time).	3–4. An adolescent needs to learn a variety of ways to cope with frustrations.
	The adolescent will set realistic goals.	4. Praise and reinforce appropriate expression of feelings and development of realistic goals. Patient Education: 1. Explain to adolescent and family that restricted mobility may cause frustration due to loss of control. 2. Explain ways to gain control.	Patient Education: 1–2. Knowing that the feelings he experiences are normal relieves the teen of some guilt and diminished self-esteem.
Anxiety related to lack of information or misinformation.	The adolescent can explain what to expect from the health care plan.	Dx: 1. Determine what the adolescent has heard or read about the disease process, treatment or procedures.	Dx: 1–4. Past experiences, misinformation and fantasies about the body and health influence adolescent's expectations of what may happen. Anxiety in-

Table continued on the following page.

NURSING CARE PLAN FOR THE ADOLESCENT WITH MUSCULOSKELETAL ALTERATION (Continued)

Nursing Diagnosis	Expected Outcome	Nursing Intervention	Rationale
		2. Assess past experiences with health care agencies and/or professionals.	creases when adolescent is not prepared.
		3. Determine what adolescent thinks will happen.	
		4. Determine how much the parents understand and have shared with child.	
		5. Utilize parents to determine things that may be anxiety-producing for the adolescent.	5. Parents may know what the adolescent fears but is unable to share with the health care team.
		Tx:	Tx:
		1. Encourage patient to ask questions and express concerns to nurse and doctor.	1. Immobilization subjects adolescent to impulses, wishes and fantasies he is ordinarily able to keep from conscious awareness with physical activity.
		2. Orient patient and family to the institution or agency's guidelines and expectations.	2. Orientation and instructions help decrease anxiety resulting from fear of the unknown or unfamiliar.
		3. Have parents and adolescent write down questions and answers received.	3–4. Knowing he will get honest answers to questions and that he is included in his health planning reduces the teen's anxiety and builds his confidence in health providers.
		4. Encourage parents and health team to include adolescent in discussions and decisions of health care.	
		5. Compliment accomplishments.	5. Reinforcements and rewards stimulate or increase learning.
		6. Help set realistic, attainable goals.	6–7. Unrealistic goals cause frustration and anger.
		7. Recognize that certain health care management tasks can be difficult.	

	Patients and parents can relate contents of educational plan.	Patient Education: 1. Explain and prepare patient for procedures, surgery and tasks in advance. 2. Use scientific terms in explanations—correlate them to lay terms. 3. Use pictures, tours and written material in education process. 4. Have adolescent demonstrate techniques he has learned. 5. Keep parents informed, provide the same education but have them assist as needed and encourage independence. 6. Utilize resource people who are experts in specialty field.	Patient Education: 1. Advance knowledge of what will happen, what the teen will feel and how he can help reduces his sense of helplessness and anxiety. 2. The adolescent can understand and use scientific terms. 3–6. Thorough instruction with return demonstrations encourages participation in care and adherence to treatment programs.
Changes in body image related to impaired mobility and disfigurement.	The adolescent will have an opportunity to discuss changes in body image. The adolescent will have an opportunity to discuss changes in life style.	Dx: 1. Assess adolescent's ability to verbalize feelings. 2. Assess family interactions and methods of giving support. Tx: 1. Encourage verbalization of feelings and fears of body changes or loss of mobility. 2. Assist in identifying adolescent's strengths. 3. Reinforce behavior that draws on patient's strengths. 4. Provide privacy.	Dx: 1–2. Psychological and social assessments are needed to determine patient's strength, support systems and ability to verbalize feelings. Tx: 1. Immobilization may cause patient to become narcissistic (focus attention on the body and its functions). 2–3. Helping the teen identify his positive features helps him look at his body alteration more realistically. 4. Everyone needs solitude and privacy, especially when working through grief.

Table continued on the following page.

THE HOSPITALIZED ADOLESCENT 1355

NURSING CARE PLAN FOR THE ADOLESCENT WITH MUSCULOSKELETAL ALTERATION *(Continued)*

Nursing Diagnosis	Expected Outcome	Nursing Intervention	Rationale
		5. Encourage expression of feelings through music, art, and writing.	5. Feelings can be expressed non-verbally. These other means may allow adolescent to remain in control.
	Family members will have an opportunity to plan ways to provide support and reinforce adolescent's strength.	Patient Education: 1. Explain to adolescent and parents that mourning over changes in body image is normal. 2. Describe ways to identify and reinforce strengths.	Patient Education: 1–2. Grief work to cope with changes in body and loss of pleasure from activity and independence can be expected.
Inability to maintain schooling and/or accomplish career goals related to hospitalization, permanent mobility changes, and environmental barriers.	The adolescent will be able to continue his education.	Dx: 1. Determine educational level, career interests and educational program. 2. Determine patient's career goals. 3. Assess parental support and interest in career choices. 4. Assess environment for potential barriers to education and vocational program.	Dx: 1–4. Career goals are developed during adolescence. Immobility may interrupt or change these. The health team must know the teen's goals to help him plan realistically for his future.
	The adolescent will have an opportunity to discuss career goals.	Tx: 1. Utilize OT, PT, PHR, school and vocational rehabilitation to assist with assessment, plans and implementation. 2. Contact school. 3. Provide quiet for studying. 4. Reinforce realistic goals and plans. 5. Assist in obtaining equipment and supplies.	Tx: 1–5. Decreased mobility may decrease motivation and ability to concentrate or solve problems. External resources can re-motivate the immobilized teen to re-establish his life style.

Depression related to impaired mobility, sensory overload and/or deprivation, decreased peer interactions.	The adolescent will have opportunities to participate in activities with peers. The adolescent will be able to modify interaction in his restricted environment.	Patient Education: 1. Reinforce restrictions on limits and assist in explaining options. Dx: 1. Determine amount of peer interactions the adolescent has had. 2. Assess environment for amount and type of stimuli available. Tx: 1. Plan activities and set up schedules with the adolescent. 2. Encourage visits from school friends. 3. Assist in getting adolescent use of a phone, a pass for a visit home, and the means to participate in activities and trips. 4. Introduce adolescent to other patients with similar problems. 5. Utilize volunteers, school teachers, chaplains, others. Parent Education: 1. Explain that decreased mobility may make a person feel sluggish, want to sleep. 2. Explain that some depression is normal but that interactions are needed.	Patient Education: 1. Understanding restrictions helps in planning and accomplishing goals. Dx: 1. Peers are important to adolescent. He fears that his absence from their social circles may result in rejection. 2. Prolonged depression and regression lead to loss of motivation and energy for dealing with decreased mobility. Tx: 1–3. Channel his energies into constructive activities. 4–5. The adolescent must establish life patterns of interacting with the environment that provide gratification. Parent Education: 1–2. Immobilization lessens opportunity to select friends and interact with peers.
Parental grief and/or guilt related to permanent deformity or restricted activities.	Parents will have opportunity to discuss feelings about child's decreased mobility.	Dx: 1. Assess parents' feelings about adolescent's restrictions and decreased mobility.	Dx: 1. Parents may attempt to relieve guilt or anger by providing close monitoring or special privileges.

Table continued on the following page.

THE HOSPITALIZED ADOLESCENT 1357

NURSING CARE PLAN FOR THE ADOLESCENT WITH MUSCULOSKELETAL ALTERATION (Continued)

Nursing Diagnosis	Expected Outcome	Nursing Intervention	Rationale
		Tx: 1. Talk with parents alone; allow them to express fears and concerns. 2. Provide support and comfort to parents. Patient Education: 1. Explain to parents that grief and guilt feelings can be expected.	Tx: 1–2. Parents need time to work through initial shock of the alteration. Patient Education: 1. Duration of grieving is related to severity and visibility of the alteration and the extent to which it interferes with adolescent's life plans.
Parental ambivalence about dependency needs of their adolescent.	The parents will have an opportunity to plan and participate in care of their adolescent.	Dx: 1. Assess previous parent and adolescent interactions and conflicts about independence and dependence. Tx: 1. Include parents in assessing and planning care. 2. Encourage parents to participate yet respect independence needs of adolescent. 3. Encourage adolescent to tell parents what he needs. 4. Talk with parents alone, provide support. 5. Do not side with parent or adolescent. Patient Education: 1. Explain adolescent developmental needs to parents. 2. Demonstrate and discuss ways to participate in care yet encourage independence.	Dx: 1. Parents may find it difficult to allow the adolescent to do self-care or monitor illness. Tx: 1. Parents may feel guilty, angry or inadequate when nurses take over some care of adolescent. 2. Parents may enjoy or feel more comfortable with a dependent adolescent as opposed to one striving for independence. 3–4. Adolescent may exhibit anger and become demanding of parents because of forced dependency. 5. Independence conflicts are at a peak during adolescence. Patient Education: 1–2. Knowledge about adolescent growth and development issues will assist parents in understanding child's behavior and providing appropriate support.

APPENDICES

APPENDIX I

AUTOSOMAL DOMINANT MODE OF TRANSMISSION

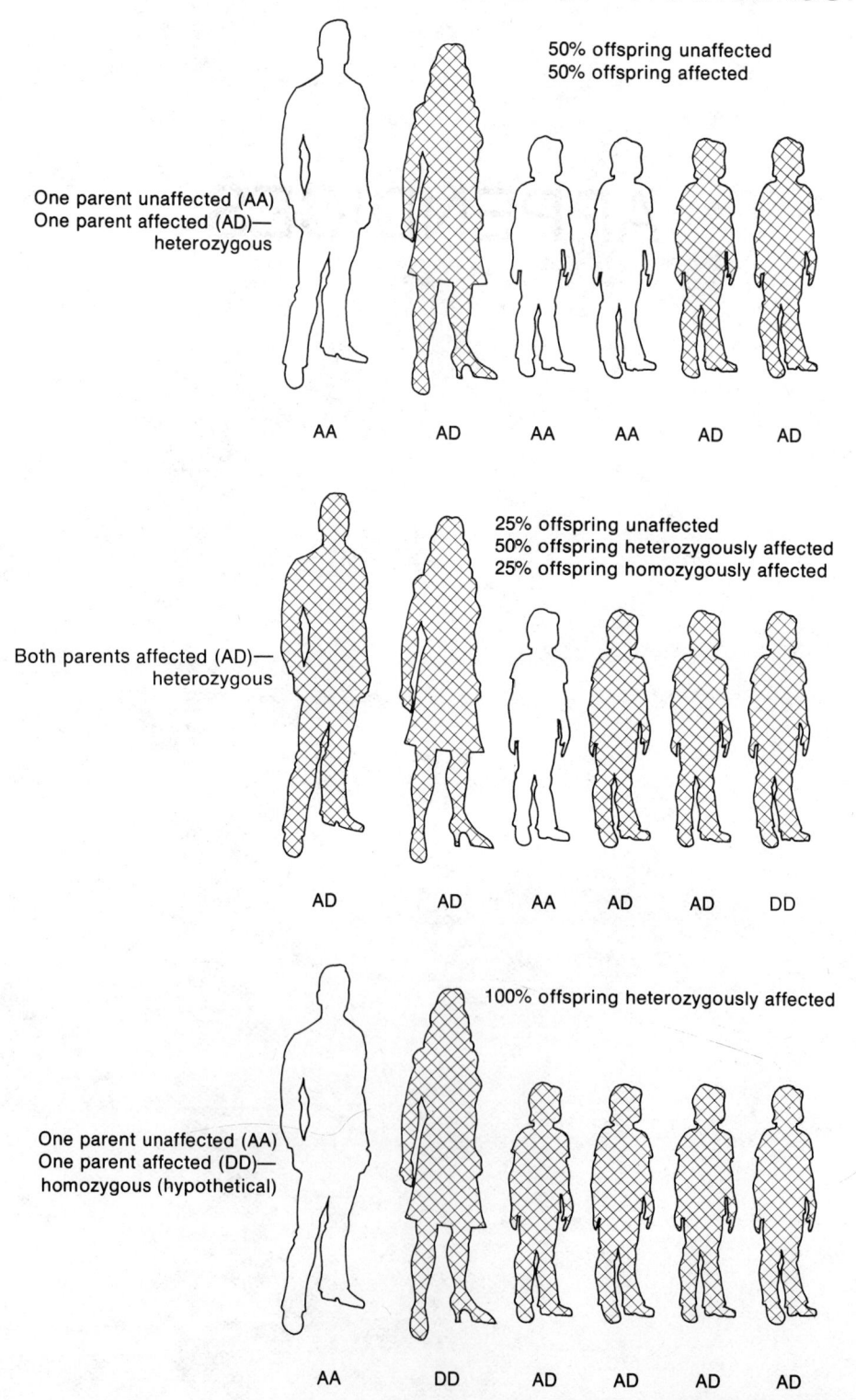

One parent unaffected (AA)
One parent affected (AD)—
heterozygous

50% offspring unaffected
50% offspring affected

AA　　AD　　AA　　AA　　AD　　AD

Both parents affected (AD)—
heterozygous

25% offspring unaffected
50% offspring heterozygously affected
25% offspring homozygously affected

AD　　AD　　AA　　AD　　AD　　DD

One parent unaffected (AA)
One parent affected (DD)—
homozygous (hypothetical)

100% offspring heterozygously affected

AA　　DD　　AD　　AD　　AD　　AD

AUTOSOMAL RECESSIVE MODE OF TRANSMISSION

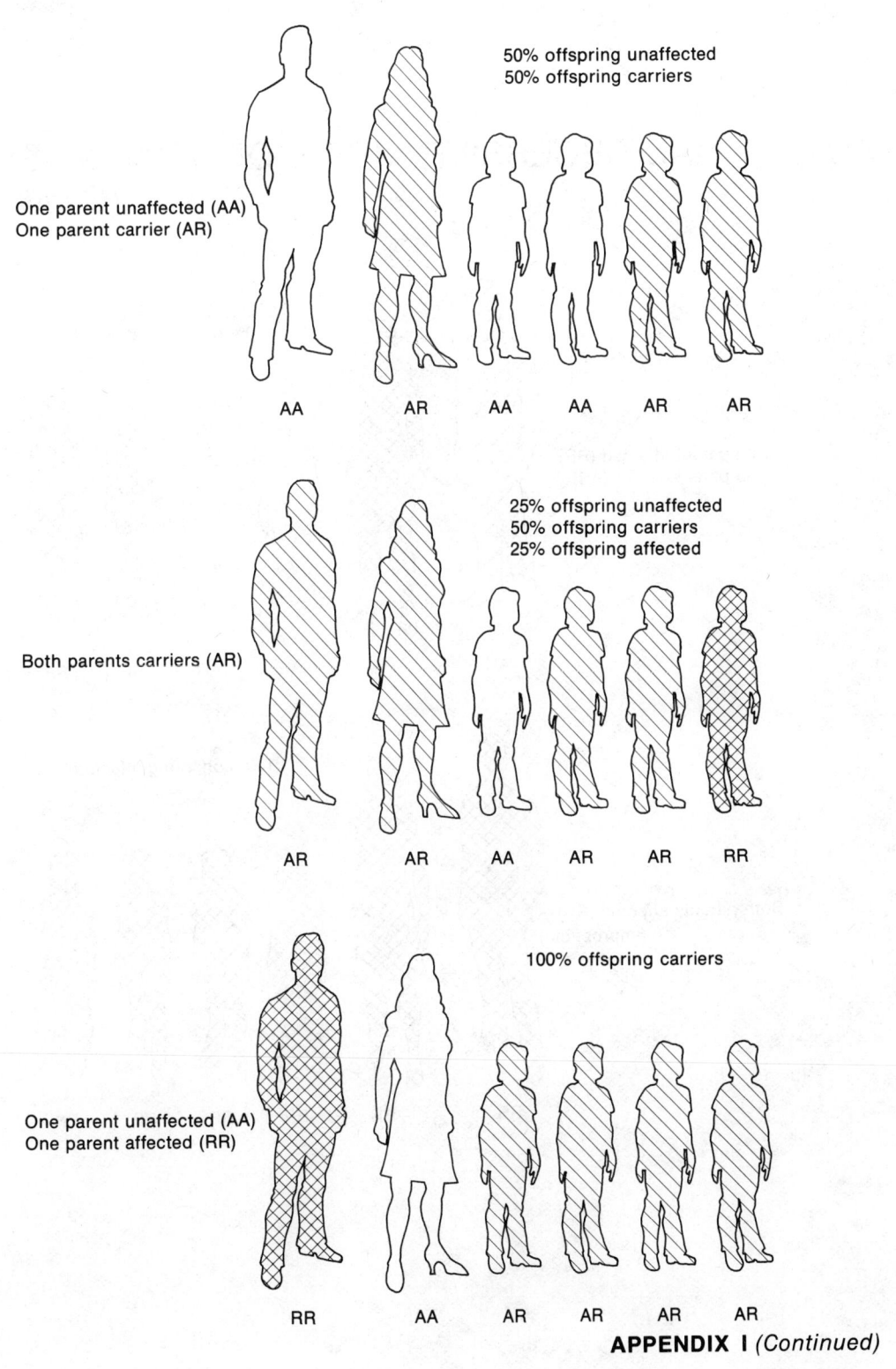

One parent unaffected (AA)
One parent carrier (AR)

50% offspring unaffected
50% offspring carriers

| AA | AR | AA | AA | AR | AR |

Both parents carriers (AR)

25% offspring unaffected
50% offspring carriers
25% offspring affected

| AR | AR | AA | AR | AR | RR |

One parent unaffected (AA)
One parent affected (RR)

100% offspring carriers

| RR | AA | AR | AR | AR | AR |

APPENDIX I *(Continued)*

AUTOSOMAL RECESSIVE MODE OF TRANSMISSION
(Continued)

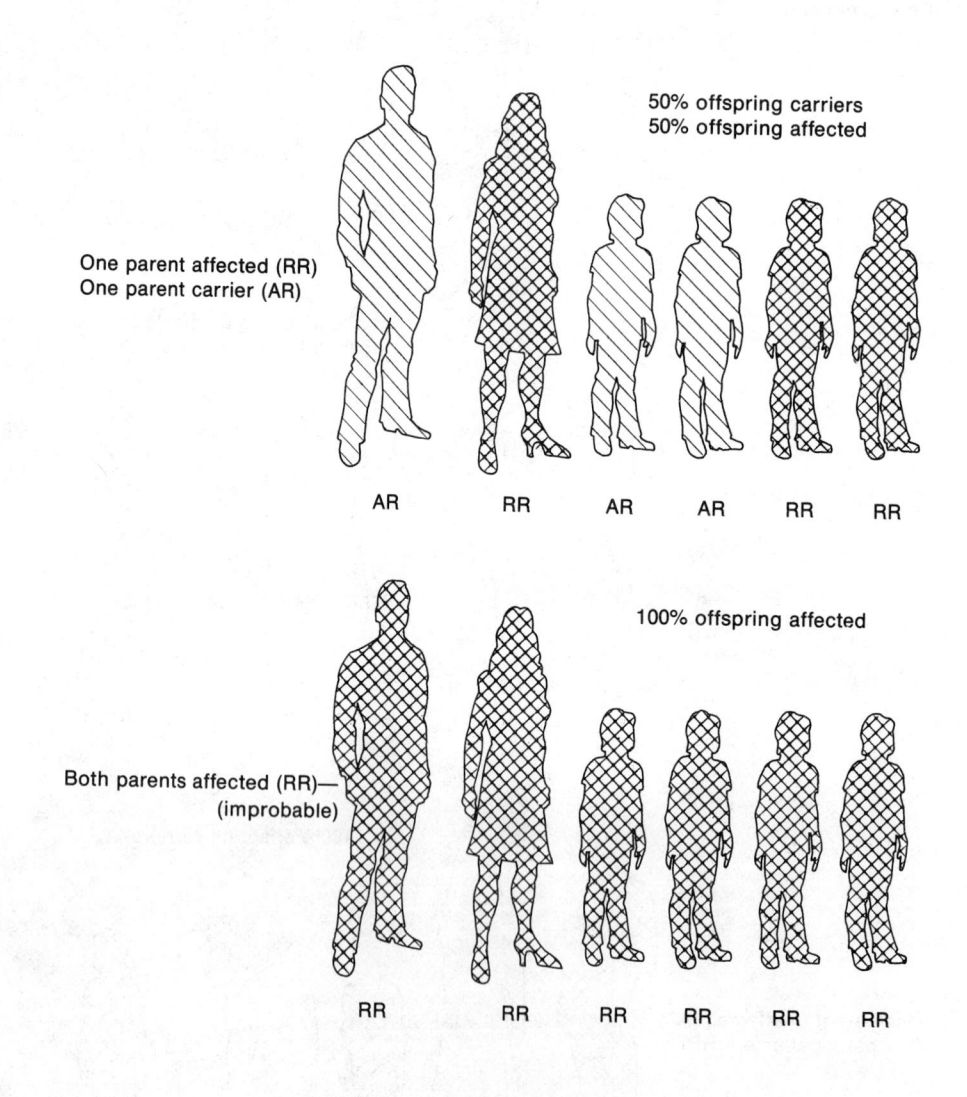

One parent affected (RR)
One parent carrier (AR)

50% offspring carriers
50% offspring affected

AR RR AR AR RR RR

Both parents affected (RR)—
(improbable)

100% offspring affected

RR RR RR RR RR RR

APPENDIX II

APPENDIX II

X-LINKED DOMINANT MODE OF TRANSMISSION

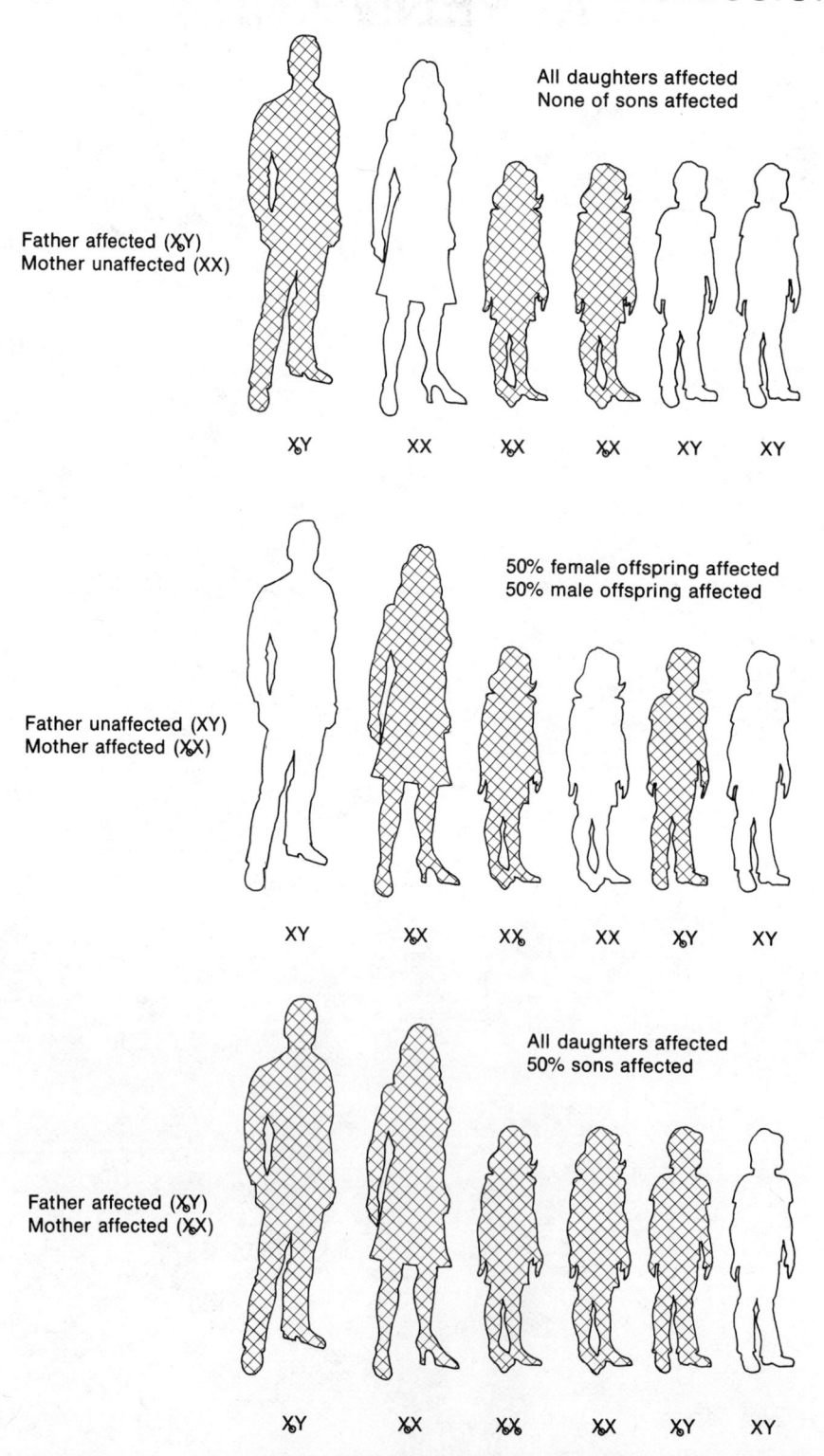

Father affected (XY)
Mother unaffected (XX)

All daughters affected
None of sons affected

XY   XX   XX   XX   XY   XY

Father unaffected (XY)
Mother affected (XX)

50% female offspring affected
50% male offspring affected

XY   XX   XX   XX   XY   XY

Father affected (XY)
Mother affected (XX)

All daughters affected
50% sons affected

XY   XX   XX   XX   XY   XY

X-LINKED RECESSIVE MODE OF TRANSMISSION

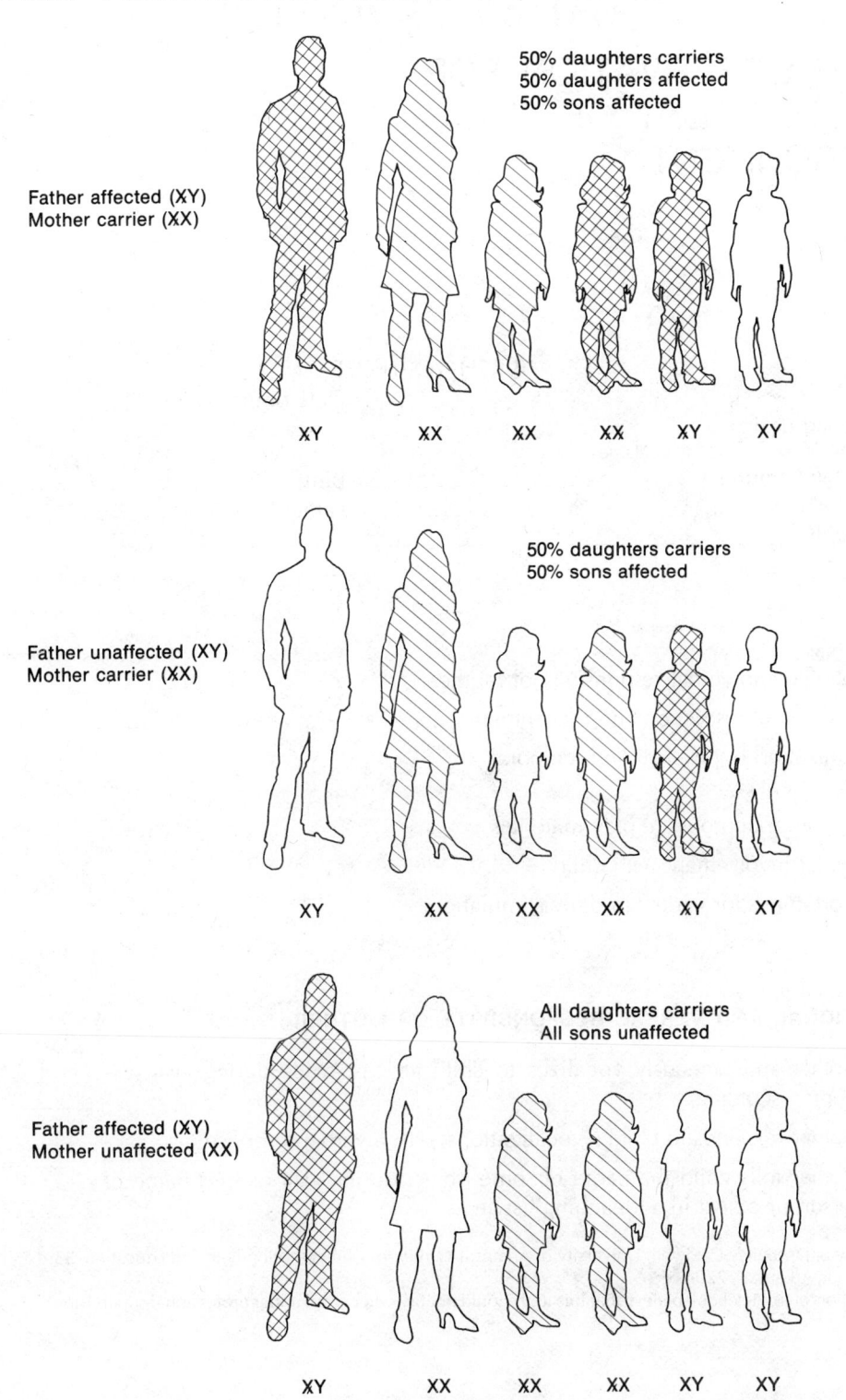

Father affected (X̸Y)
Mother carrier (X̸X)

50% daughters carriers
50% daughters affected
50% sons affected

XY XX XX XX XY XY

Father unaffected (XY)
Mother carrier (X̸X)

50% daughters carriers
50% sons affected

XY XX XX XX XY XY

Father affected (X̸Y)
Mother unaffected (XX)

All daughters carriers
All sons unaffected

XY XX XX XX XY XY

APPENDIX III
HOME OBSERVATION FOR MEASUREMENT OF THE ENVIRONMENT

BIRTH TO THREE

Date of interview_____

Child designee_____
Name

Age Sex Ethnicity

Child's birthday_____ Birth order_____

Mother's name_____ Father's name_____

Address_____

Categories	Raw scores	Percentile scores
I. Emotional and verbal responsivity of mother	_____	_____
II. Avoidance of restriction and punishment	_____	_____
III. Organization of physical and temporal environment	_____	_____
IV. Provision of appropriate play materials	_____	_____
V. Maternal involvement with child	_____	_____
VI. Opportunities for variety in daily stimulation	_____	_____
Totals	_____	_____

I. EMOTIONAL AND VERBAL RESPONSIVITY OF MOTHER

Yes No

1. Mother spontaneously vocalizes to child at least twice during visit (excluding scolding). _____ _____

2. Mother responds to child's vocalizations with a verbal response. _____ _____

3. Mother tells child the name of some object during visit or says name of person or object in a "teaching" style. _____ _____

Courtesy of Dr. Bettye Caldwell, University of Arkansas Center for Child Development and Education, 33rd and University, Little Rock, Arkansas 72204.
The authors of this textbook believe that this tool should not be used except under professional supervision.

	Yes	No

4. Mother's speech is distinct, clear, and audible. ___ ___

5. Mother initiates verbal interchanges with observer—asks questions and makes spontaneous comments. ___ ___

6. Mother expresses ideas freely and easily and uses statements of appropriate length for conversation (e.g., gives more than brief answers). ___ ___

*7. Mother permits child occasionally to engage in "messy" type of play. ___ ___

8. Mother spontaneously praises child's qualities or behavior twice during visit. ___ ___

9. When speaking of or to child, mother's voice conveys positive feeling. ___ ___

10. Mother caresses or kisses child at least once during visit. ___ ___

11. Mother shows some positive emotional responses to praise of child offered by visitor. ___ ___

Subscore ___ ___

II. AVOIDANCE OF RESTRICTION AND PUNISHMENT

12. Mother does not shout at child during visit. ___ ___
13. Mother does not express overt annoyance with or hostility toward child. ___ ___
14. Mother neither slaps nor spanks child during visit. ___ ___
*15. Mother reports that no more than one instance of physical punishment occurred during the past week. ___ ___
16. Mother does not scold or derogate child during visit. ___ ___
17. Mother does not interfere with child's actions or restrict child's movements more than three times during visit. ___ ___
18. At least ten books are present and visible. ___ ___
*19. Family has a pet. ___ ___

Subscore ___ ___

III. ORGANIZATION OF PHYSICAL AND TEMPORAL ENVIRONMENT

20. When mother is away, care is provided by one of three regular substitutes. ___ ___
21. Someone takes child into grocery store at least once a week. ___ ___
22. Child gets out of house at least four times a week. ___ ___
23. Child is taken regularly to doctor's office or clinic. ___ ___
*24. Child has a special place in which to keep his toys and "treasures." ___ ___
25. Child's play environment appears safe and free of hazards. ___ ___

Subscore ___ ___

*Items that may require direct questions.

APPENDIX III *(Continued)*

IV. PROVISION OF APPROPRIATE PLAY MATERIALS

		Yes	No
26.	Child has some muscle activity toys or equipment.		
27.	Child has a push or pull toy.		
28.	Child has stroller or walker, kiddie car, scooter or tricycle.		
29.	Mother provides toys or interesting activities for child during interview.		
30.	Provides learning equipment appropriate to age—cuddly toy or role-playing toys.		
31.	Provides learning equipment appropriate to age—mobile, table and chairs, high chair, play pen.		
32.	Provides eye-hand coordination toys—items to go in and out of receptacle, fit together toys, beads.		
33.	Provides eye-hand coordination toys that permit combinations—stacking or nesting toys, blocks or building toys.		
34.	Provides toys for literature and music.		
	Subscore		

V. MATERNAL INVOLVEMENT WITH CHILD

		Yes	No
35.	Mother tends to keep child within visual range and to look at him often.		
36.	Mother talks to child while doing her work.		
37.	Mother consciously encourages developmental advance.		
38.	Mother invests "maturing" toys with value via her attention.		
39.	Mother structures child's play periods.		
40.	Mother provides toys that challenge child to develop new skills.		
	Subscore		

VI. OPPORTUNITIES FOR VARIETY IN DAILY STIMULATION

		Yes	No
41.	Father provides some caretaking every day.		
42.	Mother reads stories at least three times weekly.		
43.	Child eats at least one meal per day with mother and father.		
44.	Family visits or receives visits from relatives.		
45.	Child has three or more books of his own.		
	Subscore		

APPENDIX III *(Continued)*

THREE TO SIX

Date of interview _____

Child designee _____
Name _____ Age _____ Sex _____ Ethnicity _____

Child's birthday _____ Birth order _____
Mother's name _____ Father's name _____
Address _____

Categories	Raw scores	Percentile scores
I. Provision of stimulation through equipment, toys, and experiences	_____	_____
II. Stimulation of mature behavior	_____	_____
III. Provision of stimulating physical and language environment	_____	_____
IV. Avoidance of restriction and punishment	_____	_____
V. Pride, affection, and thoughtfulness	_____	_____
VI. Masculine stimulation	_____	_____
VII. Independence from parental control	_____	_____
Totals	_____	_____

I. PROVISION OF STIMULATION THROUGH EQUIPMENT, TOYS, AND EXPERIENCES

Yes   No

1-12 The following are present in home and either belong to child subject or he is allowed to play with them:

1. Toys to learn colors, sizes, shapes—typewriter, pressouts, play school, peg boards, etc.
2. Toy or game facilitating learning letters (e.g., blocks with letters, toy typewriter, letter sticks, books about letters, etc.).
3. Three or more puzzles.
4. Two toys necessitating some finger and whole hand movements (crayons and coloring books, paper dolls, etc.).
5. Record player and at least five children's records.
6. Real or toy musical instrument (piano, drum, toy xylophone or guitar, etc.).
7. Toy or game permitting free expression (finger paints, play dough, crayons or paint and paper, etc.).
8. Toys or game necessitating refined movements (paint by number, dot book, paper dolls, crayons and coloring books).
9. Toys to learn animals—books about animals, circus games, animal puzzles, etc.
10. Toy or game facilitating learning numbers (e.g., blocks with numbers, books about numbers, games with numbers, etc.).

APPENDIX III *(Continued)*

I. PROVISION OF STIMULATION THROUGH EQUIPMENT, TOYS, AND EXPERIENCES (Continued)

	Yes	No
11. Building toys (blocks, tinker toys, Lincoln logs, etc.).	__	__
12. Ten children's books.	__	__
13. At least ten books are present and visible in the apartment.	__	__
14. Family buys a newspaper daily and reads it.	__	__
15. Family subscribes to at least one magazine.	__	__
16. Family member has taken child on one outing (picnic, shopping excursion) at least every other week.	__	__
17. Child has been taken out to eat in some kind of restaurant three-four times in the past year.	__	__

18-20 Child has been taken by a family member to the following within the past year:

	Yes	No
18. Airport	__	__
19. A trip more than 50 miles from his home (50 miles radial distance, not total distance).	__	__
20. A scientific, historical, or art museum.	__	__
21. Child is taken to grocery store at least once a week.	__	__
Subscore	__	__

II. STIMULATION OF MATURE BEHAVIOR

22-29 Child is encouraged to learn the following

	Yes	No
22. Colors	__	__
23. Shapes	__	__
24. Patterned speech (nursery rhymes, prayers, songs, TV commercials, etc.)	__	__
25. The alphabet	__	__
26. To tell time	__	__
27. Spatial relationships (up, down, under, big, little, etc.)	__	__
28. Numbers	__	__
29. To read a few words	__	__
30. Tries to get child to pick up and put away toys after play session—without help.	__	__
31. Child is taught rules of social behavior which involve recognition of rights of others.	__	__
32. Parent teaches child some simple manners—to say, "Please," "Thank you," "I'm sorry."	__	__
33. Some delay of food gratification is demanded of the child, e.g., not to whine or demand food unless within 1/2 hour of meal time.	__	__
Subscore	__	__

APPENDIX III *(Continued)*

III. PROVISION OF A STIMULATING PHYSICAL AND LANGUAGE ENVIRONMENT (observation items, except **45)

	Yes	No
34. Building has no potentially dangerous structural or health defect (e.g., plaster coming down from ceiling, stairway with boards missing, rodents, etc.).	___	___
35. Child's outside play environment appears safe and free of hazards (no outside play area requires an automatic "No").	___	___
36. The interior of the apartment is not dark or perceptibly monotonous.	___	___
37. House is not overly noisy—television, shouts of children, radio, etc.	___	___
38. Neighborhood has trees, grass, birds—is esthetically pleasing.	___	___
39. There is at least 100 square feet of living space per person in the house.	___	___
40. In terms of available floor space, the rooms are not overcrowded with furniture.	___	___
41. All visible rooms of the house are reasonably clean and minimally cluttered.	___	___
42. *Mother uses complex sentence structure and some long words in conversing.	___	___
43. Mother uses correct grammar and pronunciation.	___	___
44. Mother's speech is distinct, clear, and audible.	___	___
**45. Family has TV and it is used judiciously, not left on continuously (no TV requires an automatic "No"—any scheduling scores "Yes").	___	___
Subscore	___	___

IV. AVOIDANCE OF RESTRICTION AND PUNISHMENT (observation items, except **51 and **52)

	Yes	No
46. Motor does not scold or derogate child more than once during visit.	___	___
47. Mother does not use physical restraint, shake, grab, pinch child during visit.	___	___
48. Mother neither slaps nor spanks child during visit.	___	___
46. Mother does not express over-annoyance with or hostility toward child—complain, say child is "bad" or won't mind.	___	___
50. Child is not punished or ridiculed for speech.	___	___
**51. No more than one instance of physical punishment occurred during the past week (accept parental report).	___	___
**52. Child does not get slapped or spanked for spilling food or drink.	___	___
Subscore	___	___

V. PRIDE, AFFECTION, AND THOUGHTFULNESS (observation items, except **53, **54, **55, **56, **57, **58, **59)

	Yes	No
**53. Parent turns on special TV program regarded as "good" for children (Captain Kangaroo, Magic Toy Shop, Walt Disney, Flipper, Lassie, educational TV, etc.).	___	___

---

*Throughout interview this refers to *mother* OR other *caregiver* who is present for interview.

APPENDIX III *(Continued)*

V. PRIDE, AFFECTION, AND THOUGHTFULNESS (Continued)

		Yes	No

**54. Someone reads stories to child or shows and comments on pictures in magazines fives times weekly.

**55. Parent encourages child to relate experiences or takes time to listen to him relate experiences.

**56. Parent holds child close ten to fifteen minutes per day, e.g., during TV, story time, visiting.

**57. Parent occasionally sings to child, or sings in presence of child.

**58. Child has a special place in which to keep his toys and "treasures."

**59. Child's art work is displayed some place in house (anything that child makes).

60. Mother introduces interviewer to child.

61. Mother converses with child at least twice during visit (scolding and suspicious comments not counted).

62. Mother answers child's questions or requests verbally.

63. Mother usually responds verbally to child's talking.

64. Mother provides toys or interesting activities or in other ways structures situation for child during visit when her attention will be elsewhere. (To score "Yes" mother must make an active guiding gesture or suggestion to structure child's play.)

65. Mother spontaneously praises child's qualities or behavior twice during visit.

66. When speaking of or to child, mother's voice conveys positive feeling.

67. Mother caresses, kisses, or cuddles child at least once during visit.

68. Mother sets up situation that allows child to show off during visit.

Subscore ____ ____

VI. MASCULINE STIMULATION

69. Child sees and spends some time with father or father figure four days a week.

70. Child eats at least one meal per day, on most days, with mother (or mother figure) and father (or father figure). (One-parent families get an automatic "No.")

71-73 The following are present in home and either belong to child subject or he is allowed to play with them:

71. Ride toy (tricycle, scooter, wagon, bike with or without training wheels).

72. Medium wheel toys—trucks, trains, doll carriage, etc.

73. Large muscle toy (jump rope, swing, ball, climbing object, etc.).

Subscore ____ ____

APPENDIX III *(Continued)*

VII. INDEPENDENCE FROM PARENTAL CONTROL

                                                                                                          Yes   No

74. Child is encouraged to try to dress himself.
75. Child is permitted to choose some of his clothing to be worn except on very special occasions.
76. Child is permitted some choice in lunch or breakfast menu.
77. Parent lets child choose certain favorite food products or brands at grocery store.
78. Child is permitted to go to another house to play without having the caregiver accompany him.
79. Child can express negative feelings without harsh reprisal.
80. Child is permitted to hit parent without harsh reprisal.

                                                                        Subscore

                                                                       Total score

APPENDIX IV

SCORING INSTRUCTIONS FOR THE DENVER DEVELOPMENTAL SCREENING TEST

The Denver Developmental Screening Test (DDST) is a device for developmental screening in infancy and the preschool years. It has been standardized on children of Denver. The test form is reproduced in Figure 13–24.

Test Materials. Skein of red wool, box of raisins; rattle with a narrow handle; small clear glass bottle with 5/8 in. opening; bell; tennis ball; test form; pencil; 8 1-inch cube blocks, colored red, blue, yellow, green.

General Instructions. The parent should be told that the purpose is to obtain an estimate of the child's level of development and that the child will not be able to perform all test items. The test relies on observations of the child and on report by a parent who knows the child. Direct observation should be used whenever possible. Every effort should be made to put the child at ease. The younger child may be tested while sitting on the parent's lap in such a way that he or she can comfortably reach the test materials on a table. One or two test materials may be placed in front of the child while the parent is queried regarding personal-social items. The first test items chosen should assure the child an initial successful experience. To avoid distractions it is best to remove all test materials from the table except those required for the test that is being administered.

Steps in Administering the Test

1. Draw a vertical line on the examination sheet at the child's chronologic age. Place the date of the examination at the top of the age line. For children who were born prematurely, subtract the number of months of prematurity from the chronologic age. Adjust the age line appropriately and note the amount of adjustment at the top of the line.

2. The items to be administered are those in the Personal-Social, Fine Motor-Adaptive, Language, and Gross Motor sectors through which the child's chronologic age line passes. In each sector one should establish age levels at which the child passes all the items and at which all items are failed.

3. When a child refuses to do an item requested by the examiner, the parent may administer the item, provided this is done in the prescribed manner.

4. If a child passes an item, a large letter "P" is written on the bar. "F" designates a failure, and "R" designates a refusal.

5. Note is made of the child's adjustment to the examination (cooperation, attention span, self-confidence) and relationships to parent, to the examiner, and to the test materials.

6. The parent reports whether the child's performance was typical. This is recorded.

7. For retesting, use the same form with different colors for each scoring line and age.

8. Instructions for administering footnoted items are on the back of the test form.

Interpretations. Each test item is designated by a bar. The left end of the bar, the hatch mark at the top of the bar, the left end of the shaded area, and the right end of the bar designate respectively the ages at which 25 per cent, 50 per cent, 75 per cent, and 90 per cent of the reference population performed the item successfully.

Failure on an item achieved by 90 per cent of children of the same age should be considered a "delay." Performances are scored as *abnormal* if two or more sectors have two or more delays, *or* if one sector has two or more delays and one other sector has one delay and in the same sector the age line does not intersect one item that is passed; as *questionable* if any one sector has two or more delays, or if one or more sectors have one delay *and* in the same sectors the age line does not intersect an item that is passed; as *untestable* if refusals occur in numbers large enough to cause the test score to be questionable or abnormal if the refusals were to be scored as failures; and as *normal* if the performance is not abnormal, questionable, or untestable.

Suspect performances should be evaluated. They may be due to temporary factors, such as fatigue, illness, hospitalization, separation from parent, fear, and so on; chronic unwillingness to do things requested; general retardation; pathologic factors, such as deafness or neurologic impairment; or familial patterns of development.

If test results are abnormal, questionable, or untestable, the child should be rescreened a month later. Without improvement, the child should be evaluated with more extensive and refined diagnostic studies.

Caution. The DDST is *not* an intelligence test and does *not* establish a DQ or an IQ. It is a screening instrument for use in clinical practice to identify children whose development may need critical study.

The DDST form is copyrighted. Forms, kits, manuals and instructional films may be purchased through LADOCA Project and Publishing Foundation, Inc., East 51st Avenue and Lincoln Street, Denver, Col. 80216.

We are indebted to the authors for permission to include the test in this volume.

Adapted from V. Vaughan et al. Nelson Textbook of Pediatrics, W. B. Saunders Co., 1979.

APPENDIX V

RECOMMENDED DIETARY ALLOWANCES

MEAN HEIGHTS AND WEIGHTS AND RECOMMENDED ENERGY INTAKE

Category	Age (years)	Weight (kg)	Weight (lb)	Height (cm)	Height (in.)	Energy Needs (kcal)	(with range)
Infants	0.0–0.5	6	13	60	24	kg × 115	(95–145)
	0.5–1.0	9	20	71	28	kg × 105	(80–135)
Children	1–3	13	29	90	35	1300	(900–1800)
	4–6	20	44	112	44	1700	(1300–2300)
	7–10	28	62	132	52	2400	(1650–3300)
Males	11–14	45	99	157	62	2700	(2000–3700)
	15–18	66	145	176	69	2800	(2100–3900)
	19–22	70	154	177	70	2900	(2500–3300)
Females	11–14	46	101	157	62	2200	(1500–3000)
	15–18	55	120	163	64	2100	(1200–3000)
	19–22	55	120	163	64	2100	(1700–2500)
Pregnancy						+300	
Lactation						+500	

Adapted from recommended dietary allowances, 9th ed. National Academy of Sciences, Washington, D.C., 1980.

FOOD AND NUTRITION BOARD, NATIONAL ACADEMY OF SCIENCES–NATIONAL RESEARCH COUNCIL RECOMMENDED DAILY DIETARY ALLOWANCES,[a] REVISED 1980

Designed for the maintenance of good nutrition of practically all healthy people in the U.S.A.

	Age (years)	Protein (g)	Fat-Soluble Vitamins			Water-Soluble Vitamins						Minerals				
			Vitamin A (μg RE) (IU)	Vitamin D (μg)	Vitamin E (mg)	Vitamin C (mg)	Thiamin (mg)	Riboflavin (mg)	Niacin (mg)	Vitamin B-6 (mg)	Vitamin B-12 (μg)	Calcium (mg)	Phosphorus (mg)	Magnesium (mg)	Iron (mg)	Zinc (mg)	Iodine (μg)
Infants	0.0–0.5	kg × 2.2	420 1400	10	3	35	0.3	0.4	6	0.3	0.5	360	240	50	10	3	40
	0.5–1.0	kg × 2.0	400 2000	10	4	35	0.5	0.6	8	0.6	1.5	540	360	70	15	5	50
Children	1–3	23	400 2000	10	5	45	0.7	0.8	9	0.9	2.0	800	800	150	15	10	70
	4–6	30	500 2500	10	6	45	0.9	1.0	11	1.3	2.5	800	800	200	10	10	90
	7–10	34	700 3300	10	7	45	1.2	1.4	16	1.6	3.0	800	800	250	10	10	120
Males	11–14	45	1000 5000	10	8	50	1.4	1.6	18	1.8	3.0	1200	1200	350	18	15	150
	15–18	56	1000 5000	10	10	60	1.4	1.7	18	2.0	3.0	1200	1200	400	18	15	150
	19–22	56	1000 5000	7.5	10	60	1.5	1.7	19	2.2	3.0	800	800	350	10	15	150
Females	11–14	46	800 4000	10	8	50	1.1	1.3	15	1.8	3.0	1200	1200	300	18	15	150
	15–18	46	800 4000	10	8	60	1.1	1.3	14	2.0	3.0	1200	1200	300	18	15	150
	19–22	44	800 4000	7.5	8	60	1.1	1.3	14	2.0	3.0	800	800	300	18	15	150
Pregnant		+30	+200	+5	+2	+20	+0.4	+0.3	+2	+0.6	+1.0	+400	+400	+150	h	+5	+25
Lactating		+20	+400	+5	+3	+40	+0.5	+0.5	+5	+0.5	+1.0	+400	+400	+150	h	+10	+50

[a] The allowances are intended to provide for individual variations among most normal persons as they live in the United States under usual environmental stresses. Diets should be based on a variety of common foods in order to provide other nutrients for which human requirements have been less well defined.
Adapted from Recommended Dietary Allowances, 9th ed. National Academy of Science, Washington, D.C., 1980.
1 μg retinal (RE) = Vitamin A activity from 3.33 IU of retinal equivalents.

APPENDIX V *(Continued)*

ESTIMATED SAFE AND ADEQUATE DAILY DIETARY INTAKES OF VITAMIN K AND ELECTROLYTES

	Age (years)	Vitamin K (μg)	Electrolytes		
			Sodium (mg)	Potassium (mg)	Chloride (mg)
Infants	0–0.5	12	115–350	350–925	275–706
	0.5–1	10–20	250–750	425–1275	400–1200
Children and	1–3	15–30	325–975	550–1650	500–1500
Adolescents	4–6	20–40	450–1350	775–2325	700–2100
	7–10	30–60	600–1800	1000–3000	925–2775
	11+	50–100	900–2700	1525–4575	1400–4200

Adapted from Recommended Dietary Allowances, 9th ed. National Academy of Science, Washington, D.C., 1980.

RANGE OF AVERAGE WATER REQUIREMENT OF CHILDREN AT DIFFERENT AGES UNDER ORDINARY CONDITIONS

Age	Average Body Weight in kg	Total Water in 24 hrs, ml	Water per kg Body Wt in 24 hrs, ml
3 years	3.0	250– 300	80–100
10 days	3.2	400– 500	125–150
3 months	5.4	750– 850	140–160
6 months	7.3	950–1100	130–155
9 months	8.6	1100–1250	125–145
1 year	9.5	1150–1300	120–135
2 years	11.8	1350–1500	115–125
4 years	16.2	1600–1800	100–110
6 years	20.0	1800–2000	90–100
10 years	28.7	2000–2500	70– 85
14 years	45.0	2200–2700	50– 60
18 years	54.0	2200–2700	40– 50

From V. Vaughan et al. Nelson Textbook of Pediatrics. W. B. Saunders Co., 1979.

APPENDIX VI
NORMAL VALUES FOR COMMON LABORATORY TESTS

CHEMISTRY LABORATORY VALUES

Determination	Specimen	Value		
			Premature mg/dl	Full-term mg/dl
Bilirubin, total	Serum	Cord	<2	<2
		0–1 day	<8	<6
		1–2 days	<12	<8
		3–5 days	<16	<12
		Thereafter	<2	0.2–1.0
Bilirubin, direct			0.0–0.2 mg/dl	
Calcium	Serum	Newborn	3.7–7.0 mEq/l	
		Infant	5.2–6.0 mEq/l	
		Child	5.0–5.7 mEq/l	
		Thereafter	4.5–5.8 mEq/l	
Carbon dioxide, partial pressure pCO_2	Arterial blood	Infant	27–41 mm Hg	
		Thereafter		
		Male	35–45 mm Hg	
		Female	32–45 mm Hg	
Catecholamines	Urine		*Norepinephrine*	*Epinephrine*
		Neonate	2–12 µg/d	1–2 µg/d
		Infant	3–30 µg/d	1–15 µg/d
		Child	20–70 µg/d	1–15 µg/d
		Adolescent	30–80 µg/d	5–15 µg/d
Chloride	Serum	Infant	95–110 mEq/l	
		Child	101–108 mEq/l	
		Thereafter	98–106 mEq/l	

Table continued on the following page.

CHEMISTRY LABORATORY VALUES (Continued)

Determination	Specimen	Value	
Cholesterol, total	Serum	Infant	70–175 mg/dl
		Child	120–200 mg/dl
		Adolescent	120–210 mg/dl
		Thereafter	140–250 mg/dl
Creatinine	Serum		0.2–1.0 mg/dl
Fecal fat	Feces	0–6 yrs	<2 g/d
		Thereafter	2–6 g/d
Iron, total	Serum	Newborn	100–250 µg/dl
		Infant	40–100 µg/dl
		Child	50–120 µg/dl
		Thereafter	
		Male	60–150 µg/dl
		Female	50–130 µg/dl
Iron-binding capacity	Serum	Newborn	60–175 µg/dl
		Infant	100–400 µg/dl
		Thereafter	250–400 µg/dl
17-Ketogenic steroids (17–KGS)	Urine	0–1 yr	<1 mg/d
		1–10 yr	<5 mg/d
		Adult	
		Male	5–23 mg/d
		Female	3–15 mg/d
17-Ketosteroids (17–KS)	Urine	0–14 days	1–3 mg/d
		14 days–2 yrs	0–1 mg/d
		2–6 yr	0–2 mg/d
		6–10 yr	1–4 mg/d
		10–12 yr	1–6 mg/d
		12–14 yr	3–10 mg/d
		Thereafter	
		Male	9–22 mg/d
		Female	6–15 mg/d
Lead	Whole blood		<40 µg/dl
	Urine		<80 µg/dl
Oxygen pressure (pO$_2$)	Arterial blood	Newborn	65–80 mm Hg
		Thereafter	83–108 mm Hg
Oxygen, % saturation	Arterial blood	Newborn	40–90%
		Thereafter	95–98%
pH (37°C)	Arterial blood	Newborn	7.27–7.47
		Thereafter	7.33–7.43
	Venous blood		7.33–7.43
Phenylalanine	Serum	Premature/low birth weight:	2.0–7.5 mg/dl
		Full-term newborn	1.2–3.4 mg/dl
		Thereafter	0.8–1.8 mg/dl

CHEMISTRY LABORATORY VALUES (Continued)

Determination	Specimen	Value	
Phosphorus	Serum	Infant	4.5–6.7 mg/dl
		Child	4.5–5.5 mg/dl
		Thereafter	3.0–4.5 mg/dl
Potassium	Serum/plasma	Infant	4.1–5.3 mEq/l
		Child	3.4–4.7 mEq/l
		Thereafter	3.5–5.3 mEq/l
Protein-bound iodine	Serum		4.0–8.0 μg/dl
Protein, total	Serum	Newborn	4.6–7.6 g/dl
		Child	6.2–8.0 g/dl
		Thereafter	6.0–8.0 g/dl
Sodium	Serum	Newborn	134–144 mEq/l
		Child	138–146 mEq/l
		Thereafter	135–148 mEq/l
Vanillylmandelic acid (VMA)	Urine	Infant	0–2 mg/d
		Child	1–5 mg/d
		Thereafter	2–7 mg/d
Antistreptolysin O filter (ASO)	Serum	Normal	<166 Todd Units
		Recent streptococcal infection	200–2500 Todd Units
Cold Agglutinins	Serum	0–1:32	
C-reactive protein (CRP)	Serum	None detected	
Heterophile antibody mono "spot" test	Serum	Negative	

From V. Vaughan et al. Nelson Textbook of Pediatrics. W. B. Saunders Co., 1979

HEMATOLOGIC LABORATORY VALUES

	Hematocrit %	Hemoglobin g/dl	Fetal Hemoglobin % of total	Red Blood Cells (mil/mm³)	Platelets (in thousands per mm³)	Sed. Rate mm/hr.	Reticulocyte Count % of Total RBC	White Blood Count Total (in thousands per mm³)	Neutrophils %	Lymphocytes %
Cord	50–60	14–20	–	–	100–290	–	3.0–7.0	9–30	61	31
Newborn	53–65	15–22	40–70	4.4–5.8	140–300	0.2	1.1–4.5	9–30	61	31
Neonate	43–54	11–20	20–40	4.1–6.4	150–390	3–13	0.1–1.5	5–19.5	35	56
Infant	30–40	10–15	2–10	3.8–5.5	200–473	3–13	0.5–3.1	6–17.5	32	61
Child	31–43	11–16	1–2	3.8–5.5	200–473	3–13	0.0–2.0	4.8–10.8	60	30
Thereafter:										
Male	42–52	14–18	1–2	4.7–6.1	150–450	1–20	0.0–2.0	4.8–10.8	60	30
Female	37–47	12–16	1–2	4.2–5.4	150–450	1–30	0.0–2.0	4.8–10.8	60	30

NORMAL BLADDER CAPACITY AND VOIDING

Age	Approximate Capacity	Number of Voidings in 24 hrs	Average Quantity at Each Voiding in cc's
Birth	60 cc	14	30
Birth to 3 months	60–115 cc	13–14	30
3–6 months	115–150 cc	20	30
6–12 months	150–280 cc	16	45
1 year	280 cc	12	60
6 years	500–700 cc	7–8	120–150
12 years	850 cc	7–8	180–240

NORMAL ROUTINE URINALYSIS RESULTS

Appearance	Clear
Color	Pale yellow to amber
Specific gravity	1.001–1.030
pH	4.6–8
Glucose	None
Ketones	None
Protein	None
Microscopic Examination	
Red blood cells	1–2 RBC's
White blood cells	1–2 WBC's
Cast	Occasional

COAGULATION LABORATORY VALUES

	Specimen	Values	
Partial thromboplastin time (PTT)	Plasma	Premature	<120 sec
		Newborn	<90 sec
		Thereafter	24–40 sec
Prothrombin time	Plasma	Newborn	<17 sec
		Thereafter	11–14 sec
Clotting time	Whole blood		
Two tubes			5–8 min
Three tubes			5–15 min
Bleeding time	Whole blood	Premature	1–8 min
		Newborn	1–5 min
		Thereafter	1–6 min

From V. C. Vaughan et al. Nelson Textbook of Pediatrics, W. B. Saunders Co., 1979.

APPENDIX VII

INJECTION SITES

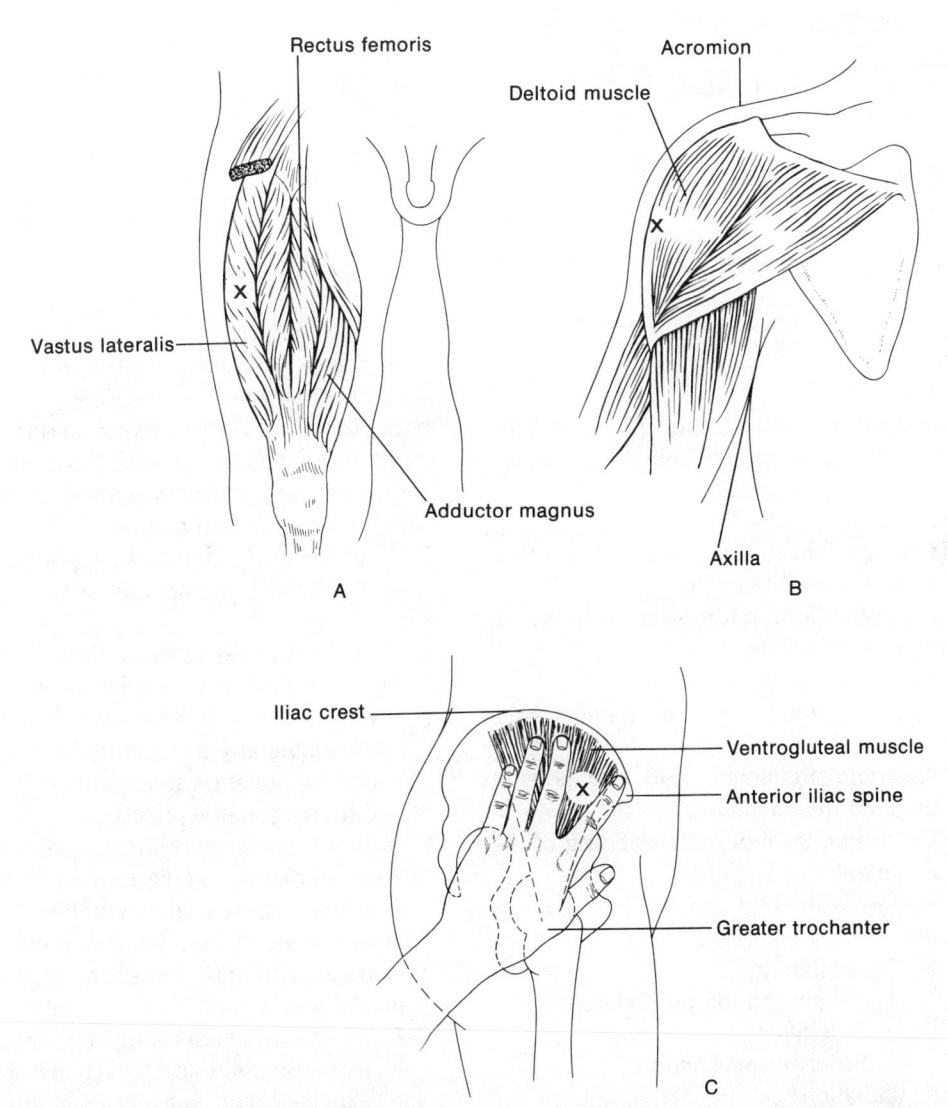

A, Vastus lateralis site. The site is located in the mid-third of the thigh and is found by dividing the thigh into thirds from the greater trochanter of the femur to just above the knee. The area of insertion within the mid-third of the thigh is found midway between imaginary lines midanteriorly and midlaterally.

B, Deltoid site. The site is located in the lower part of the upper third of the deltoid. The site of insertion is midway between the acromion and the axilla on the lateral surface of the arm.

C, Ventrogluteal site. The site is located by placing the palm on the greater trochanter, the index finger on the anterior iliac spine (this may be facilitated by flexing of the thigh at the hip); the middle finger is extended along the iliac crest as far as possible, forming a triangle. The injection is given in the center of the triangle or V formed by the hand, with the needle directed slightly upward toward the iliac crest.

APPENDIX VIII

COMBINATION TREATMENT (CHEMOTHERAPY AND RADIATION THERAPY)

Nursing goal:
Short-term:
1. To provide physical and emotional care during combined therapy to minimize side effects

Long-term:
1. To assist child to fulfill optimum level of health and well-being, or
2. To assist child to return to accustomed or improved life style

A. Pretreatment teaching
   1. Ascertain what child and parents have been told
   2. Ascertain frequency and duration of planned treatment
   3. Determine level of understanding of the treatment
   4. Review with child and family any questions:
      a. Chemotherapy
         (1) Administration procedure
         (2) Side effects
         (3) Mechanism of action
      b. Radiation
         (1) Technique
         (2) Side effects
         (3) Mechanism of action

B. Psychological and emotional preparation
   1. Determine what this therapy means to these individuals (i.e., what value has been placed on this treatment)
   2. Assess the nature of optional coping mechanisms
   3. Reinforce realistic expectations
   4. Attempt to allay anxieties and fears of treatment and/or diagnosis
      a. Provide information
      b. Provide emotional support
      c. Provide therapeutic play opportunities
      d. Encourage verbalization of fears

C. Maintain time-dose relationship:
   Provide for timely administration of chemotherapy in relationship to planned time of radiation treatments.
   Observe for side effects:

D. Skin erythema/excoriation (perianal, vulvar); stomatitis; genitourinary symptoms; diarrhea; nausea and vomiting; loss of appetite; weakness; bone marrow depression; arrhythmias; extremity pain or itching; alopecia
   1. Notify physician as appropriate
   2. Reassure child and family that these are expected and may resolve after treatment is completed
   3. Utilize nursing comfort measures and medical treatments prescribed.

E. Skin care
   1. Keep skin (especially in treatment areas, perineum, and buttocks) clean and dry
   2. Encourage exposure to air, e.g., through wearing of cotton clothing and use of light linens

3. Bathing:
   a. Tepid water only
   b. Soap in sparing amounts only when approved by radiation therapist
   c. Take care not to remove field markings
4. Maintain skin blood supply
5. No heating pads or hot water bottles applied to treatment area
6. No ice packs applied to treatment area
7. Do not expose treatment area directly to the sun or heat lamps
8. Use only baby oil, lanolin, or white vaseline for skin care in the treated area. Permission for use of other ointments, etc., must come from radiation therapist.

F. Stomatitis
1. Good oral hygiene
   a. Rinse mouth frequently with water after and between meals
   b. Use cotton swabs and hydrogen peroxide and water to clean sore gums and teeth
   c. Regular dental evaluation
2. Normal saline or viscous xylocaine gargles
3. Alter diet to minimize discomfort without diminished intake
   a. Liquid diet of tepid temperature in severe cases
   b. Pureed foods or soft diet in mild to moderate cases
   c. Use a straw for liquids
   d. Bland foods cause less irritation; butter, thin gravies and sauces make foods easier to swallow.

G. Diarrhea
1. Low residue, low fiber diet
2. Clear liquids first 12–24 hours after acute onset and gradually resume regular diet as tolerated
3. Serve liquids and foods at lukewarm temperature
4. Limit raw foods, citrus fruits, carbonated beverages
5. Observe for electrolyte depletion; include potassium-rich foods daily in diet; salt intake is usually sufficient in American diets to make up for any sodium depletion
6. Offer small amounts of food at more frequent intervals; offer liquids between meals rather than with meals
7. Give milk and milk products cautiously during therapy until any lactose intolerance is determined. (Some chemotherapy drugs produce temporary lactose intolerance.)
8. Utilize medication prescribed
   a. For severe/uncontrolled diarrhea, give at regular intervals around-the-clock until controlled
   b. For mild diarrhea, give PRN

H. Urinary symptoms
1. Increase fluid intake
2. Administer urinary analgesics and/or antispasmodics as prescribed

I. Nausea and vomiting: anorexia
1. Small frequent meals, eaten slowly
2. Serve fluids between rather than with meals; encourage liberal fluid intake
3. Serve foods tepid, cool, chilled or frozen in cubes; hot foods often stimulate or increase nausea
4. Provide rest after meals to facilitate digestion
5. Child on therapy often feels best in the morning; take this opportunity to provide a high-protein, high-carbohydrate meal
6. Cold, salty, low fat foods are usually tolerated best; avoid foods that are fatty, greasy, overly sweet, spicy, hot or that have a strong odor
7. Do not force intake of nutritionally important or favorite foods while child is nauseated; this may cause permanent aversion to the food
8. Good oral hygiene
9. Utilize medication prescribed
   a. Offer ½ hour before meals and ½ hour before treatments
   b. For severe nausea and vomiting, give around-the-clock

J. Nutrition
1. Encourage high-nutrition diet (high protein, high calorie) by teaching child and family what foods are preferable
2. Offer favored foods as much as possible
   a. Dietary consult
   b. Family may bring food from home

K. Weakness
1. Schedule daily activities in short bursts with rest periods
2. Reassure child that this is expected during therapy
3. Observe for signs of anemia and electrolyte imbalances

(Continued)

L. Diversion for long-term hospitalization (when applicable)
   1. Suggest quiet activities child might enjoy (e.g., reading, crafts, TV, music)
   2. Ask for playroom privileges or short passes for those whose condition permits
   3. Ask for weekend pass for those who are able to go home with family
M. Bone marrow depression
   1. Thrombocytopenia
      a. Observe puncture sites carefully for bleeding
      b. Observe for petechiae, bleeding gums
      c. For severe conditions, minimize punctures
      d. Give mouth care cautiously (soft toothbrush, gauze square or cotton swab)
      e. Avoid physical trauma
   2. Leukopenia
      a. Protect from infections
      b. Educate parents to monitor for signs of infection

N. Allergic reactions to chemotherapeutic agents
   1. For occurrence during infusion, discontinue drug immediately
   2. Observe child for extremity pain or itching, infusion site discoloration, urticaria or systemic signs of inflammatory response
   3. Consult doctor about use of systemic anti-inflammatory agents
O. Alopecia
   1. Educate parents to understand young child (under 5) is not disturbed by loss of hair and does not want to bother with wig; child's general reaction will be a reflection of parents' reactions
   2. Wigs are available for older children; however, some children still prefer not to bother with them

From: National Cancer Institute. Diet and Nutrition: A Resource For Parents of Children with Cancer. U. S. Department of Health, Education and Welfare, NIH Publication No. 80-2038, December 1979.

D. Smith, et al. Nursing Care of patients undergoing combination chemotherapy and radiotherapy. Cancer Nursing, April 1978, p. 133

APPENDIX VIII *(Continued)*

APPENDIX IX

CONVERSION TABLES

CONVERSION OF POUNDS TO KILOGRAMS FOR PEDIATRIC WEIGHTS

Pounds → ↓	0	1	2	3	4	5	6	7	8	9
0	0.00	0.45	0.90	1.36	1.81	2.26	2.72	3.17	3.62	4.08
10	4.53	4.98	5.44	5.89	6.35	6.80	7.25	7.71	8.16	8.61
20	9.07	9.52	9.97	10.43	10.88	11.34	11.79	12.24	12.70	13.15
30	13.60	14.06	14.51	14.96	15.42	15.87	16.32	16.78	17.23	17.69
40	18.14	18.59	19.05	19.50	19.95	20.41	20.86	21.31	21.77	22.22
50	22.68	23.13	23.58	24.04	24.49	24.94	25.40	25.85	26.30	26.76
60	27.21	27.66	28.12	28.57	29.03	29.48	29.93	30.39	30.84	31.29
70	31.75	32.20	32.65	33.11	33.56	34.02	34.47	34.92	35.38	35.83
80	36.28	36.74	37.19	37.64	38.10	38.55	39.00	39.46	39.91	40.37
90	40.82	41.27	41.73	42.18	42.63	43.09	43.54	43.99	44.45	44.90
100	45.36	45.81	46.26	46.72	47.17	47.62	48.08	48.53	48.98	49.44
110	49.89	50.34	50.80	51.25	51.71	52.16	52.61	53.07	53.52	53.97
120	54.43	54.88	55.33	55.79	56.24	56.70	57.15	57.60	58.06	58.51
130	58.96	59.42	59.87	60.32	60.78	61.23	61.68	62.14	62.59	63.05
140	63.50	63.95	64.41	64.86	65.31	65.77	66.22	66.67	67.13	67.58
150	68.04	68.49	68.94	69.40	69.85	70.30	70.76	71.21	71.66	72.12
160	72.57	73.02	73.48	73.93	74.39	74.84	75.29	75.75	76.20	76.65
170	77.11	77.56	78.01	78.47	78.92	79.38	79.83	80.28	80.74	81.19
180	81.64	82.10	82.55	83.00	83.46	83.91	84.36	84.82	85.27	85.73
190	86.18	86.68	87.09	87.54	87.99	88.45	88.90	89.35	89.81	90.26
200	90.72	91.17	91.62	92.08	92.53	92.98	93.44	93.89	94.34	94.80

APPENDIX IX (Continued)

CONVERSION FACTORS FOR TEMPERATURE

Celsius	Fahrenheit	Celsius	Fahrenheit
34.0	93.2	38.6	101.5
34.2	93.6	38.8	101.8
34.4	93.9	39.0	102.2
34.6	94.3	39.2	102.6
34.8	94.6	39.4	102.9
35.0	95.0	39.6	103.3
35.2	95.4	39.8	103.6
35.4	95.7	40.0	104.0
35.6	96.1	40.2	104.4
35.8	96.4	40.4	104.7
36.0	96.8	40.6	105.2
36.2	97.2	40.8	105.4
36.4	97.5	41.0	105.9
36.6	97.9	41.2	106.1
36.8	98.2	41.4	106.5
37.0	98.6	41.6	106.8
37.2	99.0	41.8	107.2
37.4	99.3	42.0	107.6
37.6	99.7	42.2	108.0
37.8	100.0	42.4	108.3
38.0	100.4	42.6	108.7
38.2	100.8	42.8	109.0
38.4	101.1	43.0	109.4

$(°C) \times (9/5) + 32 = °F$
$(°F) - 32) \times (5/9) = °C$
$°C$ = temperature in Celsius (centigrade) degrees
$°F$ = temperature in Fahrenheit degrees

INDEX

Note: In this index, page numbers in *italics* refer to illustrations. Page numbers followed by (t) refer to tables.

Abdomen, assessment of, 226–228
 distention of, 226
  in Hirschsprung's disease, 589
  in intestinal atresia, 584
  in volvulus, 586
 neonatal circulation and, 533
 of normal newborn, 419
Abdominal masses, midline, 562, *563*
Abdominal pain, in intussusception, 586–587
Abdominal reflex, evaluation of, 236
Abortion, elective, 107
 spontaneous, 108
 threatened, 107
Abscess, retropharyngeal, 606–607
Abuse, of adolescent, 1253–1255
Abuse, of child, 85
Abused child, care of, 88–89
 care of parent of, 89
 discharge planning for, 89–90
 family and, 84–90
Acceleration-deceleration phenomenon, in head injuries, 1109
Acceptance, parent-child-nurse relationship and, 167
 stage of preparation for death, 306
Accidents, toddler and, 758–760
Accommodation, of eyes, 206
 and vision, 962
Accommodative esotropia, 965, *965*
Acetaminophen, 343, 343(t), 821
Acetylsalicylic acid, 343, 343(t)
Achilles reflex, 238
Acid-base balances, 347, 348–349(t), 350
 nurse's role in maintaining, 353–356
Acid-base imbalance, 348–349(t)
Acidosis, 347
Acne vulgaris, 1263–1265
Acromegaly, 633
Action for Children's Television, 31
Activities, group, hospitalized child and, 300–301

Activities of daily living, of families, 256
Activity, tuberculosis and, 1310
Activity level, of children, 1076
Acute glomerulonephritis, 1117–1119, *1118*
Acute laryngotracheobronchitis (LTB), 823, 824(t)
Acute period, of burn care, 811–814
Acute polyneuritis, 1124
Acyanotic heart defects, with increased pulmonary vascularity, 538–544
 with normal pulmonary vascularity, 544–547
Adaptability, of children, 1076
 of families, 251–252
Adenitis, cervical, scarlet fever and, 929(t)
Adenoids, diseased, 941–943
Adipose cells, childhood obesity and, 1134
Admission phase, hospitalized preschooler and, 1021–1022, *1021*
 hospitalized school-age child and, 1204–1205
Adolescence, characteristics of, 1332(t)
 communicable diseases of, 1288–1293
 infectious diseases of, 1266–1270
 potential stresses during, 1249–1262, 1263–1272, 1273–1297, 1298–1313, 1314–1330
 pregnancy in, 115–125
Adolescent, abuse of, 1253–1255
 alienated, 1230
 at risk for social problems,1250(t)
 divorce and, 65(t)
 drugs and, 1228–1229
 physical examination of, 188
 family with, growth and development needs of, 1221–1225
 potential stresses in, 1226–1231

Adolescent (*Continued*)
 health of, irreversible alterations in, 1298–1313
 life-threatening alterations in, 1314–1330
 reversible alterations in, 1273–1297
 temporary alterations in, 1263–1272
 health care of, 1243
 hospitalized, 1331–1338
 interviewing, 179
 musculoskeletal alteration in, nursing care plan for, 1340–1358
 sexual activity and, 1255–1257
 sexuality of, 1227–1228, *1228*
Adolescent pregnancy, impact on health professionals, 120–124
Adolescent schizophrenic reaction, 1300–1302
Adoption, 69–72
 preparing for parenthood in, 101–102
 single parent, 71–72
 transracial, 71, *71*
Adrenarche, premature, 1114
Adrenogenital syndrome, 665–667
Adventitious deafness, 975, 975(t)
Adventitious lung sounds, 223(t)
Advocacy, of child in dysfunctional families, 80
 of poor families, 28–29
Agammaglobulinemia, 664–665
Aganglionic megacolon, 589–593
Age, gestational, appropriateness of size for, 411
 Dubowitz assessment of, 408–409, *410*, 410(t)
 large for, 443–444
 small for, 443
 variations in, 429–445
 of child, effect on parenting styles, 50–51
Agenesis, anal, 595, *595*–597

1389

Aggression, of school-age child, 1078
  of toddler, 746–748
AIDS scale, 486–487, 490
  instructions for, 488–489
Airway obstruction, upper, major burns and, 806(t)
Akinetic seizures, 1161
Alcohol, adolescent and, 1229, 1258–1259
  adolescent pregnancy and, 120
Alerting, 423
Alienated adolescent, 1230
Allen Cards, 208
Allergic contact dermatitis, 499–501, *500*
Allergic rhinitis, chronic, 995(t)
  seasonal, 995–996
Allergic salute, 987, *987*
Allergic shiners, 987, *987*
Allergic threshold, 985
Allergy, 494–497
  gastrointestinal, 506–507
  prevention of, 497–498
  skin testing in, 990
  to stinging insects, 995
Allergy-producing substances, 494(t)
Allergy-proofing, techniques of, 497(t)
Alterations, of infant health, 645–669
  attachment breakdown and, 475–476
  temporary, 493–521
Alternating strabismus, 965
Alternative family life styles, 60–75
Amblyopia, 898, 966–967
  in toddler, 738
  strabismic, 966
Amblyopia ex anopsia, 966
Ambulation, of toddler, 732–734, *732*
Amebiasis, 794
Amelia, 648
Amenorrhea, 1270–1271
American Academy of Pediatrics, guidelines for oxygen therapy, 438–439
  statement on school health education, 1071
Amputation, in bone tumor, 1318–1319
Anal agenesis, 595, *595*
  nursing responsibilities in, 597–598
Anal fissures, infant constipation and, 513
Anal membrane, imperforate, 595, *595*
Anal stenosis, 595, *595*
Anal wink, 236, 1095
Analgesia, in sickle cell anemia, 675
Anemia, Cooley's, 676
  iron deficiency, 785–788
  leukemia and, 1006
  sickle cell, 672–674
Anesthesia, 369–372, 370(t)

Anger, as parents' response to birth of infant with defect, 525
  dying adolescent and, 1315
  in parents of irreversibly ill child, 292
  in preparation for death, 306
  in school-age child, 1078, *1078*
  in toddler, 746–748
Angiotensin, in regulation of fluid and electrolyte balance, 346
Anisometropic amblyopia, 966
Ankle dorsiflexion, of newborn infant, 410
Ankle flexion, in preterm and term infant, *430*
Anogenital area, of normal newborn, 419
Anomalies, congenital, of heart, 528–558
  facial, 565–569
  musculoskeletal, 599–605
  of gastrointestinal tract, 569–599
  of genitourinary tract, 561–562
  of urinary tract, 560–565
Anorectal malformations, 595–598
Anterior pituitary hypofunction, 630–636
Antibiotics, in cystic fibrosis, 1327
  preterm infant and, 441
Anticipatory guidance. See under subjects.
Antidiuretic hormone, fluid and electrolyte balance and, 346
  oversecretion of, 352
Antisocial behavior, identifying and managing, 1100–1102
  school-age child and, 1098–1102
Anus, assessment of, 230
  imperforate, 595–596, *595*
Anxiety, in situational crisis, 276
  of parents, nurse and, 302–303
Aorta, coarctation of, 544–545
Aortic stenosis, 546–547
APGAR, family, 253, 253(t)
Apgar score, 407–408, 408(t)
Apical pulse, 317
Aplastic crisis, 674
Appearance, general, in physical examination, 193, 195
  of preschooler, 896
  of preterm infant, 430–432
  of school-age child, 1060–1063
  of term infant, 430–432
  of toddler, 732–733
Appendicitis, 1123–1124
Appliances, dental, school-age child and, 1137
Appraisal of health, 177–250
Approachability, of children, 1076
Appropriateness of size for gestational age, 411
Arboviruses, encephalitis and, 619
Arginine tolerance test, for pituitary dwarfism, 631–632
Arm and leg restraints, 322
Arm recoil, of newborn infant, 410
Arms, assessment of, 230
Arthritis, juvenile rheumatoid, 1179–1180
Arthrodesis, 1281, 1286, 1286(t)
Articulation, 1074
Ascariasis, 791
Aseptic measures, 288

Aspiration, of foreign body, 761
Aspirin, for fever, 343, 343(t)
Assessment, nursing process and, 128–129
  of adolescent, at hospital admission, 1332–1333
  of family, 251–257
  of family finances, 28
  of family religion, 34
  of family structuring of time, 26
  of infant obesity, 625
  of parent-infant attachment, 490
  of parental discipline, 42
  of parental use of punishment, 44
  of parental use of reward, 45
  of parenting capabilities, 55–59
  of potential fluid and electrolyte imbalance, 353–356
  physical, in history taking, 185–193
  of newborn, 408–420
Associative play, 162–163
Asthma, attack, 985–986
  extrinsic, 985
  intrinsic, 985
  laboratory tests in, 989(t)
  long-term management of, 990–992, 991(t)
Astigmatism, 964
Astrocytoma, cerebellar, 1190
  cerebral, 1191
Atelectasis, pertussis and, 927(t)
Athlete's foot, 1104–1105
Atopic dermatitis, 504–505
Atresia, biliary, 668–669
  choanal, 558–559
  esophageal, tracheoesophageal fistula and, 572–577, *572*
  intestinal, 584–585
  tricuspid, 550
Atrial septal defect (ASD), 538–540, *540*
  differential diagnosis from ventricular septal defect, 540
Atrophy, skin, *199*
Attachment, parent-child, assessing problems in, 482–491
  blind child and, 969
  breakdown of, 475–482
  dynamics of, 472–475, *472*
  emotional-social competency and, 461
  forming, 386–388
  infant with defect and, 525–526
  separation and, 745–746
Attention span, of children, 1077
Audiometer, 898
Audiometry, play, 213
Auditory communication, hearing impairment and, 982
Auscultation, in physical examination, 194(t)
  of abdomen, 226–227
  of chest, 221–223
  of heart, 224–225
  neonatal circulation and, 534
Authoritarian parenting style, 51(t)
Autism, 1164–1166
  education and, 1165
Autocratic parenting style, 51(t)
Automobile accidents, preschooler and, 911
  toddler and, 758–760

Autonomy, of irreversibly ill child, 828–830
  of toddler, 748
Autosomal dominant inheritance, 140
Autosomal recessive inheritance, 140–141
Aversive therapy, 1303

Babinski reflex, 422–423, *422*
  evaluation of, 238
Baby bottle syndrome. See *Milk bottle syndrome.*
Bacillary dysentery, 794–795
Back, of normal newborn, 420
Bacteremia, cellulitis and, 931(t)
  impetigo and, 931(t)
Bacterial meningitis, 616–618
  role of nurse in, 617–618
Bacterial pneumonia, in infants, 612–613(t)
  major burns and, 806(t)
  responsibilities of nurse in, 614–615
Balance, assessment of, 233
Balanced suspension, 1131–1132
Bands, 1001
Bargaining, stage of preparation for death, 306
Barium enema, in treating intussusception, 587–588
Barrel chest, 222
Basophils, 1001
Bathing, of hospitalized child, 315–316
  of newborn, 425–426
Bed confinement, school-age child and, 1121, *1121*
Bedtime, postponing by preschooler, 907
Behavior, antisocial, school-age child and, 1098–1102
  illness-seeking, *260*
Behavior, managing, of adolescent, 1249–1262
  of preschooler, 914–920
  of school-age child, 1090–1102
  of toddler, 764–769
  of 6-year-old, 1082
  of 7-year-old, 1082
  of 8-year-old, 1082–1083
  of 9-year-old, 1083, *1085*
  of 10-year-old, 1083–1084
  of 11-year-old, 1084–1085
  of 12-year-old, 1084–1085
  problem, in child, 279–282, *280*
  sex-typed, 754
  stereotyped, in blind child, 972
  wellness-seeking, *260*
Behavior modification, autism and, 1165
  childhood obesity and, 1135–1136
  hyperactivity and, 1147
  schizophrenia and, 1303
  techniques of, 281
Behavioral patterns, of newborn, assessment of, 423–424
Behavioral signs, in potential fluid and electrolyte imbalance, 355

Behaviorist approach, to problem behavior, 281
Bicycle accidents, 1108
Biliary atresia, 668–669
Bilirubin, in health assessment, 248–249
Bill of rights, child's, 54
Bill of rights, parent's, 54–55
Biopsy, in bone tumor, 1316
  muscle, in muscular dystrophy, 1323
Birth control, for adolescent, 1245–1247
Birth defects, attachment breakdown and, 475–476
Birth history, in history taking, 180(t), 183
Birth order, sibling rivalry and, 774
Birth weight, variations in, 429–445
Bisexuality, of parents, 73
Black children, sickle cell anemia in, 674–675
  vitamin D deficiency rickets in, 629
Black English, 1075
Blackhead, 1263
Bladder, palpation of, 227
  persistent infantile, 950
Bladder control, in preschooler, 899–900, *900*
  anticipatory guidance on, 900
Blalock-Taussig procedure, in tetralogy of Fallot, 550
Blennorrhea, 508–509
Blepharitis, 503
Blind child, fostering independence in, 972
Blind infant, attachment breakdown and, 477
Blindness, 967, 968–973
Blood, normal, components of, 1000–1002
Blood cells, production of, 1002, *1002*
Blood pressure, assessment of, in hospitalized child, 317–318
  neonatal circulation and, 533
  in potential fluid and electrolyte imbalance, 354
  of children, *193*
Blood specimens, in health assessment, 245, 248–249
  techniques in obtaining, 245, 248
Blood studies, in iron deficiency anemia, 786–787
Body composition, of adolescent, 1233
  of newborn, 427
  of school-age child, 1061–1062
  anticipatory guidance on, 1062–1063
Body image, adolescent, acceptance of, 1240
  blind child and, 973
  hospitalized adolescent and, 1333
  of school-age child, 1207, 1208–1209
  spinal abnormalities and, 1283
Body part perception, 233
Body proportions, of infant, 449–450

Body water, loss of, per 100 calories metabolized, 356(t)
Body water compartments, 345
Boils, 1105–1106
Bonds, human, growth of, 471–492
  father-infant, 387
  mother-infant, 386–387
  sibling-infant, 387–388, *388*
  of families, 255
Bone age, 144
Bone marrow, 1002
Bone tumors, 1316–1319
Boundaries, individual, of families, 252
Bowel control, in preschooler, 899–900
  anticipatory guidance on, 900
Bowleggedness, 231
Boys, adolescent, delinquency in, 1250
  physical development of, anticipatory guidance on, 1236
  female single parent families and, 62–63
  head circumference of, *190*
  height of, *189*
  sexual maturity in, 1234–1235, 1234(t), *1234*
  weight of, *189*
Braces, in cerebral palsy, 1160
  in Legg-Calvé-Perthes disease, 1112–1113, *1113*
  in spinal abnormalities, 1281–1286
Bradford Frame, split, for congenital hip dislocation, 604, *605*
Braille, 971
Brain dysfunction, minimal, 1144–1146
Brain stem gliomas, 1190
Brain tumor, distribution by age at diagnosis, 1001
Brazelton Neonatal Behavioral Assessment Scale, 644
Bread, preschooler diet and, 909(t)
Breast feeding, necrotizing enterocolitis and, 593
Breasts, assessment of, 224
  development of, premature, 1114
  of adolescent girl, 1234, 1235(t)
Breath sounds, characteristics of, 223(t)
Breathing, deep, nursing actions related to, 328(t)
Breathing exercises, in cystic fibrosis, 1326
Bronchial asthma, 984–995
Bronchiolitis, 607, 610–611, 608–609(t)
  nurse and, 610–611
Bronchitis, in infants, 608–609(t)
Bronchodilator, in acute asthma attack, 993
Bronchopneumonia, 611
  rubeola and, 923(t)
Bronchopulmonary dysplasia, 439
Brushfield's spots, 206
Bryant's traction, 1132, *1133*

INDEX **1391**

Buck's extension, 1131, *1129*
Budget, in preparation for parenthood, 99–100
  reprioritizing of, 711–712
Bulla, *198*
Burns, 799–817
  assessing severity of, 800–802
  major, 803–805
    complications of, 806–808(t)
  minor, 802–803, 812
  prevention of, 800, 817
  responsibilities of nurse in, 814–815
  toddler and, 760–761
Burn care, basic, 805, 808–814
Burow's solution, use of, for allergic contact dermatitis, 500, 501

Café au lait spots, 654
Calcium, imbalance of, 352–353, 351(t)
Calorie, malnutrition, severe, 627–628
  requirements of toddler, 738
Cancer, child with, dying, 1013–1014
  home care of, 1012–1013
  diagnosis of, nurse and, 1009, 1011
  distribution by age at diagnosis, *1000–1001*
Candidiasis, 1292–1293
  primary, 502(t)
Canker sores, 1138
Cannula, oxygen by, 437, *437*
Caput succedaneum, 417, *417*
Car accidents. See *Automobile accidents.*
Car seat, infant and, 428–429, 469
  toddler and, 760, *760*
Carbohydrates, hypoglycemia and, 1177, 1177(t)
  requirements of infant for, 455–456
Carbon monoxide poisoning, major burns and, 806(t)
Carbuncles, 1106–1107
Cardiac catheterization, nurse's role in, 536–538
"Cardiac infant," position in sleep of, 534
Cardiac surgery, 551–555
  nurse and, 551–555
Cardiac valve injury, in rheumatic fever, 1119
Cardiopulmonary resuscitation, of infants and small children, 343–344
Cardiovascular function, of preterm infant, 434–435
Cardiovascular pulses, 226
Carditis, rheumatic fever and, 1120–1121, 1120(t)

Care, infant, parental lack of knowledge of, 399–401
Carey Infant Temperament Questionnaire, 239, 462–463
Caries, dental, 1137–1138
Casefinder, nurse as, in dysfunctional families, 79–80
Casefinding, giantism and, 633
Cast, care of, 601, 1128–1129
  in clubfoot, 600, *601*
  in fractures, 1128
  in Legg-Calvé-Perthes disease, 1113, *1113*
  in scoliosis, 1281, 1285(t)
"Cat's eye reflex," 846, *846*
CAT scan, in hydrocephalus, 652
Cataracts, 657–658
"Catharsis hypothesis," television viewing and, 31
Catheter, care of, in total parenteral nutrition, 367
  in infant cardiac catheterization, *536*
  in pediatric urological surgery, 563–564
Catheterization, cardiac, nurse's role in, 536–538
  clean, 338(t)
  clean intermittent, 336–337, 338(t)
  urethral, 340
Celiac crisis, 834
Celiac disease, 832–835
  role of nurse in diagnosing, 833–834
Cellular fluid, shift to extracellular, 346–347
Cellulitis, 930–931(t)
  impetigo and, 931(t)
Centering characteristic, 903
Central diabetes insipidus, 1166, 1168
Central disorders, of hearing, 975–976
Central nervous system, alterations in, 648–653
Central nervous system leukemia, 1004–1005
Cephalhematoma, 417, *417*
Cereals, preschooler diet and, 909(t)
Cerebellar astrocytoma, 1190
Cerebellar function, assessment of, 233–235
Cerebral astrocytoma, 1191
Cerebral function, evaluation of, 232–233
Cerebral palsy, 1159–1161, 1159(t)
  cerebral pacemaker in, 1160
Cerebrospinal fluid, contusions and, 1111
  findings in, 617(t)
Cervical adenitis, scarlet fever and, 929(t)
Cervical traction, 1133
Chalazion, 1269–1270
Chance, concept of, 1073
Chants, of childhood, 1075
Cheating, school-age child and, 1099
Chemotherapy, in acne vulgaris, 1266
  in bone tumor, 1317
  in febrile seizures, 520(t)

Chemotherapy (*Continued*)
  in Hodgkin's disease, 1320, 1321(t)
  in intracranial tumors, 1194–1195
  in neuroblastoma, 1007–1008
  leukemia and, 1004
Chest, assessment of, 218–224
  neonatal circulation and, 534
  barrel, *222*
  funnel, *222*
  of normal newborn, 419
  pigeon, *222*
Chest circumference, in health assessment, 192
  of toddler, 732
Chest physical therapy, 328–330
Chickenpox, 924–925(t)
  Reye's syndrome and, 1196
Child, bill of rights of, 54
  deviant behavior of, 58
  diabetes and, 1171
  dying, 305–314
  examination of, 186–187
  failure-to-thrive, care of in hospital, 83
  hospitalization and, 295–305
  hospitalized, bathing and hygiene of, 315–316
    preadmission preparation of, 297–298
    restraints of, 320–324
    safety measures and, 318–325
    transportation of, 320
  impact of burn on, 814–815
  irreversible illness and, 290–291
  irreversibly ill, autonomy needs of, 828–830
    competencies of, 831
  latch-key, 1055–1056
  role of, 19
  school-age, growth and development of, 1060–1089
    interviewing, 179
    expanding world of, 1041–1047
  with cancer, 1011–1012
    dying, 1013–1014
  with defect, overprotection of, 643–644
Child abuse, identifying and diagnosing, 85, 88
  incest and, 891–892
  nursing interventions in, 85, 88–90
Childhood obesity, 1134–1136
Child-parent conflict, 270(t)
Childproofing, of home, 710–711
Childrearing, in communal families, 72–73
  in traditional nuclear families, 73
Childrearing practices, of families, 256
Child review of symptoms, in history taking, 182(t), 184
Children, adapting family resources for, 709–714
  communication with, principles of, 171–175
  future, planning for, 102–103, 713–714
  illness in, 282–295
  in dysfunctional families, 79

Children (*Continued*)
  school-age, potential stresses in families with, 1052–1059
  spacing of, 102, 713–714
    sibling rivalry and, 774
  teaching of, 265, 267–268, 266(t)
"Children of Divorce," 63
Choanal atresia, 558–559
  role of nurse in, 558–559
Chomsky, Noam, innate theory of, 150
Christmas disease, 835
Chromosomal aberrations, definition of, 140
Chronic conditions, infant and, 639–670
Chronic illness, families at risk for adapting to, 290(t)
"Chronic sorrow," of parents of child with defect, 640
Chronological approach, to study of growth and development, 143–144
Church of Jesus Christ of Latter-Day Saints, 34
Circulation, fetal, 529–530, *530*
  neonatal, 530–532, *531*
  problem in, 532–536
Circulatory alteration, toddler with, nursing care plan for, 868–875
Circulatory changes, of newborn, later assessment of, 412–413
Circulatory system, anatomy and physiology of, 529–532
Circumcision, 419
  care in, 426–427
  hemophilia and, 835
  hypospadias and, 949
Circumoral cyanosis, 413
Clean-catch specimen, collection of, 339–340
Clean intermittent catheterization, 336–337, 338(t)
Cleft lip, 565–569, *566*
  repair of, 567–568
Cleft palate, 565–569, *566*
  repair of, 568–569
  responsibilities of nurse in, 566–569
Clinics, health care, for adolescent, 1243
Clinic visit, anticipatory guidance for, 288
Clinitest, 1173
Clonus, 1162
  evaluation of, 238
Closed question(s), in history taking, 178
Clothing, of newborn, 427
Clotting, of IV, prevention of, 363
Clotting mechanism, 835, *836*
Clove hitch restraint, *323*
Clubbing, of infant fingers, 533, *533*
Clubfoot, 599–601, *600*
Coarctation of aorta, postductal, 544–545, *545*
  preductal, 544–545, *544*
Cocaine, adolescent and, 1258
Cognition, language, blind child and, 970–971
Cognitive development,
  contribution of play to, 159–161

Cognitive development (*Continued*)
  in preschooler, 903
    anticipatory guidance on, 903
  of adolescent, 1236–1238
    abuse and, 1254
    anticipatory guidance on, 1237–1238
  of school-age child, 1072–1074
    anticipatory guidance on, 1074
  stages of, 739–741
Cognitive theory, of play, 158
Cold, common, in infancy, 509–511
Colic, 515–517
Color, of skin, in physical examination, 195
  of newborn, 414
Color vision, assessment of, 209
Colostomy, in anal agenesis, 598
  temporary, in Hirschsprung's disease, 590–591, *590*
Colostomy care, 335–336, 337(t)
Coma, diabetic, 1169–1170
  in Reye's syndrome, 1196
Comedone, 1263
Comedone extractor, 1265–1266, *1265*
Communal families, 72–73
  childrearing in, 72–73
Communicable diseases, of adolescence, 1288–1297
  of childhood, 922–931
    isolation procedures for, 932
    prevention of, 923, 930
    spread of, 922–929(t), 930–931(t)
Communicating hydrocele, 584, *583*
Communication, cultural barriers to, 36–37
  family, 26–27
    expanding, 1048
  hearing-impaired child and, 982–983
  hospitalized school-age child and, 1202–1203, 1204(t)
  in family with adolescent, 1224–1225, *1225*
  mentally retarded child and, 1154
  partial sightedness and, 968
  process of, 166
  skills of, 169–171
  nonverbal, 168–169
    in families, 26–27
  verbal, 169
  with children, 171–175
  with parents, 175–176
Communication patterns, expansion of, in parenthood, 100
  of dysfunctional families, 77–78
  of normal families, 8–9
Community organizations, school-age child and, 1049
Competency approach, to study of growth and development, 143–144
Competency development, of school-age child, 1086–1087(t)
Competitive play, 163
Complications, of major burns, 811–812
Compound fracture, 1127
Concrete operations, 1236

Concrete operational period, of intellectual development, 149, 1072–1074, *1073*
Concussion, 1109–1110
  epidural hematoma in, 1111
Condom, birth control and, 1245
Conduction, in newborn, 424
Conduction loss, of hearing, 899, 976–977
Conflict, child-parent, 270(t)
  of family and peer values, 1042
Congenital aganglionosis, 589–593
Congenital anomalies, of heart, 528–558
  of respiratory tract, 558–559
  of urinary tract, 560–565
Congenital cretinism, 633
Congenital deafness, 975, 975(t)
Congenital dislocation of hip, 602–605, *603*
Congenital heart disease, nursing care plan for toddler with, 866–867
Congenital laryngeal stridor, 559
Congenital nephrotic syndrome, 839
Congenital osteogenesis imperfecta, 1142–1143
Congenital scoliosis, 1277(t)
Congenital syphilis, 667–668, 667(t)
Congestive heart failure, congenital heart defects and, 550–551
  potential, nursing care plan for, 867–868
Conjunctivitis, 507
  of rubeola, 922(t)
Conscience, developing, 906
  anticipatory guidance on, 906
Conservation, in cognitive development, 1236
Consonance, toddler
  emotional-social competency and, 744–745
Consonants, preschooler and, 902, 902(t)
Constipation, encopresis and, 1095
  of infant, 513–514
Contact dermatitis, allergic, 499–501. *500*
  primary irritant, 502(t)
Contagion, 938
Continuous positive airway pressure (CPAP), 437
Contraceptive care, adolescent and, 121–122
Contraceptive foam, 1245
Contract(s), healthy behavior and, 269
  hospitalized adolescent and, 1337
Contracting family, 15–16(t)
Contractures, Guillain-Barré syndrome and, 1125
Contusions, 1111
Convection, in newborn, 424
Convergence, vision and, 962
Convulsions, febrile, 518–520
  in head injury, 1110
  pertussis and, 927(t)

INDEX **1393**

Cooley's anemia, 676
Cooperative play, 163, 894
  of preschooler, 910, *910*
Coordination, assessment of, 233, 235
  eye-hand, in school-age child, 1066–1067, *1066*
Coordination of secondary schemata, intelligence of infant and, 458
Cord, umbilical, care of, 426
Corneal light reflex test, for strabismus, 206
Corrosives, accidental ingestion of, 820
Cortical sensory interpretation, 233
Corticosteroids, in acne vulgaris, 1266
Coryzal symptoms, in bronchial asthma, 985
Cough, in asthma, 988
  nursing actions related to, 328(t)
Counselling, of adolescents, 1247–1248
  on health promotion, 268–270
  on infant obesity, 626
  on television viewing, 33
  of dysfunctional families, 80
  problems requiring, 270(t)
  role of nurse in, 268–270
Countercurrent immunoelectrophoresis (CIE), 614
Couvade, 101
Cover test, to detect strabismus, 206
Coxa plana, 1112
Cradle cap, 426, 501, 503–504, *503*
  differential diagnosis from eczema, 503
Cranial nerves, assessment of, 233
  Guillain-Barré syndrome and, 1124
Craniopharyngioma, 1190–1191
Creative expression, contribution of play to, 160–161, *161*
Credé maneuver, in spina bifida, 650–651, *651*
Credibility, parental, reinforcing, 263–264
Cremasteric reflex, 947
  evaluation of, 236
Cretinism, congenital, 633
Cribs, hospital, safety and, 859, 860
Crisis, aplastic, 674
  celiac, 834
  familial and individual, 274–277
    in dysfunctional families, 77
    prevention of, 277–278
  hemolytic, 674
  sequestration, 674
  sickle cell, 673–674
  thrombotic, 674
Crisis intervention, suicide and, 1253
Crisis theory, in families, 252
Critical period hypothesis, child development and, 143

Croup, 823–827
  nursing care in, 824–826
Croup tent, 825, *825*
Crust, skin, *198*
Cry, of infant, nature of, 463
Cryptorchidism, 230, 947–948
  and hypospadias, 949
  role of nurse in, 947–948
Cued speech, 983
Cultural beliefs, related to health and illness, 37
Cultural influences, infant and, 464
Culture, definition of, 35
  effect on family of, 35–37
  societal, school-age child and, 1080–1081
Culturette swab, 341
Cup, infant and, 467
Curling's ulcer, major burns and, 807(t)
Cutaneous problems, 1103–1107
Cyanosis, assessment of, 195
  circumoral, 413
  neonatal circulation and, 532–533
Cyanotic defects, with decreased pulmonary vascularity, 549–550
  with increased pulmonary vascularity, 547–549
Cystic fibrosis, 1324–1329
Cytomegalovirus, infection with, 680–682
  pregnancy and, 113

Dacryocystitis, 520
Dacryostenosis, 520–521
Dactylitis, 674
Dark, fear of, in preschooler, 907, 917, 918
Data base, in documentation of health care, 130–133
  in health appraisal, 177
Data collection, nursing process and, 128
"Dating rape," 1227
Dawdling, in toddler, 748
Day care, evaluation of, 887, 887(t)
Day care centers, 885
Day care homes, 884–885
Deaf infant, attachment breakdown and, 477
Deafness, 973–983
  adventitious, 975, 975(t)
  congenital, 975, 975(t)
  nerve, 899
Death, explaining, to toddler, 843–844
  grieving process and, 308–309
  impending, of child, 1188–1189
  of preterm infant, family care after, 445
  of previous infant, attachment breakdown and, 478
  of spouse, single parent family by, 65–66
  perception of, by adolescent, 1314–1316
    by school-age child, 1184–1188
  stages of preparation for, 305–306

Debridement, in major burn wound management, 813
Decibels, 973, 974(t), 975
Declining family, 16(t)
Decompression, by nasogastric tube, 334
Deep tendon reflex responses, evaluation of, 236, *237*
Deficiencies, nutritional, signs of, 1245(t)
Deficit therapy, principles of, 357
Dehydration, 350–351
  gastroenteritis and, 622
  in infant, nursing care plan for, 701
  pertussis and, 927(t)
Delinquency, adolescent, 1250–1252
Delivery, of infant, attachment breakdown and, 480
Democratic parenting style, 51(t)
Demographic data, in health history, 179, 180(t)
Denial, dying adolescent and, 1314
  hospitalized preschooler and, 1023
  hospitalized toddler and, 853
  in family of child with genetic disorder, 678
  in family of infant with defect, 525
  response to hospitalization in young child, 299
  stage of preparation for death, 305–306
Dental care, adolescent and, 1244
  preschooler and, 896–897, *897*
  school-age child and, 1068
Dental problems, school-age child and, 1137–1138
Dentition, in infant, anticipatory guidance on, 449–450
  in preschooler, 896
    anticipatory guidance on, 896–897
  in toddler, 734
    anticipatory guidance on, 734–735
Denver Development Screening Test (DDST), 238–239, *240–242*, 644
Denver Eye Screening Test, 209, *210*
Denver Prescreening Developmental Questionnaire (PDQ), 239
Depression, in adolescent, 1303–1304
  stage of preparation for death, 306
  suicide and, 1253
Dermabrasion, in acne vulgaris, 1266
Dermatitides, of infancy, 499–505
Dermatitis, allergic contact, 499–501, *500*
  atopic, 504–505
  seborrheic, 501, 503–504, *503*
Dermatomyositis, 1324, 1322(t)
Despair, hospitalized toddler and, 853
  response to hospitalization in young child, 299

Developing person, 748–753
  preschooler, 903–906
  school-age child, 1081–1085
Development, adaptation in, 138
  adolescent, 1232–1248
    family situations and, 1250(t)
    hospitalization and, 1332, 1334(t)
  conflict in, 138
  genetic influence on, 139–141
  in hospitalized infant, 702–703
  in hospitalized toddler, 858–859
  in toddler with circulatory alteration, nursing care plan for, 873
  nurturing forces and, 141–142
  of family with toddler, 709–721
  of infant with defect, 644–645, 646–647(t)
  of language in preschooler, 901–902
  of preschooler, 894–913, 912–913(t)
  of school-age child, 1060–1089
  of sensory organs, in school-age child, 1066
  of toddler, 731–763, 758–759(t)
  of vision, assessment of, 962(t)
  ordinal position and, 142
  principles in, 136–138
  social environment and, 142
  study of, chronological approach to, 143–144
    competency approach to, 143–144
Developmental competency, in parenting styles, 51
Developmental disabilities, 1149–1166
Developmental history, in history taking, 181–182(t), 183
Developmental needs, of family with adolescent, 1221–1225
  of family with preschooler, 879–887
  of family with school-age children, 1041–1051
  of family with toddler, 719, 720
  of hospitalized preschooler, 1016–1020
  of hospitalized school-age child, 1201–1204, 1202–1203(t)
  of hospitalized toddler, 856–857(t)
Developmental Profile, The, 239
Developmental screening, 238–242, 240–242, 243
Developmental stage, of child, effect on parenting styles, 50–51
Developmental tasks, 138
  conflicts of, 719
  irreversibly ill preschooler and, 956
  of adolescent, 1240
Deviant behavior, of child, and parenting problems, 58
Diabetes insipidus, 1166–1168
  responsibilities of, nurse in, 1167
Diabetes mellitus, 1168–1179
  behavior problems and, 1175
  responsibilities of nurse in, 1169
Diabetic coma, 1169–1170

Diabetic ketoacidosis (DKA), 1169–1170
  laboratory values in, 1170(t)
Diabetic ketosis, 1170
Diaper dermatitis, seborrheic, 503
Diaper rashes, 501, 502(t)
Diaphragm, birth control and, 1246–1247
Diaphragmatic hernia, 579–581, *579*
Diarrhea, dietary measures for, 288
  gastroenteritis and, 621
  metabolic acidosis and, 350
  mild, in infant, 514–515
Diet, alterations in metabolic functioning and, 663–664
  childhood obesity and, 1135–1136
  diabetes mellitus and, 1172–1173
  in cystic fibrosis, 1327
  of infant, mild diarrhea and, 514–515
    solids added to, 465–467
  tuberculosis and, 1310
Diet therapy, in iron deficiency anemia, 787
Differentiation, family, level of, 252
Dignity, parental, 49
Digoxin, administration of, parents' questions about, 554
Diphtheria, 928–929(t)
Diplopia, 965
Direct question(s), in history taking, 178
Disbelief, as grief reaction after death of child, 308
Discharge phase, hospitalized preschooler and, 1025–1026
  hospitalized school-age child and, 1212
  hospitalized toddler and, 866
Discipline, adolescent and, 1239
  asthmatic child and, 994
  preschooler, ownership rights and, 915–916
  toddler and, 717–718
Diseases, communicable, preschooler and, 922–931
Dislocation, congenital, of hip, 602–605, *603*
Diseases, hereditary, in history taking, 185
Dissonance, toddler emotional-social competency and, 744–745
Distractibility, of children, 1077
Diuresis, in acute glomerulonephritis, 1119
Divorce, children's responses to, 63–64, 65(t)
  single parent families by, 63–65, *64*
Documentation, of child abuse, 88
  of health care, 130–133
Doll play, uses of, during examination, 187–188
Down's syndrome, 1157–1159, *1156*
  endocardial cushion defects in, 542
Drainage, postural, *326–327*, *328–329*

Drains, in pediatric urological surgery, 564
Dramatic play, 163–164
Dressing, in minor burn care, 812
Dropout, 1260
Drowning, toddler and, 760
Drowsiness, excessive, in head injury, 1109, 1110
Drugs, acute lymphocytic leukemia and, 1005(t)
  adolescent and, 1228–1229
    misuse of, 1258–1261
  epilepsy and, 1162, 1163(t)
  hepatitis and, 1292
  iron deficiency anemia and, 787–788
  leukemia and, 1005(t)
  pediatric allergy and, 496(t)
  pregnancy and, 110–112, 111(t)
  tuberculosis and, 1311, 1311(t)
Drug education, school-age child and, 1088
Dual-career family, 888–890, *889*
Dubowitz assessment of gestational age, 408–409, *410*, 410(t)
Duchenne's muscular dystrophy, 1321, 1323–1324, 1322(t)
Dunlop's traction, 1132
Dwarfism, pituitary, 630–632
Dwyer instrumentation, 1286, 1286(t)
Dying child, 305–314
  home care of, 307–308
  hospice care of, 307
  hospital care of, 308
Dysentery, bacillary, 794–795
Dysfunction, in families, 76–79
Dyslexia, 1147–1149
  responsibilities of nurse in, 1148–1149
Dysmenorrhea, 1271
Dystrophy, muscular, 1321–1324
  Duchenne's, 1321, 1323–1324, 1322(t)

Ears, assessment of, 209, 211–214
  of normal newborn, 418
Ear drops, hospitalized toddler and, 865
Eardrum, assessment of, 211–212, *212*
Eating, blind child and, 972
  toddler and, motor skills affecting, 736
Eating behavior, of toddler, 749
  guidelines for, 755(t)
Ebstein's malformation, 550
Echolalia, 1165
Ectopic pregnancy, 108–109
Ectopic testis, 947
Eczema, differential diagnosis from cradle cap, 503
  infantile, 504–505
  seborrheic, 501, 503–504
Edema, assessment of, 196
  causes of, 350
  in nephrotic syndrome, 839, 840
  major burns and, 806(t), *809*

INDEX **1395**

Education, about muscular dystrophy, 1323
　about spinal fusion, 1286
　about systemic lupus erythematosus, 1307
　autism and, 1165
　mentally retarded child and, 1153–1155
　of hospitalized preschooler about his disease, 1022–1025
　of hospitalized school-age child about his treatment, 1206–1210
　preoperative, in bone tumor. 1318–1319
Educational materials, for blind student, 971
Elbow restraint, 320–321, *322*
Elective mutism, 1053–1054
Electra complex, 905
Electrocardiogram (ECG), congenital anomalies of heart and, 535–536, *535*
Electroencephalogram (EEG), in Guillain-Barré syndrome, 1124
　in infantile spasms, 655
Electrolytes, imbalances of, 350–357
　internal transport of, 346–347
　intravenous, administering, 360–364
　maintenance dose of, calculation of, 356–357, 357(t)
　regulation of, 345–347
Electrolyte disturbances, major burns and, 807(t)
Elimination, in infant, 454–455
　in newborn, 428
Elimination skills. See also *Toilet training.*
　school-age child and, 1068
Emancipation, hospitalized adolescent and, 1331
Emergent period, of burn care, 808–811
Emerging family, 12(t)
Emotional competency, hospitalized school-age child and, 1203–1204, 1203(t)
Emotional development, of adolescent, 1238–1240
　abuse and, 1254
　anticipatory guidance on, 1238–1240
　of irreversibly ill preschooler, 957
　of normal preschooler, 903–904
　of school-age child, 1076–1081, 1086(t)
　of toddler, 743–744, *743*
　play and, 161–162
Emotional energy, of family with toddler, 722–725
Emotional needs, in total parenteral nutrition, 368
Emotional problems, in adolescent, 1239–1240
Emotional-social competency, definition of, 144, 151–155

Emotional-social competency (*Continued*)
　hospitalized preschooler and, 1017, 1018–1019(t), 1020
　infant and, 460–464
　of preschooler, 903–908
　of toddler, 743–754
Emotional space, children and, 709–710
Emotions, expression of, contribution of play to, 161
　of infant, 463
　of school-age child, 1077–1080
Empathy, in parent-child-nurse relationship, 167–168
Empyema, streptococcal pneumonia and, 943
Encephalitis, 619–621
　chickenpox and, 925(t)
　role of nurse in, 619–620
　rubella and, 923(t)
Encopresis, 1093–1095
　management of, 1095, 1101
Endocardial cushion defect, 542–543
Endocarditis, subacute bacterial, 551
Endocrine alterations, in infants, 630–636, 631(t)
En face position, 381–382
Enema, administration of, to hospitalized child, 335, 336(t)
Energy, of parents, depletion of, 722–725
Enjoyment theory, of play, 158–159
Enteric isolation, in gastroenteritis, 623
Enterocolitis, necrotizing, 593–595
Enteroviruses, encephalitis and, 619
Entitlement, in adoption, 70
Enuresis, 1091–1093
　diabetes insipidus and, 1166
　management of, 1091–1093, 1101
Environmental safety, of hospitalized child, 318–320, *319*
Enzymes, in major burn wound management, 813
Eosinophils, 1001
Ependymoma, 1192
Epidural hematoma, 1111
　in concussion, 1111
Epiglottitis, 943–945
　acute, 824, 824(t)
Epilepsy, 1161–1164
　drugs and, 1162, 1163(t)
　responsibilities of nurse in, 1162–1164
Epistaxis, 1107
Equilibrium, assessment of, 233
Erb-Duchenne paralysis, 517–518
Erikson, E., theories on psychological development, 151, 151(t), 461
Erosion, skin, *198*
Erythema, assessment of, 195
Erythema infectiosum, 922(t)
Erythema toxicum, 416
Esophageal atresia, with tracheoesophageal fistula, 572–577, *572*
　role of nurse in, 572–577
　without fistula, 575–576
　role of nurse in, 575–576

Esophageal chalasia, 517
Esotropia, accommodative, 965, *965*
Evaluation, nursing process and, 129–130
Evaporation, in newborn, 424
Eventration, 580
Evocative approach, to problem behavior, 281
Ewing's sarcoma, 1316
　distribution by age at diagnosis, 1000
Examination, of young child, techniques of, 186–187
　physical, sexual assault and, 1058–1059
Exanthem subitum, 509
Exchange transfusion, for hyperbilirubinemia, 434
Excoriation, *199*
Exercise, diabetes mellitus and, 1173
　excessive, school-age child and, 1063
　in total parenteral nutrition, 368
　school-age child and, 1065–1066
Exercises, breathing, in cystic fibrosis, 1326
　passive, spina bifida and, 650
Expanding family, 12–14(t)
Expectations, age-appropriate, for preschooler, 882
　realistic, of preschooler family members, 882–883
　unrealistic, attachment breakdown and, 478
Extended family, lack of, potential stress and, 398
Extracellular fluid, shift to cellular, 346–347
Extremities, assessment of, 230–232
　of normal newborn, 419–420
　pain in, of osteomyelitis, 1125
Extrinsic asthma, 985
Eye(s), assessment of, 205–209
　in potential fluid and electrolyte imbalance, 355
　of normal newborn, 418
Eye drops, hospitalized infant and, 696
　hospitalized toddler and, 865
Eye-hand coordination, in infant, 148
　in school-age child, 1066–1067, *1066*
　anticipatory guidance on, 1067
Eye-occiput line, 209
Eye patch, 965–966
Eye problems, in head injury, 1109, 1110
Eye safety, 899
Eye signs, of chronic asthma, 987, *987*

Face, assessment of, 204
　of normal newborn, 418
Facioscapulohumeral muscular dystrophy, 1321, 1322(t)
Failure, sense of, irreversibly ill preschooler and, 957
Failure-to-thrive families, 80–84

Falls, infant and, 469
   toddler and, 761–762
   in hospital, 859
Familial diseases, in history taking, 185
Familial dysautonomia, 677–678
Family(ies), allergy and, 497–498
   as system, 273–274
   assessment of, 251–257
   birth of infant and, 388–391, 394
   cancer treatment and, 1011–1012, *1011*
   characteristics of, shared, 8–9
   childbearing, growth and development needs of, 95–105
   communal, 72–73
   communication in, 26–27
   congenital infections and, 682
   cultural influences on, 35–37
   defective child and, 642–645
   definition of, 5
   developmental tasks of, 10, 12–16(t)
   diabetes and, 1171
   division of labor in, 389–390, 399
   Down's syndrome and, 1157–1158
   dual-career, 888–890, *889*
   dysfunctional life patterns and, 76–91
   extended, lack of, 398
   failure-to-thrive, 80–84
   functions of, 9–10
   genetic disorders and, 678–679
   growth and development of, 5–21
   health care system and, 255
   health history of, 254
   heart disease in infant and, 555–557, *555*
   historical perspective on, 6–8, 7(t)
   hospitalization of child and, 303–304, 1026, 1212
   hospitalization of infant and, 690–691
   identification of infant and, 381–383, *382*
   illness of infant and, 522–523
   infant with problems of gestational age or birth weight and, 444–445
   interdependency in, 251
   irreversible illness of child and, 290, 290(t), 831–832
   life cycle of, 10, *11*, 12–16(t)
   life-threatening illness and, 309–310
   living space of, 23
   major burns and, 815–816
   mentally retarded child and, 1153–1155
   nature of, 5, 22–27
   philosophy of, 717–721
   poverty and, 28–29
   public policy and, 34–35
   religion and, 33–34
   resources to aid, 271(t)
   roles in, 8–9, 10, 17–20
   runaway adolescent and, 1258
   significant events in, 254
   single parent, 61–67

Family(ies) (*Continued*)
   social history of, 185
   status asthmaticus and, 994–995
   structuring of time by, 25–26
   sudden infant death syndrome and, 684–685
   surgery of newborn and, 524–525
   with adolescent, potential stresses in, 1226–1231
   with infant, growth and development needs of, 381–395
      potential stresses in, 396–405
   with preschooler, growth and development needs of, 879–887
      potential stresses in, 888–893
   with school-age child, potential stresses in, 1052–1059
   with toddler, growth and development of, 709–721
      potential stresses in, 722–730
      reorganizing relationships in, 714–717
   work and, 29–30
Family circumstances, attachment breakdown and, 479–480
Family developmental framework, 251–252
Family function framework, 253
Family life styles, alternative, 60–75
Family living, adaptive process of, 20
   influential factors in, 22–38
Family planning, 102–103, 713–714, 881–882
   adolescents and, 121
Family profile, in history taking, 182(t), 184–185
Family relationships, potential stress related to, 401–404
Family strengths framework, 252–253
Family systems framework, 252
Family unit, 254
   establishing stable, 391–395
Father(s), absence of, effect on sons, 62–63
   assuming role of, 383–384, *384*
   expectant, 98–99
   identification of infant, 382, *383*
   role of, 18–19, 48
   single. See *Male single parent families.*
Father-infant bond, 387
Fear, of dark, in preschooler, 907, 917, 918
Fears, in school-age child, 1078–1079
   hospitalized, 1201
   in toddler, 746, 764–769
Febrile seizures, 518–520, 519(t)
Feeding, of infant, obesity and, 625–626
   with cleft palate or lip, 567
   of newborn, 427
   with gastrostomy tube, 334–335
Feeding difficulties, neonatal circulation and, 532
Feeding history, sudden infant death syndrome and, 683
Feet, assessment of, 231

Females, anal agenesis in, 596, *596*
Female genitalia, assessment of, 228–229, *228*
   of normal newborn, 419
Female single parent families, 62–63
Femoral hernia, palpation of, 228, *228*
Femoral rotation, internal, 783
"Fencing position," 422, *422*
Fetal alcohol syndrome, 120
Fetus, teratogenic effects on, 110–114
Fever, control of, 288
   in bacterial meningitis, 616
   in infectious mononucleosis, 1267
   in influenza, 1268
   in osteomyelitis, 1125
   in pneumonia, 615
   in seizures, relief measures, 519–520
   medications for, 343
   of infant, in common cold, 509
Fifth disease, 922–923(t)
Finances, of family, 27–28
   after birth of baby, 390
   potential stress related to, 404–405
   with school-age child, 1050
Fine motor manipulation, 452
Fine motor skills, of school-age child, 1064
   anticipatory guidance on, 1064–1066
Fingerspelling, 983
Fire safety, preschooler and, 911
First aid, emergency, 288
Fissure, skin, *198*
Fistula, tracheoesophageal, 572–577, *572*
Fit, mother-infant, 480
"Floppy baby," 635
Flow sheets, in documentation of health care, 132–133, *132*
Fluid, cerebrospinal, findings in, 617(t)
Fluids, imbalances of, 356–357
   in gastroenteritis, 622–623
   internal transport of, 346–347
   intravenous, administering, 360–364
      calculation of rate for, 362
   maintenance requirements of, 357(t)
   regulation of, 345–347
Fluid and electrolyte balance, in infants and children, 345–365
Fluid and electrolyte imbalance, 350–353
Fluid therapy, burns and, 809–811
   surgery and, 357(t), 360
Fluoride, 735, 1137–1138
   requirement of infant for, 456
Focal motor seizures, 1161–1162
Focus, in tuberculosis, 1308
Fontanel(s), anterior, in potential fluid and electrolyte imbalance, 355

INDEX **1397**

Fontanel(s) (Continued)
  assessment of, 200–201
  of head of newborn, 416, 417
Food(s), basic groups, preschooler and, 909(t)
  toddler and, 756(t)
  solid, infant diet and, 465–467
Food allergy, 506–507
Food diary, 243–244
Food guide, for adolescent, 1244(t)
Foot, of preschooler, 895–896
Forceps marks, 416
Foreign body, aspiration of, differential diagnosis from croup, 824, 824(t)
  toddler and, 761, 860
Formal operational period, of intellectual development, 149, 1237
Formal play, 164
Foster parents, 67–68
Fourth trimester follow-up, 397–398
Fracture(s), 1126–1134
  in osteogenesis imperfecta, 1142–1143
  of skull, 1111
  role of nurse in, 1127
Frejka pillow splint, for congenital dislocation of hip, 603, 604
Fremitus, 220
Freud, S., theory of play of, 157–158
  theory of psychological development of, 151, 151(t), 152
Frolich's syndrome, 1300
Frostbite, 1107–1108
Fruits, preschooler diet and, 909(t)
Functional hearing impairment, 976
Fundus, assessment of, 207, 207
Fungal infections, 791–793
Fungicides, in treatment of thrush, 508
Funnel chest, 222
Furuncles, 1105–1106

Gag reflex, assessment of, 218
Gait, assessment of, 232–233
  in head injury, 1109, 1110
Galactosemia, 662–664
  phenylketonuria and, 663(t)
Games, in concrete operations stage, 1073–1074
  parent-infant, in assessment of attachment, 484–485
Gamma globulin, in agammaglobulinemia, 665
Gas exchange, in preterm infant, 436–439
Gastric tube, child with, nursing care of, 332–335, 333
Gastritis, pyloric stenosis and, 570
Gastroenteritis, 621–624
  role of nurse in, 622–623

Gastroesophageal reflux, with hiatal hernia, 581–582
Gastrointestinal allergy, 506–507
Gastrointestinal anomalies, 569–599
Gastrointestinal considerations, in cystic fibrosis, 1327
Gastrointestinal disturbances, of infant, 513–517
  infections, 621–624
Gastrointestinal functioning, alterations in, 668–669
Gastrointestinal system, in preterm infant, 432–433
  in term infant, 432–433
Gastroschisis, 578–579, 579
Gavage feedings, necrotizing enterocolitis and, 593
Gender identity, of toddler, 753–754
  anticipatory guidance on, 754
General appearance. See Appearance, general.
Genes, 139
Genetic counselling, in cystic fibrosis, 1328
  in hemophilia, 836
  in muscular dystrophy, 1323
  in neurocutaneous syndromes, 665
  in preventing blindness, 967
  in sickle cell anemia, 674
Genetic defect, in Down's syndrome, 1157
Genetic diseases, 140–141
Genetic disorders, impact on family, 678–679
  life-threatening, of infant, 672–679
Genetic factors, sudden infant death syndrome and, 683
"Genetic grief," 672
Genetics, influence of, on growth and development, 139–141
  mendelian, 140–141
Genital herpes simplex, 1295(t)
Genitals, ambiguous, 949
  female, assessment of, 228–229, 228
  of normal newborn, 419
  male, assessment of, 229–230, 229
  of normal newborn, 419
Genitourinary tract anomalies, 561–562
Genu valgum, 231, 783, 784
  extreme, 784–785
  in toddler, 733
Genu varum, 231, 783, 784
  extreme, 783–784
  in toddler, 732
Geographic tongue, 218, 987, 988
Geographical mobility, of family, 24, 27
Geophagia, 788–789
German measles, 922(t)
Gestational age, appropriateness of size for, 411
  Dubowitz assessment of, 408–409, 410, 410(t)
  large for, 443–444
  small for, 443
  variations in, 429–445

Giantism, 632–633
Girls, adolescent, physical development of, anticipatory guidance on, 1235–1236
  delinquency in, 1250
  head circumference of, 190
  height of, 189
  sexual maturity in, 1234, 1234(t), 1234
Glaucoma, developmental, 658–659
Glioma(s), brain stem, 1190
  of optic path, 1191–1192, 1191
Glomerulonephritis, acute, 1117–1119, 1118
  impetigo and, 931(t)
  scarlet fever and, 929(t)
Glucagon, hypoglycemia and, 1177
Gluteal reflex, 236
Gluten challenge, 833
Gluten-induced enteropathy, 832–835
Goal(s), of families, 255–256
Gonadal dysgenesis, 1300
Goniotomy, for developmental glaucoma, 659
Gonorrhea, 1294(t)
Gower's sign, 1321
Grammar, 1074
Grand mal seizures, 1161
Grandparent(s), family with toddler and, 716–717, 717
  irreversible illness of child and, 294
  pregnancy and, 96–97
  role of, 19–20, 19
Granulocytes, 1001(t)
Graphesthesia, 233
Grasp reflexes, 420
Grasping, steps in learning, 452(t)
Greenstick fracture, 1126–1127, 1126
Grief, after death, 65, 308, 313–314
Griseofulvin, 792
Groos, Karl, theory of play advanced by, 157
Gross motor skills, of school-age child, 1063–1064, 1064
  anticipatory guidance on, 1064–1066
Groups, Wilms' tumor classification, 1008
Group activities, hospitalized child and, 300–301
Growth, changes in, 136
  defining, 136
  factors influencing, 138–142
  giantism and, 632–633
  of adolescent, 1232–1248
  of children, 135–156
  of family with toddler, 709–721
  of infant, 447–470, 448(t)
  of preschooler, 894–913, 912–913(t)
  of school-age child, 1060–1089
  of toddler, 731–763, 758–759(t)
  hospitalized, 858–859
  principles in, 136–138
  study of, chronological approaches to, 143–144
  competency approach to, 143–144

1398 INDEX

Growth charts, height and weight, 144
Growth failure, in infant, 632
Growth needs, of family with adolescent, 1221–1225
 of family with preschooler, 879–887
 of family with school-age child, 1041–1051
 of family with toddler, 709–721
Growth patterns, childhood obesity and, 1135
Growth retardation, intrauterine, 444
Growth spurt, in adolescence, 1233
Guidance, anticipatory. See under subjects.
Guillain-Barré syndrome, 1124–1125
 role of nurse in, 1124–1125
Guilt, in parents of irreversibly ill child, 291–292
 in preschooler, 904
Gums, assessment of, 216

H-type tracheoesophageal fistula, 576–577
Habits, development of, in infant, 147–148
Hair, assessment of, 197
 of hospitalized child, care of, 316
 of preterm infant, 432
 of term infant, 432
Hand-eye coordination, of infant, 457
Hand-foot syndrome, 674
Happiness, in school-age child, 1079
Harlequin color change, of newborn, 414
Harrington rod instrumentation, 1286, 1286(t)
Head, assessment of, 200–201
 of newborn, assessment of, 416–419
Head circumference, chart of, 413
 in health assessment, 190, 191–192
 of infant, 449
  anticipatory guidance on, 449
 of toddler, 732
 physical development and, 144
Head control, of infant, stages of, 451, 450(t)
Head injuries, 1108–1111
Head lag, of newborn infant, 410–411
Headache, of head injury, 1109, 1110
 of intracranial tumors, 1192
Health, managing of, 258–272
Health appraisal, 177–250
Health care, of adolescent, 1243
Health care clinics, for adolescent, 1243
Health care record, organization of, 130
Health education, American Academy of Pediatrics statement on, 1071
 school-age child and, 1070

Health history, of child, 179–185
 of family, 254
Health maintenance, of adolescent, 1243–1248
 of preschooler, 908–913, 912–913(t)
 of school-age child, 1085–1088
 of toddler, 754–763, 758–759(t)
 problem-solving skills in, 267–268
Health needs, personal, identifying, 258–259
Health promotion, as nursing goal, 258–262
Health status, of adolescent, irreversible alterations in, 1298–1313
 life-threatening alterations in, 1314–1330
 reversible alterations in, 1273–1297
 temporary alterations in, 1263–1272
 of infant, irreversible alterations in, 639–670
 life-threatening alterations in, 671–688
 reversible alterations in, 522–638
 temporary alterations in, 494–521
 of preschooler, irreversible alterations in, 955–998
 life-threatening alterations in, 999–1015
 reversible alterations in, 937–954
 temporary alterations in, 921–936
 of school-age child, irreversible alterations in, 1140–1183
 life-threatening alterations in, 1184–1200
 reversible alterations in, 1116–1139
 temporary alterations in, 1103–1115
 of toddler, irreversible alterations in, 828–842
 life-threatening alterations in, 843–848
 reversible alterations in, 797–828
 temporary alterations in, 780–796
Hearing, assessment of, 212–214, 213(t)
 of infant, 453
 of newborn, 423
 of preschooler, 898–899
  anticipatory guidance on, 899
 of toddler, 737–738
Hearing aids, 983
Hearing impaired, resources for, 998
Hearing impairment, 973–983
 role of nurse in managing, 980–983
Hearing loss, behavioral indices of, 981(t)
 pertussis and, 927(t)
 physical findings in, 981(t)
Hearing screening, by behavioral testing, 978–980

Hearing screening (Continued)
 in newborn, 977–978, 978(t)
Heart, anomalies of, congenital, 528–558
 assessment of, 224–226
 conduction system of, 534–535, 535
 development of, 529
Heart defects. See Congenital anomalies of heart and under specific anomalies.
Heart disease, congenital, nursing care plan for toddler with, 866–867
Heart failure, congestive, congenital heart defects and, 550–551
Heart murmurs, 225–226
Heart rate, of newborn infant, assessment of, 407
Heart surgery, 551–555
 of toddler, nursing care plan for, 869–870
Heat exhaustion, sports injuries and, 1112
Heat lamp, for diaper rashes, 501
Heat loss, in newborn, 424–425
Heat production, in newborn, 425
Heat rash, 502(t)
Hedonic theory, of play, 158–159
Heel to ear, assessment of newborn infant, 410
Height, in health assessment, 188–191, 189–190
 of infant, 447
  anticipatory guidance on, 447, 449
 of preschooler, 895
  anticipatory guidance on, 895
 of school-age child, 1060–1061
  anticipatory guidance on, 1061
 of toddler, 731–732
  anticipatory guidance on, 732
Helminthic infections, 790–791, 789(t)
Hemangiomas, strawberry, 415, 415
Hematocrit, 248
Hematologic tests, neonatal circulation and, 536
Hematoma, epidural, 1111
Hemoglobin, 1000
 measurement of, in health assessment, 248
Hemolytic crisis, 674
Hemomyoglobinuria, major burns and, 806(t)
Hemophilia, 835–838
 role of nurse in, 836–837, 837–838
Hemophilus influenzae pneumonia, 612–613(t)
Henoch-Schonlein purpura, 945–946
Hepatitis A, 1288, 1289(t)
Hepatitis B, 1288, 1289(t)
Hepatitis C, 1288, 1289(t)
Hepatitis, viral, 1288, 1292, 1289(t), 1290–1291(t)
Hereditary diseases, in history taking, 185

Hermaphrodite, 665
Hernia(s), abdominal, palpation of, 227–228
　diaphragmatic, 579–581, *579*
　femoral, palpation of, 228, *228*
　hiatal, with gastroesophageal reflux, 581–582
　inguinal, 582, *583*
　　palpation for, *229*, 230
　pertussis and, 927(t)
　umbilical, 226, 227, 582
Herpes simplex, encephalitis and, 619
　genital, 1295(t)
Herpes simplex II, 668
　congenital syphilis and, 667(t)
Herpes simplex infection, as teratogen in pregnancy, 113
Herpes zoster, 924–925(t)
Hertz, 973, 975
Heterotropia, 209
Hiatal hernia, with gastroesophageal reflux, 581–582
Hiccough reflex, 421
High chairs, in hospital, toddler safety and, 859–860
Hip, congenital dislocation of, 602–605, *603*
　　assessment for, 419
　malrotation of, 781–785
　rotation of, assessment of, 781–782, *781*
Hip spica cast, 604
"Hippie" communes, childrearing in, 72–73
Hirschsprung's disease, 589–593
Histoplasmosis, 792–793
History, in assessment of parent-infant attachment, 485–486
History taking, 177–185, 180–183(t)
　in failure-to-thrive families, 81–82, 82(t)
　pediatric, outline, 180–182(t)
Hodgkin's disease, 1319–1321
　distribution by age at diagnosis, 1001
Holophrastic speech, 742
Home, allergy-proofing, techniques of, 497(t)
　childproofing of, 710–711, *710*
　space and facilities in, children and, 709–710
　stable, establishing, 720
Home care, in cystic fibrosis, 1328–1329
　of child with cancer, 1012–1013
　of dying child, 307–308
Home Observation for Measurement of the Environment (HOME), 241, 1366–1373
Homosexual parents, 73–74
Homosexuality, adolescent and, 1256
Honesty, importance in communication, 172
Hood, oxygen by, 437, *438*
Hookworm, 791
Hordeolum, 936

Hospice care, of dying child, 307
Hospital, admission, child and, 297–298
　experiences, child and, 299–305
　physical environment, child and, 296–300
　procedures, child and, 300
　social environment, child and, 296
Hospital care, of dying child, 308
Hospital facilities, for parents of hospitalized child, 298
Hospitalization, in cystic fibrosis, 1328
　of adolescent, 1331–1338
　of child, 295–305
　　bathing and hygiene in, 315–316
　　parents and, 301–304
　　restraints in, 320–325
　　safety measures and, 318–325
　　transportation in, 320
　of infant, effects of, 689–697, 690
　of preschooler, 1016–1037
　of school-age child, 1201–1217
　of toddler, 849–875
　sensory-impaired child and, 983–984
Hot lines, parental stress and, 516
Household responsibilities, in pregnancy, 95–96
　of new parents, 399
Humor, in language, 1075
Hydatidiform mole, 108
Hydramnios, esophageal atresia and tracheoesophageal fistula and, 572–573
Hydration, in sickle cell anemia, 675
Hydrocarbons, accidental ingestion of, 820
Hydrocele, 583–584
Hydrocephalus, 651–653
　nursing management in, 652–653
　operative treatment of, 652–653, *652, 653*
Hydrostatic pressure, 347
Hydrotherapy, major burn wounds and, 813, *813*
Hygiene, of hospitalized child, 315–316
Hyperactivity, 1146–1147
　nursing and, 1146–1147
Hyperalimentation, 365–368
Hyperbilirubinemia, treatment of, 434
Hypercalcemia, 352
Hyperglycemia, 1170–1171
Hyperkalemia, 352
Hypernatremia, 350–352
Hyperopia, 963
Hyperpituitary function, 632–633
Hypersensitivity, of ill infant, attachment breakdown and, 476–477
Hypertension, major burns and, 807(t)
Hypertonic dehydration, 350
Hypervolemia, major burns and, 806(t)
Hypocalcemia, 352–353
Hypocalcemic tetany, vitamin D deficiency rickets and, 629

Hypoglycemia, 1177
Hypokalemia, 352
Hyponatremia, 350–351
Hypopituitarism, 630
Hypospadias, 948–950
　role of nurse in, 948–949
Hypostatic pneumonia, traction and, 1134
Hypothermia mattress, 343
Hypothyroidism, 633–636
　role of nurse in, 634–635, 635–636
　screening test for, 635
Hypotonic dehydration, 350–351
Hypovolemia, major burns and, 806(t)

Icterus neonatorum, 415
Identifying data, in health history, 179, 180(t)
Idiopathic diabetes insipidus, 1166
Idiopathic nephrotic syndrome, 839
Idiopathic scoliosis, 1277(t)
Ignoring approach, to extreme temper tantrums, 779
Illness, adolescent and, 1333–1335
　in children, 282–295
　　temporary, 286–289
　　irreversible, 289–294
　in preschooler, 955–956
　life-threatening, in preschooler, 999–1015
　nurse's role during, 309–312
　of newborn, attachment breakdown and, 475
　preschooler and, 937–939
　reversible, 289
　of infant, family reactions to, 522–523
　preschooler and, 937–939
　past, in history taking, 181(t), 183
Imipramine, for enuresis, 1093
Imitative learning, in infant, 148, 458–459, *459*
Immunizations, in infant, 469–470, 470(t)
　in preschooler, 912
　in school-age child, 1088, 1087(t)
　in toddler, 762–763
　record of, in history taking, 183
Immunological competence, of preterm infant, 435
Immunological functioning, alterations in, 664–665
Imperforate anal membrane, 595, *595*
Imperforate anus, 595–596, *595*
Impetigo, 930–931(t), *934*
Implantable devices, for intracranial tumors, 1195, *1195*
Incest, preschooler and, 891, 891(t)
Independence, asthmatic child and, 994
　blind child and, 972
　contribution of play to, 161
　dying adolescent and, 1315
　economic, of adolescent, 1241
　hospitalized adolescent and, 1331
　irreversibly ill adolescent and, 1299

Independence (*Continued*)
  irreversibly ill child and, 1141
  irreversibly ill preschooler and, 958
  school-age child and, 1048–1050
    anticipatory guidance on, 1049–1050, 1053
  toddler and, 748
Indirect question(s), in history taking, 178
Individual boundaries, of families, 252
Induction, in leukemia, 1004
Industriousness, irreversibly ill child and, 1141
  school-age child and, 1081, *1081*
Infancy, allergies in, 494–498
  dermatitides of, 499–505
  genetic disorders of, life-threatening, 672–679
  infectious diseases of, life-threatening, 679–682
  potential stresses during, 471–492, 493–521, 522–638, 639–670, 671–688
Infant, accepting responsibility for, 383
  altered health states in, 645–669
  attachment breakdown and, 475–477
  body proportions of, 449–450
  dentition in, 449–450
  development of, 447–470
  diet of, 465–467
  elimination in, 454–455
  emotional-social competency of, 460–464
  endocrine alterations in, 630–636, 631(t)
  examination of, 188
  family with, growth and development needs of, 381–395
    potential stresses in, 396–405
  gastrointestinal infections in, 621–624
  growth of, 447–470
  head circumference of, 449
  health of, irreversible alterations in, 639–670
    life-threatening alterations in, 671–688
    reversible alterations in, 522–638
    temporary alterations in, 494–521
  hearing in, 212, 453
  heart disease and, 555–557, *555*
  height of, 447, 449
  hospitalized, medications and, 693–697
  illness in, parents and, 526–528
  intellectual competency of, 457–460
  internalizing existence of, 381–388
  language development in, 459–460, *460*
  motor development of, 450–453
  mouth of, 449
  newborn, 406–446
  nutritional requirements of, 455–457

Infant (*Continued*)
  obesity in, 625–636
  physical competency of, 447–457
  reaction to stress of, 481
  respiratory infections in, 606–615
  sleep of, 454
  social responsiveness of, 461
  suctioning in, 332
  temperament of, 462–463
  vision of, 453, *453*
  weight of, 447, 449
  with defect, developmental stimulation of, 644–645
    family reaction to, 523–526
  with respiratory alteration, nursing care plan for, 698–705
Infant car seat, 428–429
Infant care, parental lack of knowledge of, 399–401
Infantile paralysis, 958–961
Infantile spasms, 655–657
  role of nurse in, 655–656
Infantilism, in toddler, encouraging, 727
Infection(s), bacterial, in agammaglobulinemia, 664
  burns and, 811
  cardiac surgery and, nursing care plan for, 870–871
  cleft palate and, 567
  common, 508–513
  cystic fibrosis and, 1328
  cytomegalovirus, 680–682
  gastrointestinal, in infant, 621–624
  helminthic, 790–791, 789(t)
  maternal, infant and, 112–114, 667–668
  neurological, in infant, 616–621
  parasitic, 789–795
  polio virus, 959(t)
  preterm infant and, 440–441
  respiratory, in infant, 606–616
    neonatal circulation and, 532
  rickettsial, 793–794
  sickle cell anemia and, 676
  streptococcal, rheumatic fever and, 1119
  urinary tract, 950–952
Infectious disease(s), life-threatening, of infancy, 679–682
  of adolescence, 1266–1270
  sudden infant death syndrome and, 683
Infectious mononucleosis, 1266–1267
Infectious neuronitis, 1124
Inferiority, adolescent and, 1239
  school-age child and, 1043, 1081–1082
Infiltration, of IV, prevention of, 363–364
Inflammatory processes, reversible, 1117–1126
Influenza, 1267–1269
  Reye's syndrome and, 1196
  viruses of, 1267–1268, 1268(t)
Ingestion, of poison material, hospitalized toddler and, 860
  nurse and, 861
  toddler and, 760, 818–822

Inguinal hernia, 583, *583*
  palpation for, *229*, 230
Inhalation therapy, in cystic fibrosis, 1326, 1327, *1327*
Inheritance, mendelian modes of, 140–141
Initial plan, in documentation of health care, 131, *131*
Initiative, in preschooler, 903–904
  anticipatory guidance on, 904
Injections, hospitalized infant and, 693, 696, *693*
  hospitalized preschooler and, 1023–1025
  school-age child and, 1210
Injury(ies), head, 1108–1111
  sports, 1111–1112
  toddler and, 761–762
Innate theory, of language development, 150
Insect(s), stinging, allergy to, 995
Insecticides, accidental ingestion of, 820
Inspection, in physical examination, 194(t)
Instinctive-practice theory, of play, 157
Insulin, diabetes mellitus and, 1172, 1172(t)
Insulin dependent diabetes mellitus, 1168
Insulin tolerance test, for pituitary dwarfism, 631–632
Intake and output, in potential fluid and electrolyte imbalance, 355
Integrated record, in documentation of health care, 130
Intellectual competency, definition of, 143–144, 145–150
  hospitalized preschooler and, 1017, 1018(t)
  hospitalized school-age child and, 1201–1203, 1202–1203(t)
  of infant, 457–460
  of preschooler, 900–903
  of toddler, 739–743
    anticipatory guidance on, 741
  school-age child and, 1070–1074, 1086(t)
Intelligence, of infant, 457–459
  of preschooler, anticipatory guidance on, 901
  of school-age child, 1070–1072
    anticipatory guidance on, 1072
Intelligence quotient, 900
Intelligence tests, school-age child and, 1070–1072
Interaction, of mother and infant, 386–387
Interests, of parents, parenting style and, 51, 52(t)
Interferon, 511
Interim health history, 178
Intermediate inheritance, 141
Interrelationships, in family, 254–255
Interstitial fluid, shift to vascular, 347
Intertrigo, *501*, 502(t)

INDEX **1401**

Intervening approach, to extreme temper tantrums, 778–779
Intervention, nursing, in child abuse, 88
　in failure-to-thrive families, 81–84
　in maturational crisis, 275–276
　in parenting, 58–59
　in situational crisis, 276–277
　irreversibly ill preschooler and, 957–958
　sexual assault and, 1059
Interview, problem, 178
　well-child, 177–178
Interviewing, 177–179
Intestinal atresia, 584–585
　role of nurse in, 584–585
Intestinal obstruction, Hirschsprung's disease and, 589
　Meckel's diverticulum and, 588
Intimacy, adolescent and, 1238, 1256
Intoeing, 782
Intracranial pressure (ICP), in Reye's syndrome, 1197–1198
Intracranial tumors, 1189–1195
Intramuscular injections, 693, 696, *693*
　hospitalized toddler and, 865, 874
Intrauterine device (IUD), birth control and, 1246
Intrauterine growth retardation (IUGR), 444
Intrauterine length chart, *413*
Intrauterine weight chart, *412, 413*
Intravenous fluids, administering, 360–364
Intravenous pyelogram (IVP), 951
Intrinsic asthma, 985
Intuitive stage, of intellectual development, 149, 1072
Intussusception, 586–588, *587*
　role of nurse in, 587–588
Iron, requirement of infant for, 457
Iron-binding studies, in iron deficiency anemia, 787
Iron deficiency anemia, 785–788
　diarrhea and, 785
　role of nurse in, 787–788
Irreversible alterations, in health status, of adolescent, 1298–1313
　of infant, 639–670
　of preschooler, 955–998
　of school-age child, 1140–1183
　of toddler, 828–842
Irreversible illness, 289–294
　child and, 290–291
　family and, 290
Irritability, of intracranial tumors, 1192
Ishihara plates, 209
Isolation, as punishment, 43
Isotonic dehydration, 350, 354(t)
Itching, of athlete's foot, 1105
　of scabies, 1104

IV, calculating rate of fluid administration, 362
　maintaining, 362–364
　nursing guidelines for, 358–359(t), 363
　restraint with, 360–361
　starting, 360–362
IV therapy, child on, 364, *364*

Jacket restraint, 321–322
Jargon, expressive, of toddler, 742
Jaundice, assessment of, 195
　in intestinal atresia, 584
　in normal newborn infant, 415
Jealousy, in school-age child, 1079
　psychodynamics of, 773
Jock itch, 1269
Joints, in hemophilia, 837
　in juvenile rheumatoid arthritis, 1179–1180
　in rheumatic fever, 1120
　in systemic lupus erythematosus, 1305
Jones criteria, rheumatic fever and, 1120, 1120(t)
Juvenile acquired hypothyroidism, 633–634
Juvenile diabetes mellitus, 1168
Juvenile rehabilitation, social programs for, 1251
Juvenile rheumatoid arthritis (JRA), 1179–1183
　role of nurse in, 1180–1182

Kaiser-Permanente Medical Center, Family-Centered Perinatal Program, 404
Karyotyping, 1157
Keloid, *199*
Kernicterus, 415, 433
Ketoacidosis, diabetic, 1169–1170
　long-term care in, 1176–1177
Ketodiastix, 1173
Ketosis, diabetic, 1170
Kibbutz, childrearing in, 72
Kidney(s), palpation of, 227
　urinary tract infection and, 952
　vesicoureteral reflux and, 953
Kindergarten, 886–887
Kinesthesia, 233
Klumpke's palsy, 518
Knock-knees, 231
Kohlberg, Lawrence, theory of moral development, 152–153
Koplik's spots, 216
Krebs cycle, 1196
Kübler-Ross, Elisabeth, 65
Kwashiorkor, 627
Kyphoscoliosis, thoracic, *222*
Kyphosis, 1274, 1276, *1274*
　assessment for, 232

Labor, household, after birth of baby, 389–390
　division of, 712–713
　family with adolescent and, 1223

Laboratory assessment, in potential fluid and electrolyte imbalance, 355–356
Laboratory screening, 245–250
Lacrimal drainage tract, massage of, 520–521, *520*
Lacrimal stenosis, 520–521
Language, development of, 149–150, 741–743, 901–902
　anticipatory guidance on, 742–743
　blind child and, 970–971
　contribution of play to, 160
　in infant, 459–460, *460*
　in preschooler, 902
　in school-age child, 1074–1076
　anticipatory guidance on, 1075–1076
　stages in, 150(t), 742
　theories of, 150
　sign, 983
Language acquisition device (LAD), 150
Language ability, assessment of, 233
Lanugo, 416
Large for gestational age (LGA) infant, 443–444
Laryngeal stridor, congenital, 559
　role of nurse in, 559
Laryngitis, spasmodic, 823
Laryngomalacia, 559
Latch-key child, 30, 1055–1056
　parents and, 1056
Law, pertaining to adolescent parents, 123–124
Laxatives, in treating infant constipation, 513–514
Lead poisoning, 821–822
Lead toxicity, screening for, 249
Learning, contribution of play to, 160
　imitative, of infant, 458–459
Learning disabilities, 1144–1149
Leg recoil, of newborn infant, 410
Legg-Calvé-Perthes disease, 1112–1113
Legs, assessment of, 231
Length, intrauterine, chart, *413*
Lesbians, as parents, 73–74
Lesions, skin, assessment of, 196–197, *198–199*
Letting go, by parents, of school-age child, 1048–1049, 1053
Leukemia, central nervous system, 1004–1005
　distribution by age at diagnosis, 1000
　in preschooler, 999–1006
　testicular, 1005
Lice, head, 934–936, *935*
Lichenification, *199*
Life cycle, of family, 10, *11*, 12–16(t)
　of man, eight stages of, 151(t)
Limb-girdle muscular dystrophy, 1321, 1322(t)
Lip, cleft, 565–569, *566*
Lipreading, 982, 983
Lips, assessment of, 214
Listening, communication and, 170–171
　in history taking, 178

1402　INDEX

Liver, assessment of, 227
Liver function, of preterm infant, 433
  of term infant, 433
Living space, of family, 23–26
Localizer cast, 1281, 1285(t), *1282*
Locomotion, of infant, 451, *451*
  of toddler, 735–736, *735*
Lordosis, 1274, 1276, *1274*
  assessment for, 232
Love, in school-age child, 1079
Lovemaking, of parents and infants, 471–472, *472*, *473*
Lower arm palsy, 518
Lower extremity(ies), alignment of, *733*
  traction of, 1131–1132
Lower respiratory tract infection, in infants, 607–615
Lumbar puncture, in bacterial meningitis, 617
  in contusions, 1111
  in Guillain-Barré syndrome, 1124
  positioning of child for, 324–325, *325*
Lungs, assessment of, 218–224, *219–222*
Lupus band test, 1305
Lupus erythematosus, systemic, 1304–1308
Lupus nephritis, 1306
Lying, management of, 1100–1101
  school-age child and, 1099
Lymph nodes, *200*
Lymphadenopathy, of rubella, 922(t)
Lymphatic system, 197, 200, 202–203(t)
  in toddler, 735
Lymphocytes, 1001(t)
Lymphosarcoma, non-Hodgkin's, 1195–1196

Macule, *198*
"Mainstreaming," of mentally retarded child, 1155, *1156*
Male children, effect of female single parent families on, 62–63
Male genitals, of normal newborn, 419
  assessment of, 228–229, *228*
Male single parent families, 61–62, *61*
Males, anal agenesis in, 596, *597*
Malnutrition, maternal, pregnancy and, 113
  protein and calorie, severe, 627–628
Malocclusion, 1136
Malrotation, and volvulus, 585–586
Man, developmental models of, 135–136
Mantoux test, 1309(t)
Marasmus, 627
Marijuana, adolescent and, 1228
Marital relationship, independence and, 718–719
  maintaining, 714–715
Mastoiditis, 513
Masturbation, excessive, management of, 919–920
  preschooler and, 918–920
  preschooler and, 890, 905–906

Maternal infections, infant and, 667–668
"Maternal response failure," 482
Maternicity, 387
Maturation, defining, 136
Maturational crisis, 275–276
Maturing family, 15(t)
Maturity, neuromuscular, of newborn infant, 410–411
  physical, of newborn infant, 409–410, 409(t)
Mealtime, blind child and, 972
  preschooler and, 908–909
  school-age child and, 1085–1086
  toddler and, 736
Measles, 922–923(t)
  immunization to, 762
Measuration, in physical examination, 194(t)
Measurements, in health assessment, 188–192
Meat, preschooler diet and, 909(t)
Meatal opening, assessment of, 229
Meatal stenosis, 562
Mechanical mirror model, developmental model of man, 136
Mechanical ventilation, preterm infant and, 437–438
Mechanistic world view, developmental model of man, 136
Meckel's diverticulum, 588–589, *588*
Meconium, 428
Meconium ileus, cystic fibrosis and, 1325
Medic-Alert bracelet, 1163, 1178
Medications, administration of, 288, 693–696
  to hospitalized toddler, 861–865, 874
  behavior control and, 1147
  for common cold in infant, 510–511
  hospitalized adolescent and, 1337
Medication guidelines, 1 to 3 months, *694*
  3 to 12 months, *695*
  12 to 18 months, 862
  18 to 30 months, 863
  2½ to 3½ years, 864
  3½ to 6 years, 1024
Medulloblastoma, 1190
Memory, assessment of, 232
Menarche, 1234
Mendelian genetics, 140–141
Meningitis, bacterial, 616–618
  viral, 618–619
Meningocele, 648, *649*
Meningoencephalitis, mumps and, 925(t)
Meningomyelocele, 648
Menstrual disturbances, 1270–1272
Menstrual irregularity, 1271–1272
Mental retardation, 1150–1159
  nurse and, 1150–1153
  of Sturge-Weber syndrome, 653–654
Mentally retarded child, communication skills and, 1154
  education of, 1153–1155, *1156*

Mentally retarded child (*Continued*)
  self-care and, 1154–1155
  speech and, 1154
Metabolic functioning, alterations in, 662–664
  major burns and, 807(t)
  nurse and, 662–664
Metatarsus adductus, 601–602, *602*
Microencephaly, 1156–1157
Migrant children, 68–69, 69(t)
Migrant Student Record Transfer System, 69
Milestone, developmental, in developmental history, 181–182(t), 183
Milia, of newborn, 416
Miliaria, 502(t)
Milk, infant and, 467
  preschooler diet and, 909(t)
  toddler diet and, 739
Milk bottle syndrome, 450, *450*
Milwaukee brace, 1281, 1278(t), 1284, *1281*
Minerals, requirement of infant for, 456
Minimal brain dysfunction, 1144–1146
Miscarriage, 108
  previous attachment breakdown and, 477
Mobility, blind child and, 969, 972
  partial sightedness and, 968
Model, hypothetical, of parent reaction to child with congenital malformations, *679*
Moisture, of skin, 195–196
Molding, of head of newborn, 416
Money, as source of conflict in families, 27–28
  family of adolescent and, 1222–1223
Mongolian spots, 415, *415*
Moniliasis, 508, *508*
Monitoring, in total parenteral nutrition, 367–368
Monocular strabismus, 965
Monocytes, 1001(t)
Mononucleosis, infectious, 1266–1267
Monospot, 1267
Mood, in children, 1076–1077
MOPP chemotherapy, in Hodgkin's disease, 1321
Moral development, adolescent and, 1237
  child and, 152
  preschooler and, 906
Morale, of family, during pregnancy, 97
  maintaining, after birth, 388–389
Morality, conventional, 153
  development of, contribution of play to, 161–162
  preconventional, 153
  principled, 153
Mormons, 34
Moro reflex, 420, *421*
Mosaicism, 1157

Mother(s), energy depletion in, 722
  overprotective, 727
  rejecting, 727–728
  role of, 18, 381–384, *382*
  traditional, 48
  single. See *Female single parent families.*
  never-married, 66
  working, attitudes of, 889
    effect on family, 29–30
Mother-infant bond, 386–387
MOTHERS, support group, 726
Motor development, blind child and, 969
  of infant, 450–453
  of preschooler, 897–898, *898*
    anticipatory guidance on, 898
  of school-age child, 1063–1064
  of toddler, 735
Motor skills, fine, 452
  of toddler, 736–737
Mouth, assessment of, 214, 216–218
  of infant, 449
  of normal newborn, 418
Mouth-to-mouth resuscitation, of infants and small children, 343–344
Mucus trap, 342
Multi-generational transmission process, 252
Multiple births, sudden infant death syndrome and, 683
Mummy restraint, 320, *321*
  modified, 320, *322*
Mumps, 924–925(t)
Murmur(s), heart, 225–256
  classification of, 534
  of patent ductus arteriosus, 542
Muscle tone, of newborn infant, assessment of, 407
Muscles, assessment of, 235–236
Muscle biopsy, in muscular dystrophy, 1323
Muscular dystrophy, 1321–1324
  Duchenne's, 1321, 1323–1324, 1322(t)
  facioscapulohumeral, 1321, 1322(t)
  limb-girdle, 1321, 1322(t)
  pseudohypertrophic, 1321, 1323–1324, 1322(t)
Musculoskeletal anomalies, 599–605
Musculoskeletal system, assessment of, 230–232
Mustard procedure, for transposition of great vessels, 548
Mutism, elective, 1053–1054
"Mutual adaptation," attachment breakdown and, 480
Myasthenia gravis, neonatal, 518–520
Myelomeningocele, 648
Myocarditis, diphtheria and, 929(t)
Myoclonic seizures, 1161
Myopia, 963–964
Myositis, 1322(t)
Myringotomy, for otitis media, 512–513

Nails, assessment of, 197
Nail beds, cyanosis of, neonatal circulation and, 533
Narcotic use, physical risk in adolescent pregnancy, 120
Negative recording, in documenting health care, 130
Nasogastric intubation, decompression by, 334
  nursing care in, 332–335
Nasopharynx, specimen collection from, 342
Nasotracheal intubation, in epiglottitis, 944, *944*
National Group on Classification of Nursing Diagnoses, 129
Natural consequences, as punishment, 43–44
Nausea, of intracranial tumors, 1192
Neck, assessment of, 204–205, *204*
  of normal newborn, 418–419
Necrotizing enterocolitis, 593–595
  role of nurse in, 593–595
Negativism, in toddler, 748
Neglected child, family of, 84–90
Neonatal sepsis, 620
Neonatal transition, *414*
Neonate(s). See *Newborn infant.*
Nephrogenic diabetes insipidus, 1166, 1167
Nephropathy, diabetes mellitus and, 1178
Nephrotic syndrome, 838–842
  role of nurse in, 840–842
Nerves, cranial, assessment of, 233
Nerve deafness, 899
  auditory, mumps and, 925(t)
Neuritis, diphtheria and, 929(t)
Neuroblastoma, 1006–1008
  distribution by age at diagnosis, 1001
Neurocutaneous syndromes, 653–655
Neurofibromatosis, 654–655
Neurological alteration, of school-age child, nursing care plan for, 1214–1217
Neurological examination, 232–238, 234–235(t), *237*
  of normal newborn, 420–424
Neurological infections, in infant, 616–621
  role of nurse in, 617
Neurological sequelae, of encephalitis, 620
Neurological signs, in potential fluid and electrolyte imbalance, 355
  soft, 238
Neuromuscular disorders, 517–520
Neuromuscular maturity, of newborn infant, 410–411
Neuromuscular scoliosis, 1277(t)
Neuronitis, infectious, 1124
Neuropathy, diabetes mellitus and, 1178
Neutrophils, 1001
Never-married single parent families, 66–67
Nevi, telangiectatic, 415
Nevus flammeus, 653
Newborn(s), 406–446
  chest physical therapy in, 331

Newborn(s) (*Continued*)
  examination of, 188
  hearing defects in, 977–978
  heat loss in, 424–425
  neuromuscular maturity of, 410–411
  normal, 406–429
    assessment of, 407–420
    neurological examination of, 420–424
    physical care of, 424–429
    physical maturity of, 409–410, 409(t)
Night terrors, 917, 918, 919(t)
Nightmares, 917, 919(t)
90–90 traction, 1131, *1131*
Nocturnal emissions, 1236
Nodule(s), *198*
  of acne vulgaris, 1263
Noncommunicating hydrocele, 583–584, *583*
Non-Hodgkin's lymphoma, distribution by age at diagnosis, 1000
Non-Hodgkin's lymphosarcoma, 1195–1196
Nonparalytic strabismus, 964
Non-pure tone screening, 979–980
Nonshivering thermogenesis, 425
Nonsurgical techniques, in spinal abnormalities, 1281–1286
Nonverbal communication, 168–169
  in families, 26–27, *27*
  in history taking, 178–179
  parent-infant attachment and, 482–483, *483*
Nose, assessment of, 214
  of normal newborn, 418
Nose drops, for treatment of common cold, in infant, 510
  hospitalized toddler and, 865
Nosebleed, 1107
Nuchal rigidity, in bacterial meningitis, 616
Nuclear family(ies), childrearing in, 73
  relationships to world beyond, 884–887
Nurse, allergy and, 498–499
  anesthesia of children and, 369–372
  as advocate of poor families, 28–29
  child with problem behavior and, 281–282
  communicating with children, 171–175, *173*
  communicating with parents, 175–176
  counselling in health promotion and, 268–270
  counselling of adolescents, 1247–1248
  counselling of dysfunctional families, 80
  counselling on infant obesity, 626
  counselling on television viewing, 33
  counselling role of, 268–270
  dying child and, 305–314
  family assessment and, 251–257
  health appraisal and, 177–250

Nurse (*Continued*)
  health promotion and, 258–264
  hospitalization of child and, 295–305
  hospitalized adolescent and, 1336–1338
  hospitalized infant and, 691–697, *691*
  hospitalized school-age child and, 1204–1217
  hospitalized toddler and, 849–858, 856–857(t)
  illness of infant and, 522–523
  impact of burn care on, 816–817, *816*
  infant with defect and, 523–526
  life-threatening illness and, 309–314
  oxygenation and, 325, 328
  parent-infant attachment and, 482–491
  parents of child with cancer and, 1013
  parents of child with defect and, 539, 640–642
  parents of newborn and, 397–398
  patients and, 262
  pregnant adolescents and, 121
  relationship with parent and child, 166–168
  responsibilities of, in childhood illness, 282–295, 283(t), 284(t)
  in diagnosis, of infant, 639–642
  IV therapy and, 363
  pediatric procedures and, 325–344
  restraints and, 322–324
  total parenteral nutrition and, 366–368
  traction and, 1133–1134
  urological surgery of infant and, 563–565
  role of, in identifying congenital heart defects, 539
  in irreversible illness, 828–832, 957–958
  in maintaining acid-base balance, 353–356
  in maintaining fluid and electrolyte balance, 353–356
  in preventing childhood communicable diseases, 923, 930
  in referrals, 270–271
  in school adjustment, 1047–1048
  in teaching, 264–268
  juvenile delinquency and, 1251–1252
Nursery school, 885–886, *886*
Nursing, pediatric, principles and skills of, 315–377
Nursing care. See names of specific conditions and procedures.
Nursing Care Plan, for adolescent with musculoskeletal alteration, 1340–1358
  for infant with respiratory alteration, 698–705
  for preschooler with urinary alteration, 1028–1037

Nursing Care Plan (*Continued*)
  for school-age child with neurological alteration, 1214–1217
  for toddler with circulatory alteration, 866–873
Nursing diagnosis, as part of nursing process, 128–129
Nursing implications, needs of hospitalized school-age child and, 1201–1204
  of growth and development, of children, 135
  of spinal fusion, 1286, 1287(t), 1288
Nursing intervention, as part of nursing process, 129
Nursing process, and problem-oriented recording, 128–134
Nurturing, of children, 46–47
Nurturing forces, effect on development, 141–142
Nutrients, requirement of infant for, 455–457
Nutrition, adolescent and, 1244–1245, 1244(t), 1245(t)
  altered, in infant, nursing care plan for, 700–701
  in infant with central nervous system condition, 656
  in major burn wound management, 813–814
  in preterm infant, 439–440, 439(t)
  inadequate, in adolescent pregnancy, 119
  newborn and, 427–428
  preschooler and, 908–913
  school-age child and, 1068–1070, 1085–1086, 1087(t)
  toddler and, 755–757
  anticipatory guidance on, 1070
Nutritional alterations, in infants, 624–630
Nutritional assessment, 242–245, 247(t)
Nutritional deficiencies, 1245(t)
Nutritional history, 244(t)
Nutritional requirements, in total parenteral nutrition, 365
  of infant, 455–457, 456(t)
  of preschooler, 900
  of toddler, 738–739, 756(t)
Nystagmus, of optic path gliomas, 1192

Obesity, adolescent, 1293, 1296–1297
  childhood, 1134–1136
  nurse and, 1135–1136
  in muscular dystrophy, 1323
  infant, 625–626
  nurse and, 625–626
  school-age child and, 1070
Object permanence, 739
  emotional attachment and, 473
  intelligence of infants and, 148, 457
Observation, as skill of communication, 169–170
Oepidal phase, preschooler and, 881, 905

Office visit, anticipatory guidance for, 288
Oliguria, major burns and, 806(t)
Ommaya reservoir, 1192, 1195, *1193*
Omphalocele, 577–578, *577*
  nurse and, 577–578
Oncotic pressure, 347
One-point discrimination, test for discriminatory sensation, 236
Oneida community, 72
Onlooker, type of play, 162
Open bed, for preterm infant, 435–436
Open question(s), in history taking, 178
Ophthalmoscope, in eye assessment, 206–207
Optic path gliomas, 1191–1192
Oral communication, hearing impairment and, 982
Oral contraceptive, birth control and, 1247
Oral hygiene. See also *Dental care.*
  in total parenteral nutrition, 368
Oral medications, administration of, hospitalized infant and, 693
  hospitalized preschooler and, 1023–1024
  hospitalized school-age child and, 1210
  hospitalized toddler and, 861
  schizophrenia and, 1302
Oral needs, of infant, importance of meeting, 461–462
Orbit, of eye, assessment of, 205
Orchidopexy, 948
Ordinal position, effect on development on, 142
Organic lamp model, developmental model of man, 136
Organismic world view, developmental view of man, 136
Organized supplementary play, 163
Orthodontia, 1136–1137
Orthopedic conditions, temporary, of toddler, 781–785
Orthoplast jacket, 1281, 1278(t), 1285(t), *1281*
Osmosis, 346
Osmotic pressure, 346
Osteochondritis, 1112
Osteogenesis imperfecta, 1142–1143
  congenital, 1142–1143
  nurse and, 1143
Osteogenic sarcoma, 1316
  distribution by age at diagnosis, 1000
Osteomyelitis, 1125–1126
Ostomy, care of, 591
Otitis externa, 503
Otitis media, 511–513
  pertussis and, 927(t)
  rubeola and, 923(t)
  serous, hearing loss and, 976–977
  suppurative, scarlet fever and, 929(t)

Otoscopic examination, 211–212, 899, 979
Out-toeing, 782
Outward Bound, juvenile rehabilitation program, 1251
"Overheard" technique, of teaching rules, 42
Overprotection, child with cancer and, 1012
  child with irreversible health alterations and, 643–644
  elective mutism and, 1053–1054
  irreversibly ill child and, 292–293, 293(t)
  irreversibly ill preschooler and, 957
  separation anxiety and, 770
  school phobia and, 1096
  toddler and, 727
Ownership rights, preschooler and, 914–916
Oxygen, by cannula, 437, 437
  by hood, 437, 438
  in bronchiolitis, 610
  in pneumonia, 615
  preterm infant and, 436–438
Oxygen therapy, American Academy of Pediatrics guidelines, 438–439
  hazards of, 438–439
Oxyuriasis, 791
Oxygenation, nursing skills in, 325, 328

Pacemaker, cerebellar, in cerebral palsy, 1160
Pain, hospitalized child and, 300
  hospitalized adolescent and, 1337
  of burns, 811
  of fractures, 1127
  of osteomyelitis, 1125
  perception of, in school-age child, 1207–1210, 1208(t)
  phantom, 1319
  postoperative, management of, 376
  toddler with life-threatening illness and, 844
Palate, assessment of, 218
  cleft, 565–569, 566
Pallor, assessment of, 195
Palmar reflex, 420, 420
Palpation, in physical examination, 194(t)
  of abdomen, 227
  of chest, 219–220
Palsy, cerebral, 1159–1161
  Klumpke's, 518
  lower arm, 518
Pancreas, cystic fibrosis and, 1325
Pancreatitis, mumps and, 925(t)
Pancytopenia, 1003
Papule(s), 198
  of acne vulgaris, 1263
Parallel activity, type of play, 162, 753
Paralysis, Erb-Duchenne, 517–518
  of Guillain-Barré syndrome, 1124
  of poliomyelitis, 960–961

Paralytic ileus, major burns and, 807(t)
Paralytic scoliosis, 1277(t)
Paralytic strabismus, 964
Parasitic infections, 789–795
Parent Effectiveness Training (PET), 62
Parental past, attachment breakdown and, 479
Parental roles, socialization and, 40–49
Parenteral therapy, related to surgery, 357, 360
Parents, abuse of adolescent and, 1253–1255
  abuse of child and, 89
  adolescent, law pertaining to, 123–124
    teaching parenting skills to, 123
  attachment breakdown and, 477–479
  bill of rights of, 54–55
  blindness in child and, 969
  child with cancer, and, 1009–1011
  child with cardiac condition and, 555, 556(t)
  child with defect and, 639–642
  child with epilepsy and, 1163
  child with hearing impairment and, 980
  children's play and, 164
  communicating with, 166–176
  credibility of, reinforcing, 263–264
  fatigue of, 398–399, 722–725
  foster, 67–68
  homosexual, 73–74
  hospitalized adolescent and, 1338
  hospitalized child and, 298, 301–304
  hospitalized toddler and, 850–852, 855
  illness of child and, 291–293, 939, 1142
  illness of infant and, 526–528, 527(t), 672
  infant development and, 465–470
  infant obesity and, 626
  infant with defect and, 525–526
  interests and activities of, 715–716
  irreversible illness of child and, 291–293
  latch-key child and, 1055–1056
  marital relationship of, 714–715
  prejudice and, 1055
  preschooler and, 880, 882
  relatives and, 716–717, 717
  self-esteem of, 55–57, 263
  sexual assault of child and, 1057–1059
  single, adoption by, 71–72
    families of, 61–67
  social relationships of, 715–716
  step, 67
  support structures of, 396–398
Parent-adolescent differences, 1227
Parent-child interactions, guide to assessment of, 484

Parent-child-nurse relationship, 166–168
Parent-child relationship, disturbed, 57(t)
  hospitalized infant and, 704–705
Parenthood, family philosophy and, 717–721
  preparing for, 99–102
Parenting, 39–59
  assessment of, 55–59
  definition of, 40–41
  dependence/independence in, 726–728
  disagreements about, 725–726
  goals and functions of, 45–46
  information to increase success of, 263
  of parents, in dysfunctional families, 80, 83
  principles of, 49–50
  problems of, 57–58
  shared, 48–49
  support by society for, 39–40
Parenting styles, 50–54, 51(t)
Parents Anonymous, 89
Parents Without Partners, 62
Partial sight, 967, 968
Participation, in treatment, hospitalized child and, 301
Patch, skin lesion, 198
Patellar reflex, evaluation of, 238
Patent ductus arteriosus, 540–542, 541
Pauciarticular juvenile rheumatoid arthritis, 1180
Pearson attachment, 1131, 1132
Pediatric history-taking outline, 180–182(t)
Pediatric nursing, principles and skills of, 315–377
Pediculosis capitis, 934–936, 935
Peeling agents, in acne vulgaris, 1265
Peer group, adolescent and, 1229–1230, 1229
  adolescent drug use and, 1259
  delinquency and, 1250
  hospitalized adolescent and, 1333, 1335
  irreversibly ill child and, 1140–1141
  school-age child and, 1042, 1043, 1046–1047
Peer relationships, adolescent, expanding, 1240–1241
Penis, assessment of, 229t
  of adolescent, 1235, 1236, 1234(t)
Perceptive loss, of hearing, 899
Perceptual stage, of intellectual development, 149
Percussion, in physical examination, 194(t)
  in postural drainage, 329, 329
  of abdomen, 227
  of chest, 220–221
  of heart, 224
Perforation, appendicitis and, 1123
Periosteal hinge, 1127, 1127
Peripheral impairment, of hearing, 975–977
Peritonsillar abscess, scarlet fever and, 929(t)

Permanent object, and intelligence of infant, 457
Permissive parenting style, 51(t)
Persistence, of children, 1077
"Persistent infantile bladder," 950
Person, developing, 748–753
   preschooler, 903–906
   school-age child, 1081–1085
   toddler, 749–753
Personality. See also under *Person, developing.*
   of child, parenting styles and, 50, 52–53(t)
   types of, 154(t)
Perthes' disease, 1112
Pertussis, 926–927(t)
"Petalling," of cast, 1128
Petit mal seizures, 1161
"Phantom pain," 1319
Pharyngotonsillitis, 940–941, 941(t)
Pharynx, assessment of, 218
Phenomenism, 938
Phenylketonuria (PKU), 662–664
   galactosemia and, 663(t)
   testing for, 249
Philosophy, of family, birth of baby and, 394
   parenthood and, 717–721
   values in, 718
Phobia, speech, 1053
Phocomelia, 110
Phonics, 1074
Phototherapy, for hyperbilirubinemia, 434
   for neonatal jaundice, 415
Physical assessment, in history taking, 185–193
Physical competency, 143, 144–145
   hospitalized preschooler and, 1017, 1018(t)
   hospitalized school-age child and, 1201, 1202(t)
   in infant, 447–457
   in preschooler, 895–900
   in toddler, 731–739
Physical development, contribution of play to, 159, *159*
   of adolescent, 1235–1236
   of school-age child, 1060–1070
Physical energy, of family with toddler, 722–725
Physical examination, 193–238
Physical punishment, preschooler and, 904
Physical therapy, chest, 330
   in cystic fibrosis, 1326
   in juvenile rheumatoid arthritis, 1181
Piaget, theories of intellectual development, 146–149, *147, 148, 149,* 457
   theory of play, 158
Pica, 788–789
Pigeon chest, *222*
Pill, the, birth control and, 1247
Pink eye, 507
Pinna, assessment of, 209
Pinworm, 791
Pituitary dwarfism, 630–632
   nurse and, 632
Pituitary gland, intracranial tumors and, 1195
   tumor of, 633

Placental dysfunction syndrome, 442
Placing reflex, 422
Plan, development of, as part of nursing process, 129
Plantar reflex, 420, *420*
   evaluation of, 236
Plants, accidental ingestion of, 821
Plaque, *198*
Plasma, 1000
Plasma iron studies, in iron deficiency anemia, 787
Platelets, 1000
Play, blind child and, 971–972
   cognitive development and, 159–161
   developmental characteristics of, 162–164
   health examination and, 186–188
   helping parents to promote, 164
   hospitalized child and, 300–301
   hospitalized infant and, 692
   hospitalized preschooler and, 1025
   hospitalized school-age child and, 1210–1212
   hospitalized toddler and, 858–859, *858*
   in concrete operations stage, 1073
   infant and, 148–149, 468
   irreversibly ill preschooler and, 958
   physical development and, 159, *159*
   preschooler and, 880, *880*, 910–911
   school-age child and, 1086–1087, 1087(t)
   theories of, 157–159
   toddler and, 736, 757
   socialization and, 752–753
   symbolic, 740
   types of, 162–164
   understanding, 157–165
Play equipment, accidents and, 762
Play schools, 886
Pneumococcal pneumonia, 612–613(t)
Pneumonia, 611–615
   bacterial, major burns and, 806(t)
   hypostatic, traction and, 1134
   pertussis and, 927(t)
   role of nurse in, 614, 615
   scarlet fever and, 929(t)
   streptococcal, 943
   viral, 608–609(t)
Point of maximal impulse (PMI), 224, 413–414
   location of, 534, *534*
Poisoning. See also *Ingestion, of poison material.*
   accidental, 818–820
   toddler and, 760, 818–822
   carbon monoxide, major burns and, 806(t)
   iron tablet ingestion and, 788
   lead, 821–822
Polio virus, infection from, 959(t)
Poliomyelitis, 958–961
   differential diagnosis from Guillain-Barré syndrome, 1124
Polyarticular juvenile rheumatoid arthritis, 1179–1180

Polymyositis, 1322(t)
Polyneuritis, acute, 1124
Polys, 1001
Popliteal angle, of newborn, 410
Port wine stain, 653
Positioning, of child for hospital procedures, 324–325
Postoperative nursing care, 375–377
Post-term infant, 442–443, *443*
   in cystic fibrosis, 1326
Postural drainage, 328–329, *326–327*
Posture, of newborn, 410
   of school-age child, 1062–1063, *1062, 1063*
   resting, of preterm infant, *431*
Potassium, imbalance of, 352, 351(t)
   maintenance dose of, calculation of, 357
Poverty, of families, 28–29
Preadmission preparation, hospitalized child and, 297–298
   hospitalized preschooler and, 1020–1021, *1020*
   hospitalized school-age child and, 1204–1205, *1205*
Precocious puberty, 1113–1115
Preconceptual stage, of intellectual development, 148–149, 740
Preconventional morality, 153
Pregnancy, adjustment to, 95–99
   nurse and, 99
   difficult, 108
   ectopic, 108–109
   expectant father and, 98–99
   grandparents and, 96–97
   in adolescence, 115–125, 1255
      impact on health professionals, 120–124
   interrupted, 108–109
   potential stresses during, 106–114
   preparation for parenthood in, 100–101
   psychological phases of, 98, *98*
   redistribution of household labor in, 95–96
   sexual relations and, 96
   teratogens in, 110–114
   unplanned, 106–107
Prejudice, 1055
Premature adrenarche, 1114
Premature thelarche, 1114
Prematurity. See also *Preterm infant.*
   attachment breakdown and, 476
   esophageal atresia and tracheoesophageal fistula and, 572–573
   significance for long-term development, 442
Premenstrual tension, 1272
Prenatal care, adolescent pregnancy and, 119
Preoperational stage, of intellectual competency development, 148–149, 740

Preoperational thought, preschooler and, 903
Preoperative nursing care, 373–375, 375(t)
Pre-readmission, hospitalized preschooler and, 1020–1021
Preschool program, 908
Preschool years, potential stresses during, 937–954, 955–998, 999–1015
Preschooler, age-appropriate expectations for, 882
  aggression in, excessive, 892
  behavior of, managing, 914–920
  cancer and, 1010, 1012
  developmental tasks of, 881
  examination of, 188
  family with, growth and development needs of, 879–887
    potential stresses in, 888–893
  general appearance of, 895–896
  health of, irreversible alterations in, 955–998
    life-threatening alterations in, 999–1015
    maintaining, 908–913
    reversible alterations in, 937–954
    temporary alterations in, 921–936
  hearing of, 898–899
    assessing, 212, 979–980
    impairment, 980–982
  hospitalized, 1016–1037
  intellectual competency of, 900–903
  irreversible illness in, 955–957
  peers and, 884
    perception of, 937–938
  physical competency of, 895–900
  potential stresses and, 914–920, 921–936
  vision of, 898
Present illness, in history taking, 180(t), 182–183
Preterm infant, 430–435. See also *Prematurity*.
  death of, family care after, 445
  discharge of, family care after, 445
  general appearance of, 430–432
  special needs of, 435–442
  term infant and, 430–435
Preventive health action, factors influencing, 261(t)
Primary circular reactions, intelligence of infant and, 457
Principled morality, 153
Prism telescope, for partially sighted preschooler, 968
Privacy, adolescent and, 1221–1222
  birth of baby and, 391
  school-age child and, 1049
Privilege withdrawal, as punishment, 43
Problem behavior, in child, 279–282, *280*

Problem identification, as part of nursing process, 128–129
Problem interview, 178
Problem list, in documentation of health care, 131
Problem-Oriented Medical Record, 177
Problem-oriented recording, in documentation of health care, 130–133
  nursing process and, 128–134
Problem-solving skills, 259–260
  contribution of play to, 160
  in health promotion, 267–268
Problems, of parenting, 57–58
Progress notes, in documentation of health care, 132–133, *133*
Proptosis, of optic path gliomas, 1192
Protectiveness, parental, parenting styles and, 54
Protein, malnutrition, severe, 627–628
  requirement of infant, 455
  requirement of preschooler, 900
  requirement of toddler, 738
Protest, hospitalized child and, 299
  hospitalized toddler and, 852–853
Prothrombin activator, 835
Pseudocryptorchidism, 230
Pseudohermaphrodite, 665
Pseudohypertrophic muscular dystrophy, 1321, 1323–1324, 1322(t)
Pseudostrabismus, 964, *964*
Psychoanalytic theory, of play, 157–158
Psychoanalytic world view, developmental model of man, 136
Psychological status, altered, in adolescent, 1300–1304
Puberty, delayed, 1299–1300
  onset of, 1233
  precocious, 1113–1115
Pubic hair, assessment of, 197
  development of, in boys, 1235, 1234(t), *1234*
  in girls, 1234, *1234*, 1235(t)
Public policy, family and, 34–35
Pulmonary damage, primary, major burns and, 806(t)
Pulmonary disease, cystic fibrosis and, 1325
Pulmonary edema, major burns and, 806(t)
Pulmonary embolus, major burns and, 806(t)
Pulmonary stenosis, 545–546
Pulse(s), assessment of, in hospitalized child, 317
  cardiovascular, 226
  in health assessment, 192(t)
  in potential fluid and electrolyte imbalance, 354
  neonatal circulation and, 533
Punishment, asthmatic child and, 994
  in socialization of children, 43–44
  preschooler and, 904, 946
  tantrums and, 778

Pupils, eye, recording of size of, 1109
Pushout, 1260
Pustule, *198*
Pyloric stenosis, 570–572, *570*
  nurse and, 570–572
Pyoderma, 930–931(t)

Q fever, 793

Rabies, 931–934, 934(t)
Radiation, newborn and, 424–425
  pregnancy and, 110, 112
Radiation therapy, in bone tumor, 1317
  in Hodgkin's disease, 1320
  in intracranial tumors, 1194
  in retinoblastoma, 847
Radioallergosorbent (RAST) test, 495–496
Rales, 223–224
Rape, dating, 1227
Rashes, diaper, 501
  of chickenpox, 924–925(t)
  of erythema infectiosum, 922–923(t)
  of Henoch-Schonlein purpura, 945
  of herpes zoster, 924–925(t)
  of rubella, 922–923(t)
  of scarlet fever, 929(t)
  of systemic lupus erythematosus, 1304–1305, *1304*
Reaction, intensity of, in children, 1076
Reactivity, of newborn, 423–424
Reading disorders, 1147–1149
Reason for contact, in health history, 179, 180(t)
Reasoning, in infant, 148
  prelogical, in child, 149
Reassurance, for parents, 55–57
Rectal atresia, 596, *595*
Rectal bleeding, Meckel's diverticulum and, 588
Rectal medications, hospitalized toddler and, 865
Rectal stenosis, in infant, 513
Rectum, assessment of, 230
Referrals, nurse's role in, 270–271
Reflex action, evaluation of, 236, *237*
Reflex irritability, of newborn infant, assessment of, 407
Reflexes, pathological, 238
Reflux, vesicoureteral, 952–954
Refractive errors, 961–963
Regressive behavior, of hospitalized toddler, 851
Rehabilitation period, of burn care, 814
Reinforcement theory, of language development, 150
Relationship(s), family, potential stress related to, 401–404
  parent-child, disturbed, 57(t)
  parent-infant, disturbed, 475–482
  spouse, birth of baby and, 392–394
  stimulation of, 880

Relatives, relationships with, 716–717, *717*
Reliability, of nurse, importance in communication with children, 172
Religion, of family, 33–34, 256
  assessment of, 34
Remodeling, in fractures, 1127
Renal biopsy, in nephrotic syndrome, 840–842
Renal damage, diphtheria and, 929(t)
Renal disease, 1117–1119
  chronic, 838–842
Renal dysfunction, complications of, nursing care for, 1033–1035
Renal function, of preterm infant, 435
Renal involvement, of Henoch-Schonlein purpura, 945
Renin-angiotensin system, in regulation of fluid and electrolyte balance, 346
Renocardiovascular mechanism, fluid and electrolyte balance and, 346
Reorganization, of family, infant with defect and, 525
  infant with genetic disorder and, 679
Reproductive functioning, alterations in, 665–667
Residence, family, 254
Residual vision, 967
Resistive behavior, of hospitalized toddler, 851
Resources, family, 255–256
  adolescent and, 1221–1222
  birth of baby and, 99–100, 391–392
  preschooler and, 879–880
  to aid families, 271(t)
Respect, parent-child-nurse relationship and, 167
Respiration, aiding, nursing skills in, 325, 328
  assessment of, in hospitalized child, 317
  in potential fluid and electrolyte imbalance, 354
  of newborn, later assessment of, 412–413
  paradoxical, 218–219
Respirator, poliomyelitis and, 960
Respiratory alteration, in infant, nursing care plan for, 698–705
Respiratory care, in burns, 808–809
Respiratory conditions, preschooler and, 940–946
Respiratory development, of preterm infant, 432
  of term infant, 432
Respiratory difficulty(ies), neonatal circulation and, 532
  of diaphragmatic hernia, 579–580
Respiratory distress, in preterm infant, 436
Respiratory effort, of newborn infant, assessment of, 407
Respiratory infection, in infant, 606–616
  neonatal circulation and, 532

Respiratory isolation, influenza and, 1268
Respiratory obstruction, diphtheria and, 929(t)
Respiratory rate(s), 221
  in health assessment, 192(t)
Respiratory tract, congenital anomalies of, 558–559
Responsibility, adolescent and, 1223, *1223*, 1242
  school-age child and, 1049–1050
    anticipatory guidance on, 1049–1050
  teaching to children, 712–713
Rest, preterm infant, and, 441–442
  school-age child and, 1068
  sickle cell anemia and, 675–676
  tuberculosis and, 1310–1311
Rest routines, preschooler and, 906–907
Resting posture, in preterm infant, *431*
  in term infant, *431*
Restitution, grief reaction after death of child, 308–309
Restraint, hospitalized child and, 320–324
  hospitalized infant and, 692–693, 696
  in alterations in visual functioning, 660
  IV and, 360–361
  nursing responsibilities in, 322–324
  of infant, after cleft lip repair, 568, *568*
  traction and, 1134
Resuscitation, cardiopulmonary, of infants and small children, 343–344
Retina, assessment of, 206
Retinoblastoma, 845–848, *846*
  distribution by age at diagnosis, 1000
Retinopathy, diabetes mellitus and, 1178
Retractions, 219
Retrolental fibroplasia, 438
Retropharyngeal abscess, 606–607
Reversible alterations, in health status, of adolescent, 1273–1297
  of infant, 522–638
  of preschooler, 921–936
  of school-age child, 1116–1139
  of toddler, 797–827
Reversible illness, 289
Reward, use of, in socialization of children, 44–45, 45(t)
Reye's syndrome, 1196–1199
  chickenpox and, 925(t)
  nurse and, 1198–1199
Rhabdomyosarcoma, 845
  distribution by age at diagnosis, 1000
Rheumatic fever, 1119–1122
  scarlet fever and, 929(t)
Rheumatism, juvenile, Sydenham's chorea and, 1122
Rhinitis, chronic allergic, 995, 995(t)
Rhonchi, 223–224

Rhythm method, birth control and, 1245–1246
Rickets, vitamin D deficiency, 628–630
  nurse and, 629–630
Rickettsial infections, 793–794
Rights, respect of, 54–55
Riley-Day syndrome, 677–678
Ringworm, 791–792, 792(t)
Rinne test, of hearing, 213–214
Risser cast, 1281, 1285(t), *1282*
Rituals, hospitalized toddler and, 854–855, *854*
  toddler with life-threatening illness and, 845
Rochester method, hearing impairment and, 982
Rocky Mountain spotted fever, 793–794
Role model, nurse as, 79–80, 264
Role(s), of parents, 46–49, *47*, 47(t)
Rolling, of infant, stages of, 451, 451(t)
Romberg test, of sensory equilibrium, 233
Rooming in, 696–697
  adolescent parents and, 123
  family of hospitalized sensory-impaired child and, 984
  family of hospitalized toddler and, 851
Rooting reflex, 420
Roseola infantum, 509
Roundworm, 791
Routines, hospitalized toddler and, 854–855, *854*
  preschooler and, 906
  toddler with life-threatening illness and, 845
"Rubber," birth control and, 1245
Rubella, 922(t)
  pregnancy and, 110, 112–113
Rubeola, 922(t)
Rule of nines, 800, *802*
Rules, parental, 41–43, *46*
Runaways, 1257–1258
Russell's traction, 1131, *1130*

Sadness, birth of child with defect and, 525
  birth of child with genetic disorder and, 678
  death of child and, 308
Safety, burn prevention, 800
  hospitalized child and, 318–325
  hospitalized toddler and, 859–865, 874
  of infant, 468–469, *468*
  of newborn, 428–429
  preschooler and, 880, 911–912
  school-age child and, 1087–1088, 1087(t)
  toddler and, 710–711, *710*, 758–762

INDEX 1409

Salicylates, accidental ingestion of, 820–821
  in juvenile rheumatoid arthritis, 1180
Sarcoma, Ewing's, 1316
  distribution by age at diagnosis, 1000
  osteogenic, 1316
    distribution by age at diagnosis, 1000
Scabies, 1103–1104, *1104*
Scale, skin, *198*
Scalp, assessment of, 201
  hygiene of, 503
  of normal newborn, 417–418
Scalp vein, IV insertion site, 360
Scar, *199*
Scarf sign, of newborn, 410
Scarlet fever, 928–929(t)
Schizophrenia, 1300–1303
  nurse and, 1303
School, adjustment to, 1044–1045(t)
  adolescent and, 1260–1261
  inappropriate assimilation of child in, 1053–1054
  irreversibly ill child and, 1140–1141
  life-threatening illness and, 1188
  readiness for, 907–908
    anticipatory guidance on, 908
School-age child(ren), competency development of, 1086–1087(t)
  death and, 1184–1188
  emotional development of, 1076–1081, 1086(t)
  examination of, 188
  expanding world of, 1041–1047
  growth and development of, 1060–1089
  health of, irreversible alterations in, 1140–1183
    life-threatening alterations in, 1184–1200
    reversible alterations in, 1116–1139
    temporary alterations in, 1103–1115
  hearing screening in, 980
  hospitalized, 1201–1217
  intellectual development of, 1070–1074, 1086(t)
  interviewing, 179
  language development of, 1074–1076
  potential stresses in families with, 1052–1059
  social development of, 1081–1085
  trauma and, 1107–1112
School-age years, potential stresses during, 1090–1102, 1103–1115, 1116–1139, 1140–1183, 1184–1200
School phobia, 1095–1098
  irreversibly ill child and, 1141
School program, modifying, to correct mutism, 1054(t)
Sclavotest, 1309(t)

Scoliosis, 1276–1288, 1275(t), 1277–1279(t), 1284–1286(t), *1274*
  assessment for, 232, 1280
  management of, nonsurgical, 1281–1283, 1286, 1284–1285(t)
    surgical, 1281, 1286, 1288, 1286(t)
Scrotum, assessment of, 230
Seasonal variation, sudden infant death syndrome and, 683
Seborrheic dermatitis, 501, 503–504, 502(t), *503*
Seborrheic diaper dermatitis, 503
Secondary circular reactions, intelligence of infant and, 457–458
Segs, 1001
Seizures, akinetic, 1161
  febrile, 518
  focal motor, 1161–1162
  grand mal, 1161
  infantile myoclonic, 655–657
  intracranial tumors and, 1195
  myoclonic, 1161
  of Sturge-Weber syndrome, 653–654
  petit mal, 1161
Self-awareness, development of, contribution of play to, 161
Self-care, adolescent and, 1243–1244
  blind child and, 972–973, *973*
  contribution of play to, 161, *161*
  hospitalized preschooler and, 1017
  in bracing of spinal abnormalities, 1282
  in diabetes mellitus, 1174, 1174(t)
  irreversibly ill preschooler and, 958
  responsibility for, 260–262
  retarded child and, 1154–1155
  toddler and, 736–737, 752
Self-esteem, in parents, 263
  in preschooler, 903–904
  in toddler, 748
Self-talk, 902
Sensation, testing of, 236
Sense of industry, in school-age child, 1081. See also *Industriousness*.
Sense-pleasure play, 163
Senses, of newborn, assessment of, 423
Sensorimotor period, of intellectual development, 147–148, *148*
Sensorineural losses, of hearing, 976–977
Sensory-impaired child, hospitalization and, 983–984, *984*
Sensory organ development, in school-age child, 1066
  anticipatory guidance on, 1066
Sensory stimulation, of preterm infant, 441
Sensory system, assessment of, 236
Separation, attachment breakdown and, 478
  normal, stages of, 771

Separation (*Continued*)
  of school-age children from parents, 1048–1049
  of toddler from parents, 745–746
Separation anxiety, excessive, 770–772
  in hospitalized toddler, 852–854
  in irreversibly ill child, 830–831
  in toddler with circulatory alteration, nursing care plan for, 871–872
  in toddler with life-threatening illness, 844–845
  normal, psychodynamics of, 769–770
  school phobia and, 1096
Sepsis, major burns and, 807(t)
  neonatal, 620
Septicemia, 620–621
  cellulitis and, 931(t)
  nurse and, 620–621
  osteomyelitis and, 1125
Sequestration crisis, 674
Seriation, 149
Serous otitis media, 511
  hearing loss and, 976–977
  suppurative otitis media and, 512(t)
Setting sun eyes, 418
Settling-in, response to hospitalization in young child, 299
Seventh-Day Adventists, 34
Sex, of infant, attachment breakdown and, 476
  in adrenogenital syndrome, 666
Sex education, adolescent and, 1257
  preschooler and, 881, 905
  school-age child and, 1088
Sex-role identification, of toddler, 753–754
  anticipatory guidance on, 754
Sex-typed behaviors, 754
  preschooler and, 906
Sexual abuse, of adolescent, 1254–1255
Sexual activity, of adolescent, 1255–1257
Sexual assault, adolescent and, 1227
  nurse and, 1057–1059
  possible, assessment of, 1058(t)
  school-age child and, 1056–1059
Sexual identity, of preschooler, 905–906
  anticipatory guidance on, 905–906
Sexual infantilism, 1300
Sexual maturation, of adolescent, 1233–1235
Sexual relations, pregnancy and, 96
  resumption of after childbirth, 402–403
Sexuality, development of, 152
  of adolescent, 1227–1228
  of toddler, 754
  anticipatory guidance on, 754
Shared parenting, 48–49
Shift work, family and, 29
Shigellosis, 794–795
Shiners, allergic, 987, *987*

Shock, in contusions, 1111
    of family, birth of child with genetic disorder and, 678
        birth of infant with defect and, 525
        death of child and, 308
Shoes, of toddler, 734
Sibling-infant relationship, 103–105, *104*, 387–388, *388*
Siblings, cancer and, 1011, 1014
    death among, 684–685, 1014
    epilepsy and, 1163
    fighting among, 775
    hospitalization of infant and, 690–691
    identification of infant and, 382
    illness among, 285, 939
        irreversible, 293–294, 958
        life-threatening, 310
    learning disabled child and, 1145
    nephrotic syndrome and, 842
    preschooler and, 881, *881*
    role of, *18*, 19
        assuming, 385–386, *385*
    sharing among, *723*
    sickle cell anemia and, 676
    stillbirth and, 109–110
    sudden infant death syndrome and, 684–685
Sibling rivalry, 714
    excessive, 772–776
    preschooler and, 881
Sickle cell anemia, 672–674
    nurse and, 674–676
Sickle cell crisis, 673–674
Sickle cell disease, 672–674
Sickle cell trait, 672–673
Sickledex, 248, 675
Sidearm traction, 1132
Sign language, 983
Silastic sheeting, omphalocele and, 577, *578*
Silence, communication and, 171
Silo technique, gastroschisis and, 579
    omphalocele and, 577–578
Single parent adoption, 71–72
Single parent family(ies), 61–67
    by death, 65–66
    by divorce, 63–65, *64*
    preschooler and, 906
Sinuses, assessment of, 214, *215*
Sitting, learning in, stages of, 451, 451(t)
Situational crisis, 276–277
Skeletal abnormalities, 1274–1288, *1274*
Skeletal age, 144
Skeletal growth, of preschooler, 895–896
    anticipatory guidance on, 896
    of school-age child, 1062
        anticipatory guidance on, 1062–1063
    of toddler, 732–733
Skeletal traction, 1131
Skill play, 163
Skin, assessment of, 195–197
    burns and, 799–800
    care of, in traction, 1133
    in potential fluid and electrolyte imbalance, 354–355
    of newborn, initial assessment of, 407–408

Skin, of newborn
    (*Continued*)
        later assessment of, 414–416
    neonatal circulation and, 532–533
    problems of, 1103–1107
Skinfolds, measurement of, *246*
Skinner, B. F., reinforcement theory of, 150
Skin testing, in allergy, 990
Skin traction, 1131
Skull, transillumination of, 201
Skull fracture, 1111
Sleep, of "cardiac infant," 534
    of infant, 454
    of preschooler, 906–907
    of school-age child, 1068
    of toddler, developing regularity and routines in, 750
        anticipatory guidance on, 750–751
    sudden infant death syndrome and, 683
Sleep disorders, management of, 917–919
    preschooler and, 917–919
Sleep/wake patterns, of newborn, 423˙
Sleepwalking, preschooler and, 919
Small for gestational age (SGA) infant, 443
Smell, sense of, of newborn, 423
Snacks, blind child and, 972
Snellen Alphabet Chart, 207–208, *208*
Snellen E Chart, 207–208, *208*, 898
SOAP (Subjective Objective Analysis Plan), 132
Social-affective play, 163
Social competency, hospitalized school-age child and, 1203–1204, 1203(t)
Social development. See also *Socialization.*
    contribution of play to, 161–162
    of adolescent, 1240–1243
        anticipatory guidance on, 1242–1243
    of school-age child, 1081–1085, 1086(t)
    of toddler, 743–754
Social history, family, in history taking, 185
    in assessment of parent-infant attachment, 490
Social interaction, of families, 255
Social learning theory, of language development, 150
Social relations, early, normal development of, 471–475
Social responsiveness, of infant, 461
Socialization, blind child and, 971–972
    of child, *40*
    or preschooler, 906–908
    of school-age child, 1080–1081
    of toddler, 752–753
    parental roles and, 40–49
Sodium, imbalance of, 351–352, 351(t)
    replacement of, in adrenogenital syndrome, 667
Soft neurological signs, 238

"Soft spot," 416
Soft tissues, tumors of, 1195–1196
Solid food, infant diet and, 465–467
Solitary independent play, 162
Somogyi effect, diabetes mellitus and, 1178
Sorrow, chronic, of parents of child with defect, 640
Sounds, breath, characteristics of, 223(t)
    lung, adventitious, 223(t)
    vascular, abdominal, 227
Source-oriented record, in documentation of health care, 130
Space, in home, adolescent and, 1221–1222
    birth of baby and, 391
    children and, 709–710
Spanking, 43, *44*
Spasmodic laryngitis, 823
Spasms, infantile, 655–657
Spatial perception, partial sightedness and, 968
Speech, cued, 983
    mentally retarded child and, 1154
    of hearing-impaired child, 981–983
    of school-age child, 1074
    of toddler, characteristics of, 742
    screening of, 242
Speech difficulty, in head injury, 1109, 1110
Speech disturbances, preschooler and, 916–917
Speech phobia, 1053
Speechreading, 983
Speech training, 983
Spencer, Herbert, theory of play of, 157
Spica cast, hip, 604
Spina bifida, 648–651, *649*
    exercises and, 650
Spina bifida cystica, 648–651, *650*
Spina bifida occulta, 648
Spinal abnormalities, 1274–1288
    nurse and, 1281–1286
Spinal fusion, activities after, 1287(t)
    in scoliosis, 1281, 1286, 1286(t)
Spinal tap, positioning of child for, 324–325, *325*
Spine, assessment of, 232
Spleen, palpation of, 227
Splinting, of fractures, 1128
Splint(s), in internal tibial torsion, 783
    in juvenile rheumatoid arthritis, 1181
Spoiling, of infants, 474
Sports injuries, 1111–1112
Spots, Mongolian, 415, *415*
Spot test, 1267
Spouses, importance of communication for, 880
    relationship of, after birth of baby, 392–394

Spouses, relationship of (Continued)
in family with adolescent, 1224
irreversibly ill preschooler and, 956
roles of, 17
Sputum specimen, collection of, 342
Square window, assessment of newborn infant, 410
Squatting, in tetralogy of Fallot, 550
Stabs, 1001
Staging, in neuroblastoma, 1007
in non-Hodgkin's lymphosarcoma, 1196
in Reye's syndrome, 1197
Staging laparotomy, in Hodgkin's disease, 1320
Stance, assessment of, 232
Stanford-Binet IQ test, 900–901
Staphylococcal pneumonia, 612–613(t)
Startle response, 420–421, *421*
Status asthmaticus, 993–995
Stealing, management of, 1101–1102
preschooler and, 914–916
school-age child and, 1100
Stem cell, 1002
Stenosis, anal, 595, *595*
aortic, 546–547
lacrimal, 520–521
meatal, 562
pulmonary, 545–546
pyloric, 570–572, *570*
Stents, in pediatric urological surgery, 564
Step-parents, 67
Stepping reflex, 422, *422*
Stereotyped behaviors, in blind child, 972
Stereotyping, nurse-family relationship and, 37
Sterility, orchitis, mumps and, 925(t)
Steroids, in nephrotic syndrome, 840–842
Stiff neck, in bacterial meningitis, 616
Stillbirth, 109–110
Still's disease, 1180
Stimulation, hospitalized infant and, 692–693
of infant with visual condition, 660–662
Stimuli, threshold for, in children, 1076
Stinging insect allergy, 995
Stool, in intussusception, 587
in iron deficiency anemia, 787
in necrotizing enterocolitis, 593
in volvulus, 586
Stool specimen, collection of, 342
"Stork bites," 415
Strabismic amblyopia, 966
Strabismus, 205–206, 964–966
corneal light reflex test for, 206
cover test for, 206
in toddler, 738

Strabismus (Continued)
of optic path gliomas, 1192
retinoblastoma and, 846
Strained food, infant diet and, 466
Strawberry hemangiomas, 415, *418*
Strawberry tongue, of scarlet fever, 928(t)
Streptococcal infection, rheumatic fever and, 1119
Streptococcal pharyngotonsillitis, 941(t)
Streptococcal pneumonia, 612–613(t), 943
Stress(es), family and, 274
managing, 273–313
of hospital stay, for child, 295–305
nurse and, 300–302
potential, in family with adolescent, 1226–1231
in family with infants, 396–405
in family with toddler, 722–730
in school-age years, 1090–1102
response to, in dysfunctional family, 77
in infant, 481
Stretch reflex, 421
Stridor, congenital laryngeal, 559
role of nurse in, 559
Strong families, communication in, 26
Stryker frame, spinal fusion and, 1286
Sturge-Weber syndrome, 653–654
Stuttering, preschooler and, 916–917
St. Vitus dance, 1122
Stycar Chart, 208
Stye, 936
Subacute bacterial endocarditis, 551
Substitution, behavior control of children and, 43
Sucking, of infant, importance of, 462
Sucking reflex, 420
Suctioning, in infants, 332
nursing actions related to, 328(t)
Sudden infant death syndrome (SIDS), 682–687
community follow-up, 686–687
of previous infant, attachment breakdown and, 478
Suffocation, toddler and, 761
Suicide, adolescent, 1252–1253
crisis intervention and, 1253
Superego, 906
Support systems, for mothers, 726
of irreversibly ill adolescent, 1299
of parents, lack of, 396–398
attachment breakdown and, 480
of school-age child, 1042–1043, 1046
Suppurative otitis media, 511
serous otitis media and, 512(t)
Supraglottitis, 943–945, 944
Surgery, acne vulgaris and, 1266
biliary atresia and, 668–669
bone tumor and, 1318

Surgery (Continued)
cardiac, 551–555
of toddler, nursing care plan for, 869–870
cleft lip and, 567–569
cleft palate and, 567–569
congenital hip dislocation and, 604–605
diaphragmatic hernia and, 580
fluid therapy and, 357, 360
hiatal hernia with gastroesophageal reflux and, 581–582
Hirschsprung's disease and, 590–592
hydrocephalus and, 652–653, *652*, *653*
hypospadias and, 949
intestinal atresia and, 584–585
intracranial tumors and, 1194
intussusception and, 588
malrotation and volvulus and, 586
necrotizing enterocolitis and, 594–595
nursing care before and after, 373–377
pyloric stenosis and, 571
preparation for, 373–375
tonsillectomy and adenoidectomy, 941–942
tracheoesophageal fistula and esophageal atresia and, 574, *574*
tuberculosis and, 1312
umbilical hernia and, 582
undescended testes and, 948
urological, of infant, 563–565
vesicoureteral reflux and, 953
Surplus-energy theory, of play, 157
Sutures, of head of newborn, 416
Swallowing reflex, 420
Sweat test, 1326
Sydenham's chorea, 1122
Symbolic play, of toddler, 740
Symptomatic care, teaching to parents, 288–289
Symptoms, child review of, in history taking, 184, 182(t)
Syndrome. See under name of syndrome.
Syphilis, 1294(t)
congenital, 667–668
pregnancy and, 113
Systemic lupus erythematosus, 1304–1308
Systems approach, to families, 252

Tachypnea, in problem in neonatal circulation, 533
Talipes equinovarus, 599
Tantrums, temper, extreme, 778
Tapeworm, 791
Task performance, of families, 252
Taste, sense of, of newborn, 423
Tay-Sachs disease, 676–677
Teacher, nurse and, 1047
nurse as, in dysfunctional family, 80
school-age child and, 1042–1043

Teaching, approaches to, according to child's age, 267–268, 266(t)
in muscular dystrophy, 1323
nurse's role in, 264–268
of hospitalized child, about his condition, 1022–1025, 1206–1210
preoperative, in bone tumor, 1318–1319
Tearing, 205
of dacryostenosis, 520
Teasing, by parent of infant, in assessment of attachment, 484–485
Teeth. See also *Dentition*.
assessment of, 216, *217*
caries of, 1137–1138
of toddler, 734–735
school-age child and, 1067–1068
anticipatory guidance on, 1068
staining of, by iron supplements, 788
by tetracyclines, 1266
Telangiectatic nevi, of newborn, 415
Telescope, prism, for partially sighted preschooler, 968
Television viewing, control of, by parents, 32–33
counselling by nurse about, 33
preschooler and, 883, *884*
Temper tantrums, extreme, 778
maladaptive, 776–779
of toddler, 746–748
Temperament, emotional-social development and, 153–155
of child, and parenting styles, 50, 52–53(t)
of infant, 462–463
of school-age child, 1076–1077
anticipatory guidance on, 1077
of toddler, 744–745
anticipatory guidance on, 745
traits of, 153–154
Temperature, assessment of, in hospitalized child, 316–317
in health examinations, 192–193
regulation of, in newborn, 425
skin, assessment of, 196
Temperature recording devices, electronic, 317
Temporary alterations, in health, of adolescent, 1263–1272
of infant, 493–521
of preschooler, 921–936
of school-age child, 1103–1115
of toddler, 780–796
Temporary illness, in children, 286–289
anticipatory guidance in, 286–288, 287(t)
Tension, in situational crisis, 276
premenstrual, 1272
Tension-fatigue syndrome, 987
Teratogenic agents, to fetus, 110–114
Term infant, ankle flexion in, *430*
general appearance of, 430–432
preterm infant and, 430–435
Terminal care, of dying child, 307–308
Tertiary circular reactions, 739
Testape, 1173

Testicular leukemia, 1005
Testis(es), of adolescent, 1234, 1234(t)
ectopic, 947
undescended, 947–948
Tetany, hypocalcemic, vitamin D deficiency rickets and, 629
of newborn, 353
Tetracycline(s), in acne vulgaris, 1266
staining of teeth by, 1266
Tetralogy of Fallot, 549–550, *549*
Texture, of skin, 196
of normal newborn, 416
Thalassemia, 676
Thalidomide, pregnancy and, 110
Thelarche, premature, 1114
Therapeutic play, hospitalized school-age child and, *1206*
Thermal management, of newborn, 425
Third-spacing, 347, 350
Thomas splint, 1131, *1132*
Thoracic kyphoscoliosis, *222*
Thorax, deformities of, *222*
Thrill, 224
Throat, assessment of, 218
specimen collection from, 341–342
Thrombotic crisis, 674
Thrush, 216, 508, *508*
Thyroid, assessment of, 204
Tibia, malrotation of, 781–785
torsion of, internal, 783
Tibial rotation, assessment of, *782*
Time, impact of, on family life, 24–26
structuring of, by family, 25–26
Tine test, 1309(t)
Tinea capitis, 792
Tinea corporis, 792
Tinea cruris, 1269
Tinea pedis, 1104–1105, *1105*
Titmus Vision Tester, 208
Toddler, burns and, 799–817
developmental needs of, 856–857(t)
examination of, techniques for, 188
explaining death to, 843–844
family of, establishing stable home, 720
growth and development of, 709–721
potential stresses in, 722–730
growth and development of, 731–763
hearing of, 212–213
screening, 979
health of, irreversible alterations in, 828–842
life-threatening alterations in, 843–848
reversible alterations in, 797–827
temporary alterations in, 780–796
hospitalized, 849–875
intellectual competency of, 739–743
managing behavior of, 764–779
nutritional requirements of, 738–739
overly dependent, 726–727

Toddler (*Continued*)
parenting practices and, 726–728
rejected, 727
safety of, 710–711, *710*, 758–762
sleep of, 750
speech of, 742
temperament of, emotional-social competency and, 744–745
with circulatory alteration, nursing care plan for, 866–873
Toddlerhood, potential stresses during, 764–779, 780–796, 797–827, 828–842, 843–848
Toilet training, 751, *752*
anticipatory guidance on, 751–752
blind child and, 972
encopresis and, 1094
genitourinary problems and, 947
spina bifida and, 651
unhealthy patterns of, 728–730
Tongue, assessment of, 216, 218
geographic, 218, 987, *988*
Tonic neck reflex (TNR), 422, *422*
Tonsillectomy and adenoidectomy (T & A), 941–942
Tonsils, assessment of, 218
diseased, 941–943
Tonus, 1162
TORCHS, 112
Torsional deformity, 781–783, 782(t)
Total anomalous venous drainage, 548
Total body water, 345, 346(t)
Total communication, hearing impairment and, 983
Total parenteral nutrition, 365–368
nurse and, 366–368
Touch, communication by, 172
sense of, of newborn, 423
Touch and movement interaction, of parent and child, 484
Toxoplasmosis, 679–680
pregnancy and, 112
Toys, accidents and, 762
health examinations and, 187–188
Tracheobronchitis, in infants, 608–609(t)
Tracheoesophageal fistula, esophageal atresia and, 572–577, *572*
H-type, 576–577
Tracheostomy, child with, caring for, 330–332
closing of, 332
Traction, in congenital dislocation of hip, 604
in fractures, 1129–1134, *1129–1133*
nursing care during, 1133–1134
of lower extremity, 1131–1132
of upper extremity, 1132–1133
Traction response, 420
Transfusion, exchange, for hyperbilirubinemia, 434
Transition, neonatal, *414*

INDEX **1413**

Transposition of great vessels, 547–548
Transracial adoption, 71, *71*
Trauma, school-age child and, 1107–1112
Travel, work-related, family and, 29
Treatment, discontinuing, of dying child, 306–307
Treatment phase, hospitalized preschooler and, 1022–1025
hospitalized school-age child and, 1206–1212
Trial-and-error behavior, in infant, 148
Triangling, families and, 252
Trichomoniasis, 1292–1293
Tricuspid atresia, 550
Trisomy 21, 1157
Truant, 1260
True hermaphrodite, 665
Truncus arteriosus, 548–549
Trunk incurvation reflex, 421
Trust, development of, in infant, 461
Tube, oxygen by, 437
Tube feeding, nasogastric, of infant, 333–335
Tuberculosis, 1308–1312
nurse and, 1311–1312
Tumor(s), *198*
brain, distribution by age at diagnosis, 1001
intracranial, 1189–1195
of bone, 1316–1319
of pituitary, 633
of soft tissues, 1195–1196
Wilms', 1008–1009
distribution by age at diagnosis, 1001
Tuning fork, in assessing hearing, 213
Turgor, of skin, 196
of normal newborn, 416
Turnbuckle cast, 1281, 1285(t), *1282*
Turner syndrome, 1300
Tylenol. *See Acetaminophen.*
Tympanic membrane, assessment of, 211–212, *212*
Tympanometry, 979

Ulcer, Curling's, major burns and, 807(t)
skin, *198*
Umbilical cord, care of, 426
Umbilical hernia, 226, 227, 582
Umbilical stump, 419
Umbilicus, examination of, 226
Unoccupied behavior, type of play, 162
Unrealistic expectations, attachment breakdown and, 478
Upper extremity traction, 1132–1133
Upper respiratory infection, in infants, 606
of rubeola, 922(t)

Urachal anomalies, congenital, 562
Urea cycle, 1196
Ureter(s), obstruction of, 562
reimplantation of, 953–954, *954*
Ureteral duplication, 561–562, *566*
Ureterocele, 562, *562*
Ureteropelvic junction obstruction, 562, *562*
Urethral catheterization, 340
Urethrocutaneous fistula, hypospadias and, 950
Urinalysis, 250
in urinary tract infection, 951
Urinary alteration, preschooler with, nursing care plan for, 1028–1037
Urinary incontinence, in spina bifida, 650
Urinary output, 24-hour, collection of, 340–341
storage of, 341
Urinary tract anomalies, and related conditions, 560–565
Urinary tract infection, 950–952
nurse and, 950
Urination, normal, in infant, 560
Urine, collection of, 338
clean-catch, 339–340
routine, 338–339
dark, in acute glomerulonephritis, 1117, 1118
in health assessment, 249–250
testing of, in diabetes mellitus, 1173
Urine bag, 338–340
Urine culture(s), 250
specimen for, 339–340
Urine specific gravity (USG), in gastroenteritis, 623
in potential fluid and electrolyte imbalance, 355
Urogenital problems, 946–954
Urogram, excretory, 951
Uvula, assessment of, 218

Vaccination, for influenza, 1269
Vaccine, experimental, for cytomegalovirus infection, 682
Vaginitis, 1292–1293
Values, of families, 255–256, 718
sociocultural, effect on parenting styles, 50–51
Valvar stenosis, valvotomy for, 546
Varicella, Reye's syndrome and, 1196
Vascular fluid, shift to interstitial, 347
Vascular sounds, abdominal, 227
Vasopressin, in central diabetes insipidus, 1167–1168
Vectorcardiogram, 536
Vegetables, preschooler diet and, 909(t)
Veins, scalp, as IV insertion site, 360
Venereal diseases, 1292–1295, 1295(t)
testing for, 248
Venipuncture, positioning of child for, 324

Ventilation, mechanical, in preterm infant, 437–438
Ventral suspension, of newborn infant, 411
Ventricular septal defect (VSD), 543–544, *543*
Verbal communication, 169
Verbalism, 970
Vernix caseosa, 416
Vesicle, *198*
Vesicoureteral reflux, 952–954
Vibration, in postural drainage, 330
Viral hepatitis, 1288, 1292, 1289(t), 1290–1291(t)
Viral infections, of lower respiratory tract, 608–609(t)
Viral meningitis, 618–619
Viral pharyngotonsillitis, 941(t)
Viruses, of influenza, 1267–1268, 1268(t)
Vision, assessment of, 963(t)
development of, assessment of, 962(t)
of infant, 453, *453*
of newborn, 423
of preschooler, 898–899
anticipatory guidance on, 899
of toddler, 737–738
residual, 967
Visual acuity, assessment of, 207–209, 209(t)
Visual fatigue, partial sightedness and, 968
Visual fields, assessment of, 205, *205*
Visual functioning, alterations in, 657–662
Visual handicap, 967
Visual impairment, 967–968
Visual interaction, of parent and child, 484
Visual problems, preschooler and, 961–973
Visual sensory interpretation, 233
Visually impaired, resources for, 998
Vital signs, assessment of, 192–193
in hospitalized child, 316–318
in potential fluid and electrolyte imbalance, 353–354
neonatal circulation and, 533
Vitamin D, breast-fed infant and, 456
Vitamin D deficiency rickets, 628–630
nurse and, 629–630
Vitamin K, newborn and, 427
Vitamins, accidental ingestion of, 821
requirement of infant for, 456
Vocal interaction, of parent and child, 484
Vocalization, of infant, 460, *460*
Voiding cystourethrogram (VCUG), 951, 953
Volkmann's syndrome, 1132
Volvulus, and malrotation, 585–586
Vomiting, bilious, in intestinal atresia, 584
in volvulus, 586
dietary measures for, 288
in esophageal chalasia, 517

1414 INDEX

Vomiting (*Continued*)
  in hiatal hernia, 581
  in intracranial tumors, 1192
  in Reye's syndrome, 1196
  pernicious, of pregnancy, 107
  persistent, in head injury, 1109, 1110
  pyloric stenosis and, 570
von Recklinghausen's disease, 654–655
Vowels, preschooler and, 902, 902(t)
Vulva, assessment of, 228

Walking. See also *Ambulation*.
  blind child and, 969–970, *970*
Warmth, preterm infant and, 435–436
Washington Guide to Promoting Development in the Young Child, 239, 242
Water, requirement of infant, 455
  requirement of preschooler, 900
Weaning, of infant, 467–468
Weber test, of hearing, 213
Wechsler Preschool-Primary Scale of Intelligence (WPPSI), 901
Weight, in health assessment, 188–191
  in potential fluid and electrolyte imbalance, 354

Weight (*Continued*)
  intrauterine, chart, *412, 413*
  of infant, 447, 449
    anticipatory guidance on, 447, 449
  of preschooler, 895
    anticipatory guidance on, 895
  of school-age child, 1060–1061
    anticipatory guidance on, 1061
  of toddler, 731–732
    anticipatory guidance on, 732
Weight reduction programs, adolescent obesity and, 1296–1297
Well-child interview, 177–178
Wellness, maintaining, of family with adolescent, 1221–1225
  of family with infant, 381–395
  of family with preschooler, 879–887
  of family with school-age child, 1041–1051
  of family with toddler, 709–721
  of adolescent, 1232–1248
  of infant, 447–470
  of preschooler, 894–913
  of school-age child, 1060–1089
  of toddler, 731–763
Wellness-seeking behavior, development of, *260*
Wheal, 198

Wheezing, expiratory, in asthma, 988
White blood cells, 1000–1001, 1001(t)
Whitehead, 1263
Whooping cough, 926–927(t)
"Why" questions, of children, 174
Wilms' tumor, 1008–1009
  distribution by age at diagnosis, 1001
Withdrawal, birth control and, 1245
Work, family and, 29–30
Work-related travel, family and, 29
Working mothers, family and, 25, 30
Worry, in school-age child, 1078–1079

X-linked dominant inheritance, 141
X-linked recessive inheritance, 141

Yawn reflex, 421

Z-plasty, for cleft lip, 567–568
Zinc sulfate, in acne vulgaris, 1266